PRIMARY CARE

The Art and Science
of Advanced Practice
Nursing

FOURTH EDITION

Carry Taber's today and SAVE 20%

Use promo code:
CARRYTABERS

PRIMARY CARE

The Art and Science of Advanced Practice Nursing

FOURTH EDITION

Lynne M. Dunphy, PhD, APRN, FNP-BC, FAAN
Professor and Associate Dean for Practice and Community Engagement
Christine E. Lynn College of Nursing
Florida Atlantic University
Boca Raton, Florida

Jill E. Winland-Brown, EdD, APRN, FNP-BC
Professor and Family Nurse Practitioner
Christine E. Lynn College of Nursing
Florida Atlantic University
Boca Raton, Florida

Brian Oscar Porter, MD, PhD, MPH
Clinical Development Physician
Private Biopharmaceutical Industry
and
Medical House Officer
Veterans Affairs New Jersey Health Care System—Lyons Campus
Lyons, New Jersey

Debera J. Thomas, DNS, RN, FNP/ANP
Dean and Professor
School of Nursing
Northern Arizona University
Flagstaff, Arizona

F.A. Davis Company • Philadelphia

F. A. Davis Company
1915 Arch Street
Philadelphia, PA 19103
www.fadavis.com

Printed in the United States of America

Last digit indicates print number: 10 9 8 7 6 5

Senior Acquisitions Editor: Susan Rhyner
Developmental Editor: Marcia Kelley
Director of Content Development: Darlene D. Pedersen, MSN, FNP, BC
Content Project Manager: Echo Gerhart
Design & Illustration Manager: Carolyn O'Brien

As new scientific information becomes available through basic and clinical research, recommended treatments and drug therapies undergo changes. The author(s) and publisher have done everything possible to make this book accurate, up to date, and in accord with accepted standards at the time of publication. The author(s), editors, and publisher are not responsible for errors or omissions or for consequences from application of the book, and make no warranty, expressed or implied, in regard to the contents of the book. Any practice described in this book should be applied by the reader in accordance with professional standards of care used in regard to the unique circumstances that may apply in each situation. The reader is advised always to check product information (package inserts) for changes and new information regarding dose and contraindications before administering any drug. Caution is especially urged when using new or infrequently ordered drugs.

Library of Congress Cataloging-in-Publication Data

Primary care (Dunphy)
Primary care : the art and science of advanced practice nursing / [edited by] Lynne M. Dunphy, Jill E. Winland-Brown, Brian Oscar Porter, Debera J. Thomas. — Fourth edition.
    p. ; cm.
 Includes bibliographical references and index.
 ISBN 978-0-8036-3801-3
 I. Dunphy, Lynne M. Hektor, editor. II. Winland-Brown, Jill E., 1948- , editor. III. Porter, Brian Oscar, editor. IV. Thomas, Debera J., editor. V. Title.
 [DNLM: 1. Nurse Practitioners. 2. Primary Nursing. WY 128]
 RT82.8
 610.73—dc23
                    2014031716

The contents of this textbook and the independent contributions of Dr. Porter do not represent official views of Novartis, the VA, the FDA, the NIH, or any other U.S. federal government agency.

"We are not really in doubt about the more serious of our shared aims. We know what they are. We know they are difficult. And we know that we have not achieved them."

—*John Gardner,* Excellence, *p. 155, as quoted by Martha E. Rogers,* Reveille in Nursing, *p. 1*

This book grew out of a commitment to primary-care practice and a love and valuing of nursing knowledge. Fifty years ago, in 1964, Martha E. Rogers, Chairperson of the Department of Nursing Education, New York University, came out with a small red and white volume, soft-covered and a total of 96 pages, titled *Reveille in Nursing,* published by F. A. Davis. It was a book, she was later to comment, "that scared the pants off a lot of people" (Martha E. Rogers, personal communication, June 22, 1988). F. A. Davis continues to stand on its commitment to nursing knowledge with its publication of this text. The abandonment of nursing knowledge in some primary-care nurse practitioner programs is not a trend that Martha would have favored. One can hear her saying, "Where's the *nursing* in nurse practitioner primary-care practice? 'Where's the beef?'"

What we offer here is the "beef," a text that builds on the *Circle of Caring,* a holistic, caring-based approach to primary-care practice, consistent with nursing's historical base. Unit I contains five chapters that provide the theoretical base to a caring-based primary-care practice, which is operationalized in the remainder of the text. In this first unit, in Chapter 1, we provide a theoretical model of primary-care nursing, the *Circle of Caring.* The caring base of primary-care practice is presented by Drs. Boykin and Schoenhofer in Chapter 2, as a transformative model for our health-care system. A chapter on health promotion by Drs. Dorothy Dunn and Debera J. Thomas provides a base for primary-care practice that situates the patient and family in the context of the community in Chapter 3. Chapter 4, "The Art of Diagnosis and Treatment," by Dr. Susan K. Chase, describes how primary-care practice in a *Circle of Caring* is actualized through decision making and management plans. "Evidence-Based Practice," by Dr. Angela K. Golden, provides essential information for today's care practice environment. It is essential that all clinicians be able to provide care with a good understanding of the standard of care and the ability to meet that standard in a meaningful way.

Unit II uses the traditional system-based approach to provide the essential information necessary to provide safe and effective primary care to patients. Each system-based chapter begins with "Common Complaints," a symptom-based approach to phenomena that lays out the associated differential diagnoses of each symptom-based complaint a patient may present with. Then each chapter develops these various differentials under "Common Problems." Each problem is defined and the associated epidemiology and causes are outlined, as well as the pathophysiological processes. Dr. Brian O. Porter again has provided a thoughtful and in-depth update on the pathophysiology of each disorder developed within the chapters, as well as a thorough review of diagnostic processes and management plans.

The subjective and objective manifestations of each problem are elaborated, as well as the associated diagnostic testing that might be used. A review of potential differential diagnoses is elaborated, as well as the underlying reasoning and critical thinking involved in the decision making used to reach a specific diagnosis, which then determines treatment. As consistent with our model, a holistic database is established, built on the patient's voice and experience. Management strategies, including pharmacological and surgical therapy, when indicated, are outlined. Again, as consistent with our approach, complementary therapies and psychosocial interventions are elaborated providing a holistic plan of care. Follow-up and referral are included, along with long-term management strategies, and patient education—the important teaching/learning component of caring-based primary-care practice—is also included. Tables, figures, and recurring displays are provided in each chapter in Unit II. Displays include drug charts, therapeutic procedures that a clinician in primary care might be called on to perform, risk factors, screening guidelines, differential diagnosis flowcharts, treatment standards, and guidelines, as well as sidebars on focusing the history and advanced assessment techniques. Also, we provide highlights of complementary therapies and holistically-based advanced practice nursing interventions. Included are "Nursing Situations," essentially case studies, along with abstracts of nursing-based research, and anecdotes from patients, called "The Patient's Voice." The provision of this variety of information will assist any primary-care provider, regardless of disciplinary background, in establishing and implementing a holistic, caring practice base. These features assist the student (or current practitioner) in linking ideas to practice and actualizing a *Circle of Caring.*

We gained some new and exciting contributors to Unit II, such as Dr. Susan Kelly-Weeder, PhD, FNP-BC, from Boston College, who assisted us in redrafting Chapter 8, "Eyes, Ears, Nose, and Throat Problems." Building on the excellent work of Lori Martin-Plank, PhD, FNP-BC, GNP-BC, FAANP, we added Terry South, MSN, APRN, FNP-BC to Chapter 15, "Musculoskeletal Problems." We are also pleased to have added scholar-clinician Michael Zychowicz, DNP, FNP-BC,

FAANP, FAAN, noted specialist in the area of musculoskeletal problems, to oversee and finalize this chapter. We have collaborated with another physician, Michael B. Keller, MD, MS, who added valuable contributions to several chapters, specifically the neurological and cardiac content, and will continue to add his clinical expertise in the future. Dr. Keller is the son of our faculty colleague, Dr. Kathryn B. Keller, who coauthored the cardiac chapter, her area of specialization.

Unit III begins with Chapter 20, "Palliative Care," by Susan Derby, RN, MA, GNP-BC, ACHPN, and Mary Layman Goldstein, RN, MS, ANP-BC, ACHPN, of Memorial Sloan-Kettering Cancer Center in New York City, a chapter that includes comprehensive information on pain management. We are very pleased to provide our readers with an update of the popular chapter "The 15-Minute Hour: Practical Psychotherapy for Primary Care," authored by a new contributor, Brandi Parker Cotton, MSN, Psychiatric NP and doctoral student, building on the prior work of Drs. Eliezer Schnall and Marian Stuart. New content includes motivational interviewing as well as current evidence to support practice in this area. These approaches, developed specifically for primary-care practice, will provide primary-care practitioners with additional therapeutic communication skills that will enable them to "hear" the patient's true concerns, again supporting a holistic and caring practice model. "Ethical and Legal Issues of a Caring-Based Practice" is also an essential for practice, updated by leading nurse-ethicist Dr. Jill E. Winland-Brown. Chapter 22, "The Business of Advanced Practice," has been completely redone to integrate the information and implications of the Affordable Care Act. The author of this chapter, Dr. Marcella M. Rutherford, has a PhD in nursing as well as an MBA and years of experience in medical practice administration from which to draw. We conclude with essential information in "Putting Caring Into Practice: Caring for Self." This chapter has also been completely redone, with two new authors from the University of Rhode Island: Mary Lavin, DNP, APRN, FNP-BC, and Rebecca Carley, DNP, APRN, ANP-BC. They have used a different theoretical base from which to examine caring for self, as well as some important ideas for caring for one's own health.

As long-time nurse practitioner faculty, we remain committed to providing an in-depth book with a comprehensive and holistic approach that can be used across the curriculum (and in a variety of different curricula) and that includes participation by practitioners from other disciplines, such as medicine. Primary-care curriculum content exists in master's-level and doctorate of nursing practice programs. While appropriate for either level, we, as authors, are attentive to shifting practice boundaries and feel that the articulation of a largely nursing base for primary care, rooted in caring and holistic approaches, is critical to disciplinary identity and growth. This text provides a high-level pathophysiological base, evidence-based diagnostic and management strategies, and a holistic plan of care that is consistent with this level of practice. The student is able to find a large amount of information in one text. Although we realize that graduate students will always need supplementary texts to provide the currency and depth of information that they require, we nonetheless believe that they (and their faculty!) will appreciate one large, complete text, complemented by an ever-expanding collection of ancillaries for faculty and student use.

What we also provide is the "beef"—the "beef" of caring-based, advanced practice nursing as actualized in the NP role, in the full flowering of all that primary-care practice *could* be. We are answering the call that Jean Watson sounded in her 1995 article, "Advanced Nursing Practice . . . and What Might Be":

> Such a reform calls for nursing to shift its accountability and voice from the medical cure functional tasks and institutional demands and constraints toward making itself directly accountable to the public for its caring, healing, health knowledge, skills, and practices.
> —*Jean Watson (in Watson, J. "Advanced Nursing Practice ... and What Might Be" in Nursing & Health Care, Vol. 16, Number 2, p. 81)*

It is the most exciting time for advanced practice nursing. Health-care reform is a reality. The demand for new service approaches in health care is high. The professional doctorate—the DNP—is providing primary-care practitioners of nursing with a well-grounded base of pathophysiology, diagnosis and management, and follow-up, situated in a nursing-based model. Consumers are informed and powerful. Now it is time for nurse practitioners to provide consumers with the "beef"—advanced nursing primary-care practice within a *Circle of Caring*.

There are numerous people to thank for helping this book become a reality:

Joanne P. DaCunha, our wonderful, PATIENT, always supportive, always optimistic publisher, whom we have come to know well, and who is, most of all, our friend.

Susan Rhyner, Senior Acquisitions Editor, who joins our team with a fresh eye, an innovative perspective, and infectious motivation.

Echo K. Gerhart, our new Content Project Manager, who has had to work *very* hard to keep us all in line!

Marcia Kelly, our Developmental Editor from afar, who was efficient, enthusiastic, and patient.

Kelly Boutross of Graphic World Inc., who worked tirelessly to "pull it all together" and maintained her composure at all times, even the most trying!

The entire F. A. Davis production team—*all* of whom were always patient, flexible, and terrific!

Dr. Marlaine Smith, Dean of the Christine E. Lynn College of Nursing, Professor, and caring scholar, who was quoted in this text far before she came to FAU—for her support for *all* our work.

Dr. Anne Boykin, Founding Dean of the Christine E. Lynn College of Nursing, who helped shape our vision for nursing and provides the glue that holds it together—caring.

Dr. Mary Sullivan, Interim Dean and Professor of the University of Rhode Island College of Nursing, for her support and encouragement during Dr. Dunphy's years at URI.

All of our students, past and present, who always continue to teach us as much, if not more, than we teach them!

We also acknowledge the following chapter authors of the third edition of this book, without which this new edition would not have been possible:

Sandra Allen, MSN, APRN, FNP-BC

Lisa J. Bedard, MSN, APRN, FNP-BC

Lauren Gallagher, MS, APRN, FNP-BC

Diane Gerzevitz, MSN, APRN, FNP-BC

Ruth McCaffrey, DNP, APRN, FNP, BC

Jacqueline Rhoads, PhD, RN, CCRN, ACNP-CS

Linda Hall Rothery, DNP, MSN, APRN, FNP-BC

Edwin W. Schaefer, ND, APRN, FNP-BC

Karilee Halo Shames, MSN, RN, HNC

Cathy M. St. Pierre, PhD, FNP, BC

And most of all, we acknowledge our patients, who taught us to "hear" their voices.

Lynne M. Dunphy, PhD, APRN, FNP-BC, FAAN Dr. Lynne Dunphy recently re-joined the faculty at the Christine E. Lynn College of Nursing, Florida Atlantic University, Boca Raton, Florida, in the role of Associate Dean for Practice and Community Engagement. In this role she is coordinating and directing the college's nurse-managed practices. Dr. Dunphy spent the last eight years at the College of Nursing at the University of Rhode Island, serving as the inaugural Routhier Chair of Practice and Associate Dean for External Affairs. She has been a Robert Wood Johnson Executive Nurse Fellow and was the founding nursing lead of the Rhode Island Action Coalition, dedicated to the implementation of the Institute of Medicine's recommendations for the Future of Nursing. Dr. Dunphy recently completed four years of service on the Board of the National Organization of Nurse Practitioner Faculties (NONPF).

Jill E. Winland-Brown, EdD, APRN, FNP-BC Dr. Winland-Brown was born in Boston, but raised in Pennsylvania. After high school, she went to Newport Hospital School of Nursing, Salve Regina College, Newport, Rhode Island, for her BSN, Boston College for her MS, and Florida Atlantic University for her EdD and post master's FNP. Her first teaching position was at the University of Rhode Island, after which she moved to Florida. She teaches ethics in the undergraduate program and teaches in the graduate and FNP programs. Children include his, mine, and ours, although after 30 years, all five are ours. In whatever little free time is left, her loves are the beach and tennis. Dr. Winland-Brown is also on the ANA Center for Ethics and Human Rights Advisory Board.

Brian Oscar Porter, MD, PhD, MPH Dr. Porter is a triple Board-certified and licensed Allergist and Immunologist, Internist, and Pediatrician. After completing both his MD and PhD in Immunology and Microbiology at the University of Miami School of Medicine (Miami, Florida), as well as his MPH at the Harvard School of Public Health (Boston, Massachusetts), Dr. Porter completed combined residency training in Internal Medicine and Pediatrics at the Virginia Commonwealth University Medical Center (Richmond, Virginia), followed by fellowship training in Allergy and Immunology at the National Institutes of Health (Bethesda, Maryland), where he also served as an Adjunct Intramural Investigator in the Laboratory of Immunoregulation and Principal Investigator on two NIH-based clinical and translational research protocols in primary and acquired immunodeficiency. Dr. Porter then joined the U.S. Food and Drug Administration's Center for Drug Evaluation and Research as a Primary Reviewer and Medical Officer, before transitioning into the private biopharmaceutical drug development industry as a clinical development physician focusing on biological immunotherapies and global product development strategy. Dr. Porter has held leadership roles in several companies, including Human Genome Sciences, GlaxoSmithKline, and most recently Novartis Pharmaceuticals, where he currently serves as a Global Program Medical Director* (East Hanover, New Jersey). He also continues to work actively as a clinician in the Veterans Affairs New Jersey Health Care System as a Medical House Officer* (Lyons, New Jersey). Dr. Porter credits his multidisciplinary approach to human health largely to the influence and encouragement of his mother,

*The contents of this textbook and the independent contributions of Dr. Porter fall completely outside of his current employment and do not represent official views of Novartis Pharmaceuticals, the U.S. Department of Veterans Affairs, or any other U.S. federal government agency.

Dr. Luz Sobong Porter, a nurse clinician, educator, and researcher, who always involved him in her work and remains one of his primary collaborators to this day.

 Debera J. Thomas, DNS, RN, FNP/ANP Dr. Thomas is Professor and Dean of Nursing at Northern Arizona University in Flagstaff, Arizona. Her teaching career began in 1978 at Augustana Hospital School of Nursing in Chicago, Illinois. She has held numerous faculty and administrative positions at institutions including Kent State University, Case Western Reserve University, Florida Atlantic University, University of Connecticut, and Northern Arizona University. In her free time, Debera is a potter. She prefers wheel throwing and functional ceramics and works in high fire clay. On most weekends, you can find her hiking the trails in Northern Arizona and the Grand Canyon.

Anne Boykin, PhD, RN
Founding Dean and Professor Emeritus
Florida Atlantic University
Christine E. Lynn College of Nursing
Boca Raton, Florida
Chapter 2 Caring and the Advanced Practice Nurse

Rebecca Carley, MS, DNP, RNP
Assistant Clinical Professor
University of Rhode Island
Kingston, Rhode Island
Chapter 24 Putting Caring Into Practice: Caring for Self

Susan K. Chase, EdD, RN, FNP-BC
Professor and Associate Dean
Graduate Program
University of Central Florida
Orlando, Florida
Chapter 4 The Art of Diagnosis and Treatment

Brandi Parker Cotton, APRN, MSN
Psychiatric Nurse Practitioner
Gateway Healthcare, Inc.
Pawtucket, Rhode Island
Chapter 23 The 15-Minute Hour: Practical Psychotherapy for Primary Care

Susan Derby, RN, MA, GNP-BC, ACHPN
Nurse Practitioner
Neurology, Pain, and Palliative Care Service
Memorial Sloan Kettering Cancer Center
New York, New York
and
Adjunct Faculty
New York University
School of Nursing
New York, New York
Chapter 20 Palliative Care

Dorothy J. Dunn, PhD, RNP, FNP-BC, AHN-BC
Assistant Professor
Northern Arizona University
Flagstaff, Arizona
Chapter 3 Health Promotion; Chapter 11 Abdominal Problems

Lynne M. Dunphy, PhD, APRN, FNP-BC, FAAN
Associate Dean for Practice and Community Engagement
Professor of Nursing
Christine E. Lynn College of Nursing
Florida Atlantic University
Boca Raton, Florida
Chapter 1 Primary Care in the Twenty-First Century: A Circle of Caring; Chapter 15 Musculoskeletal Problems

Angela K. Golden, DNP, APRN, FNP-C, FAANP
President, American Association of Nurse Practitioners
Owner, NP from Home, LLC
Munds Park, Arizona
Chapter 5 Evidence-Based Practice; Chapter 16 Endocrine and Metabolic Problems

Mary Layman Goldstein, RN, MS, ANP-BC, ACHPN
Nurse Practitioner
Memorial Sloan-Kettering Cancer Center
New York, New York
Chapter 20 Palliative Care

Kim S. Griswold, MD, MPH, AS, RN
Associate Professor
Department of Family Medicine
State University of New York (SUNY) at Buffalo
Buffalo, New York
Chapter 18 Psychosocial Problems

Joyce Hickey, PhDc, APRN, PMHCNS
Adjunct Faculty
College of Nursing
University of Rhode Island
Kingston, Rhode Island
Psychosocial Ancillaries

Bette K. Idemoto, PhD, RN, ACNS-BC, CCRN
Cardiovascular Clinical Nurse Specialist
University Hospitals Case Medical Center
Cleveland, Ohio
Chapter 21 Ethical and Legal Issues of a Caring-Based Practice

Jill Johnson, DNP, APRN, FNP-BC
Lead Nurse Practitioner, Louisville Market
Take Care Heath Systems
Louisville, Kentucky
Chapter 14 Women's Health Problems

Kathryn B. Keller, PhD, RN
Professor
Christine E. Lynn College of Nursing
Boca Raton, Florida
Chapter 10 Cardiovascular Problems

Michael B. Keller, MD, MS
Department of Medicine
Johns Hopkins Hospital and School of Medicine
Baltimore, Maryland
Chapter 6 Neurological Problems; Chapter 10 Cardiovascular Problems

Susan Kelly-Weeder, PhD, FNP-BC
Associate Professor
Boston College William F. Connell School of Nursing
Newton, Massachusetts
Chapter 8 Eyes, Ears, Nose, and Throat Problems

Mary Lavin, MS, RNP
Associate Clinical Professor
University of Rhode Island
Kingston, Rhode Island
Chapter 24 Putting Caring Into Practice: Caring for Self

Dianne M. Loomis, DNP, FNP-BC
Associate Clinical Professor
State University of New York (SUNY) at Buffalo
    School of Nursing
Buffalo, New York
Chapter 18 Psychosocial Problems

**Lori Martin-Plank, PhD, FNP-BC, GNP-BC,
    PhD, FAANP**
Clinical Assistant Professor, College of Nursing
University of Arizona
Tucson, Arizona
Chapter 15 Musculoskeletal Problems

Debbie J. Nogueras, PhD, MSN, ANP/FNP-BC
Associate Professor
Northern Arizona University
Flagstaff, Arizona
*Chapter 12 Renal Problems; Chapter 13 Men's Health
    Problems*

Patricia A. Pastore, MS, FNP-BC
Family Nurse Practitioner
Women's Wellness Primary Care
Veterans Administration, Western New York Health
    Care System
Buffalo, New York
Chapter 18 Psychosocial Problems

Brian Oscar Porter, MD, PhD, MPH
Clinical Development Physician
Private Biopharmaceutical Industry
and
Medical House Officer
Veterans Affairs New Jersey Health Care System–Lyons
    Campus
Lyons, New Jersey
*Chapter 1 Primary Care in the Twenty-First Century: A
    Circle of Caring; Chapter 7 Skin Problems; Chapter 8
    Eyes, Ears, Nose, and Throat Problems; Chapter 9
    Respiratory Problems; Chapter 10 Cardiovascular
    Problems; Chapter 12 Renal Problems; Chapter 13
    Men's Health Problems; Chapter 14 Women's Health
    Problems; Chapter 16 Endocrine and Metabolic
    Problems; Chapter 17 Hematological and Immune
    Problems; Chapter 19 Emergency Problems*

Marcella M. Rutherford, PhD, MBA, MSN
Dean, College of Nursing
Nova Southeastern, Ft. Lauderdale, Florida
Chapter 22 The Business of Advanced Practice

Denese Sabatino, MSN, APRN, NP-C, CCRN
Department of Critical Care Medicine
Cleveland Clinic, Ft. Lauderdale, Florida
Chapter 10 Cardiovascular Problems

Eliezer Schnall, PhD
Clinical Assistant Professor
Yeshiva University
New York, New York
*Chapter 23 The 15-Minute Hour: Practical Psychotherapy
    for Primary Care*

Savina O. Schoenhofer, PhD, RN
Professor
Alcorn State University
School of Nursing
Natchez, Mississippi
Chapter 2 Caring and the Advanced Practice Nurse

Terry South, MSN, APRN, NP-C
Spinal Pain Solutions
Harriman, Tennessee
Chapter 15 Musculoskeletal Problems

Marian R. Stuart, PhD
Clinical Professor
Department of Family Medicine
UMDNJ-Robert Wood Johnson Medical School
New Brunswick, New Jersey
*Chapter 23 The 15-Minute Hour: Practical Psychotherapy
    for Primary Care*

Debera J. Thomas, DNS, RN, FNP/ANP
Family and Adult Nurse Practitioner
Dean and Professor
School of Nursing
Northern Arizona University
Flagstaff, Arizona
*Chapter 1 Primary Care in the Twenty-First Century:
    A Circle of Caring; Chapter 3 Health Promotion;
    Chapter 11 Abdominal Problems; Chapter 12 Renal
    Problems; Chapter 13 Men's Health Problems;
    Chapter 14 Women's Health Problems; Chapter 16
    Endocrine and Metabolic Problems*

Sharon Thrush, DNP, APRN, FNP-BC
Family Practice of Palm Beach
West Palm Beach, Florida
and
Adjunct Faculty
Christine E. Lynn College of Nursing
Florida Atlantic University
Boca Raton, Florida
Chapter 8 Eyes, Ears, Nose, and Throat Problems

Jill E. Winland-Brown, EdD, APRN, FNP-BC
Professor and Family Nurse Practitioner
Christine E. Lynn College of Nursing
Florida Atlantic University
Boca Raton, Florida
*Chapter 1 Primary Care in the Twenty-First Century: A
    Circle of Caring; Chapter 6 Neurological Problems;
    Chapter 7 Skin Problems; Chapter 9 Respiratory
    Problems; Chapter 10 Cardiovascular Problems;
    Chapter 17 Hematological and Immune Problems;
    Chapter 19 Emergency Problems; Chapter 21 Ethical
    and Legal Issues of a Caring-Based Practice*

Michael Zycowicz, DNP, FNP-BC, FAANP, FAAN
*Associate Professor and Director, Master of Science
    in Nursing Programs*
Duke University School of Nursing
Duke University Health System
Durham, North Carolina
Chapter 15 Musculoskeletal Problems

Sallie Coke, PhD, APRN, CPNP, CFNP
Associate Professor
Georgia College and State University
Milledgeville, Georgia

Patricia Murray Given, PhD, RN, FNP, CCRN
Assistant Professor
The College of Staten Island – the City University
    of New York (CUNY)
Staten Island, New York

Sheila C. Grossman, PhD, APRN, FNP-BC, FAAN
Professor and Coordinator, Family Nurse Practitioner
    Track
Fairfield University
Fairfield, Connecticut

Joyce Hickey, PhDc, APRN, PMHCNS
Adjunct Faculty
College of Nursing
University of Rhode Island
Kingston, Rhode Island

Eileen McCann, DNP, BC-FNP
Assistant Professor and Program Director
Saint Xavier University
Chicago, Illinois

Geri C. Reeves, PhD, APRN, FNP-BC
Assistant Professor
Vanderbilt University School of Nursing
Nashville, Tennessee

Luann Richardson, PhD, CRNP
Assistant Professor, NP/DNP programs; Faculty
Duquesne University
McKees Rocks, Pennsylvania

Michelle Taylor Skipper, DNP, FNP-BC
Director, AGNP and FNP Concentrations
East Carolina University
Greenville, North Carolina

Jennifer K. Sofie, DNP, FNP-C, ANP-BC
Assistant Clinical Professor and DNP/FNP Clinical
    Coordinator
Montana State University
Bozeman, Montana

Terri LaCoursiere Zucchero, PhD, RN, FNP-BC
Clinical Assistant Professor
Connell School of Nursing, Boston College
Chestnut Hill, Massachusetts

CONTENTS

Chapter 8   **Eyes, Ears, Nose, and Throat Problems** *252*
Susan Kelly-Weeder, PhD, APRN, FNP-BC • Sharon Thrush, DNP, APRN, FNP-BC •
Brian Oscar Porter, MD, PhD, MPH

Chapter 9   **Respiratory Problems** *340*
Jill E. Winland-Brown, EdD, APRN, FNP-BC • Brian Oscar Porter, MD, PhD, MPH

Chapter 10   **Cardiovascular Problems** *430*
Kathryn B. Keller, PhD, RN • Denese Sabatino, MSN, APRN, NP-C, CCRN • Jill E. Winland-Brown, EdD, APRN, FNP-BC • Brian Oscar Porter, MD, PhD, MPH • Michael B. Keller, MD, MS

Nursing—The Seasons of My Life

Nursing is the spring of my life—
Each experience is fresh and new.
There's wonderment
Like flowers washed with morning dew.

Nursing is the summer of my life—
A time to perfect all I know.
There's confidence
A world where I can grow.
Nursing is the autumn of my life—
Ablaze with experience rich and glowing.
There's compassion
From richness of caring and knowing.

Nursing is the winter of my life—
A tapestry, a mosaic of all I am.
There's challenge
To find the spring again.

—Charlotte Dison, RN

Caring-Based Nursing: The Art

Advanced practice nursing is not filling the gap with medical care where it does not exist; it is filling the existing gap in health care with the core of nursing practice. . . . The core of advanced practice nursing lies within nursing's disciplinary perspective on human–environment and caring relationships that facilitate health and healing. This core is delineated specifically in the theoretic foundations of nursing. True advanced nursing practice is theory-based [and] fully integrated into the nurse's way of being and practicing.
—Marlaine Smith: The core of advanced practice nursing. Nurs Sci Q 8(1):2–3, 1995

Primary Care in the Twenty-First Century: A Circle of Caring

Lynne M. Dunphy, PhD, APRN, FNP-BC, FAAN • Jill E. Winland-Brown, EdD, APRN, FNP-BC • Brian Oscar Porter, MD, PhD, MPH • Debera J. Thomas, DNS, RN, FNP/ANP

Chapter 1

■ WHERE WE HAVE BEEN AND WHERE WE ARE GOING

This is a wonderful and exciting time to begin the study of primary care. The road ahead is brighter than ever for advanced practice registered nurses (APRNs). Our health-care system is in the process of reform. It is re-making itself. It is primary-care providers who will implement new and innovative ways of caring for patients. Education models are also in the process of being reformed; interprofessional education (IPE) and team-based approaches are becoming the required norm. APRNs will be a critical part of this reformed health-care team. Heeding the recommendations of the Institute of Medicine's report *The Future of Nursing: Leading Change, Advancing Health* (2011) that all nurses practice to their full scope of practice, states are implementing important changes in APRN practice regulations. This chapter will review the disciplines of nursing and medicine from a historical perspective, highlighting the different strengths that each brings to the care of patients. The *Circle of Caring* practice model on which this text is based will be presented as a way of making primary-care practice, which *must* incorporate aspects of what has been traditionally defined as "medical" practice, richer by the incorporation of nursing-based understanding of the patient's issues and concerns.

Currently, the American health-care system continues to struggle with fiscal realities, as well as questions of quality and access to care. Technological advancements, an aging population, chronic illnesses, and an increasingly educated and informed consumer are additional themes that color the ongoing debate over the American health-care system and, specifically, the Affordable Care Act (ACA). More than 2,000 pages long, the ACA passed both houses of Congress in early 2010, but public opinion about it remains divided.

Nonetheless, major reforms, such as the Patient-Centered Medical Home, are being implemented in many settings. At present, though, it is known that

illness continues too often to be treated episodically, outside the context of home, family, community, and people's day-to-day lives, in isolation from the trajectory of the life of the individual. The major goals of *Healthy People 2020* (U.S. Department of Health and Human Services, 2010) of increasing quality and years of healthy life and the elimination of health disparities are far from being met. Health-care reform supports changes in reimbursement that will support health promotion, disease prevention, and chronic disease management in a more meaningful way. However, these areas have not historically been priorities in a technologically driven, acute-care–oriented, specialized health-care system. Despite increasingly strong evidence of the need for strengthening health-promotion and disease-prevention strategies, including behavioral change, as well as the need for caring and interaction in the health-care provider–patient relationship, these shifts are not easily accomplished. Health-care disciplines are in the throes of change, and change is never easy. Disciplinary and professional turf battles abound as health-care reimbursement shrinks.

Increasing access to care for more of the population, though morally essential, will exacerbate this crisis, as occurred in Massachusetts after the passage of that state's health-care reform legislation. There is a rising demand for primary-care services and a decreasing supply of professionals providing these services (Health Resources & Services Administration, 2013). As the population ages and the number of older Americans swells, so will the burden of chronic illness. Increasing numbers of older adults live with *multiple* chronic illnesses; currently 87% of Americans aged 65 to 79 years live with one chronic condition, and more than 45% suffer from three or more (Bodenheimer et al, 2009). By 2020, a projected 157 million patients will suffer from chronic disease.

Cancer, mental disorders, and diabetes will increase by 50% by 2023 (Bodenheimer et al, 2009). The number of individuals with disabilities is projected to grow from about 5.1 million in 1986 to 22.6 million in 2040, or nearly 350%, even as the elderly population overall will grow by only 175% (Administration on Aging, 2012). For this reason, a range of community determinants of health, empowerment of individuals and families, and a substantially broadened role and impact of primary-care and other community-based services must be harnessed to ensure a seamless journey through the system of care throughout a person's whole life.

In the past, a portion of the burden of chronic-illness care was provided in hospitals and specialty practices, whereas today that care must be provided in primary-care settings and communities. This trend is expected to accelerate and will continue to stress the resources of primary-care systems (Decker et al, 2009). In this milieu, APRN care providers will be needed more than ever. APRNs excel in coordination of community-care services, and their nursing-based models of care support patient and family empowerment.

In a keynote address at the Centennial Conference of the National League for Nursing in 1993, Donna Shalala, former Secretary of the Department of Health and Human Services, stated that patients, families, groups, and communities are calling for the appearance of the "good fairy" in health care—someone who really hears them and their concerns, the nitty-gritty of their day-to-day experiences and struggles. Patients and their families need someone to hear why they did not take the medication that their health-care provider was so quick to prescribe, but that they just could not tolerate, could not afford, could not get to the pharmacy to pick up, or that had directions for administration that they could not understand or read; to hear why they did not have the mammogram—because they were afraid; to hear why the baby was not immunized—because putting food on the table was more important.

The Tip of the Iceberg

The health problems encountered in day-to-day practice are merely the tip of the iceberg that our health-care system, traditionally focused on the easily visible peaks above the water, has "plowed into." Reimbursement streams pay for the "tip" of this iceberg: a visit to a primary-care provider to put a diagnostic label, for billing purposes, on the symptomatology that the patient presents with, and a "treatment"—typically a pharmaceutical product—aimed at treating that symptom or underlying disease. Whether health-care reform will be able to effect meaningful changes in this current reality of the U.S. system remains to be seen. Will the ACA really be able to reverse the dysfunctional fee-for-service payment model?

The true causality of whatever brought the patient into the primary-care setting is the much larger part of the iceberg that lies under the surface. This "understructure" is built of various lifestyle issues, as well as environmental, community, socioeconomic, spiritual, family, and biological–genetic factors that have an

impact on health, often referred to as the *social determinants of health*. The nursing perspective—Donna Shalala's "good fairy"—is even more critical in today's world than it was in 1993. Nurses can and must understand the *whole* of the "patient's iceberg" (Fig. 1.1); they are educated to see both above *and* below the water and to intervene accordingly.

The classic medical model focuses on disease, an abnormality in the structure and function of body organs and systems, and is concerned with the malfunction or maladaption of biological or psychophysiological processes in the individual. In his textbook of family practice, Robert Rakel makes a distinction between the terms *disease* and *illness* (Rakel, 2011). *Illness* is "all the sensations of a patient and all the ramifications of a disorder." *Disease*, however, "is a theoretical and taxonomic concept, a useful tool that enables the healthcare provider to make inferences and predictions concerning phenomena." As such, the two concepts of illness and disease belong to two different universes of discourse: one, the world of theory, and the other, the lived experience of the patient. Benner and Wrubel (1989) also distinguish between disease and the experience of disease, or illness. *Illness* is defined as the way the sick person and his or her social network perceive and respond to disease. Illness is inextricable from the context of the patient's life, including the intersections of social, political, economic, spiritual, and cultural factors—in other words, the whole of the iceberg, which includes all of the community determinants of health.

Historically, nursing has been concerned with the whole person, the promotion of health across the life span—what Florence Nightingale referred to as "the Laws of Health." Nurses also have historically focused on people's responses to the illness experience in the

Figure 1.1 Nurses understand the *whole* of the iceberg; they are educated to see both above *and* below the water and to intervene accordingly.

context of their day-to-day lives. Much of the challenge in the role of the APRN has been the negotiation of seemingly disparate worlds: the reconciliation of an essentially holistic nursing model with a health-care system still focused predominantly on disease-oriented care. It is precisely this nexus between more discrete diagnostic categories of disease and a more holistic view of the continuum between health and illness—the iceberg—that gives nursing its identity, richness, diversity, and usefulness. Today's primary-care practitioners dwell in this nexus and must bridge these two realities—the world of disease and the world of illness, including the context of the patient's life in all its complexity. The increasing and necessary placement of APRNs into primary-care settings and teams across the health-care continuum provides nursing with the opportunity to effect change on both the micro and macro levels—in the lives of individual patients and families, as well as in the well-being of communities, including the global community.

A recent Hastings Center Report discussed the difficulty in making prevention a meaningful part of health-care reform because it involves changing behavior. The author notes that changing health behaviors involves changing habits that have "complex developmental, psychological, cultural, and socioeconomic roots" (Blacksher, 2009). In addition, health promotion and disease prevention require comprehensive policy changes and community involvement. In addition to care of the sick, the real-life, day-to-day health needs of people, their social and economic circumstances, and their communities are all part of the traditional domain of nursing practice as stated by Florence Nightingale. Nightingale understood these links and discussed them, as well as care of the sick, in her prophetic *Notes on Nursing* (1860).

Nurse historian Ellen Baer notes that the services demanded of primary-care providers today are broader in scope than those within the domain of medicine before the 1960s. Supportive functions, previously the domain of the clergy or multigenerational families and the like, are now within the purview of the primary-care provider. Likewise, the conceptual shift to health promotion, coupled with increased knowledge about healthy lifestyles, necessitates that primary-care providers be well grounded in their patients' community context. In making her case for the role of the nurse in primary care, Baer concludes: "The best reason for nurses to provide primary care is because they are nurses. Nursing's focus on people; its blend of medical, behavioral, and social science expertise; and its commitment to caring, teaching, counseling, and supporting patients are the characteristics of nursing that make nurses so uniquely qualified to provide primary health care services" (Baer, 1993).

This text provides a nursing-based approach to primary care and includes content on health promotion and disease prevention, as well as the diagnosis, management, and treatment of disease in the primary-care setting. The essentials of disease pathology and management necessary

for safe and satisfactory functioning in the clinical area are integrated into a view of the wholeness of persons, an understanding of human responses, and a repertoire of therapeutic options. This information will enable the primary-care provider, regardless of disciplinary background, to become an orchestrator of health and wellness, as well as a skilled negotiator and mediator in the space that exists between health and illness, between disease and the "lived experience of the patient" in the context of his or her community. APRNs must understand the discipline of nursing to effectively fill the gap between health and illness with true nursing care. Nurses on teams and in IPE educational settings must be confident and secure about their knowledge base and its contribution to the care of the patient.

The American Association of Colleges of Nursing (AACN) has called for all APRN preparation to take place in practice-based programs at the doctoral level—the Doctor of Nursing Practice (DNP). In 2006, the AACN *Essentials of Doctoral Education for Advanced Nursing Practice* was approved (American Association of Colleges of Nursing, 2009). Essential VIII, Advanced Nursing Practice, was further defined as a set of advanced nursing practice competencies (Table 1.1).

The DNP is a catalyst, allowing nursing to develop and expand nursing knowledge and practice through health promotion and disease prevention practices, essential for disciplinary distinction and growth (Burman et al, 2009). As noted by Burman et al, "Ultimately our vision is for NP care to be consistently 'different,'

Table 1.1   Essential VIII: Advanced Nursing Practice Competencies
1. Conduct a comprehensive and systematic assessment of health and illness parameters in complex situations, incorporating diverse and culturally sensitive approaches.
2. Design, implement, and evaluate therapeutic interventions based on nursing science and other sciences.
3. Develop and sustain therapeutic relationships and partnerships with patients (individuals, family, or group) and other professionals to facilitate optimal care and patient outcomes.
4. Demonstrate advanced levels of clinical judgment, systems thinking, and accountability in designing, delivering, and evaluating evidence-based care to improve patient outcomes.
5. Guide, mentor, and support other nurses to achieve excellence in nursing practice.
6. Educate and guide individuals and groups through complex health and situational transitions.
7. Use conceptual and analytic skills in evaluating links among practice, organizational, population, fiscal, and policy issues.

Source: American Association of Colleges of Nursing (AACN). *Essentials of doctoral education for advanced nursing practice.* 2006.

yet just as essential as physician care, leading to positive outcomes in health promotion and disease management" (2009).

■ HISTORICAL PERSPECTIVES ON ADVANCED PRACTICE NURSING

Nursing as a discipline and a profession with a theoretical base can be traced to Florence Nightingale. As long ago as 1860, Nightingale in *Notes on Nursing* proclaimed that there were laws of sickness and laws of health. There was not enough known, she wrote, about the laws of health. Nursing the "room," meaning the environment surrounding the patient, was as important as nursing the patient. She also wrote that nursing and medicine were like "cats and dogs" and should not be mixed.

The early public health nurses of Lillian Wald's Henry Street Settlement House at the turn of the 20th century were an autonomous lot, with their own vision of health and illness. They took this message directly to the community, including both working and living in this community. Lavinia Dock, one of the first Henry Street nurses, evolved a model, shown in Figure 1.2, that is much needed today. New and emerging primary-care models are attempting to recapture population-based care, health promotion, and disease prevention in more meaningful and reimbursable ways, such as team approaches and the ideas of Patient-Centered Medical Homes (PCMHs) and Affordable Care Organizations (ACOs), integrated health-care systems that cross the continuum of care.

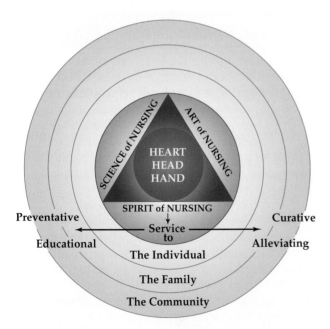

Figure 1.2 The professional equipment of the modern nurse and the scope of her responsibilities. *(Source: Dock, LL, and Stewart, IM. A short history of nursing: From the earliest times to the present day, ed 3. GP Putnam's Sons, New York, 1931, p 337.)*

Nurses' functions have always been rooted in population-based, public health approaches, and nursing has always claimed domains that were educational and preventive as well as curative. Nurses alleviated illness and actualized self and "other" through service to the individual, family, and community. As noted by Blacksher in an editorial in the *Hastings Center Report on Prevention,* "Health happens where people live, learn, love, work, and play" (2009). These activities flowed from the spirit, science, and art of nursing or the "heart, head, and hand" of nursing (a phrase popularized by Virginia Henderson [1966]). The first instances of standardized protocols, for example, evolved from the work of the early school nurses and the New York City Public Health Department. These early public health nurses enjoyed an autonomy of practice similar to that exercised by today's primary-care providers. Dock and Stewart (1920) likened the relationship between nursing and medicine to workers on a team who complement and supplement each other; the relationship is based on neither independence nor subordination but on interdependence and cooperation.

Henderson's 1966 book *The Nature of Nursing* was an attempt to provide nursing with its own explanatory model for practice. Building on her own experiences in nursing (Henderson also spent time as a public health nurse at the Henry Street Settlement) and on her understanding of physiology, she tried to place nursing on a continuum with medical care. Henderson argued that nurses had to place themselves (figuratively) "inside" patients in order to become their "counterpart, alter ego, or helper" (1966).

Martha Rogers, another nurse-theoretician, argued for the necessity of an independent basis of nursing science out of which autonomous nursing practice grows. According to Rogers, "Primary care by nurses is as old as modern nursing," citing a number of examples rooted in her early public health nursing experiences (as quoted in Hektor, 1989). She was, however, staunchly opposed to the development of the nurse practitioner role. In a 1975 position statement published in the *American Journal of Nursing,* she boldly asserted, "Not all nurses have succumbed to the blandishments of euphemisms and the increasingly blatant perfidy spawned by such terms as *pediatric associate, nurse practitioner, primary-care practitioner, geriatric practitioner, physician extender,* and other equally weird and wonderful cover-ups—designed to provide succor and profit for the nation's shamans" (Rogers). Those patients that ended up in hospitals were, in her words, "our mistakes" (as quoted in Hektor, 1989).

The early nurse practitioner "movement" evolved with little connection to academia and the flurry of nursing conceptual models and theories that proliferated throughout the 1970s and 1980s. These pioneering nurse practitioners, rooted in practice, usually in a primary-care setting, and often "trained" in certificate programs, had little patience with the abstractions of nursing theory that provided little meaning for their day-to-day practice. They needed and valued the medical model to care for their patients. Yet most remained nurses at heart, devoted to health promotion, disease prevention, and providing holistic care to their patients. Nurses in today's DNP programs bring 4 years of a nursing baccalaureate base with them, as well as practice as *nurses*. Thus, the DNP is a strong base on which to build advanced nursing practice.

Very few nursing models have addressed or attempted to make sense of the dichotomy of nurse practitioner practice and medical care. Some argue that no dichotomy exists. A number of others, however, identify the relationship between advanced nursing practice and medical practice as an issue requiring ongoing attention. Cody views medicine as still dominating nursing politically, and he states that many nurses "actually value having medical tasks delegated to them" (1994). On a more ominous note, he points out that nursing must realize what is merely delegated from another (more powerful) discipline can also be taken away. He concludes, "Only when nurses everywhere are guided by a theory base specific to nursing will nursing have achieved parity with other scholarly disciplines." In a coauthored article, Barbara Bates, MD, and Joan Lynaugh, NP, venture some thoughts on the relationship between nursing and medicine: Medicine, they speculate, is concerned with structure; nursing is focused on function (Lynaugh & Bates, 1973).

In an unpublished paper, Lynaugh discusses the respective roles of nurses and physicians in greater depth. She notes that the biomedical model of disease and cure, which swept across the Western world, seemed far more compelling and promising than nursing's holism, environmentalism, and "watchful waiting" approach to illness (Lynaugh & Bates, 1973). Nurses, she elaborates, seem to be both inarticulate in explaining their work and "touchingly confident" that altruism will eventually be rewarded. Years of medical dominance have drawn a veil over the work of nursing. Lynaugh stresses that this invisibility is serious because it compromises the public's access to good nursing care in an era in which reimbursement for care is restricted to payment based exclusively on the phenomena of interest to physicians. The power relationships among patient, nurse, and physician are complicated by economic issues, professional territoriality on all sides, and profound questions of disciplinary identity; therefore, Lynaugh suggests, adjustments in these relationships will come slowly, step by step, but inevitably. An essential component of this process is making the "invisible" work of nurses more visible. It is the part of the iceberg that is below the water that takes up so much of nursing's time and energy and is so unnamed and unseen. Demonstration of nursing's contribution to patient care is vital. This is accomplished, in part, through the clear articulation of nursing's theoretical base.

As nursing theory embraces the mode of midrange theory development and testing, with real-life clinical applications for practice, the applicability to advanced practice nursing and the utilization of theory-based practice should increase. This still begs the question, however, of an underlying theoretical basis for advanced practice nursing. It can be argued, as Burman et al do in an article titled "Reconceptualizing the Core of Nurse Practitioner Education and Practice," that "the heart and soul of nursing is health promotion both in healthy persons and those dealing with chronic illness" (Burman et al, 2009). Nursing practice as a DNP should focus more explicitly on health promotion, changing health behaviors, and chronic disease management, thus advancing a unique nursing science. These are traditional nursing domains and strengths. These authors state that advanced practice nurses "can fill the growing societal need for expert clinicians to assume major leadership roles in clinical management and evaluation of outcomes research arenas. Doctor of Nursing Practice (DNP) programs include extensive clinical practicum and have a strong focus on scholarly and evidence-based practice."

■ ADVANCED PRACTICE NURSING: MODELS OF PRACTICE

Expert practice domains of the clinical nurse specialist and nurse practitioner were originally identified by Fenton and Brykczynski in 1993 and evolved from domains identified in Patricia Benner's 1984 book *From Novice to Expert*. In 1990, these identified domains were used by the National Organization of Nurse Practitioner Faculties (NONPF), the long-time leader in education of nurse practitioners (Zimmer et al, 1990) to create a framework for primary-care nurse practitioner curricula.

In a study by Lewis and Brykczynski (1994), the authors elaborated on the practical knowledge as well as the healing role of nurse practitioners. In the discussion of their findings, the authors state that to bring about healing, nurse practitioners will go beyond the call of duty, going to schools, for example, to fight for a patient's rights, making phone calls, driving patients to appointments, and going to funerals. The practitioners in the study describe both the professional and personal satisfaction derived from their caring practices, even when the rewards of such actions were small. Lewis and Brykczynski (1994) situate their work within a caring paradigm, citing work by Sally Gadow, Jean Watson, and Madeline Leininger. They also cite the 1991 work of Benner, who, in studying the effectiveness of expert nurses, found that mere technique and knowledge were not enough, and that caring, or a certain level of human involvement, was required for expert human practice. Indeed, expert "human practice" should be a goal of all primary-care providers.

Johnson (1993) cites clear evidence of a nursing perspective in nurse practitioner practice in primary care. According to Johnson, nurse practitioner–patient dialogue incorporates the voice of medicine and the voice of the "lifeworld" (of the patient). The skilled practitioner "knows self" and how to share his or her own personal experience to either enhance the patient's progress or strengthen the provider–patient bond. An element of camaraderie was viewed as positive and not in opposition to maintaining a professional stance. *Coordination, continuity,* and *advocacy* were the major functions the nurse practitioners in this study believed they contributed to the practice. All primary-care practice needs these functions, which constitute some of the foundational ideas of a Patient-Centered Medical Home.

Swanson (1995) proposed "A Spirit-Focused Conceptual Model of Nursing for the Advanced Practice Nurse" in which she identified the core of every person, both patient and nurse, as the spirit. She describes the act of nursing as a goal-directed interpersonal relationship between the patient and nurse, based on traditional nursing process components such as assessing, planning, intervening, and evaluating. Interventions are broad based, ranging from play, music, and stories to utilization of counseling principles such as active listening and anticipatory guidance. The use of this approach in primary-care practice could be adapted by any primary-care practitioner.

The Shuler Nurse Practitioner Practice Model (Shuler & Davis, 1993) is an ambitious attempt to describe the nurse practitioner's integrated role. Building on a holistic nursing assessment, the next step is the mutual identification of unmet patient health needs to identify health problems. The treatment plan must be mutually agreeable and oriented toward self-care; disease prevention and health promotion activities are incorporated into the treatment plan. Nonpharmacological treatments, including alternative and complementary healing practices, are also integrated into the plan. These approaches are framed within the concept of functioning within a multidisciplinary team and could be seen as particularly relevant for today.

In addition, this model is seen as enhancing both the patient's and the nurse practitioner's personal movement toward wellness. Patients are encouraged to examine their lives honestly and to identify areas that are not "balanced." The patient's physical and psychological ability to participate in wellness activities is assessed; creative, uninhibited problem-solving and identification of appropriate wellness activities are pursued. The model emphasizes that the primary-care provider's personal commitment to wellness and health can have a direct impact on the practitioner's ability to influence positive patient outcomes.

Another interesting approach to nursing phenomena, not elaborated as unique for APRNs, but yet with wide applicability to the autonomy of an advanced practice nursing role, is "symptom management." This work has evolved from the University of California, San Francisco, School of Nursing Symptom Management Faculty Group (1994) and has since been revised based on research studies testing the model (Dodd et al, 2001). Proponents of this approach note that when the underlying cause of the patient's problem and the presenting symptoms are managed concurrently, patients are more likely to benefit and remain in treatment.

The Symptom Management group proposes that symptoms be viewed as subjective experiences reflecting changes in a person's biopsychosocial function, sensation, or cognition. They contrast this view of the word *symptom,* a subjective phenomenon, with the word *sign,* which is used to mean an abnormality indicative of disease, which can be observed by another person and sometimes by the patient, and is thus identified as objective. The model they propose for looking at symptoms has three dimensions:

1. The symptom experience (subjective)
2. Symptom management strategies
3. Symptom outcomes

In the revised Symptom Management Model, the nursing domains of nursing science, person, health/illness, and environment are described as having an effect on these three dimensions (Dodd et al, 2001). The model encompasses a multidimensional approach to the experience of the symptom, ways to approach the management of symptoms (always in concert with the patient and family), and outcomes that are gauged on a variety of axes.

Snyder and Mirr (1995) conceptualize advanced practice within a nursing paradigm built around human responses as a focus for nursing interventions. They identify the following foci for advanced practice nursing:

1. Self-care limitations
2. Impaired functioning in areas of rest, sleep, ventilation, circulation, nutrition, and the like
3. Pain and discomfort
4. Emotional problems related to illness and treatment, life-threatening events, or daily experiences, such as anxiety, loss, or loneliness
5. Distortion of symbolic functions reflected in interpersonal and intellectual processes such as hallucinations
6. Deficiencies in decision-making ability to make personal choices
7. Self-image changes required by health status
8. Dysfunctional perceptual orientations to health
9. Strains related to life processes such as birth, development, and death
10. Problematic affiliative relationships

Patient problems, conceptualized in this manner, are amenable to uniquely nursing-based interventions. Attention to human responses, as such, provide the missing link to much that is absent within today's contemporary health-care system. Many of these responses are tied to social determinants of health—such as where one lives and works. Our current health-care system, however, is not structured in such a way to make many of these practices sustainable: They are not coded for reimbursement.

Ryan's (2009) Integrated Theory of Health Behavior Change (ITHBC) is based on the belief that health promotion activities are an integral part of the long-term health and well-being of both healthy people and those with chronic illnesses. For health promotion to be successful, people must take responsibility for initiating and maintaining both health behavior changes and prevention behaviors. APRNs are in a position to facilitate and support health behavior changes in their patients, and therefore APRNs require knowledge of what drives people to make these changes. This is especially true in today's health-care system, which requires patients and their families to take responsibility for increasingly complex conditions in the home. This trend will continue to escalate as hospital care will be reserved for acutely ill patients.

The ITHBC can be used by APRNs to tailor interventions for individual patients in such a way that positively affects their long-term health status. Health behavior change is directly influenced by "fostering knowledge and beliefs, increasing self-regulation skill and ability, and enhancing social facilitation" (Ryan, 2009). Social facilitation involves both social influence and support, which is of particular importance to APRNs, who are in a unique position to be a source of both for their patients. New research demonstrates that health behaviors are strongly influenced by the health behaviors of those in the patient's social network. Models such as ITHBC have great relevance for APRNs in primary-care settings today.

Cumbie, Conley, and Burman's (2004) Model of Promoting Process Engagement is a patient-centered theory developed to assist APRNs to manage the care of chronically ill patients. In this model, interventions of the APRN are chosen based on each patient's needs and expectations of his or her care and are developed in collaboration with the patient. "Interventions focus on motivational strategies designed to facilitate and support individuals as they make sense of health information, engage in health promoting activities, and sustain health-related behavioral change" (Cumbie et al, 2004). People are influenced by a number of internal and external variables that cause them to either "resist or engage in beneficial health behaviors" (Cumbie et al, 2004). To promote engagement, APRNs must help patients make sense of health information so that this information can become meaningful to them.

APRNs can use the intervention structure of the model to help their patients become actively involved in managing chronic illness. Engagement strategies include patient-centered assessment followed by therapeutic interview, and communication techniques (Cumbie et al, 2004). When the patient's health–illness situation is understood, the APRN works with patients to determine their health priorities and to develop mutually agreed on health goals and a plan of action to meet these goals

(Cumbie et al, 2004). Case management, advocacy, and referral are activities of the ongoing collaborative process, which is the part of the intervention that is used to "sustain health process engagement" (Cumbie et al, 2004).

■ CHANGING MODELS OF MEDICAL PRACTICE

Changes are afoot in medical practice as well. Fiscally unsustainable, the American health-care system *had* to change. Cost-consciousness, the availability of medical information (and misinformation) on the Internet, the move from hospital to community provision of health care, multiculturalism, the growing interest in holistic care and alternative therapies, an increasingly litigious environment, and the ever-expanding use of technology— all of these factors continue to force reexamination of traditional professional roles.

Advances in therapeutics over the course of the 20th century, which are often taken for granted now, were overwhelmingly different than any that had been seen before. Medicine is able to intervene—specifically, powerfully, and radically—in the course of previously fatal diseases. No disorder, however complex, seems beyond the possibility of understanding and cure. As a result, the impact of medicine is felt far beyond the immediacies of the patient–provider encounter. Alcoholism, for example, viewed as a moral disorder in earlier times, is now a phenomenon conceptualized as a disease, with an array of both psychological and pharmacological interventions available to practitioners.

A review of the progress of medicine in combating disease is a journey from an integrated view of illness and therapeutics to one of discrete diseases with distinct causes and an armamentarium of ever-expanding and specific therapeutics. From the time of the ancient Greeks and Romans until well into the 19th century, illness was seen as an imbalance in the economy of the whole body, which could be expressed in the relationships between input or output of food, sweat, secretions, urine, phlegm, and the like. Treatment was focused on restoring harmony and balance between body and environment (a view promulgated by Nightingale, 1860/1969). Specific symptoms were not treated; instead, a systemic physiological effect was sought through such methods as inducing or facilitating sweating, febrilysis, diuresis, and/or vomiting. These interventions, it was theorized, would assist the body to recover its balance.

Throughout the course of the 19th century, however, this integrated view of disease and therapeutics was increasingly challenged by notions of discrete disease states with specific causes. Illnesses seemed less amenable to purges, bleeding, and diuretics (the so-called holistic approaches) than was previously thought. Quite late in the modern era, the first active principles of some of the oldest, most useful botanicals were isolated, and later some were even synthesized. A new dimension was added to the emerging concept of specificity of therapeutics by the discovery of sulfonamides in the late 1930s and penicillin in the early 1940s. Not only could therapy be directed at particular symptoms, but for the first time, therapeutics could become "radical," matching the power of the surgeon's knife—that is, they could eradicate the primary cause of an illness, in this case, specific microorganisms.

More highly specific measures, such as the use of antisera, the isolation of blood fractions, and the synthesis of polypeptide hormones, are products of the last few decades. Advances in laboratory analysis and diagnostic techniques confer on therapeutics the capability of effecting cure at the molecular loci of disease. The era of specific and radical therapeutics has only just begun. What seems certain is the trend toward even greater specificity in diagnosis and treatment of disease, extending to the genetic level. This will continue to have profound effects on the medical profession, on society, and on inherent power imbalances among patients, nurses, and physicians. Additionally, new diagnostic and therapeutic technologies will surely raise questions of access to care and equitable distribution among all patients.

Medicine's successes have led to a generation of physician-specialists, some of whom are far removed from the day-to-day lives of their patients. The effectiveness of modern therapeutics adds a powerful strain of reductionism and positivism to the 20th-century medical ethos. Although this has been a useful stance for the creation of effective medical interventions, when universalized to all realms of medical practice, this stance may be antithetical to the fulfillment of the more sensitive moral and social responsibilities of medicine. Care—when defined as helping the patient and family to cope, offering reassurance, educating, and relieving worry—does not require a high level of scientific sophistication, but it does require human understanding. When the physician's remuneration was meager and he or she was a member of the community, issues such as those raised above may have been negotiated more successfully between doctor and patient. The doctor of today, however, is more often a stranger with multiple competing priorities. This raises a fearful dilemma for patients: They must trust the physician because of his or her power to heal, but that trust is undermined by the fear of the physician's self-interest. Additionally, social responsibilities in a broader sense—in a public health sense—have become neglected.

Concurrently, there has been a dawning recognition of the *limits* of medical progress and its partner, technological innovation. Beginning with the AIDS epidemic in the early 1980s through the current struggle with multidrug-resistant organisms, it has become increasingly clear that not everything can be controlled solely through medical technology and the development of newer therapeutics. Overwhelming evidence exists that technological innovations are drivers of health-care costs. In numerous studies over time, some 60% of improvement in health status is

tied to socioeconomic factors, particularly education and income. With the notable exception of the health care of elders, this means that only approximately 40% of improvements in health result from medical care.

There is an increasing call for a better balance between cure-oriented and care-oriented medicine. Chronic disease continues to emerge as the most difficult and expensive kind of health problem to manage, as demonstrated in the failure of cure-oriented medicine to completely eradicate the most common causes of morbidity, such as heart disease and cancer. People are merely living with them longer; in fact, much of medicine is focused on the long-term management, rather than cure, of chronic disease. Care-oriented medicine reflects well-coordinated medical assistance to patients to enable them to manage disease combined with the marshaling of needed family and social supports—again, traditional nursing strengths and domains. Prevention as an approach can only go so far, however. In the end, sickness and death can be forestalled, but not eradicated, and the costs deferred or minimized, but not eliminated entirely. According to Daniel Callahan, "Serious progress would mean turning back the clock: learning to take care of ourselves, to tolerate some degree of discomfort, to accept the reality of aging and death, and to see our personal doctor as someone as likely to talk to as to have us scanned" (Callahan, 2009).

Medicine is not unaware of this quandary; indeed, these issues are widely discussed in medical circles and among policy makers. A loss of 60% of the nation's hospital beds has been predicted in some reports. There is a converging agreement among health-care and health-care policy experts that allopathic medicine as it has developed across the 20th century does not give the country that much health. Nine-tenths of the health of a community has to do with habits, lifestyles, environment, and genetics. Allopathic medicine only operates at the margin, yet the American health-care system has been structured on this mode of care (Commonwealth Fund Commission on a High Performance Health Care System, 2008).

Over the last decade, American health professional schools were charged with expanding the scientific base of their programs to include psychosocial–behavioral sciences, as well as population-based approaches to clinical work (Whitcomb & Nutter, 2004). The sharing of clinical teaching resources, especially in key areas of preclinical and clinical training, is mandated, as well as cross-teaching and more exploration of the roles played by various professionals, referred to as interprofessional education (IPE). Active modeling of effective team integration in the delivery of efficient, high-quality care is essential to the aims of decreased costs, increased access, and improved quality outcomes that are the hallmark of health-care reform.

In addition, effective interdisciplinary teamwork is essential to bridge the ever-widening chasm between basic science research and the implementation of that research at the bedside. Over the last 30 years, basic science and clinical research have diverged, and a divide has opened between biomedical researchers and the patients who need their discoveries (Committee on Facilitating Interdisciplinary Research, 2005). This has led to the conceptualization of *translational research* as bridging that gap. Indeed, many of the major strides in understanding disease mechanisms are not resulting in commensurate gains in new treatments, diagnostics, or prevention; conversely, important clinical questions arising at the bedside are not making their way back to the laboratory for investigation. New cures and therapies are ever more expensive to develop and "worryingly thin on the ground". The spectacular success of basic science research, largely funded by the National Institutes of Health (NIH), has led to questions regarding the mandate to apply that knowledge, as consistent with the mission of pursuing fundamental knowledge and applying it "to reduce the burdens of illness and disability" (Committee on Facilitating Interdisciplinary Research, 2005). Biomedical research was previously the domain of physician-scientists, who also cared for patients. However, advances in molecular biology in the 1970s created a new paradigm, in which clinical and basic research began to diverge. Today, the majority of biomedical research is conducted by highly specialized PhD scientists, whereas physician-scientists are a minority. In turn, translational research *demands* collaboration. Large multidisciplinary groups composed of basic scientists and clinicians, as well as bioinformaticians, statisticians, engineers, and industry experts, are needed to work together and bridge the gulf between bench and bedside. Certainly, DNPs and APRNs would be appropriate team members to participate in this enterprise and may be ideally suited to coordinate, if not lead, such teams.

Emerging trends in medicine have included more explicitly the need for relational models of care. In 1995, Dacher espoused the "Whole Healing model," which is rooted in assumptions of dynamism, holism, and purposefulness. He called for a renewed emphasis on the quality and character of the relationships that constitute the healing process—the practitioner to himself or herself, to his or her patient, to other practitioners, and to the community at large—and a careful balance between reductive and holistic perspectives. This integrated model expands the diagnostic process, for example, to include a concern with psychological, spiritual, community, and environmental issues and acknowledges the uniqueness and subjectivity of a person's life circumstances. This approach is totally consistent with a nursing-based approach.

In *Patient-Centered Medicine,* the physician authors (Stewart et al, 1995) address the need for a new method of patient care, founded in new paradigms. On the limitations of the current medical model, situated in the context of disease and curative therapeutics, the authors remind us: "A particular disease is what everyone with that disease has in common, but the illness experience of every person is unique." Patient-centered medicine encourages exploring both the disease and the illness experience, understanding the whole person, finding common ground, incorporating prevention and health promotion, enhancing the patient–doctor relationship, and being realistic. Clearly, these components have been well established in nursing models.

In 2003, the Institute of Medicine published *Health Professions Education: A Bridge to Quality.* This report on reforming education for the health professions emphasized the relationship of high-quality and safe patient care to substantive changes in the way health professionals are educated. Five core competencies were identified:

- Provide patient-centered care
- Work in interdisciplinary teams
- Use evidence-based practice
- Apply quality improvement
- Use informatics

An idea that has gained particular currency in the context of the ACA is the Patient-Centered Medical Home (PCMH). Operational characteristics of this idea include accessible, continuous, comprehensive, family-centered, coordinated, compassionate, and culturally effective care (Payne, 2009). Further statements include a definition of the PCMH as "a health care setting that facilitates partnerships between patients, their personal physicians, and when appropriate, their families."

The American Association of Nurse Practitioners (AANP) supports the concept of the PCMH. The AANP defines the medical home as "a healthcare provider group that provides patients with a single point of access to care, coordinated by a provider who has in-depth knowledge of the patient" (Riffle, 2010). But exactly *who* is that provider? *Must* it be a medical doctor? Important reimbursement decisions for the future—as well as the nature of health care—rest on the question of *which* primary-care providers are qualified and should be defined as the "leader" in this model. It will be up to APRNs in each state to work toward guaranteeing their full inclusion as leaders in various pilot projects, as the effectiveness of the PCMH is evaluated. Additionally, APRNs must *own* their own practices and outcomes in order to share full accountability with physician providers. True data on outcomes of care by APRNs will not be accurate if APRNs bill for reimbursement "incident to" the physician's practice. Being an APRN demands full professional responsibility. Increased responsibility also brings increased liability.

Medicine recognizes the need to incorporate new perspectives of practice, essentially following the long-established lead of nursing. Likewise, it is equally appropriate that nursing incorporate traditional aspects of the medical model into its continually expanding scope of practice. Patient problems, after all, are real and complex, necessitating multidimensional approaches. The *Circle of Caring* model (discussed next) is offered as a unique approach to patient problems, one that incorporates and builds on both traditional nursing and medical approaches, as well as retaining an openness to a variety of other approaches to phenomena. This model may reflect what most primary-care providers intuitively do, making more visible the so-often "invisible" work of nursing in the health-care encounter—work that is not currently coded or reimbursed but that is there and is often tremendously meaningful for the patient. In this sense, the *Circle of Caring* model may not be considered original but rather is derived from the realities of day-to-day advanced nursing practice in primary care.

■ A TRANSFORMATIVE TEMPLATE: THE CIRCLE OF CARING

Both the traditional medical and nursing models are predicated on a subjective and objective database, a labeling of the patient's problem and response, a therapeutic plan, and an evaluation of the outcome. The *Circle of Caring* model builds on these features and expands them to include the following:

- A broadened and contextualized database, more typical of a holistic nursing assessment, that gives the health-care provider a more in-depth understanding of the patient's situation, life, strengths, and weaknesses, including social determinants of health.
- A labeling of the patient's concern that more actively incorporates the patient's responses to the meaning of illness in his or her day-to-day life, as well as standard medical diagnostic language.
- A holistic and creative approach to an individualized therapeutic plan that includes nursing interventions based on evidence, including complementary therapies as appropriate, incorporated with standardized pharmacological, surgical, and other nonpharmacological interventions.
- A view of outcomes based on the patient, family, social group, and community perceptions of improvement, as well as the more traditional, quantified outcome measures such as mortality and morbidity, with emerging primary-care quality indicators and costs of care also built into these outcomes. This integrates the health of populations into the outcomes of care.

The *Circle of Caring* model is a synthesized view of the problem-solving methodology that may be used in a variety of settings—primary-care, acute-care, and community-based settings. A linear representation of the problem-solving method necessitated in practice was chosen for clarity of communication of the concepts of the model, and it is embedded in the middle of the schema (see Fig. 1.3).

This process is encircled by caring, a visual representation of the interpersonal process that occurs among the caregiver and the patient, which also reflects the family, social group, and community of the patient. The ability to provide effective and meaningful care for the patient is based on the processes of care. This is what enables the nurse to hear the patient's "call" and to fashion creative nursing responses. Care is actualized through caring processes drawn from Mayeroff (1971) and Boykin and Schoenhofer (2001): patience, courage, advocacy, authentic presence, commitment, and knowing.

A Broadened, Contextualized Database

A contextualized approach—the lived experience of the patient in the context of his or her community—is central to this model and is one that most nurses have learned in their undergraduate nursing programs. Although the patient's subjective perception of this experience is captured in the history portion of the assessment database, the *Circle of Caring* is based on hearing the patient's story in all its complexity, as well as eliciting the patient's own unique meaning of *health*. In addition, increased attention is focused on the interplay among perceptual, psychodynamic, socioeconomic, cultural, and environmental factors that have an impact on the patient's health status—in other words, increased awareness and attention to social determinants of health.

The Nature of Patient Responses

The 1995 American Nurses Association's Social Policy Statement defined nursing as the "diagnosis and treatment of human responses to actual and potential health problems." The *Circle of Caring* model may be used effectively with the traditional tool of nursing diagnosis. Boykin and Schoenhofer (2001) conceptualized the phenomenon of human responses as "calls for nursing." As such, these calls remain unique, interactional, and contextualized, and thus not amenable to any form of generic labeling. It is through coming to know people as caring persons that the nurse is able to fully hear each patient's call.

The importance of the labeling of the patient's problem (i.e., the "call for nursing"), be it in medical or nursing diagnostic terminology or in a more generic format, is that it helps to address the patient responses more effectively. Labeling thus involves the acknowledgment and knowledge of the complex interplay of perceptual, psychodynamic, socioeconomic, cultural, and environmental factors that contribute to health. APRNs are especially skilled at eliciting and understanding this complexity and at fashioning nursing-based responses that are uniquely suited to the individual.

A Creative Approach to Therapeutics

Another hallmark of the *Circle of Caring* model is its broadened approach to therapeutics. This approach should be actualized in day-to-day practice by APRNs, yet remains an especially invisible piece of nursing work. This flexible nursing-based approach entails working with

Figure 1.3 The *Circle of Caring* model.

the individual patient to tailor evidence-based interventions geared to the meaning of *health* as defined by that patient. Building on current standards of medical and nursing practice, interventions are fine-tuned for each patient, in the context of community. Although a focus of this text is to provide current evidence-based standards of care, this approach often requires care providers to make decisions through narrowly prescribed filters. As noted by Richard Payne, "there is an art to clinical practice that extends beyond hard science and numbers and often requires swift, sound, decision-making in an environment of incomplete evidence. Sometimes no formula or calculation based on quantified evidence and data can determine the appropriate action" (2009).

Alternative and complementary therapies are considered. This requires a creative approach to therapeutics that includes holistic approaches to healing, as well as a sophisticated understanding of evidence-based practice. Research in this area is proliferating as patients are calling for alternative and complementary approaches (Riffle, 2010).

In nursing as caring, the nurse is an artist who responds creatively to calls for nursing with unique nursing responses. Any taxonomy of nursing must, of necessity, have universal applicability. What distinguishes so many of nursing's interventions, however, is precisely their uniqueness and the tailoring of an individual response to each patient. This is the "artistry" of the APRN.

A broadened approach to therapeutics based on a contextualized database implies attention to the context of the patient's life, and as such the social determinants of health.

■ POPULATION-BASED APPROACHES

Outcomes: Who Decides What Is Desirable?

Outcomes-based research of today demonstrates the need to incorporate patients' perceptions as measured both objectively (by functional assessments and similar methods) and subjectively. Quality-of-life measures and, most important, the various and individualistic meanings of health and illness must be taken more fully into consideration. The *patient experience* is a frequently used measure of quality care in both the acute- and primary-care settings. Plans must be assessed according to their potential to assist patients, families, social groups, and communities to meet their goals in ways that are meaningful to them, not just as standard items on a checklist of preventive measures. The voice of an increasingly informed, information-savvy health-care consumer demands no less.

Multiple social and environmental factors on health are recognized as additional pieces of the health-care puzzle—that of public health. Social determinants of health are increasingly acknowledged as one component of the huge understructure of the primary-care iceberg discussed earlier—the "unseen" and often invisible part beneath the water.

Sometimes labeled *community-oriented primary care,* health-care approaches that account for social and environmental factors are now understood to be essential elements of a truly reformed health-care system and are also referred to as *population-based care* or *preventive care.* This holistic approach was largely abandoned by allopathic medical science in the earlier part of the 20th century in favor of technology-based interventions and medical specialization (Brandt, 1997). However, modern medicine recognizes the need for such approaches to provide more effective care with lasting effects and to deal with current health-care realities that highlight the interplay among human health and environmental and social influences (e.g., the health effects of community violence, teen pregnancy, and HIV infection). As with medicine, nursing has renewed its emphasis on population-based approaches, reaffirming its historic roots, and there is now a shared understanding of the importance of these approaches. This is an ideal climate in which to build interprofessional education—shared *core* understandings of care, but with variations in ways to implement or practice these understandings.

Much of the hope for a more responsive, more effective, and less expensive health-care delivery system seems, as of this writing (2014), to be pinned on the PCMH or, as it is described in some circles, "the medical home." Not a physical building of any kind, its architecture is "a philosophical transformation of the way that care is delivered" (Nutting et al, 2009). Patient care within a PCMH should have a whole-person orientation and be coordinated across the health-care system, replacing a fragmented, episodic health-care delivery system. New reimbursement models should reflect the added value of the PCMH to the patient by providing for continuous coordinated care and expanded access to services that fall outside of the fee-for-service system. The process of transition into a PCMH model is a lengthy and complicated one and will require a champion—someone who can allocate resources to this effort and both support

and coordinate the process of change. This process requires strong leadership and excellent organizational skills—additional areas in which APRNs excel.

Additionally, someone must lead the team of health-care providers and support staff who work with specific patient populations (e.g., diabetic patients or those with congestive heart failure). This leader might be the same person who advocates for the process of change, or it might be someone different who is focused solely on the provision of care to individual patients. Effective implementation of the PCMH model requires someone to delegate duties among the team of providers and to make decisions, along with the patient, about aspects of care such as referral to specialists. Regardless of who assumes this role, the PCMH leader must be able to move the organization forward to meet the accreditation requirements and to receive enhanced reimbursement as a PCMH practice. Similar to JCAHO or Magnet recognition programs, a PCMH practice must meet specific criteria and inspection requirements by one of four current accrediting agencies: the National Committee for Quality Assurance (NCQA); the Joint Commission (JCAHO); the Utilization Review Accreditation Committee (URAC); and/or the Accreditation Association for Ambulatory Health Care (AAHC). For example, to receive recognition as a PCMH practice by the NCQA depends on meeting specific elements in six standard categories (see Table 1.2).

Evaluation of the PCMH model is just beginning, and thus far, results are mixed. Wide-scale adoption of this model would fundamentally change the primary-care landscape. At present, the physician's skill set is not geared toward care coordination or managing transitions in care, because these functions have been historically performed by nurses.

However, the challenges in our health-care system call for creative thinking and innovative improvements in care. Various technologies will continue to emerge, and health care will continue to evolve, but the interpersonal caring base on which nursing has always been grounded will continue to be widely needed.

■ FURTHER UNDERSTANDING THE *CIRCLE OF CARING*

The *Circle of Caring* model (see Fig. 1.3) has grown out of, and is rooted in, the assumption that caring is the central concept in nursing and is uniquely known and expressed in nursing. Boykin and Schoenhofer (2001) contend that all nursing takes place within nursing situations, as "shared lived experiences in which caring between the persons of nurse and nursed enhances the process of living and growing in caring."

Watson (1988) viewed caring as an intersubjective human process based on the belief that "persons learn from one another how to be human by identifying ourselves with others or finding their dilemmas in ourselves." Boykin and Schoenhofer (2001) extended this

Table 1.2	NCQA PCMH Specific Elements and Standards
Enhance access and continuity	Accommodate patient's needs with access and advice during and after hours. Give patients and families information about medical home. Provide patients with team-based care
Identify and manage patient populations	Collect and use data for population management
Plan and manage care	Use evidence-based guidelines. Provide preventive, acute, and chronic care management, including medication management
Provide self-care support and community resources	Assist patients and their families in self-care management with information, tools, and resources
Track and coordinate care	Track and coordinate tests, referrals, and transitions of care
Measure and improve performance	Use performance and patient experience data for continuous improvement

concept and defined caring in nursing as "the intentional and authentic presence of the nurse with another who is recognized as a person living caring and growing in caring."

Mayeroff (1971) discussed the primacy of caring as a process in contrast to caring as a product, with caring viewed as an end in and of itself. Mayeroff also identified "ingredients" of caring: knowing, alternating rhythms, patience, honesty, courage, humility, trust and hope. Boykin and Schoenhofer viewed caring in nursing "as a mutual human process in which the nurse responds with authentic presence to a call from another" (2001). The caring attributes of the *Circle of Caring* are based on these—knowing, patience, authentic presence, commitment, courage, and advocacy—and are elaborated by Boykin and Schoenhofer in Chapter 2 of this text. It is the caring attributes that characterize the nurse–patient relationship, enabling healing. Healing is meant in the broadest sense of the word: it might imply a good death, for example.

Neither medicine nor nursing alone can heal the current problems ailing the U.S. health-care system. Both are needed more than ever to shape a healthful future. Both must rethink their roles, functions, and cultures.

Moving away from the hierarchical role structures of the hospital setting creates the opportunity for redefining the content and processes of clinical practice and negotiating a new and as yet undefined space. The boundaries of practice continue to expand and contract for both medicine and nursing during this transformative period. The larger questions for both professions include the following:

- How will all health-care professionals be accountable to their patients?
- Are physicians and APRNs willing to share accountability in a responsible manner?
- How can the Institute of Medicine's *Bridge to Quality* become a reality?
- How can disciplines work together in a meaningful way to achieve the goals and objectives of *Healthy People 2020*?
- How can medicine and nursing work together to achieve the triple aim of health-care reform: improving the patient experience of care (including quality and satisfaction); improving the health of populations; and reducing the per capita cost of health care?

Lynaugh, in an unpublished paper from 1989, suggests that both disciplines can occupy the same territory to the benefit of patient care; however, she notes that tension is created by proximity, stating that "physicians and nurses quarrel occasionally when they jostle each other in the narrow passageway of patient care." She makes the case, however, that tension is preferable to the distrust and ignorance that stem from silence and distance between the two disciplines. She advocates a "productive tension" and social parity between the two professions that will benefit the care of all patients. Nurses and physicians are natural allies. Both are needed, working together, for good and effective change to occur in the health-care system. Never did we need both perspectives more.

Daily in practice, primary-care providers hear the frustration of patients and families in dealing with today's health-care system. Although the technology of medical care continues to improve, the interactional and collaborative aspects of care are often underdeveloped. A *Circle of Caring* model is needed for patients, families, social groups, and communities. This model is also a way to document and describe the practice of primary-care providers, who respond to calls from patients and who imaginatively, creatively, and powerfully foster meaningful responses in the context of the situation. These responses may be fashioned on the micro level—the one-to-one clinician–patient relationship in primary or acute care—or on a macro level, as nursing-based knowledge unites with traditional public health approaches and is applied to the care of communities and populations (see Chapter 3). This transformative model, the *Circle of Caring,* incorporates the strengths of nursing, public health, and medicine, and reformulates them in a new model of care. Primary-care clinicians are the appropriate providers to demonstrate the efficacy of an integrated model of caregiving, rooted in the lived experience of the patient as experienced in the context of community. This text offers you the necessary tools to provide care in ways that will be meaningful for patients, their families, their social groups, and the larger communities in which they live.

 DavisPlus | For additional resources please visit http://davisplus.fadavis.com

References

Administration on Aging. *Aging into the 21st century.* U.S. Department of Health & Human Services. Retrieved from www.aoa.gov/AoARoot/Aging.Statistics/future_growth/aging21/health.aspx

American Association of Colleges of Nursing (AACN). Essentials of doctoral education for advanced nursing practice. 2009. Retrieved from www.aacn.nche.edu/dnp/PDF/essentials

American Nurses Association (ANA). *Nursing: A social policy statement.* ANA, Kansas City, MO, 1995.

Baer, E. Philosophical and historical bases of primary care nursing. In Mezey, MD, and McGivern, DO (Eds.), *Nurses, nurse practitioners: Evolution to advanced practice,* ed 2. Springer, New York, 1993, p 114.

Benner, P. *From novice to expert.* Addison-Wesley, Menlo Park, CA, 1984.

Benner, P, and Wrubel, J. *The primacy of caring.* Addison-Welsey, Menlo Park, CA, 1989.

Blacksher, E. Health reform: What's prevention got to do with it? Perspectives. *Hastings Cent Rep* 39(6):49, 2009.

Bodenheimer, T, Chen, E, and Bennett, HD. Confronting the growing burden of chronic disease: Can the U.S. health care workforce do the job? *Health Affairs, 28:* 64–74, 2009.

Boykin, A, and Schoenhofer, S. *Nursing as Caring: A model for transforming practice.* Jones and Bartlett and National League for Nursing Press, Sudbury, MA, 2001.

Brandt, AM. 'Just Say No': Risk, behavior, and disease in twentieth-century America. In Walters, R (Ed.), *Scientific authority and twentieth century America.* Johns Hopkins University Press, Baltimore, MD, 1997, pp 82–98.

Burman, ME, et al. Reconceptualizing the core of nurse practitioner education and practice. *Am Acad Nurse Pract* 21:11–17, 2009.

Callahan, D. Medical progress: Unintended consequences. In *Connecting American values with health reform.* A Publication of the Hastings Center, Garrison, NY, pp 12–14, 2009.

Cody, WK. Nursing theory-guided practice: What it is and what it is not. *Nurs Sci Q* 7(4):144–145, 1994.

Committee on Facilitating Interdisciplinary Research. *Facilitating interdisciplinary research.* Washington, DC: National Academy of Sciences, National Academy of Engineering, National Academy of Medicine, 2005.

Cumbie, SA, et al. Advanced practice nursing model for comprehensive care with chronic illness: Model for promoting engagement. *Adv Nurs Sci* 27(1):70–80, 2004.

Dacher, E. Reinventing primary care. *J Altern Ther Health Med* 1(5): 29–34, 1995.

Decker, J, et al. Use of medical care for chronic conditions. *Health Affairs* 28(1):26–35, 2009.

Department of Health and Human Services. *Report to Congress: National Strategy for Quality Improvement in Health Care.* Washington, DC: Department of Health and Human Services, 2011.

Dock, LL, and Stewart, IB. *A short history of nursing.* G. P. Putnam's Sons, New York, 1920.

Dodd, M, et al. Advancing the science of symptom management. *J Adv Nurs* 33(5):668–676, 2001.

Fenton, MV, and Brykczynski, KA. Qualitative distinctions and similarities in the practice of the clinical nurse specialists and nurse practitioners. *J Prof Nurs* 9:313, 1993.

Hektor, LM. Martha E. Rogers: A life history. *Nursing Science Quarterly, 2,* 63–73, 1989.

Henderson, V. *The nature of nursing.* Macmillan, New York, 1966.

Health Resources and Services Administration, Bureau of Health Professions, National Center for Health Workforce Analysis. *Projecting the supply and demand for primary care practitioners through 2020.* U.S. Department of Health & Human Services, Washington, DC, 2013.

Institute of Medicine. *The future of nursing: Leading change, advancing health.* National Academy Press, Washington, DC, 2011.

Institute of Medicine. *Health professions education: A bridge to quality.* National Academy Press, Washington, DC, 2003.

Johnson, R. Nurse practitioner–patient discourse: Uncovering the voice of nursing in primary care practice. *Schol Inq Nurs Pract Int J* 7(3):143, 1993.

Lewis, PH, and Brykczynski, KA. Practical knowledge and competencies of the healing role of the nurse practitioner. *J Am Acad Nurse Pract* 6(5):207–213, 1994.

Lynaugh, J, and Bates, B. The two languages of nursing and medicine. *Am J Nurs* 73(1):66, 1973.

Mayeroff, M. *On caring.* Harper & Row, New York, 1971.

Nightingale, F. *Notes on nursing: What it is and what it is not.* Dover, New York, 1860/1969.

Nutting, P, Miller, W, Crabtree, B, Jaen, CT, Steward, E, and Strange, K. Initial lessons from the First National Demonstration project on practice transformation to a patient-centered medical home. *Annals of Family Medicine, 7*(3), 254–260.

Payne, R. The quality mantra: Proceed carefully. *Hastings Cent Rep* 39(6):14, 2009.

Rakel, R (Ed.). *Textbook of family practice,* ed 4. WB Saunders, Philadelphia, 2011.

Riffle, K. CAM therapies for nurse practitioners. *Adv Nurse Pract.* Retrieved from http://nurse-practitioners.advanceweb.com/Editorial/content

Rogers, ME. Nursing: To be or not to be? *Nurs Outlook* 20:42–46, 1972.

Rogers, ME. The nurse practitioner movement: Pro and con. *Am J Nurs* 75(10):1834–1843, 1975.

Ryan, P. Integrated theory of health behavior change: Background and intervention development. *Clin Nurse Special* 23(4):161–170, 2009.

San Francisco School of Nursing Management Faculty Group. A model for symptom management. *Image J Nurs Scholar* 26(4): 272–276, 1994.

Shalala, DE. Nursing and society—The unfinished agenda for the 21st century. *Nurs Health Care* 14(6):4–7, 1993.

Shuler, PA, and Davis, JE. The Shuler Nurse Practitioner Practice Model. *J Am Acad Nurse Pract* 5(1):11–17, 1993.

Stewart, M, et al. *Patient-centered medicine: Transforming the clinical method.* Sage, Thousand Oaks, CA, 1995.

Swanson, C. A spirit-focused conceptual model of nursing for the advanced practice nurse. *Issues Comp Pediatr Nurs* 18:267–275, 1995.

U.S. Department of Health and Human Services. *Healthy people 2020.* International Medical Publishing, McLean, VA, 2010.

University of California, San Francisco, School of Nursing Symptom Management Faculty Group. A model for symptom management. *Image J Nurs Scholar* 26:272–276, 1994.

Watson, J. *Nursing: Human science and human care.* Appleton-Century-Crofts, Norwalk, CT, 1988.

Whitcomb, M, and Nutter D. *Learning medicine in the 21st century: The general professional education of the physician.* Carnegie Institute study: Educating doctors to provide high quality care: A vision for medical education in the United States. Association of Medical Colleges, Washington, DC, 2004.

Zimmer, P, et al. *Advanced practice nursing: Nurse practitioner curriculum guidelines.* National Organization of Nurse Practitioner Faculty, Seattle, WA, 1990.

Bibliography

Atlas, SJ. Patient-physician connectedness may affect quality of care. *Ann Intern Med* 150:325–335, 2009.

Boykin, A, et al. Aesthetic knowing grounded in an explicit conception of nursing. *Nurs Sci Q* 7(4):158–161, 1994.

Cooke, M, et al. American medical education 100 years after the Flexner Report. *N Engl J Med* 355(13):1339–1344, 2006.

Eisenberg, L. Disease and illness: Distinctions between professional and popular ideas of sickness. *Cult Med Psychiatry* 1:9, 1977.

Engebretson, J. A multiparadigm approach to nursing. *Adv Nurs Sci* 20(1):21–33, 1997.

Gordon, M. *Nursing Diagnosis: Process and Application,* ed 2. McGraw-Hill, New York, 1987.

Howie, JGR. A new look at illness in general practice: A reclassification of illness based on antibiotic prescribing. In Rakel, R (Ed.), *Textbook of family practice,* ed 4. WB Saunders, Philadelphia, 2011.

Institute of Medicine. *Health Care Quality Initiative: Crossing the quality chasm: A new health care system for the twenty-first century.* National Academy Press, Washington, DC, 2001.

Madden, M. Conceptualizations of advanced nursing practice. In Hamric, AB, Spross, JA, and Hanson, CM (Eds.), *Advanced practice nursing: An integrative approach,* ed 1. WB Saunders, Philadelphia, 1996, pp 25–41.

Mishler, EG. *The discourse of medicine: Dialectics of medical interviews.* Ablex, Norwood, NJ, 1984.

Mitchell, G. Nursing diagnosis: An obstacle to caring ways. In Boykin, A (Ed.), *Power, politics, and public policy.* National League for Nursing Press, New York, 1995.

National Organization of Nurse Practitioner Faculties (NONPF). *National Organization of Nurse Practitioner Faculties domains and core competencies of nurse practitioner practice, March 2006.* Retrieved from www.nonpf.com/associations/10789/files/DomainsandCoreComps2006.pdf

Parker, M. Exploring the aesthetic meaning of presence in nursing practice. In Gaut, D (Ed.), *The presence of caring in nursing.* National League for Nursing Press, New York, 1992.

Reed, PG. A treatise on nursing knowledge development for the 21st century: Beyond postmodernism. *Adv Nurs Sci* 17(3):70, 1995.

St. Anthony's: *ICD-10-CM: Code book for physician payment,* Vols 1 and 2. St. Anthony Publishing, Cincinnati, 2005.

Shuler, PA, et al. Providing holistic health care for the elderly: Utilization of the Shuler Nurse Practitioner Model. *J Am Acad Nurse Pract* 13(7):297–303, 2001.

Snyder, M. Defining nursing interventions. *Image J Nurs Scholar* 28(2):137, 1996.

Snyder, M, and Mirr, S. *Independent nursing intervention,* ed 2. Delmar, Albany, NY, 1995.

Spross, JA, and Lawson, MT. Conceptualizations of advanced practice nursing. In Hamric, AB, Spross, JA, & Hanson, CM (Eds.), *Advanced practice nursing: An integrative approach,* ed 4. Saunders Elsevier, St. Louis, MO, 2008, pp 33–74.

Caring and the Advanced Practice Nurse

Chapter 2

Anne Boykin, PhD, RN • Savina O. Schoenhofer, PhD, RN

The role of advanced practice registered nurse (APRN) is a special way of nursing. Although the role often blends elements of medical practice and generic primary care, it is also a form of nursing and is thus characterized by caring as a way of being, knowing, and doing. The prominent place of medical science knowledge and skill in master's and doctorate of nursing science programs to prepare APRNs may tend to obscure the fact that the educational program is intended to facilitate the development of advanced practice nursing.

The advanced practice of nursing must be firmly grounded in advanced knowledge and skill in caring. The framework presented in this text is intended to help students, faculty, and providers retain a nursing focus while addressing advanced practice in the interdisciplinary environment.

Dunphy's advanced practice nursing model, the *Circle of Caring* (see Chapter 1), introduces the term "caring process" as a pivotal element. "Process" in this model is understood to mean "unfolding" (rather than a series of cognitive or psychomotor steps or things to do, as in familiar uses such as nursing process or problem-solving process). Caring processes are ways to express your way of being and living as a caring person in the profession of advanced nursing. There is no defined set or list of caring processes; rather, there are as many caring processes as there are persons and situations.

■ CARING

Caring is the essence of being human, and nursing is a deeply human relationship; thus, caring is the essence of nursing. The meaning of caring as the essential nature of humanness cannot be encapsulated within a single limiting definition; however, caring can be understood, recognized, and developed both philosophically and practically. Caring expressed in nursing is the intentional and authentic presence of the nurse with another who is recognized as a person who is living, caring, and growing in caring (Boykin & Schoenhofer, 2001).

All human service disciplines are based on caring. Nursing is unique, however, as caring is what most directly characterizes nursing's knowledge base and service.

By contrast, in the discipline of medicine, the fundamental commitment to caring is directly characterized in the diagnosis and treatment of human structural and functional problems manifested primarily in physical terms. The nature of the APRN role permits the direct focus on care and caring that is nursing while incorporating the focus of medicine. An APRN does not practice medicine but rather draws on and transforms characteristic medical ways of practice for nursing purposes, just as the practice of holistic medicine draws on and transforms characteristic nursing ways of practice for medical purposes.

The APRN, such as the nurse practitioner, practices a specialized form of nursing practice, which means that specialized opportunities for creating situations of care call forth specialized patterns of caring. What does this mean in a practical sense? It means that the person coming for care presents with an issue that is typically viewed as being within the medical sphere. As in all nursing practice, the APRN is focused on co-creating a relationship in which care is experienced and possibilities for personally meaningful ways of living unfold. Specialized patterns of caring in the role of nurse practitioner blend knowledgeable perspectives of the health situation (diagnosis) and recommendations for characteristically medical ways of ameliorating presenting issues (treatment) with generalized patterns of nursing care. Generalized patterns of nursing care are represented in the *Circle of Caring* model as:

- Courage
- Authentic presence
- Advocacy
- Knowing
- Commitment
- Patience

Specialized patterns of care are incorporated in the uniqueness of caring processes. Knowledge of general patterns of care is important; however, that knowledge must be creatively used in actual, unfolding processes of care if the situation is to be considered nursing.

Caring is the matrix, the medium, the "stuff" within which the APRN–patient relationship is brought to life.

In this relationship, the APRN lives his or her commitment to caring by facilitating a personal connection that communicates "I acknowledge you as a caring person, one who is worthwhile and deserving of my respect, my attention, my commitment, my care." That effort to create a personal connection also communicates the practitioner's acceptance of the trust being placed in him or her as a caring person, as one who is available and able to participate effectively in the life of the other. Within the caring relationship each participant has the opportunity for enhancing personhood, that is, for living life grounded in caring and for growing in one's capacity to express caring in meaningful and satisfying ways. Knowing another as a caring person requires a commitment to entering into the world of the nursed with the explicit intention of knowing the person individually and uniquely. Entering into the world of another with caring intention requires that the practitioner know himself or herself as caring and be open to growing in the relationship. A truly collaborative relationship (in contrast to one in which the collaboration is taken at face value or in some way limited) emerges in the context of this caring intention.

The APRN's involvement with the nursed reflects themes or qualities of caring expressed as courage, authentic presence, advocacy, knowing, commitment, and patience. These themes of caring can serve as a conceptual structure or framework to assist the practitioner in examining, recognizing, and understanding the fullness of caring in practice. Though interconnected, each individual theme is addressed theoretically and then in action in a practice situation to illustrate caring processes.

Courage

Courage is a human act (Tillich, 1952). Courage comes to light in making deliberate choices resulting in acts that express who we are and what is important to us. Courage is the daily application of values, the living out of one's beliefs in spite of obstacles and challenging situations. Expressions of courage affirm our being.

This understanding of courage offers an ethical grounding for the practice of advanced nursing. It requires that, in each nursing situation, the nurse live the values held dear. The nurse risks entering each situation with the fullness of his or her being, willing to be rejected or not understood, or, perhaps equally risky, being accepted and known.

As part of courage, the nurse also understands and acts on the obligation to come to know that which matters to those seeking care. What shapes the moments the nurse has with people is the intention to know them as caring, to hear their stories, and to create nurturing responses reflective of the uniqueness of the situation. Courage manifests itself because of the nurse's deliberate choices to carry out, in a particular time and place, the beliefs that serve as the core of advanced nursing practice. Courage manifests itself in making one's nursing

vocation a commitment to these values and beliefs that undergird caring.

Authentic Presence

Nursing is communicated through authentic presence. Authentic presence is a unique way of being with others, unique in that it is a way of ordering and balancing self so as to grow in one's beauty and spirit. Such presence with self requires trust, courage, and the desire to know. One who is authentic with self and others is able to see things from the inside that others see only from the outside. There is an inner genuine awareness that is congruent with feelings, attitudes, and actions lived moment to moment. The commitment to truly know oneself frees one to be with others in authentic presence.

Authentic presence may be understood as intentionally being with another in the fullness of one's personhood. The caring that is communicated through authentic presence is the initiating and sustaining medium of nursing within the nursing situation. Nurses are called to be authentically present in nursing situations. Stories of nursing practice portray the depth of such experiences. The degree to which one knows oneself influences one's presence with others and thus the degree of commitment possible in the situation.

Advocacy

Advocacy is a way in which nurses have traditionally expressed caring. There are many opportunities for advocacy, that is, many situations in which "speaking up for" another is an important aspect of the role. From a depth of knowledge and understanding, the practitioner speaks up for the person as unique and worthwhile, for the person as having personal hopes, dreams, intentions, and preferences that are honorable. In addition, Gadow's (1990) formulation of existential advocacy calls for the nurse to advocate for alternative interpretations of the situation that arise from experience and specialized knowledge. Existential advocacy is contrasted with advocacy that is either paternalistic or consumer oriented. Paternalistic advocacy is characterized by a sense of "as the expert, I know what is best for you and your life." Consumer-oriented advocacy takes the approach that "I'll just give you the facts and options; you sort them out by yourself."

In existential advocacy, self is brought into the situation as a full partner, sharing alternative perspectives for consideration, though not insisting on them or imposing them. The patient enters into the relationship seeking to connect with the practitioner as a whole person, not just as a set of facts. When the practitioner takes the paternalistic stance (dismissive and overbearing, offering an all-or-none option) or the consumer-oriented stance (withdrawn to an objective distance, offering an essentially value-free set of options), the patient experiences the loss of an opportunity to connect with another assumed to be truly concerned, knowledgeable, and giving. When the nurse offers existential advocacy, the nursed feels truly known, respected, and connected in a way that affirms humanity and being.

Knowing

Knowing as an aspect of caring encompasses "knowing that," "knowing about," "knowing directly," and "unknowing." "Knowing that" and "knowing about" refer to descriptions and analyses of the patient's situation in the context of facts and information. Caring competence requires knowledge of facts and data points that are empirically and objectively derived. "Knowing directly" involves being deeply attuned to the person-as-person and comes through intentionality and authentic presence. "Unknowing" refers to an openness to unfolding, a humble sense that all is not yet known. The practitioner who truly embraces unknowing recognizes that what might be right or timely in general terms may be neither right nor timely for the particular person seeking care in a particular moment.

Carper (1978) described patterns of knowing fundamental to nursing: personal, empiric, ethical, and esthetic knowing. The practitioner draws on the personal way of knowing as essential intuitive knowing. Empiric knowing is an avenue for drawing on science and skilled observation. Ethical knowing prompts the practitioner to ask, "What are the personal and professional values that enter into this situation?" And thus, "What is right for this situation?" Esthetic knowing develops as the practitioner incorporates knowing gained from the other patterns in the context of fully living the situation as she or he co-creates with the nursed an integrated understanding of the unfolding whole picture.

The *Circle of Caring* is developed and strengthened as the practitioner and patient communicate their unfolding knowing of self, of each other, and of the situation. Knowing, as described briefly here, contributes to enhanced personhood, to the affirmation and growth of self and other as caring persons.

Commitment

Is there any greater act of courage than the commitment to another? Commitment is a sign of that which we value. Choosing to be a member of the discipline and profession of nursing speaks to the deep valuing and life-long commitment of service to humankind. Commitment directs obligations or what "ought to be" in particular situations. Because these commitments are so internalized as values, however, one's obligation is not experienced as a burden but as a response that is right, deliberate, conscious, and caring (Roach, 2002).

Nurses in advanced practice roles frequently face challenges to commitment. Choices made in practice reflect one's devotion to particular commitments. Often the values of an economically based health-care system, of which nursing is such an integral part, do not support or seem to be in line with the substantive nature of caring and its essential relation to practice. A struggle to preserve nursing's values often results. The APRN has the unique opportunity to demonstrate how a commitment to the values of nursing influences the outcomes of care.

The practice of advanced nursing must be firmly rooted in the values of the nurse. In addition to many essential types of knowledge and skills, he or she must be able to draw on the knowledge of nursing, especially knowledge of caring, to create environments for care that honor person-as-person and that humanize care.

Nursing always occurs in a relational context. As a human science, nursing calls for the continued commitment to understand better the lived experience of the nursed, to truly hear their stories, and to respond in ways that matter, ways that nurture and sustain persons as they live and grow in caring. Central to advanced practice is the commitment to know self and others as caring.

Patience

Patience as a key theme in caring refers to trusting people to grow in their own time and in their own way (Mayeroff, 1971). Patience is not passive but rather an active openness to "the moment alive with possibilities." Humility and courage are intimately connected to patience. The ability to remain actively engaged with the person while honoring individual circumstances and freedom of choice is an act of courage and leads to the kind of patience that communicates caring.

■ CARING PROCESSES

Below are stories of practice shared by two nurse practitioners. These stories illustrate ways in which advanced nursing practice is truly an expression of caring processes. The first story was shared by a family nurse practitioner (FNP) in practice in a family clinic in a small rural southern town.

Nursing Situation 2.1 Like a Pebble in a Pond—The Circle of Caring

The incident that I am describing involved an 18-year-old female college student—I'll call her Lucy—and her mother, Mrs. K. Lucy presented at my clinic with a history of shortness of breath and flu-like symptoms for several months. She and her mother had been to multiple health-care providers seeking a diagnosis and resolution of Lucy's problem. I had never seen this patient, so I went through the usual process of taking a history of the present illness, past medical history, social history, and a thorough physical exam. I then ordered what I determined to be the necessary tests. The outcome was a referral to a pulmonologist in a nearby city with the eventual successful resolution of her illness.

The interesting part of this story is what happened years later regarding this clinical incident. My husband and I went into a newly opened used bookstore in our community. On entering, there was no one but the owner and the two of us in the store. When the owner saw me, she came over and hugged me like a long-lost friend—it was Mrs. K! I did not even remotely recognize her and was sure she had mistaken me for someone else. She looked at my husband and stated, "She saved my daughter's life." She then began to cry as she related her feelings about the event and what had transpired. Mrs. K was embarrassed by her emotions (so was I), but she was determined to tell her story.

Mrs. K said that she had taken her daughter to multiple health-care providers seeking help for her child. She felt they did not take the case seriously and "blew her off" even as her daughter worsened. When Mrs. K and Lucy came to me, Mrs. K was desperate for help for her daughter. Mrs. K described her feelings regarding the clinical visit, grateful that I had listened and believed what she was saying. She then quoted something I had said to her that she said had given her hope and comfort. I told her that "I will do everything possible to find out what is wrong in order to help Lucy get better. We will not give up until we knew what is going on with Lucy." Mrs. K said a burden was lifted from her because at last she felt that "someone cared." Mrs. K told us that with the referral, the problem was diagnosed and resolved. It was her profound belief that I had literally saved her daughter's life. I do not remember Lucy's final diagnosis at this point in time, and I don't know how much actual assistance I was in the final resolution of her illness; but I will always remember Mrs. K's gratitude for a caring response to her feelings of helplessness while dealing with the health-care system. Mrs. K's belated description of her heartfelt feelings regarding her daughter's illness and my interventional actions made a profound impression on me as a provider. The need for a caring response to each of our patients is evident; yet, we may never know how much such caring can impact a life.

As shared by Carolyn B. Dollar, PhD, APRN-BC, FNP

In this story, the most prominent caring processes are authentic presence and commitment, as the FNP offered self in a way that truly communicated caring to this beleaguered family. The FNP's commitment to caring for the family and her courage and patience in tackling an issue that obviously had been given a "pass" by previous health-care providers who had been consulted illustrate the importance of opportunities to hear and respond effectively to calls for caring in advanced nursing practice. Referral is an act of advocacy that is frequently an element of NP practice, and when it is recognized as an opportunity for caring through advocacy, it becomes even more an integral expression of advanced nursing. The fact that the FNP offered this particular story as an exemplar of caring in advanced nursing practice makes evident the merging of knowing in past–present–future: the FNP continues to be open to knowing self and other through appreciating the mother's report of the impact of an act of caring initiated in a rather distant past.

A second story from an APRN practicing in a specialty clinic in an urban health sciences center showcases the centrality of the nurse–patient caring relationship in the midst of treatment situations involving complicated biomedical technology.

Nursing Situation 2.2 Spirited Caring

My APRN role has been a rewarding challenge. The story that I am going to share was pivotal to my development as an APRN. The story focuses on a pleasant, jolly, gem of a patient, with a warm smile—I'll call her Mrs. J. Her energy lit up the room. This independent free spirit also worked as a volunteer at the clinic. She served cookies and other baked goods to the patients undergoing chemotherapy. Her strong faith and compassion for others impressed me as a busy provider. To the nursing staff, she stood out as a patient and volunteer. Her faith helped her in aiding the sicker patients to maintain hope. Her genuine concern for others encouraged nursing staff and family members to have compassion for others. Mrs. J was always the first to ask, "How are you doing?" This unique patient was a beacon of light in a dark, sobering environment.

My favorite patient and I developed a good rapport as I saw her weekly in Coumadin Clinic. She was my first patient on my very first day. When she stepped into my office and noted my frazzled appearance, she grabbed my hands and prayed with me. Because we are in the Bible belt, I considered that to be normal. She later apologized because she did not know my religious beliefs. I assured her that her actions had calmed me and made my day go a little better. Mrs. J had been doing exceptionally well although she had been diagnosed with cancer. She had a history of Stage II breast cancer but had been in complete remission for 2 years.

One Friday, she presented to the clinic at four o'clock in the afternoon. She had been complaining of vision changes and had her son bring her to the clinic. I knew something was wrong because this independent woman always presented to visits alone. Mrs. J's primary-care provider was not available by phone, and her oncologist was out of town. She reported a headache with vision changes, which seemed strange for a woman who had undergone chemotherapy with adjuvant radiation therapy without difficulties. She explained that 4 days before this clinic visit, she experienced the worst headache she had ever had. Her clinical presentation led me to get a computed tomography (CT) scan of the head with contrast. After reading her CT, the radiologist called me immediately. He had identified a large mass that was pressing against her sulcus. At this point, I had to find her hematologist, start her on high-dose steroids, find the neurosurgeon on call, and prepare her for everything that was about to take place. I was so consumed by my actions that I nearly forgot to care for the patient.

Mrs. J demonstrated sincere compassion when I had to give her the hard news. She grabbed my hands and prayed for me and the other health-care providers. She prayed that we would make the right decisions regarding her health care. Just as we had started our relationship, we were ending it. Her demonstration of faith was a unique testament to her life. Her strength in a time of weakness showed the vigor of her faith. Though she was a devout Catholic and I am a Methodist, we had to rely on our genuine concern for each other and our beliefs in a higher being to get us through this difficult time. Compassion and faith were integral components in our provider–patient relationship.

The experience taught us that compassion and faith coupled with therapeutic communication can get you through the toughest of situations. In revisiting this story, I am reminded of the need to foster a sense of caring and respect for patients' beliefs as I mature and develop as a nurse. The patient's actions were surprising. I had been taught about putting my compassion and faith into action. However, I had never seen it done. It was affirming as an APRN to recall how we cried and laughed and came to the sobering realization that this disease might beat her. However, we had given it our best effort. This experience was beneficial to me because it was my first time being the bearer of bad news to a patient. Consumed as we are with time management, compassion and faith are not always exhibited, shared, or utilized in my daily practice. However, by revisiting this story, I am challenged to treat others as I treated my special patient. The core values that guided my practice in the past have been rekindled while reflecting on my nursing experience. Nursing is a rewarding challenge if you allow it to be.

As shared by C'Sara Strong, MSN, CFNP

This story needs no interpretation; it can be easily recognized as an exquisite example of creating a holistic fabric of caring integrating a multitude of harmonious patterns: interpersonal, clinical, and technological.

These stories of advanced nursing practice illustrate the use of caring processes. As situations are studied and relived, students, faculty, and providers discover the limitless ways caring is expressed. As nurses, we live out our personhood—our living grounded in caring—in unique and special ways. We bring to our practice our humanness, our expertise in caring, and our intention to participate fully in the life experiences of those we are privileged to nurse, and thus to bring the benefits of nursing to those seeking care.

Authors' Note: We have elected to make no notable changes to the content of Chapter 2 for this edition of the text. The words of Boykin and Schoenhofer remain as timeless and true today as they did when they were originally written in 1999. They provide an important interpretation of the *Circle of Caring* as described in Chapter 1. The miracle of changing practice and the care of patients, families, and communities through transformative advanced practice nursing remains as vital a need now as it was then. The authors wish to thank Boykin and Schoenhofer for their unfailing commitment to the art and science of caring.

 | For additional resources please visit
http://davisplus.fadavis.com

References

Boykin, A, and Schoenhofer, SO. *Nursing as caring: A model for transforming practice.* Jones & Bartlett, Sudbury, MA, 2001.

Carper, B. Fundamental patterns of knowing in nursing. *Adv Nurs Sci* 1(1):13–23, 1978.

Gadow, S. A model for ethical decision making. In Pence, T, et al (Eds.), *Ethics in nursing: An anthology.* Publ. No. 20-2294. National League for Nursing, New York, 1990, pp 52–55.

Mayeroff, M. *On caring.* HarperPerennial, New York, 1971.

Roach, S. *Caring: The human mode of being. A blueprint for the health professions.* CHA Press, Ottawa, ON, 2002.

Tillich, P. *The courage to be.* Yale University Press, New Haven, CT, 1952.

Chapter 3

Health Promotion

Dorothy J. Dunn, PhD, RNP, FNP-BC, AHN-BC •
Debera J. Thomas, DNS, RN, FNP/ANP

■ HEALTH

The ultimate goal of all health-care providers is to promote health and prevent disease. Patients share this goal. Engaging in health-promoting activities helps individuals live longer and healthier lives. To put this in perspective, the basic tenets of health must first be explored.

What is health? Several disciplines and organizations have tried to define health, and the definition continues to evolve. Many view health as the absence of disease. This definition does not account for the multidimensional characteristics integral to a human being. Humans are physical, social, spiritual, cultural, and emotional beings. To define health only as the absence of disease does not address all the dimensions that makes us human. In 1948, the World Health Organization (WHO, 1948) defined health as a "state of complete, physical, mental and social well-being"; this definition provides a more holistic view of health because it incorporates the social and mental aspects of a human being, as well as the physical dimension. In fact, this definition has not been amended since its inception in 1948. However, this definition does not account for the spiritual and cultural dimensions of a person. According to the American Holistic Nurses' Association (Mariano, 2013), health can be described as a state or process in which an individual experiences a sense of well-being, harmony, and unity of one's body-mind-spirit within an ever-changing environment. Health is therefore a state in which the physical, psychological, social, spiritual, and cultural attributes of a person are in balance, creating harmony within the body (Fig. 3.1).

The balance of each of these dimensions is an important parameter when considering health. A patient whom we care for may be physically healthy, but his or her spiritual, cultural, social, and psychological dimensions may not be balanced, and therefore the patient is not experiencing optimal health. It has been said that the whole is greater than the sum of its parts. We cannot accurately determine someone's health status without evaluating all of these attributes.

Historically, the medical evaluation of a patient was based only on physical signs and symptoms of a disease. If the patient lacked symptoms, we considered him or her healthy. We now know that this type of assessment is incomplete and does not take into account how the other attributes of a person either contribute to or subtract from health status. We also know that many patients have medical problems that have not yet presented as signs and symptoms of a disease.

When assessing a patient, it is imperative to also evaluate his or her social, psychological, spiritual, and cultural well-being, as well as the physical state. In performing a complete health assessment, the provider should ask questions related to the person's social and dietary habits; current living and work situation environment; and feelings, beliefs, values, and life satisfaction, as well as questions about his or her philosophical and spiritual beliefs.

Along with physical signs and symptoms, all these parts of a patient's history inform diagnosis and treatment plans. The focus on all component parts of a person helps to provide a more holistic view that can assist in making a more comprehensive assessment of the

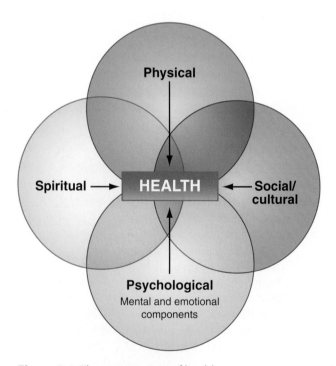

Figure 3.1 The components of health.

current health status of the patient. The determination of health is based on the synthesis of all the parameters of health and should be incorporated into all patient assessments.

■ HEALTH PROMOTION

Health promotion can be defined as activities and preventive measures that contribute to an individual's state of optimal health. Such activities and preventive measure include immunizations, fitness/exercise programs, breast self-examination, appropriate nutrition, relaxation, stress management, social support, prayer, meditation, healing rituals, cultural practices, and promoting environmental health and safety. Health and well-being are created by a balance of physical, psychological, spiritual, cultural, and social components of health. Health promotion requires a commitment on the part of the individual patient, the health-care provider, and the community. Health promotion efforts are achieved only when everyone works in partnership to achieve goals that will enhance health and well-being.

Health promotion efforts should always begin with the clinician because the clinician plays a pivotal role in educating the patient and the community about health-promoting behaviors. The clinician can help provide insight to each patient about how his or her environment can contribute to health or disease. In addition, the community must understand the impact that environment can have on individuals so that health promotion activities can be a community effort. Health-care providers play an important role by providing consultation to the community and the legislature regarding environmental health.

Consultation with influential members of the community can help in the development of legislation that can support healthy living conditions in a community. In addition, legislative efforts can help to provide funding to maintain or improve environmental health. If patients are trying to promote their own health, living conditions in the community must also be healthy to sustain and support their efforts. Basic community resources such as water and sanitation must be monitored for potential threats to health and well-being, and these resources are the responsibility of community and local government agencies. Health-care providers and patients need to work in collaboration with these agencies to ensure that elements essential to health, such as clean water and street sanitation, are maintained or improved. To be successful, health promotion must be a group effort.

Historically, health promotion has been viewed as an effort to prevent disease and illness. Most sources cite three levels of prevention: Primary prevention is the prevention of disease; secondary prevention consists of early screening and detection of disease; and tertiary prevention is the restoration of health after illness or disease has occurred. Focusing health-care efforts on all three levels of prevention is important to promoting health,

but during the last two decades, primary prevention has become the ultimate goal of health promotion.

The focus in health care during the first half of the 20th century was on care for the patient who was already ill. The prevailing belief at the time was that patients should seek health care when they were ill. During this time, most health-care practitioners cared for patients at the tertiary level by (1) preventing further insult or injury after the disease or illness had occurred, by stabilizing the patient's condition to prevent deterioration; (2) helping patients to recover from the current illness or disease through treatment; and (3) whenever possible, to help restore patients to their previous state of health.

Advancements in technology during the second half of the 20th century contributed to better diagnostic testing, helping to shift the focus of health care to secondary prevention. Providers became savvier about the importance of screening "at risk" patients at appropriate intervals for known diseases and illnesses. A focus on secondary levels of prevention led health-care providers to encourage early detection and treatment.

With the focus on screening and early detection, treatment could be instituted before overt signs and symptoms appeared, thereby preventing some of the long-term sequelae associated with illness and disease. For example, blood pressure would be checked in a patient with no symptoms of hypertension, and if elevated, a plan of treatment would be instituted. The goal was and is maintaining the patient's blood pressure within normal limits and minimizing the development of catastrophic complications such as stroke or myocardial infarction. Certain circumstances must exist for a screening test to be useful. These are summarized in Box 3.1.

In determining whether or not screening is appropriate, health-care providers should keep in mind that early signs of chronic disease often surface in midlife, that is, in persons aged 40 to 65 years. In general, the earlier

---

Box 3.1   U.S. Clinician Handbook of Preventive Services Criteria for Inclusion

1. The condition must have a significant effect on the quality and quantity of life;
2. Acceptable methods of treatment must be available;
3. The condition must have an asymptomatic period during which detection and treatment significantly reduce morbidity and mortality;
4. Treatment in the asymptomatic phase must yield a therapeutic result superior to that obtained by delaying treatment until symptoms appear;
5. Tests that are acceptable to patients must be available, at a reasonable cost, to detect the condition in the asymptomatic period; and
6. The evidence of the condition must be sufficient to justify the cost of the screening.

disease is identified, the easier it is to treat, and the more likely it is to have a successful outcome. In addition, individuals in midlife tend to focus more on behaviors to extend life and prevent disability than do younger people. Adults aged 20 to 40 years focus more on relationships, family, self-image, and career development, whereas those older than 65 spend much time responding to and coping with overt, established illness. As life expectancy increases and older adults anticipate living longer, more attention is focused on health enhancement, adding quality years to the life span of older persons.

Focusing on primary prevention enables providers to assess patients' potential risk factors, including lifestyle and genetic history, and to help them make lifestyle changes that will foster health and prevent disease and disability. Health-care providers are aware that health or wellness is best achieved through primary prevention strategies. However, when this is not possible, secondary and tertiary levels of prevention are employed. Each health-care interaction between a patient and clinician is an opportunity to promote health at the primary, secondary, and tertiary level. Optimal wellness or health for all patients is the ultimate goal.

Health-care providers can use the levels of prevention in several ways: on an individual level, with small groups (families), and with larger groups such as a community. Individual encounters with patients provide an opportunity to educate patients about their individual risk factors and changes they can make to prevent, or at least delay, the onset of disease(s) and the potential sequelae of disease (implementing primary and secondary prevention strategies). Incorporating family members into the educational process of health promotion can provide support and reinforcement for patients during the early phase of risk reduction. This incorporation of family may also serve the individual family members by educating them regarding their own risk for disease. Family members can also serve as advocates for patients by helping to synthesize the information given and providing the patient with a support system to make healthy lifestyle changes.

Health-care providers can be instrumental in developing health promotion strategies in a community. This can be accomplished by developing interventions that include identifying community groups at risk for certain diseases and developing community-wide educational programs that will educate this group about their potential risks. Community-based educational programs reach a broad audience with the potential to have a significant impact on the health status of a community (Fig. 3.2).

Expanding knowledge has increased our awareness that many diseases today can be minimized or potentially avoided with early assessment and management. The effects of diseases such as hypertension, cardiovascular disease, and diabetes on patients' lives can be minimized or avoided with early interventions. For example, most patients diagnosed with diabetes have had the disease for at least 5 years. Diabetes has serious consequences in many organ systems if it is not diagnosed early and treated aggressively. The development of a community-wide diabetes education/screening program can help identify patients who are at high risk for the disease. With early diagnosis and treatment, long-term complications associated with diabetes such as peripheral neuropathy, cardiovascular complications, and retinopathies can be minimized.

Clinicians can take a leadership position within a community by developing targeted programs for early identification and treatment. This type of wide-scale intervention can reduce morbidity and mortality rates. Early diagnosis, before signs/symptoms of a disease are present, can have a significant impact on the outcomes of disease. If patients are identified early, educated about the importance of healthy nutrition and lifestyle, and treated aggressively, the outcome may be a long and healthy life. Table 3.1 provides examples of primary, secondary, and tertiary prevention.

Risk Factors in Health Promotion

The identification of risk factors is an essential component of health promotion. Some patients have no known risk factors, whereas others have many. The key component of effective health promotion is to screen patients for potential known risk factors and intervene. Not all diseases can be prevented, and not every person with unhealthy lifestyle choices will get a particular disease, but the elimination or alteration of certain risk factors can affect disease outcomes.

Some risk factors are modifiable, whereas others are not. Nonmodifiable risk factors, including sex, age, and genetic/family history, are considered nonmodifiable because they cannot be changed in any way (at this time). Because these factors are nonmodifiable, early and aggressive identification of all risk factors should be done so that patients with nonmodifiable risk factors can make any possible changes in the modifiable risk factors and effect a more favorable outcome.

Modifiable risk factors include weight, diet, social habits, lifestyle choices, and stress. For example, 38-year-old Mr. Hart is being seen for a physical examination. He has not had a physical in 20 years. His past medical history is negative for any diseases, surgeries, or illnesses. His social history includes the use of alcohol and cigarettes; he works an average of 60 hours per week as an emergency medical technician and does not exercise. His family history reveals that his father, paternal uncle, and grandfather had all had a myocardial infarction before age 50. Mr. Hart's physical exam reveals the following: height, 69 inches; weight, 230 pounds; and a body mass index (BMI) of 34. Mr. Hart's laboratory results include a cholesterol level of 250 mg/dL, a high-density lipoprotein (HDL) of 30 mg/dL, and a low-density lipoprotein (LDL) of 160 mg/dL. Box 3.2 reviews the risk factors for heart disease for Mr. Hart.

Although Mr. Hart cannot change his age, sex, or family history, there are several factors that he can

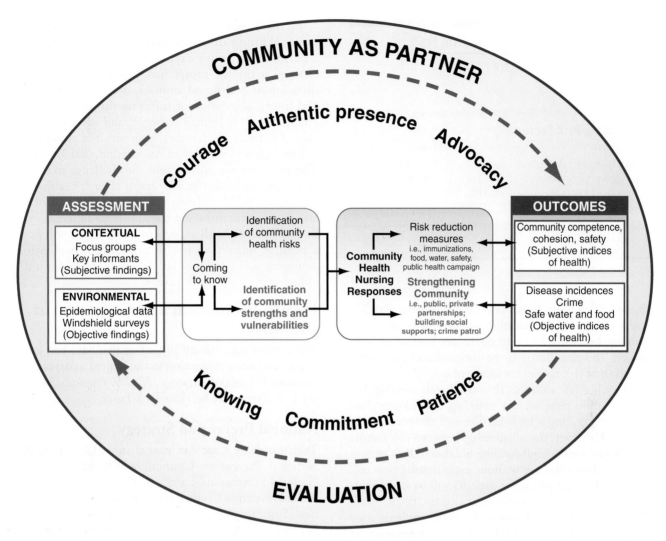

Figure 3.2 The community-based *Circle of Caring.*

Table 3.1	Examples of Primary, Secondary, and Tertiary Prevention	
Primary Prevention	Secondary Preventionv	Tertiary Prevention
Immunizations	*Screening for:*	*Treatment to prevent further sequelae of:*
Health education	Skin cancer	Cardiovascular disease
Skin cancer prevention	Oral cancer	Respiratory disease
measures	Lung cancer	Gastroenterology disease
Weight control	Breast cancer	Genitourinary disease
Seat belt use	Testicular cancer	Endocrine diseases
Violence prevention	Prostate cancer	Immunodeficiency disease
Substance abuse	Diabetes	Infectious disease
Education on:	Hypertension	Dermatological disease
Smoking, alcohol, and drugs	Cardiovascular disease	Oncology disease
Environmental hazards	Ovarian cancer	Gynecological disease
avoidance	Cervical cancer	Musculoskeletal disease
Protective hearing equipment	Fecal occult blood	Neurological disease
Protective eye equipment	Sexually transmitted infections	Psychiatric disease
Safety helmets for motorcycles,	Tuberculosis infection	Reproductive disease
skateboards, and bicycles	Pediatric developmental screening	
Nutrition counseling	Lead screening	
Exercise	Anemia screening	
Stress reduction	Height, weight, and body mass index	
Eliminate allergen exposure	screening	

Box 3.2 Risk Factors for Mr. Hart

Nonmodifiable Risk Factors
• Male sex
• Age
• Family history

Modifiable Risk Factors
• Weight
• Sedentary lifestyle
• Elevated cholesterol
• Elevated LDL and suboptimal HDL
• Alcohol consumption
• Smoking
• Stress level

change. With improvements in his diet, regular exercise, stress reduction, moderation of alcohol intake, and smoking cessation, Mr. Hart can reduce his risk for heart disease. This case illustrates the importance of early identification of risk factors for intervention.

Ongoing research has shown the relationship between certain risks such as smoking, consuming alcohol, and ingesting a high-fat diet and the presence of disease. However, the relationship between risk factors and disease can be confounding because often a person may develop a disease without experiencing any risk factors. For example, some patients will have no identified risk factors for a particular disease, yet will still develop the disease. Conversely, some patients may have several identified risk factors and yet never go on to develop the disease. Evidence-based research will continue to focus on efforts to identify as yet unknown risk factors or health-promoting determinants that could influence the outcomes for disease.

■ INFLUENCES ON HEALTH PROMOTION

Many factors influence health promotion activities today. Government initiatives, community health programs, and media attention all focus attention on the importance of health literacy, health promotion, and disease prevention.

Health Literacy

Most persons will encounter health information when they seek health care, and most persons will encounter health information that they cannot understand. More than a measurement of reading skills, health literacy also includes writing, listening, speaking, arithmetic, and conceptual knowledge. *Health literacy* is commonly defined as the degree to which individuals have the capacity to obtain, process, and understand basic information and services needed to make appropriate decisions regarding their health.

Health literacy is required when acute illness, injury, or chronic disease management necessitates that a person seek health care. Consider that nurses are charged with "the protection, promotion, and optimization of health and abilities, prevention of illness and injury, alleviation of suffering through diagnosis and treatment of human response, and advocacy in the care of individuals, families, communities, and populations" (American Nurses Association, 2010, p. 10). Therefore, nurses must accept the challenge to screen and assess for health literacy levels at each health-care encounter. By identifying those at risk for misunderstanding instructions and the ability to adhere to recommendations in all aspects of care, nurses will have a positive impact on health promotion, prevention strategies, and treatment adherence successes for individuals who seek health care.

Health Promotion and Government Initiatives

Three major government initiatives that have had great impact on health promotion in the United States are the National Prevention Strategy, *Healthy People 2020,* and the U.S. Preventive Services Task Force.

National Prevention Strategy

The Affordable Care Act passed in 2010 created the National Prevention Council, which developed the National Prevention Strategy (NPS). In 2011, the National Prevention Council released the *National Prevention Strategy: America's Plan for Better Health and Wellness,* a comprehensive plan that sets forth evidence-based and achievable means for improving health and well-being for all Americans at every stage of life. These efforts are designed to stop disease before it starts and to create strategies for a healthy and fit nation, recognizing that prevention must be part of daily life. The goal of the NPS is to transform us from a system of sick care to one based on wellness and prevention. *Healthy People 2020* is a foundational resource for the NPS Four Strategic Directions and Seven Priorities.
The Four Strategic Directions are

• Health and Safe Community Environments
• Clinical and Community Preventive Services
• Empowered People
• Elimination of Health Disparities

Within this framework, the Seven Priorities are identified to reduce the burden of the leading causes of preventable death and major illness.
The Seven Priorities are

• Tobacco-Free Living
• Preventing Drug Abuse and Excessive Alcohol Use
• Healthy Eating
• Active Living
• Injury and Violence-Free Living

- Reproductive and Sexual Health
- Mental and Emotional Well-being

Healthy People 2020

Healthy People 2020 is based on the accomplishments of four previous Healthy People initiatives: (1) the 1979 Surgeon General's Report, *Healthy People: The Surgeon General's Report on Health Promotion and Disease Prevention;* (2) *Healthy People 1990: Promoting Health/Preventing Disease: Objective for the Nation;* (3) *Healthy People 2000: National Health Promotion and Disease Prevention Objectives;* and (4) *Healthy People 2010: Objectives for Improving Health. Healthy People 2020* is the result of a multiyear process that reflects input from a diverse group of individuals and organizations.

There are nearly 600 objectives in *Healthy People 2020* with more than 1,300 measures. The topic areas were developed from experts from the following federal agencies: Administration on Aging; Agency for Healthcare Research and Quality; Centers for Disease Control and Prevention; Food and Drug Administration; Health Resources and Services Administration; Immediate Office of the Assistant Secretary for Health; Office of Public Health and Science; Indian Health Services; National Institutes of Health; Office of Global Health Affairs; Office of Minority Health; Office of Population Affairs; Office of the National Coordinator for Health Information Technology; Office of Policy, Strategic Planning, and Communications; Office of the Assistant Secretary for Preparedness and Response; President's Council on Sports, Fitness, and Nutrition; Substance Abuse and Mental Health Services Administration; Department of Agriculture; and Department of Education.

Over the course of the decade, the four foundation health measures will be used to monitor progress toward promoting health, preventing disease and disability, eliminating disparities, and improving quality of life. See Box 3.3.

Healthy People 2020 focuses on identifying, measuring, tracking, and reducing health disparities through a determinants-of-health approach. Over the past two decades, Healthy People's overarching goals have focused on disparities. In *Healthy People 2000,* the goal was to reduce health disparities among Americans; in *Healthy People 2010,* it was to eliminate, not just reduce, health disparities. In *Healthy People 2020,* the goal is expanded further to achieve health equity, eliminate disparities, and improve health for all groups. Currently, *Healthy People 2020* is assessing health disparities in the U.S. population by tracking rates of illness, death, chronic conditions, behaviors, and other types of outcomes in relation to demographic factors, including race and ethnicity, gender, sexual identity and orientation, disability status and special health care needs, and geographic location. See Table 3.2.

There are 13 new topic areas for 2020, and these are listed in Table 3.3. Each of the *Healthy People 2020*

Box 3.3 *Healthy People 2020* Foundation Health Measures

1. General health status measures such as life expectancy at birth and at age 65, healthy life expectancy, years of potential life lost, physically and mentally unhealthy days, self-assessed health status, limitation of activity, and chronic disease prevalence.
2. Health-related quality of life and well-being such as physical, mental, and social health–related quality of life, well-being/satisfaction, and participation in common activities.
3. Determinants of health, a range of personal, social, economic, and environmental factors that include biology, genetics, behavior, access to care, and environment in which people are born, live, learn, play, work, and age.
4. Disparities that include race/ethnicity, gender, physical and mental ability, and geography.

topic areas includes related evidence-based interventions and resources from U.S. Preventive Services Task Force Clinical Preventive Services, Guide to Community Preventive Services, and healthfinder.gov's Quick Guide to Healthy Living Information for Consumers. *Healthy People 2020* also hosts an online community using Twitter, LinkedIn, or one of the *Healthy People 2020* webinars. Leading health indicators reflect high-priority health issues and communicate actions that can be taken to address them. These indicators will be used to assess the health of the nation over the decade, to facilitate collaboration across sectors, and to motivate action at the national, state, and community levels to improve the health of the U.S. population.

According to the *Healthy People* initiative, *health promotion* is defined as any strategy that helps individuals make personal choices in a social context about lifestyle that will have a positive influence on the individual's health prospects. *Health protection* is defined as those interventions that are related to the environment made by regulatory bodies to protect a large population group. *Preventive services* include screening for disease, counseling, medication to prevent disease, or immunization interventions for individuals in the clinical setting. The last priority area of surveillance and data systems was essential to track all of the changes that would occur with programs focusing on meeting the goals of *Healthy People 2020.*

The *Healthy People 2020* initiatives continue to have a significant impact on primary health care in the United States. The incorporation of health-promoting and disease prevention strategies has become the foundation for primary care. It is believed that all of the goals of *Healthy People 2020* are achievable with support from individual health-care providers, local and national government

Table 3.2   Topic Areas for *Healthy People*

• Access to Health Services • Adolescent Health* • Arthritis, Osteoporosis, and Chronic Back Conditions • Blood Disorders and Blood Safety* • Cancer • Chronic Kidney Disease • Dementias, Including Alzheimer's Disease* • Diabetes • Disability and Health • Early and Middle Childhood* • Educational and Community-Based Programs	• Environmental Health • Family Planning • Food Safety • Genomics* • Global Health* • Health Communication and Health Information Technology • Health-care–Associated Infections* • Health-Related Quality of Life and Well-being* • Hearing and Other Sensory or Communication Disorders	• Heart Disease and Stroke • HIV • Immunization and Infectious Diseases • Injury and Violence Prevention • Lesbian, Gay, Bisexual, and Transgender Health* • Maternal, Infant, and Child Health • Medical Product Safety • Mental Health and Mental Disorders • Nutrition and Weight Status • Occupational Safety and Health • Older Adults* • Oral Health • Physical Activity • Preparedness*	• Public Health Infrastructure • Respiratory Diseases • Sexually Transmitted Diseases • Sleep Health* • Social Determinants of Health* • Substance Abuse • Tobacco Use • Vision

*New for *Healthy People 2020*.

Table 3.3   New and Archived Objectives for *Healthy People 2020*

Objectives Archived from *Healthy People 2010*

Archived objectives are *Healthy People 2010* objectives that are not included in the proposed set of *Healthy People 2020* objectives for data, target, or policy reasons.

Increase in counseling on health behaviors among persons at risk with a physician visit in the past year.

Reduce hospitalization rates for three ambulatory-care–sensitive conditions.

Increase the proportion of persons who have access to rapidly responding prehospital emergency medical services.

Establish a single toll-free telephone number for access to poison control centers on a 24-hour basis throughout the United States.

Increase the number of tribes, states, and the District of Columbia with state-level trauma system facilitation and coordination of statewide defined criteria.

Reduction in proportion of adults aged 65 years and older with long-term-care needs who do not have access to the continuum of long-term-care services.

Objectives New to *Healthy People 2020*

A renewed focus on identifying, measuring, tracking, and reducing health disparities through a determinant of health approach.

New topic areas: Adolescent Health; Blood Disorders and Blood Safety; Dementias; Early and Middle Childhood; Genomics; Global Health; Health-care–Associated Infections; Health-Related Quality of Life and Well-Being; Lesbian, Gay, Bisexual, and Transgender Health; Older Adults; Preparedness; Sleep Health; and Social Determinants of Health.

Source: Retrieved from www.healthypeople.gov/2020/about/new2020.aspx

agencies, and, most important, the active participation of individual patients.

Healthy People 2020 stresses the importance of each individual taking personal responsibility for his or her own health, in partnership with his or her health-care professional. For the public to have an effective role in illness prevention, individuals must work in partnership with clinicians who have been educated in health promotion and disease prevention strategies.

U.S. Preventive Services Task Force

The U.S. Preventive Services Task Force (USPSTF) is composed of private sector experts who make recommendations to the health-care community regarding clinical prevention strategies. This group was first convened by the U.S. Public Health Service in 1984 and since 1998 has come under the umbrella of the Agency for Healthcare Research and Quality (AHRQ). Their mission, as mandated by Public Law Section 915, is to conduct scientific evidence reviews of a broad array of clinical preventive services; develop recommendations for the health-care community; and provide ongoing administrative, research, and technical support to disseminate the findings.

The USPSTF meets and reviews scientific evidence for each of the current health-care screening guidelines, as well as preventive medications, immunizations, and counseling, and makes recommendations. Through consensus, the task force assigns a grade to each recommendation based on net benefits for patients and the strength of evidence for each of the current recommendations.

The result of the task force's efforts is an online *Procedure Manual* that can be used by clinicians who provide preventive services. The USPSTF *Procedure Manual* is available for distribution from several sources and has its own Web site: www.uspreventiveservicestaskforce.org/uspstf08/methods/procmanual.htm.

An evidence-based prevention resource for nurse practitioners is available at www.uspreventiveservices-taskforce.org/uspstf09/epbnursep/epbnursep.htm. The *Procedure Manual* provides recommendations for screening, including the following: cancer screening and chemoprevention strategies; screening for heart and valvular disease, infectious disease, injury and violence, mental health issues, and substance abuse; metabolic, nutritional, and endocrine screening; and pediatric screening guidelines. Nurse practitioners can use its evidence-based recommendations for clinical preventive services.

The USPSTF not only makes recommendations for screening select populations but also prioritizes services. Some recommendations are not implemented unless the provider feels that they are warranted. Thus, although guidelines are provided and recommendations are made, each health-care provider has the responsibility to assess each patient's history and risk factors and determine whether the current recommendations are appropriate for the individual patient. For example, patients who have a significant family history for a particular type of cancer may need to be screened earlier than recommended for the general population.

The work of this task force continues. Some of the current recommendations, such as lead poisoning and iron-deficiency anemia screenings, have been included as part of the well-child visits in pediatrics for many years. It is important that screening programs be continued or eliminated based on the strength of scientific evidence available and not just on tradition. If the evidence is not strong enough to support current recommendations, practices such as generalized screening for anemia and lead poisoning may need to be eliminated. This type of screening is relatively easy to do and is inexpensive but does cause trauma to the child (and often the parents), so decisions should be based on sound evidence and not just a matter of routine.

With the rapid evolution of technology in health care, it is important to be knowledgeable about current health-care information. Resources such as the NPS, *Healthy People 2020,* and the USPSTF recommendations are essential tools to help clinicians keep up to date with current best practices. All of these initiatives have Web sites that provide updates to the current printed reports. The NPS encourages partnerships among federal, state, tribal, local, and territorial governments; business, industry, and other private sector partners; philanthropic organizations; community and faith-based organizations; and everyday Americans to improve health through prevention. Initiatives such as *Healthy People 2020* and the USPSTF recommendations are excellent examples of well-researched tools that can help to enhance health promotion and disease prevention. The end result will be comprehensive care to patients with the goal of optimal health for all.

Immunization Practices

Immunization administration is one of the best examples of primary health promotion. Immunizations provide the patient's body with the ability to build up antibodies to a potential life-threatening illness before exposure to the offending agent. The guidelines for immunization continue to evolve and change over time. Currently, immunizations begin at birth and are continued throughout life. During early childhood, infants and children (birth through 6 years old) are immunized with a wide variety of vaccines, including hepatitis B (Hep B); hepatitis A (Hep A); diphtheria, tetanus, and acellular pertussis (DTaP); inactivated polio vaccine (IPV); *Haemophilus influenzae* type B (Hib); measles, mumps, and rubella (MMR); varicella-zoster virus (VZV); pneumococcal conjugate vaccine (PCV); influenza (flu); pneumococcal vaccine; and rotavirus (RV). The 2013 Advisory Committee on Immunization Practices (ACIP, 2014) recommends immunizations for children aged 7 to 18 years to protect against tetanus, diphtheria, and pertussis; meningococcal conjugate vaccine (MCV) is recommended at this age as well. At age 11 to 12, boys and girls should receive the human papillomavirus (HPV) vaccine. Either HPV4 or HPV2 may be used for females, and only HPV4 may be used for males. Teens who received MCV for the first time between age 13 and 15 should receive a one-time booster between age 16 and 18. All children should receive approximately 25 vaccines by the time they reach 5 years of age. After this point, they should continue to receive a tetanus, diphtheria, and acellular pertussis (Tdap) booster every 10 years. Recommendations for adults include annual flu immunizations, as well as pneumococcal, meningococcal, Hep A, and Hep B immunizations for those with certain risks related to their health, job, or lifestyle. Older adults should receive a VZV immunization at age 60 to prevent shingles and a pneumococcal polysaccharide vaccine at age 65 to protect them from pneumonia. The immunization schedules change periodically, so to obtain the most current information, go to www.cdc.gov/vaccines/schedules/index.html, which offers current immunization guidelines for children and adults. Table 3.4 provides a summary of immunization guidelines current as of the publication date.

Immunizations are an effective form of primary health promotion, but they are not without controversy. Over the past several years, some consumers have argued that immunizations are not safe and in fact cause diseases such as autism and attention-deficit hyperactivity disorder. To date, the etiology of these diseases has not been found to be a result of immunization administration. However, there is always the potential for vaccines to cause side effects; therefore, patient education is paramount.

Each clinician must provide patients and their families with accurate information regarding immunization administration, including potential side effects and known contraindications to immunization, and keep a copy of a written consent for each immunization on file. This consent must be obtained for each immunization given, before vaccine administration. If, after administration of a vaccine, a patient develops a significant reaction (such as very high fever, uncontrollable crying for more than 2 hours, lethargy, coma, etc.), the patient should be evaluated in a timely manner, and the potential adverse reaction to the vaccine should be reported. In 1986, the National Childhood Vaccine Injury Act required that all health-care providers report any severe adverse reactions to the Vaccine Adverse Event Reporting System (VAERS) and Centers for Disease Control and Prevention (CDC). The length of time from administration to the appearance of an adverse reaction that is a reportable event is between 7 and 30 days and is

Table 3.4 Summary of Immunization Guidelines for Children and Adults		
Pediatric (0–6 Years)	**Children (7–18 Years)**	**Adult**
Hep B Three between birth and 18 months		
DTaP Five between age 2 months and 6 years	*Tdap* One between 11 and 12 years	*Td* Every 10 years Substitute 1 dose with Tdap
Hib Four between age 2 months and 18 months		
IPV (polio) Four between age 2 months and 6 years		
MMR Two between age 12 months and 6 years		*MMR* One dose if born in 1957 or later
Varicella Two between age 12 months 6 years		*Varicella* Two doses if no evidence of immunity
	HPV (females and males) Three doses between age 11 and 12 years	*HPV (females and males)* Three doses between age 19 and 26 years if not done earlier
		Zoster One dose after age 60 years
PCV (pneumococcal) Four between age 2 months and 18 months		*PCV* One dose after age 65 years
Influenza Yearly after age 6 months	*Influenza* Yearly	*Influenza* Yearly
Hep A Two between age 12 months and 2 years	*MCV (meningococcal)* 1 between age 11 and 12 years unless in a high-risk group	
RV Two between 2 months and 4 months		

Source: Summary of Immunization Guidelines for Adults and Children (ACIP, 2014). Retrieved from www.cdc.gov/vaccines/schedules

dependent on whether the vaccine contains live virus. When in doubt, it is best to report the event.

The information regarding potential reactions for each vaccine is available in the Red Book developed by the American Academy of Pediatrics (www.aap.org) or on the CDC Web site under the Morbidity and Mortality Weekly Reports (MMWR) (www.cdc.gov/mmwr) section. To file a report on a potential reaction with the CDC, complete the VAERS form, which can be downloaded from www.vaers.org. Immunization is still one of the best methods we have for preventing illness and disease or the serious sequelae that can develop from specific diseases such as polio, diphtheria, *H influenzae,* and others. It is an example of primary prevention at its best.

Individual Influences on Health Promotion

The key to successful health promotion is the motivation and commitment of the patient. To obtain a successful outcome, the patient must be willing to make lifestyle changes. The clinician should provide patients with health education that informs them of their current risk factors, the possibility of reducing or eliminating risk factors by lifestyle changes, and the potential benefits of implementing these changes. Once the clinician has provided the information to the patient, the decision to take action rests with the patient. An ideal scenario for health promotion would involve both patient and clinician working in partnership toward mutually agreed on health goals. However, the choice to engage in this partnership is the patient's decision. For example, 36-year-old K. J. is being seen for a routine physical exam and reveals a smoking history of a pack a day of cigarettes for 20 years. She is counseled about her smoking habit and the associated risk for cardiac, respiratory, and peripheral vascular disease. She states that she understands that smoking is not good for her health but currently is not willing to quit. This scenario illustrates that despite the best efforts of the clinician, the patient still has the right to not engage in health-promoting behaviors.

Many factors can influence a patient's motivation to engage in health promotion activities, such as willingness to alter lifestyle practices, belief that making the changes will affect health, and belief that promoting health can prevent disease. All of these factors will influence whether or not a patient decides to make lifestyle changes. Several health models have been developed to identify factors that influence a patient's willingness to take action and make changes. Nola Pender's 1997 health belief model provides a framework for health-care providers to use in assessing patients' readiness to make lifestyle changes to promote their own health (Pender, 2010). Pender's model describes and defines several factors that affect a patient's decision to take action (Fig. 3.3). She divides these factors into two types: cognitive-perceptual factors and modifying factors. Cognitive-perceptual factors include items such as importance of health, perceived

control of health, and perceived barriers to health-promoting behaviors. Modifying factors include biological characteristics, situational factors, and demographic characteristics.

Pender states that all of these factors will affect a patient's willingness to take action (which she terms "cues to take action"). For example, 17-year-old Jonathan had not been consistently wearing a seat belt while riding in or driving a car until 2 months ago. His friend Kyle was involved in a motor vehicle collision (MVC) in which Kyle was seriously injured. Kyle's parents informed Jonathan that Kyle's injury could have been prevented if Kyle had been wearing a seat belt. In this situation, Jonathan has changed his perception (cognitive-perceptual factors) about the importance of wearing a seat belt (health-promoting behavior) based on interpersonal influences (his friend's involvement in an MVC). His "cue to action" was hearing that the injuries incurred by Kyle could have been avoided had Kyle been wearing his seat belt.

This scenario illustrates that although various factors can influence positive health changes, the "cues to action" for patients may vary. In this scenario, it would be interesting to find out if the MVC caused Kyle to change his behavior regarding seat belt use. It is important that clinicians strive to offer patients a variety of scenarios to promote health.

Today's focus on primary disease prevention is empowering for patients, in contrast to the situation 20 years ago, when most patients were not given the option of actively participating in their health care. Health care today provides many opportunities for patients and clinicians to optimize health through health promotion and disease prevention.

Community Influences on Health Promotion

Community efforts can also substantially enhance health promotion efforts. As described previously, the burden of responsibility regarding sanitation, hygiene, and clean water supplies rests with the local community government. A person who lives in a community that lacks appropriate waste disposal, air pollution controls, or law enforcement is exposed to greater health risks than is an individual who lives in a community in which each of these environmental issues has been effectively addressed. Unfortunately, local government agencies are faced with widening budget deficits, and many social and environmental programs are being cut in the wake of the recession affecting the United States.

Health-care providers need to work in partnership with local government agencies to ensure that healthy living conditions are a right for each citizen and not dependent on an individual's race or ethnicity, geography, or socioeconomic status. Clinicians can provide education and expertise to local government agencies for understanding the connection between effective sanitation measures and health. Each health-care provider can also alert the local

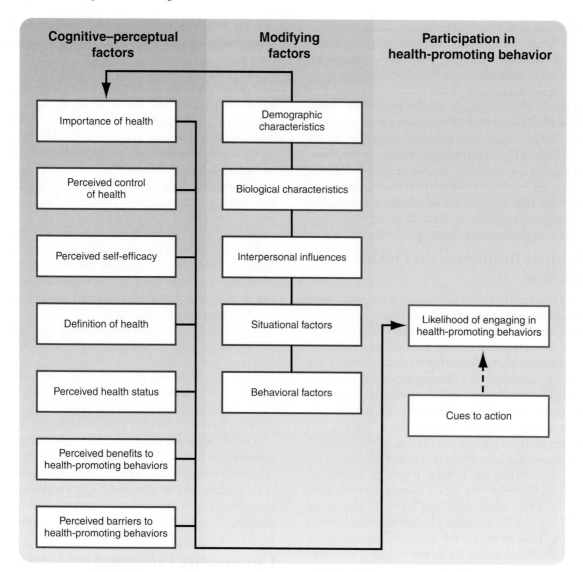

Figure 3.3 Health Promotion Model. *(Source: Pender, N. Health Promotion in nursing practice, ed 5. Prentice-Hall, Upper Saddle River, NJ, 2006.)*

community to possible outbreaks of illness and disease that can affect the greater community at large.

One of the major transitions that occurred from the earlier initiatives of *Healthy People* to *Healthy People 2000/2010/2020* was the shift from a largely federal government initiative to more involvement from local and community agencies. It was believed that this shift in responsibility would result in a significant improvement in meeting the goals of the initiative.

Community programs aimed at providing health information are one way that local communities can assist with this initiative. Offering forums for dialogue between health-care providers and local citizens is an excellent way to educate a broader audience. If these types of efforts are supported by community leaders, there will be a larger impact in the community. The development of health-promoting legislation is another way that local communities can help effect change. For example, the passage of smoking restrictions in public areas is an excellent

example of how local efforts can improve the health of the communities they serve. Legislative policies and interventions that affect the health of individuals and communities, such as housing, labor, energy, transportation, education, justice, and so forth, can be initiated by local and regional agencies. *Healthy People 2020* encourages the active participation of all civic and community agencies to help meet the goals for 2020.

Communities can also respond to the "call for action" from *Healthy People 2020* by ensuring that their citizens have equal access to health care, which is a priority for the *Healthy People* initiatives. For example, it is often difficult for indigenous populations to access health-care services in their communities because of the rural nature of the Indian Reservations. The Navajo Nation is the largest Indian Reservation in the United States, covering 27,000 square miles and spanning parts of Utah, Arizona, and New Mexico. The nearest health-care facility can be a 3-hour drive away.

In addition, many communities do not have systems in place to support the efforts of patients who have language or financial barriers to seek care in their community. Often, a disadvantaged patient's only access to care is through the hospital emergency department. At that time, tertiary measures of prevention are employed and are very costly. Community hospitals can work together with local government agencies to develop health programs/settings that will provide access to health care for all citizens, not just those who have health insurance or whose primary language is English.

The long-range goals of establishing these types of health programs are a reduction in direct hospital costs and an improvement in the quality of life for all citizens. Saving money is a major concern for both hospitals and local communities, and improving access to nonemergent health care can provide significant savings to both. Providing access to health-care services to groups of people who lack the means to access care in traditional settings will do much to improve the health disparities currently affecting our nation.

The Affordable Care Act (ACA) was signed into law on March 23, 2010, and the Supreme Court rendered a final decision on June 28, 2012, to uphold the healthcare law. The ACA puts consumers in charge of their health care, allowing for improved access to care, stability and flexibility of care, and information needed to make informed choices about their health.

The Patient's Voice 3.1

Looking Back to Move Forward, by Dorothy Dunn
Looking back I was always active, fit, and healthy.
He was born 10 pounds 14 ounces, a vaginal delivery.
"He will be obese, and we need to watch for diabetes."
Truth is that when pregnant, I was the obese one.
Now he is active, fit, and healthy, never having a weight concern.

Now I am aging, moving forward in my life span.
Menopause came and went, a beautiful passage into becoming older with grace.
Now, postmenopausal, my path has been a battle against metabolic syndrome.
As I move forward I slow, dare not to stop.
I learn I have a medical condition, a disease named obesity.
How did this happen to always being active, fit, and healthy?

Choosing to battle metabolic syndrome seemed kinder to the cruelty of being obese.
Is this what it will take to call it what it is?
Is there truth in what my path is, the obesity battle?

I can choose. I choose the path of health and well-being,
A healthy passage as I age.

Enjoy active walking, enjoy colorful eating, enjoy renewed spirit.

Looking back, I was always active, fit, and healthy. Moving forward, I will enjoy my next passage into quality years to come.

Other Influences

Health promotion strategies can be effective only when we have adequate knowledge of diseases affecting any given population. With this knowledge, individuals, families, health-care providers, community partners, and governmental agencies can work together to alleviate or minimize the impact of disease on patients. The evaluation of current health indicators is important in order to change the course of illness and disease. Evaluating and reviewing the current leading causes of death in the United States is one way to evaluate past trends. Once this evaluation is made, it can be determined whether these diseases can be prevented or reversed with lifestyle changes. The leading causes of death in this country are published by the National Center for Health Statistics. The top 10 causes of death in the United States for 2011 are listed in Table 3.5. Our current knowledge regarding all of these diseases indicates that healthy lifestyles can

Table 3.5	Top 10 Causes of Death (National Vital Statistics Report for 2011)	
Cause of Death	Statistics	Amendable to Intervention
Heart disease	596,339	Yes
Cancer	575,313	Some
Chronic lower respiratory disease	143,382	Yes
Stroke (cerebrovascular disease)	128,931	Yes
Accidents (unintentional injuries)	122,777	Yes
Alzheimer's disease	84,691	Early diagnosis to slow progression
Diabetes mellitus	73,282	Yes
Influenza and pneumonia	53,667	Yes
Nephritis, nephrotic syndrome, and nephrosis	45,731	Yes
Intentional self-harm (suicide)	35,539	Yes

indeed positively affect their outcomes. For example, heart disease has been the number 1 cause of death in the United States for many years. A healthy lifestyle can prevent or at least ameliorate heart disease in most individuals. The previously discussed health scenario of Mr. Hart is an excellent example of risk factors for heart disease. As you recall, Mr. Hart had several lifestyle factors that put him at risk for heart disease: smoking, alcohol consumption, overweight, and elevated cholesterol and LDL levels. Making different lifestyle choices could potentially help Mr. Hart to control his heart disease in order to live a long and healthy life, without the devastation of a myocardial infarction or possibly even death from heart disease.

The majority of the current top 10 causes of death could be avoided or delayed with healthy lifestyle choices, providing hope for the future health status for patients. With early health assessment and screenings, clinicians can intervene by helping patients to make healthier life choices and lowering their risk for devastating health consequences.

■ PRACTICAL EPIDEMIOLOGY

It is essential for clinicians to monitor trends in health and disease that may affect patients' health. In the role of health promoters for both their patients and the larger community, clinicians gather and contribute raw epidemiological data to various health organizations. Clinicians then consume the analyses of these data in the research reports and journals produced by these organizations.

Epidemiology is the evaluation of distribution patterns and determinants of health and disease in populations. The *focus* of epidemiology is to study the trends of disease occurrences in groups rather than in individuals. The *goal* of epidemiological studies is to discover and evaluate the trends of illness or disease in groups of

---

CASE STUDY 3.1 The Journey to Health Promotion

Delia, a 41-year-old woman, comes in for a complete physical exam. She states that she has completed the questionnaires that were sent to her in anticipation of this appointment. She shows you the completed primary health promotion questionnaire (see Box 3.4) and tells you that she has never had any health-care provider in the past ask her so many in-depth questions about her own health and well-being. She states that she realizes, after completing this assessment form, that there are many factors in her life that contribute to her health status. She relates that completing this survey has made her take a personal inventory of her patterns on an emotional, social, cultural, and psychological level; and she has begun to see how they either contribute to or detract from her current physical health. She indicates that she is willing to work with her health-care provider to begin to change some of her current health and lifestyle patterns to enhance her own health and well-being. She states that completing this questionnaire has been a very enlightening exercise for her and she is excited to begin "her journey" to balancing her life for better health and harmony.

Box 3.4   Primary Health Promotion Assessment Form

Identifying Information
Name
Date of Birth
Where were you born?
What languages do you speak?
What is your highest level of education?
Current Medical History
Past Medical History
Current Medication History
Current Medical History
Describe your current health status: _____
Has your health status changed in the past 2 years? (If yes, describe) _____
_____
What are your own personal health goals?_____
Current weight _____ BMI _____
Current height _____
Current social habits _____

Box 3.4   Primary Health Promotion Assessment Form—cont'd

Current Medication History

	Name(s)	Dosage(s)	Frequency
Prescription meds			
Nonprescription meds			
Vitamins			
Supplements			
Alternative/complementary meds			
Home remedies			
Other			

Current Social Habits

Type	Amount	Frequency	Date of Most Recent Use
Cigarettes/cigars/chewing tobacco/snuff			
Alcohol			
Illicit drug use:			
Type:			
Other: _____			

Current Health Promotion Activities

Do you currently wear a seat belt?
Consistently?
Use of sun screen protection: Lotions? Sun protection factor (SPF) no.: _____
    Clothing
    How many times/week are you out in direct sunlight?_____
    Duration of time in sun per week?_____
Helmet Use:
Do you currently wear a helmet when using a bike, scooter, motorcycle, etc.?_____
Do you consistently wear a helmet?_____
Have you ever sustained a head injury/fall related to use of a bike, scooter, motorcycle, etc.? (describe)_____

Home Hazards

Do you have lights to help you to see where you are going outside of your home?_____
Do you have paved sidewalks to your home/apt/condo?_____
Are there smoke detectors in your home?_____
Electric?_____ Battery operated?_____
Other (describe)_____
Where do you store chemicals in your home?_____
Any guns/weapons in the home?_____
If yes, type and where are they stored?_____

Work Hazards

Which type of work do you do?_____
Are you currently aware of any hazards to your health at work?_____
_____

Environmental Hazards

Do you currently feel safe where you are living?_____
Are you aware of any hazards/toxic exposures in your neighborhood? _____
Gas exposure? _____
Chemical exposure? _____
Lead exposure? _____

Continued

Box 3.4   Primary Health Promotion Assessment Form—cont'd

Current Exercise Patterns

Do you currently exercise?_____

Type of exercise: _____

How often do you exercise?_____

Duration of exercise?_____

Injuries related to exercise:_____

Leisure Time Patterns

Type of Activity	Time Spent Doing Activity	How Often	Last Time You Engaged in Activity
Reading			
Crafts			
Woodworking			
Playing sports			
Watching television			
Listening to music			
Meditating			
Journaling			
Knitting			
Sewing			
Playing a musical instrument			
Gardening			
Other			

Cultural/Religious/Spiritual Affiliations

What cultural or ethnic practices do you use for health care?

Do you participate in any religious/spiritual programs?

Type: _____

Frequency: _____

Do you practice your religion/spirituality at home?

Current Emotional Health

Describe your current emotional status: _____

_____

_____

Who are your current social supports?

When was the last time you felt happy?_____

When was the last time you felt sad?_____

When was the last time you felt angry?_____

What do you do when you are upset? Angry? _____

Dietary Health Habits

How many meals do you eat/day? _____

Do you follow any special type of diet? _____

         Describe: _____

Duration of time on this diet? _____

Do you currently have any food allergies/sensitivities?

         Describe: _____

When did each allergy start? _____

Box 3.4   Primary Health Promotion Assessment Form—cont'd

Daily servings of: _____ meats/protein _____ fruits _____ vegetables _____ fats _____ sugar _____ other

What is your favorite beverage of choice? (check all that apply)

_____ water _____ how much/day type: _____ (bottled, filtered, tap)

_____ milk _____ how much/day type: _____ (% of fat)

_____ coffee _____ how much/day

_____ tea _____ how much/day

_____ soda _____ how much/day

_____ other (describe) _____ how much/day _____

Do you have any concerns about your current weight? _____

Immunization Health

When was your last: _____ Tetanus shot

_____ Flu shot

_____ Measles, mumps, and rubella shot

_____ Hepatitis B shot

_____ Pneumococcal vaccine

_____ Tuberculosis screen

_____ Other (describe) _____

Current Life Stressors

Which of the following do you consider current stressors in your life (check all that apply):

_____ home _____ school _____ work _____ health _____ family

_____ friends _____ other (describe)

Please provide more detail regarding each of the identified stressors: _____

What do you do for yourself when you feel stressed? (check all that apply)

_____ overeat	_____ use alcohol and/or drugs	_____ avoid food
_____ yell/scream	_____ become depressed	_____ cry
_____ become physically aggressive	_____ isolate myself	_____ journaling
_____ talk with family and friends	_____ talk with no one	
_____ seek counseling	_____ use exercise as an outlet	
_____ meditate	_____ listen to music	
_____ other (describe) _____		

What is the best thing that you do for yourself? _____

What is the worst thing that you do to yourself? _____

Add any other comments that you would like:

_____

_____

_____

_____

_____

_____

---

people in order to determine cause and effect and thereby prevent further disease. For example, a single case of swine flu (H1N1) is a concern, but it is not the focus of epidemiology. Instead, increasing numbers of cases of the H1N1 virus become an epidemiological study when they occur in close proximity of time and place. When susceptible populations are studied for the presence of a particular infection or disease, distribution patterns and symptoms may begin to emerge.

When disease statistics are given, reports often refer to the prevalence and incidence rates of a certain disease. The *prevalence* rate refers to the number of cases of a particular disease at a particular point in time divided by the percentage of the population at a point in time (Table 3.6). The prevalence rate does not distinguish between *new* and *old* cases. For example, if the current prevalence rate for a disease was 1 million, it would indicate the number of new and old cases of the disease in the current population. The *incidence rate* is the number of *new* cases of a disease diagnosed at a point in time (e.g., 1 year). Prevalence and incidence rates are commonly used terms to describe disease trends, and the formula is provided in Table 3.6.

Table 3.6	Prevalence and Incidence Rates
Prevalence Rate	**Incidence Rate**
New and old cases of "B" disease at a specific point in time	New cases of "C" disease at a specific point in time
Number of cases divided by total population at specific point in time	Number of cases divided by total population at a specific point in time

Additional common terms used to study trends include *morbidity, mortality, sporadic, endemic, pandemic,* and *epidemic.* Morbidity and mortality rates are often described together. Morbidity defines the number of people who have been diagnosed with a disease divided by the number of total population at risk. The number of people who have died from a particular disease divided by the total population is the mortality (Table 3.7).

To understand the difference between morbidity and mortality, consider the human immunodeficiency virus (HIV). During 2003, the estimate for the number of persons living with HIV/AIDS in the United States was 1,185,000 (morbidity rate). During the same year, the total number of deaths from AIDS was 17,934 (mortality rate). The current rates for HIV infection indicate that significant strides have been made in improving prevention of HIV, which has in turn influenced the incidence, prevalence, morbidity, and mortality associated with the disease. More people are living longer with HIV as a result of significant advances in its medication and management.

Certain illnesses affect the population during annual predictable cycles. Terminology regarding these cycles includes *epidemic, endemic, sporadic,* and *pandemic.* For example, influenza virus is known to be prevalent during the winter season and can cause significant morbidity and mortality. The ability to predict the active cycle of this virus helps health-care practitioners to educate and inoculate patients before predicted outbreaks. These health promotion efforts are effective means of decreasing the prevalence and incidence of the influenza virus, commonly called the "flu." Each year, predictions are made regarding the number of patients who, without health promotion efforts, will experience the flu. In the

past, there have been years in which the number of patients experiencing the flu was significantly higher than expected. This is called an *epidemic* and is defined as the presence of an event (illness or disease) at a much higher rate than expected on the basis of past history.

Although the common cold appears to have some variation, it is known to be present throughout the year. Because it is considered to be present consistently throughout the year, it would be considered an endemic outbreak. *Endemic* is the term used when the presence of an event is constant at or about the same frequency as expected based on past history. A sporadic outbreak occurs when there are occasional cases of an event unrelated in space or time. For example, a gastrointestinal virus may be present in 3 patients this month, 20 patients 2 months from now, and 100 patients in 6 months. The virus is present but is not causing illness at a specific time and place. It is rare to hear of a patient having the flu during the summer season. The last epidemiological term that it is important to understand is pandemic. A *pandemic* is defined as the presence of an event in epidemic proportions affecting many communities and countries in a short period of time. For example, in 2005 to 2006, there was widespread concern regarding avian or "bird" flu. It was found in several countries in a short period of time, and there was concern that it would reach pandemic proportions by affecting many people in many countries. The purpose of all of these epidemiological terms is to clarify the significance of a particular illness or disease at a given point in time (Table 3.8).

The CDC generally monitors and reports the incidence, prevalence, morbidity, and mortality rates of diseases and specifically monitors the rates of infectious diseases. This information is distributed weekly in a report titled *The Morbidity and Mortality Weekly Report* (MMWR), which is available online at www.cdc.gov/mmwr. The report contains useful information about current infectious diseases that are a threat to local and

Table 3.7	Morbidity and Mortality Formulas
Morbidity Formula	**Mortality Formula**
Number of new cases of "D" disease divided by total population at risk	Number of deaths from "E" disease divided by total population at risk

Table 3.8	Epidemiological Terms
Term	**Definition**
Sporadic	Outbreaks of an illness/disease that occur occasionally and are unrelated in space and time
Epidemic	Presence of an event (illness or disease) at a much higher rate than expected based on past history
Endemic	Presence of an illness/disease constantly present or present at a rate that is expected based on history
Pandemic	Presence of an event in epidemic proportions affecting many communities and countries in a short period of time

global communities and provides the latest guidelines for treatment of infectious diseases. It is a helpful tool to investigate current infectious disease trends and potential health promotion practices that may minimize or eliminate the threat of infectious disease.

■ CONCLUSION

Health promotion is one of the most powerful tools available today to prevent disease and disability. Clinicians should use health promotion strategies at the primary, secondary, and tertiary levels of prevention. Each level of prevention is important, but the ultimate goal is primary prevention because it has the most significant impact on disease. Actively engaging in primary prevention strategies such as health promotion creates a wonderful opportunity for patients and health-care providers to work together as a team with the common goal of wellness and the prevention of disease. When primary prevention strategies are not feasible, *Healthy People 2020* and the U.S. Preventive Services Task Force provide clinicians with guidelines to initiate secondary prevention strategies, such as early screening and detection of illness and disease. The utilization of these guidelines and health-focused initiatives will help to improve the health of the nation. With all of the current health promotion strategies in place and a focus on disease prevention, it may be possible to eliminate or minimize the most expensive level of health promotion: tertiary prevention. As we embrace the second decade of the 21st century, we continue to build momentum on primary health promotion strategies with the goal of ensuring optimal health and wellness for all citizens.

Davis*Plus* | For additional resources please visit http://davisplus.fadavis.com

References

Advisory Committee on Immunization Practices (ACIP). *Recommendations and guidelines,* January 31, 2014. Retrieved from www.cdc.gov/vaccines/schedules/index.html

American Nurses Association. *Nursing's social policy statement: The essence of the profession,* ed 3. American Nurses Association, Silver Springs, MD, 2010.

Centers for Disease Control and Prevention. *Healthy people 2010.* Retrieved from www.cdc.gov/nchs/healthy_people/hp2010.htm

Mariano, C. *Holistic nursing: scope and standards of practice.* In B. Dossey & L. Keegan, American Holistic Nursing Association. *Holistic nursing: A handbook for practice,* ed 6. Jones & Bartlett Learning, Burlington, MA, 2013. Page 60.

National Prevention Council. *National Prevention Strategy: America's plan for better health and wellness.* Washington, DC, June 2011. Retrieved from www.surgeongeneral.gov/initiatives/prevention/strategy/report.pdf

Pender, N. *Health promotion in nursing practice,* ed 6. Prentice-Hall, Upper Saddle River, NJ, 2010.

U.S. Department of Health, Education and Welfare, Public Health Service. *The Surgeon General's report on health promotion and disease prevention.* U.S. Department of Health and Human Services. U.S. Government Printing Office, Washington, DC, 1979.

U.S. Department of Health and Human Services. *Healthy people 2000.* U.S. Government Printing Office, Washington, DC, 1996.

U.S. Department of Health and Human Services. *Healthy people 2010.* U.S. Government Printing Office, Washington, DC, 2000.

U.S. Department of Health and Human Services. *Healthy people 2020.* Retrieved from www.healthpeople.gov/2020/topicsobjectives2020/default.aspx

World Health Organization. *Constitution of the World Health Organization, 1948.* Retrieved from http://www.who.int/about/definition/en/print.html

Bibliography

Agency for Healthcare Research and Quality. *Guide to clinical preventive services, 2012.* Retrieved from www.ahrq.gov/professionals/clinicians-providers/guidelines-recommendations/guide

Clinician's handbook of preventive services, ed 2. U.S. Government Printing Office, 1998.

Dossey, B, and Keegan, L. *Holistic nursing: A handbook for practice,* ed 6. Jones & Bartlett Learning, Burlington, MA, 2013.

Resources

Agency for Healthcare Research and Quality
www.ahrq.gov
American College of Nurse Practitioners
www.nurse.org/acnp
American Academy of Family Physicians
www.aafp.org
American Academy of Nurse Practitioners
www.aanp.org
American College of Sports Medicine
www.acsm.org
www.physsportsmed.com
Centers for Disease Control and Prevention
www.cdc.gov/cdc.html

Food and Drug Administration
www.fda.gov
National Institutes of Health
www.nih.gov
National Institute of Nursing Research
www.nih.gov/ninr
National Library of Medicine
www.nlm.nih.gov
Occupational Safety and Health Administration
www.osha.gov
U.S. Department of Health and Human Services
www.hhs.gov

The Art of Diagnosis and Treatment

Susan K. Chase, EdD, RN, FNP-BC

Chapter **4**

The Affordable Care Act will likely change health-care delivery in the United States over the next few years. Central to the law is granting increased access to health-care services to people who had previously not been able to receive regular primary care. Advanced practice registered nurses (APRNs) will be central in delivering much of the primary care in the new system. APRNs are able to offer unique services in primary care for several reasons. All health-care providers are called to provide evidence-based care, which involves providing care and making treatment and screening choices based on current research findings. Further, evidence-based care works best when systems of care are established so that local protocols and tracking systems support the diagnosis and treatment decisions of providers. Nurse practitioners are able to enact evidence-based care particularly well because they bring a nursing perspective of whole-person care to patient encounters that in some settings have been more disease centered than person centered. As clinicians work with patients to plan how to improve health, they take into account more than a plan for prescription medications. They include considerations of each individual's life situation when choosing regimens that may include medication, but clinicians will also include recommendations for diet, activity, rest, stress management, and health promotion. Evidence-based practice requires more than a "diagnose and treat" mentality. There is more to do in a primary-care visit than set up a treatment plan. Treatment decisions are made based on patient values, preferences, and resources while also considering guidelines and research-based recommendations. Learning to practice primary care in an artful way such as this requires a certain kind of thinking. The kind of thinking that clinicians engage in is the subject of this chapter.

■ THE CONTEXT OF CLINICAL JUDGMENT IN PRIMARY CARE

Clinical Judgment and the *Circle of Caring*

The *Circle of Caring* model, introduced in Chapter 1, provides a framework for advanced practice nursing. It includes aspects of the more traditional medical model approach within a model that has nursing as its origin.

The *Circle of Caring* incorporates elements of the patient's experience, including the context of that experience in the patient's life and the environment in which care is delivered. It includes traditional modes of assessment, such as history taking, that are similar to those of the medical model, as well as a database for a nursing perspective, the functional health patterns, or other more holistic measures. Objective findings include physical assessment data, laboratory test data, and functional measures. The *Circle of Caring* demonstrates that the clinician uses these data as part of a data-collection process that leads to the identification of both medical diagnoses as listed in the International Classification of Diseases, 10th Revision (ICD-10) (www.cms.gov/Medicare/Coding/ICD10) and the human responses to those specific diagnoses or nursing diagnoses as listed in taxonomies such as the North American Nursing Diagnosis Association International (NANDA-I). The NANDA-I list includes consideration of problem prevention and wellness promotion and goes beyond a narrow problem-solving framework. A full understanding of the patient situation provides a basis for planning interventions based on best available evidence. Patient preferences are considered as the patient and provider together design a treatment plan that may include pharmacological measures but will also include lifestyle choices and complementary modalities to approach healing and wellness. The *Circle of Caring* reflects that outcomes of APRN practice include improved mortality and morbidity statistics for aggregates of patients; optimized use of the health-care system that provides early, relatively inexpensive treatments to prevent more expensive problems later; and improved functional status and quality of life, as judged by the patient. All of this occurs in an environment consistent with the Institute of Medicine's recommendations that all patients have access to care based on best available evidence, as well as care that takes into account the patient's preferences and values.

Not only is the *Circle of Caring* an expanded way of thinking of both the nursing and the medical clinical process, but it also denotes the way in which the APRN and patient relate to each other within this model. The APRN is able to make appropriate diagnosis and intervention selections on the basis of knowing the patient, being committed to using appropriate clinical guidelines, and having patience when working with the patient, who may be required to make substantial lifestyle change as a result of illness or risk factors. In addition, both patient and nurse exhibit courage in that they engage in this most human of endeavors, that of caring. Throughout the assessment, diagnosis, and treatment, the APRN brings an authentic presence, which is in itself humanizing and healing, and is willing to be an advocate for the patient in personal or professional realms. The *Circle of Caring* requires a balance. The nurse and patient working together need to come up with a meaningful treatment plan and a plan for follow-up support. The *Circle of Caring* depicts a complex yet rewarding practice that enriches both patient and nurse.

This chapter focuses on the process aspects of the model. The *Circle of Caring* model includes the medical model perspective that nurses with baccalaureate degrees may not have learned in an academic setting or practiced in hospital or community settings. It also includes a broader sense of nursing than practice at the baccalaureate level allows. Therefore, the APRN role includes elements from the medical realm and from an expanded nursing base.

Essential to high-quality clinical judgment is the ability of the nurse to form a link between the patient's experience of his or her health concerns and the range of diagnostic and therapeutic choices available to achieve a range of possible outcome states. The nurse must be expert at eliciting the true story of the patient and in recognizing patterns that are presented in the data so as to arrive at an appropriate diagnosis and therapeutic plan. This chapter focuses on merging the results of research with diagnostic reasoning and clinical judgment to facilitate their application by the APRN.

Purpose and Goal of Diagnostic Reasoning

From the patient's point of view, the purpose of a visit to a clinician may be to solve a physical problem. Beyond problem-solving, the practitioner must always keep in mind that every visit is an opportunity for disease prevention, for screening for high-risk problems, and for health promotion based on appropriate guidelines. The patient must know that his or her initial concerns are taken seriously and are not ignored. The APRN can establish a tone that attends to body, mind, and spirit in every visit. Diagnostic reasoning to solve problems, to promote health, and to screen for disease or illness all require a sensitivity to complex stories, to contextual factors, and to a sense of probability and uncertainty. At times, the patient will schedule a visit stating one concern, but during the visit other issues arise that become more important. Headache might be caused by a stressful job or family situation, or the patient might not want to tell the scheduler that domestic violence or a sexual concern is really what is bothering

the patient. Clinicians learn to pay attention to the "By the way, I was wondering about . . ." lead-ins to real concerns.

The mental tasks of eliciting and sorting through large amounts of data, clustering data elements into meaningful patterns, connecting patterns to reasonable diagnostic statements, considering risk factors, and selecting appropriate interventions require the highest order of cognitive processes. It is these analytical functions that distinguish advanced practice nursing and are the reason patients seek our services. The human element of caring helps elicit rich data and establish the trust necessary to encourage patients to adjust their living patterns in the short or long range.

Primary Care and Its Uniqueness

Many students come to advanced practice programs with extensive experience in acute- or critical-care nursing. They are committed to learning an expanded mode of practice but may be overwhelmed by the amount of new material that must be mastered. Even students with community health experience find that the issues faced in primary care are different from those encountered in their previous practice and require new knowledge and skills. Primary care is a new world with a different set of problems to be solved, different kinds of constraints on choices, and a different culture of care. Entering this world with sensitivity to its differences can help reduce anxiety for new advanced practice students and can explain other reactions to this new nursing setting that might arise.

The types of problems that are solved in primary care are different from those encountered in acute- or critical-care settings. Upper respiratory infections, common abdominal complaints, skin rashes, and vaginal discharges are problems not often encountered in acute-care settings. Even chronic conditions present differently in primary care. Hypertension, congestive heart failure, arthritis, or diabetes present with day-to-day management problems that are different from the crises that acute-care nurses must respond to in tertiary-care settings. Patients with psychosocial problems such as anxiety and depression frequently present with vague, nonspecific somatic complaints.

The pace of care is different in primary care. Nurses who are seeking refuge from busy acute-care duties will be surprised by the mental fatigue that comes from diagnosing and treating up to 30 different patients or families in a day. The sheer variety of possible problems faced in a day's time is exciting and interesting, but it is also challenging. The office visit allows for focused attention with an individual patient, but the former staff nurse will realize that an organized approach to obtaining and processing information is necessary because the patient will not be available to fill in missing pieces of information at the end of the day. On the other hand, the relationship with a growing family or the treatment of patients with chronic conditions will continue over years. This long-term relationship is very rewarding to both the APRN and the patient and family.

Primary care includes more than problem-solving and symptom management. It involves screening for problems as yet undetected and supporting health promotion and disease and injury prevention at every opportunity. Teaching patients of all ages about how their bodies work, risk reduction, and treatment options helps patients assume more responsibility for their own wellness. These activities support patients in increasing their health literacy so that they can be active participants in their own care. Researchers from Canada are exploring how APRNs help patients participate in their own care more actively through a concern for their comfort and for a sense of coherence in their lives (Sangster-Gormley & Frisch, 2013). Establishing trust and believing that the APRN cares about the whole person promotes true patient-centered care.

Uncertainty

Primary care and the increased autonomy that advanced practice clinicians enjoy also bring an increase in uncertainty. Patient problems are not already labeled when the nurse practitioner sees the patient. Many different conditions present in similar ways. Even the "hard numbers" of laboratory tests must be evaluated for their reliability. Once a diagnosis is made, multiple treatment approaches are available even for simple problems. Further, patients do not always carry out recommended treatment plans (Michaels et al, 2008). Many problems require lifelong lifestyle adjustment. At the end of the day, the clinician may have nagging doubts about the decisions that were made on many levels. New practitioners especially need support to develop confidence in their diagnostic and treatment-planning capabilities, but even experienced practitioners describe learning to live with the uncertainties involved in primary care. Intellectual honesty and humility are important aspects of thoughtful practice and can be cultivated, but they must be balanced with confidence that is based on experience; this serves to increase the effectiveness of the provider.

Nursing versus Medical Model

APRNs perform in both the nursing and the medical domains. The nursing domain contains consideration of individual and family responses to actual or potential threats to health. It involves helping patients cope with disease processes that may be occurring, and it anticipates human distress and works on the level of what an illness experience means to the patient. By becoming an APRN, nurses do not leave their nursing model of practice. As APRNs gain skill in the medical domain of practice, they learn new diagnostic reasoning possibilities and new treatment options for specific medical problems. These new skills are built on the nursing framework, but they do not replace the nursing basis for practice.

APRNs have been proven to be effective and efficient care providers for patients with acute and chronic health problems. The process of clinical judgment is unique in primary care because patients and their families will actually carry out the care (Elliott, 2010). Patients are actively involved in their own care, and the clinician must take that into account in designing a treatment or health promotion plan. Though much of this textbook is designed to provide a background for managing medical problems, all that the nurse has learned in caring for patients still applies. An APRN's approach to patient problems is often very individualized and, therefore, less easy to summarize in a textbook. Nevertheless, the nursing model supports and nurtures the APRN's practice. It provides the basis for the *Circle of Caring*.

Patient–Advanced Practice Nurse Linkages

A model for how the provider and patient work together in a clinical encounter is presented in Figure 4.1. Clinical judgment is not a process that happens in the mind of the practitioner alone: It happens in a dialogue that occurs between patient and provider. The quality of communication and the agreement about what the encounter is meant to accomplish will improve both effectiveness and satisfaction with the patient encounter for both parties. The model includes patient factors, provider factors, and environmental factors, all of which have an influence on the clinical judgment process (Chase, 2004).

The Patient–Advanced Practice Nurse linkage model is based on research in diagnostic reasoning in general and the particulars of the primary-care encounter. Johnson (1993) described the discourse between patient and nurse as having several phases: establishing the agenda for the encounter; eliciting information from the patient, including being alert to cues and helping to problem solve; and conducting the physical examination, including attending to comfort level, preparing and informing, and developing a plan of care and using a teachable moment. Teaching in this case is not content centered but patient centered, based on understanding the perspective of the patient. Finally, the APRN personalizes solutions based on knowing the patient. Investigating overall satisfaction with care, a large quantitative study has shown that patients are equally satisfied with care access and overall care experience when care is provided by a nurse practitioner or physician assistant compared with a visit managed by a physician in both adult and pediatric settings. Patients were more satisfied, however, with nurse practitioner and physician assistant care when rating the quality of practitioner interaction (Roblin et al, 2004). A review of the literature on nurse practitioners' communication style (Charlton et al, 2008) characterized nurse practitioner communication style as either biomedical or biopsychosocial. The biopsychosocial

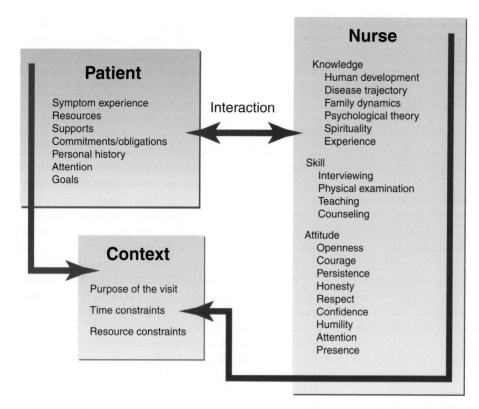

Figure 4.1 Patient–advanced practice nursing linkages. *(Source: Chase, SK. Clinical judgment and communication in nurse practitioner practice. FA Davis, Philadelphia, 2004.)*

style was associated with higher patient satisfaction and better adherence to treatment plans. A qualitative study of health outcomes achieved in a home visiting model for young disadvantaged mothers showed that the nature of the relationship between carer and recipient goes beyond protocols with a result of enhanced personhood and new possibilities developed by these young women (SmithBattle, 2009). The personal relationship between APRN and patient within which this work is done is unique.

■ THE CLINICAL PROCESS AND ITS LIMITATIONS
Human Memory Limitations

One of the most useful models available to understanding diagnostic reasoning is that of the information processing model. This model is built on the premise that the human brain has both short- and long-term memory and that these forms of memory are different from each other. Short-term memory is the processing space that can hold new pieces of information and elements of the patient history and physical data. It has the limitation of being able to hold only approximately seven "bits" of information. Much of the mental activity used in diagnostic reasoning is done to maximize the active processing space and to clustering or "chunking" cues into collections of data that can be managed together, which helps to maximize processing capacity. In contrast, long-term memory is practically unlimited. It can hold vast

quantities of facts, sensations, and experiences. To bring these facts or experiences to bear on a given situation, long-term memories must be accessible. Research has shown that the ability to retrieve a fact depends on the frequency with which the fact is brought forward for use. This is why in some cases repetitive exercises assist in cementing long-term memory. Another factor that affects retrievability of facts from long-term memory is the organization structure with which the fact is associated. Body systems and functional health patterns are systems of data organization that help busy clinicians retrieve relevant bits of information as needed.

In actuality, although the information processing model is a useful starting point, the human brain functions differently from a computer. The brain is able to sense patterns of data and to include emotional responses to experiences with human beings. The ability to empathize with a patient, to be available personally, and to be invested with the patient in maximizing health make the human decision-maker much more valuable than any computer or protocol system could ever be. If protocols were enough for effective management, the Internet or other computer system would be sufficient to provide health care to anyone with access to the system. Patients come to a health-care provider for more than a diagnosis, however. They come for a human connection. The human aspect of the nurse–patient relationship adds to, rather than detracts from, diagnostic accuracy. One researcher called this "getting alongside" (Elliott, 2010, p. 2,714) when describing ways the nurse practitioners listen to the patient's perspective on his or her problem. Technology can assist clinicians by prompting routines and in offering diagnostic and therapeutic options that might have been missed (Lee et al, 2009). The technology system, however, does not substitute for human judgment and should not become a barrier to provider–patient communication.

Critical Thinking

Diagnostic reasoning can be seen as a kind of critical thinking. *Critical thinking* has been defined as reflective thinking because the process involves questioning one's thinking to determine if all possible avenues have been explored and if the conclusions that are being drawn are based on evidence. This kind of thinking supports clinical judgment in several ways. First, it becomes a habit of mind to have humility about one's thought processes and to know that even the most experienced thinker can be mistaken. Second, it becomes a systematic way of generating creative ways of thinking about problems. Third, critical thinking returns one to an examination of the strength of evidence for a given conclusion. "Evidence" in this context means more than "hard" data such as laboratory values. Even laboratory values must be examined critically when they are used to assist diagnostic reasoning. The type of evidence that is useful includes subjective impressions of the ways patients present themselves. The patient's initial complaint may be fatigue, but any patient who describes a bone-chilling inability to generate energy for daily living (compared with a fulfilled fatigue that comes after a challenging situation is completed) is providing data the APRN can use to investigate potentially serious health problems.

Critical thinking can include creative thinking—in this sense, the APRN is creative in developing potential problem lists. A patient may complain of abdominal pain. The pattern is unclear or may indicate irritable bowel syndrome. The creative APRN will explore stress management issues as a way of generating diagnostic and therapeutic choices that could include a diet and symptom log, increased fiber in the diet, a walking program, or a quick follow-up visit to check on symptoms. Creativity may also be required in developing goals with patients for their short- or long-term problems. In addition to creative processing, critical thinking includes systematic thinking that evaluates each new piece of data as it either supports some diagnostic hypotheses or reduces the likelihood of others.

Intuition

Another kind of thinking that develops with experience is that of intuition. Research on intuition shows that it develops after long experience in the particular setting and that it is based on unconscious thought that is probably an exquisite pattern matching. The experienced clinician is reminded of a situation that occurred in the past when presented with a certain new situation. Past experience provides a picture of what will likely happen. The experienced clinician often could not list the specific data points that led to the conclusion. In fact, in some studies of computerized "artificial intelligence," experienced clinicians were asked to "think aloud" as a research device aimed at identifying the steps involved in reaching a diagnosis. Experienced clinicians reported that being asked to do that kind of thinking changed their thought process and slowed them down. Although intuition characterizes expert practice, it is not a goal in itself. Being able to reflect on one's thinking processes opens the process to analysis, sharing, and improvement (Thompson & Yang, 2009).

Developing Expertise

Benner et al (1996) have done extensive work describing differences in clinical judgment based on experience. APRN students, even those who are experts in hospital or specialty care, find it disconcerting to enter a world where they feel like novices again. Even skills that were a part of their old practice feel awkward. Their minds often do not generate ideas smoothly, and they focus on their own performance of skills more than on the patient's situation. With the experience of the clinical practicum, however, the student gains skill and by graduation is probably functioning at the advanced beginner level. Features of diagnostic reasoning used in the various stages of expertise are summarized in Table 4.1.

Table 4.1 Skill Acquisition in Advanced Practice Nursing Practice	
Skill Level	Features of Clinical Judgment
Novice	Rule-based actions, unaware of context
Advanced beginner	Sensitive to aspects of the situation, able to formulate principles, needs help setting priorities
Competent	Goal-directed actions, feeling of mastery based on experience, deliberate planning
Proficient	Sees situation as a whole, immediate grasp of meaning, recognizes patterns of normalcy or aberrance, uses maxims to guide action
Expert	Transcends rules, intuitive grasp of the wholeness of situation, creative response to particularities of situation, flexible response to situations

■ DIAGNOSTIC PROCESS OVERVIEW

Diagnostic reasoning is a process of data generation and clustering, hypothesis generation, probabilistic reasoning, pattern matching, planning, problem-solving, and critical reflection. These processes are commonly summarized by describing the steps in the nursing process or the clinical reasoning process. Research has shown that many clinicians, physicians, nurses, occupational and physical therapists, dentists, and others use a similar method. Although research that uses simulated case studies to examine methods of clinician reasoning tends to oversimplify what happens in real life, it is helpful to review a simplified description of the diagnostic process as outlined here.

Data Collection

Research has shown that expert clinicians generate a list of possible diagnoses or diagnostic hypotheses early in the clinical encounter. Further, the likelihood that the diagnostic choice will be correct is higher if the correct diagnosis is included in the initial hypothesis list. In generating hypotheses, the APRN considers a number of labels that could be associated with the initial complaint and considers potential problems for each patient based on the patient's age and demographics and the setting of the practice.

For experienced clinicians, data acquisition in history taking and physical examination is most effective if it is hypothesis driven—that is, when the information selected and gathered is related to the list of possible diagnoses. For common problems, the data collection approach becomes routine and, therefore, takes less active processing space in short-term memory. In contrast, novices tend to use a "shotgun" approach and ask a little bit about everything that might be possible, not considering which diagnoses are most likely. Hypothesis-driven data collection means that data that would confirm or disprove a specific hypothesis is specifically sought and recorded. It is not enough to note only those data that fit with one possible problem. Competing hypotheses must be ruled out by seeking nonconfirmatory data. In doing this, the clinician must be open to changing the priority list of hypotheses based on new information. For example, rhinitis may present similar to a viral infection, but if, when asked whether the symptoms have occurred before, the patient says, "Yes, I had the same thing two weeks ago," this decreases the likelihood of viral illness and increases the likelihood of allergy.

An approach to data collection that is completely symptom driven, however, can result in leaving out important concepts. The agenda for the visit includes not only the patient's agenda but also expands the visit to provide health promotion.

Hypothesis Evaluation

Data are clustered together into meaningful "chunks" of information that explain and account for the different elements of the history. Clinicians are alert to any data bits that do not fit the pattern of what is expected. They are alert to the feeling in themselves that "something is just not right here." This can indicate that the problem is more serious than initially appeared or that there are data bits that are not yet accounted for. Diagnosticians are persistent in trying to fit the pieces of data into a coherent picture. One must be on guard not to ignore discrepant data. Research has shown that "we see what we expect to see" in many cases, so an openness to the patient situation must be maintained in order to continue "seeing" all the data present.

A maxim of practice is that "common things occur commonly." Students are frequently excited to make a diagnosis for the rare or exotic condition. This can be the result of a rich experience in acute- or critical-care settings where the most serious cases were seen. In primary care, common problems predominate. The maxim that "when you hear hoof beats, think horses, not zebras" applies. In real life, "zebra" diagnoses are rare. Rare conditions can be considered with the differential list, but their lower probability must be taken into consideration.

Experienced clinicians keep their antennae raised for the most serious conditions. Abdominal pain could be from gas, but if it is from a ruptured ectopic pregnancy, a dissecting abdominal aortic aneurysm, or a ruptured appendix, immediate surgical consultation is necessary. The clinician must make it a point to collect and document data that rule out any potentially life-threatening condition.

Diagnoses are frequently interrelated. Obesity, hypertension, hyperlipidemia, and type 2 diabetes mellitus frequently occur together. When evaluating competing hypotheses, the APRN can cluster related problems together. The lifestyle recommendations for all these conditions are the same. The medication approach might differ. For nursing diagnoses, many occur together. Try to approach the core diagnosis, which, if managed appropriately, will ameliorate all the others. For instance, ineffective coping with stress can result in an array of symptoms including altered sleep patterns, constipation, difficulty concentrating, and interpersonal tension. By dealing with the underlying problem, the other problems might not need direct intervention. If the APRN focuses only on the superficial problem level, the problems may still remain. Table 4.2 summarizes habits that promote effective clinical judgment. Table 4.3 describes common errors in diagnostic thinking that are made even by experts.

Clustering history data into a likely problem list helps to focus the physical examination, laboratory test evaluation, and initial management plan. Physical examination for a problem-focused visit serves to rule in or rule out competing diagnostic hypotheses. A new hypothesis rarely emerges during a physical examination, but this might occur for a problem that the patient cannot see or that causes no symptoms, such as a skin lesion. Laboratory

Table 4.2   Habits That Support Clinical Judgment

Phase of Diagnostic Reasoning	Habits That Support Clinical Judgment
Data acquisition	Use systematic or hierarchically organized approach (general to specific). Review multiple systems.
Hypothesis formulation	Generate hypotheses early in encounter. Develop competing hypotheses. Consider life- or function-threatening problems. Consider "zebras" but recognize them as such.
Hypothesis evaluation	Recognize interrelation of diagnoses. Consider probabilities in context. Consider likelihood of altering course of problem with treatment. Rule out life- or function-threatening problems.
Problem naming	Choose most fundamental problem. Include multiple perspectives (biopsychosocial, spiritual; medical, nursing). Include illness prevention and health promotion.
Goal setting	Include patient in goal setting. Make goals explicit and realistic.
Therapeutic option consideration	Include modalities from multiple paradigms. Consider patient preferences. Consider context and cost in economic and human terms.
Evaluation	Plan for follow-up visit or phone call. Consider symptom or treatment logs or diaries. Measure and document the outcome of your practice for the individual. Report the effectiveness of your practice in the aggregate.

Source: Chase, SK. *Clinical judgment and communication in nurse practitioner practice.* FA Davis, Philadelphia, 2004, p. 43. Used with permission.

Table 4.3   Errors in Diagnostic Reasoning

Phase of Clinical Judgment	Diagnostic Errors
Data collection	Not obtaining all relevant clues Misjudging importance of clues Overemphasizing clues that favor top hypotheses Ignoring data that disconfirm working hypothesis Forgetting that some data are unreliable Ignoring pertinent negative findings
Hypothesis	Not generating enough competing hypotheses Oversimplifying Not generating hypotheses early Not including correct diagnosis on hypothesis list Failing to revise hypothesis list (premature closure) Selecting "favorite" hypotheses Generating too many hypotheses and getting lost Overestimating low-probability situations Underestimating high-probability situations

Source: Chase, SK. *Clinical judgment and communication in nurse practitioner practice.* FA Davis, Philadelphia, 2004. Used with permission.

tests also provide information that is not available any other way.

Finally, a working diagnosis is reached, even though there might still be some uncertainty. A management plan is discussed with the patient in light of mutually shared goals and guidelines for practice based on published research. Honest conversation about the patient's ability and willingness to follow treatment recommendations will result in more realistic plans.

Written instructions often help patients implement complicated treatment directions. Part of the treatment plan always includes a plan for follow-up. Patients need to know when to return for a visit and under what circumstances they should telephone. Documenting these plans in the patient record reduces the possibility of misunderstanding and places appropriate responsibility with the patient. Some patients need support in learning how to engage the health-care system in an effective way. This is one aspect of health literacy that the APRN can support.

The Diagnostic Process in Action

A simple encounter for a self-limiting acute illness might proceed like this:

A patient requests an appointment for a "sore throat." The patient is known by the APRN as a resourceful, independent young adult. Before even entering the room, the clinician draws from experience with other patients who have complained of sore throat and begins to generate a list of hypotheses. Contextual factors enter into the reasoning: It may be allergy season in that particular area, or the clinician may have seen a large number of other patients with similar complaints who have tested positive for *Streptococcus* infection. The clinician enters the room and notes the general appearance of the patient. Is the patient ill appearing, flushed, fatigued, or mildly irritated? These observations may serve to adjust the hypothesis list. The patient's story is elicited, beginning with history of present illness, along with a review of data already present in the record regarding past medical history and medications. Further questions regarding current life stresses and exposures may also serve to adjust the hypothesis list. The history narrows the hypothesis list to a short one, although experienced clinicians have ways of preventing the common diagnostic error of premature closure and work to consider alternative conditions that could also be represented by the same cluster of symptoms.

The physical exam serves to verify hypotheses and to screen out unlikely, though troubling, alternative diagnoses. The hypothesis list is narrowed further as data are weighed to see whether they fit the pattern of the highest-favored hypothesis; disconfirming data are also elicited to avoid leaping to conclusions too early. Finally, diagnostic tests may be chosen to firm up the diagnosis if the findings of the tests will have a bearing on how the patient's care is to be managed. Once findings of relevant tests have been obtained, treatment decisions are considered, including patient factors such as resources, reliability, and the risk of the patient not following through on instructions. For example, insufficiently treated strep throat could result in rheumatic heart disease. Besides prescribing medication, consider comfort measures that are likely to assist the patient and judge the appropriateness of health promotion and educational opportunities at the moment. For example, is this a good time to give the patient smoking cessation materials? Finally, a plan to evaluate the treatment plan is made. Is a follow-up appointment necessary? Would a telephone call be useful? For which date should the next "well" visit be scheduled? The list of decisions made in this rather simple example is long. Given a few data or situational changes, the management of the patient's care could be quite different, and a new-patient visit requires even deeper background data collection. Patients who present with more complex, long-term problems require even more complex decision making by the clinician. In observing the experienced clinician, many of these mental processes may not be apparent. Many of these processes occur as a kind of internal dialogue, but they occur nonetheless.

■ FOCUS ON ELEMENTS OF CLINICAL JUDGMENT

A more detailed examination of each step in the diagnostic reasoning process follows.

Focus on Data Collection: History
History of Present Illness

Taking a history is the first step in the diagnostic reasoning process. Problems cannot be found, strengths identified, or appropriate direction known without a real grounding in the life experience of the individual patient. If the patient's visit is for "episodic" care or one in which a new complaint is being addressed, the history begins with a history of present illness (HPI). There are a number of mnemonics that can help the clinician remember the essential data elements. The elements of the "OLD CART" mnemonic are listed in Box 4.1.

Immediately on hearing the chief complaint, the clinician begins to sort out diagnostic possibilities. The list

---

Box 4.1 OLD CART Mnemonic

Onset	When did this problem start? How did it start? Has it changed over time?	**D**uration	Are the symptoms constant, fluctuating, getting better or worse?
		Characteristics	How are the symptoms experienced? Dull ache, sharp pain, heat, or electrical?
	For an injury, exactly how did the injury occur (the mechanism of injury)?	**A**ggravating factors	What makes the symptoms worse?
Location	Where exactly are the symptoms experienced?	**R**elieving factors	What makes the symptoms better?
	Can a specific location be identified, or is the problem more generalized? Has the symptom moved?	**T**reatment	What have you done so far to try to help the problem?

of possibilities helps to generate questions to follow up on the HPI and in other areas of the history. Specific questions are asked that help distinguish between competing diagnostic hypotheses. For example, the question, "Do you feel the pain more often on an empty stomach or several hours after eating?" helps distinguish between ulcer and gallbladder disease. In general, asking open-ended questions helps the patient give his or her perspective and provides a richer database. An open-ended question is one that cannot be answered by a "Yes" or "No" response. Eliciting the patient's story will assist the APRN in understanding the illness experience from the patient's point of view. Frequently interrupting the patient's story distracts and places the story in the context of the examiner and not in the context of the patient's own life.

The APRN continues to clarify the patient's story until a clear picture of the illness appears. This can require patience because patients do not know which facts "fit together" to support diagnostic hypotheses. Patients may get the chronological order confused or not recall the exact onset of their problems. They may also have more than one problem and may not be able to distinguish which symptoms cluster together. At times, the picture is not completely clear at this point of history taking, but other areas of history can fill in some gaps. Periodically, the APRN can restate the emerging understanding of the story to clarify and summarize it. This summary allows the patient to clarify any misunderstandings. One important issue to address as part of the HPI is what the *patient* thinks may be wrong. Patients know their own bodies, and parents know their own children better than anyone and may have important insights to share. On the other hand, when patients share their fears, the APRN can also explain reasons why many of those fears may be unfounded. A recurring headache does not necessarily indicate a brain tumor.

Visits for periodic health screening, to establish a new patient–provider relationship, or to follow up on an existing problem do not use the HPI in the same sense unless a new problem is also identified. The APRN can ask, "What do you want to accomplish today?" or "What is the most important issue for us to deal with today?" This is particularly useful for the patient with a long list of problems or complaints. Be sure to make a plan for follow-up on other problems. Other elements of patient history are discussed in detail during the visit.

Past Medical History

Past medical history helps to refine the hypothesis list by offering new explanations for symptoms or by ruling out others. The history also gives suggestions of risk factors for other problems that are being considered. If a patient reports that his or her gallbladder was removed 10 years ago, cholecystitis is now off the hypothesis list, but abdominal adhesions might go onto the list. Past medical history is frequently divided into childhood and other illnesses, surgical history, other hospital admissions, history of trauma, pregnancies, and psychiatric diagnoses. Travel outside the United States and any possible exposure to infectious or toxic agents can be explored. Treatment for cancer in the distant past is important in that the treatments may have increased the risk of other conditions. For example, some chemotherapy agents can lead to heart failure in later years.

The history includes information regarding all medications that patients take, including prescription and over-the-counter medications, as well as vitamins and herbal remedies. Patients also need to be asked if they take any medications that have been prescribed for other members of the family. Even for patients who are well known to the practice and whose medications are listed on the chart, asking the patient what medications he or she is currently taking allows the clinician to learn what the patient remembers about the medication regimen. For patients with multiple prescriptions, it sometimes helps to use the "brown bag" method: Ask the patient to bring in all the medications he or she is taking, then go over them one by one. This helps to determine if the medications that have been ordered are really being taken. This review of medications also gives the clinician information about the patient's understanding of his or her medications and helps to determine any difficulties he or she is having with the prescribed regimen. Immunization status is part of the history. Many parents bring their child's immunization cards with them to office visits. This allows any additional immunization series to be documented. Adults often forget that they need immunizations for things such as tetanus or pneumonia.

Allergies can be discussed at this time and reviewed. The kind of reaction the medications or food caused can help to distinguish an adverse effect from a true allergy. By noting the adverse effect, one can avoid confusing it with an allergy, which is characterized by rash, hives, wheezing, or other hypersensitivity reactions.

Health maintenance practices can be questioned, as well as risk reduction techniques such as seat belt use and exercise habits.

Family History

Family history provides information for a part of the risk factor pattern for this patient. The most efficient way to represent the family history is to draw a genogram (Fig. 4.2). This method of representation can be used to record family patterns of births, ages at death, and causes of death. The genogram can also record family members with whom the patient currently lives. Try to include information for at least two generations back, as well as for any children and their health status. The genogram can be used to map difficulties such as alcoholism or the quality of relationships in the family by drawing slashes across the relationship lines that are troubled or by using thick lines to represent relationships that are strongly supportive. Judgment is required

Genogram of Family History

Figure 4.2 Genogram of family history. *(Source: Chase, SK. Clinical judgment and communication in nurse practitioner practice. FA Davis, Philadelphia, 2004.)*

to determine if this level of information is useful. If there is no room in the patient's record for a genogram, list the major diseases that have familiar patterns, such as diabetes, heart disease, arthritis, psychiatric problems, alcoholism, and cancer.

Social History

Social history in a medical model interview includes such things as work patterns. Even if the patient is retired, the type of work in which the patient had engaged is important because worksite exposures can be risk factors for many potential problems. Work background also gives the clinician a sense of how the person might handle new information and what kind of resources he or she might have at his or her disposal. Medical model histories also include the use of alcohol, tobacco, and illegal drugs. Nursing histories are more expanded in this area. Include such information as leisure time activities, risk factors and exposures, and the patient's resources and activity level. If a full functional health pattern is collected, much of this information can be recorded there. If the documentation system in use in a particular setting does not accommodate functional health patterns, expand the social history section to reflect nursing issues.

Review of Systems

This section of the history is often completed by the patient immediately before the physical exam. It is organized by body systems. Advanced Assessment 4.1 presents sample questions that can be used during the review of systems. Whenever the review is completed, it can include problems and symptoms that are current or related to past medical history and prompt the patient to report any past difficulties. This also helps remind patients of conditions they may have forgotten and can help to

refine the hypothesis list further or to screen out potential new problems. When introducing a body system, start questions in general terms and then proceed to more specific items. When documenting this section, students frequently forget that these data are appropriately recorded as subjective data because they are reported from the patient's point of view.

Functional Health Patterns

Functional health patterns, developed by Marjory Gordon, serve as a database for determining nursing diagnoses. APRNs engage in some activities that require making medical diagnoses, but their practice base is always nursing. The value that APRNs bring to a practice is an enhanced ability to assist patients with lifestyle changes and an ability to support patients as they cope with illness. The openness and thoroughness that patients report when cared for by an APRN are dependent on the APRN practicing from a database that is broader and more personal than that of the traditional medical model. Even in practice settings using a medically dominated model, the nurse has an obligation to represent nursing's contribution to care. The type of data recorded in the functional health pattern in the medical record can reflect a nursing approach.

For episodic visits, some patterns are more important than others, and the list can be prioritized accordingly. For example, for a patient with a sore throat, important data are nutrition (Is he or she able to eat and drink sufficiently?), sleep and rest (Is sleep interrupted?), activity and exercise (Does he or she feel fatigued?), and role relationship (Is he or she able to work? Are there children in the home?). Inability of the patient to carry out any normal, day-to-day function is often a "red flag"—an indicator for the APRN of a potentially serious disease process that may be developing.

The purpose of the functional health pattern is to determine the extent to which illness is affecting the person's ability to live his or her "normal" life. What accommodations must be made, even for a self-limiting condition? This is nursing's central question. What is the human response to the health problem? Advanced Assessment 4.2 presents the 11 functional health patterns and sample questions that can be used to elicit data for each functional pattern area.

At this phase of history taking, the hypothesis list is taking shape. The initial diagnostic possibilities generated are weighed as each new piece of information is gathered. Some data serve to support one hypothesis in favor of another; some data are noncontributory. Some data serve to rule out specific hypotheses. The problem list may contain physical disorders with signs or symptoms that are visible, along with other physical disorders that are presumed to be present based on the patient's story, emotional distress related to specific disorders, general emotional disorders, family or social disorders, or even spiritual distress. The patient's problem list may

Advanced Assessment 4.1   Review of Systems and Sample Questions

System	Sample Questions	System	Sample Questions
General	How is your general health? Are you sleeping restfully? Is your appetite good? Have you had any recent weight changes? Any fever, chills, or night sweats?	Chest	Any chest pain, cough, difficulty breathing, shortness of breath? How far can you walk before becoming breathless?
Skin	Any rashes, moles, itching, changes in color, easy bruising, changes in hair?	Cardiovascular	Any chest pain, palpitations?
Head	Any headache, dizziness, fainting, history of head trauma?	Gastrointestinal	Any stomach pains, indigestion, nausea, or vomiting? Any blood in your stool? Have your bowel movements changed? Any diarrhea or constipation? Any rectal itching, pain? When, if ever, was your last colonoscopy?
Neurological	Any weakness or paralysis? Any feeling of needles and pins or other loss of sensation? Any trouble walking, any seizures? Any trouble with memory or speech? Any nervousness or depression?	Endocrine	Any intolerance of heat or cold? Frequently thirsty? Do you have problems with frequent urination or getting up to urinate at night? Do you experience unusual fatigue? Have you noticed any unusual hair loss?
Eyes, ears, nose	Any eye problems, blurring, loss of vision? Any trouble hearing, ringing in ears, pain, throat discharge or itching? Any problem with runny nose, change in ability to smell, nosebleeds, or sinus trouble? Frequent sore throats, trouble swallowing, hoarseness?	Urinary	Any trouble passing urine, burning, itching, odor, frequency, loss of control or pain?
Mouth	Any mouth sores, dental problems?	Female genitalia	Any vaginal discharge, itching, or odor? When was your last menstrual period? What is the length of your cycle, the length and amount of flow? Do you engage in sexual relations with men, women, or both? What method of contraception is used? Might you be pregnant now? How many children do you have? How many times have you been pregnant? Are you having any symptoms related to menopause? Do you take any form of hormone replacement? Is your sex life satisfying?
Neck	Any pain, swelling, or stiffness in the neck?	Male genitalia	Any urethral problems such as discharge, burning? Do you do testicular self-exam? Do you engage in sexual relations with men, women, or both? What method of contraception is used? Is your sex life satisfying?
Lymph nodes	Any swelling or painful lymph nodes in armpits, groin, neck?		
Breasts	Any lumps, pain, or discharge? Do you check your breasts regularly? When, if ever, was your last mammogram?	Extremities	Any leg pain or cramping, joint pain, or stiffness? Do your feet get cold easily? Do you have vein problems? Any back pain? Have you ever had a broken bone? A bone density scan?

Advanced Assessment 4.2   Functional Health Patterns: Questions to Elicit Data

Pattern	Sample Questions	Pattern	Sample Questions
Health perception	Do you have a regular health-care provider?	Cognitive/perceptual concept	Any hearing or vision problems? Any memory changes? How do you like to learn new things? Any pain or discomfort?
Health management	How often do you go to your health-care provider? What do you do to stay healthy?	Self-perception/ self-concept	How would you describe yourself? Do you feel good about yourself? Any changes in how you feel about your body? Do you get angry or down at times?
Nutrition/metabolic	What did you eat yesterday or on a typical day? What do you drink? How is your appetite? Any skin problems?	Role relationship self-perception/ self-concept	Who lives with you? Do you have friends? What kind of work do you do? Do you have other responsibilities?
Elimination	What are your bowel and bladder elimination patterns? Do you have unexpected loss of control?	Sexuality/ reproductive Role relationship	Any problems with your sexuality? Any changes? If sexually active, do you practice safe sex? Do you use birth control? What mode of birth control do you use?
Activity/exercise	How far can you walk before feeling tired? Do you have energy to do the things you want? Do you need any assistance with feeding, bathing, toileting, dressing, getting around (activities of daily living)? Do you need any help with cooking, shopping, or cleaning (instrumental activities of daily living)?	Coping/stress tolerance	How do you cope with stress? Any use of alcohol, drugs? Do you have someone to talk things over with?
Sleep/rest	How many hours do you sleep? Any trouble falling asleep or with early wakening? Do you feel rested?	Value/belief	What is most important to you in your life? Are you religious? Any values about life that health-care providers should know? Do you have a health-care proxy (medical power of attorney) or living will (advance directive)?

contain more than one diagnosis from any of the biological, psychosocial, or spiritual realms. It may also include health risks. Further data are available to help refine the hypothesis list by performing the physical examination and ordering diagnostic tests.

Focus on Data Collection: Physical Exam

The physical exam serves to clarify diagnostic hypotheses and to detect unanticipated problems of which the patient is unaware. In primary care, there is a wide range of ways of performing the physical exam. Textbooks of

physical assessment outline a general head-to-toe model that is useful for an initial visit with a full physical exam or a periodic reassessment. In most practices, an initial patient visit is scheduled for more time, and in coding schemes the visit may be reimbursed at a higher level because of its comprehensiveness. Students in nursing or medical school learn to perform the head-to-toe exam in an organized way. In actual practice, however, clinicians must learn to focus their physical assessment skills and make the physical exam appropriate to the patient's complaint and history. If the patient complains of headache, a review of head, eyes, ears, nose, and throat and a neurological examination are indicated, as well as a skin survey. For joint pain, a review of musculoskeletal tenderness, range of motion, and strength might be indicated. The body systems that are examined depend on the working hypothesis list that the clinician has generated. Examination skills need to be organized at a general screening level, with subroutines of examination techniques that can be adapted to specific findings and complaints. Positive or negative findings that serve to refine the hypothesis list must be noted and recorded in the documentation system that is in use. At times, a condition is in evolution, and the symptoms may not be clear when the patient comes for a visit. Nonetheless, the rich data reporting from that visit—even though the diagnosis is not clear—can serve to make the diagnosis more accurate later, when the condition evolves further. Full documentation serves to protect both patient and provider. The physical examination can also be a time to provide feedback and teaching about findings and about self-care. There is some evidence that thorough physical exams are becoming more rare in medicine. An overreliance on blood, radiological, and other tests to confirm diagnoses increases costs of care and reduces contact with the patient (Sanders, 2009). The ritual of the physical exam is evidence of person-to-person attention and may be perceived as the kind of professional caring expected in a health-care visit.

Ordering Diagnostic Tests

Diagnostic tests can be used to confirm or to rule out diagnostic hypotheses or as screening devices for conditions with subtle presentations that need to be picked up early, such as lead poisoning in children. Diagnostic tests vary in their usefulness based on their sensitivity, specificity, and predictive value. When considering or evaluating a test, consider that there are patient, test, and disease factors that affect the interpretation of the tests. The prevalence of a condition is the number of cases present in a given population at a particular point in time. The incidence of a condition reflects the total number of cases during a specified time period. For example, the number of cases of flu in a year (incidence) is greater than the number of people who have the flu on a given day (prevalence). Both incidence and prevalence rates are important considerations in making accurate

diagnoses. Laboratory tests and radiographic or other imaging can assist in screening for conditions and in making diagnoses. For chronic conditions, tests are used to monitor progress in managing the condition.

No test is perfect. In a given population, a positive test result is found for some people who have the condition and for some who do not. When a patient who does not have the condition has a positive reading on a test, it is called a "false positive." On the other hand, a negative test is found with people who do not have the condition and some who do. A negative test result that occurs when the patient does have the condition is referred to as a "false negative." The sensitivity of a test is greater when it has few false negatives. Sensitivity equals the number of true positives for a test divided by the number of tested individuals who truly have the disease. The specificity of a test is greater when it has few false positives. The specificity of a test equals the number of true negatives divided by the number of all tested individuals who do not have the disease. Table 4.4 represents the relationship between test results and actual conditions.

In clinical practice, the predictive value of a test is the important consideration. Given a positive test result, what is the likelihood that the patient actually has the condition? Positive predictive value equals true positives divided by all positives. Negative predictive value equals true negatives divided by all negatives. Predictive value is in part dependent on the prevalence of the condition. If a condition is highly likely, a positive test result is more likely to be accurate. If a condition is very unlikely, a positive test result needs to be questioned, perhaps with different tests.

When deciding whether to order a test, cost, convenience, sensitivity and specificity, and risk of missing a condition are considered. One can ask whether the test result would affect the potential treatment plan. If not, the test might not be necessary. It is not appropriate to order a test merely to increase the clinician's confidence and comfort. Appropriate screening for life-threatening or life-altering conditions must be considered. Clinicians can use the Clinical Preventive Services Guidelines or other research-based guidelines for deciding on screening tests for specific patients. Always consider the individual patient's situation. For example, the age for first mammogram has changed over the years based on research data and is dependent, in part, on a strong family history or other risk factors for breast cancer.

Table 4.4 Tests: Characteristics and Diseases			
Test Reading	Disease Present	Disease Absent	Total
Positive	True positive (TP) A	False positive (FP) B	All positives A + B
Negative	False negative (FN) C	True negative (TN) D	All negatives C + D
Totals	All diseased A + C	All healthy B + D	Grand Total

Source: Chase, SK. *Clinical judgment and communication in nurse practitioner practice.* FA Davis, Philadelphia, 2004. Used with permission.

Differential Diagnosis

A differential diagnosis list is the list of possible diagnoses, usually in priority order. When clinicians discuss a case, the list of differential diagnoses is usually considered. Supports for developing a rich differential diagnosis list include several guides. One approach suggests considering the problem from the "skin in." This means that if the patient complains of chest pain, the clinician can consider all the possible causes of chest pain, beginning at the skin, and visualize all the structures in the area that could possibly be affected. For example, chest pain at skin level could indicate early herpes zoster sensitivity and pain. Below the skin, the musculoskeletal system (including the rib cage) could be causing pain, from costochondritis or from muscle strain. The clinician can consider pain below the rib cage as a source of pain. Could the patient have pneumonia, pneumothorax, or pulmonary embolus? Next is the esophagus. Could the pain be from esophagitis, gastroesophageal reflux, or hiatal hernia? Next consider the pericardium as a possible source of pain, as with pericarditis. Finally, consider cardiac pain. This "skin in" approach keeps the student from jumping to early conclusions without considering a wide range of problems. It thus avoids the common diagnostic error of premature closure.

An evolving problem list can become quite long, even on an initial visit. The Patient's Voice 4.1 describes one approach to differential diagnosis. The Patient's Voice 4.2 illustrates how the diagnosis often involves more than medical problems.

The Patient's Voice 4.1
An Advanced Practice Nurse's Approach to Differential Diagnosis

An APRN describes her approach to a new patient.

My initial diagnosis at that time, just by speaking with him, without any labs and examining him physically, was this: His diabetes was in poor control. His hypertension was in poor control. He had some rhinitis, probably allergic, but he was not having a problem. He has known unequal pupils since he had surgery and had damage to the pupillary musculature, but it does not affect his vision; if you did not happen to know that, you might be very concerned about it, you know? It is real important to put that in the problem list. He had a TUR [transurethral resection] for BPH [benign prostatic hyperplasia]. He had a real bad pars plana with secondary hip pain, and he kept going to people with back pain, and nobody ever stood him up and looked at his feet. He also had seborrheic dermatitis. The guy is an Irishman with pale skin and washed-out blue eyes, and he never used sunscreen. He had lots of skin cancers. The doctor kept calling him back to cut out the skin cancers but never told him to use sunscreen.

For this patient, the APRN goes on to describe her approach to ordering diagnostic tests. Note that the

hypotheses precede the test consideration. She describes her initial treatment plan:

OK, first thing you need is your laboratory parameters to check the problems that you have just defined. I would do blood counts, chemistries, thyroid function, glycohemoglobin, urines, PSA [prostate-specific antigen]. The first time I see a patient, I always do the whole gamut. This guy also had had a bilateral total hip replacement, so I reviewed the subacute bacterial endocarditis prophylaxis because he had never been told about it. I started him on Prinivil, an ACE [angiotensin-converting enzyme] inhibitor because he has diabetes and had previously been on Hytrin, but it was not doing the trick, and it was not protecting his kidneys. I started him on Glucotrol. He had not been on anything other than Micronase, which he quit using because he really did not know how to use the stuff. I also talked to him about his seborrhea and sunscreen.

The APRN sees the wholeness of the patient's situation. This is a different approach than treating discrete problems as they come up. The APRN's description of her approach to this patient continues:

He had had previous health care, and he thought he was doing fine. He just had never had it all put together. As far as he was concerned, he happened to have some elevated blood pressure and some elevated blood glucose, but nobody had ever put it all together in terms of the effects on the whole body. He went to someone for his glucose, and he went to somebody for his blood pressure. The guy was not a train wreck, but he had a number of problems that had been overlooked until he saw me and somebody (me) made a list. For example, he had not had a recent eye exam. For any patients with diabetes, I make sure they get an eye exam every single year. And that is how I started. His wife is also a patient of mine—a great cook, which is a tragedy for a diabetic—and he, like most husbands, will eat what he is given. So she needed some education as to what is the proper thing to eat and when and how they could cheat.

The APRN is able to pull all of this patient's concerns and problems together in a way that honors his wholeness and his family dynamics. Her concern is for preventing future problems that are likely to develop, given his pattern of risk factors. Her method of collecting data and clustering it together to form a comprehensive picture of his life results in an effective, personal plan.

The differential diagnosis list should always include any conditions that are life-, organ-, or function-threatening. An APRN describing a different patient situation stated:

I always think in terms of the most dangerous or the most serious thing first—not necessarily the most catastrophic, but the most serious problem. If I know somebody has an AAA [abdominal aortic aneurysm] and he comes in with abdominal pain and it's sensitive, well, he probably has diverticulitis, but if I blow the diagnosis and go that way and it turns out that his aneurysm is dissecting, then he is dead. So I will treat his diverticulitis, but I will get the ab-dominal ultrasound right away. I consider the most urgent, deadly thing first. Cancer can be deadly, but it usually is not an emergency. It will kill you, but it is not going to kill you to-morrow. But an AAA can blow at any time. I had someone with an aneurysm blow in here once while I had the surgeon and the OR team waiting for him in the ER. We knew we had an aneurysm that was about to blow because I put my hand on his belly and it was throbbing and the patient was hy-potensive and he was sweating. He had come in to the hos-pital because he was ready to go on vacation and just wanted to check this out before he left. So, you think of the most life-threatening situation first.

The Patient's Voice 4.2
An Advanced Practice Nurse's View of Nursing Versus Medical Problems

One pediatric APRN described her interaction with an immigrant father who brought in a 3-year-old girl with a runny nose. The father was not disciplining the child, even though she was being difficult, because he had been reported to Human Services for hitting this child previously and for hitting a well baby 8 months of age.

I see myself making a dual diagnosis—a nursing diag-nosis as well as a medical diagnosis. If the father does not discipline his child at the appropriate time in an appro-priate way, that is a knowledge deficit. So I made a nurs-ing decision there, and I intervened on the basis of that nursing decision, but I also made a medical decision, in that the child had an upper respiratory infection and I prescribed what I thought to be the appropriate medica-tion for that. So, I see myself making nursing diagnoses as well as medical diagnoses and trying to somehow mesh these two to care for the family holistically because there is no way you can care for a child without caring for the family. That is my belief.

When asked if her full response was documented in the treatment plan, she responded:

Yeah, well, it sure does not fall under "upper respira-tory infection." In this case, I did not know when the fam-ily was going to apply for insurance, so I certainly did not want to put "behavior disorder" down. Instead, I put down under my diagnosis, "knowledge deficit, re: disci-pline." In my treatment plan, I noted that I discussed dis-cipline and that I gave the father 'time out' guidelines and how to reward good behavior. I also noted that the father is coming back to me in 2 weeks to report differences in his approach to discipline and how it worked out. Nobody ever leaves my office without knowing when he or she needs to come back, and I document when I tell them to come back in my treatment plan.

Developing a Management Plan

Once the problem list has been clarified, clinical judg-ment about how best to manage those problems is ad-dressed. Although APRNs bill for services in the medical

realm, they also operate in the nursing domain. One ex-pectation for APRN students is learning to "present the patient" to their preceptor in the clinical area. This skill involves taking all the data collected in history and phys-ical assessment, organizing the content, and presenting the major findings in a coherent way to the preceptor so that the preceptor can review with the student what the treatment options are so that when the preceptor sees the patient he or she can verify and clarify the data collection and move to treatment planning. Initially, students may need to use a template to ensure that they are organized as they begin this process. With experience, the organi-zation of patient data will become more obvious. This same skill of organizing patient data is useful when com-municating with consulting providers. They need a clear summary of the case for efficient consultation.

Selection of interventions for APRNs is broader than a consideration of prescription medications. The discus-sion in Chapter 1 of Engebretson's (1997) contribution is useful to consider here. In addition, Eisenhauer (1994) has argued that different levels of nursing interventions are useful when dealing with patient problems. At the most basic level, interventions deal with symptom relief, such as ice for acute muscle pain followed by heat appli-cation for strained muscles or a prescription for pain medication. At a higher level of complexity, interven-tions address functional patterns, such as stress and cop-ing. The provider could schedule a follow-up visit to determine if a stressful condition is being managed more successfully after a brief teaching or counseling session. At yet another level, an intervention could be concerned with life patterns, such as recommending a course of rehabilitation to help a patient to regain confidence in exercising after a cardiac event. Finally, at the highest level, interventions such as spiritual support could be chosen to help patients and their families cope with life processes such as a terminal condition. This typology of intervention is useful to consider when selecting an approach to a problem. If, for example, a patient has been unable to lose weight using simple diet instruction, a higher-order intervention such as counseling may be required to address the source of the problem at a deeper level.

Evidence-Based Practice

There is an emphasis in health care today to promote evidence-based practice (EBP). In a just society, patients have equal access to the most up-to-date treatment ap-proaches and are also able to make informed choices about their treatment. To justify a treatment approach, proponents of EBP argue that there must be evidence, either from clinical trials or from case studies, that the approach is likely to benefit the patient. Obviously, it is easier to demonstrate the benefit of a certain drug that has been tested on a large number of individuals than it is to demonstrate the effectiveness of individual coun-seling. Be on guard that your own practice is not limited to medicine based on clinical trials alone. This may require clinical research to demonstrate case studies of creative nursing intervention success. A research study that investigated how clinicians used guidelines in day-to-day practice showed that practitioners seldom referred directly to guidelines when planning care. They did, however, use internalized guidelines and could discuss what they were and how they were formed. Their own and colleagues' experience were also part of forming this knowledge in practice (Gabbay & LeMay, 2004). Guidelines for practice are available from government agencies (http://guidelines.gov) or from specialty/disease-related groups such as the American Heart Association. These guidelines can form the basis for protocol development and for peer evaluation.

Outcome Considerations

In many instances, the patient's and provider's chosen outcomes for an encounter are clear. The simple, acute health problem is to be resolved. The screening measures recommended for the person's age-group are ordered to rule out the presence of nascent disease. When dealing with more chronic problems or problems that provide the patient with what may be reduced quality of life, the APRN must be more sensitive to outcome determination.

Different settings prompt a different set of concerns. The Patient's Voice 4.3 presents an APRN's approach to outcome considerations.

The Patient's Voice 4.3

An Advanced Practice Nurse's Approach to Outcome Considerations

One gerontological APRN described doing an initial evaluation on an elderly client in a residential hospice situation.

Well, I think in terms of triage—comfort is the priority for me. Is there pain? I try to address that issue, and if the patient is anxious, I try to put that on the same level as psychic pain and physical pain. I try to give my patients as much information as they can tolerate—partly what the plan is, and what we are going to do to relieve their pain and try to make their living more comfortable. So then I work from there. What are some of the problems I see in my patients? Skin problems, incontinence, risk for falls, risk for aspiration—all those kinds of things.

One APRN was treating an 85-year-old patient who had suffered a CVA [cerebrovascular accident; stroke]—and was unable to communicate. The patient also had dysphagia, which meant that she needed a feeding tube. The APRN took time to ask a pertinent question: What would this patient want?

[This patient] would occasionally have bedsores, and sometimes she had a urinary tract infection and occasionally a rash from the urination [she was incontinent]. She also had frequent respiratory infections, and it appeared that she had a very poor quality of life. She could not express herself at all, and every few months, her PEG

*[percutaneous endoscopic gastrostomy] tube would have to be replaced, which happens with most patients. So after we had replaced about the fourth one, I called the family member, and I posed the question to her this way: "Would it be her wish to continue this way?" I did not ask the family member what she wanted. I asked, "What do you think would be **her** wish?" [emphasis added] This was the first time I had ever talked to this woman, and she acted as if no one had ever posed that question to her before. She said, "Well, I want the tube back in." And I said, "Well, I understand that, but what do you think would be her wish?" It was as if she had never thought about that before. And after she thought about the situation from that perspective, it was very easy for her to come to the answer that her relative's wish would be that her tube not be replaced and that she be allowed to die. She recognized that the patient's wish would not be at all to live like that. After she thought about it and talked it over with her family members, they agreed that the tube should not be replaced, and that is what happened. Without the feeding tube, the patient died in peace. She had a peaceful death.*

This APRN asked the question that made everyone consider the meaning of the experience from the patient's point of view. In this case, the outcome of the care was a peaceful death, an outcome that can be prized.

◼ DOCUMENTATION

Preparing concise, comprehensive, and meaningful documentation of one's thoughts and activities as a provider of primary care is a skill that takes time to develop. The purposes of documentation are to record the patient's report of symptoms, past medical history, lifestyle and family factors, positive and negative findings on physical exam, and the clinician's decisions and actions. An accurate record is essential to remind the clinician of findings and actions for the next follow-up visit. In a large practice, other providers will be seeing the patient and will need the benefit of the clinician's observations and actions during previous visits. The effectiveness of a treatment plan can be judged only if the plan has been adequately described. For example, if teaching about diet was provided at one visit but not recorded, the same teaching might be repeated at the next visit, to the frustration of the patient who was looking for more new information. This frustration might be misunderstood by the next provider as a lack of cooperation with the treatment plan. Finally, documentation can serve as protection for the provider or the practice in the rare case in which litigation is brought by the patient or family. In addition, third-party payers may be auditing the patient's record to determine whether the level of the visit that was billed was justified and whether the interventions billed were actually delivered. Additional details on billing and coding are provided in Chapter 22. In the student situation, the depth and comprehensiveness of documentation can assist the preceptor or faculty in determining the student's progress in learning judgment.

SOAP Format

General principles for documentation are commonly applied using the SOAP format—*Subjective, Objective, Assessment,* and *Plan*—of charting. If other systems of charting are used, the principles still apply.

Subjective

The subjective portion of the record includes all data from the patient's report: the HPI, past medical history, family history, social history, functional health patterns data, and review of systems. The clinician can include here, in an easily visible way, current medications, immunization status, allergies to foods or medications, past hospitalizations (if appropriate), and, for women, the last menstrual period and menstrual cycle information. Even when a woman is being treated for simple problems, her pregnancy status must be known before certain medications are prescribed. It is an error to confuse physical findings noticed during the exam with subjective data from the patient. If the patient's particular way of describing a problem seems important, use the patient's exact words and include quotes. This is not necessary if the description is simple and without nuance. Develop an outline form for your documentation that includes all essential data elements in a way that is retrievable. Writing in full sentences and paragraphs does not allow for easy retrieval of data by other providers. An outline template also serves as a memory tool for the new APRN. This template is useful in organizing patient presentation for the preceptor.

Objective

The objective section of the record includes all data obtained through objective means. This is not limited to numerical data. Begin the objective portion of the record with a brief description of the overall impression of the patient. Such phrases as "tired looking," "energetic," or "worried" can convey much of the patient impression that is useful in diagnostic reasoning. Include vital signs and pertinent findings from the physical exam, as well as laboratory data. Do not record diagnostic judgments in this section—think of this part of the record as "just the facts."

At first, students are unable to focus on which pieces of data are significant to a problem and tend to include every piece of data available. All data need not be recorded, but "pertinent negatives" need to be recorded. These include data that by being normal tend to rule out a possible diagnosis. Recording pertinent negatives helps to show that a diagnosis was considered and why it was ruled out. It does not take long, however, for both the subjective and objective sections to be recorded with reasonable skill, even for advanced beginner students.

When following patients over time, flow sheets can be useful for tracking data. For example, a flow sheet can show the effect of a change in medication management of hyperlipidemia or blood pressure or track a patient's weight over months or years.

Assessment

The assessment portion is an area of documentation in which much variability can be found. The assessment must include active problems that are being managed in this visit. It can also include chronic problems that may have an impact on the treatment plan. Many practices always include a health promotion line on the problem list to remind each clinician that the visit should reflect the preventive focus of that practice. For the list to serve both patient and practitioner well, a simple diagnostic label may not be enough. For example, if the patient has hypertension that is being managed by lifestyle change and medication, the effectiveness of control of the problem can be recorded in the assessment section. Assessment is ongoing in the management of health problems. For example, a patient's problem list might read as follows: (1) hypertension (HTN) stage 1, well controlled; (2) type 2 diabetes mellitus (DM), poorly controlled; (3) obesity, unchanged. This documentation directs evaluation and intervention adjustment much more clearly than a simple list of "HTN, DM, obesity." Many practices maintain an active problem list near the front of the patient record or in a part of the electronic record. This is particularly useful when dealing with chronic conditions and is recommended. The clinician can initiate such a tool in any practice, even if a blank progress note sheet is filed at the beginning of that section of the patient's record.

When reviewing the assessment part of the record, students can evaluate their own thinking by asking themselves if all data that were used to justify the naming of a problem are included in the subjective and objective section of the note. Further, one can ask whether all data were accounted for in the assessment section. In some cases, a clear problem cannot be identified. Abdominal pain that does not fit a clear diagnostic pattern can be reported in the problem list by simply naming the complaint. The clinician can reflect diagnostic hypotheses by writing "abdominal pain, rule out (R/O) irritable bowel syndrome." Or "cough, viral bronchitis vs. allergy." Students are often reluctant to admit that they cannot name the problem. It is a mistake, however, to name a problem in error, simply to have a problem on the list. The patient will not be well served if the record fails to reveal competing diagnostic hypotheses. In primary care, uncertainty is reasonable and expected. Even if the problem is not completely specified, the problem list is the basis for the intervention schedule in the treatment plan.

Plan

The plan for treatment is most effective if it is described in detail, including specific directions for each intervention. Three general sections are included in planning: First, any diagnostic testing that is to be conducted should be listed. The results of these diagnostic tests will help to clarify the assessment but, of course, are not yet available to the provider. Second, educational approaches are to be laid out. Every visit is a teaching opportunity. Patient education might include specifics of the problems being managed, such as symptom control for upper respiratory infections, medication teaching, diet and activity recommendations, and risk reduction, such as smoking cessation information or a discussion of seat belt usage. The documentation of the plan includes details regarding any therapeutic plan that is to be carried out—including prescriptions, various therapies, counseling, activity promotion or restriction, dietary changes, or any of the therapeutics discussed earlier. When recording prescriptions, be sure to include all the data that were written on the prescription list, including number or volume of doses to be dispensed and number of refills allowed. This is important because patients may call for refills before they are due, and if a different provider takes the call, he or she may have an unclear idea of how the patient's condition had been managed. This is especially important when prescribing drugs that are prone to abuse.

Finally, the treatment plan is not complete without clear plans for follow-up. When will the patient be seen again, and under what circumstances is the patient instructed to call back? For example, when treating a viral infection, remind the patient to call back if not better in 2 days or if fever develops. By documenting your instructions for follow-up, you allow other providers to manage the patient's care better if the patient calls in when you are not available.

Plans are most effective when they include a sense of the goal of treatment. If the condition is simple and self-limiting, the goal of treatment may be obvious and need not be stated. For chronic or complex problems, however, the short- and long-term goals of therapy need to be discussed and recorded. By engaging the patient in this discussion, the choices that the patient makes in altering lifestyle and in following a treatment plan may be clearer. For example, the patient with hypertension, diabetes, and obesity might have as a goal to lose 4 pounds in a month. The planned intervention to help the patient achieve this goal might be walking three times a week and one less restaurant meal a week. The feedback on the short-term goal at the next visit can help to keep the patient motivated to sustain lifelong change.

Finally, when reviewing the documentation for personal or peer evaluation, the clinician must consider whether the note conveys the scope and tone of the visit. Does it reflect the type of visit that occurred? If the patient were to ask to see the record, would the information be clear? The APRN should write the note in such a way that the patient could agree with what has been stated. Discussions of sensitive issues such as family

problems can be left in general terms. This is a useful approach when one considers that others, such as third-party payers or lawyers, might have access to the record in the future. If the provider and the patient disagree on a treatment plan—for example, on the use of medications—the record can reflect the disagreement in nonjudgmental terms, such as "Patient requested prescription for muscle relaxants, which was discussed as being unlikely to benefit the shoulder pain described." This kind of note can assist in determining patterns of behavior or documenting difficulties over time.

Documentation is an opportunity for clinicians at all levels to review the level of their thought. In general, APRNs document visits more completely and less often have charts refused for payment by third-party payers than other clinicians do. It is best to develop a system for maintaining current, accurate records. Saving up quick scratches of notes and writing all formal patient notes at the end of a busy day is not the recommended approach. Dictation and computer systems allow for complete record-keeping and help to keep time spent on the task more manageable.

Documentation systems are usually invented by each practice. If you find that elements of your care are invisible in the record because of restrictive coding or limited space, plan a meeting with the head of the practice or clinic to discuss what you feel is missing in the record. Most systems in which APRNs work are dominated by the medical model. APRNs can ensure that contributions from a nursing perspective are not invisible by claiming credit and billing for the care actually provided. They should not agree to a system of billing "incident to" the physician, except where truly warranted. Unless APRNs "own" their practice through their own, independent billing for services, nursing-based care is lost and outcomes related to APRN practice are not captured. APRNs educated at the Doctor of Nursing Practice level should have the opportunity to shape the practice environment that they manage or share with other providers (Flanagan et al, 2009).

■ REDUCTION OF MEDICAL ERROR

The reduction of medical error and the support of patient safety are important in the health-care arena. The Institute of Medicine has called for attention to the processes and systems of care in order to reduce error and enhance safety (Kohn et al, 2000). A study of reported medical error in primary care showed that the largest number of errors was considered administrative, such as information filed in the wrong place or at the wrong time, charts not being available at the time of the visit, and lack of documentation. Errors also occurred in obtaining or processing a laboratory specimen. Some errors were reportedly due to lack of clinical knowledge or skills, such as wrong or missed diagnosis or wrong treatment choices (Dovey et al, 2005). Attention to decision making and follow-through is important to all primary-care providers. APRNs can contribute to shaping the practice in their setting by, for example, developing systems to ensure that important laboratory results are addressed in a timely manner. This is all part of quality-oriented guidelines developed for the patient-centered medical homes (PCMHs) discussed in Chapter 1. These are the health-care systems of the future, and they are still emerging. APRNs have an opportunity and an obligation to participate in and influence that emergence with their own unique knowledge base, to translate their knowledge into systems that support patient engagement.

■ EMERGING TECHNOLOGIES

The use of electronic media in all facets of the health-care process is a reality. Patients have access to information about health promotion and about specific health-care concerns from the Internet; they can also communicate with health-care providers through e-mail or Web sites. Health records are maintained electronically and made accessible to providers throughout a care delivery system. One such system, the Veterans Administration in the United States, has been a leader in the use of electronic medical records. In addition, some practices send a weekly e-mail to their patients with health-related information. This can be good for marketing as well as for providing information.

Health care providers can participate in federal incentive programs through the Affordable Care Act by adopting electronic health records and demonstrating "meaningful use" of clinical data. To participate, providers must meet specific objectives in their charting, which include lists of patient drugs, computerized order entry, maintaining an active allergy list and an active problem list, and implementing decision support systems. Nurse practitioners, along with physicians, are eligible for incentive payments if a certain percentage of their patient load is in the Medicare or Medicaid system and if objectives are met.

Another new technology, telemedicine, has the capacity to open access to health care for people at remote sites. Health insurance companies are beginning to reimburse practices for telemedicine services, which will likely increase its availability (Reed, 2005). And soon, lack of access to a computer may not be a barrier to participating in telemedicine. Many business leaders predict that the next phase of medical innovation will be the use of smartphones and a variety of mobile apps to monitor

our own health and transmit the data to our health-care providers on a regular basis or in advance of an office visit (Topol, 2012). Some speculate that it is only a matter of time until we have purchasable "body scanners" to transmit a wide variety of physical exam data to a distant location where a team of health-care providers is located. Just as in the debate over online education, some speculate that telemedicine can never achieve the same benefits as "hands-on" medical care; others feel that with adept use of technology, in some instances, clinician–patient communication may be enhanced. This debate will dominate future conversation about the value of "human touch" and the benefits of the remote practice of the APRN.

■ ETHICS

Every clinical judgment is an ethical judgment. Clinical judgment begins with respect for persons and supports each individual's autonomy. Some decisions call for balancing such principles as beneficence against autonomy, for example, as when a patient chooses not to follow a treatment plan. Truth telling by the clinician can do much to establish trust and to develop a plan the patient can accept. Ethical judgments are involved as well in the allocation of scarce resources, the most prominent for APRNs being their own time. If one patient constantly requires more time than is allotted, other patients are made to wait or are given less time for their visits. Being a patient advocate means ascertaining that the health-care system provides for each patient everything that is reasonable to which the patient is entitled; such advocacy is a role of the APRN. A survey of nurse practitioners in one mid-Atlantic state showed that 61% agreed that they sometimes weighed the needs of the patient against the interests of the managed care organization (Ulrich et al, 2003). Fidelity to the patient until the problem has been solved or resolved is another aspect of APRN practice that is based on ethical principles. One could make the case that APRNs have an ethical and professional responsibility to help design and implement systems to collaborate in the establishment of PCMHs that truly reflect the intent of that model, that "hear" the voice of the patient.

The privilege of being an APRN and entering as a partner into patients' lives to support their health and wholeness requires true human presence, clear clinical judgment, and a commitment to do one's best. The *Circle of Caring* includes patient and nurse together as they enter a relationship that has the potential to enhance the humanity of both.

References

Benner, PE, et al. *Expertise in nursing practice: Caring clinical judgment and ethics.* Springer, New York, 1996.

Charlton, CR, et al. Nurse practitioners' communication styles and their impact on patient outcomes: An integrated literature review. *J Am Acad Nurs Pract* 20:382–388, 2008.

Chase, SK. *Clinical judgment and communication in nurse practitioner practice.* FA Davis, Philadelphia, 2004.

Dovey, SM, et al. A preliminary taxonomy of medical errors in family practice. *Qual Safe Health Care* 11:233, 2005.

Eisenhauer, LA. A typology of nursing therapeutics. *Image J Nurs Schol* 26:261, 1994.

Elliott, N. "Mutual intacting": A grounded theory study of clinical judgment practice issues. *J Adv Nurs* 66:2711–2721, 2010.

Engebretson, J. A multiparadigm approach to nursing. *Adv Nurs Sci* 20:21, 1997.

Flanagan, ME, et al. The effect of provider- and workflow-focused strategies for guideline implementation on provider acceptance. *Implement Sci* 4:71, 2009.

Gabbay, J, and LeMay, A. Evidence based guidelines or collectively constructed "mindlines?" Ethnographic study of knowledge management in primary care. *Br Med J* 329(7473):1013, 2004.

Johnson, R. Nurse practitioner–patient discourse: Uncovering the voice of nursing in primary care practice. *Schol Inquiry Nurs Pract* 7:143, 1993.

Kohn, LT, et al (Eds.): *To err is human: Building a safer health system.* National Academy Press, Washington, DC, 2000.

Lee, NJ, et al. The effect of a mobile clinical decision support system on the diagnosis of obesity and overweight in acute and primary care encounters. *Adv Nurs Sci* 32:211–221, 2009.

Michaels, C, et al. Saying "no" to professional recommendations: Client values, beliefs, and evidence-based practice. *J Am Acad Nurse Pract* 20:585–589, 2008.

Reed, K. Telemedicine: Benefits to advanced practice nursing and the communities they serve. *J Am Acad Nurse Pract* 17:176, 2005.

Roblin, DW, et al. Patient satisfaction with primary care: Does type of practitioner matter? *Med Care* 42:579, 2004.

Rubin, RH. *Primary care.* WB Saunders, Philadelphia, 1995.

Sanders, L. *Every patient tells a story.* Broadway Books, New York, 2009.

Sangster-Gormley, E, and Frisch, N. Articulating new outcomes of nurse practitioner practice. *J Am Acad Nurs Pract* 25:653–658, 2013.

SmithBattle, L. Pregnant with possibilities: Drawing on hermeneutic thought to reframe home-visiting programs for young mothers. *Nurs Inq* 16:191–200, 2009.

Thompson, C, and Yang, H. Nurses' decisions, irreducible uncertainty and maximizing nurses' contribution to patient safety. *Healthc Q* 12(Spec No Patient):e178–e185, 2009.

Topol, E. *The creative destruction of medicine: How the digital revolution will create better health care.* Basic Books, New York, 2012.

Ulrich, CM, et al. Ethical conflict associated with managed care: Views of nurse practitioners. *Nurs Res* 52:168, 2003.

Bibliography

American Medical Association Physician International Classification of Diseases–9. Clinical modification. AMA, Chicago, 2005.

Benner, P. *From novice to expert: Excellence and power in clinical nursing practice.* Addison-Wesley, Menlo Park, CA, 1984.

Billings, JA, and Stoeckle, JD. *The clinical encounter: A guide to the medical interview and case presentation,* ed 2. Mosby, St. Louis, 1999.

Brykczynski, KA. An interpretive study describing the clinical judgment of nurse practitioners. *Schol Inquiry Nurs Pract* 3(2):75, 1989.

Davis, S, et al. Teaching strategies used by expert nurse practitioner preceptors: A qualitative study. *J Am Acad Nurse Pract* 5:27, 1993.

Dunphy, LM, and Winland-Brown, JE. The *Circle of Caring:* A transformative model of advanced practice nursing. *Clin Excell Nurs Pract* 2:241, 1998.

Elstein, A, et al. *Medical problem solving.* Harvard University Press, Cambridge, MA, 1979.

Gordon, M, et al. Clinical judgment: An integrated model. *Adv Nurs Sci* 16(4):55, 1994.

Lewis, PH, and Brykczynski, KA. Practical knowledge and competencies of the healing role of the nurse practitioner. *J Am Acad Nurse Pract* 6:207, 1994.

North American Nursing Diagnosis Association. *NANDA nursing diagnoses: Definitions and classification,* 1997–1998. NANDA, Philadelphia, 1996.

Radwin, LE. Research on diagnostic reasoning in nursing. *Nurs Diag* 1(2):70, 1990.

Rogers, JC, and Biggs, WS. Problem solving in family medicine. In Rakel, R (Ed.): *Essentials of family practice.* WB Saunders, Philadelphia, 1999.

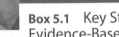

Evidence-Based Practice

Chapter 5

Angela K. Golden, DNP, APRN, FNP-C, FAANP

In health care, evidence originates from research findings used to guide clinical practice, such as decisions regarding which diagnostic tests or treatment approaches are worthwhile. Research findings are used to compile evidence for decision making in practice. Generally, evidence-based practice (EBP) refers to using research findings from multiple studies that are convincing enough to the majority of a community of scientists and providers to recommend that the findings be used for clinical decision making. EBP also involves inclusion of patient and practitioner preferences and patient values in the clinical decision-making process.

The key steps involved in determining EBP are summarized in Box 5.1. Providers during a busy clinical day will unlikely be able to go through the process described; however, they must understand the full process in order to use any abbreviated form of it. Providers must learn to compose clinical questions and to find the best evidence at the point of care quickly.

Although advanced practice registered nurses (APRNs) function primarily from a nursing framework, they also incorporate aspects of the medical model into their practice. Thus, an understanding of the major research methods used in both disciplines and the ability to apply research findings to clinical practice situations are essential. This chapter focuses on EBP across disciplines and the predominant methods used to establish evidence for practice across disciplines.

STRATEGY FOR POINT-OF-CARE EVIDENCE-BASED PRACTICE

This chapter provides specific guidelines for utilizing nursing research, evaluating evidence, and applying it to practice. But every provider needs a go-to strategy to use at the time of patient care. This strategy is based on knowledge of research and evaluation and is presented here to encourage the provider to read carefully the rest of this chapter and then apply all this information to later chapters. The point-of-care strategy is to (1) ask a clinical question, (2) have evidence resources readily available, (3) complete the search using those resources, (4) examine the results of the search, and finally (5) apply the findings to the individual patient—remembering always, as Strauss et al (2011) point out, "evidence does not make decisions." See Box 5.2 for a framework for point-of-care search strategy for EBP.

THE AIMS OF NURSING RESEARCH FOR CLINICAL APPLICATION

There are differences in perspective between nursing and biomedicine; however, the research conducted in each field has a common thread: the systematic pursuit of knowledge to answer questions of importance in the respective professions. Nursing as a discipline is concerned with the human response to health and illness; the use of a few methods to study the complexities of being human is insufficient. Because nursing focuses on the whole person, many of the questions that inform our practice are not easily answered using highly controlled, experimental methods. There is a consensus within the nursing discipline to develop not only the scientific basis of nursing through conducting research but also to develop the understanding and utilization of research by nurses at all levels of practice.

The important question to be asked when using research for evidence-based practice is "What findings constitute evidence?" Perhaps the most useful way of addressing this question is with another: "How will the

---

Box 5.1 Key Steps in Implementing Evidence-Based Practice

1. Ask the burning clinical question.
2. Collect the most relevant and best evidence from a review of the literature including published literature reviews, meta-analyses, and clinical practice guidelines.
3. Critically evaluate the evidence.
4. Integrate the best evidence with personal clinical expertise and values, as well as patient preferences, when making a practice decision or change.
5. Evaluate the change in outcomes after implementing into practice.
6. Disseminate findings.

Source: Adapted from Melnyk, BM, and Fineout-Overholt, E. *Evidence-based practice in nursing and healthcare: A guide to best practice*, ed 2. Lippincott, Philadelphia, 2010, Box 1.2, p 11.

Box 5.2   A Framework for Point-of-Care Search Strategy

1. Ask the question.
2. Select your evidence resource. Here is a list. Select two or three that will be the initial sources for your practice:
   - National Guideline Clearinghouse: www.guideline.gov
   - Cochrane Collaboration: www.cochrane.org
   - Essential Evidence Plus (formerly known as Info poems): www.essentialevidenceplus.com
   - Up to date: www.uptodate.com/home/index.html
   - DynaMed: https://dynamed.ebscohost.com
   - Smart phone or tablet options:
     - Skyscape constellation: www.skyscape.com/estore/ProductDetail.aspx?ProductId=1180
     - Pepid primary care: www.pepid.com
3. Search.
4. Examine the evidence found in your search. Think about the level of evidence the search provided (meta-analysis, systematic reviews).
5. Apply the evidence to **your** patient.

Case scenario 1: A 72-year-old man is in the office for recent onset and worsening difficulty breathing. Pulse oximetry reading was 84 (sea level) and he is complaining of difficulty completing ADLs due to the SOB even while at rest. His wife states that he is more lethargic, and this is confirmed on examination. Examination also finds peripheral cyanosis and nonpitting pedal edema that the patient did not have on his last office visit.

1. The question: What are the criteria for admission for COPD exacerbation?
2. Selected search places: National Guideline Clearinghouse (retrieved Jul 7, 2013: www.guideline.gov/index.aspx)
3. Search: National Guideline Clearinghouse. Retrieved from www.guideline.gov/content.aspx?id=43794&search=copd

Examine the evidence: This guideline lists the following that are indications for hospital admission: Marked increase in intensity of symptoms, such as sudden development of resting dyspnea; severe underlying COPD; onset of new physical signs (e.g., cyanosis, peripheral edema); failure of exacerbation to respond to initial medical management; presence of serious comorbidities; frequent exacerbations; older age; insufficient home support.

4. Explain to the patient the results found and discuss his preferences: 72-year-old man states he is willing to go to the hospital. Call for ALS transport.

Case scenario 2: A 3-year-old child is diagnosed in the clinic with AOM, mildly ill appearing, axillary temperature of 100.6°F. Child has no known allergy to medication and is otherwise a healthy 3-year-old. Child is in day care during the day at a camp; parents are migrant workers.

1. The question: What is the recommended antibiotic for AOM in a 3-year-old?
2. Selected search places: DynaMed
3. Search: Information found
4. Examine the evidence: Evidence is as follows: for children >24 months old to provide a wait-and-see approach if non-severe illness, mild otalgia, temperature less than 102.2°F (child is not severely ill and has a temperature less than 102.2°F), and follow-up can be ensured to start antibiotics if symptoms persist or worsen (this child's parents are about to move on to the next migrant camp with unknown available health care). So in the experience of the NP working in this migrant camp, the wait-and-see approach is probably not appropriate. The recommended antibiotic is amoxicillin 80–90 mg/kg per day.
5. Explain to the patient (family) the results found and discuss the family preferences. The mother states that the child had amoxicillin for one other ear infection and had pretty bad diarrhea, and she is asking if another antibiotic could be used instead because it is often difficult to have bathroom facilities while traveling to new camps. She also wonders if there is a medication that can be given just once or twice a day, because she is in the fields often very long days. With this mother's request in mind, the NP has in stock azithromycin suspension and utilizes that for this family.

Source: Retrieved July 7, 2013, from http://web.ebscohost.com/dynamed/detail?vid=3&sid=e75e6aaa-2e34-4a20-bb26-d66600e7e162%40sessionmgr4&hid=12&bdata=JnNpdGU9ZHluYW1lZC1MSVZFJnNjb3BlPXNpdGU%3d#db=dme&AN=116345&anchor=Immediate-vs—delayed-antibiotics
ADLs: activities of daily living; ALS: advanced life support; AOM: acute otitis media; COPD: chronic obstructive pulmonary disease; NP: nurse practitioner; SOB: shortness of breath.

findings be used?" This approach assumes that it is better to answer the question with the method that fits best rather than applying a few select methods to all questions. If the clinical situation requires a better understanding of what the experience of emergent cardiac catheterization is for postmenopausal women with acute myocardial ischemia, providers need to look for the form of evidence (or findings) that best suits the situation. This evidence will not be found in the results of randomized clinical trials; it will be found in studies specifically designed for understanding human experiences of health in a personal and meaningful way (such as phenomenological studies or those using grounded theory).

■ APPLYING RESEARCH-BASED EVIDENCE TO CLINICAL PRACTICE

Informed Practice?

Wide variation in practice patterns within and across provider type, specialty practice, and geographic region has been a major impetus for establishing both federal and organization-specific guidelines. Studies of decision-making processes have revealed great variation between practitioners in their approach to diagnosing and treating the same conditions. Many of these studies have demonstrated that providers who observe the same clinical situation will disagree on the assessment findings with each other, and that there is great variation in the management even when evidence-based guidelines exist.

This realization led to a search for a wider consensus on how to diagnose and treat a number of common health conditions that occurred on both national and local levels in the form of clinical practice guidelines, practice policies, and recommendations. Although some providers perceive these attempts to standardize aspects of clinical practice as stripping them of their decision making, the intent is to improve the provider's ability to make better decisions that lead to better, more reliable outcomes for patients.

Practice Standards and Guidelines

Although the terms are often used interchangeably, clinical practice standards and practice guidelines tend to originate from distinct processes, and the purpose of each is somewhat different. Standards relate to a framework for practice. Guidelines focus more on individual patient-care decisions.

Practice Standards

Unlike guidelines, *practice standards* are inflexible and are intended to be used under all circumstances. Practice standards define correct practice rather than a framework that can be tailored to fit different contexts. The American Nurses Association (ANA) has issued a definition of practice standards for nurses, which includes broad requirements for nursing practice in any setting and at any level of practice. As defined by ANA (2013), practice standards are designed to provide guidance to nurses on which to judge their practice. Two types of standards are delineated by the ANA: standards of care for clinical practice and standards of professional performance. Although considered requirements of professional practice, the ANA standards can be broadly interpreted. With respect to EBP, one obligation for nurses is to utilize research findings in practice, which may indirectly refer to the use of clinical guidelines, depending on the methods used to develop the guidelines. The American Association of Nurse Practitioners establishes the standards of practice for nurse practitioners. The standards encompass many aspects of practice, including qualifications, process of care, care priorities, and research as a basis for practice.

Practice Guidelines

Guidelines are not cookbooks taking the decision making away from providers; instead, they allow for flexibility when making individual patient-care decisions. Guidelines are intended to provide a reference point and general direction for decision making and are not to be interpreted as rigid criteria that must be followed regardless of the context in which they are being used. Nonetheless, guidelines should be followed in the majority of cases, unless there is a clear rationale for deviating from them to serve the particular needs of individuals. Tailoring care to the needs of a particular patient is a cornerstone of EBP. The usefulness of applying guidelines in clinical decision making has become increasingly recognized over the past decade and is now an expectation in the delivery of health care.

Processes Used to Design Guidelines

Just as a provider's practice is determined by current guidelines, the quality of the guidelines themselves is determined by the processes used to create them. In general, there are two approaches used to develop such guidelines: the traditional approach (also referred to as global subjective judgment) and an evidence-based approach.

The traditional approach is based on the premise that "common" practice is "correct" practice, despite the scientific evidence available either to support or refute the outcomes of such practice. Under this approach, being common is sufficient evidence that the practice is appropriate. This approach may have been useful in the past, when practice decisions were less complicated and fewer diagnostic tests or interventions were available. Today, with the complexities involved in clinical decision making, research-based evidence is required. Although elements of the traditional approach remain, the majority of guidelines are now developed from available scientific evidence.

The Agency for Health Care Policy and Research was instrumental in leading the way toward EBP, improving outcomes, and publishing national guidelines on a variety of health-care problems, such as smoking cessation, early detection and treatment of Alzheimer's disease, and caring for HIV-infected patients. The Healthcare Research and Quality Act of 1999 reauthorized this agency and renamed it the Agency for Healthcare Research and Quality (AHRQ). The mission of the AHRQ is to improve the quality, safety, efficiency, and effectiveness of health care for all Americans.

AHRQ clinical practice guidelines are being used not only as references for health-care providers but also as the framework for insurance utilization review, quality assurance, and reimbursement. In addition, adherence or nonadherence to established guidelines (such as those published by the AHRQ) has played an increasing role in influencing medical malpractice litigation outcomes.

The implementation of AHRQ guidelines in clinical practice has not been without significant challenges. Originally, the AHRQ believed that providers would modify their practices to improve care if they were provided with clinically credible and useful information and that practitioner involvement in developing the guidelines would facilitate the use of guidelines in practice. Neither of these assumptions proved accurate: Studies indicated wide variation between a practitioner's knowledge of the recommended management of a particular health problem based on the guidelines and the practitioner's actions. With further studies, a number of barriers to implementing guidelines in practice have been identified, and the AHRQ's role in supporting EBP has been redefined to include keeping relevant information in the public domain; serving as an impartial, neutral broker of the information; encouraging multidisciplinary input in all projects; advocating

for patients' perspectives and needs; and protecting special populations.

Implementing Guidelines: AHRQ Program to Address Barriers

Structurally, the AHRQ's role includes promoting initiatives focused on developing effective methods of implementing guidelines and analyzing the outcomes of care when clinical guidelines are widely disseminated and used. There are three parts to the initiatives. Evidence-based practice centers (EPCs) constitute the first part and involve a private–public partnership between the AHRQ and a variety of health-care organizations to produce evidence reports and technology assessments on several priority health-care topics. Topics to be the focus for EPC assessments are nominated by providers or others in the health-care industry and are chosen based on the selection criteria provided in Box 5.3. Final evidence reports are intended for use in practice guidelines, quality improvement programs, and the formation of policy at the state or federal level.

The second part of the AHRQ's initiative is the development of the online National Guideline Clearinghouse (NGC). The creation of the clearinghouse is a result of a private–public partnership among AHRQ, the American Association of Health Plans, and the American Medical Association. It is an electronic repository for clinical practice guidelines and provides widespread access to a number of guidelines from various professional groups. A list of the guidelines can be found at www.guidelines.gov. Box 5.4 lists examples of organizations that have supported/published EBP guidelines. Guidelines published in the NGC are required to meet established AHRQ criteria and can be accessed through

---

Box 5.3   Criteria for Inclusion of Clinical Practice Guidelines in National Guideline Clearinghouse

A clinical practice guideline must meet all of the following criteria to be included in the NGC:

1. The clinical practice guideline contains systematically developed statements that include recommendations, strategies, or information that assists physicians and/or other health-care practitioners and patients make decisions about appropriate health care for specific clinical circumstances.
2. The clinical practice guideline was produced under the auspices of medical specialty associations; relevant professional societies, public or private organizations, government agencies at the federal, state, or local level; or health-care organizations or plans. A clinical practice guideline developed and issued by an individual not officially sponsored or supported by one of the above types of organizations does not meet the inclusion criteria for NGC.
3. Corroborating documentation can be produced and verified that a systematic literature search and review of existing scientific evidence published in peer-reviewed journals was performed during the guideline development. A guideline is not excluded from NGC if corroborating documentation can be produced and verified detailing specific gaps in scientific evidence for some of the guideline's recommendations.
4. The full text guideline is available on request in print or electronic format (for free or for a fee) in the English language. The guideline is current and the most recent version produced. Documented evidence can be produced or verified that the guideline was developed, reviewed, or revised within the last 5 years.

Box 5.4   Examples of Clinical Practice Guidelines/Evidence-Based Guidelines Developed/ Published by Organizations and Agencies

Alzheimer's Association
Guideline for Alzheimer's disease management.
www.alz.org

American Academy of Allergy, Asthma and Immunology
Allergen immunotherapy: a practice parameter second update.
www.aaaai.org

American College of Physicians
Guidelines follow a rigorous development process and are based on the highest-quality scientific evidence.
www.acponline.org/clinical_information/guidelines

Faculty of Sexual and Reproductive Healthcare
Contraception for women aged over 40 years.
www.fsrh.org

Society for Acupuncture Research
Acupuncture evidence-based treatment guidelines.
www.acupunctureresearch.org

Global Initiative for Asthma
Global strategy for asthma management and prevention.
http://ginasthma.org

National Association of Pediatric Nurse Practitioners
Identifying and preventing overweight in childhood. Clinical practice guideline.
www.napnap.org

National Health Care for the Homeless Council, Inc.
Adapting your practice: general recommendations for the care of homeless patients.
www.nhchc.org

World Health Organization
WHO recommendations for the prevention of postpartum hemorrhage.
www.who.int/reproductivehealth/publications/maternal_perinatal_health/9789241548502/en

the Internet. Consistent reference to these guidelines has been used throughout this text.

A final aspect of the AHRQ's initiative involves product research and evaluation. This includes an array of research and evaluation activities aimed at the development of evidence for use in guidelines, implementation strategies, and the quality of practice when clinical practice guidelines are used (e.g., outcome-based research).

These initiatives reflect the new role the AHRQ has with respect to supporting EBP and are meant to improve the scientific basis of guidelines, decrease duplication of efforts, distribute evidence on a national level, enhance uniformity, and reinforce public and private partnerships within the health-care sector.

Development of Evidence-Based Practice Guidelines

The following are essential components of guideline development: (1) identification/clarification of the topic, (2) establishment of an expert panel, (3) a systematic review of the literature, (4) development of evidence-based tables, (5) writing a draft of recommendations based on

the evidence, (6) external review of the recommendations, and (7) final acceptance of the revised recommendations by the panel. Panel members chosen to develop guidelines will depend on the focus of the guidelines and may include physicians, nurse practitioners, clinical nurse specialists, ethicists, pharmacists, therapists, and health-care consumers.

A crucial aspect of guideline development is the review of the literature and rating of the available evidence. An adaptation of one of the most common methods of rating evidence is listed in Box 5.5.

An essential aspect in understanding the development and appropriate use of guidelines is to understand the levels of the evidence.

Research Designs for Level I Evidence: Systematic Review or Meta-analysis of Randomized Clinical Trials

Systematic reviews are considered the highest level of evidence on which to base a change in practice. Systematic reviews are also called meta-analyses. The systematic review searches for all *randomized clinical trial* (RCT)

> **Box 5.5** Quality of Evidence
>
> I. Evidence from a systematic review or meta-analysis of all relevant randomized clinical trials (RCTs), or evidence-based clinical practice guidelines based on systematic reviews of RCTs
> II. Evidence obtained from at least one well-designed RCT
> III. Evidence obtained from well-designed controlled trials without randomization
> IV. Evidence from well-designed case-control and cohort studies
> V. Evidence from systematic reviews of descriptive and qualitative studies
> VI. Evidence from a single descriptive or qualitative study
> VII. Evidence from the opinion of authorities and/or reports of expert committees

Source: Melnyk, BM, and Fineout-Overholt, E. *Evidence-based practice in nursing and healthcare: A guide to best practice.* Lippincott, Philadelphia, 2005.

---

studies that address a similar clinical question. A review of the literature allows for a compilation of all the studies to give strength to outcomes. This review is a rigorous approach and provides a high level of evidence due to the minimization of bias. The Cochrane Library has an extensive compilation of systematic reviews.

Research Designs for Level II Evidence: Single Well-Designed Randomized Clinical Trials

RCTs are increasingly considered the most respected method for establishing the cause of disease or the efficacy of a treatment/intervention. For example, the Food and Drug Administration requires evidence of a drug's efficacy from two independently conducted randomized trials before approving the drug's use in the United States. The National Institutes of Health (NIH) are increasingly funding RCTs, and agencies or organizations developing clinical guidelines now consider the evidence from RCTs to supersede findings from case-control or cohort studies.

The strength of RCTs to establish cause or efficacy lies in the ability of this design to maintain a high degree of control within experimental conditions. If there are different effects between the groups (e.g., blood pressure, the development of pressure ulcers, the prevention of pregnancy), the differences can generally be attributed to the intervention, exposure, or treatment rather than "extraneous" factors. Moreover, the random assignment of subjects into the treatment or control group allows for a high degree of confidence in making causal inferences about the effects of an exposure, intervention, or treatment.

RCTs also frequently employ the use of double-blinding to further strengthen support for identifying a cause-and-effect relationship. When RCTs are double-blind, neither the principal investigators nor the participants know who is in the control or experimental group until either significant differences are noted in a (blind) analysis of the data or the study is complete. The purpose of double-blinding is to eliminate the potential for participants in the experimental or control groups to treat themselves differently or to be treated differently by investigators.

Research Designs for Level III Evidence: Well-Designed Controlled Trials Without Randomization

Quasi-experimental research designs evaluate the effectiveness of an intervention/treatment, but subjects are not randomly assigned to either the treatment or control group. In these designs, many of the other same methods to ascertain the internal validity of the study, such as control of extraneous variables and standardization of treatment, instituted in RCTs are implemented.

Research Designs for Level IV Evidence: Well-Designed Case-Control or Cohort Studies

These types of studies are especially useful in answering clinical questions that address prognosis or causation. With this design, the study is generally initiated after the disease has developed. A group of individuals (cases) who have the disease and those (controls) who do not are selected and compared in terms of their prior exposures that are thought to be associated with the development of a particular type of disease. Case-control studies are also considered observational studies because they do not manipulate the exposure (what may also be referred to as the intervention). The course of the disease is observed without interference. The lack of control over the exposure in case-control studies (along with other observational studies) risks introducing selection bias into the study, which may confound the results. These potential shortcomings have some researchers arguing that case-control studies are essentially worthless because of the inherent potential for bias.

Despite the arguments against the value of the case-control design, it is the most commonly used epidemiological design in the medical literature today. For example, the association between unopposed estrogen use in postmenopausal women and the development of endometrial cancer was established through several case-control studies.

The Nurses' Health Study at Harvard is an example of a well-known prospective cohort study. It is a large, ongoing cohort study that enrolled more than 120,000 married female nurses who were 30 to 55 years old in 1976. The nurses completed a baseline questionnaire about a number of demographic and health characteristics. Follow-up questionnaires at 2-year intervals asked about the development of disease and any new exposures. By comparing the exposed and unexposed groups on a number of variables (e.g., those who took hormone replacements and those who did not; those who ate high-fat foods and those who did not) and the onset of disease within each group, the study has provided important information about the relationships of these variables with the development of cancer and cardiovascular disease in women.

Perhaps the most renowned example of a prospective cohort study is the Framingham Heart Study. In this study, investigators identified and examined 5,127 men and women from Framingham, Massachusetts, who were 30 to 59 years old in the 1950s. When the study was initiated, all 5,127 participants were determined to be free from coronary heart disease. Participants in the study have provided ongoing lifestyle and health status information and have been reexamined at regular intervals since 1952 for the development of coronary events. Prospective data from this study have been pivotal in identifying a number of major risk factors associated with coronary artery disease (CAD) and have been one of the sources of evidence for recommending lifestyle modifications to prevent CAD.

Research Designs for Level V Evidence: Systematic Reviews of Descriptive and Qualitative Studies

The purpose of descriptive research is to portray accurately the characteristics of a population or a clinical situation. Descriptive research can be quantitative or qualitative in design. In quantitative designs, the findings address the incidence, prevalence, or measurable characteristics of the population using descriptive statistics (frequencies, means, mode, etc.).

In qualitative designs, the population or clinical situation is displayed in a narrative format for the purpose of increasing the understanding of the various dimensions of the phenomena of interest. Common qualitative designs used in nursing research include phenomenology, ethnography, grounded theory, and historical analysis.

Research Designs for Level VI Evidence: Single Descriptive or Qualitative Studies

Case studies fall into this category. They are ranked lower owing to the likelihood of decreased objectivity. These studies describe the history of one individual or a small group of patients. Case studies are generally told in story form. The value of this study type is to alert a provider to an adverse event or a rare disease, or to add to a provider's knowledge base. It is important to recognize that no inferences can made from a case study to the general population.

Research Designs for Level VII Evidence: Opinion of Authorities and/or Reports of Expert Committees

This level of evidence is just as it states; it is the opinion of someone. This follows the traditional approach for "correct" or "common" practice and may or may not be based on strong evidence. This level of evidence should not be a sole determination of changing practice or determining the proper course of treatment. However, there are times when this is the only evidence, and it is utilized to begin treatment in rare situations that do not have higher levels of evidence.

■ EXAMPLES FROM THE FIELD: STUDIES OF IMPLEMENTING PRACTICE GUIDELINES

The clinician who uses clinical guidelines should evaluate their usefulness by examining the following major characteristics (Box 5.6):

- **Who created the guideline and what is the date of revision or origination?** Authorship and funding of the guideline may be important if there is the potential for bias. In addition, the best guideline will be created using multidisciplinary groups and follow a systematic approach as recommended by AHRQ. The guideline must be current, meaning it was created or revised in the past 2 to 3 years and used the most up-to-date evidence.

- **Are the guidelines clinically important?** To establish clinical importance, guidelines should convince you that following them will provide more benefits for your patients than whatever expected harms or costs are associated with applying them.

- **How strong are the recommendations?** This is largely determined by the strength of available evidence in making recommendations using clinical guidelines. Guidelines will grade the recommendations. This is based on the strength of the evidence the recommendation was based on. Various grading systems for the strength of the recommendations and evidence on which recommendations are based have been used to assist practitioners in determining how "strong" the recommendations are. There is no uniformity in the grading systems, requiring a provider to look at the grading system before reading the recommendations. The *Guide to Clinical Preventive Services* developed by the U.S. Preventive Services Task Force has a section describing the

Box 5.6   Answering the Questions to Determine Use of Guideline

1. Who created the guideline, and what is the date of revision or origination?
   - Authorship: Institute for Clinical Systems Improvement (private nonprofit organization)
   - Funding: The following Minnesota health plans provide direct financial support: Blue Cross and Blue Shield of Minnesota, HealthPartners, Medica, Metropolitan Health Plan, PreferredOne, and UCare Minnesota. In-kind support is provided by the Institute for Clinical Systems Improvement's (ICSI's) members.
   - Currency: March 23, 2011

2. Are the guidelines clinically important? The guideline clearly identifies the research basis and the benefits of treatment.

3. How strong are the recommendations? The guideline clearly identifies the strength of the various recommendations being made—with Class A–E and acknowledging meta-analysis and systematic reviews.

4. Are the guideline recommendations applicable to your patients? The guideline is relevant to any provider caring for children.

Source: Institute of Medicine. Clinical practice guidelines we can trust. Retrieved July 7, 2013, from www.iom.edu/Reports/2011/Clinical-Practice-Guidelines-We-Can-Trust.aspx

methodology for reviewing evidence and how the Task Force members "translated" the science into a five-point scale (with A through E ratings) to allow a quick reference for providers to determine appropriate preventative services. Some guidelines use a Roman numeral scale to define the levels of evidence or recommendations.

- **Are the guideline recommendations applicable to your patients?** Guidelines are developed for a variety of settings and for different practitioners. First, it is necessary to determine the group for which the guidelines were written (e.g., primary-care providers, specialists, or quality assurance reviewers) and whether they suit the intended purpose. Second, a determination is made on whether the individual patient has the characteristics of patients for whom the guidelines were intended. For example, if the patients you care for have a higher or lower prevalence of a disease or different set of risk factors for disease than those in the guidelines, the recommendations may not apply. The patient population for whom the guidelines are intended will likely be dictated by the sample characteristics of the studies used to develop them as evidence. Before applying recommendations to any one patient, first determine whether this patient's characteristics are consistent with those for which the guideline was intended and modify the guidelines when required (remember, they are meant to be flexible and adapted to individual needs when necessary).

- **Case study:** A 52-year-old male patient with hypertension is in the office. The patient is on a diuretic and a beta blocker with well-controlled blood pressure. The provider is trying to determine if the patient should be tested for causes of secondary hypertension. Using the Seventh Report of the Joint National Committee on Prevention, Detection,

Evaluation, and Treatment of High Blood Pressure (JNC 7), the evidence demonstrates the improved clinical outcomes associated with treating underlying causes of secondary hypertension based on several well-designed studies; however, the costs and risks of adverse outcomes associated with diagnostic tests to rule out a cause such as renal artery stenosis may be greater than the benefits when applied to the entire population. Thus, guidelines do not recommend that every person who develops hypertension undergo extensive testing. Rather, specific characteristics of patients presenting with hypertension assist us in narrowing the population to those individuals who would reap the benefits of screening beyond any potential harm of the tests. A second patient presents with new-onset elevated blood pressure. He is 28 years old with no family history of hypertension. This patient would meet the criteria in the JNC 7 for investigation of possible renal stenosis.

Study Design and the Level of Evidence

Evidence-based health care is widely supported as the new model for practice. Some suggest that the degree of evidence provided by a study is based on its method, or design. There is an increasing trend toward regarding evidence from RCTs as the only valid type of evidence appropriate for use in the practice setting. The danger in this perspective is disregarding what we have learned and can continue to learn from observational studies such as case-control and cohort studies.

The most sobering outcome of reliance on RCTs is the failure to teach providers to think and critically evaluate information. There are many circumstances in which randomization is impossible and where observational methods have provided invaluable information. Take, for instance, how we came to understand the relationship between alcohol use in pregnancy and fetal alcohol syndrome; smoking and cardiopulmonary disease; birth defects and thalidomide; the transmission of HIV and viral hepatitis; and the development of endocarditis in IV drug use. Knowledge of these associations came from observational studies. Randomizing pregnant women into experimental or control groups to either drink alcoholic beverages or not, or designing an experimental trial to determine how the transmission of HIV in humans occurs, is not ethically possible (or desirable). How we know what we know in practice must be determined through a critical appraisal of the information available. What we need is a framework for appraising the health science literature, for applying research results to practice, and for assessing sufficient degrees of evidence to change the standards of practice.

Practitioners must learn the process of research and how to evaluate the evidence. However, providers also need a way to utilize EBP at the time of patient contact.

The learning of the process must occur in the degree programs so that the point-of-care use of EBP can occur in real time.

■ USING A FRAMEWORK TO EVALUATE HEALTH SCIENCE LITERATURE

Critical appraisal of the health science literature can seem like an overwhelming task, yet it is a professional responsibility within advanced practice nursing. Using a framework for guidance can assist APRNs in taking the appropriate steps toward meeting this obligation. Some of the steps in applying the framework presented here are similar to those used for evaluating clinical practice guidelines. Two of the many sources to find literature are PubMed and CINAHL. A framework for evaluating journal articles in the health science literature is presented in Box 5.7. This framework provides an organized approach to interpreting the information found in a

---

Box 5.7   A Framework for Evaluating Health Science Literature

Learning to evaluate health science literature is critical. It can be a time-consuming process, but it is necessary to reading an article for use in practice.

1. Look at the title to determine whether it reflects your specific interest.
2. Validate that the content is relevant to your original interest and the title by reading the abstract.
3. Evaluate and determine what is being studied:
   • What are the study questions or hypotheses?
   • What are the specific variables under study?
   • How are the variables defined and measured?
4. Evaluate and determine who is being studied:
   • What are the characteristics of the study sample or subjects?
   • How were subjects selected for the study?
   • Is there an adequate sample size?
5. Evaluate and determine the type of study design and assess its validity:
   • Do the designs of the studies support the statements made?
   • Have other studies in similar (or different) samples found consistent results?
6. Evaluate and determine how data have been analyzed:
   • What are the descriptive statistics used to describe the sample characteristics?
   • Could the degree or pattern of missing data influence the results?
   • Were the inferential statistics used appropriate for the study question and design?
   • Remember that statistical tests of significance do not determine causation or clinical significance.
7. Evaluate what you have determined thus far:
   • Have you been skeptical?
   • Have you judged the quality of the literature based on the journal in which it was published?
   • Do you realize that there is no such thing as a "perfect" study?
   • How have you judged the author's treatment of contradictory results?
   • Remember that validity and reliability are crucial aspects of the study.
8. Discuss your evaluation with colleagues and seek other opinions (such as in a journal club):
   • Do your colleagues agree with your evaluation?
   • Do the results or recommendations suggest a change in your clinical practice? If so, what change is suggested and how will it be implemented?

variety of articles, be it a review of the current knowledge in an area or original research findings.

Evaluating the Evidence to Change Practice

For an example of evaluating evidence to change practice, let's look at the use of angiotensin-converting enzyme (ACE) inhibitors in patients with congestive heart failure (CHF). In the early 1990s, several clinical trials demonstrated that the use of ACE inhibitors improved clinical outcomes in patients with CHF, not only with regard to mortality but also in exercise tolerance, symptom severity, progression to left ventricular dysfunction, and fewer hospitalization rates. The consistency of the findings and the fact that they came from well-designed RCTs provided unequivocal evidence that ACE-inhibitor use was beneficial for the majority of patients with CHF. As a result, the American College of Cardiology, the American Heart Association, and the AHRQ developed clinical guidelines for the treatment of CHF that strongly encourage ACE inhibitors as standard therapy. The use of ACE inhibitors is now considered a standard of care and should be incorporated into the care of persons with CHF. For the provider at the point of care, the clinical guideline produced by these organizations provides point-of-care evidence to utilize with a patient.

Outcomes

Distinguishing between intermediate and clinical outcomes is also critical before applying research findings to practice. Outcome research has been increasingly funded in recent years. An outcome is generally considered the dependent variable of the study. Intermediate outcomes include measurements such as bone mineral density (BMD), hemoglobin levels, and eosinophil level. Clinical outcomes include measures such as the number of hip fractures, a person's functional status, peak flow values, or the number of acute asthma exacerbations experienced.

Improvement in intermediate outcomes does not necessarily lead to improvements in clinical outcomes. For example, in early studies of using fluoride to treat osteoporosis, BMD values improved greatly when given to osteoporotic women, but the number of fractures over time did not differ from those in women who were given placebos. Thus, intermediate outcomes, although important to study to gain an understanding of disease processes and treatment, should not be substituted for clinical outcome data.

■ NURSING SCIENCE: BUILDING THE EVIDENCE FOR PRACTICE

Historically, nurses have been involved in conducting research. The establishment of the National Institute for Nursing Research marked a new era by aligning nursing science with other respected institutes within the NIH. This development increased both federal funding for nursing research and the visibility of nursing science on a national level. Investment in nursing research continues to grow in terms of resources, funding, training, and the expectation for using research as the basis, or evidence, for practice. Many methods of knowing contribute to our knowledge or understanding of the world, and a combination of methods (or various ways of triangulating) will provide a clearer, more encompassing answer to questions asked within the discipline to provide the best individualized care for patients. The example (Box 5.8) of using multiple

---

 Box 5.8 Example: Integration of Evidence-Based Practice and Nursing Research–Based Practice

The management of the 8-year-old child with type 1 diabetes requires a multidisciplinary approach of which the family is an integral part. Below are two resources available to the APRN to assist in the management of the child with diabetes.

Evidence-Based Practice Guidelines

The American Diabetes Association–Professional Association supports the development of clinical guidelines for the management of diabetes. The foundation of the guideline for the management of diabetes is the recommendations made as to glycemic control. These include the following:

1. Lowering A1C has been associated with a reduction of microvascular and neuropathic complications of diabetes (A).
2. Developing or adjusting the management plan to achieve normal or near-normal glycemia with an A1C goal of <7% is reasonable if it can be achieved without excessive hypoglycemia (B).
3. A lower A1C is associated with a lower risk of myocardial infarction and cardiovascular death (B).
4. Aggressive glycemic management with insulin may reduce morbidity in patients with severe acute illness, preoperatively, after myocardial infarction, and in pregnancy (B).
5. Less stringent treatment goals may be appropriate for patients with a history of severe hypoglycemia, patients with limited life expectancies, very young children or older adults, and individuals with comorbid conditions (E).

Continued

Box 5.8 Example: Integration of Evidence-Based Practice and Nursing Research–Based Practice—cont'd

The panel rated the strength of the evidence supporting the first recommendation as "A." An "A" indicated that there was clear evidence from well-conducted, generalizable, randomized clinical trials that were adequately powered, or at the least supportive evidence from well-conducted randomized controlled trials that were adequately powered, including evidence from a well-conducted trial at one or more institutions. Evidence supporting the second through fifth recommendations were rated as "B." An evidence rating of "B" indicated that there was supportive evidence from well-conducted cohort studies. The final recommendation was given an evidence rating of "E." Evidence rated as E indicated that support for the recommendation was from expert consensus or clinical experience.

The guidelines also addressed nutrition and psychosocial assessment and care. The recommendations listed under psychosocial assessment and care are as follows:

1. Preliminary assessment of psychological and social status should be included as part of the medical management of diabetes (E).
2. Psychosocial screening should include but is not limited to attitudes about the illness, expectations for medical management and outcomes, affect/mood, general and diabetes-related quality of life, resources (financial, social, and emotional), and psychiatric history (E).
3. It is preferable to incorporate psychological treatment into routine care rather than to wait for identification of a specific problem or deterioration in psychological status (E).

Nursing Research

Sullivan-Bolyai et al (2004) conducted a study to describe the experiences of parents managing their child's type 1 diabetes with the use of continuous subcutaneous insulin infusions (CSII), commonly referred to as the insulin pump. In this qualitative study, 14 mothers and 7 fathers were interviewed and asked to describe the day-to-day experience of managing their child's diabetes. The children ranged in age from 2–11 years, and their mean age was 7.2 years of age. Parents in this study agreed that the pump was very effective in managing their child's diabetes and believed that their child's glucose was under much better control with the pump compared with using multiple daily injections (MDI). The results of Sullivan-Bolyai et al's research indicated that some parents are reluctant to change to an alternative method of achieving glycemic control for their child. But all of the parents in their study, once familiar with the device, were very satisfied with the results and reported a better quality of life after they changed methods. Another important finding was that parents reported more freedom and flexibility in their lives once their child was switched from MDI to the insulin pump. Some parents reported that once the child was placed on the insulin pump they often were tempted to impose stricter controls on their child's glucose levels.

Impact on Advanced Practice Nursing

The American Diabetes Association guidelines indicate that there is strong, reliable evidence to support interventions that assist the child with diabetes to maintain normal to near-normal glycemic levels, with less convincing evidence given to support less stringent control in very young children. Two methods currently used to achieve control are MDI and CSII, commonly called the insulin pump.

These guidelines also include a mandate for the primary-care provider to provide psychosocial assessment and care. One assessment needed is the parents' comfort with technology and resources. Technology once limited to secondary and tertiary health-care settings is now available in the community and is often managed by lay persons and caregivers.

The method used to achieve glycemic control of the child is ultimately the parents' decision. However, APRNs who care for these children and families will be influential in the education and support of these families as they make complex health-care decisions for their child. Using the guidelines as the goals for management, APRNs can provide parents with evidence-based rationales for glycemic management of their child and assist them in their choices.

Relaying information to parents based on nursing research, such as the research conducted by Sullivan-Bolyai et al, may relieve some initial hesitancy in parents about switching from MDI to SCII to manage their child's diabetes. One important consideration in using this research in practice is that the sample for the above research was described as Caucasian and well-educated. Will these same experiences be similar in other samples? However, perceptions of parents that their child's diabetes is under better control with the insulin pump and that this method has improved their quality of life can be useful to APRNs in their care of families managing this complex health condition.

This brings the evidence to the point of care, and using the providers' confidence in the evidence, their own experience with MDI or SCII, and the parents' comfort with technology demonstrates the essence of EBP.

Sources: American Diabetes Association–Professional Association. Standards of medical care in diabetes. *Diabetes Care* 2009. Retrieved October 2, 2009, from http://care.diabetesjournals.org/content/32/supplement_1/S3.full; and Sullivan-Bolyai, S, et al. Parents' reflections on managing their children's diabetes with insulin pumps. *J Nurs Schol* 36:316–323, 2004.

types of research to care for the family with a child diagnosed with diabetes demonstrates the value of multiple methods of evidence.

There are numerous other examples of nursing research that have contributed to the knowledge base of nursing. Familiarity with nursing research findings is as important for advanced practice as familiarity with medical research findings. Critically appraising studies regarding the appropriate use of results is one of the most important skills APRNs will be required to use in practice.

■ CLINICAL DECISION MAKING AND THE PATIENT'S HEALTH-CARE DECISIONS

The decisions APRNs make in practice are fundamental to the quality of care given. Eddy (1996) expresses the importance of critically evaluating the components of clinical decision making. The importance of taking into consideration the patient's beliefs and desired outcomes is basic to making any health-care decision. Eddy (1996) identified two main steps of a decision: (1) collecting and analyzing evidence (or data) on the benefits, potential harms, and costs of various options and (2) making a judgment about how to use the available evidence to achieve the health outcome desired. This step includes the provider's experience with the population of patients served and his or her knowledge of available resources in the community.

Applying analytical procedures for determining the credibility or reliability of data to be used as evidence is only one aspect of the decision-making process, however. An equal challenge in making practice decisions lies in the second part of the process, which involves making a judgment about how to use the evidence available. This second step is not a question of facts but of patient values or preferences. One of the most substantial qualities of advanced practice nursing is establishing a relationship with our patients, providing them with the most current information we can, and allowing them to make health-care decisions they determine are best for them. In this respect, Eddy (1996) further reminds us that it is not entirely important what you as a clinician prefer for your patients; rather, it is as important to understand the patient's perspective. To clarify this point, consider Ms. Jones, a 47-year-old woman

with type 2 diabetes. She is in the office for a quarterly visit. She has not met her A1C goal through metformin and lifestyle changes. The provider recognizes that the evidence supports the addition of insulin. However, the patient absolutely refuses, despite significant explanations of the benefits. With this patient's refusal, the nurse practitioner revisits the current guidelines and selects an oral medication to add to the patient's regimen. The patient agrees to add another oral medication.

There will be times, however, that what the patient desires is not appropriate. Ms. Smith, a 22-year-old, comes to the office asking for Synthroid. The patient explains that she has tried everything to lose weight and has a friend who was started on Synthroid and lost 30 pounds. The nurse practitioner does a review of systems and a physical exam and orders the appropriate diagnostics. When the patient's lab results do not confirm a need for thyroid replacement, she educates the patient about the results and does not prescribe the patient a medication just because she is asking for it. Clearly, these cases identify the use of patients' preferences when the evidence will support a change in the "best" options, while not prescribing based solely on patient preferences (Fig. 5.1).

Figure 5.1 Schematic of triangulation of evidence-based practice.

References

American Nurses Association. Practice standards. 2013. Retrieved from www.nursingworld.org/MainMenuCategories/ ThePracticeofProfessionalNursing/NursingStandards.aspx

Eddy, DM. *Clinical decision-making: From theory to practice.* Jones & Bartlett, Boston, 1996.

Melnyk, BM, and Fineout-Overholt, E. *Evidence-based practice in nursing and healthcare: A guide to best practice.* Lippincott, Philadelphia, 2005.

Melnyk, BM, and Fineout-Overholt, E. *Evidence-based practice in nursing and healthcare: A guide to best practice,* ed 2. Lippincott, Philadelphia, 2010.

Strauss, S, et al. *Evidence based medicine: How to practice and teach EBM,* ed 4. Elsevier, New York, 2011.

Sullivan-Bolyai, S, et al. Parents' reflections on managing their children's diabetes with insulin pumps. *J Nurs Scholar* 36:316–323, 2004.

Bibliography

Agency for Healthcare Research and Quality. Reauthorization fact sheet. Retrieved from http://archive.ahrq.gov/about/ahrqfact.htm

Agency for Healthcare Research and Quality. Evidence-based practice. Retrieved from www.ahrq.gov/professionals/clinicians-providers

American Diabetes Association Clinical Practice Recommendations. Retrieved from http://professional.diabetes.org/ResourcesFor Professionals.aspx?cid=84160

Facchiano, L, and Snyder, DH. Evidence-based practice for the busy nurse practitioner: Part one: Relevance to clinical practice and clinical inquiry process. *J Am Acad Nurse Pract* 24(11):640–648, 2012.

Ferrara, LR. Integrating evidence-based practice with educational theory in clinical practice for nurse practitioners: Bridging the theory practice gap. *Res Theory Nurs Pract* 24(4):213–216, 2010.

Garrish, K, et al. Factors influencing the contribution of advanced practice nurses to promoting evidence-based practice among front-line nurses: Finding from a cross-sectional survey. *J Adv Nurs* 67(5):1079–1090, 2011.

Levin, R, and Feldman, H. *Teaching evidence-based practice in nursing: A guide for academic and clinical settings,* ed 2. Springer, New York, 2013.

Melnyk, BM, et al. Nurse practitioner educators' perceived knowledge, beliefs, and teaching strategies regarding evidence-based practice: Implications for accelerating the integration of evidence-based practice into graduate programs. *J Prof Nurs* 24(1):7–13, 2008.

University of Texas Health Science Center at San Antonio. Academic Center for Evidence-Based Practice. Retrieved from http:// acestar.uthscsa.edu/acestar-model.asp

Caring-Based Nursing: The Science

The march of professionally educated nurses onto the panoramic scene in the nation's health services re-defines the boundaries of nursing practice. . . . Inter-professional collaboration is imbued with the essence of conjoined learning to provide a higher degree of service than could be offered by one profession.
—Martha E. Rogers: Reveille in Nursing. FA Davis, Philadelphia, 1964, p 77

Neurological Problems

Jill E. Winland-Brown, EdD, APRN, FNP-BC •
Michael B. Keller, MD, MS

Chapter 6

COMMON COMPLAINTS

■ CONFUSION

Confusion is not a disease process or disease state but rather a symptom. *Confusion* is an inability to think quickly or coherently. A confused patient is disoriented to time, place, or person and usually demonstrates impairment of cognitive functioning. It is usually demonstrated by inappropriate reactions to environmental stimuli and can arise suddenly or gradually and may be either temporary or irreversible. Stressful events, lack of sleep or food, or sensory deprivation may precipitate confusion. Age is not a reliable predictor; however, older adults are most at risk because of polypharmacy (multiple prescription drugs), the aging process, and the presence of chronic disease.

Differential Diagnosis

Confusion is a key sign of neurological disorders. The clinician must be diligent in determining its cause. The physical exam will provide clues. The Mini–Mental State Exam (MMSE) can help the clinician determine the degree of confusion, which helps to isolate possible causes. One major difficulty lies in disentangling symptoms of delirium from dementia. The clinician must establish whether the patient has delirium, a delirium superimposed on another condition such as Alzheimer's disease, or another neurocognitive disorder apart from delirium, such as dementia. Once the disease has been identified and treatment started, the symptom of confusion may disappear. Differential diagnoses for confusion involve almost all body systems (Differential Diagnosis Flowchart 6.1). Common causes are presented next.

Dementia

Dementia is a decline in mental functioning, affecting memory, cognition, language, and personality. An acute transient disturbance in thought process is a result of delirium, whereas persistent or more severe confusion, with or without psychomotor hyperactivity characterized by a significant timespan between symptom appearance and death, defines dementia. Clinically significant confusional states in older patients would lead the practitioner to suspect dementias such as Alzheimer's disease (AD); multi-infarct dementia as a result of cerebrovascular accident (CVA); depression, which can cause dementia; or excessive consumption of alcohol or drugs, which can also cause dementia. (AD and CVA are discussed later in this chapter.) Plassman et al (2007) estimated that in adults aged over 71 years, more than 13% are affected by dementia; this number rises to almost 40% of individuals aged over 90 years.

Patients with dementia present with an inability to focus or sustain their attention span with at least one of the following cognitive disturbances: aphasia, apraxia, and/or agnosia. The disturbance in cognitive functioning is termed a *disturbance in executive functioning,* which encompasses the following activities: planning, organizing, sequencing, and abstracting. The history and physical exam along with diagnostic studies may reveal the presence of a medical condition or drug toxicity. Screening tests listed in Table 6.1 should be followed up with a comprehensive neurological exam along with lab and diagnostic tests to rule out any reversible causes of dementia. Treatment for dementia should be disease specific. (See Common Problems sections.) Antipsychotic drugs such as haloperidol (Haldol), quetiapine (Seroquel), risperidone (Risperdal), olanzapine (Zyprexa), and aripiprazole (Abilify) can be used to reduce agitation or anxiety. Carbamazepine (Tegretol) is an anticonvulsant that may control impulsivity and aggression. Patients with panic disorders may respond to lorazepam (Ativan) or oxazepam (Serax). Referral to a specialist may help in treatment of agitation and confusion. Management goals for the family and caregivers should be supportive, specific, and consistent.

Delirium

The clinician must distinguish between delirium and dementia when evaluating confusion in the older adult. Patients with a history of delirium have a higher incidence of dementia, whereas delirium may also exist as a state by itself without any evidence of dementia. See Table 6.1 for the differences between delirium and dementia. Both, however, do share common characteristics and causes. Once the cause of the delirium is corrected, the patient should return to his or her previous state of cognitive functioning.

Differential Diagnosis Flowchart 6.1

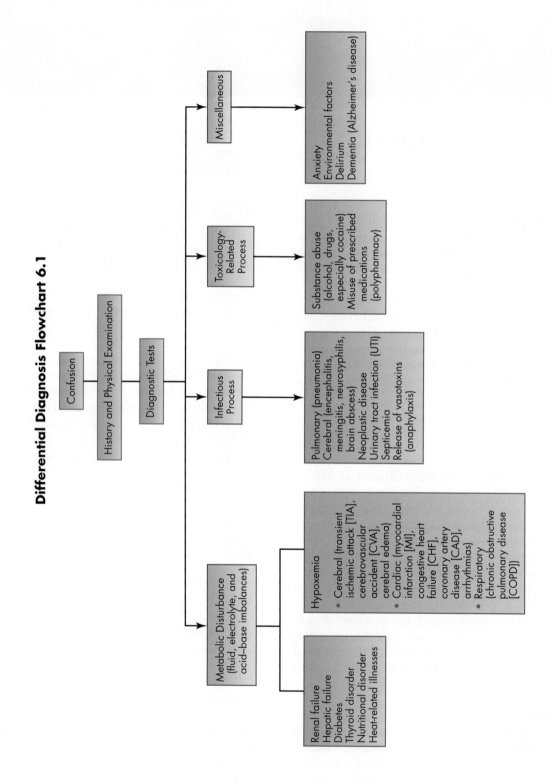

Table 6.1   Delirium versus Dementia

	Delirium (Acute Delusional State)	Dementia (Chronic)
Onset	Abrupt onset over a short period of time—days to weeks	Slowly evident over months or years
Timing	Confusion fluctuates throughout the day	Subtle decline
Duration	Hours to weeks	Months to years
Causes	A cerebral event An acute medical condition Distended bladder, constipation Sensory deprivation (poor eyesight/poor hearing) Fever, infection Actively dying Polypharmacy Adverse reaction/abrupt withdrawal of a medication, serotonin syndrome Hypoxemia Metabolic (thyroid function or organ failure) Stroke	Alzheimer's disease Parkinson's disease Motor neuron disease Medications Metabolic/endocrine disorders Trauma Infections

Symptoms	Hallmark—inattention (73%)
	Sleep–wake cycle disturbance (73%)
	Memory problems
	Psychomotor retardation (37%)
	Agitation (27%)
	Perceptual disturbances and hallucinations (26%)
	Language disturbance (25%)
		Moderate:
		   Multicognitive deficits—aphasia, apraxia, agnosia, impairment of occupational and social functioning
		Severe:
		   Incontinence, inability to perform ADLs, inability to speak more than 6 intelligible words in a day, progressive weight loss of 10% of body weight in the past 6 months

Screening tools	MMSE	SLUMS
		MoCA
		AD8 Informant interview
		MC-FAQ
		MMSE:
		   >24 early dementia
		   12–24 intermediate dementia
		   <12 severe dementia
		FAST (Functional Assessment Staging):
		Score of 7: admit to hospice
		Clock-drawing test

Treatment	Stabilize the environment; glasses or hearing aids if sensory deprivation; antipsychotics (haloperidol, chlorpromazine) if sedation is desired; for long-term prescription—risperidone, olanzapine for sedation	*Nonpharmacological interventions:*
		   Behavior Management
		   Caregiver Intervention Programs
		   Cognitive Stimulation
		   Reality Orientation Therapy
		   Recreational Activities
		Pharmacological interventions:
		   Cholinesterase Inhibitors
		   Antidepressants
		   Antipsychotics

Continued

Table 6.1 Delirium versus Dementia—cont'd		
	Delirium (Acute Delusional State)	Dementia (Chronic)
Prevention/help	Avoid illness—health promotion efforts Avoid alcohol Decrease number of medications Normalize environment Check eyeglass prescription Use hearing aids if needed	No sure way to prevent dementia; support families in ways to assist the client's brain to stay healthy longer (e.g., being physically and socially active, mind exercises) Reduce blood pressure; reduce homocysteine and cholesterol levels; control diabetes mellitus; healthy diet; cease smoking; being current on vaccines

Adapted from Alzheimer's Association. Delirium or dementia—Do you know the difference? Retrieved May 5, 2014, from www.alz.org/norcal/in_my_community_17590.asp; Blazer, DG, and van Nieuwenhuizen, AO. Evidence for the diagnostic criteria of delirium. *Curr Opin Psychiatry* 25(3):239–243, 2012; and Delirium and dementia at the end of life. Retrieved May 5, 2014, from www.medscape.org/viewarticle/499458

SLUMS: St. Louis University Mental Status exam; MoCA: Montreal Cognitive Assessment; MC-FAQ: Mini-Cog with Functional Assessment Questionnaire; MMSE: Mini–Mental State Exam.

There are many screening tools with a high degree of sensitivity and specificity to detect cognitive changes that may be used to aid the clinician in the first step toward an accurate diagnosis. These are individually available by doing a search on the Internet for each screening tool (Segal-Gida, 2013):

- MMSE
- Modified Mini–Mental State Exam (3MS)
- Mini-Cog
- Montreal Cognitive Assessment (MoCA)
- General Practitioner Assessment of Cognition (GPCOG)
- Saint Louis University Mental Status (SLUMS)
- Memory Impairment Screen (MIS)
- Clock-drawing test

Metabolic Disturbances

Fluid, electrolyte, and acid–base imbalances may be the result of metabolic problems, which can alter a patient's level of consciousness, producing confusion. The extent of the imbalance determines the severity of the patient's confusion. Typically, the patient is dehydrated and has poor skin turgor, dry skin, and a low-grade fever. Additional signs and symptoms such as dizziness, confusion, altered level of consciousness, hypotension, and coma, when evaluated with an extensive history and physical exam, will usually lead the clinician to a diagnosis. Routine laboratory tests, including electrolytes, urinalysis, chest x-ray exam, and electrocardiogram (ECG), may be performed. Treatment should be focused on restoration of appropriate fluid and electrolyte balance—specifically, correction of the primary metabolic disorder.

Infectious Process

Confusion may also be the result of an infectious process that can cause extensive tissue and organ impairment through the release of vasotoxins. If the infectious process is allowed to continue, ischemia often occurs, producing cell injury and death. Severe generalized infections (such as septicemia or bacteremia) can produce symptoms suggestive of delirium, whereas infections that affect the nervous system (such as meningitis) cause confusion, headache, and nuchal rigidity. Specific signs and symptoms of infections include fever, tachycardia, tachypnea, decreased blood pressure, confusion, and irritability. Diagnostic studies should include routine tests and those associated with the suspected infectious agent. Treatment should focus on managing the primary cause of the infection.

Tissue Hypoxia and Ischemia

Cardiovascular disorders can cause confusion as a result of tissue hypoxia and ischemia. Confusion may be insidious and may come and go, as is frequently the case. The patient typically appears ill and has significant changes in vital signs (decreased blood pressure, elevated and/or irregular pulse, and tachypnea), edema, cyanosis, reduced level of consciousness, confusion, severe headache, agitation, vomiting, and motor deficits. Diagnostic examinations should include routine laboratory testing, arterial blood gases, chest x-ray, and ECG. Treatment depends on the problem or disease identified.

Neoplastic diseases that cause confusion include systemic cancers and intracranial lesions to the brain, secondary to the extensive tissue and organ destruction caused by the invading cancers. Signs and symptoms depend on the areas of the body where the cancer is located. Extensive cerebral edema, compression, and cell injury produce ischemic states and result in cell and tissue death. This destruction impairs the circulation, increases intracranial pressure, and results in confusion, headaches, disorientation, tremors, seizures, memory loss, gait disturbances, dehydration, changes in levels of consciousness, vomiting, and sensory and motor deficits.

Diagnostic studies should include basic routine tests. Additional studies and treatment measures will vary depending on the type of cancer.

■ DIZZINESS AND VERTIGO

Dizziness is the sensation of unsteadiness and a feeling of movement within the head. *Vertigo* is the sensation of rotation or movement of the patient or the patient's surroundings. The terms are often used synonymously, but they do not have the same meaning. Vertigo may result from an inner ear disease or a disturbance of the vestibular center or pathway in the central nervous system (CNS). Dizziness is described as a feeling of light-headedness, weakness, or faintness. Loss of consciousness rarely occurs, but the feeling of faintness encourages the patient to lie down, which may cause the feelings to disappear. It is important to distinguish between vertigo and dizziness. Episodes of dizziness are brief and may be mild or severe, with an abrupt or gradual onset. Both dizziness and vertigo may be accompanied by nausea, vomiting, nystagmus, and unsteady gait. Dizziness occurs as a result of inadequate blood flow and oxygen supply to the brain and spinal cord. If other neurological symptoms occur, such as numbness or facial, arm, or leg weakness, it is more suggestive of a brainstem problem.

Differential Diagnosis

Differential diagnoses for dizziness are classified into four categories: peripheral vestibular disease, systemic disorders, CNS disorders, and anxiety states (Differential Diagnosis Flowchart 6.2). The history and physical exam are essential to pinpoint a diagnosis. Key questions to ask a patient regarding dizziness include duration, severity, and nature of the episodes and any associated symptoms such as hearing loss and weakness. Key points to assess include physical exam of the ear to rule out cerumen impaction or otitis media; hearing tests, including whisper, Weber, and Rinne; a thorough neurological assessment; and the Hallpike maneuver, to distinguish between benign vertigo and vertigo resulting from a CNS lesion. The Hallpike maneuver is performed by rotating the patient's head to one side and then lowering it slowly to 30 degrees below the bodyline. The patient should be observed for nystagmus during head rotation and vertical positioning. In patients with benign vertigo, there may be rotational nystagmus and possible severe vertigo, which usually occurs in one direction. This resolves quickly and cannot be reproduced after two to three repetitions. The clinician should suspect a central lesion when the vertical nystagmus is of a longer duration and continues with each repetition.

Peripheral Vestibular Disease

Peripheral vestibular disease accounts for up to 44% of all cases of dizziness and vertigo. Many patients who experience dizziness may have a diseased vestibular nerve. Most often the problem is located in the labyrinth of the middle ear. The problem may be caused by otoliths precipitated in the labyrinth. Signs and symptoms of vestibular disease include dizziness, nausea and vomiting, diaphoresis, difficulty with balance, vertigo, tinnitus, fluctuating hearing loss, feelings of pressure in the ear, and diplopia. Diagnostic studies include audiological evaluation, electronystagmography, magnetic resonance imaging, magnetic resonance angiography, brainstem-evoked responses, and basic laboratory screening as guided by history and physical exam. Antihistamines such as meclizine (Antivert), diphenhydramine (Benadryl), or promethazine (Phenergan) are the most commonly prescribed medications for vertigo. These agents suppress the vestibular end-organ receptors and inhibit activation of vagal responses. Patients are instructed to take the medication for a week, then to try to taper the drug slowly. Diamox is used to decrease edema in the labyrinth. Antiemetics should be considered when nausea and vomiting are severe. These agents suppress central vestibular pathways, which activate the vagal stimulus. Prochlorperazine (Compazine) orally (PO) or by suppository or trimethobenzamide (Tigan) PO or by suppository will usually bring relief to the patient. Vestibular exercises can help the patient with the symptoms of vertigo. Exercises are helpful in dislodging the otoliths. They may also help the patient acclimate to the symptoms. Exercises have been shown to decrease the duration of vertigo or produce longer symptom-free periods. The patient is instructed to reproduce the feelings of vertigo by placing the affected ear down, then assume a supine position and hold that position until the vertigo disappears. The vertigo may return when the patient sits up. The patient must repeat these maneuvers at least five times a day or until the vertigo no longer returns. Patients with persistent symptoms should be referred for assessment of nerve function. Surgery may be indicated when all else fails to relieve the vertigo.

Systemic Disorders

Systemic disorders may cause dizziness or light-headedness. Patients typically complain of light-headedness or feelings that they are about to faint or pass out. Dizziness may be aggravated by postural changes or exertion. Pallor, dyspnea, tachycardia, bounding pulse, weakness, hypotension, blurred vision, decreased breath sounds, headache, diaphoresis, and agitation suggest systemic problems. These symptoms should prompt the practitioner to look for signs of anemia, cardiovascular disease, hyperventilation, drug reactions, endocrine disorders, fluid and electrolyte imbalances, and psychiatric problems. Systemic diseases require diagnostic examination and treatment that is specific for the cause of the dizziness.

Central Nervous System Disorders

CNS disorders that disrupt the pathway between the vestibular apparatus and the brain may cause dizziness. Facial numbness, hemiparesis, diplopia, dysarthria,

Differential Diagnosis Flowchart 6.2

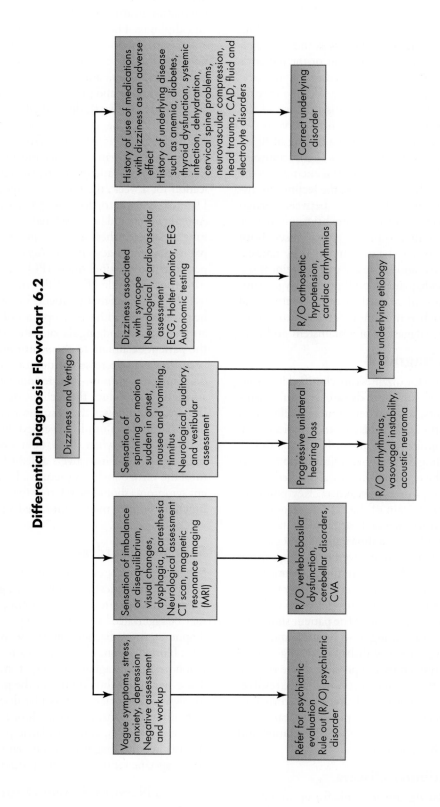

headache, nausea, and vomiting are some common signs and symptoms suggesting CNS dysfunction. Diagnostic examination and treatment depend on the underlying disorder.

HEADACHE

The most common of all human ailments is the headache. Headache may be localized or generalized and may produce mild to severe pain. About 90% of all headaches are without pathological cause.

Differential Diagnosis

Headaches may be classified into four types: muscle contraction (tension) headaches, vascular (migraine and cluster) headaches, mixed headaches (a combination of muscle contraction and vascular), and traction or inflammatory headaches. Muscle contraction headaches, often referred to as tension headaches, are either primary (without underlying pathology) or secondary (the result of pathology such as trauma, infection, arthritis, or tumor). They occur in 20% to 25% of all new cases of headaches. More than 50% of all headaches seen in primary care are muscle contraction headaches, often referred to as tension headaches. These headaches can occur at any age but are most common in young adults. Females present with the most severe cases, with underlying causes of generalized anxiety or depressive disorders. Forty percent of all patients with muscle contraction headaches have a positive family history of headaches. Any headache that is abrupt, explosive, severe, and described as the worst headache of the patient's life is suggestive of a traction or inflammatory headache and is most often due to intracranial hemorrhage, a medical emergency.

The clinician should ask questions to determine the following factors: onset; location of the headache; frequency; duration; severity; character, such as throbbing versus constant; presence of an aura; an association with sleep patterns; emotional factors; precipitating and alleviating factors; and family history. This information is essential to delineate the diagnosis and rule out other problems. Differential Diagnosis Flowchart 6.3 presents common characteristics, associated symptoms, and precipitating factors of common disorders that present with a complaint of headache. Additional information about headaches is provided later in this chapter; different types of headaches, along with their associated signs and symptoms, diagnosis, and treatment, are compared in Table 6.5 (on page 123).

PARESTHESIA AND PARESIS

Paresthesia is an abnormal sensation described as numbness or tingling, cramping, or pain without a known stimulus, felt along peripheral nerve pathways. Paresis is weakness. It may be local to a single extremity or the face, or it may involve more than one extremity. Paresis may develop suddenly or gradually and may be permanent or transient. Feelings associated with paresthesia are annoying "pins and needles" sensations that often cause the patient to touch or rub the affected area. Paresthesia is a common complaint, especially in patients with certain systemic diseases or those on certain drugs.

Differential Diagnosis

Paresthesia is usually due to damage or irritation to the parietal lobe, thalamus, spinothalamic tract, or the spinal or peripheral nerves that are the usual pathways for transmission and interpretation of sensory stimuli. It is important to explore the symptom of paresthesia by asking the patient to describe when it first began; the character, duration, and distribution of the paresthesia; and any other associated signs and symptoms such as sensory or motor loss. A medical history may reveal any neurological, cardiac, vascular, endocrine, renal, or inflammatory diseases the patient may have had or still has. Recent trauma, surgery, or invasive procedures may reveal possible causes of peripheral nerve injury. The physical exam should focus on the neurological system, assessing level of consciousness; cranial nerve function; reflexes; motor strength; and touch, pain, and temperature sensations. Skin color and the quality of all pulses should also be noted. If the patient has diabetes, symptoms of diabetic neuropathy such as a bilateral loss of pain sensation and diminished touch, temperature sensation, and proprioception may be present. They may present in a stocking-glove distribution.

The most common diagnoses associated with paresthesia symptoms are arterial occlusion, arteriosclerosis obliterans, nerve entrapment syndrome, neuropathy, transient ischemic attacks (discussed in detail later in this chapter), and herpes zoster (Differential Diagnosis Flowchart 6.4).

Arterial occlusion is a surgical emergency. An acute occlusion may be either an arterial embolism or a thrombosis. Immediate embolectomy is the treatment of choice in early emboli in the extremities and is preferably performed within 4 to 6 hours of the embolic event.

Arteriosclerosis obliterans is a disorder that involves the pathological process of atherosclerosis, which causes progressive narrowing of the arteries with subsequent obstruction of blood flow, resulting in diminished or decreased flow of blood to the legs and feet.

Nerve entrapment syndrome results from compression of a nerve pathway along the root of the nerve, which results in paresthesia or weakness. Trauma causing compartment syndrome or bruising, rheumatoid arthritis, edema, infection, prolonged standing or sitting, and tight clothing can all cause entrapment of the nerve. The compression diminishes blood supply and can result in cellular changes to the nerve pathway.

Neuropathy is usually the result of underlying diseases such as diabetes, renal failure, multiple sclerosis, cancer, collagen disease, vasculitis, thyroid disease, ingestion of toxins, or nutritional deficiency. Afferent

Differential Diagnosis Flowchart 6.3

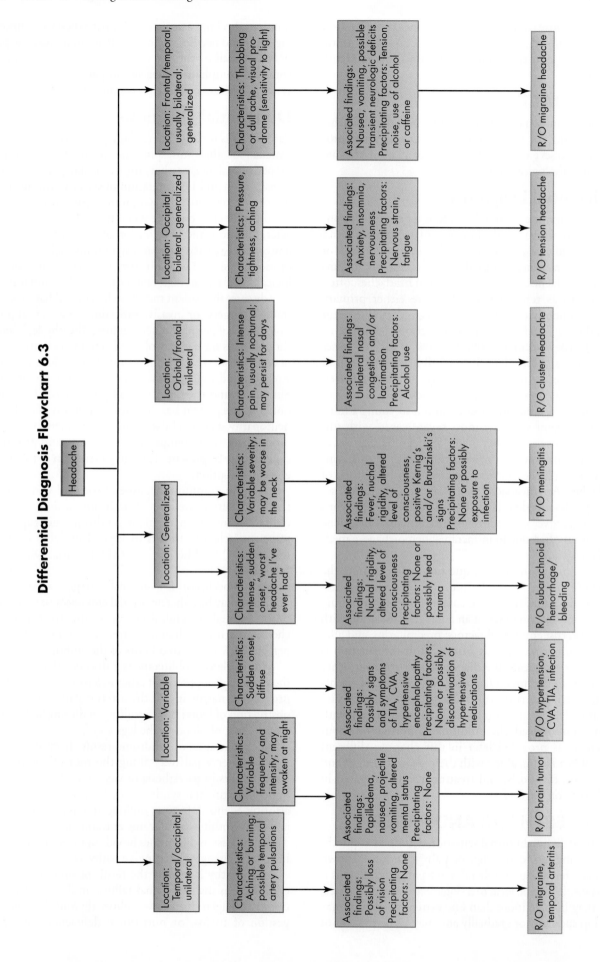

Differential Diagnosis Flowchart 6.4

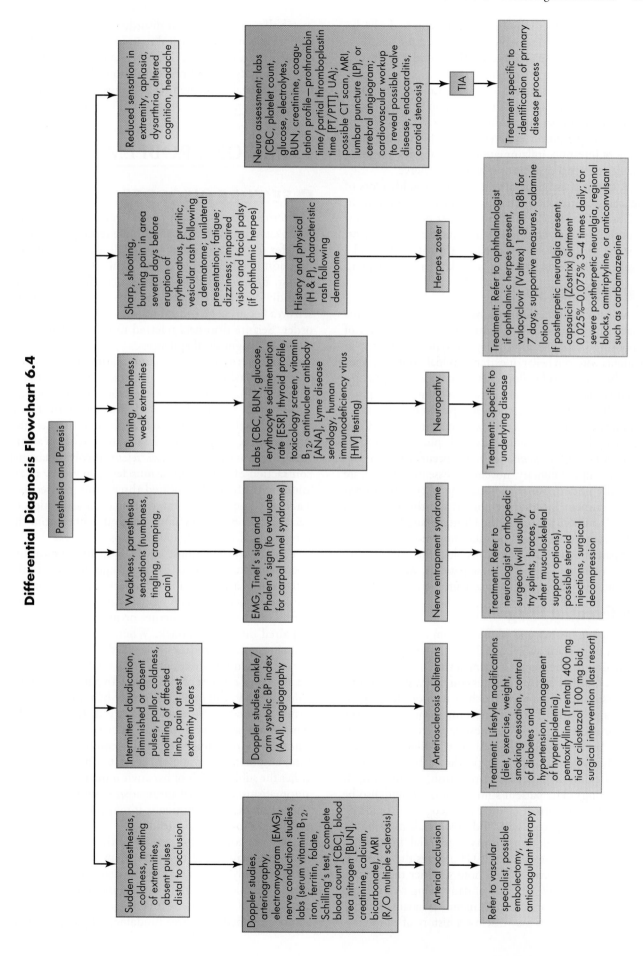

Paresthesia and Paresis

Reduced sensation in extremity, aphasia, dysarthria, altered cognition, headache

→ Neuro assessment; labs (CBC, platelet count, glucose, electrolytes, BUN, creatinine, coagulation profile—prothrombin time/partial thromboplastin time [PT/PTT], UA); possible CT scan, MRI, lumbar puncture (LP), or cerebral angiogram; cardiovascular workup (to reveal possible valve disease, endocarditis, carotid stenosis)

→ **TIA** → Treatment specific to identification of primary disease process

---

Sharp, shooting, burning pain in area several days before eruption of erythematous, pruritic, vesicular rash following a dermatome; unilateral presentation; fatigue; dizziness; impaired vision and facial palsy (if ophthalmic herpes)

→ History and physical (H & P), characteristic rash following dermatome

→ **Herpes zoster** → Treatment: Refer to ophthalmologist if ophthalmic herpes present, valacyclovir (Valtrex) 1 gram q8h for 7 days, supportive measures, calamine lotion
If postherpetic neuralgia present, capsaicin (Zostrix) ointment 0.025%–0.075% 3–4 times daily; for severe postherpetic neuralgia, regional blocks, amitriptyline, or anticonvulsant such as carbamazepine

---

Burning, numbness, weak extremities

→ Labs (CBC, BUN, glucose, erythrocyte sedimentation rate [ESR], thyroid profile, toxicology screen, vitamin B$_{12}$, antinuclear antibody [ANA], Lyme disease serology, human immunodeficiency virus [HIV] testing)

→ **Neuropathy** → Treatment: Specific to underlying disease

Weakness, paresthesia sensations (numbness, tingling, cramping, pain)

→ EMG, Tinel's sign and Phalen's sign (to evaluate for carpal tunnel syndrome)

→ **Nerve entrapment syndrome** → Treatment: Refer to neurologist or orthopedic surgeon (will usually try splints, braces, or other musculoskeletal support options), possible steroid injections, surgical decompression

---

Intermittent claudication, diminished or absent pulses, pallor, coldness, mottling of affected limb, pain at rest, extremity ulcers

→ Doppler studies, ankle/arm systolic BP index (AAI), angiography

→ **Arteriosclerosis obliterans** → Treatment: Lifestyle modifications (diet, exercise, weight, smoking cessation, control of diabetes and hypertension, management of hyperlipidemia), pentoxifylline (Trental) 400 mg tid or cilostazol 100 mg bid, surgical intervention (last resort)

Sudden paresthesias, coldness, mottling of extremities, absent pulses distal to occlusion

→ Doppler studies, arteriography, electromyogram (EMG), nerve conduction studies, labs (serum vitamin B$_{12}$, iron, ferritin, folate, Schilling's test, complete blood count [CBC], blood urea nitrogen [BUN], creatinine, calcium, bicarbonate), MRI (R/O multiple sclerosis)

→ **Arterial occlusion** → Refer to vascular specialist, possible embolectomy, anticoagulant therapy nerve fibers conduct impulses from the skin to the brain. Alterations along these nerve pathways because of disease pathology can cause paresthesia. The majority of the diseases listed involve peripheral nerves.

Herpes zoster is caused by the varicella-zoster virus, which causes an acute vesicular eruption in adults, especially in immunocompromised patients. An early symptom of herpes zoster is paresthesia, which occurs as a result of infection, inflammation, and compression along the dermatomal distribution of a spinal nerve.

A transient ischemic attack (TIA) is a sudden loss of neurological function caused by impaired blood flow to the brain. The loss of function can last from a few minutes to 24 hours; after a TIA, normal function returns. If some residual weakness remains, the patient has had a stroke. TIAs are discussed in detail later in this chapter.

■ TREMORS

Tremors are rhythmic involuntary muscle movements that result from alternate contraction and relaxation of opposing muscle groups. They are typically evident in patients with cerebellar or extrapyramidal disorders. They are also seen as side effects with certain drug regimens. Tremors are sometimes classified into seven groups: physiological, essential, toxic, cerebellar, parkinsonian, resting, and intentional. A *resting tremor* occurs in a relaxed and supported extremity and ends with purposeful movement, whereas an *intentional tremor* occurs when the patient attempts voluntary movement. Essential tremors are typically underreported because many persons do not seek treatment for mild tremors. It is estimated that at least 10 million persons in the United States have essential tremor. As the most common movement disorder, it is apparent in 1 in 20 Americans older than age 40, and 1 in 5 older than age 65. These patients, when they do present, should be referred to a neurologist.

Differential Diagnosis

A complete history and physical exam are necessary to obtain important subjective data that will provide information on the tremor's characteristics, including duration, onset of action, progression, alleviating factors, and associated symptoms (such as memory loss, agitation, and nausea). It is important to note when the tremor is present (e.g., with rest or activity), what part of the body is affected, whether it is bilateral or not, and the type of movement produced by the tremor (e.g., flexion or extension, pronation, supination, or pill-rolling). The patient's muscle tone should also be assessed: Is it normal or increased (cogwheel rigidity)? The patient's speech, gait, and posture all must be assessed. A thorough drug history is essential, including a list of any over-the-counter (OTC) drugs the patient is taking. The clinician should note whether the tremors affect the patient's activities of daily living (ADLs) and if there is any history of family members having tremors. A review of systems may disclose a history of endocrine,

metabolic, or neurological disorders. A complete musculoskeletal and neurological examination must be done to assess range of motion (ROM), mental status, strength and sensitivity, cranial nerve function, deep tendon reflexes, and gait. Differential Diagnosis Flowchart 6.5 presents common differential diagnoses of tremor.

COMMON PROBLEMS

■ SEIZURE DISORDERS

The terms *seizure disorder, convulsive disorder,* and *cerebral seizures* are synonymous with the term *epilepsy.* They all refer to recurrent paroxysmal episodes of brain dysfunction manifested by stereotypical alterations in behavior. *Epilepsy,* by definition, is a condition in which an individual is predisposed to two or more recurrent seizures because of a central nervous system (CNS) disorder. Seizure disorders referred to in this chapter include the diagnosis of epilepsy.

A *seizure* is a sudden, involuntary, time-limited alteration in behavior, including a change in motor activity, autonomic function, consciousness, or sensation, accompanied by an abnormal electrical discharge in the brain. The major behavioral feature that distinguishes seizures from usual activity is that seizures are stereotypical and repetitive. For example, a *clonic seizure* involves maximal contraction of one group of muscles followed by relaxation, with the cycle repeated three times per second. Table 6.2 presents the International Classification of Seizures and Epilepsies along with guidelines from the International League Against Epilepsy.

Partial seizures are those in which the first clinical and electroencephalographic (EEG) changes indicate initial activation of a system of neurons limited to one part of the cerebral hemisphere. A partial seizure is classified primarily on the basis of whether or not consciousness is impaired during the attack. When there is no loss of consciousness, the seizure is classified as a *simple partial seizure.* When consciousness is impaired, the seizure is classified as a *complex partial seizure.* In patients with impaired consciousness, aberrations of behavior (automatisms) may occur. Automatisms are distinguished by symptoms: eating automatisms (chewing, swallowing); automatisms of mimicry, expressing emotional state; gestural automatisms, crude or elaborate (directed toward either the subject or his or her environment); ambulatory automatisms; and verbal automatisms. Sometimes a partial seizure may not terminate; it may progress to a generalized motor seizure instead.

There is considerable evidence that simple partial seizures usually have unilateral hemispheric involvement and only rarely have bilateral hemispheric involvement; complex partial seizures, however, frequently have bilateral hemispheric involvement. Partial seizures can be classified into three fundamental groups: simple

Differential Diagnosis Flowchart 6.5

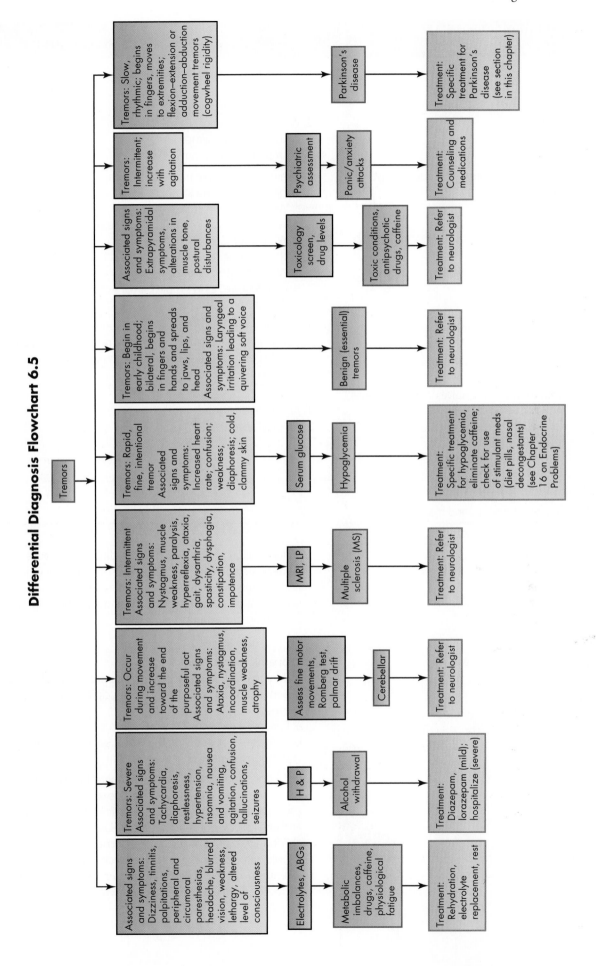

Table 6.2   International Classification of Epileptic Seizures and the International League Against Epilepsy

Seizures

I. Partial (focal, local) seizures	
A. Simple partial seizures (consciousness not impaired)	1. With motor symptoms 2. With somatosensory or special sensory symptoms 3. With autonomic symptoms 4. With psychic symptoms

B. Complex partial seizures (with impairment of consciousness)	1. Beginning as simple partial seizures and progressing to impairment of consciousness
	   a. With no other features
	   b. With features as in simple partial seizures
	   c. With automatisms
	2. With impairment of consciousness at onset
	   a. With no other features
	   b. With features as in simple partial seizures
	   c. With automatisms

C. Partial seizures evolving to secondarily generalized seizures	1. Simple partial seizures evolving to generalized seizures 2. Complex partial seizures evolving to generalized seizures 3. Simple partial seizures evolving to complex partial seizures to generalized seizures
II. Generalized seizures (convulsive or nonconvulsive) A. Absence seizures (petit mal)	1. Absence seizures 2. Atypical absence seizures
B. Myoclonic seizures	
C. Clonic seizures	
D. Tonic seizures	
E. Tonic-clonic seizures (grand mal)	
F. Atonic seizures (astatic seizures)	
III. Unclassified seizures	1. Includes all seizures that cannot be classified because of inadequate or incomplete data and some that defy classification as already described; this includes some neonatal seizures, such as rhythmic eye movements, chewing, and swimming movements

Epilepsies

I. Localization-related epilepsies	1. Idiopathic (age-related)
	   a. Benign childhood epilepsy with centrotemporal spikes
	   b. Benign childhood epilepsy with occipital paroxysms
	2. Symptomatic
	   a. Epilepsies involving the limbic system
	   b. Epilepsies not involving the limbic system (frontal, temporal, central, parietal, occipital)

II. Generalized epilepsies	1. Idiopathic (age-related) (benign neonatal familial convulsions, benign neonatal convulsions, West's syndrome [idiopathic cases], epilepsy with myoclonic-astatic seizures [idiopathic and familial cases of Lennox-Gastaut-Dravet syndrome], childhood absence epilepsy [pyknoepilepsy], epilepsy with [myo]clonic absences, juvenile absence epilepsy, benign juvenile myoclonic epilepsy [impulsive mal], epilepsy with generalized tonic-clonic seizures on awakening)

Table 6.2	International Classification of Epileptic Seizures and the International League Against Epilepsy—cont'd

2. Symptomatic
   a. Nonspecific cause (age-related) (neonatal seizures, early myoclonic encephalopathy, West's syndrome [infantile spasms, Blitz-Nick-Salaam-Krampfe], Lennox-Gastaut-Dravet syndrome)
   b. Specific cause (progressive myoclonus epilepsies such as Lafora's disease, Unverricht's disease, Unverricht-Lundborg-Hartung disease, Kufs disease, Zeman's disease)
3. Epilepsies undetermined whether focal or generalized
4. Special syndromes

partial seizures, complex partial seizures, and complex partial seizures that evolve into generalized tonic-clonic convulsions.

Generalized seizures are those in which the first clinical changes indicate initial involvement of both hemispheres of the brain. Consciousness may be impaired, and this impairment may be the initial manifestation of the seizure. Motor manifestations are bilateral. The EEG patterns are bilateral and presumably reflect neuronal discharge, which is widespread in both hemispheres.

The hallmark of an *absence seizure* is a sudden onset, interruption of ongoing activities, a blank stare, and possibly a brief upward rotation of the eye. If the patient is speaking, speech will be slowed or interrupted; if the patient is walking, he or she will stand transfixed; if eating, the food will be stopped on the way to the mouth. The attack may last from a few seconds to a half a minute.

Tonic-clonic, or *grand mal, seizures* are the most frequently encountered generalized seizures. There is a sudden, sharp tonic contraction of muscles, stridor, or a cry, and the patient falls to the ground in the tonic state. The patient lies rigid; during this state, tonic contraction inhibits respiration and cyanosis may occur. The tongue may be bitten, and urine may be voided involuntarily. This tonic stage then gives way to clonic convulsive movements lasting a variable period of time. At the end of this stage, deep respiration will occur, and all muscles will relax, after which the patient will remain unconscious for a period of time. This is known as the postictal period. After this type of seizure, the individual frequently goes into a deep sleep and may have a significant headache when awakened.

Myoclonic jerks are sudden, brief shock-like contractions, which may be generalized or confined to the face and trunk or to one or more extremities. They may occur predominantly during sleep.

Epidemiology and Causes

Seizure disorders are among the most common neurological conditions, affecting more than 2 million people in the United States. Each year, about 300,000 individuals in the United States seek medical attention because of a newly recognized seizure, representing an incidence of about 120 per 100,000. The majority of patients (75,000–100,000) presenting for treatment of seizure are younger than age 5 and have experienced only convulsions associated with a febrile illness. Each year, 50 per 100,000 individuals in the United States are diagnosed as having a seizure disorder, which is approximately 125,000 new cases each year. Although seizure disorders may start at any age, the highest incidence of seizure is among children younger than age 2 and persons older than age 65.

Men are more likely to have a seizure disorder than women. In most newly diagnosed cases, no specific cause is identified. Many factors have been implicated in the etiology of seizure disorders, such as severe head trauma, CNS infections, and stroke. Children with motor disabilities present from birth, such as those with cerebral palsy, have increased risks. Children who are mentally challenged and who may or may not have genetic disorders may have an increased risk for a seizure disorder. When both conditions coexist, 50% or more of patients affected can be expected to develop a seizure disorder by age 20. In addition, children who experience febrile seizures are at increased risk for developing a seizure disorder during their lives.

Seizure disorders frequently occur in families. The parents, siblings, and offspring of a patient with a seizure disorder are more likely (3%–5%) than the general population to have a seizure as a result of both genetic and environmental causes.

Pathophysiology

A seizure is an uncontrollable paroxysm that often includes muscular convulsions. The paroxysm is the bodily effect of abnormal repetitive firing of neurons in the brain. The motor cortex, the hippocampal formation, and the amygdaloid complex are regions that are especially susceptible to developing these abnormal firing patterns.

A great variety of disorders can initiate seizures, including drug overdose (e.g., from antihistamines, cholinesterase inhibitors, methylxanthines, muscarinic agonists, and tricyclic antidepressants), drug withdrawal (e.g., from alcohol, hypnotics, and tranquilizers), head trauma, strokes, degenerative brain disease (e.g., mesial temporal sclerosis), infections, tumors, and developmental brain defects (e.g., cortical dysgenesis and vascular malformations). The common epileptogenic feature of all these disorders is that they can cause populations of brain neurons to become hyperexcitable.

One category of disorders that cause hyperexcitable neurons includes systemic problems—fever, infection, sleep deprivation, and metabolic imbalances (hypocalcemia, hypoglycemia, hyponatremia, and hypoxia). These problems cause ionic changes throughout the body. For example, hyponatremia causes a relative increase in extracellular potassium concentrations systemically. In the CNS, increased extracellular K^+ at the neuron cell membrane lowers the threshold for triggering axon potentials, and for this reason acute hyponatremia (at levels less than 120 mEq/L) leads to seizures.

The excitability of neuron cell membranes is regulated by intramembrane molecular complexes that either actively move molecules from one side to the other (i.e., ion pumps) or control gated ion channels. Genetic defects in the manufacture of ion pumps or ion channels can cause seizures. Some of the uncommon heritable epilepsies (e.g., *generalized epilepsy with febrile seizures* and *benign familial neonatal convulsions*) are known to be caused by mutations in ion channels. It is believed that other heritable seizure disorders are caused by as yet unidentified genetic defects in ion pumps or ion channels.

The antiepileptic drugs phenytoin (Dilantin), carbamazepine (Tegretol), and lamotrigine (Lamictal) reduce the hyperexcitability of neuron cell membranes by slowing the activation of sodium channels; ethosuximide (Zarontin) decreases the activity of certain calcium channels.

Much of the excitatory activity throughout the brain is via glutamatergic synapses, and increasing the amount or the effect of glutamate in the brain predisposes a person to seizures. Normally, the amount of extracellular glutamate in the brain is minimized by astrocytes, which selectively take up glutamate. Experimental studies have shown that a brain will have seizures if its astrocytes cannot efficiently clear extracellular glutamate from the vicinity of synapses.

Glutamate depolarizes neurons by activating specific receptors that open channels for small cations, such as Na^+ and K^+. These are called *ionotropic receptors,* and the CNS contains at least three different ionotropic glutamate receptors. High brain concentrations of agonists, such as street drugs, cocaine, and angel dust (phencyclidine), may induce seizures. These agonists (chemicals) bind to a receptor and activate it to produce a biological response (the seizure).

Glutamate also activates another family of membrane receptors. These receptors alter cell metabolism and are called *metabotropic glutamate receptors.* Other types of metabotropic glutamate receptor agonists, however, have the opposite effect—activating these receptors decreases the excitability of synapses.

Much of the inhibitory transmission throughout the brain is via GABA-ergic synapses. In general, neurons using the transmitter gamma-aminobutyric acid (GABA) act to prevent the spread of abnormal bursts of neuronal discharges. Reducing the availability of GABA predisposes a person to seizures. Drugs, such as 3-mercaptopropionic acid, that interfere with the synthesis of GABA cause seizures. Vitamin B_6 (pyridoxine) is required for the biosynthesis of GABA, and vitamin B_6 deficiency can lead to seizures. Drugs that interfere with GABA receptors or with GABA binding to receptors can also cause seizures; such drugs include bicuculline, penicillin, and picrotoxin.

GABA agonists have the opposite effect—they counteract a person's tendency to have seizures. Benzodiazepines (e.g., diazepam [Valium]) are GABA agonists and are used to treat seizure disorders. Gabapentin (Neurontin) and pregabalin (Lyrica) are drugs that increase GABA. Barbiturates, which potentiate the actions of both GABA and benzodiazepines, are antiepileptic drugs. Likewise, the antiepileptic drugs tiagabine and vigabatrin both work by enhancing GABA-mediated inhibitory circuitry. Besides the GABA-ergic pathways, noradrenergic circuits (originating mainly in the reticular formation of the brainstem) also appear to play an antiseizure role, because damage to noradrenergic pathways can predispose a person to seizures.

During a seizure, brain metabolism accelerates in the affected areas. Oxygen consumption, glucose use, and lactate levels increase; free fatty acids are released into the blood; extracellular concentrations of neurotransmitters rise; and cerebral blood flow increases. Between seizures, metabolism in the affected areas drops below normal. Prolonged seizures increase the local transcription of certain genes and the synthesis of certain proteins (although the synthesis of most proteins declines). The abnormal metabolic activities associated with repeated seizures produce long-term changes in brain circuitry that make further seizures more likely. One reason for controlling epilepsy is to prevent these lasting increases in neural sensitivity.

Clinical Presentation

Subjective

The patient may or may not be aware of a seizure. He or she may wake up slightly confused, on the floor, or in a different position. The patient may have been incontinent. If an aura was present, the patient will know that a seizure took place.

Objective

The most difficult decision in evaluating a presumed seizure is determining if it was a seizure or another type of condition (such as syncope, a pseudoseizure, or a panic attack). Pseudoseizures are associated with seizure-like symptoms but are not associated with EEG changes. Up to 80% of pseudoseizures are associated with early sexual abuse, especially in females. Not all events associated with abnormal body movements are seizures. Some events may be mistaken for seizures on initial presentation but must be differentiated from them because their treatment is different. Careful and detailed history taking remains the cornerstone of accurate diagnosis of a seizure disorder. A diagnosis of seizure disorder is primarily a historical diagnosis; the initial assessment and approach to management is based on the patient's clinical history, especially on an accurate description of the event in question. Psychogenic nonepileptic seizures (PNES) are sometimes referred to as pseudoseizures, but that is not the case. PNES are similar to epileptic seizures but arise from psychological disturbances rather than abnormal electrical brain activity. They are most common in women aged 15 to 35 but may affect men.

It is often very useful to ask the patient for a description of specific attacks. This should include the last attack actually witnessed, as well as the first seizure. The setting in which the attacks occurred may be significant for differential diagnosis. A careful review of the events occurring days before the seizure is important. Points of particular interest include relation of events to the sleep–wake cycle. It is important to determine if the seizure was stimulus provoked. Many things can provoke a seizure, such as extensive sleep deprivation or use of stimulants. Questions need to be asked to determine if there is an aura associated with the seizure. The regular presence of an aura indicates that the seizure is probably localized. Obtaining a history of the patient's life, including social, behavioral, and cognitive functioning, as well as a previous health history and family history of seizure disorders or neurological disorders, is crucial. History of postictal behaviors should be elicited—how long did it take to recover to normal function? Other important questions should address any history of neonatal seizures or febrile seizures or history of previous brain injury. The clinician should also ask whether there is a personal or family history of other neurological, mental, or systemic disease.

The physical exam should take into account the interval since the patient's most recent seizure. If the exam is performed within minutes or hours of an attack, the practitioner should look for postictal signs, even of a minor grade. When the examination is performed after some time has elapsed since the last seizure, the practitioner's main objective is to determine whether there are signs of permanent nervous system dysfunction, favoring a diagnosis of symptomatic epilepsy, and if there is evidence of a focal brain lesion. The clinician should look for signs of increased intracranial pressure, although this is rather uncommon. Additional neurological signs of interest include language difficulties and possible

evidence of drug toxicity, such as nystagmus, ataxia, diplopia, or tremor.

An eye and visual examination should aim to detect papilledema and visual field loss associated with focal brain lesions. Ocular motor abnormalities may suggest involvement of the brainstem or floor of the third ventricle. Cranial nerves should be assessed to determine if neurological signs or symptoms are present. The findings on the patient's motor exam should be symmetrical. Weakness could indicate a brain lesion. A cardiovascular exam should also be performed to detect the presence of a heart arrhythmia or murmur, which may suggest a syncopal episode rather than a seizure.

Diagnostic Reasoning
Diagnostic Tests
Initial tests should be done to rule out other nonneurological causes of the seizures. Tests may include complete blood count with differential; blood glucose; serum electrolytes; liver function tests; serum calcium, urinalysis; a drug screen or blood alcohol level, if appropriate; and blood levels to assess target levels if the patient is on antiseizure medications.

Subsequent tests that may lead to the cause of the seizure disorder are EEG, computed tomography scan, or magnetic resonance imaging (MRI); lumbar puncture, if CNS infection is suspected; and ECG, if warranted.

To diagnose PNES, the gold standard is video EEG monitoring. In addition, serum prolactin levels may be drawn within 30 minutes of ictus. The levels will be elevated in generalized tonic-clonic seizures and partial complex seizures, but not in PNES. PNES must be accurately diagnosed because these patients do not require seizure medications, but rather mental health counseling.

Differential Diagnosis
The patient should be reevaluated to confirm the diagnosis and to exclude others in several situations. If the attacks are uncontrolled despite rigorous treatment and if the diagnosis of a seizure disorder has never been supported by EEG or other tests, review and repeat testing are indicated. Drug-seeking behavior, dramatic presentations with multiple attacks in public, and repeated visits to the emergency department should also invite skepticism. Common disorders such as migraine, panic attacks, and sleep apnea can develop in addition to a seizure disorder. Additional differential diagnoses are included in Differential Diagnosis Flowchart 6.6.

Management
The main principle of seizure management is to prevent the recurrence of seizures with anticonvulsant medications while avoiding adverse effects from the drugs. The clinician should refer the patient to a neurologist, who should make the decision to start treatment after a complete review of the risk of further seizures is discussed

Differential Diagnosis Flowchart 6.6

Seizure Disorders

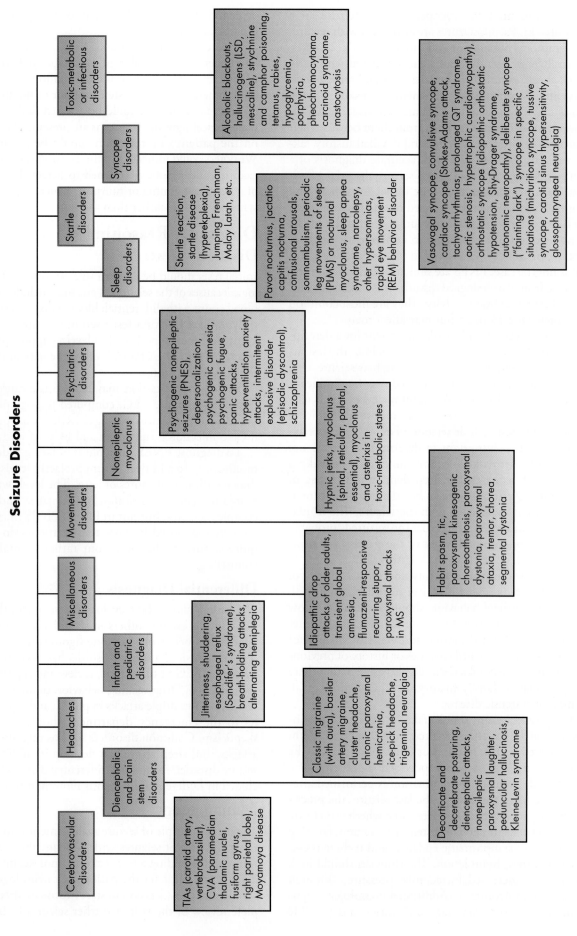

with the patient. Before initiating treatment, the type of seizure the patient experiences should be identified and classified accordingly. Typically, treatment for a single, isolated seizure episode is the identification and treatment of the underlying disorder. Antiepileptic therapy is usually not required unless the patient experiences recurrent seizure activity or a largely resistant/irreversible underlying disorder is revealed. Some structural lesions are clearly associated with recurrent seizures. These include brain tumor and arteriovenous malformation (AVM). When these conditions are diagnosed after a single seizure, there should be no hesitation in initiating pharmacological treatment; however, a much more common situation is the one in which the initial evaluation fails to reveal a specific causative factor for the seizure. Then the neurologist must carefully evaluate the risk of subsequent seizures. The choice of antiepileptic therapy must oftentimes be individualized for each patient. Choice of therapy is contingent on comorbid conditions, medication interactions, adverse side effects, patient age, and type of seizure.

Some patients have only one seizure. For these patients, the probability of a second seizure is less than 10% in the first year following the seizure and approximately 24% by the end of 2 years after the first seizure. The impact of a second seizure depends on the patient's lifestyle. Treatment may be indicated for patients who need to be able to drive or for those who face significant risk of injury or loss of self-esteem from a second seizure. The risk of recurrence is greatest in the first 2 years, so if treatment is initiated, it probably can be halted after this highest-risk period passes.

If the decision to treat is made, accurate identification of the seizure type is very helpful in choosing the drug for the best outcome. Drugs Commonly Prescribed 6.1: Seizures presents suggested medications based on the different types of seizures. Although only the first-line medications are listed, there are many drugs given in combination with these medications. Lacosamide (Vimpat) is one of these adjunctive medications used for added partial-onset seizure control. Others are not included here because a patient will initially be prescribed medications by the neurologist. Some neurologists choose to begin long-term therapy with anticonvulsant medications after a single seizure in the following situations: if the single seizure is rapidly followed by a second seizure; if an MRI or EEG shows evidence of a structural lesion such as a brain tumor, AVM, or infection; if there is a history of a seizure disorder in a sibling; or if there is a history of a brain injury or stroke.

Once the appropriate drug has been chosen based on the seizure type, serum levels should be assessed for baseline hematological and hepatic parameters. Blood levels should be checked two to three times in the first 6 months of therapy to determine if target levels have been attained and are being maintained.

Partial Seizures

The patient may resemble an intoxicated or drugged person. He or she may stare without focusing or speaking, appear to be fidgeting, make chewing movements, or smack the lips.

During the seizure:
- Do not attempt to restrain the patient.
- Gently move the patient away from dangerous objects.

After the seizure:
- Stay with the patient until the patient is fully alert.
- Reassure others that the behavior was medically caused.

Generalized Seizures

The patient may have a warning sign, cry out or scream, then fall down and rhythmically jerk arms and legs in a strong movement that cannot be stopped.

Before or during the seizure:
- Remove the patient's glasses (if wearing) and help the patient lie down in a prone position, but do not restrain.
- Clear the area of dangerous objects.
- Loosen tight clothing around the patient's neck.
- Do not force any object into the patient's mouth.

After the seizure:
- Turn the patient to one side to allow the patient's mouth to drain.
- Stay with the patient until he or she is fully awake.
- If the patient has a known seizure disorder, it is not necessary to call for medical help unless an injury has occurred, the seizure lasts longer than 3 minutes, a second seizure occurs, or the patient requests help.

Follow-up and Referral

If the seizures are controlled and blood levels are adequate, the clinician can monitor them every 6 months (twice each year) for the duration of treatment. If the seizures are not controlled with adequate doses and levels of the medication, the clinician should refer the patient to a neurologist for a second opinion and possible combination therapy.

Patient Education

Education about seizure disorders can provide the patient with understanding and a sense of control over the illness. It is necessary to recognize that to the affected individual, this condition is more than seizures. The patient and his or her family may be overwhelmed by thoughts of disability and impaired quality of life. Such factors as age at onset, duration of seizure activity, frequency, seizure type, associated neurological abnormalities, and associated environmental factors contribute to the degree of disability in each patient. Education is ongoing and should be constantly reinforced. Patients and their families should be referred to seizure literature

Drugs Commonly Prescribed 6.1   Seizures

Drug	Indication	Adverse Reactions and Prescribing Considerations
valproic acid (Depakene)	Absence seizures (petit mal) and myoclonic seizures	Optimum drug level is 50–100 mcg/mL.
divalproex sodium (Depakote)		Take with food. May cause headache, unsteadiness, blood dyscrasias, urticaria.
clonazepam (Klonopin)		Optimum drug level is 20–80 mg/mL. Potentiates CNS depression with alcohol.
phenytoin (Dilantin)	Partial or generalized seizures	Optimum drug level is 10–20 mcg/mL. May cause ataxia, blood dyscrasias, peripheral neuropathy.
topiramate (Topamax)		May cause hyponatremia, weight loss, mental fuzziness, stimulation.
carbamazepine (Tegretol)		May cause dysarthria, ataxia; may exacerbate myoclonic seizures, hyponatremia.
valproic acid		May take with food. May cause nausea and vomiting, indigestion, diarrhea, anorexia, depression, transient hair loss.
phenobarbital (Luminal)		Do not take when pregnant or breastfeeding. May decrease effectiveness of beta-adrenergic blockers, corticosteroids, digoxin, oral contraceptives, warfarin. May cause agitated mood, confusion, low blood pressure, nausea and vomiting.
primidone (Mysoline)		May cause sedation, nystagmus, irritability, megaloblastic anemia.
oxcarbazepine (Trileptal)	Partial seizures	Potentiates CNS depression with alcohol. Potentiates action of phenobarbital and phenytoin, ataxia, fatigue, gastrointestinal upset.

available through the Epilepsy Foundation of America as soon as they are diagnosed, because the well-informed patient is the best advocate for his or her own care. Using the *Circle of Caring* model and coming to know the patient and what matters most to him or her will assist in helping the patient reach his or her highest potential.

A patient with a seizure disorder lives with the fear that a seizure may strike at any moment. Persons with a seizure disorder fear dying during a seizure. They also fear personal injury. This fear is justified; therefore, health-care providers need to counsel patients regarding commonsense safety issues. Persons with a seizure disorder should take showers instead of baths and only when someone else is home. Automatic safety devices that adjust water temperature and shut off water when the shower drain is blocked can be installed. Persons with a seizure disorder should use an occupied sign on the bathroom door rather than locking it. They should swim only with a buddy who is aware of their diagnosis and knows what to do if a seizure occurs while the individual is swimming. When cooking, patients should be instructed to use the microwave or back burners on the stove and keep pot handles turned inward. They should be encouraged not to smoke, but if they must, they should never smoke when alone. Their home should be evaluated to identify any safety hazards and to develop a risk-reduction plan. Families, friends, and coworkers need to be taught what to do in case of a seizure.

Patients with a seizure disorder and their caregivers should be apprised of the risks of harm. In comparison with the general population, children and adolescents with seizure disorders have a 1,000-fold greater risk of drowning during bathing and a 70-fold greater risk of drowning while swimming. Burns tend to occur in the home and are most commonly associated with cooking, showering, and use of space heaters. Driving needs to be discussed at length. The loss of driving privilege is very serious because it restricts a patient's mobility and, therefore, independence. Each state has different laws governing the granting of driver's licenses for individuals with a seizure disorder. At the federal level, the U.S. Department of Transportation has regulations that bar anyone with a history of seizures from being licensed to drive in interstate trucking. The purpose of the driving restrictions is obvious—to protect the public. Although only six states require health-care providers to report patients who have been diagnosed with seizure disorder, all practitioners have the responsibility to advise their patients of the medical risks, legal requirements, and recommendations regarding driving. Educational and support materials are available through the Epilepsy Foundation of America.

DEGENERATIVE DISORDERS

■ AMYOTROPHIC LATERAL SCLEROSIS (LOU GEHRIG'S DISEASE)

Amyotrophic lateral sclerosis (ALS) is a progressive neurological disorder that involves destruction of the anterior horn motor cell in the spinal cord or the brainstem. The etiology is not known. It is universally fatal, though the duration of the disease is usually 5 to 6 years. If it begins with brainstem involvement, there is usually a problem with aspiration, and the course is more rapid.

Unlike in multiple sclerosis, the symptoms of ALS are symmetrical. Most commonly, it presents with a simple gait disturbance caused by weakness or a change in voice. The diagnosis is made via electromyographical studies. There is no treatment for ALS.

■ MULTIPLE SCLEROSIS

Multiple sclerosis (MS) is a chronic, potentially disabling, and demyelinating disease of the CNS that begins most commonly in young adulthood and is most frequently associated with periods of visual changes, intermittent weakness and numbness, and loss of balance. These may occur intermittently, with relapses and remissions, or may be progressive. MS is the most common cause of disability in young adults. Multiple areas of CNS or white matter inflammation, demyelination, and glial scarring or gliosis characterize MS. MS is thought to be a disorder of the T and B lymphocytes that creates an abnormal antibody that invades the CNS and attacks the myelin. There is no known cause for this change.

There are four types of MS, each with its own course and progression. The *relapsing–remitting* type of MS is characterized by acute attacks, with either a full recovery or some residual deficits between episodes. The *primary progressive* type of MS has a steady disease progression, with possibly some plateaus and remissions. *Secondary progressive* MS is a combination of the first two types, beginning as a relapsing–remitting disease but then slowly acquiring the primary progressive characteristics. The *progressive–relapsing* type of MS is a progression of the disease (including relapses and remissions, with or without recovery) on a steady downhill course, compared with the relapsing–remitting variety, in which the disease progression may stop at any point.

The clinical course of MS varies. Prognosis is a common concern. Although there are no definitive prognostic indicators, the following are general guidelines. Good prognostic indicators include minimal disability after 5 years of onset, complete and rapid remission of initial symptoms, onset at age 35 or younger, only one symptom during first year, acute onset of the first symptoms, brief duration of most recent exacerbation, long first remission, optic neuritis, or sensory symptoms. Poor prognostic indicators include late onset, chronic progressive course, motor symptoms, polysymptomatic onset, and vertigo. Patients are concerned about disability. After 15 years, 50% to 60% of patients with MS remain ambulatory, 10% to 20% need assistance devices to ambulate, and 15% to 30% are bedridden.

Epidemiology and Causes

MS occurs worldwide, but there are differences in both incidence and prevalence on the basis of race, sex, genetics, geographical location, and age at the time of probable exposure to a virus or other infectious agent. MS is most commonly diagnosed between ages 20 and 50. The first symptoms of the disease usually occur between ages 20 and 40. If the disease is diagnosed after age 50, it tends to have a more progressive course. The disease affects two to three times more women than men. It is more common among Caucasians and people of northern or central European descent. Asians and Africans/persons of African descent are at lower risk.

Some epidemiological findings suggest a relationship between MS and an unknown environmental factor, possibly a viral exposure during childhood. This exposure may lead to the entry of immune cells into the CNS, where a population of T cells becomes sensitized to a CNS antigen. After years of latency, an environmental trigger may lead to an upregulation of circulating mediators or T-cell activation that may set off an episode of demyelination and clinical disease.

The cause of MS is unknown. There are many theories on possible causes, including genetic susceptibility, autoimmune mechanisms, viral infections, and environmental factors. One leading hypothesis is that of a cell-mediated immunopathological response directed against myelin in genetically predisposed persons.

Studies have suggested that susceptibility to MS is inherited. The higher incidence in twins and in certain families provides support for this genetic susceptibility. The major histocompatibility complex on chromosome 6 has been identified as one genetic determinant for MS. Although genetic factors may contribute to an individual's susceptibility, they are neither sufficient nor necessary for development of MS. Clinical expression of the disease is likely to require additional exposure to one or more environmental factors, which are as yet undefined.

There is evidence of autoimmune mechanisms in the pathogenesis of MS. In a normal immune response, foreign antibodies are processed and presented to T-cell helpers by antigen-presenting cells and macrophages. These T-helper cells recognize foreign peptides bound to major histocompatibility complex (MHC) molecules, become activated, and release various cytokines, tumor necrosis factor, and interleukins that augment the immune response to a particular antigen. These particular class II MHC molecules are usually found only on cells involved in an immune response. In MS, class II MHC induction has been shown to occur in CNS tissue. In peripheral blood of patients with MS, several nonspecific changes are seen that are similar to those in other autoimmune diseases. Suppressor T lymphocytes are decreased in both function and number. Excessive immunoglobulin is present, especially high levels of immunoglobulin G (IgG). Suppressor cell inducers are decreased in many patients with progressive disease.

Pathophysiology

MS is a disease of the CNS stemming from the progressive patchy demyelination of axons. In MS, local immune reactions destroy CNS myelin and cause the death of oligodendrocytes. Astrocytes react to these injuries by proliferating. At the same time, many of the axons remain intact.

MS is most commonly characterized by neurological problems that periodically flare up and then abate. The symptoms reflect repeated episodes of demyelination in new parts of the white matter throughout the CNS. The specific neurological deficits of an MS patient depend on the regions of the CNS that have been affected. For example, lesions in the optic nerve produce blindness, lesions in the corticospinal tracts produce weakness or paralysis, lesions in the posterior columns produce unusual sensations or numbness, lesions in the medial longitudinal fasciculus produce double vision, and lesions in the vestibular pathways produce dizziness.

Areas of MS damage form sharply defined plaques, which are typically found around venules. MS plaques tend to be large (greater than 6 mm in diameter) and oval shaped; over time, the plaques become more and more widely distributed. Newly forming plaques, in which demyelination is not yet complete, are filled with lymphocytes, plasma cells, and macrophages. Older plaques have no myelin in their centers and contain only fibrous astrocytes and unmyelinated axons. Axon damage inevitably follows, but this appears to be a secondary phenomenon and occurs slowly. Between the plaques, myelin is also affected, although here the damage is not as dramatic.

MS plaques are the result of immune reactions, and the state of the disease is reflected in the immune indicators in the cerebrospinal fluid (CSF). When the disease flares up, the CSF has an increased number of lymphocytes (although usually less than 50/mcL). The CSF will also contain elevated levels of immunoglobulins, the majority of which are IgGs. As MS progresses, specific oligoclonal bands are found in the CSF, regardless of the current state of the disease symptoms.

It is likely that MS is an autoimmune disease, but the triggers for the immune destruction of myelin are unclear. Evidence suggests that genetically susceptible individuals develop the disease many years after exposure to certain environmental factors. One hypothesis is that these factors are viruses that happen to consist of molecules with shapes similar to regions of certain myelin molecules. Alternatively, the initial trigger may be a less specific infection that causes leakage in the blood–brain barrier and thus sensitizes peripheral lymphocytes to normal but previously unseen CNS myelin antigens.

Clinical Presentation
Subjective

The most common presenting symptoms in MS include sensory disturbances of the extremities, spasticity and weakness of legs, bladder and bowel dysfunction, ataxic gait, paresthesias in the extremities, fatigue, optic neuritis, and trigeminal neuralgia. Seventy-five percent to 95% of patients with MS experience MS-related fatigue. Exacerbations and remissions occur frequently, and signs and symptoms may indicate more than one lesion. The clinical course is variable and usually occurs in two phases, relapsing–remitting and chronic progressive. In the early phase, the patient presents with symptoms that may last from days to months and may disappear abruptly. The initial symptom is often blurred or double vision, red-green color distortion, or sometimes even blindness in one eye. The next most common complaints are speech impediments, tremors, and dizziness. The patient most often presents with the same chief complaint during the exacerbation, but some of the events will involve new symptoms. After several years, many patients enter the chronic progressive phase of MS, with a mean time from onset of the initial symptom to this phase from 6 to 7 years. In approximately 20% of patients, the disease begins in this phase; 50% of patients enter the phase within 10 years.

Objective

Clinical manifestations of MS may be transient. The patient may experience unusual sensations and have difficulty describing these. Signs and symptoms may be diverse and appear to include all the symptoms that can occur from injury to any part of the spinal cord and cerebral cortex. Symptoms tend to vary in nature and severity. Frequently, complete remission of the first symptoms occurs, but with subsequent attacks, remissions are incomplete or do not occur. The clinical manifestations depend on the areas of the CNS involved. The brainstem, spinal cord, optic chiasm, and cerebellum are common locations.

The clinician should assess the patient for common visual symptoms, including diplopia, blurred vision, diminution or loss of visual acuity unilaterally or bilaterally, and visual field defects. These symptoms may begin to manifest over a period of hours to days. Involvement of the fifth cranial nerve causes pain sensation, impairment, and diminished or lost corneal reflex. The diagnosis of MS should be considered whenever a young adult develops trigeminal neuralgia.

Limb weakness is a common sign of MS, presenting as monoparesis, hemiparesis, or tetraparesis. Fatigue out of proportion to muscle weakness is common. Fatigue may be persistent or related to physical activity or mental exertion. Fatigue interferes with ADLs in 75% of patients with MS. There may be concomitant ataxia and spasticity. Cerebellar involvement causes dysarthria, scanning speech, tremor, gait ataxia, and incoordination of limbs and trunk. Spasticity limits activities, and leg stiffness may interfere with walking or transferring. In patients with severe spasticity, there may be extensor or flexor spasms either spontaneously or on attempted movement. Spasticity may cause pain, interfere with sleep, or prevent movement.

Bladder symptoms are common, including incontinence and frequency or urgency. Patients may have a small-capacity, spastic bladder or a large, flaccid bladder with overflow incontinence. Loss of libido and erectile dysfunction are common in men with MS; in women with MS, sexual dysfunction most commonly involves lack of lubrication and failure to reach orgasm. Although bowel symptoms are uncommon, constipation may occur.

Sensory impairment and paresthesias are common. Patients may complain of tingling or numbness in the face, limbs, or trunk. A sensation of "electricity" down the back after passive or active neck flexion is called Lhermitte's sign and is indicative of a lesion in the posterior column in the cervical spinal cord. Pain is also recognized as a symptom of MS. Pain may be associated with trigeminal neuralgia, flexor–extensor spasms, tonic spasms of the limbs, and local pain syndromes such as constricting pain around a limb, burning pain, pseudoradicular pain, foreign body sensation, headache, neuralgic pain, and pain caused by pressure sores.

Patients may experience depression, euphoria, subtle aphasic manifestations, or cognitive changes. Patients may have difficulty with tasks that require processing new information rapidly, recalling newly acquired knowledge, and problem-solving. Attention deficits may be present early in MS, even before the onset of physical symptoms. In general, the longer the history of MS, the greater the attention impairment. Memory and abstract reasoning may be affected, as well as the capacity to direct attention (CDA). CDA is critical to the management of a chronic illness, and a strong CDA is necessary to learn new information, implement therapeutic self-care, and handle necessary and difficult adjustments in daily life.

Diagnostic Reasoning
Diagnostic Tests

There is no specific test for MS. The diagnosis must be based on multiple signs and symptoms with a history of remissions and exacerbations. The diagnosis is also based on the ability to demonstrate, on the basis of patient history, neurological examination, and diagnostic tests, the existence of lesions involving different parts of the CNS. An initial clinical neurological examination focused on the patient's signs and symptoms is necessary. Tests should be done to assess for increased muscle tone in legs, decreased motor strength, changes in visual acuity, bilateral clonus of ankles and knees, positive Babinski's sign, and a decreased appreciation of vibration or position sense in arms and legs. There are several instruments available to assess functional status. The Mini–Mental State Exam (MMSE) may be administered to screen for global and focal cognitive impairment.

For a diagnosis of MS to be made, two or more parts of the CNS must be involved, and signs of MS must consist predominantly of dysfunction of the optic nerve (affecting vision) or dysfunction of the corticobulbar system (affecting speech, swallowing), the corticospinal system (affecting strength), the cerebellar system (affecting gait, coordination), the medial longitudinal fasciculus system (affecting internuclear ophthalmoplegia, with diplopia and nystagmus), the spinocerebellar system (affecting balance), and the long-tract sensory system (causing position and vibratory disturbances). In addition, CNS involvement must occur in one of the following patterns: two or more episodes of exacerbations, separated by 1 month or longer and lasting more than 24 hours, with subsequent recovery (i.e., relapsing–remitting MS); a slow or stepwise progression of signs and symptoms over a period of at least 6 months (i.e., primary progressive MS); a clinical history of clearly defined exacerbations and remissions, with or without complete recovery, followed by a slow progression of signs and symptoms over a period of at least 6 months (i.e., secondary progressive MS); progression in signs and symptoms and occasional attacks (i.e., progressive relapsing MS); or no relapse or progression of attacks in the past 18 months (i.e., stable MS).

A lumbar puncture with an evaluation of CSF for the presence of immunoglobulins, lymphocytes, and oligoclonal IgG bands may provide supportive data for a diagnosis of MS. Immunoglobulin synthesis within the CSF can be expressed by formulas that adjust for passive transfer of proteins across a damaged blood–brain barrier. Oligoclonal IgG bands can be detected by electrophoresis of CSF and are present in the CSF of 90% of patients with MS, but this finding is not specific to MS. An increase in CSF basic myelin protein may confirm that an acute MS exacerbation has occurred. Elevated values (greater than 9 ng/mL) suggest demyelination.

Cortical-evoked responses or evoked potentials are of value in demonstrating clinically unsuspected lesions. Visual responses are abnormal in 75% to 97% of patients with MS. Somatosensory responses are abnormal in 72% to 87%, and brainstem responses are abnormal in 50% to 70% of patients with MS.

Magnetic resonance imaging (MRI) is a sensitive, objective measure of plaques and is used to measure the outcomes of treatment. Periodic recording of the volume and number of lesions detected in the brain by MRI can assist the clinician in monitoring the extent of the disease. Pathologically, areas of contrast enhancement observed by MRI correlate with active perivascular inflammatory damage. In addition, the MRI should be obtained as soon as possible in all patients presenting with an isolated demyelinating syndrome involving the CNS to exclude other possible neurological conditions (Level I; Filippi et al, 2011).

A clinically definitive diagnosis of MS requires either (1) evidence from history of two episodes at least 1 month apart, signs of one lesion on examination, and evidence from evoked responses or MRI of other lesions or (2) evidence from both history and neurological exam of more than one lesion. A laboratory-supported definitive diagnosis of MS requires evidence from two lesions in either history or neurological exam. If only one lesion is evident on examination or history, at least one more lesion must be evident in MRI or evoked response testing. The CSF IgG pattern and content should also be abnormal. A clinically probable diagnosis of MS requires that either history or examination, but not both, provides evidence of more than one lesion. If only one lesion is evident by history or neurological exam, MRI or evoked responses may provide evidence of additional lesions. If the collaborating neurologist is uncertain of the MS diagnosis, reevaluation of the patient may be needed.

Differential Diagnosis

Other CNS diseases may resemble MS clinically or radiologically. These are lymphomas and gliomas of the hemispheres, spinal cord, and brainstem; collagen vascular disease such as systemic lupus erythematosus (SLE); human T-cell lymphotrophic virus type I (HTLV-I); HIV infection; encephalopathy; Lyme disease; peripheral neuropathy; Behçet's disease; and sarcoidosis.

It is important to consider Lyme disease as a differential diagnosis because chronic CNS infection with *Borrelia burgdorferi* can cause spastic paraparesis, cerebellar signs, and cranial nerve palsies. Patients with Lyme disease will have a history of erythema migrans plus arthralgias or evidence of cardiac manifestations, as well as positive Lyme titers.

Patients with SLE will have a positive antinuclear antibody and anti-DNA antibody titers, as well as joint or renal involvement.

Patients with suspected MS should be tested for HIV, HTLV-I, and syphilis (human T-cell lymphoma virus) because these diseases may mimic MS. Vascular disease, tumors of the brain and spinal cord, arteriovenous malformations, and arachnoid cysts may have relapsing and remitting signs that mimic MS. MRI is usually the definitive test to rule out these causes.

Management

The principles of management include three major goals: to delay the progression of the disease, manage chronic symptoms, and treat acute exacerbations. There is no known cure for MS. Therapeutic regimens are either disease specific or symptomatic (immunosuppressive or immunomodulatory). Disease-modifying therapy should be considered early in the course of treatment, before neurological deficits have persisted for more than 6 months. Treatment decisions on individual patients should be made based on both the probability of severely disabling disease and the course of disease. Follow-up should be based on progression of disease and the treatment of symptoms and exacerbations. See Drugs Commonly Prescribed 6.2: Multiple Sclerosis.

Glucocorticoids are the mainstay of treatment for acute exacerbations. Glucocorticoids have both immunomodulatory and anti-inflammatory effects, which restore the blood–brain barrier, decrease edema, and may improve axonal conduction. The decision of whether or not to treat an acute exacerbation depends on the functional limitations of the patient, the level of patient discomfort, and objective evidence of neurological dysfunction such as profound weakness/motor dysfunction, visual disturbances, or cerebellar dysfunction. If symptoms of an exacerbation are severe enough to require treatment, IV methylprednisolone (Depo-Medrol) with or without an oral prednisone taper is administered. In sudden, severe exacerbations that do not respond to glucocorticoid therapy, the use of plasma exchange therapy may provide a benefit to patients and should be considered in refractory severe relapsing forms of MS.

Patients with relapsing–remitting MS benefit from early aggressive treatment with disease-modifying agents. The initial treatment of choice for patients with relapsing–remitting MS is either interferon 1a, interferon 1b, or glatiramer acetate. These agents have proved to be equally efficacious in the treatment of relapsing–remitting MS. Interferons are a class of cytokine that halts disease progression and inhibits the accumulation of inflammatory lesions in the CNS white matter as evidenced by MRI; interferons also reduce the number and severity of clinical relapses. Glatiramer acetate is essentially a polymer composed of four amino acid units found in myelin basic protein. It is thought to act as an

Drugs Commonly Prescribed 6.2   Multiple Sclerosis (MS)

Drug	Indication	Adverse Reactions and Prescribing Considerations
methylprednisolone (Depo-Medrol)	Exacerbation	Masks infection. Adverse effects: glaucoma, cataracts, secondary infections, hypokalemia, hypocalcemia, hypernatremia, hypertension, psychotic disorders, myopathy, osteoporosis, peptic ulcer, dermal atrophy, increased intracranial pressure, carbohydrate intolerance.
prednisolone (Deltasone)	Taper after IV therapy	As above.
interferon beta, interferon 1a (Avonex)	Relapsing–remitting MS	Adverse effects: flulike symptoms for 24–48 hours after injection (subsides after 2–3 months); treat with acetaminophen or NSAIDs.
interferon 1b (Betaseron)	Relapsing–remitting MS	As above.
azathioprine (Imuran)	Depression of cell-mediated and humoral immunity	May reduce rate of relapse; has no effect on progression of disability.
glatiramer acetate (Copaxone)	Relapsing–remitting MS resistance to interferon beta–neutralizing antibodies	Adverse effects: reaction at injection site, flushing, sweating, shortness of breath, palpitations, chest tightness, anxiety.
methotrexate (Rheumatrex)	Progressive MS	Do not give in chronic liver disease, pregnancy or nursing women, or in the presence of blood dyscrasias.
baclofen (Lioresal)	Symptomatic treatment for spasticity	May cause drowsiness and confusion.
tizanidine (Zanaflex)	Spasticity	May cause drowsiness. Do not use with clonidine (Catapres).
dantrolene (Dantrium)	Spasticity	Use with caution in patients with impaired hepatic, pulmonary, cardiac function.
diazepam (Valium)	Spasticity	Contraindicated with acute narrow-angle glaucoma; potential for abuse.
carbamazepine (Tegretol)	Tremors	Take with food; use with caution in patients with history of cardiac, hepatic, renal, or hematopoietic dysfunction.
natalizumab (Tysabri)	Relapsing–remitting MS	Monitor for progressive multifocal leukoencephalopathy.
clonazepam (Klonopin)	Tremors	Contraindicated with liver disease or acute narrow-angle glaucoma; withdraw gradually; potential for abuse.
primidone (Mysoline)	Tremors	Potentiated with alcohol and other CNS depressants; antagonizes oral anticoagulants, contraceptives, and steroids.

immunological decoy by diverting the autoimmune response away from the natural host. Other potential mechanisms include the activation of immunosuppressive regulatory Th2 cells that may effectively repress the immuno-inflammatory response.

Physicians who prescribe these medications must be thoroughly familiar with dosage, possible adverse effects, and management of those adverse effects. Patients must be taught the adverse effects, injection techniques, storage, and care of the medications. Once appropriate drug therapy has been stabilized, the clinician may monitor the patient as described under Follow-up and Referral later.

Two types of antibodies occur in patients treated with interferons: binding antibodies and neutralizing antibodies (NAbs). Binding antibodies develop at some time in 97% of treated patients and are measured by enzyme-linked immunosorbent assay (ELISA) or the Western blot technique. Many of these antibodies do not impair therapeutic effectiveness and have no known function. NAbs are formed in a minority of treated patients but are capable of reducing or abrogating the normal biological treatment effects of interferons. They are measured via a viral cytopathic effect reduction assay. There is no evidence that NAb-positive patients fare significantly worse than placebo-treated patients.

Natalizumab (Tysabri) is an effective agent in the treatment of relapsing–remitting MS; however, it is generally used only for patients whose disease course is refractory to interferons and glatiramer acetate due to the rare risk of fatal progressive multifocal leukoencephalopathy. Natalizumab administered IV monthly prevents the migration of T lymphocytes across the blood–brain barrier.

Treatment for progressive forms of MS has been less favorable to date. An assortment of prospective clinical trials have demonstrated limited efficacy with a host of treatments including pulse glucocorticoid therapy, methotrexate, cyclophosphamide, and cladribine. Further study is required before definite clinical recommendations can be made on the use of these therapies.

Symptomatic management and therapy are important in MS. Spasticity is a major cause of disability in 55% of patients with MS. Antispasmodics are listed in Drugs Commonly Prescribed 6.2. If other noninvasive therapeutic measures for spasticity have failed, the patient may be referred to a neurosurgeon for evaluation as a candidate for an implantable drug infusion pump to administer baclofen (Lioresal) intrathecally. This is highly effective because the drug can cross the blood–brain barrier. Adverse effects are minimal, and a test dose is administered intrathecally before implantation as part of the screening process for candidates.

Selective chemodenervation may be beneficial for localized spasticity in a single muscle or limb. This may be accomplished through administration of botulin (Clostridium botulinum) toxin type A (Botox). Only a specialist familiar with the use, adverse effects, and injection sites for botulinum toxin should administer this medication.

The tremors associated with MS are usually cerebellar outflow tremors. Medications recommended for the treatment of tremor are included in Drugs Commonly Prescribed 6.2.

Fatigue is a common problem in patients with MS. The existence of sleep apnea, pain, spasms, restless legs syndrome, ability to sleep, and pattern of sleep should all be investigated. Other medical problems that may cause fatigue should be excluded. Patients should be instructed to take a daytime nap and remain in a cool environment and should be educated in energy conservation techniques. A referral for occupational therapy may be beneficial for this.

Many patients with MS experience pain in the form of unpleasant sensations or overt pain. This pain can assume many forms, and the cause of new pain should be established. Acute pain includes trigeminal neuralgia, Lhermitte's sign, paroxysmal burning, extremity pain, and painful tonic spasms. Acute pain may be treated with carbamazepine (Tegretol), phenytoin (Dilantin), or valproate (Depakote). Chronic pain includes dysesthetic pain in extremities, chronic back pain, and painful leg spasms. Amitriptyline (Elavil), carbamazepine, and phenytoin may be given for chronic pain.

Providers should be aware of issues relating to complementary therapies that may be raised by patients with MS. These therapies have become so widely used that the National Institutes of Health has established an Office of Alternative Medicine that deals with therapies for all kinds of conditions. The following are frequently used complementary therapies for patients with MS: acupuncture, hypnotherapy and imagery, massage, biofeedback, tai chi, and chiropractic therapy. If referring a patient with MS to complementary therapy providers, it is important to suggest those who have an understanding of MS.

Follow-up and Referral

Follow-up and referral should occur soon after diagnosis and should be repeated initially at monthly intervals or more often as symptoms appear to assess level of functioning and effectiveness of medications, and to make dosage adjustments if needed. The patient should be instructed to contact the advanced practice registered nurse immediately for the appearance of symptoms that may signal an exacerbation. Referral to a neurosurgeon may be necessary for extreme spasticity.

Patient Education

Patients should be educated in all aspects of the disease, medications, adverse effects, complications, progression, fatigue management, pain management, diet, and exercise. The weakness that results from MS may be amenable to strengthening exercises. ROM exercise is important to prevent contractures and joint restriction. Referral to a physical therapist who has experience in the treatment of patients with MS may be beneficial. Regular exercise may change the course of the patient's response to illness by minimizing the deconditioning process and maintaining optimal levels of physical activity and functioning. The beneficial effects of prolonged activity are well documented; it can help prevent muscular atrophy and weakness, fatigue, loss of flexibility, cardiovascular deficits, depression, and sleep disturbances. It is important to balance activity and exercise to prevent fatigue. There is no conclusive scientific evidence that any diet or nutritional therapy affects the course of MS. Many of the diets available are not harmful but may be tiring because of the attention to detail required, while offering no benefit. A generally well-balanced diet is recommended.

Patients who have been diagnosed with MS may experience a wide range of emotions ranging from euphoria to depression, including helplessness, lack of hope, mental confusion, stress, and anxiety. These emotions can affect marital relationships and increase child-rearing stress. The chronic nature of MS and the inability to predict level of dysfunction contribute to difficulty in coping with chronic illness and symptoms disruptive to daily living. Patients may also experience job loss, embarrassment, exhaustion, and the feeling of making no contribution to society. It is important to teach patients health promotion behaviors to emphasize emotional and social well-being.

Patients and families should also be educated in coping with possible behavior changes and mood swings. Patients with MS have reported feelings of hopelessness, loss of control, conflict, fear, loss, and uncertainty. Education in the management of problems related to sexual dysfunction may also need to be addressed. Caregivers should be educated not to neglect their own health because coping with a chronic illness may change and stress the dynamics both within a family and within other individual relationships.

■ PARKINSON'S DISEASE

Parkinson's disease (PD) is a chronic, progressive, degenerative disorder of the basal ganglia in the CNS. The disease usually begins insidiously and eventually leads to disability. PD is the second most common neurodegenerative disorder in the elderly after Alzheimer's disease. Affecting 1% of the population older than age 50, there are approximately 1 million people in the United States suffering from PD, with 60,000 new cases diagnosed each year. It affects people in middle to later life, with a mean age at onset of 57 years. The incidence is slightly greater in men, with a 3:2 ratio of men to women. People in all ethnic groups, all countries, and all socioeconomic classes are affected. The Centers for Disease Control and Prevention's National Center for Health Statistics reports that the complications from PD account for it being the 14th major cause of death in the United States in 2010.

A *parkinsonian syndrome* (parkinsonism) is any disorder that manifests the symptoms of PD. Parkinsonism is divided into four categories: idiopathic, symptomatic, Parkinson-plus syndromes, and other heredodegenerative diseases in which parkinsonism is a manifestation. Patients with idiopathic PD make up the largest subgroup, which represents 78% of the affected population. Symptomatic and Parkinson-plus syndromes are often referred to as secondary parkinsonism when there is a known cause for the disorder such as cerebrovascular disease, drugs, infections, trauma, or exposure to toxins. Parkinsonian syndromes include heredodegenerative disorders such as Huntington's disease and other acquired degenerative diseases.

Epidemiology and Causes

The cause of PD is unknown. The pathogenesis is thought to be multifactorial, resulting from a combination of genetic predisposition, exogenous toxins, and endogenous toxins. The evidence regarding the role of heredity is conflicting. A positive family history is reported in approximately 15% of cases. It has also been reported that a higher prevalence of familial PD is revealed when an informative history is obtained.

There are many theories regarding the role of environmental factors in the development of PD. One theory has suggested increased vulnerability of "old" (i.e., aging) neurons to environmental toxins. There are also theories that have identified the following factors in the development of PD: drug-induced parkinsonism (antipsychotics, lithium), rural living, infections, exposure to heavy metals, and free radical–oxidative stress. Oxidative mechanisms are believed to be important in the pathogenesis of PD. In a normal individual, oxidative stress is balanced by antioxidative protective mechanisms naturally occurring in the brain. In patients with PD, the balance is thought to be tilted toward the oxidative stress side. Other influences, including drinking well water, farming, and industrial exposure to heavy metals, have also been associated with increased prevalence of PD.

One man's depiction of being a victim of Parkinson's disease. (Illustration by Christine Sanders.)

The role of normal aging needs to be considered. During aging, pathways lose neurons. Aging is also associated with a loss of catecholamine-containing neurons and an increase in monoamine oxidase (MAO) types A and B. In addition, there is a progressive loss of more than 60% of the dopaminergic neurons in the substantia nigra. This normal process begins at approximately age 30. There is also a decline in the striatal concentration of dopamine, an increase in the turnover of striatal dopamine, and a loss of striatal D_2 receptors. Compensatory mechanisms are thought to be responsible for the absence of PD until striatal dopamine concentrations drop below 20% of normal. The morbidity and mortality rate for PD is high; an estimated 9% of patients become disabled or die within 1 to 5 years, 21% in 6 to 10 years, and almost 38% in 11 to 15 years.

Pathophysiology

PD is a degenerative disease of the motor systems of the brain. Its neurological effects include tremor at rest, muscular rigidity, slow movements, and difficulty maintaining a steady posture. Characteristically, the motor problems of PD improve when a patient is treated with levodopa.

In Parkinson's disease, there is progressive cell loss in the substantia nigra. There are major neural connections of the substantia nigra to the basal ganglia. The full basal ganglia complex—the striatum, the globus pallidus, the subthalamic nucleus, and the substantia nigra—comprises a set of interconnected nuclei deep inside the cerebral cortex. The basal ganglia are a critical part of the motor system, with which they interact through the motor nuclei of the thalamus. The main output of the basal ganglia is a GABA-ergic inhibitory circuit from the internal segment of the globus pallidus to the ventral anterior and ventral lateral nuclei of the thalamus. This GABA-ergic circuit is itself inhibited (indirectly) by dopaminergic axons from the substantia nigra. PD depletes the substantia nigra of dopaminergic axons. As a result, the globus pallidus output remains unchecked, resulting in a blanket inhibition of the motor activity passing through the thalamus.

Besides cell loss in the substantia nigra, PD kills dopaminergic neurons in the adjacent ventral tegmental area, noradrenergic neurons in the locus coeruleus and the dorsal and medial raphe nuclei in the brainstem, and cholinergic neurons in the nucleus basalis of Meynert. In the process, PD produces a typical intracellular abnormality called a Lewy body inside degenerating neurons. Lewy bodies are spherical, insoluble clumps of neurofilaments, tubulin, synphilin, alpha-synuclein, and ubiquitin. Ubiquitin is normally used in a major intracellular degradative pathway, and evidence suggests that one metabolic abnormality underlying PD is a selective defect in this particular degradative pathway.

Clinical Presentation

Subjective

Presentation of the disease is variable. The patient may present with one or more of the six cardinal features of PD: tremor at rest, rigidity, bradykinesia or hypokinesia, flexed posture, loss of postural reflexes, and the freezing phenomenon. The major manifestations of tremor, rigidity, akinesia (or bradykinesia), and postural disturbances form the mnemonic "TRAP."

A tremor may be the reason the patient or family is seeking care and is recognized as the first symptom of PD in 70% of patients at initial diagnosis. The tremor almost always appears distally in the extremities when the extremity is motionless and as a result is termed a "resting tremor." This resting tremor disappears with action but reemerges as the limbs maintain a posture. A resting tremor is common in the chin, lips, and tongue. The resting tremor of the hands increases when the patient is walking and may be an early sign of PD before other signs are visible. Stress worsens the tremor, but resting tremors are absent during sleep. A classic presentation of PD is a characteristic motion of the thumb and forefinger called "pill-rolling."

A common subjective complaint in patients with PD is fatigue, which may be related to rigidity or bradykinesia. Progressive bradykinesia may contribute to slowness and difficulty in the performance of ADLs. Patients may also suffer from sleep disturbances, contributing to fatigue. Swallowing may be impaired in advanced disease, causing aspiration and choking.

Objective

The four common manifestations of PD may be objectively observed and evaluated by the clinician: tremor, a weak and clumsy limb, a stiff and aching limb, and a gait disorder. Rigidity is a state of increased resistance in muscle tone elicited when the clinician moves the patient's neck, trunk, or limbs. The muscle feels stiff and is difficult to move. This can appear as though the patient is having difficulty initiating movement. Rigidity is equal in all directions and is usually manifested by "cogwheeling," a ratchet-like, rhythmic contraction, especially in the hand, on passive stretching. Cogwheeling can be caused by an underlying tremor in the absence of a visible tremor. When another limb is engaged in voluntary movement, rigidity of the passive limb increases.

The patient with PD often has a flexed posture that involves the entire body. The head is bowed, the trunk is bent forward, and the back posture is kyphotic. The elbows, hips, and knees are flexed. The hands are held in front of the body. There may be hand deformities, including ulnar deviation (fingers flexed at the metacarpophalangeal joints) and striatal hand (extension of interphalangeal joints). Striatal toe (big toe dorsiflexion) and inversion of the feet may be present, along with a lateral tilting of the trunk.

The most common features of PD are slowness of movement, difficulty initiating movement, loss of automatic movement (bradykinesia), and reduction in the amplitude of movement, particularly with repetitive movement (hypokinesia). Bradykinesia has many facets depending on the body parts affected. In addition, walking is slow; patients have a tendency to shuffle, with a shortened stride length. Truncal bradykinesia causes difficulty when a patient attempts to arise from a deep chair, get out of an automobile, or turn in bed.

Loss of postural reflexes may lead to falling. Some individuals are unable to stand unassisted. As postural reflexes become impaired, the patient will collapse into a chair on attempting to sit. The *freezing phenomenon,* also called "motor block," is the transient inability to perform active movements. Most often, the legs are affected, but it may also involve eyelid opening, speaking, and writing. Freezing is transient and occurs suddenly. It typically occurs when the patient begins to walk (start-hesitation), attempts to turn while walking, or approaches a destination (target-hesitation). The patient may be fearful about the inability to handle perceived barriers such as elevator doors and heavily trafficked streets.

Other common manifestations of PD are drooling as a result of decreased frequency of swallowing, dysphagia secondary to the neuromuscular incoordination of the hypopharyngeal musculature, excessive perspiration as a result of a disorder of the hypothalamic heat-regulating mechanism and impairment of perspiration controls, constipation secondary to hypomotility of the gastrointestinal tract, orthostatic hypotension as a result of deterioration of the peripheral autonomic nervous system, and urinary hesitation secondary to autonomic dysfunction. The patient may also demonstrate a "mask-like" face (hypomimia), soft speech (hypophonia), slurred speech (dysarthria), and small, slow handwriting (micrographia).

The clinician may also perform the *pull test,* in which the examiner stands behind the patient; gives a sudden, firm pull on the patient's shoulders; and checks for retropulsion. Obtaining a specimen of the patient's handwriting and comparing it with previous samples may assist in the diagnosis. Most patients with PD exhibit behavioral changes. Personality changes become apparent as the patient becomes fearful, dependent, and anxious. Passivity, lack of motivation, and decreased attention span are common. There may also be confusion, agitation, hallucinations, and mania related to activation of dopamine receptors in nonstriatal regions. More than 50% of patients with PD experience depression, and this may precede motor symptoms.

Patients with PD commonly experience cognitive decline. The MMSE is a simple means of measuring this impairment. This exam assesses temporal and spatial orientation, digit span, and the ability to express and understand language, to follow commands, and to remember complete simple instructions. The severe type of dementia seen in patients with Alzheimer's disease is exhibited in approximately 15% to 20% of patients with PD.

The patient may be slow to answer questions and may be unable to change mental set rapidly. There may also be sensory and autonomic dysfunctions such as pain, burning, and tingling. The patient may report that these sensations diminish or disappear on moving. Autonomic dysfunctions such as cool skin, constipation, inadequate bladder emptying, difficulty in obtaining an erection, and orthostatic hypotension may be present.

Diagnostic Reasoning
Diagnostic Tests
Usually the history and physical exam lead the clinician to the diagnosis of PD. The major features of bradykinesia and akinesia—tremor with the limb at rest or resistance to passive movement of the joints (rigidity) or both of these—usually lead the clinician to the diagnosis. Genetic testing may be used in the diagnosis of PD along with other specific features such as family history and age of onset (Level B; Berardelli et al, 2013). An MRI of the brain may be performed to exclude structural brain lesions but not to demonstrate pathological changes indicative of PD. A serum calcium level may be drawn to exclude hypoparathyroidism. A transcranial sonography is not as universally used and requires some expertise in performing the exam but may differentiate PD from atypical parkinsonian syndromes, may make an early diagnosis of PD, and may detect patients at risk for PD (Level A; Berardelli et al, 2013). Single-photon emission computed tomography will help differentiate between degenerative parkinsonism and essential tremor (Level A; Berardelli et al, 2013).

There are clinical and laboratory clues that suggest that a patient with parkinsonism may have some form of the syndrome other than PD itself. PD often manifests with unilateral symptoms, whereas symptomatic parkinsonism or Parkinson-plus syndromes usually have symmetrical symptoms. Levodopa may be given on a trial basis, and one of the most important diagnostic aids is the patient's response to levodopa. Patients with PD usually have a satisfactory response to levodopa whereas other forms of parkinsonism are most likely if there is no response to levodopa.

The Queen Square Brain Bank for Neurological Disorders holds a large archive of brains donated by patients with neurodegenerative diseases, as well as neurologically normal controls. It specializes in research in PD and parkinsonian movement disorders (UCL Institute of Neurology, 2013).

Differential Diagnosis

Diagnosis is based on the clinical features of PD. These include insidious onset; slow progression; and lack of other findings to explain the symptoms, history, examination, or laboratory tests that point to some other cause of parkinsonism. PD is commonly mistaken for *essential tremor,* which is characterized by postural and kinetic tremor, not resting tremor. The most common diagnostic difficulty is recognizing progressive supranuclear palsy (Steele-Richardson-Olszewski syndrome) when the PD-like symptoms are accompanied by a supranuclear disorder of eye movements, pseudobulbar palsy, and axial dystonia. Another diagnostic error is confusion with multiple system atrophy, Shy-Drager syndrome, where there are additional symptoms of autonomic insufficiency leading to postural hypotension and widespread neurological deficits. Reversible parkinsonism may be caused by dopamine-blocking or dopamine-depleting medications such as antipsychotics, metoclopramide (Reglan), and reserpine (Serpasil). PD must be differentiated from cerebrovascular accidents, dementia, Wilson's disease, and Huntington's disease. Wilson's disease may be recognized by its onset at an earlier age than PD, the presence of other abnormal movements, gray-green Kayser-Fleischer rings in the cornea, chronic hepatitis, and increased concentrations of copper in the tissues. Patients with Huntington's disease also present with rigidity and bradykinesia, but the family history and accompanying dementia will differentiate it from PD.

Management

The principle of management is to control the symptoms of PD, because no drug or surgical approach prevents the progression of the disease. PD costs are estimated at $100 million per year in the United States, counting medications, treatment, hospitalization, loss of productivity, and disability. Because PD is one of the most expensive neurological diseases, clinicians need to work closely with families to monitor patients' conditions to help them obtain the best quality of life of which they are capable. Each patient has a unique set of signs, symptoms, and responses to medications, so treatment must be individualized. Patients also have social, occupational, and emotional needs to be considered. Treatment is lifelong; the goal is to keep patients functioning independently as long as possible.

The decision of when to initiate symptomatic treatment for PD is controversial. When the diagnosis of PD is made, it is appropriate to consider the introduction of a neuroprotective agent. *Neuroprotection* can be defined as an intervention that protects vulnerable neurons. It may also slow or stop disease progression. Some practitioners advocate early treatment to provide maximal clinical benefit. Others advocate treatment delay, to minimize the risk of developing motor complications or accelerating disease progression because of an increased concentration of oxidant radicals from levodopa metabolism. The major decision is when to introduce levodopa. The most common issues providers consider important in deciding to use symptomatic agents are threat to employability; threat to performance of ADLs; threat to the abilities to handle domestic, financial, or social affairs; and appreciable worsening of gait or balance.

Medications commonly prescribed for the management of PD are presented in Drugs Commonly Prescribed 6.3. Levodopa, a dopaminergic agent, is considered the most effective antiparkinsonian agent and has been shown to improve the symptoms of PD by 40% to 50%. Levodopa/carbidopa should also be considered to treat periodic limb movements of sleep (Level B; Zesiewicz et al, 2010).

Once levodopa therapy is started, the rule of thumb is to administer the lowest dosage that brings adequate symptom reversal. A trial period of 3 months should be given before it may be determined that the patient does not respond to the medication. Ninety percent of patients with true PD respond to levodopa. Patients may also experience the "on–off" phenomenon. After 2 to 5 years of treatment, more than 50% of patients experience fluctuations in their response to levodopa. They may also experience dyskinesia, freezing, and mental and behavioral changes. Selegiline (Eldepryl [L-deprenyl]) is an MAO-B inhibitor and is considered a neuroprotective agent. It has fewer side effects than levodopa, but the effects tend to be only moderate and provide inadequate symptomatic therapy, and thus selegiline typically is not used as monotherapy.

Dopamine agonists presumably act directly on striatal dopamine receptors and do not require metabolic conversion to an active product in order to exert effects. They are slightly less effective than levodopa but are alternative first-line agents for PD. Anticholinergic agents are centrally acting drugs and have been used to treat PD for a long time. These drugs are typically used in patients age 70 or younger in whom tremor is the dominant clinical feature and in whom cognitive function is preserved. These agents are useful for treating resting tremors; however, adverse effects—including memory impairment, hallucinations, and confusion—are common with these drugs. Adverse CNS effects of drugs used to treat PD include dysphagia, sedation, and dyskinesias. These drugs should always be discontinued gradually.

Peripheral catechol-*O*-methyltransferase (COMT) inhibitors such as tolcapone (Tasmar) and entacapone (Comtan) have been studied as adjunctive therapies to levodopa. These drugs are thought to increase the bioavailability of levodopa, thereby extending the duration of levodopa's effect. COMT inhibitors have been shown to be effective in both nonfluctuating and fluctuating patients.

Patients with severe symptoms, such as tremor, that are refractory to medications may require referral to a movement disorder neurologist or neurosurgeon for evaluation. Options of thalamotomy, pallidotomy, and deep brain stimulation may be discussed with these patients. Thalamotomy and thalamic stimulation are best for intractable tremors and drug-induced kinesias. Pallidotomy is helpful in some patients for relief of bradykinesis,

Drugs Commonly Prescribed 6.3 Parkinson's Disease

Class	Drug	Adverse Reactions and Prescribing Considerations
MAO Inhibitors		
	selegiline (Eldepryl L-deprenyl)	After several days, levodopa dosage may be reduced 10%–30%. Adverse effects: nausea, dizziness, confusion, hallucinations, dry mouth. Do not give with meperidine (Demerol) or narcotic analgesics. When given with levodopa, selegiline can increase dopaminergic effects and contribute to dopamine toxicity.
	rasagiline (Azilect)	Avoid tyramine-rich foods. Follow MAO precautions.
Dopaminergics		
	carbidopa/levodopa (Sinemet, Sinemet CR, Atamet) amantadine (Symmetrel)	Gradually titrate to relief of symptoms; may go up to 300–500 mg/day. Monitor for orthostatic hypotension. Adverse effects: dizziness, ataxia, insomnia, leg edema. Do not give at bedtime. May cause postural hypotension.
Dopamine Agonists		
	bromocriptine (Parlodel)	Potentiates alcohol and other CNS depressants. Monitor BP and mental status. Adverse effects: fluctuation of symptoms, dyskinesia, dystonia.
	pergolide (Permax)	As above.
	pramipexole (Mirapex)	As above. Titrate over 7 weeks.
	ropinirole (Requip)	As above. Taper dose over 7 days to discontinue.
Anticholinergics		
	trihexyphenidyl (Artane)	Adverse effects: memory impairment, dysphagia, rigidity. Discontinue drug gradually.
	benztropine (Cogentin)	As above.
COMT Inhibitors		
	tolcapone (Tasmar)	With carbidopa/levodopa, discontinue if no substantial benefit after 3 weeks. Increases dopaminergic side effects. Perform baseline transaminase levels, then recheck every 2 weeks for 1 year, then every 4 weeks for 6 months, then every 2 months; monitor for liver disease. Adverse effects: dyskinesias, nausea, sleep disorders.
	entacapone (Comtan)	Each dose of carbidopa/levodopa increases dopaminergic side effects: nausea and vomiting, dry mouth, postural hypotension.

tremor, and dyskinesias. All of these procedures except deep brain stimulation are destructive in nature. Deep brain stimulation is considered nondestructive and reversible. High-frequency thalamic stimulation may be effective in suppressing the rest tremor of PD. Chronic bilateral stimulation of the subthalamic nuclei or globus pallidus shows promising results as a nondestructive treatment for relief of bradykinesias, tremors, and dyskinesias. Surgical implantation of adrenal medullary tissue or fetal substantia nigra tissue is still under investigation because of mixed results.

A biotechnology company in California, the International Stem Cell Corporation, is developing stem-cell therapies that may provide therapeutic benefit through multiple mechanisms of action (International Stem Cell Corporation announces new data from Parkinson's disease program, 2013).

Follow-up and Referral

The frequency of follow-up and visits is based on the patient's response to treatment, adverse effects of medications, and disease progression. Follow-up should be early and repeated initially, especially during the introduction of a new medication or dose change. The decision for referral to a specialist should be made based on the practitioner's knowledge level and comfort treating PD and on the severity of symptoms. As the disease progresses, especially in the area of tremor, it may become necessary to refer the patient to a movement disorder neurologist or to a stereotactic neurosurgeon.

Rating scales are frequently used to evaluate and monitor a patient's response to medications. The Unified Parkinson's Disease Rating Scale (UPDRS) is a comprehensive evaluation tool that assesses mental, historical, and motor features and the complications of dopaminergic therapy. A subscale of the UPDRS is the Activities of Daily Living Scale, which assesses speech, salivation, swallowing, handwriting, cutting food, handling utensils, hygiene, turning in bed, falling, freezing, walking, tremor, and sensory symptoms.

Patient Education

Speech therapy may be beneficial to increase the voice volume; effect speech pattern modification; and assist with breathing, memory, and vocal ROM exercises. Occasional swallowing assessments and therapies may be needed to assist with problems of dysphagia and drooling.

Patients should be educated on all issues of the disease, medications, adverse effects, complications, progression of the disease, diet, sleep, and exercise. Patients with PD should be encouraged to exercise regularly. This should be focused exercise, and a referral to physical therapy may be indicated. Patients should be observed for fatigue. Exercises should include swimming, stretching, and walking. These activities can slow the secondary effects of PD. Nutrition in patients with PD is an important component in care. The patient should also be assessed for physical and psychological problems, which may interfere with eating and nutrition. Functional capacity may be limited, hindering the patient's ability to prepare meals. Special table cutlery is available with large nonslip handles that may help with eating. Fiber and fluid may need to be increased. Protein may be taken in the evening to avoid interactions between dietary protein and levodopa.

Patients must also be instructed to continue routine health maintenance and screenings. In addition, both patient and caregiver must be educated to the risk for falls in patients with decreased mobility, as well as other home safety issues. There is an increase in mortality from influenza and pneumonia among patients with PD, so guidance for immunizations must be given. Patient and caregivers may benefit from referral to a support group. Resources are listed at the end of this chapter.

■ ALZHEIMER'S DISEASE

Alzheimer's disease (AD) is a progressive, neurodegenerative condition and the most common form of dementia in the older population. One in three seniors dies with AD or another dementia. It is characterized by an insidious onset, slow progressive cognitive decline, and an array of emotional and behavioral problems that result from the cognitive decline. AD accounts for about $100 billion per year in medical and custodial expenses, with approximately $27,000 per year for each patient for medical and nursing care. In 2012, 15.4 million caregivers provided an estimated 17.5 billion hours of unpaid care, valued at more than $216 billion. This is stated in the 2013 Alzheimer's Disease Facts and Figures document from the Alzheimer's Association.

According to the American Psychiatric Association, AD is characterized by the impaired ability to learn new information or recall previously learned information and one or more additional cognitive disturbances in language (aphasia), function (apraxia), perception (agnosia), or executive function. Once considered an inevitable result of old age, recent advances in understanding AD have modified both diagnostic and treatment choices. There is a familial as well as a sporadic form of the disease. Most clinicians treat patients with the sporadic form of AD.

Alzheimer's disease was named after Dr. Alois Alzheimer, who in 1906 noticed changes in the brain tissue of a woman who had died of an unusual mental illness. She had symptoms of memory loss, language problems, and strange behavior. On autopsy, he found abnormal clumps and tangled bundles of fibers in her brain. These are now called amyloid plaques and neurofibrillary tangles.

Epidemiology and Causes

The only known cause of AD is genetic mutation, which is an abnormal change in the sequence of chemical pairs inside genes. The incidence of the sporadic form of AD in the general population rises rapidly with age. As many as 5 million Americans are currently living with AD. It affects an estimated 1 in 9 people older than age 65. AD is projected to affect nearly 16 million people in 2050, of whom 60% will be older than 85 years of age. Additional risk factors that have been identified include lower educational and occupational levels, family history, head injury, Down syndrome, and decreased estrogen levels. Because onset is often undetected, it is difficult to accurately predict duration or survival time with the disease. For 60- to 70-year-old patients with AD, the average life expectancy is 7 to 10 years after diagnosis. Alzheimer's disease is the sixth-leading cause of death overall and the fifth-leading cause of death for individuals over age 65. Over 60% of patients with Alzheimer's are expected to die before age 80 compared with 30% of people without Alzheimer's.

The relatively rare familial form of AD is considered a straightforward genetic disease. Onset is typically earlier than in the sporadic form of AD. For example, in an extended St. Louis family with the familial form of AD, the typical age at onset is 26 to 28 years. The physically fit but demented individuals in this family are considered evidence that the disease is not entirely due to age. Members of another large family from villages outside Medellín, Colombia, exhibit symptoms of AD in their early 30s. Many patients complain of severe headaches before onset of familial AD, but the progression is otherwise similar to that of the sporadic form. If a parent has the familial form of AD, offspring have a 50% chance of developing the disease.

Pathophysiology

AD is a progressive and irreversible cortical disconnection syndrome. The disease depletes the cerebral cortices of neurons, causing generalized cortical atrophy, widened cortical sulci, and enlarged ventricles. Neurons that use the neurotransmitter acetylcholine are especially susceptible to the disease; for example, the nucleus basalis (the basal nucleus of Meynert), a set of large cholinergic neurons in the telencephalon beneath the basal ganglia, is selectively depopulated of neurons. Cortical areas that are especially hard hit include the hippocampus (which loses most of its inputs and outputs), the amygdala (which shrinks as it becomes depleted), the temporal cortex, the olfactory system (including the primary sensory epithelium in the nose), and cortico–cortical (intercortical) connections.

Two pathological lesions are found in large numbers throughout the brain of an Alzheimer's patient: neuritic plaques (also called "senile plaques") and neurofibrillary tangles. Neuritic plaques are macroscopic spherical lesions found throughout the cortex (although they are relatively sparse in the primary motor and sensory areas), the hippocampus, and the amygdala. Each plaque has a core of beta-amyloid, an insoluble peptide. The core is surrounded by swollen and degenerating neurites, and these are encased in a layer of microglia and astrocytes. Excess beta-amyloid is also found diffusely throughout the cerebral cortex, the cerebellar cortex, and the basal ganglia, especially in and around blood vessels.

Neurofibrillary tangles are microscopic collections of intertwined cytoskeletal fibers that form inside neurons. The tangles are best seen in silver-stained tissue, and their density correlates with the degree of the patient's dementia. One major protein in these tangles is an aberrant form of *tau* protein (which, in its normal form, stabilizes microtubules), and patients with AD have elevated concentrations of *tau* proteins in their cerebrospinal fluid. The formation of neurofibrillary tangles immobilizes or otherwise deactivates the neuron's normally dynamic cytoskeleton and leads to the cell's death. The tangles are insoluble and remain after the neurons have degenerated.

The central biochemical problem in AD appears to be a defect in the metabolism of *beta-amyloid precursor protein*. Normally, many types of cells, including neurons, make beta-amyloid precursor protein, the function of which is not yet fully understood. When this protein

is broken down by specific secretases, the by-products include beta-amyloid peptides. There are four different forms of beta-amyloid peptide. The form identified as beta-amyloid-42 is insoluble, readily forms fibrils, and is found in neuritic plaques.

In AD, beta-amyloid peptides accumulate excessively in the brain. It is thought that abnormalities in the functioning of the secretases cause the overproduction of beta-amyloids. One current theory proposes that beta-amyloid deposition is the primary problem in AD and that intracellular neurofibrillary tangles are the consequence of the toxic effects of beta-amyloid on neurons.

Clinical Presentation

Subjective

The patient usually presents initially with complaints of memory problems. The boundary between the benign forgetfulness of age-associated memory impairment (AAMI) and the onset of AD is unclear. A complaint of memory problems must be thoroughly explored to distinguish not only AAMI but also emotional disorders, other physical insults to the brain, and early AD. Recognition of cognitive difficulty on the part of the patient or family is often related to a change in pattern: getting lost in familiar places, inability to accomplish a demanding task at work, or increasingly slow response to any cognitive challenge. Word-finding difficulty (anomia) usually occurs. Difficulties with balancing the checkbook, preparing dinner, traveling alone, or maintaining employment are frequent problems reported by family members when the disease has progressed to the point where it is noticeable to others. As the disease progresses to the middle stage, family members report difficulty with simpler tasks: choosing clothes, doing housework, and finishing chores. These behavior difficulties worsen with cognitive decline. In the later stages, the person needs help dressing, bathing, and staying continent. Eventually, the person loses the capacity to converse, walk, sit, or hold up the head. Eighty percent of patients in nursing homes with AD have behavioral problems. These may include hostility, aggression, suspiciousness and paranoia, delusions, agitation, sundowning, incontinence, and inappropriate or impulsive sexual behavior.

Objective

There is no support at present for assessing dementia in asymptomatic individuals. However, if concern about cognitive decline is expressed by the patient or family or changes in behavior or cognition are noted, this should trigger an initial assessment for dementia (Advanced Assessment 6.1).

Cognitive assessment is central to diagnosis and management of dementias and should be performed in all patients. The often heard rule of thumb that if a patient reports memory loss, he or she is not demented, has been refuted. Routine social conversation and questions that

Advanced Assessment 6.1   Alzheimer's Disease: Triggers for Further Assessment

Learning and Retaining

Is more repetitive; has trouble remembering recent conversations, events, new information appointments; frequently misplaces objects.

Handling Complex Tasks

Has trouble following a complex train of thought or performing tasks that require many steps such as balancing a checkbook or cooking a meal.

Reasoning Ability

Is unable to respond with a reasonable plan to problems at work or home, such as knowing what to do if the bathroom is flooded; shows uncharacteristic disregard for rules of social conduct.

Spatial Ability and Orientation

Has trouble driving, organizing objects around the house, finding his or her way around familiar places.

Language

Has increasing difficulty with finding the words to express what he or she wants to say and with following conversations.

Behavior

Appears more passive and less responsive; is more irritable than usual; is more suspicious than usual; misinterprets visual or auditory stimuli.

Source: U.S. Department of Health and Human Services. *Early identification of Alzheimer's disease and related dementias.* U.S. Department of Health and Human Services, Rockville, MD, 1996, AHCPR Publication 97-0703.

can be answered automatically will not elicit symptoms of early AD. Instead, ask the person such questions as "Do you remember what you did last Sunday?" or "What did you have for breakfast this morning?" The importance of maintaining the patient's dignity by examining the patient alone before interviewing others cannot be overemphasized. The patient should be informed if others are to be interviewed. It is also important to be alert to the possibility that family members at times may minimize or exaggerate their report of symptoms depending on their motives. Family members can report on the patient's ability to perform independent ADLs using the Functional Activities Questionnaire (Advanced Assessment 6.2).

The clinician should get a focused history documenting signs and symptoms related to the dementia, chronology of the problem (including onset, duration, and stepwise versus continuous progression), family history, and any condition or medications that may mimic or contribute to cognitive impairment. The physical exam should include a neurological evaluation and evaluation of any factors contributing to delirium and evidence of neglect or abuse. Neuropsychological testing can pinpoint the types and severity of impairments in language, reasoning, visuospatial, and memory deficits.

The Mini–Mental State Exam (MMSE) is a well-known, easily administered test of cognition. It should be the initial test done when trying to diagnose AD.

Within the possible scoring range of 0 to 30, the median score for adults aged 18 to 59 is 29, but the median score drops to 25 at age 80. A score of 20 to 25 indicates early-stage AD, a score between 10 and 19 indicates middle-stage AD, and a score below 10 indicates late-stage AD. Age; visual, auditory, and other physical impairments; and educational level must be taken into consideration in interpretation of test results. Another test for cognition is the Montreal Cognitive Assessment (MoCA), which may be accessed at www.mocatest.org. Functional assessment tests are also very basic screening tools. These may include the timed get up and go, a gait assessment, or the Functional Activities Questionnaire (FAQ), which may be performed by the clinician. The FAQ is also a useful measure that is reported to discriminate well at higher functional levels. There are other tests previously mentioned at the beginning of the chapter. Probably one of the easiest to administer is the clock-drawing test. Ask the patient to draw a clock face with all the numbers in place and give him or her a specific time to draw on it. Save this drawing in the patient's record and repeat this test on occasion. In addition, have the patient write a sentence and repeat this occasionally. These tests are appropriate for initial assessment. The results also provide a baseline from which any further decline can be noted quantitatively. The clinician should refer the patient to a memory disorder center or a specialist in dementing diseases if the initial assessment is suggestive of AD, particularly when

Advanced Assessment 6.2 Functional Activities Questionnaire

The Functional Activities Questionnaire (FAQ) is an informant-based measure of functional abilities. The caregiver or informant provides a score of dependent (3); requires assistance (2); has difficulty but does by self (1); or normal (0) on 10 functional items. Several other responses could be: Never did the activity but couldn't do it now (0); and Never did the activity but would have difficulty now (1).

The 10 activities are as follows:

1. Maintains financial records.
2. Collects information for IRS purposes.
3. Shops alone for necessities.
4. Does an intellectual activity.
5. Heats water and turns off the stove.
6. Cooks a healthy meal.
7. Has knowledge of what's going on in the world.
8. Carries on a conversation about something in the media.
9. Remembers medications and significant dates.
10. Arranges own travel for activities.

The sum of scores for the 10 items will range from 0–30. The higher the score, the poorer the function. It is recommended that clinicians go to the source listed below to obtain the exact FAQ and utilize this in the practice setting.

Adapted from Pfeiffer, RI, et al. Measurement of functional activities of older adults in the community. *J Gerontol* 37(3):323, 1982.

atypical presentation, severe impairment, or complex comorbidities are present.

Diagnostic Reasoning
Diagnostic Tests

Laboratory tests (complete blood count [CBC], electrolytes, blood glucose, serum calcium, and thyroid-stimulating hormone level, at a minimum) are used to rule out other conditions that may impair brain function. Structural imaging should be used in the diagnostic evaluation of every patient suspected of dementia. Noncontrast computed tomography (CT) can be used to identify surgically treatable lesions and vascular disease. To increase specificity, magnetic resonance imaging (MRI) should be used (Level I; Filippi et al, 2012). Single-photon emission computed tomography (SPECT) imaging is different from the MRI or CT scans. SPECT measures blood flow and activity patterns and can be used to differentiate AD from other possible causes. Pittsburgh compound B positron emission tomography imaging may be used to detect amyloid deposits. Studies show that this test is 86% accurate in predicting which individuals will develop AD within 2 years and 92% accurate in ruling out the likelihood of developing AD. Alzheimer's-related brain changes may occur 20 years before symptoms begin. An individual with early brain changes has preclinical AD or mild cognitive impairment (MCI) due to Alzheimer's. Those patients with symptoms have dementia due to Alzheimer's disease. Two categories of biomarkers in the blood are being studied to determine relevance for

diagnostic criteria. The first are biomarkers showing the level of beta-amyloid accumulation in the brain; the second are biomarkers showing that neurons in the brain are injured or actually degenerating. Once these biomarker tests are well established, these will be recommended for individuals with MCI to determine if they have brain changes that put them at high risk for developing Alzheimer's. These biomarkers will also be important in evaluating the effectiveness of treatment. Genetic testing is available, but its value remains controversial; less than 1% of AD cases are caused by the three known genetic mutations.

Differential Diagnosis

To some extent, the diagnosis of AD is still a process of excluding other causes of cognitive impairment (Differential Diagnosis Flowchart 6.7).

Medical conditions and drug-related adverse effects need to be ruled out in patients suspected of AD. Infection, structural CNS conditions, traumatic conditions, metabolic organic failure, and anemia need to be considered. In addition, depression, drug and alcohol abuse, drug-induced delirium, and psychosis need to be ruled out.

The patient should be assessed for deterioration from a higher level of function. Mental retardation should be ruled out. If there is no alteration in consciousness, delirium should be ruled out. Amnesia and aphasia need to be considered if multiple cognitive functions are impaired. If the course of the disease is chronic rather than subacute, the following should be excluded: Creutzfeldt-Jakob

Assessment of Alzheimer's Disease

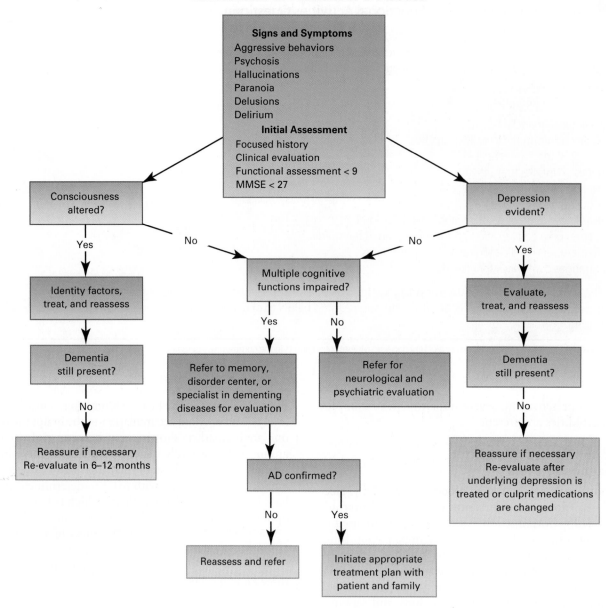

disease, tumor, nutritional deficiency (specifically vitamin B$_{12}$), drug intoxication, metabolic disorders, and so on. If there is a steady versus stepwise decline, vascular dementia should be ruled out. If there is primarily cortical dysfunction, Parkinson's dementia, Huntington's disease, trauma, vascular dementia, and so forth should be ruled out.

Many patients present with more than one problem. Delirium or depression may be superimposed on AD; PD, vascular problems, or other dementia can also co-exist with AD, complicating diagnosis.

Depression can mimic AD and is frequently mistaken for AD in older adults. Information from multiple sources—patient self-report, family members, health-care provider observations, and patient history—should be used in drawing conclusions.

The Alzheimer's Disease Management Council Clinical Consensus Panel and Scientific Roundtable proposed that the following are highly suggestive of the diagnosis of AD:

- Absence of a precipitating medical illness
- Absence of a drug-related phenomenon
- Presence of objective, well-documented, progressive, and worsening deficits in new learning and memory
- Signs of functional impairment

Management

The principles of management of AD are directed toward slowing progression of the disease pharmacologically, protecting physical health, providing emotional support, and maintaining maximum possible function through prevention or reduction of excess disability. Maintaining as much normality as possible in relationships and everyday activities may be the most effective way to prevent the development of excess disability, defined as the difference between the observed function and the actual underlying impairment.

Family members have reported that sensitivity to their distress, acknowledgment of their contributions, and information about the disease and its management have not always been dealt with adequately in encounters with primary-care providers. Both patient and family need assistance in understanding and coping with a diagnosis of AD. Most patients are eager to try approved and research-stage drugs. Support group attendance can be very helpful but must be relevant to the stage of the disease. Anxiety and depression should be recognized and treated vigorously because they probably are responsible for much of the disturbing behavior associated with AD. Legal and financial planning and discussion of future care options should take place early in the disease course.

Pharmaceutical agents may improve cognitive function or lessen some of the dementia in mild to moderate AD. Treatment with cholinesterase inhibitors should be considered at the time of diagnosis, taking into account expected therapeutic benefits and potential safety issues. (See Drugs Commonly Prescribed 6.4: Alzheimer's Disease.) The doses for the following drugs are adjusted gradually as tolerated: donepezil (Aricept), galantamine (Reminyl), and rivastigmine (Exelon). An *N*-methyl-D-aspartate (NMDA) receptor antagonist, memantine

(Namenda), has been effective in moderate to severe AD by improving cognitive function and has additive effects to cholinesterase inhibitors.

Donepezil does not prevent progression of AD, but it seems to affect the rate of decline. Patients who stop and restart donepezil will not reach the level of function that they had before stopping the drug. Therefore, if the drug is tolerated, it should be continued, because there are no clear guidelines as to when to stop it. Antidepressant drugs have shown an effect in patients with depressive symptoms. Anxious and agitated behavior may respond to anxiolytic drugs; however, use of pharmaceutical agents for noncognitive symptoms such as anxiety, depression, and insomnia should be reserved for instances where behavioral intervention is ineffective.

Because of their side effects, antipsychotics should be used with caution only for patients who exhibit persistent disruptive or dangerous behavior. Precautions include avoidance of drugs that have even a moderate anticholinergic effect and drugs that sedate, affect balance, or are known to cause confusion in older individuals. Atypical antipsychotic medications—risperidone (Risperdal), olanzapine (Zyprexa), and quetiapine (Seroquel)—are usually well tolerated. Risperidone should be avoided in patients with vascular risk factors because it may increase the risk of stroke. Federal regulations require that if antipsychotic agents are used in nursing homes, an effort should be made to reduce the dosage at least every 6 months. Alpha-tocopherol (vitamin E) may help to slow progression of AD in some patients, and an herbal extract of *Ginkgo biloba* has also been reported to have

Drugs Commonly Prescribed 6.4   Alzheimer's Disease (AD)

Drug	Adverse Reactions and Prescribing Considerations
Cholinesterase Inhibitors	
donepezil (Aricept) galantamine (Reminyl)	For mild to moderate AD. May cause diarrhea, nausea, anorexia, and weight loss.
rivastigmine (Exelon)	Rivastigmine has shown fewer side effects than the other drugs in this category.
N-Methyl-D-Aspartate (NMDA) Receptor Antagonist	
memantine (Namenda)	For moderate to severe AD. Can be used in conjunction with cholinesterase inhibitors. Contraindicated with renal impairment. Requires several weeks to show efficacy.
Anxiolytics	
buspirone (Buspar)	
Atypical Antipsychotics	
risperidone (Risperdal) olanzapine (Zyprexa) quetiapine (Seroquel)	Avoid in patients with vascular dementia or vascular risk factors. Avoid alcohol.

few beneficial effects, with few adverse effects. Research on these supplements is still ongoing.

The failure to institute timely pharmacological management in patients with AD may result in a more rapid need for institutionalization, an increase in aggression, further difficulty with ADLs, and further cognitive decline.

Given the advanced age, compromised brain function, and frequent presence of other chronic conditions in most patients with AD, close monitoring of response to any drug regimen is advisable. In addition, as the patient becomes less able to communicate physical or emotional distress, more careful observation of general health and well-being is needed.

Vigilance in regard to good nutrition, exercise, and preventive care (immunizations, dental, vision, and hearing care) should not be reduced. Patients and their families also need continued support and assistance related to changes that occur as the disease progresses. Recognition of and respect for the patient's humanity can be difficult to maintain in the face of declining cognition, leading to the unfortunate temptation to care for family members while ignoring the patient.

Follow-up and Referral

Referral to a memory disorder center is usually warranted. These centers offer multidisciplinary services ranging from differential diagnosis and access to experimental medications to counseling and support groups. They are excellent sources of accurate information on AD. Most cities have local chapters of national organizations for patients with AD and caregivers that usually offer referrals and support groups as well. Respite care, both at home and overnight in participating health-care facilities, and adult day centers provide social outlets for people with AD and a break in the constant care demands for family members. Family members must be cared for as well; if the clinician is unable to support them, it is essential to find social service agencies that will be able to help.

Patient Education

Both patient and family members need to understand the disease, its ramifications, its future course, and treatment options. Memory aids and environmental modifications can prolong independent function. Specialized communication techniques, memory training, exercise, training in the independent and basic ADLs, and therapeutic recreational activities can all contribute to improved function and quality of life as the disease progresses. Patients need information on legal and financial issues related to the capacity to make decisions, including end-of-life decisions. Driving and living alone are safety issues that arise in the earlier stages; wandering and falls become issues in the later stages. Both patient and family must deal with changes in ability, lifestyle, and relationships with others. Finally, family members need to learn how to help the patient while taking care of themselves as well.

Many patients with advanced disease are taking as many as six to eight medications daily, and many of these medications have side effects that affect cognition and result in falls. Fall precautions need to be taken at home, as well as in long-term care facilities, and clinicians should educate families regarding these at every visit.

NEUROVASCULAR DISORDERS

■ CEREBROVASCULAR ACCIDENT

Cerebrovascular accident (CVA), commonly referred to as a *brain attack* or *stroke,* is the rapid onset of neurological deficits as a result of decreased blood flow to a focal or localized area of brain tissue. Although the incidence of CVA has decreased in the past 20 years because of risk-factor management and improved treatment, it has continued to be a significant public health problem in terms of both mortality and permanent disability. CVA is the leading cause of disability in adults, incurring major economic burdens on the patient, family, and public as a result of direct medical costs and cost in lost employment. Its impact as a major health problem with demands on health-care and other support systems will continue to grow as the number of CVA survivors living with disabilities increases and the population continues to live longer. The need for continued improvement in the control of risk factors and the prevention of CVAs is critical.

There are two different kinds of CVAs—*hemorrhagic* and *ischemic.* Hemorrhagic CVAs are most often caused by intracerebral hemorrhage from ruptured aneurysms, arteriovenous malformation, hypertensive arteriolar disease, and amyloid deposition. The obstructions that cause ischemic CVAs can be caused by atherosclerosis, embolus, thrombus, hemorrhage, or vasospasm. Up to 85% of CVAs are due to ischemia. Thirty-three percent of all cases of CVAs are caused by atherosclerotic lesions and thrombosis; another 31% are attributed to emboli.

A transient ischemic attack (TIA) serves as a warning of serious underlying atherosclerotic vascular disease. It is defined as an episode of temporary, focal cerebral dysfunction due to vascular disease that lasts less than 24 hours and usually less than 10 minutes. Because most people know the seriousness of a heart attack and the necessity for early treatment, many refer to a CVA as a "brain attack" for similar reasons.

Epidemiology and Causes

CVAs are the third leading cause of death in the United States, after heart disease and cancer, and are highest in the southeastern United States. Although there are approximately 158,000 deaths from CVAs annually (1 in every 15 deaths), an estimated 795,000 people suffer a

CVA each year. Every 53 seconds, someone has a CVA. More women than men (about 3:2) die from a CVA. In reviewing long-term survival, 25% of people who have an initial CVA die within 1 year and two-thirds die within 12 years. Health costs are significant. The average health-care costs per person (inpatient and outpatient) for CVAs have been estimated to be between $8,000 and $16,500. These impressive numbers do not include the additional costs of morbidity-related expenses (lost time from work, additional nursing care, etc.). The direct and indirect costs to the nation are an estimated $53 billion. Age, sex, race, ethnic origin, and heredity have been identified as nonmodifiable risk factors for CVAs, helping to identify those at greatest risk. Compared with whites, young African Americans are at 2 to 3 times greater risk of a CVA and are 2.5 times more likely to die of one. A higher incidence of CVAs is also noted in Hispanics and Asians, particularly Chinese and Japanese, than in white Americans. For people older than age 55, the incidence of a CVA more than doubles in each successive decade. Twenty-eight percent of people who suffer a CVA are younger than age 65. An increased incidence of CVAs in some families has been noted, probably because of a genetic tendency and familial exposure to similar environmental or lifestyle risks.

Important modifiable risk factors for a CVA include hypertension, cardiac disease, diabetes, hypercholesterolemia, smoking, illicit drug use, and lifestyle factors. There is a fourfold increase of a CVA when a patient is hypertensive with a blood pressure (BP) greater than 160/95 mm Hg. Studies show that with treatment for hypertension, there is a 38% reduction in CVAs and a 40% reduction in mortality from CVAs. Atrial fibrillation is associated with a threefold to fivefold increased risk for a CVA. Other cardiac diseases related to increased risk for CVA are cardiac valve abnormalities, such as mitral stenosis or mitral annular calcification. Cardiac structural abnormalities, such as patent foramen ovale and atrial septal aneurysm, increase CVA risk. Myocardial disease, left ventricular hypertrophy, and cardiac failure also increase the risk of a CVA. People with diabetes are more prone to develop atherosclerosis, thus increasing the risk of a CVA.

Although the risk of ischemic stroke that can be attributed to lipids is uncertain, cigarette smoking increases the risk two times. Moderate use of alcohol may actually reduce the risk of a CVA, whereas heavy consumption increases the risk. Drug abuse involving substances such as cocaine, heroin, amphetamines, and marijuana has been linked to CVAs. Lifestyle factors associated with CVAs are obesity, lack of physical activity, high-fat diet, and emotional stress. Recently, studies have shown that there is no increase in risk of ischemic stroke with use of low-dose oral contraceptives. Migraine is also associated as a minor risk factor in men older than age 40. Studies have shown a link between high blood levels of homocysteine (produced from the essential amino acid methionine) and CVAs. However, treatment did not lower the incidence of a CVA. The risk of a CVA may be higher in patients with a progressing and severe stenosis of the carotid artery or in patients who have experienced a TIA. A CVA is an important complication in patients suffering an anterior myocardial infarction (MI) or in patients treated with long-term oral anticoagulants. Complicated atherosclerotic plaques in the aortic wall may contribute to a CVA.

Pathophysiology

Pathologically, there are two distinct categories of cerebrovascular accidents: ischemic and hemorrhagic.

Cerebral Ischemia

Neurons will stop functioning after less than 10 seconds of insufficient blood flow, but they will recover fully if local circulation is restored within a few minutes. After a few minutes without oxygen and glucose, however, neurons begin to die. Cerebral ischemia is caused by a reduction in blood flow that lasts for more than 4 to 5 minutes.

Transient Ischemic Attacks A brief bout of ischemia will produce neurological deficits. If the ischemia is short lived, the neurological signs and symptoms usually resolve within an hour. When the neurological problems take more than 4 hours to improve, some neuron death has probably occurred. Sudden neurological deficits that resolve in less than 24 hours are usually the result of TIAs, fleeting occlusions of cerebral arteries. People who have suffered a TIA are likely later to have a stroke.

Arterial Occlusions Neurological deficits lasting longer than 24 hours indicate that there has been significant neuron death. When the deficits are focal, the ischemic injury is probably due either to atherothromboses or to emboli. Atherosclerosis produces atheromatous plaques, gummy bulges that protrude from the inner walls of arteries. Atheromatous plaques are masses of lipids, cell debris, collagen, fibrin, platelets, and blood cells, covered by smooth muscle cells, macrophages, and lymphocytes. Plaques that fragment send embolic debris downstream, occluding smaller arteries and arterioles and producing areas of ischemia. Plaques that erode can also initiate local blood clotting. When the clot sticks to the plaque, it often grows, occludes the arterial lumen, and leads to ischemia downstream. The specific neurological deficits caused by atherosclerotic plaques reflect the locations of the areas of ischemia.

Occlusive emboli can be generated upstream some distance from the cerebral arteries. Clots and fragments of atherosclerotic plaque in the internal carotids or the vertebral arteries can dislodge and be carried into brain arteries, which then become occluded. Cardiac arrhythmias (atrial fibrillation and sick sinus syndrome), valvular diseases, prosthetic heart valves, and myocardial infarcts can generate emboli. Clots and clumps of platelets formed during angiography and cardiac surgery can become occlusive emboli. Hypercoagulability syndromes, elevated levels of blood platelets, calcified fragments of plaque and tissue, air, fat, cholesterol crystals, tumor fragments, bacterial vegetations, and foreign material (such as talc and cornstarch injected with illicit drugs) can all clog brain arteries. The occluding emboli are sometimes pushed distally in the affected arteries. This abrades the vessels walls. The injured vessels then bleed and add hemorrhagic damage to the ischemic infarction.

Decreased Brain Perfusion   Low cerebral blood flow causes syncope (fainting). If brain perfusion remains low, neurons begin to die in the areas farthest from the main arteries, that is, at the borders between regions supplied by the major cerebral arteries. Hypoperfusion ischemia leads first to loss of vision; decreased alertness; and weakness in shoulder, hand, and thigh muscles. In addition, certain hippocampal neurons are especially sensitive to a temporary loss of cerebral perfusion, and this may explain the memory deficits that occur after the hypoperfusion caused by even a brief cardiac arrest.

Cerebral Hemorrhage

The neurological symptoms of a cerebral hemorrhage result from the pressure of the hematoma. Sometimes, this pressure causes infarcts in the compressed tissue. Other times, however, there is less cell death so that when the hematoma is resorbed, the neurological deficits resolve to some degree. As a rule, the larger the hematoma, the greater and more permanent is the damage.

Epidural Hematomas   Epidural bleeding is caused by severe head injuries. Epidural hematomas are most common along the temporal cranial wall and result from tears in the middle meningeal artery. The leaking arterial blood rapidly creates a hematoma between the dura and bone. This increases the overall intracranial pressure, which in turn reduces the cerebral blood perfusion. As the hematoma enlarges, it presses on adjacent brain tissue, causing contralateral hemiparesis. Next, the increasing pressure affects the diencephalon, and the patient becomes lethargic and drowsy. When the midbrain becomes compressed against the dural rim of the tentorium, patients develop ipsilateral oculomotor nerve palsy and an enlarged pupil. Continued expansion of the hematoma compresses the contralateral cerebral peduncle, leading to ipsilateral hemiplegia. Eventually, the diencephalon and ipsilateral temporal lobe can be pushed down through the tentorial notch—such herniations compress the posterior cerebral arteries, press on the brainstem, and can be fatal.

Subdural Hematomas   Subdural bleeding is usually caused by blunt trauma that knocks the brain against the skull. Movement of the brain relative to the skull tears the thin superior cerebral veins (the bridging veins), which drain the external cerebral veins into the superior sagittal sinus. Minor repeated injuries can cause chronic venous leakage.

Venous subdural hematomas expand more slowly than the higher-pressure arterial epidural hematomas. Small, self-limited subdural hematomas are often absorbed spontaneously, but subdural hematomas can also continue to enlarge slowly without severe or clear-cut neurological symptoms, especially in the elderly. An untreated subdural hematoma will lead to permanent severe neurological deficits or death.

Subarachnoid and Intraparenchymal Hemorrhages   The remaining two classes of intracranial hemorrhages, subarachnoid bleeding and intraparenchymal bleeding, can be caused by trauma and can coexist with epidural and subdural bleeding. They can also happen without apparent external provocation.

Subarachnoid hemorrhages are caused by tears in the arteries running along the subarachnoid space at the surface of the brain. Ruptured arterial aneurysms are the most common source of subarachnoid bleeds. In the brain, these aneurysms usually occur at branch points of the large arteries, especially in the circle of Willis. A less common nontraumatic cause of subarachnoid bleeding is the rupture of a congenital arteriovenous malformation.

Cerebrospinal fluid (CSF) circulates through the subarachnoid space, and blood from a subarachnoid hemorrhage will spread quickly throughout the CSF surrounding the brain and spinal cord. In such cases, a lumbar puncture will produce CSF that contains red blood cells. In this case, the CSF will often assume a yellowish tinge referred to as xanthochromia. Xanthochromia occurs as a result of the breakdown of hemoglobin in the CSF by enzymes producing yellow-pigmented bilirubin. Ruptures of arteries in the subarachnoid space cause a sudden increase in intracranial pressure and produce severe headache, vomiting, and drowsiness.

Sudden rises in cerebral blood pressure or cerebral blood flow can rupture intraparenchymal arteries, especially when the arteries have been weakened by chronic hypertension, aneurysms, or vascular malformations. Clotting disorders, low platelet counts, anticoagulant drugs, vasoconstrictors, and eclampsia during pregnancy increase the risk for intraparenchymal bleeds. Intraparenchymal hemorrhages most often develop from ruptures of arteries to the basal ganglia and the thalamus, although hematomas also form elsewhere in the cerebral lobes, the cerebellum, and the pons. The first neurological symptoms of an intraparenchymal hemorrhage will reflect the specific location of the hematoma—for example, a basal ganglia hematoma pressing on the internal capsule will first cause contralateral motor weakness.

Clinical Presentation
Subjective

A CVA should be suspected when a patient presents with an acute onset of specific signs and symptoms. Patients presenting in the primary-care setting usually complain of weakness, numbness, or paralysis of one or both extremities on one side of the body. In addition, they usually complain of a severe headache. Impairment is seen in cognitive abilities, level of consciousness, speech, visual fields, extraocular muscle functioning, motor functioning, and gait. Cognitive changes that are exhibited by patients may indicate denial of the illness; neglect syndrome or hemiparesis; spatial and proprioceptive (awareness of body position in spaces) dysfunction; impairment of memory, judgment, problem-solving, or decision-making abilities; and decreased ability to concentrate on and attend to tasks. The patient may experience emotional lability, especially if the frontal lobe is involved. Aphasia, alexia (reading problems), and agraphia (difficulties in writing) may be apparent. Maximum neurological deficits occur at the onset with paralysis and expressive aphasia.

Objective

Information obtained during the history and physical exam assists in identifying the area of the brain involved and the etiology of the CVA and in determining whether the CVA is hemorrhagic or ischemic. Aspects of the history that are relevant are (1) the nature of the onset; (2) the nature, timing, and duration of the neurological deficit; and (3) whether the deficit is static, improving, or worsening. It is important to inquire specifically about the patient's activity when the CVA began; how the symptoms progressed; the severity of the symptoms; and whether they have worsened, improved, or remained the same. Likely findings for ischemic CVAs caused by thrombus would show that symptoms began during the day and occurred gradually and that the patient had periods of improvement between episodes of worsening. On exam, no seizures are noted, and the patient is awake

but confused. Prodromal symptoms are those associated with a TIA. Deficits increase during the first few weeks. Likely symptoms are slight headache, speech deficits, and visual problems. Patients with CVAs caused by embolus typically reveal that their symptoms began during sleep, occurred abruptly, and have progressed steadily. The patient is awake. Symptoms with a hemorrhagic stroke commonly occur during the day with activity and are abrupt in onset, with level of consciousness possibly worsening after the initial onset. Other indicators are vomiting, seizures, severe headaches, coma, and focal deficits. Symptoms also associated with a CVA are seizures or syncope. The patient may complain of feeling "drowsy and dull." The foot on the affected side may be externally rotated, a frequent finding of hemiparesis.

It is important to determine if the symptoms are transient and last no longer than 1 hour, the typical pattern in TIAs. Information can be obtained from the patient as the practitioner observes and interviews the patient for the first time. To assist in differentiating a TIA from a CVA, the patient should describe the event, what precipitated it, the associated symptoms (vision loss, diplopia, paresthesia, aphasia), and how long the event lasted. Table 6.3 presents the different pathologies of TIAs and their symptoms and diagnostic tests.

Patients with carotid atherosclerotic disease are identified by the detection of a carotid bruit or through screening examinations. Detecting the presence of a bruit is significant. Not only does it indicate atherosclerosis and ischemic heart disease, but it may also increase the risk for a CVA. In caring for a patient with asymptomatic carotid bruit, the practitioner should begin with a thorough history for the presence of coronary and peripheral vascular occlusive disease. Most important is the

Table 6.3	Pathologies of Transient Ischemic Attacks (TIAs)		
Type of TIA	Signs and Symptoms	Physical Exam	Diagnostic Tests
Carotid Artery Pathology	Paresthesia Weakness of hand, arm, face Aphasia Dysarthria Unilateral neglect Transient blindness or blurred vision in one eye Cognitive/behavioral changes (rare)	Neurological exam: Assess for carotid bruits. Assess for retinal emboli (refer for complete ophthalmological exam). Assess for temporal artery tenderness.	Laboratory tests: CBC, platelets, electrolytes, ESR, ANA, syphilis serology, toxicology screen, coagulation studies (antiphospholipid antibodies, PT/PTT, Russell's viper venom time for lupus anticoagulant) CT scan of the head (10%–20% of patients with TIA have existing infarction) MRI (more sensitive than CT) Vascular evaluation: Doppler studies of temporal and carotid vessels, transcranial Doppler studies of intracranial vertebrobasilar system, magnetic resonance angiography Echocardiography and Holter monitoring to rule out cardiac sources of emboli Transesophageal echocardiography LP CT angiography

Continued

Table 6.3	Pathologies of Transient Ischemic Attacks (TIAs)—cont'd		
Type of TIA	Signs and Symptoms	Physical Exam	Diagnostic Tests
Small Cerebral Vessel Pathology	Motor hemiparesis Hemibody sensory loss or paresthesia	As above	As above
Vertebrobasilar System Pathology	Ataxia Dizziness, vertigo Dysarthria Confusion Diplopia, hemianopia, or bilateral vision loss Unilateral or bilateral sensory or motor systems (rare)	As above	As above

identification and management of CVA risk factors. A flattened nasolabial fold and widened palpebral tissue on the same side as the hemiparesis raises the suspicion of a supratentorial lesion. (Facial droop is illustrated at www.cdc.gov/pcd/issues/2008/apr/images/07_0214_01.gif.)

The patient may be confused, agitated, or unresponsive. Difficulties may be noted in speech and cognitive abilities and an increased incidence of incontinence. The practitioner should inquire about a history of similar dysfunctions, especially within the last 2 weeks, or coexistence of cardiovascular diseases, such as hypertension, coronary artery disease (CAD), cardiac valvular disorders, atrial fibrillation, recent MI, or related disorders, such as coagulation and bleeding disorders or diabetes mellitus. A list of current medications should be obtained, including prescribed, OTC, and recreational (illicit) drugs, as well as vitamin and mineral supplements and herbal preparations. The practitioner should be attentive to the use of anticoagulants, aspirin, vasodilators, and illegal drugs, which may provide clues to the cause of the stroke or affect treatment. To complete the history, data should be obtained regarding stroke risk factors, both modifiable and nonmodifiable, with particular focus on gender, ethnic origin, age, familial history, lifestyle (obesity, physical activity, diet), and use of alcohol or cigarettes.

Assessment of visual fields may identify deficits such as horizontal defect, blindness, bitemporal hemianopsia, homonymous hemianopsia, or homonymous quadrant defect. A review of the cranial nerves (CNs) may indicate difficulties with chewing (CN V), facial paralysis or paresis (CN VII), dysphagia (CNs IX and X), an absent gag reflex (CN IX), or impaired tongue movement (CN XII).

The degree of infarction following a CVA varies depending on the severity of the reduction in blood flow, the duration of ischemia, and the adequacy of cerebral circulation.

Signs and symptoms exhibited by the patient may be localized to a particular area of the brain (see Table 6.4).

Bruits become audible when the distal lumen is narrowed to approximately 3 mm or less (about 50% stenosis). The higher the pitch of the bruit, the higher the degree of stenosis. A high-pitched bruit that fades into diastole indicates a hemodynamically important stenosis of the proximal internal carotid artery (ICA) with a residual lumen of less than 1.5 mm (75% stenosis or more). The atherosclerotic plaque commonly forms at the origin of the ICA and at the posterior aspect of the bifurcation of the carotid. The plaque narrows the lumen in a concentric fashion. Occasionally, a thrombus may form near this restricted lumen or blood may penetrate the plaque, creating an ulcer that becomes the source of formation of a thrombus.

Diagnostic Reasoning
Diagnostic Tests

The initial assessment of the patient with a possible CVA should include a CBC with platelet count, prothrombin time (PT)/partial thromboplastin time (PTT), electrolytes, blood urea nitrogen, creatinine, glucose, calcium, magnesium, sedimentation rate, ECG, and chest x-ray study.

A decreased platelet count and prolonged PT/PTT may indicate a bleeding disorder or use of anticoagulants, respectively, leading to a hemorrhagic stroke. Elevated blood glucose levels are sometimes seen in patients with hemorrhagic strokes. An elevated glucose level may be found in patients with diabetes mellitus, a contributing factor toward the development of atherosclerosis. An ECG will detect the presence of a recent MI, atrial fibrillation, or left ventricular hypertrophy, risk factors increasing the probability of a CVA. Left ventricular hypertrophy may be seen on a chest x-ray film. In addition, a high platelet count (greater than 1 million) leads to

Table 6.4	Signs and Symptoms of Occlusion of Specific Areas of the Brain	
Specific Areas	**Part of Brain Supplies**	**Signs and Symptoms of Occlusion**
Internal carotid artery (carotid system)	Anterior cerebral surfaces (2/5 of CBF)	Unilateral sensory and motor disturbances Hemiparesis, numbness, or paresthesia Visual disturbances (mononuclear blindness [amaurosis fugax], complete unilateral blindness or homonymous hemianopsia) Aphasia with left-sided lesions
Branches from subclavian into vertebral and basilar arteries (vertebrobasilar system)	Posterior cerebral surfaces (1/5 of CBF)	Ipsilateral visual field deficits Contralateral hemiplegia Bilateral motor, sensory, and visual complaints Vertigo Diplopia Dysphagia
Vertebral arteries	Parts of medulla	Contralateral impairment of pain and temperature sensation Ipsilateral Horner's syndrome (sunken eyeball, ptosis of upper eyelid, slight elevation of lower lid, constriction of pupil, narrowing of palpebral fissure, anhidrosis) Dysphagia Vertigo
Basilar artery branches	Occipital and temporal lobes, dorsal surface of thalamus, upper part of cerebellum, midbrain	Limb paralysis Nystagmus Vertigo Nausea Slurred speech Cerebellar ataxia

CBF- cerebral blood flow.

hypercoagulability, contributing to the development of a thrombus. A hematocrit greater than 60 causes increased viscosity, resulting in decreased perfusion, and can contribute to cerebral ischemia.

Practice guidelines of the American Heart Association Stroke Council recommend the use of noncontrast CT of the head in patients with suspected acute CVA to exclude a nonvascular lesion as the cause of the manifestations and determine whether the CVA is an ischemic infarction or an intracranial hemorrhage. It is also recommended for early evaluation of young adults with acute CVA.

Ideally, a neurological consultation should also be available within 30 minutes of the patient's arrival. In the practitioner's physical and neurological examination and management of the CVA, the time at onset of symptoms is particularly important to determine the proper use of thrombolytic therapy. It is strongly recommended that emergency CT be the initial brain imaging study for the emergency evaluation of a suspected ischemic CVA. A quick CT during the first hours of symptoms can detect a bleed versus a no bleed for a decision to use early clot busters. Other important information can be obtained from laboratory tests, including CBC, blood

chemistry, and coagulation profiles; pulse oximetry; and cranial CT scan without contrast. Other imaging techniques or ultrasonography can help with diagnosis but should not delay treatment. Laboratory data are used to guide intervention and to determine the etiology of the CVA.

MRI is generally recommended for patients with CVAs because it is more sensitive than CT for identifying small ischemic lesions. It also can identify hemorrhagic features, including mass effect. Echo-planar MRI diffusion and perfusion MRI may document changes within minutes, whereas conventional high-field MRI shows changes in 90% of patients after 24 hours. The changes produce increased signals in T2-weighted sequences, indicating the presence of an intraluminal clot. Other signs consist of an absence of flow void in the intracranial arteries, suggestive of occlusion. These signs can be detected almost immediately after onset. Hemorrhage can be detected through high-signal changes in T1-weighted sequences. There is no consensus regarding a method to measure the degree of stenosis from x-ray exams because of the difficulty involved with differentiating one type of lesion from the other (e.g., an atherosclerotic plaque from a thrombus or artery occlusion). Angiography is considered the test of choice. Magnetic resonance angiography, CT angiography, color duplex ultrasound, and transcranial Doppler are acceptable, noninvasive techniques to screen patients with suspected lesions.

Ischemic CVA caused by embolus has a high incidence in pregnant women. In these women, there are no specific imaging recommendations other than those related to radiation precautions. There is a potential risk of radiation-induced defects during the first trimester, when the patient may be unaware of pregnancy. Detection of an acute ischemic CVA by CT depends on the location and extent of the infarct. Large infarcts are often not documented until 3 hours after onset, but nearly 60% can be detected by 24 hours and 100% by 7 days. In hemorrhagic stroke, the CT demonstrates an irregularly hyperdense, "mottled" infarct. These signs, though subtle, can be seen within 5 hours of onset of symptoms. The most common early signs are anatomical changes, seen in the lentiform nucleus, and especially the loss of the "insular ribbon."

In hemorrhagic CVAs, an early mass effect in cerebral or cerebellar infarcts can be detected on CT within hours from onset. These effects develop before the hypodensity and are indicative of massive infarction. Calcified or hyperdense, cordlike areas in a major artery are suggestive of embolic CVAs. The use of CT with contrast for the evaluation of acute stroke is controversial and does not increase the yield. A concern exists over promoting cerebral "toxicity" when the blood–brain barrier has been disturbed in large infarcts.

An erythrocyte sedimentation rate (ESR) may be warranted in cases of unexplained CVA. If anemia is present and the history suggests ethnic or genetic predisposition to thrombosis, a hemoglobin electrophoresis may be performed. A lumbar puncture (LP) may be an additional test indicated to confirm a diagnosis of subarachnoid hemorrhage if blood is detected in the CSF when the CT is negative. Contraindications to this procedure include papilledema, thrombocytopenia, coagulation disorders, and focal neurological deficit. When common risk factors are not evident, an immune electrophoresis or fibrinogen level may be obtained. Because increased fibrinogen levels appear in early CVAs, as well as increased viscosity, this particular test can help to confirm the diagnosis. All other tests should exhibit normal findings. No laboratory test will definitively confirm the diagnosis of a CVA.

Though it is not meant to be used as a screening tool for CVA, panoramic radiography can also identify asymptomatic patients with carotid calcifications, also revealing a significant correlation with obesity because these patients typically have a high-fat diet leading to carotid blockage.

Differential Diagnosis

CT scanning and MRI assist in the differential diagnosis of CVA. A subarachnoid hemorrhage may present with a severe headache of abrupt onset with a decreased level of consciousness. In subdural hematoma, headache is the single most common symptom and is more common in older adults; however, the headache is generalized and often bitemporal. Neurological signs are usually not present for a long period of time. In most patients with a brain abscess, a headache is present, as well as neurological signs of altered level of consciousness and focal deficit, most often hemiparesis. Nausea and vomiting are frequent, along with a fever. Idiopathic intracranial hypertension (pseudotumor) shows symptoms of papilledema and diplopia, along with a headache and normal CT scan. Transient visual symptoms are present. Headache is present in most patients with brain tumor, along with seizures, weakness, and subtle cognitive changes; however, vomiting and papilledema may be present. No focal neurological signs are seen.

Arterial dissection, although occurring frequently in young adults, has an extremely important symptom of cephalic pain or headache of sudden onset, often preceding retinal or hemispheric ischemic symptoms. Carotid dissection appears initially with occipital headache or acute neck pain and is followed by ischemic symptoms of diplopia, syncope, and amaurosis fugax. Unilateral neck pain that is sudden and radiates to the ipsilateral face or eye is usually present. The headache is related to cervical manipulation, sustained exertion, or trauma. A symptom of new-onset, progressive headache appears as a major feature in temporal arteritis with some cranial symptoms of diplopia and mental sluggishness. Other symptoms are local swelling; tenderness and pulselessness of the temporal artery; and systemic symptoms of fever, anorexia, weight loss, and chills. Systemic markers of inflammation also are present. Because a headache occurs commonly in cerebral venous thrombosis and often is the only initial symptom, cerebral venous thrombosis can be differentiated easily from a CVA. No neurological deficits are seen, and it usually occurs in isolation. Common causes associated with this type of thrombosis are pregnancy and oral contraceptive use. In meningeal irritation, headache is often the most prominent feature, along with lethargy. Encephalitis is associated with a generalized headache of rapid onset, particularly when it is accompanied by confusion, altered level of consciousness, focal neurological signs, or seizures. Fever, meningismus, and signs of myalgia and fatigue are present. Changes associated with these conditions can be detected by either CT or MRI. In addition, a hemorrhagic CVA can be identified via CT, thus differentiating it from an ischemic CVA. Initial diagnostic studies should also rule out other conditions that can masquerade as a CVA (e.g., recent seizures, delirium, syncope, intoxication, suicide attempts, conversion disorders, and possible recent cocaine or amphetamine use).

Management

The main principle in the management of stroke is prevention and early recognition and treatment. Much remains to be done in order for CVAs to be recognized and managed as a medical emergency, a "brain attack."

Patients with symptoms of a possible stroke require immediate referral to an emergency department for evaluation, CT scanning of the brain, and possible use of thrombolytic therapy. In patients with a cardioembolic source of stroke, a referral to a neurologist is recommended for hospitalization and consideration of the use of heparin anticoagulant therapy. Patients with a high-grade carotid artery stenosis ipsilateral to the side of a TIA should also be considered for hospitalization and may benefit from carotid endarterectomy if they are good surgical candidates or from anticoagulant therapy if they are not. Carotid endarterectomy is established as effective for recently symptomatic (within previous 6 months) patients with 70% to 99% internal carotid artery angiographic stenosis. Symptomatic and asymptomatic patients undergoing carotid endarterectomy should be given aspirin (81 or 325 mg/day) before surgery and for at least 3 months after surgery to reduce the combined endpoint of stroke, MI, and death. Carotid endarterectomy should not be considered for symptomatic patients with less than 50% stenosis. An emergency neurosurgical consultation is indicated in the presence of an intracranial lesion caused by hemorrhage, a mass, or an increase in intracranial pressure. Patients with TIAs should be hospitalized because there is a potential risk of stroke.

Initial management of a CVA is focused on addressing the patient's airway, breathing, and circulation in order to maintain adequate tissue oxygenation. Anaerobic metabolism with depletion of energy stores can increase the extent of brain injury and worsen the outcome. In the prehospital setting, special attention is given to monitoring of the patient's oxygen status through pulse oximetry and the use of supplemental oxygen as needed. Maintaining an adequate airway is crucial, and intubation with mechanical ventilation is initiated when there is decreased level of consciousness or evidence of apparent hypoventilation. Hypotension is treated to maximize cerebral blood flow and minimize complications. Aggressive treatment of hypertension in the prehospital setting is not done in patients with known ischemic disease, because lowering the BP may precipitate hypoperfusion and injury. There is a permissive level of hypertension allowed in the days following the CVA as well. Prehospital evaluation and transport time account for significant delays in initiation of thrombolytic therapy for patients with acute CVA who require it. Aggressive CVA protocols and educational programs keyed to emergency medical services can markedly reduce the time from CVA onset to initiation of treatment.

Once the clinical presentation, the laboratory data, and the results of the CT scan are completed, if they point to a diagnosis of acute ischemic stroke, thrombolytic agents must be considered. The patient and/or family should understand that thrombolytic therapy carries at least a 6.4% risk of intracerebral hemorrhage. Intravenous thrombolytic therapy is effective in reducing the neurological deficit in some patients without CT evidence of intracranial hemorrhage who meet National Institute of Neurological Disorders and Stroke inclusion/exclusion criteria and can be treated within 3 hours after symptom onset (Level A; Edlow et al, 2013). Contraindications to thrombolytic therapy include recent head trauma in the last 3 months, previous intracranial hemorrhage, recent intracranial or intraspinal surgery, active internal bleeding, or evidence of intracranial bleed on CT scan, international normalized ratio greater than 1.7, and platelets less than 100,000. Nursing Research–Based Practice Box 6.1 describes a retrospective study that showed patients on warfarin had larger intracerebral hematomas.

It would be important for the clinician to treat and reduce sources of fever, which can accompany an infectious complication of a CVA, with antibiotics and antipyretics; to prevent recurrent seizures with anticonvulsants; and to prophylactically administer heparin, low molecular weight heparin, or heparinoids (Lovenox) to prevent deep vein thrombosis. The use of corticosteroids is not indicated in the management of cerebral edema and increased intracranial pressure due to CVA.

Once a patient's condition has deteriorated, including development of a herniation syndrome as a result of increased intracranial pressure, osmotherapy and

---

Nursing Research–Based Practice 6.1

Flaherty, ML, et al. Warfarin use leads to larger intracerebral hematomas. *Neurology* 71:1084–1089, 2008.

Among patients with intracerebral hemorrhage (ICH), warfarin use before onset leads to greater mortality. In a retrospective study, the researchers sought to determine whether warfarin use was associated with larger initial hematoma volume, one determinant of mortality after ICH. ICH volumes were measured on the first available brain scan. Univariable analyses and a multivariable generalized linear model were used to determine whether international normalized ratio (INR) influenced initial ICH volume after adjusting for other factors, including age, race, sex, antiplatelet use, hemorrhage location, and time from stroke onset to scan. Two hundred fifty-eight patients with ICH, including 51 patients taking warfarin, were included in the study. Warfarin use was associated with larger initial ICH volume, but this effect was observed only for INR values >3.0. Larger ICH volume among warfarin users likely accounts for part of the excess mortality in this group.

hyperventilation are used. Surgery is indicated to decompress and evacuate a large cerebellar infarction that compresses the brainstem, although survivors may have severe residual neurological deficits. Early ambulation and preventive measures against aspiration, malnutrition, pneumonia, deep vein thrombosis, pulmonary embolism, decubitus ulcers, contracture, and joint abnormalities are important goals in managing the patient with a CVA.

TIAs with a probable cardioembolic source may be considered for mild anticoagulation. If anticoagulation is contraindicated, antiplatelet therapy may be considered. Medical management is preferred to carotid endarterectomy for symptomatic patients with less than 50% stenosis (Level I; Berardelli et al, 2013). One of the most significant approaches to the medical management of patients with CAD with respect to CVA risk reduction has been the use of antiplatelet drugs, principally acetylsalicylic acid (ASA). Ticlopidine (Ticlid) has shown some improvement over the effects of ASA. Combination therapies, such as ASA plus dipyridamole (Persantine), are better than ASA alone. The dosage of ASA remains controversial—from 81 mg to 650 mg per day—to none at all. Clinicians disagree as to whether high or low doses are efficacious and whether ASA is more effective in women than in men. Clopidogrel (Plavix) 75 mg daily may be used in patients with TIAs to reduce the likelihood of thrombosis and microemboli.

Although ticlopidine is more effective than ASA in decreasing the risk of CVA, the cost and adverse effects are higher. Studies have shown adverse effects such as rash and diarrhea, and thus poor patient compliance. Neutropenia has been known to occur between 3 weeks and 1 month after starting treatment. CBCs should be monitored every 2 weeks for the first 3 months, with therapy continuing for a period of no longer than 6 months.

Clopidogrel (Plavix) is more commonly used than ticlopidine because of lack of neutropenia. A significant number of patients with carotid artery disease have concomitant CAD, and serum cholesterol in patients with CAD should be evaluated and treated. The hydroxymethylglutaryl–coenzyme A (HMG-CoA) reductase inhibitors, or statins, reduce the risk of both nonfatal and fatal CVAs, demonstrating a significant protective effect similar to that conferred by antiplatelet agents. The efficacy of combination therapy is still being researched.

Follow-up and Referral

Follow-up and rehabilitation focus on the return of the patient's optimum level of functioning. The patient may be assessed for the potential for rehabilitation and transferred to a rehabilitation unit. The rehabilitation process involves six major areas of focus: (1) preventing, recognizing, and managing comorbid illness and medical complications; (2) training for maximum independence; (3) facilitating psychosocial coping and adaptation by the patient and family; (4) preventing secondary disability by promoting community reintegration, including resumption of home, family, and vocational activities; (5) enhancing quality of life in view of residual disability; and (6) preventing recurrent CVAs and other vascular conditions, such as MI, that occur with increased frequency in patients with CVAs. Nursing Research–Based Practice Box 6.2 discusses patients' improved quality of life from exposure to interventions designed to increase physical activity.

Patient Education

Adjustments may need to be made in the home environment before discharge, such as building a ramp or removing a door to accommodate a wheelchair. Specific areas of teaching involve exercise and ambulation techniques, dietary requirements, recognition of symptoms of another CVA, and an understanding of the emotional lability and depression that commonly accompany a CVA. Also important are knowledge of appropriate use of medications and the time, place, and frequency of occupational and physical therapy activities. To help prevent caregivers at home from becoming overburdened and thus ill themselves, clinicians should teach caregivers to plan for respite or time away from caregiving activities

---

Nursing Research–Based Practice 6.2

Conn, VS, et al. Meta-analysis of quality-of-life outcomes from physical activity interventions. *Nurs Res* 58(3):175–183, 2009.

Interventions to increase physical activity among adults with chronic illness are intended to improve quality of life and reduce disease complications or slow disease progression. The aim of this study was to integrate quality-of-life outcomes from primary research studies testing interventions to increase physical activity among adults with chronic illness. Extensive literature searching strategies were used to locate published and unpublished primary research testing physical activity interventions. The researchers synthesized 85 samples from 66 reports with 7,291 subjects. Most design and sample attributes were unrelated to intervention effects on quality of life. Studies that exclusively used supervised center-based exercise reported larger quality-of-life improvements than did studies that included any educational/motivational content. Subjects experienced improved quality of life from exposure to interventions designed to increase physical activity. Future primary research should include quality-of-life outcomes so that patterns of relationships among variables can be explored further.

on a regular basis. Information regarding community, state, and national resources can be a welcome source of support to patients and their families. The National Stroke Association has resource information, including referral services and a quarterly newsletter. The American Heart Association provides a large variety of information regarding risk factors and referrals for assistive devices. The Easter Seal Society also may provide assistance with wheelchairs or other assistive devices. Additional listings of resources for the patient and the practitioner appear at the end of the chapter. Some communities have organizations to help with meals or transportation, along with self-help groups. Education regarding the modification and reduction of risk factors plays a significant role toward the reduction in the incidence of CVAs and TIAs. The most relevant risk factors are the control of hypertension, the use of ASA for prophylaxis in patients with a moderate to high risk of CVA or TIA, and the use of anticoagulants in patients with atrial fibrillation. In a summary of 17 treatment trials of hypertension throughout the world with nearly 50,000 patients, there was a 38% decrease in all strokes and a 40% decrease in fatal CVAs after treatment of hypertension. In the Framingham study, smoking cessation promptly reduced the risk of a CVA, with the major risk reduced within 2 to 4 years. Heavy use of alcohol also should be avoided. Moderate and heavy levels of physical activity have been associated with a decrease in chronic incidence of CVA. The physical activity is believed to exert a beneficial influence on the risk factors for atherosclerotic disease by decreasing BP, weight, and pulse rate; raising high-density lipoprotein cholesterol and lowering low-density lipoprotein cholesterol; decreasing platelet aggregability; increasing insulin sensitivity and improving glucose tolerance; and promoting a lifestyle conducive to changing diet and promoting a cessation of cigarette smoking. A diet low in fat, sodium, and cholesterol and high in fiber, fruits, and vegetables should be encouraged. Patients should also be encouraged to exercise modestly, to avoid weight gain, and to use stress reduction techniques. If the patient has atrial fibrillation, anticoagulant therapy should be initiated to prevent pooling of the blood in the atria that could promote potential microemboli.

Because treatment within 3 to 4.5 hours of onset of a stroke is critical, successful treatment depends on educating the patient and the family to recognize CVA symptoms and to contact and secure access to medical care by calling 911. Delay in treatment has been known to occur for patients who call their primary-care physician instead of 911, live alone, have onset of CVA while asleep, have onset at home rather than work, and who experience a milder severity of a CVA. Studies have documented that 38% of patients and their families did not know a single warning sign of a CVA and that 28% could identify only one sign of seizures. Thus, mild tingling or numbness of the fingers or mild gait clumsiness is attributed to a problem with the arm or leg. Patients may also feel they have dust in their eyes, when in fact they are experiencing amaurosis fugax. Patients may think such symptoms are trivial and may not seek attention, or if they do, they may not mention those symptoms to their practitioner. Older adults may simply forget that any symptoms occurred.

Education of the patient and family should include the importance of reporting any symptoms of graying, darkening, or fogging of vision; a shadow coming over the visual field; or if any episodes of peripheral numbness, tingling, or clumsiness in the upper or lower extremities (e.g., leg giving way suddenly or being weak for a short period of time) occur. Thorough teaching of high-risk patients and their families of the warning signs of a CVA, along with frequent evaluation and a careful review of symptoms by the practitioner, will assist in detecting symptomatic carotid artery stenosis and initiating treatment as soon as possible.

See the Iceberg of Stroke for the intense interactions that need to occur for a patient recovering from a stroke to achieve his or her highest potential.

■ HEADACHES

Headaches are a pain or ache in the head, sometimes restricting activity, reducing the level of functioning, and decreasing work performance. The prevalence of headaches has a great impact on society because of lost or reduced effectiveness at home, work, or school. Individual burdens result from pain, suffering, and the disabling effects of various headache syndromes. It remains difficult to gain a measure of control over headaches. Headaches pose a challenge to the practitioner to avoid underestimating their significance as an early manifestation of serious neurological disease.

Headaches may be classified into four general categories: muscle contraction headaches (tension); vascular headaches (migraines and cluster headaches); mixed headaches (a combination of muscle contraction and vascular); and traction or inflammatory headaches. A *tension headache* presents as a mild to moderate bilateral, nonpulsating, tightening pain that is not aggravated by routine physical activity. It is usually not accompanied by nausea and vomiting or photophobia. A *migraine headache* may last for 4 to 72 hours and may or may not be precipitated by an aura. It is usually of moderate to severe intensity with a pulsating quality, aggravated by routine physical activity, and accompanied by nausea, vomiting, and photophobia. A *cluster headache* usually occurs at night and may last from 15 to 180 minutes. There is usually severe unilateral orbital, supraorbital, and/or temporal pain that is accompanied on the same side of the face with sweating, lacrimation, nasal congestion, ptosis, rhinorrhea, eyelid edema, and/or conjunctival injection. A *traction or inflammatory headache* is an acute new-onset headache that has an increasing intensity; this type of headache is a medical emergency

The Iceberg of Stroke

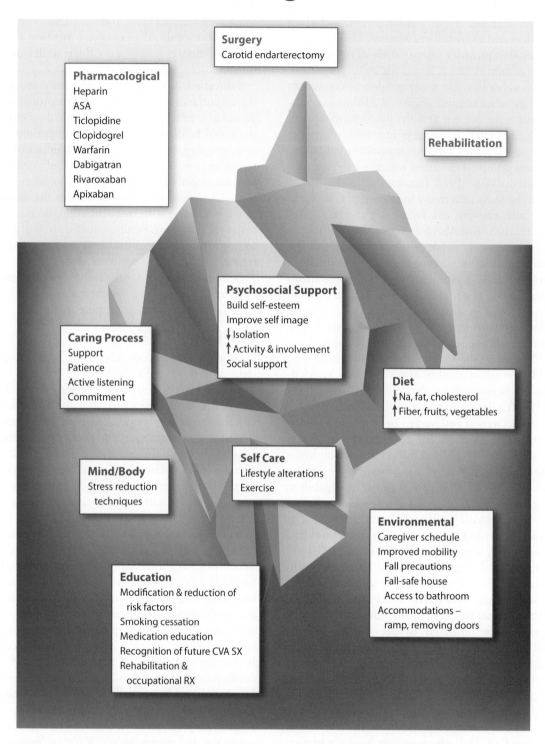

because it may be symptomatic of a more serious condition (i.e., subarachnoid hemorrhage or infection). Table 6.5 presents a comparison of the four categories of headaches. These are all considered primary headaches. Secondary headaches are a symptom of an injury or an underlying illness.

Epidemiology and Causes

More individuals complain about headaches than any other condition experienced, and they affect anyone of any age. Each year, approximately 45 million individuals complain of headaches, and more than 8 million individuals of all ages visit a health-care provider with

Table 6.5 Headaches: A Comparison of the Different Types

Type	Muscle Contraction (Tension)	Vascular (Migraine, Cluster)	Mixed	Traction or Inflammatory (Acute Headache)
Signs and symptoms	Nausea and vomiting Bilateral pressure or band-like pain	**Migraine:** Unilateral pulsating episodic pain Nausea and vomiting Photophobia Confusion Disorientation **Cluster** (associated with alcohol use): Periorbital nighttime unilateral nonpulsatile pain Photophobia Tearing Nasal stuffiness	Combination of muscular and vascular headache	New onset Usually older than age 35 Acute, constant, progressive pain that prevents sleep "Worst headache of my life"
History and physical exam findings	Sleep cycle disturbances Depression Appetite changes Relationship difficulties Recent or remote memory loss Limited neck ROM with crepitus	May be similar	May be similar	Acute onset
Diagnostic tests	MRI: lesions, trauma, hematomas CT: hemorrhage LP: to determine presence of organisms	Same	Same	Same
Treatment	Support Biofeedback Stress management Drugs: aspirin, acetaminophen (Tylenol), NSAIDs, muscle relaxants Preventive treatment	**Migraine:** Avoidance education Drugs: beta blockers, ergot alkaloids, NSAIDs, antiemetics, selective serotonin receptor agonists (sumatriptan [Imitrex]), tricyclic antidepressant (amitriptyline) **Cluster:** 100% oxygen by mask Drugs: inhaled ergotamine Preventive treatment (propranolol, amitriptyline, valproate, or lithium)	Combined approach of counseling, migraine prevention, drugs, antidepressants, and stress reduction	Refer to neurologist

this complaint annually, with the incidence decreasing with age. In the United States, some researchers estimate the annual cost of headaches, including costs of direct medical care and lost productivity, to exceed $17 billion. Headaches affect women two to three times more than men across all age-groups, with the incidence in women increasing during adolescence and peaking at menarche.

Muscular traction or a tension-type headache is a highly prevalent condition that can be disabling. It is the most common type of headache, with an estimated 80% to 90% of the population suffering from tension headaches at some period in their lives. It is found more often in women (86%) than in men (65%). Its prevalence peaks at about age 30 to 38. Tension headache occurs more frequently in whites (40%), especially with increasing educational levels (48%). Although few people who suffer tension-type headaches lose time from work, more than 40% of people affected reported decreased effectiveness at work, home, or school because of this type of headache.

Migraine headaches are the second most common type of headache. Twenty-five percent of women suffer a migraine at least once, and 8% of men are affected by migraine headaches. Racial differences in migraine prevalence are striking: African Americans and non-whites of Hispanic or other nonspecified ethnic origin are at least twice as likely as whites or Asians to be migraine sufferers. An inverse relationship exists between migraine and age. Prevalence of migraine is highest in adults younger than age 40, and lowest in those older than age 60. Migraine headaches occur in 4% to 5% of school-age children. It is not unusual for migraine headaches to begin during childhood between ages 5 and 8 years. Migraine syndromes are painful and often disabling, accounting for a loss of more than 157 million workdays to headache pain each year. In one study of patients who met the International Headache Society criteria for migraine, fewer than half had actually received a diagnosis of migraine.

Migraine headaches are often hereditary and can be traced to hormonal shifts in women. In familial migraine headaches, the cause is associated with mutations in calcium-channel genes. The causes of menstrual migraine are explained by hormonal fluctuations either before, during, or after menstruation. Falling estrogen levels can trigger a migraine that is either endogenously or exogenously induced (e.g., by a week-off [21-day] oral contraceptive pill or by hormonal replacement therapy). There are multiple and varied precipitating factors or "triggers" of migraine headaches. A migraine headache may occur shortly after or just before a period of stress. One type of migraine, sometimes known as an exertional migraine, is associated with strenuous physical activity, but in general, women who exercise regularly are less likely to get migraines or at least experience them with less severity. Some sports, however, may actually precipitate a headache, resulting in common phrases such as "swimmer's migraine" or "runner's headache." Weight lifting, cycling, and hockey have been identified as other possible culprits. Researchers believe that the relationship between exercise and sports activities and migraine is associated with increased pressure on the head or a strained neck muscle. Physical activity at high altitudes is another factor that may trigger a migraine between 6 hours and 4 days after arrival. Other factors associated with exercise may be an inadequate warm-up or dehydration. Certain foods containing tyramine or phenylethylamine are known triggers of migraine. These vasoactive substances cause both vasodilation and vasoconstriction of the cerebral vessels. Examples of vasodilator agents include alcohol and sodium nitrate. Sodium nitrate is used as a preservative and is present in processed meats and

food coloring. Vasoconstrictor agents, on the other hand, stimulate the release of noradrenalin and adrenalin, causing vascular constriction of the cerebral vessels. Caffeine is known to cause a headache after six cups of coffee are consumed. Although consuming smaller amounts of coffee may protect a person from a headache, sudden caffeine withdrawal may trigger a migraine as a result of rebound vasodilation. Monosodium glutamate (MSG) can also produce a migraine. Eighty-five percent of individuals report some sort of trigger that will kick off their headache. Table 6.6 presents common triggers of migraine headaches.

Cluster headaches, another form of vascular headaches, are named for their particular pattern of occurrence: They usually come in groups over the span of several weeks or months, then disappear for months or even years. Cluster headaches are considered to be the most painful of the headaches. They occur in middle-aged men, with the first onset between ages 20 and 30, and typically cluster on a seasonal basis, with anywhere from 3 to 18 months between headaches. Approximately 69 out of 100,000 individuals suffer from cluster headaches. A dysfunction of the hypothalamus may account for the periodicity and clocklike regularity of cluster headaches.

Table 6.6	Common Triggers of Migraine Headaches

Hormonal
• Low estrogen level, increased prostaglandin level
Environmental
• High-pitched noises, excessive sun, bright lights, weather changes, strong odors, video display terminals
Diet
• Vasodilating agents: alcohol, sodium nitrate
• Vasoconstricting agents: caffeine, tyramine (bananas, ripe cheese, nuts, pods of broad beans [Italian pole, lima, or butter beans]), chicken livers, yogurt, avocado, sour cream
Phenylethylamine
• Some cheeses, red wine, chocolate
Monosodium glutamate
• Chinese food, canned soups, frozen dinners
Artificial sweeteners
Lifestyle
• Stress, sports, swimming, cycling, hockey, weight lifting, running, inadequate warm-ups
Physical activity at high altitudes
• Cycling, climbing, skiing
Fatigue
Changes in sleep schedule
• Excessive sleep, too little sleep
Cigarette smoking
Dehydration

Older adults have fewer headaches overall. Unfortunately, about a third of those that occur are traction or inflammatory headaches that are secondary to systemic disease or primary intracranial lesions such as subarachnoid hemorrhages resulting from arteriovenous malformation (AVM) or intracranial aneurysms. These headaches require immediate medical evaluation. Other causes may be temporal arteritis and subdural hematoma.

Temporal arteritis or giant cell arteritis (GCA) affects men and women equally and occurs predominantly in adults older than age 60. Its incidence increases with age and is rare in the young. The headache from a subdural hematoma is of venous origin, typically resulting from a head injury that is usually mild and easily forgotten by the patient. It occurs predominantly in persons older than age 50 and is more common in men. The abuse of alcohol and use of anticoagulants contribute to its occurrence. It rarely is associated with a fractured skull.

The headache from subarachnoid hemorrhage commonly occurs from a ruptured intracranial aneurysm, such as a "berry" aneurysm or dissecting arterial aneurysm of the carotid or vertebral vessels. A berry aneurysm, or berry-shaped aneurysm, results from a congenital abnormality of intracranial vessels, primarily at the circle of Willis. Ruptured intracranial aneurysms are the primary cause of subarachnoid hemorrhage. Less often, a subarachnoid hemorrhage is caused by an AVM or bleeding disorder. An AVM is a congenital disorder that results in the formation of a tangled collection of dilated arteries and veins. Symptoms are usually seen in persons aged 20 to 40 years. Two-thirds of people affected by a subarachnoid hemorrhage are aged 40 to 60 years; women are affected slightly more frequently because of the higher incidence of hypertension among women. In the United States, 10 to 15 cases occur per 100,000 population per year. Activities such as lifting, straining, sexual intercourse, or emotional excitement can precipitate a hemorrhage. However, subarachnoid hemorrhage has also been known to occur during sleep.

Primary Headache Syndromes
Pathophysiology

Head Pain Inside the skull, only certain structures are sensitive to pain; these include the fold of dura between the cerebral hemispheres (the falx cerebri), the middle meningeal artery of the dura, the dural venous sinuses, and the extraparenchymal regions of the larger pial arteries. Increased pressure on and inflammation of the meninges will cause pain, and distention of or traction on the arteries will cause pain. Head trauma usually causes headaches through all these pain-inducing mechanisms.

Besides head trauma, many other medical problems can initiate a headache secondarily—CVAs (hematomas, hemorrhages, and thrombi); intracranial infections, tumors; metabolic disorders (hypercapnia, hypoglycemia, and hypoxia); sudden hypertension; changes in intracranial pressure; drugs and drug withdrawals; cranial nerve pain; and eye, ear, nose, sinus, teeth, and jaw disorders. On the other hand, in certain disorders headaches are considered to be the primary problem. The three primary headache syndromes are chronic tension-type headaches, migraine headaches, and cluster headaches.

Pain signals are transmitted from most structures in the head by branches of the trigeminal nerve (see Fig. 6.1), although pain from the back of the head and the posterior fossa of the skull are transmitted by branches of the first three cervical spinal nerves. First-order pain fibers from these nerves synapse in the brainstem and upper spinal cord, and from there, the second-order pain fibers project

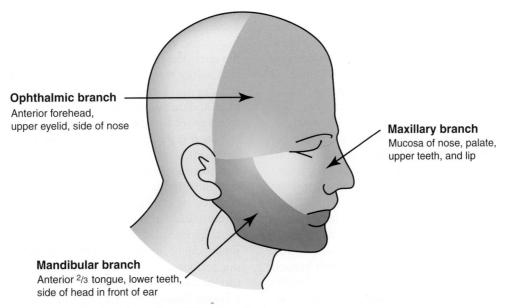

Ophthalmic branch
Anterior forehead, upper eyelid, side of nose

Maxillary branch
Mucosa of nose, palate, upper teeth, and lip

Mandibular branch
Anterior 2/3 tongue, lower teeth, side of head in front of ear

Figure 6.1 The three branches of the trigeminal nerve.

to sensory nuclei in the thalamus. Regardless of its cause, headache pain is the result of activating these trigemino-thalamic and cervico-thalamic pain circuits.

The primary headache syndromes, however, are not caused simply by the normal activation of trigeminal or cervical pain receptors inside the skull. Instead, primary headache syndromes require hypersensitization of the trigemino-thalamic or cervico-thalamic circuitry at one or more points along their route from the primary afferent axons to the thalamic sensory nuclei.

One part of this circuitry on which many headache studies have focused is the thalamus. When pain stimuli pass through the thalamus, the signals are modulated by serotonergic axons coming from the dorsal raphe nuclei in the midbrain. It is thought that an abnormal reduction in serotonergic activity in the thalamus is a part of the hypersensitization in primary headache syndromes. Among the observations consistent with this idea are the following:

• Serotonin agonists (ergotamine, dihydroergotamine, and triptans) can reduce the pain and frequency of migraines and can reduce the duration and frequency of cluster headaches.
• Increasing the effectiveness of serotonergic synapses with a selective serotonin reuptake inhibitor can reduce the frequency of tension-type headaches.
• Reserpine, a drug that depletes CNS synapses of serotonin, can precipitate migraine headaches.

Chronic Tension-Type Headaches   Chronic tension-type headaches produce mild to moderate pain that feels like a constant, bilateral head tightness and that lasts from a half hour to a week. These headaches do not pulsate, do not cause nausea, and usually are not made worse by physical activity. Chronic tension-type headaches occur repeatedly (typically many times a month), they come on gradually during the day, and they are more common in people with depression.

Although patients with chronic tension-type headaches have muscle tenderness, their headaches seem not to be caused by unusual muscle tension or contraction. Instead, in patients with this type of primary headache, the head and neck pain circuitry is hypersensitized so that normal stimuli and typical muscle strains lead to headaches. The basic cause of the hypersensitization is not known, although it is thought that chronic tension-type headaches result from abnormalities in the serotonin, norepinephrine, or dopamine pathways that originate in the brainstem and that modulate the trigemino-thalamic or cervico-thalamic pain circuits.

Migraine Headaches   Migraine headaches produce moderate to severe unilateral pain lasting from 4 hours to 3 days. These headaches throb, cause nausea, and are made worse by activity. Migraine headaches happen repeatedly (typically one to three times per month) and can be triggered by certain stimuli, most commonly alcohol, stress, menstruation, or diet.

Migraine headaches come as a set of events that unfold in a predictable pattern. First, there is a prodrome, which begins hours or days before the headache. The prodrome is often a psychological change—it can be drowsiness; depression; euphoria; hyperactivity; difficulty concentrating; irritability; or increased sensitivity to noises, lights, or smells. The prodrome is thought to reflect disturbances in the hypothalamic-limbic system.

Patients with the most common type of migraine then develop a unilateral throbbing headache, which is accompanied by anorexia and nausea (with vomiting in a third of the cases) and by a heightened sensitivity to noises, lights, and smells. The basis for the pain is a hypersensitized trigemino-thalamic circuit, which makes the normally innocuous pulsing of cerebral blood flow feel painful. The hypersensitivity can carry over to all trigeminal nerve stimuli on the same side of the head, so that normal pressures (caused by, e.g., combing, shaving, taking a shower, or wearing glasses or earrings) on the skin of the face and scalp also feel painful.

In an experimental model, migraine-like headaches can be initiated by electrical stimulation of areas in the midbrain. In this region, focal stimuli set off a cascade of specific reactions including an increase in local blood flow and a hypersensitization of the trigemino-thalamic pain circuits.

In a less common type of migraine (classic migraine), the headache is preceded by sensory phenomena called an aura. An aura is usually either a set of patterns in the visual fields or a sequence of strange feelings moving from the hand, up the arm, and onto the face. The aura coincides with a slowly spreading wave of chemical and metabolic changes that moves across the cerebral cortex from initial foci in the occipital lobe(s). As the wave reaches a region, it briefly activates the local neurons and increases the local blood flow. After the wave passes, it leaves the neurons refractory and the local blood flow decreased. It is thought that this wave contributes to the hypersensitization of the trigemino-thalamic circuits and that the wave also elicits the headache pain that follows the aura. Experimentally, it has been found that agents that reduce migraine headaches (specifically, the adrenergic agonist norepinephrine, the alpha$_2$-agonist clonidine, and the beta blocker propranolol) also stop or slow this wave of cortical depression.

Like epilepsy sufferers, patients with migraine headaches have cortical neurons that are permanently hyperexcitable. Even between migraine attacks, migraine patients experience other headaches with unusual frequency, and they can get headaches and perceptual distortions from minor visual stresses such as patterns of glare. The neuronal hyperexcitability underlying this continuous sensitivity can be inherited, and there are indications that it is due to abnormalities in certain ion channels in nerve cell membranes.

Cluster Headaches   Cluster headaches give severe unilateral pain behind the eye or temple lasting from a half hour to longer than an hour. The pain is constant, deep, and piercing and can radiate to the forehead, neck, or shoulder. These headaches do not pulsate, do not cause nausea, and usually are not made worse by physical activity. Together with the pain, there are eye or nose symptoms, such as tearing, swollen conjunctivae, runny nose, nasal congestion, eyelid droop, eyelid edema, facial sweating, or pupillary constriction. Cluster headaches come in groups that last 2 to 3 months. During one of these periods, headaches can occur as often as eight per day or as few as one every other day. Typically, a sufferer has one or two clusters of headaches per year.

Cluster headaches appear to be triggered by an abnormality in the ipsilateral circadian pacemaker, which is located in the ventral hypothalamus. The headache pain is caused by a hypersensitized ophthalmic nerve (the ophthalmic branch of the trigeminal nerve). The autonomic symptoms are caused by concurrent excitation of parasympathetic fibers running with the ophthalmic nerve. It is not known what causes these nerve problems.

Clinical Presentation

Subjective

Patients with episodic tension headaches rarely seek health care. Patients with chronic tension headaches present with symptoms of anxiety and depression but do not attribute their headaches to these symptoms. It is the astute clinician who can relate patients' subjective comments to the stress and anxiety that they are experiencing in their lives and help each patient to attribute his or her headache to that cause, thereby encouraging patients to seek treatment for the underlying stress, anxiety, and/or depression.

Two basic types of migraine headaches occur—those with aura and those without. A typical migraine without aura (previously called "common migraine") is often unilateral (60%) but may become generalized. The headache lasts 2 to 72 hours or longer and is of pulsating quality. Most patients describe the pain as intense, throbbing, or pulsating. It is moderate to severe in intensity, inhibiting or prohibiting daily activities. It can be aggravated by routine physical activity and is often relieved by sleep. During the attack, nausea and vomiting, photophobia, and phonophobia are common. Adults often experience both photophobia and phonophobia, whereas children are more likely to have one or the other.

In migraine with aura (previously called "classic migraine"), the aura develops over 4 minutes and usually lasts an hour. Following the aura may be a pain-free period lasting no longer than 1 hour before the headache pain begins. The headache may also start before or at the same time as the aura. Patients typically have one or more symptoms associated with the aura that are characteristically neural in nature, such as unilateral numbness or paresthesia of the face or extremity and speech

difficulties. Visual symptoms are common and usually occur 20 to 40 minutes before the headache. These symptoms include scotoma (blind spots), photopsia (flashing lights), fortification spectra (zigzag pattern), and diplopia. The aura phase may include additional symptoms of euphoria or depression, fatigue, hunger, and hyperosmia.

Migraine attacks may occur sporadically, with just a few headaches per year, or may be more frequent, with eight or more occurrences each month. Other symptoms may be associated with migraines, such as anorexia, constipation, pallor, dizziness, tremors, or diaphoresis. Some patients complain of cold hands or feet or experience polyuria, hunger, diarrhea, or body aches following the migraine.

The patient with a headache from a subarachnoid hemorrhage presents a picture of a sudden, abrupt, and unrelenting headache. Associated symptoms include nausea and vomiting, photophobia, and decreased level of consciousness. With small "warning leak" hemorrhages, the patient may complain of severe hemifacial pain spreading to the neck or back. The headache may have begun after exercise or intercourse.

Objective

Careful attention to the headache history is essential, including such particulars as onset, location, character, and severity; frequency and duration; associated signs and symptoms; prodromal symptoms; and precipitating factors. The practitioner should explore the patient's family and social history. Information should be sought regarding other family members who suffer from headaches, the type of headache, and the age at occurrence.

Patients with migraines usually have a parent who suffers from migraines. Information regarding the age at onset with migraines is also important because migraine frequently starts before age 20. A social history may elicit stressors or precipitating factors for the headache. Identifying the possible precipitating factors for the migraine can assist the practitioner in developing an individual prescription plan for the patient to decrease the severity or frequency of the attacks. The patient's lifestyle, dietary habits, possible job-related stress, and environmental factors should be explored. In women, information should be sought regarding the relationship of the migraine to the menstrual cycle. Headaches usually occur after ovulation and before and during menstruation. Migraines that occur before menses are considered premenstrual and associated with the premenstrual syndrome. Women are more likely to have their first migraine in the year of menarche and often cease to have migraine headaches during pregnancy. The use of oral contraceptive pills or hormonal replacement therapy should be explored. Initially, the cycle is more haphazard because of unstable blood estrogen concentration. The use of hormones for the first time may precipitate a migraine and cause the migraine to become more frequent or to be preceded by auras. Most women who suffer from migraines do not experience an aura. Discontinuing the oral contraceptive does not always resolve the problem. In patients with gynecological disorders, migraines often become more frequent and can improve when the disorder is corrected. Practitioners may consider postponing a complete medical history to a more pain-free period for the patient once more serious disorders have been ruled out. The final step of the medical history is obtaining a record of all previous work-ups and past treatments performed, including their effectiveness.

In contrast to migraine, the patient with a cluster headache experiences severe, unilateral, orbital, supraorbital, or temporal pain lasting 15 minutes to 3 hours. The pain is most commonly sharp and burning in quality. Frequently, the headache occurs at night, awakening the patient. No aura is present, and it is rare to find nausea and vomiting. Attacks commonly occur in "clusters" or groups and can last up to several weeks or even months. One of the following can be demonstrated on the affected side: conjunctival injection, miosis, ptosis and eyelid edema, nasal congestion, rhinorrhea, and forehead and/or facial sweating. Physical findings to detect a headache resulting from a subarachnoid hemorrhage are visual blurring, diplopia, fever, slight decrease in awareness, asymmetrical pupillary response, equivocal extensor plantar response, and pronator drift. Other findings from a subarachnoid hemorrhage may include decreased level of consciousness and nuchal rigidity.

Frequently, a headache is seen in patients with temporal arteritis. The intensity of GCA is severe with the quality of the pain described as deep, burning, and throbbing. A symptom specific to temporal arteritis is "claudication" of the muscles of mastication. Because of ischemia of the muscles, the patient complains of pain in the jaw on prolonged chewing. Localized tenderness of the affected artery is found. The practitioner should be alert to the potential complication of blindness. Diplopia is a common sign seen before visual impairment. Once visual impairment occurs, however, it can progress quickly to blindness in several hours. On physical exam, few abnormalities are revealed. A low-grade fever may appear. The temporal arteries may be tender and more visible or pronounced on palpation but have absent or decreased palpations.

The single most commonly occurring symptom with a subdural hematoma is headache. It is subacute and usually progresses. Characteristically, this secondary headache is generalized, is temporal, and worsens with changes in posture. It can occur during the night and may cause the patient to awaken in the morning earlier than usual. Associated symptoms are nausea, vomiting, confusion, seizures, or weakness. The practitioner should be alert to changes in personality, decreasing level of consciousness, excessive sleepiness, or sensory changes. Less common findings are focal neurological signs, such as hemiparesis or pathological reflexes. Papilledema rarely occurs because of the large volume of CSF.

Diagnostic Reasoning
Diagnostic Tests

An EEG is not useful in the routine evaluation of a patient with a headache and is not recommended to exclude a structural cause for headache. Neither a CT scan nor an MRI is warranted in adult patients whose headaches fit within the broad definition of tension or migraine headache and who have not demonstrated any recent substantial change in headache pattern, occurrence of seizures, or presence of focal neurological signs or symptoms.

A CT scan or an MRI study is recommended if the patient's headache pattern is atypical; has changed in pattern or character; or is accompanied by seizures, personality changes, or an abnormal neurological finding. Patients with migraines commonly have normal physical findings between attacks. Extensive diagnostic testing for a patient with a migraine is not warranted. A CBC, chemistry profile, and urinalysis may be obtained to rule out a systemic illness for the patient with typical migraine with no change in pattern and a normal physical exam. Nonspecific EEG abnormalities can occur; however, some of these findings are normal and others often do not require treatment.

The Headache Classification Committee of the International Headache Society has a headache classification system and operational diagnostic criteria for the different headache syndromes, divided into 14 categories. This system was designed to describe and identify headaches to allow for more accurate diagnosis and research. For example, a diagnosis of migraine with aura must include the presence of one or more fully reversible neurological (visual, motor, or sensory) symptoms. For migraine without aura, two of the following characteristics are required: unilateral location, pulsating quality, moderate to severe intensity, and exacerbation by physical activity. In addition, at least one of the following must be present: nausea or vomiting, photophobia, or phonophobia.

In an older adult patient with late-onset migraines, it is recommended that a CT scan be performed, just in case, even in the presence of a typical migraine with normal physical exam, to rule out organic disease. In a patient who has a history of migraines, the presentation of migraines can often change as the patient ages, and a headache can easily be mistaken for a migraine, overlooking a TIA. In older adults, a good indication of the need for imaging studies is an unusual presentation or change in symptoms associated with migraine.

Physical exam of patients with cluster headaches usually reveals normal physical findings. If there has been no change in the pattern or pain of the cluster headache and a normal physical exam is found, a CBC, chemical profile, and urinalysis may be completed to rule out a systemic illness.

Headaches from a subarachnoid hemorrhage should be identified quickly and an immediate CT scan performed. In a few patients with a small hemorrhage, the result may be negative. The benefit from the CT scan diminishes with time; that is, there is less sensitivity if the scan is obtained more than 7 days after headache onset. If the results are positive, an immediate neurosurgical referral is initiated.

With temporal arteritis, the ESR may be strongly elevated, from 50 to 100 mm, but it may also be normal. The C-reactive protein test (CRP) may also be elevated. These inflammatory markers, ESR and CRP, may, however, be normal and should not be used alone to rule out GCA. In this case, referral is essential, and a biopsy of the temporal artery (the gold standard) is recommended along with excision of a long segment of the artery because lesions typically are not present along the entire artery. Other laboratory findings may include anemia and an elevated alkaline phosphatase level.

A subdural hemorrhage is best evaluated by CT, which has a greater sensitivity to early hemorrhage. The CT reveals the bleeding as hyperdense, isodense, or hypodense. If bleeding is isodense, there may be a shift of midline structures without any further evidence of abnormalities on CT. MRI or angiography may be used to determine if a hematoma is present.

Differential Diagnosis

A complete history is paramount to distinguish and diagnose headaches and to rule out life-threatening events, such as subarachnoid hemorrhage or a TIA that could lead to a CVA. Patients may have more than one type of headache, so each event must be identified. A thorough history should be explored, including the family, social, and medical history. A family history may reveal migraine headaches in other family members. A social history may identify stress or other precipitating factors for the headache. A general medical history, including a review of systems, may lead to a diagnosis other than migraine headache. The clinician should explore any recent or past history of head or neck traumas and previous medical procedures contributing to a headache, such as LP, spinal anesthesia, or surgeries. Following an LP, for example, a bilateral headache may develop after 7 days. It typically worsens in 15 minutes on standing; once the patient is recumbent, the headache is relieved within 30 minutes. Possible causes of headache might be related to current medical conditions, especially hypothyroidism, hypertension, and asthma. Identifying current medications, both prescription and OTC agents, would help in distinguishing the headache. Chronic daily headaches are frequently associated with the daily use of nonprescription "pain killer" drugs, especially compounds containing 50 to 75 mg of caffeine per tablet.

Sudden onset of pain may suggest serious pathology such as subarachnoid hemorrhage, meningitis, or brain tumor. A headache that has been present over a period of years is more likely to be associated with migraine, cluster, or tension-type headaches. The character of pain in migraines also is helpful in distinguishing a migraine headache from a tension-type headache. A tension-type headache is dull and nonpulsating; it changes in intensity. Its duration may be 30 minutes to 7 days, and it is not associated with nausea or vomiting. Patients with tension-type headaches may report phonophobia or photophobia, but not both. Though tension-type headaches may limit some activities, these are generally not aggravated by physical activity and will not incapacitate the individual. Testing should include motor and sensory function to detect serious organic disease. A diagnosis of migraines with aura requires the presence of one or more fully recoverable neurological symptoms (visual, motor, or sensory). This finding helps the practitioner distinguish migraine from a progressive, organic disorder that requires further assessment. An aura that is rapid in onset and short in duration, atypical of migraine, may be caused by a paroxysmal event or specific cardiovascular disease. Prodromal signs (aura) can be differentiated from signs of a stroke by the length of the aural event, which is usually less than 60 minutes. Differentiating a migraine with aura from a TIA may be difficult. Age, for instance, may play a role in the differential diagnosis, because a TIA is rare in the young.

Some warning signs indicative of secondary problems include the following (Beithon et al, 2013):

- Progressive headaches that worsen over time
- Patient states, "This is the worst headache of my life!"
- New-onset headaches after age 50
- Persistent headache precipitated by a Valsalva maneuver
- Fever, hypertension, myalgias, weight loss, or scalp tenderness
- Neurological signs and symptoms: confusion, altered level of consciousness, changes in memory, papilledema, sensory deficits, reflex asymmetry, or gait disturbances
- Seizures

Management

Immediate hospitalization is required for the person with a severe (secondary) headache occurring suddenly with signs of meningeal irritation. A patient claim that he or she is having "the worst headache of my life" is definitely a red flag. Possible causes are intracranial hemorrhage or meningeal infection. If examination reveals evidence of symptoms or signs of increased intracranial pressure or severe intractable migraine, urgent hospitalization is indicated.

Because the majority of headaches (tension-type and migraines) can be recurrent and chronic, the principle of management is to design an individual treatment plan that identifies therapeutic goals for the patient. Goals would include strategies to avoid possible triggers and the ability to abort an attack, to obtain relief from pain and associated symptoms, and to decrease the frequency and severity of attacks.

Management for a tension-type headache is focused on the use of NSAIDs, cool compresses, and stress-reduction techniques. Aspirin and acetaminophen are recommended for acute treatment in patients with tension-type headache. Triptans are recommended as the agents of choice where prophylactic treatment is being considered in a patient with chronic tension-type headache. Drug therapy for acute headache should generally not exceed more than 2 days per week on a regular basis. More frequent treatment may result in medication-overuse chronic daily headaches.

Migraine treatment can be divided into four methods: nonpharmacological, abortive therapy, pain relief, and prophylactic treatment. Nonpharmacological measures are useful for minor migraines or as an adjunct to pharmacological treatment to prevent or decrease the severity of a headache. These methods include identifying and eliminating known triggers. Maintaining a strict schedule for sleep and meals can prevent a headache related to fatigue and hunger. It is critical to keep from getting too much or too little sleep. If exercise precipitates an attack, an adequate warm-up before working out is recommended. Biofeedback, relaxation techniques, and regular aerobic exercise are encouraged. Deep breathing, massage, and hot or cold therapy sometimes ease the pain, but excessive cold (e.g., ice packs) or caffeine can backfire.

Most migraine attacks vary in the effect on the patient's ability to function. In mild attacks, the effect is minimal. In moderate attacks, visual activities are moderately impaired. In severe attacks, however, the patient is unable to continue normal activities or can continue them only with severe discomfort. In some severe attacks, the patient is incapacitated, requiring treatment in the provider's office or emergency department.

Drug therapy should be added when these measures are not completely effective. Early treatment of migraines with effective medications improves a variety of outcomes, including duration, severity, and associated disability. It is appropriate for the clinician to take a trial-and-error approach to identify medications most successful in the relief of headaches and associated symptoms with the fewest adverse effects and minimal costs and a return to normal functioning for each patient. Some patients may require three different medications: a triptan as an abortive medication, a rescue medication for breakthrough or residual pain, and a daily preventive medication. Initially, aspirin 900 mg or ibuprofen 400 mg is recommended for acute treatment in patients with migraine. Drugs Commonly Prescribed 6.5 presents a listing of medications commonly used to treat migraines. Complementary Therapies 6.1 presents other measures that may be taken to help treat headaches.

Drugs Commonly Prescribed 6.5 Migraines: Adults

Drug	Adverse Reactions and Prescribing Considerations
Abortive	
Triptans (serotonin receptor agonists) almotriptan (Axert)	Side effects: Paresthesias, asthenia, nausea, dizziness, chest or neck tightness, heaviness, somnolence.
eletriptan (Relpax) frovatriptan (Frova) naratriptan (Amerge) rizatriptan (Maxalt) sumatriptan (Imitrex) zolmitriptan (Zomig)	Contraindicated in ischemic heart disease or other significant cardiovascular disease or cerebrovascular disease. There is a risk of rebound headache if triptans are used more than twice a week.
Ergot derivatives ergotamine 1 mg/caffeine 100 mg (Cafergot) ergotamine 2 mg/caffeine 100 mg (Cafergot supp) dihydroergotamine (DHE 45, Migranal)	Contraindicated in peripheral vascular disease, coronary heart disease, hypertension, and hepatic or renal disease. IV route preferred when rapid relief is desired.
Prophylactic Medications	
Beta blockers (Level A; Silberstein et al, 2012) propranolol (Inderal) timolol (Blocadren)	Contraindicated in asthma, sinus bradycardia, second or third atrioventricular block. Potentiated by alcohol.
metoprolol (Lopressor, Toprol)	May cause weight loss, asthenia, mental fuzziness.

Drugs Commonly Prescribed 6.5   Migraines: Adults—cont'd

Drug	Adverse Reactions and Prescribing Considerations
(Level B; Silberstein et al, 2012) atenolol (Tenormin) nadolol (Corgard) *Antidepressants* venlafaxine (Effexor XR) (Level B; Silberstein et al, 2012) *Calcium channel blockers* verapamil (Calan)	May take several months to be effective. Contraindicated in pregnancy. Adverse effects: Extrapyramidal effects, bradycardia, fatigue, weight gain, constipation, nausea, edema, muscle pain.
Antiepileptic agents (Level A; Silberstein et al, 2012) divalproex (Depakote) sodium valproate topiramate (Topamax)	Adverse effects: Asthenia, back pain, diarrhea, nausea, vomiting, dizziness, somnolence, tremor, weight gain. Has teratogenic effects. Adverse effects: Somnolence, dizziness, asthenia.

Rescue Medications

Triptans ergot derivatives (see above) *NSAIDs* ibuprofen (Advil, Motrin) ASA (aspirin) naproxen sodium (Aleve, Naprosyn)	For mild to moderate attacks. Increased risk of GI bleed with alcohol. Adverse reactions: GI upset, GI bleed.
Combination analgesics butalbital 50 mg/acetaminophen 325 mg/caffeine 40 mg (Fioricet) butalbital 50 mg/ASA 325 mg/caffeine 40 mg (Fiorinal)	For tension or muscle contraction headache. Potentiation with alcohol. Adverse effects: Drowsiness, dizziness, GI disturbances.

GI- gastrointestinal.

Complementary Therapies 6.1   Headaches

Acupuncture/acupressure
Aroma and herbal therapy
- Apply lavender oil to the temples (women).
- Apply peppermint oil to the temples (men).
- Use eucalyptus for sinus headaches.
- Drink rosemary tea or mix the essential oil in hot water and inhale.
- Take evening primrose oil 500 mg.
- Apply cold black tea bags to the eyes for 15 minutes.
- Take *Ginkgo biloba* 120–240 mg of dried extract in 2–3 doses daily.
- Take valerian (*Valeriana officialis*) 2–3 g 1–3 times per day.
Biofeedback
Diet therapy
- At the first sign of a migraine, drink 1–2 cups of strong coffee to prevent vessel dilation (effective for some individuals) or a glass of carrot or celery juice.
- To reduce throbbing and contractions, eat foods high in magnesium such as dark, leafy greens, fresh seafood, sea vegetables, nuts, whole grains, molasses.
- Eat vitamin C–rich foods such as broccoli, hot and bell peppers, sprouts, cherries, citrus.

Continued

Complementary Therapies 6.1   Headaches—cont'd

- Drink green tea.
- Avoid foods known to trigger headache: Additive and chemical-based foods (monosodium glutamate, sulfites [red wine], condiments, nitrates [aged and smoked meats]; pickled fish and shellfish; caffeine-containing foods, including chocolate; cultured foods [e.g., yogurt]; refined sweeteners); red meats; dairy products (cheese); soft drinks (the phosphorus binds up magnesium); alcohol; salty, sugary, and wheat-based foods.

Exercise

Massage or chiropractic manipulation
- Massage the temples for 5 minutes.
- Do 10 neck rolls.
- Pull ear lobes for 5 seconds.
- Rub back of ear and all around ear shell.
- Apply an ice pack to the back of the neck to reduce vasodilation or put feet in a cold water bath.

Poultices
- Rub capsaicin (Zostrix) cream on the forehead.
- Apply onion or horseradish poultices to the nape of the neck or soles of the feet.

Reflexology
- Apply pressure to the inside base of the foot and big toe 3 times for 10 seconds each.

Relaxation therapy
- Perform deep breathing.

Vitamin therapy
- Take magnesium citrate 800 mg daily.
- Take niacin 100–500 mg daily.

Other
- Avoid smoking and secondhand smoke.
- Take a coffee enema to stimulate the liver and normalize bile activity. (Bowel movements may relieve vomiting.)

For the first-choice treatment for the relief of acute attacks of cluster headaches, subcutaneous injection of sumatriptan or intranasal zolmitriptan is recommended. Oxygen inhalation is highly effective for cluster headaches when administered at the beginning of an attack with a non-rebreathing facial mask at 7 to 15 L/min. Most patients will obtain relief within 15 minutes.

Follow-up and Referral

A neurological referral should be considered in any patient with episodes of transient neurological deficits, increasing frequency and severity of unilateral headaches, or atypical auras, as well as changes in personality, excessive sleepiness, and new onset of progressive deficits suggesting a mass lesion, hemorrhage, or structural disorder. The possibility of ischemia must be carefully considered in a middle-aged or older patient with vascular risk factors who presents with a new and unexplained headache. The patient should be monitored regularly with follow-up exams. Surgical referral may be necessary for a temporal artery biopsy and definitive diagnosis or possible use of chronic steroid therapy.

Patient Education

The management of migraine is a team effort in which the patient plays an equal role. Patients must be convinced of the practitioner's interest in their complaints and commitment to their treatment. Realistic outcomes should be discussed because treatment is often ineffective or can be used for only a short period of time. Patients should be educated about the nature of migraine and given additional literature. Patients should keep a diary of any events that may be associated with an attack. This helps to identify and avoid triggers associated with a single episode and distinguish them from triggers that lead to an increase in the frequency and severity of attacks. Though clinicians may not help patients deal with endogenous triggers—endocrine factors, genetic tendencies, and psychological depression—they may help the patient identify other triggers. Exogenous triggers include foods, for example, red wine and other alcoholic beverages, aged cheese, monosodium glutamate, aspartame (dietary sweetener), and chocolate; the frequency and pattern of light; and oral contraceptives. Environmental triggers include stress and stressful family events; air travel; weather changes; odors (bad and good); and meteorological depression. Having an awareness of the triggers may help the patient avoid them, which should diminish the frequency and intensity of the attacks. The clinician should explain the importance of warming up before exercise and avoiding tight-fitting goggles, sunglasses, helmets, or other headgear and suggest that regular exercise may prevent or decrease the headaches. If exercise is found to trigger an attack, discuss the importance of adequate nutrition and fluids before and after such activities.

Women who have migraines with aura have a much higher risk of stroke with the use of estrogen-containing contraceptives compared with those without migraines. When discussing migraine therapy with women of childbearing age, the clinician should ask what method of birth control the individual is using.

Stress-management strategies and relaxation techniques are commonly taught to patients to manage frequently unavoidable family- or work-related stress and emotional problems. When pharmacological treatment is necessary, the family should fully understand the treatment. Impaired judgment may occur with severe attacks, and the patient may not remember what drugs or dosages were used. The patient should understand each medication type, its proper use, and adverse effects of the medications, including interactions with other medications and any contraindications, such as pregnancy. Ask the patient to record in a headache diary the medications used (including any OTC or other medications), dosages, response to medication, and evaluation of treatment, including adverse effects. Clinicians should advise patients not to take headache medications other than those prescribed. Excessive use of other analgesics may reduce their effectiveness. Using ergotamine and analgesics frequently can lead to rebound headaches or chronic daily headaches. Adverse effects are common, and the patient must keep the practitioner informed in case changes in medicine are needed. Patients should discuss with the practitioner if they desire to become or are pregnant.

INFECTIOUS AND INFLAMMATORY DISORDERS

■ MENINGITIS

Meningitis is an inflammation of the meningeal membranes surrounding the structures of the CNS and/or the CSF. Although meningitis is typically depicted as an acute process, syndromes of both chronic and subacute nature have been found. The common factor shared by all types of meningitis is an abnormality in the number of white blood cells (WBCs) in the CSF.

Purulent forms of acute meningitis are usually caused by three types of bacteria: *Neisseria meningitidis, Haemophilus influenzae* type B, and *Streptococcus pneumoniae.* Subacute or chronic manifestations occur with fungus, mycobacteria, spirochete, HIV, and neoplasms. Aseptic meningitis (no bacteria found in CSF) is usually associated with a virus or with noninfectious causes such as a brain tumor or CVA. Table 6.7 reviews the types of meningitis.

Epidemiology and Causes

The incidence of meningitis is 15 per 100,000, with a prevalence of 5 cases per 100,000. Since the initiation of the widespread use of antibiotics in the 1950s, the mortality figures have remained steady at 10% to 15%, and those who do survive may experience chronic long-term problems, such as brain damage, kidney disease, hearing loss, or limb amputations. Susceptibility differs with the causative organism, but generally young people, elderly people, and immunocompromised patients are at greatest risk. Fifteen percent of all cases involve adolescents and young adults. One out of seven cases among adolescents will result in death.

The majority of cases of meningitis are attributed to bacteria and viruses, with a much smaller occurrence caused by fungi or parasites. Among the viral causative agents, enteroviruses are leading in incidence. Seasonal occurrence shows a higher incidence of meningitis in the spring and fall. Infants and young children are particularly susceptible because of a lack of immunity and also because of the higher fecal-to-oral transmission that takes place in this age-group. Arboviral infection is another common source during warm months when insect vectors are in abundance. The mumps virus can also be a causative factor in unimmunized populations. Various herpes viruses have been associated with meningitis, although the incidence is low.

Meningitis caused by bacterial sources is predominantly from the organisms *H influenzae, N meningitidis,* and *S pneumoniae. H influenzae* occurs primarily in infants and young children, usually in conjunction with or following otitis media, epiglottitis, or pneumonia. *N meningitidis* is common in children aged 2 to 18. Each year in the United States, about 2,600 individuals get this highly contagious disease. High-risk groups include infants under 1 year old, individuals who are immunocompromised, travelers to foreign countries where the disease is endemic, and college students (particularly freshmen) living in dorms. Between 10% and 15% of cases are fatal. *S pneumoniae* is more frequently observed in adults with concurrent conditions such as pneumonia, sinusitis, otitis media, or endocarditis. *Staphylococcus aureus* can be a causative factor of meningitis in patients who have undergone invasive neurological instrumentation or trauma and in those with shunting of CSF.

Other organisms may be responsible for chronic meningitis syndromes and are generally rarer in occurrence than acute forms. *Mycobacterium tuberculosis*

Table 6.7   Types of Meningitis

Major Type	Description	Organism	Diagnostic Tests	Treatment
Bacterial (purulent)	Rapid onset: hours or days after exposure	**Age 3 months–18 years:** *H influenzae* *N meningitidis* *S pneumoniae* **Age 18–50:** *S pneumoniae* *N meningitidis* **Age 50 or older:** *S pneumoniae* *N meningitidis* *Listeria monocytogenes* Gram-negative bacilli	CSF Gram stain analysis Culture	**Age 3 months–18 years:** cefotaxime IV 50 mg/kg q6h **OR** ceftriaxone IV 50–100 mg/kg q12h **Age 18 or older:** cefotaxime 2g q4h IV **OR** ceftriaxone 2 g q12h IV **PLUS** vancomycin 750–1,000 mg IV q12h ampicillin 2 g IV q4h
Chronic (subacute)	Symptoms develop over months; less acutely ill	*M tuberculosis* Atypical mycobacteria Fungi Spirochetes	CSF analysis Culture	**Mycobacteria:** isoniazid (INH) IV 10 mg/kg/day rifampin IV 600 mg/day **Fungi:** amphotericin IV 0.3–0.6 mg/kg/day flucytosine IV 150 mg/kg/day **Spirochetes:** penicillin G IV 12–18 million units over 21–24 days acyclovir (Zovirax) IV 30 mg/kg/day
Aseptic (viral)	More benign type; self-limited syndrome caused primarily by viruses	Mumps virus Echo virus Herpes virus	Increased immunoglobulins in CSF	Rest, fluids; acetaminophen or ibuprofen

(tuberculosis) and *Treponema pallidum* (syphilis) sometimes produce indicators of meningitis in addition to their primary symptomatology. Other rare forms include fungal meningitis, parasitic meningitis, and rickettsial meningitis.

Pathophysiology

Meningitis is an infection that produces inflammation of the brain's meningeal membranes. Viruses, fungi, and parasites can cause meningitis, but the serious meningitides are most often caused by bacteria. Bacterial meningitis is an acute purulent infection that develops within the subarachnoid space. In adults, its signs and symptoms are fever, headache, and stiff neck, usually accompanied by vomiting, lethargy, confusion, or coma.

In developed countries, adult bacterial meningitis is usually caused by *S pneumoniae* (gram-positive cocci) or

N meningitidis (gram-negative diplococci). Both types of bacteria first colonize the nasopharynx. From the infected nasopharyngeal epithelium, bacteria then get into the underlying blood vessels. *S pneumoniae* and *N meningitidis* are both encapsulated bacteria, and their capsules protect them from phagocytosis in the bloodstream.

From the circulation, bacteria enter the CSF through the choroid plexuses in the ventricles and through injured or leaky areas of the blood–brain barrier. Bacteria can multiply rapidly in the subarachnoid space because normal CSF has few WBCs, no immunoglobulin M antibodies, and low concentrations of the complement components C3 and C4.

As the number of bacteria increases, they come in repeated contact with the brain and the meninges. Local monocytes, macrophages, astrocytes, and microglia react to components in the bacterial cell walls by making and releasing inflammatory molecules, such as cytokines, interleukin-1, and tumor necrosis factor. These molecules increase the permeability of the blood–brain barrier and attract polymorphonuclear leukocytes from the systemic circulation. Large numbers of WBCs enter the CSF and form a purulent exudate in the subarachnoid space. The exudate reduces the flow of CSF. Meningeal irritation from the exudate causes nuchal rigidity (meaning that the neck will resist passive flexion), and lumbar punctures in bacterial meningitis produce CSF with a high WBC count.

The invading leukocytes add to the concentration of inflammatory molecules, and the blood–brain barrier becomes sufficiently permeable to cause cerebral edema and significantly increased intracranial pressure. Increased intracranial pressure causes a number of neurological and systemic signs, including a depressed level of consciousness; a triad of bradycardia, hypertension, and irregular breathing; dilated nonreactive pupils; weakness in the abductors of the eyes; papilledema; nuchal rigidity; hiccupping; projectile vomiting; or decerebrate body postures. In addition, under significantly increased intracranial pressure, the mechanisms that regulate intracranial blood flow become ineffective, and systemic hypertension and hypotension will both have disproportionate effects on cerebral blood flow. Lumbar punctures (LPs) of patients with bacterial meningitis yield high CSF pressures.

Clinical Presentation
Subjective
Subjective symptoms of meningitis include headache, photophobia, and neck pain and stiffness (nuchal rigidity).

Objective
Objective signs include fever (usually high, greater than 103°F [39.4°C]) with accompanying chills, tachycardia, and tachypnea. Signs of meningeal irritation such as Brudzinski's sign (hip and knee flexion when the neck is flexed) and Kernig's sign (inability to fully extend the legs) are often present. Occasionally, opisthotonus (severe back spasm, causing arching) is observed. Altered level of consciousness is present and may include confusion, progressive lethargy, stupor, and coma. Cranial nerve dysfunction can occur, resulting in possible diplopia, deafness, facial weakness, and pupillary abnormalities.

History taking may yield clues to possible causative agents or risk factors for meningitis. Major areas to emphasize in taking the history include pertinent exposures (contacts, food consumption, sexual practices, drug use), history of extraneural disease (especially respiratory), evidence of immunocompromise, underlying systemic disorders, and travel history.

Diagnostic Reasoning
Diagnostic Tests
Initially, routine blood studies may show marked elevation of WBCs (neutrophils) in bacterial meningitis or mild elevation in viral meningitis. In addition, electrolytes, especially sodium, are evaluated for a common complication of meningitis, the syndrome of inappropriate antidiuretic hormone secretion (SIADH).

If the clinical signs and symptoms indicate the possibility of meningitis, the collaborating physician will probably refer the patient to a neurologist for LP and CSF studies. Bacterial infection is indicated by cloudy appearance of CSF, increased CSF pressure greater than 20 mm H_2O, protein levels greater than 15 mg/dL, increased neutrophils, and reduced CSF glucose compared with simultaneous serum glucose. Gram stains and cultures of CSF may assist in detecting causative organisms. An LP should not be performed if increased intracranial pressure is suspected because cerebral herniating may occur.

Imaging studies such as MRI may reveal meningeal enhancement, basilar exudate, hydrocephalus, and possible focal lesions as indicators of meningitis. Any other contributing abnormalities such as skin, lung, or sinus lesions should be investigated.

Differential Diagnosis
Many infectious and noninfectious conditions may mimic meningitis. It is also important to establish the specific type of meningitis. Some differential diagnoses include encephalitis, giant-cell arteritis, metabolic or toxic encephalopathy, systemic lupus erythematosus (SLE), and thrombotic thrombocytopenic purpura. Similarities in symptoms include headache and visual disturbances (encephalitis, arteritis), fever (encephalitis, SLE), nuchal rigidity (encephalitis), and headache (encephalopathy). Other diverse processes may also cause changes in CSF (e.g., increased neutrophils but with a normal CSF glucose).

Management
Meningitis can be a life-threatening problem. If meningitis is suspected, the clinician should refer the patient to the collaborating physician for immediate hospitalization for extensive diagnostic examination and treatment. The principal goals for managing meningitis include eliminating infection, symptomatic care, and prevention or treatment of complications.

The first goal and priority is to eliminate infection. This is achieved through the judicial use of specific antimicrobial therapy if the meningitis is bacterial in origin. If the diagnosis of bacterial meningitis is suspected, the administration of empiric antibiotics should not be delayed. Blood cultures and an LP should be performed immediately, and empiric antibiotic therapy should be initiated without delay. Antibiotic therapy should not be held if there is a delay in the performance of the LP. The choice of empiric therapy is predicated on the demographics of the patient (age, immunocompromised state, recent head trauma, basilar skull fracture). The patient's antibiotic regimen can be narrowed based on the results of cultures of the CSF. The usual course of IV antimicrobials is 10 to 14 days. Specific treatment regimens are included in Table 6.8. Although the concomitant use of corticosteroids has been reported in the care of children with meningitis, this strategy has not been studied thoroughly in adults and is not generally recommended. The main indication for the concomitant use of glucocorticoids is meningitis secondary to *S pneumoniae*. Use of these treatment regimens is thought to decrease inflammation and enhance circulation of the antibiotic.

Chronic meningitis may require prolonged intrathecal and/or IV antimicrobial therapy. Symptomatic treatment includes reduction of fever with acetaminophen and headache management with an analgesic such as codeine. The literature strongly recommends the use of acetaminophen every 4 to 6 hours. If nausea and vomiting are present, an antiemetic such as prochlorperazine (Compazine) may be used. Oversedation should be avoided because it may mask increasing intracranial pressure. Other supportive treatment includes bedrest in a quiet, darkened room, adequate liquids, and a soft, nutritious diet appropriate for the patient's age.

Several vaccines are available for the more common forms of meningitis or contributing infections. In some cases, chemoprophylaxis is advised for documented exposure. The most common preventive measures for meningitis, including vaccine for the unexposed and chemoprophylaxis if exposure has occurred, are listed in Table 6.8.

Of major concern as a complication of meningitis is increasing intracranial pressure caused by cerebral edema brought on by the inflammatory process. Early signs include drowsiness, episodes of confusion, and pupillary changes. Later signs include decreasing levels of consciousness, increase in pulse pressure, bradycardia, and respiratory changes. This serious complication requires ventilatory support, oxygen therapy, close monitoring of circulatory and respiratory status, and careful management of IV fluid replacement. Techniques such as hyperventilation and use of osmotic diuretics, such as mannitol (Osmitrol), and anti-inflammatory agents, such as dexamethasone (Decadron), help reduce intracranial pressure.

Follow-up and Referral

All patients who are suspected of having any form of meningitis should be referred to a neurologist for more definitive care. When the patient's condition is stable, the neurologist will release the patient back to the care of the primary health-care provider to continue

Table 6.8 Prevention of Meningitis			
Type	Vaccine	Indications	Chemoprophylaxis
Meningococcal	2 doses of meningococcal conjugate vaccine quadrivalent (MCV4) at least 2 months apart Single dose Meningococcal polysaccharide vaccine (MPSV4) For all of the above: may revaccinate with MCV4 every 5 years	Adults aged 55 and younger with damaged spleen or terminal complement deficiency HIV-infected persons Epidemics High-risk children aged 2 months to 10 years; all children aged 11–12 years Military personnel or travelers to endemic locations College students living in dorms (if not vaccinated after age 16) Adults aged 56 years and older	**Adults:** rifampin 600 mg q12h for 2 days **OR** ciprofloxacin 500–750 mg once For close contacts of known cases
Pneumococcal	Pneumovax: provides immunity up to 5 years	All persons older than age 2 who are immunosuppressed or who have a chronic disease Elderly, especially those in chronic-care facilities	None recommended
H influenzae	HbOC (Hib titer) PRP-OMP (Pedvax Hib)	Children aged 2 months to 5 years, especially with chronic illness and older than 18 months attending day care Children older than age 5 years, according to risk	rifampin IV 20 mg/kg/day for 4 days For household or day-care contacts, especially if younger than age 6 years

follow-up care consisting of completion of antibiotic regimen and monitoring of blood work. Any indication of a complicated course warrants close follow-up and neurological referral. Cases of uncomplicated acute meningitis such as aseptic meningitis may require only home IV antibiotic therapy after discharge. The total course of antibiotics is about 10 to 14 days. Patients with chronic meningitis or with neurological deficits require rehabilitation and continuous follow-up. The facility for this depends on the nature of the patient's needs and family resources.

Patient Education

Education regarding prevention of meningitis through available immunization or chemoprophylaxis, as well as observance for clues to impending complications, should be provided. Home management after hospital discharge should emphasize the need for assistance with routine activities for a period lasting up to several weeks to allow for complete recovery. The patient should be encouraged to have frequent rest periods and to gradually increase activities while looking for signs (e.g., shortness of breath, increased pulse) that the activity is too strenuous. The diet should be well balanced to ensure intake of nutrients such as protein and vitamin C. Soft foods may be better tolerated. Plenty of fluids should be encouraged unless other conditions are present, such as congestive heart failure or kidney disease. Two tablets of acetaminophen (Tylenol) may be given every 4 to 6 hours for pain or headache. The patient may feel more comfortable initially in a darkened, quiet room, which will prevent discomfort related to photophobia. The importance of completing the full course of antibiotic or antiviral medications exactly as prescribed must be stressed to the patient and family. The patient needs to avoid close contact with others to whom he or she may transmit germs orally. The patient needs to be taught about potential complications and when it is necessary to call the health-care provider, for example, if he or she has any signs of an upper respiratory infection, any change in alertness or awakeness, any recurrent fever, or any other sign of a worsening illness.

■ ENCEPHALITIS

Usually of viral causation, encephalitis is an acute inflammation of brain tissue, which produces inflammation, hyperthermia, altered levels of consciousness, and other focal neurological signs. Often referred to as "sleeping sickness," encephalitis may on rare occasions be caused by nonviral agents, such as bacteria. Table 6.9 presents the types of encephalitis.

Epidemiology and Causes

With more than 25 viral organisms causing the inflammation, encephalitis is relatively common, with an incidence of 15 cases per 100,000 and prevalence of 10 per 100,000. Although several thousand cases of encephalitis are reported each year, many more may actually occur because the symptoms may be mild to practically nonexistent in some patients. Arboviruses (carried by arthropods, such as mosquitos) can occur in epidemic fashion during warm-weather months. With overall mortality due to encephalitis averaging between 5% and 20% and with residual neurological deficits occurring in up to 90% of cases, treatment and supportive care become important. Although most cases of encephalitis are viral, there are many nonviral agents responsible for the other few cases of encephalitis. These include tertiary syphilis, *Rickettsia rickettsii* (responsible for Rocky Mountain spotted fever), *S aureus*, *S pneumoniae*, *H influenzae*, *Bacteroides fragilis*, *Brucella* species, *Leptospira* species, *Cryptococcus neoformans*, and *M tuberculosis*.

Table 6.9	Types of Encephalitis			
Major Type	Description	Organism	Diagnostic Tests	Treatment
Viral	Most common type; progressive altered level of consciousness, seizures, motor weakness, headache	More than 25 viral organisms, including arboviruses	Diagnosed primarily from the clinical picture	Symptomatic treatment Supportive care acyclovir 15 mg/kg q8h
Herpes simplex virus (HSV) (accounts for 10% of cases)	Sudden development of olfactory or gustatory hallucinations, prominent memory loss, bizarre behavior	HSV	CSF analysis EEG CT MRI	foscavir (Foscarnet) 20 mg/kg IV bolus, then 120 mg/kg IV q8h acyclovir 15 mg/kg q8h
Microbial	Selectively attacks CNS cells; varied signs and symptoms	Multiple bacterial organisms	Gram stain of CSF Serum antibody levels	penicillin 20 million units/day chloramphenicol 75–100 mg/kg/day divided q6h)

Encephalitis may occur at any age, but very young children and older adults are at the highest risk. There is no significant ethnic predisposition, and encephalitis occurs equally among men and women.

Pathophysiology

Encephalitis is an infection of the brain parenchyma. Typical symptoms include fever and confusion or drowsiness, which sometimes progresses to stupor and coma. Encephalitis is usually accompanied by inflammation of the meninges; therefore, headache and nuchal rigidity are also frequent symptoms. A bout of encephalitis can produce a range of specific neurological problems, including seizures, muscle weakness or paralysis, isolated cranial nerve palsies, heightened or depressed deep tendon reflexes, and papilledema. Sometimes the infection disrupts the hypothalamic-pituitary axis, and this can lead to diabetes insipidus, SIADH, or the inability to maintain a normal body temperature. When the infective agent is the herpes simplex virus (HSV), the encephalitis can cause personality changes, hallucinations, and aphasia.

Encephalitis is usually caused by a virus—in the United States, the most common cause is HSV—and the neurological signs and symptoms of encephalitis are usually preceded by other signs of viral infection, such as fever, malaise, muscle aches, rashes, gastrointestinal disturbances, or respiratory symptoms. Encephalitis viruses get into the body through a number of routes: HSVs are transmitted through person-to-person contact; enteroviruses are swallowed and invade through the gut; arboviruses are introduced by bites of insects, other arthropods, birds, and rodents; rabies enters through bites of mammals; and varicella-zoster viruses are inhaled. In most cases, the viruses replicate, a viremia develops, and virus particles get into the CNS from the bloodstream. Some viruses (rabies, HSV, and varicella-zoster), however, are carried into the CNS retrogradely inside axons.

A typical case of viral encephalitis comprises a mix of parenchymal inflammation, meningitis, cerebral edema, and hemorrhage. Throughout the brain and meninges, there is perivascular inflammation with local collections of lymphocytes, brain monocytes, microglia, and a lesser number of polymorphonuclear leukocytes. Capillary endothelial cells are injured, especially in the gray matter, causing small hemorrhages. There are areas of neuron cell death. In addition, ependymal cells can be damaged, contributing to the brain swelling.

The brain areas suffering the most damage vary from case to case. Some patients develop seizures, which can be either generalized or focal. Sometimes oligodendroglia are selectively infected, and the main damage is demyelination, which leads to focal neurological deficits. When the brainstem becomes infected, coma or respiratory failure can result. Generalized cortical edema decreases consciousness. The direct cause of these and other major symptoms of encephalitis seems to be the inflammation and immune reactions themselves because when these host responses subside, patients often recover dramatically.

Clinical Presentation
Subjective

A common presentation of viral encephalitis includes alteration in level of consciousness related to parenchymal swelling. The manifestations are usually progressive from lethargy to coma with the swelling and resultant increased intracranial pressure. Other focal neurological signs may develop, including seizures and motor weakness. Generalized headache with abrupt onset often accompanies other signs as a result of intraparenchymal bleeding and swelling. Other complaints may be nausea, vomiting, confusion, drowsiness, sensitivity to bright light, and a poor appetite.

Herpes simplex encephalitis caused by HSV may be heralded by bizarre behavior, aphasia, or hallucinations as the temporal and frontal lobes are selectively attacked by this organism. Other types of infectious agents (other herpes viruses, Lyme disease [*Borrelia burgdorferi*], varicella-zoster virus, *R rickettsii*) may produce a cutaneous rash in addition to neurological signs such as headache, seizures, or nuchal rigidity. The rash is a typical feature of many viral diseases.

Objective

Physical exam may reveal a fever, nuchal rigidity, paralysis, hyperresponsive deep tendon reflexes, and possibly a viral rash.

Diagnostic Reasoning
Diagnostic Tests

Epidemiological clues and assessment of risk factors to identify potential etiological agents should be sought in all patients with encephalitis. In addition, an LP is essential for the diagnosis. When encephalitis is suspected, the patient should be referred to the collaborating physician and to a neurologist. Cultures of body fluid specimens (e.g., from blood, stool, nasopharynx, or sputum), if clinical and epidemiological clues are suggestive, should be performed in an attempt to identify various viral, bacterial, and fungal etiologies of encephalitis. CSF testing reveals increased white blood cells (WBCs, especially mononuclear) and an increased protein level. A Gram stain of CSF may be useful for bacterial infection to provide early guidance for appropriate antibiotic treatment. Serum antibodies taken early in the infectious course and compared with a specimen drawn 1 to 3 weeks after onset of illness will reveal significant antibody increase. This may be helpful clinically to provide confirmation of a viral cause and further therapy guidance. With encephalitis caused by HSV, extensive hemorrhagic necrosis is demonstrated on CT scan and MRI.

Occasionally cell damage occurs that does not demonstrate abnormality on a CT scan or MRI.

Because changes in the CSF may not be apparent at the beginning of the infection, a repeat LP may be indicated. EEG is rarely helpful in establishing an etiology in patients with encephalitis, but it has a role in identifying patients with nonconvulsive seizure activity who are confused, obtunded, or comatose. An EEG taken in the presence of herpes simplex encephalitis often is abnormal because of localized hemorrhage and edema. MRI is the most sensitive neuroimaging test to evaluate patients with encephalitis. CT, both with and without contrast enhancement, should be used to evaluate patients with encephalitis if MRI is unavailable, is impractical, or cannot be performed. An MRI may indicate areas of demyelination or edema.

Differential Diagnoses

Because encephalitis often produces signs of meningeal irritation, the differentiating factor to consider encephalitis over meningitis is usually alteration in level of consciousness. Meningitis has an abrupt onset, and although the condition may show signs of parenchymal damage that are seen in encephalitis (e.g., memory difficulties, confusion, hallucinations, dysphasia, seizures, and focal motor/sensory deficits), these signs are usually seen late in the course of the disease compared with encephalitis, in which they are exhibited from the beginning. Photophobia and severe headache may point to acute meningitis rather than encephalitis. A preceding viral illness such as measles or mumps points to encephalitis occurring as a complication. Patient history of an animal bite in the presence of the typical symptoms may lead to suspicion regarding encephalitis caused by rabies. In addition, seasonal factors may point to an arboviral cause of encephalitis by mosquito or tick bite.

Management

A suspicion of encephalitis requires referral and patient hospitalization for definitive neurological diagnosis and treatment. The principles of treatment include inactivating and eliminating the causative organism, providing supportive care, and preventing complications.

Viral causation is treated with antiviral agents such as acyclovir (Zovirax). Antivirals are most effective when used early in the course of illness, especially before changes in level of consciousness occur. Antivirals act by suppressing replication of the virus. Vigorous supportive care for unconscious patients is necessary to prevent complications of ventilator support, catheters, IV lines, or other invasive treatment. Handling invasive equipment aseptically is essential in preventing infection. It is crucial to be alert for IV infiltration and phlebitis. The patient on a mechanical ventilator must be observed to prevent pressure necrosis, atelectasis, infection, and barotrauma.

Seizure control is achieved by the use of phenytoin (Dilantin), with dosages up to 600 mg/day for adults.

Safety must also be a consideration with these patients. Padding should be used to prevent seizure injury. Although some fever can be beneficial, occasionally extreme hyperthermia can cause seizure activity. Acetaminophen (Tylenol) is used to reduce hyperthermia and may be given as a rectal suppository if indicated. Cerebral edema resulting in increased intracranial pressure is another ominous complication of encephalitis. An osmotic diuretic such as mannitol (Osmitrol) is chosen first to reduce edema, but glucocorticoids, such as dexamethasone (Decadron), may be added if necessary. Agents used for the treatment of encephalitis are listed in Table 6.9.

Follow-up and Referral

Patients suspected of having encephalitis are referred to a neurologist for definitive care and follow-up. When the patient is stabilized, the neurologist will release the patient's care to the primary-care provider. The relative degree of neurological deficit determines the nature of follow-up care. Complete convalescence can take weeks.

Patient Education

Prevention of infection vectors through mosquito control and insect repellants should be one important focus of patient and community education. Early detection and proper removal of ticks is another important aspect. For convalescence, the importance of bedrest, fluids, and nutrition is emphasized, as well as clues to impending complications. The patient should be encouraged to take frequent rest periods and to increase activities gradually while looking for signs that the activity is too strenuous, for example, shortness of breath and increased pulse. The patient should be instructed to eat a balanced diet to ensure the inclusion of nutrients such as protein and vitamin C. Fluids should be encouraged unless contraindicated. Acetaminophen may be used for pain or a headache. The patient may feel more comfortable in a darkened, quiet room if photophobia is present. The importance of taking the antibiotics or antiviral medications exactly as prescribed should be stressed to the patient. Patients should be instructed to avoid close contact with others who may be harboring germs. If they notice any signs of an upper respiratory infection, they should seek help from their health-care provider immediately. Patients and families should be instructed to inspect the skin for ticks and to remove them intact. They should wear protective clothing to prevent tick bites. Last, patients should be instructed when to call the health-care provider, for example, if there are any changes in their level of consciousness, recurrent fever, or any other signs of a worsening illness.

■ HERPES ZOSTER

Herpes zoster, commonly known as shingles, is an infection by the varicella-zoster virus occurring along dermatomal pathways and resulting in a vesicular skin rash, especially in the intercostal areas.

Epidemiology and Causes

Varicella-zoster virus is thought to become latent after the primary infection of chickenpox; it then reactivates, usually in persons who are immunocompromised, as herpes zoster (shingles). One out of every three individuals in the United States will develop shingles. Every year, there are an estimated 1 million cases. Children may get shingles; however, the risk of disease increases as persons get older, and approximately half of all cases occur among men and women aged 60 and over. It is thought to be caused by immunosuppression that often accompanies the aging process. Four percent of patients with herpes zoster may experience a second episode but rarely a third episode.

Immunocompromised patients also have a higher incidence of complications because of their impaired ability to thwart the infectious process. In adults who have no previous history of chickenpox, exposure to the virus (usually transmitted by respiratory route or by direct contact with vesicular fluid) causes herpes zoster. In addition, patients with inflammatory bowel disease are at a significantly increased risk for developing shingles.

Pathophysiology

Varicella-zoster virus, which causes chickenpox, is also responsible for a number of neurological disorders, including encephalitis, meningitis, polyneuritis, multiple cranial neuropathies, and Reye's syndrome. Varicella-zoster virus initially infects people through the mucosa of the upper respiratory tract or the conjunctivae of the eyes. Within a week, the virus has spread throughout the body via the bloodstream, and about a week later, infections of the capillaries of the skin produce the vesicular lesions of chickenpox.

At this point, virus particles are retrogradely transported inside sensory axons to dorsal root ganglia, where the viruses remain latent for the life of the patient. Varicella-zoster virus is most often found in the sensory ganglia of the ophthalmic division of the trigeminal nerve and in the dorsal root ganglia of the mid to lower spinal cord (ganglia T3 to L2). If viruses in a ganglion are reactivated, they replicate, destroy ganglion nerve cells, and migrate through the nerves to the innervated dermatomes, where they again produce vesicular skin lesions.

The destruction of sensory neurons in a ganglion produces pain in the innervated dermatome. This pain usually precedes the skin lesions by a few days, although sometimes pain is the only symptom. Typically, viruses are reactivated in only a single ganglion at a time; therefore, the symptoms are unilateral and affect a single dermatome. When the pain does not resolve within a few weeks, the syndrome is called postherpetic neuralgia (PHN). The pain of PHN can be either constant or intermittent and worsens at night and during temperature changes. Varicella-zoster virus

that has been reactivated in the ophthalmic division of the trigeminal nerve can cause eye problems, including lesions of the cornea.

It is not known what triggers the reactivation of latent varicella-zoster viruses. The likelihood of developing this reactivation syndrome (called "herpes zoster" or "shingles") increases as a person ages and when a person's immune system becomes compromised. Herpes zoster is a frequent complication of HIV infection.

Clinical Presentation
Subjective

Initially, the patient with herpes zoster may present with unexplained pain. The pain is described as constant or intermittent, with a stabbing quality. The pain occurs along the involved dermatome, usually 48 to 72 hours before eruption of the classic vesicular skin rash. Pain acuity differs among individuals, but many patients say the pain becomes progressively worse at night or with changes in temperature. When herpes zoster is manifested along the branches of the fifth cranial nerve, herpes zoster ophthalmicus results. This condition can cause blindness and requires immediate referral to an ophthalmologist for evaluation and treatment. If the site of infection is along the trigeminal nerve, lesions will occur on the inside of the mouth, and occasionally in the external ear opening. Lesions on the eighth cranial (acoustic) nerve can cause vertigo, hearing loss, and ear pain.

Another major characteristic of the disease is the occurrence of acute neuritis along the path of the rash dermatome. PHN occurs in approximately 25% to 50% of patients older than age 60. The constant or intermittent stabbing pain worsens at night or with temperature changes.

Objective

Herpes zoster is characterized by a unilateral vesicular rash along a dermatome, most commonly a thoracic or lumbar dermatome. The rash begins as erythema, then changes to papular lesions that rapidly form vesicles. The vesicles rupture, releasing infectious fluid, and then form scabs. Occasionally the vesicles coalesce to form bullae. The skin lesions usually continue to develop for 3 to 5 days, and the entire disease course usually lasts 10 to 15 days. In some individuals, the skin lesions can persist for 30 days or longer. The pain caused by PHN may last much longer and at times may be permanent.

Diagnostic Reasoning
Diagnostic Tests

Diagnosis is made after careful review of data obtained from the history and physical exam. The characteristic appearance and distribution of the lesions along with a history of neuritis helps establish the diagnosis of herpes zoster. Usually the history and physical exam are all that is needed to make a definitive diagnosis.

If the diagnosis is questionable, a polymerase chain reaction assay, which detects the DNA sequence of the virus, may be done, along with antibody titer (which requires more than one test for comparison).

Differential Diagnosis

Other conditions with similar rashes need to be ruled out. Impetigo may present as vesicles around an area of broken skin. The scrapings of these lesions can be sent for a Gram stain, which will reveal gram-positive cocci if herpes zoster is present. Viral cultures may be done to rule out HSV or coxsackie viral infections that can appear with a dermatomal pattern.

Management

The principal goals are to manage the healed vesicles, obtain pain relief, and prevent secondary infection and other complications. Initial management of herpes zoster involves the use of antiviral agents. They reduce the impact of herpes zoster by diminishing neuritis and speeding the healing of the skin lesions. Early intervention in the treatment of herpes zoster produces the best results. Famciclovir (Famvir), acyclovir (Zovirax), or valacyclovir (Valtrex) may be used. Systemic corticosteroids such as prednisone starting at 60 mg/day and tapering over 3 weeks may assist in reducing acute pain when given in conjunction with the antiviral therapy. Lotions such as calamine and dressings soaked with Burow's solution may be used to soothe the lesions and prevent scratching or rubbing, thereby improving healing time, decreasing pain, and preventing secondary infection. Some patients find that corticosteroid cream helps as well. Some report that the pain of lesions in the thoracic area can be diminished by using a tight wrap of the chest to produce a splinting effect. The practitioner should use this method with care, especially in older adult patients or those with pulmonary disease, because the restriction (splinting) of normal breathing patterns could promote pulmonary stasis of secretions and increase the incidence of pulmonary infections. Patients with ophthalmic herpes affecting the first branch of the trigeminal nerve must be referred to an ophthalmologist because this condition may result in blindness. The patient with ophthalmic herpes will usually have a lesion on the tip of the nose.

Postherpetic neuralgia (PHN) is a persistent pain resulting from shingles that lasts more than 3 months after the disease has run its course. PHN rarely occurs in individuals under age 40, is more severe in individuals over age 50, and may occur in up to half of untreated people over age 60. Even with treatment, PHN may occur. Some clinicians think that administering systemic corticosteroids at the earliest onset of the rash reduces the risk of developing PHN. Analgesics (from nonnarcotic to narcotic agents in doses individualized for the patient) are supportive in reducing neuritis and

PHN. If PHN is present, the use of tricyclic antidepressants such as amitriptyline 25 to 75 mg taken each night may help if simple analgesics are ineffective. For additional pain relief, gabapentin (Neurontin) starting at 300 mg three times a day up to 3,600 mg daily may help. Gabapentin along with valacyclovir given to patients with acute herpes zoster reduced the incidence of PHN to almost 10% in an initial study. More research is needed in this area. Topical capsaicin cream is approved by the Food and Drug Administration for relief of PHN. There is also a capsaicin 8% patch (Qutenza), which is a one-time treatment applied in the primary-care provider's office. In about half of all patients with PHN, this patch can reduce PHN pain by about one-third. If pain is persistent, chronic PHN may respond to a regional block with or without corticosteroids. Ideally, the patient should be referred to a pain center because PHN can have devastating effects. (See The Patient's Voice 6.1.)

The Patient's Voice 6.1
Postherpetic Neuralgia
My mother died of postherpetic neuralgia (PHN).

My mother was 80 years old and had recently won the golf championship at her club. She had been a widow for 25 years and decided that she wanted to move in with me, her daughter, with her only granddaughter (age 3). We lived 4 hours away. At first she was very independent—driving around by herself and going shopping while I worked. That only lasted a few months. Then the decline began. First, she broke a wrist, which incapacitated her, and then she got pneumonia, which weakened her. Then she got "shingles" (herpes zoster), which did her in. She was diagnosed at the earliest onset of pain, yet treatment wasn't started until the vesicles erupted. She had ophthalmic herpes, so her vision was affected. She developed PHN very early, and due to the persistent pain, she became reclusive. She stopped going out, retreating to her room and eventually wouldn't get out of bed. Nothing helped the pain. I'm convinced it was because preventive treatment wasn't started early. As she became more depressed and stayed in bed, she got weaker and weaker and just gave up. She complained of shooting pain over half of her head that was worse at night, so she'd be awake all night, and sleep all day. Nobody could help; her primary-care provider, neurologist, ophthalmologist, psychologist, nor me. She died in her sleep, and I'm convinced it was the result of PHN.

I've learned two things from this experience. First, if older persons are optimally functioning, don't move them out of their familiar supportive environment. Second, treat all cases of herpes aggressively, as you don't know who is going to develop PHN. As my mom used to say, "An ounce of prevention is worth a pound of cure."

Follow-up and Referral

It is essential that any patient with ophthalmic herpetic lesions be referred to an ophthalmologist. Other follow-up would include a return visit if skin lesions become infected or if PHN is present. Referral to a neurologist may be required at any time if the patient does not respond to primary treatment plans. Patients should be referred to a pain center if PHN results in chronic persistent pain.

Patient Education

Because herpes zoster is usually treated on an outpatient basis, patient and family education is important. The clinician should encourage patients to complete the course of the antiviral agent, even if they feel the disease has abated, or especially if they feel the treatment is not as effective as they had hoped it would be. Patients should be informed that elimination of the disease could take longer than anticipated and careful medication administration and follow-up care could mean fewer complications in the long run. Patients should be instructed that the medication may be better tolerated if taken with food. If adverse effects from the treatment plan occur, patients need to keep the practitioner informed so adjustments can be made. Education on the potential for spread of the herpes zoster virus via fluid from ruptured vesicles is important. Patients should be instructed that before the rash crusts, it can release fluid that will cause an infection in others. Patients must be careful in handling dressings, linens, towels, and clothes that they have used. They should not be around children who have not been vaccinated for chickenpox or those who have not had chickenpox yet; contact with pregnant women should also be avoided. Because patients will have a low resistance to infection, they should not be around those who may have an infectious illness, such as a cold. Patients need to know that scratching the rash can lead to an infection. The clinician should pursue ways to relieve the pruritus, as mentioned previously. Patients should be instructed about the nature of the rash so that when they see it in varying stages of progression, they will not think that it is not healing. Again, the importance of completing all prescribed medications needs to be stressed. Patients need to know the reason they are taking other medications, for example, antidepressants (which may help prevent PHN), so they will continue taking them. Research has shown that the shingles vaccine Zostavax has reduced the occurrence of shingles in people aged 60 and older and offers more than a 50% protection. In addition, it reduces the incidence of PHN by almost 70%. The Centers for Disease Control and Prevention recommends a single dose of Zostavax for adults aged 60 and older, even if they have already had shingles. Immunocompromised individuals should not receive the vaccine.

■ TRIGEMINAL NEURALGIA

Trigeminal neuralgia is a distressing, painful idiopathic disorder of the trigeminal nerve (cranial nerve V). It is also known as tic douloureux (unbearable painful twitch). This excruciating facial pain is paroxysmal and lasts usually less than 3 seconds. For many individuals the severity of the pain is disabling, and patients will do almost anything to prevent triggering an episode.

The lancinating, sharply cutting pain occurs along one or more of the three branches of the trigeminal nerve. Characteristically, the painful episodes occur when specific trigger zones are stimulated by touch, chewing, talking, shaving, or environmental temperature changes. Patients often describe the pain as "electric" or "stabbing" and penetrating. The pain of trigeminal neuralgia is chronic. Although patients may experience periods of spontaneous pain remission that may last weeks or months, the pain returns with the same or greater intensity.

Epidemiology and Causes

Trigeminal neuralgia occurs more frequently in women than in men and more often in individuals over age 50. The incidence is 12 per 100,000 of the general population per year. A higher incidence of risk occurs in individuals with hypertension and multiple sclerosis (MS). These at-risk individuals are much younger than the characteristic age of patients with trigeminal neuralgia.

Most often with trigeminal neuralgia there is involvement of the muscles of the right side of the face where two or three branches of the trigeminal nerve are affected. The lower and center portions of the face are most commonly affected, and it is rare to have pain in the forehead and scalp areas.

Pathophysiology

Trigeminal neuralgia, which produces episodic paroxysms of sharp facial pain, is caused by demyelination of axons in the fifth cranial nerve, the trigeminal nerve. The trigeminal nerve has three main branches: V_1, the ophthalmic branch, transmits sensation from the eye region and forehead; V_2, the maxillary branch, transmits sensation from the midface and upper jaw; and V_3, the mandibular branch, transmits sensation from the lower jaw. The neuron cell bodies for the sensory axons in these nerves are located in the trigeminal (gasserian) ganglion, which is inside the skull along the floor of the middle cranial fossa.

Trigeminal neuralgia most often affects the mandibular or the maxillary branches of the trigeminal nerve. The problem tends to occur in middle-aged and elderly people. Patients with multiple sclerosis, another demyelinating syndrome, get trigeminal neuralgia with a higher frequency than the rest of the population.

Although it is extremely painful, trigeminal neuralgia produces no obvious neurological deficits. On the other hand, patients with trigeminal neuralgia have a general sensory hypersensitivity of the face, and 90% of sufferers have trigger points on their faces that will set off paroxysms of pain.

Trigeminal neuralgia is caused by focal demyelination of axons in the affected nerve, ganglion, or roots. Biopsy specimens of affected nerves show patches of demyelination but no significant inflammation. It has been hypothesized that, due to demyelination, axons come in direct contact with neighboring axons so that signals in one axon spread laterally to adjacent axons. A modest stimulation of the nerve will then be amplified into a massive excitation, which is interpreted by the brain as a sudden burst of pain.

Clinical Presentation

Subjective

The patient with idiopathic trigeminal neuralgia presents with complaints of severe paroxysmal pain, most commonly on one side of the face. The pain lasts for a few seconds, with no ache or pain between occurrences, and follows the trigeminal nerve distribution. The patient's history includes the onset of a painful event after trigger points have been stimulated by chewing, talking, brushing teeth, touching the face, or, in some cases, after intense physical activity, lowering of the head, and wind touching the face. The patient's history may include periods of remission with or without medical treatment.

During periods of exacerbation, the patient may be totally disabled by the severity of the pain. Patients may report refraining from eating, sleep deprivation, depression, and even suicidal tendencies, which reflect their willingness to go to great extremes to escape the severe paroxysmal pain.

Objective

On physical exam, the cranial nerves, specifically the trigeminal nerve, have normal motor and sensory function; facial muscle strength and reflexes are normal. Clinically, the cardinal signs of idiopathic trigeminal neuralgia are elicited when a facial trigger point is stimulated; the patient experiences a sharp, electric-type pain that follows the distribution of the trigeminal nerve and lasts for only a few seconds, and the patient's face grimaces. After the painful attack, there is no residual ache or pain. Facial pain, however, that is continuous and varies in intensity must be further evaluated for atypical trigeminal neuralgia that is caused by trauma, tumor, or previous facial surgery. Because of the many pathological and etiological theories regarding trigeminal neuralgia, the clinician must be alert to the characteristic symptoms of typical (idiopathic) trigeminal neuralgia. These are short periods of paroxysmal pain associated with trigger zones, pain limited to the distribution of the trigeminal nerve branches, and negative neurological findings.

Diagnostic Reasoning

Diagnostic Tests

Idiopathic trigeminal neuralgia can often be diagnosed based on clinical history that describes paroxysmal pain episodes triggered by specific activities in patients characteristically older than age 50.

Patients who have prolonged episodes of pain that increases in intensity and occurrence and are younger need to be evaluated further for pathology-related tumors, trauma, MS, and vascular compression. The tests most frequently used for the diagnosis of atypical trigeminal neuralgia are a CT scan and an MRI. The MRI is the method of choice in differential diagnoses of trigeminal nerve pathology.

Another diagnostic method for typical trigeminal neuralgia is the administration of carbamazepine (Tegretol) or a low dose of a tricyclic antidepressant. If either of these medications relieves the pain, this effect may be used to diagnose this disorder.

Differential Diagnosis

There are many causes for the general presentation of orofacial pain. These conditions can be generally categorized as inflammatory (e.g., dental pathology, sinusitis, parotitis, sialolithiasis, temporal arteritis, HSV type I), neurological (e.g., trigeminal, glossopharyngeal, or paratrigeminal neuralgia; cluster or migraine headaches; meningiomas; posterior fossa tumors), or musculoskeletal (e.g., temporomandibular joint pain, myofascial pain dysfunction syndrome). It is important, therefore, to identify whether the clinical presentation is either typical trigeminal neuralgia or some other orofacial pain cause.

Management

The major principles in the management of trigeminal neuralgia are (1) to elicit a remission by drug therapy, (2) to prevent untoward effects in patients resulting from prescribed medications, and (3) to help the patient avoid triggering painful episodes. Trigeminal neuralgia is a chronic condition that results in the need for the patient's chronic pain to be managed. In addition to interventions related to establishing remission and avoidance of painful episodes, the patient's psychological needs—related to depression, isolation, and possible suicidal tendencies—are significant areas in the plan of care.

Initially, pharmacological management is to try to initiate remission of the pain. Carbamazepine or gabapentin may block the nerve firing. The patient experiencing pain relief should stay on the medication for at least 6 months Tricyclic antidepressants such as amitriptyline can also be used to treat pain.

Patients who are taking oral contraceptives should be cautioned that the contraceptives may not be reliable when analgesic drugs are being prescribed. An alternative method of birth control must be recommended. The patient should also be warned about the hazard of driving a motor vehicle when on these drugs.

Follow-up for complications of drug therapy with anticonvulsants is essential in the pharmacological management of typical trigeminal neuralgia. If carbamazepine becomes ineffective after prolonged use or if adverse effects develop, the dosage must be gradually decreased to prevent withdrawal symptoms. Carbamazepine has many adverse effects, including nausea, vomiting, mouth ulcers, dizziness, diplopia, skin rash, blood dyscrasias (aplastic anemia, agranulocytosis, thrombocytopenia, and leukopenia), fever, and chills.

Fluoxetine (Prozac) may be prescribed for patients who experience psychological depression and difficulty coping with the pain associated with performing normal ADLs. Periods of remission and exacerbation that occur as pharmacological interventions become less effective are also very stressful for the patient.

Other therapies for trigeminal neuralgia include acupuncture, transcutaneous electrical nerve stimulation, and topical application of capsaicin (Zostrix). Some patients have reported modest pain relief after botulinum toxin injections that block the activity of sensory nerves. Patients with trigeminal neuralgia who have few or no periods of remission should be referred for surgical intervention.

The unrelenting paroxysmal pain associated with trigeminal neuralgia is frequently associated with compression of the trigeminal nerve root. Surgical intervention (rhizotomy) is performed to relieve the compression, although recurrence in 1 to 2 years is common after surgery, regardless of the surgical method chosen.

Follow-up and Referral

Because of the intense and chronic pain associated with trigeminal neuralgia, the patient may experience depression, social isolation, and suicidal tendencies. The clinician must recognize these effects of the disease and reinforce coping mechanisms the patient may use during periods of exacerbation. Referral for counseling may be required if the patient is not able to cope with the chronicity and severity of the pain. The patient experiences pain when eating and washing the face and frequently avoids these and other activities. The patient begins to lose weight and becomes dehydrated, and hygiene becomes a problem.

Patient Education

The goals of patient instruction are the avoidance of triggering painful events, pharmacological management, and coping with chronic, severe pain. Nutritional counseling should encourage intake of soft or pureed, high-caloric foods, along with increased fluids. For hygiene, the use of soft washcloths and mouthwashes should be encouraged. Patients should be educated about adverse reactions (e.g., dizziness, sleepiness, ataxia, nausea and vomiting) to their medications and about the necessity

for follow-up blood studies to detect any blood dyscrasias. Intense counseling and supportive education is a continuous process in caring for the patient with trigeminal neuralgia. Recognition of the patient's educational needs based on his or her coping mechanisms, search for pain treatment, and the status of the neuralgia will direct the clinician in establishing an individualized plan.

■ BELL'S PALSY

Bell's palsy (prosopoplegia) is a condition with an acute onset of flaccid paralysis, usually occurring on one side of the face in an otherwise healthy person. The peripheral facial palsy is self-limiting and complete recovery usually occurs in a few weeks or months in 80% to 86% of patients. Initially, the facial paralysis may be incomplete and then worsen within 48 hours after onset. The sudden experience of facial paralysis is very frightening to the patient, who usually seeks medical care immediately.

Epidemiology and Causes

The specific cause of Bell's palsy is unknown. Theories of etiology include viral infections such as herpes simplex virus type I, respiratory infections, and heredity. Approximately 40,000 individuals each year in the United States will get Bell's palsy. It does not discriminate against men or women but is less common under age 15 years or over age 60 years. A higher incidence is seen in individuals with diabetes, hypertension, trauma, toxin exposure, Lyme disease, pregnancy, and those suffering upper respiratory ailments.

A complete recovery from facial paralysis usually occurs in 3 to 6 months or no longer than 12 months. Persons at risk for incomplete recovery are those older than age 55, hypertensive, with pain other than ear pain, with complete facial paralysis, and those who have changes in lacrimation, such as involuntary shedding of tears.

Pathophysiology

Cranial nerve VII—the facial nerve—comprises both motor and sensory axons. Its efferent motor axons innervate the muscles of facial expression and its preganglionic parasympathetic axons innervate the lacrimal and nasopalatine glands and all the salivary glands except the parotid. Its afferent axons carry sensation from the taste buds of the anterior two-thirds of the tongue and from cutaneous sensory receptors of the external ear.

The various classes of axons in the facial nerve peel off group by group as the nerve makes its way through the bony canals of the skull; therefore, pressure on or lesions of the nerve at different locations will produce different deficits. Inside the skull, the facial nerve runs with cranial nerve VIII, the vestibulocochlear nerve, and pressure on the facial nerve here (such as from an acoustic neuroma) will usually cause hearing loss and vestibular problems in addition to deficits in all the motor and sensory components of the facial nerve.

Within the skull wall, the facial and vestibulocochlear nerves separate. After this, the first components to leave the facial nerve are the lacrimal and nasopalatine axons; therefore, damage to the facial nerve distal to this juncture will not affect a patient's ability to produce tears. The next components to leave the facial nerve are the taste axons and the axons to the salivary glands; therefore, damage to the facial nerve distal to this juncture will cause unilateral paralysis of all the muscles of facial expression but will not affect taste or the production of saliva.

Damage to the facial nerve inside the skull wall can be caused by skull fractures, hemangiomas, tumors, and inflammation. When the facial nerve is damaged and no structural problems are found, the condition is called Bell's palsy. Bell's palsy always produces unilateral facial paralysis, and depending on the location of the nerve lesion(s), it may also include deficits in functions of the other components of the facial nerve.

The majority of cases of Bell's palsy are preceded by systemic symptoms of a viral infection. Most cases are thought to be caused by a reactivated herpes simplex infection of the geniculate ganglion, which leads to inflammation and swelling of the nerve inside its restrictive bony canal. Reactivated varicella-zoster virus can also cause Bell's palsy; these cases probably involve demyelination of the nerve and include severe pain and sometimes hearing loss. In addition, a Bell's palsy–like facial paralysis is the most common neurological problem caused by Lyme disease.

Clinical Presentation

Subjective

Patients with Bell's palsy present with an acute onset of partial or total paralysis on one side of the face, usually involving lower motor neurons. The patient has normal ocular movements and facial sensation and often complains of loss of taste (dysgeusia), postauricular pain, abnormal sensitivity to sound (hyperacusis), and a heavy feeling in the face.

Objective

On physical exam, the motor and sensory functions along the entire facial nerve should be assessed. Bell's palsy can be diagnosed because of its acute onset and the fact that no other CNS symptoms exist. The physical assessment characteristically reveals on the affected side the absence of forehead wrinkles, wider palpebral fissure of the eye, decreased corneal reflex, Bell's phenomenon (the eyeball turns upward when the patient tries to close the eyelid), open eyelid, flattening of the nasolabial fold, narrowed lips, and loss of taste on the anterior two-thirds of the tongue. Lacrimation may or may not be affected.

A patient with Bell's palsy typically is unable to make these movements on the affected side on request: raise the eyebrow, wrinkle the forehead, close the eyelid, whistle, or retract the muscles of the mouth or chin. When talking, the patient's cheek puffs out and there is an inability to clearly pronounce words that require pursing of the lips. There appears to be a deviation of the tongue because of mouth paralysis on the affected side. The patient is unable to suck or hold fluids in the mouth but is able to swallow.

During the history, it is important to ask about pregnancy, diabetes, any recent infection such as upper respiratory infection or herpes simplex virus, and any stress.

Diagnostic Reasoning

Diagnostic Tests

Diagnosis is based primarily on patient history and clinical exam. If the history and physical exam are inconclusive for Bell's palsy, the patient should be referred for further diagnostic work-up, including a CT scan or an MRI. Evoked electromyography or electroneurography can assess the extent of nerve involvement. These tests are helpful when the patient is not recovering from the Bell's palsy as expected.

Documentation of the extent of facial function at the time of initial diagnosis and at subsequent assessments is critical to evaluate the course of the disease. Several methods to assess and document facial function are available to the clinician. Photographs, an automated computer-assisted clinimetric system, or a facial grading system may be used. Regardless of what method is used to assess facial functioning, the progression or lack of progression of the symptoms is important to differentiate Bell's palsy from other pathology.

Differential Diagnosis

Tumors, infections, trauma, drug ingestion, TIAs, CVAs, and trigeminal neuralgia may appear similar to Bell's palsy. The history and physical exam will usually provide conclusive data to support the diagnosis of Bell's palsy. Close inspection of the patient's ears and skin is done to assess for herpes zoster lesions that would indicate Ramsay Hunt syndrome, which is herpes zoster affecting the facial and auditory nerves, causing facial palsy and cutaneous herpes zoster lesions of the external ear and/or tympanic membrane. Associated symptoms include tinnitus, vertigo, and deafness.

Management

The majority of patients with Bell's palsy totally recover without treatment because the lesion is mild and a result of a conduction block. Therefore, management of a patient with idiopathic Bell's palsy is primarily directed at preventing eye injury. Loss of the ability to blink and close the eyelid subjects the cornea to drying and ulceration.

The patient is instructed to keep the eye moist by topical application of artificial tears every 30 minutes during the day and use of an ocular lubricant ointment at night. Wearing wraparound sunglasses and using a moisture shield (self-adhesive eye bubble, cellulose wrap) are ways to provide eye protection. An eye patch may be necessary if eye closure is not possible. An ophthalmologist should be consulted if the patient experiences any signs of corneal irritation or injury.

Pharmacological management of Bell's palsy is controversial because the disorder is a self-limiting condition. Some practitioners recommend treatment with acyclovir (Zovirax); others recommend prednisone to reduce inflammation and swelling. If drug treatment is chosen, the medication should be started as soon as Bell's palsy is diagnosed.

Ear pain control is essential during the first few weeks after onset of symptoms. The patient may try a variety of over-the-counter drugs, such as acetaminophen (Tylenol) and ibuprofen (Advil, Motrin). Rest and decreased auditory stimulation may lessen the effects of hyperacusis.

Follow-up and Referral

The patient should be examined at regular intervals to assess for resolution or deterioration of Bell's palsy symptoms and adverse effects of medication, if prescribed. Special attention should be given to effectiveness of eye care by the patient. If the patient's symptoms have not resolved in 6 months or if other neurological signs are evident, the patient should be referred to a neurologist. In some cases, though rarely, the patient may be advised to have surgery. Surgery may be indicated for cases in which paralysis is progressive and when incomplete involvement of some branch of the facial nerve is evident.

Patient Education

The patient with Bell's palsy is experiencing a physical and psychological crisis. The clinician provides essential teaching that supports the recovery process. The patient is in a state of shock and disbelief at the change in self-image and concern about the causes of the symptoms. Reassurance that Bell's palsy is usually a short-term condition will allay some anxiety.

To help the patient cope with self-esteem issues, the clinician may advise the patient to use cosmetic interventions to decrease objective symptoms. For example, combing hair over the affected side of the face, using make-up to emphasize the unaffected side, growing a beard or mustache, and wearing sunglasses can lessen the appearance of facial paralysis. Drinking from a plastic, spouted bottle may be easier than drinking from a cup or glass, because liquid can be squeezed into the back of the mouth.

In addition to meticulous eye care, the patient should be taught to perform oral hygiene vigorously because food becomes trapped, there is a reduced amount of

saliva, and chewing is impaired. The patient should be instructed to use a soft-bristled toothbrush, mild mouth rinses, dental floss, and an oral water-jet machine to remove food particles after each meal. Foods may also need to be spicier than normal to compensate for loss of taste. The clinician should encourage the patient to eat soft foods of high nutritional value because patients often avoid eating because of difficulty chewing and holding food in the mouth.

When muscle strength returns, facial massage and exercise can be started for 15 to 20 minutes at least twice a day. Using a cream or oil, the affected side of the face from forehead to chin should be massaged. The patient should also be encouraged to perform facial exercises, including opening and closing of eyes, winking, smiling, and showing teeth in front of a mirror.

■ GUILLAIN-BARRÉ SYNDROME

Guillain-Barré syndrome (GBS) is usually an ascending paralysis most often beginning in the legs and then progressing in an ascending fashion. It only affects about 1 person per 100,000 individuals. There is another form called the Miller Fisher variant that begins with brainstem symptoms such as ataxia, dysphonia, and dysphagia. It may be related to gastric *Campylobacter* infection. There is production of an abnormal antibody that settles on the motor neuron causing it to dysfunction. GBS may be self-limiting over days or in some cases permanent residual such as weakness may occur. Most individuals reach the stage of greatest weakness within the first 2 weeks after the symptoms appear, and 90% will reach this point by the third week. The diagnosis is made by spinal fluid analysis, which shows an elevated protein, especially gamma globulin with little or no cellular response. A nerve conduction velocity test may also help aid in the diagnosis. The treatment involves IV gamma globulin or plasmapheresis. It may progress to a chronic form, chronic inflammatory demyelinating polyneuropathy.

■ BOTULISM

Botulism is a rare paralytic illness caused by the bacterium *Clostridium botulinum* and usually enters through an infected wound or the oral route. Not pasteurizing milk or adding honey to milk puts infants at risk for infection with botulism. Home canning at elevations above 8,000 feet can fail to sterilize the media and lead to botulism. Wound botulism is on the increase due to IV drug abuse.

Symptoms begin within 72 hours of ingesting the toxin and continue for several days. The bacterium forms an endotoxin that affects nerve endings, preventing the release of acetylcholine at the myoneural junction. This causes paralysis.

The primary management of botulism is preventive. However, acute cases require supportive treatment, most often with a ventilator, and if the patient is not allergic to horse serum, trivalent antitoxin is given.

■ MYASTHENIA GRAVIS

Myasthenia gravis (MG) is a disorder of the neuromuscular junction. It is an autoimmune disease in which an antibody occupies the muscle receptor for acetylcholine. Women are more affected than men, and it occurs in approximately 10 to 15 individuals per 100,000.

The symptoms of MG are usually muscle fatigue associated with use. It affects smaller muscles, which have more acetylcholine receptors than larger muscles.

Therefore, eye movements and speech are most commonly affected. The symptoms will ameliorate with rest.

Symptomatic treatment is with anticholinesterase agents. This affords temporary relief. The major side effect is gastrointestinal irritability.

For permanent relief of the symptoms, antibody suppression is needed. This may be accomplished by giving immunosuppressant drugs. Plasmapheresis is also used to reduce antibody levels. In some patients thymectomy may help, because the thymus may be the source of the abnormal lymphocytes creating the abnormal antibodies.

 DavisPlus | For additional resources please visit http://davisplus.fadavis.com

References

Evidence-Based Practice

Beithon, J, et al. *Diagnosis and treatment of headache.* Institute for Clinical Systems Improvement, Bloomington, MN, 2013. Retrieved from www.guideline.gov/popups/printView.aspx?id=43791

Berardelli, A, et al. EFNS/MDS-ES recommendations for the diagnosis of Parkinson's disease. *Eur J Neurol* 20(1):16–34, 2013.

Edlow, JA, et al; American College of Emergency Physicians, American Academy of Neurology. Clinical policy; use of intravenous tPA for the management of acute ischemic stroke in the emergency department. *Ann Emerg Med* 61(2):225–243, 2013. Retrieved from www.guideline.gov/content.aspx?id=43762&search=emergency+department

Filippi, M, et al. Use of imaging in multiple sclerosis. In Gilhus, NE, et al (Eds.), *European handbook of neurological management,* ed 2, vol 1. Wiley-Blackwell, Oxford, UK, 2011, pp 35–51.

Filippi, M, et al; European Federation of the Neurologic Societies. EFNS task force: The use of neuroimaging in the diagnosis of dementia. *Eur J Neurol* 19(12):e131–e140, 1487–1501, 2012. Retrieved from http://www.ncbi.nlm.nih.gov/pubmed/22900895

International Stem Cell Corporation announces new data from Parkinson's disease program. *Wall Street Journal,* October 16, 2013. Retrieved from http://online.wsj.com/article/PR-CO-20131016-906505.html

Plassman, BL, et al. Prevalence of dementia in the United States: The Aging, Demographics, and Memory Study. *Neuroepidemiology* 29(1-2):125–132, 2007.

Segal-Gida, F. Cognitive screening tools. *Clin Rev* 23(1):12–18, 2013.

Silberstein, SD, et al. Evidence-based guideline update: Pharmacologic treatment for episodic migraine prevention in adults: Report of the Quality Standards Subcommittee of the American Academy of Neurology and the American Headache Society. *Neurology* 78(17):1337–1345, 2012. Retrieved from www.guideline.gov/content.aspx?id=36898&search=neurology

UCL Institute of Neurology. Queen Square Brain Bank. Updated March 22, 2013. Retrieved from www.ucl.ac.uk/ion/departments/molecular/themes/neurodegeneration/brainbank

Zesiewicz, TA, et al. Quality Standards Subcommittee of the American Academy of Neurology. Practice parameter; treatment of nonmotor symptoms of Parkinson disease; report of the Quality Standards Subcommittee of the American Academy of Neurology. *Neurology* 74(11):924–931, 2010.

Bibliography

Alzheimer's Disease

2013 Alzheimer's disease facts and figures. *Alzheimer's Association* 9(2):1–67, 2013.

Plassman, BL, et al. Prevalence of dementia in the United States: The Aging, Demographics, and Memory Study. *Neuroepidemiology* 29 (1-2):125–132, 2007.

Salamanca, S. Treatment guidelines for Alzheimer-type dementia. *Clin Advisor* 47–54, June 2011.

Cerebrovascular Accident

Anderson, D, et al. Diagnosis and initial treatment of ischemic stroke. Institute for Clinical Systems Improvement, Bloomington, MN, 2012. Retrieved from www.guideline.gov/content.aspx?id=38254&search=emergency+department

Edlow, JA, et al; American College of Emergency Physicians, American Academy of Neurology. Clinical policy; use of intravenous tPA for the management of acute ischemic stroke in the emergency department. *Ann Emerg Med* 61(2):225–243, 2013. Retrieved from www.guideline.gov/content.aspx?id=43762&search=emergency+department

Ennen, KA. Taking a second look at stroke in women. *Am Nurse Today* 8(5):12–15, 2013.

Jasmin, L. Stroke. Updated May 21, 2012. Retrieved from www.nlm.nih.gov/medlineplus/ency/article/000726.htm

Tocco, S. Identify the vessel, recognize the stroke. *Am Nurse Today* 6(9):8–11, 2011.

Delirium and Dementia

Alzheimer's Association. Delirium or dementia—Do you know the difference? Retrieved from www.alz.org/norcal/in_my_community_17590.asp

Blazer, DG, and van Nieuwenhuizen, AO. Evidence for the diagnostic criteria of delirium. *Curr Opin Psychiatry* 25(3):239–243, 2012.

Clevenger, CK. Memory maker: Clinical management of early and midstage dementia. *Adv NPs PAs* 3(9):14–17, 2012.

Delirium and dementia at the end of life. Retrieved from www.medscape.org/viewarticle/499458

Filippi, M, et al; European Federation of the Neurologic Societies. EFNS task force: The use of neuroimaging in the diagnosis of dementia. *Eur J Neurol* 19(12):e131–e140, 1487–1501, 2012. Retrieved from http://www.ncbi.nlm.nih.gov/pubmed/22900895

Halloran, L. Cognitive impairment: Pearls for practice. *J Nurse Pract* 9(4):254–255, 2013.

Segal-Gida, F. Cognitive screening tools. *Clin Rev* 23(1):12–18, 2013.

Headaches

Beithon, J, et al. *Diagnosis and treatment of headache.* Institute for Clinical Systems Improvement, Bloomington, MN, 2013. Retrieved from www.guideline.gov/popups/printView.aspx?id=43791

Headache Classification Committee of the International Headache Society. The international classification of headache disorders. *Cephalalgia* 24:1, 2004.

Milner, RL, and Haddow, SV. Giant cell arteritis. *Adv NPs PAs* 2(7): 33–35, 2011.

Scottish Intercollegiate Guidelines Network (SIGN). Diagnosis and management of headache in adults. A national clinical guidelines. Edinburgh, Scotland, November 2008. Retrieved from www.guidelines.gov/summary/summary.aspx?doc_id=13446&nbr=006857&string

Silberstein, SD, et al. Evidence-based guideline update: Pharmacologic treatment for episodic migraine prevention in adults: Report of the Quality Standards Subcommittee of the American Academy of Neurology and the American Headache Society. *Neurology* 78(17):1337–1345, 2012. Retrieved from www.guideline.gov/content.aspx?id=36898&search=neurology

Wright, WL. Assessing functional impairment during and between migraine attacks. *J Nurse Pract* 4(3):201–207, 2008.

Herpes Zoster

Davis, TL. Postherpetic neuralgia. *Adv NPs PAs* 3(9):29–31, 2012.

Janniger, CK. Herpes zoster. *Medscape.* Updated February 26, 2013. Retrieved from http://emedicine.medscape.com/article/1132465-overview

Myasthenia Gravis

Smith, C, and Stickler, D. A collaborative approach to myasthenia gravis. *Clin Advisor* 15(12):20–27, 2012.

Multiple Sclerosis

Dunmore, FR. Fatigue in multiple sclerosis. *Adv NPs PAs* 4(4):23–25, 2013.

Filippi, M, et al. Use of imaging in multiple sclerosis. In Gilhus, NE, et al (Eds.), *European handbook of neurological management,* ed 2, vol 1. Wiley-Blackwell, Oxford, UK, 2011, pp. 35–51.

Parkinson's Disease

Berardelli, A, et al. EFNS/MDS-ES recommendations for the diagnosis of Parkinson's disease. *Eur J Neurol* 20(1):16–34, 2013.

International Stem Cell Corporation announces new data from Parkinson's disease program. *Wall Street Journal,* October 16, 2013. Retrieved from http://online.wsj.com/article/PR-CO-20131016-906505.html

Zesiewicz, TA, et al. Quality Standards Subcommittee of the American Academy of Neurology. Practice parameter; treatment of nonmotor symptoms of Parkinson disease; report of the Quality Standards Subcommittee of the American Academy of Neurology. *Neurology* 74(11):924–931, 2010.

Seizures

Tocco, S. Understanding psychogenic nonepileptic seizures. *Am Nurse Today* 7(5):8–10, 2012.

Resources

Alzheimer's Disease
Alzheimer's Association
1-800-272-3900
www.alz.org
Alzheimer's Foundation of America
1-866-232-8484
http://alzfdn.org
Cerebrovascular Accident
American Heart Association
1-800-242-8715
www.americanheart.org
American Stroke Association
1-800-242-8721
www.strokeassociation.org
National Stroke Association
1-800-STROKES
www.stroke.org
Epilepsy
Epilepsy Foundation
1-800-EFA-1000
www.epilepsyfoundation.org
Multiple Sclerosis
Multiple Sclerosis Foundation
1-800-225-6495
www.msfacts.org
National Multiple Sclerosis Society
1-800-FIGHT-MS (1-800-344-4867)
http://nmss.org

Parkinson's Disease
Parkinson's Disease Foundation
1-800-457-6676
www.pdf.org
National Parkinson Foundation, Inc.
1-800-327-4545
www.parkinson.org
United Parkinson Foundation
833 West Washington Blvd.
Chicago, IL 60607
1-312-733-1893
Headache
National Headache Foundation
1-888-NHF-5552
www.headaches.org

Skin Problems

Jill E. Winland-Brown, EdD, APRN, FNP-BC •
Brian Oscar Porter, MD, PhD, MPH

Chapter 7

COMMON COMPLAINTS

■ ALOPECIA

Alopecia (baldness) can occur anywhere on the body where hair is present, although it is commonly associated with absence of hair on the scalp area. Scalp hair loss can occur in patches *(alopecia areata)* or over the entire scalp *(androgenetic alopecia).* Hair loss can occur on the eyebrows, on the beard area, or on the entire body *(alopecia universalis),* and it can be either a temporary or permanent condition.

Hair loss is a gradual process; up to 50% of scalp hair can be lost before the loss becomes clinically apparent. Alopecia is associated with emotional distress even if the hair loss is temporary *(alopecia areata).* The most common cause of permanent hair loss is androgenetic alopecia, or male-pattern baldness (common baldness). Androgenetic alopecia (AGA) has a polygenic inheritance pattern: It is inherited from both parents, not only through maternal genes—a common myth. Another common misconception is that AGA is more common in men; in reality, it occurs in both sexes. Factors that influence normal hair development and cycling include estrogens, growth hormone, glucocorticoids, thyroid hormone, retinoid, prolactin, and androgens; these factors can be adversely affected by certain medications. The most important hair growth factors are the androgens, testosterone, and its active metabolite, dihydrotestosterone. During puberty, when androgen secretion starts, hair follicles become enlarged in certain areas of the body such as the beard area, the chest, and the extremities. Androgens have the opposite effect on the hair follicles of the scalp region: They cause a decrease in the size of the hair follicles (miniaturization) and can alter the hairline on the bitemporal region and the vortex areas. Four cycles of scalp hair growth exist. The growth phase *(anagen)* of scalp hair is the longest cycle, lasting from 2 to 6 years. The majority of hair on the scalp (90%–95%) is in the anagen phase. The latent, or involution, phase *(catagen)* is the shortest cycle, which lasts only 2 to 3 weeks. The resting phase *(telogen)* lasts from 2 to 3 months. Hair is shed during the fourth phase *(exogen).* In an average person, from 50 to 150 hairs are lost daily, and the cycle is repeated. Both topical and systemic medications for hair loss affect some or all of the phases of hair growth.

Thirty-five million men in the United States experience hair loss, and 21 million women do as well. For men, 40% have noticeable hair loss by age 35 years, 65% by age 60 years, 70% by age 80 years, and 80% by age 85 years. Women tend to develop AGA 10 years later than men. Thirteen percent of women develop AGA before menopause and 75% develop it postmenopausally.

In reversible cases of nonscarring alopecia, regrowth of hair usually takes several months. Patients who are reassured of this important fact will have lessened anxiety over their condition. Two important factors that the practitioner should address in the evaluation of alopecia are (1) whether it is scarring or nonscarring alopecia and (2) whether hair loss is in a small, well-circumscribed area (alopecia areata or trichotillomania) or generalized (AGA). Based on these two general categories, the differential diagnosis is made easier for the clinician. Scarring alopecia *(cicatricial alopecia)* causes permanent hair loss and is not reversible. Hair loss from nonscarring alopecia *(noncicatricial alopecia)* can be either temporary or permanent.

Differential Diagnosis

A thorough history is important in the evaluation of alopecia. Information regarding family members—both male and female—with hair loss should be elicited. Because some medications affect hair growth factors, a review of the patient's medication history is important and should not be missed. Drugs that cause hair loss include hormones, anticonvulsants, anticoagulants, oral contraceptives, beta blockers, antimetabolites, antithyroid drugs, and excessive amounts of vitamin A or topical Retin-A.

A potassium hydroxide (KOH) and Wood's light exam is helpful in the diagnosis of tinea capitis in cases of patchy hair loss. Although most cases of tinea capitis do not fluoresce, a fungal culture can provide definitive proof of fungal infection and should be performed if suspicion is high. Some dermatologists utilize the telogen count, in which 100 hairs (only 50 hairs are needed for accuracy) are removed from different areas of the scalp and the number of hairs in telogen is counted. Telogen hairs are recognized because of the large white club on the end of each hair. The appearance of the skin on the scalp will give the practitioner a clue to the type of alopecia that is involved. In nonscarring alopecia, the scalp will have normal texture and color. In contrast, the scalp of a patient with scarring alopecia has no visible hair follicles (or no follicular openings) and is atrophied and smooth. The affected area of the scalp (or the entire scalp) is sometimes hypopigmented or hyperpigmented. Obvious scarring is seen in some patients, and some have erythema and scaling (in these cases, it is important to rule out fungal infection). Look for fine pitting of the dorsal nail plate ("hammered brass") on the physical exam.

Both systemic and nonsystemic causes are seen in nonscarring alopecia. Nonsystemic causes of alopecia include hair pulling *(trichotillomania),* excessive traction of the frontal and temporal area of the scalp (from tight cornrows or tight ponytails), trauma (both physical and chemical), radiation therapy of the head, local bacterial infection, and local fungal infection. Trichotillomania (compulsive hair pulling) is more commonly seen in children and teens. It is usually on the same side as the dominant hand and may include other than just scalp hair (e.g., eyelashes, eyebrow hair, and beards, although those hairs are usually not long enough to pull).

Systemic causes of nonscarring alopecia include alopecia areata, telogen effluvium, androgenetic baldness (common baldness), vitiligo, Hashimoto's thyroiditis, Addison's disease, systemic lupus erythematosus (SLE), hypothyroidism or hyperthyroidism, secondary syphilis, severe herpes zoster of the scalp, drug-induced alopecia (common in patients on cyclophosphamide therapy), iron-deficiency anemia, and pituitary insufficiency.

Telogen effluvium (TE)—excessive shedding of scalp hair as a result of an increased number of hair follicles entering the resting stage (telogen)—can be caused by fever and certain drugs; therefore, a search for these possible causes should be included in the history taking. TE may also be caused by stress, pregnancy and/or childbirth, extreme weight loss, and general anesthesia. TE is almost nonexistent in men. The classic signs of androgenetic baldness are thinning hairs of various diameters and lengths ("miniaturized" hairs) located in typical areas, which differ in men and women. In men, hair loss usually starts on the hairline and around the temple (bitemporal) area and the vortex or top of the head. In women, hair loss is much more diffuse and occurs mostly on top of the head. Hair loss is sometimes harder to recognize in women because of hairstyles that are used to camouflage the problem.

Alopecia areata is not an uncommon condition in primary-care practice. The cause of alopecia areata is still unknown, although an immunological mechanism is suspected. The typical patient will present with well-circumscribed patches of hair loss on the scalp or sometimes on the face, in areas such as the eyebrows or the beard area. Occasionally only one patch is seen; sometimes multiple patches of hair loss are apparent. Alopecia areata can occur once in a lifetime, or it can be a recurrent problem. Some cases become recalcitrant and are best treated by specialists. Because gray hair is spared, patients may complain of going gray overnight. In alopecia areata, when the scalp is examined closely with a magnifying lens, short, stubby hairs with tapered ends (so-called "exclamation point hairs") are seen on the periphery of the bald patch (or patches). Alopecia areata is associated with autoimmune endocrinopathies such as Hashimoto's thyroiditis, Addison's disease, and pernicious anemia.

Hair regrowth occurs after several months, with new hairs that look thinner and finer than the original hair. There is no cure for alopecia areata, but in most patients hair usually regrows spontaneously after several months. The prognosis for alopecia areata is good if it occurs after puberty: Studies have found that up to 80% of these patients will regrow hair. Occasionally, a case of persistent alopecia areata that is unresponsive to treatment is seen; these cases are best referred to dermatologists for management.

Etiology of scarring, or cicatricial, alopecia can include trauma (physical or chemical), severe bacterial or fungal infections of the scalp, scleroderma, discoid lupus erythematosus, lichen planopilaris, and excessive radiation. Early recognition and treatment of bacterial or fungal infections can help prevent or minimize the incidence of scarring. Severe local infection with either bacteria or fungi can permanently damage hair follicles and cause a patchy (and scarring) alopecia that is permanent.

When an autoimmune disease is suspected, laboratory tests include antinuclear antibodies to rule out lupus or autoimmune disorders; rheumatoid factor; and erythrocyte sedimentation rate (ESR), a nonspecific marker for inflammation. The rheumatology, or arthritis, profile is a panel of tests that may help in the diagnosis of autoimmune disorders that can cause alopecia, such as SLE and scleroderma. Scleroderma (progressive systemic sclerosis) is a multisystemic inflammatory disorder associated with sclerotic changes in the body, including the skin. The skin becomes diffusely thickened with telangiectasia. A scalp biopsy is reserved for difficult and recalcitrant cases of alopecia. For the differential diagnosis of alopecia, see Differential Diagnosis 7.1.

In addition, serum testosterone, dehydroepiandrosterone, iron, total iron-binding capacity, and thyroid function tests, along with a complete blood count (CBC), will identify most other causes of hair thinning in premenopausal women.

Differential Diagnosis 7.1 Alopecia

Type of Alopecia	Differential Diagnosis
Scarring Alopecia (Cicatricial alopecia)	Trauma (chemical, physical, heat)
	Kerion formation in tinea capitis
	Chronic discoid lupus erythematosus
	Scleroderma
	Excessive radiation to scalp
	Lichen planopilaris
	Bacterial infection of scalp
Nonscarring Alopecia (Noncicatricial alopecia)	Alopecia areata
	Drug-induced hair loss
	Trichotillomania (hair pulling)
	Telogen effluvium (after pregnancy, major surgery, major emotional stress)
	Androgenetic baldness
	Tinea capitis (with no kerion formation)
	Hypothyroidism (Hashimoto's thyroiditis)
	Systemic lupus erythematosus
	Addison's disease

A biopsy is useful in diagnosing scarring alopecia, but specimens must be obtained from the active border rather than from the scarred central zone.

Treatment

Medical treatment is available but is not a permanent solution for alopecia. Patients should be educated that total return to previous levels of hair growth is not possible, but cosmetically acceptable hair coverage is possible. Medical treatments must be used daily to maintain regrown hair. Stopping treatment will result in shedding of hair and a return to the previous levels of alopecia. Hair shedding is seen rapidly in a matter of days after stopping minoxidil (Rogaine), but is more gradual over several months with finasteride (Propecia). Propecia is for men only. Nonmedical options include hair weaves, toupees, and wigs. Wigs are either worn on top of the head or are interwoven into existing hair as a "weave." As the existing hair (to which the weave is anchored) grows, the weave must be readjusted periodically, which may impart increased stress on hair follicles. The only currently available permanent treatment for alopecia is scalp surgery with hair transplantation.

Topical treatment includes minoxidil 2% solution (Rogaine for Men or Rogaine for Women) and minoxidil 5% solution (Rogaine Extra Strength for Men), which are available over the counter (OTC). At a higher dose, oral minoxidil is a vasodilator and is used to treat hypertension. Topical minoxidil has not been found to cause lowering of systolic or diastolic blood pressure and pulse rate. The best candidates for treatment with topical minoxidil are patients with recent onset of alopecia (less than 5 years), those younger than age 50 years, and patients with smaller areas of hair loss. Up to 40% of patients who use topical minoxidil for a period of 1 year or more will experience moderate to dense hair regrowth. Minoxidil 2% solution has been shown consistently to reduce hair loss and induce new hair growth in females with female pattern hair loss (Level 2; University of Texas at Austin, 2011). Minoxidil 5% solution is more effective, but it is indicated for use by men only. The 5% solution has not produced any demonstrable improvement over that seen with the 2% solution in women. Minoxidil is used twice daily on the affected scalp area. Adverse effects include irritation, itching, dryness, scaling, and redness of the scalp; sometimes minoxidil can cause contact dermatitis. An adverse effect that is more common in women is *hypertrichosis* (excessive hair growth on the body).

Systemic treatment for alopecia with finasteride (Propecia) should not be used in women of reproductive age because this drug can cause abnormalities of the external genitalia of male fetuses. In women not of childbearing age, finasteride does not appear to be effective in treating AGA. Therefore, finasteride, once daily, is used for the treatment of androgenetic baldness in men only. Dihydrotestosterone (DHT) levels are the main issue in men because testosterone is converted to DHT by means of the enzyme 5α-reductase. Finasteride, which blocks the effects of 5α-reductase, is metabolized in the liver and should be used with caution in patients with liver disease. In men aged 60 years or older, finasteride may not be as effective as in younger men because of reduction in alpha-reductase activity. Adverse effects include decreased libido (1.8%), erectile dysfunction (1.3%), and ejaculatory dysfunction (1.2%). In most men, these sexual side effects gradually resolve with prolonged treatment.

The treatment choice is determined by the patient's age and the severity of the hair loss. For patients with hair loss of less than 50%, treatment options include corticosteroid intralesional injections, anthralin, minoxidil solution, or topical corticosteroid creams. Topical treatment with a potent corticosteroid is preferred by primary-care practitioners because it is not invasive and is simple to use, although it is not as effective as intralesional injections. Small amounts of triamcinolone acetonide 5 mg/mL (Kenalog) may be injected intralesionally into the middermal layer, spaced approximately 1 cm apart on bald patches. Hair growth is usually seen in 4 weeks. One side effect of corticosteroid use that patients and practitioners should monitor for is atrophy of the skin. Unfortunately, these injections are only a temporary solution and do not alter the underlying pathophysiology of hair loss.

■ PIGMENTATION CHANGES

The skin is the largest and most visible organ of the body. For most people, skin color is an important part of their identity as an individual. Because of the skin's visibility, conditions affecting the skin cause not only physical discomfort but also have emotional overtones. Pigmentation disorders seen in primary care include both hyperpigmentation and hypopigmentation. Either condition can be a sign of disease, or it can be considered a normal finding, depending on the rest of the clinical picture.

Melanin is a skin pigment produced by melanocyte cells that determines skin color. Although there is no difference in the number of melanocytes among the different ethnic groups, the ability of the melanocytes of darker-skinned people to produce and retain melanin (from melanosomes) is much greater than in people with lighter skin. Research has found that melanosome size is directly related to skin color: The larger the size of the melanosomes, the darker the skin color. Asians and whites have fewer and smaller melanosomes, whereas in individuals with darker skins, especially in blacks or people of African descent, melanosomes are much larger and more numerous. Darker skin gives protection from ultraviolet (UV) radiation. Studies of people with darker skin have shown that dark skin has a sun protection factor (SPF) between 5 and 13. Because of the protective aspect of darker skin, the incidence of nonmelanoma skin cancer in blacks or people of African origin is much less than in whites. Studies have shown that basal cell carcinomas are extremely rare in individuals with darker skin.

Pigmentation disorders can be clinical manifestations of diseases that include endocrine, genetic, metabolic, or nutritional problems or a malignancy. Pigmentation disorders seen in primary care include normal variations in color as a result of ethnic differences (e.g., oral hyperpigmentation in darker skins). *Vitiligo,* or the total loss of skin color in patchy areas of the body (rarely over the entire body), is recognized clinically as extremely white macules or patches that are usually located on exposed areas such as the face and the hands. More than half the cases of vitiligo occur in persons aged 10 to 30 years; vitiligo occurs equally in both sexes. It is relatively common and affects up to 1% of the population. Vitiligo is an autoimmune disorder in which the body produces antibodies against its own melanocytes. Vitiligo is associated with a higher risk of other autoimmune disorders such as thyroid disease and diabetes mellitus type 1 but not with diabetes mellitus type 2.

Skin bleaching (or lightening) creams and ointments may be used by some patients wanting to lighten their overall skin tone, particularly those from darker-skinned ethnic groups, such as Asians, African Americans, and Hispanics. These creams, typically not prescribed, are sold OTC and may be prone to misuse or overuse. In turn, their active ingredients are largely unregulated, and some preparations have been known to contain potential toxins, such as heavy metals. Patients should, therefore, be cautioned against the use of such nonprescription bleaching creams. The clinician should be sensitive to the fact that such discussions may also extend to the larger societal implications of skin color valuation as perceived on a personal level by the patient.

Differential Diagnosis

Differential diagnoses to consider in oral hyperpigmentation include Peutz-Jeghers syndrome, pigmented tumors such as melanoma, Addison's disease, heavy metal exposure, and a history of taking antimalarial medications. Peutz-Jeghers syndrome is an inherited disorder that presents with pigmented (dark brown–colored) macules on the lips and inside the mouth on the mucous membranes. It is associated with multiple polyps in the stomach, the small intestine, and large bowel, causing abdominal pain and other gastrointestinal symptoms. Patients who are suspected of having this disease need to be referred to a gastroenterologist for further evaluation.

Normal variations in pigmentation are commonly seen in the clinical area in patients with darker skin. In patients with dark skin or those of African descent, oral hyperpigmentation is considered a normal variant, but underlying pathology should be ruled out. The exception is newborn infants—oral pigmentation should not be present at this early time. The most common site of involvement is the gingivae (the gums), but other sites, such as the inside of the cheeks (buccal mucosa) and the tongue, can be involved as well. The hyperpigmented areas can range from bluish black to a deep brown in color. Another pigmentation change that is considered a normal variant in blacks or people of African descent is hypopigmentation of the midsternal area. It is more common in males; this type of hypopigmentation is seen in up to 70% of black children and in one-third of adults.

Voigt's or Futcher lines are seen in up to one-fourth of blacks or people of African descent and less frequently in Asians. These distinct lines appear down the length of each arm symmetrically, dividing lighter-colored skin anteromedially from the patient's darker skin color (the lighter shade of skin is touching the trunk). The nails of people with darker skin can be pigmented, with involvement of the entire nail plate or in longitudinal bands of streaks of darker color. Normal nail pigmentation should be bilateral and symmetrical. Any asymmetry or new onset of pigmentation should arouse the clinician's suspicion for disease, including acral melanoma. Pigmentation changes in people with darker skin do not necessarily point to pathology, but at the same time the clinician should not neglect the possibility of a disease process.

A physiological hyperpigmentation condition called *chloasma* ("the mask of pregnancy") is caused by increased levels of estrogen, progesterone, and melanocyte-stimulating hormone during pregnancy. Chloasma may also occur in 30% to 50% of women taking oral contraceptives. Areas commonly affected include the face, especially the malar region and jawline, the nipples, the genitals, and the linea nigra extending midline on the abdomen from the umbilicus to the pubis. The hyperpigmentation is worsened by exposure to sunlight, and patients should be cautioned to decrease sun exposure at this time. Treatment of chloasma can include combinations of a retinoic acid and hydroquinone, betahydroxy acid peels, and various laser and intense pulsed light photorejuvenation treatments. Chloasma can be very difficult to treat in Asian and Hispanic clients. A 24-hour skin patch test to rule out an allergy to any bleaching agent should be done before use. The cream can be applied twice a day for 2 months. The patient should be advised to avoid the eye area and to use the cream cautiously in sensitive areas such as the nose and the lips. Unfortunately, hydroquinone is labeled Pregnancy Category C, so the patient should be referred to an obstetrician for management. Certain drugs that are known to cause a diffuse hyperpigmentation (melanosis) include zidovudine and cyclophosphamide. Skin discoloration has also been reported in patients who have been taking amiodarone, chlorpromazine, and certain antimalarials. Photosensitivity reactions resulting in hyperpigmentation after sun exposure can be caused by citrus oils that are present in fruit or certain perfumes.

Although these dark patches on the face that develop during pregnancy are referred to as chloasma, *melasma* is a more general term referring to hyperpigmentation of certain areas of the skin (regardless of pregnancy status) as a result of sun exposure and hormonal influences. It is usually more common in women than in men. First-line treatments are prescription skin bleaching creams (hydroquinone) and strict sun avoidance. Studies are being done to examine the benefit of laser therapy and salicylic acid peels every 2 to 8 weeks.

Addison's disease is caused by inadequate secretion of corticosteroids as a result of partial or complete destruction (70% of cases are due to an autoimmune mechanism) of the adrenal glands. Addison's disease can cause a diffused generalized hyperpigmentation, especially on skin creases, because of increased levels of adrenocorticotropic hormone (ACTH) from the pituitary. Classic areas where hyperpigmentation is seen are skinfolds; palmar creases; pressure points such as the elbows, knees, or knuckles; inside the mouth on the cheeks (buccal area); and on scars. Symptoms of Addison's disease include generalized weakness, amenorrhea, and loss of axillary hair in women. Laboratory findings in Addison's disease include elevated serum potassium and calcium, low serum sodium, anemia, and an elevated ACTH level. Screening laboratory tests to detect autoimmune diseases include thyroid-stimulating hormone (TSH), antinuclear antibody, sedimentation rate, random blood glucose levels, vitamin B_{12} level, rheumatoid factor, and a CBC.

In patients with pigmented nevi (moles), the presence of certain unusual colors on nevi, such as blue, gray, pink, white, and black (or a variegation of color), should arouse suspicion in the clinician. Benign moles are usually a small size (less than 5 mm)—smaller than a pencil eraser—and have a well-defined border. Benign moles should be only a single shade of color—either brown, beige, or pink.

When evaluating nail pigmentation changes, symmetry and bilateral involvement of the nails and a history of no change is reassuring. A variegated color or very dark color on one solitary nail should arouse suspicion for acral melanoma. Melanomas in people with darker skin are more likely to present on the extremities (or acral area) rather than on the trunk area. The nailbeds, the palms, and the soles are sites where acral melanoma is more likely to be seen in darker-skinned people. The differential diagnoses of nail pigmentation change include acral melanoma, Peutz-Jeghers syndrome, a subungual nevus, gold therapy, Addison's disease, hemochromatosis, and a history of taking antimalarial medications. If acral melanoma is suspected, referral to a dermatologist for a nail biopsy and definitive diagnosis is imperative.

Malignant melanoma, the deadliest of all skin cancers, requires a high index of suspicion. Factors that can precipitate the appearance of acquired melanocytic nevus include immunosuppression, pregnancy, puberty, and sun exposure. Any asymmetry and changes in pigmentation, size, or surface of a mole require referral to a dermatologist. Moles that are larger than 5 mm are more likely to be atypical. Persons at higher risk for skin cancer include patients with numerous moles (50 or more countable moles), atypical and large (more than 5 mm) moles, and a family history of melanoma. The American Cancer Society mnemonic to help detect skin cancer is ABCDE: A—Asymmetry, B—Border (irregularity), C—Color (variegation), D—Diameter (greater than 6 mm), and E—Elevation or Evolving. Any patient with a suspicious mole should be referred to a dermatologist for definitive diagnosis and treatment.

■ PRURITUS

Pruritus—the sensation of itching—is perceived as unpleasant; therefore, people often seek help for this problematic symptom. Pruritus is a frequent symptom of dermatological disease; it can be acute or chronic and is sometimes so severe as to interfere with sleep and daily life activities.

Pruritus is generally caused by either local (e.g., insect bite, contact dermatitis) or systemic (e.g., uremia, hyperbilirubinemia with skin deposition of bile salts) etiology. In Hodgkin's disease, the incidence of pruritus is between 10% and 25%. Senile pruritus is common in people aged 70 years and older. Rashes or other skin lesions generally accompany the sensation of itching on the skin, although in some cases of systemic etiology, no external findings on the skin are ever located. Therefore, the finding of skin lesions or rashes is most useful in classification of the differential diagnosis of pruritus.

Differential Diagnosis

A thorough and careful history is an important step in the evaluation of pruritus. If skin findings (such as the linear shape characteristic of contact dermatitis) suggest an external causation, the history should be directed toward eliciting an external etiology. If the patient complains of generalized itching with no skin lesions, an internal or systemic causation is more likely. The presence of a generalized rash should also arouse the clinician's suspicion to drug reactions. Some systemic causes of pruritus include conditions such as allergies, drug reactions, malignancy (lymphomas and leukemias), uremia of chronic renal disease, and pruritus from obstructive biliary disease, as a result of elevated blood levels of unconjugated bilirubin. (See Focus on History 7.1.)

Pruritus is a symptom and should elicit an investigation of the possible causation. External causes of pruritus include insect bites, insect infestation (scabies, pediculosis), pinworms (more common in children), larva migrans, contact dermatitis, fiberglass dermatitis, seabather's eruption, and bacterial folliculitis. It is not uncommon for patients to deny the knowledge of insect bites (especially if the event occurred during sleep), because some insects do not have painful bites. The patient should be asked about any history of medication use, including prescriptions, hormones, vitamin supplements, and the use of nutritional and protein supplements. The history should include a review of all detergents, soaps, creams, moisturizers, cosmetics, and perfumes. A history of alternative medicines, including herbs, homeopathic remedies, and oils for aromatherapy, should also be included. Many young women who take oral contraceptives forget that

these are prescription drugs and therefore do not mention them unless the practitioner makes a special effort to elicit information about oral contraceptive use. The use of recreational substances, including chewing tobacco, marijuana, and illicit drugs, should be considered as a potential cause of pruritus. Psychiatric illness as a cause of pruritus is a diagnosis of exclusion. Skin markings are seen more often on extremities; the urge to scratch even in the absence of itch is sometimes reported. The clinician should search for symptoms of depression or mood disorder. There is frequently a history of increased stress because of personal, financial, or familial problems.

The most predominant and disturbing symptom of scabies is pruritus, especially nighttime pruritus. The clinician needs to have a high index of suspicion for scabies because it frequently does not manifest in its classic presentation. If the clinician is looking for the mites' burrows, which the patient can obliterate by scratching, the diagnosis can easily be missed. Frequently, the rash has secondary changes, including excoriation, scaling, lichenification, and occasionally nodules (nodular scabies) because of the intense inflammatory response from the mite. Even if skin lesions do not resemble those associated with scabies, the clinician should consider the diagnosis if the location of the rash is on the axilla, under the breast, on the waistline, on the penis, or between the fingers. The clinician should not assume a lack of scabies infection if the classic rash on the interdigital webs is not seen. Scabies is more common in group homes and nursing homes. The management and treatment of scabies are discussed in depth later in this chapter, under Common Problems: Parasitic Infestations.

If a pruritic rash does not respond to symptomatic treatment, a work-up for systemic diseases is in order. Laboratory tests that should be ordered if systemic disease is suspected include CBC with differential;

Focus on History 7.1	Pruritus
History	**Questions to Ask**
Insects	Have you had any exposure to mosquitoes, fleas, sand flies, ticks, or spiders? (Brown recluse and black widow bites have necrotic centers.)
Outdoors	Have you been to the beach, at a picnic, gone camping or swimming, or attended a sporting event?
Plants	Have you been in contact with plants or done any gardening?
Jewelry/metals	Any new watches, belts/belt buckles, earrings, necklace? Any contact with metals?
Occupation	What is your occupation? (Gardeners and employees of prisons, day-care centers, and schools have the potential for scabies, pediculosis, or impetigo exposure.)
Hobbies and sport participation	Any exposure to hobby paints and glues? Do you participate in any sports? (Weight lifters, athletes are prone to fungal skin infections.)
Chemical exposure	Any use or exposure to pesticides, herbicides, fertilizers, household cleaners?
Medications	Any use of topical medications such as Neosporin ointment, Benadryl topical lotion, anti-itch lotion or spray? (contact dermatitis) Any prescription medicines, over-the-counter, herbs, vitamins?
Family history	Any family members or intimate friends with the same symptoms? (scabies, pediculosis, tinea capitis)

ESR; fasting blood sugar; liver, and renal function tests; a thyroid profile or a TSH level; and a hepatitis profile. If the pruritic area is in the anus, a search for external hemorrhoids should be done. In children or in adults with small children (when pinworm infestation is suspected), a stool sample to check for ova and parasites, or a Scotch tape test, is recommended.

Dry skin, or *xerosis,* is a common finding in the elderly. It is also seen in young adults who have dry skin and are overly meticulous with personal hygiene. Use of strong deodorant soaps or daily hot baths can precipitate dry skin and worsen pruritus. Systemic causes of pruritus to consider include atopic dermatitis (eczema), psoriasis, drug reactions, urticaria (from exposure to any substance, including airborne allergens), urticarial eruptions of pregnancy, lichen planus, lichen simplex chronicus, prurigo nodularis, and a malignancy, such as Hodgkin's lymphoma, cutaneous T-cell lymphoma (mycosis fungoides), and leukemia. A history of similar pruritic lesions in the past (especially if on the same location) should bring to mind an atopic history or urticaria. Atopic skin diseases that present predominantly with pruritus include atopic dermatitis (eczema) and psoriasis. The presence of hives or a history of hives is sufficient to diagnose urticaria. It is often seen with dermatographism, which can be elicited by rubbing a blunt object or finger on the skin firmly. An immediate response is seen, with formation of whealing that resolves within a few hours.

Lichen planus can mimic psoriasis; its cause is unknown. The lesions appear with shiny flat tops that are a red to violaceous color (red violet-tinged). Other presentations include small, flat-topped papules and a netlike lesion on the buccal mucosa (reticular lichen planus), penis, and external female genitalia. Malignant oral lesions occasionally occur, but oral carcinoma is rare. Lichen planus may have several presentations and locations: Lesions may be generalized, or they may be located on the arms, trunk, mouth, and genitalia. This disease may last for months to years; it does not have a cure and is best managed by a dermatologist. See Differential Diagnosis 7.2 for the differential diagnoses of pruritus.

Treatment

The treatment of pruritus depends on making the correct diagnosis. Symptomatic treatment for dry skin consists of avoidance of strong soaps, taking shorter, tepid showers (10–20 minutes) instead of hot baths, and the use of good emollients. Mild bland soaps such as Dove, Basis, Purpose, and Neutrogena are recommended. The patient should be educated to gently towel dry the skin after showering, because rubbing the skin stimulates pruritus. To seal the moisture in the skin, applying a bland emollient such as Eucerin, Lubriderm, or Alpha-Keri immediately after dabbing the skin with the towel is helpful. Waiting too long (more than 5 minutes) after finishing a bath or shower allows moisture to evaporate. The strongest emollients are ointments that are

Differential Diagnosis 7.2   Pruritus, Scabies, and Pediculosis

Condition	Differential Diagnosis
Pruritus—Rash Present	Insect bites/pediculosis
	Burrowing insects/larvae (scabies)
	Tinea (corporis, pedis, cruris)
	Contact dermatitis
	Atopic dermatitis (eczema)
	Drug eruptions
	Transient acantholytic dermatosis (Grover's disease)
	Bullous pemphigoid
	Urticaria (hives)
	Malignancy (cutaneous T-cell lymphoma)
	Pregnancy-induced
	Psoriasis
	Miliaria (heat rash)
	Folliculitis
	Seborrheic dermatitis
	Lichen planus
	Prurigo nodularis
	Dermatographism (Darier's disease)
	Pityriasis rosea
	Dermatitis herpetiformis
	Impetigo
	Ecthyma
	Erythroderma
	Neurotic excoriation
Pruritus—No Rash Present	Uremia from chronic renal disease
	Cholestatic liver disease
	Hyperparathyroidism
	Hodgkin's lymphoma
	Polycythemia vera
	Delusions of parasitosis
Scabies	Pruritus (see above)
	Pyoderma
	Impetigo
	Ecthyma
	Furunculosis
Nodular Scabies	Urticaria pigmentosa (in young child)
	Insect bites
	Darier's disease
	Prurigo nodularis
	Secondary syphilis
Crusted Scabies	Psoriasis
	Eczematous dermatitis
	Seborrheic dermatitis
	Erythroderma
Pediculosis	Pruritus (see above)
	Dandruff
	Scabies
	Pyoderma (impetigo)

petrolatum based, followed by creams (oil in water), and then lotions (powder in water). Gels are alcohol based; they should not be used for pruritus associated with dry skin because of their drying effect. Pruritus of the scalp caused by seborrheic dermatitis (with dandruff and fine scales at the hairline, by the nares, and the ears) should be treated with ketoconazole 2% shampoo (Nizoral shampoo). The rash of seborrheic dermatitis on the hairline, nares, and ears is best treated with hydrocortisone 1% (OTC) used twice to three times a day. Fluorinated topical steroids should not be used on the face because of the risk of skin atrophy. If the etiology is an irritating external agent (such as fiberglass insulation), elimination of irritating external agents may provide clinical relief of pruritus. Treatment of scabies infection is discussed later in this chapter.

Symptomatic treatment of generalized pruritus includes classic oral H_1 antihistamines such as hydroxyzine, one of the most effective treatments for pruritus, given 3 to 4 times per day. Cyproheptadine is used 2 to 3 times per day. OTC antihistamines include loratadine once a day, diphenhydramine, brompheniramine maleate, and chlorpheniramine maleate; all can be taken every 4 to 6 hours as needed. Prescription antihistamines do not cross the blood–brain barrier and cause less (or no) sedation. These include cetirizine taken daily, fexofenadine taken twice daily, and desloratadine taken once daily.

Any patient who is on antihistamines should be warned of possible drowsiness and should be warned against driving or operating dangerous machinery until the effects of the antihistamine are known. Alcohol and other central depressants worsen this effect. For anogenital pruritus, treatment includes the use of hydrocortisone and pramoxine cream 1% or 2.5% (Pramosone) on the anogenital area. Pramoxine preparations are very effective and have a low incidence of sensitivity reactions compared with topical antihistamines and benzocaine. They are effective not only for anogenital pruritus but also for short-term relief of urticaria, insect bites, pruritus vulvae, and nummular eczema. Use of fluorinated and potent topical steroids on the anogenital area is not recommended because it can lead to atrophy and striae. Lichen planus is treated with topical and systemic steroids and retinoids, cyclosporine, and psoralens with ultraviolet A photochemotherapy; the treatment of this disease is best managed by dermatologists.

If Hodgkin's lymphoma is suspected, the clinician should perform a thorough physical exam and should especially look for painless and enlarged lymph nodes and constitutional symptoms such as generalized pruritus, weight loss, night sweats, and fever. Cutaneous T-cell lymphoma (mycosis fungoides) is a malignancy of the helper T cells of the immune system. Onset of lesions may take many years; sometimes intractable pruritus may be the only presenting symptom. The lesions are sometimes misdiagnosed as psoriasis or as nummular dermatitis (eczema) because of their similar appearance. The lesions go through several stages and can present as red and scaly plaques that mimic the appearance of psoriasis. Nodules and tumors can be present, sometimes with ulceration.

Diagnostic laboratory testing for suspected malignancy can include a CBC with differential, a peripheral smear, liver and renal function tests, ESR, a chest x-ray film, and computed tomography (CT) scan. Patients with suspected malignancy should be referred to cancer specialists.

■ RASH

The word *rash* refers to any pink or red-colored skin eruption. Words that are synonymous with rash include *exanthem* and *eruption*. Rashes are clinical manifestations of inflammation and have multiple etiologies.

Skin cells (keratinocytes) originate in the basal layer of the epidermis. These cells take approximately 28 days to mature and migrate to the surface *(stratum corneum)*. The epidermis has no blood supply of its own and is dependent on the dermis for its circulation. It is stratified into two main layers—the inner viable layer *(stratum germinativum)* and the outer layer of dead, anucleated cells, called the *stratum corneum* or the horny layer. The stratum corneum consists of up to 25 layers of flat and tightly packed anucleated cells filled with keratin. Keratin, a tough and durable protein, limits the passage of molecules into and out of the skin. Thus, this tough outer layer is relatively impermeable to many external substances and also acts to prevent the evaporation of bodily fluids. It is a protective barrier against numerous microorganisms. When the stratum corneum is damaged by inflammation (rash), it becomes more permeable to external substances, including microorganisms and chemicals. Not only do these substances and microorganisms have a greater chance of gaining entrance into the body, but therapeutic topical creams and ointments applied to inflamed skin also are more likely to be absorbed and thus increase the chance of toxicity.

The dermis, which gives the skin its elasticity and strength, is made up primarily of a complex network of collagen and elastic fibers interspersed with blood vessels, cutaneous nerves, apocrine glands, eccrine glands, the lymphatics, and the pilosebaceous units of the skin. The *dermoepidermal junction* (the topmost section of the dermis) is the interface between the epidermis and the dermis. A defect in the dermoepidermal junction results in separation of these layers and bullous formation. Inherited autoimmune diseases of the skin resulting from abnormalities of the dermis include bullous pemphigoid and epidermolysis bullosa.

Gram-positive bacterial infections such as *Staphylococcus aureus*—the causative agent of toxic shock syndrome—present with systemic symptoms such as fever, malaise, and an erythematous rash. Drug reactions can also present with a rash (e.g., erythema multiforme, urticaria). Autoimmune disorders that can cause a rash include SLE (butterfly rash), erythema nodosum, and Kawasaki disease (seen in children).

Viruses are responsible for many cases of rash and are usually self-limiting in patients with intact immune systems. Viral infections that manifest with rash and systemic symptoms such as fever and malaise include measles, rubella (German measles), hand-foot-mouth disease, erythema infectiosum, herpes simplex infection, herpes zoster, varicella-zoster (chickenpox), and roseola infantum (also known as exanthema subitum) in children.

Rashes are more difficult to see in patients with darker skins because the red to dark pink color that is associated with rash becomes less visible. Instead of the pink to red color, a rash in a person of African descent might appear as a dark brown color. Rashes on patients with darker skin can sometimes go unnoticed unless the patient complains of the problem to the clinician. The clinician must learn to use other dermatological clues besides skin color to differentiate rashes in this population. These include the history of the rash and associated symptoms, the type of lesions present (macule, papule, pustule), the texture of the lesions (flat, raised, rough), and the pattern of distribution (central versus on the extremities). See Focus on History 7.2 and Table 7.1.

Differential Diagnosis

Because the differential diagnoses of rash are so numerous, this section focuses on rashes that are associated

---

Focus on History 7.2   Rash

Onset of Skin Lesions

• When did the skin lesion(s) first appear?
• How did the skin lesion appear at onset?
• Where did the skin lesion first appear?

Spread of Skin Lesions

• Have the skin lesions spread? Where?

Change in Skin Lesions

• Has the appearance of the skin lesions changed over time?
• Have the skin lesions gotten better or worse?

Symptoms Associated with the Skin Lesions

• Are there any associated symptoms, such as itching, burning, or pain?
• Are there any systemic symptoms such as fever, anorexia, malaise, pharyngitis, or myalgia?

Treatment

• What type of self-treatment has the patient attempted?
• Has the patient seen another health-care provider for the skin lesions? What type of treatment was given? Was it effective?

Foods

• Does the patient have any food allergies or sensitivities, such as dairy, seafood, peanuts, other nuts, strawberries, tomatoes, alcoholic drinks (such as red or white wine, beer, or mixed drinks)?

Medications

• Is the patient taking any prescription medications (e.g., antibiotics such as penicillin or sulfa drugs or pain medications such as codeine) and/or OTC medications such as aspirin, NSAIDs, cold medicines, or vitamins?
• Do any of these medications contain artificial color or preservatives?

Alternative Medicines

• Is the patient taking any herbal medicines or teas, homeopathic remedies, aromatherapy, juices, or other alternative medicines?

Atopic History

• Does the patient have a history of the same rash before? What was the diagnosis? How was it treated?
• Does the patient have a family history of skin conditions or rash?
• Has the patient or family member ever been diagnosed with eczema, psoriasis, skin allergies, asthma or allergies?

Infectious Disease Exposure (any exposure up to 2 weeks before onset of rash)

• Does the patient have any exposure to other people with the same symptoms?
• Does the patient have any exposure to small children, day care, or schools?
• Has the patient had any sexual activity with a new partner (known for less than 3 months)?

Systemic Symptoms (infectious, autoimmune, malignancies, metabolic)

• Does the patient have any systemic symptoms, such as sore throat and rhinitis (viral etiology), fever, fatigue, myalgia, joint pain, nausea, night sweats, weight loss (malignancy) or weight gain (diabetes mellitus)?

Table 7.1	Skin Lesions
Primary skin lesions: 1 cm or less in diameter	*Macules* Nonpalpable; caused by changes in skin pigmentation. Example: Freckles *Papules* Elevated and palpable lesions on top of the skin. Example: Nevi (moles) *Nodules* Elevated and palpable lesions that are deeper than papules and feel harder. Example: Acne nodule
Primary skin lesions: Larger than 1 cm in diameter	*Patches* Nonpalpable; caused by changes in skin pigmentation on a larger area than macules. Example: Cafe-au-lait stain *Plaques* A superficial lesion—flat-topped, firm, and elevated; palpable, with a firm to rough surface. Example: Psoriasis *Tumor* An elevated solid mass with a hard texture; shape and borders can be regular or irregular. Can be benign or cancerous. Example: Neoplasms *Wheal* Transient elevated wheal (hive-like); pink to red color from local edema and inflammation. Borders can be regular or irregular. Example: Mosquito bite, urticaria
Primary skin lesions: Fluid-filled lesions	*Vesicle* Superficial elevated lesion with distinct borders; filled with serous fluid. Example: Herpes simplex *Bulla* A vesicle larger than 1 cm in diameter. Example: Blister *Pustule* Sizes vary. Superficial elevated lesion filled with purulent fluid. Example: Acne pustule *Cyst* Sizes vary. An elevated encapsulated lesion that is deeper than a pustule, with distinct borders. Skin on top of a cyst can be moved. Filled with fluid or semisolid material. Example: Sebaceous cyst
Secondary skin lesions	*Atrophy* A thinning of skin (epidermis and dermis); appears white or translucent. Example: Striae *Lichenification* An increase in skin markings; feels rough and thickened. Frequently caused by chronic scratching or rubbing. Example: Atopic dermatitis *Scale* Shed epithelial cells in variable sizes. Can be flat or flaky in texture; color ranges from white to yellow. Example: Seborrheic dermatitis *Excoriation* A loss of epidermis. Shapes and sizes vary and depend on the cause. Example: Abrasion *Crust* Dried exudate from blood, serum, or pus. Elevated and rough with colors ranging from gold, red or brown. Example: Scab from an abrasion *Fissure* A linear crack extending from the epidermis to the dermis. Example: cheilosis *Erosion* A loss of parts on all the epidermis; appears moist and thick, but more shallow than an ulcer. Example: Rupture of a blister caused by a burn *Ulcer* Depressed lesion due to loss of the epidermis and dermis; appears as a moist pink to red lesion with exudate. Example: Decubitus ulcer

Table 7.1	Skin Lesions—cont'd	
	Scar
	Fibrous tissue that forms as skin trauma heals, extending beyond the epidermis. Color can be red, pink, or white; scars can be hypertrophic (thickened) or keloidal (more common in darker skins).
	Keloids
	Sharply elevated bulky scar tissue that appears shiny and smooth. Formation of keloids may have a genetic component.
Vascular lesions	*Ecchymosis*
	Bleeding into the skin layers and surrounding tissue as a result of trauma or coagulation defects. Example: Bruise
	Hematoma
	A large collection of blood as a result of trauma or coagulation defects. It is frequently tender and discolored; colors change from dark blue (when new) to green, then yellow. A hematoma usually resolves in a few weeks but may take several months. If it occurs in a vital area (brain), causing increased pressure, it is drained surgically or locally. Example: Hematoma on the thigh after a car accident
	Purpura
	Skin discoloration, ranging from dark pink to purple to blue. Does not blanch with pressure. Purpura can be punctate (capillaries) to larger-sized lesions. Almost all causes of palpable purpura are serious and vasculitis must be ruled out. Example: Large bruise

with serious health consequences. Primary-care clinicians should become familiar with these rashes because of the potential for serious sequelae, including death, if the diagnosis is missed.

Cancers such as mammary Paget's disease present with a rash that looks like eczematous dermatitis of the nipple and areola. Although it is an uncommon intraepithelial adenocarcinoma, the clinician should be careful not to overlook this diagnosis. The onset is very gradual, ranging from several months to years. Early in its course, the disease is asymptomatic except for a rash. During the later stages, it is accompanied by symptoms such as pruritus, discharge, bleeding, and ulceration. The sizes of lesions can range from less than 1 cm in diameter to several centimeters. Sometimes an underlying breast mass is palpable during the later stages of the disease—a worse prognosis is associated with this ominous finding. Patients with suspected mammary Paget's disease should be referred to a breast specialist.

The usual location of the classic rash of mammary Paget's disease is on one nipple (or areola); rarely is it seen on both breasts. The skin lesion appears as an oval-shaped, erythematous scaling plaque with sharp margins. Because of the similarity in the appearance, this lesion can be misdiagnosed as eczema, psoriasis, contact dermatitis, or impetigo. Usually, the lesions of eczematous dermatitis involve both breasts and last from 2 to 3 weeks; the lesions respond to treatment with topical steroids. Contact dermatitis usually involves only one breast (sometimes both); again, the rash usually resolves in 2 weeks and responds to topical steroids. If a rash on the nipple or areolar region lasts longer than 2 weeks and

does not resolve with topical steroids, a high index of suspicion is imperative and the patient should be referred to a breast specialist for further evaluation.

Toxic shock syndrome (TSS) is an acute illness caused by toxin-producing *S aureus*. In the United States, though TSS is seen in both male and female patients, its incidence among childbearing women represents 90% of the cases of TSS. Risk factors for menstrual TSS include use of superabsorbent tampons. In these cases, symptoms begin in nearly all patients within days of the onset of a menstrual period in women who have used tampons. Risk factors for nonmenstrual TSS include surgical wounds, nasal packs, burns, catheters, postpartum period, and use of birth control methods such as the sponge and the diaphragm. The mortality rate for nonmenstrual cases is 18%, 5% for menstrual-related TSS. Severe group A beta-hemolytic *Streptococcus* (GABHS) infection can mimic TSS (except that GABHS is associated with necrotizing fasciitis) and has a higher mortality rate (30%).

TSS presents with a sudden onset of high fever (fever higher than 102°F [38.8°C]) and vomiting. It is associated with a tingling sensation of the hands and feet, myalgia, weakness, headache, and diarrhea. In severe cases, it is associated with confusion, hypotension, and shock. It is accompanied by a bright red, fine maculopapular (scarlatiniform) rash and is sometimes accompanied by petechiae and bullae. The skin on the palms of the hands and the soles of the feet is very erythematous, and in 1 to 2 weeks the palms and soles start to desquamate. Abnormal laboratory results include leukocytosis, thrombocytopenia, abnormal liver function tests, elevated levels of creatinine, and abnormally low levels of platelets (thrombocytopenia).

Complications of TSS include multisystem failure, including adult respiratory distress syndrome, acute renal failure, metabolic acidosis, disseminated intravascular coagulation, septic shock, and death. A high index of suspicion and early recognition of serious causes of rash are important to avoid potential sequelae. Patients with suspected TSS should be referred immediately to a physician or to an emergency department. Treatment consists of hospitalization in the intensive care unit for aggressive systemic antibiotic therapy and systemic supportive therapy.

■ URTICARIA

Urticaria (hives or wheals) is a common problem seen in primary care. It affects from 10% to 20% of the population at least once in a lifetime. *Urticaria* is defined as a sudden generalized eruption of pale, evanescent wheals or papules that is associated with severe itching. *Angioedema* is urticaria that involves not only edema of the dermis, as in plain urticaria, but the subcutaneous tissues as well. Angioedema and urticaria can be part of a life-threatening immunoglobulin E (IgE)–dependent anaphylactic reaction, which involves bronchospasm, laryngeal edema, and shock. If anaphylaxis is not treated and reversed immediately with subcutaneous epinephrine, it can be fatal. Angioedema associated with chronic urticaria is rarely life-threatening. In these cases, the patient will report a history of angioedema without any compromise of the throat or airway.

Urticarial wheals (hives) and angioedema are produced by the degranulation of mast cells when an offending allergen to which the patient has been sensitized is encountered. Degranulated mast cells release inflammatory factors, including histamines that increase vascular permeability and cause pruritus. On microscopic exam, the edema on the dermis is manifested by the wide separation of dermal fibers in cells from urticarial lesions, along with dilation of the venules and lymphatics. Urticaria is also associated with non–IgE-dependent reactions involving the complement cascade of the immune system. Chronic urticaria may be a symptom of an autoimmune condition.

Differential Diagnosis

The typical patient with urticaria will present with a complaint of numerous intensely pruritic hives or wheals that appear regularly at certain times of the day, then spontaneously resolve within a few hours, only to reappear again the next day. The wheals typically enlarge and coalesce, forming round to irregular shapes. Most cases of acute urticaria spontaneously resolve in 1 to 2 weeks. Because most cases of acute urticaria resolve spontaneously in 2 weeks, some authorities recommend waiting at least 2 weeks before initiating an extensive (and expensive) laboratory work-up. Laboratory results are usually normal when testing is done.

Urticaria that lasts longer than 6 weeks is classified as *chronic idiopathic urticaria*. Studies of patients with chronic urticaria have found changes in the quality of life, including sleep deprivation, social isolation, and mood changes that are on the same level as in patients with ischemic heart disease.

Urticaria is classified into several categories. *Cholinergic urticaria* accounts for one-third (34%) of all cases of physical urticarias. Factors that trigger cholinergic urticaria include exercise, anxiety, elevated body temperature (e.g., fever, exercise, sweating), or hot baths or showers. The lesions usually resolve within 30 minutes after the offending activity is stopped. The hives are small (2–4 mm), are very pruritic, are surrounded with erythema, and appear on the upper trunk and arms. *Physical urticaria* accounts for 17% to 20% of all urticarias; it occurs immediately or shortly after exposure to physical stimuli such as pressure, cold, heat, exercise, sunlight (solar urticaria), water (aquagenic urticaria), vibration, or in response to increased body temperature. Urticarial episodes resulting from exposure to these stimuli are usually of short duration; most last only 2 hours. Dermatographism occurs in 2% to 5% of the normal population and can occur with other forms of urticaria. A dermatographic reaction can be elicited by applying friction with a dull object to the skin and watching for wheal formation. The wheal (hive) lasts for a few hours, then resolves.

Some pregnant women develop an extremely pruritic eruption known as pruritic urticarial papules and plaques of pregnancy (PUPPP). These lesions appear as erythematous urticarial papules and plaques (striae distensae) that usually start on the striae of the abdomen and spread to the thighs, buttocks, and, occasionally, arms. The lesions can start at any time during the third trimester, but they are frequently seen during the last 2 to 3 weeks of pregnancy. The cause is unknown—PUPPP is not associated with increased maternal or fetal morbidity and usually resolves after delivery of the fetus. Treatment during the last trimester of pregnancy involves the use of a moderate-potency topical steroid such as triamcinolone acetonide cream 0.1% (Aristocort, Kenalog) applied two to three times daily on the skin lesions. With topical treatment, improvement of the lesions should be seen in a few days. Topical steroids should not be applied to rashes that are suspected to be of viral etiology (such as herpes simplex or varicella-zoster) because steroids can worsen them. Severe cases are best referred to an obstetrician for possible treatment with systemic steroids. There are no antihistamines that are considered absolutely safe in pregnancy, and their use should be avoided.

Treatment

The treatment for urticaria is to find the cause and to stop exposure to the sensitizing allergen. Certain drugs, such as aspirin, angiotensin-converting enzyme inhibitors, and NSAIDs should be avoided in patients with urticaria. Tight clothing should be avoided, because wheals tend to occur in areas with increased pressure or friction. Showering or bathing with hot water should be avoided because this worsens itching. Cool environmental temperatures in the home are helpful and aid in inducing sleep.

Allergens that can cause both acute and chronic urticaria include drugs; foods; food preservatives; insect bites; and bacterial, fungal, viral, or parasitic infections. If the patient is taking vitamins, herbs, and supplements that are not necessary, they should all be stopped: Even natural vitamins and herbs are not exempt. The patient can start a trial of eliminating certain highly allergenic foods such as eggs, strawberries, tomatoes, chocolate, citrus fruits, peanuts and other nuts, all vinegars and wines (sulfites), alcoholic beverages, and shellfish, although this is cumbersome and bothersome for most patients. Chronic urticaria can be caused by food dyes or food additives, such as sulfites (found in dried fruit, wines, and vinegar). Food allergens can be occasionally confirmed by the radioallergosorbent test or by skin-prick tests done by allergists. Viral infections that have been implicated in causing urticaria include herpes, hepatitis, acute mononucleosis, and rubella. Bacterial infections such as sinusitis and fungal infections have also been implicated.

In chronic urticaria, the clinical evaluation should look for underlying disease, although the etiology in most cases of chronic urticaria is never found. A careful history (including history of travel abroad) and a thorough physical exam should search for signs of chronic disease such as chronic sinusitis, a tooth abscess, a low-grade fungal infection (candidiasis), intestinal parasites, chronic hepatitis, and so on. Some screening tests that are helpful (depending on the history) include stool sample for ova and parasites, sinus x-ray films or CT scan, ESR or a C-reactive protein, CBC, liver function test, a hepatitis profile, urinalysis, and urine sample for culture and sensitivity. In most cases of chronic urticaria (which is more common in adult women in their 30s to 50s), the cause is never uncovered. Up to half of the cases of chronic urticaria and angioedema may resolve spontaneously after a period of 5 years.

The main drugs used to treat urticaria are the H_1 antihistamines, which are available both OTC (diphenhydramine, loratadine) or by prescription (hydroxyzine, fexofenadine, desloratadine, cetirizine, and cyproheptadine). The timing of administration of the antihistamine is very important—it should be tailored individually so that the bloodstream levels of the drug will peak during the times when the urticarial lesions do occur, which will differ among individuals. All antihistamines, even the so-called nonsedating prescription antihistamines, have the potential for sedation. Susceptible patients, especially elderly patients, are at higher risk for sedation and somnolence. Patients should be educated regarding

drowsiness as a potential adverse effect of antihistamine use and should be warned against driving or operating heavy machinery until the effects of the medication on the patient are known. The combination of antihistamines with other central nervous system (CNS) depressants such as alcohol, tranquilizers, and certain antidepressants will increase the risk of sedation.

Different classes of H_1 antihistamines should be tried on patients with chronic urticaria: Some patients will respond better to one type of antihistamine than to another. A combination of H_1 and H_2 antihistamines is used by some clinicians, but studies have shown only a very small increase in effectiveness. Some antihistamines (such as diphenhydramine) tend to cause more sedation than others; diphenhydramine is the main ingredient in OTC sleep aids. For patients who can tolerate its sedating effects (or avoid a problem by taking it at bedtime), diphenhydramine can be taken at 25 to 50 mg every 4 hours (maximum 300 mg daily). The classic prescription antihistamine used for pruritus and urticaria is hydroxyzine. Hydroxyzine can be given as a bedtime dose of 50 mg to reduce risks associated with daytime sedation. Cetirizine is 13% less sedating than hydroxyzine and has a rapid onset of action. The dose of cetirizine is 10 mg once daily given at bedtime. Cetirizine has been found to be especially useful for delayed pressure urticaria. Cetirizine does not cause cardiac toxicity when it is combined with other drugs such as erythromycin, imidazole antifungals, or other hepatically metabolized drugs. Fexofenadine, a nonsedating antihistamine, is given as 60 mg every 12 hours. For treatment of cold urticaria, cyproheptadine (Periactin) is given as 4 mg three times daily. The use of cyproheptadine is contraindicated in angle-closure glaucoma, concurrent use of monoamine oxidase inhibitors, prostatic hypertrophy, and elderly or debilitated patients. Because of its atropine-like actions, caution should be taken in patients with asthma, increased intraocular pressure, heart disease, hypertension, or hyperthyroidism.

Types of urticaria that should be referred to a specialist include urticaria associated with angioedema of the tongue or throat, peanut allergy, latex allergy, and urticaria that persists beyond 6 weeks (chronic urticaria). The anti-IgE monoclonal antibody therapy omalizumab (Xolair) has been proposed for the treatment of chronic urticaria, although it has not been approved by the Food and Drug Administration for this indication.

Teledermatology is the practice of dermatology from a distance and can be used in several ways. Studies evaluating teledermatology have measured the diagnostic concordance rate (DCR) and diagnostic accuracy of remote diagnoses. The DCR refers to the interrater reliability between those assessing the skin pathology. Diagnostic accuracy refers to the correct diagnosis made by the provider and the actual pathology determined via biopsy. Nursing Research–Based Practice 7.1 summarizes a recent reference that describes this emerging trend.

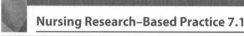

Nursing Research–Based Practice 7.1

Lowie, AM. Teledermatology: A tool for nurse practitioner practice? *J Nurse Pract* 8(8):617–620, 2012.
The emerging teledermatology technology has the potential to affect the current health-care delivery system and provide dermatology care to a greater number of patients in underserved areas. Although current research shows that the diagnostic concordance rates (DCRs) and accuracy rates are high, consultation results inherently depend on the skills and thoroughness of the provider and staff initiating the consultation, in conjunction with a thorough history and total body skin exam. Nurse practitioners have the potential to become active participants in the practice of teledermatology and ensure the provision of dermatology services to underserved populations.

COMMON PROBLEMS: PARASITIC INFESTATIONS

■ SCABIES

Human *scabies* is a highly contagious infestation that occurs mainly in children, young adults, health-care workers, and institutionalized persons of all ages. It is characterized by generalized intractable pruritus, often with minimal cutaneous manifestations. The diagnosis of scabies infection is easily missed and should be considered in patients of any age with persistent and severe pruritus. Scabies can develop into a chronic condition.

Epidemiology and Causes

Human scabies is caused by the itch mite *Sarcoptes scabiei* var. *hominis,* which infects human skin. The adult female measures 0.3 to 0.5 mm long and has a rounded body with four pairs of short legs. Scabies infestations occur worldwide and are endemic in most parts of the world. Epidemics are historically associated with war, conditions of poverty, overcrowding, poor hygiene, malnutrition, and sexual promiscuity. The World Health Organization estimates that there are about 300 million cases of scabies in the world each year. Some studies suggest 6% to 27% of the general population has scabies, but other surveys find a lower prevalence. Close personal contact is the major mode of transmission for scabies, although casual contact such as nursing care may be sufficient for transmission to occur. Institutional epidemics have been reported in which caregivers were infested. Live mites have been discovered in dust samples from the homes of infested persons, suggesting fomite transmission as a possibility.

Pathophysiology

The scabies itch mite is an aerobic organism and thus requires exposure to surface air to survive. The male mite dies shortly after mating, but the female mite may live 4 to 6 weeks. As an obligate parasite, the scabies mite burrows into the skin shortly after contact. It both resides and reproduces in human skin. The female mite can lay 2 to 3 eggs per day (up to 10–25 total) in burrows created at the base of the stratum corneum of the epidermis, traveling up to 2 mm per day. Burrows average 5 mm in length, allowing for continued exposure to surface air, but soon after egg-laying is completed, the female mite dies. Eggs hatch, and larvae emerge in 72 to 84 hours, molting at least three times before reaching adulthood. Mating of these new mites thus occurs after approximately 17 days.

Interestingly, sensitivity to *Sarcoptes scabiei* must take place for pruritus to occur. Initial sensitivity takes several weeks to develop after primary infection and is caused by a foreign body inflammatory reaction to either the mite itself or its feces. In persons who are experiencing reinfestation, pruritus may occur within 24 hours, because the immune system has been previously sensitized. Individuals who are immunocompromised or have been diagnosed with a neurological disorder such as Down syndrome, stroke, dementia, neuropathy, or spinal cord injury may be predisposed to a variant of scabies known as crusted scabies (*scabies crustosa;* previously known as "Norwegian scabies"). Scabies crustosa is characterized by scaly lesions at the sites of invasion that soon become warty and encrusted, creating a protective barrier for these mites. The number of mites infesting a patient with scabies crustosa can exceed more than a million, whereas infestation with classic scabies is usually limited to 10 mites or fewer. Half of patients with crusted scabies do not experience pruritus, reflecting the absence of key inflammatory mediators seen in classic scabies. A nodular form of scabies also exists in which firm, erythematous, dome-shaped lesions roughly 0.5 cm in size develop over the groin, buttock, and axillary areas. Histamine-mediated urticarial lesions may accompany this rash, which is intensely pruritic. In all forms of scabies, if rashes go untreated, bacterial superinfection by *Staphylococcus* species may result, worsening acute inflammation.

Clinical Presentation
Subjective

The typical patient usually presents with complaints of intense itching that is usually described as being more severe at night. Mothers may report changes in feeding patterns of children and that they are more tired and irritable than usual. Itching may be widespread but is commonly located in the interdigital web spaces, wrists, anterior axillary folds, periumbilical skin, pelvic girdle, penis, and ankles. The palms, soles, face, neck, and scalp are more frequently involved in small children. The pruritus is usually described as not responding to treatment. Many patients will complain of a rash, whereas others experience itching for months with no apparent rash. Patients are often aware of similar symptoms in family members and/or in sexual contacts. Patients presenting with the symptoms described above should be screened for possible scabies infestation. (See Focus on History 7.3.)

Objective

The earliest physical signs of scabies are small, 1- to 2-mm, red papules located in areas of the body that are most attractive to mites. Because of the intense itching, excoriations from repeated scratching, with crusting and scaling, may also be present. It may be difficult to visualize scabies mites on the skin, and the patient may complain only of incessant itchiness. Skin lesions occur at the sites of mite infestation or result from a hypersensitivity reaction to the scabies mite. Secondary skin lesions including lichenification and excoriations are the result of chronic rubbing or scratching of lesions. Secondary bacterial infections present with increased symptoms, pruritus, and crusting of lesions (secondary impetigo).

The classic scabies skin lesion is the intraepidermal burrow. Each female mite produces one burrow. In light-skinned people, burrows have a whitish color with black specks caused by fecal particles. The female mite resides at the blind end of the tunnel. She can burrow 2 to 3 mm per day. Burrows are usually distributed in areas where there are few or no hair follicles and where the stratum corneum is thin and soft.

Burrows are sometimes seen on the top of early scabetic nodules that occur in 7% to 10% of patients with scabies. Nodules vary in color from pink to brown and are 5 to 20 cm in diameter. They may become more visible after treatment.

Focus on History 7.3   Scabies

If Scabies Is Suspected

- Do you work in a nursing home or group home, in a school, or in a prison?
- Do you have any family members or sexual partners that have similar symptoms?
- Are young children displaying increased signs of fatigue or irritability?
- Have the eating patterns of children changed?

If Patient Is Complaining of Pruritus

- Where is the itching worse?
- What part of your body is itching?
- Is the itching worse at night?
- Does itching interfere with your ability to sleep?
- How long have you been itching?
- Is the itching relieved by anything? If so, what?

Diagnostic Reasoning

Clinical diagnosis of scabies is almost never made until hypersensitivity has occurred. The diagnosis is based on epidemiological history, occurrence of intractable itching, and assessment of the distribution of lesions and pruritus.

Diagnostic Tests

The practitioner should search for the presence of mites. The highest yield of mites is in burrows located on the finger webs, penis, or wrists. The Burrow Ink Test can be easily performed. To do so, rub a felt-tip pen over the suspected burrow. (Blue and green markers work best because they do not interfere with microscopic results.) Remove the excess ink with an alcohol wipe. The remaining ink concentrates in the tunnel and indicates the location of the burrow.

Once a burrow has been located, the clinician should place a drop of mineral oil over it, then scrape off the burrow using a number 15 scalpel blade. The scrapings should be placed on a slide with a drop of oil, then sealed with a cover slip. The identification of the *S scabiei* mite, its eggs, or fecal pellets is diagnostic of scabies. There are no serological tests currently available for scabies.

Failure to identify mites or their eggs or burrows does not rule out scabies infestation. If scabies infestation is suspected because of clinical symptoms, empiric treatment should be tried. Resolution of symptoms within a few days is indicative of previous scabies infection.

Differential Diagnosis

The diagnosis of scabies can be easily missed. Although there are common skin findings (e.g., burrows), the clinical picture of scabies can be extremely variable, depending on the duration of the infection and the severity of the sensitivity reaction. Variants of scabies in immunocompromised persons and persons with neurological disorders further cloud the diagnosis. Accurate diagnosis is essential for effective treatment. See Differential Diagnosis 7.2 for some differential diagnoses for scabies. It should be noted that it is possible for patients to have preexisting skin problems in addition to scabies. A thorough history can help minimize diagnostic pitfalls.

Management

With proper adherence to treatment regimens, cure rates for scabies approach 100%. However, application of medicated creams or lotions is insufficient for an affected person if the entire household is not treated and if all environmental reservoirs of the scabies mite (such as bedding, clothing, or towels) are not sufficiently cleaned with hot water and detergents. Therefore, effective care of patients with scabies involves treating the patient, his or her close personal contacts, and environment. Treating the source of the infestation and any secondary complications such as bacterial infection (secondary impetigo) or dermatitis should also be included in the management plan.

Initial management of the patient diagnosed with scabies is directed at killing all live mites. Lotions containing scabicides (such as permethrin, lindane, crotamiton, or sulfur) are commonly used. Permethrin is the first-line treatment. Antihistamines and topical steroids are helpful for pruritus. Of the products containing scabicides, lindane is the most toxic. It is rapidly absorbed through the skin and has been associated with CNS symptoms such as irritability, seizures, and, in cases of ingestion or overdose, death. Older patients, young children, and pregnant and lactating women have the greatest risk of toxicity. Therefore, the choice of scabicide should be based on the age of the patient, pregnancy status, resistance patterns, degree of toxicity, and severity of infestation. High mite populations, presence of crusts, and decreased immune status of the host make treating crusted scabies more difficult. It may be necessary to remove crusts that would protect mites from scabicides before treating.

The majority of patients require only medical treatment with a topical scabicide. A number of patients experience hypersensitivity to the mite and mite products, however, and may require the use of systemic corticosteroids to provide relief from severe pruritus. When ivermectin 200 mcg/kg is used as a single dose, it is followed by another dose 1 to 2 weeks later. This should be used in conjunction with a topical cream/lotion. Some patients may delay treatment until a secondary bacterial infection has occurred, necessitating the additional use of an antistaphylococcal antibiotic. Cephalexin or dicloxacillin for 7 to 10 days may be prescribed.

In addition, patients with extensive dermatitis lesions may obtain relief with topical corticosteroids, such as triamcinolone 0.1% cream twice daily for 7 days. Fluorinated steroids must not be used on the face or on skinfolds (intertriginous areas) because of the increased risk of skin atrophy. (See Drugs Commonly Prescribed 7.1.) Management must include a strict isolation protocol for scabies crustosa.

Follow-up and Referral

Uncomplicated scabies infestations should be followed up 1 week after the initial treatment. If generalized itching persists, hypersensitivity to remaining dead mites

---

Drugs Commonly Prescribed 7.1 Scabies

Drug	Indication	Adverse Reactions and Prescribing Considerations
Topical		
permethrin cream 5% (Elimite)	Presence of live mites (scabicide)	Mite resistance has been reported. Safe for use in children 2 months and older. May also need to treat head and neck. Apply to all areas of body from the neck down. Leave on for 8–12 hours. Repeat application in 1 week. May repeat a third time 1 week later.
lindane 19% (gamma-benzone hexachloride)	Presence of live mites (scabicide)	Potential CNS toxicity. Rapidly absorbed through skin. Do not use on infants or young children, pregnant or lactating women, or if history of seizures. Should not be used after a bath or shower or by persons with extensive dermatitis. Mite resistance has been reported. May also need to treat head and neck. *Adults:* Apply thinly to all areas of body from neck down. Wash off thoroughly after 8 hours.
crotamiton cream 10% (Eurax)	Presence of live mites (scabicide)	Reported failure rates up to 50%. Long- and short-term toxicity has not been studied. Shake well before using. Apply to all areas of body from the chin down for 2 consecutive nights. Change clothing and bed linen after 24 hours. Wash 48 hours after second application.
sulfur ointment 8%–10%	Presence of live mites (scabicide)	Extensive use suggests it is safe to use on pregnant and lactating women and young children. Malodorous and stains clothing. *Adults:* Apply to all parts of the body from neck down 3 successive days. *Children:* May need to treat head and neck also.

Drugs Commonly Prescribed 7.1 Scabies—cont'd		
Drug	**Indication**	**Adverse Reactions and Prescribing Considerations**
Systemic		
ivermectin (Stromectol)	Presence of live mites (scabicide)	Reported to be effective for common scabies refractory to topical treatment and crusted scabies in conjunction with topical cream/lotion. "Off-label" use 200 mcg/kg by mouth single dose followed by another dose in 1–2 weeks.
Others		
antihistamines	Eczematous dermatitis	Helps patient to sleep at night. Hydroxyzine, diphenhydramine: 25–50 mg at bedtime
topical corticosteroid ointment	Extensive dermatitis	For mild to moderate pruritus. Apply to areas of extensive dermatitis.
systemic corticosteroid	Severe hyper-sensitivity reaction	For severe pruritus. Prednisone: Tapered course 1–2 weeks
systemic and topical antibiotics	Secondary bacterial infection	Staph and strep are common pathogens. Risk of acute poststreptococcal glomerulonephritis in severe cases. Systemic: 7- to 10-day course

and mite products should be considered. It may be necessary to repeat the scabicide treatment, however. Patients who experience persistent scabetic nodules or crusted scabies may require advanced management and should be referred to a dermatologist.

Patient Education

Patient education is an integral part of successfully treating scabies. Patients should be instructed to trim their fingernails, to reduce the possibility of harboring mites and reinfesting themselves and others. Safety information regarding the use of scabicides should be stressed, such as not exceeding recommended exposure times, toxicity symptoms that should be reported, and the safe storage of treatment products, to prevent accidental ingestion in children. Patients should be informed that itching may continue for up to a week after successful treatment due to local irritation.

Patients should also receive instruction about treating their home environment to avoid reinfestation; they should be reminded that the scabies mite lives on humans, so environmental spraying of pesticides is not effective and therefore not recommended. Bedclothes and clothing should be washed in hot soapy water. Except in cases of crusted scabies, extensive decontamination of the environment is not necessary. Children in day care or school can return after treatment.

■ PEDICULOSIS

Pediculosis (infestation by lice) in humans has been documented for thousands of years. It is difficult to document the number of lice cases occurring annually in the United States because most states are not required to report it. It is estimated that 6 to 12 million American children are infested with head lice alone each year.

Epidemiology and Causes

Pediculosis infestations occur worldwide and are endemic in most parts of the world. Only three species of lice are known to infest humans: *Pthirus pubis* (the crab louse), *Pediculus humanus capitis* (the head louse), and *Pediculus humanus corporis* (the body or clothing louse). Lice infestations occur in people of all ages. Head lice are commonly seen in school-age children, whereas pubic lice are most often seen in sexually active young adults. Children aged 3 to 11 years are most commonly affected by head lice, with occurrence being more frequent in girls. Lice are blood-obligate parasites that obtain all their nutritional requirements from the host. Both the *Pediculus capitis* and *Pthirus pubis* lice reside and reproduce on the human host. The *Pediculus humanus corporis* louse feeds on the human host but resides and lays its eggs in clothing fibers. Body lice are increasingly rare in the United States but can be seen in communities of persons who are homeless or among persons who live in crowded conditions without the ability to wash and change clothing. Body lice are the only lice associated with disease transmission. Infected feces of the body louse can transmit typhus, trench fever, and relapsing fever. However, lice-borne outbreaks of these diseases have not been seen for many decades in the United States.

Though epidemics of pediculosis in the United States are relatively rare, outbreaks of head lice are common in elementary school settings. Outbreaks usually occur at the start of the school year and after winter and spring breaks. One explanation for the timing of these outbreaks is that they occur after children have spent extended time in the community. Close personal contact is the major mode of transmission for all types of pediculosis.

Treatments, lost wages, and school expenses total an estimated $1 billion annually, making pediculosis a major public health concern and an economic burden on families.

Pathophysiology

Pediculosis infestation can be asymptomatic or can cause few symptoms in the first 2 weeks following exposure. Sensitivity to lice must take place before pruritus can occur. Therefore, in individuals who have never been exposed to lice infestation before, it can take several weeks before clinical symptoms (e.g., pruritus) develop during the initial infestation. A foreign body inflammatory reaction ensues from the lice saliva that is injected into the skin during the insect's bite. In individuals who are experiencing reinfestation, pruritus occurs rapidly, within 24 to 48 hours, due to key inflammatory mediators including histamine.

Head lice infestation averages about 10 lice per patient. However, in severe cases they can number in the hundreds. Head lice are transmitted through close contact rather than by fomites and can survive just over 2 days off a human host, at which time they die from dehydration. Both males and females are equipped with specialized mouth parts adapted for sucking blood, as well as legs capable of adhering to human hairs. Each female head louse may lay from 7 to 10 eggs per day for a month. Pubic lice ("crab lice") lay relatively fewer eggs (up to three per day) that incubate for 1 week before hatching. Severe lice infestations may be complicated by bacterial superinfection from *Staphylococcus* species that normally colonize the skin.

Clinical Presentation

Subjective

Patients may present with complaints of intense itching in areas of the body preferred by the particular type of infesting louse. The itching is usually described as being more severe at night. Mothers may report changes in feeding patterns and that children are tired and irritable. School-age children may become inattentive and restless in class, with frequent scratching of the scalp. Some cases of pediculosis are asymptomatic or present with few symptoms.

Objective

The earliest physical signs of lice infestation are small (2–3 mm), red erythematous macules or papules that may be pruritic. Skin lesions may appear within minutes or several days after initial infestation. Some patients develop an allergic, hive-like reaction, with typical wheal and flare formation after lice infestation.

Pruritus is the hallmark of all types of pediculosis. Because of the intense itching, excoriations on the scalp, body, or pubic area (depending on the type of lice) with crusting and scaling may also be present. Fresh nits (lice eggs) on hair shafts are thought to be deposited closer to the scalp. As the hair grows (0.5 mm daily on the scalp), the nit moves further away from the scalp. Therefore, if nits are found at varying distances on the hair shafts, the infestation has been present for several weeks to months. Individual lice are difficult to see on the scalp and hair strands. They appear as six-legged, wingless insects from 1 to 4 mm in length that move extremely fast. When engorged with blood, the insect's abdomen appears dark red.

Nits (eggs) are much easier to see than live lice: The teardrop-shaped eggs are attached securely to the hair shaft by the female louse. Newly laid eggs may be tan to coffee-colored and are difficult to see. Hatched lice eggs are whitish in color and appear shiny. The cap (operculum) of the egg faces away from the scalp. Distribution of lice, itching, and lesions provides clues to the type of louse present on the host. Head lice *(P h capitis)* prefer the scalp, and crab lice *(P pubis)* infest the pubic and perianal region. However, head lice can be found in facial hairs such as eyebrows, beards, and mustaches. Crab lice and their nits can also be found in such areas as the eyelids, mustache area, axillae, or on the scalp.

Diagnostic Reasoning

Clinical diagnosis of pediculosis, body lice, or pubic lice is based on both the history of pruritus (because of a hypersensitivity reaction to the lice) and the finding of white nits or lice on the hair shaft. Sometimes, lice infestation may be picked up during a routine physical exam.

Diagnostic Tests

The practitioner should search for lice and/or nits on the area of the body where the patient is complaining of pruritus. Lice and their nits can be seen with the naked eye or with a magnifying hand lens. Gloves should be worn during this procedure. Microscopic examination is generally not required. A Wood's light exam can be done for mass screening (or individual screening), but it requires a darkened room and protective eyewear for both the clinician and the child. When the light is directed at the scalp, live nits appear with a pearl-like fluorescence, whereas empty nits do not fluoresce. The Wood's light exam is impractical in school settings and not recommended for use with young children who might be afraid of the dark. If secondary bacterial infection (impetigo) is suspected, bacterial cultures should be done with a standard culturette.

Failure to identify the presence of lice or nits does not rule out lice infestation. When suspicion is strong, based on the history and clinical presentation, the patient should be treated empirically; the relief of signs and symptoms is indicative of lice infestation. Treatment for head lice should be limited to persons who are experiencing an active infestation, which is defined as the presence of live lice. Because pubic lice are considered a sexually transmitted disease (STD), patients with this type of infestation should be screened for other STDs by rapid plasma reagin (RPR) and Venereal Disease Research Laboratory (VDRL) tests for syphilis, as well as laboratory tests for HIV infection.

Differential Diagnosis

The diagnosis of pediculosis is easily made. However, "pseudonits" (hair casts, dandruff, or sebaceous plugs) can be mistaken for nits, resulting in inappropriate treatment. A hallmark of nits is that they are firmly cemented in place and therefore do not slide easily on the hair shaft, compared with dandruff scales. Sebaceous plugs result from plugged oil glands on the scalp and (unlike nits) do not originate on the hair shaft. Secondary bacterial infection can also complicate the diagnosis. Secondarily infected skin lesions resemble impetigo lesions, with crusting and erythema. Differential Diagnosis 7.2 lists some differential diagnoses for pediculosis.

Management

Effective care of patients with pediculosis involves treating not only the patient, but also his or her close personal contacts who have been diagnosed with an active infestation. Treatment involves both medication and environmental control measures. It is important to screen all close contacts for head lice, keeping in mind that the contacts may be asymptomatic and have a small number of live lice. Treating the source of the infestation (if identified) and any secondary complications such as secondary bacterial infection (impetigo) or dermatitis should also be included in the management plan. Patients need to be reevaluated after 1 week. If live lice are present or if fresh eggs (nits) are seen close to the scalp, retreatment is necessary.

Initial management of patients who are diagnosed with pediculosis is directed at killing and/or removing lice and their nits. Shampoos and cream rinses containing permethrin, lindane, pyrethrin, and malathion are commonly used to kill lice. (See Drugs Commonly Prescribed 7.2.) Treatment history should be explored with the patient or caregiver. It is common for persons with head lice to delay seeking professional help until three to five treatment failures have occurred. Products resulting in treatment failure should not be tried again.

Of these products, lindane is the most toxic. As noted previously in the section on scabies, lindane is rapidly absorbed through the skin and has been associated with CNS symptoms such as irritability, seizures, and—in cases of ingestion or overdose—death. Lindane should not be used on older patients, any patient with a history of seizure, infants and children younger than 2 years old, or pregnant or lactating women because of an increased risk for toxicity. The pediculicide of choice should be based on the age of the patient, resistance patterns, degree of toxicity, treatment history, and, in reproductive-aged females, pregnancy status.

Manual delousing and nit removal using a fine-toothed comb is gaining popularity in the face of increasing reports of resistance to available pediculicides. In children with respiratory allergies, asthma, or compromised immune status, manual delousing methods should be considered as an initial form of treatment.

Numerous nonpesticidal treatment options have recently become available. There is limited empiric evidence, however, to support their efficacy and safety. Practitioners should caution patients against the use of home remedies that include kerosene and agricultural-grade or veterinary pesticides—such remedies are unsafe and potentially fatal.

The majority of patients with pediculosis require only pediculicide treatment or manual delousing. Some patients may delay treatment until secondary bacterial infection has occurred, necessitating the use of a topical or systemic antibiotic. Complicating staphylococcal bacterial superinfection may be treated by cephalexin or dicloxacillin for 7 to 10 days.

Children who present with pediculosis pubis (infestation by *Phthirus pubis*) in their eyelashes or hair should alert the practitioner to the possibility of sexual abuse, although intimate contact is not the only mode of transmission. Eyelash infestation can be treated by applying petroleum jelly to the eyelid margins twice daily for 10 days. Pediculosis ciliaris (eyelash infestation) may also be treated with physostigmine ophthalmic ointment 0.25% to 1% twice daily for 8 to 10 days, but this treatment may cause eye spasms in younger adults. Lice and nits should also be manually removed from the eyelashes by gently holding and sliding them off the hairs.

Follow-up and Referral

Uncomplicated pediculosis infestations do not require a follow-up. In some areas, however, the American head louse has demonstrated resistance to pyrethrin and permethrin, as well as to lindane, resulting in increased treatment failures. Follow-up in 1 week is recommended if symptoms persist; the patient or the parent can call the office to report any further symptoms. The National Pediculosis Association recommends manual delousing methods at the first sign of medical treatment failure. Because of toxicity concerns and known resistance patterns, lindane should be used only as a last resort, and prescriptions should not be

Drugs Commonly Prescribed 7.2   Pediculosis

Drug	Indication	Adverse Reactions and Prescribing Considerations
Topical		
permethrin 1% lotion OTC (Nix)	Presence of lice/nits; may use for children older than 2 months.	May need to reapply in 7–14 days. Use nit-remover products before application of permethrin. Apply to towel-dried, affected area; leave on 10 minutes, wash off.
pyrethrin 0.3% with piperonyl butoxide shampoo or gel OTC (RID, R&C shampoo)	Presence of lice/nits	May need to reapply in 7–14 days. Use shampoo for head or pubic lice, gel for body lice. Contraindicated in persons sensitive to ragweed. Apply to dry hair until wet; leave on 10 minutes, wash off.
lindane 1% shampoo	Presence of lice/nits	Possible CNS toxicity. Not recommended for children under 12 years of age or pregnant or lactating women. Apply to dry hair; leave on 4 minutes, wash off thoroughly.
malathion 0.5% (Ovide), lotion or gel	Presence of live head lice; not approved for other lice species. Lotion for use on children older than 6 years; gel safe to use on children older than 2 years	No reported resistance. Product contains 78% isopropyl alcohol and is flammable. Apply to dry hair. Use sufficient amount to thoroughly wet hair and scalp. Allow to air dry. Shampoo hair after 8–12 hours. Cover all lice on the hair and scalp. Rinse off after 10 minutes, repeat in 1 week.
benzyl alcohol 5% (Ulesfia) lotion	Use in patients older than 6 months and pregnant women	Leave on hair and scalp for 10 minutes. May repeat in 7 days if live lice are still present.
Systemic		
ivermectin (Stromectol)	Resistant pediculosis (Not FDA Approved)	For cases resistant to permethrin and malathion. 200–400 mcg/kg by mouth as a single dose followed by another dose in 1–2 weeks.

written with refills. Referrals for pediculosis infestations are usually not required.

Patient Education

Patient education is an integral part of successfully treating pediculosis. Patients and parents should be instructed not to share hats, combs, scarves, headsets, towels, and bedding. Following removal of hair and debris, combs and brushes should be washed in hot, soapy water, rinsed in hot water, and allowed to air dry.

Safety information regarding the proper use of pediculicides should be stressed, including information on not exceeding recommended exposure times, possible toxicity symptoms that should be reported, and the safe storage of treatment products in order to prevent accidental ingestion by young children. When using head lice products, patients should be instructed to cover the

eyes and rinse products out over a sink (not in the shower or bathtub) to reduce unnecessary pesticide exposure. Patients should be informed that itching may continue after successful treatment for up to a week because of the slow resolution of the inflammatory reaction caused by the lice infestation.

Patients should also receive instruction on cleaning the environment. With the exception of the body louse, lice live only on humans. Excessive decontamination of the environment is not necessary. Environmental spraying of pesticides is not effective and may be dangerous and therefore is not recommended. Bedclothes and clothing should be washed in hot soapy water and dried in a hot dryer. Normal vacuuming of carpets, rugs, upholstery, mattresses, cars, and car seats should be sufficient. Parents should devote their energy to removing lice and nits. Children in day care or school can return after treatment. Some schools have initiated a "no-nit" policy that requires parents to remove all lice and nits before a child may reenter the classroom. Parents should be instructed to screen children once a week for head lice as part of their regular hygiene routine. Early detection results in fewer transmissions and easier treatment regimens.

FUNGAL INFECTIONS

■ CANDIDIASIS

Candida, an opportunistic pathogen, causes not only superficial mucocutaneous infections but also serious disease that can be fatal, especially to the immunocompromised host. *Candida* belongs to the yeast family of fungi. There are over 20 species of *Candida* yeasts that can cause infection on humans, the most common of which is *Candida albicans. Candida* is part of the normal flora of both the oropharynx and gastrointestinal tract. In addition, up to 20% of women who are asymptomatic yield a positive culture for vaginal *Candida.* Favorable environmental factors and a weakened immune system are the two most important factors contributing to candidal infections. Certain areas of the body are also more prone to infection. Areas where there is increased heat and moisture are more likely to become infected with candidal organisms. Other synonyms for candidiasis include moniliasis and candidosis.

Risk factors for serious disease include conditions that alter cellular immunity, such as AIDS, diabetes mellitus, corticosteroid treatment, bone marrow transplant, chemotherapy, and invasive parenteral catheterization (parenteral feeding catheters are considered high risk). Broad-spectrum antibiotic therapy, including antibiotics following major surgery in normal hosts, can increase the risk of candidal infection. Only superficial cutaneous infections are discussed in this chapter.

Cutaneous infections caused by *Candida* include the following:

- Thrush, diaper dermatitis (infants)
- Oral infections: candidiasis (thrush), angular cheilitis
- Genital infections: vulvovaginitis, balanitis
- Intertriginous (skinfold) infections: inframammary area, groin, axillae, web spaces of the fingers or toes, perianal area
- Other infections: folliculitis, candidal paronychia, subungual candidiasis (beneath the nail)

Epidemiology and Causes

Although *C albicans* is the most common (60%–90%) of all yeast isolates found on the oropharynx and the genitalia, other types of *Candida* coexist in the body, including *C tropicalis, C glabrata, C krusei, C rugosa,* and other yeast strains. Unfortunately, some candidal species

(C krusei, C glabrata) are less responsive to imidazoles and have developed resistance. *Candida* infection can occur at any age and in either gender. A higher incidence of thrush is seen among patients with AIDS and in infants. No ethnic predisposition to *Candida* has been noted. Areas in the body where there is skin-to-skin contact are more prone to candidal infection. These include areas under the breast (inframammary candidiasis), between the fingers (interdigital candidiasis), between the toes, the groin, the axillae, and the genital area. Infections in these areas are collectively called *intertrigo* or intertriginous infections.

Cellular immunodeficiency states increase the risk of mucocutaneous disease. Conditions such as AIDS, diabetes mellitus, corticosteroid therapy, and immunosuppressive therapy increase an individual's susceptibility to infection to *C albicans.* Infants, who have immature immune systems, can easily become infected with *Candida* through the birth canal or through oral contact with an infected caregiver. In infants (as opposed to adults), oral candidiasis (thrush) and diaper candidiasis are considered benign findings. In adults, however, mucocutaneous candidiasis is the most common AIDS-defining condition seen. In women with AIDS, one of the earliest and most frequent opportunistic infections seen is vaginal candidiasis. Frequent episodes of vaginal candidiasis that are not accompanied by an underlying condition (e.g., diabetes, use of antibiotics, pregnancy, or oral contraceptive use) should prompt the clinician to consider HIV infection in the differential diagnosis, although most cases of candidal vaginal infections occur in normal hosts.

Vaginal infection with *C albicans* is very common; it occurs in up to 75% of women at some point in their lifetime (pregnant women and patients with diabetes are at increased risk). If left untreated, candidal vaginitis will either resolve spontaneously or will become a chronic low-grade infection. Men with diabetes, especially if uncircumcised, are at higher risk for candidal infections of the glans penis (balanitis). The uncircumcised foreskin holds heat and moisture and increases the risk of candidal overgrowth. Males become infected with *Candida* organisms from their female partners through sexual intercourse or through oral sex. In candidal paronychia, the patient will report a history of a hangnail or of minor trauma on the cuticle area before the infection. Dishwashing or frequent water exposure is sometimes the culprit.

Pathophysiology

Candida organisms cause an intense inflammatory response on the skin, which accounts for the intense erythema and pruritus commonly seen with this infection. Once *Candida* has taken hold in the skin, microscopic lesions reveal a pseudomembrane composed of masses of yeast organisms that invade the superficial layer of the epithelium. Satellite lesions are small colonies of *Candida* that have spread beyond the main lesion, which eventually enlarge and become confluent, resulting in large erythematous patches. Normal commensal flora and intact cellular immunity mediated primarily by cytotoxic T cells are the body's primary defenses against fungal overgrowth and invasive candidal infection. The use of systemic antibiotics has the potential for clearing normal microbial skin flora, and both oral and inhaled steroids, HIV infection and AIDS, malignancy, chemotherapy and other immunosuppressive drugs, diabetes mellitus, and senescence all contribute to decreased helper and cytotoxic T-cell function, increasing the likelihood of candidal skin infection.

Clinical Presentation
Subjective
Oral Candidiasis (Thrush) The patient will complain of a severe sore throat. Pain or difficulty is noted during swallowing (dysphagia), especially with acidic foods such as citrus. (See Chapter 8 for more information.)

Vaginal Candidiasis The patient, ranging in age from adolescence to middle age, typically complains of burning, itching, and irritation, either on the vulva or in both the vulva and vagina (vulvovaginitis). Sometimes, burning is noted during intercourse (dyspareunia) and during urination (dysuria). The vaginal discharge is reported as white in color, with a "cottage-cheese" or thick texture. (See Chapter 14 for more information.)

Balanitis The typical patient is a sexually active adult man who complains of a reddish rash and itching on the glans penis. It is sometimes accompanied by penile burning after intercourse. No burning is associated with urination (dysuria). Some patients will report having a female partner who is being treated for a yeast infection or who has irritative vaginal symptoms. (See Chapter 13 for more information.)

Intertriginous Candidiasis The typical patient is an obese adult who complains of a red, itchy rash that is occasionally "weepy" and moist. It is sometimes accompanied by burning. The location of the rash is the inframammary area, the groin, the perianal area, or the interdigital spaces of both the hands and feet.

Candidal Paronychia The typical patient is an adult who complains of an extremely painful fingertip that is red, hot, and swollen. A history of frequent water immersion of the hands is common.

Subungual Candida No pain or itching is associated with this infection. The typical patient is an adult who reports one or several discolored yellow fingernails for several weeks to months. Some of the nails are deformed or separate from the nailbed. A history of excessive contact with water from dishwashing, bartending, or other occupations is frequently present.

Objective
A cardinal sign of cutaneous candidal infections is a bright red rash with macules or satellite lesions seen on the borders. A cardinal symptom is pruritus and sometimes burning.

Oral Candidiasis (Thrush) The anterior and posterior pharynx (including the tongue) is frequently involved. White creamy patches are seen and can be easily scraped off with a tongue blade, leaving behind erythematous patches. The affected areas are tender to palpation and may bleed with minor trauma. In adults, the buccal mucosa, tongue, and lips may also be involved and may extend to the angles of the mouth (perlèche).

Vaginal Candidiasis The vulvar area and, in some patients, the surrounding area appear erythematous and irritated. During speculum exam, the vaginal tissue appears erythematous, with white, curd-like patches pasted on the vaginal walls. The posterior fornix of the vagina may be full of thick white discharge.

Balanitis The glans penis has small, erythematous eroded patches that are tender to touch. A different presentation is small, white round lesions on a red base on the glans.

Intertriginous Candidiasis Any area of skin on the body where there is maceration (or skin rubbing against skin) or increased heat and moisture can become easily colonized by *Candida*. These areas include the inframammary area, the axilla, the groin, the perianal area, and the interdigital areas between the fingers and toes. In some extremely obese patients, macerated skin may occur in other areas as well. The lesions appear as bright red patches with satellite lesions. The skin will appear eroded and moist and is tender to touch.

Candidal Paronychia The area around the nail (the paronychium) is bright red, swollen, and extremely tender. A purulent pocket of discharge is sometimes present; when fluctuant, this abscess will rupture and drain purulent pus.

Subungual Candida The nail is discolored and a yellow color. It can be partially or totally separated from the nailbed. No pain is associated with this condition, in contrast to candidal paronychia.

Diagnostic Reasoning
Diagnostic Tests
Skin infections caused by *Candida* yeast are generally diagnosed by their classic appearance. *Candida* yeasts are normally present in the mouth, vagina, sputum, or the stool. Candidal cultures can be obtained from skin or mucous membranes with a culturette. Because *Candida* is part of the normal flora, a positive culture from the mouth or vagina is of limited value unless confirming signs and symptoms accompany it. For vaginal candidal infections, a saline wet mount, pH paper, and KOH test are helpful in the diagnosis. (See Advanced Assessment 7.1.) The whiff test will be negative, and the vaginal pH is acidic at 4.5 or less.

Of note, although systemic *Candida* infection is not covered in this chapter, there is a rapid diagnostic test for *Candida* infections of the bloodstream that may cut patient

Advanced Assessment 7.1 Intravaginal Infections

When assessing for candidiasis, a saline wet mount (vaginal discharge) or potassium hydroxide (KOH) exam may be performed. The KOH slide exam is necessary to see candida and tinea fungus; KOH is not necessary to see yeast forms in vaginal infections. The saline wet mount works well and is faster to prepare.

The KOH examination is employed to determine the presence of mycelial fragments or budding yeast cells in a skin lesion. The test involves adding KOH solution on a glass slide, covering the slide, and applying gentle heat. The slide is examined microscopically for the fungal elements.

Performing a Saline Wet Mount Exam

1. Take a small amount of vaginal discharge from the posterior fornix of the vagina with either a long, cotton-tipped applicator or from the end of the speculum.
2. Place a small amount of the vaginal discharge in the middle of a clean, dry glass slide.
3. Add 1–2 drops of normal saline solution to the vaginal discharge and stir/mix to produce a thin, milky mixture.
4. Add a cover slip.
5. View the specimen first under low power, then at 40× magnification. Look for pseudohyphae, spores, and leukocytes.

Performing a Potassium Hydroxide (KOH) Microscopic Exam

1. Scrape an area of the rash with the edge of a clean glass slide or a no. 15 sterile scalpel blade moistened with tap water to contain scales. Transfer the scraped tissue onto a slide and add a small droplet of plain water.
2. Add 1 or 2 drops of KOH 10% solution onto the specimen slide, put on a cover slide, and warm the slide carefully for 15–30 seconds using a match, small candle, or Bunsen burner.
3. Examine the specimen under low power with minimal illumination.
4. Look for pseudohyphae and/or spores. Identify hyphae—thin tubular structures, often branching strands of uniform diameter.
5. Switch to high dry (40×–43×) magnification to confirm findings.

NOTE: Although a positive exam establishes the diagnosis, a negative test does not rule out the disease.

Microscopy Tips: Saline Wet Mount and KOH Exams

- Do not confuse a piece of hair or thread on the slide with pseudohyphae. Hairs or threads will appear as black opaque lines, whereas hyphae are translucent and colorless.
- Pseudohyphae or hyphae (the stems) have thin translucent walls that have septa dividing each segment (like a bamboo stem).
- Spores are small and oval to round in shape, seen either alone or in clusters.
- Leukocytes are round to oval and are the size of nuclei in epithelial cells.
- A large number of leukocytes are seen in candidal and trichomonal infections because of inflammation.
- Few leukocytes are seen in bacterial vaginosis (does not cause inflammation) unless there is concurrent infection with *Candida* or *Trichomonas*.
- Epithelial cells are the largest cells found on the slide. Superficial epithelial cells are the most numerous (about 90%) and appear like rounded squares.
- The presence of immature epithelial cells (from the basal and parabasal layer) indicates severe inflammation. The immature cells are smaller and have larger nuclei than superficial (mature) epithelial cells.
- Bacteria are too small to be seen on a regular microscope. They will appear as extremely small dark "specks" on the slide, under both low and high power.

mortality from 40% to 11% by diagnosing candidemia 25 times faster than a blood culture and quickly identifying the *Candida* species that is causing the infection. The test, T2 Candida, uses a polymerase chain reaction (PCR) assay to amplify *Candida* DNA in the blood.

Differential Diagnosis

The location of the skin lesions determines the differential diagnoses to be considered. Contact dermatitis lesions can appear similar to candidal lesions. Fungal infections caused by dermatophytes in other sites include nails (tinea unguium causing onychomycosis), groin (tinea cruris), scalp (tinea capitis), foot (tinea pedis), and body (tinea corporis, causing "ringworm"). For a review of the differential diagnosis of cutaneous candidiasis, see Differential Diagnosis 7.3.

Management

Most cases of mucocutaneous and vaginal candidal infections (and tinea infections) respond well to topical

Differential Diagnosis 7.3 Cutaneous Candidiasis

Type of Candidiasis	Differential Diagnosis
Thrush (oral candidiasis)	Milk curd (infants)
	Pharyngeal exudate (bacteria/viral)
Intertrigo (skinfolds)	Contact dermatitis
	Bacterial intertrigo (erythrasma)
Vaginal candidiasis	Trichomoniasis
	Bacterial vaginosis
	Contact dermatitis
Balanitis (glans of penis)	Flat genital warts
	Erythroplasia of Queyrat (Bowen's disease of the penis)
	Contact dermatitis
	Balanitis plasma cellularis (Zoon's balanitis)
Candidal paronychia (tissue surrounding the nail)	Bacterial paronychia (*Pseudomonas, Proteus*)
	Herpetic whitlow
Subungual *Candida* (under nail)	Tinea unguium (onychomycosis)

treatment with antifungal creams that are available OTC or by prescription. The formulation of the topical antifungal used will depend on the site of the infection and whether the rash is moist or dry. Powders work well with moist, macerated lesions. Creams work well in drier lesions. Solutions and sprays are alcohol based and cause burning on inflamed or macerated skin; therefore, they should be avoided on these areas. Preparations in ointment form are far more adherent than liquid, lotion, or cream forms and tend to work best for intertriginous areas. Oral formulations include suspensions and troches.

Pharmacological Therapy

Topical antifungals such as nystatin (effective for *Candida* only), clotrimazole (Lotrimin), miconazole, Monistat-Derm, naftifine (Naftin), and ciclopirox (Loprox) are effective. Most topical antifungal creams are applied twice per day for at least 2 weeks (and up to 4 weeks). The patient should be instructed to apply creams sparingly because too much cream will cause skin maceration, especially in intertriginous areas. The cream is massaged gently into the rash and the surrounding area. The patient is advised that some mild improvement in the rash is sometimes seen in a week, but frequently it takes 2 to 4 weeks until the rash is cleared. Adverse reactions are usually mild; they include erythema, local irritation, itching, burning,

and dryness. In some patients, sensitization occurs, and a true contact dermatitis results. (If so, medication should be discontinued.)

For topical treatment of severe cases of candidal vulvovaginitis, cream formulations often will yield better results than vaginal suppositories. Vaginal suppositories can become dislodged from the vagina when the patient is voiding or during defecation. For mild to moderate cases, suppositories work well and are now available for 3-day treatment. In recurrent candidal vaginitis, both partners may need treatment. Partners should abstain from sexual intercourse until both have finished treatment. If the patient does not have symptoms, treatment is not necessary. Treatment recommendations for vaginal candidiasis are listed in Table 7.2.

Some experts discourage the use of systemic therapies for cutaneous candidiasis because of the potential for adverse effects and an increase in resistance. Studies have found that the increased use of imidazoles for systemic therapy has been associated with an increase in the strains of the *Candida* species resistant to fluconazole (Diflucan). Less common candidal species such as *C glabrata* and *C tropicalis* are also more likely to be resistant to treatment with topical imidazoles. If the patient is immunocompromised, has severe vaginal or perianal candidiasis, or is unresponsive to topical medications, systemic antifungal therapy may be justified. Drug interactions may occur with many oral systemic antifungals that are available by

Table 7.2	Treatment of Vaginal Candidiasis
1-Day Treatment	Butoconazole 2% prefilled applicator in one dose
	Oral fluconazole 150 mg in one single dose
3-Day Treatment	Clotrimazole 2% applicator daily for 3 days
	Miconazole 200 mg vaginal suppository for 3 days
	Terconazole 0.8% cream one applicator full intravaginally for 3 days
	Terconazole 80 mg suppository intravaginally for 3 days
7-Day Treatment	Miconazole 2% vaginal cream intravaginally for 7 days
	Miconazole 100 mg vaginal suppository for 7 days
	Clotrimazole 1% vaginal cream, 1 applicator full daily for 7 days
	Clotrimazole 100 mg vaginal suppository for 7 days
	Terconazole 0.4% cream one applicatorful intravaginally for 7 days

prescription when given with Coumadin, phenytoin (Dilantin), and rifampin. Serious adverse events that occur with oral systemic antifungals include hepatotoxicity, angioedema, and anaphylaxis. For significant skin infections resistant to extended topical therapy, systemic antifungal treatment includes fluconazole for 10 to 14 days or itraconazole for 2 to 3 weeks. Skin infections resistant to this treatment should be reevaluated for a nonfungal or noncandidal etiology or infection by a fluconazole-resistant candidal strain in need of alternative oral or even IV antifungal treatment such as voriconazole, amphotericin B, or caspofungin. These treatments would never be prescribed in the primary-care setting because they require highly specialized care and observation.

Oral candidiasis (thrush) is treated with nystatin, which is available in suspension, pastilles, or troches. Nystatin is available in 100,000 units/mL suspension, and 4 to 6 mL (or 1 teaspoon) is given (½ dose at each side of the mouth) 4 to 5 times daily. The patient should be advised to retain the suspension inside the mouth as long as possible before swallowing. Nystatin is available in pastille form (200,000 units); the patient should be told to allow one or two pastilles to dissolve slowly inside the mouth 5 times a day for 14 consecutive days. An alternative is clotrimazole (Mycelex) 10 mg troches; the patient should be told to dissolve one troche inside the mouth 5 times daily for 14 consecutive days. Mycelex troches are also indicated for prophylaxis of thrush; the dose is 1 troche 3 times daily. Itraconazole solution (10 mg/mL) is indicated for oral candidiasis that is unresponsive to fluconazole; it is available in cherry or caramel flavor. The patient is instructed to swish 10 mL (100 mg) at a time twice daily in the mouth for several seconds before swallowing; treatment should continue for 2 to 4 weeks. Itraconazole oral antifungal medications are rated as Pregnancy Category C. Relapse frequently occurs after treatment of thrush in immunocompromised patients.

In candidal paronychia, a warm compress on the affected fingertip will enhance drainage of purulent discharge and help relieve the pain. Incision and drainage of purulent material may speed resolution and provide relief. Candidal infections of the nail (subungual candida) are best treated with systemic antifungals.

Follow-up and Referral

The patient should be seen in 2 weeks to monitor response to treatment. If there is no response to treatment, the initial diagnosis should be reconsidered or the patient should be referred to a dermatologist. If partial response is seen, treatment can be continued for another 1 to 2 weeks and the patient reevaluated. If there is poor response at that time, the patient needs a referral to a dermatologist.

Patient Education

Patients must be taught to decrease favorable environmental conditions for *Candida* such as moisture, warmth, and poor air circulation. To prevent diaper rash, the infant should be kept dry as much as possible, and the use of rubber or plastic pants should be discouraged. Baby powder with cornstarch should not be used because it will worsen the infection (*Candida* can use the cornstarch as food).

For obese patients, one method of keeping deep folds of skin apart is by using clean, dry, white tissues between the folds of skin. Educate the patient on the importance of keeping the affected area dry to assist in healing and to prevent future candidal infections. Patients may be instructed to use a hair dryer but stress that it must be kept on the "low" setting. Patients with candidal paronychia should be advised to minimize exposure of hands to water and the prolonged use of rubber gloves. If a fluctuant abscess is present, the patient should apply a warm compress to the involved finger two to three times per day to assist in drainage.

■ DERMATOPHYTOSES

Dermatophytoses, or *tinea,* are superficial skin infections caused predominantly by three fungal species: *Trichophyton, Epidermophyton,* and *Microsporum.* Transmission occurs primarily through direct contact with an infected person or animal (dogs, cats). Other modes of transmission include contact with asymptomatic carriers, who can infect family and intimate friends, or contact with soil (which is full of fungal spores). Although this route of transmission is controversial, fomites (shared objects such as combs or hats) have been implicated in spreading tinea infections. It is not uncommon to find two (or more) tinea infections in one patient. Tinea manuum often occurs in the "one hand, two feet" distribution. Tinea pedis ("athlete's foot") can occur simultaneously with both tinea unguium (onychomycosis) and tinea corporis (ringworm), as well as with other combinations. Multiple tinea infections are caused by spreading infection from one area of the body to another through scratching.

Environmental and host factors play an important role in the development of tinea infections. Favorable environmental factors that increase the chances of tinea infection include heat, moisture, and poor air circulation. Host factors include age, broken skin, broken hair shafts, and excessive moisture on the skin or nails. Tinea infections are classified by their location on the body; different types include the following:

- Tinea capitis, or ringworm of the scalp
- Tinea corporis, or ringworm of the body—also known as tinea circinata
- Tinea cruris, or "jock itch"—ringworm of the groin
- Tinea pedis, or "athlete's foot"
- Tinea manuum, or tinea of the hands
- Tinea versicolor—also known as pityriasis versicolor
- Tinea unguium (onychomycosis—covered in a separate section)

Although tinea versicolor is caused by the yeast *Pityrosporum orbiculare (Malassezia furfur)* and is not considered a classic dermatophytosis; it is also discussed in this section.

Epidemiology and Causes

The estimated lifetime incidence of tinea infections is between 10% and 20%. Tinea infections are more common in warmer climates. Individuals with diabetes are at higher risk for tinea and yeast infections. Tinea pedis, or "athlete's foot," is the most common fungal infection in the United States. Acute tinea pedis is caused by *Trichophyton mentagrophytes* var. *interdigitale,* and chronic tinea pedis is caused by *Trichophyton rubrum,* which is more common. Tinea cruris (jock itch) is more common in men and *T rubrum* is the common agent. Tinea capitis (ringworm of the scalp) is more common in children until puberty when, for unknown reasons, the incidence markedly decreases. Tinea unguium (onychomycosis) is seen more frequently in adults and elderly patients.

The most contagious of all dermatophytoses is tinea capitis (scalp ringworm). It has been known to cause epidemics in crowded conditions such as schools and group homes, as well as outbreaks among family members. Tinea capitis infections are more common in toddlers and school-age children from urban areas. The reason why tinea capitis is very contagious is because of the propensity of *Trichophyton tonsurans* to produce large numbers of infectious spores called arthroconidia. *T tonsurans* causes up to 90% of all cases of tinea capitis in the United States and Western Europe. Minor causes of tinea capitis in this country include *Microsporum canis,* a zoophilic fungi from dogs. Less common causes are *Microsporum andounii* and *T rubrum.*

Tinea barbae, an infection of the beard area, is more common in men who work with animals. Tinea manuum (tinea manus), or tinea of the hands, is relatively rare compared with all other tinea infections. Tinea manuum infection frequently occurs with tinea pedis infection. The patient infects the hand by touching or scratching an infected foot. Unlike tinea pedis, in which both feet usually become infected, in tinea manuum infection, only one hand is usually involved. Tinea versicolor (pityriasis versicolor) infection is caused by the yeast *P orbiculare* (which causes round lesions) or *Pityrosporum ovale* (which produces oval lesions); it is more common in the summertime. Tinea versicolor becomes more obvious during the summer, when tanning exposes hypopigmented macules that do not tan.

Pathophysiology

Three types of parasitic fungi are implicated in causing dermatophytic or tinea infections. *Microsporum* and *Epidermophyton* species both cause infections of the skin and nails. *Trichophyton* species cause infections not only of skin and nails but also of the hair. These fungal infections are superficial because all three types have the ability to metabolize keratin, the protein that comprises the topmost layer of body surface epithelium that normally serves as a protective barrier against microbial infection. The clinical presentation of tinea infections depends on the anatomical location and the species of fungi. Asymptomatic carriers do not show symptoms of disease but infect susceptible hosts through direct contact or by depositing spores onto fomites such as combs, brushes, or hats. Acute tinea pedis is usually caused by *T mentagrophytes* var. *interdigitale* whereas chronic tinea pedis is caused by *T rubrum* and is more common. For tinea cruris (jock itch), *T rubrum* is the most common agent.

Microscopic exam of tinea lesions reveals either acute or chronic inflammation and a sponge-like texture in the infected tissue, appropriately termed *spongiosis.* Fungal hyphae are seen on the superficial keratin layer of the epidermis. In tinea capitis, infection occurs either inside (endothrix) or outside (ectothrix) of the hair shaft. In ectothrix infections, fungal hyphae and spores invade the hair shaft, leading to destruction of the hair cuticle. Ectothrix infections are caused by *Microsporum* species (*M canis* and *M andounii*). In contrast, endothrix infections are caused by the *Trichophyton* species (*T tonsurans* in North America) and occur inside the hair shaft, leaving the hair cuticle intact. Spores (also called arthroconidia) are found inside the hair shaft, rather than on skin scrapings of surface scale in endothrix infection, also known as "black dot" tinea capitis. Because this type of infection is most common in African American children, coiling of the hair shaft may play some role in infection susceptibility.

Kerion formation sometimes results from an endothrix infection and is associated with severe inflammatory changes of the scalp consisting of nodules and boggy, exudative tissue. Secondary staphylococcal infection may complicate kerion, causing purulent drainage, with infection possibly spreading to draining lymph nodes, causing painful lymphadenitis. When it heals, it results in scarring and alopecia. A variant of endothrix infection that is uncommon in North America but more common in South Africa and the Middle East is favus infection, a severe form of tinea capitis that results in extensive hair loss and scarring.

Clinical Presentation
Subjective

Tinea Capitis The typical patient with tinea capitis is a toddler or school-age child. The parent often reports a painless bald spot. If kerion formation accompanies the infection, the child will show signs of discomfort or will complain of pain. No systemic symptoms such as fever or malaise are associated with kerion formation.

Tinea Corporis The typical patient will report a history of an erythematous round and elevated pruritic lesion that grows in size and starts to clear in the center—the classic shape of "ringworm." Sometimes, there is a history of another family member with the same infection. Some patients report a history of prior infection. The clinician should inquire about possible exposure through close contact with domesticated animals such as cats or dogs.

Tinea Cruris The typical patient is an obese adult male who complains of a pruritic rash on the groin that is spreading to the medial inner aspect of the upper thigh. Sometimes, the rash is not associated with pruritus.

Tinea Pedis The typical patient with tinea pedis is usually a male teenage athlete or an adult who comes to the clinic complaining of "athlete's foot" and strong foot odor. Most patients do not have pain with this infection unless it gets secondarily infected with bacteria, causing cellulitis. The patient reports areas of macerated soft, whitened skin between the toes. Some patients will complain of concurrent infections on the hand (tinea manuum), on the body (tinea corporis), and the toenails (tinea unguium).

Tinea Versicolor Most cases of tinea versicolor are seen in the summer because the hypopigmented spots become more visible at that time of year; they do not tan. Tinea versicolor is asymptomatic and has a very gradual onset. Rarely, a patient will complain of some mild pruritus. The typical patient is a teen or young adult, although tinea can occur at any age. People of African descent with tinea will complain of either light-colored (hypopigmentation) or dark-colored spots (hyperpigmentation). In adults, the usual sites are on the back, upper chest, arms, and sometimes the neck and face. In children, the rash is more likely to be on the face or forehead.

Objective

Tinea Capitis Three clinical presentations are seen with tinea capitis infections. One presentation is the "black dot" tinea capitis caused by *T tonsurans*. The child with "black dot" tinea capitis presents with painless patchy alopecia (either single or multiple patches). The skin on the scalp does not have erythema; the "black dot" appearance results from broken hair stubbles that remain on the scalp.

Another presentation is called "gray patch" tinea capitis. The child with this condition also presents with patchy alopecia, but the bald patches are covered with fine gray-white scales. The patch is made up of thick, keratinized skin that is grayish white in color. Broken hair shafts of different lengths are present on the surface. Because the inflammatory response is so minimal in both "gray patch" and "black dot" tinea capitis, pain, erythema, nodules, and kerion are not present.

An extremely painful and inflammatory presentation of tinea capitis is known as the kerion. The kerion looks like a bright red, boggy large "bump" on the scalp with alopecia. Purulent drainage can be expressed out of the kerion by gentle pressure, and pus can be seen oozing out of its tiny follicular openings. Kerion formation can result in scarring alopecia. The affected hair follicles atrophy and become permanently damaged; hair does not grow back, even when the scalp is healed. A permanent bald patch can result from this tinea infection if it is not treated aggressively or if the patient does not present early enough during the course of the disease.

Tinea Corporis This infection presents as the classic "ringworm" infection—it is easy to recognize in the clinical setting. The patient will present with ringlike lesions with a bright red elevated border (collarette) that is covered with scales. Tinea corporis can occur in any age-group from child to adult, and the size of the lesions can range from small to large. The patient or parent will report that the lesion has been getting bigger. Some patients have only one lesion, whereas others have numerous lesions. The lesions are usually very pruritic, but sometimes they are asymptomatic.

Tinea Cruris Tinea cruris ("jock itch") is more common in men in the summer or during warm weather. It is usually extremely pruritic, and most lesions will show some lichenification from chronic scratching. The typical lesion is round to a half-circle; lesions will spread to the inner medial upper thigh but spare the scrotum. In contrast, candidal intertrigo can infect not only the groin and thigh but also the penis and the scrotum. The color of the lesion, depending on whether it is chronic or acute, can vary from a bright red to a dull discoloration. The lesions can become macerated from infection and scratching; they may become secondarily infected with bacteria or with *C albicans*.

Tinea Pedis This infection can be seen in the clinical area in up to five different presentations. Tinea pedis is usually asymptomatic, although sometimes the patient will complain of pain from a secondary bacterial infection. The most common cause of tinea pedis is *T mentagrophytes*. The infection usually starts in the third or fourth interdigital web space and sometimes spreads to all toe webs and the soles. Other fungi that cause tinea pedis (but are less common) include *T rubrum*, *C albicans*, and *Epidermophyton floccosum*.

The most common presentation of tinea pedis is macerated white skin between the web spaces of the toes; the infection is pruritic with occasional painful fissures and can be accompanied by a concurrent unpleasant foot odor. If it becomes infected with bacteria (usually *Staphylococcus aureus*), a tender cellulitis with redness and ulceration can develop on the web space. This condition is called ulcerative tinea pedis. Moccasin-type tinea pedis is seen more often with *T rubrum* infection. Scaling and thickening of the skin is seen in a moccasin distribution on both feet.

Another presentation of tinea pedis is with an "id" eruption—a dermatophytid. Acute "id" eruptions are caused by a hypersensitivity reaction to the fungus. The "id" eruption presents as vesicles on the sides of the fingers and/or the palms of the hands. The vesicles do not contain fungus but are sterile. The patient may or may not be aware of a concurrent tinea pedis infection.

Another vesicular type of tinea pedis *(T mentagrophytes)* is associated with burning pruritus and sometimes pain. It is more likely to flare up during warm weather, forming multiple vesicles and bullae. It can become secondarily infected with bacteria, resulting in cellulitis or even lymphangitis.

Tinea Versicolor Tinea versicolor is usually asymptomatic; it is not associated with any pruritus. The patient will present with oval to round, pink or hypopigmented or hyperpigmented macules, located mainly on the back, the chest, the arms, and sometimes the neck and face. Tinea in children is more likely to present on the face, especially on the forehead. Sometimes very fine scales are visible, especially if the patient has not showered or bathed for several days; otherwise, daily bathing usually eradicates the scales.

Diagnostic Reasoning

Diagnostic Tests

Tinea infections are usually diagnosed by their clinical presentation. The classic "ringworm" lesions are fairly easy to recognize. The diagnosis can be confirmed via microscopy in the clinical area (or a specimen [skin scraping] can be sent to the laboratory in a sterile plastic cup). Fungal culture is usually not necessary except in cases where the diagnosis is in doubt or in resistant cases. The exception to this rule is for the treatment of onychomycosis (tinea unguium). Because of the length of treatment and the potential for adverse reaction from systemic antifungals, positive proof by fungal culture is necessary. Fungal cultures can take up to 2 weeks for results to become available, although if done on Sabouraud's agar or with dermatophyte test medium, results may be obtained in 3 days.

A fungal culture is recommended for onychomycosis (tinea unguium) and for tinea capitis. Because these two tinea infections are treated by long-term therapy with systemic antifungals (with a high potential for serious side effects), physician consultation is recommended. Proof of the causative agent must be provided by a positive fungal culture. Fungal cultures are also useful if the clinician is unsure of the diagnosis or if the infection does not respond to treatment. Hair bulbs and broken hair, along with scales from the active lesion, should be cultured. Specimens from the affected site should include scales and hair roots. It is important to look for spores and hyphae on the hair shaft, inside the hair shaft (endothrix), and outside the hair shaft (ectothrix) using microscopy.

To obtain a fungal culture for suspected tinea capitis, the clinician should use a dry toothbrush to brush the areas of alopecia and then impregnate the culture media with the bristles. Another method is to use a wet cotton swab, wipe it over the areas of alopecia, and then implant

it on the media. Growth is usually seen in 10 to 14 days of culture.

Microscopy is the most useful diagnostic tool to use for tinea in the primary-care setting. A small piece of skin is scraped from the active edge of the lesion and placed on a glass slide. A drop of 10% KOH is placed on the sample, which is then heated gently with a lighter or match. The slide should not be placed too close to the flame or the KOH will get too hot and boil off. The heating accelerates the effect of the KOH on the keratinized cells' walls. When the sample is ready, the hyphae will be easier to see because the cell walls have already been lysed by the KOH. If KOH is not used in this test, the examiner will not be able to see the hyphae because the keratinized cells are too thick. A Wood's light exam should be used on any area of alopecia and hypopigmentation. Some fungi fluoresce when examined under Wood's light, which emits ultraviolet (UV) light (black light). The examining room should be darkened for this exam. A characteristic color that is associated with two minor causes of tinea capitis is a blue-green or bright green color from *Microsporum canis* or *Microsporum andounii. Trichophyton tonsurans,* the most common cause of tinea capitis, does not fluoresce under a Wood's light exam.

If the tinea infection is resistant to treatment, a fungal culture is mandatory. If a secondary bacterial infection is suspected, a sample of the exudates must be taken for culture and sensitivity using a sterile culture tube.

Differential Diagnosis

Almost all tinea infections tend to have a slow and gradual onset, producing low levels of inflammation. Low levels of inflammation do not produce bothersome symptoms such as pruritus and pain. Some tinea infections have been present for months to years before the patient reports them to a health-care provider. Sometimes, tinea infections are an incidental finding during a routine physical exam.

Some tinea infections, such as tinea manuum and tinea unguium (onychomycosis), are usually asymptomatic and are tolerated by the patient for many years. Tinea infections such as tinea cruris and tinea corporis tend to be more symptomatic—the severe pruritus associated with this infection usually drives the patient to seek medical care. The differential diagnosis of various tinea infections is presented in Differential Diagnosis 7.4. Because onychomycosis is so prevalent, it is discussed separately in a subsequent section.

Management

Most cases of tinea infections (except tinea infections of the scalp and nails) respond very well to a 2- to 4- week course of topical treatment with azole-class drugs such as those listed in Drugs Commonly Prescribed 7.3. These agents should be continued for at least 1 week after the lesions have cleared. They should be applied a

Differential Diagnosis 7.4 Tinea Infections

Location	Differential Diagnosis
Scalp (tinea capitis, tinea of the scalp)	Psoriasis, seborrheic dermatitis Alopecia areata
Body (tinea corporis, "ringworm")	Atopic or contact dermatitis Psoriasis
Hands (tinea manuum)	Atopic dermatitis Dyshidrotic eczema
Groin (tinea of the groin, "jock itch")	Erythrasma Contact dermatitis Candidal or bacterial intertrigo Psoriasis
Feet (tinea pedis, "athlete's foot")	Candidal intertrigo Contact dermatitis Dyshidrotic eczema Impetigo
Nails (tinea unguium, onychomycosis)	Candidal nail infection Psoriasis of the nail Pseudomonal nail infection
Tinea versicolor (Pityriasis versicolor)	Vitiligo Pityriasis alba Pityriasis rosea

few centimeters beyond the edges of the skin lesions. Other drugs, including systemic formulations, are included in Drugs Commonly Prescribed 7.3 as well.

As noted previously, for all patients who are on systemic antifungals, physician consultation is recommended because systemically absorbed antifungal drugs can cause hepatotoxicity. A baseline liver function profile and complete blood count (CBC) should be done initially and repeated again in 4 weeks and periodically thereafter during the course of treatment. Griseofulvin can cause leukopenia and granulocytopenia. A baseline CBC and another repeated in 4 weeks are recommended. Thereafter, a follow-up CBC can be done at 4- to 6-week intervals.

The patient should be told to report symptoms such as anorexia, nausea, vomiting, malaise, dark urine, jaundice, and rash to the clinician. If the clinician suspects hepatoxicity, the offending drug should be stopped and consultation with the supervising physician is recommended.

Tinea Capitis

In tinea capitis, a kerion that looks like a honeycomb may be observed. It is an inflammatory boggy mass containing broken hairs and oozing purulent material from follicular orifices. It is a rare, delayed-hypersensitivity reaction to fungal antigens and may result in permanent hair loss. Kerion rarely needs to be treated with

Drugs Commonly Prescribed 7.3 Tinea Infections

Drug	Indication	Dosage	Comments
Topical Agents			
miconazole 2% cream	Tinea: pedis, cruris, and corporis Cutaneous candidiasis	Twice daily for 2 weeks	Tinea pedis needs longer treatment—for 4 weeks.
clotrimazole 1% cream and solution	Tinea: pedis, cruris, and corporis Tinea versicolor	Twice daily for up to 4 weeks	Tinea pedis—treat for 4 weeks.
betamethasone 0.05% and clotrimazole 1% cream and lotion (Lotrisone)	Fungal skin infections	Apply sparingly twice daily for 2 weeks Maximum: 2 weeks	Contraindications: varicella, herpes, vaccinia, other viral infections. Do not use on face. Can cause steroid atrophic changes if used too long.
terbinafine 1% cream (Lamisil AT)	Tinea: cruris, corporis, pedis Moccasin-type tinea pedis (or plantar tinea pedis)	Tinea cruris/corporis: 2 times daily for 1–2 weeks Plantar tinea pedis: 2 times daily for 2 weeks	Improvement may continue to be seen for up to 2–6 weeks after therapy.

Continued

Drugs Commonly Prescribed 7.3 Tinea Infections—cont'd

Drug	Indication	Dosage	Comments
terbinafine 1% solution (Lamisil solution)	Tinea: versicolor (pityriasis), pedis, cruris, corporis	Versicolor/pedis: Twice daily for 1 week Tinea cruris/corporis: Once a day for 1 week	Alcohol-based solution. Use only for 1 week. Apply on dry skin. Do not use spray on face, mucous membranes; avoid broken or irritated skin.
ciclopirox (Loprox) 0.77% cream, lotion	Cutaneous candidiasis and fungal skin infections (tinea pedis, corporis, cruris, versicolor)	Twice daily for 2–4 weeks	Do not use on children younger than age 10 years. Avoid occlusion.
0.77% gel	Seborrheic scalp dermatitis	Apply and massage into affected areas twice daily up to 4 weeks.	
loprox shampoo 1%	Seborrheic scalp dermatitis	Shampoo and leave on for 3 minutes, then rinse. Repeat twice weekly at least 3 days apart.	Not recommended for those younger than 16 years of age. Avoid eyes and mucous membranes.
ciclopirox 8% topical solution (Penlac nail lacquer)	Onychomycosis of fingernails and toenails	Apply thin coat once daily at bedtime.	Remove with alcohol once per week. Repeat for up to 1 year. Do not use nail polish.
ketonazole 2% (Nizoral) cream, shampoo	Tinea pedis, cruris, corporis, versicolor Cutaneous candidiasis Seborrheic dermatitis	Once daily to twice daily for 2–4 weeks or until clinical clearing.	Contains sulfites. Treat tinea pedis for 6 weeks. Seborrheic dermatitis: Use shampoo or cream for 2 weeks or till clear. Tinea versicolor: Use shampoo (1 application). Apply to damp scalp, leave for 5 minutes, rinse.
econazole 1% cream (Spectazole)	Tinea: pedis, cruris, corporis, versicolor	Tinea: once a day; others: 2 times daily	Treat tinea pedis for 4 weeks, others for 2 weeks.
sulconazole (Exelderm) 1% cream, solution	Tinea: cruris, corporis, versicolor, cream only: tinea pedis	Tinea pedis: twice daily for 4 weeks; others: once or twice daily for 3 weeks	Reevaluate if no improvement within 4–6 weeks.
naftifine 1% cream, gel (Naftin)	Tinea: pedis, cruris, corporis	Cream: once per day Gel: twice daily for up to 4 weeks	If no improvement is seen in 4 weeks, reevaluate. Wash hands after application. Not recommended for children.
nystatin cream	Cutaneous candidiasis (intertrigo)	Twice daily for 2–4 weeks	Apply liberally to affected area.
nystatin powder	Candidiasis, especially moist lesions (under breast, groin, shoes, feet, body folds)	Two to three times a day for 2–4 weeks	Good for weeping lesions under breast, in groin, body folds Irritation rare.
nystatin suspension	Thrush (oral candidiasis)	4–6 mL (1 tsp.) 4 times daily for at least 2 weeks	Retain in mouth as long as possible before swallowing.

Drugs Commonly Prescribed 7.3   Tinea Infections—cont'd

Drug	Indication	Dosage	Comments
Systemic Agents			
itraconazole (Sporanox PulsePak) (Sporanox)	Onychomycosis of toenail or fingernail, histoplasmosis, blastomycosis Tinea: capitis, corporis; recalcitrant tinea pedis infections	Toenail: 200 mg daily for 12 consecutive weeks Fingernail: total of 2 "pulses"; 200 mg twice daily for 1 week, then 3 weeks off; repeat pulse Repeat 200 mg 2 times daily again for 1 week Recalcitrant tinea pedis: 200 mg daily for 2 weeks, or 400 mg daily for 1 week Tinea corporis/severe cruris: 200 mg once daily for 1–2 weeks	Take with food; suspension form is better absorbed. Hypoglycemia with oral hypoglycemics. Numerous drug interactions; check before prescribing. Check liver function before, during, and after treatment.
terbinafine (Lamisil)	Onychomycosis of toenail or fingernail due to tinea unguium	Toenail: 250 mg once daily for 12 weeks Fingernail: 250 mg once daily for 6 weeks	Check liver function/renal function. Use with caution in patients with liver/renal disease. Clinical cure not apparent for months.
fluconazole (Diflucan)	Oropharyngeal, esophageal, systemic candidiasis	All doses once daily: Thrush: 200 mg on day 1, then 100 mg/day for at least 2 weeks Esophageal: 200 mg on day 1, then 100 mg/day for at least 3 weeks	Check liver function test. Contraindicated in patients with liver disease.
griseofulvin (ultramicrosized) Grifulvin V	Tinea capitis, onychomycosis, severe/recalcitrant tinea cruris, pedis, corporis	Tinea capitis: 500 mg once daily for 2–4 weeks Tinea corporis: 500 mg daily for 2–4 weeks Severe: 250–500 mg twice daily for 1–2 weeks Onychomycosis: 750 mg daily for 6 months Maximum: 1 g/day	Ultramicrosize formulation better absorbed. High rate of resistant strains of tinea capitis. Use with caution in patients with liver and renal disease. Monitor renal, hepatic, and hematopoietic function. Decreases effectiveness of oral contraceptives, oral anticoagulants, barbiturates.

concurrent antibiotics because a noninfected kerion can itself look exudative. It needs to be treated only if a secondary staphylococcal infection is obvious. Tinea infections of the hair and nails do not respond to topical treatment at all, unlike the other tinea infections. Tinea capitis should be treated with oral systemic antifungals, along with a topical antifungal for the local scalp lesions. A Wood's light exam should be done on all cases of alopecia on the scalp. Although some infections will fluoresce, others (*T tonsurans, T violaceum*) do not. *Microsporum canis* and *Microsporum andounii* are fluorescent. A fungal culture is necessary not only to help in the diagnosis but also to classify the species of fungi. It is important to examine the patient's close contacts, including family members (especially other children) and schoolmates. Fungal cultures on close contacts are recommended, if possible. Asymptomatic cases of tinea capitis can be treated with selenium sulfide shampoo (e.g., Selsun Blue). There is no need to wait for results of the fungal culture (which takes 2 weeks) before initiating treatment, especially if there is kerion formation.

The treatment of choice for tinea capitis is griseofulvin (Grifulvin V) 250 to 500 mg by mouth twice per day for severe cases in adults or once per day for children over 50 pounds. For children 30 to 50 pounds, 125 to 250 mg daily is recommended. Treatment duration is from 2 to 4 months or at least 2 weeks after negative cultures are obtained. Some authorities recommend against griseofulvin as the first-line drug because of its potential adverse effects. Other effective alternatives used to treat tinea capitis are oral terbinafine or itraconazole. Male patients on griseofulvin should be advised that this drug affects sperm (it is teratogenic) and to avoid fathering a child for at least 6 months after stopping the drug. Concurrent treatment with selenium sulfide shampoo 3 times per week is used as adjunctive therapy to systemic antifungals.

Tinea Corporis

Topical therapy generally works well with tinea corporis. The patient must be reminded to apply the topical agent for at least 1 week after the resolution of the lesions and to apply the cream a few centimeters beyond the edges. Concomitant short-term treatment with a mild corticosteroid such as hydrocortisone 1% (available OTC) is effective in helping to relieve itch and inflammation. In severe cases, systemic antifungals such as itraconazole or terbinafine daily are effective.

Tinea Cruris

Topical antifungal therapy is very effective for treatment of jock itch. Concomitant short-term treatment with a mild corticosteroid such as hydrocortisone 1% (OTC) is effective in helping to relieve itch and inflammation. If weeping areas are present, compresses made from Burow's solution are helpful. Use of OTC antifungal powders is helpful for prevention of future recurrences. For severe cases, a short course of a systemic antifungal such as itraconazole (Sporanox) or terbinafine (Lamisil) is effective.

Tinea Pedis and Tinea Manuum

Tinea pedis and tinea manuum are both treated with topical antifungals. Treatment of tinea pedis should emphasize moisture control: Use of drying foot powders (miconazole, tolnaftate) is very helpful. If weeping areas are present, compresses made from Burow's solution are helpful. The feet should be exposed to air as much as possible—during warm weather, the use of airy sandals or going barefoot is helpful. If socks are worn, cotton or a synthetic "wicking" blend is the best material. Socks should be changed once a day; changing socks twice a day is indicated if the patient's feet become wet in 4 hours or less. An antiperspirant spray on the soles of the feet (to be applied on normal skin only) can help

patients who are afflicted with excessively sweaty feet. Severe tinea pedis can be treated with oral agents such as itraconazole or terbinafine daily. After a short course of systemic therapy, the patient should be placed on maintenance topical therapy with a powder or a spray (miconazole, tolnaftate) to prevent recurrences.

Tinea Versicolor

Tinea versicolor is treated with topical selenium sulfide lotion (Selsun) applied daily for 7 days from neck to waist daily and then lathered for 10 minutes before rinsing thoroughly. Treatment is then done once a week for 1 month, and then once a month for maintenance. Ketoconazole (Nizoral) shampoo can also be used weekly for maintenance. The clinician must not forget to advise patients that treatment will get rid of the infection but not of the hypopigmented spots, which take longer to resolve. Patients should also be warned of the high rate of recurrence, because *Malassezia furfur* is a normal inhabitant of the skin. Exposing the hypopigmented lesions to sunlight can speed up the process in some patients. For patients who want more aggressive treatment, oral ketoconazole 200 mg daily for 1 week or 400 mg in a single dose or at weekly or monthly intervals is effective but does not prevent recurrence. Patients on oral ketoconazole should be advised not to shower for at least 12 to 18 hours because the drug is delivered to the skin by the sweat after it has been absorbed into the bloodstream. The patient should be advised that there is a risk of hepatotoxicity from oral ketoconazole. Because tinea versicolor is a superficial benign disease, this fact should be given serious consideration.

Follow-up and Referral

The patient should be seen for initial follow-up 2 weeks after initiation of therapy. For resistant cases, the clinician should make sure a fungal culture is done, or the diagnosis should be reevaluated. Resistant cases should be referred to a dermatologist for reevaluation or for more aggressive treatment with systemic antifungals. If the patient is on topical therapy only, systemic therapy can be considered. Severe tinea corporis and tinea pedis respond well to oral terbinafine or to itraconazole.

Some tinea infections have higher recurrence rates than others. Tinea versicolor (pityriasis versicolor)—although not a true tinea (because it is caused by a yeast)—has a very high recurrence rate because *P orbiculare* and *P ovale* are normal colonizers of the skin. Tinea pedis also tends to reoccur, so meticulous attention should be given to eradicating favorable environmental conditions by the patient (see discussion of tinea pedis for preventive measures). Maintenance therapy in tinea pedis with topical OTC agents in powder or spray form (miconazole, tolnaftate) is very effective in helping prevent recurrences.

If the clinician suspects that a secondary infection (cellulitis) is complicating tinea infection, a culture should be done on the purulent discharge. Empiric therapy for mild cellulitis, which is usually caused by gram-positive bacteria such as staphylococci or group A beta-hemolytic *Streptococcus,* includes oral antibiotics such as cephalexin or dicloxacillin for 7 to 14 days. For patients with penicillin allergy, either erythromycin or clarithromycin is a good alternative. Toe web infection (ulcerative type) can be due to gram-negative bacterial infection (*Pseudomonas aeruginosa, Escherichia coli,* and *Proteus*) and must be treated with systemic fluoroquinolones (i.e., ciprofloxacin). Moderate or severe cellulitis should be referred to a physician for more aggressive treatment, including IV antibiotics.

Patient Education

Patients who are on systemic antifungals must be informed of the risk of hepatotoxicity and educated on the signs and symptoms of acute hepatitis, such as anorexia, nausea, vomiting, malaise, dark urine, jaundice, and rash.

For all patients on systemic antifungals, consultation with a physician is recommended. A baseline liver function profile and CBC should be done before treatment is initiated and repeated again in 4 weeks and periodically thereafter. The patient should be told to report symptoms such as anorexia, nausea, vomiting, malaise, dark urine, jaundice, and rash. Griseofulvin decreases the effectiveness of certain drugs, such as oral contraceptives, oral anticoagulants, and barbiturates. Any woman of reproductive age who is on oral contraceptives and is prescribed griseofulvin should be warned that the contraceptive will become less effective and therefore her risk of pregnancy will be increased. The patient should be advised to see her gynecologist about using another effective method of birth control. If a patient who is on a barbiturate or an oral anticoagulant feels strongly about starting antifungal treatment, the patient should consult the physician who prescribed the original medication before starting treatment with systemic antifungals. Terbinafine is potentiated by cimetidine and is antagonized by rifampin. Itraconazole (Sporanox) is contraindicated if the patient is taking any drug that is metabolized in the liver by the CYP3A system. Itraconazole increases the blood levels of triazolam (Halcion), diazepam (Valium), digoxin, dihydropyridine class of calcium channel blockers (Norvasc, Procardia), and several other drugs. Adverse reactions to these agents include gastrointestinal (GI) upset, abdominal pain, dizziness, headache, hepatotoxicity, rash, and taste disturbance (associated with terbinafine). Blood dyscrasias including granulocytopenia and leukopenia, a lupus-like syndrome, and proteinuria are also possible adverse effects of griseofulvin. The following measures should be recommended to help prevent spread or recurrence of tinea infections:

- Tinea capitis: The parent and the child should be advised not to share combs, hats, or any headgear.

- Tinea corporis: The patient should be advised to control excessive sweat and body moisture by wearing looser clothing and to change clothing when it becomes wet or damp. After bathing, a hair dryer on the low setting may be used to dry intertriginous skinfolds.
- Tinea cruris: Cotton boxer shorts are better than tight briefs. The patient should avoid wearing tight jeans, pantyhose, or tight biker shorts.
- Tinea corporis: Some patients (especially children) may think that an actual worm is the cause of "ringworm" infections. Reassuring these patients that the infection is a fungus goes a long way in allaying anxiety.
- Tinea pedis: The patient should be advised to avoid scratching the feet because the infection can spread to the hands and to the body (tinea corporis). The patient should also avoid tight shoes and moist socks, especially socks made out of synthetic material, unless they are designed to wick away moisture. Patients who are prone to "athlete's foot" should change socks two or three times a day and expose their feet to air—they should use sandals if possible in warm weather. Absorbent nonsynthetic socks are preferred. Feet should be washed daily and dried thoroughly (a hair dryer on a low setting is helpful). Use antiperspirant spray on the soles to decrease sweating. Patients should also be advised to clean their showers with bleach and wash all white sheets with bleach. When showering away from home, shower shoes should be worn.
- Tinea versicolor: Advise the patient that exposure to sunlight will help in repigmentation of hypopigmented areas.

■ ONYCHOMYCOSIS

Onychomycosis (tinea unguium) is a benign superficial and cosmetic infection of the toenails and fingernails. Most patients tolerate tinea infections for many years. Patients who seek treatment are usually younger adults who are disturbed about the cosmetic effects of the infection. The most common etiology for onychomycosis is infection with dermatophytic fungi, but molds, yeast, and nondermatophytic fungi may be causative agents as well. Risk factors that place one at risk for onychomycosis include wearing occlusive shoes, diabetes mellitus, participation in sports, increasing age, and poor circulation of the lower extremities.

Epidemiology and Causes

Onychomycosis, or tinea unguium, is more common in adults and in elderly patients than in children. The combination of poor circulation in the lower extremities as a result of peripheral vascular disease and increasing age makes this a common problem in older adults. Toenails are more likely to become infected than fingernails. Onychomycosis is a common infection worldwide; the incidence of disease is variable and is dependent on many factors. In the United States, 20% of all adults have onychomycosis. Onychomycosis is sometimes caused by the yeast *Candida albicans*. Dermatophytic species of fungi commonly implicated in this tinea infection are *Trichophyton* species: *T rubrum, T mentagrophytes, T shoenleinii,* and several others. A zoophilic fungi that is normally found in animal species that cause onychomycosis is *T verrucosum*.

Like many infections, onychomycosis frequently has a multifactorial etiology. *C albicans* can be part of the normal flora of the mouth, the GI tract, and sometimes the vagina. The cause cannot be attributed solely to the presence of the offending organism, because most of the yeasts and fungi are ubiquitous to our environment. Molds, for example, are plentiful in soil. The soil mold *Scopulariopsis brevicaulis* is the most common nondermatophytic cause of onychomycosis. Other molds implicated in onychomycosis include the *Aspergillus* and *Alternaria* species.

Pathophysiology

Onychomycosis is classified as either primary or secondary. *Primary onychomycosis* involves invasion of the healthy nail plate. In *secondary onychomycosis,* diseased nails (e.g., from psoriasis or trauma) are involved. Factors that increase the risk of onychomycosis include a decrease in circulation, resulting from either a chronic process such as peripheral vascular disease or from an acute traumatic process, such as a fracture of the lower extremity. Abnormal enervation during spinal trauma has also been implicated. Tinea unguium can result from an extension of an infection with tinea pedis, tinea manuum, or tinea corporis.

Nail invasion can proceed in several ways. In proximal subungual onychomycosis, the pathogen enters the nailbed through the posterior nail and cuticle area, then migrates to the proximal nailbed. This form of onychomycosis is most commonly seen in immunocompromised individuals who exhibit suboptimal T-cell function. In distal and lateral subungual onychomycosis, infection starts on the distal or the lateral margins of the nail. The infection then moves toward the center of the nail until the entire nail is affected. Distal subungual onychomycosis is almost always caused by *Trichophyton rubrum*. Superficial white onychomycosis involves infection of the nail surface only and is caused mainly by *Trichophyton mentagrophytes*. Total dystrophic onychomycosis is associated mostly with chronic candidiasis, which is seen in immunodeficiency states such as AIDS.

Clinical Presentation

Subjective

The typical patient who seeks treatment for onychomycosis is either a young or middle-aged adult who is bothered greatly by the cosmetic effects of the infection. The duration of the infection can range from a few weeks to many years. Onychomycosis is an asymptomatic infection, and there should be no pain involved. Some patients will report having tried several OTC remedies with no result. The patient will complain of thickened nails or nails with cloudy, white-colored patches. Some will report nail discoloration, ranging from yellow to green or brown to black. Some patients will complain of nails that are partially detached from the nailbed (onycholysis).

Objective

Onychomycosis has several presentations. In some patients, two types can occur simultaneously. Superficial infections are more responsive to treatment with prescription topical antifungals (naftifine gel) than subungual types. (Onychomycosis infections with "subungual" as part of their name denote infection beneath the nail.) Superficial white onychomycosis involves only the nail surface but can occur with either distal or lateral subungual onychomycosis. Subungual onychomycosis can include distal, lateral, and proximal sites of infection. The first or fifth toenail is more likely to become infected than the other toes. The infected nail appears dry and has an opaque white patch with sharp borders that start on the distal, lateral, or proximal subungual portion, or occurs only on the surface (superficial white onychomycosis). As the infection persists, the nail becomes brittle and thick. The area underneath the nail accumulates chalky material made up of hyperkeratotic debris that can be scraped off easily for fungal cultures. In some patients, the white opaque areas become discolored—either yellow or brown. A green-black color indicates a bacterial *Pseudomonas* infection.

Diagnostic Reasoning

Diagnostic Tests

All cases of presumed onychomycosis must be confirmed by laboratory findings. A positive result on the fungal culture, which includes proper identification of the fungus species involved, is necessary to start treatment with systemic antifungals. Findings on the classic potassium hydroxide (KOH) exam indicating fungal infection are hyphae and spores or the classic "spaghetti and meatballs" appearance. Under the microscope, hyphae appear like translucent long tubes with septae (separate sections), and spores are small round to ovoid shapes.

Fungal Culture Fungal cultures done on Sabouraud's agar or with Dermatophyte test medium produce results in up to 3 days. The area where the samples are to be taken should be cleansed with 70% alcohol before specimen collection. Skin should be taken from the active border of the lesion. Nail samples should be taken from the subsurface of the infected nail. To obtain samples from underneath the nail, a scalpel can be used to scrape the underside of the infected nail. In proximal subungual onychomycosis, the affected part of the nail is on the proximal fold and cannot be sampled without nail removal. Nail removal is done with a bilateral digital nerve block and is contraindicated in any bleeding disorder. The patient should be referred to a podiatrist for nail removal and treatment.

KOH Exam   A laboratory exam using KOH is necessary for diagnosis, because only 50% of dystrophic nails are due to dermatophytosis. A drop of 10% KOH is placed on the sample of nail clippings and is heated gently with a lighter or match. The slide should not be placed too close to the flame, or the KOH will get too hot and boil off. The heating accelerates the effect of the KOH on the keratinized cell walls. When the sample is ready, the hyphae will be easier to see because the cell walls have already been lysed by the KOH.

Differential Diagnosis

Differential diagnosis of onychomycosis includes psoriasis of the nail, Reiter's syndrome, trauma to the nail, and congenital nail abnormalities. Onychomycosis accounts for only 50% to 60% of abnormal appearing, or dystrophic, nails. Lichen planus, eczematous conditions, and senile nailbed ischemia all may result in similarly appearing nails; however, fungal infection does not underlie such conditions, and antifungal medications would be inappropriate.

Management

Traditionally, onychomycosis of the toenail required long-term treatment with systemic antifungals and had a high recurrence rate. With the advent of newer antifungals (fluconazole, itraconazole, terbinafine), the cure rates for onychomycosis have greatly improved. Fluconazole (Diflucan) has consistently been shown to be less effective than either itraconazole or terbinafine and is not typically recommended. Removal of the affected nail is often curative.

Fingernail infection is easier to cure and has a lower rate of recurrence. The decision to treat onychomycosis aggressively must be considered carefully because it is a benign cosmetic infection. The patient's desires for treatment and his or her health history are probably the strongest determinants in deciding whether or not to treat with systemic antifungals. Other important factors include the presence of any preexisting medical problems and the past medical history. Patients who have liver disease should never be on any systemic antifungal drugs because of the high risk of hepatoxicity and liver failure. A history of infection with viral hepatitis can result in chronic infection with hepatitis B and C. A history of excessive alcohol use can result in cirrhosis of the liver or elevations in liver function tests.

Medication interactions are also problematic. Drugs metabolized by the cytochrome P450 3A enzyme system (CYP450) interact with systemic antifungals. Itraconazole potentiates the effects of many common prescription drugs, including diazepam (Valium), digoxin (Lanoxin), triazolam (Halcion), anticoagulants (Coumadin), HIV protease inhibitors (e.g., indinavir, ritonavir), methylprednisone, and verapamil. Patients who are taking vinca alkaloids (used in cancer chemotherapy) should not take itraconazole.

In addition, itraconazole requires a low gastric pH (acidic) to be absorbed. Therefore, H_2 blockers and antacids must be avoided within 2 hours of taking the drug.

Topical Therapy

Topical treatment of onychomycosis is generally not very effective (10% or less), but it is worth a try because it is not associated with any serious side effects. Good candidates for topical treatment are motivated patients with only mild involvement or with surface involvement (superficial white onychomycosis). A topical solution such as ciclopirox nail lacquer 8% (Penlac) or naftifine gel 1% (Naftin) applied twice daily may be effective when it is applied religiously to toenails for at least 6 to 18 months and to the fingernails for 4 to 6 months. Ciclopirox 8% (Penlac) is indicated for mild to moderate onychomycosis of the fingernails and toenails (without lunula involvement). Initial improvement may take up to 6 months; treatment can continue up to 48 weeks. Penlac should be applied evenly on the affected nail and surrounding 5 mm of skin once daily, preferably at bedtime. It should be applied over previous coats, then removed with alcohol once a week. Nail polish should not be used during treatment.

Systemic Therapy

For patients who desire treatment for onychomycosis, most authorities recommend systemic therapy. If concurrent tinea pedis, tinea manuum, or tinea corporis is present, it should be treated with topical antifungals, so that the source of infection is eradicated. Fingernails are easier to treat than toenails and have a higher cure rate from 50% to 70%. See Drugs Commonly Prescribed 7.3 for recommended systemic medications.

Itraconazole and terbinafine are better choices for toenail infections, which are more difficult to treat. Patients who are on H_2 blockers can also take these drugs. There is no role for griseofulvin in the treatment of toenail onychomycosis because up to 80% to 90% of patients will relapse with this drug.

Follow-up and Referral

After initiation of therapy, liver function tests should be rechecked every 4 weeks. The first follow-up visit is scheduled during the fourth week to monitor for symptoms of hepatoxicity, adverse reactions, and compliance with treatment and to obtain a liver function panel. Thereafter, the patient should be seen for follow-up every 4 to 6 weeks and liver function tests done. Resistant cases of onychomycosis should be referred to a dermatologist. Nail growth should be monitored until the nails become clinically normal.

Patient Education

The patient should avoid tight, ill-fitting shoes because they traumatize nails, especially the first toenail. Cotton socks that become moist should be changed. Patients should be encouraged to air dry their feet and wear open-toed slippers or sandals.

Patients on itraconazole and terbinafine should be advised that although mycological cure has been achieved, normal nails might not be clinically apparent until regrowth in 3 to 12 months.

BACTERIAL INFECTIONS

■ IMPETIGO

Impetigo is a highly contagious, superficial vesiculopustular infection of the skin that is commonly seen in infants and children. Impetigo spreads easily through direct contact among family members and from one child to another in the classroom or in play groups. Impetigo infection in adults is not as contagious as impetigo infection in infants and younger children. Impetigo infection typically demonstrates a mixed flora of gram-positive bacteria that includes *Staphylococcus aureus* and group A or group B beta-hemolytic *Streptococcus*. Two forms of impetigo are seen in the clinical area—bullous and nonbullous (vesiculopustular) forms. Nonbullous impetigo is the more common form, constituting approximately 70% of impetigo cases.

Epidemiology and Causes

Impetigo affects primarily infants in hospital nurseries and young children 2 to 5 years old, especially those with poor hygiene and who are in day-care groups; however, patients of all ages are susceptible. Impetigo accounts for approximately 10% of skin problems observed in pediatric practices. It is the most common bacterial skin infection and the third most common skin disease among children. Impetigo is more prevalent in hot, humid weather, when biting insects and mosquitoes are most pervasive. The trauma caused by their bites favors bacterial growth on moist skin. There is an increased incidence of impetigo in lower socioeconomic groups because of several factors, including overcrowding, lack of good personal hygiene, and a higher incidence of anemia and malnutrition. In addition, any preexisting skin disease that goes untreated (e.g., atopic dermatitis) may also predispose individuals to secondary infection. Staphylococcal impetigo may be associated with immunodeficiency disease.

Pathophysiology

The infectious process in impetigo is limited to the stratum corneum. The presence of numerous neutrophils within the blister (subcorneal blister) and the presence of gram-positive cocci are characteristic of impetigo infections. The etiological agents may be found alone or in combination. If a combination of gram-positive bacteria is causing the impetigo infection, symbiosis promotes the growth of both bacteria and produces more rapid spread.

Staphylococcus bacteria are usually noted during the very early stage of the lesions, whereas *Streptococcus* bacteria tend to predominate in the later stages. In recent years, epidemiologists have noted an etiological shift in which *Staphylococcus aureus* either alone or in combination with group A *Streptococcus* has replaced the latter as the most common causative organism Thus, chronic skin colonization with either *S aureus* or group A *Streptococcus* predisposes an individual to impetigo. Infected lesions typically result from sites of previous injury, such as insect bites. The blisters are the result of local separation (acantholysis) of the keratinocytes in the underlying epidermal layer forming the floor of the blister. Blister formation is caused by the action of epidermolytic (exfoliative) exotoxins produced by the bacteria. Group A *Streptococcus* is the primary etiological agent for a particularly severe, albeit rare, ulcerative form of impetigo known as ecthyma. Ulcer formation is also aided by coagulase-positive *Staphylococci*.

Finally, bullous impetigo is caused by *Staphylococcus aureus* infection in newborns and young children. In this condition, exfoliative toxin A causes loss of cellular adhesion in the superficial epidermis normally mediated by the protein desmoglein. This results in large blistering lesions known as bullae, which eventually drain, leaving thin, nonpurulent crusts over the entire affected skin area.

Methicillin-resistant *S aureus* (MRSA) is an increasingly common cause of impetigo. This pathogen is observed more frequently with the nonbullous form of impetigo. Over the last decade, an increasing number of community-acquired MRSA and gentamicin-resistant *S aureus* strains have been reported as causes of impetigo.

Clinical Presentation
Subjective

The most common symptom of both types of impetigo is pruritus from the lesions. The parent of a young or school-age child will complain of a red, crusty rash that is spreading or getting larger in size. The rash is usually located on the face or on the extremities. Parents or the child may report that a close friend or classmate of the patient has the same rash.

The provider should ask about the location, onset, and duration of the lesions and any associated symptoms. The clinician should also inquire if any other family member has been affected and if treatment has been effective. Fever is unusual in impetigo; but if present, it should prompt investigation for a deeper infection.

Objective

The plaques of impetigo begin as vesicles whose roofs break down, leaving shallow erosions with yellowish crusts. The lesions may be discrete or confluent in their distribution and are usually seen on the face. Early impetigo may resemble many vesicular skin conditions, such as herpes simplex. Two forms of impetigo commonly seen in the clinical area are bullous impetigo and nonbullous impetigo.

The bullous type of impetigo may present with bullae that begin as small (1–2 mm) superficial vesicles with a fragile roof that ruptures easily. Sometimes the parent or patient will deny seeing bullae because they rupture so quickly that they are not recalled by the patient or the parent. The serous fluid inside the ruptured vesicles develops into a thin, transparent, and varnish-like crust. Hence the vesicles become pustular in a matter of hours. The bullous type of impetigo is usually caused by *Staphylococcus* bacteria; it commonly occurs on the face, elbows, and knees.

In the nonbullous or vesiculopustular type, the lesions are characterized by thick, adherent, dirty yellow–colored crusts that have erythematous margins. This type of impetigo occurs more often in older children. Both bullous and nonbullous types produce symptoms such as burning and pruritus. In addition, regional lymphadenopathy is seen. When the face is involved, the cervical nodes (and sometimes the preauricular and submandibular nodes) are enlarged; when the lesions are on the upper extremities, the axillary nodes become enlarged.

A variant of bullous impetigo that is caused exclusively by *S aureus* is known as *staphylococcal scalded skin syndrome*. Exotoxins produced by the bacteria lead to bullous, sheet-like necrosis of the epidermis and cause the epithelium layer of the skin to peel off in large pieces. The "scalded skin" thus mimics a thermal burn. This serious infection is more commonly seen in children and usually begins in the intertriginous areas.

A less common form of impetigo that is ulcerative in nature is known as *ecthyma*. This form of impetigo is seen predominantly on the feet, ankles, legs, and thighs. It afflicts mostly homeless people, sewage and garbage workers, alcoholics, and neglected elderly individuals. It is a deeper version of impetigo and often results from a neglected or poorly treated superficial abrasion, or from infected insect bites. Itching is common, and autoinoculation from scratching may cause satellite lesions that are annular in form. Ecthyma presents as pruritic and tender red vesicles or pustules that are surrounded by erythema and that eventually ulcerate. Because this process is very superficial, healing often occurs spontaneously in the center of the lesion and results in scarring. The inflammatory process involves both dermal and epidermal layers. (See Table 7.3.)

During physical assessment, a thorough examination of the skin should search for erosions that are covered with moist, honey-colored crusts. Any firm and dry or dark crusts with surrounding erythema characterize a deeper form of impetigo called *ecthyma*. The physical assessment should include an examination of the head, ears, pharynx, the neck, and the regional lymph nodes should be noted for lymphadenopathy.

Diagnostic Reasoning
Diagnostic Tests

Diagnosis may be based solely on medical history and clinical presentation. Initial testing for impetigo may also include a bacterial culture and sensitivity analysis from the moist crusts of the lesions. The results of the culture

Table 7.3 Types of Impetigo

Types of Impetigo	Causative Agent	Clinical Presentation
Bullous impetigo	*Staphylococcus aureus*	Lesion starts as about 1–2 mm superficial vesicle with fragile roof, easily ruptured; ruptured vesicle forms thin, transparent, varnishlike or classic "honey-colored" crust. Becomes pustular in matter of hours; pruritic; burning sensation.
Staphylococcal scalded skin syndrome	*Staphylococcus aureus*	Variant of bullous impetigo: Epidermal necrosis caused by bacterial exotoxins, resulting in the epithelial layer peeling off in large, sheetlike pieces; mimics scalded-skin thermal burn.
Nonbullous impetigo	*Streptococcus, Staphylococcus aureus*	Lesions are thick, adherent; recurrent with dirty yellow–colored crusts with erythematous margins; pruritic and burning sensation.
Ecthyma	*Staphylococcus aureus, Streptococcus;* other infective organisms may be observed.	Pruritic tender, red vesicles or pustules surrounded by erythema; rash eventually ulcerates. Deeper impetigo resulting from inadequately treated or neglected skin infections; also seen in infected insect bites or abrasions.

and sensitivity help to assess for antibiotic resistance of the responsible pathogen. Resistance can vary from community to community. In addition, a Gram stain can be obtained; if the lesions are caused by impetigo, the stain will reveal gram-positive cocci. If herpes simplex is suspected, a viral culture can be obtained. If the patient is febrile or has systemic symptoms, a CBC with differential should be obtained.

Differential Diagnosis

The typical dirty-looking, honey-colored crust is almost pathognomonic of bullous impetigo, so much so that cultures are not necessary before treatment is started. Bullous impetigo should be differentiated from other vesicular and pustular skin conditions. Many skin diseases with weepy lesions may resemble impetigo, such as varicella-zoster virus, herpes simplex virus, eczematous dermatitis (atopic dermatitis), bullous pemphigus/pemphigoid, and contact dermatitis. The history, distribution, and morphological features of the primary skin lesions provide the best information to help in the differential diagnosis of other skin conditions.

Varicella-zoster infection (herpes zoster or chickenpox) produces a rash with widely distributed papules and vesicular lesions. The onset of the rash typically starts on the head and neck area. The lesions of herpes zoster follow a dermatomal pattern that consists of a group of uniform 2- to 3-mm vesicles on an erythematous base.

A localized group of vesicles located on a single anatomical site, with a clear to cloudy fluid on an erythematous and edematous base, helps to characterize herpes simplex lesions. These lesions are usually preceded by a prodrome of burning and tingling before the lesions erupt.

Bullous pemphigus and bullous pemphigoid are autoimmune diseases affecting the skin and causing bulla that can become eroded and infected. They should be included in the differential diagnosis for any vesicular or bullous skin disease.

Acute nummular eczema manifests as pruritic, coin-shaped plaques or papulovesicles on an erythematous base; the lesions may become exudative and crusted. Candidiasis lesions are bright red; this rash forms satellite lesions along with macerated moist patches. Candidiasis is often accompanied by pruritus and burning in the macerated areas.

Management

There are two principles of therapy in the management of impetigo: (1) Nonpharmacological measures are employed to enhance resolution and to reduce bacterial colonization on the skin surface, and (2) antibiotics are prescribed to help eradicate the responsible pathogen and to prevent recolonization and complications. Even without treatment, impetigo usually heals within 2 to 3 weeks. With appropriate treatment, lesions usually resolve after 7 to 10 days. The key to treating and preventing impetigo is practicing good personal hygiene and maintaining a clean environment.

Nonpharmacological Management

Nonpharmacological management of impetigo involves the use of solutions or substances to debride the impetiginized lesions and to expose the skin surfaces where the bacteria are present. Exudative impetigo lesions may benefit from drying compresses to remove thick crusts and desiccate (dry out) the lesions. Normal saline, plain tap water, or Burow's solution may be applied for 10 to 20 minutes, 3 to 4 times daily. Although the dehydrating effect of the compresses may help to improve the appearance of the skin lesions, disinfectant solutions are not particularly effective in treating the underlying condition.

Pharmacological Management

Pharmacological treatment of impetigo includes the use of both topical and oral antibiotics. Mild cases of non-bullous impetigo can be treated effectively with a topical antibiotic, combined with cleansing and debridement. One topical agent is mupirocin 2% cream or ointment (Bactroban) applied three times per day for 7 days. This is equivalent in efficacy to oral cephalexin. Washing with chlorhexidine (Hibiclens) is a valuable adjunct because of its bactericidal properties. The patient should be instructed to wash the affected skin areas with the bactericidal soap two to three times a day before the mupirocin cream is applied. Antibiotic creams and ointments containing neomycin may be used although neomycin can produce contact dermatitis in sensitive individuals. Sensitization usually develops after long-term use on denuded skin and is not recommended. In addition, OTC antibacterial ointments are typically too weak to kill streptococcal and staphylococcal infections, and using the ointment carelessly may actually spread the impetigo.

Another topical ointment belonging to the pleuro-mutilins antibiotic class is retapamulin (Altabax). It is specifically for impetigo caused by MRSA. Patients may be more willing to comply with this treatment because it only involves applying the ointment twice daily for 5 days. However, it is not intended for mucosal use.

Systemic antibiotics are indicated for impetigo when there are systemic symptoms such as fever or toxicity, if a large area of the skin is involved, or within the context of athletic teams or child-care or family clusters. Antibiotic therapy should cover *Staphylococcus aureus* and *Streptococcus pyogenes*. The prevalence of MRSA and macrolide-resistant *Streptococcus* are recent challenges. MRSA has been cited as being responsible for nearly 80% of all community-acquired staphylococcal skin and soft tissue infections. Penicillin therapy used to be the standard of care therapy for impetigo, but with the increasing challenge of drug resistance, this is no longer the treatment of choice. Rather, beta-lactamase–resistant antibiotics (cephalosporins, amoxicillin-clavulanate, cloxacillin, and dicloxacillin) are recommended. The drug of choice for oral antimicrobial therapy in children is cephalexin. If MRSA is suspected, the choice of antibiotic should be clindamycin, trimethoprim-sulfamethoxazole, or vancomycin. Empiric treatment depends on the prevalence and sensitivities of MRSA in the patient's geographical area. Patients with penicillin hypersensitivity should take erythromycin or clindamycin. Erythromycin, however, has not been shown to be superior to topical mupirocin cream. Because oral antibiotics have far more GI and systemic side effects than topical therapy, topical therapy is often preferred for mild to moderate infections.

Follow-up and Referral

The patient with an uncomplicated case of impetigo should be followed up in 10 days to 2 weeks after initiation of therapy. Patients who are toxic or have fever should be followed closely; consultation with or referral to a physician is recommended. Development of acute glomerulonephritis (acute nephritic syndrome) requires referral to a kidney specialist. Symptoms of this disease include the abrupt onset of proteinuria, hypertension, edema, azotemia, and red blood cells in the urine.

The majority of cases of both types of impetigo will resolve uneventfully after 10 days of treatment. Patients with recurrent impetigo should be tested for nasal carriage of *Staphylococcus aureus* bacteria with a culture of the anterior nares. If the culture is positive, treatment of the nares with topical mupirocin (Bactroban) is effective. Repeat culture should be done to confirm the patient's status. In the event of treatment failure, an infectious medicine consultation should be considered. Bullous impetigo typically resolves even without antibiotic treatment. Nonbullous impetigo generally has a good prognosis, although poststreptococcal glomerulonephritis is a possible complication of this infection.

Patient Education

The clinician plays a pivotal role in the treatment and prevention of this highly contagious skin infection through patient education and counseling. Good hand washing and personal hygiene are strongly recommended to reduce the likelihood of spread. The fingernails should be kept short so that there is less likelihood of spread to other areas of the body through self-inoculation.

Children and family members should be educated about the contagious nature of impetigo. They should be told to refrain from participation in any contact sport or activity that might spread the infection. Family members should not share personal effects such as towels, robes, razors, shavers, and so on. Bed linens should be washed with soap and hot water.

The patient should be instructed to gently clean the crusts from the lesions with antibacterial soap before applying mupirocin 2% cream or retapamulin. Nighttime application is also advised. If occlusive dressings are used, they should be discarded carefully to prevent spread of infection. If the patient is on oral antibiotics, the side effects and potential adverse reactions of the drug should be explained, as well as the importance of completing the course of antibiotic therapy to prevent the possible complication of streptococcal glomerulonephritis. Patients should be informed that good personal hygiene and cleanliness, along with prompt attention to skin trauma, will help to prevent future breakouts of impetigo. Patients should not visit hospitals or nursing homes until the infection is resolved. If MRSA is involved, patients should stay at home and not handle food until they have been on antibiotics for 24 hours.

■ FOLLICULITIS

Folliculitis is a superficial to deep skin infection of the hair follicles. Lesions can range from minute white-topped pustules in newborns to large, yellow-white tender pustules in adults. Bacteria infect the hair follicle at a superficial level, leading to erythematous papules and pustules. Although the main pathogens are gram-positive bacteria, occasional cases are caused by a fungus or by gram-negative bacilli. Folliculitis represents the start of a continuum of skin infections. Deeper infections (as complications of folliculitis) can include the furuncle (boil) or carbuncle (multiple boils), which are covered in depth elsewhere in this chapter.

Epidemiology and Causes

Folliculitis is often caused by bacteria; in particular, it is frequently caused by coagulase-negative *Staphylococcus* bacteria. Predisposing factors include diabetes, obesity, a chronic carrier state of *Staphylococci* (present in the nares, axillae, or perineum), poor hygiene, hyperimmunoglobulin E (Job's syndrome—a primary immunodeficiency disorder), exposure to chemicals and solvents (cutting oils), and chronic skin friction. However, folliculitis may have other etiologies as well. Gram-positive resident flora of the nasal mucosa and adjacent facial skin become suppressed by long-term oral antibiotic therapy and are replaced by gram-negative rods, namely *Klebsiella* and *Escherichia coli.* Thus, gram-negative folliculitis may develop in patients who are on long-term tetracycline therapy for acne or rosacea, as well as in older men who are suffering from seborrhea. Patients who have become colonized by gram-negative bacteria in the sebaceous follicles of the perioral and perinasal areas can become infected due to trauma (e.g., from shaving), resulting in a suppurative process within the hair follicle. This type of folliculitis is usually seen on the upper lip in men. In addition, antibiotic use also increases the risk of candidal folliculitis, due to clearance of the normal bacterial skin flora. Exposure to wet environments such as whirlpools or inadequately chlorinated pools, which contributes to *Pseudomonas aeruginosa* infection, also predisposes to folliculitis. In addition, chronic steroid use that compromises T-cell immunity contributes to folliculitis by *Candida albicans.*

Folliculitis most commonly occurs among middle-aged individuals (aged 40–60 years) and children, especially if they are immunocompromised or spend an extended amount of time in a prone position due to impaired mobility. Studies have found that folliculitis may be spread by fomite transmission. Intensive care units (ICUs) are the frequent origin of nosocomial outbreaks in the hospital setting. The higher incidence of folliculitis in the ICU is the result of trauma from invasive procedures performed on immunocompromised or severely ill patients. Impairment of host resistance increases a patient's risk of contracting folliculitis in the presence of virulent pathogens such as gram-negative coliform bacilli. In addition, the presence of *Malassezia furfur* (a yeast that is part of the normal skin flora in animals) has been seen among infected ICU patients. One study found the same fungus on the stethoscopes and patient care instruments of the ICU staff who had touched their pets from home.

Folliculitis may occur anywhere on the skin as a result of trauma or damage to the hair follicle from chronic irritation due to friction from clothing or blockage of the hair follicle. Occlusion of the skin with tight-fitting nylon clothing promotes infection, and symptoms may occur abruptly within 1 to 3 days. Occlusive therapy (plastic wrap) used for other diseases such as severe psoriasis allows for significant bacterial multiplication in a moist environment, which can also lead to folliculitis. Spread of bacterial infection to the surrounding skin may develop from exudative or transudative discharge from wounds, abscesses, or any type of draining lesion.

A form of sterile folliculitis called *eosinophilic folliculitis* (EF) was originally identified in an 8-month-old HIV-positive Japanese infant. On histological exam, the hair follicle in EF is invaded by eosinophils and lymphocytes. Clinically, it presents in patients with HIV as intensely pruritic papules and pustules that appear over the entire body. Successful treatment of EF with interferon-alpha 2b has been reported, but the management of this form of folliculitis requires hospitalization and patient isolation. The presence of HIV with EF lesions is a marker for advanced HIV disease, and death from opportunistic infection usually occurs within 6 months of the onset of cutaneous lesions.

Pathophysiology

Infection of the hair follicle with *Staphylococcus* or *Streptococcus* is marked by suppuration and liquefaction necrosis of the follicular base, thus termed a *pyodermal* infection. It is usually localized and results in abscess formation. Liquefaction necrosis develops when lytic enzymes released by polymorphonuclear leukocytes (PMNs) digest bacteria and cellular material. Thus, a competent immune system is required for such a response, as large numbers of PMNs are found in the central area of the abscess, along with necrotic debris. Because this inflammatory response is localized, however, folliculitis rarely causes systemic manifestations in the immunocompetent individual. Interestingly, HIV-positive patients do not display this neutrophilic response because they typically experience an eosinophilic perifollicular pustular folliculitis, as described previously.

Clinical Presentation
Subjective

Generally, the patient will present with a "bumpy rash," which can appear on any area of the body. The rash can be located on the hair follicles of the face, forehead, back of the earlobes, the neck, the shoulder, the buttocks, the torso, or the extremities. Usually, the rash is not accompanied by itching. Often there is no history of previous skin eruptions or of pertinent medical history such as diabetes. The patient is usually concerned about the cosmetic effect of the lesions. The patient may report a history of hot tub use or of borrowing a shaver or razor from a friend. The clinician should inquire about the onset, duration, and location(s) of the rash, its appearance, and whether purulent drainage was present. The patient should also be asked about any associated systemic symptoms of fever and chills.

Objective

The primary lesions in folliculitis are small pustules surrounded by 1 to 2 mm of erythema located over the pilosebaceous orifice or the ostium of the hair follicle. There is no involvement of the surrounding skin. The eyelids, face, scalp, and extremities are the most typical sites. A hair in the center of the pustule sometimes perforates the lesion. This presentation is a hallmark for diagnosis. The pustules resolve into red macules, which fade to leave postinflammatory hyperpigmented scars in susceptible persons. Folliculitis is usually asymptomatic, but it can be very pruritic and is sometimes accompanied by burning. During the physical exam, checking the vital signs, including the temperature, is important to help rule out systemic involvement. The practitioner should inspect the lesion for signs of inflammation and suppuration (erythema, swelling, pustules) and palpate the surface of the pustule for fluctuance. It is also important to palpate the adjacent lymph nodes.

Folliculitis is divided into two main types—*superficial folliculitis* and *deep folliculitis.* Follicular impetigo (Bockhart's impetigo) is a superficial form of folliculitis that presents as small, dome-shaped pustules that occur over the opening of the hair follicle. It is more common on the scalps of children. When follicular impetigo becomes chronic, it may lead to follicle destruction and consequent permanent patchy alopecia.

The distinctive forms of deep folliculitis include barber's itch, pseudofolliculitis barbae, and *Pseudomonas* folliculitis. In addition, newer diagnoses have been established based on the histological characteristic of the skin eruption, such as eosinophilic folliculitis (HIV-EF) and nosocomial folliculitis.

Barber's itch (sycosis barbae) is a chronic and recurrent staphylococcal infection of the hair follicles on the bearded area of the face in men (usually the upper lip). It is aggravated by shaving and is most commonly seen in black men. It is usually propagated by the autoinoculation of bacteria caused by shaving. A differential diagnosis of tinea barbae is similar to barber's itch, but the tinea infection is caused by a fungus. Pseudofolliculitis barbae, another differential diagnosis for sycosis barbae, is caused by hair in the beard area and posterior scalp and neck that curls toward the skin, causing an inflammatory reaction that can mimic folliculitis. It is more common in men of African American origin due to the curliness of their hair. This can become a chronic problem; the hair follicles involved can become infected with any variety of bacteria.

Pseudomonas folliculitis presents as follicular erythematous papules, pustules, or vesicles over the back, buttocks, and upper arms. Associated features include pruritus, malaise, low-grade fever, sore throat and eyes, and axillary lymphadenopathy. This type of folliculitis resolves spontaneously within 10 days.

Folliculitis decalvans is a rare disease that tends to occur in individuals who have coarse, bristly hair. The predisposing factors of this disease are still unknown. The infection begins as a localized area of follicular pustules or papules. Exudation or suppuration soon follows; as the crust accumulates, the hairs are shed. New follicles become involved at the periphery, while at the center the process eventually subsides, with scarring and permanent hair loss.

Hot tub folliculitis is caused by *Pseudomonas aeruginosa*. *P aeruginosa* is able to withstand temperatures of up to 107°F (41.6°C) and chlorine levels of up to 3 mg/L. The lesions of this variant of folliculitis are found on the trunk and lower extremities of patients who have a recent history of hot tub use. Superhydration of the stratum corneum softens this protective layer and allows the bacteria to cause infection.

There are documented cases of superficial actinic folliculitis characterized by recurrent skin eruptions occurring within 6 to 24 hours after sun exposure. Histologically, there is perivascular lymphocytic infiltration and intrafollicular accumulation of neutrophils in the upper infundibulum of the follicle; these findings indicate the presence of inflammatory response and a suppurative process.

Diagnostic Reasoning
Diagnostic Tests

A Gram stain and culture of purulent discharge is obtained by rupturing a pustule and getting samples of the exudate. The culture is useful to distinguish *staphylococcal* infections from other bacterial or fungal infections, as well as from epidermal and pilar cysts that are sterile lesions. The Gram stain is usually positive for clusters of gram-positive cocci *(S aureus)* along with a large number of PMNs. With deeper forms of folliculitis, the presence of systemic symptoms and positive blood culture require referral to a physician for hospitalization and IV antibiotics.

If fungal infection is suspected, a fungal culture or KOH microscopic exam is helpful; if results are positive, treatment should change to an antifungal agent.

Differential Diagnosis

Superficial folliculitis is differentiated from tinea barbae by using the KOH exam (see Advanced Assessment 7.1) of the affected hair or by a fungal culture. Acne vulgaris and bullous impetigo may occasionally mimic folliculitis, but the patient's age (i.e., nonadolescent) and the absence of comedones (blackheads or whiteheads) suggests a diagnosis of folliculitis. The lesions of bullous impetigo are usually larger and rupture easily, and the exudate is serous, not purulent. About 50% of HIV-infected persons with scabies have coexistent *S aureus* folliculitis.

Occasionally, follicular lesions extend more deeply, forming abscesses. Rarely, follicles covering an area several centimeters across become infected, forming large violaceous plaques. The plaque may be studded with pustules and have deep sinus tracts connecting infected follicles. Rarely, an abscess of the muscles (pyomyositis) may occur due to extension of the infectious process.

Management

Patients rarely consult a health-care provider for this minor problem except for infections that become recurrent and persistent. The goal of treatment of superficial and deep folliculitis is to make the skin inhospitable to pathogens. This includes both nonpharmacological and pharmacological approaches.

Gentle cleansing by the simple method of washing the skin twice a day with antibacterial soap (e.g., Lever 2000, Safeguard, Dial) is as important as prescription antibacterial medicines. Large pustular lesions with necrotic areas should first be cleansed with a weak soap solution, followed by soaking of (or the use of compresses on) the affected skin with saline or aluminum subacetate twice daily. When the skin is softened, the clinician can gently open the large pustules and trim away necrotic tissue. A triple antibiotic ointment (containing polymyxin B, bacitracin, and neomycin) or simply mupirocin (Bactroban) 2% can be effective when applied 2 to 4 times per day for 10 days. Clearance of nasal colonization of *S aureus* by mupirocin treatment twice daily for 5 days has been shown to reduce significantly the incidence of recurrent folliculitis. Systemic antistaphylococcal antibiotics may be ordered if the infection is resistant to local treatment or if the scalp is involved. Usually, however, systemic antibiotics are not helpful or advantageous over topical treatments. See Drugs Commonly Prescribed 7.4 for common drugs to use for folliculitis.

Follow-up and Referral

A patient who does not respond to therapy should be evaluated for possible diabetes mellitus or for chronic

carriage (in the nares, axillae, or perineum) of *S aureus*. Cultures of the anterior nares, axillae, and perineum are recommended. Topical mupirocin 2% (Bactroban) should be applied twice daily for 5 to 7 days to the sites that yielded a positive culture. Because most strains of MRSA are resistant to topical mupirocin, in cases of MRSA colonization, Altabax should be applied twice daily for 2 weeks.

More severe forms of folliculitis and rare skin eruptions such as HIV-EF should be referred to the physician.

Drugs Commonly Prescribed 7.4   Folliculitis, Acne, and Rosacea

Drug	Indication	Adverse Reactions and Prescribing Considerations
Topical		
mupirocin (Bactroban) 2% ointment or cream	Folliculitis	Consider for secondarily infected skin lesions.
azelaic acid (Azelex) cream 20%	Acne vulgaris and inflammatory Rosacea	Both bacteriostatic and bactericidal. Watch for hypopigmentation on darker-skinned patients. Wash hands after use.
sulfacetamide (Rosula) gel, wash, and cream	Acne vulgaris, rosacea, and seborrheic dermatitis	Avoid mucous membranes.
benzoyl peroxide Benzac-W 2.5%, 5%, 10% Benzac-W Wash 5%, 10%	First-line therapy for acne	2.5% as effective as 10% and less irritating. Use water-based rather than alcohol-based.
metronidazole (MetroGel 1%)	Rosacea	Will not cure rosacea but reduces inflammatory lesions.
Topical Antibiotics		
clindamycin 1% solution, lotion, gel, pledget	Acne vulgaris, rosacea	Not used alone due to antibiotic resistance. Lotion less irritating. May cause diarrhea. Avoid in patients with colitis.
Combination Topical Therapy		
clindamycin + benzoyl peroxide (BenzaClin) erythromycin + benzoyl peroxide (Benzamycin)	Acne vulgaris, rosacea Acne vulgaris, rosacea	Adults only; may bleach fabrics, avoid eyes, mucous membranes. Discontinue use if significant diarrhea occurs. Transient skin discoloration with PABA sunscreens. Caution in pregnant or breastfeeding women.
Topical Retinoids		All Pregnancy Category C unless otherwise stated.
tretinoin 0.05% cream (Renova)	Acne vulgaris	Not recommended for children younger than 10 years. Do not use on sunburned skin.
tretinoin (Retin-A) cream, gel, liquid	Acne vulgaris	Allow effects of other topical agents to subside before using.
tazarotene (Tazorac)	First-line therapy for all acne variants	0.1% strength. Women of childbearing potential, begin therapy during menses.
adapalene (Differin)	First-line therapy for all acne variants	Less sun sensitivity than Retin-A.
isotretinoin (Amnesteem)	Severe recalcitrant nodular acne or rosacea unresponsive to conventional therapy (even antibiotics)	Pregnancy Category X, must register patients in iPLEDGE program, avoid sun, monitor lipids, glucose, CBC, liver enzymes. Take with meals.

Drugs Commonly Prescribed 7.4   Folliculitis, Acne, and Rosacea—cont'd

Drug	Indication	Adverse Reactions and Prescribing Considerations
Combination Retinoid + Antibacterial		
adapalene plus benzoyl peroxide (Epiduo gel)	Acne vulgaris	Good for teenage boys because they may be more likely to use just one topical. Apply a thin film once daily after washing.
Systemic Therapies Antibiotics		
minocycline (Minocin)	Severe acne, rosacea	Take on an empty stomach with fluids.
doxycycline (Vibramycin)	Severe acne, rosacea	Monitor blood, renal, and hepatic function in long-term use. Sub-antibacterial dose doxycycline (Oracea 40 mg) is a good choice in inflammatory acne.
Hormonal Therapy		
norgestimate/ethinyl estradiol (Ortho Tri-Cyclen)	Birth control pills (BCP) for moderate acne vulgaris in females older than 15 years of age.	See Chapter 14 for all the precautions that accompany someone taking BCP.
norethindrone acetate/ethinyl estradiol (Estrostep)	BCP as above	As above
drospirenone + ethinyl estradiol (Yaz)	BCP as above	As above
Other		
ketoconazole (Nizoral) tablets	Fungal forms of folliculitis	Monitor hepatic function before and during therapy. Check the numerous drug interaction warnings.

Systemic IV antibiotics may be necessary. Referral is in order for patients with recurrent or persistent infections that do not respond to the treatment regimen.

Patient Education

The clinician should emphasize to the patient that good hygiene is essential in treating this condition. Good hand washing technique is the best approach in preventing the spread of folliculitis. Patients who are prone to folliculitis can be advised to use an antibacterial soap and to wash the affected areas twice a day with antibacterial soaps before applying topical agents. Patients should also be informed that any source of friction can predispose them to a recurrence of folliculitis.

In hospitals (especially the ICU), an emphasis on proper hand washing and proper disposal of cleaning supplies can help prevent the spread of bacteria on fomites.

Men who are prone to recurrent sycosis barbae should be advised to grow a beard (if possible) during treatment to allow complete healing. A preventive approach is the best treatment for this condition. When shaving is resumed, an electric shaver may cause fewer breaks in the skin than a razor. Patients should be cautioned to avoid borrowing or using old razor blades when shaving infected areas.

■ FURUNCLES AND CARBUNCLES

A *furuncle (boil)* is a deep bacterial infection of a hair follicle with abscess formation. Furuncles are caused almost exclusively by gram-positive *Staphylococcus aureus.* Furuncles are extremely tender to touch and appear a bright red color. The most common locations for furuncles are the scalp, neck, axilla, buttocks, groin, and thighs. Furuncles frequently become fluctuant. With the application of warm compresses, most furuncles drain pus and resolve spontaneously.

A *carbuncle* is a large, multiloculated abscess that is made up of multiple furuncles in a contiguous area. Carbuncles, which are less common than furuncles, appear as large, red, painful lumps on the skin, with multiple follicular openings. Some carbuncles can be quite large—up to 10 cm in size. Eventually, a carbuncle will spontaneously drain pus.

Epidemiology and Causes

Furuncles and carbuncles are usually caused by *S aureus* and rarely by other pathogens. In some patients, especially the immunocompromised, infection can be due to MRSA. Conditions predisposing patients to formation of furuncles and carbuncles include diabetes mellitus, poor hygiene, incarceration, obesity, and immune system defects. Chronic staphylococcal carriage in the anterior nares, axilla, and perineum also increase the risk of infection and should be explored in cases of recurrent infections. Favorable environmental conditions that predispose the individual to furuncle and carbuncle formation include areas of moisture, friction, or occluded skin. Any area of skin that is subject to friction, such as the axilla, buttocks, groin, or thighs, is at increased risk of infection.

Pathophysiology

Both furuncles and carbuncles evolve from superficially infected hair follicles (folliculitis), mediated primarily by *S aureus*. Thus, all factors that contribute to folliculitis also predispose to furunculosis and carbuncle formation. As this superficial infection extends along the hair shaft, a small, painful inflammatory nodule is formed at the follicular base that is termed a *furuncle*. Eventually, a series of abscesses form along the hair shaft involving dermal and subcutaneous layers, ultimately coalescing into a fluctuant, subcutaneous mass that develops a soft, pointed necrotic center. When the furuncle ruptures, it results in the extrusion of pus and a necrotic plug at the entrance to the follicle. A small opening or cavitation remains that eventually heals with scarring. Thus, the affected hair follicle is destroyed and does not regenerate, resulting in destruction of the hair itself.

Carbuncles ("boils") undergo a similar process, except on a larger scale. Carbuncles are made up of several furuncles that form into a large, multiloculated abscess with multiple follicular openings that eventually drain pus. Carbuncles are significantly larger than furuncles, typically involving deeper skin layers. They are more likely to occur on thicker skin, in areas such as the nape of the neck and upper back. A systemic response including fever resulting from the production of pyogenic cytokines is more common with carbuncle formation than furunculosis.

Certain risk factors are particularly associated with furunculosis and carbuncle formation. Obesity results in thick skinfolds that are closely approximated. This creates a moist environment in which bacteria are prone to reproduce. Impaired immune function from chronic steroid use, underlying systemic disease such as HIV or diabetes mellitus, or impaired neutrophil function also predispose to this condition. In particular, the presence of a bacterial virulence factor known as the Panton-Valentine leukocidin in certain strains of *S aureus* has been associated with particularly aggressive skin infections.

Clinical Presentation

Subjective

The typical patient will complain of a hot and tender, bright red bump or "boil" of several days' duration that is getting larger. Some furuncles will "come to a head" or become fluctuant and will drain spontaneously on their own. Some patients will report a history of manipulation of the furuncle or carbuncle, either by squeezing it or by puncturing it with a heated needle. Some patients will report a past history of boils and other skin infections.

Objective

Both furuncles and carbuncles are extremely tender to touch and are a bright red color. A furuncle initially appears as a small (0.5–1 cm), red, indurated nodule. As the nodule grows in size, it starts to develop a yellow-colored central plug. It begins to appear conical, with a central "nipple" that is covered by thinning skin. The pus, which is a yellow to green color, gives the "nipple" its characteristic color. Most furuncles eventually spontaneously rupture and drain pus, which hastens their resolution. As the necrotic material and pus are discharged, a small cavitation is left that heals with minimal scarring. Carbuncles initially appear as multiple furuncles that develop into a large, erythematous lump that eventually starts to drain pus from multiple follicular openings. Patients with darker skin can have permanent hyperpigmentation changes as a result of severe inflammation.

Diagnostic Reasoning

Diagnostic Tests

Although most cases of furuncles and carbuncles are caused by *S aureus*, a culture of the fluctuant lesion is still recommended. Occasional cases of MRSA are sometimes found. A CBC with differential is not necessary unless the patient has a severe case with an underlying disease such as diabetes or shows systemic symptoms such as fever.

No subsequent testing is necessary unless a patient is a staphylococcal carrier. The nares and anogenital region should be recultured after treatment with topical mupirocin (Bactroban) is finished. In resistant cases where no response is seen after 1 week of therapy, a repeat culture should be done.

Differential Diagnosis

Some skin conditions to consider in the differential diagnosis of furuncles include an epidermal inclusion cyst that is acutely inflamed. Epidermal inclusion cysts are usually located in areas of the body where there is thicker skin and a large amount of sebaceous glands, such as on the back and upper shoulders. The patient with an epidermal inclusion cyst will report a history of the cyst on the same site for months to years. In contrast, furuncles are an acute process, taking only several days to form. Another characteristic of an epidermal inclusion cyst is a cheesy white discharge with a strong odor that is present when it is expressed. A furuncle or carbuncle will have a purulent yellow to green-colored discharge when it ruptures.

Another differential diagnosis for a furuncle is a deep fungal infection of the soft tissue called *sporotrichosis*. It is more common in gardeners and other agricultural workers and is usually seen on the hands or arms. It is caused by injury from a thorn or wood splinter that has been contaminated with the common soil fungus *Sporothrix schenckii*. Because it is usually asymptomatic, patients tend to ignore it.

If the furuncle or carbuncle is located on the axilla, a differential diagnosis to consider is hidradenitis suppurativa. The lesions of hidradenitis suppurativa are also extremely tender and inflamed. Patients with this condition report a chronic history of recurrent infection in the axilla, groin, or anal region. It is a chronic disease of the apocrine glands of the axilla and groin and is associated with severe hypertrophic scarring and sinus tracts, which are not seen in furuncles or carbuncles. The classic finding in hidradenitis suppurativa that would tend to differentiate it from a furuncle or carbuncle are the numerous hypertrophic scars and sinus tracts that are found on the affected skin.

Management

Carbuncles usually must drain before healing will take place, and this usually occurs spontaneously within 2 weeks. Application of warm compresses will promote the localization and spontaneous rupture and drainage of a furuncle. No treatment with systemic antibiotics is necessary for a healthy host if no surrounding cellulitis is present. Treatment with topical antibiotics with good gram-positive coverage (e.g., mupirocin [Bactroban] or neomycin–polymyxin B [Neosporin]), applied twice per day until resolution, is satisfactory in those cases.

For furuncles or carbuncles on an immunocompromised patient (or one who is at risk for bacteremia because of a preexisting condition), systemic antibiotics are always mandatory and physician referral is recommended. In addition, incision and drainage will speed up resolution of the infection. Preexisting conditions such as diabetes or chronic steroid use (or any condition affecting the immune system) predispose a patient to more complications. These patients should be monitored very closely or referred to a physician. A furuncle (especially if it is located on the upper lip or the central area of the face) or a carbuncle located on the neck, face, or scalp should be treated with physician consultation or referred to a physician for management. Because of its proximity to the cavernous sinus, a furuncle located on the central face can spread via the venous drainage to the cavernous sinus and result in cavernous sinus thrombosis or meningitis. An occasional patient with furuncles or carbuncles will have bacteremia as a complication, with possible hematogenous spread to the heart valves (endocarditis), kidneys (perinephric abscess), joints, spine, and long bones (osteomyelitis).

If a furuncle has not come to a head by the time the patient is seen, the patient should be instructed to apply warm compresses two to three times per day until it becomes fluctuant. Systemic antibiotics are often used to treat and hasten the resolution of furunculosis. However, randomized controlled trials have failed to consistently show the benefit of such treatment. In theory, however, systemic antibiotics should lessen the risk of bacteremia. Fluctuant furuncles are ideally treated with incision and drainage. A sterile 18-gauge needle can be used to puncture the thin skin on top of a small furuncle to allow for adequate drainage of pus. For larger furuncles that are fluctuant, incision and drainage is indicated. The cavity formed by the furuncle should be packed with iodoform or petroleum jelly (Vaseline)–impregnated gauze. After a furuncle has been incised, the patient should be instructed to use warm compresses twice daily to hasten the drainage of pus.

Carbuncles frequently need incision and drainage as well to aid in recovery. Systemic antibiotics and physician referral are always indicated for the treatment of carbuncles. Systemic antibiotics with adequate gram-positive bacterial coverage (except for MRSA) include dicloxacillin, cephalexin, or amoxicillin-clavulanate. For patients with penicillin allergies, erythromycin, clindamycin, clarithromycin, or azithromycin may be used. Many strains of community-acquired MRSA are susceptible to trimethoprim-sulfamethoxazole (Bactrim) plus rifampin, clindamycin, doxycycline, or minocycline. However, particularly aggressive or extensive infections with MRSA or Panton-Valentine leukocidin–expressing strains of *Staphylococcus* may require inpatient IV antibiotic therapy (e.g., vancomycin) to ensure adequate treatment. Linezolid is also used for the treatment of MRSA. However, this antibiotic is typically used only under close physician supervision, given its potential for inducing thrombocytopenia, anemia, and neutropenia. Thus, antibiotic susceptibility testing is critical in these cases to most appropriately direct therapy.

If a patient has a history of frequent infections, a search for staphylococcal carriage is recommended. Cultures should be taken from the patient's nares, the perineum, and the anogenital region. If a patient is found to be a *Staphylococcus aureus* carrier, a daily shower with an antibacterial or benzoyl peroxide soap is recommended. Mupirocin ointment (Bactroban) should be applied three times per day to the anatomical sites where *S aureus* was cultured (nares, body folds, perineum, anogenital region) for 1 week. A repeat culture should be done to document clearance of the bacteria. This program will eliminate the staphylococcal carrier state and reduce the incidence of recurrence. There is some evidence that vitamin C supplementation (1 g per day for 4–6 weeks) may also help prevent recurrent skin infection in persons with impaired neutrophil function.

Follow-up and Referral

The patient should be seen for initial follow-up within a few days to 1 week to monitor response to therapy, compliance with treatment, and any adverse reactions. Subsequent visits can be scheduled in 7 to 10 days to monitor for continuing progress and resolution of the lesions. For carbuncles or multiple furuncles on immunocompromised patients (or patients at risk for bacteremia because of preexisting disease), a physician referral is recommended.

In addition, if a patient has systemic signs such as fever or appears toxic, physician consultation or referral is recommended. These patients frequently need multiple laboratory tests, including blood cultures, which can be done in a hospital setting, in addition to treatment with parenteral antibiotics.

Patient Education

The patient should be warned not to pop, squeeze, or to manipulate furuncles in any way, especially those that are located on the mid to upper lip or near the border of the nasolabial folds because of the risk of cavernous sinus thrombosis, which is sometimes fatal.

■ CELLULITIS

Cellulitis is a bacterial infection of the skin involving both the dermis and subcutaneous tissue, which in certain cases may result in death. Most cases of cellulitis are caused by group A beta-hemolytic *Streptococcus* or by *Staphylococcus aureus* (gram-positive bacteria). Less common bacteria that can cause cellulitis include *Haemophilus influenzae* (more common in children), *Eikenella corrodens* (human bites), *Pasteurella multocida* (cat bites), *Capnocytophaga canimorsus* (dog bites), and the *Vibrio* species (seawater-exposed injuries).

The typical lesion of cellulitis is a wide, diffuse area of erythematous skin that is warm and tender to palpation. Infection is occasionally accompanied by severe edema. Systemic symptoms such as fever, chills, and malaise may accompany some cases as well. A cellulitic infection can occasionally result in the loss of a limb.

Cellulitis may become a life-threatening event that is heralded by shock, hypotension, and toxicity. Toxic shock syndrome (TSS) and multiple organ failure resulting from both streptococcal and staphylococcal infections have been reported. The clinician must learn to differentiate between a severe case of cellulitis that is potentially life-threatening and an uncomplicated case that can be treated on an outpatient basis. Special types of cellulitis that have potentially serious consequences discussed in this chapter include erysipelas, necrotizing fasciitis, and periorbital cellulitis (see Table 7.4). Severe cases of cellulitis, such as necrotizing fasciitis, must be treated with surgical debridement in addition to parenteral antibiotics to stop the spread of rapid tissue destruction; these patients require hospitalization. Periorbital cellulitis, an emergent condition, should also be treated aggressively with parenteral antibiotics and hospitalization

to prevent permanent vision loss and extension of infection into deep cranial structures.

Epidemiology and Causes

There is usually an obvious portal of entry into the skin or mucous membranes, such as an insect bite or a wound, although in some cases there is no obvious point of entry (this is more common with recurrent cellulitis). Cellulitis may occur at any age, but some organisms are more common in certain age-groups. *Haemophilus influenzae* type B (Hib) infections are more common in children. In adults and elderly patients, *S aureus* and *Streptococcus pyogenes* are more common. In patients with diabetes mellitus or who are otherwise immunocompromised, unusual bacterial pathogens may include *Escherichia coli* and other enteric species *(Enterobacter)*, as well as *Proteus mirabilis, Pseudomonas aeruginosa, Acinetobacter, Mycobacterium fortuitum,* and *Cryptococcus neoformans.*

Any break on the skin or mucous membranes is a potential portal of entry for bacterial pathogens. Skin breaks can be caused by surgical incisions, skin tears and wounds, trauma, insect bites or stings, and animal or human bites. Preexisting skin conditions such as stasis ulcers, dermatitides (eczema, psoriasis, contact dermatitis), viral skin infections (herpes simplex, herpes zoster, or varicella-zoster), superficial bacterial infections (acne, folliculitis), and bullous diseases (bullous pemphigoid, pemphigus vulgaris, burns) all have the potential for secondary bacterial infection. The likelihood and severity of cellulitis infection is affected by three important factors: (1) virulence of the pathogen, (2) host immune status, and (3) depth of infection.

Risk factors that predispose an individual to cellulitis include conditions that affect cellular immunity and lymphatic drainage:

- Diabetes mellitus
- Lymphatic blockage
- History of recurrent cellulitis
- Postmastectomy and postsaphenous vein grafting
- HIV infection and AIDS
- Chronic steroid use
- Cancer chemotherapy
- Drug or alcohol abuse
- Peripheral vascular disease

Pathophysiology

The skin and subcutaneous tissue respond to bacterial invasion with an acute inflammatory process. An increase in vascular permeability of the microcirculation of the skin allows protein-rich fluids to leak into the interstitial tissue. This results in tissue edema, which may become chronic in recurrent cellulitis. Agents that are released into the tissue increasing vascular permeability include histamine, cytokines, platelet-activating factor, bradykinin, complement proteins, and arachidonic acid

Table 7.4	Types of Cellulitis
Erysipelas	Erysipelas is a streptococcal infection of the superficial layers of skin that does not involve the subcutaneous layers, unlike more typical cellulitis. An older name for erysipelas is "St. Anthony's fire." Despite the superficial nature of this infection, erysipelas should not be taken lightly, because it can be fatal if it is not treated promptly (especially in the very young and the elderly). Before the advent of antibiotics, a high rate of fatality was associated with this infection. Most cases of erysipelas are caused by group A beta-hemolytic *Streptococcus pyogenes*. Erysipelas is sometimes seen after an episode of strep throat. The most common sites of involvement are the face (especially the cheeks) and the lower legs. Patients usually have systemic symptoms such as high fever, chills, and malaise. Erysipelas on the face first appears as a bright red lesion by the nares that can spread rapidly within a few hours to days. An enlarging shiny, bright red, indurated plaque develops that is very warm to touch and has very sharp and distinct borders, as opposed to cellulitis, which has more diffused, flat borders. The affected skin appears shiny because of the edema from the infection.
Necrotizing Fasciitis	The hallmark of this infection is its rapid progression and the severity of the symptoms. The progress of the infection is measured in terms of hours instead of days, and the border can be seen to literally spread in just a few hours. This infection is caused by "flesh-eating bacteria," and loss of life or limb is a potential complication. Most cases of necrotizing fasciitis are caused by group A *Streptococcus* pyogenes, although several different kinds of bacteria have been implicated in these rapidly progressive infections, including *Staphylococcus aureus*, *Clostridium perfringens*, *Bacteroides fragilis*, and *Aeromonas hydrophila*. During the early phase of the infection, the lesion appears as a bright red color with edema that progresses to purpuric changes (indicated by purple color), including gangrene (indicated by black color). The patient will usually complain of severe pain at the affected site, which seems to be out of proportion to the appearance of the skin lesion. This pain is due to involvement of the fascia around the muscle and sometimes of the muscle itself (myositis). Pressure on the skin sometimes reveals crepitus due to gas production by the anaerobic bacteria *Clostridium perfringens*. Gangrene can present in a few hours, with hypotension and mental status changes regarded as particularly ominous signs.
Periorbital Cellulitis	Periorbital cellulitis is a potentially life-threatening form of cellulitis that should be treated as an emergent condition. The typical patient is a young child with erythema and edema over the affected periorbital area. The edema can be severe enough so that the entire affected side of the face is puffy. Symptoms include pain with certain eye movements because of inflamed extraocular muscles. Other symptoms include high fever, tachycardia, lethargy or mental status changes, and other systemic symptoms. On physical exam, the involved eye will lose the ability to move into certain quadrants (i.e., lateral or downward gaze) and will have an abnormal exam of cranial nerves III, IV, and VI (EOMs).

metabolites, including leukotrienes and prostaglandins. Vasodilation also occurs, giving cellulitis its characteristic bright red color and indistinct borders. In addition, during the cellular phase of inflammation, leukocytes accumulate at the site of injury and engulf particulate material such as bacteria, cellular debris, and antigen–antibody complexes. Engulfed bacteria and other cellular debris are digested inside phagolysosomes by potent hydrolytic enzymes. Interestingly, the bacterial burden in cellulitis may be low, except in cases where abscesses or skin ulcers are present.

The most predominant leukocyte during the cellular inflammatory phase is the polymorphonuclear leukocyte (neutrophil or PMN) and, to a lesser extent, basophils, mast cells, and platelets. PMNs express at least three types of granules containing proteolytic enzymes. Necrosis of normal tissue may occur during the inflammatory process due to these proteolytic enzymes, as well as reactive oxygen metabolites. Some aggressive cases of cellulitis may progress to TSS in which certain strains of *Staphylococcus* and *Streptococcus* release toxins that stimulate a massive release of inflammatory cytokines. This in turn can result in shock, multiple organ failure, and ultimately death if untreated. In addition, bacterial exotoxins have been shown to potentiate hypersensitivity responses to fungal antigens such as *Trichophyton*, the primary agent involved in tinea pedis or "athlete's foot" infection. Such responses have been shown to contribute to the pathogenesis of cellulitis in certain individuals.

Clinical Presentation

Subjective

The typical adult patient with cellulitis will complain of a tender, warm, and erythematous area of skin that is usually located on the face, neck, or extremities. The patient will usually report a history of a precipitating condition such as an insect bite or a small cut that "got infected." The patient might already have a preexisting skin condition such as acne, tinea pedis, or chronic eczema with breaks in the skin that can become the portal of entry for bacteria, although at times this is not apparent to the patient. In cases of recurrent cellulitis of the lower leg, the patient will frequently deny any trauma or injury but will report a history of repeated infections on the same leg. The size of involvement can vary from a few centimeters to a larger area, such as an entire limb. The patient will report a history of the lesion or plaque getting progressively larger over several days, but in the case of necrotizing fasciitis, the border will literally be seen to spread in just a few hours. Some patients will complain of tender and enlarged lymph nodes near the affected area. Patients with more severe cases of cellulitis or with special types such as necrotizing fasciitis, erysipelas, and periorbital cellulitis are more likely to complain of systemic symptoms such as fever and chills, lethargy, and malaise.

Objective

In adults, the lower leg is usually the most common site of infection. In cases of lower extremity cellulitis, the clinician should search for signs of tinea pedis. The clinician should look for areas of macerated or peeling skin on the interdigital area of the toes. A chronic tinea pedis ("athlete's foot") infection can become the point of entry for bacteria. In children, and occasionally in adults, the cheeks and the periorbital area are more common sites of involvement. In lighter-skinned patients, the area of skin that is infected will have a bright red color that is warm and tender to touch. In darker-skinned patients, the color will be a darker red. Sometimes extensive edema will be present, especially if an arm or leg is involved.

The red borders seen in cellulitis are flat and diffused, compared with the distinct raised border seen on an erysipelas infection. Serious signs of systemic toxicity to look for include high fever, hypotension, tachycardia, marked leukocytosis, and associated lymphangitis. If these signs are present, the patient must be treated aggressively with hospitalization and parenteral antibiotics. Referral to a physician is recommended for severe or special cases of cellulitis.

Diagnostic Reasoning

Diagnostic Tests

Most cases of mild to moderate cellulitis are diagnosed by clinical presentation and history. In the majority of cases of acute cellulitis, there is usually no discharge or obvious wound present; therefore, obtaining cultures is very difficult. If an open wound or purulent discharge is present, a culture and Gram stain should be obtained. For patients who appear ill or have systemic symptoms such as fever, a CBC and consultation with a physician is necessary. If periorbital cellulitis is suspected (swelling and redness of eyelids, limited extraocular movements [EOMs], fever), testing for EOMs should be done, along with other tests for cranial nerve function. Leukocytosis is seen in periorbital cellulitis, as well as in necrotizing fasciitis and erysipelas.

Differential Diagnosis

The site of the infection helps to guide the clinician in searching for a differential diagnosis. If a lower limb is affected, deep vein thrombosis (DVT) should be considered. It may be difficult to make the distinction between DVT and cellulitis. DVT presents as a swollen and warm limb with erythema that is tender to touch and can be very similar in presentation to acute cellulitis. A history of recent surgery, bedrest, or prolonged immobility points more toward DVT; however, DVT can occur after cellulitis, although rarely. There are usually no systemic symptoms such as fever associated with DVT. If fever is present, it points more toward the presence of cellulitis. If crepitus is noted on palpation or if violaceous bullae and intense pain are present, the clinician should rule out necrotizing fasciitis. Serious systemic symptoms that point to severe infection include hypotension, lethargy (or any change in mental status), nausea and vomiting, severe pain (points to possible fascial involvement), and a toxic appearance. If these signs are present, immediate consultation with a physician or referral to the emergency department is necessary.

Management

Treatment of cellulitis should take into consideration several factors: the severity of the infection, the site of the infection, the presence of underlying disease, and the virulence of the pathogen. Patients with diabetes are known to have a higher incidence of complications from skin infections because of chronic high levels of glucose that adversely affect the immune system and the microcirculation. Patients who are under long-term treatment with steroids or chemotherapy are also at increased risk because of immune system depression. Previous surgical procedures, such as a mastectomy or saphenous vein grafts, predispose the affected limb to cellulitis because of defective lymphatic drainage. Some sites of the body, such as the hands, feet, and the face, must be treated more aggressively to prevent any potential loss of future function. Particular care must be taken with soft tissue infections of the hand because a compartment-like syndrome can ensue in addition to destruction of complex structures.

Human bite wounds are known to have a higher rate of infection because of the large amount of anaerobic bacteria present in the mouth. Because of increased vascularity, the face and neck areas are less likely to become infected than the hands and feet. Closed-fist injuries are more likely to become infected, probably because exposed tendons and tissue that become contaminated with oral flora retract back into the skin under anaerobic conditions and allow bacteria to proliferate. Cat bites (30%–50%) are more likely to become infected (with *Pasteurella multocida*) than human bites. To a lesser extent, some dog bites (only 5%) become infected with *P multocida* or *Capnocytophaga canimorsus.* The clinician must remember that any injury that occurs in salty or brackish water has potential for infection with *Vibrio* species of bacteria. Periorbital cellulitis is potentially life-threatening and should be regarded as an emergent condition. It is seen more commonly in children than in adults.

Although *Streptococcus* and *Staphylococcus* cause the majority of skin infections, it is still important to establish the specific etiology of any infection. If purulent discharge or an open wound is present, culture and Gram stain should be obtained. Because it is difficult to culture most cases of cellulitis, diagnosis is based mostly on clinical presentation. Empiric treatment for cellulitis must provide good coverage for both staphylococci and streptococci. Good choices for uncomplicated cases of cellulitis that are not associated with human or animal bites include dicloxacillin or cephalexin for 10 to 14 days.

Patients with severe penicillin allergy are prescribed erythromycin. Infected human and animal (cat or dog) bites are best treated with amoxicillin–clavulanic acid (Augmentin) for at least 2 weeks. Physician consultation or referral is recommended in complicated cases of cellulitis. Prophylaxis (not treatment) for fresh, uncomplicated human and animal bites (less than 6 hours old) is amoxicillin–clavulanic acid for 3 to 5 days.

Management of cellulitis infection of the lower extremities requires bedrest (with bathroom privileges) and elevation of the infected leg. Patients who are at increased risk of thrombus formation should be referred to the physician for possible anticoagulation therapy.

Erysipelas is treated in the hospital with parenteral antibiotics. Necrotizing fasciitis must be treated aggressively in the hospital with parenteral antibiotics, surgical debridement, and fluid replacement.

Patients with underlying disease such as diabetes, neuropathy, arterial insufficiency, lymphatic drainage abnormalities, intermittent claudication, and a history of recent trauma on the same leg are more prone to complications and infection with unusual bacterial pathogens (gram-negative bacteria, anaerobes) and must be treated more aggressively. These cases frequently require referral and consideration for hospitalization. Unusual pathogens that may cause cellulitis include *E coli, Klebsiella, Enterobacter,* and *Pseudomonas,* which are more common in patients with impaired immune systems.

Cellulitis of vital structures such as the hand, foot, or face requires close follow-up to monitor for possible complications. Patients who are at higher risk for complications, including those with severe cellulitis and associated crush injuries, should be referred to a physician. Other patients who have a higher risk of complications include patients with preexisting diseases or conditions that affect the immune system such as diabetes, AIDS, immunosuppression, chronic steroid or IV drug use, alcoholism, a history of arterial insufficiency, and chemotherapy.

Patients who are suspected of having a complicated case of cellulitis such as possible bacteremia (fever, chills) or urgent cases such as periorbital cellulitis, necrotizing fasciitis, or erysipelas need immediate consultation with a physician or referral to the emergency department. The clinician should not rely solely on certain laboratory results such as leukocytosis before considering the seriousness of cellulitis infection. Clinical presentation and symptoms are more helpful in guiding the management of cellulitis than any laboratory test result.

For oral therapy, cefuroxime (Ceftin) can be used when *Haemophilus influenzae* is suspected. Azithromycin or clarithromycin is preferred as a macrolide over erythromycin for penicillin-allergic patients if *Haemophilus* flu is suspected. If gram-negative microorganisms are suspected, fluoroquinolones such as levofloxacin, for complicated skin infections, are typically chosen for adult patients. Clindamycin may be added to extend the spectrum of gram-positive coverage. Importantly, however, *Clostridium difficile* (C diff) colitis is particularly associated with clindamycin usage. *Vibrio* infections from seawater-associated injuries are best treated with tetracyclines, whereas cellulitis related to freshwater injuries must cover *Aeromonas* infection and include a fluoroquinolone such as ciprofloxacin combined with cefazolin. Diabetics are typically treated with Augmentin, although this may produce significant GI effects such as loose stools. Other broad-based regimens for hospitalized patients include clindamycin plus ceftriaxone, along with a fluoroquinolone. If tinea pedis infection is concurrent with cellulitis, treatment for this must be initiated using terbinafine or itraconazole (see previous section on dermatophytoses). For information on community-acquired MRSA infection, refer back to the discussion under Furuncles and Carbuncles regarding selected oral agents such as Bactrim. For significant MRSA infection, vancomycin can be used.

Follow-up and Referral

Most cases of uncomplicated cellulitis resolve with adequate antibiotic treatment. Improvement is usually obvious within 48 hours, although some cases might take 72 hours before some improvement is seen. If the patient is responding to treatment, follow-up can be done on an outpatient basis. Recurrent infections of cellulitis on a lower extremity can result in a chronic nonpitting edema. (The patient should be advised of this potential complication.) Diabetic patients should be advised to adhere to dietary and lifestyle changes (in addition to medication) to control levels of blood glucose. Good diabetic control is associated with fewer and less serious complications, including potential vascular, kidney, and eye damage.

Initial follow-up for cellulitis should be done within 48 hours or earlier for sicker patients. Improvement in signs and symptoms should be seen, including a decrease in swelling, erythema, and pain of the affected area. The borders of erythema should be receding and getting smaller. The clinician can use a marking pen (with the patient's permission) to mark some of the borders during the initial visit: This will make any changes in size easier to notice. If the patient's response is satisfactory, the next follow-up visit is usually done in 1 week (or sooner, if closer follow-up is necessary). Thereafter, the patient can be seen on a weekly basis until the cellulitis is resolved.

If the patient does not respond to treatment with oral antibiotics after 48 to 72 hours or starts to look toxic, a CBC and consultation with a physician (or referral to the emergency department) is necessary.

Patient Education

The clinician should instruct the patient to call his or her health-care provider if the infection worsens or if fever persists despite antibiotic treatment for at least 48 hours. The patient should also call the office in 3 days to report progress of simple cellulitis infection. The patient should be advised to elevate the affected limb as much as possible to decrease swelling. If the patient has chronic tinea pedis ("athlete's foot"), an OTC antifungal powder or spray should be used daily to prevent a recurrence of secondary infection with bacteria.

VIRAL INFECTIONS

■ WARTS

Warts (verruca vulgaris, plantar warts, flat warts) are skin tumors formed by infected keratinocytes, usually initiated by the human papillomavirus (HPV). Warts are identified based on their morphology (flat, mosaic, digitate, or filiform) and location on the body (e.g., the plantar, anogenital, and palmar areas).

Epidemiology and Causes

HPV is a small, double-stranded DNA virus that infects epithelial cells and causes hyperproliferation of these cells. HPV is species specific and affects only humans, with a particular tropism for epithelial cells and the mucous membranes. There are at least 150 genetically distinct human papillomaviruses (including HPV subunits). HPV type 1 typically causes plantar warts,

whereas types 6 and 11 cause anogenital warts. Certain HPV serotypes are also associated with anogenital malignancies, including cervical intraepithelial neoplasia and invasive cervical cancers. Oncogenicity of HPV appears to be determined by the viral gene products E6 and E7 proteins, which are necessary for host cell immortalization. HPV types 6 and 11 are considered either inactive or weakly capable of transformation, whereas E6 and E7 proteins in HPV types 16 and 18 are capable of producing progressive squamous epithelial neoplasia in experimental studies with mice.

In general, HPV and resultant warts can be transmitted by touch or by trauma to skin tissue such as from nail biting or shaving. Plantar warts occur at points of maximum pressure (e.g., at the heads of metatarsal bones and heels), as a thick painful callus forms in response to the pressure. In contrast, anogenital warts are usually sexually transmitted, but the route of transmission does not necessarily have to include penetrative intercourse (e.g., heavy petting, genital-to-genital contact). HPV enters through breaks in the skin or mucosa. Viral particles contained within skin cells serve as the vehicle for person-to-person transmission.

Pathophysiology

Warts (verruca vulgaris, plantar warts, flat warts) are skin tumors formed by infected keratinocytes, usually initiated by HPV infection. Infected keratinocytes form a mass that remains confined to the epidermis. A common misconception is that warts have roots. In reality, the underside of a wart is usually smooth and round. Although the wart appears to infiltrate the dermis and the subcutaneous layers, it is actually limited to the epidermis. Several types of warts form tightly fused cylindrical projections resulting in a uniform mosaic pattern that is unique to warts. This pattern is a useful diagnostic sign. The black dots seen on the surface of common warts are thrombosed capillaries that become trapped in the cylindrical, finger-like projections.

Clinical Presentation
Subjective

Patients typically complain of a wart or small "bump" (or group of bumps) that has been present for the past several weeks to many months, sometimes for years. Some patients report the same wart being treated before and then recurring on the same area. Most adult patients with common warts attempt self-treatment with OTC wart remedies, with limited to no success. Warts are usually asymptomatic. Occasional plantar warts can cause pain on weight-bearing.

Objective

Warts are small or large, fleshy or firm growths or lumps, which can be raised, fairly flat, single, or multiple, isolated, or clustered together to form a cauliflower-like shape. There are no skin lines crossing the surface, and examination with a hand lens reveals centrally located capillaries (black dots) that bleed with paring.

Common warts initially begin as smooth, flesh-colored papules. As they evolve, they become dome-shaped, gray-brown hyperkeratotic masses with black dots on the surface. Although common warts can be found on any part of the body, the hands are the most frequent site of involvement.

Filiform and digitae warts are finger-like, flesh-colored projections that protrude from a narrow or broad base.

Flat warts (verruca plana) are small (0.1–0.3 cm), slightly elevated, flat-topped papules. They are usually numerous and involve the forehead, mouth, beard, eyes, back of hands, and shaved areas. Scratching may produce a line of flat warts in the shaved areas. Flat warts range in color from pink or light brown to light yellow.

Cutaneous HPV infections (types 1, 2, 4, and 7) are more likely to be seen in children and young adults and have an incubation period of 2 to 6 months. As an individual reaches adulthood, the prevalence of cutaneous warts decreases, probably because of improved host immunity. Because these infections are usually benign, they are rarely brought to the attention of health-care providers. HPV types 5 and 8 are closely linked with a rare form of hereditary skin cancer (epidermodysplasia verruciformis).

Plantar warts occur at the heads of metatarsal bones and heels (points of maximal pressure) and appear as thick, painful calluses. This may lead to repositioning the foot while walking, causing distortion in posture, as well as producing pain in other parts of the foot, leg, or back.

Diagnostic Reasoning

Diagnostic Tests

If the clinician is unable to distinguish the lesion as a wart, a small specimen can be sent to the laboratory for identification.

Differential Diagnosis

Corns may be mistaken for warts and can be differentiated from warts by paring them with a number 15 scalpel blade. Skin lines are absent, and the black dots that are interspersed in the center of the wart will bleed with additional paring. Its mosaic pattern can be easily identified under a hand-held lens. Whereas corns have a painful, hard, translucent core, warts do not. The pain in corns is relieved when the hard central kernel is freed from the corn.

It is important to differentiate between the surface of the foot that is healing from a recent trauma and warts (black warts) that are undergoing spontaneous resolution. The black dots (thrombosed capillaries) seen on the plantar surface of a foot that has sustained a shearing injury may be confused with the black color of warts that are healing. It is hypothesized that the black color of the warts that are spontaneously healing may be part of the process of regression and may represent a specific cell-mediated immune response to HPV-infected keratinocytes.

Management

It is important to remember that most HPV lesions resolve without treatment. Therefore, initial management should be geared toward relieving pain and pressure and minimizing skin trauma and scarring caused by available therapies. Although filiform and digitate warts are relatively easy to treat, flat warts present a unique therapeutic challenge. Their duration is prolonged and they may be resistant to treatment. Because flat warts may be located in areas that are cosmetically important, treatment modalities that produce scarring should be avoided. It is important to note that therapies for HPV are usually contraindicated in pregnant women.

Therapy must be individualized because available therapies may produce unwanted effects such as pain, hyperpigmentation, scarring, damage to normal tissue, sun sensitivity, chemical sensitization, toxicity, and potential harm to pregnant women. In addition, it is important to identify previous treatment failures and successes, as well as the patient's risk factors (such as immunosuppression or lapses in therapy compliance) that may account for the failure of first-line therapy. Treatment intervals usually range from 1 to 2 weeks, but other patients may require prolonged therapy in order to eradicate more resistant lesions.

Simply covering warts with silver duct tape for 6 days at a time, then uncovering the wart, debriding it with an emery board or pumice stone, and covering it back up again a day later for repeated cycles lasting up to a month has been shown to be just as effective as pharmacotherapy. In other words, applying salicylic acid is not critical. This is an effective and inexpensive alternative therapy and might be suggested as first-line treatment.

Pharmacological Treatments

Keratolytic therapy in the form of salicylic acid plasters (Mediplast) or solution (e.g., DuoPlant, Occlusal) is a safe, nonscarring, moderately effective and low-cost OTC treatment of common warts, specifically for plantar and palmar surfaces. Once the wart is pared with a number 15 scalpel blade, pumice stone, or emery board, the area is soaked in warm water to soften the surface and to facilitate penetration of the solution. In the case of salicylic acid solution, one drop or more is applied with an applicator to cover the surface of the wart. The surface is allowed to dry and covered with a piece of adhesive tape or bandage. This will enhance the penetration of the solution.

Tape occlusion may precipitate inflammation and soreness and may necessitate periodic interruption of treatment. The patient may prefer to apply the solution at bedtime. Within a few days, a soft white keratin layer will form; this layer should be pared or abraded until pink skin is exposed. This procedure may be better accomplished by an occasional office visit. When applying keratolytic plasters (40% salicylic acid), the patient may use the same procedure outlined in the preceding text. The plaster is more useful when treating mosaic warts (a large cluster of warts). Once the plaster is cut to the size of the wart, the backing is removed and the adhesive surface is attached to the wart and secured with adhesive tape. The plaster should be removed in 24 to 48 hours, and the surface should be pared or abraded as outlined earlier; a new plaster should then be applied to the area. Although this treatment may take a few weeks, it is less irritating than the salicylic acid solution.

Chemicals such as bichloracetic acid (BCA) or trichloroacetic acid (TCA) are caustic agents that destroy warts by chemical coagulation of the proteins. These chemicals are frequently used for recurrent warts or at times as initial therapy. The clinician should pare the excess calloused skin and apply petrolatum to the surrounding area before applying the acid with a cotton-tipped applicator. BCA or TCA should be applied sparingly because both are caustic agents that can damage adjacent normal tissue. These acids are self-neutralizing, but any excess amount can be wiped away with a gauze. Repeat applications may be necessary every 7 to 10 days. A change of therapy should be considered if the patient has not improved substantially after three provider visits or if the warts have not cleared after six treatments.

Verruca plana (flat warts) are especially difficult to treat. Treatment includes applying tretinoin cream 0.025%, 0.05%, or 1% (Retin-A) at bedtime, over the entire area. Frequency of application should be adjusted to elicit a fine scaling and mild erythema. If other treatment options fail, 5-fluorouracil (Efudex 5%) can be applied one or two times a day for 3 to 5 weeks. Hyperpigmentation and recurrent warts at the site of inflammation are the limitations of this therapy.

Podophyllin resin 10% to 25% in a compound tincture of benzoin can be used for external warts. Because of the potential complications associated with systemic absorption and toxicity, it is recommended that the area of therapy be limited to 0.5 mL or less of the solution, or to no more than 10 cm of warts per session. To minimize irritation, the area should be allowed to dry and then washed off 1 to 4 hours after therapy. Podophyllin is not used for cervical warts or dysplasia and is primarily reserved for exophytic lesions. Its safety during pregnancy has not been established, and it is contraindicated for use by pregnant women.

Surgical Treatments

Although cryosurgery is very effective for common and genital warts, it may produce severe pain around the palms, feet, and nail areas. Thermal injury to nerve tissue, epithelial cells, and melanocytes can occur and cause changes in pigmentation. Therefore, light applications of liquid nitrogen are preferable. Liquid nitrogen can be stored in 1- to 2-gallon tanks for approximately 10 days. Applications can be repeated every 1 to 2 weeks. OTC home-based cryotherapy kits are now available without a prescription for use on small, isolated warts in easily accessible areas, such as the hands and fingers. Directions for these kits must be followed closely to avoid damage to surrounding normal skin and tissue. These kits should not be used for warts located in highly sensitive areas, such as the face or genitalia; consultation with a healthcare provider is warranted for such cases.

Surgical techniques such as blunt dissection or electrosurgery usually render patients wart-free with a single visit. Additional clinical training, equipment, and longer patient visits are necessary for these procedures. Blunt dissection is relatively painless if performed on areas other than the plantar or palmar surface. After preparation with local anesthesia, a plane of dissection is established by inserting the tip of a blunt-tipped scissors between the wart and normal skin. The wart is cut circumferentially and the lesion is separated from the normal tissue with short, firm strokes. After the lesion is removed, the blunt dissector is moved firmly back and forth over the area of excision, to ensure that no tissue fragments remain. Liquid nitrogen should be applied to the base using a cotton-tipped applicator. Liquid nitrogen will destroy any remaining virus.

Table 7.5 summarizes various treatment strategies for warts.

Follow-up and Referral

For the majority of common wart cases, a satisfactory response occurs after several treatments. For warts that are unresponsive or are recalcitrant to treatment, other, more aggressive treatment options are available—these are best administered by a dermatologist.

Interlesional administration of interferon (natural or recombinant) is more effective than systemic treatment. The Centers for Disease Control and Prevention does not recommend this treatment as first-line therapy because of the need for frequent office visits and the high frequency of systemic side effects. The cure rate (efficacy) is similar to that of the other therapies available. When all other treatments fail, intralesional bleomycin sulfate may be considered. Bleomycin is mixed (with 5 mL of sterile water and 10 mL of lidocaine) to form a solution, and then this solution is reconstituted with normal saline. Using a 30-gauge needle, the solution is injected into lesion to achieve blanching. The size of the wart will determine the amount of solution injected. Larger warts may require repeat injections. Leakage of the solution is unavoidable during the procedure. The cure rate is 48% (for plantar warts) to 71% (for periungual warts). A multiple-puncture method can result in a 92% cure rate. Responsive warts produce hemorrhagic eschars that heal without scarring.

Table 7.5 Warts and Their Treatment

Type of Wart	Description	Treatment
Common warts	Small, hardened growths of keratinized tissue. Warts usually grow around nails, on fingers, and backs of hands; can appear anywhere on the body.	• Silver duct tape therapy for 6 days, then repeat (see text) • Salicylic acid solution/plasters • Freezing with liquid nitrogen • Surgical excision
Flat warts (Verruca plana)	Pink, light brown or yellow; slightly elevated papules: 0.1–0.3 cm. Numerous sites: mouth, forehead, backs of hands, shaved areas (e.g., legs or beard area); may recur despite treatment. Frequently can undergo spontaneous remission. Avoid potentially scarring therapies.	• May resolve without treatment • Tretinoin cream, 0.025%, 0.05%, or 0.1%. Apply to involved areas daily; adjust treatment to produce fine scaling and mild erythema; may require weeks to months • Freezing with liquid nitrogen • Use of 5-fluorouracil (Efudex 5%) once or twice daily for 3–5 weeks produces dramatic results; may produce persistent hyperpigmentation (use ointment to minimize this adverse effect)
Filiform/digitate warts	Fingerlike, flesh-colored projections emanating from a narrow or broad base; sites: mouth, eyes, and ala nasi.	• Easiest to treat, but recurs • Shaving spreads the lesions • Retract skin and use curette drawn across base to remove wart • May use light electrocautery • Cryotherapy
Plantar warts	Lesions appear at maximum point of pressure (e.g., heads of metatarsal bones or heels) or anywhere on plantar surface; thick, painful callus forms around lesion; pain elicited on indirect pressure.	• More refractory to treatment • Remove surrounding callus with pumice stone or paring after soaking feet in warm water to soften skin • Daily application of salicylic acid liquid, film, or plaster after soaking
Black warts	Warts become black when spontaneously healing; black heel caused by sheared capillaries usually associated with trauma.	• Differential diagnosis for black heel: normal skin lines present; when area is pared with #15 blade, skin underneath is soft, and bleeds
Condyloma acuminata	Cauliflower-like wart. Usually found in anogenital region and usually sexually transmitted.	• 10%–25% podophyllin solution • Bichloracetic acid • Imiquimod cream • Cryotherapy • Intralesional injections • Laser vaporization • Refer to specialist for management of warts on anal mucosa or large collections of warts, which may be prone to profuse bleeding
Oral warts	Can be located in hard/soft palate, oral mucosa. Usually transmitted through oral–genital contact.	• Cryotherapy with liquid nitrogen • Surgical excision
Dysplastic cervical lesions	Lesions are usually subclinical. Colposcopy and biopsy for diagnosis; HPV DNA probes; PCR assays.	• CIN stages II & III: cryotherapy—lesions are frozen with liquid nitrogen every 2 weeks • Loop electrical excision • Laser vaporization • Suspicion of invasive disease: cone biopsy
HPV/koilocytosis	Pap smear indicates HPV or koilocytosis.	Refer for colposcopy and possible biopsy
Atypical squamous cells of undetermined significance (ASCUS)		Treat any underlying infections. Follow up with Pap smears every 4–6 months; if ASCUS recurs on repeat Pap smear, consider referral for colposcopy and biopsy

Need for referral to a specialist (dermatologist) is determined by several factors, including lack of response to treatment, possible cosmetic consequences (especially with warts on the face and eyelids), and the clinician's knowledge, experience, and comfort in identifying and treating specific types of warts. If the clinician is unsure of the diagnosis or if the wart is resistant to multiple treatments, the patient should be referred to a dermatologist.

Patient Education

The clinician should educate the patient on means of prevention of self-inoculation and the routes of transmission of the common warts. These measures include limiting shaving in the affected area until warts are eradicated, strategies to control nail biting, and avoidance of scratching and rubbing on the wart (see Table 7.6).

■ HERPES SIMPLEX INFECTIONS

Herpes simplex viruses are part of the Herpesviridae family and the Alphaherpesvirinae subfamily. *Herpes simplex virus* (HSV) infections are caused by two different types of viruses: HSV-1 and HSV-2. HSV-1 is associated primarily with oral infections, whereas HSV-2 is associated mainly with genital infections. Interestingly, HSV-1 genital infections are becoming more common, as are HSV-2 oral infections, probably due to oral–genital sexual contact (see Table 7.7).

Epidemiology and Causes

Both types of HSV produce identical patterns of infection. More than 85% of people worldwide are HSV-1 seropositive; however, only 20% to 40% of these individuals have a history of lesions. The National Institutes of Health (NIH) estimates that one out of four (or 45 million) Americans has genital herpes. The NIH estimates that 500,000 new cases may occur each year.

Pathophysiology

The majority of HSV-1 and HSV-2 infections are asymptomatic so that only elevated immunoglobulin G (IgG)

Table 7.6   Patient Education: Warts

About the Disease
- Warts are small growths or tumors produced by infection of normal skin tissue by the human papillomavirus (HPV). The most common areas where warts can be found include the plantar and palmar surfaces, nailbeds, hands, face, mouth, penis, vulva, cervix, and anus.
- One in four people are infected with HPV. Despite treatment, most warts will recur. Broken or abraded skin may facilitate the transport of the virus. These lesions can be spread by skin-to-skin contact, including touch, vigorous rubbing, shaving, nail biting, and sexual intercourse.
- Contrary to popular belief, warts do not have roots. The underside of a wart is smooth and round. The black dots found in the center of a wart represent broken small blood vessels (capillaries).
- Immunosuppression caused by diseases such as HIV or cancer and by organ transplants and some medications may reduce the efficacy of treatment. Cigarette smoking affects the immune system and enhances the expression of the viruses. Therefore, smoking should be discontinued.

About Treatments
- See text for information on "silver duct tape therapy."
- Treatment often involves more than one session, at 1- to 2-week intervals, and therapy may be prolonged.
- To minimize inflammation, do not apply medicated solutions, ointments, gels, creams, or plasters beyond the recommended time.
- Cryotherapy may be available in a doctor's office or as a home wart freezing and removal kit. Directions must be followed closely with home-based kits to avoid excessive damage to normal surrounding tissue.
- To improve efficacy, plasters should be cut to the size of the wart and kept in place with an adhesive for 24–48 hours. Pare or use a pumice stone to abrade the area and then reapply the plaster. The process may take a few weeks before you see results.
- Podophyllin is applied only to external warts and the area of application should be limited to 10 cm per session. To minimize irritation, the area should be allowed to dry and washed off 1–4 hours after therapy.
- Caustic acids such as bichloracetic acids or trichloracetic acid are very effective but may damage normal tissue if not allowed to dry properly. Repeat applications may be necessary every 7–10 days.
- Wash the treated area after the recommended waiting period. Always check for any signs and symptoms of infection, such as pus, severe pain, heat, redness, and swelling.
- For mild to moderate pain, take OTC analgesics.
- Pursue stress reduction activities, such as exercise, imagery, biofeedback, meditation, and yoga, and maintain a healthy diet. Decreasing stress will boost the immune system and improve healing, as well as reduce the desire to smoke, overeat, or nail bite.

Table 7.7 Herpes Simplex Infections

Infection	Location	Commonly Affected Age-group
Oral–labial herpes simplex	Lips, oral cavity	Children age 2–5 years, adults
Herpetic keratoconjunctivitis	Eyelids, periorbital area, cornea	Newborns, adults
Herpetic tracheobronchitis	Pharynx, trachea, bronchi	Older adults
Herpes simplex encephalitis	Temporal lobe of the brain	Any age, primarily adults who are immunocompromised
Herpes gladiatorum	Shoulder, neck, knuckles, areas of contact	Age 14 years and older (commonly seen in wrestlers)
Herpetic whitlow	Fingertip	Age 1 year and older
Lumbosacral herpes	Trunk or back	Adult
Herpes simplex of the buttocks	Buttocks	Adult women
Genital herpes	Labia minora, labia majora, vagina, cervix, urethra, penis, rectal area	Young and older adults, 1% of pregnant women
Eczema herpeticum	Face or any area of active or recently healed atopic dermatitis	Infants and older, commonly with a history of atopic dermatitis
Erythema multiforme	Extremities, palms, soles of feet	Age 20–30; more commonly seen in men than women

antibody titer shows evidence of previous infection. Herpes infections can occur anywhere on the skin. HSV infection has two phases: primary infection and secondary or recurrent infection. During the primary infection, the virus enters keratinocytes in the epidermis, eventually migrating to nerve endings. The virus then ascends via peripheral nerves to the dorsal root ganglion, where it enters a latent stage without active viral replication, which can last for days to years. The trigeminal ganglia are the targets of oral viral strains, whereas the sacral ganglia are the targets of genital herpes strains. Infection of the ganglia may occur within 24 hours of initial viral exposure and is essentially lifelong.

The majority of primary infections are subclinical and asymptomatic and can be detected only via an elevated IgG antibody titer. In the past several years, it has been recognized that although HSV infection is largely asymptomatic, most transmission occurs during periods of asymptomatic viral shedding. The severity of the viral infection increases with age. Herpes infection may markedly compromise nutritional intake in the elderly. HSV is spread by direct contact with active lesions, saliva, semen, or cervical secretions. In addition, HSV can be spread by patients without active disease, in whom subclinical or asymptomatic viral shedding occurs. Viral replication in the gingival epithelia facilitates oral shedding of the virus.

Symptoms may occur from 2 to 21 days after exposure. Tenderness, pain, mild paresthesias, or burning can occur before the onset of lesions at the site of inoculation. Headache, fever, muscle aches, localized pain, and tender lymphadenopathy may occur as part of the prodrome. Some patients have no prodromal symptoms. After several days, grouped vesicles on an erythematous base appear, followed by ulcers or erosions that crust over. Eventually there is a loss of crusts and reepithelialization occurs. In the moist genital region, crusts may not form; however, exudate may accumulate. Lesions typically heal in 7 to 10 days without scarring but may last up to 6 weeks or longer if they become secondarily infected with bacteria. Vesicles in primary HSV infection are more numerous and scattered than in recurrent infection.

Tissue destruction in HSV infection is mediated directly by viral replication within keratinocytes and other epithelial cells. A mononuclear cell and lymphocytic infiltrate occurs at sites of infection, consisting primarily of CD4+ T cells early on, but eventually involving equal numbers of CD8+ T cells, as well as macrophages and cytotoxic natural killer cells that attempt to clear infected host cells. The cytokines interferon-gamma and interleukin-6 are primary mediators of cytotoxic killing mechanisms. Interestingly, in animal models, nonclassic T cells endogenous to the skin and mucosal surfaces that express gamma-delta rather than alpha-beta antigen receptors have been shown to protect against severe mucocutaneous and encephalitic HSV infection.

Recurrent disease typically occurs at or near the same site of primary infection. Physical and emotional stress, fever, exposure to ultraviolet light, chapping or abrasion of the skin, immune suppression, menses, or fatigue may cause reactivation of the virus, which descends spontaneously along sensory nerve axons to the skin surface.

The anatomical site of infection and virus type affect the frequency of recurrence. Genital herpes recurs six times more frequently than oral–labial herpes. Genital HSV-2 infections recur more frequently than genital HSV-1 infections. Interestingly, oral–labial HSV-1 infections recur more often than oral HSV-2 infections.

Clinical Presentation
Subjective

The most common manifestation of HSV infection is oral–labial herpes. Primary infection with HSV may present as herpetic gingivostomatitis in children and young adults, though most commonly children aged 2 to 5 years are affected. The patient may present with fever, sore throat, hypersalivation, and painful vesicles and ulcers on the tongue, palate, gingiva, buccal mucosa, and lips. In genital herpes, early symptoms may include pain in the legs, buttocks, or genital area; genital burning or itching; vaginal discharge; and lower abdominal pressure. Within a few days, lesions appear at the site of infection. With the first episode of genital herpes, fever, headache, muscle aches, painful or difficult urination, and inguinal lymphadenopathy may also occur. HSV infections are usually oral or genital; however, any area of the body can be infected.

In elderly patients, primary infection or reactivation of oral–facial HSV-1 can be extensive. Painful oral lesions make eating difficult and can compromise nutritional status. Sometimes, superinfection with bacteria or *Candida* can further complicate HSV infection in the elderly. Of major concern in older adults is autoinoculation of the eye, causing keratoconjunctivitis, which is the most frequent cause of corneal blindness. Signs and symptoms include unilateral excessive lacrimation, edema, chemosis, photophobia, and purulent exudate. Decreased visual acuity is a bad prognostic sign.

Herpetic whitlow is an HSV infection of the fingertip. This disorder was common among health-care practitioners before the use of universal precautions. Now, herpetic whitlow is commonly found in children with a recent history of gingivostomatitis and women with genital herpes. Transmission apparently results from autoinoculation. Vesicles with a red halo may erupt on the finger. Besides generalized symptoms, a red streak may appear up the arm.

A patient with a history of atopic dermatitis who presents with vesicles on the face or areas that have recently healed is likely to have eczema herpeticum. A patient who recently had an HSV infection but now presents with iris-shaped lesions on the palms and soles of the feet most likely has erythema multiforme. HSV lesions on the back are often misdiagnosed as varicella-zoster virus (VZV), and often the correct diagnosis is not made until there is a recurrence. The primary difference on clinical evaluation is that HSV vesicles are uniform in size, whereas varicella-zoster lesions vary in size.

Both types of HSV infection can cause encephalitis. The patient presents with altered level of consciousness, personality changes, fever, and seizures. The patient may also experience smell and taste hallucinations and aphasia. Herpetic encephalitis requires immediate hospitalization and treatment with IV acyclovir (Zovirax). Herpes infections in immunocompromised patients are more severe—frequent HSV recurrences often result in chronic and nearly continuous ulcerations. Focus on History 7.4 lists some questions for eliciting information on HSV infection.

Objective

The lesions must be examined for characteristic location, appearance, and distribution. Depending on the site of lesions, the anterior and posterior cervical chains submental or the inguinal nodes should be checked for lymphadenopathy. Grouped vesicles on an erythematous base occurring in the mouth or on the face or the genitals are most likely the result of HSV infection. Vesicles on the eyelid, chemosis, or the presence of corneal dendrites require prompt referral to an ophthalmologist.

Diagnostic Reasoning
Diagnostic Tests

Viral culture is the standard method of diagnosis. HSV can be cultured from vesicle fluid or from scrapings from the base of erosion. Sampling must be done early (during the first 72 hours) in the course of the outbreak. The

Focus on History 7.4 Herpes Simplex Virus Infections

General
- When did the sores first appear?
- Have you ever had sores on the same area before?
- Before appearance of the sores, did you experience burning, tingling, pain or numbness?
- Do you have muscle aches, fever, and/or weakness?
- Are you able to swallow?
- Have you ever had this happen to you before? If so, when and how was it treated?
- Have you been around any person who may have had these symptoms?
- Do you have a history of any skin problem?

Specific Questions for Genital Herpes
- How old were you at first sexual intercourse?
- How many total sex partners have you had?
- How long have you been with your present partner?
- Have you ever had a sexually transmitted disease?
- Do you use latex condoms? If so, do you use them consistently?
- Do you engage in oral sex? Vaginal sex? Anal sex?
- Have you ever had an abnormal Pap smear?

initial viral culture may be negative, but clinical evaluation and subsequent recurrence with early culture can verify HSV infection. Viral culture differentiates between HSV-1 and HSV-2 with high sensitivity. The Tzanck smear is rapid and easily performed and can be used to identify multinucleated giant cells in vesicular fluid. The Tzanck smear does not, however, differentiate among HSV-1, HSV-2, or VZV. HSV antibodies can be detected in blood, but the serum analysis does not differentiate between HSV-1 or HSV-2. Enzyme-linked immunosorbent assay and complement fixation are available serological techniques that detect circulating antibodies with 90% sensitivity but only 50% specificity. The Western blot (currently not available in doctors' offices) is another serological technique that distinguishes between HSV-1 and HSV-2 with high sensitivity and specificity (greater than 99%). Viral culture remains the gold standard for diagnosis of HSV infection.

Differential Diagnosis

History and clinical presentation are the best guide to diagnosis. Aphthous stomatitis differs from HSV infection in that ulcerations of nonkeratinized mucosa occur. Therefore, lesions rarely appear on gingiva or hard palate, as do herpetic ulcers. Also, no fever or lymphadenopathy occurs. In addition, an aphthous stomatitis ulcer is usually solitary and larger than a herpetic ulcer. Herpangina can also mimic HSV infection. Herpangina is seen predominantly in children and infrequently seen in adults. Treatment is symptomatic for both infections. Hand-foot-and-mouth disease presents with red macules that progress to vesicles on an erythematous base. However, the extremities, in particular the hands and feet, as well as the mouth, develop lesions. Erythema multiforme can result from HSV or *Mycoplasma* infection or a drug reaction. Treatment is based on the underlying cause. Pemphigus is an autoimmune disorder that usually occurs in middle-aged patients (aged 40–60). Erosions of the oral mucosa are followed by bullae over the body.

Management

No cure for herpes exists; however, recurrences tend to be milder and of shorter duration than the primary infection. Therapy is primarily symptomatic and supportive. Nutritional intake is important, especially in elderly patients, who may benefit from using anesthetic mouth rinses. The goals for management include reduction or elimination of pain, decreased viral shedding, and healing of tissue. In cases of frequent recurrence of herpetic lesions, suppressive therapy may be needed.

Initial therapy is palliative and promotes healing. Herpetic keratoconjunctivitis requires immediate referral to an ophthalmologist to prevent blindness. For other forms of HSV infection, the practitioner can initiate management with pharmacotherapy and self-help techniques based on the location and extent of HSV infection. Acetaminophen can be used to control fever and pain. Lesions on the lip (if small) may require nothing more than applications of ice and lip ointments such as Blistex. OTC docosanol 10% (Abreva) applied 5 times daily may improve lesions. If lesions are more extensive, penciclovir 1% cream (Denavir) applied to the affected area every 2 hours while awake for 4 days promotes healing, shortens the course of the illness by several days, and substantially decreases viral shedding. Extensive oral lesions may require the use of oral anesthetics such as viscous xylocaine 2% (Lidocaine) or dyclonine hydrochloride 0.5% to 1% to control pain. In addition, acyclovir suspension 200 mg/5 mL can be used to treat the lesions directly by rinsing the mouth with 1 teaspoon and swallowing five times a day for 7 days.

Initial treatment of genital herpes requires the use of oral antiviral drugs. Valacyclovir and famciclovir have greater bioavailability and require less frequent daily dosing than acyclovir. This type of regimen makes these drugs preferable to acyclovir. Comfort measures such as warm compresses or an oatmeal sitz bath several times a day can relieve pain and promote healing. A patient with genital or urethral herpes may find it easier to urinate into the warm bath water. Every patient with HSV infection benefits from increased fluid intake and rest.

Any necessary subsequent management is based on the recurrence of symptoms. A patient with an initial negative viral culture can be told to return to the practitioner for another viral culture within the first 72 hours if symptoms recur. This procedure is important with an initial negative culture of genital herpes. A patient with genital herpes, after the first occurrence, can be given a prescription for an antiviral drug and instructed to take the medication should he or she experience the beginning of symptoms such as tingling or burning at the site. A patient with genital herpes who experiences six or more recurrent episodes per year should be placed on suppressive therapy. (See Drugs Commonly Prescribed 7.5.) Suppressive therapy will reduce outbreaks by 85%. Ultimately, there will be about a 50% reduced risk of transmission. Long-term suppressive therapy is very safe, and after a period of 5 to 7 years, many patients discontinue such therapy with no relapses.

Follow-up and Referral

Follow-up should be early and repeated depending on the extent of disease. Lesions confined to the lip area may not need to be seen unless they do not resolve. Extensive oral lesions and genital lesions should be seen on a weekly basis until resolution. As previously mentioned, herpetic lesions of the eye must be referred to an ophthalmologist immediately. Patients with herpes zoster ophthalmicus should be instructed to return to the practitioner if they experience a recurrence, until they feel comfortable in handling subsequent episodes

Drugs Commonly Prescribed 7.5   Herpes Simplex Infection

Drug	Indication	Adverse Reactions and Prescribing Considerations
Topical		
docosanol 10% cream (Abreva)	Recurrent oral–facial herpes simplex OTC	Begin at earliest sign or symptom 5 times/day
penciclovir 1% (Denavir)	Recurrent herpes labialis on the lips and face	Every 2 hours while awake for 4 days
Systemic Therapy		
amciclovir (Famvir)	Acute herpes zoster, treatment or suppression of recurrent genital herpes and treatment of recurrent herpes labialis in immunocompetent patients	Pregnancy Category B Check prescribing reference for dosage and precautions
valacyclovir (Valtrex)	Treatment of herpes zoster or herpes labialis Treatment or suppression of genital herpes in immunocompetent patients	As above
acyclovir (Zovirax)	Genital herpes, herpes zoster, varicella, herpes labialis, herpetic whitlow	As above

on their own. A patient with genital herpes may benefit from referral to a local herpes organization for information and emotional support.

Patient Education

Patient education is an integral component of the management of HSV infection. Most patients achieve relief of symptoms within 4 to 7 days of beginning therapy. Self-care techniques and instructions on the proper use of pharmacotherapy are vital. Table 7.8 provides guidelines for patient education on herpes infection.

■ ACNE VULGARIS

Acne vulgaris (commonly called "acne") is one of the most common skin conditions that the clinician will see in primary care. Acne is derived from the Greek word *acme* meaning "prime of life" because it is a disease primarily of adolescence, although it may continue into adulthood. Acne is an inflammatory disorder of the sebaceous gland and its accompanying hair follicle (or a pilosebaceous unit), with the highest incidence seen in teens and younger adults. There are approximately 5,000 pilosebaceous units on the human body. Most of them are located on the face, back, chest, and upper arms, the most common sites for acne. Acne lesions include comedones, papules, nodules, and cysts. Painful nodules and cysts are found in severe forms of acne.

Although acne is not a life-threatening illness, it has the potential for resulting not only in physical scars but in emotional trauma as well. The primary-care provider should not ignore the impact of acne on self-esteem and

identity, which are closely tied to physical appearance during the adolescent period. Many adolescents are reticent to discuss this health-care issue, and the primary care provider should be proactive about treatment in order to prevent disfiguring scarring. Most cases of acne can be treated safely in the primary-care arena. Treatment options should be offered to both the parent and the teen during routine wellness visits, as well as during episodic visits.

Common misconceptions regarding acne abound in the community. Many patients and their parents think that antibiotic treatment can result in a "quick cure." In reality, antibiotic treatment can take up to 4 to 6 weeks before visible results may begin to be seen. No connection has been found between ingestion of certain foods (fried foods, chocolate) and acne. The response rate from acne treatment tends to be slow compared with most infections treated with antibiotics. Good education regarding acne can help prevent disappointment in angry and discouraged patients who might become noncompliant because of a loss of trust in both the treatment and provider.

Epidemiology and Causes

Acne vulgaris has the highest incidence among 12- to 25-year-olds; up to 85% of this age-group is affected at one time or another. Twenty percent of all adults have some degree of acne. Sixty million Americans have active acne, with 20 million having severe acne that may cause scarring. Only 11% of acne sufferers seek advice or treatment from a professional. The incidence of acne

Table 7.8	Patient Education: Herpes Simplex Infection

- Fever, stress, sunlight, and menses can trigger recurrence of lesions.
- Burning and tingling at the site may signal recurrence of the infection. If antiviral therapy was prescribed, begin it at the first sign of infection.
- If symptoms persist beyond 10 days, see your health-care provider.

Treatment

General:
- Apply penciclovir (Denavir) 1% cream to affected area while awake every 2 hours for 4 days, or until symptoms resolve.
- Frequent hand washing, rest, and increased fluid intake are needed during any herpetic outbreak.

Lip lesions:
- Apply ice to lip lesions for 10–15 minutes as needed to relieve pain and decrease swelling.
- Lip balms (such as Blistex) may be used on the lips to prevent drying of sores and reduce pain.
- Apply lip balm sunscreen (such as Chapstick) with an SPF of 15 to lips before sun exposure.

Oral lesions:
- Apply a dental protective paste (such as Orabase) 4 times a day to prevent irritation of the lesions by the teeth.
- An equal mixture of diphenhydramine (Benadryl) syrup (12.5 mg/5 mL) and unflavored Maalox can be used as an oral rinse every 2 hours, then expectorated. Viscous xylocaine 2% (Lidocaine) 5 mL can be added to the mixture or used alone as an oral rinse before meals to decrease pain and facilitate eating.
- For those with orolabial lesions, there should be no sharing of towels, silverware, or glasses, or kissing until lesions are healed.

Genital, anal, and/or buttocks lesions:
- To soothe lesions, apply warm compresses or take a warm oatmeal sitz bath for 20–30 minutes as needed.
- A blowdryer placed on the cool setting can be used to thoroughly dry genital lesions.
- No sexual intercourse until lesions are healed. A latex condom must be used consistently to decrease viral spread.

markedly decreases as people get older. Acne occurs equally in both males and females, although it can be more severe in males. The average age at onset for Caucasians is 11 years for girls and 12 years for boys. There are some racial differences. The average age of onset is 16 years for Hispanics, 19 years for Asians, and 20 years for African Americans. Hispanic teenagers have the highest incidence of both acne and resultant scarring. Acne can recur again during adulthood and is called *adult-onset acne.* Adult-onset acne is more commonly seen in women who are in their mid-20s to 40s. Fifty percent of adult women have premenstrual flares of acne, and many women have their first flare, or worsening of existing acne, during pregnancy. The etiology of acne is interdependent on several factors, which include the following:

- An increase in production of sex hormones (androgens) in puberty and adolescence
- An increase in sebum production resulting from activation of the sebaceous glands (during puberty and adolescence) and genetic factors
- A disorder of epithelial cell "stickiness" (keratinization) and shedding (desquamation), leading to plug formation
- Proliferation of *Propionibacterium acnes* bacteria inside the hair follicles
- The host's inflammatory response

Pathophysiology

Comedones are the basic lesions of acne and are caused by a defect in desquamation at the opening of the pilosebaceous follicle. Instead of regular cellular shedding, desquamation is reduced, and shed epithelial cells become "sticky," forming plugs that block follicular openings in a process known as retention hyperkeratosis. It takes about 2 months for the accumulated shed epithelial cells, sebum, and keratin to finally produce a comedone. *Comedones* are noninflammatory lesions and are classified into two types: *closed* comedones ("whiteheads") and *open* comedones ("blackheads"). Open comedones get their black color from melanin and not from dirt, as the black color results from the oxidation of tyrosine to melanin. Tyrosine, an amino acid precursor of melanin, is a substance that is normally present in the plug material.

Enlargement of the sebaceous glands and increased sebum production triggered by adrenarche during adolescence provides a rich growth medium for the overgrowth of *Propionibacterium acnes* bacteria within the pilosebaceous follicles. *P acnes* is an anaerobic diphtheroid that is part of the normal skin flora in humans and is responsible in large part for the inflammatory response observed in acne vulgaris. *P acnes* bacteria utilize triglycerides as their primary source of nutrients by breaking down the sebum inside the affected hair follicle into its basic units—fatty acids and glycerol. Free fatty acids act as irritants and produce a sterile inflammatory response inside the sebaceous follicles. *P acnes* itself also causes a direct inflammatory response by releasing proteolytic enzymes such as hyaluronidase, as well as chemotactic factors that attract neutrophils to the site of infection.

These neutrophils extrude lysozyme, which further degrades surface epithelia, leading to rupture of the previously closed comedone. When a comedone ruptures, its contents, which include sebum, bacteria, keratin, and free fatty acids, enter the dermis and elicit a severe inflammatory response. This results in the formation of deep abscesses, which present on the skin surface as nodules and cysts. Although androgen excess may lead to acne formation, most acne sufferers do not overproduce androgens. However, their pilosebaceous glands are likely hypersensitive to these hormones and more prone to retention hyperkeratosis. Some studies have shown that the production of sebum is increased in patients with acne compared with controls of similar age, thus suggesting a possible genetic predisposition for acne vulgaris.

Clinical Presentation
Subjective

The typical patient is an adolescent male or female who has already tried self-treatment for several months with OTC products without much success. The patient might present to the clinician's office not only with numerous acne lesions but also with dry, irritated skin, a common side effect of many topical acne medications. Female patients are more likely to verbalize emotional distress over their appearance. Male patients are more likely to wait until their acne is severe before they will seek treatment from the clinician. Some patients with severe acne complain of pain and tenderness from multiple deep pustules, nodules, and cysts. Mild to moderate acne normally does not cause pain.

Objective

Mild Acne   Mild acne is composed mainly of noninflammatory comedones with occasional small papules. Commonly, there is a mixture of both types of comedones. The location of the comedones and papules will vary, from a predominantly facial involvement to other locations, such as the chest, back, and the upper outer arms. Closed comedones are small papules from 1 to 3 mm in size that are the same color as the surrounding skin, sometimes with a visible white plug. Occasionally, a closed comedone can get irritated from trauma (e.g., scratching) and become inflamed. Open comedones have a black-colored central plug. The hard plug on some comedones can be removed easily by putting firm pressure on the sides of the lesion. See the figure of the Iceberg of Acne to appreciate all the issues involved.

Moderate Acne   Moderate acne is composed mainly of inflammatory lesions such as papules and pustules. The papules range in size from a few millimeters to half a centimeter. The color of the acne papules in light-skinned patients ranges from light pink to bright red. Papules in darker-skinned patients can be red to shades of brown. Pustules are easier to recognize: They appear like pointed papules, with yellow to green-colored tops. When pustules become fluctuant, they rupture spontaneously, providing relief from pain. Resolution of a pustule is usually rapid after rupture. Scarring is more likely with larger and deeper pustules. Hyperpigmentation can be problematic, especially in patients with darker skin. (Patients with olive-toned complexions and darker tones are more likely to have this problem.) Patients who are prone to hyperpigmentation should be advised to avoid sun exposure to the face and to use oil-free sunblock on the face.

Severe (Nodulocystic) Acne   Severe acne, or nodulocystic acne (consisting mostly of nodules and cysts), always results in scar formation. The severity of acne scars is variable, from numerous atrophic pits ("pockmarks") to large, depressed scars. In patients with darker skin, keloids and hypertrophic scars can result. Severe acne is more common in males. Occasionally, fistula formation is seen in some patients. Nodules are inflammatory lesions that appear bright to dark red (or brown), depending on the patient's shade of skin. Nodules are smaller and feel harder than acne cysts. In addition, some darker-skinned patients end up with permanent hyperpigmentation changes secondary to severe inflammation, brown to black-colored macules on skin.

Acne conglobata is severe cystic acne in which nodules, cysts, and abscesses develop; lesions are predominantly located on the trunk area instead of the face. Females with acne conglobata should be evaluated for polycystic ovary syndrome. Acne fulminans is rare and is seen in young adolescent males. An acute onset of multiple painful, ulcerated acne lesions is seen, along with systemic symptoms such as fever, chills, malaise, and generalized joint and muscle aches.

Diagnostic Reasoning
Diagnostic Tests

Acne is diagnosed by its classic location and characteristic lesions. A complete history is crucial to the diagnosis and supplants the importance of most diagnostic tests, which are really only needed when an underlying condition is suspected or for cases refractory to standard treatments. For acne fulminans, a CBC, blood chemistry panel, urinalysis, and ESR can be helpful. Abnormal lab results, however, seen in cases of acne fulminans include an increase in white blood cell count (leukocytosis), an elevated ESR, anemia, and hematuria.

The Iceberg of Acne

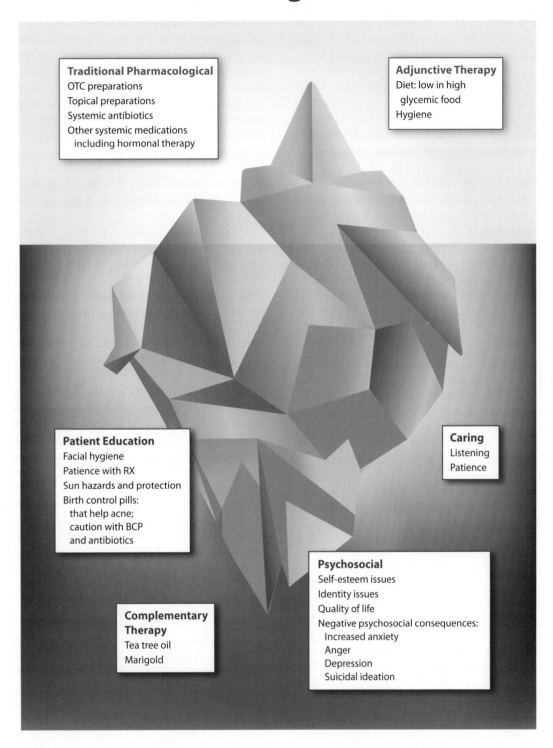

Traditional Pharmacological
OTC preparations
Topical preparations
Systemic antibiotics
Other systemic medications
  including hormonal therapy

Adjunctive Therapy
Diet: low in high
  glycemic food
Hygiene

Patient Education
Facial hygiene
Patience with RX
Sun hazards and protection
Birth control pills:
  that help acne;
  caution with BCP
  and antibiotics

Caring
Listening
Patience

Complementary Therapy
Tea tree oil
Marigold

Psychosocial
Self-esteem issues
Identity issues
Quality of life
Negative psychosocial consequences:
  Increased anxiety
  Anger
  Depression
  Suicidal ideation

If an endocrine disorder such as polycystic ovaries is suspected (e.g., in a hirsute overweight female with moderate to severe acne and amenorrhea or irregular menses), an evaluation for excessive androgen production should be done. A complete physical exam, along with laboratory tests that include serum total and free testosterone and dehydroepiandrosterone sulfate, is recommended. A pelvic ultrasound should be ordered to look for enlarged ovaries.

Differential Diagnosis

Rosacea used to be called "acne rosacea" and needs to be ruled out. Rosacea is more common in adults and older patients and is located more centrally on the face, cheeks, chin, and nose. Comedones are never found in rosacea. There is a tendency for easy flushing in response to alcohol or heat. Telangiectasia, a dilation of a small group of blood vessels, may be present. It can be accompanied by eye complaints such as excessive dryness and irritation. It is more common in patients from an Irish, Scottish, or English ethnic background. Chronic rosacea can result in rhinophyma (hyperplasia of nasal tissue) and is seen more often in older men.

"Hot-tub" folliculitis (folliculitis lesions caused by staphylococci) appears within 1 to 4 days after hot tub use (because of inadequate temperature and chlorination). Patients will complain of small red pustules that can be occasionally pruritic. Folliculitis is located on the areas of the body that have been immersed in the water, such as the lower torso, buttocks, and legs. Perioral dermatitis appears as small, erythematous papules that occur around the mouth area and the nasolabial folds. The main diagnostic clue is the location: It is seen only on the perioral area and is more common in adult females (usually 20–30 years old). Treatment is similar to that for acne rosacea. Topical steroids are contraindicated.

Management

The primary goal of acne treatment is to prevent and/or to minimize scarring and permanent pigmentation changes. Patient education is very important in acne management and should not be neglected. Mild acne is treated with topical medications only (see discussion that follows). Systemic antibiotics may be used in moderate cases of acne that are unresponsive to topical agents and are used in severe cases.

A combination of several types of acne lesions is not uncommon, but the most predominant lesions present will help in the determination of treatment choices. Other factors that help determine treatment include a higher risk of pigmentation changes (more common in patients with darker skin), a patient's refusal of systemic antibiotic treatment, and severity of the acne. Parental permission is necessary to treat patients younger than age 18 years. The popular media have suggested that tretinoin has been associated with psychotic or suicidal behavior in teens, but this has never been substantiated by rigorous epidemiological data.

Topical Treatment of Comedonal Acne

Comedones respond well to topical retinoids (Level I; Strauss et al, 2007). Synthetic retinoids such as tretinoin (Retin-A) and adapalene gel (Differin) decrease comedone formation by increasing cell turnover and decreasing epithelial cell cohesiveness. Adapalene gel seems better tolerated on sensitive skin than tretinoin, but patients with extremely sensitive skin can still develop skin irritation. Mild adverse effects include dryness, erythema, scaling, and burning. Azelaic acid (Azelex) is the least likely to irritate sensitive skin (compared with retinoids) and does not cause photosensitivity, but

practical results in the clinical area have been disappointing. Patients who are unable to tolerate topical retinoids may be good candidates for this drug.

Tretinoin has been shown to thin out the top epidermis during the first 4 weeks of treatment, and thus can be very drying and irritating. At this time, patients might notice more skin sensitivity to the elements (cold air, wind, sun) and an increase in skin photosensitivity. Sunscreen or sunblock should be used during the entire treatment period, especially during this time. The thickness of the epidermis returns to normal after 4 to 6 weeks. Topical retinoids are derivatives of vitamin A and are available in multiple vehicles in a wide variety of concentrations. They are rated as Pregnancy Category C and should not be used in pregnant women or on children.

It is important to warn patients and parents that tretinoin and, to a lesser extent, adapalene gel will cause a worsening of acne lesions during the first 4 to 6 weeks of treatment, because preexisting comedones will continue to surface during this time. Improvement should become visible by 6 to 8 weeks, however. A trial period of 2 months is generally recommended for topical retinoids, unless the patient develops contact dermatitis or other problems with the medicine. To avoid excessive skin irritation, the patient should wait for at least 10 to 15 minutes after washing and should allow the skin time to dry before applying topical acne agents. Patients with a history of eczema or with sunburned skin should not use this medicine. The patient should avoid the eyes, mouth, angles of the nose, and mucous membranes when applying this medicine. Adverse reactions include excessive skin irritation, an apparent exacerbation of symptoms, transient pigmentation changes, stinging on application to the skin, and dry skin. The effects of other topical acne agents, such as benzoyl peroxide, sulfur, resorcinol, and salicylic acid, should be allowed to subside before the application of topical retinoids. (See Advanced Practice Nursing Interventions 7.1.)

Topical Treatment of Inflammatory Acne

Patients with predominantly inflammatory lesions may respond well to topical antibiotics such as erythromycin or clindamycin, benzoyl peroxide, or a combination of benzoyl peroxide and erythromycin. Other good candidates for nonretinoid topical acne therapy include patients who cannot tolerate tretinoin or adapalene gel or patients who have concurrent eczema. All topical antibiotics are applied once or twice daily. The most common side effects include mild erythema or burning. Because topical antibiotic solutions use an alcohol base, they can cause excessive skin dryness. To avoid this problem, the clinician should tell the patient to start gradually on a once-a-day basis for 2 weeks. Monotherapy with topical antibiotics may lead to bacterial resistance with a resultant slower therapeutic effect, so switching the patient to a combination of antibiotics

Advanced Practice Nursing Interventions 7.1
Initiating Tretinoin Therapy

Start with tretinoin 0.025% (Retin-A) cream (the least irritating). Apply three to four times per week at bedtime for the first 2 weeks until the patient can tolerate a daily dose. Give this dose a trial of 6–8 weeks.

• Gradually increase to a 0.05% cream or 0.025% gel if patient can tolerate the above regimen and needs a stronger dose (if no reduction in acne lesions seen after 8 weeks).
• If there is still breakthrough of acne lesions, increase to the 0.1% cream.

   NOTE: The most potent and irritating dose of tretinoin is the 0.05% liquid formulation. Remind the patient that acne breakout is expected at weeks 4–6 of treatment, then skin will start to clear up. Tretinoin 0.05% (Renova) has been shown to decrease the effects of solar damage and is approved by the FDA for the treatment of fine wrinkles, mottled hyperpigmentation, and tactile roughness of the skin.

and benzoyl peroxide has shown an increased efficacy and reduction of the antibiotic resistance of *P acnes*. The antibiotics must be stored in the refrigerator. The combination products, available in gel form, include 1% clindamycin–5% benzoyl peroxide (BenzaClin) and 3% erythromycin–5% benzoyl peroxide (Benzamycin). Azelaic acid (Azelex), a dicarboxylic acid with bacteriostatic and keratolytic properties, is approved for acne in the 20% cream formulation. It is particularly effective in treating patients with postinflammatory hyperpigmentation or concomitant melasma.

Systemic Antibiotic and Hormone Treatment of Moderate to Severe Acne

Topical acne medicines are a much safer alternative than oral antibiotics and have less potential for adverse effects. Topical therapy has its limitations, however. Oral antibiotic treatment should generally be continued for 4 to 6 months, and maximal clinical results may not be evident before 3 to 4 months.

Good candidates for oral antibiotic treatment include patients who:

• Have a lack of response to topical medications after a trial of at least 2 to 3 months.
• Have the inability to tolerate topical acne treatment.
• Have large numbers of inflammatory lesions after several months on topical treatment.
• Have severe nodulocystic acne.
• Have large numbers of inflammatory lesions located on the back or upper outer arms (hard-to-reach areas).

• Want quick relief from inflammatory acne.
• Are at increased risk of pigmentation changes or scarring.

Oral antibiotics are the standard of care in the management of moderate and severe acne and treatment-resistant forms of inflammatory acne (Level I; Strauss et al, 2007). *P acnes* is a biofilm-forming organism, and topical treatment is recommended along with oral antibiotics. Oral antibiotics used in the treatment of inflammatory acne include doxycycline and minocycline, which are more effective than tetracycline. There is evidence that minocycline is superior to doxycycline in exerting not only an antibacterial effect against *P acnes* but a direct anti-inflammatory effect as well. Trimethoprim-sulfamethoxazole and trimethoprim are also effective in instances where other antibiotics cannot be used (Level I; Strauss et al, 2007).

One study found that treatment with minocycline resulted in faster resolution of inflammatory acne lesions than tetracycline. The starting dose of minocycline (for tetracycline-resistant acne) is 50 mg at bedtime for 1 week; then the dose is gradually increased to 100 mg at bedtime. Once improvement is seen at 4 to 6 weeks, the dose can be decreased gradually every 6 to 8 weeks. The maintenance dose of minocycline is 50 mg once a day. Adverse effects include vertigo, dizziness, and ataxia (this antibiotic affects the vestibular apparatus of the inner ear). This effect can be avoided or decreased by starting the patient on a lower dose. Rare cases of blue-gray discoloration of the skin are sometimes seen in minocycline use. Other adverse effects associated with tetracyclines include serum sickness, hepatitis, and a lupus-like syndrome.

Doxycycline and minocycline are more lipophilic and can be taken with food without affecting most of the drug's activity. Doxycycline is a good choice for patients who develop erythromycin-resistant *P acnes* infection. Doxycycline should be taken with a full glass of water (if it becomes lodged in the esophagus it can cause ulceration). Adverse reactions to doxycycline include photosensitivity, GI upset, enterocolitis, rash, blood dyscrasias, and hepatotoxicity. If the patient's occupation or hobbies include plenty of sun exposure, another drug besides doxycycline should be considered. The patient must use strong sunscreen or sunblock while on this drug in addition to avoiding excessive sun exposure.

Tetracyclines should not be used on pregnant women and patients younger than 9 years of age because of the risk of tooth discoloration and inhibited skeletal growth. Another important factor to consider is that tetracyclines are labeled by the Food and Drug Administration (FDA) as potentially reducing the effectiveness of oral contraceptives (a potential medico-legal risk). Patients on oral contraceptives should use a reliable second method of birth control, such as condoms. Adverse reactions to tetracyclines include nausea, dizziness, rash, blood dyscrasias, pseudotumor cerebri, photosensitivity, and hepatotoxicity. Antacids, dairy products, and iron- or magnesium-containing vitamins will inactivate tetracyclines because of their propensity for binding with those substances. Erythromycin is a macrolide antibiotic that prevents the production of bacterial proteins. Although erythromycin is effective, use should be limited to patients who cannot use the tetracyclines (pregnant women or children younger than age 8 years because of the potential for damage to the skeleton or teeth). The development of bacterial resistance is more common during erythromycin therapy (Level I; Strauss et al, 2007). Adverse reactions to erythromycin include nausea, GI upset, abdominal pain, anorexia, candidal vaginitis, hepatic dysfunction, rash, superinfection, and pseudomembranous colitis (rare). Because *P acnes* is quickly becoming resistant to erythromycin, this is usually considered a second-line agent.

The FDA has approved three types of birth control for acne. Norgestimate/ethinyl estradiol (Ortho Tri-Cyclen) uses estrogen combined with a progestin (norgestimate). It is available with different doses of progestin. Estrostep uses estrogen combined with a progestin (norethindrone). It is available with different doses of estrogen. Drospirenone/ethinyl estradiol (YAZ) uses estrogen combined with an artificial form of progestin (drospirenone). Although thromboembolism is an established risk for all forms of hormonal birth control, the FDA has concluded that birth control pills containing drospirenone may have an increased risk for thrombus formation compared with pills containing other progestins. Oral contraceptives are indicated for moderate acne in females who are 15 years of age or older and have acne that is unresponsive to topical medications. The female patient should have no known contraindications to hormonal therapy such as a history of thrombophlebitis or thromboembolic disorders, cerebrovascular or cardiovascular disease, breast or other estrogen-dependent neoplasms, hepatic tumor, or undiagnosed genital bleeding.

Severe

Severe acne should be referred to the dermatologist for aggressive treatment with isotretinoin, a vitamin A derivative that is indicated for severe recalcitrant nodular acne that has not responded to conventional therapy (including oral antibiotics). Isotretinoin induces sebaceous gland atrophy, normalizes follicular keratinocytes, reduces *P acnes* colonization, and has direct anti-inflammatory effects. It is one of the most potent teratogens known today (Category X) and carries huge medico-legal implications for the clinician when it is prescribed to females of reproductive age. The manufacturers of isotretinoin require all prescribers to join a program called iPLEDGE to minimize fetal exposure. The clinician should refer any female of potential reproductive age who is a candidate for isotretinoin therapy to the dermatologist for management. If the clinician decides to prescribe this drug to a reliable female of childbearing potential (physician consultation is highly recommended), the criteria for the iPLEDGE program must be adhered to. The risk and the benefits of therapy should be discussed with the female patient, including the possibility of pregnancy and contingency plans if she gets pregnant (including termination of the pregnancy).

Two negative pregnancy tests must be obtained within 1 week of prescribing the medication, and two forms of reliable contraception must be used (unless abstinence is the chosen method). Monthly pregnancy tests must be ordered thereafter. The patient must have maintained effective contraception for at least 1 month before, during, and after therapy. The most frequent adverse effect is cheilitis, which occurs in up to 90% of patients. Other adverse effects commonly seen during therapy (in up to 80% of patients) include dry skin, dry nose, dry mouth, pruritus, epistaxis, and an increase in skin fragility. The link between isotretinoin and depression remains controversial. Some state that it has been known to cause depression, psychosis, and, rarely, suicide. Because of this, the clinician may not want to prescribe this medication in patients with a history of these conditions. Patients who complain of headache should be evaluated for pseudotumor cerebri or benign intracranial hypertension. Corneal opacities and decreased night vision have also been reported while patients are on this medication. The incidence of hypertriglyceridemia is very high (one patient in four). Some patients develop elevated liver transaminases, and elevated blood sugar levels have been seen in patients with diabetes. Baseline laboratory testing, such as fasting lipids and liver function tests, should be done before treatment and follow-up testing should be done weekly (or biweekly) thereafter until the patient's response to therapy is known; then it can be done monthly.

The dose of isotretinoin is gradually increased to a maintenance dose. Only a 1-month supply of the drug should be prescribed for each visit. Isotretinoin should be taken with food. The medicine can be discontinued early if the acne nodule count is decreased by 70% or more. If the patient complains of moderate to severe myalgias, the medication must be discontinued immediately and follow-up laboratory tests must be done. After a period of 2 months or more off therapy, if persistent or recurrent severe nodular acne recurs, referral to a dermatologist is recommended. Isotretinoin will induce long-term remissions of acne in up to 40% of patients. Patients with acne fulminans should be referred and treated with prednisone, the drug of choice for this condition. For other drugs listed above, see Drugs Commonly Prescribed 7.4.

Other Medical Therapies

There are therapies other than or in conjunction with medications that may assist in the overall treatment of the patient with acne. The surgical procedure of comedone extraction is common for the treatment of comedomal acne and may be used with topical retinoids. This extraction may be done manually using a comedone extractor. Beta-hydroxy acid peels may also be effective against comedonal acne. To reduce acne scarring, fraxel, laser resurfacing, dermabrasion, and subcision or punch grafting may help. In addition, dermal augmentation with autologous or nonautologous tissue may improve the appearance of atrophic scars.

Photodynamic therapy with the use of a blue light or intense pulsed light and aminolevulinic acid may be given every other week. Results are usually apparent after the second treatment.

Follow-up and Referral

Patients should be reevaluated in 4 to 6 weeks to monitor response and potential adverse effects of acne medication. Noncompliance issues should be addressed. Topical retinoids frequently cause skin dryness and irritation if not started gradually or if used incorrectly. The role of patient education is very important in the use of topical retinoids. Most patients are not willing to try it again after they experience skin irritation and the temporary flare-up of acne seen within 4 weeks of starting therapy. Female patients on oral antibiotics or isotretinoin should be monitored for continued use of reliable methods of birth control. There is no need to wait until the acne becomes severe enough before considering referral to a dermatologist. Severe acne or moderate acne that is unresponsive to conventional treatment should be referred to a dermatologist for more aggressive treatment to minimize scarring.

By the third month of treatment, clinical improvement of acne lesions should be visible. If no improvement is seen or if the acne worsens, topical treatment with two agents or systemic therapy should be considered. The chances of skin irritation are increased when two topical agents are combined; therapy should be started slowly to minimize these effects. Systemic oral antibiotic treatment should generally be continued for a period of 4 to 6 months. Without treatment, acne lesions can last months to years.

Patient Education

Patient education is a vital and important component in acne treatment because of the long duration of treatment and potential for adverse effects (some serious). Patients and parents (if the patient is younger than 18 years) should be warned of potential adverse effects of oral acne medication (as discussed under Management). Table 7.9 presents patient education information. Patients should be encouraged to read product labels and to only use noncomedogenic (non–acne-causing) products, makeup, moisturizers, sunscreens, and so forth.

Patients on oral contraceptives for acne therapy should be aware of potential drug interactions, which include

Table 7.9 Patient Education: Acne

- Wash the face gently at least twice a day with an antibacterial soap (Dial, Lever 2000) or with a very mild soap (Dove soap).
- Wait at least 30 minutes after washing the face before applying topical acne medications in order to minimize the chance of skin irritation.
- Topical acne medications should not be used on sunburned or irritated skin, abrasions, cuts, or on eczematous skin. If these conditions are present, the medication can be temporarily stopped for a few days.
- Avoid contact with eyes, lips, angles of the nose, and the mucous membranes when applying topical acne medicines.
- Sunscreen should be used with all acne medications, especially in sunny climates and during the summer.
- Avoid oily makeup or oily hair conditioners or scalp products.
- Avoid excessive handling of the face and cradling phones on the chin.
- Avoid excessive scrubbing of the face.

decrease in their efficacy when used in conjunction with certain antimicrobials, including the tetracyclines. Oral contraceptives should not be used in breastfeeding patients.

■ ROSACEA

Rosacea is a chronic and progressive skin disorder in middle-aged and older adults that resembles acne. It is characterized by flare-ups that include three cutaneous components that may occur individually or concurrently. The first component is vascular in nature with persistent erythema primarily involving the central face. This may be followed after a period of time by the development of telangiectasia or clusters of small, superficial blood vessels. Flushing episodes may occur spontaneously. The second cutaneous component involves recurrent acneiform erythematous papules and pustules around the central face. The third component consists of connective tissue hyperplasia around the central face with discrete sebaceous gland hyperplasia (rhinophyma), consisting of persistent yellow papules particularly around the nose. Blepharoconjunctivitis may result if there is ocular involvement.

Rosacea is a lifelong condition that is usually exacerbated by sun exposure. Other environmental triggers include the following: hot or cold weather and wind; overheating during exercise; excessive alcohol ingestion or hot beverages; spicy or aged food products such as cheese; emotional stress; irritating cosmetics; hot baths, saunas, or hot tubs; smoking; caffeine; and excessive washing of the face. Rosacea and acne often look similar, may respond to the same treatments, and may coexist in the same patient.

Epidemiology and Causes

Although rosacea affects nearly 14 million Americans, fewer than 10% are diagnosed because patients confuse the symptoms with acne, sunburn, flushing, or a temporary rash. Rosacea is most common in persons aged 30 to 60 years who are of Irish, English, Scottish, Welsh, or eastern European ancestry. Women are three times more likely to develop rosacea than men, particularly the first cutaneous component. Patients sometimes have one or more close relative with the condition. Rosacea is idiopathic with no recognizable causes other than certain triggers that exacerbate the condition. Several researchers have suggested that *Helicobacter pylori,* an organism found in the stomach, may possibly be a cause, as well as the *Demodex* species of mite, which has been found in the hair follicles of patients with rosacea.

Pathophysiology

At present, the underlying pathogenesis of the vascular dilation characteristic of rosacea is not fully characterized. Inflammation, rather than infection, appears to be the primary mechanism, as shown through several lines of indirect evidence. For example, studies have failed to show consistent differences in *H pylori* seropositivity between patients with rosacea and unaffected controls. Moreover, the ability of amoxicillin-metronidazole-bismuth treatments to clear *Helicobacter* infection and improve rosacea symptoms has been attributed to the anti-inflammatory effects of metronidazole. This was similarly shown with tetracycline treatment of rosacea associated with *Demodex* mite infestations. Mite counts were not decreased with this treatment, although symptomatic improvement was evident. Moreover, the anti-inflammatory effects of tetracycline antibiotics have been well documented in the treatment of acne vulgaris.

Clinical Presentation
Subjective

Patients with rosacea usually do not seek out care because they think they have acne, sunburn, or a temporary rash. They usually present because they become intolerant of the persistent burning, itching, or stinging sensations. Patients with ocular rosacea complain of watery, irritated, or bloodshot eyes.

Objective

Initially the patient's forehead, cheek, nose, or chin may have a rosy hue without comedones. This is the central third of the face and is referred to as the "flush/blush" area. There may be inflammatory papules, pustules, and telangiectasias. Scarring is usually inapparent unless the patient also has concomitant acne. Although the lesions tend to be symmetrical bilaterally, they may also appear on only one side. Seborrhea may also be seen. If there has been

ocular involvement resulting in blepharoconjunctivitis, there will be redness of the eyelids and conjunctiva.

With prerosacea, the clinician will note a rosy-cheeked ruddy complexion on a patient who never develops the full clinical spectrum of the disease. There is no effective treatment for prerosacea, nor is any needed. Patients should just be observed for signs of developing rosacea and encouraged to use sunscreen.

There are four subtypes of rosacea classified by the pattern or grouping of symptoms:

Subtype 1: Erythematotelangiectatic rosacea—flushing and persistent redness, which may include visible blood vessels
Subtype 2: Papulopustular rosacea—persistent redness with transient bumps and pimples
Subtype 3: Phymatous rosacea—skin thickening usually with hyperplasia of the nose resulting in a large, bumpy, and bulbous appearance
Subtype 4: Ocular rosacea—ocular manifestations with dry eye, tearing and burning, erythematous eyelids, recurrent styes, and the possibility of vision loss from corneal damage

Diagnostic Reasoning
Diagnostic Tests

There is no diagnostic test for rosacea; physical assessment is the key to diagnosis. Although there is no cure for rosacea, if treatment is started early, some of the cutaneous manifestations may be prevented.

Differential Diagnosis

Differential diagnoses include adult acne, perioral dermatitis, seborrheic dermatitis, the "butterfly" rash of systemic lupus erythematosus, and steroid-dependent facial dermatoses. Acne may be a concomitant condition along with rosacea, but acne is characterized by the presence of comedones, a lack of facial flushing and telangiectasias, and a broader distribution around the face than the limited central distribution of rosacea. Perioral dermatitis is typically seen in young women, although it may occur in women aged 15 to 40 years. Multiple acneiform papules are seen around the mouth with a clear area spared directly around the lips. The small erythematous papules or pustules of perioral dermatitis lack telangiectasias. Seborrheic dermatitis usually has a scaly appearance not seen in rosacea. The erythema is without acneiform lesions and may be distributed throughout the nasolabial area, eyebrows, and scalp. The "butterfly" or malar rash of systemic lupus erythematosus lacks papules and pustules, and laboratory evaluation typically verifies the presence of antinuclear antibodies. Long-term topical steroid use on the face can result in burning erythema, sometimes associated with erythematous papules and/or scaling. When topical steroids are abruptly discontinued, a rebound flare-up of this condition typically occurs.

Management

The key to management is early diagnosis and avoidance of triggers because rosacea is a chronic condition with no known cure. Topical treatments should be the mainstay of therapy, with oral antibiotics used only for breakthrough flare-ups. Potent topical steroids should be avoided, because they may worsen the condition.

Topical Therapy

Metronidazole cream is the mainstay of therapy but may take up to 6 to 8 weeks for a therapeutic response. If metronidazole (0.75% or 1%) is not effective, topical clindamycin or erythromycin may be tried. (See Drugs Commonly Prescribed 7.4.) The same therapy is used for perioral dermatitis and topical steroid–induced rosacea.

Systemic Therapy

Antibiotics should be reserved for flare-ups or when initiating therapy with topical medications, and then antibiotics should be discontinued. Clinicians should taper the dose as soon as possible; typically patients readily learn how to taper the dosage at home. Treatment with tetracycline, minocycline, or doxycycline usually delivers a rapid therapeutic response. Antibiotic therapy is usually effective in reducing acneiform lesions, and this helps confirm the diagnosis of rosacea. These antibiotics typically work more as anti-inflammatory agents rather than antibiotics. The flushing of rosacea and the flat telangiectasias tend to persist and do not respond well to antibiotic therapy. In refractory cases, metronidazole, amoxicillin, or rifaximin may be used. Isotretinoin may succeed when other measures fail.

Other Therapies

Electrocautery with a small needle may be used to destroy small telangiectasias. Larger telangiectatic vessels may require lasers (intense pulsed light therapy). For men with rhinophyma, surgical reduction may be used to reduce the bulbous appearance of the nose.

Follow-up and Referral

Patients should be referred to a dermatologist if rosacea results in telangiectasias for electrodesiccation or laser treatment for cosmetic purposes. A dermatologist may also help patients with diffuse facial erythema due to rosacea with pulsed light therapy.

Patient Education

Patients should be taught about the events or circumstances that can trigger a rosacea flare-up and learn how to avoid them. Sunscreen with a sun protection factor of at least 15 should be used on all exposed skin surfaces when outdoors. Patients should stay cool on hot days and protect their face from cold air and wind by using a scarf. Caution should be used when exercising, and patients should be encouraged to exercise for shorter, more frequent intervals, using a cool towel around the neck and taking frequent water breaks. Gentle cleansing with fragrance-free facial cleansers should be encouraged. Proper use of topical creams and lotions should be stressed, along with the use of minimal antibiotics.

DERMATITIS

■ ATOPIC DERMATITIS

Atopic dermatitis (eczema) is not considered a distinct disease entity but is a descriptive term for a group of skin disorders characterized by pruritus and inflammation, whose distinct cause is unknown. *Eczema* is a more general term that is often used collectively to describe skin of an erythematous and inflamed appearance, reflective of a superficial pathological process. Currently, the terms *eczema* and *dermatitis* are often used synonymously in the clinical arena in a nonspecific sense. The use of the term *eczematous rash,* although also indistinct, may be helpful both diagnostically and therapeutically, because eczematous dermatitis may be classified into two major etiological categories—contact dermatitis and atopic dermatitis. Early in its presentation, atopic dermatitis is erythematous in appearance, with papulovesicular lesions that ooze and crust. At its later stages, the rash becomes a red-purple color, dries, and develops scaling and lichenification, which is exacerbated by itching resulting from its highly pruritic nature.

Epidemiology and Causes

Atopic dermatitis is a constitutional and inherited reaction, which usually begins in infancy. Interestingly, children born to older women are more likely to develop eczema than children born to younger women. For unknown reasons, the prevalence of atopic disease has risen steadily over the past 30 years, and the prevalence is now estimated at 1 in 18 or 5.5%, which amounts to 15 million people in the United States. About 10% of the U.S. population will have atopic dermatitis at some point in their lifetime. Atopic dermatitis presents more severely in childhood. Onset during the first year of life occurs in up to 50% of all patients; in 85%, onset is before age 5 years. Up to 5% of all children are affected by atopic dermatitis. Most cases (40%) resolve by adulthood, however. The remainder of patients with atopic dermatitis are affected with a chronic course of the disease that is characterized by acute exacerbation (often during times of stress) and intermittent remissions.

No ethnic predisposition has been found for atopic dermatitis, and it occurs equally in both sexes. The cause of atopic dermatitis is unknown. Family history is positive for atopy in two-thirds of all cases. Genetic predisposition may be the most important etiological factor in all-atopic conditions. A personal or family history of all or part of the "atopic triad"—asthma, allergic rhinitis, and eczema—is often present. It has been proposed that individuals with any of these three conditions have preferential production of allergen-specific immunoglobulin E (IgE) and that the presence of such antibodies should be a mandatory criterion for the diagnosis of atopic dermatitis. Such a diagnostic test, however, only establishes the diagnosis of *atopic syndrome*, not atopic dermatitis. Any patient with a history of hives (urticaria), hay fever, or rashes should be considered to have an atopic history.

All atopic individuals seem to have itchier skin, yet what seems to be unique about the atopic patient's skin is its hypersensitivity. Many factors that do not make non-atopic individuals itch will make the atopic person feel itchy. Atopic patients are known to itch seconds after experiencing a stressful event. This type of reaction is thought to be caused by neuropeptide-induced vasodilation, which produces a rise in skin temperature and erythema. Symptoms are triggered or exacerbated through the interaction between genetic predisposition and environmental factors. Environmental factors that trigger atopic dermatitis include dust mites, animal dander, pollen, microbes, pollutants, climate, and emotional stress.

Excessively hot or cold climates or excessively dry or moist environments are particularly suitable for setting the stage for the atopic process. Anything that dries the skin can aggravate symptoms: Common triggers include excessive bathing, hand washing, lip licking, sweating, or swimming. Contact with irritants such as solvents, detergents, deodorants, tobacco, cosmetics, soap, and woolen and synthetic fabrics can precipitate an exacerbation of atopic dermatitis. Heat and sweat may also be aggravating factors for atopic dermatitis. Factors that generate an increase in body temperature include hot showers or baths, overdressing, use of heating pads, and electric blankets. Patients with atopy are intolerant of heat, have difficulty with thermal sweating, and are more likely to develop heat exhaustion. It is thought that perspiration retention might be a complicating factor in atopic patients. Excessive humidity is, therefore, a problem, because it interferes with normal evaporation of sweat from the body. Improperly fitting clothes can create friction and irritate the skin, and contact with certain fabrics, most notably wool, can precipitate a flare-up. Other skin conditions or infections can also lead to an exacerbation of atopic dermatitis (eczema).

Pathophysiology

The inflammatory process in eczema causes erythema of the skin as a result of dilated blood vessels that are surrounded by inflammatory cells that migrate into the epidermis, resulting in edema both inside and in between the epidermal cells (spongiosis). The epidermal cells malfunction as a consequence, resulting in thickening of the epidermis (acanthosis), excess production of keratin, and scaling. The outer epidermal layer of the skin, the stratum corneum, normally forms an impermeable barrier that protects the living cells beneath from environmental irritants and toxins. In atopic dermatitis, this outer barrier is impaired. There is an increase in the water loss and a decrease in water binding, which leads to a brittle outer barrier. This condition is made worse by environmental factors such as physical trauma from scratching, cycles of wetting and drying, and the chemical erosion that is caused by detergents and solvents. In addition, superinfection of eczematous skin by bacterial (e.g., *Staphylococcus aureus*) or fungal (e.g., *Malassezia furfur*) species and irritation from dust mites and their dung is an important factor that worsens atopic dermatitis by potentiating the immune response. Superinfection is also much more likely in atopic dermatitis than in other forms of dermatitis such as psoriasis. Thus, infection may be thought of as both a trigger and a complication of atopic dermatitis.

Immunological abnormalities are key to the pathophysiology of the atopic response. These abnormalities can include elevated serum IgE levels, which are seen in 85% of affected individuals; hypereosinophilia; reduced cell-mediated immunity and antibody-dependent cellular cytotoxicity; slowed chemotaxis of neutrophils and monocytes; relative increase in the number of CD4-positive (CD4+) Th2 helper T cells that secrete interleukin-4 (IL-4); and a decrease in CD4+ T helper cells that secrete interleukin-2 (IL-2). Interestingly, however, in later stages of the immune reaction, Th1 helper T-cell activity, which enhances cell-mediated immunity, appears to play an increasing role. Th17 cells and their associated cytokines have also been implicated in this disease process, including in the protection against infection/colonization with superficial skin fungi and bacteria (e.g., *Staphylococcus*) containing superantigens that are thought to trigger dysregulated immune responses, resulting in eczematous lesions. However, reports in the literature are conflicting and have implicated Th17 cells in both pro-inflammatory and anti-inflammatory roles. Impairment of essential fatty acid metabolism has also been implicated as a causative factor of atopy.

Clinical Presentation
Subjective

Atopic dermatitis is characterized by an extremely low threshold for pruritus and has been referred to as "the itch that rashes." Almost always, the itch occurs before the rash appears, and scratching the rash only worsens it clinically. In fact, the cardinal sign of atopic dermatitis is severe pruritus, which is often extremely distressing in both the acute and chronic stages. In turn, the diagnosis of atopic dermatitis cannot be made without a history of pruritus, and if pruritus is absent, alternate diagnoses should be sought. The patient may report a personal or family history of other atopic conditions (asthma, allergic rhinitis). The patient usually reports a history of episodic exacerbation of similar symptoms or of a childhood rash or eczema. The clinician should inquire about any exposure to known or unknown common antigens and irritants, regardless of the history. Individuals with atopic dermatitis are not immune to contact dermatitis; in fact, they are more susceptible to irritant reactions because of their impaired epidermal barrier layer. Often, the rash is reported as better in the warmer months and worse in the fall and winter.

Objective

Atopic dermatitis usually begins as infantile eczema, with lesions affecting the cheeks, face, and upper extremities. Erythema is often seen before pruritus. The acute lesions are often excoriated, maculopapular, and inflamed. In infancy and early childhood, oozing and crusting usually characterize the erythema. As the child becomes older, the disease can go into remission or change to a flexural distribution (antecubital fossae and neck area). Flexural eczema usually lasts until about age 4 to 10 years but may continue into adulthood.

In adults, eczema presents with symmetrical lesions that are crusting and excoriated. In the early stages, lesions may be erythematous, papulovesicular, edematous, and weeping. Later the rash becomes crusted, scaly, thickened, and lichenified. Intergluteal involvement is uncommon and should raise suspicion of another diagnosis. The classic locations for lesions are noted to correspond to areas that are most accessible to rubbing and scratching. In addition, the typical flexural sites are more susceptible because they are areas that are more likely to be hot and moist. (See Advanced Assessment 7.2.)

Diagnostic Reasoning

Diagnostic Tests

Laboratory tests are usually not useful in the diagnosis of atopic dermatitis, but they can be helpful in ruling out other disorders or to confirm that a patient is prone to atopy (allergic reactions). If a viral etiology (e.g., HSV) is suspected, a viral culture should be done on the exudate and moist parts of the rash. If atopy (allergy) is suspected, a radioallergosorbent test (RAST) may be done on serum to quantify levels of allergen-specific IgE. The RAST test is usually available to primary-care clinicians, whereas the scratch (skin prick) tests are typically done only by trained allergists. However, interpretation of RAST test results requires specialized knowledge of the specificity and sensitivity of the assay, because false-positive results are not uncommon. Thus, RAST tests should not be ordered arbitrarily or as a general atopic screening tool; instead, they should be directed by a detailed patient history. RAST panels often include not only antigen-specific IgE levels but also antigen-specific IgG and IgM levels, which are not helpful in the diagnosis of atopic disease (hypersensitivity) and are, therefore, prone to misinterpretation.

Advanced Assessment 7.2   Atopic Dermatitis

Distribution

Infants: Trunk, face, extensor surfaces, scalp
Children: Antecubital fossae, popliteal fossae
Adults: Face, neck, upper chest, genital area, hands

Stages

Acute
Erosions with serous exudate
Intense pruritus
Papules and vesicles on an erythematous base
Pain, heat, tenderness

Subacute
Scaly, excoriated
Pruritus (may be intense)
Papules or plaques over an erythematous base
Secondary infection possible

Chronic
Lichenification, pigmentary changes (increased or decreased)
Pruritus
Excoriated papules and nodules
Dryness, fissuring

Other Clinical Manifestations

Keratosis pilaris ("chicken skin"): Asymptomatic follicular papules, particularly on the posterolateral aspects of the upper arms and lateral thighs
Lichenification of the skin: predilection for flexural creases
Ichthyosis vulgaris: Hyperlinear palms and soles and fishlike scales, especially on the lower legs
Dennie's sign/Morgan line: Infraorbital fold
Excessive fissuring under the earlobes, palms, soles, and fingers
Pityriasis alba: Hypopigmented asymptomatic areas on the face and shoulders
Allergic "shiners": Facial pallor and infraorbital darkening
Anterior capsular cataracts
Keratoconus: A cone-shaped cornea may develop in the second or third decade of life (in severe cases)
Facial erythema, dry skin, history of wool intolerance, nonspecific hand dermatitis, and a tendency for skin infection (commonly impetiginization of excoriated skin)

A RAST test panel may include testing for allergy to dust mites, mold, ragweed, animal dander, tree pollen, and many other allergens. RAST testing also exists for food allergens, which are often highly relevant in pediatric patients; however, true IgE-mediated food allergies are far less common in adults. Thus, RAST tests are useful for patients who are suspected of having an atopic history if ordered in a directed fashion by the patients presenting signs, symptoms, and environmental exposures (Level I; Leung et al, 2004). An atopic or allergic tendency is manifested by chronic or recurrent symptoms (in addition to dermatitis), which might include a history of allergic rhinitis (nasal congestion, chronic postnasal drip, sneezing, itchy nose) and asthma during childhood. Some patients will deny any allergic tendency but will report a history of frequent "sinus problems." The RAST test is usually positive in patients with a history of symptoms of atopic dermatitis, but it often does not correlate well with clinical symptoms. Results appear to vary with the type of allergen being tested. Another potentially helpful marker for atopy is serum IgE levels. Serum IgE levels are usually elevated during acute periods of dermatitis but may decrease during periods of remission. Higher levels of total serum IgE, however, also increase the tendency toward false-positive allergen-specific RAST test results.

Patients should be advised to stop all antihistamines for at least 2 weeks before undergoing allergen skin testing, because these medications will interfere with skin test outcomes and may lead to false-negative results. In addition, delayed-type hypersensitivity responses to epicutaneously applied antigens (as used in scratch and skin-prick tests) may be blunted in atopic skin during periods of disease activity, so scratch tests should be avoided during flare periods to avoid uninterpretable results. Alterations in cell-mediated immune responses may help explain the increased susceptibility of atopic patients to cutaneous viral infections, such as HSV, vaccinia, and molluscum contagiosum. Thus, atopic patients should be warned of their increased risk of these infections and encouraged to take measures to avoid future exposure.

If the diagnosis is confusing or if serious pathology (mycosis fungoides) is suspected, a skin biopsy can provide important information. The skin biopsy of atopic skin will reveal a thickened and hyperkeratoid epidermis, along with perivascular inflammation of the dermis. Patients with pustular superinfection should have their lesions cultured for antibiotic sensitivities if they do not heal in response to empiric therapy.

Differential Diagnosis

Both common and rare skin disorders can mimic atopic dermatitis. Common disorders include contact dermatitis, tinea infections (dermatophytosis), seborrheic dermatitis, and the early stages of mycosis fungoides (cutaneous T-cell lymphoma). In contact dermatitis, the characteristic linear or asymmetrical distribution of the skin lesions helps to distinguish this condition from atopic dermatitis. The location and characteristic ringlike, erythematous lesions with central clearing distinguish tinea corpora infections (ringworm) from atopic dermatitis. Mycosis fungoides skin lesions do not respond to topical steroids; therefore, lesions that do not respond to topical steroids after a minimum of 2 weeks of treatment should be referred for skin biopsy.

If none of the common skin disorders apply, rare systemic diseases and skin disorders that can mimic atopic dermatitis include gluten-sensitive enteropathy, acrodermatitis enteropathica, phenylketonuria, hyper-IgE syndrome, Wiskott-Aldrich syndrome, X-linked agammaglobulinemia, selective IgA deficiency, and Letterer-Siwe disease (see Differential Diagnosis 7.5).

Management

The primary aim in the management of atopic dermatitis is to control signs and symptoms because no cure exists at present. Management of dermatitis embodies the fundamental principles of dermatology: Precipitants should be eliminated, wet lesions should be dried, dried lesions should be hydrated, and inflammation should be treated with corticosteroids. The goals of management are to decrease pruritus, prevent secondary infection, and educate patients so that they can control the disease themselves. Crucial to management is a careful and systematic assessment of trigger factors. In addition, the critical importance of skin hydration cannot be overestimated, because chronic use and overuse of corticosteroids carry significant iatrogenic risks, including both local adverse effects (e.g., skin atrophy, local irritation, telangiectasias) and the potential adverse effects of systemic absorption (e.g., cataract formation, growth impairment, bone demineralization, adrenal suppression). The benefits of barrier-restoring therapies are highlighted in Nursing Research–Based Practice 7.2.

Nonpharmacological Management

Errors in bathing and moisturizing are by far the most common causes of persistent atopic dermatitis. To avoid excessive irritation and skin dryness, the patient should

Differential Diagnosis 7.5 Atopic Dermatitis

Scabies
Seborrheic dermatitis
Allergic contact
Tinea
Psoriasis
Ichthyosis
Dermatitis herpetiformis
Mycosis fungoides (cutaneous T-cell lymphoma)
Netherton's syndrome
Wiskott-Aldrich syndrome
Acrodermatitis enteropathica
Neurodermatitis
HIV infection (especially in children)
Phenylketonuria (if symptoms appear during the first year of life)
Hyper-IgE syndrome
Dermatomyositis

Nursing Research–Based Practice 7.2

Valdman-Grinshpoun, Y, et al. Barrier-restoring therapies in atopic dermatitis: Current approaches and future perspectives. *Dermatol Res Pract,* Sept-Oct. 2012. Retrieved from http://dx.doi.org.ezproxy.fau.edu/10.1155/2012/923134

Atopic dermatitis is a multifactorial, chronic relapsing, inflammatory disease characterized by xerosis, eczematous lesions, and pruritus. The latter usually leads to an "itch-scratch" cycle that may compromise the epidermal barrier. Skin barrier abnormalities in atopic dermatitis may result from mutations in the gene encoding for the protein filaggrin, which plays an important role in the formation of cornified cytosol. Barrier abnormalities render the skin more permeable to irritants, allergens, and microorganisms. Treatment of atopic dermatitis must be directed to control itching, suppress inflammation, and restore the skin barrier. Emollients, both creams and ointments, improve the barrier function of the stratum corneum by providing it with water and lipids. Studies on atopic dermatitis and barrier repair treatment show that adequate lipid replacement therapy reduces inflammation and restores epidermal function. Efforts directed at developing immunomodulators that interfere with cytokine-induced skin barrier dysfunction provide a promising strategy for treatment of atopic dermatitis. Moreover, an impressive proliferation of more than 80 clinical studies focusing on topical treatments in atopic dermatitis has led to growing expectations for better therapies.

use mild emollients that are soap substitutes (e.g., Cetaphil) instead of soap. Some patients may insist that soap is necessary for cleanliness; they can be informed of studies showing that Dove soap was the least irritating among 18 soaps and detergent bars that were tested. Reducing exposure to water will minimize the drying effects to the skin; if soap is used, it should be limited only to the axilla, groin, and feet. No other national population bathes as much as Americans, and this practice has become more ritualistic than purposeful.

Personal habits such as excessive bathing can be detrimental because bathing is an effective way to remove the skin's protective oils. Older patients should take short, lukewarm showers and avoid long, hot baths, which are extremely desiccating. The use of bubble baths and fragrance-containing oils should be discouraged. Bath oils are of minimal benefit because whatever oil remains on the skin is wiped off with toweling. Minimizing contact with cosmetics, deodorants, detergents, and solvents should be stressed. Moisturizers are useful in helping to prevent water loss and are most effective when applied immediately after patting the skin partially dry after a short shower. Atopic dermatitis patients should be cautioned against using lotions and gels, because they contain alcohol, preservatives, and fragrance. Patients with atopic dermatitis should not use agents that contain lactic acid or other alpha-hydroxy/glycolic acids that can aggravate the condition.

Ointments (which contain petroleum jelly) form an occlusive layer and are more effective in preventing water loss than lotions. For less severe conditions or in hot, humid areas, creams that do not contain fragrance and have few preservatives are acceptable (e.g., Cetaphil cream, Eucerin, Dermabase, Unibase). Humidifiers are most helpful in cold and dry climates, but they can provide an environment that is conducive to increased dust mite and mold populations. Acaricide is an insecticide that is effective against dust mites; it can be used on all fomites (pillows, beds, sofas, etc.). After application, a thorough vacuuming, preferably with a high-efficiency particulate air–filtered apparatus, must be done to remove the insecticide. Antifungal cleaners for wet and damp areas are recommended for patients who are sensitive to mold. Acaricide and other pesticides/chemical treatments have not been shown to be consistently helpful and are *not* first-line preventive treatments.

Pharmacological Management

If the skin lesions are wet, are inflamed, or have exudate, wet soaks or compresses with cool tap water, Burow's solution (1:40 dilution), saline (1 teaspoon per pint of water), or silver nitrate solution (25.5%) can be used to dry out the lesions and provide comfort. Aluminum acetate solution (Burow's solution) can be applied as a compress for 20 to 30 minutes four to six times throughout the day. OTC topical corticosteroids should be immediately applied to inflamed areas after the soak. Prescription corticosteroid cream may be needed for more severe cases.

Given that dry skin lesions are most characteristic of atopic dermatitis, petrolatum or other emollients (e.g., Aquaphor healing ointment, Eucerin cream, Keralac lotion) should be applied not only to dry eczematous lesions, but also to all noninflamed areas of the skin, in order to maintain hydration. Colloidal oatmeal baths (Aveeno) are soothing and may also be helpful with more generalized lesions.

Although antihistamines are often used to relieve pruritus, they are usually ineffective in atopic dermatitis because histamine is not the only factor responsible for the mediation of pruritus in atopic dermatitis. The sedative effect of antihistamines may be more beneficial than its antipruritic properties if used at night. Individuals with atopic dermatitis have a tendency to scratch in their sleep, so sedation at bedtime may decrease the amount of scratching during sleep. If the patient does not obtain relief from antihistamines, first generation H_1 blockers, such as ethanolamines (diphenhydramine) and phenothiazines (promethazine), are very sedating. Some tricyclic antidepressants, such as doxepin (Sinequan), have potent antihistaminic activity as well and are useful in urticaria and other forms of pruritus. An added benefit to using an antidepressant agent is the relief of depression that is not uncommonly seen to accompany atopic dermatitis. First generation sedating antihistamines are *not* generally recommended in children, however, because they have been shown to lead to daytime drowsiness and impair school performance in many cases, as well as have a paradoxical effect of inducing hyperactivity in some children. Thus, sedating patients at night for severe atopic dermatitis, urticaria, or other forms of pruritus only applies to adults.

Montelukast sodium (Singulair) at 5 to 10 mg/day may contribute to the treatment of atopic dermatitis in a patient with other forms of concurrent atopy. Montelukast is a leukotriene-receptor antagonist and inhibits eosinophil infiltration in the skin, a major histological characteristic in atopic dermatitis. Of note, however, montelukast is not FDA approved for the treatment of atopic dermatitis.

Corticosteroids are effective anti-inflammatory agents and usually are considered first-line pharmacotherapy for atopic dermatitis, although their use must always be preceded by optimal moisturizing, because restoring skin hydration is the most important step in breaking the itch-scratch cycle of atopic dermatitis. In addition, the use of emollients (e.g., petroleum jelly, Eucerin, Lubriderm) will enhance the absorption and effectiveness of topical corticosteroids. Applying topical corticosteroids after hydrating the skin (after a shower or bath) may increase their absorption up to 10-fold. A weak coal tar preparation applied over a corticosteroid ointment can also reduce itching at night.

Acute exacerbations can be treated with a potent to midstrength topical corticosteroid for a few days to quickly control acutely inflamed skin lesions, but the patient should switch to a weaker-strength agent when the lesion is under control. Medium- to high-potency topical steroids should not be used on the face or neck area because of potential adverse effects such as local irritation, atrophy of the skin, and telangiectasia. Skin atrophy is more likely to occur when potent topical corticosteroids are applied repeatedly to thin and highly absorptive inflamed skin. In some instances, hypopigmentation has been associated with the use of topical corticosteroids, especially in darker-skinned individuals, such as African Americans. Most cases of pigmentation changes are related to the underlying dermatitis, however, rather than the use of topical corticosteroids. Topical corticosteroids may also complicate treatment by masking underlying bacterial or fungal infections or impairing healing processes. Topical corticosteroids should never be used on ulcerated skin.

Systemic corticosteroids are rarely necessary for the treatment of chronic atopic dermatitis, but they may be useful for an incapacitating acute exacerbation or when large numbers of weeping lesions are present. In these rare instances, the patient may benefit from a short course of oral prednisone (40–60 mg per day for adults and 1 mg/kg per day for children). Short-term therapy with prednisone does not require tapering if it is limited to 5 to 7 days and the patient does not have a history of recent oral prednisone use. As the lesions dry, topical corticosteroids may be started. Of note, given the significant adverse effects associated with systemic corticosteroid use, such regimens should be considered a last resort and not used regularly. In some instances, the decision to use systemic corticosteroids to treat atopic dermatitis may signify the need for inpatient care to gain control of a debilitating exacerbation, particularly in pediatric patients.

When the acute inflammation subsides after 2 to 3 weeks, the patient should decrease the frequency of the topical corticosteroids and focus primarily on emollients such as petroleum jelly or Eucerin cream. The chronic use of topical corticosteroids (mid to low strength) should be limited to twice-weekly applications to any given area and should not be continued indefinitely.

Topical tacrolimus (Protopic) and the related agent pimecrolimus (Elidel), applied twice per day, have been shown to be effective and safe for use as second-line agents in atopic dermatitis (Level I; Leung et al, 2004). These are immunomodulating calcineurin inhibitors. Most patients experience a dramatic reduction of pruritus within 3 days of initiating treatment and significant improvement in quality of life. When used as long-term maintenance therapy, topical preparations reduce the number of flares of atopic dermatitis and the requirement for corticosteroid treatment (Level I; Leung et al, 2004). Of note, given limitations in the long-term safety data for these agents, including rare reports of malignancy, the FDA has issued a "black box" warning for tacrolimus and pimecrolimus, warning clinicians against continuous long-term use of these agents in any age-group and highlighting the lack of approval of these agents in children less than 2 years of age.

Aggressive treatment of atopic dermatitis may also include cyclosporine A (CyA), an immunomodulatory drug, which may be as effective as corticosteroids, with fewer adverse effects. It is indicated for patients who have failed to respond to at least one systemic therapy or in patients for whom other systemic therapies are contraindicated or are intolerable. Its use can be highly beneficial in severe cases, but renal function must be closely monitored, and treatment courses must be restricted to 8 to 12 weeks. Azathioprine (Imuran) may also be used for maintenance therapy, but hematological and hepatic function must be followed. As with systemic corticosteroids, the use of a systemic immunosuppressant, such as CyA or azathioprine, for atopic dermatitis would strongly suggest the need for inpatient care to adequately control such an exacerbation.

Omalizumab (Xolair), an anti-IgE antibody that has been developed as an immunotherapeutic biological agent, has shown benefit in reducing atopy in highly allergic individuals, although it is not FDA approved to treat atopic dermatitis. In severe cases of atopic dermatitis, phototherapy with ultraviolet B radiation or PUVA photochemotherapy (psoralens with ultraviolet A radiation) may be used as an adjunct therapy. Lesions of patients with pustular superinfection should be cultured for antibiotic sensitivities if they do not heal in response to empiric therapy. Bacterial or fungal superinfections must be treated appropriately.

Complementary Therapy

Studies indicate that certain herbs may be of value in the treatment of dermatological conditions. These include chamomile, arnica, calendula, hamamelis (witch hazel), aloe vera, cardiospermum, *Mahonia aquifolium,* oak bark, bittersweet stalk, and capsaicin. Use of these herbs should be reserved for experienced practitioners in alternative health medicine because of the potential for allergic reactions.

Follow-up and Referral

If basic management of atopic dermatitis fails, referral to a dermatologist should be prompt. More aggressive treatment by a dermatologist is necessary for patients who have severe and extensive lesions or who do not respond to usual treatment with topical and/or systemic corticosteroids. Atopic skin is very susceptible to bacterial and viral infections. These patients may develop widespread herpes infections of the skin (eczema herpeticum, which may be life-threatening in children), and they should be protected from people with active herpetic lesions. During an exacerbation, patients may contract secondary bacterial infections, and empiric therapy with erythromycin or penicillinase-resistant penicillins is sometimes necessary.

Patient Education

Patients with atopic dermatitis should be educated to be vigilant in watching for the signs of secondary bacterial infection. The patients should be told to report it immediately so that an oral antibiotic can be prescribed. Education about the importance of environmental measures in the prevention of disease exacerbation should be emphasized. House dust mites, animal dander, and pollen are all identified as potential triggers based on IgE antibodies in the bloodstream of some patients and should be addressed when educating patients. Patients can be assisted in discovering ways to reduce sweating, such as reducing the amount of bedclothes at night; avoiding occlusive, hot garments; and keeping the living areas cool. Patients should be encouraged to recognize their stress "triggers" and to find measures to reduce their stress level, such as exercise.

Because *Staphylococcus aureus* colonizes the skin of more than 90% of patients with atopic dermatitis (compared with only 5% of persons without the disease), fingernails should be kept short, smooth, and clean. This may prevent the scratching, which exacerbates the inflammation that may allow microbes to be introduced into the skin. Patients should be informed that a change in seasons will cause exacerbations of their disease, especially during the fall. Patients can be reminded to use extra care in taking care of their skin at this time by upgrading to stronger moisturizers (from lotions to petroleum jelly). Refills of their medication should be ordered before recurrence of symptoms. The provider can assist the patient in developing a simple regimen of topical steroid therapy for acute exacerbations. Patients with frequent exacerbations of skin lesions on their hands should avoid occupations that require repeated hand washing, immersion in water, or other wet conditions.

Food allergies are a common aggravating factor in up to 20% of patients with atopic dermatitis and are more common in children. A dietitian should be consulted when patients are eliminating foods from their diet, because unsupervised food restriction may lead to malnutrition.

■ CONTACT DERMATITIS

Contact dermatitis is a common condition categorized as either *irritant dermatitis* or *allergic dermatitis.* Although both of these conditions can have similar presentations, the etiology of each disease is what differentiates the two dermatitides. *Allergic contact dermatitis* is immunologically mediated, whereas *irritant contact dermatitis* is the result of repeated "insults" to atopic skin from caustic, irritant, or detergent-type substances.

Epidemiology and Causes

Almost any substance may induce a cutaneous reaction depending on its concentration, the duration of contact, and the condition of the contacted skin. The etiology of allergic contact dermatitis may be from antimicrobials such as neomycin, antihistamines, anesthetics such as benzocaine, hair dyes, preservatives, latex, or adhesive tape. The etiology of irritant contact dermatitis may be from soaps, detergents, or organic solvents. Irritant contact dermatitis accounts for about 80% of all cases of contact dermatitis.

Delayed-type hypersensitivity reactions are immunological responses to contact allergens that occur in sensitized individuals. One of the most frequent causes of allergic contact dermatitis is from plants in the *Rhus* genus, which includes poison ivy, poison oak, and poison sumac. Other common topical sensitizers include ragweed pollen, dust mites, ethylenediamine (a stabilizer in many topical creams), potassium dichromate, paraphenylenediamine (dyes), nickel (10% of females are allergic to nickel found in jewelry), rubber compounds, and benzocaine (an OTC topical anesthetic for itching or pain). It is estimated that there are more than 6 million chemicals in the environment and that approximately 3,000 of them are potential sensitizers.

Contact dermatitis accounts for 4% to 7% of all dermatology consults. Hand dermatitis affects 2% of the population at any given time, and 20% of female patients will be affected at least once in their lifetime. Contact dermatitis is more common in adults than in children, and effects are more extreme in elderly patients. Women are twice as likely as men to develop dermatitis and are at highest risk after childbirth. White Americans are affected more frequently, and fair-skinned redheads are the most vulnerable population.

Pathophysiology

Contact dermatitis is considered either allergic or irritant induced. A delayed-type hypersensitivity response (type IV immune reaction) elicits a non–IgE-mediated allergic response to specific antigens when applied to the skin, producing a local reaction characterized histologically by epidermal changes including intracellular edema, spongiosis, and vesiculation. On initial contact with the offending agent, the antigen is taken up and processed by epidermal antigen-presenting cells known as Langerhans cells. These cells present antigens to naïve, antigen-specific CD4+ and CD8+ T lymphocytes, located in regional lymph nodes that drain the affected areas of skin. Over approximately 10 to 14 days, sensitized T cells migrate from the lymph nodes to sites of antigenic exposure, where subsequent reexposure to the same antigen results in an allergic reaction mediated by cytokine release. This response with notable skin surface changes typically occurs within 12 to 48 hours of reexposure to the antigen.

Irritant contact dermatitis is the result of a direct cytotoxic effect of an irritant to the cells of the epidermis, with a subsequent inflammatory response in the dermis. The main pathological feature of contact dermatitis is intracellular edema of the epidermis, which may result in intraepidermal vesicles and bullae formation in the acute phase. In chronic cases, papules, scaling, and lichenification occur. Irritants penetrate and disrupt the stratum corneum and injure the underlying epidermis and dermis as various immune cells congregate around dilated capillaries, contributing to the inflammatory process.

Rubber-glove dermatitis demonstrates the spectrum of pathophysiological mechanisms involved in contact dermatitis. Chemical irritants used in the glove manufacturing process (e.g., thiram, mercapto derivatives) may cause an allergic dermatitis via a delayed-type T-cell–mediated hypersensitivity reaction. In addition, rubber glove components may result in a direct irritant effect on the moist skin of glove-wearers. Finally, the natural rubber protein *latex,* once widely used in medical products, may elicit a profound IgE-mediated immediate hypersensitivity response, leading to systemic anaphylaxis and even death.

Interestingly, people with venous stasis (i.e., impaired venous return with pooling of blood in distended veins, particularly in the lower extremities) are more susceptible to irritant contact dermatitis, particularly from wood alcohols such as lanolin, fragrances, topical antibiotics such as neomycin, and methylparaben preservatives. Correctly diagnosing this condition is often difficult because contact dermatitis is often indistinguishable from stasis dermatitis.

Clinical Presentation
Subjective

The cardinal symptom of contact dermatitis is a pruritic erythematous rash. Often, the patient is not aware of a previous history, but there may have been periodic episodes of pruritic rash that resolved spontaneously. The patient may or may not be able to describe the conditions or substances contributing to the dermatitis, but exposure history to known or unknown common antigens and irritants should be sought by the clinician. In allergic contact dermatitis (in contrast to atopic dermatitis), the inflammatory reaction on the skin occurs much faster, typically within 6 to 12 hours of reexposure. In contrast to allergic contact dermatitis, irritant reactions do not always occur immediately after contact with the offending substance. The response time between the initial contact with the irritant and the symptoms is variable, and the severity of the reaction depends on the concentration, amount, and length of exposure to the irritating substance.

Objective

Contact dermatitis presents with inflammation of the epidermis and is manifested by erythema (as in all types of dermatitis), but it does not present with the smooth, intact epidermal surface that characterizes hives (urticaria). The epidermal inflammation seen in acute contact dermatitis results in rough, reddened patches but without the thickening and discrete demarcation of psoriasis. The acute lesions of contact dermatitis are characterized by weeping lesions with numerous tiny vesicles on an erythematous base that is pruritic or has a burning or stinging sensation. The surrounding area in severe cases is also erythematous, with edema and increased heat in the area, making it difficult to rule out secondary bacterial infection in some cases.

Lesions in nonallergic and delayed-type hypersensitivity contact dermatitis present in similar fashion, but the typical distribution and the lack of an atopic history are the most helpful factors in the diagnosis. A clothing- or detergent-related cause should be suspected if the lesions are generalized and primarily affect the borders of the axillae, waist, and upper thighs. Reactions to toxic plants (e.g., *Rhus* or *Toxicodendron* species) follow a history of exposure. The characteristic rash is vesicular and linear (or asymmetrical) and is frequently found on the hands and ankles. *Rhus* dermatitis lesions are sometimes found on the facial area if the patient has inadvertently scratched the face with contaminated fingers. Lesions in an area where jewelry has been worn recently (e.g., neck, wrist, earlobes) may indicate a hypersensitivity to nickel. Usually, the area of skin that has been the most heavily contaminated will break out first, followed by areas of lesser exposure. The location of the rash gives the clinician the best clues to the possible etiological agent. For example, a patient with a rash on the scalp and the back of the neck might report a history of the use of a new shampoo, a new hair dye, or other scalp or hair treatments. (See Advanced Assessment 7.3.)

Diagnostic Reasoning

Diagnostic Tests

Diagnosis of contact dermatitis is based on the history of exposure to an irritant or allergen and the subsequent appearance of a rash on the exposed skin, either immediately or later on (delayed hypersensitivity). If scabies is suspected, skin scrapings can be examined under a microscope to rule out that condition. If tinea (corporis, cruris, pedis, manuum) infection is suspected, skin scrapings should be treated with potassium hydroxide (KOH) and gently heated. A microscopic exam for tinea infection should search for hyphae and spores. If bacterial infection (impetigo) is suspected, cultures should be taken from the moist areas of the rash or from the discharge. Viral cultures can be done to rule out suspected viral etiology (herpes simplex, herpes zoster).

Advanced Assessment 7.3 Contact Dermatitis

Stages

Acute
Erythema and edema
Clear, fluid-filled vesicles or bullae
Exudate, clear fluid
Distinct margins

Subacute
Lessening edema
Formation of papules
Less distinct margins

Chronic
Minimal edema
Scaling skin
Lichenification
Minimal erythema

Laboratory tests that are done by specialists (allergist) include the scratch and intradermal tests. Scratch (skin-prick) tests should not be done during an acute episode of contact dermatitis because of an increased rate of false-positive reactions. The patch test performed by a dermatologist is useful to identify specific irritants in patients with histories that are suggestive of acute contact dermatitis. Allergens that are commonly responsible for such reactions are fixed in dehydrated gel layers and taped against the skin of the patient's back for 48 hours and then removed. A final reading done at 72 to 96 hours after initial application will usually reveal any evidence of contact dermatitis. In some patients, a CBC with differential will show eosinophilia, but this blood test is neither sensitive nor necessary for the diagnosis. Skin biopsy is rarely necessary for diagnosis, particularly in the setting of a convincing contact exposure history.

Differential Diagnosis

The differential diagnosis of contact dermatitis is similar to that for atopic dermatitis and includes both common and rare disorders. Common disorders that have a similar presentation to contact dermatitis include seborrheic dermatitis, impetigo, and herpes zoster. Seborrheic dermatitis rashes, although erythematous, have a greasy and scaly appearance and appear only in certain areas of the body such as the hairline, the ears, the scalp, and the face. Impetigo, which is caused by gram-positive *Staphylococcus* or *Streptococcus* bacteria, is more common in children. A honey-colored crust is seen on top of the erythematous lesions; impetigo also does not have a linear appearance like contact dermatitis. Herpes zoster is more common in older patients, and the lesions appear as multiple small vesicles on an erythematous base. Although herpes zoster has a linear distribution, it is more likely to occur on the trunk area (contact dermatitis occurs more often on the hands or face) and will follow the path of a dermatome.

Management

The clinical challenge in the treatment of contact dermatitis is to provide symptomatic relief to the patient while attempting to identify the underlying allergic precipitant. Identifying the antigen or irritant in contact dermatitis is critical, both to eliminate or minimize the current contact and to avoid future exposure (Level I; Beltrani et al, 2006). The responsible irritant should be identified and eliminated to prevent the cycle of itching, scratching, and skin disruption, which can lead to chronic changes in the skin. A careful history of exposures is key in addition to a thorough skin examination. The effects of *Rhus* dermatitis (from poison ivy, poison oak, or poison sumac) may be lessened if the exposed skin is thoroughly rinsed in soap and water or with isopropyl alcohol, as soon as possible after exposure. Exposed clothing should be discarded.

For localized contact dermatitis with weeping lesions, treatment with moist compresses and simple drying agents or antipruritic lotions (e.g., Burow's aluminum acetate solution, Calamine lotion) applied several times a day is usually effective. For more extensive and severe cases, potent topical steroids in cream form (avoid the use of ointments on wet lesions because they can cause skin maceration) can be applied twice daily for the first few days to help decrease pruritus and inflammation. If treatment is necessary beyond 2 weeks, a less potent (mild or moderate) topical steroid may be used twice daily until the rash resolves. High-potency steroids should not be used on the face or in bodily folds (intertriginous areas) because of their ability to thin the skin and cause hypopigmentation.

Oral systemic steroids may be indicated in acute and particularly severe cases of contact dermatitis offering relief within 12 to 24 hours (Level I; Leung et al, 2004). Relatively high doses of oral prednisone can be given for 10 to 14 days (or up to 21 days in the most severe cases). Abrupt cessation of high-dose systemic corticosteroids that are given for more than 5 days' duration should be avoided. Potential adverse effects of oral prednisone therapy are more likely with long-term use and may include any of the following: suppression of the hypothalamic-pituitary-adrenal axis, hypokalemia, hypocalcemia, masking or worsening of infection, increased likelihood of secondary infection, carbohydrate intolerance and worsening of diabetes, glaucoma, cataracts, osteoporosis, dermal atrophy, skin hypopigmentation, and psychiatric disorders including depression, euphoria, or even acute psychosis. It should also be noted that even systemic steroids will likely prove ineffective if exposure to the offending allergen or irritant is not limited.

Follow-up and Referral

Follow-up and referral are determined by the patient's condition and response to therapy. Severe cases should be referred to a dermatologist or an allergist.

Patient Education

The provider should teach the patient and family about the disease and the appropriate use of medications, as well as adverse effects or exacerbations that should prompt the patient to contact the health-care provider. The mainstay of prevention is helping patients identify the agents causing the dermatitis and teaching them to avoid exposure or to use protective clothing and gloves.

■ SEBORRHEIC DERMATITIS

Seborrheic dermatitis is one of the most common skin conditions seen in primary care among adults and the elderly. It is a chronic condition that is marked by remissions and exacerbations. Seborrheic dermatitis commonly manifests in patients with HIV infection. A severe or resistant case on a patient should prompt investigation for risk factors of HIV infection. The rashes of seborrheic dermatitis are seen on skin that is rich in sebaceous glands. (It is associated with an increased production of sebum.) The affected skin is pink, edematous, and covered with yellow to brown scales and crusts. These rashes are most easily seen on the scalp, the forehead, the eyebrows, and the area surrounding the nose and the ears.

Epidemiology and Causes

Seborrheic dermatitis affects approximately 2% to 5% of the adult population. It runs in families and has a known genetic component. It may be an inflammatory reaction to *Malassezia furfur* yeasts. The occurrence of seborrheic dermatitis is most common during early infancy on the scalp ("cradle cap"), after the second decade of life, and in the elderly or immunocompromised patients. A strong association with HIV infection and AIDS is well established.

Pathophysiology

This type of dermatitis was originally defined by excess oil secretion from the sebaceous glands and is thus found on areas of the body where such glands are most concentrated, that is, in decreasing order, the scalp, face, chest, upper back, pubic area, and axillae. Interestingly, however, overproduction of sebum is not seen in all cases of seborrheic dermatitis, nor is the composition of the sebum the main factor in this condition. Skin biopsies typically reveal parakeratotic scale heaped around hair follicles and an inflammatory lymphocytic infiltrate. Thus, mild epidermal hyperproliferation has been cited as a contributing factor. However, it is not known whether this occurs in response to infection by saprophytic skin fungi or vice versa.

Malassezia furfur commonly colonizes affected individuals. Recurrence of symptoms has been linked to an increase in the number of *M furfur* organisms found on the skin surface. Fungal-specific stains of affected skin reveal large numbers of *M furfur* spores within the stratum corneum, the uppermost skin layer.

Clinical Presentation
Subjective

The typical patient is an adult male who complains of a pink, scaling rash located on the face and scalp. Seborrheic dermatitis can also be an incidental finding; some patients, especially elderly patients, are not bothered by the cosmetic effect of the rashes. The lesions are usually asymptomatic in most patients, but pruritus may be present (and is aggravated by perspiration), especially in scalp lesions.

Objective

Seborrheic dermatitis presents as scaly patches that may be slightly papular; each patch is surrounded by erythema. The lesion borders are poorly defined, and the scales may be greasy and appear yellow. The most frequently involved area is the scalp, and the condition is differentiated from common dandruff (pityriasis sicca) by the appearance of erythema, which may be minimal or moderate. The affected areas may include the forehead at the hairline, eyebrows, nasal folds, and the retroauricular and presternal areas. In more severe cases, intertriginous areas, as well as the external ear canal and umbilicus, are involved. The rashes may be more difficult to recognize in fastidious patients because daily bathing removes some of the scale.

Diagnostic Reasoning
Diagnostic Tests

Diagnosis of seborrheic dermatitis is based on clinical findings and the history. Dermatologists and allergists can test for *Malassezia furfur* using antigen-specific skin-prick or serum RAST testing. Fifteen percent to 65% of patients with seborrheic dermatitis have positive responses to skin-prick tests with *Malassezia* extracts. *Malassezia* antibodies have also been found in young adults with head and neck dermatitis. Fungal-specific periodic acid Schiff and Gamori Methenamine Silver stains identify hyphae and spores in skin scraping or biopsy samples; however, these specialized stains typically require specialist referral and are not commonly used in the primary-care setting. Rather, the diagnosis of seborrheic dermatitis is most commonly based on the characteristic appearance and distribution of the rash, as well as its response to empiric therapy.

Differential Diagnosis

Skin conditions that mimic seborrheic dermatitis include impetigo, atopic dermatitis, psoriasis, scabies, tinea capitis, and Langerhans cell histiocytosis. A history of the same rash recurring at characteristic locations on the body (e.g., the scalp and hairline, sides of the nose and upper lip, eyebrows and eyelashes, cheeks, or ears) will give the clinician the best clues to identify seborrheic dermatitis correctly. Impetigo, a bacterial infection of the skin caused by *Staphylococcus* or *Streptococcus* bacteria, has an acute onset and tends to occur on the extremities (a location not seen in seborrheic dermatitis) or on the face. The most useful distinguishing feature between atopic dermatitis and seborrheic dermatitis is the increased number of lesions on the forearms in the former, compared with the increased number of lesions in the axillae in the latter. The erythema of seborrheic dermatitis typically has a pinkish hue, rather than the bright-red appearance of psoriasis.

Seborrheic dermatitis is also associated with several chronic conditions, including Parkinson's disease, HIV infection and AIDS, phenylketonuria, cardiac failure, zinc deficiency, and epilepsy. Other dermatological disorders, such as acne vulgaris, rosacea, and psoriasis, may also be associated with these diseases, however. Importantly, florid manifestations of seborrheic dermatitis may be an early cutaneous indicator of HIV infection, and these patients may demonstrate extensive symptoms that are often resistant to therapy.

Management

The high incidence and chronic benign nature of seborrheic dermatitis present a therapeutic challenge. Mild to moderate cases do not seem to bother some patients, especially elderly patients who frequently refuse treatment or are noncompliant. Younger patients who are bothered by the cosmetic effects of the rashes on the face frequently request treatment. The therapeutic approach is aimed at managing symptoms and reducing the yeast count on the skin.

The regular use of an OTC dandruff shampoo is sufficient to control most scalp symptoms. The preparations must remain on the scalp for at least 5 to 7 minutes to be effective. Commonly used ingredients in these products include selenium sulfide, zinc pyrithione, tar, salicylic acid, sulfur, or ketoconazole. Zinc pyrithione and selenium sulfide are classified as keratolytic agents. They appear to be both fungicidal and cytostatic. The combination of sulfur and salicylic acid has keratolytic, antifungal, and antiseptic actions. Coal tar agents must be used with caution in fair-haired persons because they may cause an undesirable change in color.

Resistant seborrheic dermatitis may require a prescription shampoo. A 2.5% selenium sulfide shampoo, a ketoconazole shampoo (Nizoral shampoo), and a detoconazole shampoo are available. Keratolytic or oil-based lotions are recommended to soften heavy crusts.

A topical corticosteroid may be necessary when significant erythema is present. Hydrocortisone cream 0.5% to 1.0% (OTC) for the face or betamethasone valerate 0.1% for the scalp should be applied after cleansing. Facial application and long-term use of topical corticosteroids should be avoided because of the risk of telangiectasia and dermal atrophy. These risks are not present with the topical use of ketoconazole. Exudative lesions may require compresses of Burow's solution applied for 30 minutes three times daily. Ketoconazole shampoo every other day is recommended for resistant cases. Ketoconazole 2% cream may be applied to the affected areas twice daily when there is facial or chest involvement.

Calcineurin inhibitors that lower the activity of the immune system may be effective for recalcitrant cases although these drugs are not FDA approved for seborrheic dermatitis. Such agents include tacrolimus (Protopic) and pimecrolimus (Elidel), which are available in topical formulations. As indicated for second-line therapy in atopic dermatitis, the FDA cautions against the chronic, long-term use of these medications in any age group, given concerns over their long-term safety, including rare reports of malignancies.

Once symptoms resolve, maintenance therapy may be required with a once to twice a week application. The prophylactic use of a ketoconazole shampoo (Nizoral) once a week is safe, easy, and at times very rewarding. For a superinfection of gram-positive skin bacteria, cephalexin 7 to 10 days is required.

Because a strong association with HIV infection and AIDS is well established, treating the underlying HIV infection with effective antiretroviral therapy is often the key to resolution of the patient's skin findings.

Follow-up and Referral

Repeated secondary infections or resistance to standard management require a prompt referral to a dermatologist.

Patient Education

Patients should be reassured that seborrheic dermatitis is not contagious or progressive. They must, however, understand the chronic nature of the condition and the need for continued management. The role of emotional stress in acute flare-ups should be explained. If topical steroids are used, the patient needs to be instructed in the proper application and the potential adverse effects. A list of effective OTC preparations should be provided, so each patient can select one that meets his or her personal preferences. Daily shampooing of oily hair is recommended for the first week, decreasing to two or three times a week as maintenance therapy.

■ PSORIASIS

Psoriasis is a chronic relapsing disorder of keratin synthesis that is characterized by well-circumscribed, raised, erythematous papules and plaques, covered with silvery-white scales, usually involving extensor areas in adults such as the elbows and knees, the scalp, and, in some forms, the flexural surfaces of the body. The phrase "heartbreak of psoriasis" was coined because of the physically and emotionally disabling effects of the disease. The more commonly seen variants of psoriasis are plaque, guttate, inverse, pustular, and erythrodermic psoriasis. Inflammatory arthritis may complicate this condition in 10% to 20% of cases. Plaque psoriasis is the most common form in young adults, which presents as erythematous lesions with well-demarcated margins, topped with a thick, silvery scale. Plaque psoriasis accounts for approximately 80% of all cases of psoriasis. Guttate psoriasis is more common in children, presenting as an acute eruption of multiple, smaller plaques (less than 1 cm). Inverse psoriasis is characterized by localization of psoriatic plaques to flexural (intertriginous) surfaces. Pustular psoriasis is the most serious form characterized by widespread scaling with a sheet of superficial pustules. Erythrodermic psoriasis may be considered a separate entity or as the most severe form of pustular psoriasis, which may be life threatening and is associated with chronic immunosuppression (e.g., HIV disease). Bright-red erythema affecting a large portion of the skin surface is the most prominent feature of erythrodermic psoriasis, which may present with variable keratotic scale and the presence of pustules.

Epidemiology and Causes

Psoriasis affects almost 3 million Americans annually and 2% to 4% of the population worldwide. Psoriasis is universal in occurrence, but the prevalence varies according to geography, race, and ethnicity. Geographical variations in prevalence (e.g., almost no cases in South Americans living in the Andes, nearly 3% of the population in Denmark) reflect the influence of both genetic and environmental factors. Psoriasis is less frequent among Asians and among North and South American native peoples compared with people of European ancestry. It is also less frequent among West Africans, which may help explain the low prevalence of psoriasis among African Americans. Prevalence is highest among Scandinavians, with rates being slightly higher in northern rather than southern Sweden, further supporting the role of climate and sunlight exposure in the expression of the disease. Prevalence of the disease in the United States is about 2% to 3% overall.

Adult men and women are affected with equal frequency. The two peak ages at onset are during the late teens to early 20s and in the late 50s to early 60s. Women and adolescent girls tend to have earlier onset than males. Earlier onset is associated with a more severe disease. There is little to no epidemiological evidence that psoriasis is mediated by infectious agents.

Psoriasis has a strong genetic influence, with one-third of patients with psoriasis reporting having a relative with the disease. In family studies, when one parent is affected, 8% of offspring develop psoriasis and tend to have earlier onset. When both parents have psoriasis, the percentage increases to 41%. The mode of genetic transmission is not yet defined, however.

Environmental factors are known to precipitate the disease among genetically predisposed patients and include trauma to normal skin that results in psoriasis in areas of repeated friction (Köbner's phenomenon), infections (upper respiratory infections, *Streptococcus pyogenes*, HIV), stress, fatigue, warm humid climate, sunlight, and certain drugs (systemic corticosteroids, lithium, beta-adrenergic blockers, NSAIDs, and antimalarials). Risk factors for psoriasis are listed in Risk Factors 7.1.

Despite intensive investigation, the cause of psoriasis remains unknown, but it is deemed to be a multifactorial disease, with genetic, environmental, biochemical, and immunological origins. Psoriasis, formerly theorized as an idiopathic skin disease, is now known to be a genetically controlled, immune-mediated chronic disease. Because cutaneous lesions of psoriasis were thought to result from unregulated hyperproliferative activity in the epidermis, for decades, treatment for psoriasis was primarily suppressive and was directed toward normalizing the hyperkeratinocytic activity.

Currently, the speculation is that genetically predisposed persons may experience clonal T-cell activation in response to antigenic stimulation. Proponents of this theory advance this view based on evidence that affected persons have an increase of various human leukocyte antigens (HLAs), particularly certain class I HLAs such as HLA-B27, which is also seen in patients with psoriatic arthritis, a form of inflammatory arthritis with redness and painful swelling of joints that may co-occur with psoriasis (although not all patients with psoriatic arthritis will have active skin manifestations). In addition, psoriatic plaques are rich in activated T lymphocytes that are capable of both cellular proliferation and inflammation.

Current research is focused on the role of T cells and the ability of cytokines to influence the dermal immune response to an as yet unidentified antigen. This focus is based on the finding that the immune-modulating agent cyclosporin is capable of improving psoriatic symptoms, which led to a rethinking of disease pathogenesis. The genetic components of the disease have been the subject of extensive research. One genetic region linking susceptibility to psoriasis in some individuals has been isolated to chromosome 6, and the first non–chromosome 6 gene marker for psoriasis has been identified on chromosome 17q. Others have identified possible DNA loci on chromosomes 4, 8, and 16. Thus, a primary goal of current psoriasis research is to elucidate fully the interplay of genetic and environmental influences on the errant cellular effects seen in the disease.

Pathophysiology

Microscopic examination of psoriatic plaques typically reveals thickened stratum corneum with hyperplasia of the epidermis and little inflammation. The basic pathology of psoriasis is the uncontrolled hyperkeratinization of the stratum corneum layer of the skin. Hyperproliferation of keratins 6 and 16 (common to reactive and healing skin) predominates, whereas expression of keratins 1 and 10 (typically found in normal skin) is reduced. The psoriatic process occurs in varying degrees and results in a wide range of clinical symptoms. If increased mitosis or hyperkeratinization predominates, the result is a thick, silvery scale because of the separation of corneocytes and the presence of air in between. Despite this epidermal hyperplasia and parakeratosis, however, the granular layer of the epidermis is significantly thinned or absent. In contrast, if vasodilation predominates, the result is a diffused red and hot, slightly scaling skin. Of note, these two processes may coexist.

There are three stages to the psoriatic process: (1) an increased mitotic rate that results in rapid cellular turnover and shortened transit time for the basal layer to the stratum corneum or epidermis (3–4 days, versus a normal 28 days); (2) dilation of upper dermal capillaries with intermittent extravasation of T cells and polymorphonuclear neutrophils into both the dermis and epidermis, leading to (3) the faulty keratinization and accumulation of the stratum corneum, which clinically presents as raised papules and plaques covered with white, silvery scales. Multiple growth factors (e.g., epidermal growth factor, transforming growth factor–alpha) and cytokines (e.g., interferon-gamma, IL-2, IL-6, IL-8, and IL-17) are overexpressed in psoriatic skin. Moreover, in plaque-type psoriasis, the T cells localized to the epidermis appear to express specific clonalities with regard to their antigenic receptors, implicating unrestrained T-cell replication in the pathogenesis of the disease. Interestingly, however, psoriasis is also associated with many causes of chronic immunosuppression and may be the presenting finding in newly diagnosed HIV infection—particularly the severe erythrodermic form.

Most recently, the importance of a novel subset of CD4 T helper T cells, known as Th17 cells, has been highlighted in the autoimmune pathogenesis of psoriasis. Activated Th17 cells produce multiple cytokines, including IL-17, IL-21, and IL-22, and proliferate in response to IL-23. Several studies have demonstrated the importance of Th17 cells in fighting infection by extracellular bacteria and fungi. Thus, one theory is that dysregulated Th17 function leads to an exuberant immunoresponse to skin flora and ultimately the hyperkeratinization characteristic of psoriasis. In turn, Th17 cells have been isolated from psoriatic skin plaques. Work in this field is ongoing.

Drug-exacerbated psoriasis offers some insights into disease mechanisms. Lithium is believed to act by enhancing the release of inflammatory mediators from neutrophils. Beta blockers lead to psoriasis by decreasing cyclic adenosine monophosphate (AMP)—dependent protein kinase—an inhibitor of cellular proliferation. NSAIDs cause a buildup of the pro-inflammatory mediator arachidonic acid by inhibiting the enzyme cyclooxygenase. Antimalarials, the antifungal terbinafine, and angiotensin-converting enzyme inhibitors are also associated with exacerbation of psoriasis, although these mechanisms are unclear. Drug-induced exacerbations can be unpredictable and severe. Importantly, they are often delayed and may occur months after the start of drug use.

Clinical Presentation

Subjective

Patients with psoriasis usually present to the practitioner with concern over "itchy, red, inflamed and dry, scaly plaques that have gotten worse." Statements about the onset and course of the disease are highly variable for each individual. Symptoms usually begin gradually and are confined to only a few areas (one or both elbows, knees, buttocks, or scalp), but psoriasis can also be explosive in onset. One cause of an explosive onset is a preceding streptococcal throat infection, which can lead in 2 to 3 weeks to multiple, small, guttate lesions with a generalized distribution over the body. Once the disease appears, it follows an irregular, chronic, unpredictable course. It may remain localized to a few areas, or it may cause intermittent or continuous generalized lesions. Itching is usually not a problem in psoriasis, but it may be severe in some patients. These patients often notice blood stains on the bed linens from traumatic, inadvertent scratching of the plaques during sleep. Lesions often occur at sites of trauma (Köbner's phenomenon). A family history of psoriasis is elicited in one-third of patients, and 50% of these patients have an affected parent.

There are three tools commonly used to assess the severity of psoriasis:

- The Psoriasis Area and Severity Index (PASI) combines the assessment of plaque severity (erythema, induration/thickness, and scaling) and the skin surface area affected.

- The Dermatology Life Quality Index (DLQI) has the patient self-rate the impact of the condition on important aspects of the patient's life.
- Affected Body Surface Area (BSA) is an assessment of the overall skin area involved by percentage.

A Web site for accessing and automatically calculating disease severity scores using these tools is listed under Resources at the end of the chapter. The PASI is the most widely used tool in clinical research and practice settings.

Objective

Physical exam reveals lesions that are erythematous plaques surrounded by a thick, silvery scale (which is not easily removed), resembling mica. When these micaceous scales are traumatically removed, multiple small bleeding sites appear (Auspitz's sign). In intertriginous areas, maceration and moisture prevent dry scales from accumulating, but the lesions remain red and sharply defined.

Lesions usually are distributed symmetrically over areas of bony prominences such as the elbows and knees. Scaly plaques also occur frequently on the trunk, scalp, intergluteal cleft, and umbilicus. The latter three areas are frequently overlooked by the patient and clinician, but are important in making the diagnosis, especially in patients with associated psoriatic arthritis and limited skin lesions. The nature of such inflammatory arthritis may become apparent only after typical skin lesions are recognized.

A thorough examination of the entire skin surface is crucial, therefore, to the diagnosis and treatment of a patient with suspected psoriasis. Another helpful diagnostic feature is the Köbner's phenomenon, in which intense trauma induces formation of new skin lesions. Such isomorphic lesions can also be induced on the palms of patients whose hands are exposed to friction.

Nail involvement may include stippling or pitting of the nail plate or a yellow to red-brown coloring ("oil-staining") of the nails (nail psoriasis). An accumulation of yellow debris under the nails, simulating a tinea infection (tinea unguium), is seen in some patients. Swelling, redness, and scaling of the paronychial margins occur often and are associated with arthritis of the distal interphalangeal joints. The clinical course of this disease is characterized by chronicity and seasonal fluctuations, with improvement in the summer (due to sun exposure) and worsening in the winter as dry skin leads to epidermal injury.

Some patients with psoriasis (10%–20%) may suffer from inflammatory arthritis, although the most common form of arthritis seen in psoriasis patients is osteoarthritis. The inflammatory joint manifestations of psoriatic arthritis may occur when psoriatic skin lesions are present, or they may precede initial skin manifestations, with psoriatic arthritis being suspected in a patient with inflammatory joint disease due to a family history of psoriasis. Associated inflammatory arthritis seen in psoriasis patients typically involves the distal interphalangeal joints of the hands and feet but may also involve the vertebrae of the spine, as seen with another form of seronegative (i.e., rheumatoid factor–negative) arthritis known as ankylosing spondylitis.

The recognized clinical variants of psoriasis (plaque, pustular, guttate, inverse, and erythrodermic) are discussed in greater detail in Differential Diagnosis 7.6.

Diagnostic Reasoning
Diagnostic Tests

Initial laboratory studies include routine laboratory testing (CBC with differential and serum chemistry profile) plus serum uric acid level, antinuclear antibody titer, and rheumatoid factor. Throat culture is appropriate if *Streptococcus pyogenes* infection is suspected as the

precipitating factor (such as in guttate psoriasis). Often, the laboratory values are generally within normal limits except for the serum uric acid level, which may show elevation (hyperuricemia). In more severe variants of psoriasis, other specific tests may be ordered. An elevated erythrocyte sedimentation rate and decreased albumin levels, along with anemia, can be observed in chronic disease. Immunoglobulins are generally normal, but selective IgA and IgG deficiencies are observed in some patients. In pustular psoriasis, leukocytosis and hypocalcemia are seen.

X-ray studies of the hands are sometimes helpful to search for associated psoriatic arthritis in patients who complain of joint pains in their hands. X-ray films of patients with psoriatic arthritis will show extensive erosion and luxation of distal interphalangeal or metatarsophalangeal joints bilaterally.

Only in unusual circumstances (severe or unusual forms of the disease) are histological studies necessary to

---

Differential Diagnosis 7.6   Psoriasis

Type of Psoriasis	Clinical Presentation	Differential Diagnosis	Key to Diagnosis
Plaque Psoriasis	• Plaques with white silvery scales • Seen on knees, elbows, neck, scalp, between buttocks, or on back • Usually bilateral involvement • Intertriginous areas may be involved, but scales are absent • Positive Auspitz's sign and Köbner's phenomenon • Gradual onset, chronic course	Seborrheic dermatitis	Sharply marginated yellowish red patches with sharp borders and greasy scales. Seen on scalp, central face, eyebrows, eyelids, nasolabial folds, and external ear. Can be pruritic.
		Nummular eczema	Pruritic, coin-shaped plaques or papulovesicles on an erythematous base and uniform scaling; may become exudative and crusted. Typically seen on legs, upper extremities, and trunk.
		Lichen planus	Pruritic, flat, irregular purple papules with fine white lines and scales. Commonly seen on flexor surfaces, nails, and scalp.
		Pityriasis rubra pilaris	Generalized erythematous, red-orange lesions with diffuse thickening interspersed with areas of normal skin; the palms and soles are usually affected.
		Mycosis fungoides	Sharply demarcated, scaly, raised plaques to violaceous nodules that may ulcerate. Also known as cutaneous T-cell lymphoma.
		Atopic dermatitis	Severe pruritus; palmar markings; increased infraorbital folds, red cheeks in infancy; sides of neck, hands, and flexural surfaces most commonly affected after age 12 years.

Continued

Differential Diagnosis 7.6 Psoriasis—cont'd

Type of Psoriasis	Clinical Presentation	Differential Diagnosis	Key to Diagnosis
Pustular Psoriasis	• Lesions may be localized, appearing on the hands and feet (Barber's disease), or involve the entire skin surface (Von Zumbusch's disease) • Accompanying systemic symptoms • Onset is sudden. Pustules appear on the edges of existing psoriatic plaques and on the palms. Pruritus and intense burning sensation are present. Patient may have a fever and systemic symptoms. Systemic complications include pneumonia, congestive heart failure, and hepatitis.	Pustular dermatitis	Persistent or recurrent dry red and scaly rash; first appearance in infancy; history of dry skin since birth.
Guttate Psoriasis	• Characterized by small, red papules (<1 cm in diameter)	Secondary syphilis	Base of lesion (ulcer) is clean and smooth; edges are raised and well circumscribed. Usually occurs in genital region or on lips.
	• Discrete lesions, seen in a raindrop- or showerlike distribution, usually on the trunk and extremities • Triggered by streptococcal infection • May see Köbner's phenomenon	Pityriasis rosea	Peripheral scaling, well-demarcated, salmon-colored patch, forming a fine collarette (herald patch); followed by other lesions on trunk and proximal extremities. Christmas-tree distribution on exposed areas.
Inverse Psoriasis	• Involves the flexural area (e.g., armpit, groin)	Candidiasis	Erythematous; macerated patches with sharp, scaling border. Satellite papules and pustules that are tender and pruritic are common.
Erythrodermic Psoriasis	• Severe form of pustular psoriasis • Generalized distribution • Erythema with variable scale with fluid and electrolyte loss; chills	Drug eruption	Massive superficial dermal edema lifts the epidermis, forming necrosis, appearing as violaceous plaques or bullae; then heal with postinflammatory hyperpigmentation, e.g., Stevens-Johnson syndrome, toxic epidermal necrosis.
		Pityriasis rubra pilaris	Fine to thick scales on palms or soles; orange-red with diffuse thickening.
		Eczematous dermatitis, mycosis fungoides	See descriptions above for nummular eczema and atopic dermatitis.

diagnose psoriasis. Biopsy is seldom necessary because the clinical features of psoriasis are so distinctive. At times, an invasive biopsy may be necessary for questionable diagnoses. Biopsies should be planned to yield maximal information. When performing a biopsy, intact, nonexcoriated lesions should be sampled. If there are lesions at different stages of eruption, more than one sample is necessary. Biopsies can include partial dermal thickness procedures such as shave or curettage biopsy, or full-thickness sampling with punch or excisional biopsy.

A skin biopsy is done with the use of a local anesthetic to obtain sufficient tissue for accurate diagnosis. Skin biopsy is a "clean" procedure and should be done very simply and quickly. The standard 4 mm punch biopsy is often used and is recommended. Minimal scarring is the desired end result. A biopsy should not be performed on infected skin, on any patient with a bleeding disorder, or on any individual who is allergic to local anesthetics. The key to a good biopsy is good selection of the sample. It is often useful to take two to six samples at the first examination of complex cases. Experience is invaluable in performing good biopsies. Clinicians who are not experienced in this procedure should refer the patient to a dermatologist. (See Therapeutic Procedure 7.1.)

Of note, the sudden onset of psoriasis, in particular erythrodermic forms, may be associated with HIV; thus, the presence of underlying HIV infection should be ruled out in such patients, if unknown.

Differential Diagnosis

Often, psoriasis is mistaken for other dermatological conditions. It is not uncommon to see a patient with more than one variant of psoriasis at the same time, and the pattern may also change over time. Other skin diseases should be ruled out, especially in atypical cases that are complicated by other systemic disorders. (See Differential Diagnosis 7.6.)

The differential diagnosis for psoriasis includes the following: atopic dermatitis, nummular eczema, cutaneous T-cell lymphoma (CTCL), tinea corporis, lichen planus, seborrheic dermatitis, drug eruptions, and secondary syphilis. Hyperkeratotic eczema of the palms is a common cause of misdiagnosis.

Atopic dermatitis frequently has its first presentation in infancy or childhood. The patient has a persistent or recurrent dry, red, scaly rash and a history of dry skin since birth. Atopic dermatitis at times develops a psoriasiform appearance, especially on the legs. Nummular eczema has a characteristic morphology that helps to distinguish it from other eczematous eruptions. Initially, nummular eczema presents with tiny papules and vesicles and then assumes its characteristic clinical appearance of coin-shaped plaques. It is typically seen on the legs, but it can also appear on the upper extremities and trunk; the lesions are pruritic, erythematous, and surrounded with uniform scaling.

CTCL can be difficult to diagnose in its early stages. Early on, the rash may appear as single or multiple erythematous, scaly macules. In its subsequent stage, which may occur anywhere from 6 months to 6 years later, the development of sharply demarcated, scaly, elevated, red to violaceous plaques, known as mycosis fungoides, occurs. These plaques may coalesce to form larger plaques with annular, circinate, or serpiginous borders, or they may completely regress. The disease may further progress to brown or purplish red dermal nodules (tumors). The nodules often occur in the face, the body folds, and the inframammary area in women. The tumors can progress further to exfoliative erythroderma. Through much of the process, CTCL may resemble atopic dermatitis with diffuse erythema and scaling; a definitive diagnosis can be made by skin biopsy.

Tinea corporis (ringworm) presents as erythematous patches and plaques with central clearing and peripheral scales, crusts, vesicles, and pustules. It may spontaneously resolve or worsen with topical corticosteroid treatment. In seborrheic dermatitis, the lesions are lighter in color, less well defined, and covered with a dull yellow scale. Lesions commonly occur in a similar psoriatic distribution, including face, scalp, and central chest. Lichen planus gives rise to diagnostic difficulty if it presents as hypertrophic lesions on the legs, as penile lesions, or on the hands. It results from excessive

---

Therapeutic Procedure 7.1   The Skin "Punch" Biopsy

- Prep the area around the lesion that has been carefully selected.
- Inject 1% lidocaine slowly and superficially at several sites around the lesion, for rapid effect and minimal injury. Epinephrine may be used to control bleeding except at certain sites, given the risk of tip necrosis (nose, ears, fingertips, toes, penis).
- Punch into the skin around the lesion at a 90-degree angle to the plane of the skin, with a quick back-and-forth twisting motion, reaching in fast.
- Carefully lift out the plug and snip it at the base with sharp tissue scissors.
- Place the tissue plug in a formalin solution.
- Apply pressure with sterile gauze for hemostasis.
- Close with two sutures (4.0 or 5.0 size). (Suture removal will be determined according to the location—sutures on the face should be removed sooner than those on the extremities.)

  NOTE: Nerve damage can occur in areas where nerves are very superficial, such as the lateral aspects of fingers and the ulnar groove of elbows. Any lesions in these areas (including the face for cosmetic reasons) should be referred to a dermatologist.

scratching. In pityriasis rosea, a single herald patch occurs first; subsequent smaller eruptions follow skin lines in a Christmas-tree pattern. Pityriasis rubra pilaris presents as generalized erythematous lesions with areas of normal skin; the palms and soles are usually affected.

Drug eruptions resulting from beta blockers, methyldopa, and gold can produce psoriatic-type lesions. Intertriginous psoriasis may appear similar to candidiasis but in most cases would be distinguishable through Wood's light and KOH testing. Mycosis fungoides lesions progress to violaceous, indurated plaques and nodules, which typically begin on the thighs, buttocks, and trunk.

Management

The goal of therapy for psoriasis is to control the disease so that the patient no longer feels physically or psychologically hindered by the skin lesions. For sparse or mild lesions that do not bother the patient, no treatment may be needed. When treatment is indicated, however, the disease is controlled by decreasing epidermal proliferation and underlying dermal inflammation with topical corticosteroids and other immunomodulatory agents, along with phototherapy in some patients. Systemic agents are reserved for moderate to severe or recalcitrant cases. The chronic course of psoriasis and the lack of cure can be both discouraging and challenging for the patient and the clinician. Patients should be reassured that the therapeutic options today are much broader than in the recent past, and several new therapeutic approaches and medications, including highly effective biological therapies, are now available, as well as improvements in phototherapy and photochemotherapy.

Some patients find the presence of even a few small plaques highly objectionable because the location of the plaques in highly visible areas of the body is disfiguring or may hinder physical activity. Other patients are willing to accept the condition as bothersome but not overly impairing, particularly when they realize there is no cure. A long-term individualized plan of disease management is therefore helpful for patients with psoriasis in order to help deal with exacerbations, which frequently cause frustration or discouragement.

Topical Therapy

Topical agents are the first-line pharmacotherapeutics for psoriasis and are usually effective. If less than 20% of the body (e.g., no more than the elbows, knees, ears, and scalp) is involved, topical agents are very effective. But if more than 20% of the body is affected, systemic therapy may be required, and referral to a dermatologist is recommended. For stubborn, persistent, and widespread lesions, ultraviolet (UV) light treatment should be strongly considered. Systemic therapy in psoriasis is usually used as a last resort, because the significant effectiveness of biological agents must be weighed against their significant cost and side-effect profile.

Widely used topical agents are available both as OTC and prescription formulations. OTC emollient creams or ointments applied on the skin at least twice a day are helpful in preventing cracking and fissuring of lesions, especially those on palms and soles. Keratolytic agents, such as 1% to 5% salicylic acid preparations, may be combined with emollients to enhance absorption of other drugs, such as topical corticosteroids, through thick psoriatic lesions. Keratolytic agents may be applied twice daily.

Topical corticosteroids are widely used because they are relatively easy to apply. Those with intermediate and strong potency should be applied no more than once or twice a day. Topical corticosteroids are an appropriate treatment in cases involving 10% or less of the body surface (e.g., the face, neck, flexures, and genitalia). The plaques usually blanch and thin in response to the treatment. More potent corticosteroids may be applied to achieve complete clearing of psoriasis and are helpful in treating exposed areas of the body. However, caution is needed in corticosteroid usage, because they can cause skin atrophy and suppression of the hypothalamic-pituitary-adrenal (HPA) axis, resulting in a Cushingoid syndrome.

The effective treatment approach for exacerbations of psoriasis is to initially use "superpotent" topical corticosteroid preparations (e.g., Diprolene, Psorcon, Temovate, Ultravate) for 2 weeks and then decrease to a lesser potency agent for maintenance therapy. Superpotent corticosteroids should not be used for more than 2 weeks. Once symptoms are under control, other topical agents or a weaker corticosteroid may be substituted after gradually tapering the dose (Table 7.10).

The penetration and absorption of topical steroids will increase with occlusive dressing, but some superpotent corticosteroids should not be applied with occlusion because of increased risk of HPA suppression from systemic absorption. Ointment preparations are preferred over creams or lotions if the psoriatic scale is thick. When heavy scaling is present, gentle brushing of the psoriatic scales after warm soaks or during warm baths before applying the topical agents will increase absorption. Hard scrubbing should be avoided, however, because skin trauma can exacerbate the psoriasis.

Topical corticosteroid therapy has its shortcomings. Remission periods are often relatively short. Prolonged use produces striae and thinning of skin (atrophy), and the rebound effect is much worse, possibly converting a "stable" disease to an "unstable" one if the dose of corticosteroid is suddenly discontinued. Prolonged use of corticosteroids has been associated with suppression of the HPA axis and a Cushingoid syndrome, as noted previously.

Topical tar and anthralin are agents that can be used once a day in combination with topical steroids. Scalp involvement may benefit from use of a tar shampoo (Zetar, Sebutone, Pentrax) before the application of a topical corticosteroid. The tar shampoo is gently massaged

Table 7.10 Potency of Topical Corticosteroids for Atopic Dermatitis

Super High
betamethasone dipropionate, augmented 0.05%
clobetasol propionate 0.05%
fluocinonide 0.1%
flurandrenolide 4 mcg/sq. cm (tape)
halobetasol propionate 0.05%

High
amcinonide 0.1%
betamethasone dipropionate 0.05%
desoximetasone 0.05%, 0.25%
diflorasone diacetate 0.05%
fluocinonide 0.05%
halcinonide 0.1%
triamcinolone acetonide 0.5%

Intermediate
betamethasone valerate 0.05%, 0.12%
clocortolone pivalate 0.1%
desonide 0.05%
desoximetasone 0.05%
fluocinolone acetonide 0.025%
flurandrenolide 0.025%, 0.05%
fluticasone propionate 0.005%, 0.05%
hydrocortisone probutate 0.1%
hydrocortisone butyrate 0.1%
hydrocortisone valerate 0.2%
mometasone furoate 0.1%
prednicarbate 0.1%
triamcinolone acetonide 0.05%, 0.1%, 0.2%

Low
alclometasone dipropionate 0.05%
fluocinolone acetonide 0.01%
hydrocortisone base or acetate 1%, 1.85%, 2%, 2.5%
triamcinolone acetonide 0.025%

on the scalp and left on for a few hours and then rinsed off. Softened scales are gently removed. The scalp should be gently dried before application of the steroid lotion. Wearing a shower cap after corticosteroid application enhances absorption and improves results. Excessive combing after washing the hair should be avoided, in order to prevent trauma.

Anthralin (0.1% and 3.0% ointment) belongs to the class of trihydroxyanthracene compounds; it is used topically for psoriasis. Anthralin is an antimitotic agent capable of inhibiting DNA synthesis. Anthralin is applied once or twice a day and should be washed off after 10 to 30 minutes. It produces quick remission of plaques after several weeks of use but has a tendency to irritate and stain adjacent skin and clothing, making it less preferable than other treatment options. Paradoxically, if topical corticosteroids are added to an anthralin regimen, there may be an increased risk of early relapse.

Another topical treatment includes calcipotriene (Dovonex), a vitamin D ointment derivative. Calcipotriene produces keratinocyte differentiation and controls proliferation. It is superior to a superpotent corticosteroid and is the best treatment for mild to moderate disease. It is a major alternative to topical corticosteroid therapy for plaque-type psoriasis. Studies have found it to be effective in nearly three-quarters of patients with plaque psoriasis, with relatively minor side effects. Pulse therapy utilizes calcipotriene for 5 days and then a moderate- to high-potency topical corticosteroid for 2 days.

A topical agent with similar action to calcipotriene is tazarotene (Tazorac). It interferes with excessive differentiation and proliferation of epidermal cells and also limits the migration of inflammatory mediators to the areas of hyperkeratinization. It achieves a 60% to 70% rate and long remissions (up to 12 weeks). It is available as an ointment, cream, or lotion preparation. Like other receptor-selective retinoids, tazarotene is considered teratogenic and should not be used by pregnant women.

The topical calcineurin inhibitors tacrolimus (Protopic) and pimecrolimus (Elidel), applied twice per day, may be effective. These treatments have been particularly helpful for psoriasis in the facial and intertriginous areas where topical corticosteroid treatments (other than low-potency agents) should be avoided, given the risk of dermal atrophy. Exposure to natural sunlight improves psoriasis and permits a more enduring remission than does the use of topical corticosteroids. In some patients, topical corticosteroids may even be suspended during the summer. Although sun exposure to the point of mild erythema is helpful, sunburn exacerbates psoriasis and should be avoided.

In 1925, W. H. Goeckerman, a physician at the Mayo Clinic, achieved encouraging results with experimental use of midrange ultraviolet B (UVB) light and coal tar ointment for patients whose psoriasis did not respond to topical therapy. With some modifications of the sunbeam spectrum and combined with topicals, the traditional Goeckerman program is still being used. Crude coal tar of 1% to 2% in gel or ointment form is applied at night to the psoriatic plaques and is followed by UVB treatments. UVB treatment is continued for 4 to 6 weeks and causes remission (for up to 4 months) in 60% to 90% of patients without evidence of increased risk of skin cancer. Guttate psoriasis, in particular, responds well to UVB therapy.

A more aggressive treatment approach is photochemotherapy, or psoralen plus ultraviolet A (PUVA). It has been reported to achieve an 80% to 90% rate of remission on otherwise recalcitrant severe forms of psoriasis, such as the pustular form. The treatment inhibits mitosis by stopping DNA replication and is administered two to three times per week. PUVA involves ingestion of an oral psoralen compound (methoxsalen) before light exposure. Psoralen may be taken orally or it can be added to a bath, but "bath PUVA therapy" is not widely used in the United States. Psoralen is inactive in the body, but on the skin it is activated by UVA (long-wavelength ultraviolet A light). The eyes must be protected during exposure to UVA light because of the potential for cataract formation. Because of the significant occurrence of nausea, body malaise, phototoxic erythema, premature aging of the skin, and pruritus following administration of psoralens, the attrition rate of this treatment is high. Although it can clear chronic plaque psoriasis in 6 to 8 weeks, overexposure to UVA light can cause acute sunburn in the short term; in the long term, it can cause nonmelanoma cancer. Since the mid-1980s, the use of phototherapy has been shown to be associated with squamous cell carcinoma. In 1991, some cases of melanoma began to surface among patients who had received more than 250 courses of treatment. Therefore, careful follow-up of patients who have had PUVA therapy is crucial. Patients considered to be at increased risk for skin cancer (those with fair skin who are easily sunburned or individuals who have had previous x-ray therapy to skin) should not receive PUVA. PUVA in combination with topical agents has been found to be extremely effective (Level 1; Menter et al, 2010).

Systemic Therapy

Systemic therapy is reserved for patients with severe incapacitating disease—pustular, guttate, and/or arthritic psoriasis. It is administered only by expert specialists such as rheumatologists or dermatologists who regularly use systemic antimitotic agents, including methotrexate, etretinate, and cyclosporine.

Methotrexate is a folic acid antagonist and a cytotoxic agent that inhibits cellular proliferation. It is used in chemotherapy for cancer but is also useful in patients with severe psoriatic arthritis. Oral regimens include every other day and once-weekly dosing. If nausea is significant, intramuscular administration can be used. A therapeutic response is usually seen within 2 to 3 weeks, at which time the dose or interval should be reduced. With prolonged use, accumulative doses of methotrexate could result in hepatotoxicity, nephrotoxicity, and bone marrow depression. Coadministration of folic acid 1 mg by mouth daily effectively protects against many of the minor side effects associated with this treatment, such as stomatitis. Methotrexate is contraindicated in patients with cirrhosis of the liver or diabetes or with a history of alcohol or IV drug use.

Monitoring of blood counts, including platelets, should be done weekly, followed by monthly testing. Renal and liver function tests (baseline and follow-up) should be done. Intermittent liver biopsies are recommended because hepatic fibrosis may occur with prolonged use. Methotrexate is teratogenic and should not be given to those who are pregnant or who want to become pregnant.

Cyclosporine is an immunosuppressant that was originally used for prevention of organ rejection in organ transplant patients. Its efficacy in severe erythrodermic and psoriatic arthritis was discovered serendipitously while the drug was being tested for rheumatoid arthritis. Significant improvement and even total clearing of psoriasis becomes evident within days in some patients. Withdrawal of cyclosporine is associated with relapse within weeks. Hypertension and nephrotoxicity can develop during cyclosporine treatment, although in the vast majority of patients renal function subsequently returns to normal. Treatment with cyclosporine for more than 1 year is not recommended because it may cause prolonged immunosuppression and myalgias. Serum creatinine levels should be monitored throughout the duration of treatment because cyclosporine can cause interstitial fibrosis and tubular atrophy. Other systemic immunosuppressants such as hydroxyurea (Hydrea), azathioprine (Imuran), and tacrolimus have also been used, although these systemic agents all carry significant safety risks and their use is reserved only for cases of sufficient severity.

The most significant development in the psoriasis treatment armamentarium in recent years has been the array of immunomodulatory biological agents used for moderate to severe plaque psoriasis, psoriatic arthritis, and refractory disease. These initially included alefacept (Amevive), a recombinant CD2 antagonist fusion protein that inhibits T-cell activation, and efalizumab (Raptiva), a humanized monoclonal antibody against CD11a. However, efalizumab was withdrawn from the market by the FDA in 2009 due to its association with fatal cases of progressive multifocal leukoencephalopathy, and alefacept was voluntarily withdrawn from the market by its manufacturer in 2011. Currently, the most widely used class of biological agents for psoriasis are the tumor necrosis factor–alpha antagonists, which include the tumor necrosis factor receptor fusion protein etanercept (Enbrel), the human monoclonal antibody adalimumab (Humira), the human monoclonal antibody golimumab (Simponi), and the human-murine chimeric monoclonal antibody infliximab (Remicade). Most recently, the anti–IL-12/IL-23 human monoclonal antibody ustekinumab (Stelara), which is specific for the shared cytokine subunit p40, has proven highly effective in the treatment of psoriasis. These biological agents have been revolutionary in the treatment of moderate to severe and refractory psoriasis. However, they require laboratory monitoring and carry the risk of significant side effects, including infection and a theoretical risk of malignancy. In addition, given their significant cost, these agents are typically considered second-line therapeutics when UV light therapy fails.

An oral systemic agent, acitretin (Soriatane), is a retinoid that can be beneficial for patients with moderate to severe pustular and erythrodermic variants of psoriasis. In severe cases, etretinate can be used in combination with PUVA. About 50% of patients who are refractory to PUVA alone improve when a retinoid is added. Female patients who are treated with etretinate should be advised not to become pregnant for 3 years after ceasing treatment, because retinoids are teratogenic. Careful monitoring of blood counts, plasma triglycerides, and liver function tests is required.

Follow-up and Referral

Newly diagnosed patients and patients who have moderate to extensive skin involvement or severe disease (e.g., pustular psoriasis) should be referred to a dermatologist or psoriasis specialty treatment center. Patient support groups may be of great psychological help. Patients with recalcitrant or frequent flare-ups should be referred to a dermatologist for UV light therapy and/or systemic treatment. An ophthalmology consultation is necessary before UV therapy to rule out the presence of cataracts.

Patients with severe psoriasis are usually followed up every 2 months by a specialist or more often as required by their particular treatment regimen. Patients who exhibit symptoms of depression or poor coping skills will benefit from referral to a psychiatrist for psychological evaluation and therapy.

Patient Education

Psoriasis presents many challenges to both the patient and the health-care provider. For patients with disfiguring and uncontrollable psoriasis, education and support are central to the treatment process. The patient should be informed of available community resources and support groups. Explanation of the disease process and treatment, including potential adverse effects of medications, is very helpful. The new patient and his or her family should be reassured that the disease is not contagious or infectious.

Although the genetic aspects of psoriasis are complex and incompletely characterized, it may be explained to family members of a patient that if neither parent has psoriasis, the chances are less than 10% that another child will develop the disease. If one parent is affected, the chance of developing psoriasis increases to 15%. If both parents are affected, the chance increases to 59% that one or more children will have the disease.

The clinician should educate the patient that there are several ways of remaining in remission: Patients with psoriasis should avoid skin trauma and should keep the skin relatively dry to decrease pruritus, scratching, and scaling. They should avoid photosensitizing medications such as tetracyclines, sulfa drugs, or phenothiazines. If drugs of these types are necessary, patients should be advised to inform the prescribing physician of their psoriasis and to ask for a possible alternative. Although photosensitizing drugs should be avoided, controlled sun exposure during the summer is beneficial. The patient should be advised to use a high-SPF sunscreen to prevent sunburn. Patients should be informed to seek treatment for streptococcal infections (e.g., skin infections, sore throats) immediately. Aggravating factors for psoriasis include increased stress and alcohol.

The clinician should explain to the patient that dietary manipulations do not appear to play a role in treating psoriasis. However, healthy eating habits support a strong immune system, and nutritionists recommend a low-fat, high-fiber diet for patients. Naturopaths recommend many herbal medicines to improve psoriasis and to control or provide relief from the disturbing effects of the flare-ups. (See Complementary Therapies 7.1.) Although many persons subscribe to these therapies, there is a lack of data from randomized clinical trials to confirm their effectiveness.

An active support group for psoriasis is the National Psoriasis Foundation, 6600 SW 92nd Avenue, Suite 300, Portland, OR 97223-7195, 1-800-723-9166, www.psoriasis.org.

SKIN LESIONS: BENIGN

■ SEBORRHEIC KERATOSIS

Seborrheic keratoses are benign, warty-appearing growths that are commonly seen in older adults. These growths are usually found on the trunk, but they may also be seen on the hands and face. They develop in both sun-exposed and protected areas. See Table 7.11 for information about other skin lesions, including nevi, skin tags (acrochordons), and lipomas.

Epidemiology and Causes

The tendency to develop seborrheic keratosis is an autosomal dominant trait. Seborrheic keratosis is extremely common; it has been found in 88% of persons older than age 65 years. Of this group, approximately 50% often develop 10 or more lesions. In fact, for some individuals, lesions may number into the hundreds. The

---

Complementary Therapies 7.1

Acne

Herb	Comments
Marigold (*Calendula officinalis*)	Topical application Available as a soap Has anti-inflammatory properties
Tea tree oil (*Melaleuca alternifolia*)	Topical application twice daily

Continued

Complementary Therapies 7.1—cont'd

Eczema

Herb	Comments
Chamomile (*Matricaria recutita*)	Topical application Anti-inflammatory Contraindicated in patients with ragweed allergy
Evening primrose (*Oenothera biennis*)	Should not be taken with phenothiazines
Marigold (*Calendula officinalis*)	Topical application—ointment or cream Has anti-inflammatory properties
Goldenseal (*Hydrastis canadensis*)	Used topically by Native Americans Powdered root mixed with water to make a paste and applied to rash
Licorice (*Glycyrrhiza glabra*)	Topical application Anti-inflammatory properties
Turmeric (*Curcuma longa*)	Topical application; anti-inflammatory

Fungal Infections

Herb	Comments
Tea tree oil (*Melaleuca alternifolia*)	Topical application; antifungal properties Apply twice daily

Psoriasis

Herb	Comments
Angelica (*Angelica archangelica*)	After ingestion, expose affected area to mild sunlight Contains photosensitizers (*furocoumarin*) Possible interaction with anticoagulants and aspirin
Avena (*Avena sativa*) "Oatmeal"	Applied as an oatmeal paste
Avocado (*Persea americana*)	Cooling, soothing effect Mashed avocados are rubbed into scaling patches
Bishop's weed (*Ammi visnagae*)	Topical application Inhibits cell division Treatment may irritate the skin
Brazil nut (*Bertholletia excelsa*)	Soothing; relieves itching Contains an oil rich in thiamin and selenium
Chamomile (*Matricaria recutita*)	Topical application Anti-inflammatory Contraindicated in patients with ragweed allergy
Flax (*Linum usitatissimum*)	Need to ingest about 10–12 grams (5–6 tsp) May add flaxseeds to salads; caution as to laxative effect
Licorice (*Glycyrrhiza glabra*)	Topical application; may be more effective than hydrocortisone
Milk thistle (*Silybum marianum*)	Anti-inflammatory Taken as a tea, tincture, or in capsules
Oregon grape (*Mahonia aquifolium*)	Antioxidant
Red pepper (*Capsicum*)	Contains capsaicin Reduces scaling and redness, but can cause burning and stinging Wash hands thoroughly after applying, avoid getting in the eyes or on mucous membranes
Omega-3 fish oil	Decreases symptoms and severity of chronic plaque psoriasis and acute guttate psoriasis

Table 7.11 Other Skin Lesions

Lesion	Description	Clinical Presentation	Management
Lipoma	A lipoma is a benign subcutaneous tumor that consists of adipose tissue. Lipomas are most commonly found in older adults; usually asymptomatic. Cause is unknown.	• Rubbery smooth and round mass of adipose tissue that is compressible and has a soft to very firm texture. • May have symptoms of irritation, such as redness and tenderness. • Commonly occurs on back of the neck, trunk, and forearms.	• Observe for changes, rapid growth • Excision or liposuction • Referral to dermatologist if indicated
Nevi	Nevi (moles) are circumscribed areas of pigmentation. Types include congenital, acquired, or atypical or dysplastic (>5 mm, in diameter, with color variation and irregular borders).	• Flat or raised circumscribed area of pigmentation. • Assess for suspected melanoma (check ABCDEs: asymmetry, irregular borders, variations in color, diameter >6 mm, elevation above the surface of the skin).	• Excision • Referral to dermatologist if melanoma is suspected
Skin tags	Skin tags (acrochordons) are benign overgrowths of skin, commonly seen after middle age. Cause is unknown.	• Overgrowths of normal skin that have formed soft, polyp-like lesions that have a stalk. • Usually found on the neck, axilla, groin, upper trunk, and eyelid.	• Usually none unless patient is bothered by the cosmetic effect or irritation • If treatment is required, may include snip excision, electrocautery, or cryosurgery • Referral to dermatologist if skin tag is located on the eyelids or face or if patient has a history of keloids, diabetes, or infection, or is on high-dose steroid therapy, or if there is the possibility of a malignant lesion

lesions found on sun-exposed areas rarely increase in size, whereas seborrheic keratotic lesions in protected areas tend to be darker, have a more crumbly appearance, and may enlarge in size.

Seborrheic keratosis is more prevalent in persons with white skin. The lesions are raised, brownish gray, and appear "stuck on."

Pathophysiology

Seborrheic keratosis lesions originate from the horny layer of the epidermis and are the result of a benign proliferation of immature keratinocytes. Inspection of the lesions may reveal dark keratin plugs or firm, horny cysts on their surface. A predisposition for seborrheic keratosis appears to be inherited in an autosomal dominant pattern. These are epidermal tumors, but they are not considered malignant or premalignant because they do not undergo transformation into cancerous lesions. However, a phenomenon known as the sign of Leser-Trélat exists, which is characterized by the sudden development of multiple seborrheic keratotic lesions, along with skin tags, and acanthosis nigricans

(a darkening and mild thickening of the skin in characteristic intertriginous areas). Although the skin lesions in this condition are not considered malignant, the sign of Leser-Trélat is associated with various types of underlying malignancies, including lung and gastrointestinal cancers and, thus, is considered a neoplastic syndrome. Moreover, seborrheic keratosis has also been observed in association with certain skin malignancies such as basal cell carcinomas, occurring at different skin sites.

Clinical Presentation

Subjective

The typical patient is an older white woman who complains of the cosmetic effects of the lesion. The patient typically complains of the unsightliness of the lesion, itching, and constant irritation from friction or clothing.

Objective

Seborrheic keratotic lesions are benign, superficial epithelial growths that appear as well-defined scaly, hyperpigmented lesions with a warty or "stuck-on" appearance. They are most often found on the trunk, face, and arms. Lesions look as if they could literally be "picked off" the skin surface. Seborrheic keratotic lesions tend to grow slowly and are round to oval in shape. The lesions occasionally appear as smooth papules. The color of the lesions can range from flesh tone to dark brown in white patients. In black women, the lesions also appear as smooth, round to oval black papules on the upper part of the face (dermatosis papulosa nigra).

Diagnostic Reasoning

Diagnostic Tests

No laboratory testing is necessary to diagnose seborrheic keratosis. However, if the patient presents with an atypical lesion, diagnosis should be confirmed with a biopsy.

Differential Diagnosis

The diagnosis of seborrheic keratosis is based on the appearance of the lesion and on patient demographics (especially age). Skin lesions that can mimic seborrheic keratosis include any pigmented papule or nodule. The differential diagnoses for seborrheic keratosis include benign pigmented nevi, pigmented basal cell carcinoma, and malignant melanoma.

Pigmented nevi appear as smooth round macules or papules that do not have a warty appearance. Nevi (moles) are also seen in younger patients as well as in adults, unlike seborrheic keratosis, which appears mostly in patients aged 30 years and older. Pigmented basal cell carcinomas usually have a waxy surface with dilated blood vessels. They may be ulcerated during later stages—a feature not seen in seborrheic keratosis. Malignant melanomas can appear in younger patients; melanomas may be nodular but usually do not have a warty, stuck-on appearance. A malignant melanoma's borders can be irregular, and it can have a variegation (inconsistency) of color. Most patients with melanoma will also report a history of a changing mole.

Management

If the diagnosis is uncertain, especially if melanoma cannot be ruled out, the patient should be referred to a dermatologist for further evaluation. A skin biopsy can be done for a more definitive diagnosis.

Treatment is warranted for those lesions that are symptomatic or are unsightly to the patient. Seborrheic keratosis may be removed using liquid nitrogen therapy or mechanical methods. Results obtained with cryosurgery (liquid nitrogen) are slightly superior to those obtained using electrodesiccation with curettage; however, the choice is generally the practitioner's preference. Liquid nitrogen may produce transient hyperpigmentation or hypopigmentation. Mechanical methods of removal include curettage and snip or shave excision. (See Therapeutic Procedure 7.2.)

Therapeutic Procedure 7.2   Removal of Seborrheic Keratoses

Liquid Nitrogen

• Spray the area with liquid nitrogen or apply the liquid nitrogen with rayon–wool tipped applicators. Special care must be taken not to contaminate the reservoir of liquid nitrogen. If using applicators, dip the applicator into the reservoir only once, apply, and discard.

   NOTE: It is generally preferable to lightly freeze (underfreeze) the lesion than to freeze too deeply and risk scarring. A second application may be applied at a follow-up visit if necessary. Hyperpigmentation and hypopigmentation are possible sequelae of liquid nitrogen treatment (cryotherapy). Reactive hyperpigmentation is more common in Asians.

   NOTE: Care must be taken in treating areas where nerves are relatively superficial and can be damaged, such as the lateral aspects of the fingers and the ulnar groove of the elbows.

Curettage

• Anesthetize the area with 1% lidocaine and cleanse the area.
• Stretch the skin surrounding the lesion with the fingers of one hand.
• Using a 5-mm or 6-mm curette, scrape off the base of the keratosis with short, clean strokes.

   NOTE: If the lesion is in a critical area such as the face, lateral aspects of the fingers, ulnar groove in elbow (superficial nerve present), or if diagnosis is uncertain, referral to a dermatologist is recommended. If the lesion is in the hairline or groin, styptics or aluminum chloride may be used to control bleeding.

Snip or Shave Excision

• Anesthetize the area with 1% lidocaine and cleanse the area.
• Using iris scissors, snip off the lesion, or, using a number 11 or number 15 scalpel, shave off the lesion.
   NOTE: Control bleeding using pressure, gel foam, styptic, or aluminum chloride, if needed.
   NOTE: Treatment is for patient comfort or for cosmetic reasons only.

Follow-up and Referral

A follow-up visit is generally not necessary unless the liquid nitrogen does not completely remove the lesion. A biopsy should be performed on any keratosis that fails to respond to liquid nitrogen. Should the removal of a lesion by cryotherapy from the dorsa of the hands result in blistering, the patient should return to have the blister drained. This is accomplished by puncturing one edge of the blister with a sterile needle or with a number 11 scalpel. The top of the blister should not be removed. Infection following the application of liquid nitrogen is rare.

A biopsy or referral to a dermatologist should be done if the diagnosis is unclear and the clinician wants to rule out a pigmented basal cell carcinoma or malignant melanoma. A high index of suspicion is necessary in the diagnosis of melanoma because of its aggressive and malignant nature. Any pigmented lesion for which a clinician suspects melanoma should be evaluated by a dermatologist.

Patient Education

The clinician should inform the patient that seborrheic keratoses are a harmless and common occurrence as people age. Some people develop many lesions, whereas others will have only a few. These lesions are not caused by chronic exposure to sunlight and may develop on any exposed or protected area of the body. Color changes in these lesions are harmless, but if the clinician is unsure about the exact nature of the lesion, referral to a dermatologist is recommended.

SKIN LESIONS: PREMALIGNANT

■ ACTINIC KERATOSIS

Actinic keratosis is the most common precancerous skin lesion found in light-skinned (white) patients. *Actinic keratoses* are premalignant lesions that are also known as senile or solar keratoses. They are found on sun-exposed areas of skin that have been damaged from cumulative sun exposure. Left untreated, actinic keratosis can progress to squamous cell carcinoma with a latency period of 10 years. Estimates of progression to squamous cell carcinoma vary widely from 0.25% to 20%. Another estimate is that only 1 in 1,000 actinic keratotic lesions may progress to squamous cell carcinoma. However, up to 25% of actinic keratoses spontaneously regress without treatment. Therefore, aggressive treatment of these premalignant lesions remains controversial.

Epidemiology and Causes

Actinic keratosis is caused by the accumulation of damage to epithelial skin cells caused by chronic sun exposure. These keratoses are more common in men, probably as a result of occupational exposure (working outdoors). The most susceptible individuals are fair skinned, with a history of frequent sun exposure and evidence of other signs of sun damage, such as freckles, senile lentigines (liver spots), wrinkles, and uneven pigmentation. Actinic keratoses are found predominantly in older adults (older than age 50 years); however, occasionally they are seen in young adults with fair skin. Renal transplant patients have also been found to have an increased tendency to develop actinic keratoses. The typical patient with actinic keratoses is an elderly, fair-skinned, sun-sensitive person.

Pathophysiology

Cumulative damage from ultraviolet radiation in sunlight causes damage to the DNA in epithelial cells. The primary lesions of actinic keratosis consist of macules or plaques that are poorly circumscribed. Secondary lesions appear erythematous and scaly. Areas of skin that have actinic keratosis feel rough to the touch due to hyperkeratosis and have been likened to feeling like sandpaper. With further ultraviolet light exposure, continued cumulative DNA damage may lead to malignant transformation of epidermal cellular clones. Actinic keratoses that progress to squamous cell carcinoma tend not to be very aggressive unless they occur on the lip.

Clinical Presentation
Subjective

The typical patient is a middle-aged or older adult who complains of an irritated rough or scaly rash. Some patients also complain of pruritus, tenderness, or a stinging sensation in one or several lesions. Some patients are asymptomatic and will only complain of cosmetic concerns or uneasiness about a potential malignancy. The lesion is also typically found on a fair-skinned patient. These patients usually have some Celtic background (Irish, Scottish, English) and are light haired (blond or red haired) and blue eyed. They also tend to freckle easily and sunburn.

Objective

The lesions of actinic keratosis appear reddened, scaly, rough, or have an uneven surface. The hyperkeratosis of these lesions is characteristically hard or spiny. Actinic keratoses are found in areas of skin that have been chronically exposed to the sun, such as the face, ears, back of the neck, neckline, dorsum of the arms, and (in women) the dorsum of the legs. Palpation is generally the best diagnostic tool to use because of the typical sandpaper-like texture of the lesions. Actinic keratoses are small (0.2- to 5-mm) papules that can be flesh colored or slightly hyperpigmented. Actinic keratoses are predominantly found on the cheeks, forehead, forearms, and dorsal surface of the hands. In older men, they are also predominant on the ears and balding scalp.

Diagnostic Reasoning

Diagnostic Tests

The diagnosis can usually be made by history and physical examination. Palpating the lesion is key to the diagnosis by feeling for the scaly, rough, and uneven texture, because lesions may be better recognized by palpation rather than by visual inspection. Fluorescence with the use of a photosensitizing drug such as methyl ester of 5-aminolevulinic acid can be used as a diagnostic tool for actinic keratosis, because areas of involvement emit a pink fluorescence with a Wood's lamp or photodynamic therapy lamp.

Differential Diagnosis

Skin lesions that can mimic actinic keratosis include squamous cell carcinoma, seborrheic keratosis, and verruca plana (flat warts). Squamous cell carcinoma is characterized by an indurated plaque or nodule that is eroded or ulcerated and has a thickened scale. The lesion is found on sun-exposed skin, as is actinic keratosis. What differentiates squamous cell carcinoma from actinic keratosis is the induration and ulceration. Seborrheic keratosis lesions are highly pigmented (brown to black) and have a warty, stuck-on appearance. They can appear on both sun-exposed and protected skin. Verruca plana are caused by the human papillomavirus and appear as multiple flesh-colored to light brown warts that are from 1 to 5 mm in size. Their color and smaller size distinguish them from actinic keratoses.

Management

There is no solid evidence that removal of all actinic keratosis lesions on a patient is effective in the prevention of skin cancer. Indeed, only 1 in 1,000 actinic keratoses will progress to squamous cell carcinoma. However, it is standard dermatological practice to remove most actinic keratosis lesions. Because the lesions reside in the epithelium, therapies that separate the epidermis from the dermis are most effective and do not leave scars.

Two methods are currently available to the primary-care provider—topical therapy and surgical destruction of the lesion. Treatment may also include a combination of both methods.

Topical Therapy

Topical application of 5-fluorouracil (5-FU) cream (Efudex, Carac) may eradicate actinic keratosis, because 5-FU is selective for affecting only sun-damaged cells. The cream is applied to the lesion twice per day for an average of 3 weeks. The eyelids, folds of the nose, and lips should be avoided. Healing takes from 2 to 4 weeks and is accomplished by the replication of epidermal and adnexal cells. Patients treated with 5-FU frequently become noncompliant because the inflammatory effect (destruction of the lesion) leaves raw, tender, reddened skin in its place. If the lesion or lesions do not respond to one treatment with 5-FU, these lesions must be evaluated for potential carcinoma via skin biopsy. Some evidence shows that tretinoin (Retin-A) when used in combination with 5-FU may increase effectiveness and shorten the length of therapy. The safety and efficacy of 5-FU during pregnancy have not been established.

Imiquimod 5% cream may be used on face and scalp lesions and is applied three times weekly for 8 weeks. Other topical treatments that have been used include topical chemotherapies such as diclofenac 3% in 2.5% hyaluronan gel (Solaraze) applied twice per day for 60 to 90 days and topical retinoids such as adapalene 0.1% to 0.3% gel (applied to lesions daily for 4 weeks, and then increased to twice per day). Side effects may include erythema, pruritus, rash, and xerosis (dry skin). Some topical chemotherapeutic treatments have even been used in conjunction with phototherapy, such as aminolevulinic acid (Levulan Kerastick) in conjunction with either blue or red wavelength light. These specialized treatments typically give improved cosmesis over the more commonly used method of cryosurgery and may be preferred for facial lesions. In addition, they only require a 2-day course of therapy. A cytotoxic agent, ingenol mebutate, may also be used, which works by killing rapidly growing cells such as the abnormal cells associated with actinic keratoses. For the scalp, ingenol mebutate 0.015% gel is usually applied once a day for 3 days in a row. On the torso or extremities, 0.05% gel is applied once a day for 2 consecutive days.

Another treatment for actinic keratosis is photodynamic therapy, which uses a light-sensitizing compound that uniquely accumulates in actinic keratosis cells, where it is activated by the appropriate wavelength of light. Delta-aminolevulinic acid is a component of the heme biosynthetic pathway that accumulates in dysplastic cells. Once inside the cells, it is enzymatically converted to a potent photosensitizer. With exposure to light of an appropriate wavelength, oxygen free radicals are generated and cell death results.

Cryosurgery

Before cryosurgery is performed, informed consent must be obtained from the patient. Cryosurgery with liquid nitrogen is used most frequently for patients with solitary or few lesions. (See Therapeutic Procedure 7.3.)

With cryosurgery, the clinician must rely entirely on a clinical diagnosis because tissue is destroyed by freezing; therefore, there is no specimen available for pathological analysis. Liquid nitrogen is a rapid and effective treatment for eradicating actinic keratoses, especially in patients with one to few lesions. The liquid nitrogen probe should be applied firmly to the lesion for 10 to 15 seconds and repeated twice in one visit. The lesions will crust over and generally disappear in 10 to 14 days. A possible drawback to this procedure is the potential for hypopigmentation because a white spot may appear at the treated site.

Therapeutic Procedure 7.3 Performing Cryosurgery for Actinic Keratoses

- Liquid nitrogen applied with a cotton-tipped applicator is preferred because it causes minimal damage to the dermis.
- Using liquid nitrogen, freeze each lesion for 10–15 seconds. It may be necessary to repeat the freezing cycle a second time. The more pressure is applied to the cotton swab, the deeper the point of freeze contact or "freeze ball."
- The "freeze balls" should be approximately 1.5 times as wide as they are deep.
- If in doubt, it is better to underfreeze and to retreat lesions than to overfreeze them and leave a scar or hypopigmentation (if damage to the dermis is avoided, scarring will not occur).
- Any lesion that does not respond to liquid nitrogen must be biopsied.

   NOTE: If diagnosis of any skin lesion is in doubt, refer to a dermatologist for possible skin biopsy. The treated area will become red and swollen a few hours after treatment. A serous or blood-filled blister forms and will subsequently crust and disappear in 10–14 days. The patient should be advised not to cover the blister with any bandages and to leave the blister alone. The blister will protect the treated area until it is healed.

Other Surgical Techniques

Lesions that are isolated and thick may be amenable to surgical curettage, shave excision, or conventional excision, particularly when located on the dorsal surfaces of the upper extremities. However, there are few data that speak to the efficacy of this approach, and these techniques are typically not considered first-line interventions. Importantly, however, surgical resection is the only method of actinic keratosis removal that produces an intact biopsy sample available for histological examination and diagnostic confirmation. In addition, this method may be more appropriate for immunocompromised patients or for lesions suggestive of invasive cancer.

Follow-up and Referral

Patients on 5-FU should be followed up in 2 to 3 weeks or during completion of treatment. Adverse effects of the medication, compliance issues, and effectiveness of treatment should be noted at this time. Any skin lesions that remain after treatment with 5-FU cream for 2 to 3 weeks must be biopsied for pathological examination. Patients treated with cryosurgery are reevaluated in 2 weeks. Patients who have had excision biopsy by a dermatologist are usually seen again in 2 weeks.

   Any actinic keratosis lesion that does not respond to treatment should be referred to a dermatologist for further evaluation, including the need for a skin biopsy, even for superficial lesions. A dermatologist may remove multiple superficial lesions with an acid followed by pulsed light laser therapy or photodynamic therapy. This is effective on the face and does not result in the hypopigmentation that may result from cryotherapy. An added benefit is one of esthetic skin rejuvenation.

Patient Education

Regardless of the method of treatment, the patient should be educated regarding the need for using sunscreen and wearing of protective clothing such as a hat and a shirt with long sleeves. The hallmark of actinic keratosis

management must actually center on prevention—avoidance of excessive sun exposure is key to avoiding development of these premalignant lesions and their cancerous sequelae. In addition, the patient can also be taught the signs and symptoms of melanoma screening by using the ABCDE mnemonic: A = asymmetry, B = border irregularity, C = color change, D = diameter larger than a pencil eraser (greater than 6 mm), E = elevation from a flat lesion to a raised or evolving lesion.

   Patients treated with 5-FU should be warned that exposure to sunlight during treatment can exacerbate the inflammatory effect of the medicine. The clinician should instruct the patient that if erosions develop while using 5-FU cream, petroleum jelly can be applied to provide comfort, but the treatment must be continued for a total of 10 to 14 days. Patients should be warned to avoid prolonged sunlight exposure during and after treatment. A good-quality sun block should be worn after treatment to prevent future damage to the skin.

   Patients treated with cryosurgery should be informed that bandages are not necessary after treatment and actually impede healing. If blister formation results, the patient should be instructed to return to the office so that the blister can be drained. The patient should be advised to avoid irritation of the treated lesion with clothing or jewelry. Showering and the use of makeup are permissible. The patient should be taught to monitor for the signs and symptoms of infection (e.g., redness, purulent discharge, heat). Infection is a rare occurrence after cryosurgery.

SKIN LESIONS: MALIGNANT

■ MALIGNANT MELANOMA

Malignant melanoma is the most deadly of all skin cancers. *Melanoma* is malignancy of the skin that arises from epidermal melanocytes. Melanocytes produce *melanin,* a brown-black pigment that is responsible for skin, hair, and eye color. Almost all melanomas arise from the skin (more than 90%), but a few melanomas originate from the eye (uveal melanoma), and very few (less than 4%) do not have a primary site.

Types of melanoma are *superficial spreading* (70%–85%—characterized by extensive lateral or radial growth before vertical invasion), *nodular* (15–30%—characterized by vertical growth only), *lentigo maligna* (5%—an in situ form that may persist for years before vertical extension), and *acral lentiginous* (2%–8%—a particularly aggressive form most common in darker-skinned patients, especially when appearing on the hands or feet).

Although the majority of skin cancers in the United States are basal cell carcinoma (the most numerous type) and squamous cell carcinoma, melanoma is responsible for 75% of all skin cancer deaths. Melanoma, if discovered early enough, is a highly curable malignancy, but if the melanoma extends beyond 4 mm in depth, the prognosis is extremely poor. A 75% mortality rate is associated with this stage. Therefore, the role of primary-care clinicians in screening for this skin cancer is important and cannot be overemphasized. Screening programs that result in early diagnosis are important weapons in the armamentarium against this disease. The American Cancer Society's ABCDE mnemonic, explained in the premalignant section, is an easy tool for the clinician to remember and use to teach patients how to recognize potential melanomas and dysplastic nevi, the precursor lesion of melanoma, at an early stage.

Epidemiology and Causes

The incidence of melanoma in the United States has been rising for both men and women over the past decade, with rates of melanoma increasing annually for both white men and women, although rates have remained stead for African Americans, Hispanics, Asians, and Native Americans, in whom melanoma is much less frequent. In 2009, the Centers for Disease Control and Prevention estimated that there were 61,646 cases of melanoma and 9,199 deaths from it in the United States. Of the seven most common cancers in the United States, melanoma is the only type of cancer whose incidence is consistently increasing. In adults aged 25 to 29 years, melanoma is the most common form of cancer and the second most common among 15- to 19-year-olds. One contributing factor is the use of tanning beds among young people, because just one indoor tanning session has been estimated to increase a person's chances of developing melanoma by 20% and each additional session during the same year increases that rate by another 2%.

Several factors have been identified that increase an individual's risks of melanoma (see Risk Factors 7.2). Exposure and sensitivity to sunlight remain two of the most widely recognized risk factors. A disproportionate

Risk Factors 7.2   Malignant Melanoma
Age
Risk increases with age
Skin, Eye, Hair Color
Fair, blue or green eyes, red or blond hair
Personal History
History of skin cancer
History of dysplastic nevi; congenital nevi >20 mm
History of blistering sunburn before age 20 years
History of immunosuppression
Family History
History of melanoma
Environmental History
Excessive exposure to ultraviolet radiation/indoor tanning

number of melanoma deaths occur among whites, particularly fair-skinned individuals who sunburn easily. Whites (Caucasians) who are at highest risk come from Celtic (Irish, Scottish, English) backgrounds and have light hair (especially red hair), light eyes, and freckles. The ability of the skin to freckle in response to sun exposure is thought to be a marker of susceptibility to melanoma, although stronger risk factors for melanoma exist. Teaching patients about the proper use of sunscreen cannot be overemphasized. One study found that the risk of developing any melanoma was reduced by 50% and invasive melanoma by 73% with daily rather than discretionary use of sunscreen.

Research into the genetic component of melanoma and the presence of dysplastic nevi has found a relationship between dysplastic nevi, family history, and the development of melanoma. The finding of dysplastic nevus (one or more atypical moles) or any other type of skin cancer (such as basal cell carcinoma or squamous cell carcinoma) is thought to increase one's risks of melanoma. The number of nevi (moles) normally peaks during young adulthood (ages 20–25 years), then gradually decreases after age 50 years. Large numbers of nevi on an individual who is older than 50 years is considered to be a strong marker for increased risk of melanoma. It is estimated that 7% of the white population has at least one atypical nevus; many individuals have numerous nevi that should be monitored closely.

All melanomas should be tested for mutations in *BRAF*, a gene involved in cell growth signaling, because they appear in about half of all metastatic melanomas. Although *BRAF* is the official symbol designation, the gene is also known as *B-Raf* or *v-Raf murine sarcoma viral oncogene homolog B1*. As with other proto-oncogenes, when mutated this gene has the potential to cause normal cells to become cancerous. The benefit of identifying this mutation is in the personalization of melanoma therapy, because at least two small molecule inhibitor drugs, vemurafenib (Zelboraf) and dabrafenib (Tafinlar), have been developed to treat *BRAF* mutation–positive melanomas. This drug and others are mentioned in the treatment section.

The combination of a history of a first-degree relative with melanoma combined with the presence of one or more dysplastic nevi increases the chances of developing melanoma by up to 50% compared with the general public. Individuals in this population tend to develop multiple primary lesions at a younger age than individuals with other melanomas. In addition, large-sized nevi (more than 20 mm) are believed to be associated with increased melanoma risk. Currently, lifetime risk among all populations is estimated at 1 in 75, with fully one-third of all cases occurring in persons younger than age 45 years.

Pediatric overexposure to UV rays, especially a history of one or more blistering sunburns before age 20 years, has been linked to a dramatic increase in lifetime risk of developing melanoma. The effect of accumulated sunburn in addition to genetic predisposition may not be seen until years later, because the incidence of malignant melanoma in children is low. Intermittent intense exposures (e.g., those that may occur in occupational groups such as farmers) that result in blistering sunburn appear to be associated more with increased melanoma risk than chronic exposure.

Pathophysiology

A combination of UV exposure and genetic susceptibility is believed to be the most common mechanism for developing melanoma. Studies have linked UV radiation, particularly UVB rays, to genetic mutations in DNA in susceptible individuals, resulting in the development of abnormal pigmented lesions (dysplastic nevi). Genetic predisposition to melanoma appears to be the result of the presence of a mutated or absent tumor suppressor gene. Abnormalities have been mapped to chromosomes 1 and 9. In particular, mutations in chromosomal region 9p21, which encodes the tumor suppressor gene *CDKN2A* that produces the protein p16, have been observed in a large proportion of both familial and spontaneous melanomas, as well as the previously discussed mutations in the *BRAF* gene, which are seen in over half of all melanomas. Germline mutations in the gene *CDK4* have also been observed. Individuals in these susceptible groups tend to develop melanoma at multiple primary sites at an earlier age. Another strong genetic association is observed in the autosomal recessive condition xeroderma pigmentosum. Persons affected with this inherited disorder lack a critical DNA repair mechanism that corrects UV light–associated cross-linked DNA nucleotides. This results in multiple DNA breaks in response to cumulative UV light exposure and a resultant high level of sun-associated skin cancers.

Atypical nevi are precursors to malignant melanoma. They differ histologically from benign nevi in that they are disorganized and carry higher potential for transformation into malignant tissue. Initially, the tumor remains confined to the epidermis. If left untreated, it spreads into the subcutaneous fat. Metastasis occurs in the regional lymph nodes and occasionally into distant sites such as the lungs, liver, bone, brain, and other viscera. Microscopic lesions of superficial spreading-type melanoma have large, atypical pigmented cells of variable colors in the epidermis and the papillary dermis and lymphocytes. Nodular melanoma lesions have multiple tumor cells that form a nodule in the dermis, with invasion to the deeper dermal layers. Metastases to distant sites result when tumors invade through dermal lymphatics or blood vessels. The most commonly affected target organs are the lung, liver, and brain.

In the absence of metastasis, the four primary prognostic factors for melanoma are patient age and gender, tumor thickness, and tumor location. Worse prognoses are seen in older men with thicker tumors located in an axial distribution, as opposed to on the extremities. In addition, the relative importance of certain prognostic factors also depends on tumor stage. In earlier disease limited to the skin, tumor thickness and the presence of ulceration are key. However, in more advanced disease, along with the presence of ulceration, the degree of nodal involvement is the most important factor.

Clinical Presentation
Subjective

The typical patient is an adult who is concerned about a large mole that has changed in appearance. A change in characteristics of a mole is a frequent observation made by melanoma patients. Some patients who come in do so in response to a concerned family member, typically a spouse, who has advised them to have the mole checked. The patient typically will report having had the same mole for many years. A family history of melanoma or skin cancer may be reported by some patients. There are usually no symptoms associated with the majority of cases of melanoma; however, some patients present with a pruritic, ulcerated, or bleeding mole.

Objective

Most melanomas appear on sun-exposed areas of skin. The back and the neck are the most common sites in men, and the legs are more common in women. In blacks and Asians, the feet, fingers, nailbeds, eyes (uveal tract), and mucous membranes are more common sites.

Melanoma often presents as an asymmetrical lesion with an irregular border, notching, and a diameter greater than 6 mm. The tumor often exhibits variegation in color, with admixtures of blue, red, tan, brown, black, and white. Rarely, tumors appear as amelanotic. Early nodular tumors, for example, are typically flat and may lack most of the typical characteristics of melanoma. As the tumor advances, an increase in thickness causes elevation into a firm nodule (in nodular melanoma). Atypical nevi bear many of the same characteristics of a true melanoma, including irregular, ill-defined borders; color variegation; and large size (more than 6 mm). The emphasis on larger lesion size as an increased risk factor for melanoma is not always accurate because early melanomas can be smaller than 6 mm in diameter. Distinguishing between malignant melanoma and benign nevi can be difficult and often requires a skin biopsy.

Nailbed or subungual melanoma may be observed in older patients and is most commonly found on the thumb or great toe. This variant of acral lentiginous melanoma may present similarly to an ungual fungal infection, because discoloration of the nailbed known as longitudinal melanonychia may distort the nail itself. Posterior nailbed involvement called Hutchinson's sign is an ominous physical finding associated with advanced disease.

Diagnostic Reasoning

Diagnostic Tests

Following a thorough physical exam including full-body skin inspection, suspicious lesions should be biopsied under local anesthesia by a dermatologist. Excisional biopsy is the preferred method if melanoma is suspected because measurement of thickness can be made along with staging, as a predictor of prognosis and guide for treatment. Thickness or depth of the melanoma is one of the critical factors in determining both prognosis and choice of therapy. Traditionally, the Breslow depth classification system has been used as a prognostic factor, complemented by the Clark staging system of tumor invasiveness, as described in Table 7.12. In addition, the American Joint Committee on Cancer classification system has been developed to take into account tumor thickness, mitotic rate, ulceration, and invasiveness (localized tumor versus nodal or distant metastases) as key prognostic factors.

If biopsy pathology reveals only atypical nevi, removal of the lesion by excisional biopsy is sufficient treatment. A patient who has dysplastic nevi should receive regular skin surveillance. Skin exams are usually done at 6-month intervals by the dermatologist. A patient diagnosed with melanoma should be referred to a dermatologist or an oncologist for excision of the melanoma and its margins.

Subsequent testing may include a lymph-node biopsy via computed tomography (CT)–guided needle aspiration. Sentinel node biopsy and lymphatic drainage mapping have been shown to identify more occult metastases, employing a technique that identifies the lymph node that specifically drains the area of skin that contains the melanoma. This node, called the *sentinel node,* is excised and examined for melanoma cells. If any cancer cells are present, the remaining nodes in the area are dissected. If biopsy of the sentinel node is negative,

Table 7.12	Skin Cancer Classification Systems

Malignant Melanoma

The American Joint Committee on Cancer (AJCC) has an ongoing collaborative staging system in process. (See www.cancerstaging.net)

The TNM (tumor, node, metastasis) system adopted by the AJCC uses both Clark and Breslow's methods to clinically stage malignant melanomas (MMs). The extent of the tumor is determined only after excision.

The presence or absence of lymph node involvement is the most important predictor of survival.

• Clark's Levels—describes the lesion based on the invading depth into the dermis and subcutaneous fat and is related to the metastatic potential of the lesion.

Level I (in situ)	Confined to epidermis
Level II	Extends through the basement membrane and into the papillary dermis (upper)
Level III	Extends into the papillary dermis (lower)
Level IV	Extends into the reticular dermis
Level V	Invades the subcutaneous tissue

• Breslow's method—describes tumor thickness by measuring the distance from the dermis to the deepest level of involvement. The thicker the lesion, the higher the incidence for metastasis. Measured in millimeters (mm).

Non-Melanoma Staging System

Stage	Criteria
0	Squamous cell carcinoma in situ, or Bowen's disease Involves only the epidermis
I	Less than 2 cm deep No spread to lymph nodes or organs
II	More than 2 cm deep No spread to lymph nodes or organs
III	Spread to muscle, bone, or cartilage and/or regional lymph nodes No spread to organs
IV	Spread to organs, e.g., lungs or brain

metastasis is unlikely and recurrence rates are low. If metastatic disease is suspected, however, a thorough physical exam, laboratory tests, x-ray films, and CT scans are done to identify distant sites of metastases.

Differential Diagnosis

Differentiating between melanoma and benign or premalignant lesions can prove challenging, even for dermatologists. Although the majority of atypical nevi and melanomas fit the ABCDEs of melanoma, an occasional lesion will escape early detection. The differential diagnosis for melanoma includes pigmented skin lesions such as benign nevi, solar lentigines, and seborrheic keratoses.

Seborrheic keratoses are benign lesions that are common in elderly and older adult patients. The lesions are light to dark brown and appear as soft, wart-like growths, located mainly on the trunk. In contrast, melanoma is usually located on sun-exposed areas such as the neck, the back, or the legs. Solar lentigines (liver spots) are pigmented (light to dark brown) macules that appear on sun-exposed areas such as the dorsum of the hands and arms. Benign nevi (moles) are round to oval, with regular borders; most are less than 5 mm in diameter. The color is evenly distributed in a benign nevus; it is asymptomatic.

Management

A high index of suspicion is necessary because it is often hard to distinguish atypical nevi from melanoma or from normal nevi. If a clinician suspects possible melanoma or dysplastic nevi, referral to a dermatologist is necessary. There are four treatments available for melanoma: biological therapy, chemotherapy, radiation, and surgery.

If the melanoma lesion is discovered early enough (at less than 4 mm in diameter and with superficial involvement only), the chance of a complete cure with excision is good. Management will depend on the staging of the lesion (see Table 7.12). In situ melanomas require excisional margins of at least 0.5 cm. Melanomas measuring less than 2 mm in thickness require at least a 1-cm circumferential surgical margin, whereas thicker tumors need at least 2-cm margins. Lymph node dissection is required when there is evidence of draining lymph node involvement on clinical exam, but its ability to improve outcomes is unclear when performed empirically.

Nonmetastatic melanomas that have not spread beyond their site of origin are often curable. Melanomas with a Breslow thickness of 2 mm or more are curable in a significant proportion of patients, but the risk of lymph node and/or systemic metastasis increases with increasing thickness of the primary lesion. Some melanomas that have spread to regional lymph nodes may be curable with wide local excision of the primary tumor and removal of the involved regional lymph nodes.

In addition to excision of the lesion with its margins, patients with metastatic disease are treated with several modalities. One of the main treatments is chemotherapy with dacarbazine, cisplatin, and vincristine or a combination of these agents. Only 15% to 30% of patients respond to chemotherapy with a reduction in tumor size. Unfortunately, the response to chemotherapy is typically short term. Fewer than 5% of patients will experience a remission of their disease. If the melanoma is located on a limb, high-dose chemotherapy via isolated limb perfusion is available. In this technique, the circulation of the affected limb is isolated by tourniquet at the root of the limb. High-dose chemotherapy is infused and is limited to the affected limb only, minimizing adverse systemic effects from the chemotherapy.

External beam radiation to treat melanoma is usually reserved for palliative treatment. For metastatic lesions of the lung, brain, or viscera that cause pressure on tissue, radiation therapy is used to reduce the tumor's size and provide relief from pain.

Administration of biological therapy such as high-dose interferon and interleukin-2 in high-risk patients (to prevent recurrence) has shown some promise. In addition, therapies directed at specific gene mutations as mentioned above have also shown promise. Although melanomas that have spread to distant sites are rarely curable, the small molecule serine/threonine protein kinase inhibitors vemurafenib (Zelboraf) and dabrafenib (Tafinlar), as well as the fully human monoclonal antibody biological therapy ipilimumab (Yervoy), which is an antagonist of the cytotoxic T-cell inhibitory factor CTLA-4, have demonstrated improvements in progression-free survival of metastatic melanoma patients in large studies. Combination therapy with both biological therapy and chemotherapy continues to be studied.

In addition, vaccines that stimulate immune function against tumors are being developed and tested. Despite chemotherapy, the melanoma patient with extensive metastasis has a life expectancy of about 6 to 8 months.

Follow-up and Referral

The patient identified as being at increased risk for developing melanoma should be referred to a dermatologist for increased surveillance, including regular physical exams and full skin and mucosal surface inspection. Ophthalmological exam may also be indicated in the metastatic patient without a readily identifiable primary tumor (e.g., a patient with melanomatous liver metastases but no primary skin tumor), given the propensity for melanoma to develop in the pigmented uveal cells of the eye. The patient who wishes to participate in clinical trials for melanoma can obtain information on current studies from the oncologist. Hospice and palliative care should be offered for consideration to the patient and his or her family.

Patient Education

Prevention of all skin cancers should start early during infancy, especially in individuals with Celtic backgrounds or with a positive family history for skin cancer. Prevention remains the most important intervention, and early diagnosis significantly improves treatment outcomes. Thus, early detection is made easier to remember with the ABCDE mnemonic. The patient should avoid staying out in the sun during the hottest part of the day, high-SPF sunscreens should be applied on a daily basis, and hats or headgear are useful in helping to protect the scalp and the back of the neck. The hazards of tanning beds need to be discussed with all patients. Wearing loose-fitting long-sleeved shirts and pants provides some protection from the sun and is equivalent to wearing a sunscreen if the skin is entirely covered. Unfortunately, although the level of evidence regarding preventive teaching is at Level III, most clinicians think it is crucial and will continue to aggressively teach about self-examination and give preventive advice (Early detection of cancer, 2012).

Survivors of melanoma need to be informed of their increased risk of a second primary tumor or of recurrence of the previous lesion. Any change in an existing lesion or any new pigmented skin lesion should be reported to the patient's primary-care clinician and dermatologist. Likewise, patients should be urged to report any swelling in the lymph nodes of the neck, axilla, or groin area.

◼ NONMELANOMA SKIN CANCERS

The two most common forms of nonmelanomatous skin cancer in humans are basal cell carcinoma and squamous cell carcinoma. *Basal cell carcinoma* is a malignant tumor of the skin that originates from the basal cells of the epidermis. It is a slow-growing and locally invasive tumor that rarely metastasizes. It represents the beginning of a continuum of skin cancers in both severity and mortality. *Squamous cell carcinoma,* a malignant tumor originating from keratinocytes, can invade the dermis and occasionally metastasize to distant sites. Avoidance of excessive sun exposure is an important factor in preventing these skin cancers. In addition, screening programs are important in the early recognition and diagnosis of these skin cancers, because they are highly curable when discovered in their early stages.

Epidemiology and Causes

The incidence of basal and squamous cell carcinoma is expected to rise in the United States during the next decade because of the increase in the older adult population and a longer overall life expectancy. The exact incidence of basal cell and squamous cell carcinoma is not known, because physicians are not required to report cases of nonmelanoma skin cancers. However, more than one out of every three cancers are skin cancers, and the vast majority are basal cell carcinomas. There are an estimated 2,500 deaths annually from basal and squamous cell carcinomas.

Basal cell carcinoma is the most common malignancy seen in humans, accounting for approximately 75% of all skin cancers. Rarely, basal cell carcinoma results from basal cell nevus syndrome, an inherited autosomal dominant disorder. Patients with this disorder tend to have multiple sites of basal cell carcinoma at a younger age; it is associated with bone cysts, palmar skin pits, and frontal bossing (a protuberance of bones of the skull—particularly those under the skin of the forehead).

Squamous cell carcinoma is the second most common skin cancer, accounting for an estimated 20% of all skin cancers. Bowen's disease is an intraepidermal

squamous cell carcinoma that can be induced by exposure to inorganic trivalent arsenic or inhaled mustard gas, in addition to chronic sun exposure. It affects mostly older white men.

The most important risk factor for both basal cell and squamous carcinoma is chronic accumulated sun exposure. Therefore, these skin cancers are typically seen in older adults and elderly patients. In particular, midrange ultraviolet light in the UVB part of the spectrum is believed to be more cancer inducing than UVA rays. Individuals most at risk are those patients of Celtic background (Irish, Scottish, English) who are fair haired (red haired or blond), blue eyed, and freckled and who sunburn easily. In addition, men are twice as likely to develop basal cell carcinoma and three times as likely to develop squamous skin cancers compared with women. Other conditions that increase the risk of squamous skin carcinoma include immunosuppression, a history of exposure to ionizing radiation, exposure to arsenic and polycyclic aromatic hydrocarbons (paint thinners, organic solvents), treatment with psoralens and UV light (PUVA therapy, used for psoriasis), and infection with oncogenic human papillomavirus (HPV). Squamous cell carcinomas are also seen with increased frequency in areas of damaged skin resulting from chronic inflammation, burns, old scars, or chronic ulcers. (See Risk Factors 7.3.)

Pathophysiology

The majority of basal and squamous cell carcinomas are the result of DNA damage in skin cells that have been

Risk Factors 7.3   Nonmelanoma Skin Cancer

Age
Risk increases with age
Gender
Male
Skin, Eye, Hair Color
Fair; tendency to tan poorly and burn quickly Blue eyes, red or blond hair
Personal History
History of skin cancer History of basal cell nevus syndrome History of precancerous lesions, including actinic keratosis History of burn scars or areas of skin damaged by chronic   inflammation or ulcers History of immunosuppression
Environmental History
Excessive exposure to ultraviolet radiation Exposure to arsenic, polycyclic aromatic hydrocarbons,   or radiation

exposed to many years of UV radiation from sunlight. The damage is cumulative and is mediated primarily by defects in DNA repair mechanisms in response to mutational cross-linking by UV light. Such cumulative damage is particularly important in the development of basal cell carcinoma, particularly within skin containing a high concentration of sebaceous glands. Several forms of basal cell carcinoma are seen clinically, including nodular, sclerosing, and superficial forms. The nodulo-ulcerative type is the most common, with well-differentiated tumor cells that may extend from the dermal–epidermal interface into the dermis and subcutaneous fat. Superficial basal cell carcinoma appears similar to dermatitis with erythema and scaling bordered by a fine rim. The origins of these tumors appear to be multifocal, with multiple small nodules arising from different epidermal foci. The sclerosing, or morpheaform, type of basal cell carcinoma is highly aggressive with a high rate of recurrence, presenting as a white plaque with palpable fibrosis and poorly circumscribed margins. Histologically, these tumors consist of spindle cells invading the dermal skin layer. If left untreated, basal cell carcinomas continue to grow and invade surrounding cartilage, bone, and soft tissues. Basal cell carcinomas rarely metastasize to distant sites, however.

In contrast, squamous cell carcinoma is considered more dangerous than basal cell carcinoma because of its faster rate of growth and its more aggressive tendency to metastasize. The precursor lesion of most squamous cell carcinomas is a skin lesion called actinic keratosis, a relatively common finding in older white patients. Actinic keratosis results from accumulated chronic sun exposure and is found only on sun-exposed skin. Actinic keratoses are premalignant lesions involving the uppermost layer of the epidermis and have a very low potential for malignancy (estimated at 1%–5% chance). In situ squamous cell carcinoma (Bowen's disease) involves the full thickness of the epidermis and is the earliest form of squamous cell carcinoma. Interestingly, in contrast to basal cell carcinoma, more recent excessive UV light exposure, rather than cumulative lifetime exposure, correlates best with the development of squamous cell skin cancer, particularly in areas with few sebaceous glands. Invasive squamous cell carcinoma is characterized by penetration through the epidermis and into the dermis, with a rate of metastasis of approximately 5%, primarily to the regional lymph nodes. Lesions that metastasize at a higher rate include those located on the lips, the ear, or at sites of trauma such as old scars and chronic wounds (ulcers). Larger lesions (more than 2 cm in diameter or more than 4 mm in depth) and patients on immunosuppressive therapy also have a higher rate of metastasis.

As observed in melanoma, any underlying condition affecting the capacity for DNA repair increases the risk of developing basal cell and squamous cell carcinoma, for example, the rare autosomal recessive condition xeroderma pigmentosum in which individuals lose the ability to repair UV light–induced DNA cross-linking damage, resulting in multiple DNA breaks and malignant transformation of skin cells. UV light exposure has also been correlated with mutations of specific oncogenes and tumor suppressor genes, including *p53* (seen in more than half of all basal cell carcinomas and up to 90% of squamous cell carcinomas) and the human patched gene. Such mutations result in dysregulated programmed cell death (apoptosis) and uncontrolled proliferation of epidermal cellular clones.

Several other mechanisms also contribute to the development of keratinocyte and basal cell skin cancers. Epidermal antigen-presenting Langerhans cells suffer direct damage from UV radiation, compromising the ability of the immune system to recognize and clear tumor antigen-expressing cancer cells. Systemic glucocorticoids also contribute to immunosuppression and have been shown in some studies to more than double the risk of nonmelanoma skin cancer. In fact, intact immunosurveillance is key to the prevention of cutaneous carcinomas, because basal cell carcinoma is 10 times more likely to develop in chronically immunosuppressed organ transplant recipients, whereas squamous cell carcinoma is up to 250 times more likely to occur. Although these tumors tend to develop at least 2 years after the transplant, they are more aggressive, more likely to occur at multiple sites, and begin to develop at a younger age than in nontransplanted, immunocompetent individuals.

Several types of pro-inflammatory cytokines have been identified in affected skin including tumor necrosis factor–alpha and IL-10. Prostaglandin synthesis also appears critical to this process, and selective cyclooxygenase-2 (COX-2) inhibitors have been shown to confer a protective effect against basal cell and squamous cell carcinoma in mouse models. HPV infection is well associated with the development of anogenital squamous cell carcinoma—particularly by serotypes 16 and 18. In immunosuppressed individuals, the development of cutaneous warts and nonmelanoma skin cancers appears to be correlated. In addition, keratoacanthoma (a fast-growing hyperkeratotic nodular lesion indistinguishable from well-differentiated squamous cell carcinoma) has also been associated with HPV infection. However, the specific role of HPV in additional forms of keratinocyte skin cancers remains controversial, and further research to explore this relationship is ongoing.

Clinical Presentation
Subjective

A typical patient with nonmelanoma skin carcinoma is an adult or elderly patient who presents with complaints of a spot or a bump that is getting larger or a sore that is not healing. The skin lesion may be pruritic or asymptomatic.

Objective

Basal cell carcinomas typically appear in areas of skin that are chronically exposed to the sun, such as the face, ears, cheeks, nose, and the neck. Nodulo-ulcerative basal cell carcinomas are characterized by elevated papules that have a pearly appearance, with some crusting. When the crusts are removed, a small amount of bleeding ensues. On close examination, telangiectatic blood vessels are seen on the border of the lesion. A central ulceration is seen during the later stages of basal cell carcinoma lesions. Basal cell carcinoma lesions may be the same color as the patient's skin or have areas of variegated color such as blue, black, or brown.

Squamous cell carcinomas are typically found on sun-exposed areas, such as the lips, the tips of ears, nose, the upper cheeks, the scalp (in bald men), the dorsa of the hands and forearms, and the shins in women. Smokers are prone to cancerous lesions on the lips and tongue. The most common presentation of squamous cell carcinoma is a firm papule with a scaly (keratotic) rough surface with irregular borders. These lesions may even present as cutaneous horns, with columnar hyperkeratosis atop an erythematous base. Later on, the surfaces of squamous cell carcinoma lesions tend to bleed easily (become friable) with minor trauma and appear eroded with ulcerations. The typical lesion of Bowen's disease appears as a solitary, slowly enlarging erythematous, red-brown hyperkeratotic plaque that has a slight scaling and minimal crusting. Similar lesions in the anogenital region known as Bowenoid papulosis have been associated with oncogenic HPV strains.

The presence of actinic keratosis lesions on patients is considered a marker for excessive sun exposure. Recognition of actinic keratosis, a precancerous skin lesion, is important because treatment during this stage is very simple. Typical actinic keratosis lesions appear on sun-exposed surfaces and are pink to red or sometimes brown. In contrast to basal cell carcinomas, where only one or a few lesions are present at a time in most patients, actinic keratosis lesions typically are present in greater numbers. Lesions vary in size from 2 mm to 1 cm in diameter. These numerous lesions are also located on chronically sun-exposed areas such as the face and the head, the back of the neck, the dorsum of the hands and arms, and the upper shoulders.

Diagnostic Reasoning

Diagnostic Tests

Suspicious lesions (if not located on the face) can be biopsied by an experienced primary-care clinician or referred to a dermatologist. Because basal cell carcinomas rarely metastasize, staging of the lesions is not necessary. Squamous cell carcinomas, however, have a higher rate of metastasis and may require staging based on the pathologist's report. Other important factors that determine staging include tumor characteristics, spread to regional lymph nodes, and metastasis to other organs (see Table 7.12).

Differential Diagnosis

The differential diagnosis of nonmelanoma skin cancer includes seborrheic keratosis, eczema, solar lentigo, and actinic keratosis. In contrast to squamous and basal cell carcinoma, seborrheic keratosis lesions predominantly appear on nonexposed areas such as the trunk in older adult patients and do not appear erythematous or scaly. A patient with eczema will report an atopic history and recurrence of lesions on the same location that resolve with treatment on steroid creams in 2 weeks. Solar lentigo lesions are found in older adults on sun-exposed areas of skin; these "liver spots" appear as multiple smooth, flat brown macules (like enlarged freckles) that are from 1 to 3 cm in size.

Management

Management of nonmelanoma skin cancers is dependent on several factors: size and depth of the invasion, location, cosmetic concerns, and metastasis to other sites. Squamous cell carcinoma has an overall rate of remission of up to 90% after therapy.

Almost all cases of basal cell carcinoma and most cases of squamous cell carcinoma require only simple excision under local anesthesia. Some primary-care practitioners and dermatologists elect excisional biopsy at the time of initial diagnosis; this procedure is both diagnostic and curative. Alternative methods for removal of small basal and squamous cell carcinomas include electrodesiccation and curettage, cryosurgery (liquid nitrogen), and laser surgery.

Mohs microsurgery has the highest cure rate for both basal and squamous cell carcinomas. This precise technique involves the surgical removal and simultaneous microscopic examination of small layers of skin, with removal of only the smallest amount of tissue necessary to eradicate the tumor (until disease-free margins are confirmed). This technique involves less scarring and is particularly suited for treatment of tumors in places of cosmetic importance, such as the face. Skin grafting may be necessary in addition to tumor removal.

In addition to surgical excision, lymph node dissection and systemic chemotherapy are used to treat large and invasive squamous cell carcinomas that have metastasized. External beam radiation is used as the primary treatment on tumors that are large or located in areas of skin that make surgery difficult, or in elderly or debilitated patients who are poor surgical candidates. External beam therapy is also used as adjuvant therapy in lesions with high risk of recurrence or in cancers that have metastasized.

Topical therapies are also used for superficial forms of basal cell carcinoma, including imiquimod cream (used five times weekly), topical 5-fluorouracil (5-FU), and photodynamic treatment (used for both nodular and superficial forms) utilizing a photosensitizer with blue wavelength phototherapy to create reactive oxygen species. Similar approaches are being used for squamous cell carcinoma, for example, imiquimod for in situ Bowen's disease. Premalignant actinic keratosis is also typically treated with topical chemotherapy (e.g., 5-FU cream) or cryotherapy with liquid nitrogen. Other treatment options include dermabrasion, shave excision, electrodesiccation and curettage, and laser therapy.

Recurrence rates for both basal cell and squamous cell carcinomas after treatment range from 5% to 50%. Rates vary with tumor characteristics and treatment modality, and most recurrences occur within 3 years after treatment. Mohs microsurgery is an option for recurrent lesions; it has a particularly high curative rate in lesions that have recurred after other types of treatment.

Follow-up and Referral

Referral to a dermatologist or oncologist is necessary for all suspicious skin lesions, including nonmelanoma skin cancers. The majority of patients require only simple excision of the skin lesion, with follow-up to monitor skin healing by the dermatologist or practitioner who performed the procedure. Subsequent follow-up includes complete physical exams with skin exams every 6 to 12 months or more often if there is any sign of new or changing skin lesions or recurrence at the primary site. The patient who has been diagnosed with any type of skin cancer is at increased risk of developing more skin lesions in the future or of recurrences of the primary lesion.

Patient Education

The American Cancer Society recommends annual skin exams for all adults aged 40 years and older. The importance of careful examination of the skin on an annual basis in certain patients cannot be overemphasized. This includes patients with a family history of melanoma, multiple nevi, a history of sunburns and frequent sun exposure, and persons who work in certain occupations or avocations, such as farmers, gardeners, and sailors. Unfortunately, research has shown that a large proportion of primary-care practitioners do not routinely document findings related to the skin on physical exams. Patients of all ages should be taught the importance of monthly skin self-exams and to report any changes in preexisting skin lesions (see Table 7.13).

The patient should be instructed to report any changes in existing moles or the development of new or rapidly growing lesions. Survivors of nonmelanoma skin cancer should be informed of increased risk of developing a second lesion or of recurrence of the original lesion. Approximately 80% of lifetime exposure to UV radiation occurs before age 20 years in the majority of patients. Strategies to avoid sun exposure should be discussed with all patients at every physical exam, particularly with parents of infants, young children, and

Table 7.13	Patient Education: Skin Self-Exam
\multicolumn{2}{l}{• Once a month, perform a skin self-exam. Record your initial exam, then note any changes with each subsequent exam. Use the table below as a guide for your exam.}	
Head	Looking in a mirror, carefully inspect your head. Using a comb or hair dryer, carefully part your hair and inspect your scalp.
Face and neck	Looking in a mirror, carefully inspect your entire face and neck, including the nose, lips, and ears.
Arms and hands	Holding up each arm, carefully inspect each arm and hand, including the underarms and back of your upper arms (a mirror may be needed). Holding up each hand, carefully inspect the front and back of each hand and wrist, including the areas between each finger and the fingernails.
Chest, torso, and front of the legs	Standing and looking in a full-length mirror, carefully inspect your chest (including breasts), torso, and front of the legs.
Back, buttocks, and back of the legs	Standing and looking in a full-length mirror, turn so that you can carefully inspect your full back, buttocks, and back of the legs (a hand mirror may also be needed).
Ankles and feet	Sitting and propping each foot on a chair or stool at a comfortable height, carefully inspect the tops and bottoms of both ankles and feet, including the areas between the toes and the toenails.
Genitalia	Sitting and using a hand mirror, carefully inspect the genitalia.

adolescents. Patients and their families should be advised of the following preventive strategies:

- Avoid sun exposure from 11 a.m. to 4 p.m.—the time of the most intense UV radiation.
- Wear protective clothing (tight-weave fabric, long-sleeve shirt, and wide-brimmed hat).

- Wear large-framed, wraparound sunglasses with 99% to 100% UV absorption.
- Apply a sunscreen with an SPF of at least 15 as directed, even on hazy days; reapply sunscreen as needed.
- Avoid the use of tanning beds and sun lamps.

 DavisPlus | For additional resources please visit
http://davisplus.fadavis.com

References

Evidence-Based Practice

Beltrani, VS, et al. Contact dermatitis: A practice parameter. National Guideline Clearinghouse. 2006. Retrieved from www.guideline.gov/summary/summary.aspx?doc_id=13606&nbr=006967&string=

Early detection of cancer. In *Guidelines for preventive activities in general practice,* ed 8. Royal Australian College of General Practitioners, East Melbourne, Australia, 2012, pp 60–72. Retrieved from www.guideline.gov/search/search.aspx?term=skin

Leung, DY, et al. Disease management of atopic dermatitis: An updated practice parameter. National Guideline Clearinghouse. 2004. Retrieved from www.guideline.gov/summary/summary.aspx?doc_id=6872&nbr=004210&string=

Menter, A, et al. Guidelines of care for the management of psoriasis and psoriatic arthritis. Section 5. Guidelines of care for the treatment of psoriasis with phototherapy and photochemotherapy. *J Am Acad Dermatol* 62(1):114–135, 2010. Retrieved from www.guideline.gov/search/search.aspx?term=skin

Strauss, JS, et al. Guidelines of care for acne vulgaris management. 2007. Retrieved from www.guideline.gov/summary/summary.aspx?doc_id=10797&nbr=005625&string=

University of Texas at Austin, School of Nursing, Family Nurse Practitioner Program. *Treatment of female pattern hair loss in primary care.* University of Texas at Austin, School of Nursing, May 23, 2011.

Bibliography

General

Fauci, AS, et al. *Harrison's principles of internal medicine,* ed 18. McGraw-Hill, New York, 2011.

Halloran, L. New treatments in dermatology. *J Nurse Pract* 8(8):665–666, 2012.

Kravitz, M. Essential dermatology toolbox. *J Nurse Pract* 8(8):667–668, 2012.

Lowie, AM. Teledermatology: A tool for nurse practitioner practice? *J Nurse Pract* 8(8):617–620, 2012.

Papadakis, M, et al. *Current medical diagnosis and treatment.* 2013. McGraw-Hill, 2013.

Scheinfeld, NS. Skin disorders in older adults: Cutaneous signs of normal aging. *Consultant* 51(12):933–936, 2011.

Atopic Dermatitis

Valdman-Grinshpoun, Y, et al. Barrier-restoring therapies in atopic dermatitis: Current approaches and future perspectives. *Dermatol Res Practice,* Sept-Oct 2012. Retrieved from http://dx.doi.org.ezproxy.fau.edu/10.1155/2012/923134

Alopecia

Monroe, JR. After 15 years, still losing hair, only faster. *Clin Rev* 23(4):13–14, 2013.

Cellulitis

Beltrani, VS, et al. Contact dermatitis: A practice parameter. National Guideline Clearinghouse. 2006. Retrieved from www.guideline.gov/summary/summary.aspx?doc_id=13606&nbr=006967&string=

Blome, C, et al. Measuring patient-relevant benefits in pruritus treatment: Development and validation of a specific outcomes tool. *Br J Dermatol* 161(5):1143–1148, 2009.

Leung, DY, et al. Disease management of atopic dermatitis: An updated practice parameter. National Guideline Clearinghouse. 2004. Retrieved from www.guideline.gov/summary/summary.aspx?doc_id=6872&nbr=004210&string=

Impetigo

Lewis, LS. Impetigo treatment and management. Medscape Drugs, Diseases & Procedures. Updated March 20, 2013. Retrieved from http://emedicine.medscape.com/article/965254-treatment#aw2aab6b6b3

Melanoma

US Preventive Services Task Force. Screening for skin cancer: US Preventive Services Task Force recommendation statement. 2009. Retrieved from www.guideline.gov/summary/summary.aspx?doc_id=13695&nbr=007029&string=

Pediculosis

Caruthers, KL, and Jennings, PR. Head lice—Getting down to the nit of things. *Adv NPs PAs* 3(8):12–14, 2012.

Psoriasis

Cottrill, RR. Psoriasis: A review of diagnosis and management. *Adv NPs PAs* 4(5):20–26, 2013.

Spencer, JM. Actinic keratosis. Medscape, April 15, 2013. Retrieved from http://emedicine.medscape.com/article/1099775-overview

Skin Cancers

Bruner A, and Schaffer, SD. Diagnosing skin lesions: Clinical considerations for primary care practitioners. *J Nurse Pract* 8(8):600–604, 2012.

Gouley, A. Melanoma staging. *Adv NPs PAs* 4(5):31–32, 2013.

Johnson, SR, and Taylor, MA. Identification and management of malignant skin lesions among older adults. *J Nurse Pract* 8(8):610–616, 2012.

Resources

American Academy of Dermatology
www.aad.org
American Cancer Society
www.cancer.org
Centers for Disease Control and Prevention
www.cdc.gov
National Alopecia Areata Foundation
(415) 472-3780
www.naaf.org
National Cancer Institute
www.nci.nih.gov
The National Eczema Society
www.eczema.org
Online resource for herpes and HPV
www.herpes.org
National Institute of Allergy and Infectious Disease
www.niaid.nih.gov
National Institutes of Health
www.nih.gov
National Pediculosis Association
www.headlice.org
National Psoriasis Foundation
6600 SW 92nd Ave., Suite 300
Portland, OR 97223
(503) 244-7404, (800) 723-9166
www.psoriasis.org

Others
Information on dermatological drugs
www.nsc.gov.sg/brochures.html
American Society of Dermatology
www.asd.org
Psoriasis Tools
Psoriasis Area Severity Index (PASI) Calculator
http://pasi.corti.li
Dermatology Life Quality Index (DLQI)
www.dermatology.org.uk/quality/dlqi/quality-dlqi-questionnaire.html
Case presentations to educate practitioners—International Dermoscopy
    Society (IDS)
www.dermoscopy-ids.org
Free dermoscopy training is also available at:
www.dermlite.com/cms/en/learn/for-professionals/video-course.html
http://dermoscopic.blogspot.com
http://dermnetnz.org/procedures/dermoscopy.html

Eyes, Ears, Nose, and Throat Problems

Chapter 8

Susan Kelly-Weeder, PhD, FNP-BC • Sharon Thrush, DNP, APRN, FNP-BC • Brian Oscar Porter, MD, PhD, MPH

COMMON COMPLAINTS

This section briefly introduces common complaints involving the eyes, ears, nose, and throat that are frequently encountered in the primary-care setting. Several of these conditions are further expanded in the section on common problems.

■ DRY EYE

Dry eye is a relatively common syndrome that affects a significant portion of the U.S. population, especially those older than 40 years of age, and may be more prevalent in Asian and Hispanic populations. It is characterized by inadequate tear production. Dry eye occurs as a result of (1) mechanical abnormalities that interfere with the spread or maintenance of tears over the eyeball surface, (2) lacrimal gland malfunction, or (3) mucin deficiency. Mechanical abnormalities include abnormalities of eyelid structure and function and protrusion of the eyeballs; they may also result from the misuse of contact lenses.

Dry eye commonly affects both eyes and is often described as "a feeling of sand in the eyes," especially when blinking. The eyes feel hot, irritated, and gritty and may redden. The patient may present with complaints of blurred vision, lack of tears, or excessive tearing, burning, itching, foreign body sensation, sensitivity to light, and loss of glossy appearance of the cornea. The complaint worsens with smoky or dry environments, such as hot air heating systems, or with excessive computer use.

Differential Diagnosis

Differential diagnosis of dry eye includes, but is not limited to, the following:

- Conjunctivitis
- Blepharitis
- Contact lens complications
- Exophthalmos
- Ectropion
- Bell's palsy
- Medicamentosa
- Sjögren's syndrome
- Age-related changes
- Hormonal changes
- Systemic vitamin A deficiency
- Drug action

■ EXCESSIVE TEARING (EPIPHORA)

Excessive tearing is often a case of paradoxical tearing, that is, a response to dry eye. It is an especially common complaint in elderly patients and in individuals with allergies. A healthy eye is a wet eye; however, a continuously wet eye with uncontrolled tearing signals a malfunction due to a variety of possible causes. The complaint of excessive tears may be related to dryness of the eye. If there is a malfunction of the lacrimal apparatus or nervous control of the lacrimal apparatus, eyes that were dry may tear inappropriately. The eye may also water secondary to an irritant. Excessive tearing is frequently related to allergy, infection, trauma, pain, or structural abnormalities, as in ectropion. Eyes can also water as a result of eyestrain that may be sustained, for example, with prolonged computer use, which can also lead to pain that spreads to the neck, shoulders, and back. The patient may complain of "excess tears," when in reality the tears are a discharge secondary to some form of red eye. Sensitivity to preservatives in certain eyedrops and contact lens solutions can also cause this relatively common problem. Excessive tearing may also occur secondary to a blockage in the drainage system from the accumulation of discharge from conjunctivitis. Frequently, excess tearing will lead to increased irritation and even more tearing, so it is necessary to break this cycle to treat the symptom effectively.

Differential Diagnosis

Differential diagnosis of epiphora includes, but is not limited to, the following:

- Allergens
- Dry eye syndrome
- Viral or bacterial conjunctivitis

- Blocked lacrimal duct
- Ectropion
- Trauma (e.g., foreign body or corneal abrasion)
- Environmental pollutants
- Glaucoma

This subject is dealt with in detail later in the chapter.

■ EYE PAIN

The most important thing for the clinician to know in the case of eye pain, and in dealing with eye problems in general, is when to refer the patient to an ophthalmologist. The liability and potential for human suffering related to damage to vision are high.

Table 8.1 presents conditions associated with any eye pathology that require immediate referral to an ophthalmologist.

Because of the subjective nature of the pain experience, the presentation of eye pain might mean a variety of things. In addition, it is important to differentiate whether the pain is coming from the eye itself or from one of the surrounding structures. The most common cause of eye pain is trauma.

Differential Diagnosis

Differential diagnosis of eye pain includes, but is not limited to, the following:

- Referred pain (trauma, headache, sinusitis, temporomandibular disorders [TMDs], herpes zoster ophthalmicus, postherpetic neuralgia, tumors, stroke, trigeminal neuralgia)
- Eyelid disorders (hordeolum, trauma, blepharitis)
- Conjunctivitis, corneal abrasions, ulcerations, foreign body, ultraviolet light overexposure, overuse of contact lenses or computer use
- Pain with swelling (orbital cellulitis)
- Pain with eye movement (scleritis, episcleritis)
- Deep pain (uveitis, glaucoma)

Table 8.1	Conditions Requiring Immediate Referral to an Ophthalmologist

Patient complains of severe and sudden vision loss or sudden severe nontraumatic eye pain.
Physical exam reveals:
- Corneal ulceration
- Suspected herpes zoster ophthalmicus
- Hazy cornea
- Irregular pupil
- Elevation of fundus on funduscopic exam
- Papilledema
- Limbal flush
- Muscle paresis
Management issues:
- Conditions requiring steroid therapy
- Patient not improving with conservative therapy

■ RED EYE

Red eye, a common ophthalmic problem encountered in the acute and primary-care settings, is a nonuniform redness of the conjunctiva from hyperemia, which can be diffuse, localized, or peripheral, or may encircle a clear cornea. The most common condition is viral conjunctivitis (pink eye), which is benign; other causes of red eye include bacteria, allergies, chemical irritations, or minor eye irritation from inadequate sleep, overuse of contact lenses, environmental irritants, or excessive rubbing. Some conditions are benign; others may threaten vision and require the immediate attention of an ophthalmologist.

Differential Diagnosis

Differential diagnosis of red eye includes, but is not limited to, the following:

- Conjunctivitis
- Hordeolum (stye)
- Glaucoma
- Iritis
- Corneal abrasions
- Dry eyes, keratitis sicca
- Subconjunctival hemorrhage

Differential Diagnosis 8.1 presents a comparison of the selected differential diagnoses for red eye.

■ VISUAL DISTURBANCES AND IMPAIRED VISION

Patients often come to the primary-care setting with symptoms related to changes in their vision. The list of differential diagnoses of impaired vision is quite lengthy; however, a number of conditions occur commonly and should be well known to the clinician.

Common visual disturbances include "floaters" and flashing lights. These subjective complaints usually have different causes. The visualization of floaters is usually due to contraction of the vitreous humor, which is a common sequela of the aging process (degenerative vitreous changes, or syneresis). This may also result from tear-film debris or from material in the vitreous. Floaters are usually unilateral and are often seen when looking at a bright background. Floaters that appear gradually and become less noticeable over time are usually benign and require no treatment. Floaters that appear suddenly, especially if bilateral, may warrant further evaluation. *Photopsia,* or flashing lights, is the subjective sensation of sparks or flashes of light induced by mechanical or electrical retinal stimulation. Any patient who complains of seeing flashing lights should be evaluated immediately for retinal tear or detachment. Monocular photopsia may occur secondary to cataracts, migraine headaches, epilepsy, vertebral basilar insufficiency, retinitis, retinal hole, detachment of the retina, or retinal microembolization. In addition, a condition seen especially among

Differential Diagnosis 8.1 Red Eye

Assessment	Bacterial Conjunctivitis	Allergic Conjunctivitis	Viral Conjunctivitis	Iritis	Acute Glaucoma
Discharge	Purulent, thick Crusted lids in morning	Stringy mucoid	Watery	Rare	None
Visual acuity	Normal	Normal	Normal	May be decreased if iritis is severe	Decreased
Pain	Sandiness	Itching and burning	Itching	Moderate pain	Severe pain
Conjunctival abnormalities	Moderately heavy, diffuse	Mild, diffuse	Moderate, diffuse	Moderate, around cornea	Anterior chamber may appear narrow with penlight exam
Pupillary abnormalities	None	None	None	Poor light reflex	Middilated nonreactive or sluggish
Photophobia	No	No	No	Yes	Mild
Bilateral involvement	Sometimes	Usually	Often, highly contagious	No	Sometimes
Intraocular pressure	Normal	Normal	Normal	Normal	Increased
Preauricular lymph nodes	Not palpable	Not palpable	Palpable	Not palpable	Not palpable
Other symptoms	Occurs in fall and winter	Rhinorrhea, sneezing, watery eyes, occurs in the fall and spring	Upper respiratory infection	May have connective tissue disease	Nausea, vomiting, and headache

women 55 to 65 years of age is vitreous detachment, causing a fluid-filled, optically empty space between the vitreous and the retina.

Differential Diagnosis

Differential diagnosis of impaired vision includes, but is not limited to, the following:

- Refractive errors
- Cataracts
- Glaucoma
- Diabetic retinopathy
- Macular degeneration
- Retina detachment
- Vitreous hemorrhage
- Central retinal artery or vein occlusion

Differential Diagnosis 8.2 presents a comparison of the selected differential diagnoses for impaired vision.

■ EAR PAIN (OTALGIA)

Ear pain in general is a common clinical complaint. Ear problems are often caused by an infection. However, in the absence of physical signs in the structures of the ear,

other causes of ear pain need to be ruled out, such as dental abscesses, sinus infections, temporomandibular joint (TMJ) disease, or mastoiditis. Otalgia can be bilateral or localized to one ear. Ear pain may also have a seasonal affinity such as in otitis externa, which is more common in the summer months, or sinus infections, which may be more common during peak allergen season. Ear pain associated with acute and chronic otitis media are frequently associated with eustachian tube disorder, especially in the pediatric population.

Differential Diagnosis

Differential diagnosis of ear pain includes, but is not limited to, the following:

- Otitis externa
- Acute otitis media
- Otitis media with effusion
- Eustachian tube dysfunction
- Barotrauma
- Ceruminosis
- Dental disease
- TMJ dysfunction

Differential Diagnosis 8.2   Impaired Vision

Diagnosis	Patient Age	Subjective Assessment	Objective Assessment	Urgent Treatment Required
Refractive Error				
Myopia	Teenager	Painless progressive loss of vision (PPLV)	No change in fundal exam	No
Presbyopia	Older than 40	PPLV; may have blurred vision	No change in fundal exam	No
Cataracts	Older adults	PPLV	Vision decreased Opacity may be apparent, cloudy lens, decreased view of fundus	No
Macular degeneration	Older adults	PPLV Decreased central vision	Decreased central vision Blood, lipid exudates on fundal exam	Usually not
Diabetic retinopathy	Related to length of time patient has had diabetes and any comorbid conditions	PPLV	Vision will usually not improve with pinhole test Varies with stages of retinopathy Dot-blot hemorrhages Microaneurysms, lipid exudates Infarcts in nerve fiber layer	Usually not
Chronic glaucoma	Usually older than 40, but may occur in younger patients	PPLV Halo around lights	Decreased peripheral field of vision, decreased central vision is a later sign Increased intraocular pressure, increased cup-to-disc ratio Normal chamber angle	Usually not
Acute glaucoma	Usually 50–85	Sudden onset Severe eye pain, vomiting, headache	Conjunctiva may be infected Steamy cornea, pupil may be fixed, partially dilated, narrow chamber angle	Yes

- Perforated tympanic membrane
- Sinus disease
- Cervical lymphadenopathy

IMPAIRED HEARING

Hearing loss is the decreased ability or complete inability to hear. It may involve the middle ear, which indicates a mechanical or conductive problem (usually implying a reversible problem), or the inner ear, which indicates a nerve or sensorineural problem. Hearing loss may have both conductive and sensorineural components. Often cerumen (ear wax) impaction is present. Many types of hearing loss can be improved with hearing aids; however, only 10% to 15% of patients who could benefit from a hearing aid actually use one.

The prevalence of hearing loss increases after age 40 years. Hearing loss affects approximately 25% of all adults aged 65 to 74 years and 50% of all adults older than age 85 years. Sensorineural hearing loss increases with age. The degenerative decline starts at age 20 years. Ethnicity and gender are not significant. Hearing loss is a universal phenomenon of aging, with an increased incidence in individuals with a family history of hearing loss.

Differential Diagnosis

Differential diagnosis of hearing loss includes, but is not limited to, the following:

- Presbycusis
- Noise exposure
- Ototoxic drugs
- Eustachian tube dysfunction
- Cerumen impaction

- Chronic middle ear infection, effusion
- Otosclerosis
- Tympanosclerosis
- Cholesteatoma
- Trauma
- Congenital disorders

■ TINNITUS

Tinnitus is a subjective perception of noise when in reality no environmental noise is present. It may be intermittent, continuous, or pulsatile (synchronous with heartbeat). It has been variously described as the sound of escaping air, the sound of running water, or the sound heard inside a large seashell or as a buzzing, ringing, or humming noise. Tinnitus also has been described as a roaring or musical sound. It may be unilateral or bilateral.

Recent estimates suggest that as many as 40 million Americans are affected by tinnitus. Approximately 90% of patients with hearing loss experience some tinnitus, and approximately 1% of the population suffers from chronic tinnitus.

Differential Diagnosis

Differential diagnosis of tinnitus includes, but is not limited to, the following:

Subjective Tinnitus

- Otologic: Hearing loss, Ménière's disease, acoustic neuroma
- Ototoxic medications or substances
- Neurological: Multiple sclerosis, head injury
- Metabolic: Thyroid disorder, hyperlipidemia, vitamin B_{12} deficiency
- Psychogenic: Depression, anxiety, fibromyalgia

Objective Tinnitus

- Vascular: Arterial bruit, venous hum, arteriovenous malformation, vascular tumors
- Neurological: Palatomyoclonus, idiopathic stapedial muscle spasm
- Patulous eustachian tube

■ MOUTH SORES

Problems of the oral cavity and throat account for approximately 20% of visits to primary-care providers. Although the mouth may be thought of as merely a receptacle for food and a vehicle for speech, several anatomical structures within the oral cavity may be the foci of disease. The oral cavity is lined by the buccal mucosa, which is rich in mucous glands. The mucous glands of the lips open into the oral cavity. The mouth cavity communicates with the pharynx posteriorly. The floor of the mouth contains the tongue and the openings of submandibular and sublingual salivary glands.

Specific lesions of the oral and buccal mucosa are immunogenic, inflammatory (most commonly aphthous ulcers), or traumatic or may be caused by a localized malignancy. Painful inflammatory lesions may occur in isolation, or they may be associated with a generalized disorder of other mucous membranes or skin. The patient's history is important because it indicates whether the lesions are acute or chronic, single or multiple, and primary or recurrent.

Differential Diagnosis

Differential diagnosis of mouth sores includes, but is not limited to, the following:

- Food or drug allergies
- Chemical irritation
- Dry mouth
- Mechanical or thermal injury
- Infections (bacterial, viral, fungal)
- Host immunosuppression
- Nutritional deficiency

■ HOARSENESS

Hoarseness is a common complaint; the term describes a voice with harsh quality and low pitch. Use of the term can also include weakness, raspiness, or simply a change from the usual voice quality. Hoarseness suggests an abnormality in voice production at the level of the larynx. It is a common symptom that may occur in both men and women at any age. Changes in the voice are part of the natural process of aging. In elderly men, the voice becomes weaker and higher in pitch as a result of muscle atrophy and increased stiffness of tissues. In women, the same changes occur, but the pitch of the voice becomes lower because during menopause, mucoid edema accumulates in the submucosa of the vocal folds. More severe edema and polyps may occur in women who smoke. Hoarseness is a cardinal sign of laryngeal cancer, which is most commonly seen in men 50 to 70 years of age.

Differential Diagnosis

Differential diagnosis of hoarseness includes, but is not limited to, the following:

- Infection
- Inflammation
- Overuse
- Vocal cord pathology (polyps, nodules, tumors)
- Vocal cord paralysis
- Muscle atrophy (aging)
- Gastroesophageal reflux disease
- Chronic allergies

Differential Diagnosis 8.3 presents a comparison of the differential diagnosis of hoarseness.

■ SORE THROAT

Sore throat is defined as discomfort or pain in the throat that is most intense when swallowing. It can be associated with sore mouth, especially if there is a viral infection such as herpes simplex virus (HSV) that erupts as

Differential Diagnosis 8.3   Hoarseness

Infectious	Neurological	Traumatic	Neoplastic
Viral laryngitis Bacterial tracheitis or laryngitis Papillomatosis	Dystonia Neuromuscular disease Laryngeal nerve involvement by thyroid, pulmonary, or esophageal causes	Vocal cord nodules or polyps Smoke inhalation Esophageal reflux Chronic cough	Vocal cord cancer Supraglottic cancer with muscle invasion

lesions that can cause soreness in both anatomical locations. Sore throat can be part of a generalized upper respiratory infection or a specific infection localized in the pharynx. The most common causes of sore throat are streptococcal and viral infections, such as those of rhinovirus. Each year in the United States, pharyngitis is responsible for 40 million visits to health-care providers, and viral pharyngitis is one of the most common causes of absence from work or school.

Differential Diagnosis

Differential diagnosis for sore throat includes, but is not limited to, the following:

- Streptococcal pharyngitis
- Tonsillitis
- HSV
- *Gonococcus*
- Candidiasis
- Aphthous ulceration
- Influenza virus
- Rhinovirus, adenovirus, Epstein-Barr virus, coxsackievirus
- Mycoplasma

COMMON PROBLEMS

LID PATHOLOGY

■ BLEPHARITIS

Blepharitis is an inflammation of the eyelids and margins. There are two forms of blepharitis: (1) a nonulcerative form associated with seborrhea of the face and scale and (2) an ulcerative form that may involve the lash follicle and the meibomian glands of the eyelid. Secondary infections may develop with either form, and recurrences are common and frequently persistent. Both types may coexist.

Epidemiology and Causes

Blepharitis is the most common ocular disease, affecting males and females equally. Nonulcerative blepharitis is occasionally seen in those with trisomy 21 and tends to affect people with psoriasis, seborrhea, eczema, allergies, and lice infestations. Poor hygiene is implicated, as well as poor nutritional status, immune suppression, acne rosacea, and yeast infections. Exposure to chemical or environmental irritants, as well as the use of eye makeup and contact lenses, may contribute to the development of this disorder.

Pathophysiology

Although difficult to discern without a full ophthalmological exam, the localization of blepharitis speaks to the differentiation of affected structures. Anterior blepharitis typically affects the eyelash hair follicles along the eyelid's anterior lamella, whereas posterior blepharitis involves inspissation and inflammation of the meibomian gland orifices (meibomianitis) along the tarsal plate. Seborrheic gland dysfunction, along with accelerated shedding of skin cells, appears to be the primary insult resulting in inflammation in the nonulcerative form, in which an oily crust envelops individual eyelash cilia (seborrheic blepharitis). The inflammatory, noninfectious skin disorder known as acne rosacea, which commonly affects the central face, is another common etiology of blepharitis in the younger population. Blepharitis may also be a manifestation of an allergic process such as a contact dermatitis if a foreign irritant comes into contact with facial skin. In contrast, underlying infection by skin flora, most notably *Staphylococcus aureus*, produces an ulcerative form that may become chronic, extending to the conjunctivae and cornea, known as blepharoconjunctivitis—a condition with a strong potential to affect eyesight.

Clinical Presentation
Subjective

Both forms of blepharitis may present with complaints of itching and burning, and foreign body sensation in the eye. Sensitivity to bright lights and tearing may also be present. Presentation may be unilateral or bilateral.

Objective

Lid margins are edematous and erythematous. Inspection with a magnifying glass may reveal scaling, erythema, and ulcers. Nonulcerative blepharitis may present with scales along the lid margins that are easily removed. With ulcerative blepharitis, there may be pustules at the base of the hair follicles that may crust and bleed. The lashes become thin and break easily. Use gloves to palpate the lid margins and lid for masses and palpate for preauricular lymphadenopathy.

Diagnostic Reasoning

Diagnostic Tests

With any eye problem, it is vital to evaluate visual acuity. Any alteration in visual acuity may indicate a potentially serious underlying problem that warrants further investigation. If there is a discharge, a culture and sensitivity should be considered. Referral for patients with blepharitis should occur in the following situations: visual loss, moderate to severe pain, chronic redness of the eye, corneal involvement, recurrent blepharitis, and when patients fail to respond to therapy. Any lesion in or around the eye that does not respond to conventional therapy within 1 month should be referred to a specialist for possible biopsy. Persistent inflammation and thickening of the eyelid margin may indicate squamous cell,

basal cell, or sebaceous cell carcinoma. Sebaceous cell carcinoma has a 23% fatality rate; up to one-half of potentially fatal sebaceous cell carcinomas resemble chronic, benign inflammatory disease, particularly chalazion and blepharoconjunctivitis.

Differential Diagnosis

Persistent inflammation and thickening of the eyelid margin may indicate squamous cell, basal cell, or sebaceous cell carcinoma masquerading as blepharitis. Carcinoma may also mimic styes or chalazion.

Management

Any swelling or inflammation of the eyelid that does not resolve promptly (within 1 month) with treatment should be evaluated further. Therapeutic Procedure 8.1 describes the management of various forms of blepharitis.

Follow-up and Referral

The clinician should reevaluate the patient in 2 weeks; if symptoms are improving, the patient should be reevaluated in 2 months. As noted, if there is no resolution in

Therapeutic Procedure 8.1   Blepharitis

Type	Description	Treatment
Nonulcerative Blepharitis	This type of blepharitis may be persistent and treatment is aimed at improving hygiene.	Eyelid hygiene with dilute 1:1 no-tears shampoo (baby shampoo) and water using a soft washcloth or cotton balls. Warm, moist compresses to provide comfort and serve to open meibomian glands and facilitate drainage. The patient should apply compresses for 20 minutes, then rest for at least an hour. Patients should be advised that eyelid hygiene may be required for life, and that symptoms may recur if treatment is discontinued. Advise the patient to discontinue the use of eye makeup and contact lenses.
Staphylococcal Blepharitis/ Ulcerated Lesions	Infectious blepharitis should be treated with topical antibiotic ointments that adhere to the eyelid margins more effectively than drops.	Bacitracin or erythromycin 0.5% ointment can be prescribed and applied on the eyelids one or more times daily or at bedtime after gentle cleansing and using warm compresses. Treatment may continue for 1 or more weeks. The frequency and duration of treatment should be guided by the severity of the blepharitis. For resistant staphylococcal infections, a quinolone antibacterial ointment is appropriate or a sulfacetamide/ corticosteroid combination that, like erythromycin, has been shown to be effective against staphylococci. The combined corticosteroid is useful in decreasing both inflammation and symptoms. Use of the two agents combined has been shown to increase patient compliance. Blephamide is available in an ophthalmic suspension and in an ointment, both containing the same concentrations of active ingredients (10% sulfacetamide/ 0.2% prednisolone).
Severe Blepharitis	Associated with rosacea.	Oral doxycycline 100 mg PO twice daily or tetracycline 250 mg PO four times daily is appropriate. These are prescribed for several weeks and then tapered. Continued hygienic measures as above.

1 month, the patient should be referred to an ophthalmologist. Vision changes and pain in the eye also warrant referral. Blepharitis may be difficult to resolve, and recurrences are common. Hordeolum, loss of lashes, or misdirection of the eyelashes (trichiasis), scarring, and corneal infection may occur.

Patient Education

Patients should be encouraged to wash their hands often and dry them with clean towels to prevent reinfection or transfer of bacteria or virus to other persons. In addition, patients should be advised to avoid environmental irritants, to use hypoallergenic soap and makeup, and to exercise care in use of contact lenses. The clinician should educate the patient as to the chronic and recurrent nature of this disorder and the need for vigilance in adherence to the treatment plan until the blepharitis is completely resolved. Long-term eyelid hygiene—gently cleansing with diluted baby shampoo daily—is required to control this disorder. Eye makeup should not be used until resolution of the disorder, and then the patient should switch to hypoallergenic makeup. A blepharitis fact sheet is available from www.med.nyu.edu/patientcare/library/article.html?ChunkIID=12013.

■ HORDEOLUM/CHALAZION

A *hordeolum,* also known as a *stye,* is an acutely presenting, erythematous, tender lump within the eyelid. This condition involves an inflammation/infection of the eyelid margin affecting the hair follicles of the eyelashes (external hordeolum) or the meibomian glands (internal hordeolum) and may evolve into a chalazion. A *chalazion* is a granulomatous infection of a meibomian gland, presenting in the form of painless swelling on the eyelid. Initially, a chalazion may be tender and erythematous before evolving into a nontender lump. Blepharitis is frequently associated with chalazia.

Epidemiology and Causes

These are common eyelid disorders that affect men and women equally. The cause is often a blockage in a duct of the meibomian gland leading to the eyelid surface; secondary infection may be present, again, commonly with *Staphylococcus.* This duct obstruction results in inflammation that may manifest as a hard mass (chalazion), infection of the sebaceous glands of the eyelash (external hordeolum), or infection of posterior margin of the eyelid (internal hordeolum). Previously unresolved blepharitis, poor hygiene, immunosuppression, and underlying chronic diseases all contribute to the development of eyelid disorders. Again, skin conditions such as acne rosacea or seborrheic dermatitis may also predispose the individual toward the development of a hordeolum.

Pathophysiology

Hordeolum and chalazia are various manifestations of the inflammatory response at the eyelids, exhibiting both microscopic (accumulation of fluid and cells at the inflammatory site) and macroscopic (redness, swelling, heat, pain, and loss of function) hallmarks of inflammation. An internal hordeolum is a suppurative infection of the oil-secreting meibomian glands within the tarsal plate of the eyelid that may evolve into a chalazion. An external hordeolum occurs with infection of the more superficial anteriorly located glands of Zeis or Moll found at the eyelid margin. With a stye (hordeolum), the eyelid may manifest a classic inflammatory reaction; however, a chalazion results from an obstruction of the meibomian gland with a granulomatous response and is typically painless. The blockage of the gland's duct at the eyelid margin results in the release of the gland's contents into the surrounding eyelid soft tissue, and a lipogranulomatous reaction ensues, producing a pea-sized nodule within the eyelid. Occasionally, a chalazion may also become secondarily infected with *Staphylococcus aureus.*

Clinical Presentation
Subjective

Hordeolum presents as a localized tender inflammation of the eyelid (external) or redness at the margin of the eyelid, with swelling (internal). In addition, patients may experience itching or scaling of the eyelid, chronic redness, and eye irritation, leading to localized tenderness and pain.

Chalazion commonly presents as a slow-developing, painless hard mass, with inflammation and possible involvement of the surrounding tissue.

Objective

The clinician should evaluate visual acuity. With chalazion, inversion of the eyelid will reveal a red, elevated mass that may become quite large and press against the eye, causing nystagmus and distortion of vision. With a hordeolum, there is erythema and localized tenderness with palpation; there may also be drainage from the lesion on the margin of the lid. The clinician should also palpate for preauricular adenopathy.

Diagnostic Reasoning
Diagnostic Tests

Hordeolum and chalazia are usually diagnosed by their appearance. If drainage is present, culture the drainage. If the conditions persist, referral for biopsy may be indicated.

Differential Diagnosis

As noted previously, any inflammation or swelling that does not resolve within 1 month with treatment should be referred. Squamous cell, basal cell, or sebaceous cell carcinoma may mimic other disorders of the eyelid. As noted previously, sebaceous cell carcinoma, according to some reports, has a 23% fatality rate. Up to one-half of these potentially fatal carcinomas may resemble benign inflammatory disorders. A concurrent and predisposing blepharitis may be present.

Management

Therapeutic Procedure 8.2 describes the various treatments of hordeolum and chalazion.

Follow-up and Referral

Any patient with visual change or pain should be referred to an ophthalmologist. Recurrence of hordeolum/chalazion is likely without proper lid hygiene. If there is no improvement in 1 month, refer for evaluation.

Patient Education

The clinician should explain the recurrent nature of the disorder and the need for vigilance, and begin treatment at the first sign of recurrence. The practitioner should explain that staph (*S aureus*) infections are contagious and instruct the patient and family members not to share towels or washcloths. The patient should use clean cloths for each warm compress to the eye and be sure to wash his or her hands frequently.

■ DRY EYE

Lacrimal disorders may be acquired or congenital. Acquired disorders may be systemic, such as Sjögren's syndrome; may reflect a more local infectious process, as in some forms of conjunctivitis; or may be related to trauma, such as in facial nerve (cranial nerve [CN] VII) palsy. It has been shown that patients with chronic dry eye experience increased activation of T cells. These T cells produce cytokines that may result in a neural signal to the lacrimal gland that disrupts production of natural tears; this process leads to a decrease in the patient's own tears, to tissue damage in the lacrimal glands and on the ocular surface, to recruitment of additional T cells, and, therefore, to increased cytokine production.

Certain medications, such as anticholinergic agents, beta-adrenergic blockers, and antihistamines, decrease tear production because the lacrimal gland is stimulated by the parasympathetic system. Mucin deficiency may also be caused by certain medications, such as those listed here, as well as by vitamin A deficiency, by certain forms of chronic conjunctivitis, or as a result of the aging process. Consequently, tear production decreases with aging, especially in women during menopause, so this is a frequently encountered complaint. In addition, patients may have a diminished blink rate due to working at a computer or a microscope, which can cause evaporative loss.

Epidemiology and Causes

Dry eye is a common disorder affecting a significant percentage (approximately 10%–30%) of the population, especially those older than 40 years. In the United States,

---

Therapeutic Procedure 8.2 Hordeolum/Chalazion

Initial Treatment of Hordeolum	At the first sign of inflammation and pain, warm compresses should be applied to reduce inflammation and increase blood supply and potentiate spontaneous drainage. Gently scrub the eyelids with a 1:1 dilution of baby shampoo and warm water two to four times a day, or directly apply diluted baby shampoo with a cotton-tipped applicator and then rinse with warm water. Follow with gentle massage of the eyelid. Blepharitis, if present, should be treated. Eye makeup should be discontinued until infection resolves. Contact lenses should not be used during treatment. *The hordeolum (stye) should not be squeezed.*
Infection or Inflammation	Erythromycin ophthalmic ointment or sulfacetamide (Sulamyd) ophthalmic ointment can be applied four times a day or ciprofloxacin ointment (Ciloxan, Cipro) can be applied three times a day. Use a thin application to the lid margin with a cotton-tipped applicator.
Resistant or Recurrent Hordeolum *Basal cell carcinoma or sebaceous cell carcinoma of the eyelid can be misdiagnosed clinically as a recurrent hordeolum or chalazion.*	A course of oral antibiotics that is effective for *Staphylococcus* and *Streptococcus* organisms, such as Cephalexin (Keflex, Keftabs), can be prescribed.
Chalazion (Unresolved) *A chalazion that persists for more than 4 weeks needs referral to an ophthalmologist for incision and drainage, biopsy, or injection directly with glucocorticoids.*	Warm compresses and gentle massage of the swelling in the lid with a 1:1 dilution of baby shampoo and warm water may help to open the blocked meibomian duct.

an estimated 3.23 million women and 1.68 million men, a total of 4.91 million people, aged 50 years and older are affected. The frequency of this condition internationally closely parallels that of the United States. However, the frequency and the clinical diagnosis of dry eye are greater in the Hispanic and Asian populations.

Keratoconjunctivitis sicca associated with Sjögren's syndrome is a type of dry eye that affects 1% to 2% of the population, and 90% of those affected are women. Approximately 1% of the U.S. population is affected with Sjögren's syndrome, and it affects 15% of patients with rheumatoid arthritis.

Pathophysiology

A genetic predisposition to Sjögren's syndrome–associated keratoconjunctivitis sicca is evidenced by a high prevalence of human leukocyte antigen B8 in these patients. This is associated with a chronic inflammatory state, producing autoantibodies (antinuclear antibodies [ANAs], rheumatoid factor [RF]) and inflammatory cytokine release and focal lymphocytic infiltration (CD4 T cells and B cells) of the lacrimal and salivary glands, with eventual degeneration and apoptosis of the lacrimal glands and conjunctiva. The result is dysfunction of the lacrimal gland, decreased tear production, loss of response to neural stimulation, and less reflex tearing. Cytokine release inhibits neural function and may also convert androgens into estrogens, resulting in meibomian gland dysfunction. Both androgen and estrogen receptors are located in the lacrimal and meibomian glands. At menopause, there is a decrease in circulating sex hormones, possibly affecting the secreting function of the lacrimal gland. Deficiency of mucin synthesizing genes may be a factor in dry eye syndrome development as well. Vitamin A deficiency, Stevens-Johnson syndrome, and ocular cicatricial pemphigus may contribute to loss of goblet cells and promote dry eye syndrome.

Clinical Presentation

Dry eye commonly affects both eyes and is often described as "a feeling of sand in the eyes," especially when blinking. The eyes feel hot, irritated, and gritty and may become reddened. The patient may present with complaints of blurred vision, lack of tears, burning, itching, foreign body sensation, sensitivity to light, and loss of glossy appearance of the cornea. The triad presentation of burning, itching, and a foreign body sensation in the eye is sometimes referred to as *keratoconjunctivitis sicca* (KCS). This symptom is frequently associated with the diagnosis of Sjögren's syndrome, a systemic disorder affecting all secretory glands that is often associated with rheumatoid arthritis.

Untreated or severe KCS may result in inflammation, erosion, and eventually keratinization of the cornea and/or conjunctiva, and may even cause blindness. A correlation does not always exist, however, between the failure of tear production, leading to dry eye, and

inflammatory or degenerative changes to the surface of the eye. Accessory glands in the palpebral conjunctiva may secrete sufficient tears to prevent corneal damage.

Subjective

Careful history taking (Focus on History 8.1) includes inquiries about current medication usage, especially the overuse of artificial tears, in which the ocular surface develops toxicity to active ingredients or preservatives in lubricant formulations. Consider vision-threatening issues such as cataracts, macular degeneration, and glaucoma and attendant medication usage for these conditions. Past medical history about coexisting connective tissue disorders, rheumatoid arthritis, Parkinson's disease, rosacea, and thyroid abnormalities will help the clinician to formulate a diagnosis. A family history of rheumatoid arthritis may contribute to the diagnosis. In the review of systems, dry mouth (xerostomia), muscle or joint pains, and heat or cold intolerance are significant findings.

Objective

The physical exam of the eyes must always include visual acuity, which may be normal. The exam may reveal a mechanical, infectious, and/or traumatic cause for the complaint of dry eyes. If one of these conditions is revealed, once it is treated, the dry eye complaint should resolve. The conjunctiva may be infected and dull, and the lids and surrounding tissues may be erythematous due to frequent rubbing. The lacrimal apparatus will be nontender; and in the case of keratoconjunctivitis sicca or Sjögren's syndrome, the mucous membranes of the mouth will be dry. Examination of the eyes with fluorescein staining and slit lamp may reveal punctuate lesions of the conjunctiva.

Diagnostic Reasoning

Frequently the complaint of dry eye is a subjective finding with few or no cues in the physical exam, and a clinical diagnosis will require referral to a specialist for

---

Focus on History 8.1　Eye Complaints

- Onset of symptoms (sudden or gradual)
- Change in vision (sudden or gradual)
- Pain
- Photophobia
- Mechanism of injury (if pertinent)
- Discharge characteristics
- Use of contact lenses (type, wearing schedule, and care)
- Current medication(s)
- Past history of eye problems
- Exposure history (new cosmetics, contact with person with an eye infection, travel, work environment, etc.)
- Systemic complaints (fever, genital discharge, rash, joint pains, etc.)

specialty examination and testing. Occasionally the patient will complain of excessive tearing (epiphora) or inappropriate tearing, which may be reflexive due to poor neural control of the lacrimal apparatus from dry eyes.

Diagnostic Tests

In addition to slit-lamp examination, a Schirmer test to quantify lacrimal secretions may be done. Laboratory tests to rule out an autoimmune disease include an erythrocyte sedimentation rate, ANA, and RF. If discharge is associated with the complaint, it should be cultured.

Differential Diagnosis

Differential diagnosis includes conjunctivitis, blepharitis, contact lens complications, exophthalmus, ectropion, Bell's palsy, medicamentosa, Sjögren's syndrome, age-related and hormonal changes, and systemic vitamin A deficiency.

Management

It is not unusual that the patient's contact lens prescription may need to be altered or that the self-care regimen may need to be addressed. Elimination of systemic medications that may have contributed to the condition should be considered. A patient with chronic complaints of dry eye or conjunctivitis may need to be referred to an ophthalmologist. Reports in the literature have associated the relief of dry-eye symptoms with the institution of estrogen replacement therapy in postmenopausal women. Most cases of dry eye are best managed symptomatically. However, when the complaint of dry eye is persistent and unrelieved by self-care measures, referral is necessary.

The principles of treatment for dry eye are based on the severity of the condition and the 2007 Report of the International Dry Eye Workshop (Level I) (Management and therapy of dry eye disease, 2007).

The first level of treatment provides education and suggests environmental and dietary modifications. It includes elimination of offending systemic medications; the introduction of artificial tear substitutes, lubricants, gels, and ointments; and possibly eyelid therapy. Wearing wraparound sunglasses to keep wind from drying the eye surface, using a humidifier in the home, and avoiding rubbing the eyes are methods patients can use to overcome dry eye. Specific pharmacological measures include application of ocular lubricants such as an ophthalmic ointment of petrolatum, lanolin, and mineral oil (Duratears Naturale) as needed, which is especially helpful for use with soft contact lenses, or a 1 to 2 drops of 1% polyvinyl alcohol preservative-free ophthalmic solution (HypoTears) as needed. Sodium chloride 2% or 5% ophthalmic solution (MURO 128) may be used (1–2 drops) every 3 to 4 hours, reducing frequency as inflammation subsides. Transient stinging may occur on instillation.

The second level of care is instituted if the first level is not effective. This includes the use of specific pharmacological measures, including ocular lubricants, nonpreserved artificial tear substitutes, and anti-inflammatory agents such as topical cyclosporine A, topical corticosteroids, or topical/systemic omega-3 fatty acids. Topical cyclosporine ophthalmic emulsion (Restasis) is used to treat chronic dry eye. It contains a very small concentration of cyclosporine, which is believed to inhibit the activation of T cells. T cells disrupt normal tear production in the lacrimal glands. Improving lacrimal gland function is believed to result in increased tear production and resultant relief of inflammation and further damage. Temporary punctal plugs may be warranted after inflammation has resolved. Punctal plugs are painlessly inserted and act as a sort of dam that prevents tears from draining into the puncta and into the nasolacrimal duct. Several studies have demonstrated positive subjective and objective findings as to the efficacy of punctual plugs in the treatment of dry eye syndrome. Moisture chamber spectacles have been in use for many years; however, there is limited evidence in the literature for the efficacy of this treatment.

The third level of treatment is instituted when the previous levels have failed to adequately treat the symptoms. The therapies at this level consist of use of autologous serum, special contact lenses, and permanent punctual occlusion. The final level includes the institution of systemic anti-inflammatory agents and possible surgical intervention to correct abnormalities of the lid. Other surgical procedures may include grafting of mucous membranes or possible transplantation of a salivary gland duct.

Follow-up and Referral

Supportive measures such as listening to the patient's fears associated with vision changes or the possible systemic causes of dry eye are both therapeutic and compassionate. Arranging for prompt referral to an ophthalmologist for accurate diagnosis and specialized treatments promotes a patient's confidence in the primary-care clinician.

Patient Education

In general, the prognosis for visual acuity in patients with dry eye syndrome is good. However, complications of decreased visual acuity and blindness can occur, and patients need to seek medical advice should visual acuity diminish or if the current regimen has lost effectiveness or the symptoms worsen. Table 8.2 summarizes several environmental modifications that patients can make to minimize the symptoms and recurrence of dry eye.

Omega-3 fatty acid deficiency, especially reduced levels of docosahexaenoic acid (DHA) and eicosapentaenoic acid (EPA), have been linked to dry eye syndrome. Dietary intake of these compounds is generally lower than the recommended daily intake; therefore, it is important to encourage patients to increase their dietary intake of DHA- and EPA-rich foods (e.g., salmon, tuna, mackerel, anchovy, halibut, and scallops). Regular use of lubricating drops or ointments and consistent use of prescribed ocular medications should be stressed.

Table 8.2   Ocular Self-Care for Dry Eye
Keep home humidity between 30% and 50%.
Cleanse humidifier frequently with 1:10 bleach solution. Rinse well with fresh water.
Wear wraparound sunglasses, especially on windy days.
Wear goggles when swimming.
Use a preservative-free artificial tears preparation or bathe your eyes in an herbal therapy solution made with Eyebright (*Euphrasia officinalis*) when irritated.
Avoid blowing hot air from hair dryer in the eyes.
Take frequent rest periods away from computer or microscope work.
Stop smoking.

A helpful link for patient information on a variety of ocular disorders is www.emedicinehealth.com/script/main/art.asp?articlekey=60170.

■ EXCESSIVE TEARING (EPIPHORA)

Excessive tearing is often a case of paradoxical tearing; that is, it is a response to dry eye. It is an especially common complaint in elderly patients and in individuals with allergies. Anatomical abnormalities such as ectropion, entropion, lower lid laxity, and lacrimal pump weakness due to Bell's palsy may lead to structural and functional problems in the distribution and drainage of tears. Lacrimal obstruction that limits normal drainage into the lacrimal ducts is a significant contributor to the problem. Obstruction can be associated with thickened discharge secondary to infection, tumor, trauma, or autoimmune diagnoses. The eye may water excessively secondary to irritation from contact lenses, medications, or irritants in the environment as a protective mechanism; or excessive tearing may be related to allergy, infection, trauma, or pain. The patient may complain of "excess tears," when in reality the tears are a discharge secondary to some form of red eye. Sensitivity to preservatives in certain eyedrops and contact lens solutions can also cause this relatively common problem. Frequently, excess tearing will lead to increased irritation and even more tearing, so it is necessary to break this cycle to treat the symptom effectively. As mentioned previously, a healthy eye is a wet eye; however, a continuously wet eye with uncontrolled tearing signals a malfunction due to a variety of possible causes.

Epidemiology and Causes

Epiphora is a common problem and will become more widespread as the population ages. Because epiphora is frequently associated with "dry eye," the epidemiological statistics are similar.

Pathophysiology

Tears are made up of several layers, and each layer has a role to play in the maintenance of a stable tear film. The outer layer is a lipid layer, which forms a superficial layer of the tear film. The intermediate layer is an aqueous layer derived from the main lacrimal gland. The inner layer is a mucin layer derived from goblet cells. During blinking, a suction effect draws the tear film into the lacrimal apparatus. In the case of facial nerve palsy, the loss of the blink reflex allows tearing to occur without any anatomical obstruction. This is also an issue with prolonged computer use accompanied by decreased blink reflex; the eyes become dry and may reflexively tear excessively. A malfunction of the lacrimal apparatus or neural control of the lacrimal apparatus may also cause eyes to water inappropriately.

Clinical Presentation
Subjective

A complete history, which should include any trauma and infections that could be vision threatening, needs to be elicited. If the patient complains that clear tears run down the cheek, it may signal that there is an obstruction of the lacrimal system. If the complaint is of "watery eyes," with tears collecting or welling up in the lower eyelid pouch, the problem may be associated with poor tear quality or poor tear distribution. The complaint of blurred vision, diplopia, photophobia, or eye pain may herald a serious condition. Allergic causes for excessive tearing are common, and frequently the source of the allergen is identified early during the history. Past medical history of seasonal allergies, asthma, or other atopic diseases, as well as a family history of atopic conditions, contributes to making an accurate diagnosis. The review of systems addresses systemic symptoms such as fever, headache, upper respiratory complaints, sore or itchy throat, cough or wheeze, dizziness, malaise, and skin changes.

Objective

The physical exam will focus on visual acuity and careful examination of the structures in the eye and the surrounding tissues, looking for edema, redness, discharge, rashes, and any structural abnormalities. Careful examination for foreign bodies or corneal irritants is essential. Most practice environments have access to a slit lamp and fluorescein staining or use of the slit lens on the ophthalmoscope, which can demonstrate damage in the anterior structures of the eye. In addition, signs of allergies such as pale, boggy mucous membranes in the nose, dry skin, or eczematous changes may be present.

Diagnostic Reasoning
Diagnostic Tests

Diagnostic testing would rarely be done in primary care with the exception of slit-lamp examination. However, the clinician should be aware that ophthalmologists will use a variety of tests to determine tear quality, quantity, and flow. The dye disappearance test is one such test. A drop of fluorescein dye is placed in both eyes in the inferior fornix, and the tear meniscus height is measured after 5 to 10 minutes. This is an easy test for assessing whether there is an excretory problem with the tearing or not. There are other dye tests that look at whether fluid drains into the inferior meatus and into the lacrimal sac. Lacrimal irrigation and probing can demonstrate a punctual or canalicular problem. Occasionally, computed tomography scanning of the lacrimal drainage system can be done.

Differential Diagnosis

Presentation of acute unilateral epiphora with red eye and pain suggests foreign body or corneal abrasion. Irritating bilateral epiphora may be due to allergies, dry eye syndrome, environmental pollutants, glaucoma, or viral conjunctivitis. Blocked lacrimal duct and bacterial conjunctivitis is usually unilateral. Ectropion may be unilateral or bilateral, whereas the development of lid laxity associated with aging is usually bilateral.

Management

Treatment of excessive tearing secondary to trauma or infection includes the use of topical antibiotics. Steroid eyedrops and anesthetic drops should not be used, because they may retard healing and increase the risk of infection. If, on physical exam, a foreign body is visualized, it should be removed by saline flushes. If it cannot be removed with flushes, referral is necessary. Eye rest is important, but patching may be too uncomfortable and is not advised. Corneal abrasions should be reevaluated in 24 hours. If corneal erosion is suspected or there has been no relief in the excess tear production and the pain level is unchanged or worsens, the patient needs to be referred immediately for evaluation by an ophthalmologist. It is important to communicate this information to the patient, and again, timely referral to specialists is essential.

Treatment of allergic causes for excessive tearing (allergic conjunctivitis) consists of cold compresses for comfort and relief of itch, topical antihistamines, topical NSAIDs, mast cell stabilizers, and systemic antihistamines. Occasionally it will be necessary for consultation with an allergy specialist for allergy testing and recommendations for treatment. See Drugs Commonly Prescribed 8.1 for approved medications for allergic and other forms of conjunctivitis.

Follow-up and Referral

The patient with chronic epiphora should have an ophthalmological consultation to evaluate and consider treatment with possible surgical correction. Individuals with conjunctivitis should be reevaluated after a course of antibiotic therapy or after 2 weeks of instituting

Drugs Commonly Prescribed 8.1 Conjunctivitis		
Allergic Conjunctivitis	Mast Cell Stabilizers	Drugs
	Block a calcium channel essential for mast cell degranulation, stabilizing the cell and thereby preventing the release of histamine and related mediators.	lodoxamide 0.1% (Alomide) nedocromil 2% (Alocril) pemirolast 0.1% (Alamast)
	Antihistamines	
	Combat the histamine released during an allergic reaction by blocking the action of the histamine on the tissue.	emedastine 0.05% (Emadine) levocabastine 0.05% (Livostin)
	Combination Mast-Cell Stabilizers and Antihistamines	olopatadine 0.1% (Patanol) azelastine 0.05% (Optivar) ketotifen fumarate 0.025% (Zaditor) epinastine 0.05% (Elestat)
	Nonsteroidal Anti-Inflammatory Agents	ketorolac 0.5% (Acular)
	The mechanism of their action is thought to be due to the ability to inhibit prostaglandin biosynthesis; thereby, they have an analgesic and anti-inflammatory action.	

Drugs Commonly Prescribed 8.1   Conjunctivitis—cont'd

Bacterial Conjunctivitis	Antibiotics	Drugs
Usual organisms: *Streptococcus pneumoniae, Haemophilus influenzae,* group A *Streptococcus, S aureus,* pseudomonads	First-line therapy: Treat empirically with broad-spectrum topical agents. High levels of the agent are delivered directly to the site of infection. The level of concentration exceeds what is normally achieved in body tissues by oral or parenteral routes. Most agents available as ointments or solutions.	sodium sulfacetamide (Bleph 10, Cetamide, AK-sulf) erythromycin ointment (E-Mycin) azithromycin ophthalmic (AzaSite) bacitracin (AK-Tracin, Baciguent) ciprofloxacin (Ciloxan) trimethoprim and polymixin B (Polytrim) tobramycin (Tobrex) neomycin (Mycifradin) ofloxacin (Ocuflox) levofloxacin (Quixin) besifloxacin (Besivance) gentamicin (Genoptic, Ocumycin)
Chlamydial Conjunctivitis	**Antibiotics**	**Drugs**
Common in developing nations. Leading cause of blindness in these nations.	*Systemic antibiotics in addition to topical agents are necessary. Sexual partners should be evaluated for infection and treated simultaneously.*	azithromycin 1 g as a single dose or doxycycline 100 mg twice daily for 7 days
Viral Conjunctivitis	**Antibiotics**	**Drugs**
	Usually not recommended unless there is a secondary bacterial infection. Lubrication for comfort.	Ocular lubricants: artificial tears (Refresh, Celluvisc, Murine) 1–2 drops 4–8 times a day
	Antiviral Agents	
	Herpes simplex conjunctivitis requires systemic or topical antiviral agents. *Any patient with HSV or herpes zoster ophthalmicus (varicella zoster virus) eye disease needs to be seen by an ophthalmologist.*	pyrimidine (thymidine) ophthalmic sol. *(may have toxic reaction)* Oral antivirals: Acyclovir (Zovirax) PO. *Start therapy within 72 hours to prevent postherpetic neuralgia.*

pharmacological measures for allergic problems. Referral to an allergist may be appropriate.

If symptoms worsen before the next scheduled visit, the patient should be reevaluated as soon as possible. The presentation of acute epiphora suggests a corneal abrasion or a foreign body, and the patient should be followed up in 24 to 48 hours.

Patient Education

Patients need to be attentive to changes in pain or discharge and should understand general expectations as to how quickly symptoms should resolve. In addition, they should be alert as to when to seek medical intervention. Vision loss is a very concerning issue, and problems of red eye with visual changes must be addressed promptly. Hygienic measures, such as washing hands, using separate washcloths, and disposing appropriately of dressings,

should be stressed. Washing hands before applying eyedrops or ointment is essential to prevent infection or cross-contamination of a bacterial infection. Patients need to know that there are surgical options to manage changes in eyelid structure that have caused epiphora during the aging process. If the excessive tearing is paradoxically associated with "dry eye," consistent, appropriate use of topical cyclosporine emulsion will eventually bring both symptoms under control. It may take several weeks for the full effect to be realized.

■ RED EYE/CONJUNCTIVITIS

Conjunctivitis is an inflammation of the conjunctiva (mucous membrane) covering the front of the eye. The conjunctiva protects the eye against foreign materials and microorganisms. "Pink eye" refers to non-*Neisseria* bacterial conjunctivitis. Although most conjunctivitis is self-limiting, a few types may lead to permanent vision impairment if not promptly diagnosed and treated. It is essential for the clinician to be able to distinguish between types of conjunctivitis. Differential Diagnosis 8.1 presents a comparison of selected differential diagnoses for red eye.

Epidemiology and Causes

Conjunctivitis is the most common of all eye disorders, affecting all ages. Males and females are equally affected; there are no specific ethnic predispositions. Risk factors are numerous, including trauma from wind, heat, smoke, cold, chemicals, and foreign bodies. Common causes of conjunctivitis include infectious agents (which may be bacterial, viral, or fungal), as well as toxicity (from an inciting agent of some sort) and allergy. Sexual transmission and ophthalmia neonatorum (transmission from passage down the birth canal) are associated with *Chlamydia, Neisseria gonorrhoeae,* and herpes simplex virus (HSV) I. Trachoma, the leading cause of blindness in developing nations, is caused by *Chlamydia trachomatis;* it is spread by direct contact with eye, nose, and throat secretions from affected individuals or contact with fomites (inanimate objects), such as towels or washcloths, that have had similar contact with these secretions. Flies can also be a route of mechanical transmission. Untreated, repeated trachoma infections result in entropion—a painful form of permanent blindness in which the eyelids turn inward, causing the eyelashes to scratch the cornea. Children are the most susceptible to infection because of their tendency to frequently get dirty, but the blinding effects or more severe symptoms are often not felt until adulthood.

Most forms of conjunctivitis, depending on the organism, may be transmitted by contaminated towels, washcloths, or the patient's own hands. Noninfectious conjunctivitis may be drug-induced as a result of chronic irritation from use of eye medications over a long period of time. A chronic inflammatory conjunctivitis may develop similarly, secondary to irritation from contact lens use, seen most commonly with soft lenses but occasionally with hard lenses. A family history of atopy is a risk factor for certain types of allergic conjunctivitis.

Pathophysiology

A hallmark of conjunctival inflammation is hyperemia of the ocular and palpebral surfaces, with injection of this cell layer by engorged, superficial capillaries. Contact with viruses, bacteria, or allergens is the most common cause of inflammation of the conjunctiva. There is also an idiopathic form of conjunctivitis associated with certain systemic diseases such as thyroid disorders and infectious monoarthritis (formerly known as Reiter's syndrome). The most common causative bacterial agents include *Staphylococcus aureus, Streptococcus pneumoniae,* and *Haemophilus influenzae. Neisseria gonorrhoeae, Moraxella catarrhalis,* and *Chlamydia* are responsible for

a particularly virulent hyperacute bacterial conjunctivitis. Viral agents implicated are adenovirus serotypes 3, 4, 7 (which cause pharyngitis with conjunctivitis), adenovirus serotypes 8 and 19 (which cause epidemic keratoconjunctivitis), adenovirus 11, coxsackievirus A24, enterovirus 70 (which causes acute hemorrhagic conjunctivitis), primary or recurrent HSV (usually type I), and herpes zoster (which spreads down the optic nerve), as well as molluscum contagiosum. *Chlamydia trachomatis* (trachoma) causes adult inclusion conjunctivitis, as well as ophthalmia neonatorum. *Chlamydia oculogenitalis* (which causes inclusion conjunctivitis) and *Chlamydia lymphogranulomatis* (which causes lymphogranuloma venereum) are also sexually transmitted causative agents.

Allergic (atopic) conjunctivitis may be linked to a systemic humoral or local histaminic response to an inciting environmental allergen. Certain autoimmune phenomena such as Sjögren's syndrome or Wegener's granulomatosis may also be involved. The conjunctivitis may be (1) seasonal, also called hay fever conjunctivitis, which is usually caused by grass pollens in May and June and by ragweed pollen in August and September; (2) vernal keratoconjunctivitis, which usually occurs in childhood and youth in individuals with a family history of atopy, is recurrent in warm weather, and is associated with large "cobblestone" papillae lining the posterior pharynx in those with a history of chronic atopy; or (3) an atopic keratoconjunctivitis that usually occurs in the late teen years.

Clinical Presentation
Subjective

Symptoms will vary with the cause, but cardinal symptoms of conjunctivitis are itching, watering, and redness of the eye. There may be a foreign body sensation and/or a sense of fullness around the eyes. Bacterial infections such as *S aureus* may produce significant thick, yellow, sticky exudate of the eyelids. This profuse exudate occurs especially in the morning, and patients may complain that their eyelids "are stuck together" when they wake. Bacterial infections usually begin unilaterally whereas viral infections often appear in both eyes at once. Adenovirus conjunctivitis causes a foreign body sensation and minimal pruritus and exudate but profuse tearing. This type of conjunctivitis is often bilateral; preauricular adenopathy is common, along with systemic symptoms typical of a virus, such as fever, myalgia, and the like. Other family members may be affected. Associated upper respiratory tract infection symptoms may point to a viral cause. Visual loss, photophobia, and severe eye pain may suggest corneal involvement. The clinician should ask the patient about any history of allergens and potential contacts, including mention of symptoms of sexually transmitted diseases. Chlamydial causality tends to present bilaterally, with minimal pruritus and moderate to profuse tearing and exudate. Allergic conjunctivitis also presents bilaterally, with severe pruritus, moderate tearing, and no exudate.

Objective

Use gloves when examining the eyes of a patient with suspected conjunctivitis. The first step in the examination is testing of visual acuity in both eyes, as well as in each eye when tested separately. On inspection, there will be hyperemia and tearing. The clinician needs to determine the amount of inflammation involved, and it is important to note where the inflammation is in regard to the pupil, whether it is local or diffuse, and whether it is symmetrical or asymmetrical in one or both eyes. If exudate is present and is thick and copious, the cause is probably bacterial or chlamydial. There may be eyelid swelling. The clinician needs to examine the eyelids, lashes, and surrounding skin for abnormalities. Areas of lymphoid tissue hyperplasia that appear as dome-shaped elevations with blood vessels on their surface are called follicles; these are present in many types of conjunctivitis. If follicles are prominent in the upper tarsus, this is usually indicative of a viral etiology such as adenovirus or *Chlamydia*. Minute elevations with vascular cores that may coalesce to form large papillae occasionally form secondary to inflammatory process. These may be present on the superior tarsal plate in cases of vernal keratoconjunctivitis, adenovirus, or HSV.

Preauricular nodes often represent a viral etiology, such as HSV or adenovirus, and in chlamydial infections and in *N gonorrhoeae*. The nodes are less prominent and more tender to palpation in patients with conjunctivitis of bacterial etiology. Subconjunctival hemorrhage may be seen in bacterial conjunctivitis or enterovirus 70 conjunctivitis.

Assess papillary response for equality and reactivity to light and accommodation. Failure to react appropriately is indicative of a more serious problem and should be referred to an ophthalmologist for evaluation.

Corneal involvement, which often manifests as eye pain, decreased visual acuity, and photophobia, may be present; it may manifest as punctate epithelial lesions. The potential for corneal involvement is increased in cases of adenovirus, vernal keratoconjunctivitis, and *N gonorrhoeae*. The presence of a membranous film that covers and adheres to the entire surface of the conjunctival epithelium is usually associated with epidemic keratoconjunctivitis, HSV, *S pneumoniae,* and *N gonorrhoeae.* If the membrane is removed, a bleeding surface is left behind.

Diagnostic Reasoning
Diagnostic Tests

The clinician should always check visual acuity first. Additional testing in routine cases of conjunctivitis is usually not necessary. A dilated pupil exam should be performed in patients with hyperemia accompanied by proptosis, optic nerve dysfunction, decreased visual acuity, diplopia, or anterior chamber inflammation. Fluorescein staining may be indicated to rule out corneal involvement or keratitis. Use blue penlight illumination to observe for corneal scratches, corneal dendrites (which represent HSV), or corneal ulceration. The clinician should use anesthetic drops before staining the eye. If *N gonorrhoeae* is suspected or conjunctivitis has failed to respond to treatment or in cases of ophthalmia neonatorum, membranous conjunctivitis, and prolonged, severe conjunctivitis, Gram stain and culture should be done. In cases of suspected *Chlamydia* or herpes, the clinician should perform specific cultures and/or a fluorescent antibody test.

In persistent cases of conjunctivitis, referral to an ophthalmologist is essential so that scrapings, cultures, and smears can be taken. Conjunctival biopsy is occasionally useful in refractory or atypical conjunctivitis and is always done in cases of suspected neoplasm. When a hypopyon (a layer of white blood cells) or hyphema (a layer of red blood cells) in the anterior chamber is detected on examination, an immediate referral to an ophthalmologist is required, because this may reflect infectious keratitis/endophthalmitis or penetrating eye trauma.

Differential Diagnosis

In *bacterial conjunctivitis,* signs and symptoms include itching and tearing, either bilaterally or unilaterally, with a moderate amount of mucopurulent (yellow-green) discharge. There is a moderate amount of conjunctival hyperemia, with a shiny red appearance to the lower lids. There is no pain, nor are there any visual disturbances. The cornea is clear; there is no preauricular adenopathy. Bacterial conjunctivitis most commonly occurs in the winter and fall.

In *allergic conjunctivitis,* there is bilateral itching, with a watery discharge. The patient may have a history of atopy. The conjunctiva and lids are swollen and reddened. This is a seasonal occurrence, most common in fall and spring, and may be accompanied by sneezing, rhinorrhea, and throat itching.

Viral conjunctivitis should also be ruled out. The patient with this type of conjunctivitis typically complains of itching, burning, and increased tearing. The conjunctiva is brilliant red, diffuse, and peripheral. There is a watery mucoid discharge, with a moderate amount of mucoid debris. The patient may also have conjunctival edema, follicles on the palpebral conjunctiva, and lid edema. Preauricular adenopathy may also be present. There are usually signs of an upper respiratory tract infection or a history of recent contact with another person with red eye.

In *iritis,* the patient presents with marked conjunctival injection, mainly around the cornea; it is unilateral, without discharge. The patient has moderate to severe pain and photophobia. The vision is blurred, pupils are constricted, and pupillary response to light is poor. Iritis requires a prompt referral to an ophthalmologist.

Keratoconjunctivitis, as discussed earlier in this chapter in the section on dry eye—in which the lack of an adequate tear film to cover and protect the cornea and conjunctiva causes a nonspecific irritation, with burning, redness, dryness, the sensation of foreign body, and generalized eye pain—should also be ruled out.

Other conditions that may present as red eye include the following:

Blepharitis, as discussed earlier in this chapter, is an inflammation involving the structures of the lid margin, with redness, scaling, and crusting. It commonly affects older adults, and is usually secondary to either chronic staphylococcal infection or seborrheic dermatitis. Treatment includes warm eyelid compresses and eyelid scrubs with dilute baby shampoo two to four times per day. Chronic cases may require antibiotic ointment.

Pterygium, a conjunctival degeneration that results in an opacity that partially covers the cornea, is most commonly seen at the 3 and 9 o'clock positions. There is conjunctival injection and tear filming; the opacity is usually slow growing and may eventually obstruct the vision. Pterygium is most commonly seen in persons with excessive exposure to ultraviolet light, windy conditions, or dusty surroundings. Treatment includes artificial tears to alleviate irritation, protective eyewear to be worn when outside, and surgical removal of the opacity if visual disturbance occurs.

Subconjunctival hemorrhage—the sudden onset of painless red eye without any other associated symptoms—is usually caused by trauma, excessive straining, coughing, or hypertension. No treatment is needed if the cause can be found. The patient should be reassured that resolution will take place in 2 to 4 weeks.

The signs and symptoms of *herpes zoster ophthalmicus* include eye pain (which may be severe), tearing, photophobia, mucoid discharge, and moderate conjunctival hyperemia. The cornea may be clear or cloudy. Vesicles may or may not be present. Symptoms are usually the result of reactivation of latent zoster infection because of stress or infection. Patients with herpes zoster ophthalmicus should be immediately referred to an ophthalmologist.

Signs and symptoms of *corneal abrasion* include pain, foreign body sensation, photophobia, tearing, and conjunctival hyperemia. The patient will usually have a history of scratching the eye, contact lens irritation, or actual trauma. The clinician should stain the eye with fluorescein and use cobalt blue filter light or slit lamp to inspect the eye for foreign objects or scratches. Treatment includes antibiotic drops or ointment for 5 days. Patching is not usually necessary. The patient should avoid wearing contact lenses until the abrasion heals. The clinician should follow up daily until symptoms are resolved.

With acute closed-angle *glaucoma,* the patient will have a sudden onset of severe pain and blurred vision, with nausea and vomiting. The patient will report seeing rainbow halos around lights. There will be corneal cloudiness, with diffuse conjunctival hyperemia. The pupil of the affected eye will be moderately dilated and completely unresponsive to light. Any patient with glaucoma should be referred to an ophthalmologist immediately. Corneal disease or foreign body may be ruled out with fluorescent staining. The patient who presents with acute glaucoma is usually older; more visual loss is present, pain is more severe, and there may also be headache and nausea. Uveitis (iritis, iridocyclitis, choroiditis) usually presents with more severe eye pain, photophobia, blurred vision, injection in the limbus area, and deposits in the cornea. All of these are ocular emergencies; patients should be referred to an ophthalmologist immediately to avoid permanent vision loss.

The more typical task for the clinician is to decide which type of conjunctivitis is involved, an essential task before treating the patient. See Differential Diagnosis 8.1 for a comparison of the selected differential diagnoses for red eye.

Management

Treatment will depend on etiology. In general, visual acuity should be assessed and recorded. Do not patch the eye. Although steroids sometimes help with irritation, clinicians should not routinely order topical steroids, but rather refer the patient to an ophthalmologist, especially if there is an ulcer, keratitis, or suspected herpes or if the conjunctivitis worsens in 24 hours. Any purulent material or debris should be removed from the conjunctival area. Lubrication of the eye with artificial tears is recommended, or frequent cleansing by lavage. With blepharitis or conditions that are accompanied by discharge, the patient should be instructed to clean the lid margins with a dilute no-tears shampoo and discontinue wearing contact lenses (if any). Compresses are often effective for local relief; they should be warm in cases of infective conjunctivitis and cold in cases of allergic or irritative conjunctivitis. The patient should be cautioned to avoid spreading the conjunctivitis (or persistent reinfection) through autoinoculation. Pharmacological therapy will depend on the identified or suspected causative agent (see Drugs Commonly Prescribed 8.1: Conjunctivitis).

Follow-up and Referral

Given the potential for unresolved conjunctivitis to be vision threatening, patients with red eye that does not resolve as expected with standard therapy should be referred to an ophthalmologist in a timely fashion for further diagnostic studies and therapeutic management.

Patient Education

The clinician should instruct the patient to instill medication in the outer aspect of the lower lid. It may be best to use ophthalmic solution during the daytime and then to apply a thin film of ointment before sleep. The clinician should explain that secretions may remain infectious for at least 48 hours after the start of treatment. Conjunctivitis is highly contagious; therefore, the patient should take care when coming in contact with other members of the household, especially infants, children, older adults, and pets. Spread of conjunctivitis may be prevented by using effective hand washing, avoiding touching the eyes, and not sharing towels and washcloths. The clinician should instruct the patient to avoid autoinoculation: The patient should not touch the medication applicator to the eye, and should use separate eyecups for each lavage. No contact lens usage is allowed until the infection is resolved.

VISUAL DISTURBANCES AND IMPAIRED VISION

■ REFRACTIVE ERRORS

Normal vision is dependent on a clear image being projected through the cornea, aqueous humor, lens, and vitreous humor onto the retina. All of these structures must be clear to provide a clear retinal image, and the optic nerve must be healthy to transmit an accurate image to the visual cortex in the occipital lobe of the brain. Refractive errors result in blurred vision due to aberrations in how external light is reflected into the eye.

Epidemiology and Causes

Refractive errors that are incompletely corrected or not corrected are the most common cause of visual impairment. Approximately 45% of the U.S. population has some degree of refractive error.

Pathophysiology

In order to transmit an external image into the eye, parallel rays of light enter the cornea, which are bent by the cornea and lens to converge on the retina. The macula of the retina is responsible for central visual acuity and, thus, is the most important portion of the retina for distinguishing visual details, such as when reading. The patient perceives a blurred image when light rays do not converge on a common point on the retina. Light-ray convergence in front of the retina causes myopia or nearsightedness. If light rays converge posterior to the retina, the patient is hyperopic or farsighted. If light rays focus on two separate lines rather than a single point, the patient has astigmatism.

Clinical Presentation

Refractive errors have a gradual onset and are not usually accompanied by pain or redness. Often, if the refractive error is in only one eye, no problem is perceived unless something happens to the other eye.

Diagnostic Reasoning

A simple "pinhole test" can be administered in the primary-care setting to determine if the diminished visual acuity is the result of a refractive error or the presence of organic disease. A pinhole test is performed by creating pinholes 0.5 to 2 mm in diameter in a stiff paper card. The patient is asked to look through one of the pinholes one eye at a time. If the visual acuity improves without the use of corrective lenses, the diminished acuity is a refractive error. If there is no improvement, the diminished acuity is organic. This is because the pinhole card blocks peripheral light waves, which are most distorted by a refractive error.

Management

Corrective lenses (eyeglasses or contact lenses) must be ordered to correct refractive errors. Accurate prescriptions for such lenses may be obtained from appropriately trained and equipped clinical vision experts, such as optometrists or ophthalmologists.

Follow-up and Referral

Accurate diagnosis and characterization of refractive errors requires referral to an optometrist, ophthalmologist, or other qualified clinician, with the appropriate equipment to measure refractive errors. These referrals are needed to obtain prescriptions for effective corrective lenses, as well as to screen for other common eye problems, which may also be contributing to decreased visual acuity.

Patient Education

Patients should be encouraged to use corrective lenses for all activities that require optimal visual acuity, such as reading, driving, or operating machinery. Proper care of eyeglasses and contact lenses should be discussed with all patients.

■ CATARACTS

A *cataract* is any opacity of the natural lens of the eye. It may or may not be associated with visual impairment or functional consequences, and may be localized or generalized. More than 90% of cataracts are age related. Other causes of cataracts include congenital, metabolic, and traumatic etiologies, such as excessive exposure to sunlight (ultraviolet B [UVB] rays) without protective lenses over time. In the United States, cataract surgery is the most common surgical procedure performed under Medicare, is most commonly done in an outpatient setting, and is effective in improving vision in 95% of patients treated.

Epidemiology and Causes

Cataracts remain one of the leading causes of blindness worldwide. An estimated 17 million people have become blind from cataracts, mainly in third world countries.

More than 50% of all people aged 65 to 75 have cataracts; 92% of all patients older than age 75 have some opacities, and 46% of this group have significant vision loss, defined as 20/30 or worse. These percentages are equally distributed between males and females, as well as across ethnic groups.

Risk factors for cataract formation include aging and predisposing diseases such as diabetes, uveitis, intraocular tumor, medication usage (such as corticosteroids, inhaled, nasal, or oral) over time, excessive exposure to sunlight (UVB rays) over time, trauma (blunt or penetrating), excessive exposure to heat (e.g., glass blowers, welders), radiation exposure, and electrical injury. Smoking has been identified as a risk factor for cataracts, along with family history, excessive alcohol intake, poor dietary habits (lack of antioxidants), and atopic dermatitis.

Pathophysiology

The transparency of the human lens results from the highly ordered nature of its composite stratified epithelia, which contain a high density of cytoplasmic proteins called crystallins. Normally, the lens is a naturally clear, biconvex structure located behind the cornea and supported by zonules. Over time, the crystalline lens becomes fibrotic, hardened, and dehydrated, in turn progressively opacifying and transforming into a cataract. Contained within the lens capsule is a central nucleus surrounded by a cortex. The lens is avascular, deriving its metabolic needs from the aqueous and vitreous humors. Early in life, the lens is pliable and can change its shape as connecting zonules anchored to ciliary bodies place varying degrees of stress on the lens through involuntary contraction and relaxation. These changes in lens shape result in accommodation, allowing objects to come into focus at varying distances.

Aging alters the biochemical and osmotic balance required for lens clarity, as does the hyperglycemia of uncontrolled diabetes mellitus. Fluctuating visual acuity and rapid-onset nearsightedness known as a "myopic shift" caused by alterations in the glucose, electrolyte, or water balance within the lens are early symptoms of diabetes mellitus. Moreover, unlike the other endothelia in the body, the lens cannot shed nonviable cells. Thus, as the lens ages, it loses both its pliability and its clarity. These changes are thought to occur because of damage from oxidation, a biochemical process set in motion when a highly reactive form of oxygen (an oxygen radical) forms within the cells of the lens itself. In addition to senescence, several other cataract risk factors are thought to increase oxidative damage, including alcohol consumption, sunlight (UVB) exposure, and tobacco smoking, which has been attributed to more than 20% of the cataracts in the United States. Additional well-recognized risk factors include excessive lead exposure and systemic corticosteroid use. Moreover, healing fibrosis from ocular trauma is a primary etiology of acquired cataracts, whereas secondary cataracts may also result from other forms of ocular inflammation that extend to the lens, including uveitis, topical anticholinesterase preparations, and radiation therapy used to treat ocular tumors.

There are three subtypes of cataracts, categorized by anatomical localization: nuclear sclerotic, cortical spoking, and posterior subcapsular. Many patients have a combination of these subtypes. The size, density, and location of the cataract determine its effect on vision and the most appropriate method of surgical intervention/lens replacement. Nuclear cataracts are characterized by significant nearsightedness and a slow, indolent course. In contrast, cortical cataracts do not significantly impair vision. Posterior cataracts, on the other hand, create a subcapsular haze and a severe glare in bright light. They are strongly associated with systemic steroid use and progress much faster than the nuclear form (months rather than years). Regardless of anatomical type, immature cataracts are those that do not obscure the red retinal light reflex on funduscopy. In contrast, mature cataracts obscure the red reflex with significant visual impairment, and hypermature cataracts are characterized by liquefaction of the cortical lens with mobility of the nucleus.

Clinical Presentation
Subjective

The patient with cataracts may or may not present with visual changes and/or functional impairment. Cataracts produce a gradual, painless, progressive loss of vision; many patients are unaware of vision problems. For example, with monocular (asymmetrical) cataracts, reduced vision may only be apparent when the less affected eye is covered. Age-related cataracts tend to be bilateral in nature and may manifest as blurred or distorted vision, with complaints of a glare when driving at night or in bright light, or the patient may present after a fall, injury (e.g., hip fracture), or accident due to decreased visual acuity. Because of the increase of yellow-brown pigment in the lens, color perception is also affected.

The increased density of the lens nucleus results in nearsightedness that may require frequent eyeglass prescription changes. Myopia, or nearsightedness, may result from nuclear cataracts. The term "second sight" refers to older adults who abandon their reading glasses related to this phenomenon; however, as the cataract worsens, so does their vision. Mononuclear diplopia (double vision in one eye) is a cardinal refractive error associated with cataracts. Cataracts in patients younger than age 60 should raise suspicion of an underlying systemic or localized eye disease.

Objective

In some patients, opacity will be apparent on inspection, but this is not always the case. Decreased visual acuity, often manifested as asymmetry, is the most common objective finding associated with cataracts. Mature or "ripe" cataracts eventually produce a gray or white pupillary reflex known as leukoria, although a dense posterior subcapsular cataract may produce reduction in vision without altering the pupillary reflex. Cataracts are best evaluated by slit-lamp evaluation after pupillary dilation, a procedure that is usually performed by an ophthalmologist.

Diagnostic Reasoning

Diagnostic Tests

A visual acuity of 20/30 or worse that is not corrected with glasses, with concurrent observation of opacity, confirms the diagnosis of cataracts. In family practice, cataracts should be classified according to types based on visual impairment using Snellen far and near visual testing. Cataracts are classified as follows:

- Type I is characterized by visual acuity better than 20/40 in the affected eye/eyes.
- Type II is characterized by visual acuity of 20/40 or worse in the affected eye/eyes.

Cataracts do not produce an afferent pupillary reaction (Marcus Gunn pupil); if abnormal pupillary reactions are present, other ocular pathology must be ruled out. In these cases, biomicroscopic (slit-lamp) exam or careful ophthalmoscopic exam should establish the diagnosis.

Visual quality assessment tests such as the Glare test may assist in the diagnosis or assessment of retinal/macular function. Increased intraocular pressure and/or an increased cup-to-disc ratio with significant cupping should raise the suspicion that glaucoma is contributing to the vision loss.

Differential Diagnosis

Cataracts remain the most common cause of decreased visual acuity in adults. Among patients suspected of having cataracts, the following causes of visual impairment should be ruled out: (1) error of refraction, (2) corneal opacities, (3) glaucoma, (4) retinopathy, and (5) age-related macular degeneration. Any sudden change in vision or sudden vision loss should be treated as an emergency and referred to an ophthalmologist immediately. Cataracts are gradual in onset; they develop over time. Macular degeneration usually presents as a slow, progressive loss of central vision, but may also manifest with symptoms of acute vision loss and distortion (metamorphopsia) resulting from leakage from abnormal subretinal vessels. Open-angle glaucoma produces a slow, painless visual field loss that usually begins peripherally and often (although not always) presents with increased intraocular pressure and/or an increased cup-to-disc ratio and cupping. Diabetic retinopathy may also contribute to vision loss; funduscopic exam will usually reveal dot-and-blot hemorrhages, microaneurysms, exudates, dilated and torturous vessels, and neovascularization of the disc and retina. Cataracts often obscure the fundus, however, making assessment difficult.

Opacities may be a surface opacity of the cornea (scarring), lens opacities, tumor, retinal detachment, or gliotic retinal scars. In elderly patients, visual impairment is usually the result of multiple factors, including cataracts and macular degeneration, to name a few. Cataracts develop sooner in diabetic patients because metabolic imbalances predispose the lens to cataract formation.

Management

The role of the clinician will involve referral to an ophthalmologist. Although surgery is the only definitive treatment for cataracts, the patient may manage at first with monitoring and frequent eyeglass prescription changes. The decision regarding at what point to have surgery should be determined by the patient and the ophthalmologist together. Surgery may be indicated when the cataract interferes with the optic nerve and retina, not allowing visualization in cases of patients with diabetes, macular degeneration, and glaucoma. Surgery should be discussed when changes in eyeglasses no longer help, when quality of life is jeopardized, and when it is thought that the surgery will be effective. Current cataract surgery is a relatively safe outpatient procedure.

Patients who are scheduled for cataract surgery may be referred to their primary health-care provider for a preoperative health assessment. However, among healthy adult patients scheduled for cataract surgery under local anesthesia, no routine preoperative medical testing is necessary. For patients with risk factors or co-morbid conditions, a physical exam, electrocardiogram, electrolytes, and urinalysis may be required. Causes for concern are the presence of diabetes mellitus, hypertension, ischemic heart disease, certain pulmonary disorders, and the use of anticoagulants. Any patient with uncontrolled diabetes runs the risk of postoperative vision loss related to diabetic macular edema, which causes the retinal vessels to leak, leading to swelling of the visual center. If possible, anticoagulant therapy should be discontinued before surgery. Systemic hypertension may place the patient at risk for intraocular hemorrhage during or after surgery. All medications, intolerances, and allergies should be reviewed, especially in elderly adults, who make up the bulk of patients that undergo this procedure.

Two surgical techniques are currently used—phacoemulsification and extracapsular cataract extraction. In both surgeries, an incision is made into the eye, and the central anterior lens capsule is removed. In phacoemulsification, the surgeon makes a 2- to 4-mm incision and inserts an ultrasonic vibrating needle that breaks the cataract into small pieces, which are then aspirated through the needle's central bore. The smaller incision and smaller sutures used in phacoemulsification make it the preferred method for cataract removal. In extracapsular surgery, the surgeon makes a 10- to 14-mm incision, and the entire lens nucleus is loosened from the cortex and removed through the incision. In both cases, the surgery continues with removal of the residual lens cortex and insertion of an intraocular lens. The incision may be self-sealing or closed with sutures. More than 95% of patients achieve visual acuity of 20/40 or better after surgery.

After surgery, the patient should have a protective eye shield in place and topical antibiotic and steroid ophthalmic medications. Lifting and bending should be avoided for several weeks, until cleared by an ophthalmologist. Bilateral cataract surgery is common and often indicated because of better visual acuity outcomes, although optimal timing of the second surgery remains controversial. Cataract surgery has been shown to be highly cost-effective, given the reduction in comorbidities and injury associated with progressive visual impairment.

Follow-up and Referral

As noted, these patients need early referral and monitoring by an ophthalmologist. The most important job for the clinician is to rule out any acute threat to vision and to encourage referral for more gradual cases of deteriorating vision loss. Education about the advances in surgical techniques and reassurance may be important aspects of care before referral. Comprehensive preoperative assessment is important, including psychosocial aspects of care, such as who will drive the patient to and from the surgery and assist him or her during the postoperative period.

Patient Education

Some of the educational and adaptive measures have been mentioned previously. In addition, the patient will need to have his or her vision reevaluated several weeks after the surgery for a new prescription for corrective lenses. Use of wraparound ultraviolet protecting glasses in sunny climates may slow progression of cataracts.

The use of antioxidant vitamins has been suggested as a method to decrease the risk of cataract development; however, inconsistent results have been noted in both observational and intervention studies (Level I) (Wang et al, 2013; Zhao et al, 2014). The American Optometric Association currently supports dietary increases in vitamins C and E because large proportions of the population do not get 100% of the recommended daily intake for these vitamins. It is prudent to discuss dietary sources of these nutrients with patients in an effort to decrease their risks. Vegetables rich in antioxidant nutrients such as beta-carotene, the precursor of vitamin A, and vitamins C and E—any yellow, orange, or dark green, leafy vegetables—may help prevent the oxidation process that can contribute to and worsen cataracts. Carrots contain carotenoids, which have been documented to provide preventive effects against cancers, cardiovascular diseases, and cataracts. Likewise, magnesium and manganese appear to play a role in cataract prevention. Enzymes that contain these minerals assist in the disposal of proteins damaged by oxidation. These proteins are known to contribute to eye clouding. Catnip and other mints contain both these essential trace minerals, as well as flavonoids (see Complementary Therapies 8.1).

Complementary Therapies 8.1

Supplement	Indication	Considerations and Adverse Effects
Bilberry (Vaccinium myrtillus)	Cataracts Macular degeneration	80–160 mg (standardized extract) PO 2 or 3 times daily. Boosts oxygen and blood delivery to the eye. Protects the cells in the eye from free-radical damage and boosts oxygen delivery to the retina. *May require adjustment of antidiabetic drugs. May inhibit platelet aggregation and may have additive effects with warfarin (Coumadin). Do not use with bleeding disorders.*
Vitamin C	Cataracts Macular degeneration	500–1500 mg PO daily (may cause diarrhea at higher doses). Antioxidant. Prevents lens damage from cigarette smoke and UV light. Slows the progression of macular degeneration.
Beta-carotene	Cataracts	25,000 IU PO daily. The body converts beta-carotene to vitamin A, which maintains a healthy lens. *High doses have been associated with an increased risk of lung cancer in smokers. May also interfere with the absorption of lutein. Do not exceed the recommended dose on label.*

Complementary Therapies 8.1—cont'd

Supplement	Indication	Considerations and Adverse Effects
Vitamin E	Cataracts Macular degeneration	400 IU PO daily. Research has shown that people taking vitamin E supplements cut their risk of cataracts in half. Protects against free-radical damage and decreases risk of late-stage macular degeneration. Slows progression of macular degeneration. *Patients taking warfarin (Coumadin) or other anticoagulants should check with their clinician before taking vitamin E supplements because there is a risk of internal bleeding.*
Zinc	Cataracts Macular degeneration	25 mg PO daily. Boosts the effectiveness of vitamin A. Critical in the functioning of the retina and macula and slows vision loss in those with macular degeneration. *Many drug interactions with the use of zinc.*
Quercetin	Cataracts	400–500 mg PO 3 times a day. Blocks an enzyme that leads to sorbitol accumulation that contributes to cataract formation in diabetes. *May competitively inhibit quinolone antibiotics by binding to the DNA gyrase site on the bacteria.*
Alpha-lipoic acid	Cataracts	100 mg PO daily. Increases effectiveness of vitamins C and E in protecting the lens from UV damage.
70% (rubbing) alcohol and white vinegar	Otitis externa	Equal parts rubbing alcohol and vinegar are mixed and then one dropper full is instilled in each ear after swimming. May prevent otitis externa. May also be effective in changing the pH in the ear canal making it less hospitable to *Pseudomonas*.
Bilberry	Sore throat	80–160 mg (standardized extract) PO 2–3 times daily. Decreases mild inflammation in mucous membranes. *May need to adjust antidiabetic drugs.*
Slippery elm (*Ulmus rubra*)	Sore throat	Lozenge: 1 every 4 hours (dissolve in mouth). Tea: 1 tsp. slippery elm bark powder in 2 cups of boiling water; let it stand for at least 10 minutes, then drink 1–2 cups daily. (May add sugar.) Mucilage is the major chemical compound that restores the mucous coating of irritated mucous membranes. *Pregnant women and nursing mothers should not use because safety data are lacking.*
Lemon balm (*Melissa officinalis*)	Oral herpes simplex and mouth sores	Tea: 2–3 tsp dried leaves in ⅔ cup of boiling water; steep for 5–10 minutes. Apply to lesions with a cotton ball after cooling. Also available in a cream as Herpilyn or Phyto-Pharmica Cold Sore Relief (formerly Herpalieve). Apply to sores 3 or 4 times daily at first sign of prodrome. Maximum length of use 14 days. Mechanism of action unknown, but may keep herpes virus from attaching to cells. *May potentiate barbiturates. May interfere with thyroid hormone replacement therapy. Do not use in pregnancy. Avoid use with glaucoma.*
Lysine	Oral herpes simplex and mouth sores	1,000 mg PO 3 times daily with meals at the first sign of outbreak for as long as outbreak lasts. For those prone to herpes outbreaks, maintenance dose is 500 mg daily. Lysine competes with arginine needed for herpes replication. *Do not use in pregnancy. May increase supplemental calcium absorption and decrease urinary calcium loss.*

Continued

274   UNIT II   Caring-Based Nursing: The Science

Complementary Therapies 8.1—cont'd

Supplement	Indication	Considerations and Adverse Effects
Nasal irrigations/ nasal douche/ Neti Pot	Sinusitis/postnasal drip/ allergies/cold prevention	Mix ¼–½ tsp noniodized salt with 8 oz. warm water or use Alkalol nasal douche solution diluted 1:1 with warm water. Fill Neti Pot or nasal douche apparatus with solution. Stand over the bathroom sink and, with head tilted back and to one side, let the solution flow into the nose and out the opposite nostril or down the back of the throat. Repeat on other side. Saline solution can help increase the speed and improve coordination of the cilia that line the nasal mucous membranes so that they may more effectively remove the bacteria, allergens, and other irritants that cause sinus problems. Alkalol is made of natural ingredients and essential oils that include menthol, peppermint, eucalyptol, wintergreen, cinnamon, and a few others. No prescription needed. It is very refreshing and can be used full strength as a gargle to soothe sore throats. *Do not swallow. Safe for use in pregnancy.*

Sources: Micozzi, MS. *Fundamentals of complementary and alternative medicine,* ed 4. Saunders-Elsevier, St. Louis, 2011.
Lindquist, R, et al. *Complementary and alternative therapies in nursing,* ed 7. Springer, New York, 2014.

Lutein and zeaxanthin, which are nutrients found in green leafy vegetables and other foods including eggs, have been reported to reduce the risk of age-related macular degeneration (AMD) and cataracts. These compounds are found in large quantities in the retina; they are carotenoids that filter light and act as antioxidants in the eye. Studies have reported that lutein and zeaxanthin improve visual performance. Current recommendations for individuals with intermediate AMD include lutein 10 mg, zeaxanthin 2 mg, zinc 25 mg, vitamin C 500 mg, and vitamin E 400 IU per day.

GLAUCOMA

Glaucoma is defined as a group of diseases characterized by progressive damage to the optic nerve, resulting in optic nerve atrophy and blindness, most typically associated with elevated intraocular pressure. Glaucoma is classified as open-angle glaucoma and angle-closure glaucoma (classically referred to as closed-angle or narrow-angle glaucoma). These classifications are based on the anatomy of the anterior chamber. Both types of glaucoma may be present in the same eye (referred to as combined-mechanism glaucoma). Glaucoma is further differentiated as primary or secondary (associated with an ocular condition or a systemic process). There is also a congenital form of glaucoma seen in infants. Open-angle glaucoma is more commonly seen and is characterized as a chronic form of the disorder that, before loss of peripheral visual fields, is strikingly asymptomatic. It has an excellent prognosis if treated early and appropriately. Angle-closure glaucoma, on the other hand, may have subacute and chronic components, but it is most associated with acute episodes of significant eye pain, redness, and acute visual loss, which, if untreated, may rapidly lead to permanent blindness.

Epidemiology and Causes

Glaucoma affects approximately 4% of all individuals older than age 40. Primary open-angle glaucoma (chronic glaucoma) is the most prevalent form of glaucoma and accounts for 90% to 95% of all cases. Angle-closure glaucoma (acute glaucoma) is not as common; it affects approximately 100 per 100,000 of the population (approximately 0.1%). Glaucoma is the second-leading cause of blindness among white Americans and the most common cause of blindness in African Americans. Chronic open-angle glaucoma usually occurs after age 40 years but can occur at any age. Angle-closure glaucoma tends to occur in people aged 55 to 70 years. African Americans have a higher incidence of chronic open-angle glaucoma. Angle-closure glaucoma is more prevalent in people of Asian descent, as well as in those with Eskimo ancestry, especially among the Inuit. Chronic open-angle glaucoma occurs equally in males and females. Angle-closure glaucoma occurs more frequently in females.

Increased intraocular pressure, positive family history, older age, and being of African American descent place an individual at increased risk for glaucoma. Older African Americans have a higher prevalence of glaucoma and a more rapid progression of the disease. Specifically, myopia (nearsightedness) and diabetes may both contribute to the development of chronic open-angle glaucoma, whereas hyperopic (farsighted) eyes and a small cornea contribute to angle-closure glaucoma.

Glaucoma may also develop secondarily as a result of a number of ocular and systemic diseases or medication use. The use of steroid therapy (topical, inhaled, or systemic) may lead to increased intraocular pressure. Antidepressant drugs or other anticholinergic drugs and emotional stress may contribute to an acute episode, as may childbirth, sneezing, laser therapy or surgery, and IV overhydration. Increased pressure in the anterior chamber that is uncorrected will, over time, impair peripheral visual fields, destroy central vision, and ultimately destroy the optic nerve. Increased intraocular pressure, optic nerve atrophy, and visual field loss make up the classic triad of glaucoma.

Pathophysiology

The ciliary body of the eye produces aqueous humor, which circulates from the posterior chamber to the anterior chamber and then exits through the trabecular meshwork. In primary open-angle glaucoma (in which no secondary cause is identified), elevated intraocular pressure is almost always caused by obstruction of the outflow channels, especially the trabecular meshwork; however, overproduction of aqueous humor may also occur. The manner in which the trabecular meshwork is obstructed is a matter of debate, but it probably involves changes in the biochemical makeup of the cells lining this meshwork. These changes appear to occur with aging. In addition, secondary glaucoma may result from increased intraocular pressure caused by ocular trauma or inflammation such as uveitis, chronic steroid use, vasoproliferative retinopathy, and recurrent retinal hemorrhages.

The specifics regarding how intraocular pressure leads to optic nerve atrophy are also debated. One theory is that intraocular pressure causes direct mechanical damage and loss of retinal ganglionic cell axons known as "cupping." Others theorize that intraocular pressure impairs the small-vessel circulation that provides nutrients to the optic nerve and extracellular matrix. Glutamate toxicity and processes involved with runaway apoptosis leading to axonal loss are also currently being investigated. It is critical to recognize, however, that optic atrophy may occur in the absence of increased intraocular pressure. Traditionally, elevated intraocular pressure has been defined as greater than 21 mm Hg. Ocular hypertension has also been identified in the absence of optic nerve atrophy. Thus, other pathophysiological processes leading to progressive, irreversible vision loss also function in primary open-angle glaucoma; increased intraocular pressure by itself must be considered only a risk factor, rather than the definitive glaucomatous etiology. Work is also underway to identify the gene products and functions associated with inherited forms of open-angle glaucoma, which typically occur before the age of 40 years, known collectively as juvenile glaucoma.

Angle-closure glaucoma, which may be either acute or chronic, is less common than open-angle glaucoma and is caused by anatomical narrowing of the anterior chamber angle, a factor that is fundamentally determined by genetics and becomes more likely with advanced age. This narrowing is primarily related to the size of the eyeball and lens. Specifically, angle-closure glaucoma results from the forward displacement of the iris toward the cornea, with narrowing of the iridocorneal angle resulting in an obstruction of outflow from the anterior chamber. Acute angle-closure glaucoma occurs when there is an acute closure of the iridocorneal angle with a sudden, severe rise in intraocular pressure, often well above 40 mm Hg, which is highly symptomatic. Permanent vision loss may result if this condition is not treated within 24 hours of onset.

Clinical Presentation
Subjective

Generally, patients are asymptomatic until optic nerve damage is quite advanced. Chronic open-angle glaucoma has a gradual onset, with slow, painless bilateral peripheral vision loss and poor night vision. Frequent changes in refractory prescription may be a common presenting symptom. In later stages, symptoms may include seeing halos around lights and further visual loss. Acute angle-closure glaucoma has a rapid onset, with unilateral pain and pressure, blurred vision, seeing halos around lights, and photophobia, followed by loss of peripheral vision, subsequently followed by central vision loss. A headache may be present and possibly nausea and vomiting as well. Chronic angle-closure glaucoma is as insidious in onset as open-angle glaucoma. Its fundamental mechanism relates to the anatomical narrowness of the anterior chamber angle. Often patients have a history of vague discomfort about the eyes and intermittent blurring of vision.

Objective

The physical exam in most patients with chronic glaucoma will most likely be unremarkable. In later stages, the eyeball may be hardened. Visual acuity may or may not be affected. Visual field abnormalities to confrontation will be present only in very late, profound cases. A Marcus Gunn pupil (afferent pupillary defect) may be present.

In acute angle-closure glaucoma, intraocular pressure rises rapidly to very high levels. The eye becomes red and painful, the cornea may have a "steamy" appearance, and vision is severely blurred. There may be a pupil that is mid-dilated and immobile. Findings on funduscopic exam may show a pale optic disc with excavated cupping and a shallow anterior chamber; there may be an increased cup/disc ratio related to atrophy and asymmetry on comparison with the other eye. Visual acuity is severely affected because visual field defects are common. In many cases, the clinician can detect a shallow anterior chamber and narrow angle with the flashlight test: In this test, a penlight is held at the temporal limbus of the eye and the degree of illumination is noted. A narrow angle is suggested if the nasal half of the iris is in the shadow. Dilation of the pupil with mydriatic agents tends to narrow the angle further, which can lead to an acute attack, as can dim light or darkness, and physical or emotional stress. The primary-care provider should closely monitor patients with a family history of angle-closure glaucoma or hyperopia accompanied by a history of eye ache, headache, and blurred vision.

Diagnostic Reasoning

One of the most important aspects of glaucoma in the primary-care setting is screening. The U.S. Preventive Services Task Force has found good evidence that early treatment of adults with increased intraocular pressure detected by screening reduces the number of persons who develop small visual field defects, and that early treatment of those with asymptomatic glaucoma decreases the number of persons whose visual field defects progress.

In general, tonometry readings are recommended as part of every eye exam, although the measurement of intraocular pressure by any form of tonometry has been shown to be an imperfect, insensitive screening tool for glaucoma. Nonetheless, tonometry readings are recommended as part of every annual eye exam after age 40 years, either in the primary-care setting or by an ophthalmologist or optometrist, with any visual changes requiring further evaluation by an ophthalmologist.

At the present time, guidelines for glaucoma screening by the primary-care practitioner have not been firmly established. Improvement in the diagnostic skills for the early detection of glaucoma in the primary-care setting, coupled with clear guidelines for referral to an ophthalmologist, will have significant economic and health implications. Multiple testing methods requiring specialized equipment and training are available, including pneumotonometry, which uses a puff of air against the eyeball, or the more accurate method of applanation tonometry, in which the cornea is directly observed while pressure is placed against it. Normal intraocular pressure is typically considered to be 8 to 21 mm Hg. In all chronic forms of glaucoma (open- or closed-angle glaucoma), intraocular pressure may or may not be elevated, whereas in an acute exacerbation of angle-closure glaucoma, symptomatic pressures may be as high as 40 to 80 mm Hg. However, increased intraocular pressure alone is not diagnostic, because many patients with open-angle glaucoma consistently have intraocular pressure within the normal range.

Diagnostic Tests

The diagnosis of glaucoma is not made on the basis of a single test but on the finding of characteristic degenerative changes in the optic disc and defects in visual fields. Tonometry to measure intraocular pressure is essential, though not diagnostic. In chronic, closed-angle glaucoma, there may or may not be elevation of intraocular pressure. Normal intraocular pressure is 12 to 22 mm Hg. In chronic, open-angle glaucoma, there may be normal or elevated intraocular pressure, whereas in an acute exacerbation of angle-closure glaucoma, intraocular pressure may be as high as 40 to 80 mm Hg. However, increased intraocular pressure alone is not required for the diagnosis of glaucoma because many patients with open-angle glaucoma consistently have intraocular pressure within the normal range.

Physical diagnosis relies on gonioscopic evaluation of the angle by an ophthalmologist. Gonioscopy determines the angle of the eye's anterior chamber and thus enables the examiner to differentiate between open-angle and angle-closure glaucoma; the angle is normal in open-angle glaucoma, although this often narrows with aging. Visual inspection of the angle is done using a special lens (goniolens) at the slit-lamp biomicroscopy. The two primary types of disease—open-angle glaucoma and angle-closure glaucoma—are classified according to the anatomy of the anterior chamber angle. Both types of the disease may be present in the same eye.

The appearance (e.g., color and contour) of the optic nerve and findings on visual field examination are the most important clues to diagnosis. Pathognomonic changes indicate glaucoma. Funduscopic examination of the optic nerve reveals changes in the cup and neuroretinal rim relatively early in the disease, indicating the possibility of open-angle glaucoma. Particularly significant are the size of the cup relative to the optic nerve, any thinning or nicking of the disc rim, and the presence of disc hemorrhages. Visual field examination, which requires specialized equipment, detects defects in the field of vision that are characteristic for glaucomatous damage to the optic nerve relatively early in the disease.

Testing of visual fields using confrontational finger motions to test where the patient's fields are compared with the examiner's is unreliable for diagnosing glaucoma. There are specialized tests that can be performed by an ophthalmologist or optometrist for visual field assessment, including automated perimetry, Goldmann perimetry, or tangent screen testing. Pachymetry, which is a method of measuring corneal thickness, may also be done by an ophthalmologist. Thinner corneas are at higher risk for the development of primary open-angle glaucoma.

Differential Diagnosis

Conjunctivitis and uveitis will be ruled out because of other symptomatology the clinician may observe in cases of glaucoma, specifically visual changes. Vascular disease may also produce funduscopic changes; however, these changes will be more hemorrhagic in nature. Medications such as steroids, amphetamines, and chlorpromazine can all increase intraocular pressure. Many ocular and systemic conditions are associated with the development of glaucoma; in addition, the use of topical, systemic, and inhaled corticosteroids may increase intraocular pressure, depending on dose and duration of treatment.

Management

Once nerve damage has occurred, it is irreversible; thus, the goal of treatment is to prevent progression of damage and to protect the optic nerve from pressure. Glaucoma is a disease of pressure; adequate lowering of intraocular pressure by one means or another almost always stops optic nerve damage.

Traditionally, open-angle glaucoma is managed pharmacologically for as long as possible, with laser or surgical treatment reserved for glaucoma that cannot be controlled by medication alone. The choice of medication regimen is usually made by an ophthalmologist. The goal of pharmacological therapy is to decrease and control intraocular pressure. (See Drugs Commonly Prescribed 8.2: Glaucoma.)

Beta blockers are usually first-line therapy, but sometimes prostaglandin analogs may be used as first-line therapy or added soon after beta blockers are started. Treatment compliance with multiple doses of eyedrops daily is often poor in open-angle glaucoma; however, newer topical agents require less frequent dosing (once daily for prostaglandins). If medications do not control pressure, surgical options include laser or external trabeculectomy. Laser therapy is often effective only in the first several years after surgery and then the pressure begins to build again. The timing of surgery has not been shown to influence visual outcomes, and surgery imparts greater risk for future cataracts; therefore, medications should be tried first. Target intraocular pressure that therapy attempts to achieve must be decided on an individual basis. If one medication is not sufficient to lower the intraocular pressure, a second medication from a different class may be added. It should be noted that occasionally localized or systemic reactions to the medication may occur and the patients should be instructed as to what to look for. Other systemic medications that the patient may be taking must be taken into consideration.

Drugs Commonly Prescribed 8.2   Glaucoma

Classification of Medication	Mechanism of Action	Drugs
Cholinergic	Pupillary constriction to open the angle and allow aqueous humor to escape.	pilocarpine (Isopto, Pilocar, Pilostat) *Contraindicated in conditions in which pupillary constriction is to be avoided.*
Beta blocker	Reduces the production of aqueous humor.	timolol (Timoptic), betaxolol (Betoptic), levobunolol (Betagan), carteolol (Cartrol), metipranolol (Betanol) *Additive effect in patients who are on an oral beta blocker. Contraindicated in asthma, sinus bradycardia, second- or third-degree atrioventricular block, overt CHF.*
Prostaglandin analog	Decreases intraocular pressure by increased ureo-scleral outflow (drainage).	bimatoprost (Lumigan), latanoprost (Xalatan), travoprost (Travatan) *Can cause conjunctival hyperemia, iris pigment color changes, uveitis, and macular edema.*
Carbonic anhydrase inhibitor	Reduces aqueous humor production.	brinzolamide (Azopt), dorzolamide (Trusopt), echothiophate (Phospholine), physiostigmine (Eserone sulfate ophthalmic). *Caution in patients with nephrolithiasis, diabetes, hepatic disease, and a history of sulfonamide sensitivity.*
Alpha-adrenergic agonist	Inhibits aqueous humor production.	epinephrine and dipivefrin (Propine), apraclonidine (Iopidine), brimonidine (Alphagan). *Avoid in patients with grade 2 or 3 heart block, CHF, chronic obstructive pulmonary disease, asthma, or pulmonary edema.*
Systemic medications	Reduces production of aqueous humor.	acetazolamide (Diamox), dichlorphenamide (Sulfonamide), metazolamide (Sulfonamide)

CHF- congestive heart failure.

Angle-closure glaucoma may be either acute or chronic and is less common than open-angle glaucoma. Angle-closure glaucoma is caused by anatomical narrowing of the anterior chamber angle, a factor that is determined by genetics and becomes more likely with advancing age. The narrowing is primarily related to the size of the eyeball and lens. Specifically, angle-closure glaucoma occurs when there is an acute closure of the iridocorneal angle, with a sudden, severe rise in intraocular pressure, often well above 40 mm Hg, which is symptomatic. Acute angle-closure glaucoma requires emergency treatment, or total blindness will follow within 2 to 5 days. Medications are administered during the acute attack to lower intraocular pressure so that surgical intervention can occur. Acetazolamide (Diamox) and intravenous mannitol with a topical miotic, such as pilocarpine, may be administered, followed by laser iridotomy or peripheral iridectomy. Bedrest should be maintained until the attack is broken.

Follow-up and Referral

Patients with glaucoma should be referred to and followed by an ophthalmologist. Nonetheless, as the primary-care provider, the clinician needs to understand what medications the patient is receiving as well as how often the patient should be monitored by an ophthalmologist (every 3–4 months for life). The clinician needs to be alert to possible signs and symptoms of exacerbation. There is always potential for loss of vision and possible blindness if acute glaucoma attacks are not treated promptly and consistently.

Patient Education

Careful and lifelong follow-up is essential for patients with glaucoma, especially periodic checks of intraocular pressure and eye exams. The need to take medications as ordered, to be aware of adverse effects of medications prescribed, and to recognize changes (such as sudden changes in vision) that warrant a call to the health-care provider is essential for all patients with glaucoma. The clinician may need to teach the patient how best to instill the eyedrops. If vision is severely compromised, a caregiver will need to be taught as well. Any sign of eye infection, especially fever, should be reported. In addition, the knowledge that certain medications, such as systemic steroids, may interfere with glaucoma control is essential. Support and counseling may also be necessary. In the case of open-angle glaucoma, patients need to know that they will most likely need bilateral treatment because the second eye is at risk for the same disease process.

■ DIABETIC RETINOPATHY

Diabetic retinopathy is a noninflammatory disorder of the retina that develops in patients with diabetes mellitus. It is typically divided into three stages: (1) background diabetic retinopathy, (2) preproliferative diabetic retinopathy, and (3) proliferative diabetic retinopathy.

The initial evaluation for a patient with diabetes mellitus should include a referral to an ophthalmologist for a comprehensive eye evaluation, with particular attention to the aspects relevant to diabetic retinopathy.

Epidemiology and Causes

Approximately 6.6% of the population aged 20 to 74 have diabetes mellitus; approximately 25% of individuals with diabetes have some form of diabetic retinopathy. Most patients with diabetes will eventually develop some form of retinopathy. Diabetic retinopathy accounts for approximately 10% of new cases of blindness each year and is the leading cause of new cases of legal blindness among Americans aged 20 to 64.

The peak incidence of type 1 diabetes mellitus is between ages 12 and 15; the peak incidence of type 2 diabetes mellitus is between ages 50 and 70. Almost all patients with diabetes will develop background diabetic retinopathy after they have had diabetes for at least 20 years. Two-thirds of patients with type 1 diabetes who have had the disease for at least 35 years will develop proliferative diabetic neuropathy, and one-third will develop macular edema. The proportions are reversed for patients with type 2 diabetes.

Diabetes mellitus type 1 occurs about equally in males and females, whereas type 2 is more common in women. Predilection for type 1 diabetes is higher among Anglo Americans (African Americans have the lowest incidence); however, certain groups, such as the Pima Indians, have a 35% incidence rate of diabetes mellitus type 2.

The longer the patient has had diabetes mellitus, the greater the likelihood that he or she will develop retinopathy. In addition, poor glycemic control translates into end-organ damage, including retinopathies, in patients with either type 1 or type 2 diabetes. Pregnancy, renal disease, systemic hypertension, smoking, and elevated serum lipid levels (associated with an increased risk of retinal lipid deposits) are all risk factors for the development of retinopathy.

Pathophysiology

The key insult driving diabetic retinopathy is uncontrolled hyperglycemia. The precise mechanism by which this causes retinal damage is unclear, but there are several prevailing hypotheses that likely contribute to varying degrees. Hyperglycemia is known to contribute to the dysregulation of retinal blood flow. In the setting of systemic hypertension, increased shear stress on retinal blood vessels drives the release of vasoproliferative factors (e.g., vascular endothelial growth factor, insulin-like growth factor–1, basic fibroblast growth factor, hepatocyte growth factor) that stimulate neovascularization of the retina, optic nerve, and iris. The buildup of sorbitol (a by-product of glucose metabolism by the enzyme aldose reductase) in retinal cells is believed to increase intracellular osmolality, causing fluid shifts (cellular edema) and subsequent retinal damage. In hyperglycemic states, free amino acids, serum, and tissue proteins may all become irreversibly glycosylated. These end products are thought to cross-link with collagen fibers within the extracellular space, initiating microvascular complications. Retinal microthromboses composed of platelets and fibrin have also been proposed to stimulate neovascularization, as the body attempts to compensate for decreased retinal blood flow. Moreover, several other risk factors have been identified, including certain genetic predispositions and enzymatic allelic variants, serum hypertriglyceridemia, anemia, and hormonal fluctuations associated with pregnancy.

In the case of background diabetic retinopathy, retinal pericytes and the microvascular endothelium are damaged early in the disease process, leading to vascular permeability and basement membrane thickening (similar to the histopathological changes seen in diabetic nephropathy). This predisposes retinal capillaries to microaneurysms and the retinal surface to thickening with deposits of proteinaceous and lipid material (hard exudates). If the macula is affected (i.e., macular edema occurs), vision may gradually blur and progress to profound visual loss if left untreated. In the preproliferative phase, multiple cycles of cellular death and renewal lead to venous beading, tortuous venous dilation, and intraluminal cellular proliferation, along with platelet, erythrocyte, and fibrinogen aggregation, which ultimately results in vascular occlusion. Upstream of such lesions, flame-shaped and blot hemorrhages occur; downstream, microvascular infarcts present as "cotton wool spots" or soft exudates on funduscopy. Finally, the proliferative phase is characterized by neovascularization on the retinal surface, optic nerve, and iris. These fragile vessels may be venous or arterial in origin and may extend into the vitreous chamber, attaching to the posterior pole of the vitreous in a fine fibrous mesh. This network places stress on the retinal surface as the fibers contract. As a result, hemorrhage into the vitreous body and even retinal detachment may occur, requiring both vitrectomy and laser photocoagulation.

Clinical Presentation

Subjective

The patient will complain of visual changes as the disease progresses but is usually asymptomatic in the early stages.

Objective

Changes will be noted on funduscopic exam. In background diabetic retinopathy, microaneurysms, intraretinal hemorrhage, macular edema, and lipid deposits may be apparent. As the disease progresses, nerve fiber layer infarctions ("cotton wool" spots), venous beading and dilation, edema, and, in some cases, extensive retinal hemorrhage will be noted. In the proliferative form of diabetic retinopathy, new blood vessel proliferation (neovascularization) may be seen on the retinal surface, optic nerve, and iris.

Diagnostic Reasoning

Diagnostic Tests

A thorough eye exam should be done, including an assessment of visual acuity and documentation of the status of the iris, lens, vitreous, and fundus. Fluorescein angiography will demonstrate retinal nonperfusion, retinal leakage, and proliferative diabetic retinopathy.

Differential Diagnosis

A history of diabetes, especially if present for more than 10 years, correlated with observable changes on funduscopic exam, establishes the diagnosis. Other causes of retinopathy include hypertensive retinopathy, radiation retinopathy, and retinal venous obstruction.

Management

The first goal for patients at risk for microvascular complications, including diabetic retinopathy, is prevention. Risk is significantly increased for patients with blood sugar levels above 200 mg/dL. The most significant preventive measure is to keep blood sugar under control. The American Diabetes Association sets an acceptable level of glycated hemoglobin or HgbA1C at less than 7%. In patients who have their blood sugar under adequate control, the incidence of diabetic retinopathy is far lower and the onset in those who do develop this disease is later. All patients who carry the diagnosis of diabetes mellitus must be referred to ophthalmology on diagnosis.

Similarly, patients with diabetes and hypertension should strive to maintain as normal a blood pressure as possible to prevent the development of end-organ damage. Because many patients have both disorders, vigilance is especially important in this subset of patients.

The only pharmacological agent that has been found to slow the progression of diabetic retinopathy is lisinopril, an angiotensin-converting enzyme inhibitor.

Laser surgery is recommended for patients with proliferative diabetic retinopathy and for patients with clinically significant macular edema.

Diabetic retinopathy patients should be followed by an ophthalmologist, who can decide when to treat the disorder with laser treatment (focal and panretinal photocoagulation); in certain cases, cryoretinopexy can be used to decrease the neovascular stimulus and to treat proliferative diabetic retinopathy. Vitrectomy may be considered for patients with severe proliferative diabetic retinopathy, traction retinal detachment involving the macula, and nonclearing vitreous hemorrhage (this surgical option should be considered after 1 month for a vitreous hemorrhage that has decreased the vision to the 5/200 level or worse).

Follow-up and Referral

All patients with diabetes mellitus should be monitored annually by an ophthalmologist. The patient with background retinopathy should be followed at least every

6 months, and patients with proliferative retinopathy should be seen at least every 3 to 4 months. Patients with active proliferative retinopathy should be seen approximately every 8 weeks.

Glaucoma, cataracts, retinal detachment, vitreous hemorrhage, and disc edema (papillopathy) are all common in patients with diabetic retinopathy, even in its early stages. Cataracts, especially, are common in patients with diabetes. If the patient has retinopathy, he or she should try to postpone the cataract surgery as long as possible because cataract surgery can sometimes worsen diabetic retinopathy.

Patient Education

Obviously, this is a critical area. Patients with diabetes, as well as those with hypertension, need to be educated regarding the need to keep their disease under maximal control to decrease the incidence of complications. Creating an alliance with the patient and family is essential in encouraging lifestyle changes. Working with the patient over time and being there for the patient are essential. Patients should be educated about the importance of ophthalmological evaluation and follow-up. Patience, advocacy, and commitment are all important qualities in working with these patients. Optimism and emphasis on the possibility for change, even if just to prevent further disease progression, are essential characteristics.

■ MACULAR DEGENERATION

Macular degeneration, or low vision, as it is sometimes referred to, is a disease of aging and is the leading cause of blindness in patients older than 60 years. Risk factors associated with macular degeneration are shown in Risk Factors 8.1. Macular degeneration is a condition characterized by slow, progressive atrophy and degeneration of the retina. This condition is called "dry" macular degeneration. Occasionally, new blood vessels develop under the retina in the macula, causing a sudden distortion or loss of central vision. This condition is known as "wet" age-related macular degeneration; it presents as a sudden decrease in vision that should be referred immediately to an ophthalmologist. There is often a progression from "dry" to "wet" macular degeneration. The macula is the most sensitive and central portion of the retina, a nerve-rich area essential for sight. For largely unknown reasons, after age 60, the macula begins to break down. As it degenerates, central vision and fine detail perception deteriorate. Patients typically cannot read well (if at all), see facial details, read signs, or carry out ordinary daily visual activities.

Epidemiology and Causes

A recent study reported that 30% of individuals aged 75 and older have some form of age-related macular degeneration (AMD), and 7% of those aged 75 and older have an advanced form. Recent studies estimate that 8 million Americans are considered to be at risk for developing

Risk Factors 8.1   Macular Degeneration

Caucasian race
Female gender
Age older than 60
Cigarette smoking
Family history
Macular degeneration gene (complement factor H)
Other risk factors that are unproved, but documented in some studies, include the following:

• High serum cholesterol/obesity
• Low serum carotenoid levels
• Exposure to ultraviolet light
• Hypertension
• Light-colored eyes
• Farsightedness
• Past cataract surgery

advanced AMD in the next 5 years, and 1.75 million are currently affected with the advanced form of the disease. AMD is the leading cause of blindness in older North Americans.

Pathophysiology

Research in mice has provided a few genetic-based clues to the pathogenesis of AMD and has suggested that inflammatory dysfunction may have a role in pathogenesis. Growth factor, choriocapillary endothelial damage, and key inflammatory cytokines are likely involved. Most recently, genetic research has shown that mutations in the gene for complement factor H on chromosome 1 are strongly associated with AMD, supporting a possible inflammatory etiology of AMD.

Clinical Presentation

Subjective

The clinician's main task is to determine if the problem is an acute one, needing referral for immediate treatment, or a more routine one. Determining whether the onset of the visual impairment has been acute or gradual will assist the clinician in making this determination. Likewise, the severity of the visual loss is also important. Severe and sudden visual loss should be referred immediately to an ophthalmologist. Vitreous hemorrhage, retinal detachment, uveitis, retrobulbar optic neuritis, and vascular occlusion generally present in this manner. A gradual progressive change is more indicative of changing refractive error, cataract, glaucoma, diabetic retinopathy, and macular degeneration.

Objective

First, visual acuity must be evaluated, with the patient wearing any assistive lenses. If vision is less than 20/20, it should be checked by the pinhole test. Vision that

Nursing Research–Based Practice 8.1

Moore, LW, and Miller, M. Older men's experience living with severe visual impairment. *J Adv Nurs* 43(1):10–18, 2003.

Mr. Nesbitt is a 78-year-old widower who has been in your practice for 15 years. You have managed his hypertension and mild congestive heart failure for the past 5 years, and he has been following all your advice, including walking 1 mile every day, weather permitting. He was recently diagnosed with age-related macular degeneration (AMD), and his visual loss has been progressive. He has always been very active in community events since the death of his wife and spends several hours each day at the local Senior Center where he entertains the other seniors by playing the piano during lunchtime. He usually drives himself the 2 miles across town to the center and has been doing all of his own grocery shopping, cooking, and tending to his house and yard. He has a large garden and shares his produce with his neighbors. He tearfully admits that his children have been after him to stop driving and to give up his home and move to an assisted living facility. He says he has not had any accidents and that he stays close to the center line when he drives and he knows the route by heart. "I could get there blindfolded," he jokingly remarks. As to moving he says, "Why would I do that? I know where everything is, and I haven't had any problems. My kids can help me. If they put me in a home, I might as well be dead." Mr. Nesbitt has 2 sons aged 50 and 49. Both of these men have jobs that take them out of town a good portion of the week. Both work in the family business started by their father. One son is divorced with two teenage boys, and the other is married with four children and one grandchild.

This past week both sons called asking you to bring Mr. Nesbitt to his senses and to take away his car keys, relating that he has had two near misses in the past 2 weeks. They say that he refuses to listen to reason and that his reason for the near misses is that he "got distracted by a pedestrian jay walking and by a school bus."

Consider the issues in this case based on the findings in this small study.

A phenomenological approach was used to investigate the experience of severe visual impairment in eight older men with macular degeneration. Data were gathered through audiotaped interviews and analyzed using a modified Giorgi method. The aim of the study was to gain an understanding of severe visual impairment from the perspective of older men with macular degeneration. The eight participants were recruited from a local agency for people with vision loss, and they were 68 to 87 years old with macular degeneration in both eyes. The duration of the macular degeneration ranged from 6 months to 2.5 years. Interviews were conducted in participants' homes, and spouses were present in four of the interviews. The six central themes that emerged were as follows: (1) abilities and inabilities, (2) cherishing of independence, (3) creating strategies, (4) acknowledging the progression of visual impairment, (5) confronting uncertainties and fears, and (6) persisting with hope and optimism.

One interesting finding in this study was that the theme of uncertainties encompassed skepticism about their diagnosis and treatment. Acceptance of the fact that there is no successful treatment for AMD is very hard for most individuals, and persisting with hope and optimism is interesting in the face of severe progressive visual loss and mistrust of how their case is managed.

corrects with the pinhole test implies an uncorrected refractive error. The clinician should then evaluate the external structure of the eye. The lids, conjunctivae, pupils, and extraocular movements should be checked. Acute angle-closure glaucoma presents with an unreactive pupil, for example. A Marcus Gunn pupil implies damage to the optic nerve. In addition, conjunctival injection is present with trauma, corneal problems, iritis, acute angle closure, glaucoma, and hyphema.

The funduscopic exam is normal in patients with refractive errors. If dense, cataracts may make it hard to visualize the retina, but otherwise the exam is normal. Patients with glaucoma have increased cupping of the optic disc (a normal cup-to-disc ratio is 0.5 or less). Increased cupping is cause for referral to an ophthalmologist. Retinal hemorrhages, hard exudates, "cotton wool" spots, or neovascularization indicates diabetic retinopathy. If the fundus is difficult or impossible to view, suspect vitreous hemorrhage, especially in diabetic patients

with sudden visual loss. Yellow round spots (drusen) may be indicative of early macular degeneration. Clumps of pigment irregularly interspersed with depigmented areas of atrophy in the macula are more typical of a later phase of the disorder.

Diagnostic Reasoning
Diagnostic Tests

Analysis of central vision may be done with an Amsler grid to locate macular blind spots and areas of distortion and wavy lines. Measurement of contrast sensitivity with specially designed tests for low vision may reveal the degree of loss of retinal sensitivity (contrast) and indicate the potential success or failure of optical magnifying devices.

Differential Diagnosis

As previously discussed, visual impairment may be associated with a variety of conditions. The task of the clinician is to know when to refer for ophthalmology evaluation and treatment and which conditions can be treated in primary care. The characteristics of the associated symptoms and physical findings in the problem of visual loss require focused history and excellent physical exam skills.

Management

There are no proven strategies for preventing AMD, nor are there any treatments for the initial stage of early disease. Some evidence has shown that in the intermediate stage of the disease, oral intake of high-dose antioxidant vitamins and zinc supplements modestly decreased the risk of developing severe vision loss.

Thermal laser photocoagulation may be used to treat certain forms of wet AMD. However, its use is of limited value for lesions in the central macula area. Wet AMD is also treated with injections directly into the eye (intravitreal) by a retinal specialist or ophthalmologist (see Drugs Commonly Prescribed 8.3: Wet Acute Macular Degeneration). The medication used belongs to the class of drugs called anti–vascular endothelial growth factor (anti-VEGF) therapies. These drugs reduce the growth of abnormal blood vessels and may slow leakage from blood vessels. Large-scale clinical trials have demonstrated that these drugs preserved and even improved visual acuity. There are four drugs in this class: the monoclonal antibodies ranibizumab (Lucentis) and bevacizumab (Avastin); the nucleic acid VEGF inhibitor pegaptanib (Macugen); and the receptor fusion protein

aflibercept (Eylea). These drugs are expensive and may not readily be covered by medical insurance.

A number of clinical trials are also investigating potential alternative treatments for AMD, such as submacular surgery, photodynamic therapy, and irradiation. Antioxidants and other plant chemicals (phytochemicals) have been shown to protect against the development of macular degeneration.

Follow-up and Referral

Refer the patient to a rehabilitation source where the outcome of the disease can be evaluated, daily living needs can be assessed, and visual aids may be offered. Sources may include ophthalmologists who provide low-vision services in their practices; optometrists who are trained to offer low-vision remediation; agencies for the visually impaired (either private or state supported); institutions that offer services for veterans; and organizations such as the American Academy of Ophthalmology, the American Optometric Association, the National Eye Institute, and Lighthouse International. A team approach is useful in rehabilitation, and the primary-care provider is part of the team. Because the loss of vision can be especially debilitating, quality of life needs to be assessed during routine primary-care visits. Vision loss increases the risk of falls and may limit the patient's ability to live on his or her own. Depression rates are high in cases of vision loss, and screening in primary care for signs of depression is important. A psychosocial assessment with a multidisciplinary team

Drugs Commonly Prescribed 8.3	Wet Acute Macular Degeneration		
Drug	**Indication**	**Dosage**	**Adverse Effects**
aflibercept (Eyla) *VEGF-receptor fusion protein*	Wet AMD (FDA approved)	2-mg intravitreal injection once a month for 3 months, then every 2 months	*Severe:* Allergic reaction including hives, difficulty breathing, and facial swelling; retinal detachment; endophthalmitis
bevacizumab (Avastin) *Anti-VEGF monoclonal antibody*	Wet AMD (unapproved)	1.25-mg intravitreal injection once a month (off-label use)	*Moderate:* Eye pain; eye redness; sudden vision changes, including flashes of light; photophobia; severe headache with confusion
pegaptanib (Macugen) *Nucleic acid VEGF inhibitor*	Wet AMD (FDA approved)	0.3-mg intravitreal injection every 6 weeks	*Mild:* Watery eyes; blurred vision; pain at injection site; edema of eyelid
ranibizumab (Lucentis) *Anti-VEGF monoclonal antibody*	Wet AMD (FDA approved)	0.5-mg intravitreal injection every month	

should be arranged to explore resources and monitor quality of life.

Patient Education

Recognition of the signs of advanced AMD is crucial for the success of treatment in preventing visual loss. Self-monitoring of central vision in both eyes using an Amsler grid may be useful in detecting subtle visual changes or distortion, as well as monitoring changes in vision once they have been detected. A hallmark of AMD is visual difficulties in low light.

Smoking cessation and improvement of cardiovascular risk factors are important variables in the progression of AMD. Patients should be instructed as to rehabilitation resources in the community and encouraged to take advantage of programs specifically targeted for AMD.

Optical aids include spectacles with and without prisms, hand magnifiers, stand-mounted magnifiers, and telescopes. As with any type of rehabilitation, time and patience are needed to determine the appropriate remedial lens for the patient. Working with the patient until he or she understands how to use the device is an important part of patient education. In addition, patients may be taught practical skills such as folding money in such a way that the denomination is more apparent, as well as techniques for grooming and for identifying medications. The goal is to use "whatever works" for each patient (see The Patient's Voice 8.1).

The Patient's Voice 8.1
Macular Degeneration

My mother, who is 78, called me in a panic because she could not see out of one eye. The ophthalmologist agreed to see her right away. When we met with the doctor after her exam, he told us that she had been diagnosed with macular degeneration 4 years ago. She had never told a soul! "I couldn't stand the thought of being a burden." That's what she told me. If only I'd known, maybe we could have done more to slow down the disease. Now, if anything happens to her other eye, I don't know what we'll do. This will change everything about how my mother lives and will affect everyone in the family.

EAR PROBLEMS

◼ HEARING LOSS

Exposure to loud noises, either occupationally or recreationally, is a risk factor for hearing loss, as are ototoxic drugs (e.g., aminoglycoside antibiotics, aspirin, and quinine). Allergies and other causes of eustachian-tube obstruction may also contribute to hearing loss. Risk factors for cerumen impaction specifically are ear canal hairs, hearing aids, bony growths secondary to osteophyte or osteoma, and previous episodes of impacted cerumen. Chronic middle ear infections (otitis media)

also are a contributing factor in the development of hearing loss.

Epidemiology and Causes

Approximately 17% (36 million) of American adults 45 to 64 years old have a hearing impairment. Among older Americans, hearing impairment is present in 30% of 65- to 74-year-olds, and 47% of adults who are 75 years old or older have some form of hearing impairment. Men are more likely than women to experience hearing loss.

Pathophysiology

Sensorineural hearing loss is defined as a lesion in the organ of Corti or in the central pathways, including the eighth cranial nerve (CN VIII) and auditory cortex. Age-related hearing loss, termed *presbycusis,* is a form of sensorineural hearing loss. After age 50, hair cells in the organ of Corti tend to degenerate. A capillary-fed layer of stratified epithelium known as the *stria vascularis* that secretes endolymph and promotes the sensitization of hair cells in the cochlea may atrophy. This first affects perception of high-frequency sounds and then progresses to affect hearing of lower-frequency tones. Sensorineural loss may also be a result of Ménière's disease (discussed later in this chapter) or be noise induced. Other causes of hearing loss include tumors, genetic predisposition, ototoxicity related to a variety of medications, syphilis, and metabolic disorders, such as hypothyroidism. Hearing loss also may be due to an inner ear fistula, usually secondary to pressure changes or trauma. Viral syndromes, especially mumps, may also affect hearing.

Conductive hearing loss is a lesion involving the outer and middle ear to the level of the oval window that may result from a variety of structural abnormalities. Cerumen impaction, a reversible form of hearing loss, is a common cause in all age groups. Perforation of the tympanic membrane, middle ear fluid, damage to the ossicles from trauma or infection, otosclerosis, tympanosclerosis, cholesteatoma, middle ear tumors, temporal bone fractures and injuries related to trauma, or congenital problems may all cause conductive hearing loss.

Clinical Presentation

The most important task, and frequently a difficult one, is to determine whether the hearing loss is sensorineural (which is usually irreversible) or conductive (which is often reversible). Another important piece of data is whether the loss is unilateral or bilateral. Presbycusis produces a typical high-frequency loss that is bilaterally symmetrical. Ménière's disease causes fluctuating hearing loss, usually unilateral, associated with tinnitus and vertigo. Acoustic neuroma (schwannoma), a rare tumor of cranial nerve VIII, causes unilateral constant or progressive hearing loss, possibly associated with headache. With a tumor of the acoustic nerve, there will most likely be neurological changes, such as facial weakness and tingling and loss of taste and dysphagia, in addition to hearing loss.

Subjective

Hearing loss is not a distinct clinical entity; it is a symptom or sign of multiple medical conditions. Patient complaint terminology is more diversified than for many other medical conditions. A patient may report having "difficulty hearing," which may be associated with pain, pressure, discomfort, vertigo, or loss of balance. Or the patient may complain of tinnitus, dizziness, blockage, popping, pressure, crackling, distant sounds, or stiffness. The clinician should question the patient as to how long he or she has noticed a hearing loss and whether it is partial or complete. Does the patient think both ears are affected? Is there a family history of hearing loss? The clinician should inquire whether the patient has ever had any injury or surgery to the ears and if he or she has had any serious illnesses or tuberculosis (which might have required treatment with ototoxic drugs). The review of systems should focus on the neurological system, including cranial nerve function (e.g., facial weakness or tingling, loss of taste, or dysphagia). The social and occupational history should include specific questions regarding noise or toxin exposure and any blast-related injuries, including a history of hunting and/or target shooting. A complete history of prescription and over-the-counter (OTC) medication use should be obtained.

Objective

The physical exam should include otoscopic examination to inspect the external auditory canal and middle ear. The clinician should note any redness, foreign objects, discharge, scaling, lesions, and cerumen (ear wax). There may be a significant accumulation of cerumen, especially in elderly patients. The tympanic membrane should have no perforations and should be a translucent pearly gray. Changes in the tympanic membrane may be consistent with conductive hearing loss.

The clinician should perform Weber, Rinne, and Schwabach tests to determine whether hearing loss is primarily conductive or sensorineural. Unexpected findings from the three tuning fork tests must be integrated to differentiate clinically what is occurring. Conductive hearing loss occurs when sound transmission is impaired through the external or middle ear. Sensorineural hearing loss occurs because of a defect in the inner ear that leads to distortion of sound and misinterpretation of speech.

For office testing, use the Weber test first. A vibrating 512-Hz (or higher-frequency) tuning fork is placed midline on the patient's skull. Normally, the sound should be equal in both ears. In sensorineural loss, the sound in the unaffected (or less affected ear) is louder. In conductive loss, the sound is louder in the affected ear.

The Rinne test can also be done in the office. A vibrating tuning fork is placed on the mastoid process. When the sound fades away, the fork is promptly placed (without restriking it) over the external auditory meatus.

Normally, via air conduction, the sound can be heard for twice as long as in bone conduction. In sensorineural loss, the ratio remains the same, whereas in conductive loss, the ratio is closer to 1:1, or even reversed.

In the Schwabach test, a vibrating tuning fork is placed over the mastoid process of the patient and then the examiner and the results are compared. In sensorineural loss, the patient's bone conduction is present for a shorter time than the examiner's; in conductive loss, the patient's bone conduction persists for a longer time.

Diagnostic Reasoning

Diagnostic Tests

Often, the patient needs to be referred for audiometry. Audiometry includes pure tone and speech testing, as well as impedance (middle ear pressure) testing. Both types of hearing loss may fluctuate, making audiometric results variable from test to test. Marked conductive loss on one ear may be difficult to exclude (mask) when testing the opposite ear. Computed tomography (CT) and magnetic resonance imaging (MRI) scans are used to detect tumors such as acoustic neuromas and glomus tumor, as well as damage from traumatic injuries.

The various mechanical obstructions, be they wax or tumor or fluid associated with infection/inflammation, that lead to conductive hearing loss may be visualized. CT scan and/or MRI may be needed to demonstrate tumors and cholesteatoma. Cholesteatoma may sometimes be identified by perforation that is located near the margin of the eardrum.

Differential Diagnosis

The differential diagnosis for hearing loss includes conditions that cause either sensorineural or conductive loss. Aging is associated with the sensorineural presbycusis. However, other possible conditions need to be ruled out. Sensorineural loss may also have the etiology of otoxicity, exposure to loud noises, an autoimmune issue, an acoustic neuroma, or possibly Ménière's disease. Conductive hearing loss may be explained simply by cerumen accumulation or impaction (cerumenosis) or a foreign body in the external canal, otitis externa, chronic otitis media, middle ear effusion, otosclerosis, a vascular anomaly, or cholesteatoma. To treat hearing loss properly, the etiology must be accurately identified.

Management

Many types of conductive loss are reversible; sensorineural causes tend to be irreversible. In cases of conductive hearing loss caused by cerumen buildup, cerumen disimpaction may be necessary. The recommended procedure is as follows: Use a 1:1 mixture of 3% hydrogen peroxide and warm mineral oil. Place three drops in the external ear and wait 1 hour. Then attempt to lavage the ear with warm saline. Direct the saline toward the canal wall, not toward the drum. An alternative method is to put three drops of warm olive oil in each ear to soften the wax, then flush with warm 3% hydrogen peroxide. Cerumenolytic agents such as 6.5% carbamide peroxide (Debrox) are effective; docusate sodium liquid may also be used. These agents should not be used in the presence of a perforated tympanic membrane or infection. Press gently but firmly behind the ear, then in front of the ear. Pull the lobe up and down to work the wax out. Dry the ear canal after the irrigation with a hair dryer on low, if one is available. Advise the patient who has cerumen buildup but may not be complaining of hearing loss to use Debrox for 1 week before returning for an ear irrigation as described above.

If not performed properly, cerumen removal may cause damage to the external auditory meatus, perforation of the tympanic membrane, and/or otitis media. Consider steroid/antibiotic otic solution (Cortisporin otic), four drops 3 or 4 times daily for 5 to 7 days after prolonged irrigation and trauma to the canal. Consider cerumenolytic installation 2 times daily for 5 days monthly in recurrent, resistant cases. Do not disimpact the ear if tympanic membrane perforation is present. If hearing loss is caused by infection, treat as appropriate (see section on otitis media/externa under Common Ear Problems). The cause of the hearing loss in cases of sensorineural loss must also be identified correctly to treat it properly. Noise damage is a common cause of hearing loss in the United States. Although this type of hearing loss is not reversible, it is preventable. Hearing loss related to the use of ototoxic medications (especially certain antibiotics) needs greater recognition. This etiology should be suspected when hearing loss, dizziness, and tinnitus occur during the course of treatment with certain medications. In this case, the patient should stop the medications. Salicylate toxicity, for example, is reversible. In cases resulting from metabolic causes, such as hypothyroidism, the underlying disorder should be treated.

Follow-up and Referral

Patients should be referred to an ear, nose, and throat specialist if perforation is present, as well as in cases of damage to the ossicles, tympanosclerosis, otosclerosis, tumor, and temporal bone injury. Referral to an audiologist for further evaluation may be appropriate. Patients who are suspected of having Ménière's disease should be referred to an ear, nose, and throat specialist and an audiologist for appropriate diagnostic testing and treatment. In the case of perilymphatic fistula, diagnosis should be based on evidence or history of injury to the ear (including barotrauma during diving), and referral to a specialist is indicated. Acoustic neuromas should be referred for surgical treatment.

For cases of sudden, sensorineural hearing loss with no apparent cause, high doses of steroids (80 mg per day of prednisone or equivalent) are sometimes used. Any patient who presents with this type of acute hearing loss should be referred to a specialist for treatment.

Patient Education

In cases of presbycusis, although no specific treatment will reverse the process, it is important to educate and support the patient so that no further damage will occur; for example, exposure to excessive noise and ototoxic drugs should be avoided. Severe nerve deafness, particularly when associated with tinnitus, may produce severe depression and isolation and occasionally even lead to suicide. Clinicians should inquire as to daily activities and social interaction. Teach the patient lip-reading if appropriate, and instruct family members to speak clearly, facing the patient. Encourage the purchase of hearing aids. Consult a telephone equipment company about special audio equipment that is available.

Permanent hearing loss is common in cases of sensorineural hearing loss and may also occur with conductive hearing loss. Patients need to be counseled about follow-up with audiometry and the need to use hearing aids. Middle ear problems may progress to chronic ear problems such as perforations and/or cholesteatoma, which will adversely affect hearing.

As a prevention strategy, as well as in cases of occupational or recreational hearing loss, the patient must be counseled to always use protective devices. It is also important to teach the patient to equalize ear pressure when diving and to chew gum while in airplanes. Decongestants might be indicated. If an upper respiratory infection is present, the patient should avoid flying and/or diving.

■ TINNITUS

Tinnitus is a subjective perception of noise when in reality no environmental noise is present. It may be intermittent, continuous, or pulsatile (synchronous with heartbeat). Risk factors include hearing loss, labyrinthitis, Ménière's disease, otitis media or externa, otosclerosis, ear-canal blockage (from ear wax or a foreign body), a history of high or low blood pressure, head trauma, anemia, hypothyroidism, hyperthyroidism, or allergies. Chronic exposure to noise, especially high-pitched sounds, may damage the cilia and auditory hair cells, causing tinnitus. Certain medications may contribute to tinnitus, some with reversible effects (salicylates, quinine, alcohol, and indomethacin [Indocin]) and others with irreversible effects (kanamycin, streptomycin, gentamicin, and vancomycin).

Epidemiology and Causes

Recent estimates suggest that as many as 40 million Americans are affected by tinnitus. Approximately 90% of patients with hearing loss experience some tinnitus, and approximately 1% of the population suffers from chronic tinnitus. Tinnitus is strongly associated with aging. Experts estimate that 15% of Americans have experienced tinnitus that lasts longer than 5 minutes and that 155 million have sought medical care for tinnitus. About 6% of that number report being incapacitated by tinnitus. The peak range of patients with tinnitus is 40 to 70 years. Patients in their 70s have a 25% to 30% risk of developing tinnitus. Men have a higher risk of developing tinnitus, and whites experience tinnitus in greater numbers than blacks.

Pathophysiology

Tinnitus is classified in several different ways. In addition to the subjective and objective classes as presented in the common complaints section of this chapter, tinnitus may also be divided between vibratory and nonvibratory tinnitus. Vibratory tinnitus is caused by transmission to the cochlea of vibrations from adjacent tissues or organs. Nonvibratory tinnitus is produced by biochemical changes in the nerve mechanism of hearing. Subjective tinnitus, which is more common, is heard only by the patient. Objective tinnitus can be heard by an examiner through a stethoscope placed over the head and neck structures near the ear.

The causative mechanism is poorly understood. Theories include injured cochlear hair cells discharging repetitively and stimulating auditory nerve fibers in a continuous cycle, spontaneous activity in individual auditory nerve fibers, hyperactivity in the auditory nuclei in the brainstem, or a reduction in the usual suppressive activity of the central auditory cortex on peripheral auditory nerve activity.

Clinical Presentation

Subjective

Most patients are not bothered by tinnitus when they are surrounded by the usual sounds of everyday life. However, when they are in an unusually quiet location, the perception of tinnitus may be profound. In more extreme cases, tinnitus may interfere with their lives, affecting concentration and sleep and causing severe depression in the worst cases. Tinnitus that manifests as a continuous and unbearably loud sound has led a few patients to self-destruction.

Patients have variously described tinnitus as the sound of escaping air or running water or the sound heard inside a large seashell or as a buzzing, ringing, or humming noise. Tinnitus also has been described as a roaring or musical sound. It may be unilateral or bilateral.

Other presentations commonly seen include a stiff neck and pain aggravated by activity that produces the tinnitus, accompanied by vertigo, nystagmus, hearing loss, and pain that radiates down the arms. Weakness, confusion, and feelings of unsteadiness (orthostatic hypotension) may also occur, especially when the patient stands up quickly. These symptoms may be indicative of atherosclerosis as a causative factor.

Complaints of ear fullness, itching, and hearing loss along with the tinnitus may be caused by a foreign body

obstruction, such as cerumen (ear wax) impaction; obstruction should always be ruled out. Bilateral, high-pitched tinnitus may occur with severe hypertension (diastolic blood pressure exceeding 120 mm Hg). The patient may have associated symptoms of headache, numbness, nausea, and vomiting.

The patient may describe a sudden onset of vertigo, unilateral or bilateral hearing loss, dizziness, nausea or vomiting, and nystagmus. Labyrinthitis may be considered.

Objective

In addition to usual vital signs, the blood pressure should be evaluated via orthostatic measurements. Physical exam will include gross hearing tests, as well as the Weber and Rinne tuning fork tests to detect conductive or sensorineural hearing loss. A thorough otologic exam should be done. Auscultation of the upper part of the neck near the ear of the affected side may detect a bruit and palpation may reveal a weak pulse. Vascular studies may need to be considered. Cardiovascular evaluation including electrocardiogram may detect changes associated with atherosclerotic disease. Neurological exam should be done to rule out other deficits.

Diagnostic Reasoning

Diagnostic Tests

Laboratory studies are necessary to confirm possible underlying causes of tinnitus. A complete blood count (CBC) should be done to rule out anemia or infection. Metabolic studies need to be done to rule out thyroid disease, hyperlipidemia, vitamin B_{12} deficiency, zinc deficiency, or electrolyte abnormalities. If drainage from the ear canal is evident, a culture should be obtained. MRI may reveal pathology in detail; this is currently the diagnostic procedure of choice. If the patient cannot tolerate MRI, CT scan with dye enhancement is an alternative. Special tests to determine the presence of middle ear fluid may be considered, such as tympanometry, acoustic reflex measurement, or acoustic reflectometry. Because of the association of depressive disorders in severe tinnitus, screening for psychological disorders should be done.

Differential Diagnosis

Tinnitus may arise from cardiovascular and system disorders (hypertension and anemia). Nonpathological causes include acute anxiety and presbycusis. The patient experiencing tinnitus may also present with multiple symptomatology; those symptoms may alert the practitioner to the underlying cause. For example, hearing loss and tinnitus accompanied by vertigo, facial paralysis, headaches, nausea, vomiting, and papilledema may occur with acoustic neuroma. An early symptom of acoustic nerve (CN VIII) tumor is unilateral tinnitus. Occasionally, anemia may produce mild, irreversible tinnitus. In this case, the patient may complain of dim vision, syncope, and the associated signs of anemia, such as fatigue, weakness, exertional dyspnea, and tachycardia, that accompany the tinnitus.

Bilateral, high-pitched tinnitus may occur with severe hypertension (diastolic blood pressure exceeding 120 mm Hg). The patient may have associated symptoms of headache, numbness, nausea, and vomiting.

In Ménière's disease, low-pitched tinnitus, along with vertigo and fluctuating hearing loss, may occur. Tinnitus accompanied by bleeding from the ear canal can be caused by trauma. Purulent drainage and pain with tinnitus may be caused by infection. Other presenting symptoms of tinnitus may be fever, chills, and dizziness.

Management

Elimination of possible offending medications (such as aspirin-containing products and NSAIDs) is a priority. Tinnitus usually cannot be treated successfully. However, management of symptoms and treatment of the underlying disorder (if one can be identified) may help. Overall, learning to cope with the tinnitus is the best approach. Avoidance of risk factors such as excessive noise whenever possible is advised. Some experts suggest supplementation with vitamin A, vitamin C, cyanocobalamin, and nicotinic acid or with magnesium or copper.

Protective earplugs may need to be worn. Tinnitus-masking devices can match the frequency range and intensity of the tinnitus, producing a level of noise that will help block out the tinnitus without interfering with hearing. The device fits in the ear like a hearing aid and presents a more pleasant sound. Regular relief may be obtained by masking the tinnitus with background noise. Hearing aids are also helpful in tinnitus suppression: they help to amplify environmental sounds, thereby obscuring tinnitus. For patients who find the noise intolerable, biofeedback may be needed to help with psychological problems that can develop from the near-constant feeling of distress.

Although there is no medication to help tinnitus, oral antidepressants have proved to be effective in reducing symptoms. Nortriptyline (Elavil), at an initial dose of 50 mg orally at bedtime, may be considered. Meclizine HCl (Antivert, Bonine) is the most commonly used vestibular suppressant. Diazepam (Valium), usually in low doses such as 2 mg, may be a valuable adjunct therapy to treat an acute attack of vertigo, as well as being effective for those with anxiety. If chronic vertigo and dizziness accompany the tinnitus, vestibular rehabilitation should be considered.

Patients with tinnitus related to otitis media or other infections should be treated with antibiotics for an adequate duration, with careful monitoring of serum peak and trough levels. This will also prevent loss of vestibular function and deafness from antibiotic therapy with aminoglycosides. If medical management does not resolve ear infections, surgical intervention—with myringotomy and possible tube placement—may need to be considered. Referral to an otorhinolaryngologist should be initiated.

Follow-up and Referral

Referral to an audiologist should be initiated for a patient with tinnitus and hearing loss. If vertigo, nausea, and vomiting accompany the tinnitus, the patient should be referred to an otorhinolaryngologist.

Patient Education

General measures might include playing background music during the daytime and before sleep. Patients should be advised to quit smoking and to cut back on caffeine, chocolate, and salt intake. Fatigue may increase tinnitus; therefore, patients need to be encouraged to rest during the course of the day. Chewing gum or swallowing should be encouraged during descent on airplanes to promote eustachian tube opening with deglutition (swallowing).

■ MÉNIÈRE'S DISEASE

Ménière's disease (Ménière's syndrome, endolymphatic hydrops) is a peripheral sensory disorder of both the labyrinth (semicircular canal system) and cochlea of the inner ear. Endolymphatic volume and, in turn, pressure are increased due to unknown etiology, resulting in both vestibular (proprioceptive, balance-related) and auditory dysfunction, characterized by recurrent attacks of tinnitus (ringing or buzzing in the ears), vertigo (a sense of whirling or spinning in space), and progressive hearing loss. Although Ménière's disease is not life-threatening, if untreated, acute attacks typically recur over the course of many years.

Epidemiology and Causes

Well-documented incidence figures for Ménière's disease are not available, but it is estimated that 46 new cases per 100,000 occur annually in the United States. Prevalence is estimated at 1,150 per 100,000. Age at onset is anywhere from 30 to 60 years, with most cases developing during the fifth decade of life. The disease is rare both in young children and in adults older than age 70. Some studies indicate that white Americans of European descent are at an increased risk of developing the disease. Both sexes are affected nearly equally, but some studies have reported slightly higher rates in women.

Stress, allergies, high salt intake, and exposure to high noise levels for periods of many years have all been cited as risk factors.

Pathophysiology

The precise cause of Ménière's disease is not fully established, but marked edema of the membranous labyrinth is typically observed at autopsy, and endolymphatic hydrops has been established as the defining pathological finding in the disease. Theories have implicated the inflammatory response of the inner ear to a variety of insults, including blunt trauma; viral infection; allergies; reduced or negative middle ear pressure; and various vascular, endocrine, and lipid disorders. Migraine headache and autoimmune conditions, including systemic lupus erythematosus, rheumatoid arthritis, and certain thyroid disorders, also predispose to Ménière's disease. A genetic predisposition has also been identified in 8% of people affected.

Dilation of the endolymphatic system may lead to rupture of the membranous labyrinth. This engorgement has been associated with excessive endolymph production, decreased resorption of fluid in the endolymphatic sac, and hypoplasia of the vestibular aqueduct. Resultant mixing of the endolymph and perilymph is thought to cause degeneration of both vestibular and cochlear neuroepithelial sensory hair cells, which are particularly sensitive to ionic changes from the potassium-rich endolymph, resulting in vertigo, tinnitus, and hearing loss. Compression of the vestibular portion of CN VIII by an enlarged blood vessel is yet another etiological theory.

Clinical Presentation

Subjective

Acute episodes of Ménière's disease last anywhere from 20 minutes to 3 hours and are characterized by sudden attacks of nausea; emesis; pallor; diaphoresis; dizziness (spatial disorientation); vertigo; roaring tinnitus; and increased pressure, fullness, and hearing loss in the affected ear. Patients typically refer to any vestibular symptomatology as "dizziness." Rapid movement aggravates all proprioceptive symptomatology, and patients often report a history of falls or accidents during acute episodes. The frequency and severity of attacks may decrease over time, and hearing may improve immediately after an acute attack. However, some episodes have been known to last for more than 24 hours. Overall, low-frequency hearing loss is typically progressive, with bilateral involvement in 10% to 50% of cases. Patients may also experience motion-related imbalance without vertigo between acute attacks. Complete hearing loss in advanced cases of Ménière's disease is associated with a cessation of vertiginous episodes.

Objective

On inspection, otoscopic examination typically demonstrates no apparent abnormalities, unless underlying otitis media is present. Dilation of the inner ear endolymphatic system is apparent only at autopsy. Spontaneous nystagmus is often observed after preventing eye fixation by having the patient wear 40-diopter glasses (Frenzel lenses) during the period of observation.

Diagnostic Reasoning

Diagnostic Tests

Diagnosis of Ménière's disease is based on a careful history, neurological assessment, and response to empiric therapy, because no specific diagnostic testing exists. The American Academy of Otolaryngology and Head and Neck Surgery has established diagnostic criteria requiring two distinct episodes of rotational vertigo lasting at least 20 minutes each, along with sensorineural hearing loss and either tinnitus or a perception of aural fullness. Thus, both the Weber and Rinne tests typically elicit findings characteristic of a sensorineural hearing defect. Sound lateralization to the nonaffected ear occurs when a 512-Hz tuning fork is placed midline on the top of the head (Weber test), and air conduction is superior in duration and volume to bone conduction (positive Rinne test). Audiometry also demonstrates low-frequency sensorineural hearing loss, as well as impaired speech discrimination. Both cold and warm caloric responses are typically reduced in the affected ear, as demonstrated by electronystagmography (ENG) or direct patient observation (while wearing 40-diopter Frenzel lenses), and the direction of the fast phase of nystagmus is variable. These findings are not diagnostic for Ménière's disease, however. Vestibular function tests are used to evaluate CN VIII function; however, these findings are questionable in patients taking sedative drugs of any kind.

Differential Diagnosis

Ménière's disease is a diagnosis of exclusion. Thus, numerous disorders that mimic its clinical picture must first be ruled out. Otitis media (OM) is evaluated through otoscopic examination and culture of otic fluid. If middle ear infection is present, the tympanic membrane is typically erythematous and either edematous or retracted, with altered bony landmarks and a diminished cone of light reflex. Bubbles or an air/fluid level may be seen directly behind the membrane, and mobility is reduced or absent on insufflation with a pneumatic otoscope. OM and Ménière's disease are not mutually exclusive conditions, however, because negative middle ear pressure associated with serous otitis media may be a contributing factor to Ménière's disease. OM may also precipitate a viral infection of CN VIII known as vestibular neuritis (benign recurrent vertigo), which presents as recurrent vertiginous episodes lasting several hours, which may be accompanied by severe vomiting and nausea. Vestibular neuritis may also be idiopathic, but in these patients (unlike those with Ménière's disease), auditory impairment is rarely noted. Secondary or tertiary syphilis can also affect CN VIII and is ruled out via a variety of immunological tests specific for its causative agent *Treponema pallidum*, such as the microhemagglutination (MHA), fluorescent treponemal antibody (FTA), and treponema immobilization (TPI) assays. Acute viral or bacterial infection of the labyrinth may also present with similar symptoms; however, pathogenic microorganisms are not associated with Ménière's disease because it is not of infectious etiology. Discrete lesions of the central nervous system (CNS), such as tumors or infarcts of the brain and cerebellum, as well as degenerative nervous disorders such as Parkinson's disease, multiple sclerosis, and Alzheimer's disease, may be ruled out via CT and MRI. Hypothyroidism may also mimic Ménière's disease and is ruled out through measurement of both free and protein-bound thyroid hormone levels (thyroxine [T_4] and triiodothyronine [T_3]), as well as pituitary thyroid-stimulating hormone (TSH).

Benign positional vertigo (benign paroxysmal vertigo) is a more common diagnosis than Ménière's disease of vestibular dysfunction in elderly patients who complain of dizziness. It is characterized by paroxysmal vertigo accompanied by nystagmus when lying down, turning over in bed, or tilting the head backward. The Nylen-Bárány maneuver is used to make this diagnosis: The patient is reclined rapidly from a sitting to supine position with the head tilted to one side, and the neck is hyperextended 30 degrees below the horizontal for at least 10 seconds, off the end of the examination table. The maneuver is then repeated with the head tilted to the opposite side. In this benign condition, nystagmus lasting between 15 and 45 seconds is observed after each maneuver, following a brief 1- to 5-second latent period. In contrast to Ménière's disease, benign positional vertigo does not present with hearing loss or tinnitus.

Presbycusis, the most common cause of sensorineural hearing loss in the elderly, is distinguished by high-frequency rather than low-frequency hearing loss as revealed by audiometric testing. Serum glucose levels should be evaluated to rule out hypoglycemic disorders, and hemoglobin and hematocrit are measured to assess anemic conditions, if suspected. Lipid disorders affecting cerebral blood flow and, in turn, vestibulocochlear function may be ruled out via serum lipid studies. Other cerebral and cardiovascular disorders, such as transient ischemic attacks, vertebrobasilar ischemia, or subclavian steal syndrome, may lead to CNS ischemia and vertigo, thus mimicking Ménière's disease. However, syncope (fainting) and generalized weakness are also usually observed. Angiography is used to rule out such disorders, if suspected. Another common cause of a vestibular and auditory dysfunction is iatrogenic, drug-induced ototoxicity from many commonly used drugs, including aspirin; potent diuretics; quinine; tetracyclines (especially minocycline); many cancer chemotherapies, such as *cis*-platinum; and aminoglycoside antibiotics, including gentamicin, neomycin, kanamycin, and streptomycin. If use of these medications is not prolonged, ototoxicity may be reversible once drug intake has stopped. Sedative side effects of many medications, as well as undesirable multidrug interactions, are a common cause of dizziness, especially in elderly patients, who are at an increased risk of polypharmacy-related sequelae. In the adult patient, acoustic neuroma, causing compression of the auditory portion of CN VIII, is one of the most important diagnoses of auditory dysfunction to rule out because these tumors may be life-threatening if untreated. MRI and auditory brainstem response audiometry are used to detect such neoplasms. Finally, psychiatric diagnoses should be a major consideration if examination and laboratory findings rule out systemic disease and specific organ involvement as the cause of vestibulocochlear dysfunction. Psychiatric illness is the second most common etiology of dizziness in elderly patients after peripheral nervous system disorders. Common conditions include depression, anxiety, panic attacks, somatization disorders, alcoholism, and other forms of substance abuse. A proper psychiatric evaluation, which may include drug screens of the urine and blood, is necessary to rule out such illnesses.

Management

Acute attacks are best treated by calm bedrest with the eyes closed and protection from falling. Attacks rarely last longer than 4 hours. Pharmacotherapy, if necessary, is directed at symptomatic relief because no medications are known to affect this nonspecific disease process. A low-salt diet (less than 1,000 mg/day) is considered first-line therapy to reduce endolymphatic pressure and volume, along with a mild diuretic such as chlorothiazide (Diuril) 500 mg/day orally (PO) and potassium supplements to counter diuretic-induced hypokalemia. Caffeine avoidance and tobacco cessation are also suggested to avoid vasoconstriction of the labyrinthine system. However, as with salt restriction, the efficacy of these therapies is based primarily on anecdotal evidence.

Acute attacks are managed with a combination of antimuscarinics or anticholinergics and vestibulosuppressive histamine (H_1) blockers from various classes. The muscarinic antagonist atropine 0.2 to 0.4 mg IV or the anticholinergic scopolamine (Transderm Scop 0.33 mg/24 hours—1 transdermal disc or portion thereof applied behind the affected ear for at least 3 days) or glycopyrollate (Robinul) 2 mg PO 2 times daily may be used to relieve vertigo, nausea, and emesis. Other agents with antihistaminic, antimuscarinic, and sedative effects used for acute attacks include betahistine 8 to 16 mg PO 3 times daily (not currently available in the United States), promethazine (Phenergan) 12.5 to 25 mg IV given slowly, diphenhydramine (Benadryl) 50 mg IV given slowly, and droperidol (Inapsine) 1.5 to 2.5 mg IV given slowly. GABA-ergic anxiolytics such as diazepam (Valium) 5 to 10 mg IV given slowly may also be used to sedate patients during severe episodes, but it should be noted that sedatives will affect the outcome of all vestibular function tests. Oral maintenance therapies include meclizine (Antivert, Bonine) 25 to 100 mg at bedtime or in divided doses, promethazine (Phenergan) 12.5 to 25 mg PO every 4 to 6 hours, dimenhydrinate (Dramamine) 50 mg PO 3 or 4 times daily, metoclopramide (Reglan) 10 mg PO 2 times daily, or diphenhydramine (Benadryl) 25 to 50 mg PO every 4 to 6 hours, not to exceed 300 mg/day. Of note, these treatments are most effective for vertiginous symptoms, whereas tinnitus and hearing loss are less affected.

If conventional treatment fails, intratympanic perfusion with dexamethasone may prove effective, especially if an underlying autoimmune disorder is present. As a last resort, if Ménière's disease progresses bilaterally, streptomycin or gentamicin ablation therapy may be appropriate to reduce unbearable vestibular symptoms. An aminoglycoside antibiotic is administered over a course of several days to weeks, to intentionally damage the neuroepithelium of the vestibular centers in the inner ear, thus reducing related symptomatology. However, hearing must be carefully monitored both during and after this treatment to avoid damage to auditory structures. Disabling symptoms of Ménière's disease may require surgical intervention, typically used in 5% to 10% of all cases. For patients with normal hearing ability, decompression of the endolymphatic sac may be accomplished by surgically draining excess endolymph into the mastoid or subarachnoid space. Alternatively, the vestibular nerve may be transected intracranially. For patients whose hearing ability has degenerated and is deemed unsalvageable, the cochlea itself may be decompressed (via cochleocentesis) or directly perfused with streptomycin. A more radical surgery is labyrinthectomy of the affected ear, a procedure that entirely ablates vestibular function.

Follow-up and Referral

If symptoms do not worsen, patients may return for follow-up in 3 to 6 weeks. However, patients should return for reevaluation immediately if disabling symptoms such as tinnitus, vertigo, nausea, or emesis persist. Hearing loss, in particular, must be carefully monitored for progression because this is a telltale sign of an underlying, potentially life-threatening acoustic neuroma. Patients often report that previously consulted clinicians failed to take this condition seriously when they first presented with symptoms. Thus, close follow-up care of the patient with Ménière's disease provides emotionally beneficial validation, as well.

Progressive bilateral hearing loss may result from Ménière's disease, leading to chronic tinnitus, deafness, and disabling vertigo. Accidental injuries related to vestibular dysfunction may occur in the work or home setting, and patients often report an increasing inability to function productively at their present jobs in the face of progressive disease. Failing to diagnose an underlying acoustic neuroma is a potentially life-threatening complication.

Referral to a specialist is necessary if symptoms worsen with treatment. Advanced diagnostic procedures such as ENG or specialized vestibulocochlear function tests require referral to a neurologist. A physician consultation is also needed in cases involving persistent emesis, convulsions or seizures, syncope, or fever. New, unexplained symptoms (which are often due to multidrug interactions or adverse effects of medications) also require referral to a specialist for diagnosis and treatment. Streptomycin ablation therapy and surgical interventions should be directed by a qualified specialist only, because the risk of serious sequelae is significant, including permanent hearing loss.

Patient Education

Patients must be encouraged to stop smoking because this aggravates all otic disorders. Stress levels should be monitored and controlled. Salt intake should be reduced to a maximum of 1 g/day to lessen the severity of future attacks. All ototoxic medications should be avoided, and polypharmacy (multiple prescription drug usage) should be evaluated with the aid of a specialist.

Patients should be instructed to return for further evaluation if symptoms worsen or acute episodes increase in frequency. Patients need to understand that treating Ménière's disease pharmacologically is difficult, and acute attacks are best managed with quiet bedrest and careful protection from falls. To avoid accidental injuries and minimize symptoms, patients should not drive, climb ladders, work near dangerous machinery, walk without assistance, read, or look at glaring lights during these episodes. Food intake should also be reduced during acute attacks to lessen nausea and vomiting.

■ OTITIS EXTERNA

Otitis externa is an inflammation of the membranous lining of the auditory canal and/or contiguous structures of the outer ear. The term refers to a wide spectrum of both acute and chronic inflammatory processes that may be diffuse, localized, or invasive in nature. This disorder is largely benign and self-limiting, albeit painful. Invasive otitis externa (malignant otitis externa, necrotizing otitis externa) is a potentially life-threatening disease, however, if left untreated.

Epidemiology and Causes

Ear pain, in general, is a common clinical complaint, accounting for 2% to 3% of all family practice office visits. Specifically, otitis externa is 10 to 20 times more likely to occur during the warmer summer months than in cooler seasons. Adults older than 50 years of age are at the greatest risk of developing invasive otitis externa, particularly if they are immunocompromised from medications, such as steroids, or if they have chronic diseases such as cancer or diabetes mellitus. No ethnic predispositions to otitis externa have been documented. Men and women are affected equally.

Immunocompromised persons on steroid therapy or individuals with chronic conditions such as diabetes mellitus are at a greater risk for developing infectious otitis externa and, in particular, invasive disease. Deep tissue invasion may be related to decreased polymorphonuclear neutrophil function and/or microvascular disease associated with diabetes. Steroid use specifically increases the likelihood of otomycosis, which is significantly more prevalent in the tropics and southeastern

United States, but as a whole, environmental changes are the most common risk factors for otitis externa. When the pH of the auditory canal shifts from acidic to alkaline or an increase in temperature and/or humidity occurs, the auditory canal becomes conducive to pathogenic colonization. In fact, excess moisture from any cause may predispose the external ear to infection. *Pseudomonas* infections, in particular, commonly result from the mild ear canal trauma associated with excessive swimming in hot, humid weather, especially in polluted water, hence the common name "swimmer's ear." Highly chlorinated pool water can also contribute to this disorder because it can dry out the ear canal, creating a potential portal of entry for bacteria and fungi. Inadequate cerumen (ear wax) production removes another critical nonspecific barrier to infection. In addition, patients with seborrhea have an increased risk of otitis externa resulting from seborrheic dermatitis caused by their excess sebum production. Manual picking of the ear; foreign bodies in the auditory canal; and the prolonged use of ear plugs, hearing aids, or cotton swabs may all contribute to local irritation of the external ear, as well. Other risk factors include previous ear infections, as well as skin allergies, particularly those to hair sprays and dyes that may enter the ear canal and cause contact dermatitis. In fact, dermatitic processes often precede microbial infection of the auditory canal because they create a potential portal of entry through the skin for pathogens.

Pathophysiology

Inflammation of the external ear is most commonly caused by microbial infection. Pathogenic colonization of the external ear is prevented by a number of immune and anatomical mechanisms. The keratinizing squamous epithelia of the ear canal continually sloughs, and the hair follicles that line the outer third of the canal rhythmically sweep laterally, acting as a natural cleansing mechanism and mechanical barrier to the accumulation of matter in the auditory canal. The production of viscous, hydrophobic cerumen in the auditory canal maintains an acidic pH and repels moisture, both of which antagonize bacterial growth. In addition, the presence of competing, nonpathogenic endogenous microbial flora inhibits the overgrowth of more virulent bacteria along the auditory canal. If any of these protective mechanisms is compromised, pathogenic colonization by bacteria or fungi normally found in the auditory canal may occur, resulting in acute otitis externa.

Bacterial agents of infectious otitis externa include *Pseudomonas aeruginosa,* which is the most common cause of diffuse infection and accounts for nearly all cases of invasive otitis externa, and *Staphylococcus aureus,* which typically causes a localized lesion stemming from an infected hair follicle, although it may cause the diffuse form as well. In addition, group A *Streptococcus pyogenes* is associated with localized disease, presenting

as a folliculitis or, more frequently, as outer ear erysipelas. Polymicrobial infection has also been noted in up to one-third of cases of diffuse disease, and the anaerobic bacteria *Bacteroides* and *Peptostreptococcus* have been cited in up to one-fourth of cases. Commonly identified fungal agents include *Aspergillus niger* (which typically causes focal lesions but may occasionally lead to invasive disease with bony involvement in immunocompromised patients), *Pityrosporum,* and *Candida albicans.* Hyperkeratotic processes such as eczema, psoriasis, and contact or seborrheic dermatitis can also lead to outer ear inflammation. Chronic otitis externa may result from inadequately treated otitis media with continuous serous or exudative drainage from the middle ear into the auditory canal.

Additional risk factors, if not direct causes of otitis externa, include local skin maceration and traumatic injury. The anatomy of the outer ear, which includes the tragus and conchal cartilage, serves as a physical barrier to foreign body entry into the outer ear canal. However, excessive cleaning of the ear with cotton swabs or other devices may leave small pieces of foreign matter in the canal, where they eventually disintegrate due to the canal's acidic pH, serving as a nidus of infection. This irritation in turn leads to pruritus, and excessive scratching of the ear canal only aggravates this cycle of epithelial damage and infection by creating physical access through this protective barrier. Excessive moisture in the external canal, particularly associated with swimming or humid environments, acts in a similar manner, leading to maceration and breakdown of the skin with subsequent bacterial infection.

Necrotizing otitis externa (formerly known as malignant otitis externa) is the most severe infectious form of external otitis in which bacterial infection extends from the skin of the auditory canal into the soft tissues, cartilage, and bone in the temporal region or base of the skull (i.e., skull osteomyelitis). Multiple cranial nerves may become involved, increasing morbidity, and death may result from septic thromboemboli to vessels of the brain if inadequately treated. *Pseudomonas aeruginosa* remains the most common infectious agent in such severe disease, although invasive fungal disease in immunocompromised individuals may also extend to multiple tissues.

Clinical Presentation
Subjective

The most common presenting complaint of patients with otitis externa is an acute, often severe otalgia of sudden or gradual onset, which may present bilaterally. Pain may worsen at night and disturb sleep, and it is exacerbated by pulling the pinna or earlobe or by applying pressure to the tragus. In severe cases, chewing may also elicit otic pain. Severe pain is common in invasive disease. In its early stages, the affected ear may feel full or obstructed, and a temporary conductive hearing loss related to luminal occlusion on the affected side is common if edema is severe. The affected ear may also be pruritic. A purulent discharge may be evident in bacterial disease, and systemic symptomatology such as fever or chills, although rare, may accompany cases of infectious etiology. Chronic otitis externa usually presents with dryness and pruritus of the ear canal. The ear canal may be slightly red and edematous, and there is usually an absence of cerumen.

Objective

A classic sign of acute otitis externa is tenderness on traction of the pinna and/or pain on applying pressure over the tragus. The clinician should instill several drops of benzocaine/antipyrine (Auralgan) otic solution before attempting examination in patients in acute distress. This solution should not be used in cases of suspected ruptured tympanic membrane, however.

On otoscopic examination, the auditory canal typically appears edematous and erythematous, preventing full visualization of the external canal and tympanic membrane; there also may be accumulation of purulent drainage in cases of bacterial infection. Diffuse cases present with nearly complete involvement of the auditory canal, whereas localized processes are recognized as focal lesions (pustules or furuncles) anywhere along the auditory canal or external ear structures. Sebaceous secretions in the ear canal are usually evident in patients with seborrhea, but cerumen production among patients is variable, depending on etiology. Fluid may be apparent in infectious cases. *Pseudomonas* infection produces a copious green exudate, whereas *Staphylococcus* infection presents as a yellow crusting in the midst of a purulent exudate. Fungal infections present as a fluffy white or black malodorous carpet of growth, and allergic reactions are characterized by scaly, cracked, and/or weepy tissue. Granulation tissue spreading out from the primary site of infection and eroding into the temporal bone, outer auricle, or through a perforated tympanic membrane is indicative of frank invasive disease.

Except in invasive disease or cases related to chronic otitis media, head and neck lymphadenopathy typically is not detected. Invasive disease may also be accompanied by tenderness of the temporomandibular joint (TMJ).

Diagnostic Reasoning

Diagnostic Tests

Laboratory tests are rarely needed if symptomatology clearly fits the classic clinical picture of otitis externa. However, any fluid from the ear may be cultured and, if microorganisms are detected, tested for antibiotic sensitivity. This may be particularly important in determining alternative treatment approaches for patients who do not respond promptly to empiric antibiotic therapy or those with chronic otitis externa, particularly with purulent exudates indicative of bacterial infection. Cultures and antibiotic sensitivity testing are also important for immunocompromised patients because their disease may be caused by rare pathogens or even by endogenous, typically nonpathogenic microbial flora. Fungi and mycobacteria should be ruled out, in particular. The erythrocyte sedimentation rate may be elevated, although this finding has not been thoroughly studied. Soft tissue or bony involvement in malignant disease may be assessed by CT and MRI scans. The temporal bone is the first bone to be affected. It is important to remember that at least one-third of bone mineral must be lost before radiological changes become apparent. Plain films and gallium or technetium-99 bone scans may also detect bony involvement, but these imaging techniques are less desirable because they lack specificity and, in the case of x-ray films, sensitivity.

Differential Diagnosis

In the absence of visible changes in the auditory canal and tympanic membrane, otalgia from referred pain associated with other disorders must be ruled out. These disorders include TMJ dysfunction, dental disease, neurological disorders such as trigeminal and glossopharyngeal neuralgia, parotitis (paramyxoviral infection) secondary to mumps, or, rarely, tumors of the middle ear and auditory meatus. Chondrodermatitis chronicus helicis may cause an otalgia similar to otitis externa in elderly patients, manifesting as an extremely tender nodule of the inner ear helix. TMJ dysfunction and dental disease may be specifically ruled out via dental x-ray films to demonstrate alterations in joint morphology or dentition. Mumps may be diagnosed serologically by measuring antibody titers; but in general, a thorough head and neck examination, complete with cranial nerve testing, typically will differentiate among the aforementioned causes of ear pain.

Otitis media may be distinguished from otitis externa by changes in the tympanic membrane that are characteristic of middle ear infection, including erythema, edema, and a significant lack of mobility on insufflation with a pneumatic otoscope. Moreover, movement of the tragus fails to elicit pain in middle ear infection. Otitis media should be suspected if continuous discharge from the middle ear is evident for more than 10 days, and x-ray films may aid in ruling out this diagnosis. Otitis externa and otitis media may occur concurrently. A systemic dermatological condition, such as seborrheic dermatitis, psoriasis, or erythroderma, may manifest as otitis externa.

Alternative pathologies to rule out through otoscopic examination include other dermatological disorders such as impetigo, herpes zoster infection, and even insect bites. Serious cranial infections requiring aggressive therapy must also be considered. Mastoiditis is characterized by fever, spontaneous rupture of the tympanic membrane, tenderness, edema, and erythema posterior to the auricle, as well as by palpable preauricular and anterior cervical lymph nodes. The mastoid process is exquisitely painful in mastoiditis, unlike otitis externa. Meningitis typically presents with fever, diffuse headache, altered mentation, vomiting, and cervical stiffness. A recent history of upper respiratory tract infection (URI) may be a clue to these and other infectious processes, including sinusitis and otitis media. Blood in the auditory canal may indicate temporal bone fracture or the presence of an invasive tumor. Carcinoma should be ruled out if invasive disease is suspected through the biopsy of apparent granulation tissue, which in otitis externa will demonstrate necrotizing vasculitis with no evidence of malignant cells. Other noninfectious diagnoses that may be ruled out through biopsy include primary skin and cartilage disorders such as sarcoidosis, discoid lupus, and trauma-related perichondritis of the pinna. Perichondritis may also be of infectious origin caused by *P aeruginosa,* as confirmed by culture. Excessive cerumen buildup may also lead to a feeling of fullness or stuffiness in the ear, as well as pain and hearing loss. Otoscopic examination performed before and after irrigation of the auditory canal will rule out cerumen impaction. Gouty tophi may also affect the external ear, but they are usually painless. Rarer infectious conditions that should be ruled out by special stains, cultures, and antigen/antibody tests in refractory cases include tuberculous otitis (diagnosed by acid-fast stain for *Mycobacteria*), leprosy (diagnosed by acid-fast stain for *Mycobacteria*), and syphilitic otitis (diagnosed by rapid plasma reagin [RPR] and Venereal Disease Research Laboratory [VDRL] tests and dark-field microscopy to identify the causative agent *Treponema pallidum*).

Management

Because the predominant symptom of otitis externa is pain, alteration in comfort is a primary focus of care. Medical management of the disease should focus on alleviating pain promptly.

- Local application of heat to the outer ear can offer some relief of pain.
- Some patients get relief with application of an ice pack to the outer ear.
- Nonprescription pain reliever such as aspirin or acetaminophen (325–650 mg PO every 4 hours as needed; maximum daily dose 4000 mg/day) or an NSAID such as ibuprofen (400–600 mg PO every 4–6 hours as needed to a maximum dose of 1.2 g/day).
- In cases of extreme pain, Tylenol with codeine # 3 or acetaminophen/hydrocodone 5 mg PO every 8 hours may be prescribed for the first 24 to 48 hours.
- Keep the ear dry. No swimming or submersion of the ear under water for 4 to 6 weeks.
- Treatment of otitis externa involves three basic steps:
  1. Gentle cleaning of the ear canal to remove all cerumen, exudate, and epidermal debris using a cotton pledget or irrigation with warm tap water. (Irrigation should be done cautiously until tympanic membrane perforation has been ruled out.)
  2. Evaluation of otic discharge and edema of the auditory canal and tympanic membrane.
  3. Selection of an appropriate local medication once the etiology has been identified.

Occasionally, the pustules or furuncles associated with localized otitis externa may require surgical drainage before initiating pharmacotherapy.

Diffuse bacterial otitis externa may be treated empirically. Several preparations are available for use. (See Drugs Commonly Prescribed 8.4: Bacterial Otitis Externa.)

Common topical otic preparations approved by the U.S. Food and Drug Administration (FDA) include acetic acid/aluminum acetate, acetic acid/hydrocortisone, ciprofloxin/hydrocortisone, ciprofloxin/dexamethasone, neomycin/polymixin B/hydrocortisone, and ofloxacin. Liquid ophthalmic preparations of gentamicin and tobramycin may be used otically to cover both *Pseudomonas aeruginosa* and *Staphylococcus aureus*. If the ear is edematous, a small cotton plug soaked in an otic preparation should be inserted. An absorptive 1-inch cotton wick or sponge may be inserted into a highly edematous ear canal by gentle twisting if luminal occlusion prevents the passage of otic preparations. Antibiotic drops may then be placed on the wick for the first 2 to 3 days of treatment, until swelling subsides. After this, drops should be placed directly into the ear canal.

Cases that are refractory to initial therapy or involve auricular cellulitis require systemic antibiotic treatment covering both *Staphylococcus* and *Pseudomonas*. Systemic antibiotics are also indicated in the case of specific host factors such as diabetes or in an immunosuppressed patient. Diffuse and localized otitis externa may need to be treated with multiple systemic antibiotic choices:

- First generation cephalosporins or penicillins with relatively narrow coverage such as cephalexin (Keflex) 250 to 500 mg PO 4 times daily and dicloxacillin 250 to 500 mg PO 4 times daily.
- Second generation cephalosporins such as cefuroxime (Ceftin) 250 to 500 mg PO 2 times daily or Omnicef 300 mg PO 2 times daily, or beta-lactamase–resistant penicillins such as amoxicillin/clavulanate (Augmentin XR) 1000 mg PO 2 times daily based on the amoxicillin component, which have broader-spectrum coverage.
- Fluoroquinolones such as ciprofloxacin (Cipro) 500 mg PO 2 times daily or levofloxacin (Levaquin) 500 mg PO 4 times daily with similarly broad coverage.
- Ceftazidime (Ceftaz, Fortaz) 2 g IV every 8 to 12 hours or a combination of tobramycin (1–1.5 mg/kg IV every 8 hours with dosage adjusted by monitoring serum levels and renal function) and ticarcillin (3 g IV every 4 hours). These regimens, however,

Drugs Commonly Prescribed 8.4　Bacterial Otitis Externa

Drug	Indication	Prescribing Considerations and Adverse Reactions
Drugs Safe to Use With Perforated Tympanic Membrane (TM)		
ciprofloxacin 0.3% and dexamethasone 0.1% (Ciprodex otic)	Antibiotic and steroid	Not recommended <6 months >6 months: 4 drops in affected ear 2 times daily for 7 days
ofloxacin 0.3% (Floxin otic)	Antibiotic	6 months–13 years: 5 drops to affected ear daily for 7 days Adults: 10 drops to affected ear for 7 days
Drugs Not Safe to Use With Perforated TM		
ciprofloxacin 0.2% and hydrocortisone 1% (Cipro HC otic)	Antibiotic and steroid	Not recommended <1 year >1 year: 3 drops in affected ear 2 times daily for 7 days
chloroxylenol 1 mg, pramoxine HCl 10 mg, hydrocortisone 10 mg/mL (Cortane B aqueous)	Antibacterial/antifungal + topical anesthetic + steroid	Children: 3 drops in affected ear 3 times daily for 7 days Adults: 4–5 drops in affected ear 3 times daily for 7 days
colistin 3 mg, neomycin 3.3 mg, hydrocortisone acetate 10 mg, thonzonium bromide 0.5 mg (Cortisporin-TC otic)	Antibiotic + steroid + surfactant	5 drops in affected ear 3–4 times daily for 10 days only

carry a significant risk of nephrotoxicity, ototoxicity, and bleeding diatheses. An alternative to IV therapy is the oral quinolone ciprofloxacin 750 mg 2 times daily, which is generally well tolerated and has a high cure rate in complicated disease.

- Patients who are immunocompromised from steroid therapy or who have chronic disorders such as diabetes, as well as patients with invasive bony involvement, may require surgical debridement of the affected area to drain abscesses and remove sequestered collagen. This therapy is usually followed by 4 to 6 weeks of IV antipseudomonal therapy.

- In the overwhelming majority of patients who present with chronic otitis externa, the condition is caused by persistent fungal infection. The ears are often dry and scaling. The treatment of fungal infections differs mainly in the choice of antimicrobials.

- Careful cleaning of the auditory canal is done. Then a single dusting of sulfanilamide powder is applied, followed by an otic suspension such as hydrocortisone/acetic acid otic (VoSol) solution, or acetic acid/aluminum acetate (Otic Domeboro). Four drops are placed in each affected ear 4 times daily for 7 to 10 days.

- Topical fungicide preparations containing nystatin or clotrimazole are increasingly accepted, although these agents are not available solely as otic preparations. If this treatment is planned, a referral to an ear, nose, and throat (ENT) specialist should be considered. In chronic cases of otitis externa from fungal infection, systemic antifungals such as fluconazole, ketoconazole, or griseofulvin may be considered. Clotrimazole solution is available over the counter and should be used as 4 drops in each ear daily. Ketoconazole cream may be placed into the external canal by a trained specialist using an operating microscope and a syringe with a blunt needle. About 1 inch of cream is needed to fill the canal, and it should be removed a week later.

- Steroidal therapies such as 0.1% triamcinolone solution or cream may be applied 3 or 4 times daily to relieve eczematous or psoriatic lesions.

- When otitis externa has been determined to be secondary to otitis media, therapy should be directed toward the underlying middle ear infection.

- Pharmacotherapy for chronic otitis externa is directed by extensive antibiotic sensitivity testing after the infectious organisms have been cultured and identified in the laboratory.

Follow-up and Referral

Acute otitis externa is commonly cured after 7 to 10 days of treatment. A follow-up appointment to assess the effects of treatment may be scheduled after 1 week of therapy for uncomplicated cases. If an ear wick has been placed, the patient should return in 2 days for removal and canal cleaning. The patient should be instructed to call if symptoms do not begin to subside in 48 hours.

Immunocompromised patients with invasive disease and any patient receiving IV antibiotic therapy require daily follow-up during hospitalization, and periodic appointments are recommended for up to 1 year after the discontinuation of treatment. Otherwise healthy patients with invasive disease who do not respond to treatment promptly should also be monitored closely; these patients should undergo further evaluation and diagnostic procedures as necessary. CT and MRI scans remain abnormal for many months after clinical resolution of invasive disease; thus, serial nuclear medicine scans (gallium scans) may be preferable in evaluating treatment efficacy during follow-up, because recurrence of infection may be as high as 10% within 6 months after treatment.

A common complication in the management of otitis externa is dermatitis medicamentosa. Neomycin, an antibiotic commonly found in otic preparations, is known to cause skin reactions and ototoxicity; however, these complications may be minimized by limiting the duration of pharmacotherapy. The use of neomycin-containing agents in cases in which the tympanic membrane is ruptured is controversial because neomycin may be toxic to middle ear structures if applied directly. Otitis externa may also lead to severe furunculosis (boil formation) or cellulitis (deep-tissue infection) within the ear canal. Invasive otitis externa is a potentially life-threatening complication of poorly treated diffuse and localized disease that must be detected early. Fever, excruciating pain, and the presence of friable granulation tissue are ominous signs of this sequela. Other serious cranial infections may result from inadequately treated otitis externa, including meningitis, mastoiditis, parotitis, and osteomyelitis of either the temporal bone or the base of the skull. Cranial nerve (CN) palsies affect 20% to 30% of patients with invasive disease, most commonly involving CN VII and, if disease progresses unchecked, CNs IX, X, XI, and XII.

Invasive otitis externa, cellulitis, bony involvement, and all complicating cranial infections must be referred to a specialist for immediate treatment. Patients who are immunocompromised from steroid therapy, diabetes, or other chronic illnesses should be referred to an otorhinolaryngologist to fully evaluate the extent of disease.

Patient Education

Patients should avoid getting water in the ears for at least 4 to 6 weeks after symptoms subside because moisture from any source can trigger a recurrent episode of infection. Shower caps or ear plugs should be worn when bathing, and swimming should be prohibited entirely for at least 1 month after an acute episode (cotton balls impregnated with petroleum jelly may be used as temporary ear plugs). For persons who are particularly susceptible to repeated infections, a 2% acetic acid solution may be used prophylactically to acidify the ear canal (2–3 drops in each ear, 2 times daily and after any contact with water in which the ears become wet). (See Complementary Therapies 8.1.)

Patients should be instructed in the proper method of cleaning the ears (with a soft cotton pledget) and warned never to use swabs, sticks, or chemical agents to clean the auditory canal. Patients should understand that a small amount of ear wax is necessary to prevent infection in the auditory canal and that excessive cleaning can be harmful. Clinicians should instruct patients or family members as to how to instill topical drops.

The importance of keeping the ear canals dry for at least 4 to 6 weeks, both during and after an acute episode, should also be stressed. The clinician should also discuss the importance of avoiding strong jets of water from showerheads or dental water-jet systems. Alternative or complementary therapies such as candling have not been shown to be efficacious and may in fact cause harm.

■ OTITIS MEDIA

Otitis media (OM) is an inflammation of the structures within the middle ear. Otitis media with effusion (OME) involves the transudation of plasma from middle ear blood vessels, leading to chronic effusion in the absence of the signs and symptoms of acute infection. Acute otitis media (AOM), also referred to as suppurative OM or purulent OM, denotes the presence of fluid in the middle ear in association with local or systemic illness, including otalgia, otorrhea, and fever. Recurrent OM is characterized by the clearance of middle ear effusions between acute episodes of otic inflammation. Chronic OM is present when inflammation persists for more than 3 months, typically related to tympanic membrane perforation with either intermittent or persistent otic discharge. Seventy-five percent of children experience at least one episode of OM by their third birthday. Almost half of these children will have three or more episodes of OM during their first 3 years. Measures to prevent AOM in infants and young children should be discussed with parents at well-child visits. Preventive measures include avoidance of tobacco exposure, exclusive breastfeeding for the first 6 months of life or longer, and annual influenza vaccine and pneumococcal conjugate vaccine for all children according to the updated immunization schedules. Although OM is primarily a disease of infants and young children, it can also affect adults.

Epidemiology and Causes

Ear pain, in general, is a common clinical complaint, accounting for 2% to 3% of all family practice office visits. Specifically, the incidence rate of OM increases during the winter months, when the climate is colder. Although AOM is most common in very young children, elderly adults also have a significant risk of developing disease because of decreases in natural immunity. Native Americans, particularly Navajos, and Native Alaskans have higher prevalence rates than the general population. A smaller increase in rate is also seen in white Americans of European descent. Men and women are affected equally, although OM tends to be rare in adults.

Factors contributing to eustachian tube dysfunction leading to OME include allergies, sinusitis, rhinitis, and pharyngitis, all of which cause swelling of the membranous lining of the eustachian tube. However, the most significant precipitating event is a recent or concurrent URI, attributed most often to influenza type A (*Influenzavirus,* in family Orthomyxoviridae), respiratory syncytial virus (*Pneumovirus,* in family Paramyxoviridae), or adenovirus. URI is thought to contribute to host immunosuppression and the loss of ciliated epithelium in the eustachian tube; in turn, bacterial adherence to the membranous lining is increased. Anatomical abnormalities that can lead to direct blockage of the eustachian tube include hypertrophy or chronic inflammation of the adenoids (pharyngeal tonsils), cleft palate, deviated nasal septum, and nasopharyngeal tumors. Perforation of the eardrum from direct blunt trauma, swimming or diving accidents, or sudden outward pressure or suction (such as from a kiss over the ear), may create a portal of entry for bacteria directly into the middle ear. Certain genetic conditions such as Down syndrome (trisomy 21) also predispose an individual to middle ear infections. Both active and passive smoking have been associated with an increased risk of all forms of OM, and crowded or unsanitary living conditions, along with a family history of OM (particularly in the same household), are also contributing factors.

Pathophysiology

AOM results when bacterial infection by nasopharyngeal microorganisms follows eustachian tube dysfunction in which the narrowest portion of the tube (the isthmus) becomes obstructed. Inflammation results primarily in response to bacterial products, including endotoxins and cell-wall components, creating in effect a middle ear abscess. Pressure from this buildup of pus may impinge on the fine blood vessels supplying the tympanic membrane, weakening its structure, reducing tensile strength, and eventually causing perforation or rupture of the eardrum to facilitate draining of inner ear fluid. Fortunately, in the absence of underlying immunocompromise, this structure typically begins to heal spontaneously within hours and may be fully healed by 1 or 2 weeks with complete restoration of baseline hearing capacity. OME is caused by a transudation of plasma fluid through engorged blood vessels resulting from the loss of eustachian tube patency, caused either by swelling of the membranous lining or direct anatomical blockage of the eustachian tube. Swelling of the mucosa is particularly

common in the presence of an antecedent viral URI or acute allergy attack. Effective drainage of middle ear fluid is thus prevented, and negative pressure develops in the middle ear cavity, further drawing in fluid.

Streptococcus pneumoniae (implicated in 40%–50% of AOM cases) is the most frequent pathogen isolated from middle ear effusions in adults, because the currently available polyvalent streptococcal vaccines cover only 60% to 70% of these isolates. In turn, the increasing administration of the childhood pneumococcal vaccine covering 7 serotypes (Prevnar), as well as the separate 23-serotype Pneumovax vaccine used in high-risk and elderly patients, has yet to affect incidence rates of AOM. Other common organisms include nontypable *Haemophilus influenzae* (10%–30% of cases), which are not covered by the *Haemophilus influenzae* type b (Hib) vaccine, and *Moraxella (Branhamella) catarrhalis,* the vast majority of which express the beta-lactamase gene and are resistant to first-line penicillin and cephalosporin antibiotics. These organisms are thought to reach the middle ear from the upper respiratory tract via aspiration or reflux. *Staphylococcus aureus* and *Streptococcus pyogenes* are far less common causative agents, particularly since the introduction of sulfonamide antibiotics such as trimethoprim-sulfamethoxazole (Bactrim).

Up to half of AOM cases are attributed to viral infections originating in the nasopharynx and extending to the middle ear via the eustachian tube, including rhinovirus, adenovirus, coronavirus, influenza, and respiratory syncytial virus. In fact, nearly 40% of documented influenza cases in children younger than 3 years of age are complicated by AOM, adding to the impetus for widespread flu vaccination. *Mycoplasma* and *Chlamydia pneumoniae* are also rare causes of OM. *Chlamydia trachomatis* is typically seen only in infants younger than 6 months; in developing countries, unusual agents such as *Mycobacteria tuberculosis, C. diphtheriae,* parasites (*Ascaris*), or fungi (*Blastomycoses, Candida, Aspergillus*) may be identified.

OME may be viral in origin but is usually attributed to beta-lactamase–producing bacterial strains that are resistant to first-line antibiotic therapies. Importantly, middle ear effusions often last for weeks to months after an AOM clears; thus, OME may simply reflect part of the natural history of a resolved episode of AOM. Recurrent OM typically results from bacterial infection due to anatomical abnormalities that repeatedly compromise eustachian tube patency. Chronic OM may also be caused by any of the bacteria associated with AOM, as well as *Escherichia coli* and *Proteus,* but *P aeruginosa* and *S aureus* are the most commonly isolated pathogens in the chronic suppurative form.

Clinical Presentation
Subjective

The patient with OME will typically complain of stuffiness, fullness, and a loss of auditory acuity in the affected ear only. Pain is rare, but patients may describe popping, crackling, or gurgling sounds when chewing, yawning, or blowing the nose. Very rarely, patients may experience vertigo (a sense of whirling or spinning in space) or ataxia, if inner ear complications such as labyrinthitis are present. Although patients are typically afebrile, a recent history of viral URI or either allergic or vasomotor rhinitis is common.

In contrast, AOM usually presents with marked "deep" ear pain and fever, as well as unilateral hearing loss, otic discharge, and a recent history of URI. Some patients may also experience dizziness (space disorientation), vertigo, tinnitus (ringing in the ears), vomiting, or nausea. Pain typically subsides if the tympanic membrane ruptures because this relieves middle ear pressure. In these cases, patients also usually complain of otic discharge. Recurrent OM is characterized by the clearance of middle ear effusions between acute episodes of inflammation.

Chronic OM typically presents with a history of repeated bouts of acute otitis media, followed by a period of continuous or intermittent otorrhea lasting for more than 3 months. Pain is seldom a complaint, as hearing loss (related to tympanic membrane perforation) is the primary concern. Risk factors for AOM include enrollment of a child in day care, presence of tobacco smoke in the home, and residing in communities where antibiotic-resistant forms of *S pneumoniae* are endemic.

Objective

Examination of the external ear in patients with OME is typically unremarkable; however, the mucous membranes of the nasal and oral cavities may be infected or edematous, confirming a recent history of URI. The eardrum may be dull but usually is not bulging, and eardrum mobility typically decreases on pneumatic otoscopy. When examining a patient with AOM, the use of Auralgan otic solution (a combination analgesic and anesthetic agent—contraindicated in cases of perforated eardrum) may be needed to facilitate the examination if the patient is experiencing pain. The tympanic membrane may be amber or yellow-orange, or the membrane may be infected and pinkish gray to fiery red in color. The tympanic membrane is typically full or bulging in acute cases, with absent or obscured bony landmarks and cone light reflex.

Although the auditory canal usually shows no abnormalities, a discharge from the middle ear may be present if the tympanic membrane has perforated as a result of the collection of middle ear fluid and subsequent inflammatory response. Otorrhea may be purulent or mucoid, depending on the stage of inflammation; polymorphonuclear neutrophils are prominent in the early stages of bacterial infection. Otoscopic examination in chronic OM usually reveals a perforated, draining tympanic membrane and possibly invasive granulation tissue. Chronic, foul-smelling otorrhea is typical of anaerobic bacterial infection, and a chronic, grayish-yellow suppuration may

indicate the development of a cholesteatoma from the degenerative products of invasive epithelialization (involuted squamous epithelia and keratin debris) at the site of infection. In rare cases, bullae formed between layers of the tympanic membrane (bullous myringitis) caused by certain viruses or *Mycoplasma pneumoniae* are seen, and multiple perforations of the tympanic membrane are characteristic of tuberculous otitis.

On palpation, in cases of acute infection, lymphadenopathy of the preauricular and posterior cervical nodes is common. If OM is complicated by an acute mastoiditis, tenderness over the mastoid will be elicited, because the bony architecture of the middle ear is continuous with the mastoid process.

Diagnostic Reasoning
Diagnostic Tests

Laboratory tests are rarely needed if symptomatology clearly fits the classic clinical picture of OM. However, if confirmation is desired, pneumatic otoscopy will demonstrate decreased or absent tympanic membrane mobility in serous, acute, or chronic OM with effusion. Tympanometry may be useful if fluid buildup behind the middle ear is suspected in the absence of other clinical signs; a flat tympanogram is consistent with restrictive disease of the middle ear cavity. A complete blood count is usually not indicated; however, patients with AOM may demonstrate a leukocytosis, particularly if they are febrile. Cultures of tympanocentesis fluid are not indicated in serous OM and are of little practical value in acute disease unless the patient is immunocompromised or infectious complications such as mastoiditis are evident. In subacute, recurrent, or chronic cases of OM, however, cultures and antibiotic sensitivity testing are helpful in guiding alternative treatment approaches. If cultures are obtained, fungi and mycobacteria should be specifically ruled out. Conventional sinus x-ray films and CT scans (which can reveal mucosal thickening in the middle ear space) may be helpful in evaluating patients with effusion and particularly patients with recurrent infection.

Pure-tone audiometry may be helpful both before and after treatment; Weber and Rinne tuning-fork tests typically will reveal conductive, as opposed to sensorineural, hearing loss. Sound lateralization to the affected ear occurs when a 512-Hz tuning fork is placed midline on the top of the head (Weber test), and bone conduction is superior in duration and volume to air conduction (negative Rinne test).

Differential Diagnosis

OM must be distinguished from otitis externa, which is inflammation of the auditory canal and/or external ear, including the pinna and tragus. These structures are usually not affected in OM, and otitis externa typically does not involve the tympanic membrane. Otitis externa resulting from furunculosis, local skin maceration, or trauma from a foreign body or direct blunt force must be ruled out. Exacerbated pain on manipulation of the tragus, pinna, or earlobe is a telltale sign of external ear inflammation. Barotrauma may also mimic OM, with transient middle ear effusion resulting from air travel or drastic increases in altitude, such as when driving up mountains. TMJ syndrome pain is similar to the pain of AOM. Patients may complain of ear pain when in fact the pain is being referred from the TMJ. Mastoiditis presenting without middle ear infection should be considered when no physical signs of middle ear involvement are evident. Referred otalgia from TMJ dysfunction or dental abscesses may be ruled out by dental x-ray films. Parotitis secondary to mumps (paramyxoviral infection) may be ruled out via serology studies (antibody titers), if suspected. Nasopharyngeal neoplasm must be ruled out through biopsy in cases of unilateral recurrent, chronic, or refractory OM. Rarer infectious conditions, which should be ruled out by special stains, cultures, and antigen/antibody tests, include tuberculous otitis (order an acid-fast stain for *Mycobacteria*), leprosy (order an acid-fast stain for *Mycobacteria*), and syphilitic otitis (order RPR and VDRL tests, and dark-field microscopy to identify the causative agent *Treponema pallidum*). Excessive ear wax buildup (cerumen impaction) with or without infection may also lead to a feeling of fullness or stuffiness in the ear, as well as pain and hearing loss. Otoscopic examination is performed before and after irrigation of the auditory canal to rule out this disorder.

Management

Uncomplicated cases of OM are likely to be self-limited and may require no specific intervention other than pain and symptomatic relief (see Therapeutic Procedure 8.3); however, pharmacological treatment of complicated or recurrent OM is indicated to prevent permanent anatomical changes of the middle ear and subsequent hearing loss. Changes in characteristics of auditory stimuli related to middle ear pathology lead to sensory or perceptual alterations. In the unfortunate instance when middle ear infection leads to permanent comorbidity, loss of auditory perception may affect a patient's lifestyle, communication patterns, socialization, and self-concept. Other identifiable clinical problems include alteration in comfort and an increased potential for injury related to hearing loss. Interventions should focus on moving the patient toward acceptance, identifying effective communication patterns, and recognizing support mechanisms and resources for coping with hearing loss. Fortunately, the vast majority of OM cases never reach this advanced stage.

In cases of OME, watchful waiting is indicated, with monthly exams to monitor for resolution. If the effusion is unresponsive to medical treatment and persists for longer than 12 weeks, a 10-day course of an antibiotic should be considered in addition to a referral to an otolaryngologist. Antibiotic choice needs to be individualized; however, for the patient who is not penicillin allergic and has not recently been exposed to antibiotics, amoxicillin (80–90 mg/kg/day) is a reasonable choice. For patients who have had antibiotics in the last month, a beta-lactamase stable agent (e.g., amoxicillin/clavulanate) or a second or third generation cephalosporin would be a good choice. Studies have indicated that prolonged (more than 10 days) treatment of OME has not shown an advantage over a 10-day course of therapy. Some studies suggest the addition of prednisone; however, the most recent recommendations from the American Academy of Pediatrics suggest that steroid medications are not recommended for treatment of OME in a child of any age (Level I) (Lieberthal et al, 2013; Waseem et al, 2014). Studies have not borne out the effectiveness of decongestants or antihistamines, although these may be of some benefit in patients with comorbid allergic rhinitis.

Although there is an increasing trend to observe uncomplicated AOM in children for the first 48 to 72 hours rather than prescribe early antibacterial treatment in the hopes of self-limited resolution (see Nursing Research–Based Practice Box 8.2), antimicrobial therapy in adults is largely the norm. Selection of an agent to treat AOM requires consideration of several factors, including the patient's age, OM history, drug hypersensitivity, prior antimicrobial response, and associated illnesses. For children aged 6 to 24 months, observation and systemic analgesics without the use of antibacterial agents is an option for selected children with uncomplicated AOM, based on diagnostic certainty, age, illness severity, and assurance of follow-up. In children older than 24 months, many cases of AOM may resolve and do not require antibiotics, as long as the symptoms are manageable with systemic analgesics, the child has access to reevaluation at 48 hours, and symptoms do not persist. If signs and symptoms of AOM persist in spite of using systemic analgesics for 48 to 72 hours, the child should be reassessed and antibiotic treatment should be considered. Given that the majority of AOM cases occur in pediatric patients, pharmacotherapeutic approaches for AOM in both children and adults are summarized in Therapeutic Procedure 8.3.

Follow-up and Referral

Patients with OME should be reevaluated 4 to 6 weeks after treatment because the full clinical course of the disease may last up to several weeks. Monthly otoscopic or tympanometric exams should be done as long as OME persists. Patients with AOM should be seen for follow-up in 48 to 72 hours if symptoms have not resolved. Otherwise, a follow-up appointment may be scheduled several days after the completion of pharmacotherapy. Most patients experience spontaneous closure of a ruptured tympanic membrane and recovery of normal hearing within 4 weeks of treatment. Otoscopic exam should be done 4 weeks after diagnosis. If symptoms persist, consider changing the antibiotic regimen to cover

Therapeutic Procedure 8.3   Initial Pharmacotherapy of AOM in Pediatric Patients

Indication	Drug	Dose	Prescribing Considerations
Otherwise healthy with mild symptoms	Acetaminophen (Tylenol) Ibuprofen (Motrin, Advil)	10–15 mg/kg/dose PO every 4 hours as needed (**max 75 mg/kg/day**) 5–10 mg/kg/dose PO every 6–8 hour as needed (**max 40 mg/kg/day**)	For ages 6–24 months, observation with the use of systemic analgesics *without* the use of antibacterial agents is an option for selected children with uncomplicated AOM, based on diagnostic certainty, age, illness severity, and assurance of follow-up. If older than 24 months, most cases of AOM resolve and do *not* require antibiotics, as long as symptoms are manageable with systemic analgesics, the child has access to reevaluation at 48 hours, and symptoms do not persist. If signs and symptoms of AOM persist in spite of using systemic analgesics for 48–72 hours, reassess and consider treatment with antibiotics.
***No* day-care attendance and *no* antibiotics within 90 days**	Amoxicillin	**Standard Dose:** 40–45 mg/kg/day PO in 3 divided doses • ≥2 years old: treat for 5 days • <2 years old: treat for 10 days	High risk factors increase the risk of resistant *Streptococcus pneumoniae* (*S pneumoniae*)
Day-care attendance and antibiotics within 90 days	Amoxicillin	**High Dose:** 80–90 mg/kg/day PO in 3 divided doses • ≥2 years old: treat for 5 days • <2 years old: treat for 10 days	Amoxicillin retains the best activity of all oral β-lactam agents against *S pneumoniae,* including penicillin intermediate resistant strains
β-lactam allergy	The incidence of cephalosporin cross reactivity with penicillin allergy is less than 2%. Consider allergy testing when infection resolves to confirm penicillin allergy.		
Penicillin allergy (mild, nonanaphylactic)	**Cefuroxime axetil**	30 mg/kg/day PO in 2 divided doses • ≥2 years old: treat for 5 days • <2 years old: treat for 10 days	Due to poor taste of cefuroxime suspension, recommend tablets if possible, can be crushed and put into a palatable fluid
	Cefprozil	30 mg/kg/day PO in 2 divided doses • ≥2 years old: treat for 5 days • <2 years old: treat for 10 days	Compared with cefuroxime, liquid cefprozil has a better taste but inferior coverage of *Haemophilus* and penicillin intermediate resistance–*S pneumoniae*
Penicillin allergy (severe, anaphylactic) or cephalosporin allergy	**Clarithromycin**	15 mg/kg/day in 2 divided doses for 10 days	TMP/SMX and macrolides are inferior options due to high resistance rates and clinical failure rates

Continued

Therapeutic Procedure 8.3 Initial Pharmacotherapy of AOM in Pediatric Patients—cont'd

Indication	Drug	Dose	Prescribing Considerations
	Trimethoprim/ sulfamethoxazole (TMP/SMX)	6–12 mg TMP/kg/day PO in 2 divided doses • ≥2 years old: treat for 5 days • <2 years old: treat for 10 days	Consider referral to otolaryngologist for tympanocentesis
	Azithromycin	10 mg/kg/day PO on the first day and 5 mg/kg/day PO for 4 days	

Failure of Initial AOM Treatment in Pediatric Patients

Indication	Drug	Dose	Therapeutic Considerations
Failure of standard dose amoxicillin	**Amoxicillin PLUS**	40–45 mg/kg/day PO in 3 divided doses for 10 days	The combination is recommended to provide a high dose of amoxicillin (for penicillin intermediate resistance–*S pneumoniae*) and regular dose of amoxicillin-clavulanate (for coverage of β-lactamase–producing *H influenzae* and *M catarrhalis*) without excessive clavulanate (>10 mg/kg/day), which may lead to increased incidence of diarrhea
	Amoxicillin-clavulanate (use 7:1 formulation) (2 separate prescriptions should be given)	45 mg/kg/day PO in 3 divided doses for 10 days (based on amoxicillin component)	
Failure of high-dose amoxicillin	**Amoxicillin-clavulanate** (use 4:1 formulation)	40 mg/kg/day PO in 3 divided doses for 10 days (based on amoxicillin component)	Due to poor taste of cefuroxime axetil suspension, recommend tablets if possible, can be crushed and put into a palatable fluid
	Cefuroxime axetil	30 mg/kg/day PO in 2 divided doses for 10 days	
	Cefprozil	30 mg/kg/day PO in 2 divided doses for 10 days	
β-lactam (penicillin) allergy	**Clarithromycin**	15 mg/kg/day PO in 2 divided doses for 10 days	Therapeutic options for these patients are very limited; consider referral to otolaryngologist for tympanostomy Macrolides and TMP/SMX are less efficacious than amoxicillin-clavulanate; there is significant macrolide resistance in *S pneumoniae*
	TMP/SMX	6–12 mg TMP/kg/day PO in 2 divided doses for 10 days	
	Azithromycin	10 mg/kg PO first day then 5 mg/kg/day x 4 days	

Treatment of AOM in Adults

Indication	Drug	Dose
AOM	Amoxicillin	500 mg every 8 hours OR 875 mg 2 times daily for 10 days
β-Lactamase–resistant AOM	Amoxicillin-clavulanate (Augmentin) Cefixime (Suprax)	875 mg 2 times daily for 10 days 400 mg daily for 7 days
AOM in penicillin-allergic patients	Macrolides Azithromycin (Zithromax) Clarithromycin (Biaxin)	500 mg day 1, then 250 mg daily for 4 days 500 mg every 12 hours for 7 days

Drugs to Avoid in AOM

Cephalexin	No activity against penicillin intermediate resistant–*S pneumoniae* No activity against *Haemophilus influenzae/Moraxella catarrhalis*
Cefaclor	No activity against penicillin intermediate resistant–*S pneumoniae* Marginal activity against *Haemophilus influenzae/Moraxella catarrhalis*

Therapeutic Procedure 8.3   Initial Pharmacotherapy of AOM in Pediatric Patients—cont'd

Cefixime	No activity against penicillin intermediate resistant–*S pneumoniae* Excellent activity against *Haemophilus influenzae*
Ceftriaxone	Routine use of this agent is not recommended due to potential for increased resistance to third generation cephalosporins. May be an option in severe cases who have failed therapy, in immuno-suppressed patients, or in neonates. **Note: 3 days of IM/IV therapy recommended** (single dose not as effective in eradicating penicillin-resistant *S pneumoniae*)
Clindamycin	No activity against *Haemophilus/Moraxella* spp. (Clindamycin may be an option for *S pneumoniae* in severe penicillin-allergic patients)
Erythromycin	Poor activity against *H influenzae* Significant macrolide resistance in *S pneumoniae*

Nursing Research–Based Practice 8.2

Siegel, RM, et al. Treatment of otitis media with observation and a safety-net antibiotic prescription. *Pediatrics* 112(3):527–532, 2003.

J. S. is a 2-year-old child who presents to the pediatrician's office with a temperature of 101.8°F. Her mother reports that for the past 2 days she has been tugging on her right ear, producing a moderate amount of yellow nasal drainage, and has been very irritable. On physical exam you discover that the tympanic membrane is erythematous, is bulging, and has decreased mobility. The mother states that the child's appetite is normal and denies any vomiting or diarrhea. The child's history is negative for previous ear infections, congenital syndromes, and prematurity. Immunizations are up to date, and no one else in the family has experienced these symptoms. The mother states that the child started attending day care 2 weeks ago.

Your diagnosis is acute otitis media (AOM). What treatment plan would you develop for this patient? How would you explain your diagnosis and treatment plan to the mother? What instructions would you give the mother to assist her in caring for her child?

A quasi-experimental study design was conducted to evaluate the treatment options of AOM. The aim of the study was to determine if parents in the United States would wait at least 48 hours before deciding whether to fill a safety-net antibiotic prescription (SNAP) for the treatment of uncomplicated acute otitis media in children aged 1 to 12 years. Pain control was the treatment of choice for all 194 participants in the Cincinnati Pediatric Research Group's study. After criteria had been met and consent forms were signed by the parents, the SNAP was given with instructions to wait 48 hours before filling the prescription and to treat the symptoms with acetaminophen, ibuprofen, and anesthetic otic drops. Patients were contacted on day 10 with a telephone interview and were questioned about the treatments given. Initial data and the 10-day telephone interview information were entered into the researcher's Internet Web site. The findings showed that 175 participants completed the 10-day interview. Of the 175 participants, 31% had filled the SNAP, and 78% of the parents were satisfied with acetaminophen treatment alone. Sixty-three percent of the parents were willing to treat future acute otitis media episodes with pain mediation rather than with immediate antibiotics.

beta-lactamase–producing organisms. Chronic OM requires monthly follow-up to assess the efficacy of treatment and monitor for recurrence of infection.

If medical management does not clear the infection, inner ear effusion persists, or OM episodes recur, referral to an ENT specialist for potential surgical evaluation is indicated. Common surgical procedures include myringotomy (incision of the eardrum to allow draining and relieve fluid buildup in the middle ear) or tympanostomy (insertion of tubes across the eardrum into the inner ear to drain pus or serous fluid). Tonsillectomy and/or adenoidectomy may also be used as secondary prevention measures. All infectious sequelae of contiguous cranial structures, as well as invasive complications requiring excision such as a cholesteatoma, require referral to a specialist.

OME can lead to irreversible conductive hearing loss if middle ear structures are permanently damaged from effusion-related pressure changes. If AOM is poorly treated or is present in an immunocompromised patient, it may lead to OME; chronic OM; otitis interna (labyrinthitis); vertigo; ataxia; or several acute, subacute, and chronic infections of adjacent cranial structures, including mastoiditis, petrositis, meningitis, and epidural, subdural, or brain abscesses. Other complications include perforation of the tympanic membrane, cholesteatoma, facial nerve palsies, lateral sinus thrombophlebitis, and otitic hydrocephalus.

Although the clinical course of OME may last for several weeks, patients should be referred to a specialist for impedance audiometry testing and further evaluation to rule out nasopharyngeal tumors and other anatomical eustachian tube obstructions if hearing loss persists beyond 6 weeks, extends bilaterally, or reaches more than 20 decibels. Patients with AOM may require referral to a specialist if vertigo or ataxia develops, if a ruptured tympanic membrane fails to close, if symptoms worsen after 3 to 4 days of treatment, or if significant hearing loss is present.

Patient Education

Swimming should be avoided until the infection clears because immersion in water may lead to otitis externa, complicating the middle ear infection. The ear canal should be kept as dry as possible. Tympanic membrane perforation can be avoided by not using cotton swabs or sharp objects of any kind to clean the ears. Traumatic injuries to the middle ear should be avoided as well to prevent perforation. In all cases, especially those in which the tympanic membrane is perforated, blowing of the nose should be avoided. If the nose must be blown, it should be done as gently as possible.

All patients and their families should be encouraged to stop smoking because smoking aggravates all forms of otic inflammation. Folk remedies such as "sweet oil" should also be avoided. Patients should be instructed to return to the clinic for further evaluation after 48 hours if symptoms of AOM have not ameliorated. Explain that OM per se is not contagious but that predisposing URIs may be passed from person to person. Bedrest or reduced activity may be suggested in severe cases until fever and pain subside, and the importance of completing the full regimen of all antibiotic therapies should be emphasized. Instruct patients to keep the ear canal dry during the course of infection, and demonstrate the proper method of cleaning the ear canal without chemical agents, sharp objects, cotton swabs, or a finger.

COMMON NOSE AND THROAT PROBLEMS

■ EPISTAXIS

Commonly called a "nosebleed," *epistaxis* is a hemorrhage of the nasal mucosa resulting from the traumatic or spontaneous rupture of superficial veins and/or arteries, located most often on the anterosuperior portion of the nasal septum known as Little's area (Kiesselbach's triangle or Kiesselbach's plexus). Epistaxis is a physical sign rather than a disease. Therefore, after the initial management of bleeding, a thorough evaluation is essential to determine its underlying cause.

Epidemiology and Causes

Although actual prevalence statistics for epistaxis are undocumented, it is an extremely common condition. Approximately 10% of the population experiences at least one significant nosebleed over a lifetime. Epistaxis most commonly occurs in children younger than age 10 years and in adults older than 50 years. Minor, self-limited epistaxis is twice as common in children as it is in adults. In contrast, posterior epistaxis is more common in elderly patients. No ethnic predispositions are apparent. Men and women are affected equally by nosebleeds, although some predisposing clotting disorders such as hemophilia may be expressed predominantly in males.

Excessive dryness of the nasal mucosa in poorly humidified environments or at high altitudes weakens nasal vessels, predisposing them to rupture. Septal deviation may thus contribute to epistaxis through the disproportionate exposure of one side of the nose to dry environmental air. Coagulopathies may be associated with chronic disorders such as cirrhosis, renal disease, cancer (especially Hodgkin's disease), and hypertension. As a whole, however, coagulopathies and neoplasms are associated with only 10% of cases of epistaxis. Vascular diseases such as hereditary hemorrhagic telangiectasia and arteriovenous nasal malformations are also risk factors. Medications that prolong bleeding time (e.g., warfarin, aspirin) contribute to all types of bleeding disorders, as does cocaine abuse (snorting), which leads to septal perforation. Prolonged use of nose drops is also a risk factor because it may lead to reflex nasal inflammation, known as rhinitis medicamentosum. In an elderly patient, arteriosclerosis is a contributing factor, specifically for posterior hemorrhage epistaxis. Many nutritional deficiencies and febrile infectious disorders may also predispose an individual to nosebleeds, including scurvy (extreme vitamin C deficiency) and rheumatic, scarlet, or typhoid fever.

Pathophysiology

More than 90% of nosebleeds result from local irritation related to trauma or inflammation, occurring most often in the absence of any anatomical abnormality. Trauma to both nasal polyps and the well-vascularized watershed area of the nasal mucosa known as Kiesselbach's plexus is perhaps the most common direct cause of nosebleed, particularly from picking of the nose (epistaxis digitorum) or forcible injury related to blunt trauma. Kiesselbach's plexus marks the anastomosis of three major blood vessels of the nasal cavity: the septal branch of the anterior ethmoid artery, the septal portion of the superior labial branch of the facial artery, and the lateral nasal branch of the sphenopalatine artery. Similarly, posterior epistaxis most commonly originates from rupture of the posterior wall and choanal branches of the sphenopalatine artery. Vascular disease accounts for up to one-fourth of posterior bleeds, and rupture of an intracranial or cervical vascular aneurysm must also be considered as a potentially life-threatening etiology.

Spontaneous rupture of weakened vessels may also result from acute or chronic sinusitis, upper respiratory infection, and drying or crusting of the nasal mucosa from viral or allergic rhinitis. Foreign bodies lodged in the nasal airways are another common source of vessel injury.

Inhaled drugs of abuse (e.g., cocaine and snorted heroin) chronically dry and aggravate friable nasal mucosa, predisposing to epistaxis. Anticoagulant medications such as warfarin (Coumadin) and heparin may also predispose to nosebleeds by inhibiting natural clotting pathways, and alcohol intake has been implicated as an independent, albeit far from universal, epistaxis risk factor. Malignant growths in the nasal cavity or paranasal sinuses may erode into blood vessels and present with epistaxis as their sole manifestation. An exceedingly rare cause of nasal bleeding is the presence of nasal ectopic endometrium (nasal endometriosis). Familial blood dyscrasias such as hemophilia A (factor VIII deficiency), hemophilia B (factor IX deficiency or Christmas disease), and von Willebrand disease (the most common genetic bleeding disorder), as well as hereditary hemorrhagic telangiectasia (Osler-Weber-Rendu disease), are examples of inherited conditions that may be complicated by significant epistaxis.

Clinical Presentation

Subjective

The patient with recurrent minor anterior epistaxis typically presents with a history of several episodes over several weeks. If blood loss has been extensive, patients may report light-headedness or shortness of breath. In addition, a rapid heartbeat may be detected, and the patient may report blackened stools (melena) that are discolored from clotted, swallowed blood. Posterior epistaxis may be asymptomatic or may present with hemoptysis (coughed-up blood), nausea, hematemesis (blood-streaked vomitus), or melena.

Objective

Prominent blood vessels are typically seen traversing the anterior septum, and a small amount of clotted blood may be visible. If the patient is actively bleeding from the front of the nose, blood is typically bright red, and localizing the bleeding source may be difficult. The second most common site of hemorrhage (after Little's area) is the anterior end of the inferior nasal turbinate. Epistaxis originating deeper in the nose may produce either bright red or dark blood. Usually only one bleeding site exists, but if multiple sites or a diffuse ooze are evident, an underlying systemic bleeding disorder is likely. If the source of hemorrhage is located in the posterosuperior nasal cavity, the bleeding is termed *posterior epistaxis*. In these cases, blood loss will extend into the pharynx as well, and clotted blood and brown to red throat discoloration may be evident. The most common sites of posterior bleeding are just under the posterior half of the inferior nasal turbinate or the roof of the nasal cavity. Patients with significant blood loss may demonstrate pallor, particularly in the face. Palpation of the paranasal sinuses may reveal tenderness if underlying sinusitis or malignancy is present. Likewise, percussion

of the paranasal sinuses may demonstrate tenderness in sinusitis-related or malignancy-related cases.

Diagnostic Reasoning

Diagnostic tests are rarely called for when bleeding can be managed, and most episodes of epistaxis are not recurrent. A variety of diagnostic tests are helpful in determining the underlying cause of nasal hemorrhage. Laboratory tests exist for deficiencies of most clotting factors, but factor VIII and factor IX deficiencies are clearly the most commonly observed and tested for. In the past, bleeding times were monitored to help diagnose platelet-related coagulopathies. Because the test is labor intensive and results vary among laboratory technicians, it is rarely performed. Today a more sophisticated test called platelet function assay detects the ability of the platelets to work, not just the number of platelets. A prolonged bleeding time (more than 7 minutes) may reflect platelet-related coagulopathies (e.g., von Willebrand's syndrome or thrombocytopenia), whereas a prolonged prothrombin time (PT) or partial thromboplastin time (PTT) is characteristic of clotting factor disorders. Hemophilia A (factor VIII deficiency) and hemophilia B (factor IX deficiency) produce a prolonged PTT, whereas disorders of the extrinsic clotting pathway (factor VII deficiency) result in a prolonged PT. A CBC including hemoglobin, hematocrit, and mean corpuscular volume may offer insight into the chronicity of the condition. Radiological (x-ray) examination of the nasal cavity and paranasal sinuses may identify masses, including neoplasms or foreign bodies, as well as sinusitis if mucosal thickening or air–water levels are apparent. CT scan of the head may also be done with greater sensitivity for detecting structural and soft tissue abnormalities.

Differential Diagnosis

For the patient with recurrent minor epistaxis, bleeding of nasal cavity origin must be distinguished from bleeding due to chronic sinusitis. In addition, nasopharyngeal or paranasal sinus tumors should be ruled out via x-ray films, as previously described. Differentiation among posterior epistaxis, hemoptysis, and hematemesis is critical if signs of anterior nasal bleeding are inapparent. In the absence of respiratory or gastrointestinal findings, a diagnosis of posterior epistaxis can be assumed if visual evidence exists for a posterior source of bleeding, if the majority of bleeding has occurred into the pharynx, or if anterior nasal packing fails to control hemorrhage.

Management

Specific treatment should be based on the underlying cause of epistaxis. If the etiology is undetermined, interventions should be geared toward alleviating anxiety related to symptoms of an unknown etiology, as well as stopping the bleeding. If the cause of epistaxis is found to be traumatic injury from nose picking and/or dry and cracked mucosa, advanced practice nursing interventions should be focused on educating the patient in self-care.

No pharmacological treatments to control acute nasal bleeding are available; however, any medication regimen that prolongs bleeding time should be reevaluated in the light of recurrent epistaxis. Initial treatment of uncomplicated anterior epistaxis consists of applying firm, continuous pressure for 10 to 15 minutes to both sides of the nose, immediately superior to the nasal alar cartilages. Patients should breathe through the mouth during this treatment period and must not release pressure to "sneak a peek" at the bleeding nares. To reduce vascular pressure, the patient should be seated upright with the head bent forward. Patients with no underlying medical problems may be treated at home, with directions to sit upright, minimize physical activity, and rest with the head elevated 45 to 90 degrees at night. Elderly or debilitated patients with epistaxis may require inpatient care, however, because of the increased risk of immunosuppression and anemia.

Recurrent minor epistaxis can be treated between episodes of active bleeding with vasoconstricting agents and/or chemical cauterization. A small piece of cotton or nasal pledget soaked in a topical vasoconstricting agent (such as 0.25% phenylephrine, 1:1,000 epinephrine, 0.1% xylometazoline, or 4% cocaine solution) should be applied to the nasal vestibule and pressed against the bleeding site for 5 to 10 minutes. Epinephrine should be avoided in hypertensive patients or those with coronary artery disease, and cocaine should be avoided in children. An ice pack may also be placed over the nose. Almost all venous anterior nosebleeds are stopped in this manner, but the treatment may need to be repeated. If this treatment fails, chemical cauterization of the bleeding site may be necessary. The mucosa should first be anesthetized with a cotton ball soaked in 4% cocaine, 4% lidocaine, or 2% lidocaine viscous preparation, held over the bleeding site for several minutes. Alternatively, 2% lidocaine jelly may be used. A bead of chromic acid, 25% to 50% trichloroacetic acid solution, or a silver nitrate stick is then applied directly onto the bleeding vessels with firm pressure for 30 seconds, which will allow for limited, shallow cautery of the bleeding site. Thermal or bipolar electrocautery may be required in cases of deeper lesions involving larger vessels; however, indiscriminate cauterization of a large area should be avoided.

If bleeding does not stop, anterior nasal packing should be placed to fill the entire nasal fossa. Layers of ½-in. × 72-in. gauze impregnated with petroleum jelly should be inserted in folding layers with a nasal speculum and bayonet forceps, extending as far back as possible to the posterior nasal choanae, while retaining the gauze ends at the nares. Each layer should be pressed firmly against the preceding one without disturbing the walls of the nasal cavity, with the folded ends alternating front and back in an accordion pattern. Typically, the entire 72-in. strip will be accommodated, if properly placed. A 2-in. × 2-in. gauze pad is then taped over the nostrils to prevent the anterior packing from dislodging and to catch dripping blood. Anterior packing should be removed within 2 to 3 days. The gauze inserts may be impregnated with an antibiotic cream or ointment to minimize bacterial growth and reduce odor. In addition, oral antibiotics may be administered if infection is suspected; however, the benefit of systemic antibiotics as a prophylactic measure (although common in practice) has not been confirmed by well-designed clinical trials. Recently, user-friendly nasal tampons have entered the market that are simply inserted in the nares in desiccated form and rehydrated by bathing them in 10 to 20 mL of saline or an antibiotic-containing solution (e.g., bacitracin). Posterior sources of bleeding require more complex treatment by a qualified specialist because this type of bleeding is usually more severe and difficult to control. Treatments include posterior nasal packing, sphenopalatine ganglion nerve block, and even surgical ligation of the compromised vessels. Nasal balloon-packing systems are an alternative to nasal packing, but they must not be overinflated and should be removed within 24 to 36 hours. Importantly, any form of nasal packing tends to be particularly painful for the patient once the local anesthetic has worn off, and oral or parenteral opioid analgesics should be considered. OTC analgesics such as acetaminophen may not be potent enough, whereas NSAIDs are best avoided because of their tendency to impair platelet function, which may lead to further bleeding.

All underlying medical conditions that might contribute to epistaxis should also be appropriately treated (e.g., platelet transfusions or clotting factor administration for coagulopathies). Iron supplements may be given if significant blood loss has occurred. If leukemia or another source of bone marrow immunosuppression is suspected as a causative factor of epistaxis, nasal packing should be avoided because of the increased risk of infection. In these cases, topical thrombin or hemostatic substances (Oxycel cotton or Gelfoam) should be first-line treatment.

Follow-up and Referral

Follow-up is not indicated for minor cases of nosebleed from local trauma or inflammation; however, the treatment of recurrent epistaxis should be monitored for effectiveness. Hemodynamics and blood loss should also be monitored in severe cases that require hospitalization. In the event of severe hemorrhage, anemia or even hypovolemia may develop. Various treatment modalities for epistaxis may also have important sequelae: Cocaine and lidocaine always present risks of toxicities when they are used. In addition, prolonged nasal packing may lead to infection of the nasal cavity, sinusitis, or impaired gas exchange, if poorly monitored. Excessive trauma during nasal packing or cauterization can result in septal hematoma, abscess, or perforation. External nasal deformities may also result from pressure necrosis from the anterior portion of nasal packing. Balloon-packing systems may result in mucosal pressure necrosis if the balloons are overinflated. Likewise, if the anterior portion of a two-balloon system breaks, the posterior balloon may migrate posteriorly down the airway and cause obstruction. Some patients experience vasovagal episodes during nasal packing and may pass out.

All cases of anterior epistaxis that are recurrent, particularly severe in blood loss, or refractory to vasoconstrictive or cauterization therapy should be referred to a specialist or emergency department, as appropriate. Hypovolemic or anemic patients require physician referral to evaluate the need for transfusion. Electrocautery for recurrent epistaxis caused by deep lesions should be performed only by a qualified specialist. Any elderly or debilitated patient who requires hospitalization for epistaxis should also be referred to a specialist. The management of posterior epistaxis requires a specialist because treatment modalities may include ganglionic nerve blocks, posterior nasal packing, and vessel ligation. Coagulopathy-related and malignancy-related epistaxis require specialized treatment related to the underlying disorder. Finally, infections resulting from nasal packing may necessitate referral to a specialist, especially if the patient is febrile.

Patient Education

Patients who have been treated for epistaxis should not blow their nose and should avoid sneezing for at least 12 hours after an acute episode to avoid dislodging the protective blood clot. Increased environmental humidity in the home also helps to prevent acute attacks, especially during the winter months. Petroleum jelly applied liberally to the nares promotes mucosal hydration, which helps prevent drying and cracking of the nasal mucosa. If nasal probing is persistent, the patient's fingernails should be cut to avoid mucosal trauma. Proper nasal pinching techniques should be demonstrated to enable patients to administer self-care at home for minor episodes of epistaxis. The importance of maintaining nasal mucosal hydration should be stressed, as well as the need to avoid nasal probing and vigorous blowing of the nose. The ability of certain medications to contribute to bleeding disorders (e.g., antiplatelet effects of aspirin, anticoagulant therapies such as warfarin) should also be discussed. Patients should be told not to swallow blood because this may upset the stomach, resulting in nausea, vomiting, or "gagging" (inhalation of blood into the trachea and bronchi). Patients should not talk during episodes of active bleeding for the same reason, and alcohol and hot liquids should be avoided after an acute attack.

■ RHINITIS

Rhinitis (coryza) is an inflammation of the nasal mucosa characterized by nasal congestion, rhinorrhea, sneezing, pruritus, and/or postnasal drainage. Its etiology is varied, but in general, it is categorized as either allergic or nonallergic rhinitis. Allergic rhinitis may be either seasonal or perennial. Nonallergic rhinitis may be (1) infectious, (2) irritant related (often in the workplace), (3) vasomotor, (4) hormone related, (5) associated with medication use or overuse (rhinitis medicamentosum), or (6) atrophic (seen primarily in geriatric patients). It may be acute or chronic, but the most common forms are viral rhinitis and perennial or seasonal ("hay fever") allergic rhinitis.

Although rhinitis is often a benign and self-limited disorder, poorly controlled allergic rhinitis may contribute to sleep loss, absenteeism from work or school, secondary daytime fatigue, learning impairment, decreased overall cognitive functioning, decreased long-term productivity, and decreased quality of life. In addition, poorly controlled rhinitis may lead to the development of other related disease processes, such as sinusitis, nasal polyps, OME, hearing impairment, aggravation of underlying asthma, and sleep apnea.

Epidemiology and Causes

Although the actual prevalence of acute rhinitis is undocumented, it is extremely common, occurring at least as frequently as the common cold. Moreover, an estimated 40 to 50 million U.S. adults suffer from some form of chronic rhinitis; some sources quote cumulative frequencies of 42% of the population of the United States by age 40. Specifically, the incidence of seasonal allergic rhinitis parallels pollen production, increasing in the fall and spring and peaking in the winter. Other forms of rhinitis may last year-round if they are caused by perennial allergens such as dust or house mites. Allergic rhinitis occurs in all age-groups, most commonly in adults aged 30 to 40 years, but it is rare in adults older than age 50. Onset of symptoms typically occurs between ages 10 and 20 years.

Nonallergic infectious rhinitis may be acute or chronic. Acute rhinitis is usually viral and self-limiting, whereas chronic rhinitis may be associated with bacterial sinusitis and may have associated allergic or mucociliary disturbances as predisposing factors. Rhinitis medicamentosum affects primarily young to middle-aged adults (correlating with medication use), and atrophic rhinitis affects primarily older adults, although the onset of symptoms may begin as early as puberty.

Most forms of rhinitis appear to have no ethnic predispositions. Hispanics, Asians, and African Americans seem to be particularly susceptible to atrophic rhinitis, however. In contrast, the incidence of this form is low in natives of equatorial Africa. Viral and atrophic rhinitis affect women more often than men, whereas most other forms affect both sexes equally.

Viral upper respiratory tract infections (URIs) occur more frequently in families with young children, whereas exposure to offending allergens is the primary risk factor for allergic rhinitis. The most common irritants implicated in the seasonal form are pollen and mold spores. Dust mites; insect debris (cockroaches, locusts, fish food); tobacco smoke; and animal dander, dried saliva, and urine are most common for the perennial form of allergic rhinitis. Immunosuppression secondary to illness or drug/medication use and a family history of allergic disease (e.g., eczema and/or asthma) are also risk factors for allergic rhinitis. Vasomotor rhinitis is aggravated by low humidity, sudden temperature or pressure changes, cold air, strong odors, emotional stress, cigarette smoke, and other nasal irritants. Use of nasal decongestants more frequently than every 3 hours or for periods longer than 3 weeks is the primary risk factor for the development of rhinitis medicamentosum. In some patients, certain drugs may precipitate rhinitis: Antihypertensive agents are the most frequently cited culprits. Angiotensin-converting enzyme inhibitors, beta-adrenergic antagonists, certain anti-inflammatory agents, guanethidine (Ismelin), clonidine (Catapres), hydralazine (Apresoline), prazosin (Minipress), chlordiazepoxide (Librium), amitriptyline (Elavil), or even aspirin can be a contributing factor. Oral contraceptive use and estrogen replacement therapy have also been implicated as risk factors for rhinitis, along with a family history of rhinitis and septal/anatomical obstruction. In addition, ingestion of certain foods may precipitate rhinitis in susceptible individuals. Illicit drug use such as cocaine snorting may precipitate rhinitis.

Pathophysiology

Viral rhinitis stems from an acute catarrhal response caused by viral replication in the nasopharynx, resulting in varying degrees of nasotracheal inflammation. Strongly associated with viral upper respiratory tract infection (URI or the "common cold"), the primary etiological agents of viral rhinitis include rhinovirus, influenza virus, parainfluenza virus, respiratory syncytial virus, coronavirus, adenovirus, echovirus, and coxsackievirus. When viral sinusitis is also present, the condition is collectively referred to as rhinosinusitis. The vast majority of rhinosinusitis is due to viral infection, but bacterial superinfection may complicate a small percentage of these cases. Anatomical defects or obstructions anywhere along the nasopharyngeal tract may predispose to infection by impairing physiological nasal drainage.

In contrast, allergic rhinitis results from immunoglobulin E (IgE)–mediated type I hypersensitivity to airborne irritants affecting the eyes, nose, sinuses, throat, and bronchi. IgE antibodies, elicited by repeated allergen exposure, bind to eosinophils and basophils in the bloodstream and their mucosal counterparts known as mast cells. These leukocytes subsequently degranulate, releasing chemoinflammatory substances, including histamine, leukotrienes, prostaglandins, slow-reacting substance of anaphylaxis, and erythrocyte chemotactic factor, which results in increased vasodilation, capillary permeability, mucus production, smooth muscle contraction, and

eosinophilia. On rare occasions, food allergies may be the cause. In addition, chemical or particulate airborne irritants may cause direct mucosal inflammation in the absence of IgE production or immune hypersensitivity.

Vasomotor rhinitis is a chronic, noninfectious process of unknown etiology without accompanying eosinophilia, characterized by periods of abnormal autonomic responsiveness and vascular engorgement unrelated to specific allergens. Fluctuations and reductions in estrogen associated with menses, hormonal birth control preparations, pregnancy, and menopause may all predispose to nonallergic rhinitis. Rhinitis medicamentosum is a rebound condition secondary to medication overuse. In some patients, it is caused by certain antihypertensive medications via undefined mechanisms, but most often mucosal inflammation results from the use of topical nasal decongestants such as phenylephrine (Neo-Synephrine) for greater than 3 to 4 days, which leads to secondary vasodilation, repeated small-vessel coagulation, and eventual fibrosis. Bacterial infection is thought to play a role in the development of atrophic rhinitis, in which the nasal epithelia and bones progressively atrophy, resulting in distinct morphological changes.

Clinical Presentation
Subjective

Viral rhinitis is typically accompanied by malaise, headache, sore throat, and occasionally fever. Patients with allergic rhinitis usually complain of itching in the nasal passages, conjunctivae, and roof of the mouth, as well as epiphora (stringy, watery ocular discharge). Sneezing, coughing, and a sore or burning throat commonly present in both viral and allergic rhinitis.

In contrast, patients with vasomotor rhinitis (noninfectious rhinitis without eosinophilia) rarely display any of the aforementioned symptoms. However, watery rhinorrhea, nasal congestion, "nasal" speech, and forced mouth-breathing are common complaints of patients with viral, allergic, vasomotor, or medication-related rhinitis. The onset of congestion is rapid in vasomotor rhinitis; patients typically complain of a pronounced, watery postnasal drip, as well as persistent nasal obstruction that may switch sides with each attack. Rhinitis medicamentosum patients may present with increased heart rate and elevated blood pressure because of the effects of sympathomimetic decongestants. Patients with atrophic rhinitis may complain of nasal congestion, a thick postnasal drip, frequent clearing of the throat, anosmia (impaired olfaction), a constant foul odor in the nose, and severe epistaxis (nosebleeds).

Objective

On inspection, the nasal mucosa typically appears erythematous in viral rhinitis, and throat inspection may reveal pharyngitis or laryngitis, characterized by erythematous and edematous pharyngeal mucosa or vocal cords. If the viral rhinitis is complicated by a secondary bacterial infection, the nasal discharge may be greenish yellow, which is indicative of purulence. In allergic rhinitis, the mucosa are pale, are boggy (edematous), and may take on a bluish hue. Yellowish, gray, or erythematous mucosa may also be seen. Gray-blue to yellow-tan nasal polyps may present with chronic perennial rhinitis. The conjunctivae are usually inflamed (allergic conjunctivitis), with the palpebral conjunctiva being particularly edematous (chemosis) and "cobblestoned" in appearance, owing to chronically infected blood vessels. Dark circles under the eyes ("allergic shiners") may be apparent, along with excess wrinkles under the lower eyelid (Dennie lines). In both viral and allergic rhinitis, the external nose may appear erythematous, with a transnasal crease resulting from repeated upward wiping and nose wrinkling (nasal salute). The nasal turbinates and palatine or pharyngeal tonsils (adenoids) may also be enlarged. The nasal mucosa in patients with vasomotor rhinitis will range from bright red to bluish in hue, and again, the nasal turbinates may be swollen. The mucosa in patients with rhinitis medicamentosum is also infected and edematous. In contrast, the mucosa in patients with atrophic rhinitis usually appear crusted with dried mucus or blood from repeated bouts of epistaxis, although the nasal passages typically remain patent.

The nasal mucosa in patients with viral rhinitis appears particularly friable. If present, nasal polyps are typically soft, edematous, and nontender. The external nose may be tender from repeated sneezing in patients with viral and allergic rhinitis. Some patients with rhinitis medicamentosum may present with dry and rubbery mucosa. On auscultation, wheezing breath sounds may reflect concurrent asthma associated with allergic rhinitis.

Diagnostic Reasoning
Diagnostic Tests

Laboratory tests are not typically indicated for uncomplicated cases of viral rhinitis, allergic rhinitis, or rhinitis medicamentosum. However, if an exudate is present in a colored or translucent nasal discharge, a Giemsa- or Wright's-stained smear should be prepared, along with a CBC to characterize the disease process. Leukocytosis or the presence of polymorphonuclear neutrophils in the discharge reflects an infectious disorder other than a typical viral URI. Eosinophilia in the discharge is indicative of allergic rhinitis. Peripheral eosinophil count and serum IgE levels have low predictive values; however, intradermal skin testing of minute amounts of allergens may be helpful if the diagnosis of allergic rhinitis is in doubt. Vasomotor rhinitis tends to be a diagnosis of exclusion because nasal smears and skin tests are typically negative, and no family history of allergic disorders is expected. Hormonally related rhinitis and rhinitis medicamentosum are diagnosed primarily through patient

history, once other common forms of rhinitis have been excluded. Atrophic rhinitis may be confirmed by nasal mucosal biopsy. Histopathology will demonstrate transformation of ciliated pseudostratified columnar epithelia into the stratified squamous form. In addition, the lamina propria will be decreased in thickness and vascularity, and bacterial culture of nasal secretions may also be helpful.

Differential Diagnosis

Acute or chronic sinusitis resulting from bacterial infection of the facial sinuses may also inflame the nasal mucosa. Sinus x-ray films demonstrating mucosal thickening, air-fluid levels, or opacification are effective at ruling out this disorder, as are cultures or smears of sinus aspirates to identify the infectious organisms present. Physical exam may rule out nasal foreign bodies, nasal polyps, or a deviated septum as causes of mucosal inflammation or congestion. Cocaine snorting, inhalant abuse (sniffing, huffing), and other forms of substance abuse should also be ruled out through a detailed patient history and, if appropriate, serum drug screens. Chronic inflammatory conditions such as sarcoidosis may be ruled out via biopsy, which would reveal granulomatous (histiocyte/macrophage) inflammation of the nasal mucosa. Hormonal changes associated with pregnancy and hyperthyroidism or hypothyroidism may also lead to nasal vasodilation and inflammation. Such conditions are ruled out through a careful physical exam, detailed patient history, and hematological hormone screens.

Management

With all types of rhinitis, much of the treatment regimen will focus on the relief of symptoms and self-care measures, although environmental issues must also be addressed.

Viral rhinitis is treated symptomatically, because viral URIs are predominantly self-limited. The following list outlines adult dosages:

- Fever and headache may be treated with acetaminophen 325 to 650 mg PO every 4 hours as needed (daily maximum dose 4,000 mg/day). Aspirin is not recommended because it may increase viral shedding. Rhinorrhea may be treated with oral decongestants such as pseudoephedrine (Sudafed) 30 to 60 mg PO every 3 to 4 hours as needed or topical preparations such as phenylephrine (Neo-Synephrine) 0.25% to 0.5% nasal spray one to two sprays in each nostril every 3 to 4 hours as needed for no more than 3 to 4 days.
- Intranasal ipratropium (Atrovent) 0.03% two sprays in each nostril 2 to 4 times daily as needed may also relieve excessive runny nose.
- Persistent coughs may be treated with dextromethorphan 15 to 30 mg PO every 3 to 4 hours as needed, but prescription codeine 10 to 15 mg PO every 3 to 4 hours as needed usually proves to be the only consistently effective cough suppressant.

For allergic rhinitis, avoidance or reduced exposure to offending allergens is the primary method of treatment because acute attacks are typically self-limited if not continually aggravated by allergen. Newer generation oral antihistamines designed to be less sedating are now the first-line short-term treatment of choice for allergic rhinitis. These work best for early symptoms of allergy such as sneezing, watery eyes, and ocular pruritus. However, intranasal corticosteroids have traditionally been considered the best means of controlling the longer-term symptoms of allergic rhinitis, including nasal congestion and discharge. In fact, meta-analyses have suggested that intranasal corticosteroids are the best overall first-line treatment for allergic rhinitis. It should be stressed, however, that intranasal steroid therapy may require 2 or more weeks of continuous daily use before symptomatic relief is apparent. Systemic steroids have significant side effects and tend to be discouraged for such a common condition. A newer class of medication, leukotriene receptor antagonists, has been approved for allergic rhinitis. Randomized controlled studies have shown montelukast (Singulair) to be as effective as loratadine (Claritin) in the symptomatic relief of allergic rhinitis.

Vasomotor rhinitis is also treated symptomatically, albeit at times unsatisfactorily, with environmental humidification using a vaporizer or humidified central heating system. Rhinorrhea may also be treated with systemic oral decongestants such as pseudoephedrine (Sudafed) 30 to 60 mg 3 or 4 times daily as needed. Congestion may also improve with topical saline nasal sprays. Thorough cleaning of the nose and restoration of nasal patency may be achieved using a powered device such as a Grossan nasal irrigator or a Neti pot. Intranasal ipratropium (Atrovent) 0.03% two sprays in each nostril 2 to 4 times daily as needed or azelastine (Astelin) two sprays in each nostril 2 times daily may also relieve symptoms. Rhinitis medicamentosum or "rebound rhinitis" is characterized by nasal congestion without rhinorrhea following the short-term use of topical vasoconstrictive medications. This condition can be remedied by immediately stopping all topical decongestant use. The condition typically resolves after 2 to 3 weeks.

- Oral antihistamine-decongestant preparations or short courses of topical nasal steroids may provide symptomatic relief.
- A short course of systemic steroids such as prednisone 30 mg PO daily for 5 days may be needed if other treatments prove ineffective.

Atrophic rhinitis may be treated with bacitracin ointment applied intranasally 2 or 3 times daily until the nasal crusting and foul odor are eliminated. Expectorants such as guaifenesin 400 mg PO every 4 hours as needed, physiological saline solutions as a nasal spray, regular use of a Neti pot or other means of nasal douching, or electric nasal irrigators (e.g., Grossan) may provide symptomatic relief. (See Complementary Therapies 8.1.) Menopausal women may be helped by systemic estrogens. See Drugs Commonly Prescribed 8.5: Rhinitis for more information.

Drugs Commonly Prescribed 8.5 Rhinitis

Drug	Indication	Dosage	Prescribing Considerations
Antihistamines—First Generation			
diphenhydramine (Benadryl)	Allergic rhinitis	25–50 mg PO every 4–6 hours; maximum 300 mg/day Children: 6–12 years: 12.5–25 mg PO every 4–6 hours; maximum 150 mg/day	Must use 3–5 hours before anticipated exposure or on a regular basis as long-term therapy. **Adverse effects:** CNS sedation, GI upset, anticholinergic effects (dry mouth, blurred vision), additive CNS-depressant effects of alcohol, sedative, hypnotics. Use with caution in older adults.
chlorpheniramine maleate (Chlor-Trimeton)		2–4 mg PO every 4–6 hours Children: <2 years not recommended; 2–5 years—1 mg PO every 4–6 hours; 6–11 years—2 mg PO every 4–6 hours	Must use 3–5 hours before anticipated exposure or on a regular basis as long-term therapy. **Adverse effects:** CNS sedation, GI upset, anticholinergic effects (dry mouth, blurred vision), additive CNS-depressant effects of alcohol, sedative, hypnotics. Use with caution in older adults.

Drugs Commonly Prescribed 8.5 Rhinitis—cont'd

Drug	Indication	Dosage	Prescribing Considerations
azelastine HCl (Astelin)	Seasonal rhinitis	(137 mcg/spray) two sprays per nostril 3 times daily Children: <5 years not recommended; 5–11 years—1 spray/nostril twice daily	Intranasal **Adverse effects:** Bitter taste, somnolence, CNS sedation, GI upset, anticholinergic effects (dry mouth, blurred vision), additive CNS-depressant effects of alcohol, sedative, hypnotics. Use with caution in older adults. Pregnancy Category C.

Antihistamines—Second Generation

Drug	Indication	Dosage	Prescribing Considerations
desloratadine (Clarinex) (Clarinex RediTabs)	Seasonal allergic rhinitis	5 mg PO daily dissolved on the tongue Children: <6 years use different formulation; 6–11 years—2.5 mg PO daily	**Adverse effects:** Pharyngitis, dry mouth, somnolence, headache, fatigue. Pregnancy Category C. Not recommended for nursing mothers.
loratadine (Claritin)	Rhinitis	10 mg PO daily Children: <2 years not recommended; 2–5 years—5 mg PO daily; >6 years—10 mg PO daily or 5 mg PO twice daily	**Adverse effects:** Headache, mild drowsiness. Not as effective as first generation; use in patients who cannot tolerate sedation.
cetirizine (Zyrtec)	Rhinitis	10 mg PO daily Children: <2 years not recommended; 2–6 years—2.5 mg PO daily; maximum 5 mg/day >6 years—5–10 mg PO daily	Somewhat more sedation than others, but less than first generation. Not as effective as first generation; use in patients who cannot tolerate sedation. **Adverse effects:** Drowsiness, somnolence, dry mouth, pharyngitis. Not recommended for pregnant women or nursing mothers.
fexofenadine (Allegra)	Rhinitis	60 mg PO 2 times daily or 180 mg PO daily Children: 2–11 years—30 mg PO twice daily	Not as effective as first generation; use in patients who cannot tolerate sedation. **Adverse effects:** Headache, back pain, viral infection, dizziness. Pregnancy Category C.
olopatadine (Patanase)	Seasonal allergic rhinitis	665 mcg/spray Two sprays per nostril 2 times daily Children: <6 years not recommended; 6–11 years—1 spray per nostril 2 times daily	Avoid eyes. Monitor for nasal mucosal changes. **Adverse effects:** Bitter taste, headache, epistaxis, throat pain, nasal ulceration, somnolence. Pregnancy Category C.

Continued

Drugs Commonly Prescribed 8.5   Rhinitis—cont'd

Drug	Indication	Dosage	Prescribing Considerations
Decongestants (Monotherapy)			
pseudoephedrine HCl (Sudafed)	Nasal congestion	30–60 mg PO every 4–6 hours; maximum 4 doses/day	Should not be used for longer than 3–4 days. Decongestant only. Can cause CNS excitation, hypertension, and palpitations. *Use with caution in elderly patients and those taking beta blockers. Contraindicated in patients with diabetes, benign prostatic hyperplasia (BPH), hypertension, monoamine oxidase (MAO) inhibitors, cardiac disease.*
Decongestants (Combination Therapy)			
NSAID and sympathomimetic (Advil Cold and Sinus)	Rhinorrhea, sinusitis, flu	One to two tablets every 4–6 hours; maximum 6 tablets/day	Should not be used for longer than 3–4 days. Take with food. *Use with caution in patients with hypertension, diabetes, glaucoma, BPH, and those taking beta blockers.*
diphenhydramine HCl (Benadryl) 25 mg and pseudoephedrine HCl (Sudafed) 60 mg	Rhinorrhea, nasal congestion	One tablet every 4–6 hours	Should not be used for longer than 3–4 days. *Do not use with MAO inhibitors or in patients with bronchospasm, hypertension, diabetes, BPH. Potentiates the effects of alcohol, sedatives.*
loratadine (Claritin) 10 mg and pseudoephedrine 50 mg (Claritin-D 24 Hour)	Rhinitis, sinusitis with congestion, allergic rhinitis	One tablet daily	Should not be used for longer than 3–4 days. Do not crush or chew. *Contraindicated in patients with glaucoma, BPH, hypertension, coronary artery disease (CAD). Use with caution in elderly patients and those taking beta blockers.*
fexofenadine HCl 60 mg and pseudoephedrine 120 mg (Allegra-D)	Seasonal rhinitis with nasal congestion	One tablet 2 times daily	Should not be used for longer than 3–4 days. Extend tab. Avoid giving with food.
Antihistamine and Sympathomimetic			
			Avoid other sympathomimetics. *Contraindicated in patients with glaucoma, BPH, or hypertension, and those taking MAO inhibitors.* **Adverse effects:** Palpitations, hypertension.
clemastine fumarate 1.34 mg and phenyl propanolamine HCl 75 mg (Tavist-D)	Rhinorrhea, nasal congestion, common cold	One tablet every 12 hours	Should not be used for longer than 3–4 days. Sustained release tablets. Do not crush or chew.

Drugs Commonly Prescribed 8.5 Rhinitis—cont'd

Drug	Indication	Dosage	Prescribing Considerations
			Use with caution in patients with hypertension, CAD, diabetes, and those taking MAO inhibitors, beta blockers, and CNS depressants, as well as in older adults.

Intranasal Corticosteroids

Drug	Indication	Dosage	Prescribing Considerations
beclomethasone dipropionate (Beconase AQ)	Decrease nasal inflammatory reaction	42 mcg/spray: one or two sprays per nostril 2 times daily	Available in aerosol and metered pump. May eliminate need for antihistamines or decongestants. Must be used regularly; onset of action in 2 or more days; use decongestant before application if necessary. **Adverse effects:** Local irritation, increased rhinorrhea, localized fungal infection.
budesonide (Rhinocort Aqua)	Decrease nasal inflammatory reaction	32 mcg/spray 2 sprays per nostril once daily Maximum dose 4 sprays per nostril once daily	Aerosol. May eliminate need for antihistamines or decongestants. Must be used regularly; onset of action in 2 or more days; use decongestant before application if necessary. **Adverse effects:** Local irritation, increased rhinorrhea, localized fungal infection. Caution with CYP3A4 inhibitors (e.g., ketoconazole). Pregnancy Category B.
ciclesonide (Omnaris)	Decrease nasal inflammatory reaction	50 mcg/spray: 2 sprays per nostril daily	Aerosol. May eliminate need for antihistamines or decongestants. Must be used regularly; onset of action in 2 or more days; use decongestant before application if necessary. **Adverse effects:** Local irritation, increased rhinorrhea, headache, pharyngitis, localized fungal infection. Respiratory TB. Pregnancy Category C.
fluticasone propionate (Flonase)	Allergic rhinitis	50 mcg/spray: 2 sprays per nostril daily or 1 spray per nostril 2 times daily	Available in metered pump. Maintain regular regimen. Monitor for visual changes. **Adverse effects:** Local irritation, increased rhinorrhea, localized fungal infection. Caution with CYP3A4 inhibitors (e.g., ketoconazole). Pregnancy Category C.

Continued

Drugs Commonly Prescribed 8.5   Rhinitis—cont'd

Drug	Indication	Dosage	Prescribing Considerations
triamcinolone acetonide (Nasacort)	Allergic rhinitis	55 mcg/spray: 2 sprays per nostril once a day	Available in aerosol or metered pump. Maintain regular regimen. Monitor for visual changes. **Adverse effects:** Headache, viral infections. Pregnancy Category C. It is unknown if drug accumulates in breast milk; however, other corticosteroids are excreted in breast milk. Nursing mothers should use with caution.
mometasone furoate (Nasonex)	Allergic rhinitis	50 mcg/spray: 2 sprays per nostril once daily	Begin 2–4 weeks before start of pollen season. Maintain regular regimen. Monitor for visual changes. **Adverse effects:** Local irritation, increased rhinorrhea, localized fungal infection. Caution with CYP3A4 inhibitors (e.g., ketoconazole). Pregnancy Category C.
Anticholinergic			
ipratropium bromide nasal spray 0.03%, 0.06% (Atrovent)	Prevention of rhinorrhea	21 mcg/spray: 2 sprays per nostril 2–3 times daily 42 mcg/spray: 2 sprays per nostril 2–3 times daily	Does not relieve itching or nasal blockage. **Adverse effects:** Epistaxis, pharyngitis, nasal dryness. Avoid in patients with BPH, glaucoma. Pregnancy Category B.
Mast Cell Stabilizer			
cromolyn sodium (Nasalcrom)	Prevention and relief of nasal allergy symptoms	5.2 mcg/spray: 1 spray per nostril 3 or 4 times daily; maximum 6 sprays/nostril/day	Regular use required. Do not use to treat sinus infection or asthma.
Other Categories			
Leukotriene receptor agonist (Singulair)	Seasonal rhinitis	4 mg or 5 mg chewable tabs PO once daily	Monitor with potent CYP450 inducers and with drugs metabolized by CYP2C8. **Adverse effects:** URI

Desensitizing immunotherapy may be an option for allergic rhinitis that is refractory to pharmacological treatment. Patients receive subcutaneous injections of purified allergen weekly at a dosage that increases with each treatment. The interval between injections is lengthened once a maintenance dose is reached. This treatment regimen may last up to 3 to 5 years, but it should not be continued past 12 months if symptoms are not improving; cure rates may be as low as 20%. In addition, to reduce the risk of anaphylactic reactions,

antigen injections must never be given intravenously. Occasionally, surgery is recommended if the etiology of refractory or recurrent rhinitis is anatomical, including nasal polypectomy for obstructing lesions or septoplasty if septal deviation is significant enough to interfere with the benefits of medication.

Follow-up and Referral

A return visit should be scheduled in 2 to 3 weeks to review patient education, adherence to the treatment plan, and effectiveness of prescribed treatments. After this, quarterly or biannual visits are recommended, depending on the patient's comfort level and general state of health.

Complications of most forms of rhinitis include serous OM (extension of nasal infection into the ear), acute or chronic sinusitis, and repeated or disseminated respiratory infections. Allergic rhinitis may lead to restless sleeping and chronic fatigue, and asthma may complicate allergic attacks. Rhinitis medicamentosum may be complicated by physical addiction to topical nasal decongestants, because relief periods shorten and severity of rebound congestion increases with each use. Thus, stopping the use of these drugs becomes especially difficult for the addicted patient.

Physician referral may be necessary for allergen skin testing, allergen immunotherapy, or nasal irrigation. The diagnosis and treatment of certain sequelae such as chronic sinusitis or high fever may also require physician referral. Surgical referral is necessary if anatomical obstructions of the nasal cavity (e.g., nasal polyps or a deviated septum) are etiological or complicating factors.

Patient Education

Viral rhinitis is best avoided by limiting exposure to persons with an acute URI. Allergic flare-ups are best prevented by avoiding exposure to environmental irritants. Many preventive steps may be taken. Windows and doors should be kept closed to reduce pollen entry into the household, and high-efficiency particle air (HEPA) filters are helpful in removing allergens from ambient air. Pet traffic from outside should be minimized because this may transport pollen indoors, and patients should avoid being outside on excessively sunny or windy days. Allergic attacks to mold spores can be prevented by avoiding piles of leaves during the fall months, by wiping down household surfaces where mold grows with bleach solutions, using HEPA filters, and reducing ambient humidity to 30% to 40%. Allergic attacks caused by perennial antigens such as dust or mites can be minimized by thoroughly cleaning or removing all carpets, drapes, curtains, and fabric-covered or stuffed furniture from the house, as well as by damp mopping, floor waxing, and dusting of all surfaces with a damp cloth. Stuffed animals, feather pillows, rubber mattresses, and box springs should either be covered with plastic or removed and replaced with synthetic materials, such as polyester. Chenille bedspreads, quilts, or comforters should be avoided, and bedding should be washed weekly. The use of air conditioning with frequent filter changes, rather than open windows, to cool automobiles or homes is recommended. Patients who are allergic to animal dander should bathe their pets often and restrict them from the bedroom or from the house altogether. Prophylactic use of 4% cromolyn sodium nasal spray (one spray in each nostril 3–6 times/day at regular intervals) before known antigen exposure may prevent allergic flare-ups but is ineffective once an attack is underway. Ophthalmic cromolyn sodium preparations are also available for the symptom of itchy eyes (1 to 2 drops can be instilled in each eye 4 to 6 times/day). Vasomotor rhinitis is also best avoided by limiting exposure to environmental triggers, and rhinitis medicamentosum can be prevented by diligently monitoring topical nasal decongestant use.

Patients with allergic rhinitis should be taught to avoid allergens and to observe the onset, duration, and progression of symptoms so that they can correlate their flare-ups to environmental conditions and thus better guide self-treatment. Emphasize all preventive and prophylactic measures, particularly the importance of keeping bedrooms allergen-free. Patients with all forms of rhinitis should understand the reasoning behind limiting nasal decongestant use, as well as the appropriate use of prophylactic cromolyn sodium sprays. It is also critical to explain that symptomatic relief from topical nasal steroid preparations may not be evident until 2 weeks into therapy. All patients should be instructed to arrange for further evaluation if clear rhinorrhea becomes purulent.

■ SINUSITIS

Sinusitis is an inflammation of the mucous membranes of one or more of the paranasal sinuses: frontal, sphenoid, posterior ethmoid, anterior ethmoid, and maxillary, with the latter two sinuses most often affected. This inflammation may be classified as (1) acute, which is characterized by an abrupt onset of infection and posttherapeutic resolution of symptoms lasting no more than 4 weeks; (2) subacute, in which a purulent nasal discharge persists despite therapy and lasts from 4 to 12 weeks; or (3) chronic, which occurs with episodes of prolonged inflammation with repeated or inadequately treated acute infection lasting greater than 12 consecutive weeks.

Epidemiology and Causes

The frequency of upper respiratory tract infections (the "common cold") accounts for the frequent occurrence of sinusitis in the general population. Researchers have estimated that 0.5% of all colds are complicated by bacterial infection of one or more of the paranasal sinuses. Acute bacterial sinusitis accounts for 16 million clinical visits annually, whereas chronic sinusitis is classified by the U.S. Public Health Service as the most common chronic disease in the United States and is estimated to account for more than 2 billion dollars a year in healthcare costs. Sinusitis affects adults of all ages, males and females equally, with no specific ethnic predisposition.

Mucosal inflammation and congestion from a viral URI that lasts more than 7 to 10 days is a primary risk factor for sinusitis (especially for maxillary sinus involvement), particularly during the autumn, winter, and spring seasons. Smoking; exposure to air pollution; persistent coughing; sneezing against a closed mouth; exposure to cold, damp outdoor weather or dry indoor heat; sudden changes in temperature; injury to the nose or sinuses from foreign bodies (e.g., nasogastric tubes or nasotracheal intubation) or trauma; nasal polyps; and chronic use of OTC or prescription decongestants may all impair mucociliary function, which can lead to mucosal inflammation, blockage of the sinus ostia, hypo-oxygenation of the sinuses, and transudation of fluid because of negative sinus pressure. Dental abscesses with oroantral fistulae extending into the paranasal sinuses can introduce pathogenic microorganisms; this etiology is associated with 10% to 15% of acute sinusitis cases. In addition, particularly during the summer months, airborne allergens, as well as swimming, diving, and jumping into contaminated water without holding the nose, are also common mechanisms for sinusitis to develop; allergic rhinitis is seen in 25% of sinusitis cases. Traveling in an airplane while suffering from a URI may predispose an individual to develop sinusitis. Recurrent or persistent bacterial infection resulting from blockage of nasociliary sinus drainage via the sinus ostia has been particularly associated with subacute and chronic sinusitis. Mechanical blockage may result from anatomical abnormalities such as a deviated septum, adenoidal hypertrophy, nasal polyps, reduced ostial diameter, and sinus or nasal neoplasms. Half of all asthmatic patients suffer from some form of sinusitis as a result of their inflammation-prone, hypersensitive airways. Furthermore, mucosal immunoglobulin A (IgA) deficiency, immobile cilia syndrome (Kartagener's syndrome), and cystic fibrosis also contribute to decreased mucociliary clearance and persistent sinus infection resulting from stasis. Chronic inflammatory diseases such as sarcoidosis and Wegener's granulomatosis also predispose patients to mucosal inflammation. In particular, diabetic, HIV-infected, malnourished, or other chronically immunocompromised patients may develop severe, invasive sinus disease.

Pathophysiology

Infection by nonendogenous pathogens and bacterial invasion of the sinuses by normal nasal or pharyngeal microbial flora are the primary causes of acute sinusitis. The vast majority (more than 95%) of acute sinusitis cases are caused by the same viruses associated with uncomplicated URIs. However, many of these patients do not seek primary-care interventions. Viral sinusitis (more accurately termed *viral rhinosinusitis*) is most commonly caused by the following five viruses, which collectively account for 80% of all URIs: rhinovirus (30%), coronavirus, adenovirus, echovirus, and coxsackievirus, as well as respiratory syncytial virus, parainfluenza virus, and influenza virus.

Viral rhinosinusitis is the main predisposing factor for acute bacterial sinusitis, which complicates about 2% of all cases. During these episodes, mucosal secretions from sinus goblet cells increase in volume and viscosity. The nasal mucosa also swells in response to viral

replication, creating an anatomical barrier to the steady outflow of nasal secretions. Nasal polyps, foreign bodies, allergen-induced mucosal swelling, and altered sensorium affecting nasal clearance and coordinated swallowing reflexes are other potential mechanisms of impaired nasal outflow. Moreover, the act of sneezing creates a tremendous pressure in the nasopharynx up to 60 to 80 mm Hg, capable of forcing fluid not only out the nares, but from the nasal cavity into the sinuses as well, transporting viruses and bacteria into these ideal environments for microbial replication. Here the normally ciliated pseudostratified, columnar epithelium lining the sinuses is eroded as infecting organisms proliferate, resulting in a loss of mucociliary clearance through sinus ostia (bony openings) and the ostiomeatal complex located in the anterior ethmoid region, which serves as a common drainage pathway for the frontal, maxillary, and ethmoid sinuses. Blockage of the ostiomeatal complex and/or impairment of ciliary function is thought to underlie all forms of sinusitis.

The only consistently reliable method of identifying causative organisms in acute sinusitis is direct sinus aspiration, which typically is performed only in controlled research trials or by ENT specialists because of its invasive nature. The most common bacterial pathogens isolated in acute sinusitis are *Streptococcus pneumoniae*, seen in nearly 40% of all cases, particularly during the summer and fall; *Haemophilus influenzae*, implicated in nearly 30% of all cases, especially in winter and spring; and, to a far lesser extent, *Moraxella (Branhamella) catarrhalis*, a far more common pathogen in children. Thus, the infectious agents of sinusitis closely pattern those of AOM. *Streptococcus pyogenes* (especially group A beta-hemolytic *Streptococcus*) and *Staphylococcus aureus* have each been identified in 5% of sinusitis cases studied, with *S aureus* most frequently isolated in intracranial complications. The specific role of bacteria, fungi, and viruses in chronic sinusitis is hotly debated. *S aureus*, gram-negative rods, and, in up to half of cases, anaerobic bacteria (including *Peptostreptococcus* and *Bacteroides*) are most often implicated. Polymicrobial infection is also more common in chronic than acute sinusitis. *S aureus* and *Pseudomonas aeruginosa* are the most common causes of cystic fibrosis–related and nosocomial sinus infection associated with nasal or endotracheal intubation and nasogastric feeding tubes.

In the immunocompromised host, gram-negative aerobic bacteria must be considered, as well as the fungi *Aspergillus fumigatus* and *Mucor* species, both of which may cause severe, rapidly invasive sinusitis in diabetic or otherwise chronically immunocompromised patients. More common than invasive fungal sinusitis, however, is allergic fungal sinusitis occurring in atopic individuals in which the nasal and sinus mucosa undergo an IgE-mediated type I hypersensitivity response to airborne fungal spores or fungal proliferation facilitated by obstructed sinus outflow. Dematiaceous (brown-pigmented) molds account for more than 75% of these cases, and *Aspergillus* is implicated in 10% to 20% of cases. The sinuses become filled with allergic mucin consisting of necrotic cellular debris, eosinophils, and fungal hyphae. If neither a hypersensitivity response nor an invasive sinusitis ensues, fungal colonization may result in unilateral chronic sinusitis characterized by formation of a dense fungal ball with sclerosis of the surrounding bone.

Clinical Presentation

Subjective

During the early stages of sinusitis, patients typically report a gradual onset of symptoms, including recurrent or chronic dull, constant pain over the affected sinuses (because of expanding purulent inflammation); as sinusitis progresses, pain increases and becomes characteristically throbbing. Typically, pain over the cheeks and upper teeth is correlated with maxillary sinus involvement; pain over the eyebrows indicates frontal sinus involvement; and pain over or behind the eyes indicates ethmoid sinusitis. Pain is exacerbated by coughing and sudden head movements. Specifically, frontal sinus pain may worsen with recumbency, whereas maxillary sinus pain may worsen when the patient is erect. Ethmoidal sinusitis is associated with retro-orbital pain. Notably, however, subacute and chronic sinusitis are often painless, as are some cases of acute sinusitis. These cases typically develop after at least 2 weeks of viral URI symptoms (such as a cough from postnasal drip, purulent nasal discharge, and headache). All types of sinusitis may present with nasal congestion (stuffiness), mucopurulent rhinorrhea (runny nose), a feeling of pressure inside the head, cough (in some cases), sore throat (in some cases), eye pain from ethmoid involvement, malaise, and fatigue. In particular, acute sinusitis is strongly predicted by maxillary toothache, a poor response to nasal decongestants, and a colored nasal discharge. Such patients usually report yellow-green or even blood-stained rhinorrhea, voice nasality, anosmia because of edematous nasal turbinates, early morning periorbital edema, fever and chills (in 25%–50% of cases), and a headache that is worse in the morning or when bending forward. These patients also sometimes report a nonproductive cough and disturbed sleep. Subacute or chronic sinusitis patients typically report a persistent cough or cold-like symptoms that may last from several weeks to several months, as well as a headache or feeling of pressure specifically across the cranial midline. Fever is less common, and most patients have a past history of responding poorly to sinusitis pharmacotherapy. Other symptoms include a thick postnasal discharge (postnasal drip), "popping" ears, excessive tearing, toothache-like cheek pain, difficulty chewing, and halitosis. Immunocompromised patients may present with more subtle signs and symptoms, because leukopenia may limit the inflammatory response to infection.

Objective

On inspection, purulent nasal secretions (recognized by polymorphonuclear neutrophils in a Giemsa-stained nasal smear) and total opacification of affected sinuses on transillumination (e.g., through the supraorbital or maxillary bony ridges) are strongly predictive of acute sinusitis. Although only one in four patients with decreased transillumination typically has a sinus infection, complete light transmission rules out an active sinus infection. A nasal speculum should be used to examine the anterior nasal passages. A red, swollen nasal mucosa indicates infection; a pale mucosa that appears swollen, with watery secretions, points to allergic sinusitis or rhinitis. Purulent secretions seen coming from inside the middle meatus are characteristic of sinusitis. Black or necrotic material may be seen in mucormycosis-related rhinorrhea in immunocompromised patients. Ethmoid sinus involvement may result in chemosis (eyelid mucous membrane edema), proptosis, conjunctival injection, extraocular muscle palsy, or orbital fixation.

On palpation, the affected sinuses may be exquisitely tender to palpation. Sphenoid sinusitis presents as tenderness over the vertex or mastoids, ethmoid sinusitis as retro-orbital or nasal bridge tenderness, maxillary sinusitis as cheek or dental tenderness, and frontal sinusitis as tenderness of the forehead. In the event of maxillary sinusitis related to a dental abscess, percussion over the affected sinus will produce marked tenderness in the teeth and gums.

Diagnostic Reasoning

Diagnostic Tests

It is important for the clinician to put the emphasis on clinical signs and symptoms for initial diagnosis and avoid unnecessary diagnostic tests. Even though laboratory tests and x-ray films are not needed for typical presentations of sinusitis, anteroposterior, lateral, and particularly occipitomental sinus x-ray exams can be done if symptoms show no improvement after 4 to 5 days of pharmacotherapy. Air-fluid levels, mucosal thickening beyond 4 mm, or complete opacification of the sinuses on any of these views is strongly suggestive of sinusitis. However, it should be noted that such mucosal thickening as well as impaired sinus transillumination on physical exam have both been observed in healthy, asymptomatic individuals who do not meet the criteria for acute sinusitis. In turn, the positive and negative predictive value of these diagnostic tests has consistently been questioned in the literature.

A CBC to detect leukocyte elevation may be indicated if an infectious etiology is suspected in acute sinusitis; however, leukocytosis is rarely observed in chronic sinusitis. Stains or cultures of nasal and throat secretions do not correlate with the causative agents of sinusitis because the nasopharyngeal mucosa is widely colonized by a diverse array of endogenous, nonpathogenic microbial flora. However, the presence of at least 10,000 organisms/mL on Gram stain of sinus aspirates may confirm the presence of local sinus infection. Allergic skin testing may be necessary if the patient history suggests allergic disease (e.g., allergen exposure, seasonal attacks), and these patients often demonstrate peripheral eosinophilia and elevated total or allergen-specific IgE levels. Culture and microscopic examination of sinus aspirates, sinus mucosal biopsy, or flexible fiberoptic rhinoscopy by a well-trained specialist is typically needed only for subacute, chronic, or suspected fungal sinusitis cases that are refractory to several courses of empiric pharmacotherapy or when intracranial extension is suspected. Chronic sinusitis, in particular, is characterized by a morphological change of the ciliated sinus epithelia to a hypertrophied, stratified squamous form that is evident on biopsy.

Although sinus CT scans may demonstrate mucosal thickening and osteomeatal occlusion in a large number of people with uncomplicated viral URI, this type of imaging may be helpful in cases of chronic sinusitis, infection that has spread into orbital or intracranial regions (e.g., orbital cellulitis or brain abscess), or for an immunocompromised host, to fully evaluate the disease process. Sinus MRI is superior for soft tissue discrimination but is poor at visualizing bony structures. Thus, MRI tends to be reserved for suspected sinus neoplasia or extension of sinus disease into intracranial soft tissues.

Differential Diagnosis

Myofascial pain that is unrelated to infectious causes may mimic the pain from acute sinusitis, but pain from other myofascial disorders is typically more diffuse and does not progressively worsen. Uncomplicated dental abscesses may produce a similar pain, but the pain will not extend into the maxillary sinus on physical exam. Patients with migraine, cluster headache, or trigeminal neuralgia also present with fascial and cranial pain, but, again, the sinuses will be nontender to palpation, and the accompanying signs and symptoms of inflammation will not be observed in these patients. Allergic rhinitis, vasomotor rhinitis, rhinitis medicamentosa, mechanical nasal airway obstruction, acute viral URI (persistent viral rhinitis), and chronic inflammatory conditions such as sarcoidosis or Wegener's granulomatosis may all present with nasal congestion or pain. If these cases are uncomplicated by sinusitis, no signs of sinus inflammation will be detected on examination.

If a patient has had an URI for at least 7 days, the presence of two or more of the following signs and symptoms will confirm the diagnosis of sinusitis: colored nasal drainage, poor response to decongestant, facial or sinus pain (particularly if aggravated by postural change or Valsalva maneuver), and headache. In addition, a documented history of prior episodes of sinusitis, a fever higher than 102°F (38.9°C), and tooth pain accompanying these findings all support a diagnosis of sinusitis. Viruses may produce all of the clinical manifestations described; however, patients who meet the 7-day criteria described in the preceding text are more likely to have bacterial sinusitis than a viral URI.

Management

It is important to realize that because the vast majority of acute sinusitis cases are caused by viruses rather than bacteria, antibiotics are largely unhelpful. Their indiscriminate use for symptom complexes failing to meet the aforementioned diagnostic criteria for bacterial sinusitis offers no medical benefit, wastes financial resources, and is potentially harmful in that it encourages widespread antibiotic resistance in common nasopharyngeal flora. With this in mind, antimicrobial therapy usually cures acute uncomplicated bacterial sinusitis, although recurrence is not uncommon. Adjunctive measures may also be used to enhance mucociliary clearance, countering the main risk factor for the development of sinusitis. Saline nasal spray may be helpful in improving sinus drainage, but dedicated sinus irrigation two or more times a day with an adequate volume of saline to fully flush the sinuses has been shown to significantly relieve symptoms even without antimicrobial therapy. Patients are instructed to infuse their sinuses using a warm isotonic or hypertonic saline-filled bulb syringe expressed into each nare, followed by immediate drainage of the liquid over a sink to remove both infectious organisms and excess mucus. A number of commercial saline sinus irrigation systems with balanced salt solutions are currently available. However, homemade preparations may be made by mixing 1 teaspoon of salt with 8 ounces of warm water; noniodized salt should be used, because iodine is a known mucosal irritant. A cool-mist, ultrasonic humidifier (cleaned daily with a 1:10 solution of bleach and water) may also assist in thinning sinus secretions and facilitating drainage. Smoke and other environmental pollutants should be avoided. Fluid intake should be increased, and heated mist from a facial sauna, steam bath, shower, or hot, moist towels wrapped around the face may help relieve sinus and nasal pain by liquefying secretions.

Oral analgesics may also be used for pain (e.g., ibuprofen [Motrin, Advil] 400–600 mg every 6–8 hours as needed, acetaminophen [Tylenol] 650 mg every 4–6 hours as needed, or a stronger combination of acetaminophen 300 mg/codeine 30 mg [Tylenol 3] one to two tablets every 4–6 hours as needed). In general, nonprescription medicated nose drops and sprays should be avoided, and prescription nasal sprays should be taken no longer than 3 to 4 days at a time because long-term use can lead to rebound nasal congestion (rhinitis medicamentosum) and addiction. Phenylephrine (Neo-Synephrine; one to two upright sprays in each nostril 3–4 times daily as needed) or the stronger oxymetazoline (Afrin; one to two upright sprays in each nostril 2–3 times daily as needed) may be helpful in adults. Pseudoephedrine (Sudafed) 30 to 60 mg every 4 to 6 hours as needed is an oral alternative but tends to be less effective than topical preparations. Expectorants such as guaifenesin 200 to 400 mg every 4 hours as needed and iodinated glycerol 30 to 60 mg PO 4 times daily as needed are used to liquefy sinus secretions and facilitate drainage. Anti-inflammatory topical steroids in nasal spray preparations such as fluticasone 0.05% (Flonase), mometasone (Nasonex), or triamcinolone (Nasacort), all at two sprays in each nostril daily, used for 2 to 3 weeks are becoming increasingly popular; however, randomized controlled trials have been inconsistent with regard to their effectiveness. In fact, steroid therapy has actually been shown to increase viral load in acute viral rhinosinusitis. Oral antihistamines should be avoided unless an allergic component is evident because they tend to dry the mucosa, thicken purulent sinus fluids, and slow mucosal drainage, although some studies have suggested their efficacy in symptomatic relief of uncomplicated viral URIs.

Although localized sinus infection may be self-limited, antibiotic and symptomatic therapy may be considered appropriate for suspected bacterial sinusitis to prevent disease progression and complications. Empiric antibiotic therapy for 5 to 10 days covering the most common etiological agents should be instituted before the identification of causative organisms because symptoms may progress while laboratory confirmation is awaited. In adults, common choices include narrow-spectrum antibiotics such as amoxicillin (Amoxil) 500 mg to as high as 1 g PO 3 times daily, trimethoprim/sulfamethoxazole (Bactrim) 160 mg/800 mg one double-strength tablet PO 2 times daily, or doxycycline 100 mg PO 2 times daily. In light of increasing resistance of *Streptococcus pneumoniae, Haemophilus influenzae* (up to 50% of strains), *Moraxella catarrhalis,* and virtually all *Staphylococcus aureus,* one of the following beta-lactamase–resistant alternatives may be considered: amoxicillin/clavulanate (Augmentin XR) 1,000 mg/125 mg PO 2 times daily, clarithromycin (Biaxin XL) 1,000 mg PO daily, cefaclor (Ceclor; second generation cephalosporin) 500 mg PO every 6 hours, cefpodoxime (Vantin; third generation cephalosporin) 200 mg PO 2 times daily, cefdinir (Omnicef; third generation cephalosporin) 600 mg PO daily, levofloxacin (Levaquin) 750 mg PO daily, or moxifloxacin (Avelox) 400 mg PO daily. In fact, current treatment guidelines for acute bacterial sinusitis in adults consider first-line therapy to be amoxicillin either with or without clavulanate, depending on whether risk factors for antibiotic resistance are present (e.g., high endemic rates of penicillin-resistant *Streptococcus pneumonia,* antibiotic use within the last 30 days, severe infection with systemic symptoms such as fever ≥ 102°F, age >65 years, recent hospitalization, or immunocompromised status). Penicillin-allergic or cephalosporin-allergic patients are usually steered toward an oral quinolone or trimethoprim/sulfamethoxazole as first-line therapy. Immunocompromised hosts typically require broad-spectrum coverage for gram-positive and gram-negative organisms and possibly empiric antifungal therapy. Tetracyclines do not cover *Streptococcus pneumoniae,* however, and erythromycin, penicillin, and first generation cephalosporins do not cover *Haemophilus influenzae.* Acute infections that fail to

clear after one course of antibiotic therapy are often treated with a second course from a separate antibiotic class for 14 days.

Antibiotics against anaerobic organisms such as *Peptostreptococcus* and *Bacteroides* are typically required for subacute and chronic sinusitis, with regimens lasting up to 3 to 4 weeks or even as long as 6 weeks for refractory chronic cases. Antibiotic regimens include amoxicillin/clavulanate (Augmentin XR) 1,000 mg/125 mg PO every 12 hours or cefuroxime (Ceftin; second generation cephalosporin) 250 to 500 mg PO 2 times daily. For penicillin-allergic patients, antibiotics include clarithromycin (Biaxin XL) 500 mg PO daily or clindamycin (Cleocin) 300 mg PO every 6 hours; for documented gram-negative infection, one of the fluoroquinolones (e.g., levofloxacin or moxifloxacin) should be prescribed at the doses mentioned previously. Patients requiring three or more antibiotic courses will likely benefit from referral to an otorhinolaryngologist for further diagnostic work-up. Similarly, serious invasive fungal sinusitis often requires surgical debridement and inpatient intravenous antifungal therapy with amphotericin B (1 mg/kg IV daily) or, if not tolerated due to rigors, chills, or hypotension, a liposomal amphotericin preparation (Abelcet; 5–7.5 mg/kg IV daily). In contrast, allergic fungal sinusitis calls for sinus drainage and systemic corticosteroids for 2 to 4 weeks followed by topical steroid therapy, because the benefits of antifungal therapy have not been clearly demonstrated. Fungal balls associated with sinus colonization must be removed surgically, because neither steroids nor antifungals have been shown to be effective in relieving obstruction.

Maxillary sinus puncture and aspiration may be needed to relieve pain in any form of sinusitis that fails to subside following pharmacotherapy, and patients with subacute or chronic sinusitis may require surgery to remove damaged mucosal tissue or to correct anatomical obstructions of the sinus ostia such as recurrent nasal polyps. In addition, complementary therapies may be considered in the treatment of patients with chronic sinusitis. Several studies indicate that vigorous exercise, for example, has been shown to improve nasal function (through vasoconstriction and decreased nasal resistance) in healthy patients, as well as those with allergic rhinitis. The same benefits may also result in patients with chronic sinusitis. Some patients with particularly severe chronic disease have reported trying acupuncture, herbal therapies, biofeedback, and self-help groups.

Prompt treatment of all respiratory infections can prevent acute sinusitis complications, and surgery to correct anatomical blockages of the sinus ostia (e.g., deviated septum or nasal polyps) may prevent chronic sinusitis. When sinus inflammation is connected with an allergy, desensitization by a trained allergist should be considered. Recurrent attacks of sinusitis can sometimes be prevented by the routine use of a humidifier and/or air conditioner. Nose drops or sprays should be discarded after use during an acute episode, however, and should never be shared to avoid person-to-person transmission of infectious organisms.

Follow-up and Referral

Patients should be reevaluated for symptomatic improvement in 48 to 72 hours, and a return visit should be scheduled for 10 to 14 days from the initial assessment. If symptoms fail to improve with pharmacotherapy, the patient should be evaluated for antibiotic resistance, allergic contributions, or immunological abnormalities. Sinus x-ray films may remain abnormal for up to 2 months after the resolution of acute sinusitis, so follow-up films to document improvement are not usually indicated until at least 6 weeks after initial therapy. Immunocompromised patients with sinusitis should be monitored daily in an inpatient setting.

Although complications are relatively uncommon, visual impairments, ophthalmoplegia, orbital or facial cellulitis, severe fever, aphasia, abducens palsy (CN VI deficit), seizures, altered mental status, osteomyelitis of the frontal or maxillary bones, and focal swelling over the frontal bone are all reflective of localized extensions of bacterial infection. Rare but potentially life-threatening complications that require a high index of suspicion include meningitis, subdural empyema, epidural abscess, cavernous sinus thrombosis, and other CNS complications.

Patients should be referred to a specialist if their sinusitis is allergic or immunological, refractory to antibiotic therapy, recurrent, or associated with unusual opportunistic infections, or when the infection is adversely affecting their quality of life. In addition, when sinusitis is associated with chronic OM, bronchial asthma, nasal polyps, recurrent pneumonia, immunodeficiency, allergic fungal disease, granulomas, or multiple antibiotic resistances, the patient should be referred to an allergist or an otolaryngologist.

Patient Education

Patients should be instructed to be wary of worsening symptoms after the institution of pharmacotherapy. Patients should also be informed of potential complications and should be instructed to contact the practitioner at once if telltale signs such as periorbital swelling develop. The clinician should stress the importance of avoiding contact with all contributing factors (e.g., cigarette smoke or airborne allergens), as well as the exacerbating side effects of nonprescription antihistamine use. Patients should make sure that OTC decongestant preparations do not contain antihistamines, and they should drink plenty of fluids to thin nasal secretions.

■ STOMATITIS AND GLOSSITIS

Stomatitis is a generalized inflammation of the oral mucous membranes characterized by erythema and/or vesicular or ulcerative lesions. *Glossitis* is an acute or chronic inflammation of the tongue that shares many of the same etiologies as stomatitis. Either of the two may present alone, although glossitis often accompanies stomatitis, and clinicians often group the two conditions together under the latter designation. In general, both disorders are classified according to their etiology, which is extremely variable.

Epidemiology and Causes

A variety of types of stomatitis are seen in adults; these include oral candidiasis, aphthous stomatitis (aphthous ulcers, or "canker sores," often reoccur, and may be referred to as recurrent aphthous stomatitis [RAS]), secondary herpetic stomatitis/herpes labialis, Vincent's stomatitis (acute necrotizing ulcerative gingivitis, or "trench mouth"), allergic stomatitis, nicotinic (cigarette-related) stomatitis, denture-related stomatitis, angular stomatitis, pseudomembranous stomatitis, and parasitic glossitis (black hairy tongue, anthracosis linguae). Glossitis is also a common symptom of systemic skin diseases such as erythema multiforme (Stevens-Johnson syndrome) and pemphigus vulgaris. Herpetic stomatitis and RAS occur commonly, as do nicotinic and denture-related stomatitis. Other causes are less commonly seen.

Herpes simplex virus (HSV) infection in the United States is widespread. According to recent estimates, up to 20% of the adult population may be secreting herpes simplex type 1 or 2 viruses at any given time. The prevalence of HSV-specific antibodies indicative of past or dormant HSV infection is up to 30% in higher socioeconomic strata and may approach 100% in lower socioeconomic groups. In general, prevalence of infection is estimated to be between 20,000 and 70,000 per 100,000. Oral candidiasis most commonly occurs in immunocompromised adults, such as patients with HIV infection or in cancer patients after chemotherapy and/or radiation therapy. Nicotinic stomatitis and denture-related stomatitis are common. Most other forms are rare among adults. Mouth sores may affect adults of all ages. Specifically, Vincent's stomatitis is seen among adolescents and adults aged 20 to 40 years, whereas denture-related stomatitis affects primarily elderly patients.

Chronic mouth-breathing dries the tongue and oral mucosa, and hot foods or beverages may lead to thermal injury. Chemical irritation may result from spicy, acidic, or salty foods such as potato chips and pickles, as well as from peroxide-containing mouthwashes, toothpaste, and other dental care products. Viral, bacterial, and fungal infections, prolonged radiation or chemotherapy treatments, long-term corticosteroid or antibiotic use, chronic metabolic diseases such as diabetes, emotional or physical stress, anxiety, depression, premenstrual tension, advanced age, low socioeconomic status, and malnourishment may all contribute to host immunosuppression and in turn to the development of stomatitis/glossitis. Systemic autoimmune or inflammatory diseases also predispose patients to these conditions. Pregnancy has been associated with erythema multiforme. Tobacco smoking and chewing (dipping snuff) clearly can lead to nicotinic stomatitis, whereas ill-fitting dentures, recent dental work, repeated biting during convulsive seizures, and poor oral/dental hygiene contribute to mechanical injury–related inflammation of the oral cavity and tongue. Occupational or domestic exposure to chemical irritants or allergens are risk factors, as are resective gastrointestinal surgery involving the ileum and malabsorptive disorders of the ileal mucosa such as sprue (villous atrophy), both of which impair vitamin B_{12} absorption, contributing to angular and other vitamin deficiency–related forms of stomatitis. In fact, anemia of any type is a risk factor. Repeated emesis secondary to bulimia may inflame the oral mucosa and erode the posterior (lingual) surfaces of the teeth because of repeated exposure to stomach acid in the vomitus. In addition, anorexia, bulimia, and off-and-on ("yo-yo") dieting may lead to malnourishment, vitamin deficiencies, or immunosuppression.

Prior HSV infection is the primary risk factor for all secondary manifestations of herpes simplex infection. In addition, any factors that lead to immunosuppression may be considered contributing factors. Specifically, fever, physical and/or emotional stress, excess sun exposure, menstruation, common colds, gastrointestinal upset, and dental work that excessively stretches the mouth, as well as other underlying systemic illnesses, may be considered precipitating factors. Intercourse with multiple sexual partners and unprotected sex (failure to use barrier protection, e.g., condoms during intercourse or oral sex or latex dental dams during oral sex) increase the likelihood of HSV transmission from infected sexual partners.

Pathophysiology

In general, excessive dryness of the oral cavity; food and drug allergies; chemical irritation; mechanical or thermal injury; bacterial, fungal, and viral pathogens (e.g., coxsackievirus causing hand-foot-and-mouth disease, varicella-zoster virus causing oral and lingual vesicular lesions, primary HIV infection); host immunosuppression; and nutritional deficiencies of iron, folate, riboflavin (B_2), niacin, pyridoxine (B_6), and cyanocobalamin (B_{12}) are all risk factors that can cause stomatitis and glossitis. Aphthous ulcers are one of the most common types of oral lesions, yet their pathogenesis is poorly defined. Stress, hormonal fluctuations, inflammatory bowel disease, and antimetabolite chemotherapies all predispose a patient to aphthae. Specifically, the spirochete *Borrelia vincentii* and certain fusiform *Bacillus* bacterial species are strongly associated with Vincent's stomatitis, although some cases are of indeterminate etiology. If complicated by HIV infection and left untreated, this condition may progress to necrotizing stomatitis. Nicotinic stomatitis results directly from the chemical irritants in tobacco. Denture-related stomatitis results from the mechanical injury caused by ill-fitting dentures. Angular stomatitis is symptomatic of the vitamin deficiencies discussed in

the preceding text, and pseudomembranous stomatitis has been associated with numerous chemical irritants and bacterial pathogens.

Parasitic glossitis is caused by several mycoses of the tongue, including *Cryptococcus linguae-pilosasae* and *Nocardia lingualis* co-infection. The use of systemic antibiotics is well known to clear normal microbial flora from the oral cavity and, in fact, the entire gastrointestinal tract, thus facilitating fungal overgrowth caused by the lack of endogenous microbial competition. In addition, both oral and inhaled steroids are known to compromise cellular immunity within the oral cavity—the main defense mechanism against fungal overgrowth and infection. HIV infection and AIDS, malignancy, chemotherapy, diabetes mellitus, and age-related decreases in natural immunity may all contribute to immune suppression as well, increasing the likelihood of fungal overgrowth and viral reactivation of HSV.

Erythema multiforme is a widespread immune-mediated inflammatory reaction of the skin and in the advanced stages can involve the mucous membranes, including the oral cavity. This condition may be caused by different types of infection (e.g., HSV, *Mycoplasma*, *Streptococcus pyogenes*), drug allergies (e.g., anticonvulsants, sulfonamides, allopurinol), as well as collagen vascular disorders. However, oral involvement in erythema multiforme, as well as its extreme forms (Stevens-Johnson syndrome, toxic epidermal necrolysis) will never be isolated to stomatitis, because these are systemic, life-threatening conditions. In contrast, the etiology of pemphigus vulgaris is unknown, but flaccid bullae typically begin in the oropharynx as superficial epidermal layers separate from their base. A similar appearing blistering disorder, bullous pemphigoid, only rarely presents with isolated oral lesions; but as this disease progresses, roughly one-third of individuals may demonstrate oral involvement. A number of inherited disorders of the epidermis and dermis known collectively as epidermolysis bullosa may also involve the oral mucosa in their moderate and severe forms. Finally, a wide array of autoimmune disorders such as systemic lupus erythematosus may also present with mucosal ulcerative lesions.

Clinical Manifestations
Subjective

In general, patients with stomatitis may complain of excessive dryness of the mouth; halitosis; difficulty speaking or swallowing; minor to severe oral pain; or bleeding, swollen, or erythematous gums; as well as constitutional symptoms (including fever, malaise, headache, and weight loss) that may be secondary to infection or malnourishment. Additionally, patients with Vincent's stomatitis may complain of excess salivation. Patients with secondary herpetic stomatitis usually report a 24- to 48-hour prodrome consisting of a burning sensation in the mouth, followed by the appearance of 1- to 2-mm vesicular lesions, initially fluid-filled bullae, which then evolve into ulcerated lesions, which eventually crust over the course of several days. These frequently appear around the lips. Although most patients report only one to two recurrences per year, 5% to 25% of patients suffer more than one attack per month. Patients may also report itching and burning in the mouth, particularly in cases of allergic stomatitis. In contrast, parasitic glossitis is usually painless, whereas anemia and niacin deficiency lead to lingual pain.

Objective

The mouth and the tongue (if also inflamed) often appear bright red and swollen, either at the tip and edges (from vitamin deficiencies or mechanical injury) or over the entire glossal surface. Depending on the cause of inflammation, the tongue may be ulcerated (from niacin deficiency, streptococcal infection, erythema multiforme, or pemphigus) or smooth and pale (from iron, folate, or B_{12} deficiencies). Vincent's stomatitis causes necrotic ulceration of the interdental gingival papillae and oral mucous membranes, characterized by a purulent, gray exudate. Allergic stomatitis causes intense, shiny erythema and slight swelling of the mucosa and tongue. Nicotinic stomatitis presents with centrally erythematous white nodular elevations, and pseudomembranous stomatitis produces a membrane-like exudate coating the oral mucosa. Inflammation and external fissuring of the corners of the mouth are characteristic of angular stomatitis. Parasitic glossitis presents with hypertrophied (1-cm) filiform papillae that color the dorsum of the tongue dark brown or black. In contrast, syphilis and mouth-breathing result in white patches on the tongue. Erythema multiforme presents with polymorphous disseminated macular, papular, nodular, vesicular, bullous, and target (bull's-eye–shaped) lesions of the skin and mucous membranes. Pemphigus is also characterized by disseminated thin-walled bullae throughout the skin and mucosa, which, when ruptured, leave raw patches. The lesions of pseudomembranous stomatitis cannot be scraped off with a tongue blade, whereas the lesions of parasitic glossitis are easily broken. Anterior cervical or jaw lymphadenopathy may be felt in cases that are related to autoimmune or systemic inflammatory disease.

Inspection of the oral mucosa of patients with HSV infection reveals individual or groups of 1- to 2-mm vesicular lesions that evolve into ulcers, apparent after the prodromal period (24–48 hours, characterized by pain, tingling, burning, and itching preceding vesicle formation), particularly on the gingivae, hard palate, buccal mucosa, and tongue. If observed at a later stage of healing (4–10 days after vesicle formation), oral lesions may appear ulcerated but crusted over. Herpes labialis presents as similar clusters of open vesicular lesions in the labial area, particularly at the mucocutaneous border, with erythematous bases and possibly crusting, if the lesions are in an advanced stage of healing. Palpation of the oral mucosa may demonstrate edema or tenderness, aiding in the identification and characterization of oral lesions. Anterior cervical or jaw lymphadenopathy may be felt in both conditions.

Although not directly related to HSV infection, back percussion to the posterior lungs may reveal the dull tones of pulmonary consolidation characteristic of lung infections (e.g., tuberculosis) common to HIV infection, AIDS, or other immunocompromising disorders that often underlie the reactivation of HSV infection. Likewise, chest auscultation may reveal signs such as crackles, crepitus, or wheezing, which may indicate the presence of systemic inflammatory disease or pulmonary infections secondary to an underlying immune disorder.

Oral candidiasis may exhibit diverse clinical patterns, and some patients exhibit more than one form. Factors that affect clinical presentation are the immune status of the host, such as the presence of HIV or a history of organ transplant, as well as the oral mucosal environment, for example, the impaired salivary function seen in Sjögren's syndrome, postradiation xerostomia, or age-related atrophy, and whether the person is dentate or edentulous (more common) and a nonsmoker or smoker (more common). Pseudomembranous candidiasis, also known as "thrush," is recognized by the development of creamy white plaques that resemble cottage cheese or curdled milk. When these plaques are scraped off, an erythematous mucosa is exposed. There is also an erythematous candidiasis, in which the oral mucosa appear fiery red and the mouth feels like it has been "scalded with a hot beverage." This form often follows broad-spectrum antibiotic therapy but is also associated with immunosuppression and xerostomia. Breath mints, cinnamon gum, mouthwash, or toothpaste can cause allergic reactions that mimic this form of candidiasis; so the patient's history is very important in differentiating the clinical picture because treatment will vary accordingly.

Chronic hyperplastic candidiasis, or candidal leukoplakia, is the least common form of oral candidiasis. Patients have a white patch (leukoplakia) that cannot be scraped off. Some researchers believe that this is a candidiasis superimposed on a preexisting leukoplakia lesion. Hairy leukoplakia is associated with Epstein-Barr virus (EBV). These white mucosal lesions do not rub off and may appear as faint vertical streaks or thick, furrowed areas of leukoplakia. *Candida* is present without the tissue's normal inflammatory reaction to the fungus. Hairy leukoplakia has been reported in organ and bone marrow transplant recipients and, on rare occasions, in immunocompetent patients. However, its presence strongly suggests HIV infection in an individual with no other signs of immune suppression. HIV patients with hairy leukoplakia frequently develop AIDS within 2 years of the lesion onset. Other conditions leading to an inflamed appearance of the oral mucosa include systemic or local vasculitis and oral neoplasia; the latter (oral or glottic cancer) often presents as a single, painless lesion. Biopsy is needed to rule out these conditions if lingual or mucosal lesions are chronic or recurrent. Measles (roseola paramyxovirus infection) also leads to erythematous patches with bluish white centers on the lingual and buccal mucosa, known as Koplick's spots. However, this systemic infection is accompanied by a skin rash, cough, and coryza 24 to 48 hours after the appearance of these distinctive oral lesions.

Diagnostic Reasoning

Diagnostic Tests

Stomatitis or glossitis may result from multicausal phenomena. However, detecting the primary underlying problem is key to effective management. A CBC may reflect bacterial infection if polymorphonuclear neutrophils are elevated or viral infection if lymphocytes and mononuclear leukocytes predominate. Biochemical tests, special cellular stains, and cultures are used to identify most causative microorganisms, along with specific serologies such as the RPR test for the syphilitic agent *Treponema pallidum*. Serum levels of iron, folate, riboflavin, niacin, or cyanocobalamin may reveal nutritional deficiencies that can cause stomatitis and glossitis. Autoimmune disorders are diagnosed through a wide array of serologies (e.g., antinuclear antibody test for systemic lupus erythematosus).

Herpetic stomatitis caused by HSV may be ruled out via serum levels of anti-HSV antibodies, viral culture, or a Tzanck smear of lesional scrapings, which will present as multinucleated giant cells with intranuclear inclusions. Concurrent genital lesions are common in herpetic infection, as is also the case with Behçet's disease, a neutrophilic inflammatory disorder treated with topical and systemic steroids, which does not appear infectious. Non–*Candida*-related pseudomembranous stomatitis may be distinguished from oral candidiasis by negative findings for the fungus on Gram stain or more appropriately 10% potassium hydroxide wet mount of lesional scrapings. Oral candidiasis, as well as lichen planus, may resemble nicotinic stomatitis. Lichen planus may be ruled out by biopsy, which demonstrates hyperkeratosis, irregular acanthosis, and lymphocytic dermal band–like infiltrates. Biopsy is also indicated in the case of suspected neoplasia.

Viral culture and serological tests may rule out measles and other viral infections, including infectious mononucleosis (EBV infection), warts (papillomaviruses), prodromal primary HIV infection, and severe cases of chickenpox (varicella-zoster infection), which may also present with vesicular lesions of the oral cavity, pharynx, and larynx.

Differential Diagnosis

The primary goal of the differential diagnosis for mouth sores is to determine their precise cause because etiology of these lesions is so variable. Although the aforementioned hematological screens (CBC and nutrient levels) and serological tests may be used to detect specific pathogens or nutritional deficiencies, the signs and symptoms elicited from patient history and physical exam provide the most useful information in determining the cause of mouth sores. For example, self-induced vomiting associated with bulimic disorders should be ruled out through a careful patient history. Similarly, physical exam can rule out aphthous stomatitis, which, unlike the other forms listed, produces characteristic shallow, grayish, nonvesicular ulcers surrounded by a ring of hyperemia and covered with a fibrinous yellow membrane. Pregnancy epulis (pregnancy gingivitis) results from hormonal changes and may be confused with other forms of stomatitis. However, hyperplasia is usually limited to the interdental papillae, and pyogenic granulomas may form. "Geographic tongue" (benign migratory glossitis), which may be confused with pathological forms of glossitis, presents as continuously changing areas of loss and regrowth of filiform papillae with thickened white borders surrounded by red patches, creating a map-like appearance of the tongue. Geographic tongue is considered to be a harmless, normal variant requiring no treatment.

Management

Most cases of stomatitis are effectively treated with outpatient care unless severe or resulting from an underlying disease requiring inpatient care (e.g., advanced syphilis). For example, if severe dehydration secondary to oral pain and dysphagia is present, parenteral fluids may be required.

- All behaviors or conditions contributing to lesion formation should be stopped or corrected (e.g., smoking, eating hot or spicy foods, or wearing ill-fitting dentures).
- Underlying causative infections should be treated appropriately, but treatment specific to oral inflammation is primarily symptomatic and pharmacological.
- Baking soda or salt water rinses three or more times a day (½ tsp. salt or sodium bicarbonate in 8 oz. water) may be sufficient to relieve mild discomfort. Alternatively, oral rinses of half strength 3% hydrogen peroxide solution (1:1 with water) may be used.
- Liquid antacids such as attapulgite (Kaopectate), aluminum hydroxide (Amphogel), or magnesium hydroxide (Maalox) may effectively relieve pain when taken 4 times daily.
- Equal amounts of antihistaminic elixirs such as diphenhydramine (Benadryl) may be mixed with liquid antacids (1:1) and used as an oral rinse to reduce inflammation.
- Nonprescription analgesics such as acetaminophen (Tylenol) 650 mg every 4 to 6 hours may be used to relieve mouth pain.

- A viscous solution of 2% lidocaine may be applied to oral lesions every 3 hours as a topical anesthetic or used as a gargle or swish and spit (15 mL) before meals and every 3 hours as needed.
- Severe attacks in adults may require topical gel–based 0.1% triamcinolone (Kenalog) or fluocinonide applied at bedtime and, if needed, 3 times daily after meals.
- Anti-inflammatory oral steroid "bursts" may be appropriate in severe cases of stomatitis and glossitis, but all oral medications should be monitored for toxicity because significantly more absorption than expected may result from open oral ulcers. In addition, steroids would not be indicated in immunosuppressed patients or those with viral infections, although antiviral medications such as amantadine (Symmetrel) may be appropriate. For cases of HSV, ice cubes applied locally for an hour to newly formed lesions may prove helpful; likewise, drinking cool liquids and sucking on frozen juice bars may reduce discomfort.
- Pharmacological preparations for HSV may be helpful such as Valtrex 1 g 2 times daily for 2 days or Famvir 500 mg 2 times daily for 5 days.
- High fluid intake and antiseptic mouthwashes (without alcohol, which may be irritating and painful) may help prevent secondary bacterial infection.

In cases of candidiasis, antifungal agents should be used in conjunction with antibiotics and oral hygiene.

- Nystatin (Mycostatin, Nilstat), a polyene antibiotic, is formulated for use as a pastille (lozenge) or suspension 400,000 to 600,000 units PO (swish and swallow) 4 times daily. Because it is not absorbed across the gastrointestinal tract, the drug must remain in contact with the organism and must be reapplied several times a day.
- Clotrimazole (Lotrimin, Mycelex), an imidazole agent, is not well absorbed and must be administered at least 4 times daily as a 10-mg trouche.
- Ketoconazole (Nizoral) 200 to 400 mg PO daily for 7 to 14 days, another imidazole, is absorbed across the gastrointestinal tract and provides systemic therapy by the oral route. It should not be used routinely for routine oral candidiasis, however, because of possible drug interactions and potential liver toxicities. The triazole agent fluconazole (Diflucan) 200 mg PO on the first day, then 100 mg daily for 7 to 14 days, is well absorbed systemically and only rarely causes liver toxicity, although other drug interactions, as well as drug resistance, have been documented.
- Hydrocortisone-iodoquinol (Vytone) cream can be used to ease the discomfort of angular cheilitis. It combines the anti-inflammatory and antipruritic effects of hydrocortisone with the antifungal and antibacterial properties of iodoquinol.

- In terms of hygiene, toothbrushes should be changed frequently. A patient with candidiasis who wears dentures or partials must also treat the appliances to combat the infection.

Treatment of erythema multiforme requires eliminating exposure to the offending agent in the case of drug hypersensitivity or specific treatment to the underlying infectious agent (e.g., acyclovir for HSV infection). Specialist care by a dermatologist and close inpatient observation are required for severe cases that risk progression to Stevens-Johnson syndrome or toxic epidermal necrolysis. Vincent's stomatitis requires oral penicillin V potassium (Pen-Vee K; 250–500 mg every 4–6 hours) to fight infection, as well as significant fluid intake of at least four to six glasses of nonacidic fruit juice or water per day. Severe gangrenous stomatitis requires IV antibiotic treatment and debridement of wounds. Autoimmune disorders such as systemic lupus erythematosus, bullous pemphigoid, and pemphigus vulgarus are primarily treated with systemic corticosteroids. The mucosal lesions of lupus may be treated with topical or intralesional steroids if located on the lips, whereas lesions of the oral cavity respond to antimalarials, provided no drug hypersensitivity manifests. However, for recalcitrant cases, increasingly potent immunosuppressive medications may be necessary. Treatment of any of these disorders typically requires specialist care and rapid referral.

Dehydration and malnutrition can result from altered eating habits due to oral pain. Secondary bacterial infections may complicate any type of ulcerative oral lesion. Recent scarification of lesions may progress to facial space infection, tonsillar or cervical lymph gland infection, involvement of the vocal cords, bronchial tubes, rectum, vagina, and even sepsis. Thus, oral surgery may be needed to trim away rough, highly inflamed, infected gum tissue. Glossitis may become chronic if inadequately treated, and severe gangrenous or necrotizing stomatitis seen in severe HIV-infected cases may lead to death if untreated.

Follow-up and Referral

As for difficult to treat and refractory cases, stomatitis and glossitis due to underlying systemic disorders, such as autoimmune conditions, require specialist referral to guide further management.

Patient Education

The importance of proper oral hygiene and healthful nutritional habits should be stressed to all patients. Patients should be instructed to brush their teeth with a soft-bristled toothbrush at least twice daily and to floss regularly (once a day, if possible). Patients should also wear protective headgear whenever bicycling, skating, or playing contact sports, to prevent cases of trauma-related tongue injury. Increased fluid intake during treatment should be encouraged, as should maintaining the recommended medication regimen while avoiding hot, spicy, salty, or acidic foods, and carbonated or alcoholic beverages. Patients may be instructed to drink through a straw if lesions are particularly painful. A liquid diet may be recommended during the first 2 to 3 days if pain is severe. Milk, liquid gelatin, yogurt, ice cream, and custard are usually well tolerated. Severe cases of Vincent's stomatitis may even call for at-home rest during the first few days of treatment.

The contagious nature of pathogen-related forms of stomatitis or glossitis should be emphasized. The most effective means of avoiding secondary manifestations of reactivated HSV infection, for example, is to refrain from behaviors that put the individual at risk of HSV infection or reinfection—most notably, unprotected sex with multiple partners and physical contact with persons who have active herpetic lesions. Kissing and oral sex should be avoided if an individual is actively infected, and frequent hand washing during active flare-ups of herpetic lesions will aid in preventing autoinfection and viral transmission. It is also helpful to inform patients of the high prevalence rate of HSV infection to reduce the stigma commonly associated with herpes. Early treatment of primary or secondary HSV infection may also help to prevent stomatic or labial involvement. Wearing zinc oxide-containing sunscreens on the lips and face helps to prevent herpes labialis flare-ups when exposed to excessive sunlight.

In the long term, the most effective means of avoiding stomatitis is to refrain from risk behaviors such as smoking, eating hot or spicy foods, drinking alcohol, and practicing poor dental hygiene. Avoiding exposure to affected persons, especially in the case of HSV, as well as avoiding exposure to allergens, chemical irritants, or foods that seem to trigger attacks, is also recommended. Care should be taken to fit all dentures and dental prostheses properly to prevent mechanical injury; for cases related to bruxism (tooth grinding), a night-guard prosthesis with removable splints to reduce biting pressure on tooth surfaces may reduce damage to dentition, in turn, preventing related inflammation. Early treatment of viral, bacterial, and fungal infections may prevent stomatic and glossal involvement. Wearing protective headgear during bicycling, skating, and contact sports could prevent trauma-related injury in the mouth.

■ PHARYNGITIS AND TONSILLITIS

Pharyngitis and *tonsillitis* denote generalized inflammatory processes of both infectious and noninfectious etiology, involving the pharynx and pharyngeal tonsils, respectively. Most virally related cases are self-limited, with spontaneous recovery, although other infectious cases may require antibiotic or antifungal therapy. Pharyngitis and tonsillitis may occur independently of one another; however, they often co-occur, sharing a common etiology, clinical course, and treatment regimen. Many cases of pharyngitis and virtually all cases of tonsillitis are contagious.

Epidemiology and Causes

About 8% of all patient visits in the ambulatory care setting each year are for complaints of sore throat. Viral pharyngitis related to respiratory tract pathogens occurs most often in the colder fall and winter months. Influenza infection typically occurs in epidemics between December and April. The incidence of group A beta-hemolytic streptococcal infection pharyngitis typically increases from 10% of cases reported in the fall to 40% in the winter and spring. Herpangina is known to peak in the summer and fall. Allergic pharyngitis may also peak seasonally during the summer months. Although infectious (bacterial and viral) pharyngitis and tonsillitis tend to occur most frequently in young children aged 5 to 10 years, both conditions may occur at any age. Streptococcal infection most frequently affects patients younger than age 25; however, it may occur sporadically in older adults. Infectious mononucleosis (primarily caused by Epstein-Barr virus [EBV]) is also common in adolescents and young adults and is rarely seen in the elderly. Pharyngitis associated with the postnasal drip of sinusitis most often affects adults. No ethnic predispositions have been reported for either pharyngitis or tonsillitis.

Men and women are affected equally by both conditions. URI is a common predisposing factor for the development of viral pharyngitis. The postnasal drip associated with URI or sinusitis may also contribute to irritant-related pharyngitis. The risk of all forms of infectious pharyngitis (viral, bacterial, and fungal) is increased in immunocompromised persons who are afflicted by chronic illnesses, including diabetes mellitus and white blood cell dyscrasias such as agranulocytosis or acute leukemia. Work-related stress and excessive alcohol consumption have also been implicated as a cause of decreased resistance to throat infection. In general, close living quarters, such as military barracks, schools, and day-care centers, increase the risk of person-to-person transmission of the infectious agents causing both pharyngitis and tonsillitis. EBV transmission typically requires intimate person-to-person contact between susceptible persons and symptomatic viral shedders (hence its nickname of "kissing disease"). Young adults and adolescents from higher socioeconomic backgrounds in developed countries who have not been exposed to EBV in their childhood are most susceptible. Persons with pharyngitis related to *Neisseria gonorrhea, Treponema pallidum* (syphilis), *Chlamydia*, or herpes usually have a history of receptive oral intercourse with an infected sexual partner. Sexual abuse may be a factor in these cases as well. Bisexual and homosexual men and patients with anogenital gonorrhea are the groups most frequently affected by gonorrheal pharyngitis. Adult cases of *Corynebacterium diphtheriae* occur almost exclusively in nonimmunized individuals. Recent contact with a wild animal (especially through a bite) is the major risk factor for the development of *Francisella tularensis* infection. Excessive antibiotic use has been associated with candidal infection and an overgrowth of *Candida* (thrush) in the oropharynx; tobacco and particularly marijuana smoking have also been implicated.

Pathophysiology

In up to 40% of pharyngitis cases, no causative agent is identified. Definitive diagnosis of an infectious agent is difficult, because the nasopharynx is a nonsterile environment normally colonized by an array of nonpathogenic flora. However, the current literature suggests that in adults, upper respiratory tract viruses are the most common cause of infectious pharyngitis, accounting for 30% to 50% of all cases: rhinovirus, coronavirus, adenovirus, influenza viruses A and B, parainfluenza virus, coxsackievirus (herpangina and hand-foot-and-mouth disease), enterovirus, and respiratory syncytial virus (RSV). Rhinoviruses and influenza viruses inflame the oral and nasopharyngeal mucosa via direct invasion and colonization, but the specific pathogenic mechanisms of other viruses is not well understood. Members of the herpes family of viruses are also common causative agents, including EBV and in immunocompromised hosts, cytomegalovirus (CMV), HSV, and reactivated herpes zoster. EBV, which infects pharyngeal B-lymphocytes and disseminates throughout the entire lymphoreticular system, is the primary causative agent of infectious mononucleosis, accounting for 1% to 2% of all pharyngitis cases. However, CMV causes up to 20% of all infectious mononucleosis cases. Primary infection with HIV may also cause pharyngitis owing to rapid retroviral replication; thus, HIV risk factors should always be assessed.

Bacterial agents typically cause an exudative pharyngitis, which represents roughly 20% of all cases of sore throat. Group A beta-hemolytic *Streptococcus pyogenes*, which accounts for 10% to 20% of adult pharyngitis cases, invades and multiplies within the pharyngeal mucosa, causing an intense inflammatory response known as "strep throat." Collectively, *Streptococcus* bacteria are characterized into groups based on cell-wall antigenicity. Clinically relevant groups include A, B, C, D, and G. Group A is the most important cause of pharyngitis because it may lead to the most serious complications, including heart valve damage that may occur many years after systemic infection known as acute rheumatic fever. More than 80 serotypes of *Streptococcus* have been identified. The most clinically significant strain is based on the M protein, which is the major virulence factor of group A beta-hemolytic *Streptococcus pyogenes*. M protein is antiphagocytic, because it blocks activation of the alternative complement pathway. An immune response to bacterial M protein stimulates long-lasting type-specific anti-M antibodies that adhere to individual bacteria and facilitate their phagocytosis (i.e., opsonization), protecting patients against subsequent exposure to bacteria of the same M-protein serotype. The amount of time needed for patients to mount a protective immune response is unclear. In the past, it had been suggested that treatment of group A *Streptococcus* be delayed so that a protective immune response could be mounted, but this practice has since been refuted, and rapid treatment is now the standard of care. Importantly, *S pyogenes* strains are becoming increasingly virulent, and the incidence of subsequent acute renal insufficiency due to postinfectious glomerulonephritis has increased over the past 15 years. Reports of bacteremia, deep tissue cellulitis, and systemic toxic shock–like syndrome mediated by *Streptococcal* exotoxins are also well characterized, with pharyngitis often recognized as the presenting complaint.

Other bacterial agents of pharyngitis include *N gonorrhoeae* (especially in young, sexually active adults), *Haemophilus influenzae, Streptococcus pneumoniae, T pallidum, Staphylococcus aureus,* and *Corynebacterium diphtheriae* and *C hemolyticum* (both often associated with epiglottitis and a potentially obstructive fibrinous gray membrane adherent to the posterior pharynx). The relative importance of atypical organisms known to cause bronchitis including *Chlamydia pneumoniae, C trachomatis,* and *Mycoplasma pneumoniae* as pharyngitic agents is controversial. Studies have demonstrated markedly varied prevalence rates (0%–20%), and nasopharyngeal colonization by these organisms may be asymptomatic.

Noninfectious etiologies of pharyngitis may include trauma, allergies, collagen vascular diseases such as Kawasaki's syndrome, autoimmune blistering diseases such as pemphigus, chemical or drug-induced damage, and severe dehydration. Tobacco and particularly marijuana smoking are major contributing factors to noninfectious pharyngitis related to chemical irritation, and exposure to allergens such as dust and pollen increases the risk of allergic pharyngitis, typically associated with a past history or family history of atopy. Severe drug reactions mediated by both type I immediate hypersensitivity and type III antibody–antigen immune complex reactions may extend in their most serious form to the oropharynx, as well as other mucosal sites. Both low humidity and mouth-breathing may contribute to dehydration-induced mucosal inflammation.

In contrast, tonsillitis (which may involve the posterior pharyngeal tonsils as well as the more anterior adenoid glands) is foremost a disorder of infectious etiology. It is characterized by inflammation, swelling, and purulent exudation of these lymphoid tissue collections that directly drain the colonized or infected nasopharynx. The spectrum of causative agents in this disorder is similar to that described for pharyngitis, including bacteria and upper respiratory tract viruses. Acutely, it is most often caused by group A *Streptococcus* infection, and a chronic form may also result from repeated *Streptococcus* infections. Streptococcal tonsillar infection always has the potential for progressing to peritonsillar or tonsillar abscess requiring aggressive management (incision and drainage followed by antibiotic therapy).

Clinical Presentation
Subjective

Most patients with pharyngitis and/or tonsillitis report mild to severe throat pain or the sensation of a "tickle" or pruritus in the throat. Infectious mononucleosis, adenovirus, and especially group A *Streptococcus* pharyngitis ("strep throat") tend to cause the most painful sore throats, with fever. Many patients also describe their throats as feeling swollen, with a "lump" in the back of the throat that persists despite repeated swallowing. A history of dysphagia (difficulty swallowing) is also common with throat inflammation, particularly from *H influenzae* infection, and hoarseness is often associated with *C pneumoniae*. Laryngitis and cough are commonly associated with viral infection, although fever occurs only occasionally. In contrast, chills and fever are common with bacterial infection, although cough and rhinorrhea are rarely present. Group A *Streptococcus* infection usually produces a fever higher than 101°F (38.3°C); the patient may be tachycardic, and there is usually pharyngeal exudate. As with viral infections, streptococcal symptomatology is rapid in onset; in contrast, in viral disease systemic symptoms are few. Allergic pharyngitis, on the other hand, does not present with fever, but is recognized most readily by a persistent postnasal drip, paroxysmal sneezing, itchy, watery eyes, rhinorrhea, and a mild sore throat that typically worsens with recumbency. Malaise, generalized aches and pains, and headache may also be reported in both conditions. Infectious mononucleosis is famous for its gradual onset of low-grade fever and marked fatigue and severe sore throat. Anorexia and nausea may also be present. Influenza infection is characterized by an abrupt onset of fever ranging from 100°F to 104°F (37.8°C to 40°C), myalgias, and headache, which last for about 3 days, followed by 3 to 4 days of cough, rhinorrhea, and pharyngitis, and finally a 1- to 2-week convalescent period with persistent cough and malaise. Geriatric patients with influenza may also present with gastrointestinal symptoms such as nausea, vomiting, and diarrhea. Reactivated herpes zoster infection is characterized by painful prodromes before active flare-ups. In contrast, HSV infection does not usually cause a sore throat. Moreover, primary or secondary syphilitic lesions tend to be painless. Gonococcal pharyngitis may be asymptomatic. Severe cases of tonsillitis may also present with ear pain and sometimes with cough or vomiting.

Objective

On inspection, the inflamed throat typically appears erythematous, although color may vary. Conjunctivitis is often associated with adenovirus and other respiratory viruses, whereas mucosal exudates and enlarged tonsils occur only occasionally. EBV-related infectious mononucleosis, however, may present with an exudative tonsillitis (in about 50% of cases), in addition to palatal petechiae and exanthem. The 1- to 2-mm vesicular lesions of herpes simplex infection may extend from the pharynx to the lips, gingivae, buccal mucosa, and tongue. Reactivated herpes zoster infection typically presents with 2- to 4-mm vesicular lesions unilaterally on the tongue, lip, and buccal mucosa. Herpangina presents as 1- to 2-mm oral vesicles or ulcers on the pharynx, tonsils, soft palate, pillars, uvula, and posterior buccal mucosa. Hand-foot-and-mouth disease presents with oral lesions co-occurring with exanthem on the hands and feet. Maculopapular rashes on the extremities of young adult patients may be indicative of many types of infection, including *C hemolyticum*, HIV, enteroviruses, or *T pallidum* (syphilis).

Exudates and enlarged tonsils are common findings in bacterial infections. Streptococcal infection produces a characteristic white to yellow exudate and may be accompanied by a sandpaper-like, scarletiniform rash. *Mycoplasma*-related cases may be clinically indistinguishable from streptococcal infections. *C diphtheriae* presents with a characteristic grayish pseudomembrane overlying the pharyngeal mucosa, tonsils, epiglottis, uvula, or even the nasal cavity. The nonvesicular lesions of primary syphilis are 5 to 15 mm in size and appear indurated or "healed up," extending to the lips, tonsils, or tongue. Secondary syphilitic nonvesicular lesions (2–10 mm) arise symmetrically on all parts of the oropharynx and mouth. Candidal infections produce thin, white, nonvesicular, diffuse or patchy (3–11 mm) exudative ulcers on all parts of the oropharyngeal mucosa. In most inflammatory conditions of the throat, the pharyngeal mucosa and tonsils are edematous, particularly with group A beta-hemolytic streptococcal infection. This is true of allergic pharyngitis as well, although erythema of the pharynx is minimal. Tonsillitis presents with readily noticeable swollen lymph glands located bilaterally between the fauces of the posterior pharynx.

Bacterial pharyngitis commonly presents with significant tender lymphadenopathy of the draining anterior cervical lymph nodes. This finding also occasionally occurs in viral infections such as infectious mononucleosis or primary HIV infection. However, 90% of infectious mononucleosis cases present with posterior cervical lymphadenopathy. Hepatosplenomegaly is also a common finding. Tonsillitis usually presents with swollen lymph glands on either side of the jaw.

Diagnostic Reasoning
Diagnostic Tests

Inasmuch as most cases of pharyngitis and tonsillitis are self-limited, laboratory work-up and identification of causative organisms through culture is unnecessary if the patient's clinical picture is consistent with influenza, the common cold, or irritant-induced throat inflammation. However, bacterial and viral cultures of throat swabs may be appropriate for more complicated cases or those requiring pharmacotherapy such as with herpes virus or streptococcal infection. Herpangina and hand-foot-and-mouth disease are diagnosed via coxsackie-positive viral cultures and positive serologies. For exudative cases of pharyngitis, the Rapid (10-minute) Streptococcal Antigen (Rapid Strep) Test is used to detect group A streptococcal antigens and diagnose infection. Increased antistreptolysin O (ASO) titers are also observed, but treatment may blunt this antibody response. Rapid Strep Tests are highly specific (90%) and sensitive (80–90%) when used judiciously. A Rapid Strep Test to guide antibiotic therapy is considered appropriate for any patient with two or three of the following criteria: fever above 100.5°F (38.1°C), tonsillar exudate, tender anterior cervical lymphadenopathy, and the absence of cough. Patients meeting three or four of these criteria may be empirically diagnosed with group A *Streptococcus* and treated immediately. Throat swab cultures of the posterior pharynx and tonsils—the current "gold standard" test for the diagnosis of *Streptococcal* infection—are sent rather than the Rapid Strep Test for patients meeting fewer criteria and considered to have a low pretest likelihood of infection (less than 20%). Patients with an intermediate pretest likelihood of *Streptococcus* infection (20%–50%) who present with sore throat and only two of the associated criteria are given the Rapid Strep Test first and, if positive, may avoid a throat culture. However, if the result is negative, it must be followed up by a throat culture which typically displays greater sensitivity than the Rapid Strep Test. During the summer and fall, the false-positive rates of Rapid Strep Tests may approach 50%. In turn, the recommended diagnostic approach is less aggressive at this time than during the winter or spring. During the summer and fall, no testing is recommended for patients with a sore throat who meet only one of the associated criteria unless the patient is at high risk for *Streptococcus* infection due to immunocompromising illnesses such as diabetes mellitus or HIV, has a history of rheumatic fever, or is presenting during a community outbreak of *Streptococcus* infection. If possible, household members should also be screened because treated patients may be reinfected via contact with asymptomatic carriers in the home.

Immunofluorescence staining or viral throat swab cultures are used to detect herpes virus infection. A special Tzanck smear of any ulcerative exudative lesion is used to diagnose HSV and herpes zoster; multinucleated giant cells with ballooning degeneration represent a positive finding. Infection by the many types of herpes viruses (including HSV, EBV, and CMV) may also be diagnosed by serological tests detecting virus-specific antibodies. Convalescent titers may be necessary for proper interpretation. Pharyngeal, endocervical, and urethral cultures on Thayer-Martin agar can specifically detect gonorrheal growth, if suspected in high-risk patients. Syphilis is diagnosed via serology and, if disease is in its secondary stage, by dark-field microscopy of lesional scrapings that demonstrates *T pallidum* spirochetes. *C pneumoniae* and *C trachomatis* are typically evaluated via serology, although cultures and titers are not recommended initially, because the relative contribution of these pathogens to throat inflammation remains highly controversial. Suspected *Candida* infections are diagnosed via a potassium hydroxide (KOH) wet mount or Gram stain of pharyngeal exudates, which will demonstrate spores and budding hyphal yeast forms, as well as by yeast cultures for speciation if needed. Nonspecific heterophile antibody tests, such as the Monospot test, are used to diagnose infectious mononucleosis related to EBV, although this test decreases in sensitivity when used at the extremes of age. A CBC may be done in any case of infectious pharyngitis. An increase in granulocytes indicates bacterial infection, and a documented lymphocytosis (50% lymphocytes, of which at least 10% show atypical morphology) strongly supports a viral etiology. The presence of eosinophils in a Gram stain of nasal secretions or a nasal mucosal scraping is strongly indicative of allergic pharyngitis. Radiological evaluation of the posterior pharyngeal wall may be appropriate to detect retropharyngeal processes if abscess formation is suspected.

Differential Diagnosis

Although the entire oropharynx may be involved during many infectious processes, certain microorganisms have a greater propensity for affecting the oral cavity, resulting in stomatitis, before pharyngeal involvement. Pharyngitis from postnasal drip secondary to rhinitis or sinusitis may be ruled out via nasal cavity examination and sinus x-ray films. Epiglottitis due to *C diphtheriae* is an important consideration in nonimmunized (or inadequately immunized) individuals; it should be ruled out carefully by history and general presentation, including inability to swallow, with resultant drooling and inability to speak. Examination of the oral pharynx may trigger sudden glottic spasm and risk of occlusion of the airway. Examination of the throat should take place in a facility that could support severe respiratory compromise that may result from dislodging the pseudomembrane from the posterior pharynx. Pharyngeal or tonsillar malignancy requiring surgical removal of the affected tissues must be ruled out via biopsy if malignancy is suspected.

Infection with group A *Streptococcus* causes intense mucosal inflammation because of bacterial extracellular factors such as pyrogenic exotoxin and streptolysin O. A major virulence factor is the streptococcal cell-wall M protein (with 80 serotypes), which has antiphagocytic properties; particular serotypes appear to correlate with the occurrence of rheumatic fever and glomerulonephritis, which can lead to acute renal failure. Patients may be sicker and more febrile with bacterial infection, but this is not always the case. When challenged with an infectious agent, numerous factors are brought into play, including the host's defense mechanisms, microbial virulence, quantity of infectious inoculum, and the host's susceptibility.

Management
Pharmacological Management

Most cases of pharyngitis and tonsillitis in otherwise healthy patients are entirely manageable with home care and/or antibiotics. For allergy-related forms of throat inflammation, contact with environmental irritants including tobacco smoke should be minimized, and patients may be treated symptomatically with a combination of antihistamines and decongestants as described for allergic rhinitis. In general, for infectious forms, patients should limit their physical activity until symptoms of pharyngitis and tonsillitis have subsided. Daily fluid intake should be increased to 8 to 12 glasses (2–3 quarts) of fluids such as water or nonacidic juices. Bedrest is recommended if fever is present, and regular physical activity should be resumed only after 2 to 3 days of normal temperature readings. Viral pharyngitis requires only symptomatic care, and antibiotics are never indicated (other than selected antiviral therapies). In fact, many cases of bacterial pharyngitis are self-limited as well (such as those caused by atypical organisms). However, cases of group A *Streptococcus* and *N gonorrhoeae* merit rapid antibiotic treatment to prevent significant sequelae in both the short and long term. In addition, cases caused by *C diphtheriae, H influenzae,* or influenza virus may require hospitalization because of the risk of life-threatening complications. Fungal infections also typically require antimycotic therapy.

Throat pain may be significantly relieved by the following measures:

- Voice rest
- Ambient humidification, saline nasal sprays, viscous xylocaine
- Various types of gargles taken as needed, including hot or cold double-strength tea or a warm saltwater solution (1 teaspoon of noniodized salt in 8 ounces of water)
- A regularly cleaned cool-mist, ultrasonic humidifier to increase ambient air moisture, which may be useful in relieving feelings of dryness or tightness in the throat
- Nonprescription throat lozenges or sprays (e.g., Cepastat, Chloraseptic) containing topical anesthetics such as phenol may also alleviate minor pain
- Nonprescription analgesics such as acetaminophen or aspirin (325–650 mg every 4–6 hours as needed) to relieve intermediate pain, and codeine preparations (30–60 mg PO every 4–6 hours as needed) to possibly relieve more severe pain
- Warm, moist compresses applied 4 times daily for at least 30 to 60 minutes at a time to relieve enlarged, tender cervical lymph glands (see Complementary Therapies 8.1)

Viral infections tend to be treated symptomatically, as described previously. Influenza symptoms may be relieved within the first 2 days of symptoms by prescribing amantadine (Symmetrel; 100 mg PO 2 times daily) for documented cases of influenza A, but this drug may also cause insomnia, dizziness, drowsiness, or difficulty concentrating. Thus, the dosage for elderly patients is reduced to once a day. Oseltamivir (Tamiflu; 75 mg PO 2 times daily for 5 days) may be similarly given within the first 48 hours of symptom onset to reduce duration of illness and symptom severity, as well as prophylactically in high-risk individuals during peak flu season at once-daily dosing.

Antibiotic therapy for group A streptococcal pharyngitis has been shown to shorten the clinical course of disease and reduce lymphadenopathy, fever, and pain (after 1–3 days of therapy), prevent suppurative complications and autoimmune sequelae such as rheumatic fever, and decrease person-to-person spread of infection. Empiric antibiotic therapy may be instituted before receiving culture results in certain clinical situations to prevent rheumatic fever, cardiac sequelae, and acute renal insufficiency due to poststreptococcal glomerulonephritis. Studies have demonstrated, however, that delaying treatment for 48 hours in anticipation of culture results does not significantly affect the reduction in autoimmune sequelae provided by antibiotic therapy. In cases of fever under 100.5°F (38.1°C) without an associated tonsillar exudate or anterior cervical lymphadenopathy, neither throat swab culture nor antistreptococcal therapy is recommended because a false-positive culture may lead to unnecessary antibiotic therapy. If fever greater than 100.5°F (38.1°C) accompanies a tonsillar exudate and tender anterior cervical adenitis, antistreptococcal therapy should be instituted immediately because a false-negative culture could delay critical treatment. This is especially important for patients younger than 25 years of age. If a similar fever occurs with only one of the other two physical signs, antibiotic therapy should be instituted only for culture-positive patients. High-risk factors favoring immediate empiric treatment include a past history of acute rheumatic heart fever or related cardiac damage, a scarlatiniform rash, a diabetic or other immunocompromised state, a documented exposure to group A *Streptoccocus* within the past week, or the presence of a known epidemic within the community.

Adults are typically given a 10-day course of penicillin V potassium (Pen-Vee K; 500 mg PO 2 times daily or 250 mg PO 4 times daily) or benzathine penicillin (Bicillin; 1.2 million units IM once) as an alternative to prolonged oral medication. If the patient is allergic to penicillin, erythromycin (250 mg PO daily) is recommended. If the patient fails to respond to antibiotic therapy, tests for infectious mononucleosis and streptococcal antibiotic sensitivity should be performed. A 10-day course of amoxicillin/clavulanate (Augmentin; 40 mg/kg PO daily based on the amoxicillin component, in divided doses 2 times daily), erythromycin ethyl succinate (50 mg/kg PO daily in divided doses 3 times daily), or erythromycin stearate (1 g PO daily) have all been shown to be effective for penicillin-resistant beta-lactamase–producing organisms, whereas tetracycline or trimethoprim-sulfamethoxazole preparations (Septra, Bactrim) should be avoided.

N gonorrhoeae infection calls for ceftriaxone (Rocephin; 125 mg IM once), along with empiric treatment for *C trachomatis* (azithromycin [Zithromax] 1 g PO once or doxycycline 100 mg PO 2 times daily for 7 days), given its propensity for co-infection. Extensive throat infection with *Candida albicans* (thrush, pharyngitis, esophagitis) requires antifungal treatment such as fluconazole 200 mg PO daily once, followed by 100 mg PO daily for 2 weeks total. *M pneumoniae* and *C pneumoniae* are both treated with erythromycin 250 to 500 mg PO 4 times daily for 10 days, depending on the specific preparation.

Surgical Management

Surgical removal of the pharyngeal tonsils (tonsillectomy) and/or adenoids (adenoidectomy) is absolutely indicated if tonsillar inflammation leads to airway obstruction associated with any of the following: cor pulmonale (right-sided cardiac hypertrophy), dysphagia, or weight loss. Tonsillectomy may also be indicated if active flares recur more than three times a year, if the patient experiences mild dysphagia, if the tonsils remain chronically hypertrophied after a bout of infectious mononucleosis, or if the patient has a history of rheumatic fever with heart damage due to recurrent tonsillitis. However, in these situations, the indication for surgical intervention is relative and must be evaluated further. It should also be noted that lymph glands normally swell during episodes of active inflammation as part of the body's normal immune response. In turn, tonsillectomy is not indicated for colds, asthma, allergic rhinitis, focal infections, fever of unknown origin, cervical lymphadenopathy, or enlarged tonsils without obstructive symptomatology.

Follow-up and Referral

Most cases of pharyngitis and tonsillitis are self-limiting, and symptoms tend to improve in 2 to 3 days. If symptoms fail to improve within this time, patients should return for a follow-up appointment. Throat cultures for *Streptococcus* may be repeated on completion of therapy to confirm resolution of any infectious processes. This is not recommended, however, for asymptomatic patients who have completed a 10-day therapeutic regimen for streptococcal infection or for patients whose symptoms improve within 5 days of antibiotic therapy because clinical resolution is typically the best measure of therapeutic success.

Group A *Streptococcus* pharyngeal or tonsillar infections may lead to scarlet fever or autoimmune rheumatic fever if not treated with antibiotics or if antibiotic therapy is discontinued before a full 10-day course. These

patients should be referred to a specialist. In areas where group A streptococcal infection is endemic, the probability of developing rheumatic fever is 0.3%. With epidemic pharyngitis, the risk increases to 3%. Rheumatic heart disease may develop after rheumatic fever in an adult patient with recurrent streptococcal infection or a history of poorly treated streptococcal pharyngitis as a child or young adult. This may lead to severe sequelae such as calcification of the mitral valve and/or other heart valves, as well as to the destruction of cardiac myocytes, which is attributed to cross-reacting antistreptococcal antibodies. Even when acute rheumatic fever is treated appropriately with prophylactic antibiotic therapy, 4% of patients may develop debilitating cardiac sequelae and 1% may develop severe class IV rheumatic heart disease. Chest pain is a key indicator of cardiac complications. Hematuria resulting from poststreptococcal glomerulonephritis may occur 1 to 3 weeks after acute pharyngeal or tonsillar infection because antibiotic therapy has not been shown to protect against this immune complex–mediated complication.

Cases caused by *C diphtheriae,* if left untreated, may lead to epiglottitis, which can obstruct breathing and may prove fatal if the pseudomembrane dislodges and chokes the patient as it is inadvertently swallowed. Spread of infectious organisms from the pharynx to the lungs may lead to pneumonia and severe respiratory complications. Infections of the posterior oropharynx may also ascend to the nasopharynx, leading to sinusitis and rhinitis—inflammation of the mucous membranes of the sinus and nasal cavities. The middle ear is another possible target of disseminated pharyngeal infection because the nasopharyngeal (eustachian) tube acts as a conduit for the spread of microorganisms. OM may occur in more than 20% of adenovirus infections. A less common complication of bacterial pharyngitis is septic jugular vein thrombophlebitis, which may occur several days after the initial sore throat. Patients with this complication are typically teenagers or young adults who experience an increase in neck pain and tenderness, as well as swelling of the jaw angle.

Liver function tests (e.g., serum aspartate aminotransferase [AST], serum alanine aminotransferase [ALT], serum bilirubin, platelet count, and the Coombs' autoantibody test) should be performed for all cases of suspected infectious mononucleosis to diagnose serious sequelae, including hepatitis (ALT or AST levels of more than 1,000 units/L; bilirubin levels of more than 10 mg/dL), hemolytic anemia, granulocytopenia, and thrombocytopenia. Airway obstruction may also occur in patients with infectious mononucleosis as a result of pharyngeal swelling. Such complications may require treatment with a corticosteroid such as prednisone (60–80 mg PO daily in divided doses, tapered over 1–2 weeks). Splenic rupture related to trauma is also a serious risk for all patients with infectious mononucleosis who have marked hepatosplenomegaly (liver and spleen enlargement).

Tonsillitis that goes untreated or fails to resolve with treatment may lead to grossly swollen, suppurative cervical adenitis, OM, or a peritonsillar abscess of the surrounding throat area, characterized by increasing unilateral ear and throat pain ipsilateral to the affected tonsil, dysphagia, drooling, trismus, erythema, and edema of the soft palate with fluctuance on palpation. Suppurative sequelae such as these may require surgical drainage and/or tonsillectomy. Repeated attacks of acute tonsillitis may lead to a chronic condition with a recurrent sore throat and greatly enlarged tonsils, which may complicate breathing and become potentially life-threatening; these cases also require surgical intervention.

All patients developing suppurative or retropharyngeal sequelae should be referred to an otolaryngologist. The physical exam and treatment of *C diphtheriae* infection is also highly risky and must be supervised by a qualified specialist. Surgical interventions such as tonsillectomy or abscess drainage require surgical referral.

Patient Education

Both pharyngitis and tonsillitis may be prevented by avoiding contact with persons with actively inflamed throats, particularly with URIs. Throat swabs from household members of patients should also be cultured to identify and treat carriers simultaneously in an effort to prevent the development of clinical disease and prevent reinfection. Toothbrushes should be replaced as soon as a sore throat develops because they may harbor causative microorganisms, and all eating and drinking utensils should be cleaned thoroughly and should not be shared. Food and washcloths also must not be shared during a period of active infection. It is critical to keep all immunizations up to date, particularly the diphtheria-pertussis-tetanus (DTaP, Tdap) vaccine that confers immunity against *C diphtheriae*. If a sexual partner is suspected of being infected with a sexually transmitted agent, sexual contact should cease until a proper diagnosis and any applicable treatment have been completed. In general, oral intercourse between persons of either gender should be performed only using a form of latex barrier protection, such as a condom during fellatio or a dental dam during cunnilingus, to avoid orogenital transmission of infectious organisms. Environmental irritants such as tobacco and marijuana smoke, pollution, dust and other allergens, and low-humidity environments should be avoided to prevent noninfectious forms of pharyngitis.

Warm compresses applied to relieve enlarged, tender cervical lymph nodes can be effective; however, patients must be cautioned not to burn the skin inadvertently. Although the use of aspirin during viral infections in adults has not been linked to the development of Reye's syndrome (as is the case in children), NSAIDs should be used cautiously if patients suffer from ulcers or other gastrointestinal disorders. Heavy lifting and contact sports must be prohibited for all patients with infectious mononucleosis because these activities carry a high risk of splenic trauma and rupture. Patients must be instructed to finish their entire course of antibiotics or antifungals to avoid complications from latent infection such as glomerulonephritis or myocarditis. In cases involving dysphagia, patients may be instructed on how to maintain a healthy liquid or soft food diet (e.g., milkshakes, soups, and high-protein diet or instant breakfast drinks) for a few days until the pain subsides. Patients who demand prescriptions for antibiotics in the absence of a throat culture confirming disease of bacterial origin should understand the rationale for using antibacterials versus other types of medication.

■ HOARSENESS

Hoarseness is a common complaint; the term describes a voice with harsh quality and low pitch. The term can also indicate weakness, raspiness, or simply a change from the usual voice quality. Hoarseness is the symptom, whereas *dysphonia* is the diagnostic term. Hoarseness suggests an abnormality in voice production at the level of the larynx. It is a common symptom that may occur in both men and women at any age. Changes in the voice are part of the natural process of aging. In elderly men, the voice becomes weaker and higher in pitch as a result of muscle atrophy and increased stiffness of tissues. In women, the same changes occur, but the pitch of the voice becomes lower because during menopause mucoid edema accumulates in the submucosa of the vocal folds. More severe edema and polyps may occur in women who smoke. Hoarseness is a cardinal sign of laryngeal cancer, which is most commonly seen in men 50 to 70 years of age. Psychogenic dysphonia may present with a monotonous and bizarre aberration of vocal sounds.

Epidemiology and Causes

Hoarseness affects approximately 20 million people in the United States at any given time, and about one in three people will become hoarse at some point in their lifetimes. Hoarseness is frequently the result of a viral infection of the larynx (laryngitis). Usually, acute laryngitis affects individuals aged 18 to 40 years; however, children aged 3 years and older have been clinically observed with laryngitis. In women, the prevalence of hoarseness not associated with infection is 50% higher than it is in men. Professional teachers, performers, aerobics instructors, telemarketers, and the elderly are at risk.

Pathophysiology

Vocal cord inflammation and edema as a result of an infectious process (usually viral) result in vocal fold movement that is asymmetrical with reduced mucosal waves and incomplete vibratory closure. In the process of phagocystosis, the vocal folds become more edematous and vibration is adversely affected. The phonation threshold pressure may increase to a degree that generating adequate phonation pressure in a normal fashion becomes difficult, thus elicting hoarseness. Gastroesophageal reflux disease (GERD) may also contribute to inflammation and edema of the vocal cords. Laryngeal tumor may present as hoarseness.

Clinical Presentation
Subjective

Onset of the problem is an important key to the diagnosis. A 1-day complaint is unlikely to be caused by cancer, whereas hoarseness persisting for 1 year is unlikely to be the result of an acute infection. Hoarseness that persists for greater than 3 weeks requires a work-up for chronic laryngitis. Associated conditions should be ascertained. Sore throat and otalgia often accompany hoarseness in malignant tumor of the larynx or pharynx. Chronic pain often suggests more serious underlying disease than acute onset of pain. Dysphagia or odynophagia accompanying hoarseness indicates the presence of disease affecting the pharynx or esophagus. Cough suggests irritation of the endolarynx or pulmonary disease. Hemoptysis is more serious, suggesting a malignant process of the pharyngeal, laryngeal, or pulmonary areas. Fever and oral, nasal, or otalgic discharge suggest an infectious process.

Voice use and lifestyle should be reviewed. A professional singer or weekend football fan can suffer voice overuse and abuse. An individual who smoked two packs of cigarettes per day for 45 years may have irritation or malignancy. A scratchy throat the morning after eating spicy foods suggests a diagnosis of GERD, as does chronic clearing the throat throughout the day. Previous head or neck surgery history may be a factor affecting the laryngeal nerve, as well as recent intubation or radiotherapy to the neck. The use of asthma inhalers may also produce hoarseness, and chronic exposure to pollutants may contribute as well.

Objective

A complete examination of the head and neck is necessary. Nasal drainage and excess mucus may indicate sinusitis. Tonsillar erythema or exudates indicates viral or bacterial infection. Ear canal erythema or exudate suggests infection. A normal ear exam, despite the complaint of otalgia, may be seen in patients with cancer of the pharynx or larynx. The clinician should inspect and palpate the oral cavity including the buccal mucosa, the floor of the mouth, and the tongue with a gloved hand. Palpate the neck and lymph nodes for masses. Infections often feel warm, tender, tense, or fluctuant. Malignancies typically are hard masses that may be fixed to underlying tissue. Inspect and palpate the neck anatomy, including tracheal alignment. A thorough head, eyes, ears, nose, and throat (HEENT) exam looking for evidence of infection may be essentially negative.

Diagnostic Reasoning
Diagnostic Tests

Infections cause elevated white blood cell counts. Culture and sensitivity of oral or otalgic discharge can reveal the organism responsible for the infection and guide antibiotic therapy. If hoarseness persists for more than 4 weeks and is clearly not caused by infection, referral to an otolaryngologist for laryngoscopy is required. An adequate laryngeal exam should visualize the base of the tongue, epiglottis, pyriform sinuses, false vocal cords, subglottic larynx, and true vocal cords. Use of stroboscopy improves detection of small lesions by "freezing" the vocal cords (making them appear immobile) during vibration. Adequate examination of structures may require general anesthesia, which is necessary for palpation and biopsy of any abnormalities. Routine use of CT scanning is neither cost effective nor necessary. If vocal cord paralysis is seen, CT scans from the skull base to the aortic arch are required to assess the recurrent laryngeal nerves. Thyroid tumors are the most common cause of bilateral vocal cord paralysis; esophageal and pulmonary tumors are common causes of left-sided vocal cord paralysis.

Differential Diagnosis

Differential diagnosis of hoarseness includes viral infection, which is the most common etiology, inflammation from overuse, vocal cord pathology (polyps, nodules, tumors) especially in smokers, adverse effects from medicines, vocal cord paralysis, muscle atrophy (aging), GERD, and chronic allergies.

Differential Diagnosis 8.3 presents a comparison of the differential diagnosis of hoarseness.

Management

The causes of nearly all cases of hoarseness are benign or self-limited conditions. Recent guidelines for the management of hoarseness have been developed by the American Academy of Otolaryngology–Head and Neck Surgery Foundation and are reviewed here:

- Review current medications that may be causing the symptom.
- Use common sense to avoid vocal excess and irritants such as inhaled smoke.
- Completely rest the voice. Avoid whispering because this strains the larynx.
- Avoid antihistamines because they serve to dry the mucous membranes.
- There is no benefit in using antibiotics to treat acute laryngitis.
- Imaging studies should not be performed before visualizing the larynx with laryngoscopy.
- Use of humidified air especially at night and during dry seasons may be helpful.
- Encourage increased oral fluids.

- Treatment with antireflux medication should not be undertaken in the absence of signs or symptoms of significant GERD and prior evaluation by laryngoscopy.
- Voice therapy, typically one or two sessions per week for 4 to 8 weeks, is a well-established intervention for patients of all ages who have hoarseness.
- Use of an amplifying device during heavy voice use can reduce hoarseness.
- Oral steroids are not recommended.

In the case where the "show must go on" and voice rest is impossible, if laryngeal examination rules out vocal fold hemorrhage or abrasion, it is usually safe to manage vocal fold edema temporarily with oral or parenteral steroids. A long-acting vasoconstrictor such as oxymetazoline (Afrin) may be applied directly to the laryngeal mucosa to reduce edema further. These measures do not promote healing, nor do they prevent further damage to the vocal cords.

Follow-up and Referral

For repeated and recurrent episodes of hoarseness, vocal hygiene and voice therapy should be considered, especially in professionals who must rely on their voice. Screening for contributing conditions (such as underlying allergies, chronic sinusitis, or GERD) should be pursued. As noted earlier, if hoarseness persists for more than 2 weeks, further evaluation by an ENT specialist is warranted.

Patient Education

Because hoarseness is generally self-limited, instructions to stop smoking and rest the voice are essential to facilitate improvement. Humidification and adequate fluid intake will help healing of inflamed tissues. Avoid cough and cold preparations that have antihistamines in the formulation because they will have a drying effect. Patients should return within 2 weeks to evaluate resolution of hoarseness. Patients should be instructed that persistent or chronic hoarseness requires evaluation by an ENT specialist for laryngoscopic visualization.

■ TEMPOROMANDIBULAR JOINT DISEASE

Temporomandibular joint (TMJ) *disease* is a collective term that refers to disorders affecting the masticatory musculature, the temporomandibular joint and associated structures, or both. The terms *craniomandibular disorders* (CMDs) and *temporomandibular disorders* (TMDs) are synonymous with the more familiar term *temporomandibular joint (TMJ) disease.* Most current research favors the phrase *temporomandibular disorder* (TMD). Although TMD has been traditionally viewed as one syndrome, it is actually a cluster of related disorders in the masticatory system that has many features in common. The most common presenting symptom is pain in the muscles of mastication, the preauricular area, and/or the TMJ. Chewing, bruxism (clenching, grinding, or gnashing of the teeth during nonfunctional movements of the mandible), or other jaw functions tend to aggravate the pain. TMDs are considered to be a subclassification of musculoskeletal disorders.

Epidemiology and Causes

Symptoms of TMD in individuals are common, yet not every person with symptoms would be considered to have the disorder. Epidemiological studies in specific populations show that about 75% have at least one sign of joint dysfunction (joint noise) and about 33% have at least one symptom (face or joint pain). It is estimated that only 5% of these individuals are in need of treatment for TMD. For many patients, TMD can be mild and self-limiting; for others, it may progress to chronic pain and discomfort, which will require consultation with multiple professionals over many years.

Signs and symptoms of TMD generally increase in frequency and severity from the second through the fourth decade of life. The majority of patients are between ages 15 and 45, with a mean age at onset of 35. The vast majority of patients with TMD (84%) are women, yet some data demonstrate that men have symptomatology but do not present for treatment. Symptoms may be self-limiting or may fluctuate over time, as suggested by the declining incidence with increasing age. The lack of a universally accepted classification scheme with diagnostic criteria makes it difficult to accurately determine the prevalence of TMD.

Because TMDs are diverse and multifactorial, a universal etiology does not exist. It may be more appropriate to differentiate contributing factors into predisposing, initiating, and perpetuating categories. *Predisposing factors* increase the risk of orofacial pain or TMD development. *Initiating factors* cause the onset of the disorder, and *perpetuating factors* interfere with healing and complicate management. Contributing factors are not necessarily etiological; they may be the result of the disorder instead.

Predisposing factors include biomechanical, genetic, or psychological factors that increase the chances of an individual developing TMD. Initiating or precipitating factors generally fall into two main categories— macrotrauma as a result of a single event, or microtrauma in the form of repetitive adverse loading of the masticatory system. Perpetuating factors include personality, social, emotional, and cognitive factors that are often related to the stresses of daily living. The dividing line between categories is not always clear-cut. Some initiating factors (e.g., bruxism) may also act to maintain the disorder after onset. Differential Diagnosis 8.4 and Table 8.3 present contributing factors to TMD.

Pathophysiology

The TMJ is one of the most complex joints in the body. It is a synovial, encapsulated joint that is stress bearing.

Differential Diagnosis 8.4
Temporomandibular Disease

- Sinusitis
- Myofascial pain
- Arthritis (rheumatoid arthritis, osteoarthritis, gout, septic, psoriatic, Lyme)
- Parotid gland pathology
- Otitis media and otitis externa
- Temporal arteritis
- Neuralgia
- Foreign body or cerumen in the ear canal
- Mastoiditis
- Dental abnormalities
- Headaches (cluster, migraine, tension, vascular)
- Psychogenic pain
- Mood disorders (depression, anxiety)
- Tumors of the head, neck, or brain
- Myopathies

The TMJ differs from other joints in the body in that its articular surfaces are covered with fibrocartilaginous tissue rather than with the chondrocartilage found in other joints. The articular disc separates the upper and lower joint spaces. Pain from the TMJ arises from injury to the retrodiscal tissue or the capsular ligament. Locking of the joint may occur secondary to jaw malocclusion and, most commonly, anterior disc dislocation. However, several variations of articular disc displacement have been noted with the condition, as joint laxity from underlying connective tissue disorders and even asymmetrical body alignment from poor posture have been cited as risk factors. Dental manipulation of the jaw and degeneration of the TMJ from rheumatoid arthritis or osteoarthritis often underlie extracapsular joint dysfunction, because misalignment of the TMJ places pressure

on nearby ear structures, resulting in otalgia (ear pain), tinnitus, vertigo, hearing loss, and tongue pain.

TMJ pain may also be intracapsular in origin and involve the masticatory musculature, known as TMJ myofascial pain syndome or simply TMJ syndrome. Similar to all skeletal muscles, the TMJ muscles are susceptible to muscle splinting, spasm, or inflammation. Pain that originates in the orofacial area may be referred to other areas, such as the neck, shoulders, and head, and TMJ syndrome often coexists with fibromyalgia. However, pain from the masticatory musculature is usually related to mandibular dysfunction. Abnormal chewing patterns, chronic tension of the jaw musculature, and facial trauma all predispose to muscle dysfunction. Stress-related jaw clenching and psychogenic nocturnal bruxism (unconscious nighttime teeth grinding) have also been strongly associated with TMJ syndrome. The importance of psychological stress in the development of this disorder is further bolstered by the observation that a worse prognosis is associated with a diminished capacity for supportive interpersonal relationships.

Clinical Presentation
Subjective

Patients may present with several complaints that lead to the suspicion of TMD or with only one symptom. The most common presenting symptom is pain (89%), followed by jaw noise (85%) and limited jaw movement (40%). Ear symptoms account for 28% of clinical presentations. Only 4% of patients present with obvious jaw dislocation.

Pain is usually localized in the muscles of mastication, the preauricular area, and/or the TMJ. Chewing or other jaw functions frequently aggravate the pain. Patients may complain of poorly localized pain in the face or head, which is dull, unilateral, centered in the temple, above and behind the eye, or in and around the ear. Other less obvious symptoms may include tinnitus, sinus symptoms, a foreign body sensation in the external

Table 8.3   Factors Contributing to Temporomandibular Disorders

Biomechanical Factors	Macrotrauma	Psychological Factors	Systemic Medical Conditions	Microtrauma	Habits
Past injuries	Contact sport	Personality	Rheumatic	Oral parafunctional	Bruxism
Skeletal malformations	Motor vehicle accident	Social	Hormonal		Nail biting
Postural imbalances	Whiplash	Emotional	Infectious		Gum chewing
Occlusal factors		Cognitive	Nutritional		
Cervical disorders		Anxiety	Metabolic		
		Depression Mental disorders Substance abuse			

ear canal, decreased hearing, neck or shoulder pain, visual disturbances, limited jaw opening, and popping or grating joint sounds. Patients may present with a history of trauma to the TMJ or cervical disc area (such as whiplash).

Several questionnaires have been developed to assist the health-care professional in screening for TMD. Any patient who presents with symptomatology (complaints of orofacial pain, headaches, ear pain, or tinnitus) should be screened for TMD by asking questions such as the following: Do your jaw joints make noise? Does using your jaw—such as chewing, talking, and/or yawning—cause you pain or difficulty? Have you had jaw joint problems before, and were you tested? When moving your jaw, does it ever get "stuck," "lock," or "go out"? Is opening your mouth difficult, or does it cause pain? Do you ever have pain in the head and neck area, such as the face, ears, temples, and/or forehead? Has your jaw, neck, or head ever been injured? If so, when? Do you clinch or grind your teeth at night or during the day? If you have tinnitus, does the ringing sound change in any way as you open and close your mouth while applying external pressure to the joint? Do you have frequent headaches, neckaches, or toothaches?

Objective

Because many of the presenting symptoms of TMD may be secondary to underlying medical conditions, a complete examination should be done in order to exclude metabolic, nutritional, neurological, or hormonal etiologies. Visual acuity should be assessed. Special attention should be directed to observation of the patient's balance, gait problems, or unusual habits. The muscles of mastication and the TMJ should be palpated using a bimanual technique. Muscles to be palpated include the masseter, temporalis, medial pterygoid, digastric, and mylohyoid. Tenderness, enlargement, swelling, and unusual texture should be noted. Cervical muscle groups should also be palpated to differentiate craniocervical disorders. The oral exam may reveal ground-down teeth, which would indicate bruxism.

Next, the TMJ should be examined with the mouth in the closed position, which will allow palpation of the lateral aspect. On opening of the jaw, assessment of mandibular range of motion and TMJ sounds can assist with diagnosis. A mandibular opening of less than 40 mm is considered restrictive; the mandible may deviate to one side or the other when opened (asymmetrical opening). Joint sounds may be described as clicking, popping, or crepitus. Pain may also be elicited with mandibular movement and should be noted.

Diagnostic Reasoning

Diagnostic Tests

Initial testing for diagnosing TMD may first include ruling out other underlying medical conditions. Laboratory testing should include CBC with differential, platelets, chemistry panel, erythrocyte sedimentation rate, rheumatoid factor, and thyroid-stimulating hormone. Radiographical imaging (x-ray films) may be helpful in confirming a clinical diagnosis of TMD. The clinician must remember that even if anatomical changes are found, imaging results rarely have any bearing on clinical outcome. Imaging testing is confirmatory at best, but the diagnosis may be made via history and clinical exam alone. Films are best reserved when dental anomalies are suspected or severe symptoms are refractory to conservative treatment. A transcranial view (lateral oblique projection) is the most common film taken of the TMJ. This view is useful for identification of gross osseous pathology and degenerative or traumatic changes of the joint; however, it is subject to distortion and shows only the lateral one-third of the condylar head and may not be sensitive enough to detect condylar displacement.

Subsequent testing should most likely be ordered by the dentist, otolaryngologist, or oral surgeon on referral of the patient. This could include panoramic films, CT, or MRI. CT provides the clearest picture of the osseous structures, and, with contrast, can help visualize the soft tissue of the head and neck; however, it is not useful in the diagnosis of disc displacement of the TMJ. MRI visualizes the soft tissues of the joint without radiation and the injection of contrast dye. MRI can be used to determine disc position and morphology. MRI may also show arthritic changes in the TMJ. Moreover, disc displacement seen on MRI may also be observed in asymptomatic patients, so these findings should never guide therapy alone. Diagnostic injections with anesthesia, synovial fluid analysis, or biopsy of suspicious areas by the specialist may be useful for differentiating diagnosis.

Differential Diagnosis

Because of the extensive list of contributing factors and potential symptoms, it may be difficult to arrive at a diagnosis of TMD. Accurate diagnosis is essential and has traditionally been the weak link in the chain of management of TMD. Disorders of the intracranial structures should be ruled out initially because they may be life-threatening and require immediate attention. New or abrupt onset of pain, progressively more severe pain, interruption of sleep by pain, and systemic symptoms such as weight loss, ataxia, fever, and neurological symptoms (e.g., seizures, paralysis, vertigo) are characteristic of intracranial disorders. Differential Diagnosis Table 8.4 presents common differential diagnoses for TMD.

Management

Effective care of patients with TMD involves understanding and treating the whole patient via an individualized program. A multidisciplinary approach is frequently indicated. Contributing factors must be addressed rather than concentrating on eliminating signs and symptoms.

The goals for management are similar to those of any musculoskeletal condition—reduction or elimination of pain and restoration of acceptable mandibular function. Complete resolution of TMD may not always be possible, however, as in the case of permanent damage to joint structures. In these cases, the term "cure" or "treatment" has been abandoned for the term "management."

Initial therapy should be reversible and is designed to be palliative and to promote healing. Acute disc displacement or active trigger points may require rapid treatment/referral. In general, however, the practitioner can initiate management with conservative therapies such as self-help techniques and pharmacotherapy.

One of the most significant contributions toward management of TMD can be made by adjustment in diet consistency, education and alteration of oral parafunctional habits, and application of ice (for acute symptomatology) or moist heat (for chronic symptomatology). On occasion, self-treatment alone may control signs and symptoms; specific recommendations are listed under Patient Education.

Physical therapy may be employed, primarily as an adjunct to other therapeutic modalities, in an attempt to relieve pain of musculoskeletal origin and restore normal masticatory function. Physical therapy for TMD may include electromodalities and therapeutic exercises as prescribed by a physical therapist. Behavioral therapy is indicated for patients with behavioral and emotional problems and/or noxious habits that accompany TMD. Stress relief and pain control methods such as counseling, hypnosis, biofeedback, and guided imagery are safe and noninvasive.

Pharmacotherapy can be beneficial in controlling pain and inflammation associated with TMD. Careful monitoring of the patient's tolerance to prescribed medications, as well as the effectiveness of the drug, is indicated. To avoid potential abuse of any drug that may produce dependence, dosing at regular intervals for a definite period of time is preferred, as opposed to as-needed dosing. Drugs Commonly Prescribed 8.6 presents the drugs that are commonly used to treat TMJ disease. Injection of trigger points with anesthetic agents

Drugs Commonly Prescribed 8.6 Temporomandibular Joint Disease (TMD)

Drug	Indication	Dosage	Comments
Tricyclic Antidepressants			
amitriptyline (Elavil)	TMD (chronic)	25 mg 3–4 times daily or 75 mg at bedtime Begin with low nightly dose and increase	May result in decreased orofacial pain, improvement in sleep disorders, and promotion of muscle relaxation and decreased bruxism. *Contraindicated within 14 days of use of MAO inhibitors and acute post–myocardial infarction (post-MI). Monitor serum levels with concomitant use of drugs metabolized by CYP450.* **Adverse effects:** Anticholinergic effects, drowsiness, dry mouth, arrhythmias, etc.
Benzodiazepines			
clonazepam (Klonopin)	TMD (acute)	0.5 mg 3 times daily Use as a short course of 1–2 weeks only	For relief of acute pain secondary to masticatory muscle spasm or TMD pain. *Contraindicated with severe liver disease and acute narrow-angle glaucoma. Monitor for suicidal tendencies. Potentiates many CNS effects. Caution with drugs that inhibit CYP3A.* **Adverse effects:** CNS effects, especially depression. Pregnancy Category D. Not recommended for nursing mothers.

Drugs Commonly Prescribed 8.6   Temporomandibular Joint Disease (TMD)—cont'd

Drug	Indication	Dosage	Comments
diazepam (Valium)	TMD acute and chronic	2–10 mg 2–4 times daily	*Contraindicated with acute narrow-angle glaucoma. Potentiates ETOH.* **Adverse effects:** CNS depression, ataxia, memory impairment.
Nonopioid Analgesics			
acetaminophen (Tylenol)	TMD chronic	1,000 mg 3 times daily	May relieve orofacial pain.
ibuprofen (Motrin, Advil)	TMD chronic	400–800 mg 3–4 times daily	May help inflammatory pain.
naproxen (Aleve)	TMD chronic	220 mg every 12 hours	*Contraindicated with aspirin allergy. Do not use in third trimester of pregnancy. Increased risk of GI bleed with concomitant use with ETOH.*
Muscle Relaxants			
cyclobenzaprine HCl (Flexeril)	TMD acute	5–10 mg 3 times daily	May relieve muscle spasm. Use with physical therapy (PT) modalities. *Contraindicated acute post-MI, arrhythmias, heart block, and other conduction disturbances. Not recommended with liver disease, urinary retention, glaucoma. Potentiates anticholinergics. Can precipitate hypertensive crisis with MAO inhibitors.* **Adverse effects:** Drowsiness, blurred vision, dry mouth, dizziness. Nursing mothers and Pregnancy Category B.
Corticosteroids			
methylprednisolone (Medrol, Solu-Medrol)	TMD acute and severe	Start slow Do not use for longer than 2–3 weeks Dose pack	*Used only for short term in severe unrelenting pain in the TMJ related to inflammatory conditions. Potentiated by CYP3A4 inhibitors. May antagonize anticoagulants. Need to monitor International Normalized Ratio (INR).* **Adverse effects:** Susceptiblitiy to infection, glaucoma, cataracts, electrolyte imbalances.

may be beneficial; however, it is most likely that this would be done by the specialist (dentist or oral maxillofacial surgeon) to whom the patient has been referred.

For the majority of cases of TMD, any necessary subsequent management will be initiated and followed by the dentist, otolaryngologist, or oral surgeon to whom the patient has been referred. Most of the therapies employed by these practitioners are not considered part of initial therapy for TMD because they are irreversible procedures. These therapies include orthodontics, prosthodontics, occlusal equilibration, or surgery. Wearing an intraoral appliance with an occlusal appliance or splint may be recommended, generally by a dentist. At the present time, this type of therapy is highly controversial and may not be considered an option by many practitioners although it may be indicated for patients with gross structural changes in the alignment of the TMJ. Surgery, including arthroscopic surgery or arthrotomy, may be recommended by an oral maxillofacial surgeon. Surgery may be indicated in patients who do not respond to nonsurgical therapy and who have disabling pain or dysfunction related to TMD. (See The Iceberg of TMD.)

Follow-up and Referral

The decision to refer a patient with TMD to a specialist should be made based on the individual practitioner's knowledge level and comfort in treating TMD. Once other systemic conditions have been ruled out, the practitioner may choose to begin initial management of

The Iceberg of TMD

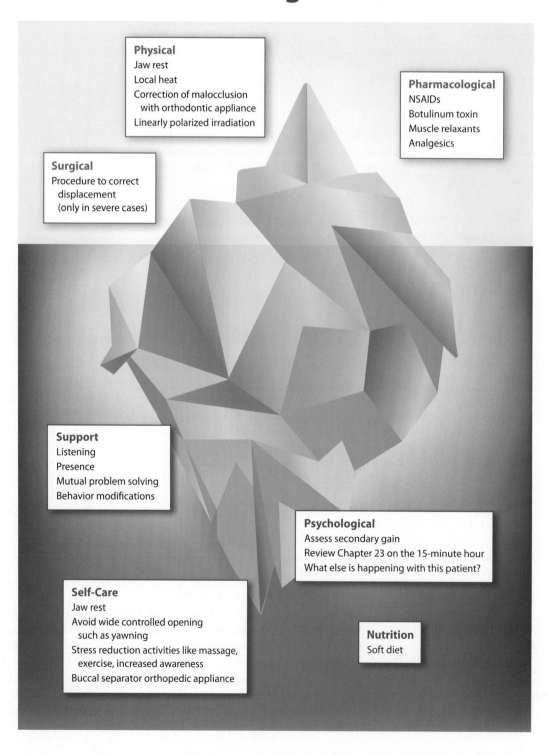

Physical
Jaw rest
Local heat
Correction of malocclusion
 with orthodontic appliance
Linearly polarized irradiation

Pharmacological
NSAIDs
Botulinum toxin
Muscle relaxants
Analgesics

Surgical
Procedure to correct
 displacement
 (only in severe cases)

Support
Listening
Presence
Mutual problem solving
Behavior modifications

Psychological
Assess secondary gain
Review Chapter 23 on the 15-minute hour
What else is happening with this patient?

Self-Care
Jaw rest
Avoid wide controlled opening
 such as yawning
Stress reduction activities like massage,
 exercise, increased awareness
Buccal separator orthopedic appliance

Nutrition
Soft diet

TMD symptoms. Follow-up should be early and repeated (e.g., in 1–2 weeks initially, and then monthly), especially if pharmacotherapy is ordered. If there is any uncertainty about the diagnosis, referral should be made at this time to a dentist or otolaryngologist or to an oral maxillofacial surgeon who is knowledgeable in the treatment of TMD. If initial therapy is unsuccessful or if advanced management is indicated, appropriate referrals should be undertaken.

Patient Education

Home care and patient education is an integral component to the management of TMD. The majority of patients achieve relief of symptoms with conservative therapy, including self-care techniques. Patient information for management of TMD includes the following recommendations:

- Limit jaw function by eating softer foods, taking smaller bites, and not opening wide when eating. Avoid foods such as apples, corn on the cob, hard breads, raw vegetables, steak, and so on.
- To help reduce stress, strive for a nutritionally balanced diet and an active exercise program.
- Ice packs can be used for acute pain and muscle spasm. Place an ice pack over the temple area and side of the face for 10 minutes, three or four times a day. For chronic pain, moist heat should be used following the same guidelines.
- Disengage your teeth—the rule is "lips together, teeth apart."
- Do not chew gum or ice.
- Sleep on your back with a pillow under your knees. Do not use firm, full pillows under your head. Orthopedic pillows can be helpful in reducing head and neck pain. Do not sleep on your stomach.
- When talking on the telephone, do not support the receiver with your shoulder.
- Prevent wide-opening when yawning. Do not sit with your chin resting on your hand.
- Practice good posture. If you must sit for long periods of time, try to stand and move around frequently to stretch your muscles.

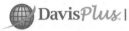 DavisPlus | For additional resources please visit http://davisplus.fadavis.com

References

Evidence-Based Practice
Lieberthal, AS, et al. The diagnosis and management of acute otitis media. *Pediatrics* 131(3):e964–e999, 2013. doi:10.1542/peds.2012-3488

Management and therapy of dry eye disease: Report of the Management and Therapy Subcommittee of the International Dry Eye WorkShop (2007). *Ocul Surf* 5(2):163–178, 2007.

Wang, SY, et al. Glaucoma and vitamins A, C, and E supplement intake and serum levels in a population-based sample of the United States. *Eye* 27(4):487–494, 2013.

Waseem, M, et al. Otitis media treatment and management. Medscape. Updated April 25, 2014. Retrieved from http://emedicine.medscape.com/article/994656-treatment

Zhao, LQ, et al. The effect of multivitamin/mineral supplements on age-related cataracts: A systematic review and meta-analysis. *Nutrients* 6(3):931–949, 2014.

Bibliography

General
Bjelakovic, R, et al. Mortality in randomized trials of antioxidant supplements for primary and secondary prevention: Systematic review and meta-analysis. *JAMA* 297(8):62–63, 2007.

Domino, F, et al. *The 5-minute clinical consult 2010*, ed 18. Lippincott Williams & Wilkins, Philadelphia, 2009.

Gaby, AR. Natural remedies for herpes simplex. *Altern Med Rev* 11(2):93–101, 2006.

Goroll, AH, and Mulley, AG. *Primary care medicine: Office evaluation and management of the adult patient*, ed 6. Lippincott Williams & Wilkins, Philadelphia, 2009.

Institute for Clinical Systems Improvement. 2009. Retrieved from www.icis.org/guidelines_and_more/gl_os_prot

Lindquist, R, et al. *Complementary and alternative therapies in nursing*, ed 7. Springer, New York, 2014.

Mazzanti, G, et al. Inhibitory activity of Melissa officinalis L. extract on herpes simplex virus type 2 replication. *Nat Prod Res* 22(16):1433–1440, 2008.

Micozzi, MS. *Fundamentals of complementary and alternative medicine*, ed 4. Saunders-Elsevier, St. Louis, 2011.

Moser Woo, T, et al. *Pharmacotherapeutics for nurse practitioner prescribers*, ed 3. FA Davis, Philadelphia, 2011.

National Library of Medicine. Complementary and alternative medicine. 2014. Retrieved from www.nlm.nih.gov/medlineplus/complementaryandalternativemedicine.html

National Library of Medicine. Herbal medicine. 2014. Retrieved from www.nlm.nih.gov/medlineplus/herbalmedicine.html

Rakel, R (Ed.). *Conn's current therapy 2010*. WB Saunders, Philadelphia, 2009.

Seller, RH. *Differential diagnosis of common complaints*, ed 5. WB Saunders, Philadelphia, 2008.

Arcangelo, VP, and Peterson, AM (Eds.). *Pharmacotherapeutics for advanced practice: A practical approach*, ed 3. Lippincott Williams & Wilkins, Philadelphia, 2013.

Visual Disturbance
Age-Related Eye Disease Study 2 Research Group. Lutein/zeaxanthin for the treatment of age-related cataract: AREDS2 randomized trial report no. 4. *JAMA Ophthalmol* 131(7):843–850, 2013.

Chew, EY. Nutrition effects on ocular diseases in the aging eye. *Invest Ophthalmol Vis Sci* 54(14):42–47, 2013.

Davila, E, et al. Sensory impairment among older U.S. workers. *Am J Public Health* 99(8):1378–1385, 2009.

Finger, RP, et al. Treatment patterns visual acuity and quality of life outcomes of the WAVE study. *ACTA Ophthalmologia* 91(6):540–546, 2013.

Huang, HY, et al. Multivitamin/mineral supplements and prevention of chronic disease: 2006. Retrieved from www.library.nhs.uk/cam/viewResource.aspx?resID=277286

Larkin, GL. Retinal detachment 2006. Retrieved from www.emedicine.com/emerg/Topic504.htm

Moore, LW, and Miller, M. Driving strategies used by older adults with macular degeneration: Assessing the risks. *Appl Nurs Res* 18:110–116, 2005.

Moore, LW, and Miller, M. Older men's experiences of living with severe visual impairment. *J Adv Nurs* 43(1):10–18, 2003.

Nootheti, S, and Bielory, L. Risks of cataracts and glaucoma with inhaled steroid use in children. *Comp Opthalmol Update* 7(1):31–39, 2006.

Patel, PJ, et al. Optimizing individualized therapy with bevacizumab for neovascular age related macular degeneration. *Retina* 2012, Vol 32(6): 3214–20.

Sharts-Hopko, N. Low vision and blindness among midlife and older adults: A review of the nursing literature. *Holis Nurs Pract* 23(2):94–100, 2009.

Tufail, A, et al. Bevacizumab for neovascular age related macular degeneration (ABC trial) multicentre randomized double masked study. *BJM* 340:2459, 2010.

USPSTF Recommendations: A summary of recent health care findings from an independent panel of experts. *Am J Nurs* 105(2):88–89, 2005.

Glaucoma

Bell, JA. Glaucoma, primary open angle 2008. Retrieved from www.emedicine.medscape.com/article/1206147

Glaucoma: Early detection can minimize vision loss. *Mayo Clin Health Lett* 23(7):1–3, 2005.

Noecker, RJ, and Kahook, MY. Glaucoma, angle closure, acute. 2009. Retrieved from http://emedicine.medscape.com/article/1206956

Richards, J, and Lichter, P. Update on glaucoma genetics. 2005. Retrieved from www.glaucoma.org/research/update_on_glauc_l.php

Screening for glaucoma: Recommendation statement. *Am J Nurs Pract* 9(9):49–50, 52–55, 2005.

Shetty, R, et al. Glaucoma drainage devices 2008. Retrieved from http://emedicine.medscape.com/article/1208066

U.S. Preventive Services Task Force. Screening for glaucoma: Recommendation statement. *Ann Fam Med* 3(2):171–172, 2005.

Red Eye

Eye Center. Excessive tearing (epiphora). Retrieved from www.theeyecenter.com/educational/0026.htm

Farina, GA, and Mazarin, GI. Red eye evaluation 2006. Retrieved from http://emedicine.medscape.com/article/1216540

Kopes-Kerr, B, and Alper, BS. Allergic conjunctivitis. *Clin Advis* 125–127, 2007.

Lloyd, A, and Pinto, GL. Common eye problems. *Clin Rev* 19(11):24–30, 2009.

Marlin, D. Conjunctivitis, bacterial. 2009. Retrieved from http://emedicine.medscape.com/article/1191730

Practical pearls for managing red eye 2007. Retrieved from www.pri-med.com/PMO/Activity.aspx?activity=388&StepInd

Scott, IU, and Luu, K. Conjunctivitis, viral. 2009. Retrieved from http://emedicine.medscape.com/article/1191370–overview

Dry Eye

American Academy of Opthalmology Cornea/External Disease Panel, Preferred Practice Patterns Committee. Blepharitis 2008. Retrieved from www.guidelines.gov/summary/summary.aspx?doc_id=13500

American Academy of Opthamology Cornea/External Disease Panel, Preferred Practice Patterns Committee. Dry eye syndrome 2008. Retrieved from www.guidelines.gov/summary/summary.aspx?doc_id=13503

Bhargava, R, et al. A randomized controlled trial of omega-3 fatty acids in dry eye syndrome. *Int J Ophthalmol* 6(6):811–816, 2013.

Dosa, L. Topical cyclosporine improves tear production 2003. Retrieved from www.medscape.com/viewarticle/463701

Dunne, M, and Sumner, D. EGFR inhibitors: Toxicities and strategies for effective management 2008. Retrieved from http://cme.medscape.com/viewarticle/579711

Foster, SC, et al. Dry eye syndrome 2009. Retrieved from http://www.emedicine.medscape.com/article/1210417

Gilbard, JP. The diagnosis and management of dry eyes. *Otolaryngol Clin North Am* 38(5):871–885, 2007.

Gupta, A, et al. Occult thyroid eye disease in patients presenting with dry eye symptoms. *Am J Opthamol* 147(5):919–923, 2009.

Lowery, RS. Blepharitis, adult 2009. Retrieved from http://emedicine.medscape.com/article/1211763

Nilufer, I, et al. Is there a relationship between pathologic myopia and dry eye syndrome? Released before published. Retrieved from FAU journals at OVID Full Text. doi:10.1097/ico00000000000033

Pflugfelder, SC. The VIEW II: Halting progression of dry eye disease CME 2009. Retrieved from http://cme.medscape.com/viewarticle/704768

Rocha, EM, et al. Hormones and dry eye syndrome: An update on what we do and don't know. *Curr Opin Ophothalmol* 24(4):348–355, 2013.

Eye Pain

Fadel, HJ, et al. 58 year old man with fever and right eye pain. *Mayo Clinic Proc* 81(9):1238–1240, 2006.

Gaeta, TJ, and Valcich, D. Scleritis. 2008. Retrieved from http://emedicine.medscape.com/article/809166

Verma, A. Corneal abrasion. 2008. Retrieved from http://emedicine.medscape.com/article/1195402

Hearing Impairment

Fitzpatrick, E, et al. A retrospective study of cochlear implant outcomes in children with residual hearing. *BMC Ear Nose Throat Disord* 2006. Retrieved from www.biomedcentral.com/1472–6815/6/7

Ibekwe, TS, et al. Correlating the site of tympanic membrane perforation with hearing loss. *BMC Ear Nose Throat Disord* 9(1), 2009. Retrieved from www.biomedcentral.com/1472–6815/9/1

Lin, Y-S. Management of otitis media–related diseases in children with a cochlear implant. *Acta Oto-Laryngol* 129(3):254–260, 2009.

Malmstrom, J. Gerontologic nurse practitioner care guidelines: Assessing and managing hearing deficits in the older adult. *Geriatr Nurs* 26:57–59, 2005.

Stachler, RJ. Clinical practice guidelines: Sudden hearing loss. *Otolaryngel Head Neck Surg* 146:1–35, 2012.

Valentino, RL. Chronic dysfunction of the eustachian tube. *Clin Advis* 21–25, 2009.

Williams, ME. Examining the ears, nose, and oral cavity in the older adult patient. 2007. Retrieved from http://cme.medscape.com/viewarticle/556144

Otitis Externa

Handzel, O, and Halperin, D. Necrotizing (malignant) external otitis. *Am Fam Physician* 2003. Retrieved from www.aafp.org/afp/AFPprinter/20030715/309.html

Lee, S, and Rosh, A. Otitis externa. 2009. Retrieved from http://emedicine.medscape.com/article/763918

Rosenfeld, RM, et al. Clinical practice guideline: Acute otitis externa. *Otolaryngol Head Neck Surg* 134(4S):S4–S23, 2006.

Walton, L. Otitis externa. *BMJ* 344:1756–1833, 2012. doi:10.113/bmje3623

Otitis Media

Acuin, J. Chronic suppurative otitis media. *BMJ Clinical Evidence* 2:507, 2007.

Coco, A: Cost-effectiveness analysis of treatment options for acute otitis media. *Ann Fam Med* 5(1):29–38, 2007.

Donaldson, JD. Middle ear, acute otitis media, medical treatment. 2008. Retrieved from http://emedicine.medscape.com/article/859316

ICSI Health Care Guideline. Diagnosis and treatment of otitis media in children. 2008. Retrieved from www.icsi.org

Lee, KY. Pediatric respiratory infections by *Mycoplasma pneumoniae*. *Expert Rev Anti Infect Ther* 6(4):509–521, 2008.

Lieberthal, AS, et al. The diagnosis and management of acute otitis media. *Pediatrics* 131(3):e964–e999, 2013.

National Guideline Clearinghouse. Evidence based clinical practice guidelines for diagnosis and management of acute otitis media. Retrieved from www.guideline.gov/summary.aspx?doc_ID=6009&NB

Prymula, R, et al. Pneumococcal capsular polysaccharides conjugated to protein D for prevention of acute otitis media caused by both *Streptococcus pneumoniae* and nontypable *Haemophilus influenzae*: A randomised double-blind efficacy study. *Lancet* 357:740–748, 2006.

Ramakrishnan, K, et al. Diagnosis and treatment of otitis media. *Am Fam Physician* 76(11):1650–1658, 2007.

Rovers, MM, et al. Antibiotics for acute otitis media: A meta-analysis with individual patient data. *Lancet* 368:1429–1435, 2006.

Smith-Vaughan, H, et al. Measuring nasal bacterial load and its association with otitis media. *BMC Ear Nose Throat Disord* 2006. Retrieved from www.biomedcentral.com/1472–6815/6/10

Vernacchio, L, et al. Management of acute otitis media by primary care physicians: Trends since the release of the 2004 American Academy of Pediatrics/American Academy of Family Physicians Clinical Practice Guideline. *Pediatrics* 120(2):281–287, 2007.

Yano, H, et al. Detection of respiratory viruses in nasopharyngeal secretions and middle ear fluid from children with acute otitis media. *Acta Oto-Laryngol* 129(1):19–24, 2009.

Tinnitus

Daugherty, JA. The latest buzz on tinnitus. *Nurse Pract* 32(10):42–47, 2007.

Gudex, C, et al. Effectiveness of a tinnitus management programme: A 2-year follow up study. *BMC Ear Nose Throat Disord* 9:6, 2009. Retrieved from www.biomedcentral.com/1472–6815/9/6

Pray, J, and Pray, S. Tinnitus: When the ears ring. 2005. Retrieved from www.medscape.com/viewarticle/506920

Ménière's Disease

Gates, GA, and Verrall, AM. Validation of the Meniere's disease patient-oriented symptom-severity index. *Arch Otolaryngol Head Neck Surg* 131(10):863–867, 2005.

Kim, HH, et al. Trends in the diagnosis and the management of Meniere's disease: Results of a survey. *Otolaryngol Head Neck Surg* 132(5):722–726, 2005.

Morrison, AW, et al. Familial Meniere's disease: Clinical and genetic aspects. *J Laryngol Otol* 123(1):29–37, 2009.

Pray, SW: Meniere's disease. Retrieved from http://medscape.com/viewarticle/509085

Radtke, A, et al. Screening for Meniere's disease in the general population—The needle in the haystack. *Acta Oto-Laryngol* 128(3):272–276, 2008.

Epistaxis

Kucik, CJ, and Clenney, T. Management of epistaxis. *Am Fam Physician* 71(2):305–311, 2005.

Rhinitis/Sinusitis

Adriaensen, GF, and Fokkens, WJ. Chronic rhinosinusitis: An update on current pharmacotherapy. *Expert Opin Pharmacother* 14(17): 2351–2360, 2013.

Chow, AW, et al. IDSA clinical practice guideline for acute bacterial rhinosinusitis in children and adults. *Clin Infect Dis* 54(8):1041–1045, 2012.

Conboy-Ellis, K, and Braker-Shaver, S. Intranasal steroids and allergic rhinitis. *Nurse Pract* 32(4):44–49, 2007.

Dowdee, A, and Ossege, J. Assessment of childhood allergy for the primary care practitioner. *J Am Acad Nurse Pract* 19:53–62, 2007.

Huntzinger, A. Guidelines for the diagnosis and management of rhinosinusitis in adults. *Am Fam Physician* 76(11):17–33, 2007.

Litvack, JR, et al. Olfactory function and disease severity in chronic rhinosinusitis. *Am J Rhinol Allergy* 23(2):139–144, 2009.

Rosenfeld, RM, et al. Clinical practice guideline (update): Adult Sinusitis. 152(2 suppl): S1–S39, 2015.

Russell, PT, and Bekey, JR. Oral antibiotics and the management of chronic sinusitis: What do we know. *Curr Opin Otolaryngol Head Neck Surg* 2013. Retrieved from FAU Journals at OVID. doi:10.1097/MOO.0000000000000022

Sheikh, J. Rhinitis, allergic. Retrieved from http://emedicine.medscape.com/article/134825

Sutter, AD, et al. Predicting prognosis and effect of antibiotic treatment in rhinosinusitis. *Ann Fam Med* 4(6):486–499, 2006.

Valet, RS, and Fahrenholz, JM. Allergic rhinitis: Update on diagnosis. *Consultant* 49(10):610–613, 2009.

Witt, CM, et al. Homeopathic treatment of patients with chronic sinusitis: A prospective observational study with 8 years follow up. *BMC Ear Nose Throat Disord* 9:7, 2009. Retrieved from www.biomedcentral.com/1472–6815/9/7

Zagaria, M, and Buonanno, A. A patient-oriented approach to the management of allergic rhinitis. *Clin Rev* 15(9):59–69, 2005.

Oral Lesions

Astroth, J. The links between oral and systemic health. *Clin Advis* 12(3):19–23, 2009.

Atenburg, MD, and Zouboulis, CC. Current concepts in the treatment of recurrent aphthous stomatitis. 2008. Retrieved from www.medscape.com/viewarticle/582101

Burgess, JA. Painful oral lesions: What to look for, how to treat, part 1. *Consultant* 1497–1500, November 2006.

Harris, DJ, et al. Putting evidence into practice: Evidence-based interventions for the management of oral mucositis. *Clin J Oncol Nurs* 12(1):141–152, 2008.

Rivinius, C. Burning mouth syndrome: Identification, diagnosis and treatment. *J Am Acad Nurse Pract* 21:423–429, 2009.

Studdiford, JS, et al. HIV-related oral lesions: Clues for early diagnosis. *Consultant* 182–184, March 2009.

U.S. Preventive Services Task Force. Screening for oral cancer: Recommendation statement. November 2013. Agency for Healthcare Research and Quality, Rockville, MD. Retrieved from www.ahrq.gov/clinic/3rduspsf/oralcanrs.htm

Pharyngitis

Aung, K, et al. Pharyngitis, viral 2009. Retrieved from http://emedicine.medscape.com/article/225362–overview

Brown, AJ, and Vega, C. Rapid strep test most cost-effective for pharyngitis workup in adults CME/CE. Retrieved from www.medscape.com/viewarticle/528883

Hoyle, C. Make your strep diagnosis spot on. *Nurse Pract* 10:47–51, 2009.

Matthys, J, et al. Differences among international guidelines: Not just academic. *Ann Fam Med* 5(5):436–443, 2007.

National Guideline Clearinghouse. Pharyngitis 2006. Retrieved from www.guideline.gov/summary/summary.aspx?doc_id=10630

Simon, HK. Pharyngitis 2008. Retrieved from http://emedicine.medscape.com/article/967384

TMJ

Buescher, JJ. Temporomandibular joint disorders. *Am Fam Physician* 76(10):1477–1482, 2007.

Emshoff, R, et al. Low-level laser therapy for treatment of temporomandibular joint pain: A double-blind and placebo-controlled trial. *Oral Surg Oral Med Oral Pathol Oral Radiol Endodontol* 105(4):452–456, 2008.

Chapter 9

Respiratory Problems

Jill E. Winland-Brown, EdD, APRN, FNP-BC • Brian Oscar Porter, MD, PhD, MPH

COMMON COMPLAINTS

■ COUGH

Each year more Americans seek medical treatment for a cough than for any other complaint. In the United States, the treatment costs for these visits exceed $1 billion annually. Cough is the body's natural protective mechanism for clearing the airways of secretions and irritants. Cough may be associated with a number of conditions, disorders, and diseases that alter pulmonary secretions (bronchitis, pulmonary edema), increase sensitivity of the cough receptors and airways (asthma), directly stimulate the receptors (aspiration), indirectly stimulate receptors (reflux), or affect psychological health. Cough may be associated with the following conditions: asthma, chronic obstructive pulmonary disease (COPD), bronchiectasis, cystic fibrosis, pneumonias, tuberculosis (TB), lung cancer, interstitial lung disease (ILD), cardiac tamponade, pharyngitis, and gastroesophageal reflux disease (GERD), to mention the most common.

In extreme cases of debilitation or in certain neuromuscular conditions, the cough mechanism may be impaired. There are times when the cough mechanism should be supported to clear the airways of unwanted irritants and times when it should be suppressed. These issues are discussed in relation to the underlying condition that initiates the cough mechanism.

Differential Diagnosis

The differential diagnosis of cough requires a comprehensive history and assessment to provide appropriate treatment and management. One patient may present with the complaint of a dry, hacking cough of sudden onset *(acute cough);* another may present with a cough of longer duration. A *chronic cough* is defined as one that lasts longer than 8 weeks. Many patients try over-the-counter (OTC) measures for a chronic, nagging cough and delay seeking treatment or seek treatment only when the cough becomes productive or when there is blood in the sputum.

A diagnosis can be made about 80% of the time via a thorough history by exploring with the patient the following details regarding the onset and nature of the cough:

• When did the cough first start? What factors may have prompted the cough (e.g., recent respiratory infection or exposure to noxious agents)? Is there a seasonal pattern? Is it related to work or hobbies?
• When does the cough occur—on arising, at bedtime, during exercise, or throughout the night?
• What factors seem to stimulate the cough or make it worse? Is the cough aggravated by exposure to certain chemicals, body position, exercise, or cold air? Does the person have any reactive airway disease?
• Has the patient identified any factors that seem to provide relief from the cough, such as sitting upright or avoiding exposure to certain agents? What measures have been tried to alleviate the cough?
• What is the quality of the cough—is it dry and hacking, wet, raspy, deep, or throaty?
• Is the cough productive or unproductive? If the patient produces sputum with the cough, ask the patient to describe the amount of sputum produced per day (e.g., 1 tsp, 1 tbsp, etc.), the color (e.g., yellow, gray, green, brown, clear, white, blood-tinged), and consistency (e.g., thick, ropy, frothy, or tenacious). When is the productive cough most productive?
• Does the patient cough more when lying supine? Is the cough 24/7?

In addition, it is essential to find out if the patient has signs and symptoms associated with the cough, such as pedal edema, dizziness, chest pain or tightness as with reactive airway disease, fatigue, dyspnea, hoarseness, fever, tachypnea, chills, heartburn, wheezing, and hemoptysis. In describing dyspnea, it is best for the patient to use a continuum scale similar to the pain scale that can describe today's dyspnea versus previous dyspnea on a scale of 0 to 10. Research indicates a vertical analog scale is best for patients to "plot" this and keep a diary or record of this until their next visit. The patient should be asked to describe in detail the onset of the associated signs and symptoms. Standard data regarding the patient's medical history should be recorded, including hospitalizations, surgeries, and major illnesses, particularly recent illnesses and respiratory allergies. The patient's lifestyle should be explored, such as occupation and work history; hobbies; exposures to noxious agents; and use of alcohol, tobacco, and other substances. Patients should also be asked about the use of marijuana, because it is now legal in several states, as well as the use of electronic cigarettes that contain nicotine. The most common cause of chronic cough is cigarette smoking, which triggers the cough reflex by direct bronchial irritation.

The patient needs to be asked about the use of prescription and OTC drugs. Certain antihypertensive drugs such as angiotensin-converting enzyme (ACE) inhibitors and beta blockers can cause hypersensitive airways, producing wheezing and a cough. Other drugs such as nitrofurantoin (Macrobid, Macrodantin) may cause interstitial fibrosis and associated cough. All patients taking nitrofurantoin (Macrobid) should be monitored for changes in lung function. Some individuals who are prone to certain autoimmune disorders seem to be more susceptible to lung disease after taking these antibiotics.

For the physical exam, focus on the following:

- Check the ears for cerumen or hairs impinging on the tympanic membrane, which may cause cough (Arnold's reflex).
- Examine the nose for discharge, edema, polyps, and sinus tenderness. In the throat, look for cobblestoning of the oropharynx, which suggests postnasal drip.
- Palpate the neck, including both anterior and posterior cervical node chains, for enlarged lymph nodes or masses.

A complete assessment of the thorax and chest should be done to rule out cardiac or pulmonary problems. If the patient has not coughed during the visit, ask the patient to reproduce the cough and listen to its sound and character. The lungs should be auscultated, especially for crackles (rales) and rhonchi. The patient should be asked to produce a forced expiration while the practitioner checks for wheezes. Generally crackles, which are fluid, do not clear with cough; but rhonchi, which are mucus, do clear after the patient is asked to cough and clear the airways. The presence of heart murmurs, gallops, and carotid bruits should also be assessed. Any of the following conditions may cause cough:

- **Postnasal drip:** This common problem is most often associated with allergic or vasomotor rhinitis and less often with sinusitis. Patients often describe a sensation of tickling or trickling in the back of the throat.
- **Postinfection:** After a bout with the flu or viral illness involving the respiratory tract, patients may have a cough for 8 or more weeks because of bronchial hyperreactivity.
- **COPD:** Chronic bronchitis, the most common type of COPD, is defined as a chronic productive cough that persists for 3 months of the year or longer for 2 or more successive years. Most smokers eventually develop chronic bronchitis.
- **Asthma:** Asthma is a reversible obstructive pulmonary disease, a reactive airway disease, and is often accompanied by cough and wheezing. The cough may be productive or dry.

- **GERD:** In most cases, cough associated with GERD is thought to be caused by stimulation of the distal esophagus, but in a small percentage of cases, it may be due to microaspiration.
- **Drugs:** Cough occurs in about 10% of patients who take ACE inhibitors, such as captopril and enalapril. A complete history of prescribed and OTC drugs, including any herbal preparations, should be taken.
- **Occupational and environmental factors:** Exposure to air pollution, industrial dust and pollutants, secondhand smoke, and other pollutants may cause chronic cough.
- **Other possible causes of cough:** Tumors (bronchogenic or mediastinal), pulmonary embolism, aortic aneurysm, heart failure, aspiration, bronchiectasis, TB, sarcoidosis, foreign body obstruction, diaphragmatic irritation (which may be seen in ascites), lung abscess, *Pneumocystis jirovecii,* and psychogenic factors.

In most cases, the underlying cause can be determined from a history and physical exam, but it may be necessary to consider the judicious use of one or more of the following diagnostic aids in conjunction with the differential diagnosis process. For example, if one suspects TB, a Mantoux purified protein derivative (PPD) (tuberculin intradermal skin test) should be placed in the forearm and read 48 to 72 hours later by a qualified staff member at a second visit. Information on interpreting the PPD results is given later in this chapter. Another blood test that may be used to detect TB is an interferon-gamma release assay such as the QuantiFERON-TB Gold Test, which only requires a single patient visit. A positive result on either screening test should be followed up with a chest x-ray (CXR) film. For patients who are immunocompromised, the TB skin test may have to be repeated because of T-cell anergy against TB antigens.

Spirometry is helpful to determine the presence of obstructive or restrictive lung disease. A CXR film should be taken if there are signs and symptoms of pneumonia, TB, possible tumor, aspiration, foreign body, or ILD or even if the patient is just not recovering as expected. This follow-up CXR may pick up a hidden tumor that would otherwise have been missed. Sinus films may be useful to rule out sinusitis when the patient presents with a history of chronic postnasal drip and chronic sinus infections.

Computed tomography (CT) scanning of the chest can detect small peripheral lung nodules, evaluate coin lesions (solid, cystic, or calcified), and distinguish the chest wall from areas of pleural or parenchymal disease. Chest vessels can be separated from lymph nodes and other solid, nonvascular structures. The CT scan has replaced bronchography in diagnosing bronchiectasis. CT scan may help to better delineate endobronchial, parenchymal, or mediastinal masses. High-resolution chest CT scan, ventilation–perfusion scan, or pulmonary angiography is indicated when pulmonary thromboembolism is suspected.

A complete blood cell count and differential is helpful in diagnosing a bacterial infection. Fungal serology should be done to identify coccidiomycosis, histoplasmosis, and aspergillosis if the history of exposure is positive or if the patient has AIDS or is immunosuppressed.

Treatment

Because a cough is a symptom, treatment should be directed toward resolving the underlying cause(s) and removing any identified triggers. In patients with chronic cough who are weak and debilitated, the goal is to reduce complications from uncontrolled, forceful coughing, such as fractured ribs, pneumothorax, aspiration, exhaustion, sleep deprivation, and post-tussive syncope.

With severe, acute coughing that disrupts sleep and causes pain or extreme fatigue and weakness, it may be necessary to treat with antitussives, but these drugs have a limited role and should only be used on a short-term basis and only at night, because you want the patient to expectorate during the day. Nonnarcotic agents such as dextromethorphan or pseudoephedrine/brompheniramine/dextromethorphan may be used every 3 to 4 hours as needed. In addition, benzonatate (Tessalon) may be effective. When sleep or eating is interrupted by persistent cough, the preferred choice is codeine, 8 to 30 mg every 3 to 4 hours, but only on a short-term basis. (Patients with terminal lung cancer and patients with cystic fibrosis at the end of life should receive codeine in sufficient doses to keep them comfortable.)

Decongestants and antihistamines, alone or in combination, are indicated in cases of allergic rhinitis and postnasal drip. Antihistamines are most useful for those who have allergic upper airway disease but are usually avoided in asthmatic individuals because they may thicken secretions and inhibit expectoration. Intranasal steroid sprays or aerosols such as beclomethasone (Beconase) or fluticasone (Flonase) may also be useful when used on a consistent basis.

Expectorants are intended to decrease sputum viscosity and are used when the patient has a productive cough and needs help in clearing the airways. Suppression of a productive cough, however, may lead to complications such as obstructive pneumonia, because the patient may not be able to clear the airways and lungs of sputum. Although expectorants may work for some cases, increasing the patient's water intake to 3 to 4 L/day is the most cost-effective means of helping to liquefy secretions, as long as the patient can manage the volume and does not have heart failure or some other disorder in which this volume of water could compromise health. Guaifenesin (Mucinex), which is available without a prescription and in inexpensive generic brands, helps to break up mucus. Patients must be reminded to drink plenty of fluids if taking this medicine. Some practitioners prefer to give an expectorant during the day and a cough suppressant at night, so that the patient may sleep.

Two herbal remedies are currently used but have not been thoroughly researched in randomized controlled trials. Horehound has been suggested as a cough suppressant, and licorice has been said to calm coughs and have expectorant qualities. Caution should be taken with licorice, however, because it may increase the blood pressure.

Encouraging the patient to stop smoking should be a priority, given the effects of cigarette smoke on destroying the mucociliary structures of the airway lining and reducing the body's natural ability to clear mucus and respiratory pathogens. A chronic cough may not disappear in ex-smokers for a year or more after smoking cessation. Smoking cessation techniques are listed later in the chapter.

Patients with GERD, whose cough reflex can be triggered by the reflux of acidic stomach contents, usually respond to a course of antireflux therapy, which includes antacids, histamine-2 receptor blockers, or proton pump inhibitors. The benefits may not be noticed for several weeks, however.

Educating the patient and family about potential environmental and occupational factors that precipitate a cough is essential. Explore ways to avoid exposure to irritants. If a family member smokes, the dangers of secondhand smoke should be explained to the patient and family. Adequate hydration (increasing fluids) and adequate room humidification may also help reduce coughing. Breathing in the steam from a hot shower may also be effective.

■ DYSPNEA

Like pain, *dyspnea* is a perceived sensation that may vary among patients, which is why using a scale from 0 to 10 is recommended. Patients with dyspnea usually describe a sense of difficult breathing or inability to get sufficient air into or out of the lungs. Dyspnea may also be described as a feeling of breathlessness, suffocation or smothering, air hunger, and labored breathing. In many cases of dyspnea, the respiratory rate is rapid; cough may be present, depending on the underlying disease or cause of the dyspnea. Dyspnea may be caused by a number of different health problems. Some individuals may experience exercise-induced dyspnea or exercise-induced bronchospasm. In an older patient, dyspnea is the major atypical presentation for ischemic heart disease and myocardial infarction and is considered a frequent anginal equivalent. Dyspnea in aging patients may be difficult to evaluate when there are associated comorbidities.

Dyspnea is one of the most commonly occurring complaints for which patients seek help from health-care providers. Dyspnea, or shortness of breath, is estimated to be the third most frequent reason for seeking medical attention. Although dyspnea occurs primarily in patients with respiratory and cardiac disorders, it may also occur in other conditions such as lung neoplasms with metastasis, neuromuscular myopathies, neuropathies, spinal cord lesions, diaphragmatic disorders, and panic disorders. In patients receiving hospice care, it is the second most common symptom secondary to pain.

Differential Diagnosis

In the majority of cases, dyspnea is a result of cardiac or pulmonary decompensation. There are several symptoms associated with dyspnea, such as tachypnea (rapid breathing), orthopnea (dyspnea relieved in the sitting or upright position), and paroxysmal nocturnal dyspnea (sudden episodes of acute dyspnea at night). The causes of dyspnea are often complex. The common causes and precipitants of dyspnea follow:

- Pulmonary: COPD, asthma, pulmonary parenchymal disease, ILD, pulmonary hypertension, severe kyphoscoliosis, exogenous mechanical factors (ascites, massive obesity, extensive pleural effusion)
- Cardiac: Congestive heart failure (CHF), pulmonary venous congestion (mitral stenosis, mitral regurgitation)
- Hematological: Severe chronic anemia
- Psychogenic: Anxiety and panic disorders

Dyspnea may be acute or chronic, and patients with COPD may have both acute and chronic dyspnea. It is important to do a complete work-up to determine the underlying cause of the dyspnea so that appropriate treatment can be initiated. Dyspnea caused by acute anxiety may mimic cardiopulmonary decompensation, and patients with pulmonary hypertension may have episodes that resemble anxiety-related dyspnea. Onset of dyspnea at rest, accompanied by a sense of chest tightness, a feeling of suffocation, and an inability to "get air in," is a common presentation of anxiety-related dyspnea. In the absence of heart and lung disease, a history of multiple somatic complaints, emotional difficulties, no activity limitations (exercise intolerance), and dyspnea unrelated to activities provides evidence for psychogenic-related dyspnea.

About 75% of cases of dyspnea are caused by respiratory conditions that may be acute or chronic. The majority of other causes of dyspnea are cardiac in origin. It is important to explore with the patient the details of the onset and character of the dyspnea. The clinician should note whether the patient has dyspnea at rest or on exertion. Standard questions include the following: (1) How many flights of stairs did the patient climb before dyspnea occurred (e.g., one-flight dyspnea)? (2) How many blocks did the patient walk before dyspnea occurred (e.g., one-block dyspnea)? (3) How many feet did the patient walk before dyspnea occurred (e.g., 100-feet dyspnea)? The rate of the patient's speech during exercise can provide good clinical information.

Exploring when the dyspnea first occurred and what the patient was doing at the time is essential. Specific questions should be directed toward precipitating factors and factors that alleviate the dyspnea. Questions should explore potential environmental exposure (e.g., recent travel) or exposure to agents (e.g., through occupation or hobbies) that aggravate the dyspnea. Paying attention to other signs and symptoms that may be associated with the dyspnea, such as cough, peripheral edema, dizziness, wheeze, fever, chest pain, heartburn, leg pain, and paresthesias, is also critical.

A complete physical exam should be done, with particular attention directed to the pulmonary and cardiovascular systems. The examiner should check for tachycardia, tachypnea, fever, mixed venous oxygen saturation (SvO_2), and hypertension. The quality of breath sounds (increased, decreased, or absent) should be noted, along with the presence of crackles, rhonchi, wheezes, egophony, and fremitus. Bronchial lung sounds heard at other than the normal locations (tubular sounds) are common with acute bronchitis. Assessment should include checking for third and fourth heart sounds, murmurs, friction rubs, jugular venous distention, pedal edema, and calf tenderness. A visual analog scale (0 = no dyspnea; 10 = worst dyspnea ever had) or the Borg scale for perceived exertion with a score of 6 to 20 (6 = no exertion; 20 = very, very hard exertion) are useful in assessing the degree of dyspnea, as previously mentioned. The scales can be used again on the patient's next visit to compare outcome effects of treatments. The scales can also be good for patient self-management.

Diagnostic tests are guided by data from the history and physical exam and the suspected causes of the dyspnea. Chest x-ray films are useful in ruling out tumors, TB, pneumonia, and other major pulmonary disorders. A complete blood count (CBC) with differential should be done to rule out anemia and infection. A blood chemistry profile is done if a metabolic acidosis is suspected and to differentiate anion-gap acidosis from nonanion-gap acidosis. Oximetry to measure the saturation level of oxygen may be useful in assessing whether the patient may be dyspneic because of hypoxemia. If the O_2 saturation level is less than 90%, arterial blood gas (ABG) analysis should be done. Levels of dyspnea have not been found to correlate well with physiological measures.

If there is suspicion of carbon monoxide (CO) exposure, a carboxyhemoglobin (COHb%) level should be obtained. COHb% levels of 4% to 15% may be found in heavy smokers. Levels above 20% may cause dyspnea and headache; levels greater than 40% may cause seizures and death.

Peak expiratory flow rate is a simple, inexpensive test that can be done with a handheld flow meter in the office or at the bedside. This test determines the degree of expiratory airflow obstruction in patients with asthma and COPD. Full spirometry is useful in determining whether the patient has obstructive, restrictive, or mixed (obstructive and restrictive) lung disease (see under Cough). Diffusion capacity should be checked if ILD is suspected. If the patient uses a flow meter at home, he or she can determine whether it is necessary to come into the office for further evaluation and possible treatment.

Treatment

Initial treatment is directed at helping the patient find relief from the shortness of breath by removing the underlying cause and contributing factors. Subsequent management is directed at prevention and assisting the patient with management of chronic dyspnea in conditions such as COPD or ILD. In cases of dyspnea caused by hypoxemia, supplemental oxygen may be indicated. In cases of shunting, the cause of the shunting must be corrected. For subsequent management, see the sections on asthma, chronic bronchitis and emphysema (COPD), and interstitial lung disease.

For treatment of dyspnea related to cardiac disorders such as CHF, refer to Chapter 10. Appropriate diuretics to relieve fluid overload may improve breathing, and supplemental oxygen may be necessary in some cases.

For anxiety-related dyspnea, psychiatric referral may be needed if other simple measures have been tried without good results. Dyspnea caused by rapid overbreathing during anxiety attacks can be corrected through patient education. Until the patient learns a rebreathing technique, it may be helpful to prescribe short-term use of anxiolytics such as buspirone HCl 20 to 30 mg/day.

■ HEMOPTYSIS

Hemoptysis is defined as expectoration of blood. The patient often reports coughing up blood or sputum that is streaked or tinged with blood. In addition, hemoptysis may be manifested as fresh (bright red) or old (dark red or black) blood or, in the case of bleeding from an infected lung cavity, it may present as slow oozing or frank bleeding. In cases of profuse hemoptysis, blood clots may be expectorated. The patient should note if the blood is from the nasal cavity, which may only be from severe irritation or dehydration.

Differential Diagnosis

About 80% of hemoptysis cases have inflammatory causes such as bronchitis, bronchiectasis, pneumonia, and TB. Less common causes may include neoplasms that damage a pulmonary vessel and rupture a pulmonary artery or persons with cystic fibrosis who have a good amount of damage to lung parenchyma. Use of pulmonary artery balloon catheters has increased the incidence of pulmonary artery rupture. Cardiovascular causes of hemoptysis include left ventricular failure, mitral stenosis, pulmonary embolism or infarct, primary pulmonary hypertension, and aortic aneurysm. Clotting defects may also cause hemoptysis. Bleeding may occur anywhere in the respiratory tract, including the nose, sinuses, and mouth.

About 95% of pulmonary blood circulation is supplied by the pulmonary artery and its branches, which is a low-pressure system. Bronchial circulation, a high-pressure system, originates from the aorta and usually provides about 5% of the blood to the lungs, mostly to the airways and supporting structures. When bleeding occurs, it usually arises from the bronchial circulation, unless trauma or erosion has affected a major pulmonary vessel. Pulmonary venous bleeding is modest and occurs in pulmonary venous hypertension, especially in conjunction with left heart failure.

The patient usually presents with a complaint of "coughing up" blood. To most people, the presence of blood in the sputum or coughing up blood is a frightening experience, and most will seek immediate medical attention. As in differential diagnosis of dyspnea and cough, a similar line of questioning should be pursued regarding onset, amount, aggravating and alleviating factors, and the presence of other associated symptoms such as dyspnea, cough, dizziness, fatigue, and chest pain. Bronchopulmonary bleeding may present as hematemesis (vomiting of blood). The patient may swallow blood during the night and may vomit blood on arising.

The history and physical exam are focused along the same lines as for the complaints of cough and dyspnea. In addition, if the examiner suspects that the hemoptysis is due to a pulmonary neoplasm, the exam should focus on the pulmonary system and lymph node enlargement.

Further diagnostic tests may be indicated, depending on the results of the history and physical examination. The common causes of hemoptysis will direct the laboratory tests. If hemoptysis occurs in patients aged 45 years or younger, it is likely caused by mitral stenosis, TB, bronchiectasis, or lung abscess. For patients older than age 45 years, common causes of hemoptysis include bronchogenic carcinoma, bronchitis, TB, and pulmonary embolus with infarction. In massive hemoptysis (loss of more than 600 mL of blood in 24 hours, which may occur in lung cancer, TB, bronchiectasis, and lung abscess), the condition is life-threatening and constitutes a medical emergency. There may be time to do only chest radiographs and a CBC before emergency surgery or bronchoscopy.

For nonemergency cases, in which the sputum is tinged or streaked with blood, there is time to do the essential tests to identify the cause of hemoptysis. In addition to chest x-ray films and a CBC, sputum should be cultured for acid-fast bacilli if TB is suspected. For suspected pneumonia or lung abscess, sputum for culture and sensitivity should be done. Patients who present with hematemesis may also have hemoptysis caused by aspiration; a chest x-ray film is indicated for these patients.

Patients with a history of thromboembolism may be taking anticoagulants. If so, clotting times should be checked to rule this out as a cause of the hemoptysis.

Because of the exertion (forceful expiratory maneuvers) required by the patient during spirometry, measurement of lung volumes during periods of active hemoptysis is not recommended.

Treatment

Massive hemoptysis requires immediate treatment, surgery, or bronchoscopy. During this time, prevention of aspiration and keeping the airway open are of utmost importance. Endotracheal intubation may be necessary. Supplemental oxygen and replacement of blood loss may be necessary, depending on the blood pressure, pulse, ABG results, and hemoglobin count.

Treatment of chronic hemoptysis is directed toward the underlying cause. When the cause is inflammation, as in chronic bronchitis, TB, and bronchiectasis, the patient must be educated to stop smoking, comply with use of prescribed medications (e.g., antibiotics, bronchodilators), perform deep breathing and coughing exercises every 2 to 4 hours regularly, and avoid exposure to secondhand smoke and other noxious agents that might precipitate cough.

Education of the patient and family regarding the causes of the hemoptysis is essential. The patient needs to know what factors may precipitate the hemoptysis and how it can be prevented. The patient should be taught to note any change in the color, amount, and consistency of the blood expectorated. Any sudden increase should be reported to the health-care provider immediately for prompt medical attention.

COMMON PROBLEMS

■ UPPER RESPIRATORY INFECTIONS

Upper respiratory infections (URIs) include some of the most common infectious diseases encountered and account for millions of visits to health-care providers annually. The majority of URIs are caused by viruses. Bacteria cause about 25% of the cases. For the average adult, URIs are a source of discomfort, disability, and loss of time. For young children, the immunocompromised, and older adults, these infections may be a cause of morbidity and serious illnesses. In children and older adults, as well as adults with underlying respiratory diseases, these viral infections are frequently complicated by bacterial superinfections.

Epidemiology and Causes

Influenza (the flu), the common cold (viral rhinitis or acute coryza), and acute laryngitis are some of the more frequently occurring URIs that the practitioner will need to manage. Infections such as acute epiglottitis and respiratory syncytial virus (RSV) infection occur predominantly in infants and younger children but may occur as a life-threatening infection in adults. RSV infection can cause severe cases of pneumonia and lower respiratory tract disease in older, institutionalized adults and adults with suppressed immune status. Acute epiglottitis can result in complete or partial airway obstruction (Table 9.1).

Influenza epidemics occur every year in the United States, with typically 5,000 to 250,000 cases annually. In some years with more severe outbreaks, as many as 40,000 deaths have occurred. Most of these deaths occur in older persons, particularly those with underlying pulmonary or cardiac disease. Infants and very young children also appear to be at greater risk for influenza-associated morbidity and mortality. Although influenza and colds may occur at any time, most cases occur during the winter and spring months. Acute laryngitis is generally associated with a viral URI and often persists for a week or more after other symptoms have cleared. The incubation period for most URIs of a viral nature is 1 to 4 days.

Table 9.1   Acute Epiglottitis

Acute epiglottitis is a life-threatening, rapidly progressing cellulitis of the epiglottis that may cause complete airway obstruction. Epiglottitis begins as a cellulitis between the tongue base and the epiglottis; the epiglottis is then pushed posteriorly. The epiglottis becomes swollen and threatens airway patency. Epiglottitis is more common and more severe in young children, but it may occur in older children and adults.

Clinical Manifestations
Epiglottitis in adults should be suspected when odynophagia (pain on swallowing) seems severe compared with pharyngeal findings. Other findings include dyspnea, drooling, and stridor.

Diagnostic Reasoning
Direct viewing of the epiglottis with a tongue blade and lighting should never be attempted because immediate laryngospasm and airway obstruction may result. It is recommended that children and adults be transported to the operating room (OR) while sitting up for visualization of the epiglottis with a fiberoptic laryngoscope, with preparations made for immediate airway control. The epiglottis will appear swollen and erythematous ("cherry red"), and an uncuffed endotracheal tube should be inserted.

Management
Acute epiglottitis requires emergency care for adequate airway control. No painful or stressful procedures should be performed on these patients unless preparations are in place for a planned intubation, such as in the OR.

The patient with epiglottitis will require hospitalization for IV antibiotics such as cefuroxine (Ceftin), ceftriaxone (Rocephin), or ampicillin/sulbactam (Unasyn). Dexamethasone (Decadron) should also be administered IV and tapered as signs and symptoms resolve. Continuous pulse oximetry and careful monitoring of the patient's airway are critical. Patients who develop hypoxemia and respiratory distress will require intubation.

Community-acquired respiratory tract infections caused by *Streptococcus* account for more than 20 million primary-care provider visits annually and are a major reason for work and school absenteeism.

Pathophysiology

The common cold (coryza) is caused by viruses spread through direct inhalation of airborne droplet sprays aerosolized by the infected person while speaking, coughing, or sneezing, as well as hand-to-face transmission after handling fomites serving as reservoirs of infection. Hand-to-hand transmission, however, is probably the most common mode of transmission in adults, underscoring the importance of frequent hand washing in the prevention of new cases. Numerous serotypes of rhinoviruses, adenoviruses, coronaviruses, coxsackieviruses, and parainfluenza viruses are associated with the common cold. The ability of the majority of these viruses to mutate readily ensures their ability to consistently evade host immune mechanisms. The number of rhinovirus serotypes, for instance, currently stands at more than a hundred. Following infection, individuals develop immunity to a specific viral strain but are susceptible to repeated infection by the same parent virus after only minor changes in surface proteins or polysaccharides.

Symptoms of congestion, rhinorrhea, and sneezing result directly from inflammation and edema of upper airway mucosal surfaces. The cough reflex may be triggered by this same mucosal inflammation in the posterior pharynx. After acute infection, postviral cough may persist for as long as 6 to 8 weeks due to postnasal drip—the persistent drainage of thin mucus down the posterior pharynx resulting in direct pharyngeal irritation.

Classic flu is caused by the orthomyxovirus influenza type A and, to a lesser extent, influenza type B, both being enveloped RNA-based viruses. In addition to the viral rhinitis symptoms of the common cold, influenza infection further leads to generalized muscle aches and pains, fatigue, significant fever, and rigors (chills). Influenza infection may also develop into frank viral pneumonia (lower airway infection), which may be further complicated by bacterial superinfection, particularly with *Staphylococcus aureus*. These additional manifestations and high potential for complicated disease underscore the importance of widespread yearly vaccination against influenza.

Repeated yearly vaccination is required because the influenza virus is capable of mutating its major surface proteins—hemagglutinin (H) and neuraminidase (N)—rendering protein-specific host antibody defenses ineffective and allowing for viral adherence and entry into host epithelial cells. Each year, a vaccine is developed using influenza proteins from the most likely serotype combination to lead to widespread infection for that year, as determined by complex disease modeling algorithms based on extensive Centers for Disease Control and Prevention (CDC) and World Health Organization epidemiological data. However, each vaccine is, in essence, a best guess, which may or may not provide adequate protection against the year's primary strain. In addition, other strains of the virus not covered by the vaccine may also cause numerous infections in any given year.

Given concerns in recent years for the potential spread of other forms of influenza, including H5N1 influenza (avian or bird flu) and H1N1 influenza (swine flu), significant efforts are also being directed toward developing safe and effective vaccines against these forms of the disease. Throughout history, the most widespread and devastating flu-related pandemics have been traced back primarily to these novel forms of the virus (in particular, avian flu). On an annual basis, however, classic influenza results in far greater morbidity and mortality each year than these other forms. For the last 40 years, widespread pandemics of avian flu and H1N1 influenza have largely been avoided through multinational public health measures. Clinical trials are underway with Vaxart, an influenza vaccine tablet. Although patient trials are being performed, the long-term effects of this drug are not known.

Most cases of laryngitis (inflammation of the vocal cords with extreme hoarseness and temporary voice loss) and croup (any combination of laryngotracheobronchitis with edema leading to airway obstruction with characteristic stridorous breathing) are caused by parainfluenza virus, RSV, influenza virus, coxsackievirus, rhinovirus, and adenovirus. Laryngitis may also be caused by group A beta-hemolytic *Streptococcus pyogenes, Haemophilus influenzae,* and *Moraxella catarrhalis*. These same viral and bacterial agents, along with *Neisseria gonorrhoeae* and Epstein-Barr virus (causing infectious mononucleosis), are also common causes of pharyngitis (see full discussion in Chapter 8).

RSV and influenza A (and less so influenza B) are the most common causes of bronchiolitis in children and adolescents, but adults tend to experience infection in the larger airways (i.e., acute bronchitis). Since the advent of widespread vaccination against *H influenzae* type B (Hib vaccine) and *Corynebacterium diphtheriae* (DTaP vaccine), epiglottitis occurs only rarely in the United States (see Table 9.1). Bacterial tracheitis is a serious purulent infection of the subglottic trachea caused primarily by *S aureus,* with a toxic clinical presentation requiring hospitalization and IV antibiotic therapy.

Clinical Presentation

The onset of influenza is usually abrupt, with fever, chills, malaise, myalgia, headache, nasal stuffiness, sore throat, and sometimes nausea. A nonproductive cough is usually present and occurs early in the course of illness. The fever may be as high as 103°F (39.4°C) in adults and typically lasts 3 to 5 days. Subjective findings in the person with the common cold include headache, myalgia, nasal congestion, watery rhinorrhea, sneezing, and a "scratchy throat." Laryngitis results in an inflammation of laryngeal mucosa and the vocal cords. Symptoms include hoarseness, aphonia, and, occasionally, pain when swallowing. Physical findings in cases of URIs are usually minimal, with normal assessment findings on chest auscultation. Cervical lymphadenopathy may be present.

Diagnostic Reasoning
Diagnostic Tests

Diagnosis of influenza tends to be more accurate during epidemics. A successful presumptive diagnosis requires appropriate symptoms at the right time of the year and a knowledge of patterns of influenzal illnesses around the world. If necessary, the diagnosis can be confirmed via virology studies (e.g., nasal and pharyngeal cultures, cells from nasopharyngeal washings stained with monoclonal antibody fluorescence stains, and complement fixation studies on paired serum samples). Diagnosis of colds and laryngitis typically are based on the subjective presentation of the patient except when the etiological agent in laryngitis is thought to be bacterial. In these situations, the practitioner should perform a throat culture to rule out group A beta-hemolytic streptococcal infection. Leukocytosis found on a CBC with differential may help to diagnose a bacterial infection.

Differential Diagnosis

Other conditions that need to be ruled out include allergic rhinitis; atypical *Mycoplasma* pneumonia, infectious mononucleosis; *Chlamydia;* and possibly mumps, rubeola, and cytomegalovirus. Close attention to epidemiology (e.g., current outbreak in the community) is important. Contact the CDC or the local health department in your community to help determine the type of disease outbreak.

Management

Management of influenza and the common cold is generally symptomatic and is directed toward relief of symptoms and prevention of secondary infections. Antibiotics are not indicated for influenza or colds unless a secondary bacterial infection occurs. Mucopurulent rhinitis frequently accompanies the common cold and is not an indication for antimicrobial treatment. Although antibiotics are often viewed by the layperson as a viable treatment for a cold or the flu, these drugs have no effect on viruses and if taken injudiciously may produce resistant organisms. In the past, clinicians ordered antibiotics in about half of the cases of URI, which is thought to have contributed to the current antimicrobial-resistant crisis (Level I; Demeter et al, 2009). Health-care providers continue to prescribe antibiotics 50% or more of the time to adults and children with viral infections.

Generally, most patients with influenza should rest at home until symptoms decrease in severity. The older patient or the patient with an underlying chronic illness may require hospitalization for influenza. In addition to rest and fluids, antipyretics and analgesics are recommended. Cough suppressants with codeine may be necessary for adequate cough control. If the practitioner is reasonably

confident that the virus in question is type A influenza, the patient may benefit from an antiviral drug. Widespread amantadine (Symmetrel) and rimantadine (Flumadine) resistance among influenza A virus strains has made this class of medications less useful clinically. Therefore, amantadine and rimantadine are not recommended for antiviral treatment or chemoprophylaxis of currently circulating influenza A virus strains. The majority of currently circulating influenza viruses are susceptible to the neuraminidase inhibitor antiviral medications oseltamivir (Tamiflu) and zanamivir (Relenza). Antiviral treatment is recommended as early as possible (within 48 hours of symptom presentation) for patients with confirmed or suspected influenza who have severe, complicated, or progressive illness; who require hospitalization; or who pose a risk for influenza-related complications. Oseltamivir, both as a pill and liquid form, is approved for the treatment of influenza in persons aged 2 weeks and older and for chemoprophylaxis to prevent influenza in patients 1 year of age and older. Zanamivir, as a powder that is inhaled, is approved to treat flu in people aged 7 years and older and to prevent influenza in patients aged 5 years and older. Zanamivir is not for persons with respiratory problems, such as asthma or COPD. Both medications are usually prescribed for 5 days for individuals in primary care, although people hospitalized with the flu may need the medication for longer than 5 days. Rest, fluids, and antipyretics are also useful in controlling the discomfort associated with a cold. Decongestants such as pseudoephedrine (e.g., Sudafed) are widely used and may help control rhinorrhea and nasal congestion. These should be used only for 3 days due to rebound effects and should not be used in the presence of hypertension. Nasal sprays such as phenylephrine (Neo-Synephrine) or ocular decongestants such as oxymetazoline (e.g., OcuClear, Visine LR) are rapidly effective. Patients should be cautioned to use them only for a few days, because chronic use leads to rebound congestion. Intranasal ipratropium (Atrovent) has also been approved for significant rhinorrhea associated with URIs. Vitamin C and zinc lozenges with echinacea are currently popular "remedies" that are sold as OTC therapies. Despite numerous randomized trials, the evidence of effectiveness of zinc lozenges in reducing the duration of colds is lacking. The efficacy of vitamin C supplements to decrease the incidence of colds or to shorten the duration has also not been demonstrated. The only exception may be for the patient who has a possible vitamin C deficiency. Several small studies have shown that black elderberry syrup shortens the duration of flu-like illnesses by up to 4 days.

Treatment of laryngitis includes complete voice rest, steam inhalations, codeine or nonnarcotic cough suppressants for cough and pain, and a liquid or soft diet. If throat cultures are positive for group A beta-hemolytic *Streptococcus,* penicillin should be prescribed, if the patient is not allergic to penicillin. Erythromycin should be used for infections associated with *M catarrhalis* or

H influenzae. For particularly toxic bacterial infections such as bacterial tracheitis, blood cultures may be appropriate to rule out bacteremia.

For the management of croup, racemic epinephrine and dexamethasone are indicated and intubation may be needed in extreme cases. Bacterial tracheitis requires IV antibiotic therapy with nafcillin or an appropriate cephalosporin, or, if methicillin-resistant *S aureus* is suspected, vancomycin or linezolid. Because of impaired oral intake, all such infections, other than the common cold, may lead to dehydration requiring oral or IV rehydration therapy. In addition, hypoxemia based on pulse oximetry or blood gas analysis should be addressed with supplemental oxygen therapy. Bronchodilator therapy is often used as well, but randomized clinical trials do not consistently demonstrate its efficacy.

Follow-up and Referral

The duration of an uncomplicated case of influenza is 1 to 7 days; the prognosis is excellent. Frequent complications do occur, however, including acute sinusitis, otitis media, purulent bronchitis, and pneumonia. Influenza causes necrosis of some respiratory epithelium, predisposing the infected person to secondary bacterial infections. The interaction between bacteria and influenza is bidirectional, with bacterial enzymes activating influenza viruses. If a fever persists for more than 4 days, if the white blood cell count rises to 12,000 cells/mcL or higher, or if the cough becomes productive, bacterial infection should be ruled out or verified and treated.

The most common complication of influenza is pneumonia; most fatalities result from bacterial pneumonia. The patient with bacterial pneumonia will experience gradual improvement of symptoms for 2 to 3 days and then develop cough and purulent sputum. Pneumococcal pneumonia is the most common bacterial pneumonia associated with influenza, but staphylococcal pneumonia is the most serious. Primary viral influenza pneumonia is the least common but has a high mortality rate among pregnant women and patients with rheumatic heart disease. The patient develops symptoms of influenza that become increasingly severe. Respiratory distress is often sufficient to require mechanical ventilation.

Most cases of the common cold and laryngitis are self-limiting. Complications of a cold may include pharyngitis, sinusitis, otitis media, tonsillitis, and chest infections. Unless symptoms of these complications are present, antibiotic therapy is not indicated. The patient with laryngitis needs to maintain voice rest until hoarseness and aphonia have resided. Any vigorous use of the voice such as shouting or singing may foster the formation of vocal cord nodules.

Patient Education

There currently is no immunization for the prevention of colds. Research has demonstrated that the best method of preventing transmission of infected droplets is through frequent hand washing, particularly in daycare facilities and congregate adult living facilities. During the cold and influenza seasons, the person with a chronic illness or a compromised immune status should be advised to avoid crowded, close situations and other persons who have obvious symptoms.

Trivalent influenza vaccine provides partial immunity (in approximately 86% of patients vaccinated) for a few months to 1 year. The vaccine's antigenic configuration changes yearly. It is based on the prevalent strains of the previous year, the viruses that are currently being seen in other parts of the world during the current year, and the estimated antibody response in persons previously infected with or vaccinated against these viruses. Vaccination in October or November of each year is recommended for all persons older than 65 years of age; nursing home residents; adults and children with underlying conditions, including heart, pulmonary, malignant, and some metabolic diseases; and health-care workers. High-risk children have a particularly low influenza vaccination rate annually, which is of significant concern. Vaccination is also encouraged for members of any large groups who may be the principal vectors of influenza in their community such as schoolchildren, children in day care, college students, military personnel, and employees of large companies. Low-income minority populations typically have lower vaccination rates than other populations. Medicare covers the cost of influenza and pneumococcal vaccination. Recent research has shown that obtaining yearly influenza vaccination can be influenced by the health-care provider's recommendations and phone calls offering encouragement and reminders. *Healthy People 2020* has set a goal of vaccinating 80% of noninstitutionalized adults aged 18 to 64 years annually; currently 25% receive the annual flu vaccine. HP 2020 has also set the goal of vaccinating 90% of high-risk adults aged 18 to 64 years; currently 39% of this population receives the annual flu vaccine. For adults aged 65 years and older, the 2020 goal of annual vaccination is 90 % (currently 67%). For health-care workers, in 2012 to 2013, the vaccination rate was only 72%, although for health-care workers in occupational settings that require vaccinations, the rate was 96.5%. The practitioner may keep abreast of current epidemiological trends in influenza epidemics and changes in vaccine recommendations by accessing the Web site for the CDC at www.cdc.gov.

■ ASTHMA

Asthma is a chronic, inflammatory, obstructive disease of the airways. It may occur at any age and may be characterized by wheezing (airway spasms), tightness in the chest, breathlessness (dyspnea), and cough. The signs and symptoms may remit spontaneously or exacerbate in response to intrinsic (stress) or extrinsic (environmental) triggers. The severity of asthma is highly unpredictable, ranging from mild attack to complete airway obstruction and death. Many pediatricians use the term *reactive airway disease* rather than "asthma," because some parents have a negative connotation of the word "asthma."

Epidemiology and Causes

Asthma affects more than an estimated 100 million people worldwide, and the number is increasing rapidly. In the United States, more than 34 million Americans have been diagnosed with asthma, or reactive airway disease, at some point in their lives. It has been estimated that 8.2% of noninstitutionalized adults and 9.5% of children currently have asthma. African Americans have asthma-related mortality rates that are higher than the rates for Caucasians. Despite newer antiasthmatic drugs, asthma is responsible for more than 134 million days of restricted activity and about half a million hospitalizations annually. In the United States, 5,500 deaths each year are attributable to asthma. Despite current prevention efforts, the incidence of asthma continues to increase every year.

Clinical practice guidelines were last updated in 2007 by the National Asthma Education and Prevention Program, which is part of the National Heart, Lung, and Blood Institute. This document is known as the Expert Panel Report 3 (EPR-3). These evidence-based practice guidelines include ways to help patients control their asthma signs and symptoms and improve their quality of life.

Although the exact cause is unknown, three principal triggers for exacerbations of asthma have been identified:

- Allergens and environmental factors: Allergens may include inhaled substances, such as molds, pollens, dust, animal dander, cosmetics, and tobacco smoke; food additives with sulfite preservative agents; and medications, especially beta blockers and aspirin or aspirin-containing drugs.
- Infections: Upper respiratory infections are common precursors to an asthma attack. Viral infections commonly precede an asthma episode.
- Psychological factors: Stressful events at work or home or a series of crises may precipitate an asthma attack. Many times, stressors may be overlooked or dismissed.

Inflammation of the airways contributes to bronchial hyperreactivity, airflow limitation, and the resultant characteristic signs and symptoms of asthma: wheezing, breathlessness, chest tightness, and cough. The stage is then set for acute bronchoconstriction, airway edema, mucous-plug formation, airway narrowing, and bronchial obstruction.

Pathophysiology

Asthma is a chronic inflammatory disease characterized by reversible hyperreactivity of the bronchi and bronchioles to a variety of stimuli. Genetic predisposition, allergy, environmental factors, stress, and infectious agents are factors that play a role in the etiology of asthma. Immunologically mediated inflammation, the major pathological mechanism of this disease, involves mast cells, eosinophils, lymphocytes, neutrophils, and macrophages, which may directly infiltrate the airway at both smooth muscle and basement membrane layers. These cells release a variety of mediators that stimulate bronchoconstriction, vasodilation, edema formation, and increased mucus production, including histamine, interleukins, leukotrienes, tumor necrosis factor, bradykinin, thromboxanes, fibroblast growth factor, and prostaglandins.

In particular, CD4+ T-helper (Th) cells bearing a Th2 phenotype (predominantly humorally mediated immunity) and resistant to apoptotic killing produce interleukin (IL)–3, IL-4, IL-5, and granulocyte-macrophage colony-stimulating factor after being stimulated by the offending allergen, which, in turn, upregulates the allergic response and airway hypersensitivity. Th1 T cells (predominantly cell-mediated immunity) have been implicated to a lesser extent. Eosinophils are a rich source of leukotrienes that directly cause contraction of bronchial smooth muscle and increase vascular permeability. Activated B lymphocytes transform into plasma cells, synthesizing large amounts of immunoglobulin E (IgE) antibody that binds and activates tissue mast cells and eosinophils. Mast cell-bound IgE molecules then become cross-linked by environmental allergens, which activates histamine release and further IL-4 and IL-5 production, thereby provoking bronchial smooth muscle contraction and vasodilation.

With each acute exacerbation of asthma, inflammatory mediators incite a structural remodeling of the airways. The alveoli remain largely unaffected, because this is not a parenchymal disease. Rather, airway remodeling entails thickening of the bronchial and bronchiolar mucosa, submucosa, and smooth muscle layers, which contributes to the persistence of disease. Increased collagen is deposited below the basement membrane, while the loose areolar connective tissue found between epithelial and smooth muscle layers also hypertrophies. Therefore, prevention of acute episodes, which minimizes the amount of remodeling, is key to the proper treatment of asthma.

Asthma is an obstructive pulmonary disease with hypoxia as the universal finding during acute exacerbations. With acute bronchospasm, residual volume increases in the lungs and peak expiratory flow rate diminishes. Inflammation and constriction of the bronchioles increase airway resistance, decrease inspiratory capacity and expiratory volumes, and lead to ventilation–perfusion mismatching and altered arterial blood gas concentrations. As a result of hyperventilation, respiratory alkalosis and hypocapnia are common findings with each episode. As an acute attack resolves, narrowing in the larger airways tends to reverse first, whereas the peripheral airways remain most constricted. If such an attack progresses, however, and fails to reverse, respiratory acidosis and an elevated arterial carbon dioxide concentration typically result, signaling impending respiratory failure. Indeed, severe irreversible bronchoconstriction and inflammation, termed *status asthmaticus,* can be fatal.

Clinical Presentation

The clinical presentation varies and depends on whether the patient is currently experiencing an acute attack or is seeking help to manage chronic asthma. It is important to note that not all people with asthma wheeze and that not everyone who wheezes has asthma.

Subjective

During an acute attack, the patient may present with a complaint of breathlessness and may be unable to talk or may be able only to blurt out short sentences. There may be profuse sweating and a complaint of air hunger. In patients who are severely obstructed, there may be no wheezing; only cough may be present.

The patient may present complaining of wheezing, persistent and recurrent cough, difficulty breathing, and/or tightness in the chest, particularly at night or in the early morning. Endurance problems during exercise may occur. Ninety percent of individuals with asthma report that exercise exacerbates their respiratory symptoms.

Any single symptom or combination of symptoms may occur, and symptoms are usually worse at night. The disease spectrum varies from a few mild episodes in a lifetime to daily debilitating symptoms. Food additives, particularly metabisulfite (used as a food preservative), certain dairy products, and, for some individuals, monosodium glutamate, may also cause symptoms. An extreme emotional state such as excessive laughing and/or crying may precipitate or exacerbate an attack.

Objective

Reversible airflow limitation and diurnal variation as measured by peak flow meter are objective signs and symptoms of asthma. Variability between morning and evening peak expiratory flow (PEF) may reflect airway hyperresponsiveness and indicate asthma instability and severity. Nasal discharge, mucosal swelling, frontal tenderness, nasal polyps, and allergic "shiners"—dark discoloration beneath both eyes—should be noted. The clinician should also check for manifestations of allergic skin conditions such as eczema. Wheezing during forced exhalation is no longer considered a reliable indicator. It may be absent between attacks and may be obscured during acute attacks related to diminished breath sounds.

Audible inspiratory and expiratory wheezing may be heard. The patient may be using accessory muscles of breathing (scalene and sternocleidomastoid) and sitting upright. Auscultation of the chest may reveal inspiratory and expiratory wheezes.

Diagnostic Reasoning

Expiratory airflow measurements are essential to the differential diagnosis of asthma. The essential elements to consider in making the diagnosis of asthma are listed in Table 9.2. In addition, asthma should always be considered as a possible etiology in a patient with a chronic cough (Level I; Demeter et al, 2009).

Differentiating asthma from other diseases is usually not difficult, particularly with the aid of pulmonary function tests (PFTs), a complete history, and laboratory test results. Spirometry is recommended for the diagnosis of asthma. A common feature of asthma is nocturnal awakening with one or more of the following symptoms: dyspnea, cough, and wheezing. Persistent wheezing localized to one area of the lung, with paroxysms of cough, is indicative of endobronchial disease such as foreign body aspiration, neoplasm, or bronchial stenosis. Acute left ventricular heart failure may initially present as asthma (wheezing), but the findings of moist, basilar crackles, gallop rhythms, and other signs of heart failure exclude the diagnosis of asthma.

Allergic rhinitis and eczema often accompany a diagnosis of asthma. Concurrent treatment for these conditions is critical. Effective treatment of allergic rhinitis

Table 9.2	Essential Elements to Consider When Diagnosing Asthma
History	• Cough (especially nocturnal) • Recurrent wheeze (absence does not rule out asthma) • Recurrent episodic dyspnea • Recurrent chest tightness
Symptoms worsen in relation to specific factors	• Airborne chemicals or dust • Animals with fur or feathers • Changes in weather • Exercise • Gastroesophageal reflux • Sensitivity to aspirin, other NSAIDs, and sulfites • Dust mites in house (mattresses, furniture, carpets) • Menses • Mold/pollen • Nighttime (patient awakens) • Nonselective beta blockers • Pollen • Smoke (tobacco, wood, etc.) • Strong emotional expression (laughing or crying hard) • Viral infection/rhinitis/sinusitis
Reversible (at least partially) airflow limitations with diurnal variability Exclusion of alternate diagnosis	• Variation in peak expiratory flow rate of at least 20% between first morning measurement (before taking an inhaled, short-acting beta-adrenergic agonist) and early afternoon measurement (after using the inhaler)

(discussed in Chapter 8) is critical as another mode to prevent triggering acute asthma attacks.

Diagnostic Tests

To establish the diagnosis of asthma, episodic symptoms of airflow obstruction must be present, airflow obstruction must be at least partially reversible, and the provider must have ruled out any alternative diagnoses. Spirometry measurements are helpful in diagnosing and then evaluating the management of the disease. Forced vital capacity (FVC) and forced expiratory volume in 1 second (FEV$_1$) are helpful measurements. Prebronchodilator and postbronchodilator PFTs, including spirometry and diffusing capacity, to determine the response to bronchodilators are essential in the differential diagnosis and subsequent management of asthma. The diagnosis is made by demonstrating the reversibility of the airway obstruction from the pre- and post-PFTs. Reversibility is defined as a 15% or greater increase in the FEV$_1$ after two puffs of a beta-adrenergic agonist have been inhaled. When spirometry is nondiagnostic, bronchial provocation testing may be useful with histamine, methacholine, or exercise.

A chest x-ray film may show only hyperinflation but may include thickening of the bronchial wall and diminished peripheral lung vascular shadows.

Arterial blood gas (ABG) analysis is included in the initial work-up to establish a baseline and to determine the degree of hypoxemia and the need for supplemental oxygen. The results of the ABG analysis and spirometry, along with the clinical history and findings on exam, are triangulated to classify the severity of the asthma, as shown in Table 9.3.

A CBC with differential, with special attention to the sedimentation rate and eosinophil count, is done.

Table 9.3 Classification of Asthma Severity

Classification	Clinical Features Before Treatment	Daily Medication Required to Maintain Control
Mild intermittent	• Intermittent symptoms less than once a week, brief exacerbations (lasting from a few hours to a few days)* • Nighttime asthma symptoms less than twice a month • Asymptomatic and normal PEF between exacerbations • PEFR or FEV$_1$: >80% predicted; PFT variability >20%	• Intermittent reliever medication taken as needed only; inhaled short-acting beta-2 agonist or cromolyn before exercise or allergen exposure • Intensity of treatment depends on severity of exacerbation • No daily medication needed
Mild persistent	• Symptoms more than 2× per week but less than 1× per day, may be several times at night/month • Exacerbations may affect activity and sleep • Nighttime asthma symptoms more than twice a month • PEFR or FEV$_1$: >80% predicted; PFT variability 20%–30%	• One daily controller medication: low-dose inhaled corticosteroids; cromolyn/nedocromil; leukotriene modifiers • Inhaled beta-2 agonists as needed
Moderate persistent	• Symptoms daily, but not continual, nighttime symptoms more than once a week, but not every night • Exacerbations affect activity and sleep • Daily use of inhaled short-acting beta-2 agonist • PEFR or FEV$_1$: 60%–80% predicted; PFT variability >30%	• Daily controller medications: combination inhaled medium-dose corticosteroid and long-acting bronchodilator (especially for nighttime symptoms); cromolyn-nedocromil; leukotriene modifiers
Severe persistent	• Continuous daily symptoms, frequent nighttime symptoms • Frequent exacerbations • Physical activities limited by asthma • PEFR or FEV$_1$: ≤60% predicted; PFT variability >30%	• Inhaled beta-2 agonists as needed • Multiple daily controller medications: high-dose inhaled corticosteroid, long-acting bronchodilator, cromolyn/nedocromil; leukotriene modifiers; may need long-term corticosteroids • Inhaled beta-2 agonist as needed

Source: National Asthma Education and Prevention Program (NAEPP). Expert Panel 3 Summary Report 2007: Guidelines for the diagnosis and management of asthma. NIH publication no. 08-5846. US Department of Health and Human Services, Public Health Service, National Institutes of Health (NIH), National Heart, Lung, and Blood Institute (NHLBI), Bethesda, MD.

*The presence of one of the features of severity is sufficient to place a patient in that category.

Levels of nasal eosinophils, serum eosinophils, and IgE are assessed to determine the allergic status of the patient. Intradermal skin testing may be indicated if the allergic status is significant.

Infections often precede an asthma attack. If infection is suspected (because of a productive cough with colored sputum), a sputum test for culture and sensitivity should be done.

When persistent asthma is present, the EPR-3 recommends that skin testing or in vitro radioallergosorbent tests be done to determine sensitivity to allergens to optimize treatment and prevention.

Differential Diagnosis

Airflow obstruction may result from foreign body aspiration or viral infections, as well as a variety of underlying pulmonary infections, such as aspergillosis, TB, hypersensitivity pneumonitis, or habitual cough. Hyperventilation syndrome, mitral valve prolapse, recurrent pulmonary emboli, congestive heart failure, and chronic obstructive lung disease may mimic asthma. In addition, for some sensitive patients, cough may be secondary to the use of certain drugs, such as ACE inhibitors, beta blockers, aspirin, and NSAIDs. One key feature to making the diagnosis of asthma is the reversibility of the obstructive phenomenon.

Management

If the patient has never been diagnosed with asthma, the clinician may want to make an initial referral to a pulmonologist. An aggressive approach to asthma management is recommended to improve symptoms in the short term, prevent recurrence of symptoms, and/or manage a potentially chronic problem—all with the goal of improving the patient's quality of life by achieving and maintaining control of symptoms. The principles of management include the following:

- Identification of factors that exacerbate the condition
- Daily monitoring of PEF with a symptom record (see Asthma Attack Trigger Diary at http://davisplus.fadavis.com)
- Written instructions on managing an acute asthma attack
- Intensive education and follow-up, emphasizing joint decision making

Initial and subsequent management of asthma is aimed at first removing all identified triggers or precipitants. The step therapy approach is a guide to assist the provider in working with the patient to make the best treatment decisions. As a rule, the highest appropriate step should be used to gain early control. The therapy should be "stepped up" if control is not maintained. The clinician should always review the patient's medication technique, adherence, and control of triggers at each visit. The stepwise approach, according to the severity of the asthma, is shown in Treatment Flowchart 9.1.

Asthma management can require daily pharmacotherapeutics with inhaled corticosteroids, long-acting beta-2 agonists, and/or leukotriene antagonists. In patients with other comorbidities, management may be complicated. Daily medications for those with mildly persistent to severe asthma may significantly reduce and control symptoms, leading to improved quality of life.

In the management of chronic asthma, ABG analysis (in hospital) and PFTs (in primary care) are done periodically to measure how well the patient is responding to treatment. The patient can be taught to use a handheld peak flow meter to measure the peak expiratory flow rate (PEFR) and gauge response to treatment. Several peak flow rate readings should be done when the patient is stable to establish a baseline (or "personal best"). This baseline can be used as a benchmark for guiding therapy. Once the patient's condition is stabilized, the daily PEFR monitoring can be done by the patient. If the PEFR reading is less than 80% of the patient's personal best, adjustments in medications or lifestyle may be necessary.

Inhaled corticosteroids are the treatment of choice as anti-inflammatory controller therapies, above other classes of inhaled medications and theophylline. Recent genetic and epidemiological studies appear to imply that certain individuals (especially of African American ethnicity) have a negative reaction to long-term beta-agonist bronchodilators, such as salmeterol. These individuals seem to do worse on long-term beta-agonist therapy. Salmeterol (Serevent) is no longer used as a single agent because of safety concerns regarding increased morbidity and mortality when used without an accompanying corticosteroid. When used in combination with an inhaled corticosteroid (Advair Discus, Symbicort), however, such combinations are extremely effective at improving lung function in patients with moderate to severe asthma.

See Drugs Commonly Prescribed 9.1 for medications for asthma.

Follow-up and Referral

Step down therapy gradually if review of patient's status at 1- to 6-month intervals suggests reduction of treatment is warranted. Smoking cessation for patients with asthma is a must. (For more information on smoking cessation, see Smoking Addiction later in this chapter.) In addition, the patient should avoid exposure to secondhand smoke. Family members also need to be educated about the hazards of secondhand smoke. Regular visits to their primary-care provider can be combined with appropriate referrals to specialists as necessary.

The use of immunotherapy in asthma remains controversial, and its effectiveness has not been well established. For most patients, avoidance of the allergens and triggers, along with the appropriate use of medications, is adequate therapy. If avoidance of certain allergens is impossible and medications fail, referral to an allergist for immunotherapy may be indicated. However, unless the patient's symptoms are exacerbated by exposure to

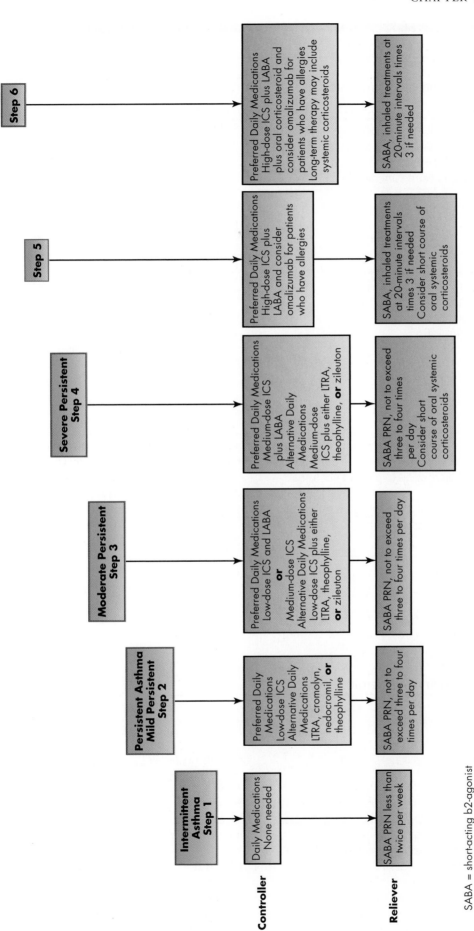

SABA = short-acting b2-agonist

ICS = inhaled corticosteroid

LTRA = leukotriene receptor agonist

LABA = long-acting b2-agonist

Step up to the next step if control is not achieved. First, however, review patient medication technique, and control (avoid all allergens or other trigger factors).

Step down to the next step when asthma is well controlled for 3 months.

Review RX every 3–6 months.

Adapted from the National Heart, Lung, and Blood Institute, Asthma Education and Prevention Program. Expert Panel Report 3 (EPR-3): Guidelines for the Diagnosis and Management of Asthma, 2007.

Treatment Flowchart 9.1 Asthma

Drugs Commonly Prescribed 9.1   Asthma

Drug	Indication and Formulation	Adverse Reactions and Prescribing Considerations
Short-Acting Beta-2 Agonists		
Provide smooth muscle relaxation.	First-line defense for acute attack; may be used prophylactically prn before exercise. Increased need (usage) indicates need to change treatment regimen.	Adverse reactions: Tachycardia, palpitations, tremor, hypokalemia Use with caution in elderly patients.
albuterol (Ventolin, Proventil)	Syrup: 2 mg/5 mL	As above 2–4 mg PO 3–4 times daily. May increase dose gradually to maximum dose of 24 mg/day.
	Metered-dosage inhaler (MDI) 90 mcg/puff Dry powder inhaler (DPI) 200 mcg/puff Nebulizer 5 mg/mL (0.5%)	2 puffs q4–6h prn 2 puffs tid–qid prn, 2 puffs 5 minutes before exercise 1.25–5 mg (0.25–1 mL) in 2–3 mL of NS q4–8h; may be mixed with cromolyn or ipratropium nebulizer solution
pirbuterol (Maxair)	MDI	As above 200 mcg/puff 2 puffs tid–qid prn
Long-Acting Beta Agonists		
	Appropriate for patients with moderate to severe asthma. Use before sleep to prevent nocturnal attacks. May be helpful in preventing exercise-induced asthma.	Should not be used without inhaled corticosteroids. Should not be used as a rescue inhaler. Should not be used in place of anti-inflammatory therapy.
Anticholinergics		
ipratropium bromide (Atrovent)	MDI: 17 mcg/puff Nebulizer: 0.02% (500 mcg in 2.5 mL) for oral inhalation	Do not give to patients with glaucoma or benign prostatic hypertrophy. 2 puffs qid, max. 12 puffs/day May precipitate heart attack, palpitations. Not for primary treatment of acute attack. 500 mcg tid–qid
Combination Beta-2 Agonist and Anticholinergic		
	May use when second aerosol bronchodilator needed.	When used in combination, overall effect is increased.
Combivent	Ipratropium bromide 18 mcg and albuterol (as sulfate) 90 mcg MDI	Use with caution with other anticholinergics and sympathomimetics. 2 puffs qid Maximum: 12 puffs/day
Leukotriene Receptor Antagonists		
	Long-term control. Prophylaxis and treatment of chronic asthma	NOT FOR ACUTE ATTACK

Drugs Commonly Prescribed 9.1 Asthma—cont'd

Drug	Indication and Formulation	Adverse Reactions and Prescribing Considerations
montelukast (Singulair)	Prophylaxis and chronic treatment 4 mg or 5 mg chewable tablets, 10 mg tablet Oral granules 4 mg/packet	Monitor with potent CYP450 indices May take 10 mg/night
zafirlukast (Accolate)	Prophylaxis and chronic treatment of asthma 10 mg and 20 mg tablets	Take at least 1 hour before meals OR 2 hours after meals May take 20 mg twice daily
cromolyn sodium (Intal)	MDI: 0.8 mg/puff Nebulizer: 20 g/2 mL	Adverse reactions: Bronchospasm, throat irritation, bad taste. 2 puffs 10–60 minutes before exposure to precipitants Acts as a mast cell stabilizer. May use qid
nedocromil sodium (Tilade)	MDI: 1.75 mg/puff	As above May use 2–4 puffs qid

Inhaled Corticosteroids

	Maintenance treatment of asthma and prophylactic treatment in asthma	
beclomethasone (Beclodisk)	Not for acute attack 40 or 80 mcg/puff	Rinse mouth after use. Avoid excessive use. Max. 10 puffs/day
budesonide (Pulmicort)	Dry powder delivery system 90, 180, or 200 mcg inhaler (800 mg max per day)	Monitor infections; susceptible to oral candidiasis. Rinse mouth after use. Avoid excessive use.
fluticasone (Flovent)	MDI: 44, 110, 220 mcg/puff DPI: 50, 100, 250 mg dose	Monitor infections; susceptible to oral candidiasis. Rinse mouth after use. Avoid excessive use.
flunisolide (AeroBid, Bronalide)	MDI: 250 mcg/puff	Has mint flavor. Contains menthol. Initially 2 puffs bid, max: 8 puffs/day

Combination Inhaled Corticosteroid and Long-Acting Beta-2 Agonist

fluticasone and salmeterol (Advair Diskus)	Moderate to severe persistent asthma	100, 250, or 500 mcg fluticasone per dose plus 50 mcg salmeterol per dose dry powder 1 puff twice daily
budesonide and formoterol (Symbicort)	Moderate to severe persistent asthma	80 or 160 mcg per dose plus 4.5 mcg formoterol per dose inhalation 2 inhalations twice daily

Systemic Corticosteroids

	For long-term treatment of severe persistent asthma. Short courses or "bursts" effective for establishing control when initiating therapy or during a period of gradual deterioration.	

Continued

Drugs Commonly Prescribed 9.1 Asthma—cont'd

Drug	Indication and Formulation	Adverse Reactions and Prescribing Considerations
methylprednisolone (Medrol) prednisolone prednisone (Deltasone)		Use with caution in patients with TB, hypothyroidism, cirrhosis, ulcerative colitis, etc. May mask infection May cause hypokalemia, hypernatremia; glucose intolerance; bone demineralization Give 7.5–60.0 mg/day in a single dose or qid as needed for control. Short "burst" 40–60 mg/day as a single dose or in two divided doses over 3–10 days; tapering not necessary.
Methylxanthines		
theophylline (Theo-24)	100, 200, 300, 400 extended-release capsules Long-acting bronchodilator for use in moderate and severe persistent asthma. Occasionally used for mild persistent asthma (step 2). Advantage is that bid level can be measured, and theophylline may have some anti-inflammatory properties.	Not for use in acute attack. Many drug interactions; contraindicated in seizure disorders, arrhythmias, active peptic ulcer disease. **Adverse reactions:** Nausea, headaches, irritability, restlessness, convulsions, diuresis To maintain steady state, keep serum concentration levels between 5 and 15 mcg/mL

an allergen and the allergen can be confirmed by skin-prick testing, it is unlikely that immunotherapy will be effective.

Patient Education

A list of reasonable expectations (see Table 9.4) for patients with asthma should be reviewed with the patient and family. If there are problems in certain areas, spend time exploring potential triggers that might be removed or problematic areas such as noncompliance or improper use of inhalants.

The patient and family should be educated about the following areas for self-care management:

- Basic asthma facts.
- When and how to use a short-acting beta-2 agonist inhaler before exercising. (There may only be exercise-induced asthma.)
- How to recognize early symptoms of an exacerbation and how to initiate a predetermined plan of action.
- Role of medications (long-acting and short-term) and the critical role for anti-inflammatory controller medication regimens to reduce the rate of acute attacks.
- Skills for inhaler (spacer) and daily peak flow meter monitoring (for patients with moderate to severe persistent asthma). Although some medications have

"built-in" spacers, spacers are universally recommended for metered-dose inhalers to obtain maximum benefit.
- Use of a nebulizer if necessary. Nebulizers may be necessary when patients cannot take in adequate breaths.
- Environmental control.
- Avoidance measures.
- Importance of pneumococcal and annual influenza vaccination.

Patient and family education is essential for control of triggers and recognition of warning signals. An Asthma Attack Trigger Diary may be used (see DavisPlus at http://davisplus.fadavis.com).

Reinforcement of medication use and proper use of the handheld flow meter should be reviewed at each visit. It should be mentioned that rescue courses of systemic glucocorticoids may be needed at times to prevent acute attacks, although recurrent attacks indicate that a greater degree of controller medication is warranted. Once patients have been followed for some time and have learned self-management, most patients with no cognitive impairment can be instructed on the proper use of glucocorticoids to prevent acute attacks.

Patients may ask which inhaled corticosteroid is the best. Research has shown that if equipotent doses are

Table 9.4   Reasonable Expectations for Patients With Asthma

When entering into a treatment plan, the patient with asthma expects to:
- Be able to participate fully in any activity.
- Be able to sleep through the night.
- Be free of severe symptoms day and night.
- Be satisfied with asthma care.
- Have the best possible pulmonary function.
- Need fewer or no emergency visits or hospitalizations due to asthma.
- Not miss work or school because of asthma.
- Use fewer medications with minimal adverse effects.

The provider is responsible for the following:
- Asking patients about their concerns and issues at each visit.
- Continually teaching and reinforcing key educational points.
- Ensuring ongoing and open communication with the patient and family.
- Reviewing short-term goals agreed on at the initial visit.
- Reviewing the asthma action plan for worsening symptoms and exacerbations.
- Reviewing the daily self-management plan and steps the patient needs to take.
- Supplying patients with appropriate educational materials for self-management and prevention.

severe acute asthmatic attack. The risk factors for fatal asthma are shown in Risk Factors 9.1.

Patients with any of these risk factors need additional teaching time so that they can learn self-management techniques to reduce risk factors to the extent possible. An algorithm for self-management that is similar to the one shown in Treatment Flowchart 9.2 should be reviewed with the patient and family. It is extremely important that the patient be trained to use the handheld peak flow meter and learn to determine the predicted (personal best) PEFR. During exacerbations, the patient should compare a current reading to the baseline PEFR as a guide to determine how severe the attack is and to gauge medication use accordingly.

The value of the algorithm as a guide for the patient and family as to when to seek emergency help should be emphasized. A family member should be educated as to how to handle an acute attack, in case the patient becomes severely hypoxic and cognitively impaired.

A caring relationship among the provider, the patient, and family may prove pivotal to effective disease management and improved quality of life. Self-care is an essential component of treatment.

Scant data exist on the prevalence of complementary therapy for asthma. One national survey study estimated that 59% of 4,741 respondents in the United Kingdom had tried some form of complementary therapy. The three adjunct therapies most frequently used in the United Kingdom were breathing techniques, homeopathy, and herbal preparations. Even less research exists on the effectiveness of these therapies, so patients and families should be cautioned about their judicious use. The

used, the efficacy is the same. The key difference is in the delivery technique. With the dry powder inhaler, age is a factor. Providers must spend time teaching the proper technique and observing a return demonstration. One of the adverse side effects of inhaled corticosteroids was believed to be their effects on growth rate in children. Research has shown that this is a very small but definable risk. In a study of 943 children who were followed for 25 years, there was only a ½-inch decrease in growth rate, which occurred in the first 2 years of treatment. Nonetheless, it must be cautioned that all individuals should be on the lowest dose of inhaled corticosteroids possible.

Another question commonly asked is which pets are hypoallergenic. There are many Web sites that promote costly specialty pets that are purported to be nonallergenic, but in reality, there are *no* hypoallergenic pets. Using commonsense measures such as keeping pets out of the bedroom and wiping down cats with a wet washcloth every night to help control dander may help; however, in some cases, removing pets from the home completely may be the only recourse.

The patient and family should be educated to the fullest extent possible to permit self-management and prevention of acute fatal attacks. Although asthma is a chronic disease, patients may die from a particularly

Risk Factors 9.1   Risk Factors for Fatal Asthma

- Comorbidity (cardiovascular or pulmonary disease, such as COPD)
- Current use of, or recent withdrawal from, systemic glucocorticoids
- Difficulty perceiving airflow obstruction or its severity
- History of sudden severe exacerbations
- Hospitalization or emergency care for asthma within past month
- Illicit drug use
- Low socioeconomic status and urban residence
- Prior intubation for asthma
- Sensitivity to *Alternaria*
- Serious psychiatric disease or psychosocial problems
- Three or more emergency visits for asthma in the past year
- Two or more hospitalizations for asthma in the past year
- Use of three or more canisters of inhaled, short-acting beta-2-adrenergic agonists per month

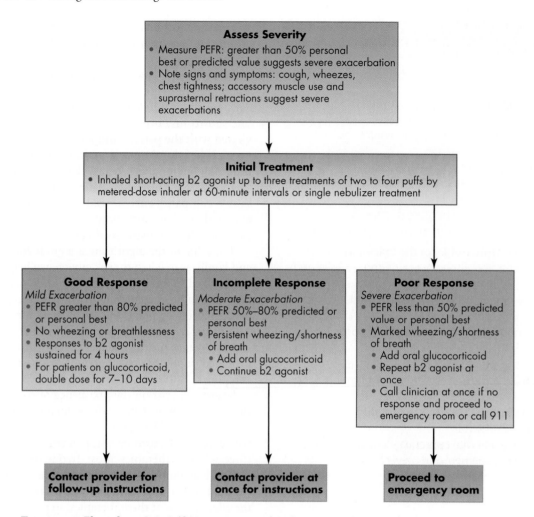

Assess Severity
- Measure PEFR: greater than 50% personal best or predicted value suggests severe exacerbation
- Note signs and symptoms: cough, wheezes, chest tightness; accessory muscle use and suprasternal retractions suggest severe exacerbations

Initial Treatment
- Inhaled short-acting b2 agonist up to three treatments of two to four puffs by metered-dose inhaler at 60-minute intervals or single nebulizer treatment

Good Response
Mild Exacerbation
- PEFR greater than 80% predicted or personal best
- No wheezing or breathlessness
- Responses to b2 agonist sustained for 4 hours
- For patients on glucocorticoid, double dose for 7–10 days

Incomplete Response
Moderate Exacerbation
- PEFR 50%–80% predicted or personal best
- Persistent wheezing/shortness of breath
  - Add oral glucocorticoid
  - Continue b2 agonist

Poor Response
Severe Exacerbation
- PEFR less than 50% predicted value or personal best
- Marked wheezing/shortness of breath
  - Add oral glucocorticoid
  - Repeat b2 agonist at once
  - Call clinician at once if no response and proceed to emergency room or call 911

Contact provider for follow-up instructions

Contact provider at once for instructions

Proceed to emergency room

Treatment Flowchart 9.2 Self-Management of Asthma Exacerbations

use of breathing exercises and devices such as the inspiratory pressure threshold device has been studied in COPD but less so in asthma. More research is needed in this area.

Nutritional therapies have been used in the treatment of asthma. It is known that certain foods may precipitate an asthma flare. To treat asthma, Moses Maimonides, the noted 13th-century physician, prescribed a spicy, herbal mixture of chicken broth that contained herbs such as fennel, parsley, oregano, mint, and onion. Hydration from such a robust broth is also a helpful component in asthma treatment. Onions and garlic have been known to have some protective effect against allergic reactions.

Strong coffee was a widely used treatment for asthma in 18th-century Europe and continues to be used as an effective bronchodilator today. Although drinking teas has never been particularly favored as an asthma treatment, tea leaves were the original source of theophylline, which means "tea leaf." Some literature cites the use of eucalyptus (as a decongestant/cough suppressant), lycopene (for exercise-induced asthma), vitamin B_{12} and vitamin C, and goldenseal, but evidence-based research lists them only as level C, so caution should be exercised when discussing these with patients.

■ CHRONIC BRONCHITIS AND EMPHYSEMA (CHRONIC OBSTRUCTIVE PULMONARY DISEASE [COPD])

There are two primary forms of lung disease—obstructive and restrictive. *Obstructive lung diseases* are those in which the expiratory flow rate is impaired. *Restrictive lung diseases* are those in which the lung volumes are reduced due to musculoskeletal disorders, tumors, lung resection, or interstitial lung disease (ILD). Obstructive lung diseases are further classified as reversible (such as asthma) and irreversible (such as chronic bronchitis and emphysema). The American Thoracic Society (ATS) has defined *chronic bronchitis* as a clinical disorder characterized by excessive mucus secretion in the bronchial tree. It is manifested by chronic or recurrent cough (with or without sputum production), present on most days for a minimum of 3 months of the year, for at least 2 successive years. In addition, dyspnea with or without wheezing is present. Whereas more than 14 million Americans have been diagnosed with COPD, an equal number are probably afflicted but not diagnosed.

Epidemiology and Causes

Chronic bronchitis and emphysema are grouped together as *chronic obstructive pulmonary diseases.* The ATS defines *chronic obstructive pulmonary disease* (COPD) as a disease state characterized by the presence of airflow obstruction due to chronic bronchitis or emphysema. Asthma is not classified as COPD but is sometimes referred to as a reversible obstructive condition, whereas emphysema is irreversible. Chronic bronchitis is usually irreversible, but it may be partially reversible if there is a bronchospastic component and a significant response to bronchodilators. The prevalence and mortality rates for chronic bronchitis and emphysema increase with age. COPD is the third leading cause of death in the United States; there are almost 140,000 deaths due to COPD annually in this country.

Morbidity and mortality are higher in persons with low incomes and less education. It is difficult to estimate the prevalence of chronic bronchitis because there is considerable overlap of conditions: Some patients have all three (asthma, chronic bronchitis, and emphysema), and some have two of the three conditions.

Several studies have established certain predisposing and risk factors for morbidity and mortality from COPD. The established and probable risk factors for COPD are shown in Risk Factors 9.2.

Cigarette smoking is responsible for 80% to 90% of the cases of COPD, and it is also the risk factor most amenable to modification for preventing or delaying the development of COPD. Educational intervention at an early age can help reduce smoking and some other risk factors, such as occupational exposure, exposure to air pollution and allergens, and respiratory infections. If certain genetic risk factors are present, the patient should be educated about periodic baseline testing for pulmonary function and about routine checks to prevent respiratory infections and reduce risks to the extent possible. The probability of a person developing COPD within 10 years can be calculated using the Tecumseh Index, in which points are allotted for the three major risk factors of age, number of cigarettes smoked per day, and FEV_1 as a percentage of the value predicted. Stopping smoking at any age has some beneficial effect for lung function even though there may be permanent damage to lung tissue.

Pathophysiology

COPD is a progressive disease characterized by airflow limitation that is not fully reversible. The disease process

---

Risk Factors 9.2   Risk Factors for COPD

Established risks:

- Age
- Male gender
- Cigarette smoking
- Reduced lung function
- Occupational exposures
- Air pollution
- Alpha$_1$-antitrypsin phenotypes

Probable or possible risks:

- Infections of the respiratory tract
- Allergic conditions
- Bronchial reactivity
- Climate
- Poor socioeconomic resources
- Alcohol intake
- Poor diet and inadequate nutrition
- ABO, ABH secretor, cell phenotypes
- Impaired immune function
- Familial factors

---

involves a combination of the pathological mechanisms of emphysema and chronic bronchitis. In addition, hyperreactivity of the airways is a common feature. Thus, COPD is a disease of both the lung parenchyma and the small airways (bronchioles).

Emphysema is characterized by destruction of alveolar walls due to an imbalance of proteinase–antiproteinase enzymatic activity. In healthy lung tissue, protective antiproteinases counteract protein-degrading enzymes secreted by white blood cells. In rare cases, a genetic condition called alpha-1 antitrypsin deficiency may play a role in causing COPD. People who have this condition have low levels of alpha-1 antitrypsin, a protein made in the liver. Chronic inflammation, caused by long-term cigarette smoking or chronic exposure to lung irritants, for example, repeatedly recruits white blood cells to the alveoli. In contrast to the atopic processes of asthma, the lymphocytic infiltration of COPD consists predominantly of CD8+ T cells, rather than CD4+ T-helper cells. Neutrophil and monocyte-/macrophage-derived proteinases progressively degrade the alveolar walls, overcoming antiproteinase defenses. Overdistended, hyperinflated, less elastic alveoli are the result of the recurring injury over time. Weak elastic recoil of alveoli leads to air trapping, increased residual lung volume, reduced expiratory flow, and retained carbon dioxide. Individuals experience hypercapnia but can maintain adequate oxygenation early on in the disease process.

Desensitization of the central respiratory receptors to P_{CO_2} occurs with long-term hypercapnia. Under normal circumstances, P_{CO_2} accumulation in the blood stimulates individuals to breathe independently. However, persons who endure long-term states of hypercapnia lose this normal respiratory stimulus to breathe. Hypoxia becomes the stimulus for breathing instead of P_{CO_2}. Hypoxia is sensed by peripheral chemoreceptors in the arteries, such as the carotid bodies. The individual who has endured hypercapnia for a prolonged period of time begins to rely on low oxygen levels to drive breathing. Consequently, supplemental oxygen must be used judiciously in these individuals because of their hypoxic drive to breathe. High levels of supplemental oxygen, as well as respiratory depressants of any kind (e.g., sedatives, narcotics), can suppress the hypercapnic individual's hypoxic drive to breathe independently.

Cigarette smoking is the major environmental risk factor for development of COPD. Although smoking cessation slows progression of the disease, reversal of pathological changes does not occur. There is a proven causal relationship between cigarette smoking and COPD; however, there is marked variability in the pulmonary function of persons with similar smoking histories. This has led to investigation into genetic risk factors for COPD. As mentioned earlier, one such genetic risk factor is alpha-1 antitrypsin deficiency. Alpha-1 antitrypsin is a major antiproteinase enzyme that can counteract alveolar destruction. Individuals can inherit different genetic mutations that lead to variable degrees of deficiency of this enzyme. Individuals with complete absence of alpha-1 antitrypsin have an increased susceptibility to emphysema and develop the disease early in life.

Compared with emphysema, chronic bronchitis is the more common pathological mechanism involved in COPD. Airflow obstruction in chronic bronchitis is caused by bronchiole edema, hyperplasia of mucus-producing goblet cells, and bronchiole smooth muscle hypertrophy. Clinically, chronic bronchitis presents as a long-term cough or recurrent sputum production, primarily on morning awakening, extending over 3 months for a period of at least 2 years. Individuals with hypoxia and cyanosis have problems with ventilatory obstruction and suboptimal oxygenation of the blood. In chronic bronchitis, long-term hypoxia leads to pulmonary vasoconstriction, which can result in pulmonary hypertension. This increased pulmonary resistance against the right ventricle can lead to right ventricular failure or cor pulmonale. Chronic hypoxia also stimulates renal erythropoietin, which initiates and perpetuates red blood cell synthesis in the bone marrow, thereby increasing hemoglobin concentration and hematocrit, which makes the right ventricle hypertrophic from pumping more viscous blood into a constricted pulmonary artery.

Acute exacerbations of chronic bronchitis are highly characteristic of this disease. Increased purulent sputum production and worsened shortness of breath are the hallmark of such episodes, which may also be accompanied by fever and increased oxygen requirements for patients on supplemental oxygen. Although viral bronchitis requiring only supportive care is the most common etiology of such exacerbations, bacterial involvement must be considered with increased sputum production lasting more than a week or new chest x-ray findings. *Streptococcus pneumoniae* is the most common agent, followed by *Haemophilus influenzae* and *Moraxella catarrhalis*, similar to the causative agents of sinusitis and community-acquired pneumonia. Antibacterial therapy is often instituted empirically, however, without the need for cultures or Gram stain evidence.

The respiratory symptoms of COPD logically follow patterns of pulmonary neuromuscular anatomy, because bronchiole smooth muscle is innervated by beta-2 adrenergic and cholinergic nerve receptors. The bronchiole constriction in COPD is largely cholinergically mediated. For this reason, blockade of cholinergic receptors by anticholinergic drugs enhances the ability of bronchioles to dilate in COPD. Increased mucus production is also counteracted by these agents. In contrast, beta-receptor activation mediates bronchodilation, as reflected in the therapeutic benefits of inhaled beta-agonist drugs. Inhaled and oral steroids, on the other hand, function by decreasing overall airway inflammation mediated largely by T cells.

There is a normal age-related decline in pulmonary function: The forced expiratory volume in 1 second (FEV_1) declines by 0.02 to 0.04 L per year. Cigarette smoking accelerates the decline by twofold to threefold. Though smoking cessation slows the rate of decline, it will not reverse most pathological changes. Pulmonary function patterns and physical findings for various pulmonary conditions are shown in Table 9.5. The PFT results reflect the underlying pathology of the condition.

It is common for patients to have mixed lung disease (both restrictive and obstructive). For example, patients with chronic bronchitis may also present with a restrictive ILD such as sarcoidosis. In cases like this, all lung volumes would be reduced, the diffusing capacity would be reduced, and the arterial blood gases (ABGs) would be abnormal (showing hypoxemia and possibly carbon dioxide retention).

Age and FEV_1 are the strongest predictors of mortality in COPD (Table 9.6). High mortality rates occur when COPD is complicated by respiratory infection (acute bronchitis exacerbations) or cor pulmonale from chronic pulmonary hypertension. These conditions increase risk for ventilation–perfusion mismatch, hypoxemia, hypercapnia, respiratory acidosis, and respiratory failure.

Clinical Presentation
Subjective

The typical smoker who develops COPD may be asymptomatic for 10 to 20 years except for more frequent colds, persistent morning cough, and upper respiratory infections. Men, in particular, may wait until the dyspnea becomes severe before seeking medical help or may seek help only when they need antibiotics for a chronic

Table 9.5   Pulmonary Function and Physical Findings in Obstructive and Restrictive Lung Diseases

Parameters	Asthma	Chronic Bronchitis	Emphysema	Restrictive Disease
Forced Vital Capacity (FVC)	Normal	Normal to increased	Normal to increased	Decreased
Residual Volume (RV)	Normal; increased during attacks	Increased	Increased	Decreased or normal
Total Lung Capacity (TLC)	Normal to increased	Normal	Normal to increased	Decreased
RV/TLC	Normal to increased	Increased	Increased	Normal
Expiratory Flow Rates	Normal to decreased	Normal to decreased	Normal to decreased	Normal to increased
FEV_1/FVC	Normal to decreased	Decreased	Decreased	Normal to increased
Bronchodilator Response (% change)	>15%	0%–15%	None	None
Diffusing Capacity	Normal to increased	Normal to decreased	Decreased	Normal or decreased (depends on type of disease)
Pao_2	Normal; decreased during attack	Decreased	Normal in mild to moderate disease; decreased in severe disease	Normal or decreased
$Paco_2$	First decreased, then increased during acute attack	Increased	Normal until advanced disease, then increased	Normal or decreased; increased in very advanced disease
Breath Sounds	Marked decrease during acute attacks If $FEV_1 = 0.5$ L or less: absent	If $FEV_1 = 1$ L: barely audible		Normal or decreased in pneumonia, atelectasis
Crackles (rales)	Coarse crackles during infections	Coarse crackles during infections	Fine crackles may be present	Varies with type of restrictive disease
Wheezes (rhonchi)	High-pitched; continuous	Forced expiratory wheezes	No	No

productive cough. They may ignore symptoms of fatigue, shortness of breath, and cough because of embarrassment. Older persons may attribute the shortness of breath and fatigue to functional decline related to aging. The onset of COPD is typically in the fifth decade or later with a 20-pack-year smoking history (number of packs of cigarettes per day times number of years).

With advanced disease in which chronic bronchitis predominates, pulmonary hypertension may result from chronic alveolar hypoxia, and cor pulmonale develops. Patients with these signs and symptoms are often called "blue bloaters" because of the edema and cyanosis that accompany their condition. A complete blood count (CBC) with differential may reveal polycythemia secondary to the increased erythropoietin stimulation of

increased red blood cells to compensate for the chronic hypoxemia.

Patients who primarily have emphysema ("pink puffers") have severe dyspnea but usually present with relatively normal ABGs that are maintained because of high minute ventilation. As the disease progresses, dyspnea increases because the diffusing capacity is severely reduced. These patients often appear very thin and may have the typical "barrel chest" resulting from hyperinflation.

A patient with an acute exacerbation of chronic bronchitis may present with cough and increased sputum that is thick and colored (yellow, brown, gray, or green); fever may also be present. Sudden onset of cough with minimal sputum, chills, fever, and myalgia is more indicative of a viral infection. Remember that older adults

Table 9.6	Severity of COPD Based on the Pulmonary Function Measures: Forced Expiratory Volume in 1 Second (FEV₁)
Stage 1:	
Mild COPD	$FEV_1/FVC < 0.7$ $FEV_1 \geq 80\%$ predicted
Stage 2:	
Moderate COPD	$FEV_1/FVC < 0.7$ FEV_1 50%–79% predicted
Stage 3:	
Severe COPD	$FEV_1/FVC < 0.7$ FEV_1 30%–49% predicted
Stage 4:	
Very severe COPD	$FEV_1/FVC < 0.7$ $FEV_1 < 30\%$ predicted or <50% predicted with chronic respiratory failure

Source: Adapted from Global Initiative for Chronic Obstructive Lung Disease (GOLD). COPD diagnosis and management at-a-glance desk reference. Updated February 2013. Retrieved July 1, 2013, from www.goldcopd.org/guidelines-copd-diagnosis-and-management.html

often have blunted responses to infection due to a decreased immune response.

Patients with COPD usually present with a complaint of chronic productive cough (chronic bronchitis) and increasing shortness of breath or dyspnea on exertion (emphysema). Associated symptoms may include fatigue, weakness, hemoptysis, loss of appetite, nausea, and dizziness. By the time there is dyspnea on exertion, the disease is usually well advanced. Patients may report having to sleep sitting up or with three or more pillows to relieve dyspnea. They may report awakening during the night with severe dyspnea (paroxysmal nocturnal dyspnea), which is relieved by sitting upright.

Objective

The physical findings will vary depending on the severity of the COPD. Physical findings are often not significant in mild to moderate COPD. In emphysema or mixed disease, the chest exam may indicate hyperinflation. There may be flattening of the diaphragm, tachypnea, and use of the accessory muscles of respiration (scalene, sternocleidomastoids). In hyperinflation, the predominant palpable or auscultatory cardiac contraction may be noted in the epigastrium rather than in the left intercostal space. On auscultation, breath sounds are distant and are not augmented much with deep breathing. End expiratory wheezes may be heard on forced expiration. Patients with a bronchospastic component may have inspiratory and expiratory wheezes. Measurement of forced expiratory time is useful to determine if airway

obstruction is present. When auscultating the lungs, have the patient take a full inspiration, then listen while the patient exhales through the mouth until airflow stops. Normal duration is 3 seconds, but in COPD the time is prolonged because of airway obstruction.

Coarse crackles may be present during an acute exacerbation. Neck vein distention, especially during expiration, may occur as a result of increased intrathoracic pressure. The patient's feet and ankles should be examined for edema that may occur as the disease progresses and cor pulmonale develops. The nailbeds should be examined for clubbing (hypertrophic osteoarthropathy), which often occurs in patients with pulmonary pathology. Other causes of clubbing are atrioventricular shunt, subacute bacterial endocarditis, inflammatory bowel disease, and biliary cirrhosis.

During the physical exam, the patient's ability to follow commands and respond to questions should be documented. Changes in mental status may be caused by hypoxemia or hypercapnia rather than dementia. Fatigue is a common finding.

Diagnostic Reasoning

The diagnostic approach to the patient is directed at assessment of the type of obstructive disease (primarily bronchitis, emphysema, or mixed) and whether it is reversible or irreversible. The possibility of underlying restrictive disease must be eliminated. Patients who have chronic bronchitis and have smoked for 20 years or longer should be evaluated for lung cancer.

Diagnostic Tests

Initial Testing The initial diagnostic evaluation should include PFTs (spirometry, diffusing capacity, and ABGs). The standard PFTs should include prebronchodilator and postbronchodilator testing to determine if there is a significant response to bronchodilators. The diagnostic criterion for COPD is an FEV_1/FVC ratio that is less than 70%. The FEV_1 (percent of predicted value) is the most useful parameter to assess severity of obstruction (see Table 9.6). The American College of Physicians' Guidelines recommend spirometry in the diagnosis of patients exhibiting symptoms but not in those who are asymptomatic.

Even though bronchitis and emphysema usually occur together in most patients, it is important to distinguish the severity of the bronchitis and the emphysema and to identify how much of a bronchospastic component is present in order to direct treatment appropriately. In chronic bronchitis and emphysema, narrowing of the airways is present that usually results in an increase in airway resistance and a decrease in maximal expiratory flow rates. In emphysema, the loss of elastic recoil accounts for a decrease in the caliber of the airways (from loss of radial traction on the airways). The elastic recoil properties of the lung serve as a major determinant of the expiratory flow rates. Maximal expiratory flow rates represent a complex and dynamic interplay among airway caliber, elastic recoil pressures, and airway collapsibility. As a result of the altered pressure-airflow relations in COPD, the work of breathing is increased in bronchitis and emphysema. The maldistribution of inspired gas (through ventilation) and blood flow (through perfusion) is always present to a degree in COPD. When the mismatching is severe, it is reflected in the ABGs as hypoxemia or hypercarbia.

Chest radiography will appear normal in patients with early COPD. In patients with chronic bronchitis, chest x-ray films may reveal increased lung markings in the lower lobes and peribronchial thickening. In patients with emphysema, the radiograph may show hyperinflation (low flat diaphragm, enlarged retrosternal space), hypovascularity, areas of hyperlucency and bullae formation, and a small cardiac silhouette. Chest computed tomography (CT) scans are used to evaluate the extent and distribution of emphysematous cysts for possible surgery. In recurrent bronchitis, CT scans may be used to rule out bronchiectasis.

Laboratory tests should include a CBC and differential. The hemoglobin, hematocrit (Hct), and red blood cell count should be evaluated to rule out anemia or polycythemia. Serum alpha$_1$-antitrypsin levels should be checked in patients who develop COPD at an early age (younger than 45), those with clinical emphysema who have not smoked, and those with a family history of young onset of COPD. A blood chemistry profile is done to assess the electrolyte (K, Na, Cl) and nutritional status (total protein, albumin) and to rule out renal or liver problems.

For an exacerbation of chronic bronchitis, sputum should be tested via Gram stain. Sputum culture and sensitivity is done to confirm the findings of the Gram stain. The Gram stain is the best clinical method for diagnosing an acute exacerbation because the bacteria can be seen and quantified. Patients with COPD often are colonized by low numbers of bacteria, including *S pneumoniae, H influenzae,* and *M catarrhalis,* which will grow in culture even though they are not present in sufficient numbers to be seen with Gram stain. If the Gram stain shows neutrophils but no bacteria in a patient with chronic bronchitis, the acute exacerbation is probably viral or chlamydial, even when the sputum culture yields *Haemophilus* or *Pneumococcus.* A negative Gram stain indicates that such culture results represent bacterial colonization rather than a true infection.

An electrocardiogram (ECG) should be done if the patient has not had a baseline test and especially if there are signs of cardiac disease or in advanced COPD. Atrial arrhythmias are common in older adults and in pulmonary patients of any age. ECG changes in pulmonary disease include peaked P waves in leads II, III, and aV$_F$ and changes associated with right ventricular hypertrophy. Cardiac abnormalities may have implications for the drugs selected to treat the COPD.

Assessing degree of functional status and quality of life of patients with COPD should be done initially to determine the potential for rehabilitation and to direct appropriate therapy. The SF-36 Health Survey is a valid, reliable tool used worldwide to assess physical and emotional health and is recommended for patients with chronic illnesses such as COPD. The tool is widely available.

Subsequent Testing   Annual spirometry, CBC with differential, chemistry profile, and chest radiographs should be done to measure the patient's decline in pulmonary function and to screen for other lung diseases that may be related to smoking. Gram stain, culture and sensitivity test of sputum, and ABG analysis are done as needed during acute exacerbations. Pulse oximetry is a noninvasive test that can be done in the office to screen for hypoxemia. An oxygen saturation of 90% or less at rest warrants monitoring ABGs. The ATS recommends ABG monitoring for hypoxemia and hypercapnia in patients with advanced disease—those with an FEV$_1$ less than 50% of the predicted value.

Differential Diagnosis

Acute bronchitis, asthma, bronchiectasis, bronchogenic carcinoma, acute viral infection, normal aging of lungs, occupational asthma, sleep apnea, and chronic sinusitis are all conditions that need to be ruled out to make a diagnosis of COPD and emphysema. In young adults, cystic fibrosis needs to be ruled out. Patient history and PFT results (including decreased FEV$_1$ with concomitant reduction in FEV$_1$/FVC ratio), as well as poor or absent reversibility, will assist in making the diagnosis of COPD.

Management

It is essential to diagnose COPD early in patients, because the estimated direct medical costs of COPD annually are more than $18 billion. This fact highlights the economic importance of prevention and of interventions aimed at early diagnosis and delaying disease progression. After the initial diagnosis is made, education of the patient and family is critical for therapy to be effective. The patient and family need to understand that although COPD is not a curable disease, with proper management and smoking cessation, the symptoms can be controlled and quality of life improved. A nursing research study (Nursing Research–Based Practice Box 9.1) is provided that shares the importance of collaborative partnerships in caring for patients with COPD due to the myriad of problems experienced with these patients.

Smoking cessation improves declining lung function and is the single most important intervention to slow the rate of lung function decline regardless of disease severity (Level I; University of Michigan Health System, 2010). After 5 years without cigarettes, the lung function returns to almost that of a nonsmoker. Patients should be urged at each clinic visit to stop smoking; family

---

Nursing Research–Based Practice 9.1

Kirkpatrick, P, et al. Research to support evidence-based practice in COPD community nursing. *Br J Community Nurs* 17(10):486, 488–492, 2012.

Evidence-based practice (EBP) is a requirement of nurses through the generation of evidence to implementing it, in a bid to improve clinical practice. However, EBP is difficult to achieve. This paper highlights an approach to generating evidence for enhancing community nursing services for patients with chronic obstructive pulmonary disease (COPD) through a collaborative partnership. A district nurse and two nursing lecturers formed a partnership to devise a systematic review protocol and perform a systematic review to enhance COPD practice. This paper illustrates the Joanna Briggs Institute (JBI) systematic review process, the review outcomes, and the practitioner learning. Collaborative partnerships among academics, researchers, and clinicians are a potentially useful model to facilitate enhanced outcomes in EBP and evidence application.

---

members should also be encouraged to do the same if they smoke. For more information on smoking cessation, see Smoking Addiction later in this chapter.

Pharmacological Therapy

Although only supplemental oxygen has been shown to improve the mortality associated with COPD, pharmacotherapy has a significant role in reducing its associated morbidities and improving quality of life. A stepwise approach to therapy, similar to that for asthma and hypertension, is used. Drugs most commonly used for management of COPD symptoms are beta-2 agonists, anticholinergics, combination short-acting beta-2 agonists plus anticholinergics in one inhaler, xanthines, inhaled glucocorticosteroids, and systemic glucocorticosteroids. Antibiotics are warranted in the presence of a prolonged illness, especially with purulent sputum.

Inhaled Beta-2 Agonist Bronchodilators Inhaled short-acting beta-2 agonists (beta-adrenergic agonists) are the first line of therapy in the Global Initiative for Chronic Obstructive Lung Disease (GOLD) Stage I. The major goals of therapy are to prevent bronchospasm with long-acting bronchodilators and to use "rescue" medication to alleviate acute episodes of bronchospasm. Each episode of acute bronchospasm causes permanent remodeling of the bronchioles; therefore, prevention of these episodes is critical. Inhaled short-acting beta-2 agonists (albuterol [Proventil, Ventolin], pirbuterol [Maxair Autohaler]) are prescribed as "rescue" medication for intermittent symptoms of acute shortness of breath. Patients may experience adverse reactions from beta-2 agonists that include tremors, nervousness, and dysrhythmias. Long-acting beta agonists are not first-line therapy but may be used for maintenance therapy to prevent acute bronchospastic episodes. They should not be used without inhaled steroids.

Inhaled Anticholinergic Bronchodilators Inhaled anticholinergic bronchodilators such as ipratropium bromide (Atrovent) are recommended for maintenance therapy in COPD. Bronchospasm in COPD has been found to be mainly cholinergically mediated; therefore

anticholinergic inhalers are effective. These drugs are well tolerated by older adults and are not systemically absorbed. Ipratropium is taken routinely, usually two puffs four times a day. A long-acting anticholinergic agent in a dry powder form such as tiotropium (Spiriva) may be effective and is inhaled only once daily. As a scheduled bronchodilator, tiotropium offers significant advantages to patients whose symptoms are not controlled by albuterol. Tiotropium is the recommended therapy for GOLD Stage II along with albuterol as a rescue medication. Many tiotropium studies have shown a reduction in the use of rescue medication, as well as a reduction of COPD exacerbations (Level I; Freeman et al, 2007). Some inhaler medications for COPD contain a combination of an anticholinergic and a beta-2 agonist bronchodilator that act synergistically. Formoterol plus ipratropium, albuterol, or a combination may also be used in Stage II. These are also recommended in Stages III and IV, along with the addition of an inhaled corticosteroid. A combination of inhaled corticosteroid and long-acting beta-2 agonist is fluticasone and salmeterol (Advair Diskus). Patients seem to do better with one inhaler rather than two.

Corticosteroids The primary role of inhaled glucocorticoids in COPD is as an anti-inflammatory agent. The dosing of inhaled corticosteroids such as beclomethasone, budesonide (Pulmicort), and fluticasone (Flovent), among others, should be individualized. Good inhaler technique with a spacing device and frequent mouth rinsing are advised to avoid oral candidiasis. Combination corticosteroid and beta-2 adrenergic agonist inhalers are effective to counteract bronchoconstriction and inflammation.

In rare cases, systemic corticosteroids may be used in the management of an acute exacerbation for no more than 10 to 14 days. However, the potential risks associated with this treatment, including immunosuppression, hypertension, and hyperglycemia, necessitate that it be used with caution. Some studies have shown that for acute COPD exacerbations, systemic corticosteroids are effective in reducing treatment failures (Level I; Quon et al, 2008). Some clinicians report that 15% to 20% of patients respond both subjectively (perceived dyspnea) and objectively (FEV_1 and improved exercise performance) with low-dose long-term systemic steroids, although this is not a widely accepted treatment. Rather, systemic steroids should be used only when the other drugs have failed and when there is an acute exacerbation with a bronchospastic component to the COPD. Patients who are likely to respond to steroids are those who have blood and sputum eosinophilia, positive allergy skin test results, elevated levels of serum IgE, and a history of allergy and bronchodilator response. Before starting oral steroids, baseline spirometry should be done; then the patient may take oral prednisone 40 mg daily for 1 to 2 weeks. Spirometry is repeated, and an improvement in FEV_1 of 15% indicates a positive response. The dose should then be tapered to a low daily or alternate-day maintenance dose of 7.5 to 15 mg. The adverse effects of systemic steroids are well known (e.g., gastric ulcer, osteoporosis, masked infections, secondary infections), and the patient should be monitored carefully for adverse reactions.

Beta-2 adrenergic agonists and anticholinergic and corticosteroid medications are available in metered-dose inhalers and dry powder inhalers. Use of these inhaler devices requires patient education. The clinician should observe a patient demonstration of proper inhaler technique because there are differences in the technique used with each type of dispenser. Many patients have difficulty mastering the proper inhaler technique to gain optimal pulmonary delivery of medication. Spacers can be used with some inhalers to enable better delivery of the drug. Nebulizers can also be used to facilitate delivery of some inhaler medications. Regardless of the method used, ongoing patient education is essential to ensure proper inhalation of the medication.

Xanthines Aminophylline or theophylline may be used as a fourth-line drug if the beta-2 agonists, the anticholinergic drugs, and the inhaled corticosteroids are not effective. These preparations have a very narrow therapeutic index, and blood levels should be monitored closely for toxicity. The therapeutic levels are 5 to 15 mcg/mL. The therapeutic benefit may be the result of improved muscle contractility and decreased muscle fatigue. Therapy should be initiated with low doses, then increased gradually because of the narrow therapeutic range. Xanthines interact with other drugs commonly taken by patients with COPD, including cimetidine (Tagamet), erythromycin, ciprofloxacin (Cipro), and beta blockers, among others. If the patient is taking a xanthine, it is safer not to use these drugs to avoid drug toxicity.

Antibiotics Antibiotics are often needed for acute exacerbations of chronic bronchitis when purulent sputum is present. There is little to no evidence for the use of chronic suppressive antibiotic therapy, and this practice has fallen out of favor. Most pulmonologists recommend the empiric use of antibiotics to treat acute episodes when the cough increases and the character and the amount of the sputum change (increase in amount, color, and consistency), even in the absence of fever, pulmonary infiltrates, and leukocytosis. For empiric therapy, the antibiotic should be effective against the three most common pathogens (*S pneumoniae*, *H influenzae*, and *M catarrhalis*), stable against the effects of beta-lactamase, and convenient to take with few adverse reactions. The choice of antibiotic should also depend on local bacterial resistance patterns and individual risk of *Pseudomonas aeruginosa* infection. Patients with COPD who have had a fairly stable course (few hospitalizations) and have not been exposed to many antibiotics typically respond well to therapy. Oral antibiotic options include doxycycline (100 mg every 12 hours), trimethoprim-sulfamethoxazole (160/800 mg every 12 hours), a cephalosporin such as cefpodoxime (200 mg every 12 hours), a macrolide such as azithromycin (500 mg the first day followed by 250 mg for 5 days), a fluoroquinolone such as ciprofloxacin (500 mg every 12 hours), and amoxicillin-clavulanate (875/125 mg every 12 hours). Some practitioners prescribe antibiotics for a period of 3 to 7 days. Some studies have shown that 5 days are as effective as 7 days with fewer side effects. Immunocompromised patients with a turbulent course should be treated carefully with the right antibiotic, even if it is the most expensive, to prevent respiratory failure and admission to an intensive care unit. Persistent gram-negative infection may require prolonged IV antibiotic administration.

Diuretics Diuretics may be necessary when there is evidence of cor pulmonale (right heart failure). Often the triad of prerenal azotemia, hypernatremia, and low cardiac output develops in cor pulmonale, and loop diuretics may be used. Small doses of furosemide (Lasix) and potassium chloride supplements are used in conjunction with a sodium-restricted diet.

Mucolytics and Expectorants Inhaled aerosols of water, saline, steam, or other agents do not improve mucociliary clearance or expectoration. Oral expectorants such as guaifenesin (Humibid, Robitussin) are usually ineffective. Chest physiotherapy and keeping the patient well hydrated is the most cost-effective way to clear the lungs.

Home Oxygen Because hypoxia leads to pulmonary hypertension and increases the work of the right ventricle, low-flow oxygen may help prevent or deter development of cor pulmonale. In addition, of all the therapies mentioned, only supplemental oxygen has been shown to reduce the mortality rate associated with COPD. Requirements for home oxygen include (1) a PaO_2 of 55 mm Hg or less or an oxygen saturation (SaO_2) below 85% and (2) a PaO_2 of 55 to 59 mm Hg if any of the following is present: erythrocytosis (Hct of 56% or more), cor pulmonale (P wave more than 3 mm in leads II, III, and aV_F), edema, or congestive heart failure. The goal of therapy is a PaO$_2$ of 60 mm Hg or SaO$_2$ of 90%, which usually can be accomplished with 1 to 2 L of oxygen per minute for 15 hours per day. The patient should be reevaluated with ABGs or oximetry at 1, 3, and 6 months, then annually. In advanced disease, supplemental oxygen has been shown to reduce the number of hospitalizations and increase the quality of life in individuals.

Surgery

Although surgery will not cure COPD, some patients have benefited from one of three surgical procedures with an improved quality of life. Because of the typically poor pulmonary state of the patient, any surgery is extremely risky and should be performed using an epidural or spinal anesthesia rather than general anesthesia. A bullectomy involves resection of a bulla, which may be effective in reducing the patient's dyspnea. Lung volume reduction surgery involves resecting 20% to 30% of the lung to reduce hyperinflation. Exercise capacity may be improved, but it is highly unlikely that life expectancy would be improved because of the advanced nature of the disease. A lung transplant has been shown to improve the quality of life, functional capacity, and exercise performance. The 2-year survival rate for lung transplantation is 75%. The decision for surgery should be made with the specialist and involve the entire family.

Follow-up and Referral

Patients who are unstable and those with severe disease should be seen monthly. If the patient is stable, an annual visit would be the minimum. If the patient is on theophylline, the blood levels should be monitored every 6 to 12 months once the patient is on the desired dose. If the patient is on home O$_2$, ABGs should be checked whenever there is any condition change or, at a minimum, semiannually. It is important to monitor oxygen saturation (pulse oximetry) more frequently.

Follow-up for the patient with COPD includes the development of a close and supportive relationship with the health-care provider. Because smoking cessation is the single most effective way to reduce the progression of COPD, the patient should be asked about this at every visit.

Patient Education

Patients with COPD should avoid extremes in temperature and humidity when possible and limit their exposure to areas that have high levels of air pollution. Smoking should not be allowed in the home, car, or other confined places. Occupational exposure to fumes, vapors, dusts, and irritants may aggravate symptoms of dyspnea and bronchospasm. High altitude and air travel can pose problems for hypoxemic patients. Arrangements can be made with the airlines in advance for patients requiring oxygen.

Most lung infections are viral, so avoiding contact with crowds during flu season and limiting exposure to people with colds may help. In the fall, patients with COPD should receive influenza immunizations with polyvalent vaccine from early October through mid-November. Obviously patients with comorbid conditions such as COPD should be treated for a viral infection as soon as possible. Oseltamivir (Tamiflu) is an abortive antiviral that helps shorten the duration and decrease the severity of influenza symptoms if used within the first 48 hours of symptom onset. Polyvalent pneumococcal vaccine should also be given. For people older than age 65, reimmunization every 5 years is appropriate. Respiratory therapy and oxygen equipment used in the home should be routinely cleaned to prevent bacterial colonization and subsequent infection.

Pulmonary rehabilitation should be considered for all patients with functional impairment (Level I; University of Michigan Health System, 2010). Physical rehabilitation is also recommended because it can not only deter functional decline but also help the patient and family to maintain a positive outlook. Often, the best exercise for patients with mild to moderate obstructive disease is an individualized walking program. Physical therapy may also be beneficial; the therapist should prescribe specific breathing exercises, arm exercises, and others that will promote general physical reconditioning. Walking aids have been shown to support the diaphragm and ease the difficulty of breathing while walking. During attacks, use of slow, pursed-lip breathing may help to decrease respiratory rate, reduce bronchospasm, and relieve dyspnea. Effective cough techniques and chest physiotherapy are also recommended.

Many patients with COPD find support groups helpful for them and their spouses or caregivers. These support groups are usually sponsored by local chapters of the American Lung Association, and they are usually listed in the phone book. Other patients have used forms of meditation or guided imagery to help relieve dyspnea and anxiety.

Patients with chronic illness such as COPD often are depressed. The Beck depression scale can be used to screen for depression. Use of the selective serotonin reuptake inhibitor antidepressants in patients with lung disease is considered safe and may improve sleep, quality of life, and functional status.

Health-care providers should have a frank discussion with patients and their families regarding end-of-life care, such as advance directives and health-care surrogates. Copies of all documents should be kept in the chart, as well as with patients' families and attorneys. See the Iceberg of COPD figure for additional patient education.

Nursing Research–Based Practice Box 9.2 is an example of how patient teaching by the provider can make a difference in improving patient outcomes.

The Iceberg of COPD

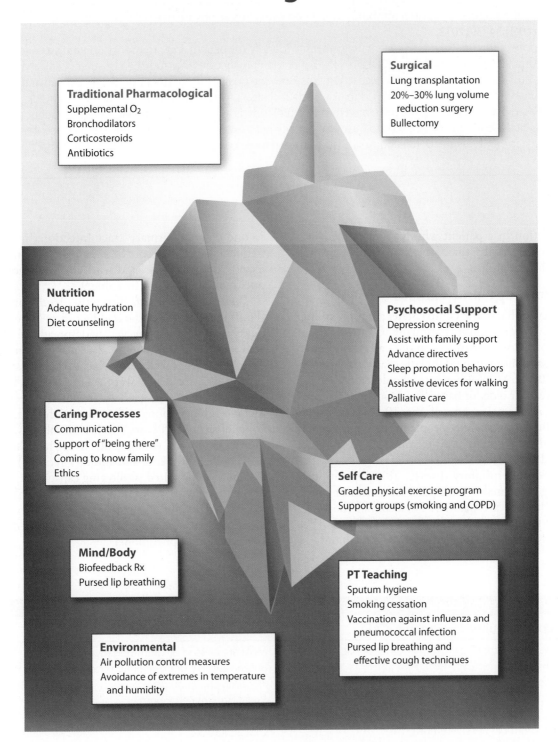

Traditional Pharmacological
Supplemental O_2
Bronchodilators
Corticosteroids
Antibiotics

Surgical
Lung transplantation
20%–30% lung volume
   reduction surgery
Bullectomy

Nutrition
Adequate hydration
Diet counseling

Psychosocial Support
Depression screening
Assist with family support
Advance directives
Sleep promotion behaviors
Assistive devices for walking
Palliative care

Caring Processes
Communication
Support of "being there"
Coming to know family
Ethics

Self Care
Graded physical exercise program
Support groups (smoking and COPD)

Mind/Body
Biofeedback Rx
Pursed lip breathing

PT Teaching
Sputum hygiene
Smoking cessation
Vaccination against influenza and
   pneumococcal infection
Pursed lip breathing and
   effective cough techniques

Environmental
Air pollution control measures
Avoidance of extremes in temperature
   and humidity

■ PNEUMONIA

Pneumonia is typically an acute inflammation of the lung parenchyma, usually infectious in origin. The lung tissue typically becomes consolidated as alveoli fill with exudate. Gas exchange may be impaired as blood is shunted around nonfunctional alveoli. The timely diagnosis and appropriate management of pneumonia in patients is critical because of the morbidity associated with bacterial etiologies, as well as the increased mortality among older patients and those with underlying pulmonary disease. Community-acquired pneumonia (CAP) occurs outside the hospital or is diagnosed within 2 days after

Nursing Research–Based Practice 9.2

Stanley, T, et al. Patient and provider attributes associated with chronic obstructive pulmonary disease exacerbations. *J Nurse Pract* 9(1):34–39, 2013.

The purpose of this quality improvement project was to identify key patient and provider attributes associated with chronic obstructive pulmonary disease (COPD) exacerbations in primary care. The study demonstrates clinical quality scholarship undertaken at the point of service to patients. Both the quality improvement processes applied and the outcomes measured have led to new ways of thinking about clinical problems routinely encountered in medical homes. Evidence-based practice, such as that generated through this study, is a means for improving care for patients, providers, and communities. Addition of these skills to the nurse practitioner's existing skill set of providing patient-centered care, patient advocacy, and service coordination will ensure an even more competent nurse practitioner and improve patient outcomes.

hospitalization in a patient who has not resided in a long-term care facility for 2 weeks or more before the onset of the symptoms.

Epidemiology and Causes

It is estimated that in the United States almost 5 million people develop pneumonia annually. Of these, about 1.3 million persons with pneumonia are admitted to hospitals, and more than 90,000 die each year. Approximately 70% to 80% of patients who develop CAP are aged 60 years or older or have a coexisting medical condition. CAP remains one of the 10 leading causes of mortality among elderly people in the United States today and is frequently the terminal event in older adults and those debilitated by chronic diseases, particularly chronic respiratory disease. This population is increasing, thus making adequate treatment of pneumonia a health-care priority. Nosocomial (hospital-acquired) pneumonias account for approximately 15% of all hospital-associated infections; pneumonia is second only to urinary tract infections in terms of frequency among hospitalized patients. The most common pathogens associated with CAP and nosocomial pneumonia are shown in Table 9.7.

Pneumocystis jirovecii (formerly *carinii*) pneumonia (PCP) remains one of the leading causes of death in patients with AIDS. However, widespread use of highly active antiretroviral therapy and antibiotic prophylaxis based on CD4 T-cell counts has led to a dramatic decline in PCP incidence over the last 10 years. For pneumonia in general, however, other vulnerable populations include infants younger than 6 months old, children younger than age 5 years, smokers, alcoholics, residents of nursing homes, young adults living in close quarters (e.g., college students and military recruits), and any patient with impaired swallowing capacity or cough reflex who is at risk for aspiration. Geographical location, the winter season, occupation, travel history, and pet or animal exposure are other factors associated with the development of pneumonia.

Table 9.7 Common Causes of Pneumonia	
Community-Acquired Pneumonia (CAP)	**Nosocomial Pneumonia**
Streptococcus pneumoniae (70% of all cases of bacterial pneumonia)	Most are caused by gram-negative bacteria.
Pneumococcal pneumonia (25%–35% of all CAP)	Enteric aerobic gram-negative bacilli
Staphylococcus aureus	*Klebsiella pneumoniae*
Klebsiella pneumoniae	*Pseudomonas aeruginosa*
Moraxella catarrhalis (less common)	*Staphylococcus aureus* (gram-positive)
Atypical pneumonias:	Oral anaerobes
Mycoplasma pneumoniae (second most common cause of CAP)	*Legionella pneumoniae* (which travel in cooling systems, condensers, and shower heads)
Legionella pneumoniae	
Chlamydia pneumoniae	
Fungi	
Oral anaerobes	
Viruses	

Pathophysiology

Pneumonia is an infection of the alveoli, distal airways, and interstitium of the lungs and, thus, predominantly a parenchymal disease. A pathogen, such as a bacterium, virus, fungus, or parasite, reaches the lower respiratory tract in sufficient number or with sufficient virulence to overwhelm the innate defenses of the respiratory tract. The inflammatory response is set in motion, which increases capillary permeability and attracts neutrophils, lymphocytes, platelets, and fibrinogen to the site of infection. Tissue fluid extravasates into the interstitial space from the pulmonary capillary bed, forming an exudate with a higher protein content than typical transudative fluid. As this exudate develops, an increasing amount of cellular debris accumulates, impeding optimal oxygen diffusion from the alveoli to capillaries with resultant hypoxemia. Vital capacity, lung compliance, residual capacity, and total lung capacity are diminished, and ventilation–perfusion mismatch occurs.

The spongy consistency of the lung tissue becomes fluid filled and infiltrated by several lineages of white blood cells depending on the infective agent involved, including neutrophils, lymphocytes, and macrophages, as well as red blood cells and fibrin. Because of these changes, the area of pneumonia is often referred to as a consolidative focus, which is typically dull to percussion on physical exam. Pneumonia may be classified as lobar pneumonia, interstitial pneumonia, miliary pneumonia, or bronchopneumonia. Figure 9.1 shows some parenchymal changes in pneumonia. Lobar pneumonia involves an entire lobe of the lung, whereas interstitial pneumonia is a patchy or diffuse inflammatory process throughout regions of the interstitium. Miliary pneumonia consists of numerous discrete lesions resulting from hematogenous spread of infection, and bronchopneumonia is a patchy consolidation involving one or several lobes. Moreover, inflammation can also extend into the pleural space, causing a parapneumonic effusion or inflammation of the pleural membranes, known as pleuritis or pleurisy.

Possible routes of infection include aspiration, aerosolization, hematogenous spread from a distant infected site, and direct spread from a contiguous infected site. Aspiration pneumonia occurs most often in postoperative, stroke, comatose, or otherwise mentally altered patients with an impaired swallowing reflex. Although *Streptococcus pneumoniae* remains the most common causative agent in aspiration pneumonia, anaerobic bacteria and gram-negative bacilli (i.e., gastrointestinal flora) must also be considered. Hematogenous spread to the lungs can take place in endocarditis, from IV central catheter line infection, or from infection at other sites such as the urinary tract. Aerosolization, the most common means of infection, is the route by which most bacteria, *Mycobacterium tuberculosis,* fungi, and viruses reach the lungs.

In adults, the most common organisms involved in CAP include viruses, *S pneumoniae, Moraxella catarrhalis, Haemophilus influenzae, Legionella pneumophila,* and methicillin-sensitive *Staphylococcus aureus,* whereas nosocomial (hospital-acquired) pneumonia raises concerns for *Pseudomonas aeruginosa* and methicillin-resistant *S aureus* (MRSA). Of note, increasing numbers of community-acquired MRSA infections are being reported, particularly among elderly nursing home residents, resulting in severe cases of necrotizing pneumonia. Extremely virulent strains of *S aureus* expressing the Panton-Valentine leukocidin toxin, which induces necrotizing pneumonia, are also surfacing in young adults with the same condition.

Streptococcus pneumoniae

The most common cause of CAP is the gram-positive bacteria *S pneumoniae,* also referred to as pneumococcal pneumonia. *S pneumoniae* is one of the leading causes of illness and death worldwide for young children, older adults, and persons with chronic, debilitating pathology. The pathogenesis of pneumococcal pneumonia has been extensively studied and serves as a prototype for the management of other bacterial pneumonia.

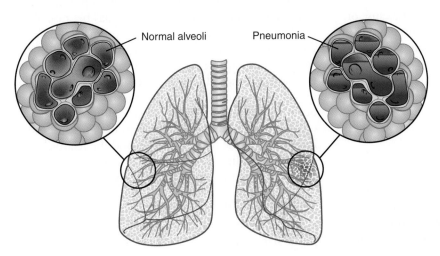

Figure 9.1 Parenchymal changes in pneumonia.

Pneumococcal pneumonia occurs as a result of infected mucus or inhalation of organisms that have colonized in the nasopharynx. *S pneumoniae* can be recovered from the nasopharynx of approximately 40% of healthy adults. In the normal host, the bacteria are inactivated by opsonization with immunoglobulins and complement. Persons with defects in host-defense mechanisms (e.g., inadequate immunoglobulin production or deficiency, impaired phagocytic function, autoimmune disease, immunosuppression, or impaired mucociliary clearance) have a far greater susceptibility.

The lower lobes are most commonly infected because of the effects of gravity. On inhalation, the pneumococcus establishes itself in the alveoli, spreading rapidly through the pores of Kohn. Pneumococcal pneumonia typically includes four responsive stages of infection: engorgement, red hepatization, gray hepatization, and resolution. During engorgement, alveolar capillaries become congested, bacteria and exudate pour into alveoli from alveolar capillaries, and the bacteria multiply without inhibition. There is continued engorgement of the capillaries, with diapedesis of erythrocytes giving the lungs the gross appearance of liver (red hepatization). As the leukocyte count increases in the exudate, it compresses the capillaries and causes the lung tissue to assume a gray color (gray hepatization). At this point, phagocytosis is achieved by polymorphonuclear leukocytes. The presence of opsonizing antibody enhances the ingestion of the bacteria. The stage of resolution is reached when the pneumococci have been destroyed and macrophages are seen within the alveolar spaces, where they lyse and absorb exudate. There often may be pleural involvement from contiguity to parenchymal lesions or by way of the lymphatics. As in the alveoli, there is an outpouring of fluid, followed by polymorphonuclear leukocytes and fibrin. The structure of the pleural space has fewer surfaces suitable for phagocytosis than do the alveoli. Control of the infection in the pleural area is more dependent on heat-stable (specific antibody) than heat-labile (complement opsins) antibodies.

Haemophilus influenzae

H influenzae, a gram-negative bacterium, is the cause of the second most common CAP. It may occur in healthy individuals, as well as in patients with chronic, debilitating diseases and chronic alcohol abuse. Development of *H influenzae* pneumonia follows colonization of the upper respiratory tract. During viral infection epidemics, there is often an increase in the incidence of *H influenzae* pneumonia.

Legionella pneumophila

L pneumophila, a gram-negative bacteria, was identified in 1976 as a causative agent of pneumonia (Legionnaires' disease) during an American Legion convention in Philadelphia. The bacteria thrive in aquatic environments. The source of human infection has been associated with contaminated air-conditioning systems and showerheads. Within the hospital setting, contaminated respiratory tubing and equipment may serve as a source of *L pneumophila*. The bacilli enter the lungs by aspiration, direct inhalation, and hematogenous dissemination. In the normal host, it is thought that the bacilli are cleared by the mucociliary process. This would explain the high incidence of the disease in patients with impaired mucociliary clearance (e.g., smokers, alcoholics, and older adults). Legionnaires' disease may occur in explosive outbreaks if large numbers of susceptible people are exposed to an infectious aerosol. Because of the low communicability of the disease, secondary cases should not occur.

Staphylococcus aureus

S aureus rarely causes pneumonia in healthy, young adults. Local pulmonary or systemic defense must be compromised before the organism can produce pneumonia. *S aureus* accounts for 2% to 9% of CAP in older adults or in patients with concomitant conditions, such as diabetes, chronic renal failure, bronchiectasis, or lung cancer, or with risk factors such as residence in a chronic-care facility or IV substance abuse. Infections may also occur in previously healthy adults following a viral influenza with residual impaired bronchopulmonary mechanism.

Viral Pneumonia

Viral infections account for 5% to 15% of cases of adult CAP. Most viral infections are restricted to the upper respiratory system and tend to cause self-limiting symptoms. Some patients, particularly those with influenza infections, may develop pneumonia. Influenza may result in a primary viral pneumonia or, more commonly, a secondary bacterial pneumonia. Secondary pneumonia is most frequently caused by *S pneumoniae* and *S aureus*. Viral infections are transmitted by hand-to-hand contact or by aerosols (sneezing, coughing). The frequency of influenza as a cause of both CAP and nosocomial pneumonia increases in the winter months.

Mycoplasma Pneumonia

Mycoplasma pneumonia is also known as primary atypical pneumonia or "walking pneumonia" because of the predominance of constitutional symptoms. *Mycoplasma pneumoniae* is a class of bacterial L-forms, which are the smallest known free-living organisms. Children older than age 5 years and young adults are at greatest risk for developing mycoplasmal pneumonia. Outbreaks can occur in populations living in close proximity, such as colleges, military bases, and prisons. Because of the long incubation phase of 2 to 3 weeks and the relatively low communicability, *Mycoplasma* pneumonia tends to move through the community slowly.

Chlamydia pneumoniae

C pneumoniae has only recently been recognized as a pulmonary pathogen. *C pneumoniae* is a gram-negative bacterium. Little is known about the mode of transmission and pathogenesis. The clinical features are similar to those caused by *M pneumoniae*. Adult-onset asthma subsequent to infection with *Chlamydia* pneumonia has been documented. Recurrent infection is common.

Anaerobic Pneumonia

Anaerobic pneumonia may occur in both the community and the hospital setting. *Prevotella melaninogenica,* anaerobic streptococci, and *Fusobacterium nucleatum* are commonly isolated anaerobic bacteria. Aspiration of oropharyngeal secretions normally occurs during sleep in healthy individuals but rarely causes disease. Individuals who are predisposed to aspiration of larger amounts of oropharyngeal secretions are at risk for anaerobic pneumonia. Alcoholism is the most frequent predisposing factor; others include dysphagia, cerebrovascular accidents, seizures, and general anesthesia. Periodontal disease, which increases the number of anaerobic bacteria, is also associated with anaerobic infection. Pneumonia typically develops in dependent zones. Although body position at the time of aspiration determines which lung zones are dependent, anaerobic pneumonia most often develops in the posterior segments of the upper lobes and the superior and basilar segments of the lower lobes. The onset of symptoms is usually insidious. Empyema, lung abscess, or necrotizing pneumonia may be present by the time the patient seeks medical attention.

Nosocomial Bacterial Pneumonias

Nosocomial bacterial pneumonias are most frequently caused by gram-negative organisms such as *Pseudomonas aeruginosa, Klebsiella pneumoniae, Escherichia coli, Serratia, Proteus,* and *Enterobacter.* However, *S aureus* (especially MRSA), *S pneumoniae,* and *H influenzae* are frequently being reported among elderly nursing home residents. As in CAPs, bacteria invade the lower respiratory tract by aspiration of oropharyngeal organisms, inhalation of aerosols containing bacteria, or by hematogenous spread from a distant body site. Patients at high risk for developing nosocomial bacterial pneumonia include postoperative patients, particularly those undergoing thoracoabdominal procedures, patients with endotracheal incubation and/or mechanically assisted ventilation, depressed level of consciousness, an episode of large-volume aspiration, underlying chronic lung disease, and patients aged 70 and older. Nosocomial pneumonia has a mortality rate of about 30%. Hospital-acquired pneumonia in patients on mechanical ventilation has mortality rates of about 48%. Patients who develop acute respiratory distress syndrome have a mortality rate greater than 68%.

Pneumocystis jirovecii Pneumonia

P jirovecii pneumonia (PCP) is an AIDS-defining opportunistic infection that was once seen in as many as 65% of HIV-infected individuals and remains a major identifiable cause of death in AIDS patients. Disease in adults represents reactivation of latent infection, because almost all people are infected with the fungus *P jirovecii* (originally characterized as a protozoan and named *P carinii,* followed by *P jirovecii*), during the first decade of life. Most cases of PCP occur when the CD4-positive T-lymphocyte count has fallen below 200 to 250 cells/mcL. Pathologically, alveolar membranes become thickened, and mononuclear cell interstitial inflammation occurs as the disease progresses.

Cytomegalic Inclusion Virus Cytomegalic inclusion virus (cytomegalovirus [CMV]) is a causative agent of pneumonia in immunocompromised patients. CMV is a type of herpes virus that results in latent infections and reactivation with shedding of the infected viruses. Pathologically, CMV produces an interstitial pneumonia that ranges from a mild disease to a fulminant course resulting in pulmonary insufficiency and death.

Clinical Presentation

Although pneumonias may be classified as two different syndromes, typical and atypical, according to the clinical presentation, they are very similar. The characteristics of the clinical manifestations do have some diagnostic value.

Subjective

The "typical" pneumonia syndrome is that which is seen in pneumococcal pneumonia, as well as in pneumonia caused by *H influenzae* and *S aureus* (Table 9.8). The syndrome is characterized by a sudden onset of fever, cough, and chest pain. Generally, patients with a productive cough are more likely to have a bacterial infection. Patients with pneumococcal pneumonia produce sputum that has a characteristic rusty coloration; purulent sputum may also be evident. Fevers may run as high as 106°F (41.1°C), with peaks observed in the afternoon or evening. The chest pain tends to be pleuritic in nature and increases in intensity during coughing or

Table 9.8	Typical Pneumonia Syndrome Associated With Pneumococcal Pneumonia
Subjective Findings	**Objective Findings**
Sudden onset of fever (may be blunted in older adults)	Crackles
	Dullness on percussion
Productive cough	Bronchophony, egophony, whispered pectoriloquy
Rust-colored or purulent sputum	Pleural friction rub (severe consolidation)
Pleuritic-type pain	Decreased or absent breath sounds
Splinting	Dense, homogenous shadows in one or more lobes on x-ray
Chills	
Myalgia	

on inspiration. Patients often feel cold; about half experience teeth-chattering, shaking, and chills. Myalgia is a common complaint and may extend to tenderness in the calves and thighs. Severe myalgia, particularly when accompanied by vomiting, should strongly suggest the possibility of bacteremia. Respiratory and non-respiratory symptoms are less commonly reported by older patients with pneumonia. The reduced prevalence of symptoms in older patients is most pronounced for the febrile response (chills and sweats) and for pain (myalgia, headache, and chest pain). Although the older adult may present with attenuated symptoms, this should not be misconstrued as an indication that such patients are less ill.

"Atypical" pneumonia is typically produced by *M pneumoniae* but can also be caused by *L pneumophila, C pneumoniae, P jirovecii,* and viruses. The atypical pneumonia syndrome is characterized by a more gradual onset, dry "hacking" cough, fever, and prominence of constitutional symptoms (e.g., pounding headaches, coryza, sore throat, shaking chills, and myalgia).

Pneumonias caused by anaerobic infections usually present with subacute or chronic constitutional and pulmonary symptoms. A chronic cough that produces purulent sputum is reported by the majority of patients. From 30% to 60% of patients report putrid sputum. This finding is considered to be virtually diagnostic of an aerobic infection and is associated with the development of tissue necrosis and cavitary lesions. Patients also present with chest pain that is dull or pleuritic in nature, hemoptysis, anemia, leukocytosis, and weight loss.

Patients with PCP present with fever, sweats, weight loss, nonproductive cough, decreasing exercise tolerance, and dyspnea on exertion. The median duration of symptoms is 1 month. Tachypnea is universal and is worsened by activity.

Objective

Physical examination of a person with typical pneumonia syndrome usually reveals an acutely ill patient who complains of chest pain and often splints on one side of the thorax. In some patients, crackles and dullness to percussion may be the only abnormality, particularly early in the disease. This finding may correlate with the period of outpouring of fluid into the alveoli. A second group of patients shows the classic signs of consolidation: egophony, bronchophony, whispered pectoriloquy, bronchial breath sounds, and dullness on percussion. In patients with severe consolidation, crackles may be absent or minimal; a leathery pleural friction rub may be heard over the area of chest tenderness. Finally, a third group of patients has one or more areas of dullness, inspiratory crackles, and diminished breath sounds, a sign of mucous plugs in the smaller bronchioles. Objective findings in atypical pneumonia tend to be less pronounced. Fine to medium crackles may be heard early or at the very end of the inspiratory cycle. Dullness on

percussion and crackles or wheezing are more likely to be observed later in the disease. Frank consolidation, pleural friction rubs, and pleural effusions are less common than in a typical pneumonia.

Although there is no "typical" syndrome of nosocomial pneumonia, one or more of the following clinical findings are present in most patients: fever, leukocytosis, purulent sputum, and a new pulmonary infiltrate on chest x-ray film. These findings must occur more than 48 hours after admission to the hospital to be considered suggestive of nosocomial pneumonia.

Auscultation of the lungs is generally negative in patients with PCP, although fine crackles may occasionally be heard. Mucocutaneous lesions such as oral thrush, hairy leukoplakia, and Kaposi's sarcoma are common and suggest the presence of underlying HIV-related immunodeficiency in previously undiagnosed individuals. Physiologically, patients manifest arterial hypoxemia.

Diagnostic Reasoning
Diagnostic Tests

Initial Testing Although a specific etiological diagnosis is optimal in the management of CAP, limitations in diagnostic testing make this difficult. The responsible microbe is not identified in approximately 50% of patients, even when extensive diagnostic tests are performed. The three most helpful tests used in the initial establishment of a diagnosis of pneumonia include the chest radiograph, leukocyte count, and Gram stain of sputum specimens.

The chest x-ray study is important for three reasons. First, it may help distinguish whether the pneumonia is bacterial or viral in nature. Lobar infiltrates strongly suggest a bacterial infection. A bacterial pneumonia will show dense homogeneous shadows involving one or more lobes. Diffuse interstitial infiltrates are suggestive of a viral, *Mycoplasma,* or *Chlamydia* infection. Lateral and anterior-posterior views are necessary to evaluate lesions lying directly behind the heart.

A second reason for a chest x-ray study is to rule out a pleural effusion, a complication occurring in approximately one-third of pneumococcal pneumonia patients. It is important to note that chest x-ray films may be normal in patients who are unable to mount an inflammatory response or early in an infiltrative process. Follow-up chest x-ray films are needed to see if the infiltrate clears completely. Younger patients and those with only single-lobe involvement tend to have earlier resolutions.

Finally, cavities may be seen on chest x-ray films in patients with pneumonia caused by anaerobes, *S aureus, S pneumoniae* serotype III, *Mycobacterium tuberculosis,* aerobic gram-negative bacilli, and fungi. Cavities occur when necrotic material is discharged into airways, resulting in a necrotizing pneumonia (multiple small cavities, each less than 2 cm) or lung abscess (one or more cavities greater than 2 cm). Anaerobic abscesses are located in dependent segments, are most frequently seen in the right lung, and have air–fluid levels. Typical and atypical tuberculosis produce unilateral, well-drained, upper-lobe fibrocavitary disease. Cavities are rarely produced by *H influenzae*, *M pneumoniae*, viruses, and other serotypes of *S pneumoniae.*

Although pulmonary infiltrates on x-ray films are considered suggestive of a nosocomial pneumonia, findings tend to be very nonspecific. Conditions such as an atelectasis, pleural effusion, pulmonary thromboembolism, and pulmonary edema may mimic nosocomial pneumonia on x-ray evaluation.

It may not always be practical or feasible to obtain a chest x-ray study, so good clinical judgment is essential. Factors that have been found to be predictive of pneumonia infiltrates on chest films include fever above 100°F (37.8°C), tachycardia, locally decreased breath sounds, and sputum production. Chest x-ray films may be normal when the patient is unable to mount an inflammatory response (e.g., in agranulocytosis), is in the early stages of an infiltrative process, or in PCP associated with AIDS.

To help identify the patients who need hospitalization, a complete blood count (CBC) with differential should be done. The count may aid in differentiating between bacterial and viral pneumonia. Although there is no clear distinction, total white blood cell counts of more than 15,000 suggest a bacterial infection. A differential cell count is not a reliable indicator of causation. Leukopenia may be seen in severe infections, as well as in alcoholics, older adults, and malnutrition. Blood cultures are indicated only for patients who require hospitalization or for cases of suspected nosocomial pneumonia.

A Gram stain of sputum remains the only diagnostic tool available to all practitioners at the onset of therapy. Caution needs to be exercised in the evaluation of a sputum specimen because expectorated material is frequently contaminated by pathogenic bacteria that colonize the upper and lower respiratory tracts without causing disease. Large numbers of epithelial cells (more than 25 per low-power field) reflect contamination of the specimen with oral contents and mandate that another specimen be collected. If the sputum has been properly collected, polymorphonuclear leukocytes can be readily seen with a Gram stain and the characteristic lancet-shaped, gram-positive diplococci associated with pneumococcal pneumonia are generally seen in abundance.

Gram stains are seldom useful in patients with atypical pneumonia because sputum is scant and most organisms that cause this syndrome cannot be detected by a Gram stain.

Acid-fast staining of sputum should be done when mycobacterial infection is suspected. (See Advanced Assessment 9.1.)

A sputum culture is less valuable than a Gram stain for providing a causal diagnosis in bacterial pneumonia. Approximately 50% of patients with pneumococcal pneumonia have negative sputum cultures, even when large numbers of organisms are present on Gram stain. Sputum cultures are also negative in 35% to 50% of cases of proven *H influenzae* pneumonia. Isolation of the causative agent in atypical pneumonia is rare.

Sputum cultures may be valuable in the diagnosis of subacute and cavitary pneumonia. Mycobacteria grow well on culture media, and it has been estimated that sputum cultures can detect as few as 10 acid-fast bacilli per milliliter of concentrated sputum. For a more in-depth discussion of the use of sputum cultures for the isolation of mycobacteria, refer to the section on tuberculosis.

The usefulness of fungal cultures varies with the organism and the stage of the disease. Chronic forms of coccidiomycosis and blastomycosis may yield positive cultures in 70% to 100% of cases if multiple specimens

---

Advanced Assessment 9.1   Sputum Stains

Sputum Stain	Organism
Gram stain	*S pneumoniae* (gram-positive, lancet-shaped diplococci) *H influenzae* (gram-positive coccobacilli) *S aureus* (gram-positive tetrads and grape-like clusters)
Acid-fast stain	Mycobacterial infection
Direct fluorescent antibody (DFA) stain	Viral respiratory culture
Fluorescent antibody: sensitivity diminished with concurrent use of inhaled pentamidine	*Legionella* infection
Wright-Giemsa stain: frequent false-positive and false-negative results	PCP
Gomori's methamine silver	Fungal growth
Periodic acid-Schiff stain	

are collected. Accurate positive cultures are not found in patients with histoplasmosis until the disease is in the chronic, cavitary stage. Fewer than 50% of patients with cryptococcosis have positive sputum cultures.

Expectorated sputum is usually collected in patients with a productive, vigorous cough, but may be scant in those with atypical pneumonia syndrome, in older adults, and in patients with altered mental status. If the patient is not producing sputum and can cooperate, respiratory secretions can be induced with ultrasonic nebulization of 3% saline solution. The use of more invasive procedures to induce sputum in the patient who is unable to produce a sputum specimen carries risks that must be weighed against the potential benefits. In patients who do not require hospitalization or in hospitalized patients who are not severely ill, the need to establish an accurate microbial diagnosis may not be crucial, and empiric therapy can be started on the basis of clinical and epidemiological evidence alone. Patients who are hospitalized with CAP and are seriously ill or those who acquire a nosocomial pneumonia clearly need to have a specific causal diagnosis established. In these patients, it may be necessary to obtain specimens from the lower respiratory tract by fiberoptic bronchoscopy, transtracheal puncture, or percutaneous transthoracic lung puncture. Of these invasive procedures, fiberoptic bronchoscopy is currently the preferred technique for obtaining lower respiratory secretions. Specimens obtained by bronchoscopy should be tested with Gram and acid-fast stains, *Legionella* direct fluorescent antibody, and Gomori's methenamine silver stains and should be cultured for aerobic and anaerobic bacteria, *Legionella*, mycobacteria, and fungi.

Diagnostic testing for CAP with *S pneumoniae* may include a pneumococcal urinary antigen test that can detect a protein common to all pneumococcal serotypes. Within 15 minutes, this test can demonstrate the presence of pneumococcus in unconcentrated urine. This can facilitate more immediate decisions about antibiotic therapy. However, the sensitivity of this test varies, and it is a complement to sputum and/or blood culture. Urinary antigen testing is also available for the gram-negative bacteria *L pneumophila* (but only for serogroup 1, which may not capture all forms of the disease), as well as the fungus *Histoplasma*.

Subsequent Testing　If the pneumonia is severe enough to require hospitalization, at least two blood samples should be obtained for culture, as well as CBC and serological analysis of sodium, urea, nitrogen, creatinine, and glucose. Liver and enzyme tests should be included if hepatic disease or malnutrition is suspected. Serological studies are sometimes helpful in defining the etiology of certain types of pneumonia. An immunoglobulin M or immunoglobulin G titer obtained by indirect immunofluorescence may be diagnostic of *M pneumoniae* or *C pneumoniae*. A *Legionella* titer or a urinary antigen test may help confirm Legionnaires' disease.

Pulse oximetry is indicated if the patient presents with respiratory distress, dyspnea at rest, or tachypnea or if the chest x-ray film shows multilobar pulmonary infiltrates. A blood gas analysis should be performed if the patient has known carbon dioxide (CO_2) retention, exacerbations of asthma, or COPD. Typically, an SaO_2 of less than 90% or a PaO_2 of less than 60 mm Hg indicates a need for supplemental oxygen. These threshold values must be modified if the patient is chronically hypoxemic.

Differential Diagnosis

Acute bacterial pneumonia should be differentiated from acute bacterial bronchitis. Both of these respiratory infections will cause fever and a productive cough. On auscultation, however, a patient with bronchitis will have clear lung sounds except for a few scattered rhonchi and possibly tubular sounds. In comparison, the patient with bacterial pneumonia will likely have crackles, dullness to percussion, and abnormal breath sounds. Cavitary forms of pneumonia need to be differentiated from pulmonary tuberculosis and systemic mycoses, particularly coccidiomycosis and histoplasmosis. Likewise, the patient who presents with symptoms of PCP and a history of fever, weight loss, and pulmonary symptoms should be concurrently evaluated for tuberculosis, lymphomas, and brucellosis. Signs and symptoms secondary to central or endobronchial growth of a primary lung cancer will mimic those of a bacterial pneumonia (e.g., productive cough, fever, cough, dyspnea, hemoptysis). The practitioner needs to be aware of any occupational or environmental hazards to which the patient is exposed. For example, workers who develop berylliosis through exposure to beryllium (found in ceramics, high-technology electronics, and alloy manufacturing) may present with an acute pneumonia or, more commonly, with a chronic interstitial pneumonia. Exposure to moldy hay can result in symptoms of pneumonia (e.g., coughing, fever, chills, malaise, and dyspnea) within 4 to 8 hours after exposure. This disease (known as "farmer's lung") may become chronic.

Severe acute respiratory syndrome (SARS) should also be ruled out. Patients should be questioned about travel to an area with known transmission of SARS, as well as close contact with a person who has SARS. The causative agent is a coronavirus. Symptoms include a fever greater than 100.5°F (38°C), cough, or respiratory distress. The diagnosis is via enzyme-linked immunosorbent assay or reverse transcriptase–polymerase chain reaction assays. Treatment is supportive care. The identification is critical from a public health standpoint rather than from the need of initiating SARS-specific care, which remains supportive.

Management

The initial task in the management of patients with CAP is to determine whether the person can be treated on an outpatient basis or whether hospitalization is required.

The use of hospital services is costly and may further impair the patient's health because of the risk of nosocomial infections. The majority of patients with CAP with no comorbidity can be treated successfully as outpatients. Most patients, even those treated initially in a hospital, prefer outpatient treatment.

The decision to hospitalize a patient with CAP may be the single most important decision during the entire course of the illness (Level I; Burman & Wright, 2007). Scoring systems are helpful in determining the site-of-care decision. The Pneumonia Outcomes Research Team's Pneumonia Severity Index (PSI) is a risk-assessment tool used to determine the need for hospitalization of patients with pneumonia. The PSI uses calculations to categorize patients into five severity classes based on age, comorbidities, physical examination, and laboratory findings. Outpatient care can usually be recommended for patients in classes I, II, or III. However, patients suffering from substance abuse or severe psychosocial problems or those lacking social support may require hospitalization despite their PSI classification. The PSI calculator may be found at http://pda.ahrq.gov/clinic/psi/psicalc.asp, and the Community-Acquired Pneumonia Prognostic calculator may be found at www.ursa.kcom.edu/CAPcalc/default.htm.

The CURB-65 criteria to determine the severity of CAP is an objective, easy tool to remember. This severity-of-illness scale (shown in Table 9.9) will help determine where treatment will take place. In addition, known risk factors for CAP-associated mortality and complications are summarized in Risk Factors 9.3.

Antimicrobial therapy represents the mainstay of treatment for patients with suspected or confirmed pneumonia. Additional management is supportive in nature and includes the use of analgesics for relief of chest pain and

Risk Factors 9.3 Risk Factors for Mortality or Complications From Community-Acquired Pneumonia

Age: Older than 65 years
Presence of coexisting illness:

- Chronic pulmonary disease
- Diabetes mellitus
- Chronic renal failure
- Congestive heart failure
- Chronic liver disease of any etiology
- Previous hospitalization within 1 year of the onset of pneumonia
- Suspicion of aspiration
- Altered mental status
- Postsplenectomy state
- Chronic alcohol abuse or malnutrition

Abnormal physical findings:

- Respiratory rate above 30 breaths/min
- Diastolic BP 60 mm Hg or below and/or systolic BP 90 mm Hg or below
- Temperature above 101°F
- Evidence of extrapulmonary sites of disease (e.g., septic arthritis, meningitis)
- Decreased level of consciousness or confusion

Abnormal laboratory findings:

- WBC count <4 × 106/L or >30 × 106/L
- Pao2 <60 mm Hg or Paco2 >50 mm Hg on room air
- Hemoglobin <9 g/dL
- X-ray showing more than one lobe involvement, pleural effusion, evidence of rapid spreading
- Severe electrolyte or renal abnormality not known to be chronic (e.g., BUN >50 mg/dL, creatinine >1.2 mg/dL, sodium <130 mEq/L)

Table 9.9	CURB-65 Criteria for Community-Acquired Pneumonia (CAP)	
Clinical Factor		**Points**
Confusion (new disorientation)		1
B**U**N >19 mg per dL		1
Respiratory rate (≥30 breaths/min)		1
BP (systolic <90 mm Hg or diastolic ≤60 mm Hg)		1
Age ≥65 years		1

Scoring:
- 0–1: Low risk—consider home treatment
- 2: Short, in-patient hospitalization or closely monitored outpatient treatment
- ≥3: Severe pneumonia, hospitalize and consider ICU

Adapted from Ebell, MH. Outpatient vs. inpatient treatment of community-acquired pneumonia. *Am Fam Physician* 73:1425–1428, 2006. Retrieved July 1, 2013, from www.aafp.org/afp/2006/0400/p41.html

myalgia, antipyretics to control fever, increased fluid intake (typically at least 3 liters over 24 hours), restricted activity or bedrest, a position of comfort (usually upright) to facilitate breathing, and humidified air to relieve irritated nares and pharynx. Expectorants may be indicated to decrease sputum viscosity and clear airways if a productive cough is present. Although many promote the use of expectorants, it bears repeating that the best and most cost-effective way to liquify secretions for ease of coughing and eliminating the secretions is hydration with water. Patients experiencing a dry, nonproductive cough may benefit from a cough suppressant with codeine.

Patients requiring hospitalization need to have ongoing assessment for any indications of impaired respiratory status. Patients who manifest arterial hypoxemia will require supplemental oxygen therapy to attempt to maintain PO_2 above 80 mm Hg. In the past, chest physiotherapy had been widely used to mobilize secretions. However, percussion and postural drainage probably offer no added benefit to the patient who has an uncomplicated pneumonia without underlying pulmonary disease.

Community-Acquired Pneumonia

The Infectious Diseases Society of America has recommended specific therapy for CAP. The clinician must note whether the patient had recent antibiotic therapy or not and determine what coexisting diseases are present, such as COPD or congestive heart failure. Treatment Standards/Guidelines 9.1 summarizes the empiric treatment of the patient with CAP (Level I; Mandell et al, 2007). In addition, treatment guidelines from 2011 are cited. In the past, macrolides were used for monotherapy, but these are now avoided because approximately 25% of *S pneumoniae* strains are naturally resistant to all macrolides. Preferred monotherapy for CAP includes doxycycline or a respiratory quinolone. These are the most cost-effective way to optimally treat CAP. No increased resistance is noted with extensive use. These are well tolerated in oral and IV forms and are ideal for IV-to-oral switch monotherapy in terms of patient compliance, safety, and cost. Highly penicillin-resistant *S pneumoniae* strains are a rare cause of CAP because most *S pneumoniae* strains remain susceptible to ceftriaxone. Avoid using proton-pump inhibitors (PPIs) for gastric protection when using respiratory quinolones for CAP drug therapy because they may alter drug levels. Either stop the PPI or use a histamine-$_2$ receptor (H_2) blocker for the duration of therapy. However, there is conflicting evidence as to the relative safety of using PPIs and H_2 blockers.

Treatment regimens for community-acquired MRSA pneumonia should typically start with vancomycin, until sensitivities are back, which may indicate susceptibility to Bactrim. Most recently, guidelines have established

Treatment Standards/Guidelines 9.1   Empiric Antimicrobial Choices for Community-Acquired Pneumonia (CAP)

Patient Profile	Antimicrobial Agent
Uncomplicated CAP	
Without recent antibiotic therapy (ATBX)*	macrolide azithromycin (Zithromax) clarithromycin (Biaxin) erythromycin OR doxycycline (Vibramycin)
With recent ATBX†	Respiratory fluoroquinolone moxifloxacin (Avelox) levofloxacin (Levaquin) OR azithromycin or clarithromycin PLUS High-dose amoxicillin (Amoxil) OR azithromycin or clarithromycin PLUS High-dose amoxicillin–clavulanate (Augmentin)
Patient with CAP plus influenza	A respiratory fluoroquinolone OR A beta-lactam IV ceftriaxone (Rocephin) IV cefotaxime (Claforan)
Patient with community-acquired methicillin-resistant *S aureus* (MRSA) pneumonia	vancomycin (Vancocin) OR Linezolid (Zyvox)

*ATBX antibiotic therapy within the last 3 months.

†Use a different class of antibiotic not chosen previously.

Sources: Adapted from Mandell, L, et al. Infectious Diseases Society of America/American Thoracic Society consensus guidelines on the management of community-acquired pneumonia in adults. *Clin Infect Dis* 44(Suppl 2):S27–72, 2007; and Struble, K. Community-acquired pneumonia empiric therapy. Medscape, 2011. Retrieved July 1, 2013, from http://emedicine.medscape.com/article/2011819-overview

linezolid (Zyvox) as an effective alternative therapy for susceptible vancomycin-resistant infections and CAP.

■ NOSOCOMIAL PNEUMONIA

Antimicrobial therapy is the mainstay of therapy for nosocomial pneumonia, as well as for anaerobic/cavitary pneumonia and PCP, but recommendations are less specific. Treatment for nosocomial pneumonia, like treatment of CAP, is usually empiric. Because of the high mortality rate associated with nosocomial pneumonia, treatment must be started as soon as pneumonia is suspected. Empiric therapy for nosocomial pneumonia in patients who are not in an intensive care unit (ICU) may consist of a beta-lactam antimicrobial agent against *Pseudomonas aeruginosa* such as ceftazidime (Fortaz), piperacillin-tazobactam (Zosyn), ticarcillin-clavulanate (Timentin), or imipenem-cilastin (Primaxin). *Staphylococcus aureus* has become increasingly methicillin resistant. Such strains are resistant to all beta-lactam antibiotics and can be resistant to erythromycin, clindamycin, and the fluoroquinolones. Vancomycin should be prescribed when methicillin-resistant organisms are the possible cause of pneumonia.

Empiric therapy for patients with ICU-associated or ventilator-associated pneumonia should be a combination of antibiotics directed against the most virulent organisms, such as *P aeruginosa, Acinetobacter,* and *Enterobacter.* The most common regimen is a broad-spectrum beta-lactam (an antipseudomonal penicillin, a third generation antipseudomonal cephalosporin, or imipenem/cilastin) plus an aminoglycoside. If the causative pathogen is isolated, it may be possible to switch to a regimen with a narrower spectrum.

The therapy for anaerobic/cavitary pneumonia depends on the pace of the illness and the degree of clinical toxicity. Clindamycin (Cleocin) is effective for most patients with anaerobic pulmonary infections and is the drug of choice. Antituberculosis therapy should also be initiated if the clinical suspicion is high. Treatment of other causes of chronic cavitary pneumonia may be postponed until a diagnosis is established.

Nursing home residents should get a respiratory fluoroquinolone alone or Augmentin plus a macrolide. MRSA CAP has been seen in nursing home patients, as well as particularly sick young adults. In these patients, vancomycin is the IV treatment of choice, with Linezolid as the alternative for MRSA treatment. Sensitivities may reveal additional susceptibilities, though, allowing for narrowing of therapy.

Refer to Chapter 17 for the therapy of *Pneumocystis jiroveci* pneumonia (PCP).

Subsequent Management The advent of antimicrobial therapy has greatly decreased complications that were commonly seen before the use of antibiotics. Pneumonia that is associated with bacteremia, leukopenia, or multiple lobe involvement increases the likelihood of complications and of death. The mortality rate for patients older than age 65 years with bacteremia and involvement of more than three lobes is approximately 60%. Complications that do occur are more frequently found in patients with underlying chronic diseases.

The radiographic resolution of CAP is complete in half of patients after 2 weeks and in two-thirds of patients after 4 weeks. Follow-up x-ray studies should be done within 3 to 6 months for all patients who smoke or who are older than age 40 years. If an abnormality has not cleared on follow-up films, the patient should be evaluated for a possible cancer.

Pleural effusion represents the most common complication seen in patients with pneumonia. Fluid can be detected radiographically in the pleural space of more than 40% of patients hospitalized with pneumonia. In most cases, the amount is so small that needle aspiration is unsuccessful. If fluid is removed it typically is not purulent, nor can microbes be seen on a Gram stain.

Fluid that is purulent and has a gram-positive stain or has a pH less than 7.1 is indicative of an empyema. *Streptococcus pneumoniae, Streptococcus pyogenes,* and anaerobic pneumonias are associated with most cases of empyema. It is critical that the infected material be removed from the pleural space by means of a thoracentesis, needle aspiration, or thoracotomy. If this treatment is delayed, the patient is likely to require a prolonged hospital stay. Lung abscesses develop infrequently in *S pneumoniae* but often occur as complications of pneumonias caused by gram-negative bacteria (e.g., *Klebsiella*), anaerobic bacteria, and *S aureus.* Drainage of the abscess is essential to prevent further necrosis of the lung tissue. Prolonged antimicrobial therapy is critical for the successful treatment of this complication.

Delayed resolution results from persistent infection and is seen on x-ray studies as residual consolidation. Delayed resolution occurs most often in the patient who is older, malnourished, or alcoholic or who has COPD. Progression of infiltrates in spite of antimicrobial therapy is a poor prognostic sign.

Metastatic infections that do occur tend to develop in the meninges, pericardium, heart valves, and skeletal system. Although these complications occur less frequently with antimicrobial therapy, persons with compromised health status remain at risk for the development of these infections. Possible metastatic infections include arthritis, pericarditis, endocarditis, and meningitis. Patients who develop arthritis will experience swollen, red, and painful joints. Purulent exudate may be aspirated from the joints. Meningitis caused by *S pneumoniae* produces purulent cerebrospinal fluid. Patients with pneumococcal pneumonia who become disoriented, confused, or somnolent should have a lumbar puncture.

Criteria for hospital discharge include the resolution of fever, an ability to take medications orally, no need for supplemental oxygen, no progression of an infiltrate seen on chest x-ray films, a decrease in the leukocyte count, and the presence of social and family support.

Follow-up and Referral

Patients considered well enough for outpatient treatment do not need to be closely monitored unless symptoms worsen in spite of antibiotics. The patient should be contacted within 24 to 48 hours of starting therapy and should be scheduled for an office visit at 1 week and 4 to 6 weeks after the initial evaluation.

X-ray resolution of CAP is complete in 50% of patients after 2 weeks and in two-thirds of patients after 4 weeks. Examination at the second follow-up should include a chest x-ray film if clinical symptoms have not resolved. X-ray evaluations should be done for all patients who smoke. If an abnormality has not cleared on follow-up films, the patient should be evaluated for a possible cancer.

Smoking cessation is essential if respiratory health is to be maintained. Patients may be most receptive to antismoking counseling while they are still ill or recovering from pneumonia. The follow-up examination provides an opportune time for patient education. Pneumococcal and influenza vaccines should also be given at this time if indicated.

Patient Education

Influenza vaccine is strongly recommended for those older than age 65 years and persons of any age who are at risk for adverse complication from influenza. A vaccine against the 23 most common serotypes of *S pneumoniae* has been available since the early 1980s. The Advisory Committee on Immunization Practices recommends that it be administered to persons older than age 2 years who have any of several underlying conditions (e.g., COPD, splenectomy, organ transplants) and to all persons aged 65 or older. *Healthy People 2020* objectives target the vaccination of 90% of persons over 65 years old at risk for pneumococcal pneumonia by 2020. Currently, the percentage of adults over 65 years old who receive this vaccination has been estimated at approximately 60%. Despite the availability of the vaccine, it is underutilized. The increasing prevalence of multiantibiotic resistance of pneumococci makes immunization of high-risk individuals of utmost importance. For the very elderly patients and those who are institutionalized, revaccination every 5 years is indicated. Vaccine use tends to increase when efforts are made to raise awareness and promote the benefits of vaccination. The practitioner may obtain current and relevant data on pneumococcal vaccines, incidence rates of CAP and hospital-acquired pneumonia, drug therapy, and other pertinent information by contacting the CDC, the National Institute on Aging, and the National Foundation for Infectious Diseases.

■ TUBERCULOSIS

Tuberculosis (TB) is one of the oldest human diseases. It is an infectious disease, most frequently caused by *Mycobacterium tuberculosis* in humans. In early writings, TB was called "consumption" because of its tendency to produce great wasting in its victims. During the 18th and 19th centuries, it was known as the "white plague." TB is the leading cause of death worldwide from any single infectious agent. The pandemic of HIV infection and the emergence of drug-resistant TB have worsened the global problem of TB.

Epidemiology and Causes

TB had once been considered to be under such good control that a possibility of eradication of the disease in the developing countries was considered to be an obtainable goal. However, it is estimated that 15 million persons in the United States alone are infected with *M tuberculosis*. Worldwide, the majority of infected persons are living in developing countries; about 75% of these infected people are younger than age 50 years. Each year, 3 million people worldwide die from the disease. TB is the most common HIV-associated opportunistic infection in many developing countries. Currently the highest estimated case rates occur in Africa.

According to the CDC, in the United States the number of reported TB cases in 2011 was the lowest recorded since national reporting began in 1953. In addition, since the 1992 TB resurgence peak in the United States, the number of TB cases reported annually has decreased. TB disproportionately affects patients belonging to racial and ethnic minorities. The prevalence is three times higher in urban than in rural populations. Case rates are approximately 10 times higher in African American populations and about five times higher among Native Americans and Hispanics. TB among foreign-born residents of the United States accounts for approximately 60% of the national total. A factor in the increase of TB among foreign-born persons is the changing trends in countries of origin. Immigration has been increasing from Asia and Latin America, where TB rates are 5 to 20 times higher than those in the United States. Currently, the foreign-born population is concentrated largely in California, New York, Florida, Texas, and New Jersey.

Overall, approximately 10% of persons infected with *M tuberculosis* will develop clinical TB sometime during their lifetimes. About 5% of infected persons will manifest the disease within 1 year of infection. The remaining persons who develop the disease will have a delayed onset of TB, typically at a point of declined protective immunity, such as occurs in silicosis, diabetes mellitus, and diseases associated with immunosuppression, for example, HIV infection and immunosuppressive drugs. Susceptibility to TB is also greater during the first 2 years of life, at puberty, and during adolescence.

Geographically, the largest increases in reported TB cases have been in areas such as New York and Florida, which, in addition to having large foreign-born populations, also have a large number of AIDS cases. Outbreaks of drug-resistant TB (resistant to at least one anti-TB drug) and multidrug-resistant TB (resistant to isoniazid and rifampin) have occurred in hospitals, prisons, shelters for the homeless, nursing homes, and AIDS residential facilities.

The genus *Mycobacterium* includes the causative agents of TB and leprosy. Mycobacteria are aerobic, asporogenous, nonmotile, acid-fast rods. Of the 58 species of the genus *Mycobacterium,* the members of the TB complex (*M tuberculosis, M bovis, M africanum,* and *M microti*) are closely related, based on DNA homology studies. The TB complex does not occur in nature and depends on host transmission for its survival. *M tuberculosis* is the major cause of human disease. Disease due to *M bovis* is rare in the United States. *M africanum* is a common cause of TB in Africa, and *M microti* is a pathogen for rodents.

Pathophysiology

Mycobacteria tuberculosis (TB) strains vary in virulence due to differences in the bacteria's genetic makeup. Similarly, persons display varying susceptibility to TB infection due to genetically conferred resistance, age, and comorbid conditions (e.g., chronic illness, immunosuppression). *M tuberculosis* is most commonly transmitted from person to person by droplet nuclei that are aerosolized by coughing, sneezing, or speaking. Transmission from an infected individual to another is influenced by the intimacy and duration of contact, the degree of infectivity of the patient, and the shared contact environment. Patients with acid-fast staining organisms in their sputum are most infectious to others.

After *M tuberculosis* organisms are inhaled, some are expelled by the ciliated epithelium, and only a small fraction reaches the alveoli, leading to primary infection. There, alveolar macrophages attempt to phagocytose and contain the bacteria; however, virulent strains can multiply rapidly and overcome these macrophages, countering their oxidative bactericidal mechanisms. Nonetheless, activated macrophages react by releasing inflammatory mediators such as interleukin-12 and tumor necrosis factor–alpha, which contribute to fever, anorexia, and weight loss. Macrophages also stimulate the recruitment of T lymphocytes to the area of infection. Helper T (CD4+) and cytotoxic killer T (CD8+) lymphocytes are also integral in the effort to kill bacteria, as activated macrophages and T lymphocytes form granulomas, or tubercles, in an effort to confine bacterial growth by walling off the mycobacteria.

Within these tubercles, multiplication of the organisms is inhibited by low oxygen content and low pH. T lymphocytes release inflammatory mediators that neutralize the bacteria contained in the tubercle's central necrotic area known as the caseum because of its cheese-like appearance on gross inspection. In a minority of cases, highly virulent strains of *M tuberculosis* may cause rapid infection, invading lung parenchyma, bronchioles,

and blood vessels. Hemoptysis, a frequent clinical sign of active infection, may reflect the erosion of a granuloma into a pulmonary blood vessel. Old granulomas eventually calcify, identifiable as one or more Ghon complexes on chest x-ray film. Known as latent TB infection (LTBI), viable bacteria may remain dormant in these lesions for decades, only to be reactivated when the fine balance between host immunity and bacterial pathogenesis is tipped in favor of the mycobacteria. This results in secondary infection known as reactivation TB, seen typically in chronically ill or otherwise immunosuppressed individuals.

Mycobacteria can also spread via lymphatics or hematogenously, resulting in disseminated infection. Extrapulmonary sites of tuberculous infection include the lymph nodes, pleura, bones, meninges, peritoneum, pericardium, and genitourinary tract. Solid organs may be seeded at multiple tiny foci, taking on a millet-seed–like appearance on gross inspection termed *miliary tuberculosis.* Such pathological findings have been noted as far back as the 1700s. Today, the term *miliary TB* has been extended to encompass all forms of progressive, disseminated TB infection but is still seen most often in children younger than 1 year of age.

When testing for TB, persons with previous exposure or infection develop a positive cell-mediated (type IV) delayed-type hypersensitivity skin reaction as a result of previously sensitized helper T lymphocytes (CD4+) that are attracted to the testing site when a small amount of mycobacterial antigen (purified protein derivative [PPD]) is injected intradermally (also known as a tuberculin skin test [TST]). Reactions of this type typically require 48 to 72 hours to develop and are classified based on the degree of skin induration (rather than erythema) at the site of injection in relation to specific population norms.

In addition to the PPD skin test, two interferon-gamma release assays (IGRAs) may be used. The QuantiFERON®-TB Gold In-Tube test (QFT-GIT) and the T-SPOT® (T-Spot) are whole-blood tests that can aid in the diagnosis of TB but do not help differentiate LTBI from tuberculosis disease.

M tuberculosis organisms are aerobic and therefore particularly attracted to the apical segments of the upper lung lobes where high oxygen concentration favors their proliferation. Although the upper lung zone is the most common site of accelerated growth of the bacilli, there may be a later progression at distant sites in the body. The kidneys, brain, and bones are the most common sites of distant progression.

Individuals may continue to discharge mycobacteria into the environment from pulmonary tubercles until multiple-drug therapy is instituted to drive bacteria into a dormant state or eradicate infection completely. Although mycobacteria are almost always found in the bone marrow, liver, and spleen when disease occurs, uncontrolled multiplication of the bacilli in these organs is rare. Immunosuppressed individuals, particularly those with T-lymphocyte deficiencies and compromised cell-mediated immunity (e.g., persons living with HIV), are highly susceptible to TB.

Clinical Presentation

Subjective

TB may mimic or occur concurrently with pneumoconiosis, pneumonia, bronchiectasis, sarcoidosis, lung abscess, neoplasm, or fungal infections. It is common for the onset to be insidious, with symptoms of anorexia, fatigue, digestive disturbances, a slow weight loss, irregular menses, and a lack of stamina. Persons may complain of being unable to complete a day's work. This pattern of onset will continue for several weeks or even months, when a low-grade elevation of temperature appears characteristically in the afternoon.

Pulmonary TB is characterized principally by a productive cough, purulent sputum, and repeated occurrences of coryza-like symptoms with rhinorrhea and nasal congestion. The cough progresses slowly over weeks or months to become more frequent and associated with the production of mucoid or mucopurulent sputum. The cough is usually due to sloughing of small caseous lesions within the presence of exudate in the bronchi. Sputum is characteristically yellow but is not tenacious or foul smelling. Hemoptysis is a common symptom in patients with necrotizing or cavitary lesions. Blood usually appears as small streaks in the sputum. Dyspnea is uncommon in pulmonary TB and usually indicates extensive parenchymal involvement, massive pleural effusion, or other underlying cardiopulmonary disease.

A less frequently seen pattern of onset may be that of an acute febrile illness with an abrupt onset of high fever, chills, tachycardia, and weakness. A productive cough is seen, along with myalgia and sweating. Erythema nodosum may occur with the acute onset of symptoms. These patients may have paid no attention to milder symptoms that have preceded the acute episode. This is a common finding in the uneducated, in alcoholics, or in older adults.

Less frequent modes of onset include pleuritic pain and hoarseness. Pleuritic pain, usually unilateral, tends to be accentuated by coughing or deep inspiration. Hoarseness is usually a result of involvement of the larynx and may be accompanied by severe pain. Constitutional symptoms tend to be general in nature and consist of night sweats, fatigue on exertion, weight loss, and malaise.

In obtaining the health history, the clinician must keep in mind the chronicity of TB and the insidious nature of the onset of symptoms. Patients should be questioned about exposure to anyone with an open case of TB. Potential sources of exposure include the family and coworkers. Other significant disclosures obtained from a health history include a past diagnosis of pneumonia with recurrence, pleurisy, uncontrolled diabetes, alcoholism, malnutrition, and occupational exposures to quartz dust or silica. Other risk factors that should be taken into account are drug abuse, country of origin, corticosteroid use, and gastrectomy.

Objective

A complete examination of any patient suspected of having TB should always be performed. Although pulmonary TB is the most common form of TB, the clinician needs to be cognizant of any indications of extrapulmonary TB. Examination of the chest will usually provide the primary indications of pulmonary TB. Rhonchi, crackles, wheezing, and bronchial breath sounds may be heard on auscultation but may have no radiographic counterparts. Dullness on percussion is commonly associated with pneumonic lesions. Persons with long-standing disease may manifest asymmetrical lung expansion, displacement of the trachea, and muscular atrophy. Although there are no specific changes related to pulmonary function, in patients with extensive parenchymal involvement, the vital capacity and other lung volumes may become decreased.

The patient should be examined for any evidence of present or past extrapulmonary TB in such structures as the genitourinary tract, lymph nodes, bones and joints, peritoneum, larynx, eye, abdominal organs, and neurological system (Table 9.10). Physical findings may include hepatomegaly, splenomegaly, and generalized lymphadenopathy. Abnormal behavior, headaches, and seizures may herald TB meningitis. Meningitis occurs frequently in infants and small children as a complication of early infection, but it may be seen in any age-group. Bone and joint involvement, most often seen in older adults, may result in arthritis, osteomyelitis, fever, and localized pain. The lower spine and weight-bearing joints are most often affected by skeletal TB. Genitourinary TB may present as recurrent urinary tract infections with no growth of common pathogens, pyuria without bacteriuria, pelvic inflammatory disease, amenorrhea, infertility, and perianal fistulas.

Diagnostic Reasoning

Diagnostic Tests

Initial Testing The tuberculin skin test (TST) remains the standard test for determining infection with *M tuberculosis* but does not distinguish between active and latent infection. The TST tends to have a strong positive predictive value, but poorer negative predictive value. Skin testing on a patient suspected of being infected may easily be done in an office or clinic setting. It is useful as an epidemiological tool to identify infected and especially recently infected people for preventive therapy and contact tracing. The American Thoracic Society (ATS) has developed criteria for tuberculin testing.

Table 9.10	Clinical Indicators of Extrapulmonary Tuberculosis	

Extrapulmonary Sites	Clinical Manifestations
Genitourinary tract	Recurrent urinary tract infections with no growth of common pathogens Pyuria without bacteriuria Unexplained hematuria Irregular menses, amenorrhea, pelvic inflammatory disease, infertility Epididymitis Induration of the prostate
Bone and joints (lower spine and weight-bearing joints most common site)	Arthritis, osteomyelitis Fever and localized pain
Meninges	Headaches, convulsions Abnormal behavior
Peritoneum	Ascites, fever
Pericardium	Pericarditis
Lymph nodes	Hilar or mediastinal lymphadenitis Cervical and supraclavicular lymphadenopathy

Persons for whom tuberculin testing is routinely indicated are listed in the Screening Recommendations/Guidelines 9.1.

The most accurately and widely used method for skin testing is the Mantoux technique of injecting intermediate-strength PPD intradermally (TST). The reaction to intradermally injected tuberculin is the classic example of a delayed cellular hypersensitivity reaction. These reactions begin at 5 to 6 hours after injection and are maximal at 72 hours. In older adults or in persons who are being tested for the first time, the reaction may develop more slowly and may not peak until after 72 hours. Older adults should be checked initially at 72 hours, and then 1 and 2 days later. A number of factors related to a decreased ability to respond to the tuberculin are included in Table 9.11. These factors do not negate testing in these situations because only a fraction of infected persons with these conditions may have falsely nonreactive results. If the lack of reaction to the testing is suspected to be a false response, a repeat TST should be done. If generalized inability to respond is suspected, it may be necessary to test delayed hypersensitivity using several other antigens to which the person has had a likely exposure. Anergy should be suspected if the person fails to respond to any of the antigens. Many infectious disease specialists think that anergy testing is no longer useful, because patients may

Screening Recommendations/Guidelines 9.1
Guidelines for Tuberculin Screening

- A person with signs and/or symptoms of current TB
- Close contact with known TB cases
- Persons with HIV infection
- Persons who inject illicit drugs
- A person from a medically underserved or high-risk minority population
- A resident or employee in a prison or long-term care facility
- An employee in a health-care facility
- Infants, children, and adolescents exposed to adults in high-risk categories (use of IGRAs for children less than 5 years of age is not established)
- Foreign-born persons arriving within 5 years from countries that have high TB incidence or prevalence (use IGRAs for persons with recent BCG vaccination)
- Persons on long-term high dose corticosteroid therapy (use TST rather than IGRA)
- Persons on immunosuppressive therapy (use TST rather than IGRA)
- Persons with medical conditions that increase the risk of TB: chronic renal failure, diabetes, hematological disorders, cancer of the head or neck, body weight less than 10% of the ideal body weight, silicosis, gastrectomy, jejunal bypass

Adapted from Catanzaro, A. The diagnosis of TB in an era of diminishing incidence of TB. Retrieved July 1, 2013, from www.thoracic.org/sections/chapters/thoracic-society-chapters/ca/current-news/resources/2DXTB.pdf and cdc.gov/tb/publications/factsheets/testing/IGRA.htm

Table 9.11	Factors Contributing to a Decreased Response to Tuberculin Skin Testing

Infections:
- Viral: measles, mumps, chickenpox, HIV infection
- Bacterial: typhoid fever, brucellosis, typhus, leprosy, pertussis, recent or overwhelming *M tuberculosis* infection
- Fungal: South American blastomycosis
- Live virus vaccinations: measles, mumps, polio
Nutritional factors: severe protein depletion
Diseases affecting lymphoid organs: Hodgkin's lymphoma, chronic lymphocytic leukemia
Drugs: corticosteroids and other immunosuppressive agents
Age: newborns, older adults
Stress: surgery, burns, mental illness, graft-versus-host reactions

have selective anergy to TB but not to other antigens, so they are not helpful in ruling out TB.

As mentioned above, the IGRAs only require a single patient visit to conduct the test and the results can be available within 24 hours. The widely used bacille

Calmette-Guérin (BCG) vaccination does not cause a false-positive IGRA test result, given its greater specificity. Limited data are available on the use of IGRAs for children younger than 5 years of age and immunocompromised persons.

It is possible to obtain an inaccurate interpretation of the patient's tuberculin response when the administration of the skin test is done incorrectly. Factors that may contribute to an inaccurate reading of the test include improper handling of the tuberculin, improper administration technique, and inaccurate reading of tuberculin test (e.g., by an inexperienced reader). To minimize reduction in potency by adsorption, tuberculin should never be transferred from one container to another, and skin tests should be given soon after the syringe has been filled. Tuberculin should be kept refrigerated and stored in the dark as much as possible. The TST (0.1 mL) should be injected into the volar or the dorsal surface of the forearm, away from veins and into intact skin, free of lesions. The injection should be made just beneath the surface of the skin, with a one-quarter- to one-half-inch 27-gauge needle and a tuberculin syringe. A discrete, pale elevation of the skin (a wheal) 6 to 10 mm in diameter should be produced when the injection has been done correctly. If the first test was improperly administered, another test dose can be given immediately, but in a site several centimeters from the original injection.

Tests should be read 72 hours after injection, using good lighting with the forearm slightly flexed at the elbow. The basis of reading the test is the presence or absence of induration, which is determined by inspection and palpation. The diameter of the induration is measured transversely to the long axis of the forearm and recorded in millimeters. The size of the TST reaction has nothing to do with erythema, but is based solely on induration, because it is a type IV T-cell–mediated immune response. Because immunity from BCG wanes over time, if it has been many years since the vaccination, a TST may be performed and accurately read. To avoid any questions about the results, however, the IGRA test is preferred.

Persons with sensitivity to tuberculin are known as reactors. The definition of a tuberculin reaction size that is indicative of an infection with *M tuberculosis* is influenced by the dose, dilution, and nature of the tuberculin preparation being used, immunological factors, and the relative prevalence of tuberculin sensitivity resulting from infection with *M tuberculosis* and that resulting from other mycobacteria in the population being studied. Reactions caused by infections with mycobacteria other than *M tuberculosis* (cross reactions) are common in many parts of the world. Generally, a reaction to *M tuberculosis* will be a larger reaction than would be seen in a cross reaction. Guidelines for the classification of reactions to intradermal Mantoux tests have established three categories of positive reactions (5-, 10-, and 15-mm induration) based on the patient's immunosuppressive status, risk factors for exposure, and probability of cross reaction (see Table 9.12). A positive reaction in any patient represents only the presence of TB infection. In the United States, a positive TST without clinical TB infection (negative chest x-ray findings and no symptoms) should be treated to minimize the possibility of reactivation (secondary) TB. Standard regimens are INH for 9 months (least hepatotoxic regimen), rifampin for 4 months, or rifampin plus pyrazinamide for

Table 9.12 Interpretation of Tuberculin Skin Testing	
Diameter of Induration	**Positive Results**
>5 mm	• Persons with HIV infection or persons with risk factors for HIV infection and unknown HIV status • Persons who were recently exposed to clinically active TB, persons with organ transplants • Persons with chest films indicating healed TB
>10 mm	• Recent arrivals (<5 years) • Foreign-born persons from high-risk countries in Africa, Asia, Latin America • Medically underserved low-income populations and high-risk racial or ethnic minority populations • IV drug abusers • Residents and employees of high-risk congregate settings: prisons and jails, nursing homes and other residential settings for elderly people and/or AIDS patients, homeless shelters • Mycobacteriology laboratory personnel • Persons with medical conditions known to increase the risk for TB: diabetes, renal failure, silicosis, immunosuppressive therapy, hematological disorders (e.g., leukemia, lymphoma), gastrectomy, 10% or more below ideal body weight
>15 mm	• All other persons

2 months (but this is the most hepatotoxic regimen). Liver function test (LFT) screening is needed while the patient is on therapy.

Subsequent Testing In patients in whom there is a clinical suspicion of TB, the first diagnostic step should be a combination of a standard anterior-posterior and lateral chest x-ray film and a sputum examination for mycobacteria. The initial radiographic manifestation of an initial infection in the adult or a child is usually parenchymal infiltration accompanied by ipsilateral lymph node enlargement. The parenchymal lesions may be seen in any portion of the lung, but are seen most commonly in the apical and posterior segments of the upper lobes or in the superior segments of the lower lobes. Lesions may be dense and homogeneous, with lobar, segmental, or subsegmental distribution. Patients with HIV disease tend to have atypical radiographic findings. These patients tend not to have cavitations, and infiltrates are less likely to occur in the upper lobes. Cavitations are also seen infrequently in older patients and in those who may be immunosuppressed. Hematogenous TB is characterized by diffuse, finely nodular, uniformly distributed lesions on the chest x-ray film. The term *miliary* is applied to this appearance, because the nodules are about the size of a millet seed (approximately 2 mm in diameter).

Chest x-ray films that show no change in findings over a 3- to 4-month interval can generally be interpreted as showing a past TB infection or another disease. The use of a single chest x-ray film as a guide to the nature or the stability of the underlying disease is questionable. The words "old" and "fibrotic" are not accurate terms to use when interpreting a single chest x-ray film. Any persistent infiltrate in an older person should be considered suggestive of TB. This form of TB is often missed in older adults, especially among patients residing in a nursing home.

In pulmonary TB, examination of sputum provides the most convenient method of identifying the presence of bacilli, in terms of low cost, widespread availability, ease of performance, and reliability. The patient must be instructed to produce material brought up from the chest by coughing. A series of at least three single specimens on different days should be collected from patients who have a productive cough. When a patient is unable to produce an adequate amount of sputum, it is possible to obtain by gastric lavage the bronchopulmonary secretions that the patient has unknowingly swallowed during the night. Gastric aspiration is done following a period of fasting for 8 to 10 hours; it should be performed before the patient arises. About 50 mL of gastric contents is required for this test, which is best performed in the hospitalized patient.

It is possible to induce sputum production by inhalation of hypertonic saline. These specimens will be thinner and more watery than sputum produced spontaneously. Sputum induced by this method may produce a violent and uncontrolled cough, so special methods of air control may be indicated. Occasionally, a pooled specimen, collected over a period of 10 to 24 hours, may be helpful if the methods previously described are not effective or appropriate. This type of specimen is more subject to contamination and is best collected in an institutional setting.

Bronchial washings obtained with fiberoptic bronchoscopy may be indicated in patients who are unable to produce sputum or in those who are thought to have TB despite negative culture reports. When extrapulmonary TB is suspected, it is necessary to collect less common clinical specimens from sources such as urine; peritoneal, pericardial, and pleural fluids; bones and joints; and lymph nodes.

The detection of acid-fast bacilli (AFB) in stained smears examined by direct microscopy provides the first evidence of the presence of mycobacteria in a clinical specimen. It is estimated that 50% to 80% of patients with pulmonary TB will have positive sputum smears. The sputum smear is the easiest and quickest procedure and provides the practitioner with a preliminary confirmation of the diagnosis. The smear also provides the practitioner with a quantitative estimate of the number of bacilli being excreted by the patient. These estimates should be described as rare, few, or numerous. The lowest concentration of organisms that can be detected by microscopic examination is 10 per milliliter of sputum. For direct microscopy of sputum, the most widely used method is the Ziehl-Neelsen staining method.

All clinical specimens suspected of containing mycobacteria must be inoculated onto culture media. Culture yield seems to be associated with the clinical presentation of the patient. One study reported that patients with cavitary disease tend to have a higher rate of positive cultures than do patients with focal infiltrates. The cultures should be incubated at 37°C and examined at weekly intervals. The time from the laboratory's receipt of the specimen to the report of the culture is usually 3 to 6 weeks. In rare situations, such as repeated contaminated specimens or patients with positive Gram stains and negative cultures, guinea pig inoculation may be necessary.

Susceptibility of tubercle bacilli to various anti-TB drugs may be determined via either the direct or the indirect test. The direct drug-susceptibility test is performed by using clinical specimens of AFB, which are inoculated directly onto a drug-containing culture medium. Growth is then compared with growth on a non–drug-containing medium. An indirect test is performed by using a subculture from the primary isolation as the inoculum. Although the direct test is preferred, because it is more representative of the bacterial population of the patient, the indirect test may be useful when the initial smear is negative but the culture is positive, when growth on the control medium is inadequate for a reliable test, or when a reference culture is submitted by another laboratory. In the past, the previously untreated patient with newly diagnosed TB was started on chemotherapy without prior drug-susceptibility testing. Recommendations for drug-susceptibility testing have been modified because of the emergence of drug-resistant bacilli and are discussed in the section on clinical management.

Differential Diagnosis

Difficulties in a differential diagnosis arise when the tubercle bacilli cannot be isolated by smear or culture and in situations in which other diseases such as carcinoma or pulmonary mycosis exist. Pulmonary lesions of small extent, particularly the solitary nodule or coin nodule, need to be differentiated from early carcinoma of the lung, pulmonary infarction, localized pulmonary fibrosis, and pneumonia of fungal, viral, mycoplasmal, or bacterial origin with delayed clearing or resolution. In extensive forms of pulmonary TB, bronchopneumonia and lobar pneumonia must be considered. The acute cavitary forms of TB must be differentiated from lung abscess. Other chronic pulmonary diseases that frequently are characterized by cavity formations include the systemic mycoses, particularly coccidiomycosis and histoplasmosis.

Pulmonary TB of hematogenous origin must be differentiated from other types of infection that may manifest in similar fashion: silicosis, berylliosis, asbestosis, sarcoidosis, diffuse interstitial fibrosis, scleroderma, metastatic neoplasms, or alveolar cell carcinoma. From the perspective of clinical manifestations, the advanced practice registered nurse (APRN) must consider other conditions that may cause prolonged or obscure fevers, such as lymphoma, brucellosis, and HIV infection.

Management

The development of specific chemotherapeutic agents revolutionized the prognosis of TB and TB infection, making the disease truly curable and preventable. Drug treatment of TB should be viewed as both a personal health measure intended to cure the ill patient and as a public health measure intended to interrupt transmission of tubercle bacilli in the community.

Initial Management

In patients in whom the clinical and radiographic findings suggest a diagnosis of TB and the sputum examination reveals the presence of mycobacteria, a working diagnosis can be made and anti-TB chemotherapy can be started. For patients in whom TB is suspected but whose smear results are negative, an alternative is to begin therapy and wait for culture results. Initiating chemotherapy in the absence of a definitive diagnosis is a valid approach, but caution needs to be exercised in doing so in patients with HIV infection and multidrug resistance. X-ray findings in patients with AIDS are often atypical and may be indicative of a range of diagnostic possibilities. A presumptive diagnosis of TB in these patients may be more speculative.

The main goal of therapy is to eliminate all tubercle bacilli from the patient while avoiding the situation of clinically significant drug resistance. The treatment consists of administering multiple drugs that the organism is susceptible to, adding new drugs to the regimen when it is suspected that treatment is not working, providing the maximum therapy in the shortest amount of time, and insisting on patient compliance. While curing the individual patient, the transmission of *M tuberculosis* to other persons needs to be minimized.

The current minimal acceptable duration of treatment for all children and adults with culture-positive TB is 6 months. The initial phase of a 6-month regimen should consist of a 2-month course of isoniazid (INH), rifampin (RIF), pyrazinamide (PZA), and ethambutol (EMB) or streptomycin in children who are too young to be monitored for visual acuity, until the results of drug-susceptibility studies are available, unless there is little possibility of drug resistance (e.g., less than 4% primary resistance to INH in the community and the patient has had no previous treatment with anti-TB medication, is not from a country with a high prevalence of drug-resistant TB, or has no known exposure to a drug-resistant case). The second phase of therapy should consist of INH and RIF for a total of 4 months (daily treatment or two to three times per week). Therapy should be prolonged if the response is slow or otherwise suboptimal.

An alternative regimen for persons who cannot take PZA (e.g., pregnant women) consists of a 9-month regimen of INH and RIF. Ethambutol should also be included until the results of the susceptibility studies are available unless there is little possibility of drug resistance. Drug resistance is most common in HIV patients and immigrants. If INH resistance is confirmed, rifampin plus PZA plus ethambutol should be continued for a minimum of 6 months. For rifampin resistance, INH plus ethambutol should be used for 18 months or INH, PZA, and streptomycin for 9 months. In HIV patients, rifabutin should always be used because rifampin interacts with protease inhibitors and nonnucleoside retroviral inhibitors.

Adverse reactions and prescribing considerations for the common TB drugs are shown in Drugs Commonly Prescribed 9.2.

Directly observed therapy (DOT) should be considered for all patients because of the difficulty in predicting which patients will adhere to a prescribed regimen. When TB is initially diagnosed, the practitioner should explain to the patient about the disease, the treatment, and the necessity of completing the recommended therapy. If DOT is considered to be indicated, the patient and the practitioner should agree on a method that ensures the greatest rate of adherence and maintains confidentiality. DOT may require an outreach worker to go

Drugs Commonly Prescribed 9.2   Tuberculosis

	Adverse Reactions and Prescribing Considerations
FIRST-LINE TB DRUGS	All must be taken on an empty stomach to facilitate absorption—if unable to comply, may take medicine with food that does not contain fat or oils (may ease nausea).
isoniazid (INH or H)	May cause peripheral neuropathy (pyridoxine may be given prophylactically). May be associated with increased risk of seizures in patients with epilepsy. May be hepatotoxic (potentiated by rifampin).
rifampin (RIF, RMP, or R)	May cause thrombocytopenia. Commonly causes rash without itching during the first few weeks; usually resolves on its own. May cause an elevation in bilirubin which usually resolves in 10 days; potentiates INH hepatotoxicity.
pyrazinamide (PZA or Z)	May cause rash. May be hepatotoxic. If the patient will not take due to tablet size, PZA syrup may be substituted.
ethambutol (EMB or E)	Periodic vision screens required, given ocular toxicity (optic neuritis).
streptomycin (SM, STM, or S)	Use with caution in patients with mild to severe kidney problems. Periodic hearing screens required, given aminoglycoside-related ototoxicity.
SECOND-LINE TB DRUGS	Choice of agent should be guided by resistance testing.
aminoglycosides (e.g., amikacin [AMK], kanamycin [KM])	Use with caution in patients with mild to severe kidney problems. Chronic use may cause ototoxicity (audiologic and vestibular dysfunction).
polypeptides (e.g., capreomycin, viomycin, enviomycin)	Capreomycin may cause nephrotoxicity.
fluoroquinolones (e.g., ciprofloxacin [CIP], levofloxacin, moxifloxacin [MXF])	Commonly causes nausea, vomiting, or other gastrointestinal symptoms. May also cause tendinitis/tendon rupture. Associated with QTc prolongation.
thioamides (e.g., ethionamide, prothionamide)	Gastrointestinal side effects may occur. Central nervous system and psychiatric effects.
cycloserine (only antibiotic in its class)	Gastrointestinal side effects may occur.
p-aminosalicylic acid (PAS or P)	Potential cause of drug-induced hepatitis.

into the community and administer each dose of medication to the patient. Many patients can, however, receive the treatment at a center agreed on by the practitioner and the patient. Common community settings include TB clinics, community health centers, migrant clinics, homeless shelters, jails or prisons, nursing homes, schools, drug treatment centers, hospitals, HIV/AIDS clinics, or occupational health clinics. In some situations, a responsible person other than a health-care worker may be able to administer the chemotherapy. Possible resources in the community include correctional facility personnel, social and welfare caseworkers, clergy, teachers, and reliable volunteers. Adequate medication adherence is critical to the complete clearance of all infectious

organisms and to the prevention of drug-resistant strains of TB. See Box 9.1 for information about multidrug-resistant TB.

HIV infection and other factors that compromise a patient's immune system are important considerations when practitioners select the most effective regimen. These factors are particularly important with drug-resistant TB because of the potential for rapid disease progression and death when patients receive inadequate treatment. DOT and experienced TB/HIV caregivers are considered to be critical to the effective treatment of both conditions. Given the propensity for rifampin to upregulate and induce the hepatic cytochrome p450 metabolic pathway, the dosage of several antiretroviral

Box 9.1 Drug-Resistant Tuberculosis: MDR-TB and XDR-TB

MDR-TB
Multidrug-resistant TB: Tuberculosis resistant at least to isoniazid and rifampin

XDR-TB
Extensively drug-resistant TB: Tuberculosis resistant to both isoniazid and rifampin, as well as fluoroquinolones and at least one of the injectable second-line anti-TB agents (kanamycin, capreomycin, or amikacin)

Principles of Treatment
The principles of treatment for both MDR-TB and XDR-TB are the same, focused on antimicrobial sensitivity testing and the selection of active agents.

Given resistance to second-line agents, XDR-TB has a higher mortality rate due to a reduced number of effective treatment options.

Treatment lasts for a minimum of 18 months and may last for years.

medications must be increased when administered with rifampin. However, substituting rifabutin (Mycobutin) for rifampin (Rimactane, Rifadin) allows for the concurrent administration of anti-TB and antiretroviral drug regimens, with no dose adjustments in the latter. Currently, most guidelines indicate that HIV-infected patients should be treated for a total of 9 months and for at least 6 months following sputum conversion. In general, intermittent anti-TB therapy is not recommended for TB/HIV–co-infected patients. See the recommendations for the treatment of TB and antiretroviral dose adjustments among HIV-infected patients in Chapter 17.

Effective therapy for TB is essential for pregnant women. Untreated TB represents a greater hazard to a pregnant woman and her fetus than does treatment of the disease. Initial treatment should consist of INH and RIF. Ethambutol (Myambutol) should also be included unless primary INH resistance is unlikely. Streptomycin should not be prescribed for pregnant women because it may cause congenital deafness in the fetus. PZA is recommended by international TB organizations for use in pregnant women. In the United States, PZA is not currently recommended because it has not been determined if there is a risk of teratogenicity. Breastfeeding does not need to be discouraged because the small concentrations of anti-TB drugs in breast milk are not adequate to produce toxicity in the newborn. TB during pregnancy is not an indication for a therapeutic abortion.

Regimens that are adequate for treating adults with pulmonary TB should be effective in treating extrapulmonary disease. Bacteriological evaluation of extrapulmonary TB may be limited by the relative inaccessibility of the disease site. Response to treatment often must be

judged on the basis of clinical and radiographic findings. Surgery may be necessary to obtain specimens for diagnosis and to treat such processes as constrictive pericarditis. Corticosteroid therapy has been shown to be of benefit in preventing cardiac constriction from TB pericarditis and in decreasing the neurological sequelae of TB meningitis.

Subsequent Management

Today, the majority of patients with TB may undergo treatment and remain in their own home settings. There may be specific patient situations that mandate the need for hospitalization of the patient with TB. Some of the indications include very ill patients who have no responsible person at home to provide care, patients with advanced pulmonary disease with highly positive sputum smears or severe extrapulmonary disease, or the presence of associated medical problems that require hospitalization.

Adults should have measurements of serum bilirubin, hepatic enzymes, blood urea nitrogen (BUN), and creatinine and a CBC, including platelet count, before starting chemotherapy for TB. Visual acuity and red-green color perception tests are recommended before initiation of ethambutol, and a serum uric acid level should be measured before starting PZA. Patients should be advised to report symptoms suggestive of drug toxicity. For INH-containing regimens, symptoms of concern are anorexia, nausea, vomiting, fatigue or weakness, dark urine, icterus, rash, paresthesias of the hands and feet, fever, and abdominal tenderness. Routine monitoring of laboratory tests for evidence is not recommended, but monthly questioning for symptoms of drug toxicity is indicated. Patients with known liver disease or heavy drinkers may need to have periodic LFTs. Appropriate laboratory tests are mandatory if symptoms of drug toxicity develop.

Periodic examination of the patient is necessary to observe for changes in symptoms, signs, body weight, and temperature. The single most important laboratory test is the bacteriological examination of bronchopulmonary secretions. A progressive fall in the number of AFB in weekly or biweekly specimens is a good indicator of effective chemotherapy. Periodic laboratory checks of blood, urine, visual acuity, eighth-nerve function, renal function, and hepatic function are desirable based on the severity of the illness and the drugs being administered. Patients should be questioned closely for any symptoms of drug toxicity, as well as the level of adherence.

It is not necessary to restrict physical activity and require bedrest for most patients. Bedrest may help make patients who are experiencing fever, night sweats, anorexia, and bouts of coughing more comfortable. Patients who present with a history of fever should have a normal temperature within 2 to 3 weeks after the initiation of chemotherapy. It may be necessary to suppress the cough reflex in patients who are experiencing severe coughing. Codeine and hydrocodone are the most useful for temporary treatment. If the patient is producing thick and tenacious secretions, suppression of the cough reflex is not desirable. These patients should be instructed in adequate hydration and air humidification and prescribed an expectorant. Chest pain may manifest if the patient develops pleuritis. Occasionally chest pain may be caused by a fractured rib resulting from hard coughing. An instillation of a local anesthetic about the rib fracture is preferred over the older method of strapping the chest. Coughing resulting in occasional episodes of streaked or bloody sputum requires no specific treatment other than managing the cough. There may be significant hemoptysis with bronchogenic spread of the TB; however, it tends to be self-limiting. In advanced chronic cavitary TB, fatal pulmonary hemorrhage or shock can occur if large pulmonary arteries or Rasmussen's aneurysm slough or ulcerate.

Follow-up and Referral

The response to anti-TB chemotherapy in patients with positive bacteriology is best evaluated by repeated examinations of sputum. Sputum cultures should be done at least once monthly until sputum conversion is documented. After 2 months of treatment with regimens containing both INH and RIF, the majority of patients should convert to negative cultures. Patients whose sputum cultures have not become negative after 3 months of treatment should be carefully reevaluated and referred to a pulmonologist. Drug-susceptibility tests should be repeated, and treatment should be administered or continued under direct observation. If organisms are found to be resistant, the treatment regimen should be modified to include at least two drugs to which the organisms

are susceptible and administered using DOT. For patients whose sputum no longer contains *M tuberculosis,* at least one further sputum smear and culture should be performed at the completion of therapy. X-ray evaluations during treatment are less important than sputum examination. A chest x-ray film at completion of treatment will provide a baseline comparison for any future films.

Shortness of breath in a patient without underlying pulmonary disease is suggestive of complications of pulmonary TB and requires further diagnostic inquiry. Sudden breathlessness may be a symptom of acute pleurisy with pleuritic pain, a pleural effusion, spontaneous pneumothorax, a massive extension of the TB, or an atelectasis. Patients who have coexisting emphysema or pulmonary disease may become dyspneic with only minimal involvement of the lungs.

Preventive Therapy

The ATS has identified risk groups for whom preventive therapy is indicated (see Table 9.13). Patients infected with *M tuberculosis* who do not have the active disease still harbor organisms. In turn, prophylactic or preventive treatment of latent TB infection significantly reduces the probability of reactivation TB later in life. INH given for 9 months is effective in asymptomatic adults (300 mg per day) or children (10–14 mg/kg per day up to 300 mg per day) with LTBI infection demonstrated by a positive TST reaction. Concurrent pyridoxine administration (25–50 mg per day in adults and 1–2 mg/kg daily in children) may reduce the potential for neuropathic complications associated with INH, and adjustments with intermittent dosing (900 mg twice weekly) or an overall shortened duration (6 months)

Table 9.13 Groups for Whom Preventive TB Therapy Is Recommended	
Group	Comments
The following high-risk groups should be given treatment if their reaction to the Mantoux tuberculin skin test (PPD) is ≥5 mm:	
1. Persons with known HIV infection and those suspected of having HIV infection (persons with risk factors for HIV infection whose status is unknown)	HIV-infected persons who are at high risk for TB but have negative skin tests should be considered for preventive therapy.
2. Close contacts of persons with newly diagnosed infectious TB	Household members and other close contacts have a 2%–4% chance of developing TB within the first year of exposure to the index case. The risk for very young children and adolescents may be twice that of the adult. People who do not develop TB disease within the first year will continue to be at risk for the disease throughout their life. Children should be treated, even if their initial skin tests are negative. Skin testing should be repeated after 3 months of INH therapy. If the skin test becomes positive, INH preventive therapy should be continued for a total of 9 months.
3. Persons with fibrotic changes on chest x-ray exam consistent with old TB	

Continued

Table 9.13   Groups for Whom Preventive TB Therapy Is Recommended—cont'd

Group	Comments
4. Recent tuberculin skin test converters	A skin test conversion is defined as an increase in induration of 10 mm or more within 2 years for those younger than age 35 years and 15 mm or more for those age 35 years or older.
5. Persons with medical conditions that increase the risk of TB with a PPD 10 mm or greater	
• Diabetes mellitus	The risk for this group may be 2–4 times that of the general population. Particularly at risk are poorly controlled insulin-dependent diabetics.
• Prolonged therapy with adrenocorticosteroids	TB that develops during corticosteroid therapy tends to be disseminated or presents in an obscure fashion. Prednisone (or equivalent) given daily at 15 mg or higher for 2–3 weeks markedly reduces tuberculin reactivity.
• Immunosuppressive therapy	Persons receiving other forms of immunosuppressive therapy are at an increased risk for TB.
• Hematological and reticuloendothelial diseases	Diseases such as leukemia and Hodgkin's disease may be associated with suppressed cellular immunity and an increased risk of TB.
• IV drug users known to be HIV-negative	Persons injecting illicit drugs may be at increased risk of TB even if not infected with HIV.
• End-stage renal disease (ESRD)	Persons with ESRD are predisposed to developing extrapulmonary TB with disseminated disease. Because these patients may be anergic, a documented history or positive skin test is an indication for preventive INH therapy unless they have been treated previously.
• Clinical conditions associated with substantial rapid weight loss or chronic malnutrition	These conditions include intestinal bypass surgery for obesity (which carries an increased risk for disseminated TB), postgastrectomy, chronic peptic ulcer disease, chronic malabsorption syndromes, chronic alcoholism, and carcinomas of the oropharynx and upper gastrointestinal tract that prevent adequate nutritional intake. The postgastrectomy state may increase the risk of developing TB even without weight loss.
Persons in the following groups who are younger than age 35 years and have a positive tuberculin skin test (≥10 mm):	
• Foreign-born persons from high-prevalence countries	These countries include those in Latin America, Asia, and Africa that have a high prevalence of TB. Recent arrivals (<5 years).
• Medically underserved low-income groups, especially high-risk racial or ethnic minority populations	These groups include African Americans, Native Americans, Hispanics, Asians, and Pacific Islanders.
• Residents of facilities for long-term care	These residents include those in correctional facilities, nursing homes, and mental health facilities. Staff of such facilities should also be considered for preventive therapy.
• Residents and staff of high-risk congregate settings (nursing homes, jails, homeless shelters)	
• Migrant farmworkers	
• Children younger than 4 years of age	
• Mycobacteriology laboratory personnel	

Table 9.13	Groups for Whom Preventive TB Therapy Is Recommended—cont'd
Group	**Comments**
• Persons with clinical conditions that make them high risk	HIV infection, substance abuse, recent infection with *M tuberculosis* (within past 2 years), previous TB, silicosis, prolonged immunosuppressive therapy, low body weight (<90% of normal), ESRD, chronic malabsorption
Persons with no known risk factors for TB may be considered for therapy if their reaction to the tuberculin test is ≥15 mm. This group should be given lower priority than the groups listed above.	

Source: Adapted from Chapter 6 of the CDC Curriculum: Preventive therapy: Treatment of TB infection. Retrieved July 1, 2013, from www.cdc.gov/tb/education/corecurr/pdf/chapter6.pdf

may be used for adult patients with medication adherence issues. For patients intolerant of INH or in whom INH-resistant LTBI is suspected, rifampin may be used as an alternative in adults (600 mg per day for 4 months) or children (10–20 mg/kg per day for 6 months).

All persons with known HIV infection or suspected of having HIV who have positive TST results should receive preventive therapy for TB. HIV-infected persons who are at high risk for TB but have negative skin tests should also be considered for preventive therapy. Preventive regimens are similar to those for non–HIV-infected individuals. However, a full course of daily INH (9 months) or rifampin (6 months) is recommended, with the latter reserved for suspected cases of INH-resistant, rifampin-sensitive LTBI.

Household members and other close contacts have a 2% to 4% risk of developing TB within the first year of exposure to the index case. The risk for very young children and adolescents may be twice the risk of the adult. People who do not develop TB disease within the first year will continue to be at risk for the disease throughout their lives. Children should be treated even if their initial skin tests are negative. Skin testing should be repeated after 3 months of INH. If the skin test becomes positive, INH preventive therapy should be continued for a total of 9 months.

Persons with medical conditions such as diabetes, long-term use of adrenocorticosteroids, use of immunosuppressive therapy, IV drug use, hematological disease, end-stage renal disease, and conditions associated with rapid weight loss or chronic malnutrition are also at risk for TB. Other risk groups include foreign-born persons from high-prevalence countries (Asia, Africa, Latin America); medically underserved groups, especially high-risk racial or ethnic populations (African Americans, Native Americans, Hispanics); and residents of long-term care facilities (e.g., prisons, nursing homes, mental health facilities).

Bacille Calmette-Guérin (BCG) vaccination is an antimycobacterial vaccine developed from an attenuated strain of *Mycobacterium bovis*. Millions of persons worldwide have been vaccinated with BCG. It is not currently recommended because of multiple factors, including its variable effectiveness against pulmonary TB. BCG vaccination in the United States should be used only after consultation with the local health department. The BCG vaccination should not be used in persons with impaired immune responses.

Because BCG vaccination has been widespread in the majority of countries outside the United States, the clinician will undoubtedly encounter patients who may be at risk for TB who have been vaccinated. Previous vaccination with BCG typically results in tuberculin test conversion, producing a reaction that may be difficult to distinguish from a natural mycobacterial infection. A large reaction to PPD tuberculin in BCG-vaccinated persons, especially among persons from countries with a high prevalence of TB, should be considered indicative of a possible TB infection, and the patient should be evaluated appropriately. Reasons for not assuming that a large reaction to tuberculin testing is due to the BCG vaccination include the following: (1) conversion rates after vaccination may be much less than 100%, (2) the mean reaction size among vaccines is often less than 10 mm, and (3) TB sensitivity tends to wane after vaccination.

To keep abreast of changes in treatment recommendations for TB, visit the Division of TB Elimination Web site at www.cdc.gov/nchstp/tb.

Patient Education

The necessity of educating the patient and the family about the disease, treatment, and importance of completing the recommended regimen is critical to the management of TB. The patient and family should understand the information and continue to be provided with reinforcement and encouragement throughout the course of therapy. Patients should be offered the option of participating in DOT. For patients who are administering their own medications, strategies that may be helpful for improving adherence include use of a weekly pill dispenser, marking off each day on a calendar as medicine is taken, taking pills at the same time every day (e.g., with breakfast or at coffee break), and asking a friend or family member to remind the patient to take pills.

Patients are typically considered to be infectious for about 2 to 3 weeks after initiation of drug therapy. If the patient is being cared for at home, he or she should not go to work or school. These patients should be instructed in controlling the spread of tubercle bacilli in microdroplets by using good hygienic measures, appropriate ventilation, and avoiding close contact with family and friends. Patients should sleep in a separate room until no longer considered infectious. Patients should be taught to always cover their mouths when they cough, sneeze, or laugh. Used tissues should be placed in a plastic or paper bag and discarded. If the weather is warm enough, patients should be instructed to place a fan in an open window to blow out air that may be contaminated with TB. Opening other windows in their room will help pull in fresh air.

Patients should be asked to identify any people who may need to be tested for TB infections, including coworkers, family members, and friends. All close contacts will need to undergo tuberculin skin testing and may require preventive INH therapy. Assurance should be provided to the patient and family by stressing that the majority of properly treated patients with TB are cured.

Some problems associated with TB among foreign-born patients stem from communication barriers, cultural and cognitive dissonance between practitioners and patients, and gaps in provider training. Education needs to be targeted to patients, providers, and community workers.

There are excellent TB control strategies available to the public from the CDC. Patients may access these guidelines at www.cdc.gov and obtain guidelines written in an easily understood manner.

However, the problems of multidrug-resistant TB and issues of compliance with therapy among all populations remain a significant challenge for health-care providers. Practicing within a *Circle of Caring* enables the provider to approach these problems in a meaningful way.

■ LUNG CANCER

Lung cancer arises from the epithelium of the respiratory tract. The four major histological types are squamous-cell (epidermoid) carcinoma, small-cell (oat-cell) carcinoma, large-cell carcinoma (including giant-cell and clear-cell carcinoma), and adenocarcinoma. Squamous-cell carcinoma is named for the resemblance of cells to the epidermis of the skin. These cells usually contain the skin protein called keratin. Squamous-cell carcinomas arise most often from the bronchial lining and may grow to obstruct air passages. Adenocarcinoma, the most prevalent carcinoma of the lung of both sexes, resembles poorly formed glandular tissue. It may be difficult to determine whether an adenocarcinoma is a primary lung cancer or a metastatic tumor from elsewhere in the body. Fifty-five percent to 60% of adenocarcinomas are

located in the periphery of the lung, not obviously related to any bronchus. Many organs in the body can develop adenocarcinoma that may metastasize to the lungs. Large-cell carcinomas, also called undifferentiated carcinoma, are characterized by a collection of poorly formed large cells that have abundant cytoplasm. These tumors may exhibit a glandlike structure and produce mucin.

Small-cell lung carcinomas (SCLCs) (oat-cell, intermediate, and combined carcinomas) are characterized by very small cells with scant cytoplasm. SCLC is a very rapidly growing tumor that usually metastasizes to distant tissue while the tumor is quite small. The clinical effect of SCLC is much different from that of the other three forms of lung cancer, which is why lung cancers are usually classified in terms of small-cell and non–small-cell lung carcinomas (NSCLCs) (Table 9.14).

Because the lung area is so large, tumors may go undetected for some time. Early symptoms such as coughing and fatigue are so common that patients often attribute these symptoms to other causes, rather than lung cancer. Because of this, early-stage lung cancer (Stages I and II) is difficult to detect, and most patients are diagnosed at Stages III and IV.

Epidemiology and Causes

Lung cancer is preventable, common, and lethal once it comes to clinical attention, and it is relatively resistant to current therapeutics. Lung cancer is the most frequent cause of cancer death in men and women in North America and accounts for 28% of all cancer deaths. In 2013, the National Cancer Institute at the National Institutes of Health reported that more than 228,190

Table 9.14	Cellular Classification of Lung Cancer	
Major Classification	**Subclassification**
Small-cell lung carcinomas (SCLCs)	• Oat-cell carcinoma • Intermediate-cell carcinoma • Combined small-cell carcinoma (with squamous-cell carcinoma or adenocarcinoma)
Non–small-cell lung carcinomas (NSCLCs)	• Squamous-cell (epidermoid) carcinoma Well-differentiated Moderately well-differentiated Poorly differentiated • Adenocarcinoma Well-differentiated Moderately well-differentiated Poorly differentiated Bronchoalveolar • Large-cell carcinoma Giant-cell Clear-cell

people were diagnosed with lung cancer and 159,480 of them died from it. Eighty-six percent of patients die within 5 years. The death rate for women is now higher than from any other cancer because of increased cigarette smoking by women and because they may be more susceptible to the carcinogenic effects of tobacco smoke than are men. In every ethnic group, men still have higher lung cancer incidence and mortality rates than women, although women are rapidly closing the gap. African American men have the highest lung cancer incidence and mortality rates. Lung cancer is the leading cause of cancer death in most racial and ethnic groups of women except Native American, Filipino, and Hispanic women. New lung cancers and lung cancer deaths peak in individuals aged 55 to 65 years old.

Tobacco use, especially cigarettes, is the main cause of the progressive rise in mortality from lung cancer. Ninety percent of the lung cancer cases in men and 70% in women are attributed directly to cigarette smoking. The risk of lung cancer increases with the duration of smoking, with earlier age at onset of smoking, and for smoking unfiltered or high-tar cigarettes. Of continued note are the effects of environmental tobacco smoke, also called secondhand smoke, sidestream smoke, involuntary smoke, or passive cigarette smoke. Exposure to secondhand smoke is thought to increase the risk of dying from lung cancer by 30%.

Lung cancer also occurs in association with occupational and environmental exposure to carcinogenic agents from sources other than smoking. Environmental or occupational risk factors associated with lung cancer include benzpyrene and radon, mustard gas, and nickel and chromium particles associated with uranium mining, asbestos, arsenic fumes, radiation, and nuclear bombs. The combination of cigarette smoking and environmental exposure produces an additive effect such that smokers exposed to asbestos increase their risk of lung cancer 92 times.

Pathophysiology

The bronchial walls have three layers: an epithelial lining, a smooth muscle layer, and a connective tissue layer. The epithelial lining of the bronchi contains single-celled exocrine glands (the mucus-secreting goblet cells) and ciliated cells. High columnar pseudostratified epithelium lines the larger airways, changing to columnar cuboidal epithelium in the bronchioles. It is hypothesized that at sites of segmental bronchial bifurcations, airflow and mucus production are altered and bronchial epithelium becomes very susceptible to injury. Carcinogenic agents, such as tobacco smoke, are likely deposited and absorbed in these areas. Particle size in environmental tobacco smoke is smaller, and inhaled particles may travel to peripheral lung regions more readily than with mainstream smoke. This is thought to explain the excess of peripheral adenocarcinomas seen in passive smokers.

Cigarette smoke contains tumor initiators, promoters, and cocarcinogens. DNA-mutating agents in cigarettes produce alterations in both oncogenes (a class of genes that encodes proteins involved in normal cell-growth processes) and tumor-suppressor genes. Multiple genetic events occur, first resulting in dysregulated growth and eventually in a malignant cell. These alterations include bronchial epithelial changes progressing from squamous cell alteration, or metaplasia, to carcinoma in situ. Repeated carcinogenic irritation to the bronchial epithelium may cause increased rates of cellular replication. Healthy ciliated cells are replaced with a proliferation of basal cells, resulting in hyperplasia, dysplasia, carcinoma in situ, and invasive carcinoma.

Small-Cell Lung Cancer

SCLC, which accounts for 15% of lung cancers, invades the submucosa and is centrally located, developing around a main bronchus as a whitish gray growth that invades surrounding structures, eventually compressing the bronchi externally. SCLC results from smoking more so than NSCLC, grows more rapidly, and metastasizes earlier than NSCLC. SCLC is also more responsive to chemotherapy than NSCLC. The most striking difference between small-cell carcinoma and other forms of malignant lung neoplasms is the aggressiveness of this tumor, resulting in a more rapid growth and early local and distant metastasis via the lymphatic and blood vessels. Oat-cell carcinoma, one of the three types of SCLC, is composed of cells with round to oval nuclei. The tumors are soft in consistency and have shiny gray cut surfaces. The more common intermediate cell type is characterized by cells with larger, more vesicular, fusiform or spindled nuclei. The third type is the combined type, in which small-cell carcinoma is combined with another cell type. The most important variant is the small-cell and large-cell, which is regarded as small-cell carcinoma for treatment purposes. It lacks sensitivity to radiation and chemotherapy but retains the aggressiveness of the "pure" small-cell carcinoma.

Non–Small-Cell Lung Cancer

NSCLC comprises approximately 85% of all primary lung carcinomas in the United States. The tumor suppressor gene p53 has been reported to be associated with human cancer more commonly than any other gene. The gene is mutated in about 60% of all cases of NSCLC. It encodes for a protein with a central role in the regulation of transcriptional events in the cell nucleus, particularly in response to DNA-damaging agents, such as ionizing radiation and a variety of other carcinogens. The central role of normal p53 protein has led to its description as the "guardian of the genome." Although many efforts to improve survival have focused on expanding indications for both radiotherapy and surgery, little progress has been made.

Squamous-Cell Carcinoma Squamous-cell carcinoma is the second most common lung cancer, accounting for

25% to 35% of cases. It is more common in men than in women and occurs almost entirely in cigarette smokers.

These tumors arise from the basal cells of the bronchial epithelium and usually present as masses in the segmental, lobar, or mainstem bronchi. The tumors tend to be bulky and invade cartilage and the adjoining lymph nodes. Based on the degree of differentiation, these tumors are divided into three subtypes: well-differentiated, moderately well-differentiated, and poorly differentiated tumors. Well-differentiated tumors may show epithelial pearl formation, whereas poorly differentiated tumors are characterized by keratinization. Because it is a relatively slow-growing tumor, several years may elapse between the development of a carcinoma in situ and clinical detection. Metastases of squamous-cell carcinomas are initially to hilar and mediastinal lymph nodes and then to the liver, adrenals, bones, and brain.

Adenocarcinoma Adenocarcinoma, which represents 35% to 40% of all lung cancers, is the most prevalent carcinoma of the lung in both sexes and in nonsmokers. It forms acinar or glandular structures. Histologically, this tumor is divided broadly into well-differentiated, moderately well-differentiated, poorly differentiated, and bronchioalveolar types. They arise from the bronchial epithelium and may form in lung scars or fibrous tissue. Adenocarcinoma usually presents as a non-small cell lung cancer in the peripheral portion of the lungs, although rapidly progressive multifocal disease may be present at diagnosis. Although adenocarcinomas are usually slow-growing tumors, they invade lymphatics and blood vessels early, and thus produce early metastases; nearly half are considered to be unresectable at the time of diagnosis. Grossly, central cavitation is uncommon. Areas of metastasis commonly include the brain, liver, bone, and adrenal glands. Patients with adenocarcinomas may have an associated history of chronic interstitial lung disease such as scleroderma, rheumatoid arthritis (RA), recurrent pulmonary infections, and other necrotizing pulmonary disease.

The bronchoalveolar subtype of adenocarcinoma represents approximately 2% to 4% of all lung cancers. Often, it is associated with prior lung disease leading to fibrosis, including repeated pneumonias, idiopathic pulmonary fibrosis, asbestosis, scleroderma, and Hodgkin's disease. There is little correlation with this type of cancer and smoking. Bronchoalveolar carcinoma commonly arises in the periphery of the lung and it grows in a scale-like fashion along the alveolar septa. Grossly, these tumors may be categorized as solitary, multinodular, or diffuse. The solitary, well-differentiated bronchoalveolar cell carcinoma has a much better prognosis than the other forms; diffuse and multinodular forms usually are not amenable to therapy.

Large-Cell Carcinoma

Large-cell carcinoma, also called undifferentiated carcinoma, is the least common type of lung cancer,

representing approximately 5% to 10% of cases. It is classified into two types: clear-cell carcinoma and giant-cell carcinoma. Large-cell carcinomas include all tumors that show no evidence of differentiation to small-cell carcinoma, squamous-cell carcinoma, or adenocarcinoma. These tumors tend to form large, bulky, somewhat circumscribed and necrotic masses in the major or intermediate-sized bronchi or in the periphery, invade locally, and disseminate widely. The giant-cell variant of large-cell carcinoma is composed of huge, multinucleated, bizarre cells that are frequently associated with an extensive inflammatory cell infiltration. These tumors are usually large and peripheral and are very aggressive, highly malignant, and most often found at a late stage. These lesions show an ability to metastasize widely, with a predilection for the small intestine. Table 9.15 summarizes the characteristics of the types of lung cancer.

Clinical Presentation

Past history of a patient with suspected lung cancer must include any history of chronic respiratory problems, as well as any prolonged exposure to environmental carcinogens. Habits must be assessed to determine the patient's risk of developing lung cancer. Smoking history includes the age when smoking started, the average number of packs smoked per day, and the number of years smoked. The type of tobacco (cigar, cigarette, snuff, or chewing tobacco) used by the patient must be determined. A positive family history of lung cancer may indicate that the patient is at a slightly higher risk to develop lung cancer. The genetic link, however, is not clear. A review of systems reexamines all pertinent present and past symptoms that relate to the chief complaint and usually completes the health history.

Clinical manifestations of lung cancer are dependent on the location of the tumor and the extent of spread. Ten percent to 25% of patients are asymptomatic at the time of diagnosis. Symptoms may be divided into four categories: intrathoracic or local–regional symptoms, symptoms resulting from extrathoracic involvement, nonspecific systemic symptoms, and paraneoplastic syndromes. Some cases of lung cancer are picked up during a routine chest x-ray study done for other reasons, for example, a preoperative physical for an unrelated surgery, or for a work physical, and so forth.

Intrathoracic or Local–Regional Symptoms

Subjective The most common symptoms of local–regional disease are ambiguous and insidious; they include cough, sputum production, dyspnea, chest pain, hemoptysis, wheezing, postobstructive pneumonia, and pleural effusions. Cough resulting from bronchial irritation occurs in 60% of patients and often is attributed to a cold. The cough frequently goes away after a few days and returns intermittently. Cough may be produced by a small tumor acting as a foreign body or by ulceration

Table 9.15   Characteristics of Lung Cancer

Lung Cancer Type	Tumor Type	Growth Rate	Metastasis	Manifestations	Treatment
SCLC	• 15%–20% • Neuroendocrine cells: Oat-cell carcinoma Combined small-cell (with squamous-cell carcinoma or adenocarcinoma)	Very rapid	Very early, via lymphatic and blood vessels	Obstruction of main bronchus; associated with paraneoplastic syndrome	• Not resectable • Treated with chemotherapy and radiation
NSCLC	• Squamous-cell (epidermoid) carcinoma • 25%–35% • Keratin-producing cells: Well-differentiated Moderately well-differentiated Poorly differentiated	Slow	Hilar and medi-astinal lymph nodes, liver, adrenals, bone, brain	Most often in cigarette smok-ers; bulky mass in main stem bronchi	• Stage I and II: Resectable • Stage III: Chemotherapy and radiation • Stage IV: Chemotherapy (Refer to Table 9.18 for staging)
	• Adenocarcinoma • 35%–40% • Columnar cells: Well-differentiated Moderately well-differentiated Poorly differentiated Bronchoalveolar	Slow to moderate	Early and most frequently via lymphatic and blood vessels to brain, liver, bone, adrenal glands	Form glandular structures in scar or fibrous tissue; single distal pul-monary nodule	• Stage I and II: Resectable • Stage III: Chemotherapy and radiotherapy • Stage IV: Chemotherapy
	• Large-cell carcinoma • 5%–10% • Undifferentiated cells: Giant-cell Clear-cell	Rapid	Early and wide-spread to small intestine	Large, bulky necrotic masses in major or intermediate-sized bronchi or in periphery	• Stage I and II: Resectable • Stage III: Chemotherapy and radiotherapy • Stage IV: Chemotherapy

of the bronchial mucosa. Severe paroxysms of coughing may lead to cough-induced rib fractures, rupture of an emphysematous bleb, or cough syncope. Cough and sputum production are not specific symptoms because the majority of lung cancer patients also suffer from chronic bronchitis and emphysema due to cigarette smoking; however, a change in the character of the cough, a change in the quality and quantity of sputum, or unresponsiveness to previously effective therapy (e.g., bronchodilators, antibiotics, steroids) should raise the suspicion that a tumor is present.

Many patients with lung cancer experience dyspnea as a result of multiple disruptions in physiological function of the respiratory system. Dyspnea has been reported in 26% to 60% of patients presenting with NSCLC and is often an ominous development, signifying intrathoracic

extension or dissemination. Some patients may have dyspnea resulting from underlying pulmonary disorders such as pulmonary fibrosis or COPD. These patients may experience difficulties in airway clearance associated with excessive tracheobronchial secretions, thick tenacious secretions, muscle weakness, and chest pain. Central lung cancers cause dyspnea by means of obstruction, with or without postobstructive pneumonitis. Large pleural effusion or paralysis of a hemidiaphragm resulting from phrenic nerve involvement may also cause dyspnea. The assessment of dyspnea should include a description of the onset, duration, magnitude, and precipitating events. It is especially important to identify any interventions the patient has discovered that are helpful in relieving the dyspnea. Usually the chest radiograph in dyspneic patients demonstrates a sizable effusion, atelectasis of a lobe or entire lung, or clear evidence of intrapulmonary dissemination.

Chest pain with deep inspiration or coughing may be reported, as well as fatigue and anorexia. Chest pain in lung cancer may indicate local invasion of the pleura, ribs, and nerves. Pain may be dull, constant, and debilitating or intermittent and sharp, varying with the respiratory cycle. It may localize to the chest wall, or it may radiate to the midback, scapula, shoulder, or arm on the side of the tumor. The pain is usually a dull intermittent ache lasting from minutes to hours on the same side as the tumor and is not related to cough or respiration. Intercostal retractions, supraclavicular retractions, and/or use of accessory muscles on inspiration indicate obstruction to air inflow, whereas bulging interspaces on expiration are associated with outflow obstruction; either may be an indication of tumor. It is important to distinguish the chest pain that accompanies direct contiguous chest wall extension from painful rib metastases that are anatomically remote from the primary lesion.

Chest discomfort can be associated with atelectasis. Atelectasis develops in the patient with lung cancer secondary to mechanical obstruction of the airways, compression of lung tissue, and shallow breathing patterns. When the tumor obstructs the airway, it prevents or reduces alveolar ventilation to a region of the lung and produces atelectasis in that region. The size of the atelectic area depends on the size of the obstructed airway and the degree of obstruction. Localized compression of lung tissue occurs with large tumors and with large pleural effusions secondary to metastases.

Hemoptysis is seen in up to 30% of patients and occurs when the tumor erodes the epithelial layer or invades a blood vessel. It occurs more often in squamous-cell carcinoma and large-cell carcinoma than in SCLC. Typically, hemoptysis consists only of blood-streaked sputum, which is sometimes erroneously attributed to chronic bronchitis. The quantity of blood is usually small, but it can become massive and life-threatening. Hemoptysis usually prompts the patient to seek medical attention and is suggestive of endobronchial tumor. Inspection very seldom reveals any changes in the chest wall. Palpation may reveal lymph node enlargement.

Nonspecific Systemic Symptoms

Systemic symptoms of lung cancer include generalized weakness and fatigue, anorexia, cachexia, weight loss, and anemia. These nonspecific signs and symptoms are common in both SCLC and NSCLC. Weight loss, which usually (but not always) is accompanied by anorexia, occurs in more than one-half of the patients, and generalized weakness occurs in one-third. Fever and anemia occur in about 20% of patients. Fever generally is not considered to be paraneoplastic in patients with lung cancer; if present, it usually is associated with a documented infection or liver metastases.

Table 9.16 presents a summary of these clinical manifestations of lung cancer.

Objective Auscultation may reveal wheezing if an airway is partially obstructed. The wheezing is usually monophonic and localized and does not disappear after a cough. Wheezing may be heard on both inhalation and exhalation. Absent or decreased breath sounds can be heard when normal lung tissue is replaced by tumor or when the patient has a pleural effusion. Percussion reveals diminished resonance over lung tissue affected by a large tumor, pleural effusion, or pneumonia (consolidation). Decreased tactile fremitus may be associated with pleural effusion and tumors of the pleural cavity, whereas increased tactile fremitus may indicate a lung mass.

The most frequent peripheral sign of lung cancer is clubbing of the fingers, which at times is associated with

Table 9.16	Clinical Manifestations of Lung Cancer
Nonspecific systemic manifestations	Weakness
	Fatigue
	Fever
	Anorexia
	Cachexia
	Anemia
	Symptoms associated with paraneoplastic syndromes
Intrathoracic or local-regional manifestations	Cough
	Dyspnea
	Hemoptysis
	Wheezing
	Chest pain
	Stridor
	Hoarseness
	Vocal cord paralysis
	Hiccups
	Atelectasis
	Pneumonia
	Pancoast's syndrome
	Horner's syndrome
	Pleural effusion
	Pericardial effusion
	Superior vena cava syndrome
Manifestations resulting from extrathoracic involvement	Bone pain
	Headache
	Dizziness
	Lymphadenopathy
	CNS disturbances
	Gastrointestinal disturbances
	Jaundice
	Hepatomegaly
	Abdominal pain

generalized hypertrophic pulmonary osteoarthropathy (HPO), also known as Bamberger-Marie disease. HPO often resembles RA. The clinical syndrome consists of swelling of the soft tissues of the terminal phalanges, with curvature of the nails, pain and swelling of the joints, and periostitis of the long bones, with elevation of the periosteum and new bone formation. The incidence of HPO, almost exclusively in patients with NSCLC, has been reported to be from 2% to 12%. It occurs only rarely, if ever, in small-cell tumors. Its occurrence is distributed equally among the other three major cell types of NSCLC. Removal of the pulmonary lesion may give dramatic remission of the arthralgia and peripheral edema.

Physical examination evidence for surgical nonresectability includes hoarseness, facial edema, arm pain, or changes in mental or emotional status. Hoarseness suggests vocal cord paralysis caused by recurrent laryngeal nerve compression by the tumor. Facial edema suggests compression of the superior vena cava by the tumor. Superior vena cava syndrome occurs when a lung tumor, usually SCLC, presses on the superior vena cava, partially or completely occluding it and impeding venous return from the head, neck, arms, and upper chest. Symptoms are related to venous obstruction, airway obstruction, and increased cerebral venous pressure. The most common symptoms include edema of the face, neck, arms, and upper torso. The conjunctiva may also be engorged. If the compression is untreated, neurological symptoms related to increased intracranial pressure may ensue, including headache, dizziness, visual disturbances, and occasionally alterations in mental status. Associated upper airway obstruction or signs of cerebral edema are very poor prognostic signs.

Tumor compression of the cervical sympathetic nerve plexus causes Horner's syndrome, which consists of unilateral ptosis, miosis, and ipsilateral anhidrosis (lack of sweating due to extension of the tumor into the paravertebral sympathetic nerves). Horner's syndrome is often associated with radiographic evidence of destruction of the first and second ribs. Pancoast's syndrome, manifested as arm and shoulder pain, suggests invasion of the brachial nerve plexus by a superior sulcus tumor. In addition, there may be muscular atrophy and decreased range of motion in the arm and shoulder; the patient may walk supporting the elbow of the affected arm.

Symptoms Due to Extrathoracic Involvement

Extrathoracic metastatic spread most often occurs in the lymph nodes, brain, bones, liver, and suprarenal glands. Bone pain caused by metastasis occurs in approximately 25% to 40% of patients although pathological fractures are rare. Neurological symptoms resulting from intracranial metastases are present in 3% to 6% of patients. These include hemiplegia, epilepsy, personality changes, confusion, speech defects, gait disturbances, or only nonspecific headache. Symptoms that relate to liver

involvement (right upper quadrant pain) are less common or nonspecific (e.g., nausea, weight loss, anemia). Rarely, jaundice, ascites, or an abdominal mass is the major complaint. Neck, muscle, or subcutaneous tissue masses are present infrequently. Involvement of adrenal glands often is asymptomatic, and most adrenal metastases are discovered incidentally, either during staging evaluation or at autopsy. If symptomatic, it presents with unilateral pain in the flank, abdomen, or costovertebral angle. Although adrenal metastases are fairly common, signs of adrenal insufficiency are rarely seen.

Paraneoplastic Syndromes

Associated with lung cancer are approximately 21 identified syndromes that meet the usual definition of the term *paraneoplastic*. Approximately 2% of patients with lung cancer seek medical advice for systemic symptoms and signs not related to metastatic spread of the tumor, the so-called paraneoplastic syndromes shown in Table 9.17. The major categories of paraneoplastic

Table 9.17	Paraneoplastic Syndromes Associated With Lung Cancer
Type of Cancer	**Associated Paraneoplastic Syndrome**
SCLC	• Ectopic adrenocorticotropic hormone (Cushing's syndrome) • Inappropriate antidiuretic hormone secretion • Lambert-Eaton myasthenic syndrome • Atrial natriuretic factor • Hyperpigmentation
NSCLC	• Humoral hypercalcemia • Hypertrophic pulmonary osteoarthropathy • Nephrotic syndrome • Hypoglycemia • Gynecomastia • Nonbacterial thrombotic endocarditis
All Lung Cancers	• Hypercoagulable state • Disseminated intravascular coagulation • Erythrocytosis • Granulocytosis • Neurological and myopathic syndromes (dementia, limbic encephalitis, optic neuropathy, sensory neuropathy, sensorimotor peripheral neuropathy) • Dermatological syndromes (acanthosis nigricans, acquired ichthyosis, dermatomyositis)

syndromes include endocrine, neurological, cardiovascular, skeletal, and cutaneous manifestation.

Paraneoplastic syndromes are often the first indication of the presence of a tumor and may antedate the demonstrable tumor by a period ranging from months to years. SCLC is associated with paraneoplastic syndromes more frequently than the NSCLCs. The majority of metabolic manifestations are the result of secretion of endocrine or endocrine-like substances by the tumor.

Hyperadrenocorticism, in association with ectopic secretion of adrenocorticotropic hormone, is a frequently observed hormonal syndrome in lung cancer, particularly with SCLC patients. It manifests as severe weakness, weight loss, edema, hypertension, hypokalemia, and hyperglycemia. The syndrome of inappropriate antidiuretic hormone secretion, seen in 5% to 10% of all SCLCs, results from antidiuretic hormone secretion by the tumor and is associated with symptoms of water intoxication (anorexia, nausea, and vomiting). Symptoms include hyponatremia and low serum osmolality, characterized by mental status changes, lethargy, seizures, and confusion. Hyponatremia resulting from the secretion of atrial natriuretic factor also can occur in some patients.

Hypercalcemia may be caused by bony metastases or excessive secretion by the tumor (usually a squamous-cell tumor) or parathyroid hormone–related protein, so-called humoral hypercalcemia of malignancy. Although squamous-cell carcinoma is most commonly associated with hypercalcemia, other histological types can cause the syndrome as well. An accompanying hypophosphatemia is also frequently found. Clinically, the hypercalcemic patient may have somnolence, irritability, confusion, or coma, as well as anorexia, nausea, vomiting, constipation, and weight loss. The Eaton-Lambert myasthenic syndrome occurs in about 6% of patients with SCLC. This pseudomyasthenic syndrome is thought to be an autoimmune disorder in which the release of acetylcholine by the motor nerve terminals is impaired. Symptoms include proximal limb muscle weakness and fatigue (especially in the pelvis, thighs, arms, and shoulders), peripheral paresthesia, dry mouth, dysphagia, diplopia, ptosis, difficulty chewing, and double vision.

Diagnostic Reasoning

Early detection is the key to successful resection of the NSCLC tumors, but mass screening programs have failed to affect mortality rates. The histological cell type and the stage of the disease are the major factors that influence choice of therapy for individuals. The currently accepted system for the staging of lung cancer is the tumor-node-metastasis (TNM) classification presented in Table 9.18. This system is a code in which T denotes the extent of the primary tumor (ranging from T0 to T4), N indicates the nodal involvement (ranging from N0 to N3), and M describes the extent of metastasis (M0 or M1). The stage of disease (also in Table 9.18) is based on a combination of clinical (physical exam, radiological, and laboratory studies) and pathological (biopsy of lymph nodes, bronchoscopy, mediastinoscopy, or

Table 9.18 Lung Cancer Staging	
Tumor-Node-Metastasis (TNM) Stage Grouping for Lung Cancer	
Occult cancer	TX N0 M0
Stage 0	Tis N0 M0
Stage I	T1 N0 M0; T2 N0 M0
Stage II	T1 N1 M0; T2 N1 M0
Stage IIIA	T1 N2 M0; T2 N2 M0; T3 N0 M0; T3 N1 M0; T3 N2 M0
Stage IIIB	Any T N3 M0; T4 Any N M0
Stage IV	Any T Any N M1
TNM Definitions of Primary Tumor (T) Characteristics in Lung Cancer	
Primary (T)	
TX	Primary tumor cannot be assessed, or tumor proved by the presence of malignant cells in sputum or bronchial washings but not visualized by imaging or bronchoscopy.
T0	No evidence of primary tumor.
Tis	Carcinoma in situ.
T1	A tumor that is 3.0 cm or less in greatest diameter, surrounded by lung or visceral pleura and without evidence of invasion more proximal than the lobar bronchus (e.g., not in the main bronchus). (*Note:* The uncommon superficial tumor of any size with its invasive component limited to the bronchial wall, which may extend proximal to the main bronchus, is also classified as T1.)

Table 9.18	Lung Cancer Staging—cont'd
T1a	Tumor 2 cm or less in greatest dimension.
T1b	Tumor more than 2 cm but less than 3 cm in greatest dimension.
T2	A tumor with any of the following features of size or extent: more than 3.0 cm in greatest dimension; involving the main bronchus, 2.0 cm or more distal to the carina; invading the visceral pleura; associated with atelectasis or obstructive pneumonitis that extends to the hilar region but does not involve the entire lung.
T2a	Tumor more than 3 cm but less than 5 cm in greatest dimension.
T2b	Tumor more than 5 cm but less than 7 cm in greatest dimension.
T3	A tumor of any size with direct extension to the chest wall (including superior sulcus tumors), diaphragm, mediastinal pleura, parietal pericardium; a tumor in the main bronchus less than 2.0 cm distal to the carina but without involvement of the carina; associated atelectasis or obstructive pneumonitis of the entire lung.
T4	A tumor of any size that invades any of the following: mediastinum, heart, great vessels, trachea, esophagus, vertebral body, carina; or tumor with a malignant pleural effusion.
Regional Lymph Nodes (N)	
NX	Regional lymph nodes cannot be assessed.
N0	No regional lymph node metastasis.
N1	Metastasis in ipsilateral peribronchial and/or ipsilateral hilar lymph nodes, including direct extension.
N2	Metastasis in ipsilateral mediastinal and/or subcarinal lymph node(s).
N3	Metastasis in contralateral mediastinal, contralateral hilar, ipsilateral or contralateral scalene, or supraclavicular lymph node(s).
Distant Metastasis (M)	
M0	No (known) distant metastasis.
M1	Distant metastases present; specify sites.
M1a	Separate tumor nodule(s) in a contralateral lobe, tumor with pleural nodules or malignant pleural (or pericardial) effusion.
M1b	Distant metastasis (in extrathoracic organs).

Note: Most pleural effusions associated with lung cancer are due to tumor; however, there are a few patients in whom multiple cytopathological examinations of pleural fluid are negative for tumor. In these cases, fluid is nonbloody and is not an exudate. When these elements and clinical judgment dictate that the effusion is not related to the tumor, the effusion should be excluded as a staging element and the patient should be staged as T1, T2, or T3.

paramedian sternotomy or other type of thoracotomy) staging.

The diagnostic approach for SCLC is the same as that for NSCLC, but the staging system is different. SCLC staging still focuses on disease extent but broadly classifies it as limited state (limited to one hemothorax with hilar and mediastinal nodes that can be included within a radiation therapy port) or extensive stage disease. The TNM staging system is not typically used for SCLC staging. The anatomical detail of the TNM classification system is unnecessary because surgical resection is not a recommended treatment modality.

Diagnostic Tests

Initial Testing A complete blood count (CBC) should be ordered because anemia may be associated with lung cancer, along with a basic metabolic panel and hepatic panel checking for abnormalities in Na, K, Ca, and liver enzymes, and a prothrombin time, partial thromboplastin time, and platelet count to assess for coagulopathies. An electrocardiogram (ECG) should be done, as well as baseline pulmonary function tests (PFTs). Anterior-posterior and lateral chest x-ray films remain the simplest method for identifying patients with lung cancer. The heart and other thoracic structures obscure large portions of the lung tissue, so it is important to evaluate both a frontal and a side view. The chest x-ray film may demonstrate asymptomatic lung cancer and is almost always abnormal when the patient is symptomatic. A tumor nodule must be at least 2 to 3 mm before it is visible on the chest radiograph. Associated atelectasis, postobstructive pneumonitis, abscess, bronchiolitis, rib erosion, pleural effusion, or bulky mediastinal lymphadenopathy may be identified on radiographs, thus raising a suspicion of primary lung malignancy. The four most common types of lung cancer usually present with slightly different chest radiographic patterns, but there is so much overlap that only biopsy and histological examination provide reliable evidence about the cell type. Mediastinal changes on radiograph may suggest lymphadenopathy or pleural effusions, and an elevated diaphragm may be seen with phrenic nerve involvement.

A chest computed tomography (CT) scan with infusion of contrast material has become widely accepted as the primary cross-sectional modality for evaluation of the thorax and is recommended to stage NSCLC. The CT scan should extend inferiorly to include the liver and the adrenal glands. Because of its earlier metastases and unresectability, staging for SCLC is less useful for treatment and prognosis. A contrast-enhanced chest CT scan will (1) characterize the size and location of the primary tumor and its relationship to other thoracic structures, (2) identify pathologically enlarged hilar and mediastinal lymph nodes, (3) identify satellite and other ipsilateral or contralateral pulmonary nodules, and (4) identify potential metastases to the liver and adrenal glands, both common metastatic sites.

Cytological evaluation of sputum, bronchial washing, bronchial brushings, and fine-needle aspirations have a high diagnostic value, but the positive and negative predictive values of each, as well as their accuracy of diagnosis, depend on sampling error, tissue preservation, processing quality, and observer experience. Sputum cytology remains a simple test with a positive predictive value that can approach 100%, but it has a sensitivity rate of only 10% to 15%. If a diagnosis can be established through collective sputum cytology, invasive tests often can be averted. Automated sputum screening is currently being evaluated and may play an increasingly important role in early diagnosis. The highest yield occurs in patients with large, centrally located tumors. It is much less helpful in diagnosing peripheral lesions because relatively few cells are released from the lesion, and those that are released rarely get to the central airways. Early-morning sputum samples are collected for 3 to 5 days; deep coughing is recommended because coughing dislodges cancer cells into the sputum.

Flexible fiberoptic bronchoscopy is an essential and standard technique for the evaluation of patients with pulmonary neoplasms. It remains the most important procedure for determining the endobronchial extent of disease. The extent and operability of the tumor are assessed by observing the site of the tumor and extent of airway involvement. When lesions are visible endobronchially, bronchial washings have a diagnostic yield of approximately 90%; bronchial brushings and bronchial mucosal forceps biopsy samples provide diagnosis of tissue in nearly 98% of visualized tumors. Under fluoroscopic control, transbronchial forceps biopsies, brushings, and washings can diagnose peripheral, parenchymal lesions up to 80% of the time. The visual assessment of the primary tumor can also provide a clinically useful estimate of the probability of tumor complications such as airway obstruction, postobstructive pneumonia, or hemoptysis.

Transthoracic percutaneous fine-needle aspiration (fine-needle aspiration biopsy) is used when lung lesions cannot be visualized by bronchoscopy but are accessible percutaneously. A needle guided by CT or fluoroscopy is inserted into the lesion for aspiration of cells. This procedure is most suitable for peripheral pulmonary nodules. Pneumothorax is the most common complication, with an increased risk in the patient with COPD. A positive pleural fluid cytology proves the spread of malignancy to the pleural space. Thoracentesis and pleural biopsy combined provide up to a 90% diagnostic yield in patients with malignancy.

Mediastinoscopy is an invasive procedure used for the diagnosis and staging of lung cancer. A biopsy is recommended if mediastinal lymph nodes are found on chest CT scan that are greater than 1.0 cm for the patient with clinically operable NSCLC. The patient with lymphadenopathy on chest CT scan will most likely have positive nodes on biopsy. Anterior cervical mediastinoscopy allows direct visualization and biopsy of mediastinal nodes with less risk than an exploratory thoracotomy.

Video-assisted thoracoscopic surgery is used for the staging and diagnosis of lung cancer when less invasive techniques fail to yield a diagnosis. Small thoracotomy incisions are made through which thoracoscopic instruments are inserted. Visualization of the chest and mediastinum and assessment of pleural effusions are superior to that achieved using older scopes, which may help improve diagnostic accuracy.

Thoracoscopy is useful for pleural evaluation but less useful for evaluating the lung. It is more than 90% sensitive for the diagnosis of pleural-based malignancies and peripheral lung nodules, with a specificity of 99%. With a thoracoscope, the mediastinum can be entered and nodes biopsied. Thoracoscopy affords the potential for more complete staging of patients with suspected mediastinal nodal spread and it has become a valuable adjunct to cervical mediastinoscopy and anterior mediastinotomy. There is a concern, however, about seeding the thoracoscope entrance site with tumor cells.

Subsequent Testing A head CT scan or brain magnetic resonance imaging, with and without infusion of contrast material, is recommended only in patients who have signs or symptoms of central nervous system disease. The finding of an isolated adrenal mass on ultrasonographic or CT exam requires biopsy to rule out metastatic disease if the patient is considered to be potentially resectable. NSCLC metastasizes to the adrenal glands in 18% to 38% of cases. A bone scan should be performed only in patients who complain of bone pain or chest pain or who have an elevated serum calcium level or an elevated serum alkaline phosphatase level. It is estimated that between 9% and 15% of patients with newly diagnosed NSCLC have bony metastases at presentation, with the vertebral bodies most commonly being affected. Finally, the finding of an isolated hepatic mass on ultrasonographic or CT exam requires a biopsy to rule out metastatic disease if the patient is otherwise considered to be potentially resectable.

Differential Diagnosis

The symptoms of lung cancer develop gradually in most cases and are often attributed by the patient to a smoker's cough or cold and by the patient's health-care provider to tracheobronchitis, pneumonia, influenza, pulmonary infarction, or lung abscess. Thus, it is common for a patient to delay seeking medical attention for several months from the first recognizable onset of symptoms. Several additional months of symptomatic treatment and antibiotics frequently pass before the health-care provider establishes the correct diagnosis. Much of the initial diagnostic task is to differentiate if this is a primary tumor or a metastatic cancer. This is evaluated on biopsy. Other differential diagnoses include tuberculosis, lymphoma, *Mycobacterium avium* complex, sarcoidosis, or a foreign body aspiration that has been retained.

Management

Active patient participation in decision making respects the fundamental ethical and legal doctrine of autonomy and is especially important for the patient with unresectable NSCLC, because the prognosis is often poor and symptom palliation is a central concern. Fewer than half of patients with lung cancer are candidates for resection, and only a small percentage of these are cured, so most patients with the disease require some form of palliation. Therapy should include efforts to slow the growth of the tumor and to treat complications as they arise, but above all, symptoms should be relieved.

Surgery

Surgical resection offers the best chance of cure for lung cancer. The patient with stage I or II NSCLC is routinely resected via a thoracotomy. Pneumonectomy (removal of a whole lung) and lobectomy (removal of a single lobe) are the most common of these surgical procedures. The nature of the tumor dictates the procedure, whereas pulmonary function determines if the patient can withstand the procedure. Pneumonectomy is required when the tumor or lymph nodes involve proximal structures such that a lung-conserving operation will not allow complete resection. Lobectomy is the most common resection performed for lung cancer. Such a resection allows removal of the primary tumor, associated disease, and lymph node–bearing areas while leaving a significant amount of residual functional parenchyma. Survival is equivalent for patients undergoing lobectomy or pneumonectomy for all stages of disease when a complete resection is performed. For lesions close to the lobar orifice, an adequate margin of resection often cannot be achieved. In such circumstances, a portion of the main bronchus must be included with the resection. This type of resection is termed *sleeve resection,* and it is performed as a parenchyma-sparing procedure avoiding pneumonectomy.

Very limited resection in the treatment of lung cancer has been reserved for patients with extremely poor pulmonary function who could tolerate no more than a very limited resection because of their underlying medical condition or low pulmonary reserve. Limited resections include segmentectomy, wedge resection, or lumpectomy. Segmental resection is the removal of a lung segment, and wedge resection is the removal of a small, V-shaped wedge of lung tissue. Lesions that reside more deeply within the pulmonary tissue often are not amenable to wedge resection and may require precise, local excision with laser or electrocautery assistance (e.g., lumpectomy). These techniques are used to preserve as much lung tissue as possible, and they are performed for the removal of small tumors located close to the surface of the lung. The guiding principle of surgical therapy in lung cancer is to remove the tumor completely, leaving as much functioning pulmonary tissue as possible. The aim of most operations is curative, and procedures that leave gross tumor are not warranted. Resection is abandoned if the tumor extends beyond the lung, when pleural seeding is evident, or when fixed mediastinal nodes are present.

Patients with stage I disease have a 50% to 80% 5-year survival and patients with stage II disease have a 25% to 50% survival at 5 years. However, 75% of patients present with advanced disease and significant comorbidities. Treatment decisions should consider symptom control, quality of life, the patient's value or meaning of life, and the patient's perceptions and attitudes about a specific treatment.

Chemotherapy

Neoadjuvant chemotherapy involves giving antineoplastic drugs before surgery or radiation therapy. Adjuvant chemotherapy involves administering antineoplastic drugs after surgery or radiation therapy. Given that chemotherapy for advanced disease is marginally beneficial and noncurative, its use must be governed judiciously, with each decision evaluated individually for each patient.

Current chemotherapeutic approaches consist initially of defining new combinations of established chemotherapeutic agents that may act synergistically (Table 9.19). In addition, new drugs with novel mechanisms of action are also being investigated, both as single agents and, subsequently, as agents to be used in combination with established drugs.

Non–Small-Cell Lung Cancer Chemotherapy Chemotherapy modestly improves median survival with distant metastatic NSCLC compared with best supportive care, but it is not curative.

If a patient has Stage I disease, there is no agreement on the role of adjuvant chemotherapy. It is more widely used with patients with Stage II and IIIA disease. Patients with Stage I and N0 Stage II disease treated with multidrug platinum-based chemotherapy show improved survival of 3 months at 5 years. Because of the toxicity, risks versus benefits must be discussed with the patient and family. Newer drugs with less toxicity are currently being studied. With patients in advanced stages, chemotherapy has shown to improve the patient's quality of life by decreasing bothersome symptoms.

For patients with Stage III lung cancer that cannot be removed surgically, chemotherapy is typically combined with definitive high-dose radiation treatments. In Stage IV lung cancer, chemotherapy is typically the main treatment, because radiation is used only for palliation of symptoms. Chemotherapy usually consists of a combination of dugs including cisplatin (Platinol)

or carboplatin (Paraplatin) plus docetaxel (Taxotere), gemcitabine (Gemzar), paclitaxel (Taxol), vinorelbine (Navelbine), or pemetrexed (Alimta).

The newest developments in lung cancer treatment are targeted treatments. Whereas chemotherapy drugs cannot differentiate between normal cells and cancer cells, targeted therapies are designed specifically to attack cancer cells by attaching to or blocking targets that appear on cancer cell surfaces. Patients with advanced lung cancer with certain molecular biomarkers may receive treatment with a targeted drug alone or in combination with chemotherapy. Some of these targeted treatments include erlotinib (Tarceva), bevacizumab (Avastin), and crizotinib (Xalkori).

Small-Cell Lung Cancer Chemotherapy Combination chemotherapy is capable of effecting high objective response rates in SCLC. Furthermore, the simultaneous administration of multiple agents is superior to the sequential administration of the same drugs. Chemotherapy is most effective in SCLC with an 80% to 100% response in limited-stage disease (50%–70% complete response) and 60% to 80% response in extensive stage disease (15%–40% complete response). Remissions last a median of 6 to 8 months. If the cancer recurs, the median survival time is 3 to 4 months. Among the regimens, cisplatin plus etoposide (Toposar or Vepesid) is the current treatment of choice for many reasons. In the setting of relapsed SCLC, the combination of cisplatin and etoposide is capable of producing objective response rates of equal to or more than 50% in patients who have experienced a recurrence after cyclophosphamide-based therapy. No other drug combination has yielded response rates of this magnitude in a similar setting. Further, in previously untreated patients, cisplatin plus etoposide yields excellent overall response rates and survival results that are equivalent to cyclophosphamide- or doxorubicin-based regimens, albeit with less host-related toxicity. Cisplatin plus etoposide is particularly well suited for the simultaneous administration of radiotherapy, given its lower incidence of toxicity and the putative radiation-sensitizing effect of both drugs. Thus, for many clinicians, cisplatin plus etoposide has become the de facto standard induction regimen for the patient with SCLC. Occasionally, some may use carboplatin (Paraplatin) plus irinotecan (Camptosar).

Radiation

The basic indication for radiation therapy is inoperability; in addition, radiation is sometimes used to help prevent metastasis to the brain as prophylactic cranial irradiation. Radiation therapy can modify the natural course of the disease, relieve distressing symptoms, and produce an apparent cure in an occasional patient. Long-term results, however, have been generally disappointing. One-year and 5-year overall survival rates range from 25% to 55% and from 4% to 10%, respectively.

Table 9.19	Chemotherapeutic Agents Used to Treat Lung Cancer
Small-Cell Lung Cancer	**Non–Small-Cell Lung Cancer**
cisplatin* (Platinol) plus etoposide* (Vepesid, Toposar) carboplatin (Paraplatin) plus irinotecan (Camptosar)	*Localized disease:* cisplatin* (Platinol) or carboplatin* (Paraplatin) plus docetaxel* (Taxotere), gemcitabine (Gemzar), paclitaxel (Taxol and others), vinorelbine (Navelbine and others), or pemetrexed (Alimta). *Targeted treatments:* erlotinib (Tarceva) bevacizumab (Avastin) crizotinib (Xalkori)

*Current treatment of choice.

It is used as adjunctive therapy after surgery to improve tumor control, and it is used as palliative therapy to control symptoms in others.

Non–Small-Cell Lung Cancer Radiation Radiation therapy is commonly offered to the patient with inoperable NSCLC when the cancer has not spread beyond the thorax. In this case, the asymptomatic patient or the patient who is still functioning at a high level is most likely to benefit. In addition, radiation therapy is used to shrink the tumor and control symptoms in the patient with inoperable lung cancer and to prevent brain metastasis. Treating the tumor with radiation therapy may relieve hemoptysis, shoulder and arm pain, chest pain, and dyspnea. It can be used in superior vena cava obstruction to reduce the tumor size and alleviate obstruction. Although there are currently no data that demonstrate a survival advantage for postoperative adjuvant therapy in patients with completely resected Stage II disease, regardless of whether the patient receives radiation therapy alone or radiation therapy and chemotherapy, most of these patients are treated with postoperative radiation therapy to decrease local recurrence. Unfortunately, prevention of local recurrence has not been shown to translate into survival benefit. The patient with a malignant pleural effusion or with distant metastatic disease is not appropriate for definitive thoracic radiotherapy.

Small-Cell Lung Cancer Radiation SCLC is quite sensitive to both radiation and chemotherapy. In limited-stage SCLC, the addition of both radiation and chemotherapy can increase the 5-year survival rate from about 11% to 20%. Most oncologists consider thoracic radiation therapy in combination with chemotherapy for limited-stage disease to be the standard of care. The major contribution of thoracic irradiation is local tumor control, and local control of the intrathoracic tumor is a sine qua non for cure. Thoracic radiation therapy does reduce the risk of dying of SCLC but at the price of increased toxicity. Concurrent or alternating treatment schedules appear to improve response rates over sequential chemotherapy and radiation therapy, although toxicity is more intense with concurrent therapy.

A summary of the treatment of NSCLC is shown in Treatment Flowchart 9.3.

Follow-up and Referral

When lung cancer is first detected, the patient should be referred to a specialist for staging and treatment decisions. The patient who has been successfully treated for lung cancer needs to be followed routinely. The goal of monitoring patients with unresectable lung cancer in complete remission is to detect symptomatic progression of their disease that may benefit from therapeutic intervention or symptom management. However, the great majority of patients with unresectable Stage III and Stage IV disease will not achieve a complete remission, or, if achieved, the duration of remission will be short.

A history and physical examination should be performed every 3 months during the first 2 years, every 6 months thereafter through year 5, and yearly thereafter. For the patient treated with curative intent, there is no clear role for routine x-ray evaluation in the asymptomatic patient and for those in whom no interventions are planned. A yearly chest x-ray film to evaluate for potentially curable second primary cancers may be reasonable. CT of the chest/abdomen, bronchoscopy, CBC, and routine chemistries, including liver function tests, should be performed only as indicated by the patient's symptoms. These tests do not appear to detect asymptomatic recurrent disease with a high frequency.

Patient Education

Assessment of learning needs and provision of information is likely to be of paramount importance for the patient at the time of initial biopsy, between diagnosis and definitive treatment, and at discharge. These are highly stressful times for patients, and they may be easily overwhelmed by the information regarding treatment options. It is important to assess what level of participation in the decision-making process is desired by the patient because that will help direct informational interventions and can reduce anxiety and psychological distress. This is particularly important for patients who have a choice between two treatment options or are deciding between participating in a clinical trial or receiving standard therapy.

Smoking cessation, never initiating smoking, and avoidance of occupational and environmental exposure to carcinogenic substances are recommended as effective interventions to reduce the risk of a second primary lung cancer in the curatively treated patient. For the patient with distant metastatic disease, the outlook is poor, and smoking cessation has little effect on overall prognosis but may improve respiratory symptoms. A tapering nicotine patch or other delivery system has been proved to increase the odds of smoking cessation when combined with behavioral interventions.

Recommendations for lifestyle change are the same for the patient with a history of lung cancer as for those who have no previous history of lung cancer. Epidemiological studies also suggest that people who consume relatively large amounts of fruits and vegetables have a lower risk of both cancer and cardiovascular disease. Antioxidant vitamins contained in fruits and vegetables prevent carcinogenesis by interfering with oxidative damage to DNA and lipoproteins; however, the use of antioxidants and/or chemopreventive agents for lung cancer (retinoic acid, beta-carotene, and selenium) is investigational.

When medical care for the patient with lung cancer shifts from curative to palliative, the patient and family must choose a care setting. Home or hospice care can provide familiar surroundings, feelings of normalcy, involvement of family, and a more comforting situation as they participate in readiness for death activities. Although

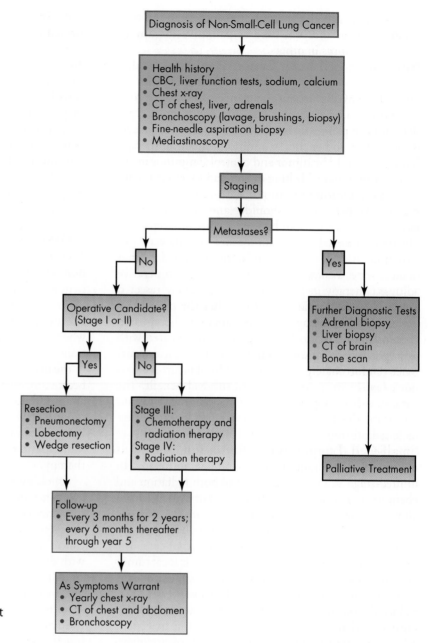

Treatment Flowchart 9.3 Treatment of Non–Small-Cell Lung Cancer

hospice has proved to be an extremely effective model for terminal care, referrals to a hospice often are not made until the final days of life. The difficulty lies in predicting when death will occur, because Medicare reimbursement requires that a hospice patient have a life expectancy of 6 months or less. Many states now have an "open access" model that allows for patients seeking curative care to still receive hospice services. Supportive resources for self-care should be provided as required by the individual situation. Patients will be able to manage less self-care as the disease progresses, and family members will require education with demonstration of care techniques and opportunities for questions and verbalization of feelings about caring for the one who is ill. Within the *Circle of Caring* model, collaborative planning is essential in

helping the patient and family make informed choices and live in the moment.

■ INTERSTITIAL LUNG DISEASE

Interstitial lung disease (ILD) encompasses nearly 200 clinical disorders that affect the epithelium, the endothelium, or both cell surfaces of alveolar wall and satellite structures, including terminal and respiratory bronchioles. ILD comprises a heterogeneous group of diseases that cause inflammation and fibrosis of the lower respiratory tract. The term *pulmonary fibrosis* is also applied to these diseases because fibrosis of the lung is the ultimate result of ILD. The term *interstitial* is misleading in that most of these disorders have extensive alteration of alveolar and airway architecture as well. *Diffuse parenchymal lung disease* is, perhaps, a more appropriate descriptive term for this heterogeneous group of lung diseases, because the term *interstitium* usually refers to the microscopic anatomical space bounded by the basement membranes of epithelial and endothelial cells. The entire lung parenchyma is affected, however, in ILD.

The ILDs have many common features, including similarity of patient symptoms, comparable appearance of chest x-ray films, consistent derangements in pulmonary physiology, and typical histological features. Four different infections may be associated with the cause or onset of most of the various diseases: disseminated fungus (coccidioidomycosis, blastomycosis, histoplasmosis), disseminated mycobacteria, *Pneumocystis* pneumonia, and certain viruses.

Although all of the diffuse ILDs share the common morphological characteristic of an abnormal lung interstitium, a satisfactory classification has been elusive because about 150 individual diseases have a component of interstitial lung involvement, either as primary disease or as a significant part of a multiorgan process, such as a collagen-vascular disease. Generally, ILDs are classified according to the type of agent that caused the lung injury. About one-third of patients with ILD have an identifiable agent responsible for inducing lung injury; however, the large majority of patients have disease attributable to no known cause. Therefore, ILDs are classified as those with a known cause and those with an unknown etiology; each of these groups is further subclassified according to the presence or absence of granuloma in interstitial or vascular areas.

Epidemiology and Causes

As many as 81 of every 100,000 Americans have some form of ILD. For patients with usual interstitial pneumonia, there is a slight male predominance with occurrence between ages 55 and 60. There is a slightly younger age distribution associated with some of the other ILDs (age 40–45 for respiratory bronchiolitis–associated ILD and age 45–55 for nonspecific interstitial pneumonitis). ILDs of known cause can be divided into several major subcategories. By far the largest group comprises occupational and environmental inhalant diseases; these include diseases resulting from inhalation of inorganic dusts, organic dusts, gases, fumes, vapors, and aerosols. Other categories include ILDs caused by drugs, irradiation, poisons, neoplasia, and chronic cardiac failure. The major subgroups within the category of unknown causes are idiopathic pulmonary fibrosis (IPF) and connective tissue (collagen vascular) disorders with ILD, including rheumatoid arthritis (RA), systemic lupus erythematosus (SLE), progressive systemic sclerosis, polymyositis-dermatomyositis, and Sjögren's syndrome. Systemic vasculitides often have granulomas in tissue and include a variant of polyarteritis nodosa called allergic granulomatosis, lymphomatoid granulomatosis, and hypersensitivity vasculitis.

Seven major entities that are most frequently associated with diffuse ILD are (1) idiopathic pulmonary fibrosis, (2) bronchiolitis obliterans organizing pneumonia, (3) connective tissue (collagen vascular) diseases (SLE, RA, progressive systemic sclerosis, and polymyositis-dermatomyositis), (4) systemic granulomatous vasculitides (Wegener's granulomatosis [WG], lymphomatoid granulomatosis, and allergic angiitis and granulomatosis), (5) drug-induced pulmonary disease, (6) sarcoidosis, and (7) hypersensitivity pneumonitis.

Pathophysiology

ILD denotes a diverse group of conditions characterized by the common pathological finding of pulmonary fibrosis and similar clinical presentation of restrictive lung findings (i.e., dyspnea on exertion and chronic nonproductive cough). The term *interstitial* used to describe this group of diseases is misleading because inflammation and fibrosis affect bronchioles, alveoli, and capillary endothelia, as well as the interstitium of the lower respiratory tract. Thus, a more illustrative term for this disease is *pulmonary fibrosis*. Sarcoidosis, hypersensitivity pneumonitis, pulmonary fibrosis in connective tissue disorders (e.g., SLE, RA, tuberous sclerosis, scleroderma), and occupational pulmonary diseases are all categorized as ILDs. Tissue injury and acute inflammation are believed to be the initial pathological processes. In some conditions, such as sarcoidosis, the inciting antigen is unknown, whereas occupational pulmonary diseases are caused by repeated inhalation of environmental irritants, inorganic and organic dusts, fumes, or gases. For most ILDs, including idiopathic conditions, cigarette smoking is a primary risk factor.

In the majority of ILDs, there is a perpetuation of the inflammatory process with repeated tissue injury and aberrant wound healing with subsequent remodeling of the lung architecture. Infiltration of the lung parenchyma by various combinations of immune cells mediates this process, including neutrophils, lymphocytes, plasma cells, eosinophils, basophils, mast cells, and alveolar macrophages. Cytokine production (e.g., granulocyte colony-stimulating factor, transforming growth factor–β1, interleukin (IL)–1β, IL-8, tumor necrosis factor–alpha) drives these inflammatory and wound-healing processes. Regions of chronic inflammation can develop granulomas consisting specifically of discrete masses of lymphocytes, macrophages, and fibroblasts. In turn, fibroblast proliferation and differentiation into myofibroblast forms (i.e., cells with both fibroblast and smooth muscle cell features) lead to fibrosis (collagen deposition) or scarring of the lungs and the development of cystic airspaces known as "honeycombing."

Such pathological pulmonary tissue becomes less compliant and increasingly rigid, with consequential impedance of ventilation and gas exchange, characteristic of a progressive, minimally reversible restrictive lung disease. Diffusion capacity also worsens with increasing fibrosis of the lung parenchyma. In turn, ventilation–perfusion mismatch, hypoxemia, and pulmonary vasoconstriction develop, and increased resistance on the right ventricle may lead to cor pulmonale (right ventriculomegaly). Hypercarbia typically manifests only in end-stage disease. Total lung capacity, functional residual capacity, residual volume, and forced expiratory volumes (FEV and FEV_1) are all commonly decreased on pulmonary function testing; however, because fibrotic lung tissue is stiffer with greater elastic recoil, rapid exhalation of a major portion of the expiratory volume may be seen, as reflected in a normal or increased FEV_1/FVC ratio on pulmonary function tests (PFTs)—a key feature distinguishing restrictive from obstructive pulmonary disease.

Interestingly, recurrent dysregulated wound healing rather than neutrophilic or immune cell–mediated inflammation has been cited as the primary pathophysiological mechanism in ILD, potentially explaining the ineffectiveness of anti-inflammatory and immunosuppressive treatments in many forms of ILD. Lung tissue biopsy is not required for the diagnosis of ILD, which may be made from a combination of clinical and radiographic findings (including PFTs and certain serum markers of underlying connective tissue disease). However, the extent of lung fibrosis observed histopathologically is perhaps the most accurate prognostic indicator for this condition. In turn, much investigation has shifted toward antifibroblast therapies for ILD aimed at decreasing pulmonary collagen deposition.

Clinical Presentation

The typical patient with ILD presents with an insidious onset of dyspnea on exertion, often accompanied by fatigue and cough. This breathlessness has no other obvious cause such as asthma, obstructive airway disease, bronchitis, or heart failure. Although emphasis is usually given to this most common presentation of patients with ILD, the provider must recognize the variability of clinical presentations. Dyspnea is a virtually constant finding in patients with IPF, but it is by no means so consistent in other ILDs. Less common but important and sometimes misleading presentations include the following:

• Fatigue in the absence of dyspnea
• Dry cough without other respiratory symptoms
• Predominant systemic symptoms (e.g., fever, weight loss)
• Abnormal-appearing (90%) chest x-ray film in the absence of symptoms
• Incidental abnormalities of PFTs (discussed in testing)

Respiratory signs such as pleuritic chest pain, visceral chest pain, wheezing, or hemoptysis do not usually occur. Half of the patients have mucus hypersecretion and expectoration. This occurrence has been correlated with glandular hypertrophy in the airway mucosa and accumulated mucus in the airways. Patients with more advanced ILD may have clubbing and cyanosis. Clinical manifestations specific to the various types of ILD are discussed in Table 9.20.

Diagnostic Reasoning
Diagnostic Tests

Initial Testing The symptoms of ILD are similar regardless of the underlying cause. In addition, the symptoms of lung involvement are nonspecific and could

---

Table 9.20	Interstitial Lung Diseases

Interstitial Pulmonary Fibrosis
A syndrome progressing from alveolitis to interstitial inflammation to fibrosis of the lungs.
Pulmonary Manifestations: Presents with dyspnea, cough, fatigue, adventitious crackles sounding like Velcro, tachypnea, finger clubbing, abnormal PFTs.
Management: No curative medical therapy. Nonspecific anti-inflammatory agents and immunosuppressive drugs are generally ineffective; other treatment options include cytotoxic agents and antifibrotic agents (colchicine or penicillamine).

Bronchiolitis Obliterans Organizing Pneumonia (BOOP)
A disease characterized by masses of granulation tissue in the lumens of small airways with patchy organizing pneumonia distal to these obstructions.
Pulmonary Manifestations: Presents with cough, flu-like illness, inspiratory crackles, expiratory squeaks, restrictive ventilatory defect, and abnormal diffusing capacity; chest x-ray film shows patchy alveolar infiltrates often with a ground-glass appearance.
Management: Corticosteroid therapy.

Collagen Vascular Diseases
• **Systemic Lupus Erythematosus:** Chronic, multisystem inflammatory disease of connective tissue that involves the skin, joints, serous membranes (pleura, pericardium), kidneys, hematological system, and CNS.
Pulmonary Manifestations: May present with pleuritis with or without effusion, diaphragmatic dysfunction with reduced lung volume, acute lupus pneumonitis, diffuse alveolar hemorrhage, diffuse interstitial disease, pulmonary hypertension, and pulmonary thromboembolism.
Management: NSAIDs, corticosteroids, immunosuppressive agents (cyclophosphamide [Cytoxan]), plasmapheresis (severe cases).

Table 9.20   Interstitial Lung Diseases—cont'd

- **Rheumatoid Arthritis:** Chronic, systemic disease characterized by recurrent inflammation of the diarthrodial joints and related structures.
  Pulmonary Manifestations: Abnormal PFTs with reduced diffusing capacity and restrictive mechanics, pulmonary nodules, BOOP, pleuritis with or without effusion, ILD.
  Management: Rheumatoid lung disease responds very poorly to drug therapy; a trial of prednisone is usually given but fewer than 10% of patients have a measurable response.
- **Progressive Systemic Sclerosis (Scleroderma):** A disorder of connective tissue characterized by fibrotic, degenerative, and occasionally inflammatory changes in the skin, blood vessels, synovium, skeletal muscle, and internal organs.
  Pulmonary Manifestations: Presents with dyspnea, bibasilar crackles, reduced lung compliance, pleural thickening, and pulmonary fibrosis on x-ray, abnormal PFTs, pulmonary hypertension, recurrent aspiration pneumonia.
  Management: No specific drugs or combination of drugs have been proved effective; in general, corticosteroids are not beneficial, and only a few patients respond to penicillamine (Cuprimine) therapy.
- **Polymyositis-Dermatomyositis:** Diffuse inflammatory myopathies of striated muscle, producing symmetrical weakness, usually most severe in the proximal muscles.
  Pulmonary Manifestations: The three types of lung disease classically described are interstitial pneumonitis, aspiration pneumonia due to esophageal dysmotility, and pneumonia secondary to hypoventilation as a result of respiratory muscle involvement.
  Management: Corticosteroids; cyclophosphamide (Cytoxan).

Systemic Granulomatous Vasculitis

- **Wegener's Granulomatosis:** Characterized by a triad of (1) necrotizing granulomatous vasculitis of the upper and lower respiratory tracts, (2) glomerulonephritis, and (3) variable degrees of vasculitis of small arteries and veins.
  Pulmonary Manifestations: Upper respiratory tract lesions include sinusitis, otitis media, nasal septal ulceration. Pulmonary manifestations vary from focal granulomatous vasculitis to diffuse alveolitis and capillaritis that may present as alveolar hemorrhage. Pulmonary function tests reveal a restrictive pattern.
  Management: Cyclophosphamide (Cytoxan) and prednisone; azathioprine (Imuran) and methotrexate (Folex, Rheumatrex) are alternative agents.
- **Lymphomatoid Granulomatosis:** A systemic disease consisting of angiocentric lymphoid granulomatous vasculitis, primarily of the lungs, with frequent involvement of the kidneys and skin.
  Pulmonary Manifestations: Presenting symptoms are usually cough, dyspnea; chest x-ray reveals multiple, bilateral, ill-defined or nodular densities that may cavitate.
  Management: Cyclophosphamide (Cytoxan) and corticosteroids; chemotherapy regimen if recurrence with malignant lymphoma.
- **Allergic Angiitis and Granulomatosis (Churg-Strauss Syndrome):** Rare disorder characterized by necrotizing angiitis of the lungs, heart, skin, and CNS with involved organs containing infiltration with eosinophils.
  Pulmonary Manifestations: Presents with an allergic history, often with asthma; chest x-ray abnormalities may range from patchy densities to large bilateral nodular infiltrates; cavitation is rare.
  Management: Corticosteroids, prednisone, azathioprine (Imuran), cyclophosphamide (Cytoxan), plasma exchange.
- **Drug-induced Pulmonary Disease:** Iatrogenic and adverse complications of various drugs (cytotoxic agents, antibiotics, immunosuppressives).
  Pulmonary Manifestations: Hypersensitivity pulmonary disease with dyspnea, nonproductive cough, lung crackles, tachypnea, diffuse linear streaks and densities in lower lung zones on x-ray.
  Management: Discontinuation of the drug or reduction in drug dosage in conjunction with corticosteroid therapy.
- **Sarcoidosis:** A multisystem syndrome of unknown etiology, involving complex cellular immune pathways; it most frequently affects the lung.
  Pulmonary Manifestations: Lung most common organ affected; PFTs reveal a restrictive pattern and small lung volumes; tissue biology demonstrates characteristic granulomas.
  Management: Corticosteroids, and other drugs such as hydroxychloroquine (Plaquenil), methotrexate (Folex).
- **Hypersensitivity Pneumonitis (Allergic Alveolitis):** Caused by inhalation of a variety of organic dusts. Dusts can be derived from animal dander and proteins; from fungi that contaminate vegetables, wood bark, or water-reservoir vaporizers; and from dairy and grain products. Colorful, descriptive names for the diseases underscore the frequent occupational nature of exposure.
  Pulmonary Manifestations: In acute form of disease, respiratory and systemic symptoms develop explosively within 4–6 hours after dust is inhaled and consist of dyspnea, cough, chills, fever, and malaise. Symptoms abate in 12 hours. With each reexposure, the acute episode occurs again. The acutely ill patient is dyspneic with inspiratory crackles in lower lung zones. Chest x-ray film shows fine, diffuse alveolar filling and variable interstitial streaks, PFTs are abnormal.
  Management: Avoidance of inhaled substance, corticosteroids (prednisone).

suggest many other causes, including obstructive lung disease, heart disease, or pulmonary vascular disease. The first symptom of ILD is usually progressive dyspnea on exertion or a nonproductive cough. The patient initially notices dyspnea only during heavy exertion; but in very advanced stages of the disease, dyspnea occurs at rest.

The occupational and environmental history is the single most helpful tool to determine whether a respiratory problem may be related to an occupational or environmental exposure (see Focus on History 9.1). A careful history must include a detailed chronological account of the patient's employment activities, social activities, travel, immune status, pets, hobbies, and environment. A thorough review of the patient's past medical history, along with current and previous medications, is also important. The goal of these questions is to determine whether the patient has been exposed to agents known to cause ILD. Many patients have an occupational history that includes exposure to one or a variety of toxic inhalation products, and this may add uncertainty to the precise onset of symptoms and may suggest the contribution of several etiological factors. The temporal relationship to the exposure may be obvious in some cases, but in others a low-grade exposure may provoke chronic illness without acute flares after exposure. The latency may be extremely long (e.g., more than 20 years for asbestosis) so that it is mandatory to take a detailed occupational history, including summer jobs and hobbies, in all patients with suspected ILD. Moreover, a history of smoking is associated with an increased risk for the development of IPF. Finally, the occurrence of familial cases of IPF suggests that genetic factors may modulate responses to causative agents.

Dyspnea in the patient with ILD is the result of increased work of breathing caused primarily by the stiffness of the lungs and by excessive minute ventilation. Hypoxemia, often aggravated by exercise, may amplify the sensation of dyspnea by carotid body stimulation. Unfortunately, patients do not always know what toxins they were exposed to, and exposures to toxins may be easily overlooked so that considerable investigation may be required. For example, fungi in cooling systems or birds in the home may be a source of allergens that can elicit hypersensitivity pneumonitis. History of medication use is also critical to diagnosing ILD. Patients who have been using drugs (e.g., nitrofurantoin) for years may not report them as medications on routine questioning. Mineral oil taken as a laxative or nose or ear drops also may not be considered medications.

Diseases in other organs may present as ILD, so a detailed review of systems is important. With occupational lung diseases, the physical exam is generally unrevealing about specific cause. It is most helpful in ruling out nonoccupational causes of respiratory symptoms or diseases such as cardiac problems or connective-tissue diseases. Chronic heart disease may present as ILD with dyspnea, cough, crackles, and interstitial-type

Focus on History 9.1 Taking an Occupational and Environmental History

General health history	• Does the patient think symptom/problem is related to anything at work? • When was the onset of symptoms, and how are they related to work? • Has the patient missed a day of work, and why? • Prior pulmonary problems • Medications • Cigarette use
Current or most relevant employment	• Job or process: title and description • Type of industry and specific work • Name of employer • Years employed
Exposure information	• General description of job process and overall hygiene • Materials used by worker and others • Ventilation/exhaust system • Use of respiratory protection • Are other workers affected? • Industrial hygiene samples and Occupational Safety and Health Administration (OSHA) data
Environmental nonoccupational factors	• Cigarettes • Diet • Hobbies • Pets
Specific workplace exposures	• Fumes/dust/fibers • Gases • Metals • Solvent • Other chemicals: plastics, pesticides, corrosive agents • Infectious agents • Organic dusts: cotton, wood • Physical factors: noise, repetitive trauma • Radiation • Emotional factors, stress
Past employment	• List jobs in chronological order • Job titles • Exposures • Military service

abnormalities on the chest x-ray film. Malignancies of virtually any organ system may spread to the lungs and present as ILD. The manifestations of the collagen-vascular diseases (e.g., rashes, Raynaud's phenomenon, fevers, arthralgias, muscle weakness) may give important clues on history taking. Dysphagia or regurgitation may relate to either recurrent aspiration or collagen-vascular disease, especially scleroderma. The connective-tissue diseases may be difficult to rule out because the pulmonary manifestations occasionally precede the more typical systemic manifestations by months or years. Patients with AIDS complicated by pneumocystosis or lymphocytic interstitial pneumonia may first present with an insidious onset of dyspnea and fatigue, as do patients with other ILDs. Therefore, sexual orientation and other possible risk factors for AIDS should be identified.

Abnormalities on the chest x-ray film may be the first clue to the presence of ILD; however, the patient with ILD may be asymptomatic with normal or abnormal chest x-ray results, or may be symptomatic with normal or abnormal chest x-ray results. The initial abnormality on the chest x-ray film is usually described as ground glass or a hazy appearance of the lungs. As disease progresses, diffuse abnormalities are found bilaterally. Pulmonary opacities (infiltrates) are usually described as small nodules (nodular), lines (reticular), or both (reticulonodular). Nodules are most commonly found in granulomatous diseases and hypersensitivity pneumonitis. The development of reticular densities is thought to be the result of edema, infiltration, or fibrosis of the septa in the periphery of the lung. A common characteristic of ILD is a progressive worsening in the opacities, with the development of honeycomb lung. The honeycomb-like appearance is created by the cyst-like spaces that characterize the pathology of advanced ILD. Many ILDs have unique radiographic presentations. For example, WG is associated with lower lobe cavities and nodules, and sarcoidosis is associated with swelling of the lymph nodes of the hilum of the lung (hilar lymphadenopathy). The hila are composed of the pulmonary arteries and their main branches, the upper lobe pulmonary veins, the major bronchi, and the lymph nodes.

High-resolution computed tomography (HRCT) has become widely used for evaluating ILDs. In addition, HRCT is unsurpassed in the detection and localization of pericardial and pleural fluid collections. HRCT examines only 1 mm of lung at each level, thus revealing some of the lung parenchyma's delicate architecture. Several signs of ILDs may be noted on HRCT. The most common are interface signs—the thickened and irregular appearance of the normally smooth interface of lung parenchyma with bronchi, blood vessels, and visceral pleura. Although HRCT is an exceptional tool for evaluation of parenchymal lung disease, it is important to note its limitations. It cannot be used to study the entire thorax; conventional CT must be used to avoid missing abnormalities between images. Some HRCT findings may be difficult to interpret without a conventional CT image to use for reference.

Serological tests for antinuclear antibodies and rheumatoid factor are positive in 20% to 40%, although rarely diagnostic, and antineutrophil cytoplasmic antibodies may be diagnostic in some settings.

A transbronchial biopsy has become the leading invasive tool for evaluating and treating patients with a wide spectrum of pulmonary disorders. In addition, the technique of bronchoalveolar lavage through the fiberoptic bronchoscope into a segmental or smaller bronchus provides a means to sample the cellular and soluble components of the lower respiratory tract. The area beyond the bronchoscope is washed with saline. The saline that is then aspirated back through the bronchoscope contains a small number of cells. The cells that are recovered include many from the alveoli and are representative of the cells associated with the inflammatory process. This procedure has aided in the diagnosis, pathogenesis, and assessment of activity of ILDs.

PFTs measure lung volumes and airflow with a spirometer. Whether the patient is symptomatic or not, PFTs should be performed to establish that disease is present, to determine its severity, and to monitor response to treatment. The sensitivity and specificity of these tests to diagnose the various ILDs is low, however. Routine spirometry values and lung volumes are often initially normal, as are resting blood gas measurements; only after exercise are gas-exchange abnormalities evident. The evaluation of the patient during exercise, although not constituting a direct measurement of respiration, gives more information than static measurements of lung volume or diffusing capacity regarding ventilation, blood flow, gas exchange, and control of breathing. PFTs usually show a purely restrictive defect in most patients with ILD. Obstructive lung disease develops gradually in some patients and more commonly in some diseases (sarcoidosis, hypersensitivity pneumonitis).

The compliance of the lungs decreases as lung involvement progresses. This is caused, in part, by fibrosis of the pulmonary parenchyma and the formation of cystic airspace. Diffusion capacity of the lung (DLCO) is a good reflection of alveolar capillary surface area. Destruction of lung parenchyma results in a reduction in DLCO as ILD progresses. An abnormal DLCO may be the earliest evidence of ILD found on standard PFTs.

The use of the thoracoscope in combination with standard surgical instruments has led to the designation video-assisted thoracic surgery or video-assisted thoracoscopy (VATS). VATS provides the same access to the hemithorax as both thoracoscopy and thoracotomy. VATS procedures are particularly useful for obtaining lung biopsies in patients with diffuse ILD. With VATS, the visualization of the lung is better than it is with a limited thoracotomy, and more areas of the lung can be sampled.

Transbronchial lung biopsy involves passing a forceps or needle through the bronchoscope. A specimen is obtained with forceps or aspirated through a needle. Pleural biopsy is useful in diagnosing granulomatous disease or malignancy of the pleura and should be performed only if these two diseases are suspected. If a specific diagnosis is not made by transbronchial biopsy, an open lung biopsy is indicated. Open lung biopsy is the most definitive way to diagnose and stage the disease so that appropriate prognostic and therapeutic decisions can be made. Depending on the age of the patient and the potential risks of the surgery in a compromised patient, empiric therapy may be initiated.

Differential Diagnosis

When confronted with a patient with unexplained dyspnea and fatigue, the differential diagnosis is immense. Pulmonary, cardiac, hematological, renal, neuromuscular, and even endocrine diseases may present with exercise intolerance of dyspnea. A complete work-up of these systems is required to determine the correct diagnosis. Some of the conditions that give rise to dyspnea, diffuse pulmonary infiltration, and granulomatous reaction include the following: extrinsic allergic alveolitis, asbestosis, silicosis, berylliosis, lymphoid granulomatosis, connective-tissue diseases, certain drugs, miliary TB, lymphoma, leukemias, PCP, and coccidiomycosis.

Management

Management of most ILDs is difficult, and different approaches are taken depending on the specific entity. Regardless of etiology, end-stage fibrosis is irreversible and untreatable. An extensive and aggressive diagnostic evaluation early on, even in the patient with relatively few symptoms, is recommended. Early clinical intervention in patients who are more likely to develop lung disease could be of considerable benefit for the patient. A good example is the identification and assessment of disease progression in diffuse lung disease found in systemic sclerosis. The first course of action when faced with a patient with ILD is to determine whether exposure to environmental agents or drugs is the cause and to discontinue the exposure. Therapeutic dilemmas arise because discontinuation of such drugs as tocainide or amiodarone may result in life-threatening dysrhythmias. Second, the best chance for therapeutic success begins with the correct diagnosis. Finally, in cases in which specific medication is employed, such as prednisone or cytotoxic agents, there is usually suppression rather than cure of the primary process. Many patients with ILD are older adults, so the decision to treat them with immunosuppressive drugs should not be taken lightly, because the toxicity and adverse effects of these medications can be substantial. In addition, anti-inflammatory and immunosuppressive treatments may be ineffective because of recurrent dysregulated wound healing rather than neutrophilic or immune cell–mediated inflammation.

Investigational studies are looking at a shift toward antifibroblast therapies for ILD aimed at decreasing pulmonary collagen deposition.

Initial Management

Corticosteroids may be initiated in the therapy for ILD. A trial with them is reasonable, even for the patient who is in an advanced stage of the disease with relatively acellular and fibrotic changes in lung tissue. The best predictor of ultimate steroid responsiveness and a better prognosis is early benefit following the initial 1 to 2 months of steroid therapy. The dosage and duration of corticosteroid therapy depend on the specific disorder, but in general relatively high doses are used for the first 6 weeks (1–2 mg/kg per day, or 60–100 mg/day) over the ensuing 3 months. A period of 3 to 6 months is often required to determine the steroid responsiveness of fibrosing alveolitis, although patients with sarcoidosis and cryptogenic organizing pneumonia may respond much more quickly with lower dosages. Certain processes, such as idiopathic pulmonary fibrosis, commonly require therapy for 12 months or longer.

Subsequent Management

For the patient who is not well controlled with or responsive to corticosteroids, additional immunosuppressive therapy may be considered. Cyclophosphamide (Cytoxan), an alkylating drug, is a potent immunosuppressant and seems to be effective in patients with ILD who are not helped with corticosteroids. If improvement in the lung disease is documented after 3 months of this therapy, it should be continued for a 12-month interval. Azathioprine (Azasan, Imuran) has been used as an alternative to cyclophosphamide. Penicillamine (Cuprimine, Depen) has been used in some patients, with the rationale that it might prevent the cross-linking of abnormal collagen being synthesized in the interstitium and prevent or retard fibrosis. Exercise tolerance may be significantly improved with supplemental oxygen.

Because the pulmonary vascular bed is impaired by progressive fibrosis, pulmonary hypertension and cor pulmonale can develop; right-sided congestive heart failure can be difficult to control. Judicious use of diuretics is advised, for a significant decrease in intravascular volume may be deleterious for lung perfusion. Digitalis or antidysrhythmic drugs may be required, although adequate oxygenation is probably the best treatment for heart failure in this situation. Some patients may also develop obstruction to air flow and be troubled with wheezing and coughing that may respond to bronchodilators. Because infection may occur during immunosuppressive therapy, it is important to maintain a high index of suspicion and to treat infection aggressively. Prophylactic use of pneumococcal and influenza vaccines is encouraged. Finally, lung transplantation may be an option for patients with refractory disease limited to the chest.

Follow-up and Referral

Reassessment of disease activity is generally performed at 3, 6, 12, and 24 months and more often if needed. Responsiveness is defined as a decrease in symptoms: radiographic improvement, physiological improvement, or no further decline in clinical, radiographic, or physiological parameters. The patient should be followed for signs of infection that are masked by immunosuppressive drugs, pneumothorax, or development of lung cancer, which occurs in 5% to 10% of patients. The patient on steroids must be monitored closely during times of illness or stress and during steroid tapering or withdrawal. The patient should be encouraged to wear a medical identification bracelet. In view of exercise-related hypoxia, the patient should be assessed for benefit of supplemental oxygen during exercise. Patients with a collagen vascular disorder must be regularly assessed for progression or exacerbations of their chronic illnesses. For example, patients with RA require rest, joint protection, daily heat and exercise, and psychological support. Community resources such as a home care nurse, homemaker services, and vocational rehabilitation may be considered. Self-help groups may be beneficial for the patient. These diseases require the collaborative and integrated approach as emphasized in the *Circle of Caring* model.

Specialized testing should be undertaken and the patient referred to a pulmonologist if no specific cause of dyspnea or cough can be found; if the symptoms exceed the physiological or radiographic abnormalities identified; if empiric management (with bronchodilators, diuretics, smoking cessation) resulted in an atypical or unsatisfactory clinical outcome; if the patient needs an impairment or disability evaluation for workers' compensation or any reason; if specialized cardiopulmonary testing (e.g., lung biopsy) is needed; or if a therapeutic immunosuppressive or cytotoxic drug trial is contemplated.

Patient Education

Patients with ILD must be educated about the nature of their illness, the related diagnostic tests, and the treatment regimen for their particular type of lung disease (see Table 9.21). For example, avoidance of exposure to antigens is paramount for those with hypersensitivity pneumonitis. All patients must be advised and assisted to stop cigarette smoking to prevent further lung damage. In many cases, the most comprehensive patient education occurs within the context of a pulmonary rehabilitation program.

The need to reduce repeated admissions into expensive ICUs brought about the proliferation of formal inpatient and outpatient pulmonary rehabilitation programs in the United States for patients with chronic lung disease. The target population for these programs has been severely disabled patients with COPD or ILD, who require a broad range of comprehensive services to keep

Table 9.21	Educational Content for the Patient With Interstitial Lung Disease

- Respiratory anatomy and physiology
- Pathophysiology of interstitial lung disease
- Respiratory diagnostic tests:
  Chest x-ray
  PFTs
  Exercise tests
  Bronchoscopy
  HRCT
- Self-care measures:
  Pulmonary medications
  Diet
  Fluid intake
  Smoking cessation
  Environmental control
  Signs of infections
- Chest therapy:
  Relaxation and guided imagery
  Breathing retraining
  Controlling dyspneic episodes
  Postural drainage
- Progressive exercise conditioning:
  Walking programs
  Treadmill or bicycle exercise training
  Arm or leg range-of-motion exercises
- Respiratory equipment:
  Oxygen therapy
  Handheld nebulizer

them clinically stable and out of the hospital for long periods of time. Appropriate patients with all levels of respiratory impairment, not only the severely disabled, should be referred to such programs.

Each program has criteria for referral that generally include the following patient characteristics: dyspnea on exertion, inability to carry out selected activities of daily living, repeated hospitalizations or need for home care services, time lost from work or school, and desire for educational update of self-care techniques. Moreover, the following laboratory features are inclusion criteria for pulmonary rehabilitation: reduced vital capacity in restrictive disease, reduced expiratory flow rates, hypercapnia, and hypoxemia at rest or during exercise.

The team teaches self-care educational content and implements a program of bronchial hygiene and physical conditioning, based on needs identified during the initial assessment. Group and individual instruction and counseling are provided by a variety of personnel. Patient progress is evaluated using respiratory assessment parameters and teaching–learning tools. A final evaluation with recommendations for long-range treatment is forwarded to the referring clinician.

■ SLEEP APNEA

Sleep apnea is defined as a temporary pause in breathing during sleep that lasts at least 10 seconds to as long as 90 seconds. For a confirmed diagnosis, this should occur a minimum of five times an hour. The three patterns of apnea are central, obstructive, and mixed. Central apnea occurs when both airflow and respiratory efforts are absent. *Central apneas* are a result of an absence of neural output from the brainstem's respiratory centers, which leads to a lack of inspiratory effort. The respiratory center in the brain fails to respond to elevated carbon dioxide concentrations. In contrast, during *obstructive sleep apnea* (OSA), respiratory efforts persist although airflow is absent at the nose and mouth. Airflow obstruction occurs when the tongue and the soft palate fall backward and partially or completely obstruct the pharynx. Finally, many adult patients exhibit mixed apneas in which both central and obstructive patterns occur.

Each apnea results in progressive asphyxiation until an arousal from sleep occurs, with a subsequent restoration of upper airway patency and airflow. A patient then usually returns to sleep quickly, resulting in another occlusion of the upper airway. Apnea and arousal cycles occur repeatedly, as many as 200 to 400 times during 6 to 8 hours of sleep. Sleep hypopnea is a period of hypoventilation, or decreased airflow, defined as a 50% reduction in thoracoabdominal movements, with a 4% fall in oxygen saturation lasting at least 10 seconds during sleep. OSA/hypopnea is present when the respiratory drive is intact but the upper airway intermittently becomes obstructed during sleep. The *respiratory disturbance index* (RDI) (also called the apnea/hypopnea index)—the number of apneas plus hypopneas per hour of sleep—may be used to define and quantify the severity of OSA. The RDI is obtained by dividing the total number of events throughout the entire night by the total sleep time in hours. An index greater than 5 is abnormal, although it probably does not become clinically significant until it reaches 20. In general, as the RDI increases, so does the severity of symptoms.

Patients with OSA may experience a number of potentially adverse physiological and neurobehavioral problems. Consequences of OSA are the result of daily exposure to abnormalities in breathing during sleep and result in long-term morbidity in the neurobehavioral and cardiovascular domains. Sleep-disordered breathing is an independent risk factor for the development of hypertension and, subsequently, left ventricular dysfunction. The patient with combined coronary artery disease (CAD) and OSA may have an increased cardiac risk because of worsening of the relationship between myocardial oxygen demand and supply as a result of apnea-associated hypoxemia and activation of the autonomic nervous system (Table 9.22).

Moreover, cardiac dysrhythmias, usually occurring during apneic episodes, have been reported to be a

Table 9.22	Possible Consequences of Sleep Apnea
Pulmonary hypertension	
Systemic hypertension	
Cardiac dysrhythmias	
Right or left ventricular failure	
Right ventricular hypertrophy	
Myocardial infarction (increased risk of)	
Stroke (increased risk of)	
Nocturnal angina	
COPD (exacerbation of)	
Insulin resistance	
Endothelial cell dysfunction	

significant complication of OSA. In a 2013 long-term study of 10,701 adults conducted by the Mayo Clinic Sleep Disorders Centers, people with sleep apnea had a higher risk of dying from sudden cardiac arrest (Gami et al, 2013). In addition, sleep quality may be influenced by apnea-associated activation of the central nervous system (CNS) (arousals) and ischemia-associated arousals. Timely diagnosis and treatment of CAD, as well as sleep apnea, is necessary for these patients.

OSA can cause mild pulmonary hypertension, even in the absence of pulmonary disease. Sustained pulmonary hypertension, often associated with clinical evidence of right ventricular failure, has been observed in about 20% of OSA patients. It is hypothesized that repetitive hypoxemia during sleep may lead to vascular remodeling in susceptible patients and thus cause pulmonary hypertension during the day. Further, because the patient with OSA is often obese or has pathological lung function resulting in abnormalities of daytime arterial blood gas (ABG) values, pulmonary vasoconstriction is another mechanism inducing pulmonary hypertension.

Epidemiology and Causes

Sleep apnea is an extremely common clinical disorder; as such, it has major public health implications. Unrecognized and untreated OSA in the general adult population, most of whom are in the most productive period of their lives, contributes to significant and disabling psychomotor deficits. An estimated 40 million Americans are chronically ill with various sleep disorders, and 38,000 cardiovascular deaths annually are directly attributable to OSA; yet the vast majority of Americans with sleep disorders remain undiagnosed and untreated. This, in turn, costs billions of dollars in accidents in the home, at the workplace, and in traffic.

Approximately 4% of women and 9% of men have significant OSA. OSA is most prevalent in men older than age 50 and in postmenopausal women, probably related to hormonal changes, although it is seen in younger people as well. Usually men have a significantly higher pharyngeal and supraglottic resistance than women, which makes them more susceptible to pharyngeal collapse and OSA and may contribute to the male predominance of the syndrome. Pharyngeal resistance increases with age in normal men, possibly related to greater body weight, and it is widely believed that the risk of developing OSA increases with age in men. This assumption, however, is far from conclusive. Moreover, once a disorder is labeled as predominantly a male condition, clinicians may be less likely to think about it in women and, hence, less likely to refer women to sleep disorder centers. Compared with OSA, central sleep apnea syndrome is uncommon. In most sleep laboratories, patients with central sleep apnea syndrome constitute fewer than 10% of patients tested. The division between central and obstructive sleep apnea is not as clear-cut as it might appear because many patients with central sleep apnea present with clinical features more suggestive of OSA. It is possible that in some patients upper airway occlusion triggers a central, rather than an obstructive, apnea. Support for this notion comes from the finding that some patients with central sleep apnea can be successfully treated with nasal continuous positive airway pressure (CPAP).

The cause of OSA is poorly defined but appears to be multifactorial; upper airway tract malformation, oropharyngeal muscle dysfunction, and abnormal respiratory drive each play a greater or lesser role. A number of recognized anatomical abnormalities are associated with narrowing of the upper airway and predispose patients to OSA. Conditions associated with facial dysmorphism or mandibular abnormalities show a predisposition to OSA and include adenotonsillar hypertrophy, choanal atresia, micrognathia (small mandible), retrognathia, macroglossia, nasal septal deviation, and craniofacial dysostosis. Micrognathia is particularly associated with OSA because a small or retropositioned mandible places the base of the tongue closer to the posterior pharyngeal wall and interferes with the efficiency of the genioglossus muscle in keeping the tongue out of the narrowed pharynx.

There is increasing evidence that sleep apnea has a familial distribution. Relatives of a person with sleep apnea have approximately twice the normal risk of having sleep apnea. Most adult patients with OSA, however, have no specific skeletal or soft tissue lesion obstructing the upper airway, but they often have a small, congested oropharyngeal airway. Symptoms of sleep apnea are present two to six times more frequently in family members of affected patients than in a control population.

Obesity and alcohol consumption are well recognized as aggravating factors. One possible explanation for the relationship between obesity and OSA is that the upper airway is narrowed in the obese patient as a result of increased fat deposition in the pharyngeal walls. Fat in the neck plays the largest role. Neck (or collar) size is the best indicator of the presence of sleep apnea. Approximately 30% of snoring males with a collar size larger than 17 inches will have OSA. Neck size in women is less well investigated, but when it is over 16 inches, it increases the risk for sleep apnea. Another possible explanation for this relationship is the fact that the obese patient often has smaller lung volumes, particularly functional residual capacity, than the nonobese patient; this, in turn, can indirectly influence upper airway size and contribute to upper airway narrowing. About 16% of patients with sleep apnea, however, are not obese. Any factor that interferes with the arousal mechanism, such as alcohol consumption, could lead to more profound and prolonged apneas. Alcohol, which reduces upper-airway muscle tone, and sedatives or hypnotics, which reduce the arousal mechanism, exacerbate OSA. There is considerable evidence that OSA carries a substantial morbidity and mortality, particularly from cardiovascular complications.

Pathophysiology

Sleep is divided into two states—rapid eye movement (REM) sleep and non–rapid eye movement (NREM) sleep. NREM sleep is further divided into four stages, based on changes in the electroencephalogram (EEG) pattern. Normal sleep begins with Stage I, which is characterized by slow eye movements, usually preceding sleep onset. Stage II involves further slowing of the EEG, with the presence of sleep spindles and slow eye movements. Stage III is manifested by low-frequency delta waves with occasional sleep spindles but no slow eye movements. Finally, Stage IV is characterized by high-voltage delta waves. REM sleep is characterized by desynchronized, low-voltage, fast activity that occurs about every 90 minutes beginning after 1 to 2 hours of NREM sleep. The normal adult sleeper alternates between NREM sleep and REM sleep approximately every 90 minutes throughout the night.

Typically, during the lighter stages of NREM sleep, the breathing pattern is irregular because of the decrease in respiratory drive associated with the stimulatory effect of wakefulness and decreased metabolic rate associated with sleep. In the deeper stages of NREM sleep, breathing is typically very regular; however, overall ventilation is reduced compared with that during wakefulness. During REM sleep, the respiratory drive is irregular because of the transient decrease in ventilatory response to chemical and mechanical stimuli. The influence of sleep on the upper airway is similar to its effects on other skeletal muscles, resulting in a general loss of muscle tone and a reduction in tidal volume and minute volume. The sleep structure of the patient with OSA is characterized by the loss of physiological REM/NREM alternation, as well as by a deficit of REM and slow-wave sleep. This can be caused by sleep fragmentation as a result of the high amount of arousals related to respiratory events.

Central Sleep Apnea

Etiological factors of central sleep apnea are found mainly in disturbances in the respiratory control system in the brainstem. The cause of such disturbances of the breathing control system remains unclear in most cases, however. Central apneas are commonly seen in altitudes where hypoxemia induces hyperventilation with associated alkalosis. Cheyne-Stokes respiration with central apneas may also occur in the patient with congestive heart failure. Neurological diseases affecting the brainstem may cause breathing pattern disorders in sleep. Well-known neurological diseases such as arteriosclerosis in the older adult, infarctions, tumors, hemorrhage, trauma with damage of this region, encephalitis, poliomyelitis, or other infectious diseases may cause central apnea during sleep, even though no abnormalities of breathing patterns are present during wakefulness. If the neural pathways from medullary respiratory groups to motor neurons of the ventilatory muscles are interrupted, the metabolic control of breathing may be disturbed. This may occur after cervical cordotomy.

Obstructive Sleep Apnea

The underlying pathophysiology of sleep apnea is complex and not fully understood. However, it is generally accepted that patency of the upper airway is dependent on the action of oropharyngeal dilator and abductor muscles, which are normally activated in a rhythmic fashion during inspiration. The available evidence indicates that in OSA, the site of upper airway obstruction is the pharynx and that obstruction of the pharynx

during sleep is a result of an imbalance between the forces that serve to dilate the pharynx and those that promote pharyngeal closure. The upper airway is subject to collapse when the force produced by these muscles for a given cross-sectional area of the upper airway is exceeded by the negative airway pressure generated by inspiratory activity of the diaphragm and intercostal muscles. Upper airway obstruction can occur if the suction pressure is too high or if the counteracting forces of the dilating muscles are too weak, for any given suction pressure.

The subsequent obstructive apnea results in progressive and sometimes profound hypoxia and hypercapnia. These apnea-associated changes in P_{O_2} and P_{CO_2} stimulate ventilation, resulting in increasing inspiratory efforts. Eventually the progressive hypoxemia and hypercapnia and/or the associated increase in inspiratory effort result in arousal of the patient. With this usually transient arousal occurs augmentation of upper airway dilator muscle activity to an extent proportionately greater than the simultaneous augmentation of diaphragm activity. This leads to deocclusion of the pharynx and restoration of airflow. During the subsequent brief period of ventilation, P_{O_2} rises and P_{CO_2} falls. The rapid resumption of sleep, however, results in reocclusion of the upper airway. This cycle of events may recur hundreds of times each night, triggering repeated arousals that may contribute to many of the clinical features of OSA (Fig. 9.2).

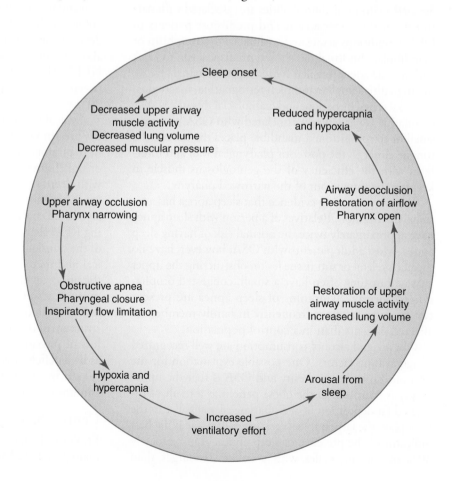

Figure 9.2 Pathogenesis of obstructive sleep apnea.

Clinical Presentation

Subjective

The diagnosis of OSA is not difficult to make: the symptoms are typical, and the major risk factor is relatively obvious. Patients with sleep apnea have both nighttime and daytime symptoms (Table 9.23). Hypersomnolence is the single most important presenting symptom of sleep apnea and frequently identifies which patient will require and accept specific therapy.

Hypersomnolence is not tiredness, fatigue, or lassitude; it is clear-cut, uncontrollable sleepiness. It develops over a long period and is first experienced by a patient as sleep onset when attention is not demanded (e.g., when watching television, sitting in a college lecture, or waiting at a traffic light). Eventually, more alerting situations are affected, such as long-distance driving or quiet conversation. Daytime symptoms include a morning headache (from hypercapnia) and neuropsychological disturbances, including falling asleep while performing purposeful activities. These episodes can occur during work or social functions and can lead to embarrassment, domestic discord, decreased work productivity, loss of employment, and an increased incidence of accidents. The patient may complain of nocturnal restlessness, frequent urination or enuresis, and choking.

The patient usually reports impaired intellectual performance, such as decreased concentration, ambition, and memory loss. Patients with sleep apnea also report limiting social contact because of their fear of sleepiness and falling asleep. Personality changes such as irritability and moodiness are seen in about 50% of patients, and more severe psychiatric disturbances such as major depression and psychosis have been reported. Sexual dysfunction is common (e.g., diminished libido, even though men with apnea can obtain an erection). Persons with sleep apnea may note nocturnal palpitations or skipped heartbeats. OSA is characterized by loud snoring that is repeatedly interrupted by episodes of complete upper airway obstruction and resolves with temporary arousal. The snoring of OSA is both loud (it can be heard in an adjacent room) and habitual (it occurs nightly). Hypoxemia and hypercarbia of varying degrees frequently accompany apnea or hypopnea. It is not uncommon for some patients to regularly desaturate to oxygen saturation levels below 70% and, occasionally, below 60%. Apneas and hypopneas often result in arousal from sleep, which then terminates the breathing disturbance and results in a surge in blood pressure (BP). Once aroused, the CNS can respond appropriately to the partial or complete closure of the pharynx with a brief contraction of the pharyngeal dilating muscles. This restores upper airway patency and permits resumption of airflow, with subsequent reversal of the hypoxemia and hypercarbia. Arousals often last for only 1 to 3 seconds and are not recognized by the patient. Occasionally, during the arousal that terminates the apneic event, the bed partner may witness arm flailing or other gross movements.

On awakening in the morning, the patient is often completely unaware that he or she aroused several hundred times during the night. It is believed that recurrent arousals and the consequent sleep disruption are the causes of many of the daytime symptoms and effects of sleep apnea. Automobile accidents have been reported to occur 2.0 to 2.6 times more frequently among patients with OSA than among other individuals, a consequence that contributes to many unnecessary and costly days in the hospital.

Clinically, patients with central sleep apnea usually show less daytime sleepiness than do patients with other types of apnea. Sleep disruption, frequent awakening, shortness of breath after awakening, and signs of right heart failure such as peripheral edema are observed quite often. The patient with central sleep apnea tends to have a normal body weight. Psychiatric symptoms such as depression may occur as well. As in obstructive apnea, oxygen desaturation and consequent hemodynamic disorders may be observed.

Table 9.23	Conditions Presenting With Excessive Daytime Sleepiness

- Sleep apnea syndrome
- Narcolepsy
- Idiopathic hypersomnia
- Periodic limb movements in sleep
- Psychiatric disorders
- Drug and alcohol dependency
- Insufficient sleep syndrome
- Circadian disorders (jet lag, shift work)
- Obesity-hypoventilation syndrome (Pickwickian syndrome)
- Hypothyroidism
- Seizure disorder
- Depression

Objective

The predominant clinical manifestations of OSA reflect the risk factors: obesity (particularly of the upper body), increased neck size, crowded oropharynx (tonsillar hypertrophy and enlargement of soft palate [uvula] and tongue, as well as lateral peritonsillar narrowing), retrognathia, and micrognathia.

Diagnostic Reasoning

Diagnostic Tests

OSA should be suspected whenever hypersomnia and snoring coexist. The recording of specific historical details from the patient and his or her spouse is crucial to the diagnosis, particularly because the patient sometimes does not realize the severity of the sleepiness. This is perhaps because he or she finds it socially unacceptable or has slipped into it so gradually. Initial testing may take the form of determining how easy it is for a patient to fall asleep or, alternatively, how difficult it is for the person to remain awake. This type of testing may include both subjective and objective assessments. Two common subjective assessments of sleepiness are the Stanford Sleepiness Score (SSS) and the Epworth Sleepiness Scale (ESS). The SSS is used to record the degree of sleepiness experienced by a patient at a given time and does not necessarily relate to his or her overall propensity to fall asleep. It is an introspective measure of sleepiness where the patient rates his or her alertness on a 7-point scale at different times during the day. If the score falls below a 3 when he or she should be feeling alert, a serious sleep deficit exists. The SSS can be found at www.stanford.edu/-demet/sss.html. The ESS measures sleepiness as a reflection of a patient's tendency to fall asleep during eight specific nonstimulating situations. Each situation is scored from 0 to 3. A total score of 10 is considered abnormal. The ESS can be found at www.stanford.edu/-dement/epworth.html.

The definitive test for sleep apnea is an overnight polysomnogram. This all-night recording of the patient's sleep, performed in a sleep center, is the gold standard for identifying the presence, type, and severity of sleep apnea. The standard raises two major problems, however. First, the test is not accessible to many patients because it is limited to specialized sleep centers; second, it is expensive. The polysomnograph is a multichannel recorder that records the patient's eye movements, airflow, respiratory movements, leg movements, EEG readings, pulse oximetry, electrocardiograph (ECG) readings, and snoring. From such records, apneas, hypopneas, and snoring-related arousals are scored. The RDI is calculated from the number of apneas plus hypopneas per hour. Recently, multichannel devices that record a limited number of parameters (e.g., respiratory movements, airflow, snoring, pulse oximetry, and ECG) have been introduced for home studies, which may be comparable to a full polysomnogram.

The development of large numbers of limited diagnostic systems in recent years represents a recognition of the logistical problems involved in gaining access to large sleep centers. Unfortunately, there is no uniformity among these devices, and the only consistent variable common to all such systems is the oxygen saturation level. Most offer some measure of respiration, based either on nasal flow or chest bands. In the patient with OSA, the polysomnogram demonstrates frequent episodes of apnea with corresponding periods of oxygen desaturation as demonstrated by pulse oximetry. The effort to breathe remains intact during the periods of OSA, as evidenced by the movement of the lower chest and abdomen.

If the polysomnogram is negative for OSA in the patient with significant daytime sleepiness, a multiple sleep latency test (MSLT) should be performed in a sleep center to rule out narcolepsy. The MSLT is performed the day after the polysomnogram. The patient is instructed not to take any medications such as sedatives and certain antidepressants for 2 weeks before the test. The patient is allowed to take four or five 15- to 20-minute naps 2 hours apart. Healthy subjects have a sleep latency of 10 to 20 minutes in the MSLT. A test is considered consistent with excessive daytime sleepiness if sleep onset occurs within 5 minutes. The presence of two sleep-onset REM episodes in the appropriate clinical setting is diagnostic of narcolepsy.

The syndrome of periodic limb movements (PLMs) (also known as nocturnal myoclonus or periodic leg movements) consists of stereotypic periodic leg (or arm) movements during sleep that may or may not be associated with arousals. If enough arousals occur, sleep may be so fragmented that daytime sleepiness results. Because patients with narcolepsy frequently have PLMs, any patient with excessive daytime sleepiness and PLMs on a polysomnogram should be questioned carefully concerning narcoleptic manifestations.

An otolaryngological exam should be performed. In addition, screening with a home nocturnal pulse oximetry has a high negative predictive value if no desaturations are seen. Erythrocytosis is common. A hemoglobin level and thyroid function tests should also be performed.

Differential Diagnosis

A number of disorders present with excessive daytime sleepiness (see Table 9.23). Drug addiction and depression can masquerade as sleep apnea, especially in the older adult patient, in whom a number of apneas during sleep may be considered normal. Certain diagnostic tests, such as ABGs, thyroid function testing, PFTs, the ECG, and chest x-ray exam, are routinely indicated to determine the potential cause, presence, or severity of signs of hypoxic exposure occurring as the result of repetitive apneas during sleep. A recording of the patient's usual amount and pattern of sleep may be instructive.

Management
Obstructive Sleep Apnea

Currently, the first line of treatment for OSA is medical management. The treatments for OSA include the following:

- General measures: Avoidance of alcohol, sedatives, and hypnotics; weight loss; and other (less effective) measures, including pharmacological agents, oxygen therapy, and nasal dilators
- Specific measures: Position therapy, positive airway pressure (CPAP, bi-level systems, auto-CPAP), and oral appliances

OSA and its treatment are highly dependent on patient behavior. Clinicians have both an opportunity and a responsibility to advise patients of the profound influence that their behavior can have on disease severity and outcome. For patients who cannot tolerate medical treatment or who do not desire long-term medical therapy, surgical treatment of sleep apnea should be considered.

Elimination of Risk Factors A reasonable first step in the management of the patient with sleep-disordered breathing is to identify and subsequently eliminate, or avoid, the risk factors. The adverse effects of alcohol on upper airway stability during sleep and the arousal response to chemical stimuli mandate that the patient with OSA be instructed to abstain from alcohol. Although not invariably associated with OSA, obesity is usually present in this patient population. Weight reduction may result in significant improvement in OSA and sleep quality, and may obviate the need for further therapeutic interventions. Efforts in this regard represent a major, lifelong therapeutic challenge, best approached by utilizing the multidisciplinary resources of the physician, nutritionist, psychologist, and a peer support system. It is difficult to accomplish and maintain weight loss, but it is very beneficial to patients with sleep apnea when they do so. Benefits of weight loss in obese patients with sleep apnea include reduced RDI, reduced BP, and optimal CPAP pressure; improved pulmonary function, daytime ABGs, polycythemia, sleep structure, and oxygen saturation; elimination of snoring; and prevention of relapse after surgical treatment.

The relationship between sleep in the supine position and augmentation of snoring and sleep apnea in some patients is apparent. It has been hypothesized that the effects of gravity in promoting posterior movement of the tongue with apposition against the posterior pharyngeal wall are magnified in the supine position. Although manipulation of the sleeping position is not an effective therapy for the majority of patients with sleep-disordered breathing, it may be all that is needed in selected patients. It has been suggested that there may be a decreased incidence of sleep-disordered breathing events during sleep in the lateral decubitus position. Position therapy can be accomplished by sewing pockets for one or two tennis balls in the back of patients' sleeping attire in an attempt to prevent them from assuming the supine position. Devices to train people to sleep in the lateral position have been described.

Devices That Maintain Upper Airway Patency CPAP administered through a nasal mask has become the most common treatment for OSA. Nasal CPAP also effectively reduces or eliminates mixed apneas, including both the central and obstructive components. A continuous flow of air is delivered from a blower unit to a tightly fitting nasal mask held in place by head straps. Nasal CPAP acts as a pneumatic splint preventing collapse of the upper airway in all phases of respiration. The device is used for the entire sleep period every night. The optimal CPAP pressure is determined by technologists during polysomnography. Typically, 5 to 20 cm H_2O is

the pressure needed to abolish apneas, snoring, and oxyhemoglobin desaturations in all positions and during REM sleep. Although CPAP use is associated with few serious complications, it does elicit a number of complaints. Minor adverse effects of CPAP include feelings of suffocation, nasal drying or rhinitis, ear pain, difficulty in exhaling, mask and mouth leaks, chest and back pain, and conjunctivitis. Most of these can be alleviated.

Newer automatic CPAP devices continuously adjust the positive pressure to the required levels. In the automatic CPAP mode, the positive pressure is maintained as long as ventilation remains stable; however, any respiratory disorder results in a progressive increase in the pressure. If a breathing disturbance has not occurred for more than 4 minutes, the positive pressure decreases again. For many patients who use it at home regularly, CPAP quite dramatically eliminates apneas and hypopneas, improves sleep architecture, and reduces daytime sleepiness, even for those with mild sleep apnea. The effectiveness of CPAP is limited, however, by incomplete patient compliance.

Oral Appliances Oral appliances are an effective noninvasive alternative to CPAP in patients with mild to moderate sleep apnea. Although oral appliances are effective in some patients with OSA, they are not universally effective. There are major design differences in the numerous oral appliances that are now available, and this may have an impact on their success and compliance rates. A novel anterior mandibular positioner has been developed with an adjustable hinge that allows progressive advancement of the mandible. This appliance may be an effective first-line treatment for the patient with mild to moderate OSA and may be associated with greater patient satisfaction than CPAP. For these devices to treat sleep apnea effectively, the mandible should be advanced to 50% to 75% of the maximal forward protrusion of the jaw. In most patients, dental appliances lessen but do not abolish OSA and snoring. In many patients treated with an oral appliance, the RDI still remains high, with more than 20 events per hour after treatment. The side effects of oral appliances include excessive salivation, dental misalignment, and pain in, or damage to, the temporomandibular joint. Several pulmonologists believe that oral appliances are just as effective as CPAP in treating sleep apnea.

Surgical Management

Surgery for OSA is designed either to bypass the obstructing region of the upper airway or to modify the upper airway in such a fashion that it is less likely to lose patency. The obstruction may result either from a wide variety of structural aberrations, such as nasal deformity, nasal polyps, hypertrophic tonsils and/or adenoids, craniofacial disproportion, neoplasms, or, as in most cases, no detectable anatomical abnormalities. Accordingly, a variety of surgical procedures have been applied to the management of these patients.

Extensive excision of soft tissue in the oropharynx, termed *uvulopalatopharyngoplasty* (UPPP), was developed to improve pharyngeal function during sleep. The procedure involves a bilateral tonsillectomy and a submucosal resection of redundant tissue. A variable portion of the posterior margin of the soft palate and the uvula is also removed and the palatopharyngeus muscle may also be resected. In the absence of weight gain or other confounding factors, a success rate of 50% has been sustained for at least 1 year postoperatively. However, even OSA patients who are UPPP failures often have substantial reduction in snoring after surgery, despite persistent apnea. A repeat polysomnogram is necessary to assess the therapeutic outcome of surgery. The success rate in patients undergoing UPPP appears to be partly related to the location of the obstructing tissue: Patients with retropalatal obstruction removal experience better results than those with retroglossal obstruction removal. The preoperative presence of tonsils has been associated with improved success of UPPP.

The patient undergoing surgical reconstruction of the airway for OSA, such as UPPP, often has coexisting medical problems, especially cardiovascular disease, which can complicate treatment. The uncertainty regarding the proper predictive parameters for surgical success greatly limits optimal patient selection. Further, a significant number of patients have difficulty at induction and intubation for general anesthesia. Men with increased neck circumference and associated skeletal deformities should be evaluated carefully and considered for fiberoptic intubation.

Laser-assisted uvulopalatoplasty is a procedure to treat snoring in the outpatient setting. The procedure entails reshaping the palate and tonsillar pillars in one to seven serial sessions under local anesthesia. Each session lasts approximately 15 minutes and is generally well tolerated; the incidence of complications is low. The procedure is successful in reducing snoring in 90% of patients. However, the success rate in patients with OSA is not yet clear.

A variety of maxillofacial and nasal surgical procedures may be performed to normalize the bony relationships of the maxilla and mandible to minimize the likelihood of airway collapse during sleep. Many of these procedures are preceded by UPPP and, if the results are unsatisfactory, a second stage involving mandibular advancement is undertaken. These procedures require a great deal of surgical and orthodontic expertise, along with careful consultation with anesthesia services and pulmonary medicine.

Nasal surgery has been performed on patients with OSA in an effort to reduce the predisposition to collapse during sleep. A nasal septoplasty is performed if gross nasal septal deformity is present. The definitive therapy is a tracheostomy. Because of the drastic nature of this procedure, it is limited to patients with life-threatening arrhythmias or severe disability who have not responded to conservative therapy.

Central Sleep Apnea

Medical treatment is ineffective in the patient with central sleep apnea. Implantation of a diaphragm-pacing device is an aggressive measure, the efficiency of which has not been proven by long-term clinical trials. Diaphragm pacing may precipitate upper airway occlusion during sleep due to dyssynchrony between activation of the diaphragm and the upper airway and laryngeal dilators. Thus, tracheostomy is often performed concomitantly with diaphragm pacing. These difficulties, in conjunction with the resource-intensive nature of the procedure and subsequent care, have made this technique one that is infrequently employed in the clinical setting of central sleep apnea.

The use of a timed bi-level system (BiPAP) device is able to normalize blood gases during sleep. The BiPAP prevents development of severe pulmonary artery hypertension during sleep. BiPAP delivers a higher airway pressure during inspiration (when the airway is most likely to be occluded) and a lower airway pressure during expiration (patient exhales against less resistance). Cardiac dysrhythmias decrease significantly. Improvement of the respiratory situation and of the hemodynamics using a timed BiPAP device may reduce the mortality rate in these patients. Bilevel systems are more expensive than conventional CPAP systems, however, and the algorithms to adjust the inspiratory and expiratory pressures are essentially empiric. Consequently, bi-level systems are typically reserved for patients who cannot tolerate CPAP, especially for those who experience difficulties with exhalation or chest pain as a result of the hyperinflation produced by the applied positive pressure.

Follow-up and Referral

In recent years, COPD and sleep apnea syndrome have been found to coexist in many patients, who are at increased risk of respiratory insufficiency. The detection of small airway disease may be difficult in OSA patients because this syndrome is associated with various pulmonary function abnormalities resulting from obesity and upper airway obstruction. Both of these factors can be responsible for airway obstruction. Patients with both disorders frequently have marked hypoxemia, hypercapnia, and pulmonary hypertension, so they should be referred for investigation of both COPD and sleep apnea. The patient with this so-called "overlap syndrome" is at a higher risk of developing respiratory insufficiency and pulmonary hypertension than the patient with "pure" OSA. Finally, hypoxemic stress is placed on the coronary circulation during sleep that may contribute to nocturnal mortality in the patient with COPD.

Patient Education

Because CPAP is a safe and effective treatment of OSA, it is important to improve patient compliance with regular CPAP use. Only 75% of patients continue to use

CPAP after 1 year, citing the noise, interference with positioning, and complaints of bed partners. Systematically collected data on family members' learning needs and descriptions of the psychosocial impact of CPAP technology treatments on family function and quality of life are essential to developing a comprehensive protocol for teaching and counseling for CPAP therapy. The effect of group patient education sessions on compliance with CPAP therapy has proved to be a simple and effective means of improving treatment of OSA. Nasal discomfort and lack of perceived benefit are possible characteristics of patients with poor compliance; these patients might benefit from education sessions and emotional support. The personal contact and teaching, along with interaction with other OSA patients, may provide an atmosphere of encouragement and support.

Counseling may be needed concerning the potential loss of employment because of poor performance or poor decision making related to profound fatigue from sleep deprivation. Problems of depression, extreme sleepiness, and the effects of hypoxia on cognition pose special difficulties for teaching these patients; their family members must be educated. Family problem-solving skills for managing equipment, overcoming psychosocial barriers to regular nightly use, and eliminating the physiological side effects of CPAP such as oral dryness are important skills and knowledge for this patient population. Home follow-up programs could help patients to eliminate reported physiological adverse effects of CPAP treatments, monitor cardiac stability, and provide ongoing education and family function assessment as evidenced in other follow-up programs. A follow-up program would be cost-effective when quality of life is considered or when compared with hospital admissions for traffic accidents or the severe cardiovascular sequelae associated with OSA.

Teaching must include nutrition counseling. Weight loss may be curative, but because 10% to 20% of body weight loss is required, many patients give up. Strict avoidance of alcohol and hypnotic medications must also be stressed. One of the developmental objectives from *Healthy People 2020* is to reduce the proportion of vehicular crashes caused by persons with excessive sleepiness. Educating patients to be aware of this and to take corrective action is an important role of the health-care provider.

■ SMOKING ADDICTION

A pack-a-day smoker takes more than 70,000 puffs per year. Each puff delivers a rich assortment of chemicals into the lungs and blood. Each puff also reinforces the habit a little more and augments the establishment of secondary reinforcers, such as the sight and smell of cigarettes, the lighting procedure, and the milieu and context of a meal with a cup of coffee or a cocktail. Nicotine fulfills all the criteria of a drug addiction: compulsive use, psychoactive effects, withdrawal symptoms, and

drug-reinforcing behavior. Tolerance and physical dependence, manifested by an abstinence-mediated withdrawal syndrome, contribute to the strong control exerted by nicotine on smoking behavior. Although nicotine is the most popular suspect for the reinforcing agent in tobacco, there are other possibilities. Tar and carbon monoxide are the two most likely contenders. Tobacco use is the leading preventable cause of disease, disability, and death in the United States, particularly cardiovascular disease, cancer, and lung disease. Cigarettes are responsible for one in every five deaths in the United States. In addition, 8.6 million people suffer with a serious illness caused by smoking. For every person who dies from smoking, 20 more suffer from at least one serious tobacco-related illness. Besides the loss of life and the reduction in the quality of life, billions of dollars in medical expenses a year can be directly attributed to cigarette smoking.

There are hazards for nonsmokers who breathe the smoke of others' cigarettes (passive smoking or environmental tobacco smoke). *Environmental tobacco smoke* (ETS) is defined as a combination of the smoke emitted by a burning cigarette, cigar, or pipe and the smoke exhaled by smokers. Passive smoking is associated with a modestly increased risk of lung cancers and possibly other cancers and has been classified by the Environmental Protection Agency as a known human carcinogen. Exposure to ETS causes about 3,000 deaths from lung cancer per year in nonsmoking U.S. adults and damaging the respiratory health of hundreds of thousands of children who live in homes with a parent who smokes cigarettes. It has been estimated that between 150,000 and 300,000 cases of respiratory illness occurring in infants and children up to 18 months of age may stem from exposure to ETS, which increases the risk of lower respiratory tract infections.

Epidemiology and Causes

Substantial gains have been made in reducing smoking prevalence in the United States, although still almost one in four Americans smoke. More than 430,000 deaths per year in the United States are attributed to tobacco use. At the current rate, an estimated 5 million persons younger than age 18 will die prematurely from a disease related to smoking. At the cost of $50 billion per year for medical expenses, this problem is epidemic in proportion. The initiation of smoking by adolescents is now of great concern, but smoking also has become an important issue of women's health. Despite the publicizing of health risks, women continue to start smoking and to persist at high rates.

Although the reduction in overall smoking prevalence represents a major victory for public health, there are many groups within the population that have not experienced these gains. For example, low socioeconomic status and low educational attainment are now the primary predictors of smoking status in the United States and

Canada. Although there have been some important strides made in the reduction of smoking among the U.S. population, there are important target groups that continue to smoke at disproportionately high rates. These groups have been less likely to experience the benefits of tobacco control efforts.

Some forms of smokeless tobacco (plug, leaf, and snuff) have increased. "Dipping snuff," the placing of a coarse, moist powder between the cheek and gum, which results in the direct absorption of nicotine and other carcinogens through the oral tissue, has caused great concern. Oral cancer occurs more frequently among snuff dippers, as well as among pipe and cigar smokers, compared with nonusers of tobacco.

The use of tobacco products is a complex, learned behavior that is woven into the fiber of daily life and is linked to how the smoker deals with the world. Numerous daily activities, thoughts, and emotions serve as powerful cues to smoke. Such conditioned ties become paired with positive neuroregulatory effects of nicotine to reinforce the addictive process. Personal characteristics such as education level, belief in one's ability to change, and coping skills are determinants of tobacco use. Similarly, environmental factors such as the level of acceptance of smoking in the home, peer group, workplace, and community norms influence smoking behavior.

The tobacco industry's drive for profits is the root cause of why cigarette smoking continues to thrive in the United States despite towering and irrefutable evidence that it is a health hazard and a form of drug addiction. Legislative initiatives to control cigarette smoking in the United States are appreciated but not as stringent as they should be. Millions of dollars are spent every day on tobacco advertising. The estimated 3,000 children and youths who become regular smokers each year suffice to ensure an enduring supply of adult smokers. Bans on smoking in the workplace and in some restaurants have done little to discourage smokers from smoking.

Pathophysiology

When cigarettes are smoked, approximately 4,000 chemicals and gases are inhaled into the lungs. Many carcinogens have been isolated from cigarette smoke; 3,4-benzpyrene is the most dangerous. At least 43 other components have been identified as carcinogens, cocarcinogens, tumor promoters, tumor initiators, and mutagens. The primary active (and addictive) ingredient in tobacco is nicotine. In its purest state, nicotine is an extremely toxic, clear, oily liquid with a characteristic odor. At low doses, it acts as a stimulant; at high doses, it depresses the central nervous system (CNS).

Nicotine enters the body through a variety of routes. Inhalation of smoke from a cigar, cigarette, or pipe is perhaps the most common route. During smoking, some absorption of nicotine occurs through the membranes of the mouth, throat, and bronchi, as well as the alveoli of the lungs. In the case of snuff and chewing tobacco, nicotine reaches the bloodstream by absorption through the mucous linings of the mouth, nose, and throat.

Inhalation is the quickest and most effective delivery method. It is estimated that 90% of the nicotine that reaches the alveoli of the lungs in each breath is absorbed into the blood. Although an average cigarette contains from 15 to 20 mg of nicotine, only 1 to 2 mg from each cigarette smoked is actually delivered to the mouth. About 25% of the nicotine is immediately carried to the brain, where it easily crosses the blood–brain barrier and interferes with normal brain biochemistry. In humans, 60 mg of nicotine is a lethal dose.

Acute Effects of Nicotine Use

Outside the CNS, nicotine affects the transmission of nerve signals by mimicking acetylcholine. It occupies receptor sites at the synapses and prevents the transmission of nerve impulses from neuron to neuron and from neuron to muscle cells. Smoking exerts its deleterious effects primarily on the cardiovascular and pulmonary systems (Table 9.24). Nicotine, a direct adrenergic agonist, causes the release of epinephrine, which increases heart rate, systemic vascular resistance, and blood pressure. Smoking directly increases coronary vascular resistance, especially at sites of atherosclerotic plaques and stenosis. Inhaled cigarette smoke also exerts a negative inotropic effect on the myocardium, possibly due to the binding of carbon monoxide (CO) to cytochrome oxidase and myoglobin, resulting in increased myocardial oxygen consumption and decreased oxygen delivery. These changes are accompanied by the constriction of the blood vessels beneath the skin, a reduction in the motility in the bowel, and a loss of appetite.

CO, a component of tobacco smoke, is present in cigarette smoke in similar concentrations as in automobile exhaust. CO has a binding affinity for the hemoglobin molecule 250 times greater than that of oxygen, thereby reducing the smoker's oxygen-carrying capacity. In heavy smokers, as much as 15% of circulating hemoglobin may be bound to CO, reducing the oxygen-carrying capacity of the blood. In addition, CO shifts the oxyhemoglobin dissociation curve to the left, inhibiting the release of oxygen. The half-life of the COHb complex is 4 hours when the individual is breathing room air. The heart's need for oxygen is increased because of the sympathetic stimulatory effect of nicotine. Because the blood's oxygen-carrying capacity is reduced, the heart must pump more rapidly to adequately supply tissues with oxygen.

The effects of smoking on the respiratory system are diverse. The irritating effect of the smoke causes hyperplasia of cells, including goblet cells, which subsequently results in increased mucus production. Hyperplasia reduces airway diameter and increases the difficulty in clearing secretions. Smoking is known to disrupt mucociliary function and its ability to clear particles from

Table 9.24 Effects of Tobacco Smoke

Cardiovascular Effects	Respiratory Effects
Increased myocardial oxygen consumption	Decreased mucociliary clearance
Increased heart rate	Bronchospasm
Increased systemic vascular resistance	Cough
Decreased myocardial inotropic activity	Sputum accumulation
Decreased myocardial oxygen supply	Decreased circulating immunoglobulin levels
Carboxyhemoglobin (reduced available hemoglobin)	Decreased neutrophil chemotaxis
Coronary artery vasospasm	Decreased pulmonary macrophage count and adherence
Oxyhemoglobin dissociation curve shifted to the left	Altered T-lymphocyte immunoregulatory activity
	Decreased natural killer lymphocyte activity
	Decreased function of alpha$_1$-antitrypsin

the peripheral airways before any abnormality in pulmonary function is measured; smoking may cause actual loss of ciliated cells. Smoking also produces abnormal dilation of the distal air space, with destruction of alveolar walls. Many cells develop large, atypical nuclei, which is considered a precancerous condition. Smoking also alters pulmonary immune defense mechanisms by depressing neutrophil chemotaxis, decreasing immunoglobulin levels, reducing natural killer lymphocyte activity, decreasing macrophage adherence, and altering immunoregulatory T-lymphocyte activity.

In the CNS, nicotine activates receptors within the brain. Stimulation of the brain is seen by changes in EEG patterns, reflecting an increase in the frequency of electrical activity. This is part of a general arousal pattern signaled by the release of the neurotransmitters norepinephrine, dopamine, acetylcholine, and serotonin. Heavy tobacco use, resulting in high levels of nicotine in the bloodstream, eventually produces a blocking effect, as more and more receptor sites are filled. The result is a generalized depression of the CNS. When the blood levels of nicotine reach a critical point, the brain's vomiting center may be activated.

Chronic Effects of Nicotine Use

The chronic effects of nicotine include the development of tolerance and chemical dependence. These phenomena cause the user to consume greater quantities of nicotine for longer periods than the user had originally planned and thus endanger the user's health. Dependence on nicotine is quickly established in the majority of those who use it. Although psychological dependence may occur as well, the development of physical dependence, the establishment of tolerance, and the presence of withdrawal symptoms have all been demonstrated. Nicotine withdrawal symptoms include dysphoric or depressed mood, insomnia, irritability, frustration, anger, anxiety, poor concentration, restlessness, decreased heart rate, and increased appetite.

To understand better the neuropsychopharmacological basis of why people smoke, researchers performed positron emission tomography scans on smokers and abstainers and found that smokers had 40% less of a brain enzyme known as monoamine oxidase B (MAO B). The mechanisms of MAO inhibition by cigarette smoke are not known. The enzyme breaks down dopamine, a neurotransmitter associated with feelings of pleasure. Given that nicotine stimulates dopamine release and that dopamine produces pleasurable effects, it is significant in reinforcing and motivating smoking behavior. Therefore, smoking seems to create a self-perpetuating cycle: Less MAO B leads to more dopamine, which leads to more pleasure, which leads to more smoking, which leads to less MAO B, and so on. The researchers proposed that reduction of MAO B activity may synergize with nicotine to produce the diverse behavioral and epidemiological effects of smoking. The myriad of diseases associated with cigarette smoking are shown in Table 9.25.

Clinical Presentation
Subjective

Demographic, anthropometric, physiological, and laboratory features that distinguish cigarette smokers from nonsmokers reflect both baseline differences between these groups and the effects of smoking. Smokers drink more alcohol, coffee, and tea than do nonsmokers. Their weight and BP are slightly lower and their heart rate is slightly faster than those of nonsmokers. Women who smoke are at increased risk for early menopause, decreased bone density, and osteoporosis. Smoking has also been shown to decrease fertility in those attempting pregnancy and to impair uteroplacental function, which adversely affects the fetus during pregnancy. Further, sudden infant death syndrome is two to four times more common in infants whose mothers smoked during pregnancy. Smokers have impaired maximum exercise performance and impaired immune systems compared with nonsmokers. A markedly increased number of pulmonary alveolar macrophages is present in smokers, and the function and metabolism of these cells are abnormal.

Table 9.25 Diseases Associated With Cigarette Smoking

Cardiovascular	• Atherosclerotic cardiovascular disease (CAD; carotid vascular disease; mesenteric, renal, iliac disease; abdominal aortic aneurysm) • Coronary artery spasm • Arrhythmias • Peripheral vascular diseases (thromboangiitis obliterans, deep vein thrombosis, pulmonary embolus)
Endocrine	• Altered hormone secretion • Graves' disease • Antidiuresis • Goiter
Gastrointestinal	• Peptic ulcer disease (gastric, duodenal) • Gastroesophageal reflux disease • Chronic pancreatitis • Crohn's disease • Colic adenomas
Genitourinary	• Glomerulonephritis • Benign prostatic hypertrophy
Immune/musculoskeletal	• Rheumatoid arthritis • Osteoporosis
Infectious	• Tuberculosis • Pneumococcal infection • Meningococcal infection
Integumentary	• Skin wrinkling • Psoriasis
Malignancies	• Respiratory tract malignancies • Lung cancer (squamous-cell, adenocarcinoma, large-cell, small-cell) • Laryngeal cancer • Oral cancer • Others (esophagus, pancreas, bladder, uterine, cervical, breast, kidney, anus, penis, stomach, liver, leukemia)
Pediatric	• Effects on children of parental smoking (asthma, rhinitis, otitis, pneumonia, increased risk for child to begin smoking)
Psychiatric	• Depression • Schizophrenia
Reproductive	• Premature ovarian failure • Decreased sperm quality • Pregnancy-related diseases (prematurity, premature rupture of membranes, spontaneous abortion) • Fetal-/infant-related diseases (low birth weight, impaired lung growth, sudden infant death syndrome, febrile seizures, reduced intelligence, behavioral disorders, atopic disease or asthma)
Respiratory	• COPD • Asthma • Eosinophilic granuloma of the lung • Respiratory bronchiolitis • Goodpasture's syndrome • Sleep apnea • Pneumothorax
Sensory and head and neck	• Loss of olfaction • Loss of taste • Cataracts • Periodontal disease

In smokers, the ratio of high-density lipoprotein cholesterol to low-density lipoprotein cholesterol is reduced.

A causal association is present between smoking and coronary heart disease, atherosclerotic peripheral vascular disease, cerebrovascular disease, lung and laryngeal cancer, oral cancer, esophageal cancer, COPD, intrauterine growth retardation, and low-birth-weight babies. In addition, smoking is considered by many to be the probable cause or a contributing cause for other conditions such as unsuccessful pregnancies; increased infant mortality; peptic ulcer disease; and cancers of the bladder, breast, pancreas, uterus, and kidney (see Table 9.25). Smokers are at risk for increased fractures, premature wrinkling, gingival recession, dental caries, periodontal disease, cataracts, and glaucoma. Depression is twice as common among those who smoke than in people who have never smoked and has been linked to increased smoking initiation and to failures in smoking cessation efforts. A strong association also exists between smoking and other substance abuse disorders, especially alcohol. Clinical manifestations of these specific diseases, though beyond the scope of this chapter, are all clinical manifestations, directly or indirectly, of cigarette smoking.

Objective

The smoker usually demonstrates many observable signs of tobacco addiction. The smell of tobacco smoke lingers on the individual's clothing and on his or her skin and hair. The breath and sputum often smell of stale tobacco and the fingers and nails are often stained from tobacco use. Use of smokeless tobacco may manifest in periodontal disease, a gum disease that may result in the loss of teeth, abrasive damage to the enamel of the teeth caused by the tobacco during processing, and oral cancer. The patient may also have lumps in the jaw or neck area; color change in lumps inside the lips; or white, smooth or scaly patches in the mouth or throat or on the lips or tongue. A patient who smokes may present with a red spot or sore on the lips or gums or inside the mouth that does not heal or difficulty or abnormality in speaking or swallowing.

Signs of cardiopulmonary disease often accompany tobacco addiction. A productive cough, dyspnea, wheezing, and fatigue should alert the clinician to respiratory problems related to smoking. Frequent bouts of pneumonia, influenza, and bronchitis, as well as chronic diseases such as emphysema, interstitial lung disease (ILD), or chronic airway obstruction, often result from cigarette smoking. Cardiovascular signs of smoking including tachycardia, cardiac dysrhythmias, increased blood pressure, decreased peripheral blood flow, and angina must all be assessed to determine the risk for and extent of cardiovascular disease.

Nicotine dependence is related to the amount and duration of smoking and manifests as withdrawal symptoms. These signs and symptoms begin within a few hours of the last cigarette, peak 48 to 72 hours later, and return to baseline within 3 to 4 weeks of quitting. Criteria for nicotine dependence disorder are published in the *Diagnostic and Statistical Manual of Mental Disorders*. They include dysphoric or depressed mood, insomnia, irritability or anger, frustration, anxiety, concentration difficulties, decreased heart rate, and increased appetite or weight gain.

Diagnostic Reasoning

Asking the patient about smoking status and recording this information in the medical record takes only an additional 15 seconds and serves as a reminder to the practitioner to discuss the problem with each smoker. In spite of this, only 20% of smokers receive any medical quitting advice during visits to health-care providers. All patients should be asked if they use tobacco and should have their tobacco-use status documented on a regular basis as a new vital sign. It is unfortunate that teens generally do not seek medical care, because they would benefit the most from hearing about smoking cessation. This is the age-group that all providers should try to reach with this information. Several questionnaires measuring self-reported tobacco dependence have been used. The six-question Fagerstrom Test for Nicotine Dependence (FTND) predicts the level of nicotine dependence and may help predict smoking cessation success, as well as influencing nicotine replacement dosages. The FTND can be accessed at www.outcometracker.org/library/FTND.pdf.

Diagnostic Tests

Laboratory assays of smoking-related biochemical compounds such as thiocyanate, cotinine, nicotine, and carboxyhemoglobin (COHb) can be performed to verify smokers' reports of smoking status or abstinence. There are four potential sources of objective information to determine whether or not a person has smoked: urine, blood, breath, and saliva.

A urine sample can be assayed for the constituents of the cigarette smoke itself or for excretion products that are associated with the physiological effects of smoking. Nicotine excretion in smokers correlates well with the number of cigarettes smoked and inversely with pH of the urine. Urine metabolites of epinephrine can also be measured; however, a potential for false-positive results related to severe anxiety exists.

Carbon monoxide (CO) is found in the blood of those who smoke and combines to form COHb. A value of 2% suggests that smoking has occurred. However, one must take environmental and occupational sources of CO into account. Although COHb increases proportionally with number of cigarettes and varies with nicotine content, discretion is necessary in interpreting the data.

The determination of mean alveolar CO partial pressure makes it possible to determine the COHb levels of the blood with a high degree of correlation. Also, by subtracting expired CO from inspired CO, it is possible to determine if a smoker is an inhaler. Smokers have higher levels of both expired CO and thiocyanate. To measure CO, the patient is instructed to inhale deeply and to hold his or her breath for 10 to 15 seconds before expiring with full force through the inflow valve of the monitor (EC_{50} monitor). Levels of 9 parts per million (ppm) or lower are considered to indicate non-smoking status.

Cotinine is a major metabolite of nicotine and is a useful marker. A sample of at least 3 mL of unstimulated saliva is collected in a plastic cup. The presence of nicotine (as reflected in cotinine levels) in saliva can be determined by gas chromatography and an alkali flame ionization detector, but it is difficult to distinguish a pattern of smoking. Moreover, nonsmokers who have ingested cigarette smoke passively may also have nicotine in their saliva.

Differential Diagnosis

The best way to rule out differential diagnoses is to ensure that, for every patient at every clinic visit, tobacco-use status is queried and documented. The cause of a smoker's cough and dyspnea must be explored to rule out other explanatory causes such as lung cancer, ILD, allergies, and infections. Unfortunately, many patients with symptoms of cough, dyspnea, sputum production, and changes in pulmonary function testing not only are smokers but also suffer from some form of lung disease or disorder. Smokers tend to have unique laboratory findings such as increases in Hct, total white blood cell count, and platelet count. They may also have decreases in leukocytes, vitamin C levels, serum uric acid, and albumin.

Management

The changing face of health-care delivery in the United States indicates the need to incorporate smoking cessation as a regular part of clinical care, particularly in the current managed care environment. The Agency for Healthcare Research and Quality (AHRQ) has an extensive review and synthesis of the outcome of smoking cessation strategies, as well as recommendations for the delivery of smoking interventions in clinical practice (Level I; Agency for Healthcare Research and Quality). The Practice Guideline's key findings emphasize the importance of offering cessation treatment to every smoker at every office visit. Patients who are counseled to quit are 1.6 times as likely to attempt quitting as those who receive no counseling. The Guideline proposes a series of recommendations for primary-care clinicians, smoking cessation specialists, and health-care administrators and purchasers of health insurance, as well as specific strategies for carrying out each of the recommendations (http://www.ahrq.gov/professionals/clinicians-providers/ guidelines-recommendations/tobacco/clinicians/references/ quickref/index.html). Clinicians aiding patients in smoking cessation should remember the Five A's: **A**sk, **A**dvise, **A**ssess, **A**ssist, and **A**rrange, as shown in Treatment Flowchart 9.4.

The goal of every practitioner ought to be to change clinical culture and practice patterns to ensure that every patient who smokes is offered treatment. It is essential to provide a brief but effective smoking cessation intervention for all tobacco users at each clinical visit.

Initial Management

Smoking Cessation Programs Once the patient has been identified as a smoker, it is important to advise him or her of the need to quit. This should be done after the patient's chief complaint has been addressed. The patient's response will determine the proper strategy to pursue. The patient must be informed of how unhealthy smoking is. Pregnant smokers should be strongly encouraged to quit throughout pregnancy. Because of the serious risk of smoking to the pregnant smoker and fetus, pregnant smokers should be offered intensive counseling treatment. Patients should choose a quit date, usually within a month. This will provide a chance to develop effective alternative behaviors to smoking. Periods of extreme stress or depression are not optimal times to attempt smoking cessation.

Before initiating a smoking cessation program, the clinician must know which state of smoking cessation the client is in at that time. This is the first step of the provider-initiated smoking cessation program. Most smokers transition through five stages of behavioral change in their attempts at cessation—precontemplation, contemplation, preparation, action, and maintenance. By understanding the smoker's stage of behavior and readiness to change, the clinician can better assist him or her to achieve a successful cessation.

Smokers in the *precontemplation stage* have no desire to quit in the next 6 to 12 months. These individuals usually benefit from motivational interventions that increase awareness of the adverse affects of smoking. Smokers who are giving serious thought to and are interested in quitting but are not yet ready to do so are in the *contemplation stage*. These smokers also will benefit from motivational counseling emphasizing the negative effects of smoking. Smokers who are serious about quitting and have taken the initial steps toward cessation are in the *preparation phase*. Individuals in this stage benefit from interventions that assist them in quitting. These interventions include providing information about nicotine replacement and developing behavior modification skills.

During the *action stage,* the smoker quits smoking. The action stage lasts from several weeks to 6 months after cessation, which is a common time of relapse. Because of the likelihood of relapse during this stage, interventions should address relapse prevention, including congratulating successes and rewarding positive behavioral changes with more frequent contacts by the clinician. When a smoker has abstained from cigarettes for

Treatment Flowchart 9.4 Smoking Cessation Strategies

6 months, the *maintenance stage* begins. Most successful quitters relapse and recycle through these stages three or four times before attaining long-term abstinence; some may take several years to move through these stages until abstinence can be maintained.

Effective smoking cessation requires behavior modification. The behavior of smoking is usually linked to a variety of triggers (e.g., stress, foods or beverages, driving). When a patient is able to recognize the triggers, healthy alternative behaviors can be substituted. It is crucial to develop alternative coping strategies to overcome the urge to smoke. Such strategies include deep breathing and relaxation exercises, chewing gum, exercise, drinking water, sucking on a piece of sugarless candy, and eating carrots or celery sticks.

Patients with any chronic health problem need support from their clinicians, their families, and other persons. The clinician can help the patient handle particularly difficult triggers and can treat any underlying behavior problems, such as anxiety or depression. The family can provide invaluable positive reinforcement to the patient during this time. If there are other smokers in the patient's household, the clinician should encourage them to quit smoking at the same time as the patient. It is very difficult for a person to refrain from smoking in the long term when a spouse or a family member continues to smoke. Many patients benefit from the support of groups such as Nicotine Anonymous, the American Lung Association's Freedom from Smoking program, and the American Cancer Society's Freshstart program.

Hypnosis   The goal of hypnosis in smoking cessation is to enable the smoker to achieve an altered state of consciousness that enhances the ability to quit. However, the hypnotic trance is generally not measurably different from deep muscle relaxation. The effects of hypnosis are often short-lived. Controlled trials of hypnosis have generally not documented long-term efficacy for smoking cessation. Hypnosis is of low reliability, with published quit rates ranging between 0% and 88%. Although it is of uncertain value, hypnosis remains a commercially popular stop-smoking method. The primary advantage of hypnosis is that it may be an attractive alternative for people who have failed to quit with other methods.

Aversion Conditioning   Aversion conditioning is based on the premise that smoking is a learned response that can be extinguished by creation of an association between smoking and a negative sensation. Among the aversion techniques utilized for smoking cessation are electric shock; nausea-inducing drugs; hot, smoky air treatments; and rapid smoking. High quit rates were reported in some of the early smoking cessation trials using aversion conditioning; however, these high rates may be attributed, in part, to factors related to patient selection, because arguably only the most highly motivated persons are willing to undergo therapies such as electric shock or the breathing of hot, smoky air. In addition, aversion conditioning techniques may represent a health hazard.

Subsequent Management

Pharmacological Approaches   Although some smokers may need antidepressants or anxiolytics, it is difficult to predict who will benefit from these adjunctive therapies. Bupropion (Zyban) is an antidepressant and smoking deterrent. Bupropion is a weak inhibitor of the neuronal uptake of norepinephrine and dopamine but has no effect on serotonin. Its dopaminergic and noradrenergic activities are responsible for its efficacy in smoking cessation, with the dopaminergic activity affecting areas of the brain having to do with the reinforcement activity affecting nicotine withdrawal. Bupropion appears to have no effect on patient depression scores, so it is unlikely that the mechanism for the efficacy of bupropion is through its antidepressant effects. Bupropion is well tolerated, with the most frequent adverse effects being headache, insomnia, and dry mouth. Antidepressants are associated with a small risk of seizure. Moreover, patients with a history of severe head trauma, eating disorders, recent myocardial infarction, unstable heart disease, or active alcoholism should not take bupropion.

The dosage of 300 mg per day (150 mg per day for 3 days followed by 150 mg twice a day) is begun 1 to 2 weeks before smoking cessation. It is important for the steady-state plasma levels of bupropion to be reached (usually within 8 days) before smoking cessation is begun. This dosing schedule has been found to lead to less weight gain during the medication phase. The duration of treatment is usually 7 to 12 weeks. For maintenance therapy, bupropion SR 150 mg twice a day for up to 6 months should be considered. As with the nicotine replacement products, behavioral modification therapy should coexist. For heavily addicted smokers, nicotine replacement therapy and bupropion can be coadministered concurrently.

Varenicline (Chantix) is a nicotinic acetylcholine receptor partial agonist used as a smoking cessation aid, and it is also recommended that therapy begins 1 week before a target quit date is set. Smoking cessation aids are listed in Drugs Commonly Prescribed 9.3.

Health-care providers need to be aware of the nuances of smoking cessation. For example, individuals often experience constipation during cessation, as the gastrointestinal system adjusts to withdrawal from the stimulating effects of nicotine. The use of a bulk-forming agent such as Metamucil, increased dietary fiber, and increased fluids will alleviate the problem. A form of exercise, such as walking, is an excellent, affordable stress reliever. A walking program also assists with reducing the expected mean weight gain of 5 to 7 pounds that occurs with smoking cessation. Nicotine is an appetite depressant, and once its effects have cleared from the body, food tastes better.

Drugs Commonly Prescribed 9.3 Therapies for Smoking: Prescribing Considerations

Drug	Dosage	Advantages	Disadvantages
Transdermal Patch		**Continuous Delivery**	**Expensive**
Nicoderm CQ (worn 24 hr/day)	21 mg/day for 4–6 weeks, then 14 mg/day for 2–4 weeks, then 7 mg/day for 2–4 weeks	Less instruction required than gum	Risk of insomnia or nightmares
Gum (nicotine polacrilex)		**Useful on "As Needed" Basis**	**Requires Good Dentition**
Nicorette	2 mg/piece; max 30 pieces/day 4 mg/piece; max 24 pieces/day	Provides oral gratification Patient control Delayed weight gain	Risk of mouth irritation Dyspnea, nausea Risk of developing dependence
Nasal Spray		**Useful on "As Needed" Basis**	
Nicotrol (10-mL bottle)	0.5 mg/spray; 2 sprays; maximum 40 doses/day for 3 months	Rapid delivery	Risk of nasal and throat irritation Runny nose Watery eyes
Inhaler			
Nicotrol inhaler	13 mcg/puff; 6–16 cartridges/day for 3 months	Mimics smoking behavior	Risk of cough, irritation of mouth and throat
Lozenge			
Commit	2 mg (if first cigarette smoked >30 min after waking) 4 mg (if first cigarette smoked within 30 min of waking) max. 20 lozenges/day, dissolve over 20–30 min; minimize swallowing		May cause hiccoughs, heartburn.
Other			
Bupropion hydrochloride (Zyban)	150 mg/day for 3 days, then 150 mg bid for 7–12 weeks (possibly up to 6 months)	Nonnicotine, less weight gain	Risk of seizures, headache, dry mouth, insomnia
Varenicline (Chantix)	0.5 mg/day for 3 days, then 0.5 mg bid for 4 days, then 1 mg bid for 12 weeks, take with a glass of water after eating	Nonnicotine	Nausea Risk of serious neuropsychiatric symptoms including depression, altered mood and behavior, and suicidality

Nicotine Replacement Therapies Nicotine is the drug of choice to assist smoking cessation. The nicotine patch, gum, and lozenges are available over the counter (OTC), and nicotine nasal spray and inhalers are available by prescription (see Drugs Commonly Prescribed 9.3).

Increased access through OTC availability has substantially increased the number of quitters in the United States. Evaluations of the efficacy of nicotine gum through 12-month follow-up suggest that the gum improves smoking cessation rates by approximately 40% to

60% compared with control interventions. Efficacy is increased when nicotine gum use is combined with an intensive psychosocial intervention. The efficacy of the nicotine patch overall appears to be somewhat stronger than that for the gum. The patch has been found to double the 6- to 12-month abstinence rates over those yielded by placebo interventions.

The cost of the patch remains relatively high, however, which places this cessation strategy out of the reach of some smokers. Although the manufacturer of nicotine gum has developed a series of strategies for increasing access to nicotine replacement therapy among underserved populations, it is not clear if the penetration of such programs can match the need for an effective strategy among lower-income and other underserved groups.

The gum must be correctly chewed to a softened state and then placed in the buccal mucosa. Clients should not eat for 15 minutes before or during use of the nicotine gum. A piece of gum should be chewed intermittently over a 30-minute period. Initially, one piece is chewed every 1 to 2 hours over 6 weeks with a maximum of 24 pieces in 24 hours. Time intervals for gum use are gradually increased to 2 to 4 hours for 3 weeks, then every 4 to 8 hours for 3 weeks. Fewer than 10% of patients will become dependent on the gum although many will require long-term use (1–2 years) to maintain abstinence. Nicotine absorption is decreased by acidic foods and beverages, which should be avoided during use. Irritation and trauma to the oral mucosa, teeth, and dental work can occur. Many patients experience jaw ache, gastrointestinal discomfort, hiccups, and cardiostimulation.

Nicotine patches are applied every morning and worn for 24 hours per day. Patches are usually indicated for 8 to 12 weeks to promote long-term abstinence. Patients should be instructed to change the application site daily to minimize skin irritation. The highest-dose patch should be considered if the patient smokes more than 20 cigarettes per day and has no active cardiovascular disease. Because a dose–response effect has been found, researchers recommend that a higher nicotine dose is more effective for smoking cessation. The adverse effects of the patches include skin reactions, insomnia, vivid dreams, and myalgias. If vivid dreams or insomnia occur, the patient should be instructed to remove the patch before going to bed and then to apply a new patch on arising.

The nicotine nasal spray (Nicotrol nasal spray) delivers nicotine in a more rapid manner and thereby serves as a better substitute than nicotine gum or a nicotine patch. The device is similar to nasal antihistamine sprays. The nasal spray delivers 0.5 mg of nicotine per spray. Smokers are instructed to use one to two doses per hour for 3 months for up to 40 doses per day. The nasal spray delivers nicotine more rapidly than gum, patch, or inhaler but less rapidly than cigarettes. Peak levels occur within 4 to 15 minutes and are about two-thirds of those associated with cigarettes. Patients initially experience nasal and throat irritation, rhinitis, sneezing, coughing, and watering eyes. Tolerance to these effects develops in the first week. The spray may cause serious dysrhythmias, elevated blood pressure, and angina in post–myocardial infarction patients. Use of the spray is not recommended in patients with several other chronic diseases, including asthma, peptic ulcer disease, chronic nasal disorders, severe renal impairment, liver disease, diabetes, and hyperthyroidism.

Researchers have found that the use of a nicotine patch with a nicotine nasal spray is significantly more effective for long-term smoking cessation than with either alone. The results suggest an increased efficacy in prevention of relapse with more intake of nicotine or by combining different types of nicotine replacement therapies. The combination of a nicotine patch and nicotine nasal spray may be successful not only because of the high level of substitution but also because of the opportunity to respond quickly to the smoker's need. Researchers have suggested that using a patch for 5 months with a nicotine nasal spray for 1 year provides a more effective means of stopping smoking than using a patch alone.

The nicotine inhaler (Nicotrol inhaler) is a plastic rod with a nicotine plug that provides a nicotine vapor when puffed on. Each active cartridge contains approximately 10 mg of nicotine and 1 mg of menthol. The menthol is added to decrease the throat irritation caused by the nicotine. Although the device is designed as an inhaler, this label is a misnomer because the device does not deliver a significant amount of nicotine to the lungs; rather, the device delivers nicotine buccally. This occurs whether smokers use deep or shallow puffs. Each cartridge lasts about 20 minutes and provides the nicotine equivalent of about two cigarettes. Patients use 6 to 16 cartridges per day for 3 months, then taper for 6 to 12 weeks as needed. The most common adverse effects are cough and irritation in the mouth and throat. The inhaler has the potential to assist in the smoking cessation process not only by providing nicotine replacement but also by mimicking the behavioral aspects of smoking. Such a device clearly blurs the line between cigarette and nicotine-delivery device, however. In effect, the patient is brand switching (i.e., switching from his or her usual brand of cigarette to a smoke-free nicotine-delivery device) even though the effort required to obtain nicotine from the inhaler is greater than that required from a cigarette. Combining the nicotine inhaler with the nicotine patch may increase the efficacy over using the patch alone because the inhaler would serve to supplement the nicotine provided by the patch and mimic smoking behavior.

Follow-up and Referral

As with any serious medical problem, follow-up is essential after the initial intervention. A supportive phone call the week after the quit date can be made by a healthcare worker with the reinforcement of the self-help materials that have been provided. Office follow-up by the clinician at 1 and 3 months after the quit date can help the patient who has quit smoking to cope with persistently difficult triggers or situations; this support can help the patient who may have relapsed get back on the right track. In the case of relapse, the client should be assisted to set another quit date, revisit the reasons for quitting, and begin the process again. Assure patients that stable abstinence is commonly achieved only after five or six attempts.

Patient Education

For years, cigarette smoking was viewed as largely a social or psychological habit. As such, the ability to quit was considered a measure of personal motivation and willpower. Motivation to stop smoking, combined with sufficient psychological resources, was seen as a driving force behind successful cigarette abstinence. Thus, if smokers could be educated about the health risks of cigarette smoking, they could theoretically become sufficiently motivated and psychologically empowered to quit. Unfortunately, the anticipated benefits of achieving smoking cessation through education were overoptimistic and simplistic. More than 80% of current smokers indicate they would like to quit but cannot. Educational programs to aid smoking cessation have produced disappointing results and high long-term failure rates. Only about 4% of smokers are able to quit each year. Nonetheless, it is helpful to give the patient some age-specific smoking cessation literature.

It is important to understand the meaning of smoking to the individual patient, to hear the "patient's voice" (see The Patient's Voice 9.1). Assisting the patient in ceasing smoking involves an empowerment process that enhances the patient's motivation and self-esteem. The provider can facilitate this process by providing available cessation information to both the patient and the family. There must be a family-focused emphasis, with shared commitment and participation. Providers can encourage patients to identify daily stressors and assist them to reframe situations and develop alternative coping strategies. Equally important is developing an enhanced self-efficacy, which includes accepting and believing in the ability to succeed. Providers need to ask how the patient usually deals with stress and give simple, usable alternative coping strategies. A telephone hotline with recorded messages that empower and encourage can be an effective way to manage and overcome the desire to smoke. Information about the rewards of smoking cessation, such as improved health with lower blood pressure and improved circulation and lung functioning, should be provided. Individuals who cease smoking report more energy, enhanced taste and smell, money saved, freedom from addiction, feeling better about oneself, and better performance in sexual and sports activities. Smokers older than age 55 years should be informed that despite many years of smoking, smoking cessation will improve their health. They will enjoy a better quality of life as ex-smokers and their risk for lung and other smoking-associated cancers will be reduced. Smokers die 5 to 8 years earlier than persons who have never smoked. Additional rewards for older adults can be the satisfaction of being a positive role model for other family members and making a contribution to the improved health of their grandchildren. To enhance recovery from nicotine addiction and prevent relapse, both individual and group cessation counseling and education must include a family focus.

The Patient's Voice 9.1
Battleground

"What is it with you and your cigarettes, anyway?" I angrily thought to myself after yet another heated debate with my father about smoking. As usual, he had been defending cigarettes as a source of pleasure, saying he always enjoyed smoking. He was against federal attempts to regulate levels of nicotine or restrict access. After smoking for 60 years, he quit last year, when the severity of his lung disease nearly took his life. Why couldn't I make him understand that cigarettes were killing people?

He must have sensed my frustration or read my mind, because as his O_2 concentrator clicked off and on, he looked at me and said softly, "You know, Snicklefritz, it was cigarettes that saved my life many times during the war." My father rarely talks about THE WAR. He was a combat infantryman, a machine gunner, part of the Fifth Division known as "Roosevelt's Red Devils." He started slowly . . .

"At night we were the point. Machine gunners never got relieved. The cold was the worst. You couldn't imagine the cold. Raining—below freezing. We would take turns sleeping. You couldn't sleep for more than an hour. You had to rely on your buddies to wake you up. You had to keep moving to keep from freezing. Many only lasted one night and had to be sent back because their feet were frozen. I think we lost more men to cold that winter than from enemy fire.

"I remember standing up one night with tracers going by my head, yelling 'Go ahead and shoot me—put me out of my misery!' My buddy had to pull me down. He said. 'Have a cigarette—calm yourself!' We had to cover our heads with raingear to keep anyone from seeing to light up and give away our positions. You can't imagine the warmth and comfort in one cigarette. We were worried about living through the night.

"There were times warmth of a cigarette was the only thing that kept us alive. We were short of supplies that winter, but they always kept us in cigarettes. Even our K-rations came with a pack—I'll give them that."

As he talked, I tried to imagine, to understand, the inhuman conditions he was describing and the meaning cigarettes held for him. As I listened to my father's story and watched him pull his arms to his chest and cup his hands to his face, as if he were holding something as precious as life itself, I finally heard what he had been saying for years. I began to feel my anger slipping away—anger with my father for smoking all those years and for nearly dying before my 3-year-old son had a chance to come to know him.

I felt my eyes fill with tears, not for the suffering my father had experienced during the war, but for the suffering he experienced because his daughter, the nurse, never understood.

— Shirley Countryman Gordon, from "Nightingale Songs." Publication of Florida Atlantic University College of Nursing.

 DavisPlus | For additional resources please visit http://davisplus.fadavis.com

References

Evidence-Based Practice

Agency for Healthcare Research and Quality. Treating tobacco use and dependence: Quick reference guide for clinicians, 2009. Retrieved from http://www.ahrq.gov/professionals/clinicians-providers/guidelines-recommendations/tobacco/clinicians/references/quickref/index.html

Burman, ME, and Wright, WL. Diagnosis and management of community-acquired pneumonia: Evidence-based practice. *J Nurse Pract* 3(9):633–649, 2007.

Demeter, PL, et al. Cough. In *Pulmonary (acute and chronic)*. Work Loss Data Institute, San Diego, CA, 2009, pp 28–43. Retrieved from www.guideline.gov/content.aspx?id=15495&search=asthma

Freeman, D, et al. Efficacy and safety of tiotropium in COPD patients in primary care—The SPiRiva Usual CarE (SPRUCE) Study. *Respir Res* 8:45, 2007. doi:10.1186/1465-9921-8-45

Gami, AS, et al. Obstructive sleep apnea and the risk of sudden cardiac death: A longitudinal study of 10,701 adults. *J Am Coll Cardiol* 62(7):610–616, 2013. Retrieved from www.sciencedirect.com/science/article/pii/S0735109713022511

Mandell, LA, et al. Infectious Diseases Society of America/American Thoracic Society consensus guidelines on the management of community-acquired pneumonia in adults. IDSA/ATS Guidelines for CAP in adults. *Clin Infect Dis* 44(Suppl 2):S27–S72, 2007.

Quon, BS, et al. Contemporary management of acute exacerbations of COPD. *Chest* 133(3):756–766, 2008.

University of Michigan Health System. *Chronic obstructive pulmonary disease.* University of Michigan Health System, Ann Arbor, MI, 2010.

Bibliography

General

American Psychiatric Association. *Diagnostic and statistical manual of mental disorders,* ed 5 (DSM-5). American Psychiatric Association, Washington, DC, 2013.

Longo, DL, et al (Eds.). *Harrison's principles of internal medicine,* ed 18. McGraw-Hill, New York, 2011.

McPhee, SJ, and Papadakis, MA. *Current medical diagnosis and treatment.* Appleton-Lange/McGraw-Hill, New York, 2010.

Asthma

Bernstein, JA. Allergic rhinitis and asthma: How to help patients control environmental triggers. *Consultant* 52(7):508–514, 2012.

Bernstein, JA. Allergic rhinitis and asthma: Role of environmental determinants. *Consultant* 52(7):490–497, 2012.

Chronic Bronchitis and Emphysema (COPD)

Kirkpatrick, P, et al. Research to support evidence-based practice in COPD community nursing. *Br J Community Nurs* 17(10):486, 488–492, 2012.

Menn, P, et al; KORA Study Group. Direct medical costs of COPD—An excess cost approach based on two population-based studies. *Respir Med* 106(4):540–548, 2012.

Stanley, T, et al. Patient and provider attributes associated with chronic obstructive pulmonary disease exacerbations. *J Nurse Pract* 9(1):34–39, 2013.

Yawn, BP. Pulmonary practice pearls for primary care physicians. *J Family Practice* 1(1). Retrieved from http://newsletter.qhc.com/JFP/COPDlandingpage.html

Dyspnea

Newsham, K. Evaluating dyspnea in the athletic patient. *J Nurse Pract* 9(5):288–294, 2013.

Pneumonia

Struble, K. Community-acquired pneumonia empiric therapy. Medscape, 2011. Retrieved from http://emedicine.medscape.com/article/2011819-overview

Sleep Apnea

Gami, AS, et al. Obstructive sleep apnea and the risk of sudden cardiac death: A longitudinal study of 10,701 adults. *J Am Coll Cardiol* 62(7):610–616, 2013. Retrieved from www.sciencedirect.com/science/article/pii/S0735109713022511

Tuberculosis

Catanzaro, A. The diagnosis of TB in an era of diminishing incidence of TB. Retrieved from www.thoracic.org/sections/chapters/thoracic-society-chapters/ca/current-news/resources/2DXTB.pdf

Centers for Disease Control and Prevention. Core curriculum on tuberculosis: What the clinician should know. Updated July 9, 2013. Retrieved from www.cdc.gov/tb/education/corecurr

Resources

American Cancer Society, Inc.
www.cancer.org
American Sleep Apnea Association
www.sleepapnea.org
American Sleep Association
www.americansleepassociation.org
National Sleep Foundation
http://sleepfoundation.org

Asthma and COPD (selected Web sites)

Allergy, Asthma, and Immunology Online
http://allergy.mcg.edu/physicians/manual/manual.html
www.nhlbi.nih.gov/guidelines/asthma
American Academy of Allergy, Asthma, and Immunology
www.aaaai.org
American College of Allergy, Asthma, and Immunology
www.acaai.org

Asthma and Allergy Foundation of America
www.aafa.org
Asthmacontrol.com—a GlaxoSmithKline Web site offering two
   questionnaires for asthma control tests
American Lung Association
www.lungusa.org
National Institute of Allergy and Infectious Disease
www.niaid.nih.gov
Cancer Care, Inc.
www.cancercare.org
www.cancer.gov and *http://cancernet.nci.nih.gov*
National Institutes of Health
National Heart, Lung, and Blood Institute
www.nhlbi.nih.gov
National Library of Medicine
www.nlm.nih.gov

CDC's SARS Web site
www.cdc.gov/ncidod/sars/infectioncontrol.htm
CDC H1N1 Flu Web site
www.cdc.gov/h1n1flu
Patient Education (selected Web sites):
www.betterhealth.com
www.cdc.gov
www.medscape.com
Smoking Cessation
American Lung Association
www.lungusa.org
www.meds.com/pdq/small_cellpro.html
Smoking Cessation Behavior Modification
www.clc.gov/tobacco/how2quit.htm

Cardiovascular Problems

Chapter 10

Kathryn B. Keller, PhD, RN • Denese Sabatino, MSN, APRN, NP-C, CCRN • Jill E. Winland-Brown, EdD, APRN, FNP-BC • Brian Oscar Porter, MD, PhD, MPH • Michael B. Keller, MD, MS

COMMON COMPLAINTS

■ CHEST PAIN

Although chest pain is often associated with cardiovascular problems, it may also have pulmonary, gastrointestinal, musculoskeletal, neurological, psychogenic, or idiopathic causes. If the chest pain is related to coronary artery disease, the incidence increases after age 35 in men and after menopause in women. See Nursing Research-Based Practice Box 10.1 for a discussion of women's decisions to seek treatment for the symptoms of potential cardiac illness. In individuals up to 50 years of age, chest pain occurs more frequently in men, and then equally in men and women older than 50 years.

Differential Diagnosis

Obtaining a focused health history and physical exam is essential for accurate assessment and appropriate treatment for a patient with chest pain (see Differential Diagnosis Flowchart 10.1). Critical components of the history include appraisal of the major symptoms of heart disease, including chest pain, dyspnea, syncope, and heart failure. The clinician should ask patients in all age-groups about tolerance of exercise, especially whether exercise provokes any of the aforementioned complaints. The history of the present illness of the person with chest pain should focus on personal risk factors for cardiovascular disease.

The clinician should obtain a complete chest pain symptom analysis including location, quality, duration, aggravating or relieving factors, and associated symptoms or signs. In particular, localized, fleeting, and moving pain is rarely indicative of serious cardiac pathology. Anxiety and bereavement can cause diffuse pain and chest tenderness lasting for hours. Costochondritis is often described as localized, and it can be replicated with arm movement or pressing on the area of tenderness.

In contrast, the discomfort of angina pectoris is classically described as a diffuse, retrosternal sensation, often with radiation, and a heavy, burning sensation, usually lasting more than 1 minute but less than 10 minutes.

Exertional symptoms are usually more common in individuals with fixed atherosclerotic lesions. In assessing the person with known angina pectoris, it is critical to ascertain if there has been a change in the symptom pattern because this may indicate an alteration in vessel patency such as that found in accelerated atherosclerosis or vessel spasm. The word "pain" should be used with caution in taking the history of a person with suspected myocardial ischemia because the patient may deny that pain is present but may agree that tightness, burning, fullness, or other sensations more aptly describe the complaint.

The terms *unstable angina, preinfarct angina,* and *crescendo angina* are synonyms used to describe the condition in which there is a new onset of cardiac ischemic chest pain at rest but without evidence of acute myocardial infarction (MI). Reports of symptoms at rest are

---

Nursing Research–Based Practice 10.1

Turris, SA. Women's decisions to seek treatment for the symptoms of potential cardiac illness. *J Nurs Scholars* 41(1):5–12, 2009.

Cardiac disease is the number one killer of Canadian women, and therapies are often highly time dependent. Consequently, understanding the forms of knowledge that women draw on to understand and interpret their symptoms of a potential cardiac event may be important in relation to efforts to reduce treatment-seeking delay. Data for this grounded-theory study were drawn from in-depth interviews with 16 women who went to one of two emergency departments for the treatment of symptoms indicating potential cardiac illness. The basic social process of maintaining integrity explained the women's interpretations of, and actions in relation to, their symptoms. Decisions about treatment seeking were influenced primarily by the context of the women's lives as mothers, daughters, and wives and only secondarily by the women's interpretations of and conclusions about their symptoms. Four ways of knowing are shared to explain their decisions to seek treatment.

Differential Diagnosis Flowchart 10.1

Chest Pain

Location: Substernal; may radiate to jaw, neck, arms, and back
Characteristics: Aching, squeezing, pressure, heaviness, burning; usually subsides within 10 minutes
→ **Aggravating factors:** Eating, physical activity, smoking, cold weather, stress, anger, hunger, lying down
Alleviating factors: Rest, nitroglycerin
→ R/O angina

Location: Across chest; may radiate to jaw, neck, arms, and back
Characteristics: Pressure, burning, aching, tightness; may be accompanied by shortness of breath, diaphoresis, weakness, anxiety, or nausea; sudden onset; usually lasts 1/2 to 2 hours
→ **Aggravating factors:** Exertion, anxiety
Alleviating factors: Narcotic analgesics (morphine)
→ R/O acute myocardial infarction (MI)

Location: Substernal; may radiate to neck, left arm
Characteristics: Sharp and may be accompanied by friction rub; sudden onset
→ **Aggravating factors:** Deep breathing, supine position
Alleviating factors: Sitting up, leaning forward, anti-inflammatory agents
→ R/O pericarditis

Location: Retrosternal, upper abdominal, or epigastric; may radiate to back, neck, shoulders
Characteristics: Excruciating, tearing; may be accompanied by blood pressure differences between right and left arm; sudden onset
→ **Aggravating factors:** None
Alleviating factors: Analgesics
→ R/O dissecting aortic aneurysm

Location: Over lung area
Characteristics: Stabbing; may be accompanied by cyanosis, dyspnea, or cough with hemoptysis; sudden onset
→ **Aggravating factors:** Inspiration
Alleviating factors: Analgesics
→ R/O pulmonary embolus (PE)

Location: Lateral thorax
Characteristics: Severe; may be accompanied by dyspnea, increased pulse rate, decreased breath sounds, or deviated trachea; sudden onset
→ **Aggravating factors:** Normal respiration
Alleviating factors: Analgesics, chest tube insertion
→ R/O pneumothorax

Location: Lower chest or upper abdomen
Characteristics: Sharp, severe
→ **Aggravating factors:** Eating a heavy meal, bending, lying down
Alleviating factors: Antacids, walking, semi-Fowler's position
→ R/O hiatal hernia

Location: Epigastric
Characteristics: Burning feeling after eating; may be accompanied by hematemesis or tarry stools; sudden onset; usually subsides in 15–20 minutes
→ **Aggravating factors:** Lack of food, highly acidic foods
Alleviating factors: Food, antacids
→ R/O peptic ulcer

Location: Anywhere in the chest
Characteristics: Sharp, continuous or gradual; chest may be tender to the touch; gradual or sudden onset
→ **Aggravating factors:** Movement, palpation
Alleviating factors: Time, analgesics, heat applications
→ R/O costochondritis

Location: Anywhere in the chest
Characteristics: Dull or stabbing pain; usually accompanied by hyperventilation or breathlessness; sudden onset; may last less than a minute or for several days
→ **Aggravating factors:** Increased respiratory rate, stress, anxiety
Alleviating factors: Slowing of respiratory rate, stress relief
→ R/O acute anxiety

more likely to be associated with coronary artery vasospasm, a condition usually seen in patients with coronary atherosclerosis. The combination of two mechanisms of lumen narrowing leaves the patient at considerable risk for an acute coronary syndrome; in these cases, rapid and accurate assessment is vital to ensure appropriate disposition and treatment.

About one-third of patients with angina pectoris will have simultaneous dyspnea caused by transient increase in pulmonary venous pressures that accompanies ventricular stiffening during an episode of myocardial ischemia. The presence of diaphoresis with chest pain is particularly worrisome, often indicating a significant drop in cardiac output during the episode of pain and subsequent decreased perfusion of the skin. In contrast to the patient who complains of anginal pain, the patient who is experiencing an acute MI often complains of anginal-like chest pain that lasts in excess of 20 minutes but occasionally waxes and wanes during that period. The pain is frequently accompanied by dyspnea, diaphoresis, nausea, and dizziness. The pain may radiate to the neck, jaw, shoulder, or arm (left side more than right). Patients show extreme variation in the amount of pain experienced with an MI, from complaining of a "vise around the heart" to apologizing for seeking assistance with "just a bit of indigestion that will not clear up." In particular, women, older adults, and people with diabetes mellitus are likely to have minimal or atypical symptoms with an acute MI. A more detailed discussion of the pain of angina and MI is provided in the sections on treatment of those conditions later in the chapter.

■ PALPITATIONS

Palpitations are commonly reported by the individual who has or is at risk for heart disease. *Palpitations* are defined as the awareness of the beating of one's heart and may be benign or pathological in nature. When questioning the patient with palpitations, the clinician should obtain a detailed description of the sensation. If the patient reports a sensation of a strong but regular rhythmic beating of the heart after stress or exertion, this likely indicates a normal physiological response to the increased catecholamine production. If there is a report of skipped or missed beats, particularly with the sensation that the heart "stopped" momentarily, this may indicate the presence of an atrial or ventricular ectopic beat.

Differential Diagnosis

Atrial ectopic beats are most often benign, occurring with excessive caffeine, alcohol, or tobacco use. On occasion, atrial ectopic beats occur with cardiac pathology, sometimes as a precursor to a supraventricular rhythm such as multifocal atrial tachycardia or atrial fibrillation. This is most likely in the patient with chronic obstructive pulmonary disease (COPD) or rheumatic heart disease and valvular dysfunction.

Ventricular ectopic beats are somewhat more likely to indicate cardiac pathology than atrial ectopy. If the patient is at high risk for or has known heart disease, the clinician must carefully assess the complaint of palpitations because ventricular ectopy may indicate increased risk for sudden cardiac death.

Another variation on the presentation of palpitations is the patient who complains of a sudden onset of a very rapid heartbeat or fluttering of the heart. The etiology may be a supraventricular or ventricular tachycardia, often with equally rapid and unpredictable cessation of the rhythm, or a rhythmic paroxysm. Although this type of rhythmic sensation is usually regular, such as in paroxysmal supraventricular tachycardia or ventricular tachycardia, it may also be irregular, such as in intermittent atrial fibrillation. In any case, the clinician should query the patient carefully about cosymptoms such as chest pain related to decreased coronary artery filling and increased myocardial oxygen demands, as well symptoms associated with low cardiac output.

Diagnostic testing should be directed by information obtained in the health history and physical exam. As with cardiac-related syncope, thyroid function (thyroid-stimulating hormone), blood chemistries, hemoglobin, and hematocrit should be evaluated to help rule out thyroid disorder, electrolyte imbalance, or anemia as a possible, though less common, cause of palpitations. Ambulatory cardiac monitoring (Holter monitoring) until at least one event is recorded is most helpful in ascertaining the presence of a potentially lethal cardiac rhythm disturbance. Echocardiography may be necessary to assess cardiac outflow tract patency and to help rule out valvular stenosis or hypertrophic cardiomyopathy.

Intervention should be directed at the underlying cause of the palpitations. For example, if a rhythm disturbance such as recurrent supraventricular or ventricular tachycardia is the cause, treatment directed at eliminating this is warranted. In any event, the clinician should consult with a physician or cardiologist who has expertise in this area to ensure patient safety and optimal outcome.

Differential diagnoses of palpitations are presented in Differential Diagnosis Flowchart 10.2.

■ SYNCOPE

Syncope is loss of consciousness that occurs abruptly as a discrete episode and usually lasts for a short period of only a few minutes. The implied pathology is decreased cerebral blood flow caused by a marked decrease in cardiac output. Approximately one million people are affected by syncope in the United States every year. Whereas some of these episodes are explainable and of noncardiac origin (e.g., fluid loss, dehydration, emotional stress), the vast majority of these episodes are cardiovascular in origin. Cardiac-related syncope is an ominous sign associated with high rates of mortality. A syncopal episode may be the only warning sign of impending sudden death. One of the most common cardiac causes of

Differential Diagnosis Flowchart 10.2

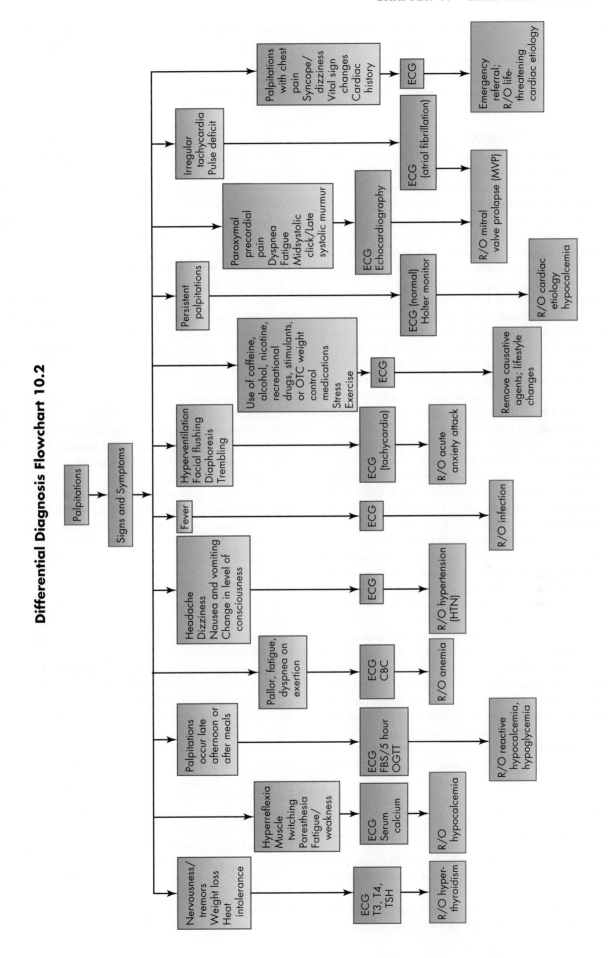

syncope is cardiac arrhythmias (Level I; Heart Rhythm Society, 2013). A wide range of conduction disturbances can precede a syncopal event and may include tachycardia-bradycardia syndrome (sick sinus syndrome), supraventricular and ventricular tachycardias, heart blocks, and bradycardia.

Differential Diagnosis

Cardiac outflow tract blockage, such as the obstruction that may occur in hypertrophic cardiomyopathy and aortic valve stenosis, can also produce syncope. This is most often seen in response to increased activity or stress when the outflow tract blockage impedes the increase in cardiac output needed to meet the increased demands for oxygen. This leads to syncope that typically lasts for a few seconds and ends when the "rest" of the syncopal episode helps balance supply and demand.

Presyncope, a state of light-headedness, feeling faint, and muscular weakness, is most often cardiovascular in origin. The etiology is usually the same as for syncope. In contrast, *vertigo* is when the person has the sensation of staggering or veering in a certain direction or of spinning. The sensation can often be reproduced by a change in head position. In vertigo, the cause is usually something other than decreased cerebral blood flow, often an inner ear disturbance, for example.

Diagnostic testing for cardiac-related syncope should be directed by the information obtained in the health history and physical exam. Blood chemistries, thyroid-stimulating hormone, hemoglobin, and hematocrit should be checked to help rule out electrolyte imbalance, thyroid disorder, or anemia as a possible, though less common, cause of syncope. Ambulatory cardiac monitoring until at least one event is recorded is most helpful in ascertaining the presence of a potentially lethal cardiac rhythm disturbance. Echocardiography may be necessary to assess cardiac outflow tract patency and to rule out valvular stenosis or hypertrophic cardiomyopathy. A tilt-table test may be performed to assess for orthostatic syncope.

Intervention in cardiac-related syncope should be directed at the underlying cause. If a rhythm disturbance (as described previously) is the cause, treatment should be directed at eliminating the conduction disorder. Ablation, an internal cardiac defibrillator, and/or a permanent pacemaker may be indicated depending on the type of arrhythmia. In any event, the clinician should consult with a cardiologist to ensure patient safety and an optimal outcome.

■ DYSPNEA: SHORTNESS OF BREATH

Dyspnea, or shortness of breath, is a highly subjective complaint, yet it is one of the most common cardiac symptoms. The challenge to the clinician is to determine its etiology. As with any complaint, the patient with dyspnea should be asked about precipitating factors, quality, duration, alleviating factors, and the length of time needed to relieve the symptom after discontinuing the precipitating event. In addition, dyspnea may be an anginal equivalent, especially in older adults and individuals with diabetes.

Patients with a chief complaint of dyspnea vary markedly in presentation; however, because this is a subjective complaint, the patient's report should be taken as fact. As with the complaint of pain, the discomfort and degree of dyspnea represents the patient's reality; however, correlating the complaint with physical findings may help to establish the cause of the dyspnea, thus leading to an effective plan of intervention (Level I; Institute for Clinical Systems Improvement, 2012).

Differential Diagnosis

Dyspnea has a number of possible causes. With left-sided cardiac outflow tract blockage, such as in severe aortic stenosis or obstructive cardiomyopathy, dyspnea likely arises from the decrease in cardiac output. When dyspnea is associated with recurrent myocardial ischemia, as in angina pectoris, the shortness of breath is likely caused by an increase in pulmonary vascular pressure, coupled with a transient decrease in cardiac output. In right-sided cardiac problems, such as tricuspid and pulmonic valvular dysfunction, the complaint of dyspnea usually arises from increased pulmonary pressures and resistance to cardiac emptying of the right ventricle. Another common cause of dyspnea is pulmonary disease, such as COPD, asthma, pleural effusion, pneumothorax, pulmonary embolus, or pulmonary hypertension secondary to interstitial lung disease or pulmonary fibrosis. Other noncardiac causes of dyspnea are severe anemia and metabolic acidosis (i.e., Kussmaul's respirations), obesity, physical deconditioning, and anxiety or emotional distress.

The patient's assessment of the severity of dyspnea may differ from the objective findings. For example, some patients who have been observed to have rather marked difficulty breathing have little complaint of breathlessness, whereas other patients who have few objective findings will describe marked difficulty breathing. In addition, when asked about difficulty breathing, one patient may admit to feelings of suffocation, in that getting sufficient air in and out of the lungs is a problem, whereas others will describe a need to take deep breaths.

Dyspnea is a poorly sensitive and nonspecific marker for cardiovascular disease. Factors contributing to the complaint of breathlessness in the absence of heart disease include poor conditioning and exercise intolerance related to inactivity and obesity. The patient usually reports that the onset of this type of dyspnea accompanies increased activity and resolves rapidly when the activity ceases. In any event, in cardiovascular disease, dyspnea is usually a result of increased stiffness in the lungs caused by increased pulmonary blood volume or pulmonary congestion. This is usually found in conditions with poor cardiac output, such as heart failure (HF), recurrent myocardial ischemia, poorly controlled hypertension, valvular dysfunction, and heart disease.

When dyspnea is the complaint, it is essential for the clinician to assess the change in the patient's ability to perform average daily activities. In particular, dyspnea often is first detected by the patient as the inability to talk during exertional activities. Pinpointing the onset of the symptoms and concurrent events may be helpful in determining its etiology. In addition, asking about cosymptoms such as wheezing and weight gain is crucial because dyspnea is the most common presenting complaint in HF.

Orthopnea is shortness of breath that begins when the patient has been in a supine position. The patient usually compensates for this sensation by sleeping on an increased number of pillows, hence the use of the qualifying term *three-pillow orthopnea*. When the person slides off the pillows, shortness of breath reoccurs, causing the person to awaken. Orthopnea is usually caused by HF as a result of increased right-sided heart pressure, which increases after the patient has been supine for a few hours, mobilizing fluid that pooled in the extremities during the waking, more active hours.

Paroxysmal nocturnal dyspnea is shortness of breath that occurs 1 to 2 hours into sleep, concurrent with redistribution of body fluids and a subsequent rise in left atrial pressure. The person awakens suddenly with significant difficulty breathing. He or she usually stands or sits up until symptoms are relieved in about 10 to 30 minutes. As with orthopnea, the diagnosis of HF should be considered.

■ LEG ACHES

Leg aches associated with peripheral vascular disorders are caused by impaired blood flow to the extremities. Peripheral vascular disease (PVD) affects the arteries and veins. When the disease is arterial, it is usually the result of accumulated fatty streaks and fibrous plaques (high levels of low-density lipoproteins). Venous problems relate to venous incompetence secondary to valve obstruction, leading to chronic venous insufficiency and varicose veins.

Differential Diagnosis

Patients presenting with leg aches may have a number of disorders other than PVD, so a thorough history and physical exam must be performed to rule out thrombosis, phlebitis, polycythemia, anemia, Raynaud's disease, and Buerger's disease. Because some of the contributing factors to PVD may be smoking, high blood pressure, and diabetes, these problems must be addressed and underlying conditions managed. Both peripheral arterial disease and peripheral venous disease are discussed in more detail later in the chapter.

■ PERIPHERAL EDEMA

Peripheral edema is the accumulation of fluid within the interstitial spaces of the extremities. When the edema involves the lower extremities, it is a symptom of an underlying disorder; it may be caused by cardiac conditions (e.g., heart failure, chronic venous insufficiency, or thrombophlebitis); by renal or hepatic disease; or by trauma, tumors, or inflammation. Peripheral edema occurs equally among men and women.

Differential Diagnosis

Peripheral edema is usually diagnosed via the history and physical exam, although laboratory findings assist in determining the cause of the edema. Specific diagnostic tests the clinician should order include complete blood count, urinalysis, serum chemistries, and a thyroid profile. X-ray studies may be ordered if trauma or osteomyelitis is suspected, and a chest x-ray film should be ordered to assess the heart and lungs. A computed tomography scan may help to assess the edema distribution and pinpoint the extent of venous and lymphatic obstructions. An electrocardiogram is essential for assessing cardiac function, and Doppler studies may be ordered to evaluate for deep vein thrombosis. It is essential that the underlying cause be identified and treated, or the peripheral edema will remain, possibly causing tissue ischemia from compressed and diminished arterial circulation. Differential diagnoses of peripheral edema are presented in Differential Diagnosis Flowchart 10.3.

COMMON PROBLEMS

■ HYPERTENSION

Hypertension (HTN) is one of the most common chronic health problems seen in the primary-care setting, with approximately one in three adults affected. Treatment thresholds for HTN vary in different demographics, such as adults aged 18 to 59 years without major comorbidities or patients 60 years or older who have diabetes, chronic kidney disease (CKD), or both conditions. See Table 10.1 for the breakdown of HTN per the Joint National Committee (JNC 8) guidelines.

The JNC 8 guidelines provide updated recommendations on the thresholds used to initiate pharmacological treatment for hypertension. Under the most recent guidelines, in adults over 60 years of age, pharmacological treatment is initiated to lower blood pressure to a systolic blood pressure of less than 150 or a diastolic blood pressure of less than 90 (Grade A). In adults younger than 60 years of age (including those with diabetes), pharmacological treatment is initiated at a systolic blood pressure of greater than 140 or a diastolic blood pressure of greater than 90. The initial pharmacological agent used in the general non–African American population may be a thiazide diuretic, an angiotensin-converting enzyme (ACE) inhibitor, an angiotensin receptor blocker (ARB), or a calcium channel blocker. In the African American population, initial treatment may consist of either a calcium channel blocker or a thiazide diuretic (ACE inhibitors

Differential Diagnosis Flowchart 10.3

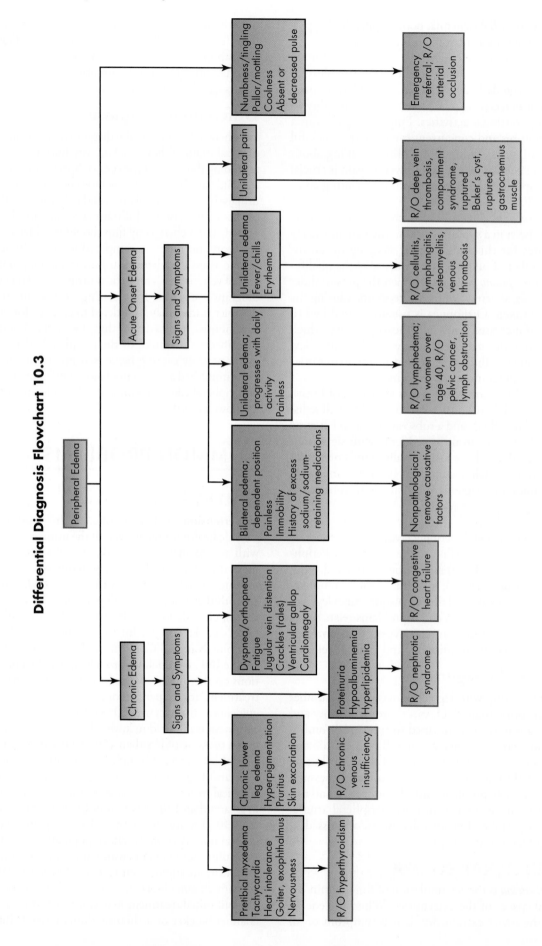

Table 10.1 Classification of Blood Pressure for Adults Aged 18 Years or Older

JNC 8 Guidelines suggest several new recommendations as to goal BP:
- In patients aged <60 years, treatment initiation and goals should be 140/90 mm Hg
- In patients aged >18 years with either chronic kidney disease or diabetes, goal should be goal of 140/90 (ADA cites goal of 140/80).
- In patients aged 60 years and over, start treatment when SBP > or equal to 150/ DBP >or equal to 90 and treat to under thresholds.
- In nonblack patient with HTN, initial treatment can be a thiazide-type treatment, CCB, ACE inhibitor or ARB; in the black population, initial therapy should be a thiazide-type diuretic or CCB.
- In patient aged 18 years or more with CKD, initial or add-on therapy should be an ACE inhibitor or ARB, regardless of race or diabetes status.

A key point to note in the JNC 8 is that although the targets have been loosened, the new guidelines do not mean that providers should ease up on treatment for patients who are doing very well based on JNC 7 guidelines. If JNC 7 is working, clinicians do not have to necessarily change the treatment plan and allow higher BPs. The study simply notes that if treatment can consistently get patients' SBP below 150, health outcomes are improved.

Additional interesting treatments to possibly speak to may include renal denervation as a promising therapy in the treatment of resistant HTN.

have been shown to be less effective in this population). In patients with chronic kidney disease, pharmacological treatment should be initiated to lower blood pressure to a systolic blood pressure of less than 140 and diastolic blood pressure less than 90. The initial agent of choice in patients with CKD should be an ACE inhibitor or ARB.

After the initiation of pharmacological treatment, the blood pressure should be reevaluated within a month. If the goal blood pressure is not attained, up-titration of the dose of the current pharmacological agent may be required. Alternatively, the addition of a pharmacological agent from another class may be added. If blood pressure goals are not obtained with the use of two blood pressure agents, a third agent may be added. Failure to respond to a triple-therapy regimen may require a referral to a hypertension specialist. Of note, beta blockers are no longer recommended as initial pharmacological agents in the primary treatment of HTN. In addition, ACE inhibitors and an ARB should not be used together in combination therapy.

More than 95% of patients with elevated blood pressure (BP) have primary, or essential, HTN, with no single identifiable cause; this type of HTN results from the interplay of multiple genetic and environmental factors, including lifestyle influences. Less than 5% of patients, therefore, have secondary HTN, a specific, possibly reversible, cause of elevated BP such as certain cardiac, renal, and endocrinological problems or the use of vasoconstricting medications.

After decades of a steady reduction in rates of HTN-related diseases, researchers have reported a recent leveling off of coronary heart disease rates, coupled with a slight increase in end-stage renal failure and age-adjusted stroke rates. These changes are likely caused by a number of factors, including a growing aging population; however, the role of undetected untreated and inadequately controlled

HTN contributes significantly. Considering this, the clinician should be committed not only to the detection and treatment of HTN but also to its prevention. When a patient develops HTN, primary prevention measures have not been successful. The clinician must aggressively monitor the patient and encourage his or her participation in the management.

There is a specific listing for Heart Disease and Stroke in the *Healthy People 2020* objectives, because cardiovascular disease is so prevalent in our population. The goal is to improve cardiovascular health and quality of life through the prevention, detection, and treatment of risk factors; early identification and treatment of heart attacks and strokes; and prevention of recurrent cardiovascular events. These objectives have been modified and new ones developed. The clinician is strongly encouraged to review the U.S. Department of Health and Human Services Web site for the most up-to-date *Healthy People 2020* information cited in the bibliography. There are 23 total objectives, out of which 6 relate to BP.

Epidemiology and Causes

HTN occurs in one out of three Americans or 31% of the population of the United States (about 67 million persons). Historically, HTN has been more prevalent in males and particularly black males. However, this gender gap is narrowing and appears to be influenced by age. For persons under 45 years of age, men are affected more than woman, whereas in persons 65 years of age and older, more woman than men have HTN. Recent statistics show that among African Americans more women than men are hypertensive and that black women are more hypertensive than black men. African Americans continue to experience HTN more often and at an earlier age than whites or Latinos. The prevalence of hypertension continues to increase with age. Results from the Framingham Heart Study demonstrate that among middle-aged and elderly persons the residual lifetime risk of developing HTN is 90%. HTN can lead to ischemic heart disease, heart failure, diabetic hypertension, chronic kidney disease, and cerebrovascular disease. An increase in body mass index (greater than 30 kg/m²) contributes to high BP and cardiovascular disease. Today, 122 million Americans are considered overweight or obese, a situation that is reaching epidemic proportions. Although this is dismal news, a study from the National Health and Nutrition Examination Survey (NHANES) demonstrates an improvement in BP control by 50% among Americans with HTN.

The onset of diastolic HTN, with or without systolic elevation, after age 60 is unusual. If this is found, the diagnosis of new-onset secondary HTN should be considered. In particular, renovascular disease is a common cause of new-onset diastolic HTN in this age-group.

Primary HTN is a result of the interplay of a number of genetic, environmental, and lifestyle issues. HTN is more common among individuals whose parents or other close family members have HTN. In these individuals, diminished ability to excrete excessive sodium, coupled with long-term high dietary sodium intake, appears to be a predisposing factor to increased peripheral vascular resistance and rise in BP.

Pathophysiology
Pathophysiology of Essential Hypertension

The term *essential hypertension* describes high BP that has no identifiable etiology after thorough clinical examination excludes possible secondary causes. Although etiology is unknown, endothelial dysfunction is the key pathophysiological process involved in essential HTN. The arterial endothelium is an important regulator of vascular tone, vascular structure, thrombosis, and inflammation. Endothelial dysfunction is central to a wide array of cardiovascular disorders, including HTN, atherosclerosis, and myocardial ischemia. Vascular tone is maintained by endothelium-derived mediators such as nitric oxide, endothelin-1, and angiotensin II. Nitric oxide, a major vasodilator, counteracts the potent vasoconstrictors endothelin-1 and angiotensin II, which regulate normal vascular tone. In essential HTN, there is an imbalance in the vasodilator and vasoconstrictive substances secreted by the endothelium. Plasma levels of nitric oxide are diminished, whereas levels of endothelin-1 and angiotensin II are elevated. Reasons for this imbalance have not been elucidated, and it is not clear whether endothelial dysfunction precedes or is the result of HTN.

Other investigations have found that renin levels are markedly abnormal in some hypertensive individuals, despite normal renal function. Renin oversecretors experience constant cycling of the renin-angiotensin-aldosterone cascade, which raises blood volume and BP. Low renin secretors, in general, are salt-sensitive hypertensive individuals. Ingestion of sodium increases water reabsorption into the bloodstream, which raises blood volume and BP. The cause of renin imbalance in some persons with essential HTN is unknown. Measuring plasma renin levels in patients with refractory hypertension may assist in clinical diagnosis and treatment.

HTN is a common disorder that occurs with aging in industrialized societies. Data from the Framingham Heart Study suggest that even individuals who are normotensive at 55 years of age still have a 90% lifetime risk of developing HTN. There is a particular rise in systolic BP that progresses throughout life, with a difference of 20 to 30 mm Hg between early and late adulthood. Worldwide epidemiological evidence demonstrates that age-related HTN is uncommon in societies where individuals maintain lower body weight, consume less sodium and more potassium, and engage in greater levels of physical activity. These findings indicate that high BP is influenced by environmental and lifestyle factors and is not an inevitable consequence of aging. Smoking, obesity, and stress are examples of modifiable lifestyle factors that raise BP.

Genetic and ethnic influences also play a role in the development of HTN. Persons with a family history of HTN are four times more likely to suffer HTN than those with no family history of the condition. Studies show that the genetic contribution to essential HTN is complex, and multiple genes are likely involved. Most genetic effects involve gene–gene interactions and gene–environment interactions. Genes that encode components of the renin-angiotensin-aldosterone system are being extensively studied. Results of this line of investigation have implicated mutations in the angiotensinogen gene and angiotensin-converting enzyme (ACE) gene.

Studies of HTN in African Americans demonstrate that ethnicity is related to HTN susceptibility and plays a role in the efficacy of specific types of drugs. Morbidity and mortality due to HTN and HTN-related disorders are more common in blacks than in Caucasians and non-Hispanic Americans. HTN also seems to follow a more malignant course in African Americans. Compared to whites with HTN, African Americans have an increased risk of left ventricular hypertrophy, heart failure, and renal failure.

HTN has localized and systemic adverse effects. Locally, high BP creates a shearing force against the arterial walls, which injures the endothelium and accelerates development of atherosclerosis. Endothelial injury initiates a detrimental localized reaction of vasoconstriction, inflammation, platelet aggregation, and fibrin and lipid deposition—the rudiments of arteriosclerotic plaque formation. Target organs that are damaged by HTN include the heart (left ventricular hypertrophy and coronary artery disease resulting in angina or acute myocardial infarction), the kidneys (chronic renal insufficiency), the brain (transient ischemic attacks [TIAs], cerebrovascular accidents [CVAs], and increased risk of dementia), the eyes (retinal hemorrhages and hypertensive retinopathy), and the peripheral arteries (peripheral vascular disease).

The role of altered sodium excretion by impaired epithelial cells in the kidney may be a factor in the development of HTN. Other contributors include aging, sympathetic nervous system overactivity, toxins, and low nephron numbers.

Metabolic syndrome with its resultant insulin resistance and increased insulin levels may lead to increased sympathetic activity and hypertensive states. An additional overlooked cause of essential HTN is sleep apnea with its associated activation of sympathetic and renin-angiotension systems.

In summary, the etiology and pathophysiology of essential HTN are incompletely understood. It is a complex, multifactorial disorder that involves genetic and environmental factors, diet and lifestyle practices, imbalances in vasoactive substances, and dysfunction of the arterial endothelium.

Pathophysiology of Secondary Hypertension

Secondary HTN is elevated BP due to an identifiable, underlying condition. Detection of secondary HTN is critical in order to reverse the source of the pathological process and prevent hypertensive target organ damage. Less common than essential HTN, secondary HTN has an overall frequency of 5% to 10% in primary-care practices. Secondary HTN is often distinguished from essential HTN by certain assessment findings, such as age at onset younger than 30 years or older than 50 years, BP higher than 180/110 mm Hg at diagnosis, significant target organ damage at diagnosis, hemorrhages and exudates on funduscopic examination, renal insufficiency, left ventricular hypertrophy, accelerated or malignant HTN, and poor response to therapy. Resistant HTN is often due to unexplored, reversible secondary causes.

Reversible causes of secondary HTN include obesity, obstructive sleep apnea, renovascular disease, chronic steroid therapy, Cushing's syndrome, primary hyperaldosteronism, pheochromocytoma, coarctation of the aorta, thyroid disease, parathyroid disease, and excess alcohol intake. Secondary HTN can also be drug induced, and a thorough history of the patient's medications, including herbal supplements, over-the-counter (OTC) agents, and any illicit drug use is essential. Common drugs that can cause HTN include NSAIDs, cyclooxygenase-2 (COX-2) inhibitors, sympathomimetics such as decongestants and anorectics (diet pills), oral contraceptives, erythropoietin, cocaine, amphetamines, steroids, tacrolimus, cyclosporine, and herbal ephedra supplements. Licorice, smoking, and chewing tobacco also raise BP.

"White Coat" Hypertension

"White coat" HTN with a prevalence of 12% to 18% is a transient rise in BP experienced by a patient when in the clinical or hospital setting, most likely due to anxiety. This condition of "pseudohypertension" is common in primary-care practice. The "white coat" effect can lead to overestimation of BP and prescribing of unnecessary antihypertensive treatment. In addition, the patient's transiently high BP can be misinterpreted as ineffectiveness of antihypertensive therapy. Care must be taken to use the appropriate sized BP cuff. If too small a cuff is used, this will artificially increase the readings. Obese patients or those with large arms need to have a cuff that is large enough to measure BP accurately. Patients with "white coat" HTN are more accurately assessed through the use of ambulatory BP monitoring, which provides an automated 24-hour recording of the patient's BP during normal daily activities that can be reviewed by the clinician. Alternatively, the patient may be instructed to measure and record intermittent BP readings over several weeks with reliable, consistent equipment for later review.

Masked Hypertension

Masked hypertension is defined as HTN that is present during daily life and yet absent in clinical assessment. Studies conducted by the National Institutes of Health state that masked hypertension may be present in as high as one out of every seven to eight individuals with normal clinical or office BPs.

Risk factors identified for masked hypertension are smoking, alcohol use, lack of physical activity, and work-related and physiological stressors. Clients who are at high risk for masked hypertension have a higher incidence of cardiovascular events and subsequently a higher risk of mortality and morbidity due to missed opportunities to treat.

Ambulatory blood pressure monitoring (ABPM) or home BP self-monitoring by the client who is at high risk is a cornerstone to optimizing outcomes. Without active patient participation and buy-in, this prognostically challenging condition will go untreated.

Pathophysiology of Malignant Hypertension (Hypertensive Emergency)

Malignant HTN has been noted in up to 1% of patients diagnosed with central hypertension. Malignant HTN is diagnosed when a patient presents with severely elevated BP in the range of ≥180 mm Hg/110 mm Hg and evidence of acute target organ damage. Although the terms are often used interchangeably, *hypertensive emergency* or *hypertensive crisis* denotes this process acutely. If not treated with immediate parenteral antihypertensive therapy in an acute-care setting, a hypertensive emergency may prove fatal. In contrast, a significantly elevated BP alone with *no evidence* of target organ damage does *not* constitute an emergency and is classified as *hypertensive urgency.* Hypertensive urgencies may be treated with oral agents over a period of 24 to 48 hours to achieve stabilization. An isolated finding of severely elevated BP can be reduced over the course of hours with oral medications in an outpatient setting. In hypertensive emergency, acute target organ damage most commonly involves the neurological, cardiac, or renal systems. Acute cerebrovascular events, papilledema, acute myocardial ischemia or infarction, pulmonary edema, aortic dissection, acute renal failure, epistaxis, states of catecholamine excess, and preeclampsia/eclampsia are conditions associated with severely elevated BP. A patient presenting with acutely severe BP elevation requires a thorough clinical examination that includes funduscopy, electrocardiogram (ECG), urinalysis, serum creatinine measurements, and chest x-ray study. A computed tomography scan of the head to rule out stroke may be necessary. Evidence of target organ damage includes the following:

- Papilledema, hemorrhages, or exudates on funduscopic examination
- Change in mental status or neurological deficits on physical examination
- Dementia
- ECG consistent with myocardial ischemia or infarction
- Chest x-ray film showing heart failure or aortic dissection
- Renal dysfunction evidenced by hematuria, proteinuria, and elevated serum creatinine

The primary-care provider should refer patients with hypertensive emergency to an acute-care setting for appropriate diagnostic testing, monitoring, and treatment.

Clinical Presentation

Subjective

Typically the diagnosis of HTN is made after several routine office visits with the patient complaining of no symptoms. Occasionally, if the BP is extremely elevated, the patient may present with a headache that occurs on awakening and is located in the occipital area.

Objective

A systematic approach should be used when assessing the person with or at risk for HTN. The assessment should include two measurements of BP in both arms, with the patient preferably seated with both feet on a flat surface (crossing legs may increase the systolic blood pressure (SBP) by 2–8 mm Hg), back supported with the arm at heart level (may increase the diastolic blood pressure [DBP] up to 6 mm Hg). Avoid conversation with the patient during the reading, and use the appropriate size cuff (too large will provide a falsely low BP, too small will provide a falsely elevated BP). When elevated BPs are obtained, a bilateral assessment for confirmation should be obtained when not contraindicated (e.g., by the presence of an atrioventricular shunt, postmastectomy status, etc.). BP should be taken again after the patient has stood for at least 2 minutes. The higher readings should be recorded. In groups such as the elderly, the obese, and patients with arrhythmias, certain criteria should be noted. In the elderly, the clinician should note that an auscultatory gap is common; this is

usually associated with vascular disease and results in an underestimation of SBP. The obese client will often have short upper arm length relative to upper arm width; in this instance a wrist cuff may be used. Place the wrist at heart level to avoid the potential for error. In clients with very irregular arrhythmias such as atrial fibrillation, the BP varies beat to beat, so the provider should measure the BP several times and average the readings. In the client with severe bradycardia, the provider should deflate the cuff more slowly to prevent underestimating SBP and overestimating DBP.

The National Institute for Health and Clinical Excellence (NICE) guidelines state that a diagnosis of primary HTN should be confirmed with 24-hour ABPM or sequential home BP readings. Twenty-four–hour ABPM is indicated to rule out "white coat" or "masked" hypertension, to uncover apparent drug-resistant hypertension, and to identify hypertensive symptoms while the patient is being treated with hypertensive medication.

When a person has been diagnosed with or is suspected to have HTN, assessment should include a focused health history and physical exam, staging of BP elevation, and investigation for evidence of hypertensive target organ damage (TOD). This exam should include funduscopic examination, palpation of the chest for point of maximal impulse (PMI) or auscultation of the heart, abdominal assessment for bruits or widened aortic diameter and enlarged kidneys, examination of the carotid arteries for bruits, palpation of peripheral pulses, and a neurological examination (Level I; Calhoun et al, 2008). See Advanced Assessment 10.1 for assessment areas to evaluate in persons with HTN. Evidence of TOD includes retinopathy, which may appear as arteriolar narrowing, arteriovenous nicking, hemorrhages, or exudates. A bruit may be auscultated over either carotic artery, indicating stenosis. The chest may demonstrate a displaced PMI and/or an S_4 heart sound indicating left ventricular hypertrophy (LVH). Auscultation of an S_4 heart sound is associated with decreased elasticity of the left ventricle that occurs in LVH. The patient should also be evaluated for the presence of heart failure, a known sequela of long-standing HTN. An S_3 gallop, pulmonary crackles, jugular venous distention, and peripheral edema are signs of heart failure. A bruit heard in the abdomen may indicate an aneurysm or renal artery stenosis. Palpation of a widened aortic pulsation is associated with abdominal aortic aneurysm. Diminished peripheral pulses and sensation in the lower extremities can indicate peripheral arterial disease. Neurological exam can reveal deficits associated with TIAs or a CVA.

The history should include a thorough investigation of cardiovascular risk factors such as age, gender, postmenopausal status, diet, activity level, alcohol and caffeine use, smoking, dyslipidemia, diabetes, family history of heart disease, and current medications. Some medications, such as NSAIDs or OTC cold remedies, may exacerbate BP elevation. Excess use of alcohol is often the source of

Advanced Assessment 10.1   Hypertension

Assessment	Common Findings
Blood Pressure Measurement	
Proper technique:	SBP >140 mm Hg (see Table 10.1 for specifics) (depends on age)
Cuff size has a bladder length of 80% and a width of at least 40% of arm circumference Rest for 5 minutes before measurement.	DBP >90 mm Hg
Patient in a sitting position, arm resting at level of the heart with feet on flat surface, legs uncrossed. Average 2 readings at least 2 minutes apart (if >5 mm Hg difference, obtain additional readings)	
Physical Exam	
Height, weight, BMI	Obesity (BMI >27), especially with central or truncal pattern
Waist measurement	Men: >39 inches Women: >34 inches
Funduscope	Hypertensive retinopathy (arteriolar narrowing, arteriovenous nicking, hemorrhages, exudates, papilledema)
Carotid arteries	Bruits
Neck veins	Distention
Thyroid	Enlargement Nodules
Cardiac	PMI and apex displaced laterally; greater than one intercostal space S_3, S_4 heart sounds Murmur or mitral regurgitation
Lungs	Crackles Bronchospasm
Abdomen	Bruits, masses, abnormal aortic pulsations Enlarged kidneys
Extremities	Absence of peripheral arterial pulsations Bruits Edema
Diagnostic Tests	
Urinalysis	Proteinuria
BUN/Creatinine	Increased
CBC	May show anemia
Potassium	Increased or decreased
Blood glucose	May be increased
Triglycerides, HDL, LDL	Increased
12-lead ECG	May show target organ damage
BNP	Hormone released by the ventricle indicative of increased myocardial demands

refractory HTN. Culture and ethnicity should be assessed within the history as well. Compared with Caucasians, African Americans have a higher risk of HTN, diabetes mellitus, and renal impairment, which requires aggressive management of BP and specific drug therapy.

Particular care must be taken when assessing an older patient with HTN. If severe vessel rigidity is present in the brachial artery, the BP cuff may be unable to compress the calcified vessel well, leading to a falsely high pressure. This phenomenon is known as *pseudohypertension*. Although it may raise the BP by 30 mm Hg or more, it does not by itself represent a disease state.

Diagnostic Reasoning

Diagnostic Tests

Diagnostic testing of a patient who has or is suspected of having HTN should focus on the evaluation of target organs and concurrent conditions, as well as on excluding certain causes of secondary HTN. Additional testing may be indicated, particularly when concurrent diseases such as diabetes mellitus or hyperlipidemia are present.

The ECG is an important screening tool to assess for cardiac target organ damage in the hypertensive patient. It can be used to assess the presence of left atrial enlargement, left ventricular hypertrophy, myocardial ischemia or infarction, premature ventricular contractions, and atrial fibrillation. Left atrial enlargement is one of the earliest ECG findings associated with HTN. An echocardiogram is useful to detect the presence of increased left ventricular wall thickness and hypertrophy.

Differential Diagnosis

The key to differential diagnosis is to determine the underlying etiology of the HTN, whether it is essential or secondary, for instance, and to assess the degree of HTN (prehypertension, HTN, malignant or benign, etc.). A presumptive diagnosis is made if the average of at least two seated BP measurements on at least two or more visits exceeds either 90 mm Hg DBP or 140 mm Hg SBP in adults older than age 18.

Management

The key to HTN management is not only the reversal of HTN-related disease trends but also the prevention of target organ damage. The following are public health approaches to achieve a downward shift in the distribution of a population's BP, thus potentially reducing morbidity, mortality, and the lifetime risk of an individual becoming hypertensive.

- Develop community health programs to stress reducing calories, saturated fat, and salt in processed foods.
- Encourage food manufacturers and restaurants to reduce the sodium in the food supply by 50% over the next decade.
- Increase community/school opportunities for physical activity.

- Address the diversity of racial, ethnic, cultural, linguistic, religious, and social factors in the delivery of community services to increase the community's receptiveness to use of public health services.
- Improve opportunities for treatment and control of HTN. Health-care providers can help break down barriers to the diagnosis and treatment of HTN. Examples include nursing and work-site clinics and offering health services on evenings and weekends, which increase the likelihood of those who work during the weekday hours having access to care.

Patient-specific goals include the following:

- An awareness regarding the risks involved in prehypertension. Teens and young adults with high normal BP are at markedly increased risk of developing HTN in their fourth and fifth decades of life. Behavioral therapies such as a program of regular aerobic exercise and a diet that is lower in fat and sodium and higher in potassium should be initiated to help avoid HTN.
- Knowing one's own body mass index. This should serve as a guide to weight loss rather than just looking at ideal body weight.
- Improving HTN control in persons already diagnosed. Many with HTN have a BP greater than 140/90 mm Hg (see Table 10.1 for specifics), demonstrating inadequate control.
- Reducing cardiovascular risks. Many patients with HTN will have additional modifiable cardiovascular disease risk factors such as diabetes mellitus, hyperlipidemia, tobacco use, and inactivity; therefore, a comprehensive plan to treat HTN must also address these issues.

The use of lifestyle modifications (Table 10.2) should be a part of every patient's regimen to prevent or treat elevated BP (Level I; Calhoun et al, 2008). The clinician should work with the patient on a plan of lifestyle modification and medications as needed to lower the BP as much as is tolerated without symptoms. In patients with diabetes mellitus, the American Diabetes Association shares a target SBP of less than 140 mm Hg and has a target DBP of less than 80 mm Hg. Note that this diastolic threshold differs from the JNC 8 guidelines' goal DBP of less than 90 based on the lack of quality randomized control trials supporting the benefit of a goal DBP less than 90 in patients with diabetes. For patients with CKD and proteinuria, the therapeutic plan should be very individualized with attention to balancing side effects of medications (hypotension or worsening renal disease) with BP goals. Renal impairment should compel the clinician and patient to work together to maintain meticulous BP control to minimize the development of nephropathy. In addition to public health programs, community-affiliated programs, including parish-based programs and neighborhood and work-site health promotion events, should be utilized to assist patients.

Table 10.2	Lifestyle Modifications to Manage Hypertension

- **Weight reduction:** Maintain normal body weight (BMI, 18.5–24.9 kg/m^2) (weight reduction lowers BP by 5–20 mm Hg).
- **Adopt DASH (Dietary Approaches to Stop Hypertension) eating plan:** Consume a diet rich in fruits, vegetables, and low-fat dairy products with a reduced content of saturated and total fat (DASH diet lowers BP by 14–18 mm Hg).
- **Dietary sodium reduction:** Reduce dietary sodium intake to no more than 100 mmol (2.4 g sodium) per day (lowers BP by 2–8 mm Hg).
- **Physical activity:** Engage in regular aerobic physical activity such as brisk walking (at least 30 minutes per day, most days of the week) (lowers BP by 4–9 mm Hg).
- **Moderation of alcohol:** Limit consumption to no more than two drinks (1 oz. or 30 mL of ethanol, e.g., 24 oz beer, 10 oz wine, or 3 oz 80-proof whiskey) per day for most men and to no more than 1 drink per day for women and lighter weight persons (lowers BP by 2–4 mm Hg).
- **Stop smoking and/or use of other tobacco products.**
- **Understand hot-tub safety:** When combined with heat, antihypertensive drugs may cause vasodilation resulting in dizziness, light-headedness, fainting, reduction of cerebral blood flow, with the potential for falling and risk of injury.
- **Maintain adherence to pharmacotherapeutic plan:** When medication regimen is not adhered to, BP will rise.
- **Monitor for drug-induced hypertension:** Drugs that may induce HTN include NSAIDs, antidepressants, glucocorticoids, oral contraceptives, hormone replacement therapy, and OTC medications that contain decongestants.

Special Considerations for Older Adults

Nearly one-half of all adults aged 65 years and older develop isolated systolic hypertension (ISH), defined as an SBP above 160 mm Hg with a normal DBP (86 or below) as a consequence of atherosclerotic thickening of the vessels. More than two-thirds of persons older than age 65 develop HTN in general. Given its frequency, the development of ISH is often viewed as an unavoidable part of aging, but clinicians should be aware that behavior-based therapies used to avoid and treat HTN can also help minimize age-associated increases in BP. Historically, older adults with HTN have not received the emphasis on treatment that was merited. Present-day guidelines now stress the importance of treating HTN in older adults. Older adults benefit greatly from the treatment of ISH, yielding significant reduction in congestive heart failure and cardiovascular and cerebrovascular disease.

Even in persons older than 50 years of age, SBP greater than 140 mm Hg is a much more important cardiovascular disease risk factor than DBP. Even patients with a normal BP at age 55 still have a 90% lifetime risk for developing HTN. In a patient with a BP of 115/75 mm Hg, the risk of cardiovascular disease doubles with each incremental increase of 20/10 mm Hg.

Pharmacological Therapy

Lifestyle modifications should be used for patients at risk for HTN. No antihypertensive drug therapy is indicated if there is no compelling indication other than potential risk factors. Monitoring for drug-induced hypertension is essential before the initiation of pharmaceutical therapy. Pharmaceuticals such as NSAIDs, glucocorticoids, antidepressants, oral contraceptives, hormone replacement therapy, and OTC medications must be investigated before treatment. The use of alcohol and tobacco must be reviewed. The presence of sleep apnea must be assessed. For most patients with newly diagnosed HTN, therapeutic lifestyle changes should be tried for 1 month. If not effective in lowering the BP after 1 month, add pharmacological therapy. In the general nonblack population, including those with diabetes, initial antihypertensive treatment should include any one of four classifications of HTN medications—a thiazide-type diuretic, calcium channel blocker, ACE inhibitor, or angiotensin receptor blocker. Any of these may improve cardiovascular outcomes.

When it comes to thiazide diuretic therapy, use chlorthalidone 12.5 to 25 mg/day. A second choice is hydrochlorothiazide. These both have been shown to improve cardiovascular outcomes. Thiazide diuretics are first-line proven antihypertensive drugs. These agents are useful in the presence of ISH, as well as being inexpensive and efficacious. They are also helpful for patients with osteoporosis because they help preserve bone density. Thiazide diuretics are well documented for reducing stroke and cardiovascular-related mortality and morbidity; however, the clinician should choose antihypertensive therapy with concurrent disease or comorbid conditions in mind.

Beta blockers are no longer used as initial treatment for the hypertensive patient.

Examples of antihypertensive drugs that can be used in patients with concurrent diseases include choices from the following groups:

- **Angiotensin-converting enzyme inhibitors**
  (ACEIs—drugs with generic names ending in *-pril*, such as captopril, enalapril, and lisinopril) are effective in the presence of heart failure and myocardial infarction (MI) with systolic dysfunction to help limit myocardial remodeling. These should be ordered when certain comorbid conditions including renal insufficiency and diabetes mellitus are present and may assist in preserving or enhancing renal function (Level I; Michigan Quality Improvement Consortium, 2011).

- **Angiotensin II receptor blockers** (ARBs) are helpful in antihypertensive individuals with comorbid conditions such as heart failure and type 2 diabetes. Because they have a higher cost than ACEIs and because long-term research is lacking, ARBs should be reserved for patients who develop a cough when taking ACEIs.
- **Beta blockers** (drugs with generic names ending in -*lol,* such as metoprolol) are no longer commonly recommended for the primary management of HTN but may be used in the presence of angina, post-MI (to reduce cardiac workload and enhance rhythm stability), atrial tachycardia (to blunt tachycardia response), migraine headache (nonselective for reduction in frequency and severity of headache), and essential tumor (nonselective). These drugs may help to reduce the tremor resulting from blockage of beta-2 receptor sites.
- Long-acting dihydropyridine (DHP) **calcium channel blockers** (CCBs) are suggested for black clients of African or Caribbean descent who are younger than age 55, for patients with ISH, and for patients with HTN and stable angina pectoris.
- **Alpha-adrenergic antagonists** (alpha blockers) are usually effective in patients with benign prostatic hyperplasia because they facilitate bladder emptying by decreasing prostate size.

Additional drugs may include combination drugs, such as ACEIs and CCBs, ACEIs and diuretics, ARBs and diuretics, centrally acting drug and diuretics, and diuretics and diuretic agents. (See Drugs Commonly Prescribed 10.1.)

Initial therapy should consist of a low dose of the agent chosen. If the agent is well tolerated but BP control has not been achieved, the dose should be increased.

Small doses of two agents from different classes may have a synergistic effect in lowering BP while avoiding the problems of higher doses of either agent given alone and may possibly give additive therapeutic benefit (see Drugs Commonly Prescribed 10.1). These combination products may be appropriate for first-line antihypertensive therapy. In particular, a very low dose (12.5 mg) of chlorthalidone has the ability to potentiate the effect of other agents without producing negative metabolic effects.

If treatment continues to be ineffective, substitute another drug from a different class or add a second agent from a different class. If the desired effect has still not been achieved, continue to add drugs from other classes. A cardiologist should be consulted if the HTN remains uncontrolled.

Choosing the Best Drug Certain patient characteristics, including ethnicity, may influence the choice and efficacy of an antihypertensive agent. A common perception is that the best antihypertensive effect for African Americans and older adults with HTN can be achieved by using a combination of diuretics and CCBs. This should not be viewed, however, as a contraindication to

using ACEIs or ARBs. Indeed, these drugs may offer significant benefit when concomitant disease is present or poses significant risk. ACEIs and ARBs may be used in all groups; however, when these drugs are used in older adults and African Americans, higher doses may be needed, and a longer period of time may elapse before the onset of action is seen. ACEIs and ARBs should not be prescribed together.

An agent with once daily dosing (24-hour activity with at least 50% of action in the last 12 hours) is recommended. (See Drugs Commonly Prescribed 10.1.) The clinician should prescribe a once-daily dose, especially if patient adherence is a problem. This provides the patient with persistent, smooth control of HTN, and adherence to drug therapy is improved. In addition, with longer-acting formulas, there is less risk of hypertensive rebound resulting from a missed dose, providing protection against risk of stroke, MI, or sudden death from cardiac arrest induced by a dramatic increase in BP.

In certain clinical situations, some medications should be used with caution or are contraindicated because they may have unfavorable effects on comorbid conditions. (See Drugs Commonly Prescribed 10.1.) The JNC 8 guidelines stress that if the patient's medications are working, they should not be changed just because new guidelines are in place.

Age-Related Concerns Certain age-related physical changes predispose older adults to difficulty with HTN drug therapy. Because this group benefits significantly from control of HTN, the appropriate drug should be chosen with care and with consideration of particular factors including loss of baroreceptors, which increases the risk for postural HTN. As a result, BP should be measured with the patient in both standing and sitting positions. In addition, older adults should be instructed to change position slowly while on antihypertensive medication.

The Beers criteria is a clinical tool developed to assist clinicians in improving medication safety in older adults. The clinician should consult the Beers criteria for potentially inappropriate medication use in older adults (see www.americangeriatrics.org/health_care_professionals/clinical_practice/clinical_guidelines_recommendations/2012).

The force of myocardial contractility decreases with age, leaving older adults more sensitive to hypertensive medications with negative inotropic effects, such as beta blockers. Because of lower circulating volume, diuretics, which are particularly effective antihypertensive agents for this age-group, should be used in lower doses. Older adults usually have decreased renal excretory capacity; therefore, smaller doses of medications are required. The adage "Start low and go slow" should be followed. The dose titration of antihypertensive drugs should be monitored closely with every dose adjustment.

Concurrent Use of Select Medications Through their sodium-retaining effect, NSAIDs can negate the BP-lowering effects of select antihypertensive medications

Drugs Commonly Prescribed 10.1   Hypertension

Medications Preferred in Specific Comorbid Conditions

Diabetes*	ACEI or ARB For metabolic syndrome, ACEI or ARB or CCB
Chronic kidney disease	ACEI or ARB
Heart failure	ACEI or ARB, mineralocorticoid receptor antagonist, beta blocker, diuretic (loop preferred) For LVH, ACEI or ARB, CCB
High-risk CAD	Beta blocker or CCB for angina ACEI or CCB for asymptomatic atherosclerosis
Post-MI	ACEI or ARB, beta blocker
Recurrent stroke prevention	Any effective antihypertensive

*To reduce risk for major CV events and slow progression of CKD in adults with diabetes not on dialysis with urine albumin <30/24 hour, the blood pressure goal is <140/90. If urine albumin is >30/24 hour, the goal is ≤130/80.
†Initial combined therapy should be used cautiously in those at risk for orthostatic hypotension.

Drug Classification	Indication	Adverse Reactions and Prescribing Considerations
Diuretics		
Thiazide diuretics (e.g., chlorthalidone)	First-line diuretic to treat hypertension. Thiazide diuretics are indicated in the management of hypertension, either as the sole therapeutic agent or to enhance the effect of other antihypertensive drugs in more severe forms of hypertension.	Use with caution in severe renal disease, which may precipitate azotemia, and in patients with impaired hepatic function. Contraindicated in patients with anuria, hepatic coma, or precoma; or known allergy or hypersensitivity to these products or other sulfonamide-derived drugs. Hypokalemia, hyperuricemia, and rise in blood lipids may occur. Occasional urticaria and skin rash; postural hypotension; gastrointestinal (GI) distress; loss of appetite; impotence; vertigo. Thiazide diuretics are less effective when creatinine is ≥1.8.
Loop diuretics furosemide (Lasix)	Loop diuretics are more potent than thiazides in promoting diuresis; however, they are less effective than thiazides in BP management. Indicated for the treatment of mild-to-moderate hypertension and in the management of edema associated with congestive heart failure. Also beneficial in the management of HTN associated with hepatic and renal disease, including the nephritic syndrome. Will likely remain effective in patients who have creatinine ≥1.8.	May cause hypokalemia, hyponatremia, low magnesium, dehydration, postural hypotension, tinnitus, hyperuricemia leading to gout, increased sensitivity to sunlight. Hypertensive patients who cannot be adequately controlled with thiazides will probably also not be adequately controlled with furosemide alone.
Aldosterone receptor blockers spironolactone (Aldactone)	Weak antihypertensives. Potassium-sparing diuretics are indicated for the treatment of HTN or edema in patients who develop hypokalemia. Aldosterone antagonists block the effects of serum aldosterone and therefore are better at regulating Na+ and water homeostasis and maintaining stable intravascular volume.	The use of potassium-sparing agents is often unnecessary in patients receiving diuretics for uncomplicated essential HTN when such patients have a normal diet. May cause nervousness, skin rash, increased sensitivity to sunlight, confusion, irregular heart rhythm, shortness of breath, lethargy, and weakness. Hyperkalemia risk is increased with the use of ACE/ARB. Use with caution in cases of renal impairment.

Continued

Drugs Commonly Prescribed 10.1   Hypertension—cont'd

Drug Classification	Indication	Adverse Reactions and Prescribing Considerations
Beta-Adrenergic Blockers		
carvedilol, metoprolol (Toprol XL)	Not indicated as first-line management of hypertension unless compelling indications such as acute coronary syndrome or heart failure is present. May be used in combination with other antihypertensive agents, especially thiazide-type diuretics. Beta blockers are a component of core measures in the client after an ACS.	May cause sinus bradycardia, atrioventricular block, hypotension, shortness of breath, depression, dizziness, fatigue, vivid dreams, diarrhea, nausea/vomiting, increased triglycerides, increased sexual dysfunction, pruritus, skin hyperpigmentation, alopecia, xerosis, and urticaria. Use with caution in patients with COPD, asthma, and PVD. May increase the risk of developing type 2 diabetes.
Angiotensin-Converting Enzyme Inhibitors		
enalapril, lisinopril (Zestril)	Use alone or in combination with thiazide diuretics. Effective for the patient with comorbidities of heart failure, MI, left ventricular dysfunction, renal insufficiency, glomerulosclerosis. Diabetes with nephropathy may likewise benefit. May be effective in the prevention of stroke. ACEIs are a component of Core Measures in the client after an ACS.	May exacerbate hyperkalemia and increase the risk of angioedema. Avoid in pregnancy. May cause a chronic cough. When dosed with aldosterone receptor blocker, may cause orthostatic hypotension, sinus tachycardia, fatigue, dizziness, syncope, headache, hyperkalemia. Renal adjustment is indicated in renal insufficiency. Do not dose in the presence of bilateral renal artery stenosis.
Angiotensin II Receptor Blockers		
losartan (Cozaar) **Calcium Channel Blockers** Nondihydropyridines— diltiazem, verapamil (Calan) Dihydropyridines— amlodipine, felodipine (Plendil)	Most potent antihypertensive agent routinely utilized. May be useful for the treatment of stable angina pectoris, especially the dihydropyridines. CCBs may be effective in the management of angina from coronary artery spasm. Effective in reducing cardiac muscle burden and lessens myocardial demand for oxygen.	Use with caution in HF and 2nd- and 3rd-degree heart block (unless pacer in place). All CCBs potentiated with grapefruit juice. May cause lower extremity edema. Avoid in patients with recent MI. May cause peripheral edema, headache, dizziness, flushing, palpitations, fatigue, nausea/vomiting, abdominal pain, and drowsiness. Caution in acute heart failure, renal, or hepatic impairment.
Alpha-Adrenoceptor Blockers		
prazosin, doxazosin, terazosin (Hytrin)	Use with comorbidities of benign prostatic hyperplasia, prostatism, as well as in dyslipidemia. May be used alone or in combination with diuretics, beta-adrenergic blocking agents, calcium channel blockers, or ACEIs.	Do not use as first-line or "solo" agents. A higher rate of stroke and heart failure is associated (ALLHAT). Alters lipid metabolism by decreasing LDL-C and VLDL-C. May cause mild sexual dysfunction, dizziness, light-headedness, headache, drowsiness, fatigue, nausea/vomiting, peripheral edema, nasal congestion, palpitations. May cause complication years later during cataract surgery by leading to floppy iris syndrome during eye surgery.
Centrally Acting Agents		
clonidine, methyldopa, reserpine (Catapres)	Effectively lower BP by decreasing central sympathetic outflow.	May cause drowsiness, impotence, dry mouth, increased respirations, increased GI motility, miosis, decreased LVRL. Less common effects are depression and Coombs-positive anemia (with alpha-methyldopa). Abrupt withdrawal may lead to a rebound HTN.

Drugs Commonly Prescribed 10.1   Hypertension—cont'd

Drug Classification	Indication	Adverse Reactions and Prescribing Considerations
Direct Vasodilators		
hydralazine, minoxidil, isordil	Good for hypertension in pregnancy. Injectable hydralazine is used as a first-line agent in the treatment of hypertensive emergencies. Direct vasodilators play an important role in the treatment of severe heart failure.	May cause peripheral edema, headache, tachycardia, angina, hirsutism, mastalgia, and bullous rash, as well as orthostatic hypotension.
Combination Drug Therapy		
ACE/CCB amlodipine + benazepril (Lotrel) enalapril-felodipine (Lexxel) trandolapril-verapamil (Tarka)	Effective with atrial tachycardia or fibrillation, especially the nondihydropyridines, diabetes type 1 and 2. CCBs may be useful in Raynaud's syndrome, as well as ISH, and those at high risk of CAD. The nondihydropyridines such as verapamil and diltiazem have been shown to reduce CV mortality, proteinuria, and diabetic nephropathy progression independent of ACEI use.	
ACE/Diuretics benazepril-hydrochlorothiazide (Lotensin HCT) captopril-hydrochlorothiazide (Capozide) enalapril-hydrochlorothiazide (Vaseretic) fosinopril-hydrochlorothiazide (Monopril/HCT) lisinopril-hydrochlorothiazide (Prinzide)	As above.	See above.
ARBs/Diuretics candesartan-hydrochlorothiazide (Atacand HCT) eprosartan-hydrochlorothiazide (Teveten HCT) irbesartan (Avalide) losartan + hydrochlorothiazide (Hyzaar) olmesartan-medoxomil (Benicar)	Use alone or in combination with other antihypertensive agents. ARBs are an alternative to ACEIs in patients who develop a chronic cough secondary to ACE inhibitor usage. Attention must be paid to the exact cause of the cough and assessment as to etiology to identify possible worsening of heart failure. As above.	Avoid use in pregnancy. May exacerbate hyperkalemia, angioedema, renal impairment. Diarrhea, dyspepsia, orthostatic hypotension, syncope, dizziness, insomnia, angioedema, vasculitis, hyperkalemia, hyponatremia, elevated hepatic enzymes, hyperbilirubinemia, decreased hematocrit and hemoglobin. See above.

Continued

Drugs Commonly Prescribed 10.1   Hypertension—cont'd

Drug Classification	Indication	Adverse Reactions and Prescribing Considerations
telmisartan-hydrochlorothiazide (Micardis) valsartan-hydrochlorothiazide (Diovan HCT)		
Centrally Acting Drugs and Diuretic methyldopa-hydrochlorothiazide (Aldoril) reserpine-chlorthalidone (Diupres)	As above.	See above.
Diuretic Combination spironolactone-hydrochlorothiazide (Aldactazide) combination HCTZ and triamterene (Dyazide)	Used to treat fluid retention and hypertension.	May exacerbate hyperkalemia, metabolic acidosis, gynecomastia, gout, renal and hepatic impairment. May cause GI disturbances. Useful in patients with refractory HTN. Use in patients with need for potassium-sparing diuretic. Do not use potassium supplements or other diuretics. Advise patients to obtain emergency medical help if any signs of an allergic reaction occur: hives; difficulty breathing; swelling of face, lips, tongue, or throat. May cause numbness, muscle pain or weakness; uneven heartbeat; drowsiness, restless, or light-headedness; changes in urination pattern; shallow breathing; tremors, confusion; nausea, stomach pain, low fever, loss of appetite, dark urine, clay-colored stools, jaundice.

such as ACEIs and diuretics. In addition, use of vasoconstricting medications such as decongestants (e.g., pseudoephedrine, phenylpropanolamine, caffeine) and drugs of abuse (e.g., cocaine, amphetamines) can cause persistently elevated BP readings in spite of intervention. Excessive alcohol use may also prevent many antihypertensive medications from achieving full therapeutic effect. In addition, one of the first manifestations of alcohol withdrawal is BP elevation. Nicotine and many of the chemically active, vasoconstricting substances ingested with cigarette smoke can also contribute to inadequate BP control.

On occasion, a given clinical condition necessitates the use of a drug such as cyclosporine, erythropoietin, or certain antidepressants known to cause BP elevations. In this case, the antihypertensive therapeutic agent must be chosen with care and an adequate dose prescribed.

Concurrent health problems that are inadequately treated may also affect the BP. The normal pain response includes vasoconstriction; therefore, inadequate control of both acute and chronic pain can cause a rise in BP.

Follow-up and Referral

For the patient on lifestyle modification, a follow-up visit should be scheduled every 3 to 6 months to determine effectiveness and adherence to the regimen. If ineffective, pharmacological therapy should be initiated. HTN can be controlled only if the patient is motivated. Using the *Circle of Caring* model and involving the patient in his or her own care may assist in increasing motivation.

After initiation of antihypertensive therapy, a follow-up visit should be scheduled in 2 to 3 weeks for a BP check or even in 1 to 2 weeks for an electrolyte or side-effect check. Once the BP goal is reached, visits can be scheduled every several months. More frequent visits may be needed if comorbid conditions exist. Serum potassium and creatinine levels should be monitored several times per year. Lifestyle modifications need to be stressed at each visit, particularly with vigorous promotion of tobacco avoidance. Low-dose aspirin therapy should be initiated when BP control is achieved. If aspirin therapy is started when the patient is still hypertensive, there is a potential risk of hemorrhagic stroke. Because the majority of MIs occur in the morning, aspirin should be administered at night. If a patient is on two HTN medications, one should be given in the morning and one in the evening.

Patient Education

A patient-directed interdisciplinary team approach is critical to successful HTN care. This team should include representatives from nursing, pharmacy, medicine, and nutrition for the continued education of the patient and family and therapeutic monitoring during antihypertensive therapy. Education is stressed to improve patient adherence to behavioral and pharmacological therapy.

Numerous factors influence the efficacy of HTN therapy. Certain issues should be considered when HTN persists. Nonadherence to therapy is the most common reason for persistent HTN. The most common reasons for nonadherence are (1) lack of perceived benefit of the intervention, (2) difficulty with provider follow-up, and (3) adverse effects of medication. The clinician must work with the patient to develop a plan of care that will meet therapeutic goals and fit with the patient's needs. Choosing well-tolerated drugs for intervention and continually acting as the patient's advocate and coach for lifestyle changes are critical.

Using the *Circle of Caring*, the patient will be involved with the clinician in addressing diet, exercise, tobacco use, and every modifiable risk factor that may be positively changed. Family may be an important component of the *Circle of Caring* and should be present when patient teaching occurs. Many times a successful regimen is spearheaded by a conscientious family member.

The Framingham Scoring System is helpful to the clinician to evaluate the risk of patients for having an acute coronary event in the next 10 years. At a patient's annual visit, this risk assessment may be done by the clinician as a teaching tool to encourage patients to change behaviors such as smoking, exercise, and diet. The clinician can "plug in" the patient's numbers and discuss the results with the patient. The scoring system is found at www.nhlbi.nih.gov/guidelines/cholesterol/risk_tbl.htm. Note that this scoring tool takes into consideration neither persons over age 79 years nor family history.

Also recommended is the Clin Calc Pooled Cohort Risk Assessment equation to predict the 10-year risk for a first atherosclerotic cardiovascular disease (ASCVD) event. If a patient's assessed risk is greater than 7.5%, it is recommended that the clinician initiate lipid-lowering therapy. This calculator is found at http://clincalc.com/Cardiology/ASCVD/pooledCohort.aspx. Clinicians might

want to use both assessment tools with patients to gain their commitment to make changes.

Oral contraceptives may increase BP, and the risk of HTN increases with the length of use. BP should be monitored regularly in women taking oral contraceptives. If a woman becomes hypertensive while taking oral contraceptives, the clinician should advise the patient to consider other forms of birth control.

The frequency of erectile dysfunction (ED) is significantly higher in men who are hypertensive than in men who are normotensive. If ED occurs, the antihypertensive medication should be discontinued and treatment restarted with another agent. Hypertensive men should be advised that there is a lower risk of ED in men who are physically active, not obese, and nonsmokers. Therefore, these lifestyle modifications should be encouraged for all men to forestall ED.

Because some older adults develop postural hypotension with hypertensive drug therapy, the clinician must insist that these patients change position slowly while on HTN medication and that they sit on the edge of the bed for several minutes before standing. In addition, patients with postural hypotension should be urged to avoid volume depletion by drinking adequate quantities of water. Lifestyle modifications cannot be stressed enough. Teaching at every visit should reinforce the suggestions listed in Table 10.2.

■ DYSLIPIDEMIA

Dyslipidemia, also referred to as *hyperlipidemia,* is a general term for elevated concentrations of any or all of the lipids in the plasma. A major risk factor for cardiovascular disease (CVD), increased lipid levels positively correlate with a growing risk of acute coronary syndrome (ACS). In 2013, the American College of Cardiology (ACC) and the American Heart Association (AHA) released guidelines recommending consideration of statin therapy to those millions of Americans who do not currently have CVD but who have a 7.5% or greater risk for stroke or heart attack. This risk is calculated using an updated equation from the AHA/ACC panel that includes race, gender, age, total cholesterol, high-density lipoprotein, blood pressure (BP), use of BP meds, diabetes mellitus (DM), and smoking. The risk calculator may be found at http://myamericanheart.org/cvriskcalculator.

The AHA/ACC recommend that the clinician begin a discussion determining the best therapy for each unique patient situation. These recommendations from the AHA/ACC are changing the way clinicians view traditional treatment guidelines. Previously, clinicians focused on achieving a target low-density lipoprotein (LDL). However, there have been no clinical trials that have supported using LDL levels as an indication for prescribing statins.

Epidemiology and Causes

The correlation between dyslipidemia and coronary events is well documented. Elevated lipid levels present the greatest risk factor for the development of coronary artery disease (CAD). In the United States, CVD claims the lives of approximately 815,000 men and women each year. The Framingham Heart Study (the largest ongoing cohort study of heart disease in the United States) has documented that 40% of participants who developed a myocardial infarction (MI) had a total cholesterol (TC) level between 200 and 250 mg/dL. A patient with a TC level greater than 259 mg/dL is three times more likely to develop CAD than a patient with a level less than 200 mg/dL. It is important to recognize that dyslipidemia is only one of the many factors that increase the risk of developing CAD. The greater the number of risk factors present, the greater the probability of developing clinically significant CAD.

Pathophysiology

Dyslipidemia is a heterogeneous metabolic disorder that involves levels of lipids and lipoproteins that increase risk of atherosclerosis. Lipoproteins are molecules that carry cholesterol in the bloodstream. Lipoproteins differ in size, density, and atherogenicity and are divided into several classes—very low density lipoprotein (VLDL), intermediate-density lipoprotein (IDL), low-density lipoprotein (LDL), lipoprotein (a) (Lp[a]), and high-density lipoprotein (HDL). Atherogenesis is mediated by the lower density lipoproteins: Lp(a), VLDL, IDL, and LDL. These small LDL particles migrate into the inflamed region of the blood vessel wall where they are oxidized and phagocytosed by macrophages to form foam cells, ultimately leading to the formation of fatty streaks and atherosclerotic plaques. LDL cholesterol (LDL-C) is the specific type of cholesterol that constitutes the lipid core of arteriosclerotic plaque deposits. In clinical analyses, Lp(a), LDL, IDL, and VLDL are combined into the single fraction of LDL. Desirable levels of LDL are dependent on the existence of other CVD risk factors. (See Table 10.3 for all lipid levels.) Triglycerides (TGs) are large lipid molecules formed from dietary fats that also contribute to atherogenesis. To prevent cardiovascular disease, the desirable TG level is less than 150 mg/dL.

Atherogenic forms of cholesterol–lipoprotein complexes include all types of non-HDL cholesterol- and triglyceride-transporting proteins: LDL, IDL, Lp(a), and VLDL. Total cholesterol in the blood arises both from ingested fats and from synthesis in the liver. The measurement of total blood cholesterol is based on LDL-C, TG, and HDL-C. The following equation is used to calculate total cholesterol: $TC = LDL\text{-}C + TG/5 + HDL\text{-}C$. The desirable level of total cholesterol in the blood is less than 200 mg/dL.

HDL cholesterol (HDL-C) is excreted from the body and not deposited on the arterial walls. HDL removes excess cholesterol from blood vessels and delivers it back to the liver through reverse cholesterol transport. Once in the liver, cholesterol is excreted into the intestine as bile. HDL also plays a protective role by blocking the

Table 10.3 Serum Lipid Levels	
Classification Level	Laboratory Value
Total Cholesterol (mg/dL)	
Desirable	<200 mg/dL
Borderline high	200–239 mg/dL
High	>240 mg/dL
Triglycerides (mg/dL)	
Normal	<150 mg/dL
Borderline high	150–199 md/dL
High	200–499 mg/dL
Very high	>500 mg/dL
HDL (mg/dL)	
Low	<40 mg/dL
High (optimal: cardioprotective)	>60 mg/dL

oxidation of LDL, which, in turn, inhibits atherogenesis. A low HDL level (≤40 mg/dL) is considered a cardiovascular risk factor, whereas a high level of HDL-C (≥60 mg/dL) is considered cardioprotective. An HDL-C level less than or equal to 60 mg/dL is a negative cardiovascular risk factor, subtracting one factor from the total number of CVD risk factors.

Primary goals of treatment of dyslipidemia are (1) lowering elevated LDL, (2) lowering elevated TG, and (3) raising suboptimal levels of HDL in order to prevent CVD development. Table 10.3 shows lipid values and classifications according to the Guidelines of the National Cholesterol Education Program, National Institutes of Health, and the National Heart, Lung, and Blood Institute. Dyslipidemia can also arise as a result of a genetic disorder, such as familial hypercholesterolemia. Behavioral factors, such as dietary consumption of fats and a lack of physical activity, also play a role. Moreover, dyslipidemia can be part of a constellation of abnormalities known as metabolic syndrome. Metabolic syndrome is characterized by abdominal obesity, glucose intolerance, insulin resistance, hyperinsulinemia, dyslipidemia, and hypertension (HTN).

It is important to assess patients for secondary causes of dyslipidemia before instituting lipid-lowering treatment. Treatment of the primary disorder can correct the dyslipidemia. Secondary causes of dyslipidemia include obesity, diabetes mellitus, hypothyroidism, nephrotic syndrome, end-stage renal disease, hepatic disorders, excessive alcohol consumption, estrogen administration, Cushing's syndrome, and glycogen storage disease. Certain drugs can cause lipid abnormalities such as thiazide diuretics, steroids, beta blockers, HIV protease inhibitors, isotretinoin, and growth hormone.

Clinical Presentation
Subjective

Typically, the patient may present without symptoms when diagnosed with dyslipidemia. Often, however, concurrent problems such as HTN or CAD exist.

Objective

The clinician, on noting an abnormal lipid profile, may be the first to diagnose dyslipidemia in the unsuspecting patient. Physical examination may reveal a carotid bruit and corneal arcus. In some forms of dyslipidemia, yellowish skin deposits of cholesterol called xanthomas may occur. These deposits commonly occur around the eyelids (xanthelasma) and extensor tendons. Interestingly, even with effective lipid-lowering therapy, these deposits tend not to regress.

Diagnostic Reasoning

Diagnostic Tests

The fourth Adult Treatment Panel guidelines from the National Cholesterol Education Program (ATP IV NCEP) of the National Heart, Lung, and Blood Institute was released in November 2013. Previous guidelines recommended specific LDL and non-HDL cholesterol targets for patients with CVD to maintain, with some suggesting LDL levels lower than 100 mg/dL and others proposing levels less than 70 mg/dL. The latest ACC/AHA guidelines state that there is no evidence from trials to support treatment to a specific LDL target. These guidelines identify four groups of primary and secondary prevention patients on whom to concentrate efforts aimed at reducing CV events:

- Patients with atherosclerotic cardiovascular disease (ASCVD)
- Patients with LDL levels greater than or equal to 190 mg/dL such as those with familial hypercholesterolemia
- Patients with diabetes aged 40 to 75 years with LDL between 70 and 189 mg/dL and without evidence of ASCVD
- Patients without evidence of CVD or DM but who have LDL levels between 70 and 189 mg/dL along with a 10-year risk of ASCVD greater than or equal to 7.5% as determined by the CV risk calculator

It is recommended that the first two groups use high-intensity statins and the last two groups use moderate-intensity statins.

Differential Diagnosis

Some potential causes of secondary dyslipidemia are listed in Table 10.4. Elevated TC levels may be present in CAD, type II familial hypercholesterolemia, idiopathic hypercholesterolemia, obstructive jaundice, biliary cirrhosis, hypothyroidism, von Gierke's disease, pregnancy, uncontrolled DM, other pancreatic disease, chronic nephritis, glomerulosclerosis, and obesity. Decreased TC levels may be present in malabsorption, starvation, anorexia nervosa, liver disease, severe cell damage, HTN, chronic anemia, and drug therapy with agents such as adrenal corticotrophic hormones and antibiotics.

Elevated TG levels may be present in liver disease, alcoholism, nephrotic syndrome, renal disease, hypothyroidism, uncontrolled DM, pancreatitis, gout, glycogen storage

Table 10.4	Potential Causes of Secondary Hyperlipidemia	
Causes	**Lipid Abnormality**
Inactivity	HDL ↓
Alcohol abuse	TG ↑, HDL ↑, LDL ↑
Diabetes mellitus	TG ↑, HDL ↓, TC ↑
Hypothyroidism	TG ↑, TC ↑
Thiazide diuretic use (high dose)	TC ↑, LDL ↑, TG ↑
Beta blocker use (high dose)	LDL ↑, HDL ↓
Chronic renal insufficiency	TC ↑, TG ↑

disease, MI (increased levels may last for 1 year), metabolic diseases related to endocrinopathies, von Gierke's disease, stress, high-carbohydrate diet, and HTN. Decreased triglyceride levels may be present in malnutrition, hyperthyroidism, exercise, and malabsorption syndrome.

An elevated HDL level may be associated with chronic liver disease or chronic intoxication, long-term aerobic exercise or other vigorous exercise, and estrogen and birth control pills. A decreased HDL level may be caused by hypertriglyceridemia, hypothyroidism, end-stage liver disease, diabetes mellitus, obesity, chronic inactivity, uremia, and homozygous Tangier disease.

An increased LDL level may be the result of familial hypercholesteremia and secondary causes such as a diet high in cholesterol and saturated fat, nephrotic syndrome, chronic renal failure, pregnancy, porphyria, diabetes mellitus, multiple myeloma, steroids, and estrogens. A decreased LDL level may be the result of malnutrition and malabsorption syndromes.

An increased VLDL level may be caused by familial hyperlipidemia and secondarily by alcoholism, obesity, diabetes mellitus, chronic renal disease, pancreatitis, pregnancy, estrogen, birth control pills, and progestins. A decreased VLDL level may be the result of malnutrition and malabsorption syndromes.

Management

To determine if a patient should be on a statin, the clinician should ask the following four questions; if any response is *yes*, the patient is a potential candidate (Page, 2013):

1. Does the patient have a history of any of the following?
   a. ACS
   b. MI
   c. Stable or unstable angina
   d. Coronary or arterial revascularization
   e. Stroke, transient ischemic attack
   f. Peripher arterial disease of artherosclerotic origin
2. Does the patient have an LDL level of greater than or equal to 190 mg/dL? (indicative of familial hypercholesterolemia)
3. Is the patient 40 to 75 years of age with DM?

4. Is the patient 40 to 75 years of age with a CV risk score of greater than or equal to 7.5%?

For patients with ASCVD who are under age 75 years, high-intensity statin therapy should be used to reduce their LDL-C levels by 50%. For patients older than 75 years, use moderate-intensity therapy. A moderate-intensity statin therapy should be used for patients with DM aged 40 to 75 years, because the goal is to reduce their LDL-C levels by 30% to 49%. If these patients have a 10-year CV risk greater than 7.5%, use high-intensity therapy. In addition, for patients aged 40 to 75 years without CVD or DM, but who have a CV risk score greater than 7.5% and an LDL level anywhere from 70 to 189 mg/dL, moderate-intensity therapy is also acceptable. See Drugs Commonly Prescribed 10.2 for classifications and dosages of statins.

If patients do not fall into any of the previous categories, additional factors should be considered, such as family history of premature ASCVD in a first-degree relative; high-sensitivity C-reactive protein greater than 2 mg/dL; presence of calcification on a coronary artery calcium scan; and an ankle-brachial index less than 0.9.

Diet

A cholesterol-lowering diet is recommended for all Americans. Diets very low in total fat or in saturated fat, however, may lower HDL-C as much as they do LDL-C. A sensible nutritional approach is the best recommendation. Most nutritionists advocate reducing total fat to 25% to 30% of daily calories and saturated fat to less than 7% of daily calories. Dietary cholesterol should be limited to less than 200 mg/day. This regimen will replace fat, particularly saturated fat, with carbohydrate, usually resulting in fewer total calories consumed and facilitating weight loss in overweight patients. The Mediterranean diet has been shown to decrease cholesterol levels in some patients.

Pharmacological Therapy

For years, diet has been the cornerstone of treatment for hyperlipidemia; however, recent studies have demonstrated that diet alone is often insufficient in lowering cholesterol.

The 3-hydroxy-3-methylglutaryl coenzyme A (HMG-CoA) reductase inhibitors (medications with generic names ending in -statin) are the first-line drugs of choice in the majority of patients.

Baseline liver function tests (LFTs) should be done before prescribing statins. There is no evidence from the Food and Drug Administration to support routine monitoring of LFTs during statin therapy unless clinically indicated. The clinician should caution patients about use of statins with other hepatotoxic drugs and alcohol. Other adverse effects include muscle weakness and, in extreme cases, rhabdomyolysis with significant elevations in serum creatine phosphokinase (creatine kinase) levels. Gastrointestinal complaints include dyspepsia and abdominal pain.

Once the initial dose of statin medication is prescribed, the clinician considers whether to increase the dose or add another agent if the statin does not seem to be effective. Although some practitioners recommend them, there is lack of evidence to support the use of fibrates, niacin, and fish oil to treat hyperlipidemia. Lifestyle counseling should occur at the initial and follow-up visits as the foundation for statin therapy and may improve the patient's overall risk.

Drugs Commonly Prescribed 10.2 presents information on the different levels of statin therapy along with specific dosages. Therapies are either categorized as low, moderate, or high intensity.

Follow-up and Referral

The clinician should be very well equipped to treat the patient with hyperlipidemia. If treatment goals are not reached, consultation with a cardiologist may be indicated. Consultation with a nutritionist may be recommended if the patient cannot follow or understand a cholesterol-lowering diet.

Patient Education

It is important for the clinician to provide ongoing support and reinforcement to patients undertaking both dietary and pharmacological therapy for dyslipidemia. Many patients do not like to take medications and feel that diet alone is sufficient to keep them "under control." Sometimes, showing the patient the lab results and having a discussion about what the numbers mean, especially the ratio of HDL to TC, in terms of the risk of having an MI, is an effective way to get the patient to take a hard look at potential benefits of combined therapy. Calculating the patient's CV risk score will facilitate the conversation about the possible need for statin therapy. In addition, discussing the patient's Framingham Heart Score to predict the risk of having an acute coronary event might help to motivate a patient in adhering to a diet, exercise, and drug treatment program. Using the *Circle of Caring* model, patients can be encouraged through the highs and lows that typically occur when initiating long-term changes.

■ METABOLIC SYNDROME

Metabolic syndrome refers to a cluster of specific cardiovascular disease (CVD) and diabetes risk factors where the underlying pathophysiology is thought to be related to insulin resistance. Because the term *metabolic syndrome* has been imprecisely defined, clinicians should evaluate and treat all CVD risk factors without regard to whether a patient meets the criteria for diagnosis of the metabolic syndrome. The clinician needs to be cognizant of new information pertaining to this syndrome, because a new definition typically appears every few years. Metabolic syndrome has been characterized by a combination of atherogenic and diabetogenic factors. Increased body mass index (BMI), elevated systolic blood pressure (BP),

Drugs Commonly Prescribed 10.2 Hyperlipidemia

Drug	Effect on Lipids	Adverse Reactions and Prescribing Considerations
HMG-CoA Reductase Inhibitors (Statins)		
High-Intensity atorvastatin (Lipitor) 40–80 mg rosuvastatin (Crestor) 20–40 mg	Decreases LDL. Increases HDL. Decrease TGs.	May cause myositis (especially in patients taking fibrates or niacin). Do not use with gemfibrozil. Take in the evening.
Moderate-Intensity rosuvastatin 10 mg (Crestor) atorvastatin 10–20 mg (Lipitor) pravastatin (Pravachol) 40 mg simvastatin (Zocor) 20–40 mg lovastatin (Mevacor) 40 mg		Do not give to patients with active or chronic liver disease. Monitor LFTs before initiating therapy.
Bile Acid Sequestrants		
cholestyramine (Questran and Questran Light) colesevelam (WelChol) colestipol (Colestid)	Decreases LDL anywhere from 10%–25%. Increases HDL 5%–10%. TG: Same or increased.	Mix with liquids. GI symptoms are common, with constipation and gas. Use psyllium to prevent. Contraindicated with dysbeta-lipoproteinemia. Do not give with TG >400 mg/dL.
Cholesterol Absorption Inhibitor		
ezetimibe (Zetia)	Decreases LDL 15%–20%.	May be given with a statin or fenofibrate. May cause back pain, arthralgia, diarrhea, abdominal pain, fatigue, cough. Give 2 hours before or 4 hours after bile acid sequestrants. Monitor warfarin.
Combination Therapy		
Statin plus calcium channel blocker atorvastatin + amlodipine (Caduet)	All lower LDL, increase HDL, and lower TGs.	May cause edema, dizziness, palpitations, flushing, fatigue, constipation, dyspepsia, abdominal pain, drowsiness, myopathy, elevated liver enzymes, rhabdomyolysis with renal dysfunction. Monitor liver function before start of therapy. May increase serum levels of digitalis, BCP.
Statin plus cholesterol absorption inhibitor simvastatin + ezetimibe (Vytorin) Statin plus niacin lovastatin + niacin (Advicor) simvastatin + niacin (Simcor)	All lower LDL, increase HDL, and lower TGs.	Caution with moderate to severe liver disease. May cause headache, myalgia, extremity pain, myopathy, rhabdomyolysis, elevated serum transaminases. Avoid fibrates, alcohol, grapefruit juice. May potentiate vasoactive drugs; monitor warfarin, antidiabetics. May cause flushing, headache, pain, pruritus, dyspepsia.
liptruzet (ezetimibe/ atorvastatin)	Lowers LDL by approximately 10% more than atorvastatin, but this may not translate to better patient outcomes.	Muscle pain, tenderness for weakness, increased fatigue, or elevations of liver enzymes.

hypertriglyceridemia, hyperglycemia, and low levels of protective high-density lipoprotein cholesterol are found in affected persons. Any three of these conditions occurring together usually establish the diagnosis (see Table 10.5). The etiology is unknown; however, environmental, genetic, and behavioral factors contribute to the development of metabolic syndrome, particularly physical inactivity and excess body fat. Elevated BMI is apparent as central obesity, with the affected individual demonstrating an "apple shape" or high waist circumference. Metabolic syndrome is also a proinflammatory and prothrombotic disorder causing endothelial injury, as evidenced by elevations of the inflammatory marker C-reactive protein, increased platelet aggregation, and increased fibrinogen levels. In addition to hyperglycemia and deranged lipid metabolism, peripheral tissues are resistant to insulin. The pancreas oversecretes insulin to overcome tissue resistance, which results in hyperinsulinemia. Obesity enhances insulin resistance and predisposes the individual to type 2 diabetes mellitus.

Obesity is believed to contribute significantly to the development of metabolic syndrome. The National Cholesterol Education Program (NCEP) recommends obesity as the primary target for intervention. Abdominal obesity is defined as a high waist-to-hip ratio. Weight loss improves serum lipid profiles, reduces BP, decreases insulin resistance, and ameliorates glucose intolerance.

■ CORONARY HEART DISEASE (ATHEROSCLEROTIC CORONARY ARTERY DISEASE)

Coronary heart disease (CHD), also referred to as coronary artery disease (CAD), is the leading cause of death in the United States, responsible for more than one in four, or approximately 600,000, deaths per year. Mortality from CAD has declined over the years because of patient education regarding risk factors and early recognition and treatment of symptoms; management of existing problems such as hypertension (HTN), dyslipidemia, and diabetes; and improved technologies such as thrombolytic drugs.

Epidemiology and Causes

Risk factors for CAD are classified as nonmodifiable, modifiable, or contributing and are listed in Risk Factors 10.1. Nearly 13 million Americans have CAD, and the incidence increases with age. More than 10 times the number of women die from atherosclerotic cardiovascular disease each year than from breast cancer.

Angina is the number one symptom of CAD. The narrowing of the coronary arteries as a result of atherosclerosis causes angina. A thrombus, coronary artery vasospasm, aortic stenosis, aortic insufficiency, severe HTN, or idiopathic subaortic hypertrophic stenosis may also cause angina. Angina is the presenting symptom in CAD in 38% of men and 61% of women. Middle-aged and older men and postmenopausal women are most prone to developing angina. Variant angina may occur in patients with normal coronary arteries who have cyclically recurring angina at rest that is unrelated to effort. The pain of unstable angina tends to last longer and have greater intensity than the pain of stable angina.

Pathophysiology of Arteriosclerosis and Coronary Artery Disease

The coronary arteries provide arterial blood flow that supplies oxygen and nutrients to afford optimal myocellular function of the heart. The coronary arteries dilate via release of vasoactive substances to further augment oxygen delivery to keep pace with changing metabolic demands.

Table 10.5	Components of Metabolic Syndrome
Risk Factor (three required for diagnosis)	**Defining Level**
Abdominal Obesity	*Waist Circumference*
Men:	>40 inches
Women:	>35 inches
Triglycerides HDL-C	*>150 mg/dL*
HDL-C (cardioprotective)	
Men:	<40 mg/dL
Women:	<50 mg/dL
Blood Pressure	*≥130/ ≥85 mm Hg*
Fasting Glucose	*>110 mg/dL*

Adapted from www.americanheart.org/presenter.jhtml?identifier=456

Risk Factors 10.1   Coronary Artery Disease (CAD)

Category	Risk Factors
Nonmodifiable	Male gender
	Increasing age
	Family history of CAD
	African American ethnicity
Modifiable	Hypertension (>140 mm Hg SBP and/or ≥90 mm Hg DBP, depending on age)
	Smoking
	Sedentary lifestyle
	Hyperlipidemia
	For women: natural or surgical menopause without estrogen replacement therapy; oral contraceptive use combined with cigarette smoking
Contributing	Diabetes mellitus
	Obesity
	Stress

In addition, the lumen of each coronary artery needs to be patent in order to maintain optimal tissue perfusion. In CAD, arteriosclerotic plaque hinders optimal blood flow and dilation of the coronary arteries. Coronary arteries become obstructed and incapable of vasodilation, which severely impedes perfusion of the myocardium. During physical exertion, when increased blood flow is required, coronary artery blood flow becomes insufficient for the oxygen demands of the myocardium.

This coronary insufficiency, in turn, leads to ischemia of heart muscle. Ischemia creates anaerobic conditions for the myocardium, particularly if acute occlusion results. Anaerobic metabolism yields inadequate energy (approximately 5% of normal) for myocardial demand, allowing for less than a 20-minute period of tissue viability after occlusion. Lactic acid is created as a waste product, leading to localized tissue acidosis. Because lactic acid is irritating to muscle tissue, lactic acid buildup is the source of chest pain in ischemic heart disease. The term *angina pectoris* means chest pain due to ischemia of the heart muscle. If myocardial ischemia is prolonged, myocardial infarction (MI) ensues. Thus, if untreated, CAD progresses to ischemia of the heart muscle or angina pectoris, which can then lead to MI.

Atherosclerosis (arteriosclerosis) is a systemic disease affecting all arteries of the body. If CAD is diagnosed, it is likely that arteriosclerosis is present throughout all arterial systems. Likewise, if vascular disease is identified in target end-organs, CAD is likely to already be present. The process of arteriosclerosis begins with endothelial injury, which can be incited by a number of etiological agents. Free radicals, HTN, hyperglycemia of diabetes, and hyperlipidemia have been found to be agents of injury to arterial endothelial cells. Endothelial injury provokes an inflammatory reaction that attracts T cells, macrophages, monocytes, and platelets to the site. White blood cells secrete mediators, such as interleukins, tumor necrosis factor–alpha, and C-reactive protein (CRP), which perpetuate the inflammatory reaction. Platelets aggregate and form microthrombi. Inflammation is now thought to be the major force that drives atherosclerosis. This idea is supported by findings of elevated levels of *high-sensitivity C-reactive protein (hs-CRP)*, an inflammatory marker, in individuals with coronary arteriosclerosis.

Inflammation of the endothelium depletes nitric oxide, a major vasorelaxant of the arterial muscle wall. This depletion results in a net vasoconstrictive effect. Other pro-inflammatory mediators stimulate proliferation of vascular smooth muscle within the arterial wall, which intensifies the vasoconstrictive effect further. Concurrently, macrophages within the vessel wall engulf and ingest low-density lipoproteins, forming "foam cells." Disruptions of the arterial endothelium by inflammation, lipid-laden macrophages, platelets, and vasoconstricting mediators are the initiating events of arteriosclerosis or atherogenesis.

In the process of atherogenesis, an initial fatty streak on the arterial wall evolves over time, serving as a nidus for fibrin deposition to become a fibrous, calcified plaque. *Arteriosclerosis* means "hardened arteries," which is an apt term for the rigid arteries resulting from long-term plaque formation. Arteries lose significant vasodilation capacity and are lined by calcified arteriosclerotic plaque. The lipid-rich, calcified plaque becomes brittle and unstable, easily rupturing with mechanical stress. When disruption of the plaque occurs, this induces platelet aggregation and activation of the coagulation cascade. A thrombus forms at the site that can embolize, lodge in, and obstruct the lumen of narrowed arteries. In patients who die of unstable angina or MI, pathological studies find that death occurs as a result of ruptured plaque with associated thrombosis. Obstruction due to thrombosis is the most common cause of ischemia in *any* arterially supplied region of the body. Common sites of arteriosclerosis are the coronary arteries, cerebral arteries, and peripheral arteries of the lower extremities. Consequently, ischemia-prone regions of the body are the myocardium, brain, and lower extremities. Prolonged, severe episodes of ischemia can lead to acute coronary syndrome, ischemic stroke, and peripheral arterial insufficiency.

Clinical Presentation
Subjective

In most patients, CAD develops many years before the patient is aware of its existence. Because collateral circulation develops, the patient is usually unaware that anything is wrong unless other concomitant conditions are present, such as dyslipidemia or HTN. Typically, symptoms of CAD are not reported until 75% of the coronary artery is narrowed. Eventually, if CAD is uncorrected, the patient will usually present with exertional angina, which should lead the clinician to suspect CAD. Associated symptoms may include radiation of the discomfort to the left arm and jaw, nausea, shortness of breath, and lightheadedness (syncopal episodes). It should be noted that not all patients present with these "typical" symptoms. Please review the differential diagnosis section.

Objective

The clinician should note all the peripheral pulses; auscultate for carotid bruits; note jugular venous distention; take the blood pressure sitting, lying, and standing; and examine the skin condition for evidence of decreased perfusion. The history should include a detailed description of other risk factors that are present, which will guide further assessment for resultant problems such as angina. (Pertinent questions related to angina are covered later in this chapter.) Because atherosclerosis is a widespread problem, patients with CAD also have a much higher incidence of peripheral vascular disease and cerebrovascular disease than other individuals. The clinician should assess for other symptoms that suggest vascular insufficiency such as intermittent claudication or transient ischemic attacks.

Diagnostic Reasoning

Diagnostic Tests

An electrocardiogram (ECG), stress test, nuclear scanning, and angiography may be ordered to determine the extent of the CAD and to identify which vessels are affected. ECGs are discussed in detail in the section on MI.

An exercise ECG, or a stress test, may be ordered to detect and evaluate CAD. Carefully controlled and supervised exercise increases the myocardial oxygen demands, which assists in evaluating the coronary arteries' ability to meet the increased demands successfully. When the patient is unable to achieve a vigorous level of exercise, a dipyridamole thallium-201 test may be used. It may produce false-positive readings, especially in women, and in cases of certain drugs and electrolyte imbalances. A stress test is contraindicated in acute cardiovascular disease (CVD) (e.g., MI, unstable angina, or heart failure) because the heart cannot respond to an increased demand for oxygen.

Nuclear scanning (technetium-99m ventriculography) studies the motion of the left ventricular wall and measures the ventricle's ability to eject blood, referred to as the ejection fraction (normally 55%–75%). When ischemia is present because of a narrowed coronary artery, the segment of the myocardium that artery serves exhibits diminished wall motion (hypokinesis) or contractility that is represented as pooled blood within the ventricular and atrial chambers.

Contrast-enhanced computed tomography (CT) scan imaging is a noninvasive imaging method of assessing overall "plaque burden," the extent to which atheromatous plaque undermines the integrity of an artery wall. Estimating "plaque burden" can assess the risk of atheromatous plaque rupturing and causing ischemia. This CT scan, also termed *CT calcium scoring,* can evaluate the overall burden of calcified atherosclerotic plaque.

A cardiac catheterization with angiography for coronary artery visualization is performed, commonly after the patient is stabilized in acute coronary syndrome (ACS) or if there is high suspicion of ACS. Visualization of the coronary arteries confirms diagnosis of CAD and can evaluate the extent of stenosis of coronary arteries.

Ultrasonography can be used with cardiac catheterization to add diagnostic information. Intravascular ultrasonography (IVUS) used during cardiac catheterization measures "plaque burden" through real-time intraluminal imaging of vessel walls. IVUS can also be used to assess plaque regression when the patient is on antilipemic drug therapy.

Because arteriosclerosis is a chronic inflammatory condition, the biomarker CRP is commonly elevated in individuals with CAD. CRP is an acute-phase inflammatory protein produced by the liver and by the smooth muscle cells within arteriosclerotic coronary arteries. An elevated level of hs-CRP has been shown to be an independent predictor of risk of MI, stroke, peripheral arterial disease, and sudden cardiac death. Measurement of hs-CRP adds to the total cardiac risk assessment of the patient and should not be solely relied on as a confirmatory test.

Epidemiological studies show that an elevated level of the amino acid homocysteine is an independent risk factor for arteriosclerosis and CAD. Homocysteine requires folic acid, vitamin B_6, and vitamin B_{12} for its metabolism. This amino acid accumulates in the blood and injures the endothelium when there are inadequate levels of the B vitamins and folate for its proper metabolism. Therefore, elevated serum homocysteine levels add to the cardiac risk assessment of a patient. Research has shown that reducing homocysteine levels with vitamins does not reduce the risk of heart disease.

Differential Diagnosis

Differential diagnoses for CAD include gastrointestinal, pulmonary, or cardiac problems that are not related to ischemia. Gastroesophageal reflux disease, esophageal spasm, or biliary colic can present with symptoms similar to MI or angina. Patients with CAD or MI often present with epigastric pain that is misinterpreted as "heartburn" or related pain. This misinterpretation is often the reason for a patient's delay in obtaining prompt medical evaluation.

Patients with anxiety or panic attacks often present to the emergency department with symptoms that mimic angina or MI. Extreme stress can precipitate chest pain, dizziness, dyspnea, and hyperventilation, all of which mimic the symptoms of angina or MI. Costochondritis, a musculoskeletal problem, can also present as chest pain that may be misinterpreted as CAD by patients. The pain of costochondritis can usually be reproduced by pressing on the sternum and costochondral regions of the chest.

Persons with diabetes may experience angina or silent MI with minor symptoms or no symptoms at all. Diabetes causes nerve related damage that blunts heart pain. Patients with CAD may experience nausea and vomiting, dyspnea, epigastric pain, diaphoresis, or dizziness with no complaint of chest pain. These symptoms are referred to as "anginal equivalents." Women experiencing angina or MI commonly present with "anginal equivalents" rather than with chest pain. Historically, clinicians have underestimated the risk of CVD in women. Atypical presentation of ACS in women contributes to lack of early recognition of cardiac symptoms by both patients and clinicians. Women classically delay seeking medical care for ischemic symptoms, which contributes to their overall higher morbidity and mortality with cardiac events.

Pneumothorax, pneumonia, pericarditis, pulmonary embolism, mitral valve prolapse, and aortic dissection are other less common causes of chest pain. The diverse causes of ischemic chest pain (angina) must be determined. Because chest pain is so often the impetus to the diagnosis of CAD, the pain characteristics that drive the differential diagnoses need to be carefully assessed. In a young, otherwise healthy adult, reproducible point tenderness is likely musculoskeletal chest wall pain and not ischemic.

Pleuritic pain worsens on inspiration and is likely from lung pathology such as pneumonia, especially if accompanied by fever and productive cough. Clinicians need to have a high level of suspicion and to complete a thorough cardiac risk assessment to rule out MI in all patients complaining of chest pain or "anginal equivalents."

Management

The principles of management include establishing the diagnosis, controlling the symptoms, and preventing the disease progression that may lead to MI or sudden death. During a cardiac catheterization, fibrinolytic agents may be infused directly into an occluded coronary artery in an attempt to restore coronary blood flow. Other therapeutic approaches may include balloon angioplasty, stent placement, and coronary artery bypass graft. Presently there are two types of stents in use—bare-metal stents (BMS) and drug-eluting stents (DES). With both types of stents, anticoagulation is begun immediately. DES require a longer duration of anticoagulation therapy than BMS (Level II; Brar et al, 2008).

Risk-Factor Modification

Risk-factor modification is essential to stop the progression of CAD. This involves aggressive lowering of lipid levels (which is discussed in the Dyslipidemia section), strict glycemic control in patients with diabetes (see Chapter 16), aggressive antihypertensive therapy (discussed in the Hypertension section), smoking cessation (see Chapter 9) and cessation of all tobacco use, and modifying the lifestyle to include regular exercise, stress reduction, and a heart-healthy diet (less than 300 mg cholesterol/day and 7% or less of total calories from saturated fatty acids).

Complementary Therapies 10.1 presents suggested vitamin, mineral, and herbal supplementation for various cardiovascular disorders.

Complementary Therapies 10.1   Cardiac Conditions

Agent	Indication	Adverse Reactions and Considerations*
Hawthorn	Angina, CHF, CAD, functional cardiovascular disorders, hypertension (in diabetes), orthostatic hypotension	May cause abdominal discomfort, agitation, arrhythmia, diaphoresis, dizziness, dyspnea, fatigue, headache, palpitations, sleeplessness, rash. Caution with: HTN medications (may increase risk of hypotension); antilipemic agents (additive effects); calcium channel blockers (additive vasodilation); cardiac glycosides and vasodilators (additive vasodilation). Monitor BP, coagulation panel, heart rate, lipid profile.
Magnesium	Arrhythmia, acute MI, CAD, HTN, mitral valve prolapse	May cause areflexia, asthenia, cardiac arrhythmias, cardiac arrest, drowsiness, hypermagnesemia, hypotension, loss of tendon reflexes, polydipsia, respiratory paralysis. Caution with aminoglycosides (increased risk of muscular weakness and paralysis); antibiotics (decreased effects); antidiabetic agents (increased absorption); antihypertensive agents (additive effects). Monitor alkaline phosphatase, blood glucose, BP, calcium levels, coagulation panel, cortisol, LFTs, ECG, parathyroid hormone.
Beta-glucan	Antioxidant, CVD, heart protection during CABG, hyperlipidemia, HTN	May cause dizziness, flushing, headache, hypertension or hypotension, inflammatory airway disease, keratoderma, nausea, polyuria, urticaria, vomiting. Caution with diabetic agents (additive effect); antihypertensive agents (additive effect); antilipemic agents (additive effect). Monitor blood glucose, BP, lipid profile, WBC count.
Selenium	Antioxidant, cardiomyopathy, CVD prevention, circulation	May cause digitalis dysfunction, garlic-like breath odor, hepatorenal dysfunction, irritability, loss or thickening of hair and nails, metallic taste, muscle tenderness, nausea/vomiting, nervous system abnormalities, skin lesions, thrombocytopenia, tremor, weakness. Caution with barbiturates (increased sedation); HMG-CoA reductase inhibitors and niacin (decreased efficacy).

Continued

Complementary Therapies 10.1 Cardiac Conditions—cont'd

Agent	Indication	Adverse Reactions and Considerations*
Vitamin B₆	Angioplasty, CVD, CHD risk reduction, coronary restenosis, homocysteine reduction	Prolonged excessive use may cause neuropathy. Monitor vitamin B₆ levels.
Vitamin B₁₂	Angioplasty, CHD, coronary restenosis, homocysteine reduction, orthostatic tremor (restless legs syndrome)	Monitor vitamin B₁₂ levels.
Vitamin C	Atherosclerosis, circulation, ischemic heart disease, MI risk reduction	In large doses may cause abdominal cramps, diarrhea, nausea, skin rashes. In diabetics, may cause falsely elevated blood glucose readings. Caution with iron (increased iron levels); warfarin (in high doses, lowers prothrombin time). Monitor vitamin C levels.
Vitamin E	Angina, arterial elasticity, atherosclerosis, CVD, CHF, dyslipidemias, intermittent claudication, DVT	May cause abdominal pain, blurred vision, diarrhea, fatigue, headache. Increased risk of mortality with high doses with history of severe CVD (CVA or MI). Caution with anticoagulants/antiplatelets (increased risk of bleeding); chemotherapy (interfere with effectiveness). Monitor coagulation panel (with high doses), vitamin E levels. Discontinue use 2 weeks before dental or surgical procedures.
Flaxseed Oil	CVD, HTN, hyperlipidemia	May cause abdominal discomfort, anaphylaxis, bleeding, bowel obstruction, constipation, diarrhea, dyspnea, hypoglycemia, hypotension, mania, nausea/vomiting, increased risk of prostate cancer, pruritus, skin rash, sneezing, stuffy nose, seizures, watery eyes. Contraindicated with hypertriglyceridemia. Caution with anticoagulants/antiplatelets (increased risk of bleeding); antidiabetic agents (increased risk of hypoglycemia); antihypertensives (increased risk of hypotension); antilipemic agents (decreased effects on triglycerides); furosemide (decreased absorption of furosemide). Monitor alkaline phosphatase, blood glucose, coagulation panel, inflammatory markers, lipid profile, prostate-specific antigen (PSA), red blood cells, triglycerides.
Garlic	Anticoagulant, atherosclerosis, familial hypercholesterolemia, hyperlipidemia, HTN, prevention of MI, PVD	May cause anorexia, bleeding, burning inside the mouth, chills, constipation, diarrhea, dizziness, diaphoresis, dyspepsia, dyspnea, fever, flatulence, halitosis, hyperglycemia or hypoglycemia.
	#24- NNRTI is Non-Nucleoside Reverse Transcriptase Inhibitor	Contraindicated with concurrent use with isoniazid, NNRTIs, or protease inhibitors, inflammatory bowel disease, pregnancy, and lactation. Caution with anticoagulants/antiplatelets (increased risk of bleeding); antidiabetic agents (altered effects); antihypertension agents (additive effect); antilipemic agents (additive effect); contraceptives (decrease effectiveness); some HIV/AIDS meds (decreased levels of NNRTIs and PIs).
	#25 Protease Inhibitors	Monitor blood glucose, coagulation panel, lipid profile, urinary allylmercapturic acid.
Lycopene	CAD, HTN	May cause abdominal pain or cramps, anorexia, diarrhea, flatulence, nausea/vomiting. Monitor androgen, lipid profile, PSA.

Complementary Therapies 10.1 Cardiac Conditions—cont'd

Agent	Indication	Adverse Reactions and Considerations*
Coenzyme Q10	Adjunct to statin therapy, angina, cardiomyopathy, cardioprotection during surgery, CHF, CAD, hyperlipidemia, HTN, MI	May cause bleeding, diarrhea, dizziness, dyspnea, fatigue, flu-like symptoms, GI upset, headache, heartburn, hyperglycemia or hypoglycemia, hypotension, insomnia, irritability, loss of appetite, nausea/vomiting, photosensitivity, pruritus, rash, thrombosis, thyroid hormone alterations. Caution with antidiabetic agents (altered effects); antihypertensives (additive effect); antilipemic agents (additive effects); corticosteroids (decreased effects); warfarin (decreased anticoagulant effects). Monitor blood glucose, BP, coagulation panel, LFTs, lipid profile, T_4/T_8 ratio.
Calcium	HTN	May cause abdominal pain, arrhythmias, calcium deposits in heart and kidney, chalky taste, confusion, constipation, GI irritation, headache, irritability, MI, nausea/vomiting, nephrotoxicity, polydipsia, polyuria, renal calculi, skin reactions, urinary incontinence. Caution with calcium channel blockers (decreased effects); levothyroxine (decreased effectiveness of levothyroxine). Monitor bone mineral density, calcium levels, renal function tests.
Red Yeast Rice	CHD, hyperlipidemia	May cause bloating, dizziness, flatulence, GI discomfort, headache, kidney damage. Caution with alcohol (increased risk of liver damage); gemfibrozil and niacin (increased risk of myopathy); HMG-CoA reductase inhibitors (increased risk of adverse effects); protease inhibitors (altered effects). Monitor LFTs, kidney function.

*Chart does not list all information. For an extensive review, see Ulbricht, C. *Davis's pocket guide to herbs and supplements.* FA Davis, Philadelphia, 2011.

Pharmacological Therapy

Pharmacological agents are used to control the symptoms of angina and to prevent subsequent events (see discussion in the Acute Coronary Syndrome section). Most clinicians recommend low-dose daily aspirin (81–325 mg) to decrease the incidence of a first MI in middle-aged men and women. Coated aspirin is recommended for individuals with gastric problems. The dose should be decreased if there is a tendency to bruise. There is still controversy regarding dosage and concomitant use if patients are on other anticoagulants.

Follow-up and Referral

Patients need to understand the chronicity of this disease and be committed to frequent follow-ups for control of risk factors. The clinician should refer the patient to a cardiologist for a stress test and for any further cardiac work-up indicated by the results.

Patient Teaching

On each visit, the clinician should stress risk-factor modification. The lifestyle modifications listed in Table 10.2 for managing hypertension are good activities for overall cardiovascular health.

■ ACUTE CORONARY SYNDROME

Acute coronary syndrome (ACS) is a term used for the disorders of myocardial ischemia—stable angina, unstable angina, variant angina (Prinzmetal's), or myocardial infarction (MI). ACS refers to acute conditions; however, stable angina is covered in this section. Although angina pectoris (chest pain related to ischemia of the myocardium) is described as chest discomfort, the pain may radiate elsewhere. *Stable angina* (chronic exertional) is a diagnosed condition of myocardial ischemia that is predictable in pattern and frequency and controlled with medication.

Unstable angina is myocardial ischemia that is newly diagnosed or previously diagnosed angina that has changed in pattern, frequency, or severity. Unstable angina is commonly a forerunner of acute MI. Table 10.6 presents the types of angina and their characteristics.

A *myocardial infarction (MI)* is necrosis or death of part of the myocardium as a result of prolonged ischemia

Table 10.6	Types of Angina
Type of Angina	Characteristics
Stable	Chest pain: Transient episodes related to activities that increase myocardial oxygen demand. Duration: Typically lasts 3–15 minutes. Associated signs and symptoms: Nausea, vomiting, shortness of breath. Relief: Rest and/or nitroglycerin tablets.
Unstable	Chest pain: More severe and brought on with less exertion; may occur at rest. Duration: Prolonged. Associated signs and symptoms: Nausea, vomiting, shortness of breath, diaphoresis. Relief: Not relieved by rest and/or nitroglycerin tablets; relieved by morphine.
Variant (Prinzmetal's)	Chest pain: Episodes unrelated to activities that increase myocardial oxygen demand. Duration: Cyclic; often occurs during sleep (most common in early morning hours); pain intensifies quickly and lasts longer than that of stable angina. Associated signs and symptoms: Palpitation, syncope, bradycardia. Relief: May subside with exercise.

(an insufficient supply of oxygenated blood). The location and extent of the infarction determines the prognosis in addition to the speed with which reperfusion is supplied to "cut-off" areas. Because the use of early reperfusion therapy increases the likelihood of survival and improves left ventricular function, the patient with a suspected MI should be assessed rapidly and prompt, appropriate care provided. The Iceberg of Myocardial Infarction figure explores many facets involved with a patient with an MI.

Epidemiology and Causes

Each year, an estimated 640,000 Americans have a new coronary attack (defined as first hospitalized MI or coronary heart disease death) and almost 280,000 have a recurrent attack. It is estimated that an additional 150,000 persons have a silent MI every year. Approximately every 34 seconds, an American has a coronary event; every minute, an American will die of one.

The mortality rate is approximately 30% for a severe MI. More men than women experience MIs; however,

after menopause this gap dramatically closes. The majority (55%) of MIs occur in individuals who are older than 65 years of age. Eighty percent of patients who die from an MI are older than age 65. Men have about a 20% chance of having an MI or coronary artery disease (CAD). MIs are more common in Western societies. African Americans have a higher incidence of MI due to the higher incidence of hypertension (HTN) in that population.

The contributing factors for an MI include the same risk factors as for CAD (see Risk Factors 10.1), as well as tachycardia, left ventricular hypertrophy (LVH), anemia, increased platelet aggregation, and abuse of illegal substances.

Pathophysiology

Acute coronary syndrome (ACS) is a broad term to describe a continuum of disorders that arise from coronary artery occlusion. ACS is either an episode of angina pectoris or an MI. In both angina and MI, decreased myocardial perfusion occurs because of coronary artery narrowing caused by thrombus formation subsequent to rupture of atherosclerotic plaque. In stable angina, coronary occlusion causes a brief ischemia that is treatable and reversible. In unstable angina, coronary occlusion leads to ischemia with high risk for MI. When ischemia is prolonged, MI occurs. The two types of MI are classified according to their electrographic changes—non–ST-segment elevation MI (NSTEMI) and ST-segment elevation MI (STEMI). NSTEMI indicates an infarction caused by a *nonocclusive* thrombus that *partially* interrupts perfusion of the myocardium and results in an infarction affecting only part of the myocardial wall, rather than full thickness. STEMI is caused by an *occlusive* thrombus that leads to complete *transmural* MI—an infarction of the full thickness of the myocardial wall. The majority of MIs are due to nonocclusive thrombi that cause partial wall infarctions.

After myocardial ischemia occurs, anaerobic metabolism becomes the predominant form of energy production in the affected cardiac tissue. Anaerobic metabolism yields low energy that can sustain the heart tissue only for a maximum of 20 minutes. Death of myocardial tissue (infarction) occurs as energy requirements are not met, thus underscoring the importance of acute beta blocker therapy in the management of MI to decrease cardiac workload and myocardial oxygen demand. Moreover, lactic acid, a waste product of anaerobic metabolism, is noxious to surrounding cells, further disrupting cell function.

The pharmaceutical treatment of ACS is directed primarily at dissolution of the intracoronary thrombus by antiplatelet therapy (e.g., aspirin, glycoprotein IIb/IIIa receptor antagonists), anticoagulant therapy (e.g., heparin), and relief of symptoms by antianginal (e.g., nitroglycerin, beta blockers, supplemental oxygen therapy) and analgesic (morphine sulfate) medications. After MI

The Iceberg of Myocardial Infarction

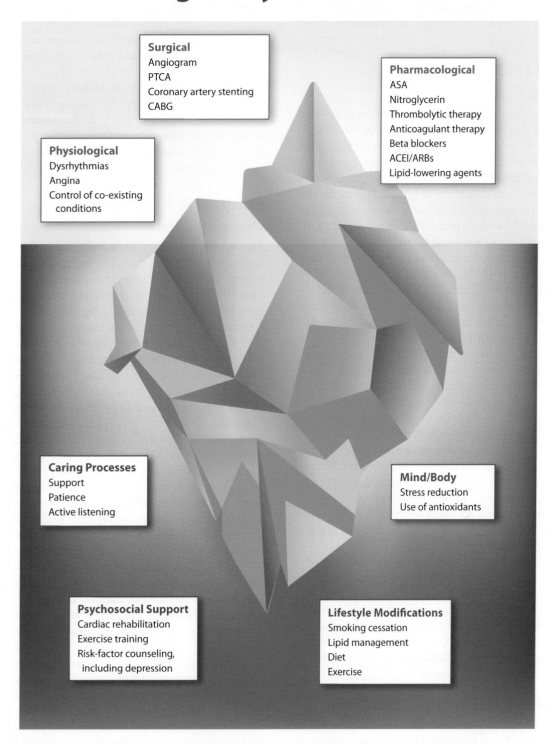

Surgical
Angiogram
PTCA
Coronary artery stenting
CABG

Pharmacological
ASA
Nitroglycerin
Thrombolytic therapy
Anticoagulant therapy
Beta blockers
ACEI/ARBs
Lipid-lowering agents

Physiological
Dysrhythmias
Angina
Control of co-existing
   conditions

Caring Processes
Support
Patience
Active listening

Mind/Body
Stress reduction
Use of antioxidants

Psychosocial Support
Cardiac rehabilitation
Exercise training
Risk-factor counseling,
   including depression

Lifestyle Modifications
Smoking cessation
Lipid management
Diet
Exercise

is confirmed, urgent evaluation for salvage of viable myocardial tissue is initiated through reperfusion treatments based on coronary angiographic studies.

An infarcted region of the myocardial wall is an area of necrosis that disrupts the conduction system and decreases the strength of the heart muscle as a mechanical pump. Arrhythmias and heart failure are common sequelae of MI. The more damage to the heart muscle, the greater the risk of heart failure. *Papillary muscle rupture* is also a common complication that results from MI. Heart valve leaflets are attached to papillary muscles via stringlike membranous attachments called chordae tendineae. Disrupted papillary muscles and ruptured chordae tendineae cause valvular dysfunction that may manifest as a heart murmur due to turbulent blood flow. MI of the left ventricle (LV) with papillary muscle rupture can cause dysfunction of the mitral valve, and mitral regurgitation is a common complication of left ventricular MI.

Clinical Presentation

Subjective

With angina, the patient will complain of chest discomfort that may be described as pressure, tightness, burning, or heaviness. The pain may radiate to the arms, chest, back, neck, jaw, or teeth. Patients frequently describe the discomfort as indigestion because it may be accompanied by nausea or vomiting. Shortness of breath and diaphoresis may also be present, either at rest or with physical activity. The patient may also be anxious, light-headed, and tachycardic. The pain may frequently occur after meals because of increased oxygen consumption during the meal, or it may be brought on by psychological stress. Rest and nitroglycerin, either sublingual (SL) or spray, may relieve the symptoms of stable angina. The patient may be in denial and will often rationalize that the symptoms are caused by indigestion or overexertion.

In acute MI, the patient often complains of angina-like chest pain lasting more than 20 minutes but occasionally waxing and waning during that period. Often, dyspnea, diaphoresis, nausea, and dizziness are also reported. Radiation of the pain to the neck, jaw, shoulder, or arm (left more often than right) is usually described. The degree of distress with these symptoms varies greatly, however, from the patient who complains of an "elephant standing on my chest" to the patient who is apologetic for seeking assistance with "just a bit of indigestion that will not clear up." In particular, women, older adults, and persons with diabetes mellitus are likely to have minimal or atypical symptoms with an acute MI.

About 15% of patients suffer a painless MI that may be detected on a future ECG or on autopsy or if the patient presents with other symptoms that prompt the clinician to question the possibility of an MI. This occurs more often in an older patient or a patient with diabetes or HTN. In this instance, the patient may complain of dyspnea, general upper abdominal pain, exacerbation of heart failure, or acute confusion.

Objective

In a patient with angina, the clinician may auscultate a transient third (S_3) or fourth (S_4) heart sound, a transient mitral regurgitant murmur, and/or a carotid arterial bruit. The patient should be asked to describe the pain in terms of its quality, location, radiation, precipitating factors, alleviating factors, and associated signs and symptoms during the attack. In addition, the patient may appear dyspneic and be diaphoretic.

In a patient with an MI, the clinician may observe pallor; cool, diaphoretic skin; crackles on auscultation; a third (S_3) or fourth (S_4) heart sound; murmurs; edema of the extremities; and possibly neck vein distention. In addition, the patient may have a low-grade fever. The presence of diaphoresis with chest pain is particularly worrisome, often indicating a significant drop in cardiac output during the episode of pain and subsequent decreased perfusion of the skin.

The cardiac exam should include inspection, palpation, and auscultation. As with any physical exam, the cardiac exam should begin with the general survey, in which the clinician begins to develop a picture of the overall health status of the patient and continues to gather diagnostic clues.

Diagnostic Reasoning

Diagnostic Tests

The best laboratory tests to rule out MI are cardiac-specific troponin I and T (cTnI and cTnT). Cardiac troponins are cardiac proteins released from dead heart muscle, and they are not detected in the blood of healthy individuals. Troponin levels rise within the first 2 to 4 hours after MI and remain elevated for 7 to 10 days.

Serum cardiac enzymes, which include the specific MB isoenzyme of serum creatine phosphokinase (CPK), are also released from necrotic heart muscle after MI. The CPKmb isoenzyme level rises within 4 to 8 hours after MI and generally returns to normal by 48 to 72 hours. The other cardiac enzymes (rarely used) are serum glutamic oxaloacetic transaminase and lactate dehydrogenase. These become elevated much later in the course of MI and are not indicators of acute MI.

A blood level of the CPKmb fraction remains elevated in the blood more briefly than cardiac troponin. Therefore, episodes of recurrent ischemic discomfort and recurrent MI are more readily diagnosed with a rise in cardiac troponins. The prolonged elevation of cardiac troponins does not allow recognition of repeat episodes of acute MI within the first few days after the initial insult. The rise in CPKmb fraction correlates better with infarct size than does troponin level. If the diagnosis of MI remains uncertain, serum cardiac biomarkers should be measured on admission, at 6 to 9 hours after admission, and again after 12 to 14 hours.

Myoglobin is a muscle protein that rises in the blood within only a few hours after MI. It is one of the earliest serum cardiac markers to rise after MI; however, it is nonspecific for cardiac muscle death and can rise with skeletal muscle injury. Blood levels return to normal within 24 hours of infarction and cannot be relied on for diagnosis of MI.

Other laboratory tests, which include complete blood count (CBC), erythrocyte sedimentation rate (ESR), serum electrolytes, blood urea nitrogen (BUN), and serum creatinine, should be drawn. Leukocytosis is a nonspecific indicator of myocardial injury. White blood cell counts often reach levels of 12,000 to 15,000/mcL.

ESR, a general indicator of inflammation, also rises after MI and remains elevated for several days.

After the patient is stabilized, echocardiography and cardiac catheterization with angiography are procedures that give clinicians significant prognostic information. Echocardiography can be done to detect wall motion abnormalities, right and left ventricular function, valvular or septal defects, and LV ejection fraction. Echocardiography is a noninvasive procedure that is easily performed in most emergency departments; however, it is not recommended as a reliable diagnostic test of MI. When the patient is assessed angiographically, coronary artery occlusion can be estimated along a scale called the Thrombolysis in Myocardial Infarction (TIMI) grading system. The TIMI scale grades coronary artery occlusion from grade 0, indicating complete occlusion, to grade 3, indicating full perfusion of the coronary artery with full normal flow.

In addition, radionuclide imaging can detect reversible ischemic regions or fixed infarcted areas. Radionuclide substances are distributed in proportion to myocardial blood flow. This type of myocardial perfusion imaging reveals a "cold spot" during the first few hours after MI. However, it cannot distinguish acute MI from the scarring of the myocardium from an MI suffered in the past.

12-Lead Electrocardiogram Although chest pain can be caused by a number of conditions, assessing for life-threatening cardiac conditions such as angina and acute MI is critical. In the emergency clinical setting, a 12-lead ECG can reveal myocardial ischemia, STEMI, NSTEMI, or arrhythmias.

An ECG should be performed promptly: The presence of an ST-segment elevation greater than 1 mm in contiguous leads usually indicates acute coronary artery occlusion, usually from thrombosis. In addition, clinically significant ST-segment elevation largely dictates reperfusion therapy. The ECG will further delineate the location of the MI and its corresponding coronary artery.

Ischemic and injured cells have an altered action potential and altered patterns of depolarization and repolarization. Infarcted cells have no action potential and cannot conduct impulses through dead tissue, which leads to changes in the ECG.

Myocardial ischemia is demonstrated by enlargement and inversion of the T wave caused by altered late repolarization. The ischemic area remains depolarized when adjacent areas have returned to the resting state. Myocardial injury is demonstrated by ST-segment changes. With epicardial injury, injured cells depolarize normally but repolarize more rapidly than do normal cells. This causes an elevation in the leads facing the areas of injury. In endocardial injury, the ST segment is more likely to be depressed (usually 1 mm or more) in the leads facing the injury. The decision to proceed with thrombolytic therapy is based in large part on the presence of ST-segment elevation in two or more ECG leads. Because of the absence of depolarization of the cells in the area of an acute MI, Q waves show up about 1 to 3 days after the infarction. Electrical impulses cannot travel through dead tissue and are deflected away, causing an abnormal Q wave. An abnormal Q wave is usually 0.04 seconds wide and 25% or greater in depth than the R wave is tall. Figure 10.1 shows the typical ECG changes seen with cardiac damage.

At times, myocardial perfusion halts temporarily, then is reestablished in a relatively short period of time. This may be the result of vessel spasm or sudden drop

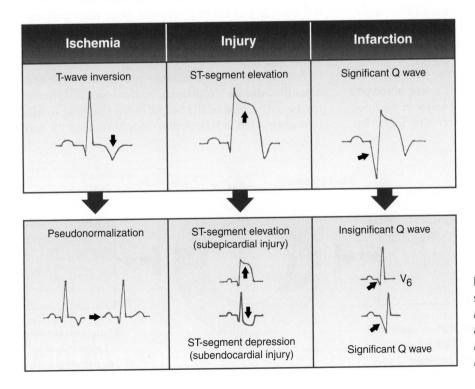

Figure 10.1 Typical ECG changes seen with cardiac damage. *(Source: Lipman, B, and Cascio, T. ECG assessment and intervention. FA Davis, Philadelphia, 1994. Reprinted with permission.)*

in BP, such as with severe blood or fluid loss. In this situation, a small portion of subendocardial tissue is damaged, yet adjoining myocardial tissue remains viable. As a result, ECG changes are present but differ significantly from those in a classic transmural MI. Q waves do not form because electrically active tissue backs up the area of infarction. Because tissue injury, ischemia, and infarction are subendocardial rather than oriented toward the epicardium, as in transmural MI, injury pattern is reflected in ST-segment depression. The ECG changes are transient—present only during the acute event and during tissue healing. Thus, if not found during the acute presentation, a non–Q wave MI may never be diagnosed. The terms Q–wave and non–Q wave MI are now referred to as NSTEMI or STEMI (as previously defined). There may be a temptation to think of a non–Q wave MI/non–STEMI as a "small heart attack" with limited long-term sequelae. These patients have well-demonstrated risk for future MI and other cardiac events, particularly during the next 3 to 6 months. The majority of patients with non–Q wave MIs are older adults (aged 70 or older) with a history of prior MI and congestive heart failure (CHF). Figure 10.2 illustrates the difference between NSTEMI and STEMI ECG changes.

The 12-lead ECG presents 12 leads, or "views," of the heart, to detect myocardial damage. Leads I, II, and III are the three standard (bipolar) leads. Leads aV_R, aV_L, and aV_F are augmented or unipolar leads; the chest or precordial leads (V_1 to V_6) view the heart in a horizontal plane. Figure 10.3 shows the normal ECG wave configuration of a normal 12-lead ECG.

By identifying the leads that contain the ECG changes, the location of the myocardial damage and its corresponding coronary artery can be determined (Table 10.7). However, the identification of these abnormal views should be the last step in interpreting a 12-lead ECG. If the clinician is not systematic in an interpretation approach, errors can be made. For instance, if the presence of a left bundle branch block (LBBB) is not observed, these changes may be interpreted as Q-waves in the inferior leads or ST elevation in the precordial leads. An

LBBB prevents a true look at the area because the normal path of depolarization is blocked and does not directly travel down the normal conduction pathway. This results in a distorted view, and the typical LBBB ECG changes are observed instead. Therefore, after determining the rate and rhythm of the ECG, observing for LBBB is the second step. However, the clinician needs to keep in mind that an LBBB could result from the acute ischemic process of an MI. If this is a new ECG change, it should be noted and incorporated into the clinical picture.

The 12-lead ECG can also provide information about axis deviation, which is the third step in systematic interpretation. Electrical axis is, for all practical purposes, synonymous with the wave of myocardial depolarization. Healthy myocardial tissue depolarizes in a predictable pattern, thus recording in the ECG a predictable electrical axis. The normal wave of depolarization travels down the heart and to the left. This normal axis shows as a positive QRS complex in lead I and lead aV_F. This is because the net ventricular forces travel toward the pole of lead I and down toward the pole of lead aV_F.

With cardiac disease, the wave of depolarization swings away from areas of damage or necrosis, creating axis deviation, or a change from the norm. When the axis is shifted to the left, the QRS complex is positive in lead I and negative in lead aV_F. Left axis deviation is subdivided into normal left axis deviation (NLAD) and abnormal left axis deviation (ALAD). NLAD is often seen in the presence of LVH. ALAD is seen in a block of the anterosuperior division of the left bundle branch, often referred to as a left anterior fascicular block (LAFB). ALAD is also seen in Q-wave inferior-wall MI and a right apical pacemaker. Right axis deviation (RAD) is seen in a block of the posterior inferior division of the left bundle block, often referred to as a left posterior fascicular block (LPFB). RAD is also caused by an extensive Q-wave lateral-wall MI and may be seen in right ventricular hypertrophy (RVH).

Axis deviation is occasionally present in the absence of cardiac disease. In pregnancy, the heart is shifted in the cavity because of the height of the diaphragm. This may cause a left axis deviation. In addition, adults with

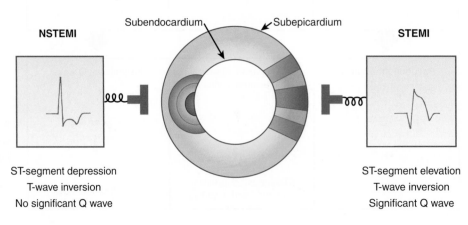

NSTEMI

ST-segment depression

T-wave inversion

No significant Q wave

Subendocardium · Subepicardium

STEMI

ST-segment elevation

T-wave inversion

Significant Q wave

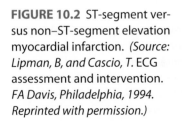

FIGURE 10.2 ST-segment versus non–ST-segment elevation myocardial infarction. *(Source: Lipman, B, and Cascio, T. ECG assessment and intervention. FA Davis, Philadelphia, 1994. Reprinted with permission.)*

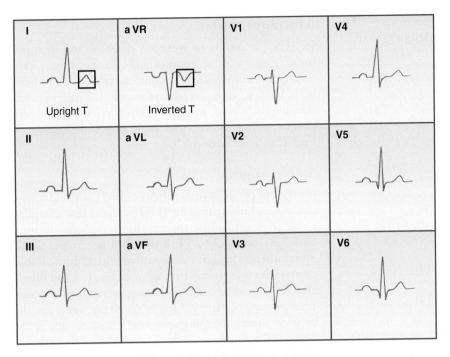

FIGURE 10.3 The normal 12-lead ECG. *(Source: Lipman, B, and Cascio, T. ECG assessment and intervention. FA Davis, Philadelphia, 1994. Reprinted with permission.)*

Table 10.7 Location of Myocardial Infarction

Location of MI	Leads	Reciprocal Changes	Coronary Artery Affected
Anterior	V_2–V_4	II, III, aV$_F$	Left anterior descending (LAD)
Anteroseptal	V_1–V_3	None	LAD
Anterolateral	I, aV$_L$, V_4–V_6	II, III, aV$_F$	LAD, left circumflex
Inferior	II, III, aV$_F$	I, aV$_L$	Right coronary artery (RCA) in 80%–90%, left coronary artery (LCA) in 10%–20%
Posterior	V_1–V_3	R wave greater than S wave, depressed ST segment, elevated T wave	RCA, left circumflex
Lateral	I, aV$_L$, V_5–V_6	V_1–V_2	Left circumflex

abdominal obesity may demonstrate left axis deviation. In infants and children and tall, thin adults right axis deviation is normal. Advanced Assessment 10.2 presents a quick quadrant method for determining axis deviation.

The 12-lead ECG may also provide information about heart chamber enlargement. Chamber enlargement, or hypertrophy, is usually a consequence of obstruction of blood flow out of the affected area of the heart. For example, left atrial hypertrophy is a common consequence of mitral valve stenosis because the atrium must generate excessive pressure, thereby becoming enlarged, as a result of forcing open a stiff, diseased valve. The following are the typical ECG findings associated with chamber enlargement:

1. Right atrial hypertrophy (RAH), also known as P pulmonale
   • Peaked P wave in leads II, III, aV$_F$, V_1
   • P wave more than 2.5 mm in leads II, III, aV$_F$

2. Left atrial hypertrophy (LAH), also known as P mitrale
   • Notched P wave more than 0.10 seconds in leads II, III, aV$_F$
   • Prominent negative P terminal in V_1 (more than 1:1)

3. RVH
   • Reversal of R wave progression in the precordial leads
   • Although not routinely seen, RVH may be seen in patients with chronic obstructive pulmonary disease (COPD)

4. Left ventricular hypertrophy (LVH), which uses the Estes Scoring System:
   • 3 points for any or all of the following: voltage of 25 mm or more (S wave in V_1 or V_2); R wave in V_5 or V_6 and/or voltage of 20 mm or more (R or S wave in leads I, II, III, aV$_F$, aV$_L$)
   • 1 point for secondary ST-segment T-wave changes if the patient is taking digitalis

Advanced Assessment 10.2   Assessing Axis Deviation

The quadrant method is a rapid, accurate way of assessing electrocardiogram (ECG) electrical axis. Although it does not yield an exact degree measurement, such as obtained when using an ECG ruler, this method can be done without the use of special equipment. When using the quadrant method, do the following:

• Examine leads I and aV$_F$ for the presence of a positive or negative QRS complex.
• Determine the results as follows:

   Normal axis: Positive complex (tall R wave) in leads I and aV$_F$
   Left axis deviation: Positive complex (tall R wave) in lead I; negative complex in aV$_F$
   Right axis deviation: Negative complex in lead I, and positive complex (R wave) in aV$_F$
   Extreme right axis deviation: Negative complex in lead I and aV$_F$

• 3 points for secondary ST-segment T-wave changes if the patient is not taking digitalis
• 3 points for an abnormal P terminal in V$_1$
• 2 points for left axis deviation
• 1 point for an RS interval of more than 0.09 seconds
• 1 point for ventricular activating time in V$_5$; 0.05 seconds or more in V$_6$

If the patient has 4 points, there is the probability of LVH; 5 points is a strong indication of LVH.

The final step in interpretation is identifying the leads that contain ECG changes and assessing for myocardial damage. If the determination of an LBBB has not been made before this last step, the interpretation will be flawed. However, even if the clinician is unable to accurately read the 12-lead ECG due to an LBBB, the clinical context of the situation needs to be noted and appropriate interventions implemented. If an acute STEMI is suspected, additional diagnostics should be obtained and may include left heart catheterization.

Differential Diagnosis

Differential diagnoses for angina may include an acute MI, esophagitis, esophageal spasm, peptic ulcer, gastritis, cholecystitis, costochondritis, pericarditis, aortic dissection, pulmonary embolus (PE), pulmonary HTN, pneumothorax, anxiety, and panic disorders.

Differential diagnoses for MI include pericarditis, myocarditis, acute aortic dissection, pneumothorax, PE, acute cholecystitis, esophageal spasm, unstable angina, biliary tract disease, and panic attack.

Management

In ACS, the goal is to promptly diagnose and treat the underlying condition appropriately. In the primary-care setting, the clinician can attempt to stabilize the patient with ASA and nitroglycerin. However, the patient experiencing ACS needs to be transferred to a hospital emergency medical setting, preferably one with access to a cardiac catheterization lab.

Stable Angina

If a patient presents with ischemic chest pain, and nitroglycerin and rest relieve the chest pain, the result implies stable angina. Chronic anginal pain is typically of short duration, usually 3 to 5 minutes, but it may last up to 30 minutes or longer. For a patient with chronic stable angina who is currently having an attack, rest and nitroglycerin should be ordered. Nitroglycerin may be given as an SL tablet or spray. One tablet or one spray should be used under the tongue every 5 minutes for three doses. If the pain has not been relieved after three doses, the local emergency medical services system should be called and the patient transported immediately to the emergency department.

After the patient's chest pain has been relieved, a beta blocker and/or long-acting nitrate may be prescribed. Beta blockers decrease myocardial oxygen demand by interfering with the effects of the sympathetic nervous system on the beta-1 receptors in the heart. Long-acting nitrates, topical or oral, may be added to the beta blocker regimen to increase myocardial oxygen supply by coronary artery vasodilation. Many beta blockers may be used such as atenolol, metoprolol, nadolol, or propranolol.

Long-acting nitrates, topical or oral, may include the nitroglycerin transdermal patch or paste in varying strengths. The patch should be in place for 12 hours and removed for 12 hours to prevent intolerance. At present the use of hydralazine is being looked at as a way to inhibit nitroglycerin paste intolerance. Isosorbide dinitrate is another good long-acting nitrate that is taken orally. Long-acting nitrates may be taken daily as prophylaxis to prevent recurrent angina.

All patients with diagnosed angina should be placed on daily aspirin therapy to help prevent coronary thrombosis. Aspirin (ASA) 81 to 325 mg daily may be taken (use coated ASA if gastric problems exist). Ticlopidine with food may be ordered for patients who are allergic to aspirin or those with a history of gastrointestinal bleeding.

Unstable Angina

With unstable angina, the goal is to diagnose the underlying condition and treat appropriately. If rest and nitroglycerin do not relieve the chest discomfort, the patient must be immediately transported by ambulance to the emergency department for further evaluation. Treatment Flowchart 10.1 presents the management of unstable angina.

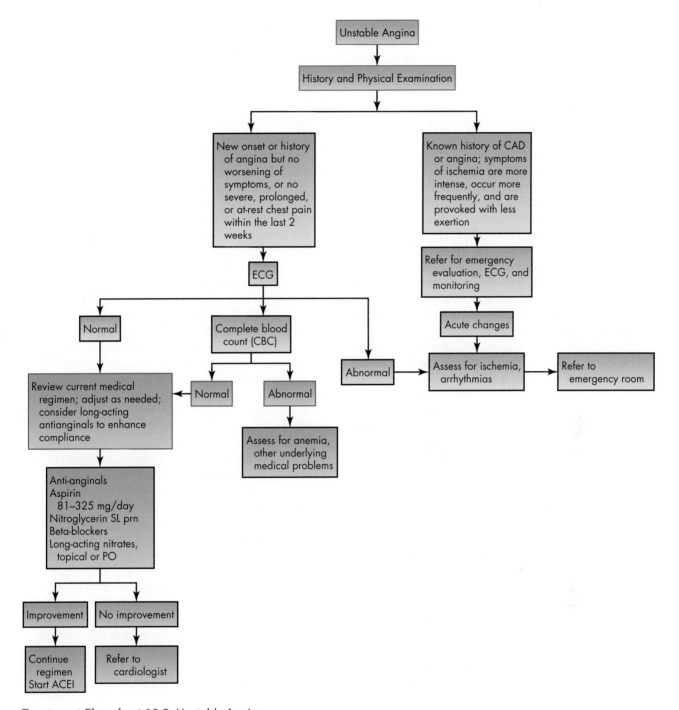

Treatment Flowchart 10.2 Unstable Angina

Variant (Prinzmetal's) Angina

Prinzmetal's angina is an atypical form of angina pectoris that occurs as a result of vasospasm of otherwise normal coronary arteries. Pain is experienced at rest, and an ECG, when taken during the attack, will indicate ST-segment elevation rather than depression. This ECG change will abate when the patient is treated with nitroglycerin (see previous section) and drugs that influence calcium metabolism. A calcium channel blocker such as verapamil HCl may be used in treatment.

Myocardial Infarction

The goal of management is to salvage the ischemic myocardium before it becomes necrotic by reperfusing the area as soon as possible. After that, the goal becomes directed at preventing future attacks.

If an MI is suspected at the time of a clinical visit, a 12-lead ECG should be done promptly. Immediate interventions of rest, aspirin, and nitroglycerin administration should be implemented. Nitroglycerin can be administered sublingually as a tablet or spray. If relief is not achieved within 2 to 3 minutes after the initial dose of nitroglycerin, a second or third dose can be given at 5-minute intervals for a total of three doses. One or more inches of nitroglycerin gel (Nitropaste) may also be used to vasodilate and lower BP, because this topical form of nitroglycerin may be easily removed by wiping off the skin to stop its effects. Similarly, in an advanced clinical setting, an adjustable IV nitroglycerin drip may be used if appropriate nursing and medical supervision is available. A 162- to 325-mg aspirin tablet can also be administered in the ambulatory clinical setting. Aspirin exerts an antiplatelet effect, and nitroglycerin decreases preload and coronary spasm, thus contributing to the overall beneficial effect in an acute MI. The patient should initially chew and swallow one aspirin. The 325-mg dosage should not be exceeded, because that will negate the platelet effect. This initiation of thrombolytic therapy given at the time of onset (within 70 minutes) of the symptoms, before hospitalization, has lowered the mortality rate of patients.

The patient should then be transferred to an emergency medical setting. The clinician should begin an IV, provide oxygen, and monitor the patient until the emergency medical system can be activated. Once the patient is stabilized, emergency care clinicians can determine if the patient is a candidate for reperfusion treatment with thrombolytic agents or primary percutaneous coronary intervention (PCI). They should be used only for patients with acute MI associated with STEMI or with LBBB with suspected acute MI. Thrombolytic agents, such as alteplase (recombinant tissue plasminogen activator [tPA]), reteplase (rPA), or tenecteplase (TNK), are most effective when administered early in the course of an MI. The first thrombolytic agent, streptokinase, is not commonly used because it is a non–fibrin-specific agent. For the best therapeutic effect, thrombolytics should be administered within the first 3 hours (ideally 30 minutes) of presentation of symptoms of MI. Studies have shown that thrombolytic therapy can be of benefit up to 12 hours after initial presentation of symptoms of MI. Alternatively, thrombolytic therapy can be combined with antiplatelet agents known as glycoprotein IIb/IIIa inhibitors.

Cardiac catheterization with angiography can decipher whether or not the patient is a candidate for reperfusion therapy, percutaneous transluminal coronary angioplasty (PTCA), coronary artery stenting, or coronary artery bypass grafting. Immediate coronary angiography and primary PCI, which includes stenting of the infarct-related artery, have been shown to be more effective than thrombolysis if done within 90 minutes for STEMI. This 90-minute time frame is referred to as "door to balloon" time and is managed only in specialized centers. Stenting may be done in conjunction with administrations of the platelet glycoprotein IIb/IIIa antagonist abciximab in patients with acute MI.

The American Heart Association (AHA) has published guidelines for the management of patients with acute MI.

Developed from consensus of nursing and medical experts and evidence-based health care, the AHA recommends the following for a person with suspected MI:

- Community systems, including primary-care providers, should work together to ensure prompt initial care of the patient with suspected MI. Once the patient enters care in the emergency department, initial evaluation should occur within 10 minutes.
- The following care should be provided immediately: Administration of oxygen via nasal prongs; sublingual nitroglycerin unless SBP is less than 90 mm Hg and heart rate is less than 50 or more than 100 beats per minute; adequate analgesia with morphine sulfate or meperidine; and aspirin (ASA) 162 to 325 mg PO (Level II; O'Gara et al, 2013). The ASA should be administered regardless of whether or not thrombolytic therapy is being considered. Chewable ASA has a more rapid effect and is preferred. In addition, some clinicians will give a loading dose of clopidogrel (300–600 mg). Nitroglycerin should not be given for the patient who has received phosphodiesterase inhibitor therapy in the prior 24 hours.
- Clinically significant ST-segment elevation largely dictates reperfusion therapy by use of thrombolytic therapy or primary PTCA. When thrombolysis is used, heparin is usually given for 48 hours to ensure continued vessel patency. A viable alternative to unfractionated heparin (if no renal or hepatic impairment is present) is a low molecular weight heparin such as enoxaparin sodium (Lovenox).
- If LBBB is present on ECG and the clinical scenario is consistent with acute MI, the same level of care should be offered. Patients with presentations suggestive of MI but without ST-segment changes should not receive thrombolysis, because it may cause more harm.
- The patient should be hospitalized and placed on continuous ECG monitoring for rhythm disturbances. Serial 12-lead ECGs should be obtained and results correlated with clinical measures of myocardial necrosis such as creatine kinase (CK) or CPK isoenzymes and troponin T or I.
- Aspirin therapy should be continued; the use of heparin should also be considered in the presence of a large anterior MI or LV mural thrombus because of increased risk of embolic stroke. Initially, the dosage for aspirin should be 325 mg/day, with anywhere from 81 to 325 mg given once per day after discharge ad infinitum.
- If no contraindications are present, Core Measures should be implemented. Core Measures as put forth by the Joint Commission include the following: aspirin on arrival and discharge, angiotensin-converting enzyme (ACE) inhibitor or angiotensin receptor blocker (ARB) for left ventricular systolic dysfunction (LVSD) beta blocker therapy as tolerated, and statins

prescribed as indicated on discharge. Beta blocker therapy and ACE inhibitor therapy should be initiated promptly because the use of these products is associated with reduced mortality and morbidity after MI. Beta blocker therapy should be continued indefinitely, with ACE inhibitor use being most appropriate for patients with LV dysfunction characterized by systolic ejection fraction less than 40% or in the presence of heart failure. Beta blockers exert their beneficial effect in patients with an MI by reducing myocardial oxygen demand, reducing myocardial wall stress, and antagonizing the arrhythmogenic effects of catecholamines. ACE inhibitors reduce the progressive ventricular dilation and remodeling after an MI, and in some studies have been shown to reduce myocardial reinfarction (for an unknown reason). ACE inhibitors also reduce the incidence of heart failure, thus reducing mortality in patients with large myocardial infarcts and in patients with left ventricular dysfunction.

- Ongoing care includes a goal of reducing LDL cholesterol to less than 100 mg/dL using diet, exercise, and, if necessary, drug therapy. This is in keeping with an overall plan to reduce or eliminate all cardiac risk factors, including inactivity, tobacco use, and obesity.
- Coronary artery bypass surgery is not usually done during an evolving MI unless the patient has a serious complication such as acute severe mitral regurgitation with or without papillary muscle rupture, acute septal rupture, or a free wall rupture that might be associated with a pseudoaneurysm, refractory cardiogenic shock, or recurrent severe ischemia postinfarction that cannot be managed with drugs and PTCA.

Follow-up and Referral

As previously stated, patients with unstable angina should be referred to the emergency department and a cardiologist for a complete evaluation. Patients with stable angina may be managed by the clinician with either beta blockers and/or long-acting nitrates with nitrolingual tablets or spray as needed for emergency and prophylactic use. Patients should be followed every 3 months to determine their adherence to risk factor modification strategies. From the instant the clinician suspects a patient is experiencing an acute MI, the patient must be immediately transported to the emergency department and be evaluated by a cardiologist. The clinician may follow the patient after hospitalization. When the cardiologist discharges the patient from his or her care, the clinician may become involved in the follow-up care. The cardiologist should have already referred the patient to a cardiac rehabilitation program before discharge. The clinician should take an active role in encouraging the patient to adhere to the prescribed program.

On discharge, a review of the aforementioned Core Measures should be implemented. In addition to a beta blocker (and, if indicated, an ACE inhibitor), the patient should be prescribed nitroglycerin (SL tablet or spray) with

instructions on when to take it and how to store it. The patient should also be taking a daily enteric-coated aspirin of at least 81 mg, as well as a statin cholesterol-lowering drug. For patients with residual myocardial ischemia or with significant left ventricular dysfunction, a longer-acting nitrate such as isosorbide (Isordil) should also be considered. Research has shown that with the addition of a diuretic, there has been a decrease in mortality.

Patient Education

Patients should be taught about their medications, usage, adverse effects, and how to take nitroglycerin prophylactically. In addition, the clinician should stress that nitroglycerin tablets should remain in the light-resistant bottle in which they are packaged and not be put in another pill box or remain in areas that are or could become warm and humid. Once opened, the bottle must be dated and discarded after 6 months.

The clinician should assist the patient to reduce CAD risk factors and factors that exacerbate angina. The patient should be placed on a low-fat diet, with minimal calories if weight reduction is necessary. Coexisting conditions such as HTN, anemia, hyperthyroidism, and CHF should be managed aggressively. The clinician should encourage the patient to enter a cardiac rehabilitation program of safe exercise and risk-factor modification. The clinician should also encourage the patient to adhere to activity limitations determined by exercise tolerance testing and to stop smoking and/or using other tobacco products. Patients should be taught to use nitroglycerin prophylactically before any stressful physical activity such as sexual intercourse. Anxiety and fear often accompany anginal attacks because the patient may fear the onset of an MI. Patients and their families should be allowed to express their fears and concerns and should be collaborative partners in necessary lifestyle changes. As with all cardiac conditions, family members should learn cardiopulmonary resuscitation.

Patient teaching after the patient has experienced an acute MI involves aggressive risk factor modification to prevent a recurrence. Lifestyle modifications should be stressed as stated in Table 10.2. Patients should be referred for cardiac rehabilitation to improve exercise tolerance, cardiac symptoms, blood lipid levels, and psychosocial well-being. Exercise training through cardiac rehabilitation increases the arterial oxygen saturation and improves the oxygen uptake by the peripheral tissues, thereby improving the efficiency of oxygen transport and use by the peripheral tissues, resulting in a decrease in the cardiac output required to perform exercises.

There are three phases of cardiac rehabilitation: Phase I begins in the early in-hospital postinfarct phase with range-of-motion exercises progressing to an increase in the activities of daily living. Phase II is a structured outpatient program of exercise training and risk-factor counseling and education. Phase III establishes a lifelong pattern of regular aerobic exercise and further modification of risk factors; it is usually undertaken in a community wellness center. The Patient's Voice 10.1 shares one person's experience of having an MI.

At every visit to the office, the patient should be educated about risk-factor modification, such as smoking cessation, lipid management, control of coexisting conditions such as diabetes mellitus and HTN, stress reduction, and the use of antioxidants.

■ HEART FAILURE

Heart failure is a condition in which cardiac output is insufficient to meet the body's demands. Each patient presents differently because there are various causes and stages of heart failure. The patient with left ventricular failure (LVF) presents with symptoms of pulmonary origin due to a backup of hydrostatic pressure into the pulmonary arterial system. Right ventricular failure symptoms occur as a result of hydrostatic pressure buildup in the venous system. Clinical manifestations of systemic edema occur with right ventricular failure. Biventricular heart failure can cause a combination of these clinical manifestations. Clinicians use the term *heart failure* to describe all types of conditions in which cardiac supply is less than metabolic demand. Previously patients with heart failure were generally hospitalized, but many now may be managed at home. Early identification of patients at risk for heart failure and patient education is key, not only for the prevention of the disease but also for the quality of life of these patients.

Epidemiology and Causes

Heart failure, unlike other cardiac disorders, has been increasing in incidence and prevalence, especially in the

---

The Patient's Voice 10.1
Myocardial Infarction

It was 4:30 A.M. . . . Damn, what a case of indigestion . . . . Have to get to the golf course. . . . It's the first day of the seniors' tournament, and employees will be there early. Driving to work, the indigestion seemed to be subsiding. Arrived at work and started getting things organized for the day's events. Started pulling kegs of beer to be placed around the course when the pain started coming back and I got nauseated. Pain getting worse now. Now it's starting to feel like someone is sitting on my chest. Someone called the paramedics. I'm in the ambulance now. I'm sweating, feeling clammy, . . . chest pain continues. We get to the hospital. The people there ask if I'm allergic to anything. Pain is getting worse. They're sticking tubes and needles in me. A doctor tells me I'm having a heart attack . . . and not to worry, they have it all under control. Not worry—what does he think! Then he tells me he's going to give me a clot-busting drug. I'm trying to listen, but I really don't understand what's going on. The chest pain is starting to go away. I'm only 40 . . . I can't be having a heart attack! This isn't happening to me!

---

older adult population. The Centers for Disease Control and Prevention estimates that 5.7 million people in the United States suffer from heart failure, with more than 400,000 new cases each year. The incidence is increasing because of the use of newer medications and technologies that have increased survival at the expense of increased morbidity. Heart failure is the most common discharge diagnosis in patients older than age 65; it is diagnosed in 10% of the population by the time they reach age 75 years. The annual mortality rate is as high as 60%, and the 5-year survival rate for patients with severe heart failure is about 50%. Approximately 280,000 patients each year die of heart failure. The cost for care and evaluation of patients with heart failure exceeds $34.4 billion in resources each year.

Heart failure may occur acutely, or it may occur after a cardiac abnormality has been present for years, when an increased demand is placed on a heart in an already compensated state and there is further deterioration. It is critical for the clinician to identify not only the underlying cause of heart disease but also the precipitating cause of the heart failure. Prompt treatment and elimination of precipitating causes may save the patient's life. Table 10.8 presents causes of heart failure and their effects on the heart. Nursing Research–Based Practice Box 10.2 shares some reasons why elders delay responding to heart failure symptoms.

Ongoing research is being conducted to explore the neurohormonal hypothesis of heart failure. This research began with the discovery that angiotensin-converting enzyme (ACE) inhibitors and possibly beta blockers were better in reducing mortality than potent afterload-reducing drugs. In the neurohormonal model, active molecules that are released in heart failure are toxic to the myocardium. Currently, noradrenaline, angiotensin, vasopressin, endothelin, and tumor necrosis factor–alpha are being studied for their relationship to heart failure. Clearly, heart failure involves a number of complex physiological changes that are progressive. Because of the increasing incidence of heart failure, new theories are being generated to explain the elusiveness of this disease process to intervention and cure.

Pathophysiology

Heart failure is a constellation of clinical manifestations that result from the heart's inability to pump adequate amounts of blood to meet the demands of peripheral body tissues. It can result from a dysfunctional ventricle that is unable to eject an adequate amount of blood (*systolic dysfunction*) or from the inability of the ventricle to fill with a sufficient amount of blood (*diastolic dysfunction*). There are numerous etiologies of heart failure; however, ischemic heart disease and long-standing hypertension (HTN) are common underlying causes. Ischemic heart disease causes diminished coronary perfusion of the myocardium, which weakens strength of contractility of the ventricles. HTN creates excess mechanical stress on the ventricles, resulting

Table 10.8   Precipitating Causes of Heart Failure

Precipitating Causes	Effect on the Heart
Infection	Increases demand on the heart secondary to fever, tachycardia, hypoxemia, and increased metabolic demands.
Anemia	Increased cardiac rate to meet peripheral oxygen demands leads to increased cardiac demand.
Pulmonary edema	Increased pulmonary arterial pressure leads to increased right ventricular afterload.
Pregnancy, thyrotoxicosis arrhythmias	Adequate tissue perfusion in these conditions requires increased cardiac output. Tachyarrhythmias decrease diastole and lead to cardiac ischemia. Loss of "atrial kick" leads to increased atrial pressures. Abnormal intraventricular conduction can lead to decreased cardiac output, which will lead to further attempts to compensate. Any arrhythmia that alters the formula: cardiac output = heart rate × stroke volume has the potential to increase demands on an already decompensated heart.
Rheumatic heart disease and other forms of myocarditis	Alterations in cardiac output increase cardiac demand secondary to infectious or inflammatory processes.
Infective endocarditis; physical dietary, environmental, and emotional excesses	Valvular damage, fever, and inflammatory processes increase cardiac demand. Electrolyte disturbances, alteration in medication regimen, excessive heat or humidity, overexertion.
Systemic HTN	Sudden elevation of arterial pressure leads to increased systemic vascular resistance and increased cardiac workload.
MI	May lead to impaired ventricular function.

Nursing Research–Based Practice 10.2

Jurgens, CY, et al. Why do elders delay responding to heart failure symptoms? *Nurs Res* 58(4):274–282, 2009.

Elders with heart failure (HF) are at risk for frequent hospitalizations for symptom management. Repeated admissions are partly related to delay in responding to HF symptoms. The purpose of this study was to describe contextual factors such as prior illness experiences and social/emotional factors related to symptom recognition and response among elders hospitalized with decompensated HF. Seventy-seven patients completed several questionnaires. Median duration of early symptoms of HF decompensation was 5 to 7 days, but dyspnea duration ranged from 30 minutes to 90 days before action was taken. Longer dyspnea duration was associated with higher physical symptom distress. Sensing and attributing meaning to early symptoms of HF decompensation were problematic. The physical symptom experience and the cognitive and emotional response to HF symptoms were inadequate for timely care seeking for most of this older age sample.

in the structural change of hypertrophy and eventual left ventricular dilation. Factors that increase risk of heart failure include obesity, valvular disorders, coronary artery disease (CAD), anemia, diabetes mellitus, chronic renal insufficiency, myocarditis, dysrhythmias, thyrotoxicosis, pulmonary embolism (PE), sleep apnea, alcohol abuse, substance abuse, and chemotherapeutics. There are also differences in susceptibility to heart failure associated with gender, race, and genetic background.

Regardless of etiology, heart failure provokes hemodynamic changes, neurohormonal stimulation, vasoactive substance secretion, and cardiac structural alterations (myocardial remodeling)—all of which have systemic consequences. Heart failure may be described as *systolic* versus *diastolic* dysfunction, *right-sided heart failure* versus *left-sided heart failure*, *right ventricular* versus *left ventricular failure*, or *forward* versus *backward failure*. These contrasting terms are descriptions that illustrate the different pathophysiological mechanisms of heart failure for academic purposes. However, clinically, most patients with heart failure exhibit a combined clinical presentation of the preceding descriptions.

The terms *systolic dysfunction* or *forward failure* describe the same process in heart failure. In *systolic dysfunction* and/or *forward failure*, the diminished ejection of blood from a weakened ventricle sets off a detrimental cascade of events. The weakened ventricle cannot pump sufficient blood volume forward into the arterial system, which results in decreased cardiac output and hypoperfusion of organs. Hypoperfusion of the arteries and kidney stimulate a *neurohormonal response*, which attempts to increase circulation. Blood pressure (BP) drops in the hypoperfused arteries, and this drop is sensed by baroreceptors, pressure sensors within arterial walls. Baroreceptors stimulate the *sympathetic nervous system* to constrict the arteries in efforts to raise BP. Hypoperfusion of the kidneys stimulates renin, which provokes the *renin-angiotensin-aldosterone cascade.* Renin circulates in the bloodstream, and when it reaches the liver, angiotensinogen is released. Angiotensinogen circulates, and when it reaches the lungs, this proenzyme is converted to angiotensin I. Within the lungs, a key reaction occurs; angiotensin I is converted to angiotensin II by ACE.

Angiotensin II acts in various ways to raise BP further and increase blood volume. Angiotensin II is a potent vasoconstrictor that directly incites peripheral arterial vasoconstriction. It also stimulates the adrenal gland to secrete aldosterone, a hormone that acts at the nephron to increase sodium and water reabsorption into the bloodstream and to excrete potassium. Angiotensin II also directly provokes genetic changes within cardiac myocytes to promote hypertrophic remodeling. Increased BP and blood volume, increased peripheral vascular resistance, and myocardial hypertrophy are the net results of sympathetic stimulation and activation of the renin-angiotensin-aldosterone cascade. These effects, although compensatory mechanisms, raise blood volume and peripheral resistance, which increase workload on the weakened heart pump. As the ventricle endures greater workload, further systolic dysfunction occurs, and the neurohormonal mechanism is cyclically activated. This cycle increases blood volume and leads to fluid overload and further deterioration of systolic function.

Diastolic dysfunction or *backward failure* describes an abnormality of filling, distensibility, or relaxation of the ventricles. There is elevated filling pressure in the left and/or right ventricle, which causes backward buildup of hydrostatic pressure into the atria. In left ventricular diastolic dysfunction or backward failure, there is a backup of hydrostatic pressure into the left atrium and, in turn, the pulmonary venous system, which results in the extravasation of fluid into the pulmonary interstitium. If hydrostatic pressure builds to high levels, pulmonary capillary wedge pressure increases; high amounts of fluid build in the pulmonary interstitial spaces, which is called *pulmonary edema.* Clinical manifestations of fluid in the pulmonary interstitium are dyspnea, cough, orthopnea, paroxysmal nocturnal dyspnea, and crackles heard on auscultation of the lungs. The classic sign of pulmonary edema is *pink, frothy sputum. Orthopnea* is a term that describes the inability of the patient to breathe comfortably while lying supine. As a patient endures diastolic dysfunction or backward failure, the backup of pulmonary fluid in the interstitial spaces creates breathing difficulty. Patients breathe easier with the head of the bed elevated because this position disperses fluid downward into the lung bases. Patients often report needing two or three pillows to breathe comfortably,

termed *two-or-three-pillow orthopnea.* Frequently patients report awakening in the middle of the night feeling breathless or awakening due to a "nightmare." This nighttime hypoxia due to fluid accumulation in the pulmonary tissues is *paroxysmal nocturnal dyspnea* (PND).

Left-sided heart failure or *left ventricular failure* (LVF) is the most common type of heart failure. Most often the left ventricle (LV) becomes dysfunctional due to long-standing hypertension. Systemic hypertension increases resistance against the LV, thereby increasing workload. This leads to left ventricular hypertrophy, and eventually the LV decompensates into failure. In addition, the LV is vulnerable to ischemic insults due to coronary artery disease and may endure MI. One of the most common sites of arteriosclerosis is the left anterior descending artery, a branch of the left main coronary artery, a major supplier of the LV. Repeated ischemic episodes can lead to weakening of the LV with eventual failure. LVF can occur as systolic dysfunction (forward failure) and/or diastolic dysfunction (backward failure) as described previously. The classic clinical presentation of LVF involves the pulmonary signs and symptoms of exertional dyspnea, cough, orthopnea, PND, crackles heard on auscultation, and the hemodynamic finding of elevated pulmonary capillary wedge pressure. These symptoms are a result of the buildup of hydrostatic pressure backward into the pulmonary vasculature due to a failing LV. Ejection fraction (EF) is decreased in LV systolic dysfunction to less than 50% of total ventricular volume (normal EF ranging from 55%–70%). In contrast, in diastolic dysfunction, EF may be normal or even increased to greater than 70%, representing the need for the LV to eject a larger proportion of its total blood volume during systole to compensate for reduced diastolic filling.

Right-sided heart failure or *right ventricular failure* most commonly occurs as a result of LVF. The same cardiac muscle comprises both right and left ventricles, which endure biochemical and hemodynamic stresses during heart failure. Therefore, in the clinical setting, often manifestations of right- and left-sided heart failure appear together. The right ventricle (RV) can undergo systolic dysfunction (forward failure) and/or diastolic failure (backward failure) in the same manner as the LV. In right-sided heart failure, the classic signs and symptoms are due to backup of hydrostatic pressure into the venous system. Venous congestion of the superior vena cava is reflected in the classic sign of jugular venous distention. Venous congestion of the inferior vena cava is reflected in the gastrointestinal system as hepatomegaly, splenomegaly, and peritoneal edema *(ascites).* Depending on the position of the patient, peripheral edema is apparent as either sacral edema or ankle edema.

Isolated right ventricular failure can also occur due to pulmonary disease. The term *cor pulmonale* is used to describe right-sided heart failure, which is a result of a pathological pulmonary process, such as pulmonary fibrosis, recurrent pulmonary emboli, or other phenomena leading to pulmonary hypertension due to arterial vasoconstriction in the pulmonary vascular bed. Chronic hypoxia is a common cause of pulmonary arterial vasoconstriction. The high pulmonary arterial pressure leads to increased resistance against the RV. The RV hypertrophies in response to the increased workload initially. However, eventually the hypertrophic RV decompensates from the excess workload, leading to right ventricular failure. This syndrome is then called *cor pulmonale.*

The most common cause of right-sided heart failure, however, is initial left-sided heart failure. In this case, right-sided heart failure does not occur in isolation, but rather results from a failure of forward cardiac output. This leads to vascular congestion in the pulmonary arterial bed with increased capillary wedge pressure, which is eventually transmitted to the RV, thus compromising its function as it attempts to pump against this increased resistance.

Heart failure evokes the secretion of vasoactive substances and cytokines, which initially help the body adapt to changes from reduced cardiac output. However, in chronic heart failure, these substances cause further myocardial damage and impairment of cardiac function. When cardiac muscle contraction is weakened, *endothelin,* a potent vasoconstrictor, is secreted by the arterial endothelium in response to a drop in BP. Although endothelin helps the body compensate by raising BP, chronic secretion increases afterload and resistance against the heart pump. Another substance, *tumor necrosis factor–alpha* (TNF-α), is found in the circulation and heart muscle during heart failure. TNF-α is an anorexigenic cytokine that also increases wasting of lean body mass. Two important vasodilator peptides are released with dilation of the atria and ventricles in heart failure: *atrial natriuretic peptide* (ANP) and *brain natriuretic peptide* (BNP). These are natural diuretic substances that counteract the excess water reabsorption and fluid overload caused by activation of the renin-angiotensin-aldosterone cascade in response to decreased cardiac output, by stimulating the excretion of sodium and water. Circulating serum BNP level is a useful indicator of the degree of heart failure, compared with a baseline value obtained in the absence of acute cardiac decompensation. Heart failure severity has traditionally been described with the symptom-based New York Heart Association (NYHA) classification system. The newer American College of Cardiology/American Heart Association (ACC/AHA) guidelines supplement this with a staging system describing the progressive phases of heart failure. The two systems are complementary, with the NYHA system describing symptom severity and the ACC/AHA system providing a framework for a stage-based therapeutic approach. Patients who present with a past medical history of HTN, diabetes mellitus, CAD, previous exposure to cardiotoxic drugs, or a strong family history of cardiomyopathy may be screened using the following tools as put forth by the NYHA and ACC/AHA.

NYHA Classification of Heart Failure Severity:
  I. Patients with asymptomatic heart failure
  II. Patients with heart failure symptoms with significant exertion
  III. Patients with heart failure symptoms with minor exertion
  IV. Patients with heart failure symptoms at rest

ACC/AHA Staging Criteria of Heart Failure:
  A. Patients at risk for developing left ventricular dysfunction
  B. Patients with left ventricular dysfunction who have not developed symptoms
  C. Patients with left ventricular dysfunction with symptoms
  D. Patients with refractory end-stage heart failure

By utilizing a combination of the NYHA heart failure class and the ACC/AHA heart failure stages, a more exacting assessment and subsequent management plan can be afforded. The following are examples of combining the two systems:

- A patient with minimal or no symptoms but a large pressure gradient across the aortic valve or severe obstruction of the left main coronary artery is classified as Function Capacity I, Objective Assessment D.
- A patient with severe anginal syndrome but angiographically normal coronary arteries is classified as Functional Capacity IV, Objective Assessment A.

Clinical Presentation
Subjective

The patient with heart failure will present complaining of symptoms related to the pulmonary system, central nervous system (CNS), and generalized systemic and organ systems.

Complaints related to the pulmonary system are cough, orthopnea, dyspnea, dyspnea on exertion, and paroxysmal nocturnal dyspnea. Orthopnea refers to dyspnea that is positional. The patient feels more dyspneic in a recumbent position but obtains relief by sitting or standing. The number of pillows that the patient sleeps on can grade the severity of orthopnea. Two related symptoms are dry nocturnal cough, seen early in heart failure, and dyspnea in the left lateral decubitus position. As heart failure progresses, the degree of dyspnea increases. If the progression is gradual, the patient may not be aware of the dyspnea. Assessment of the patient during activity may be necessary to elicit this symptom. Paroxysmal nocturnal dyspnea occurs as a result of hypoxia from the accumulation of fluid in the pulmonary interstitium. The patient is usually not aware that he or she is hypoxic and may describe paroxysmal nocturnal dyspnea as awakening during sleep because of a "nightmare" or extreme shortness of breath. The clinician must have a high level of suspicion because the description of paroxysmal nocturnal dyspnea varies from patient to patient. Slight relief may be noted with sitting, standing, or inspiration of fresh outdoor air. When severe coughing and wheezing are associated with this symptom, the condition is sometimes referred to as *cardiac asthma*. Patient symptoms related to the CNS range from delirium, insomnia, anxiety, and headache all the way to hallucinations and unresponsiveness.

Patient complaints of systemic and organ symptoms are many. Patients may complain of fatigue and generalized weakness, which are associated with low cardiac output and may occur at rest or with increased activity. These symptoms may also be caused by blood volume depletion and electrolyte imbalance secondary to overdiuresis. Patients may also notice a decreased urine output during the day, as well as nocturia that is the result of enhanced renal filtration secondary to recumbency. During the waking hours, renal filtration of sodium and water is decreased in the heart failure patient. Nocturia may not be present if concurrent renal failure is present. The patient may also complain of peripheral and dependent edema. Patients may present with ascites; fullness; nausea; vomiting; constipation; upper abdominal pain; anorexia; or conditions related to liver, spleen, and intestinal congestion. They may also report light-headedness, near-syncope, or syncope. In addition, the patient may be confused or have difficulty concentrating, an impaired memory, headache, insomnia, or anxiety. Some patients may present with chest pain.

Objective

A complete physical exam is necessary to diagnose the condition and determine the etiology of heart failure and provide the clinician with enough information to optimize intervention techniques. On general inspection, the clinician may note breathlessness, dyspnea on exertion, peripheral cyanosis (as a result of low cardiac output), pallor in extremities, and distended peripheral veins. There may be jugular venous distention along with abnormal pulsations. A skeletal deformity (as seen in Marfan's syndrome) may be noted. In addition, the patient may have dependent edema, jaundice (suggesting hepatic congestion), ascites, or anasarca.

Vital signs may show tachycardia; pulsus alternans (a weak pulse alternating with a strong pulse); atrial fibrillation, which may contribute to heart failure; rapid, shallow respirations at rest or with minimal exertion; and possibly Cheyne-Stokes respirations during sleep. Cheyne-Stokes respirations are crescendo-decrescendo patterns of respiratory swings terminating in apnea. Cheyne-Stokes respirations are caused by the prolonged circulation time from the heart to the brain. Verification of this type of sleep disturbance would need to be obtained from either a family member or health-care provider who has observed the patient during sleep.

On cardiac assessment, the clinician may note lateral and downward shift in the point of maximal impulse secondary to cardiac enlargement, the presence of a third heart sound (S_3) in adults older than age 40 (increased likelihood by 11-fold), and the sudden development of the murmurs of mitral or tricuspid regurgitation.

When performing a lung assessment, the clinician may note crackles (rales), generally heard bilaterally in the bases or in the most dependent regions of the lungs on inspiration. Wheezing may also be present, as well as pleural effusion (stony dullness, or shifting of dullness with position changes is characteristic of percussion with pleural effusion). In evaluating these symptoms, the clinician should also consider arterial embolism, which is present in 4% of patients with primary dilated cardiomyopathy.

Diagnostic Reasoning
Diagnostic Tests

The clinician should initially order laboratory tests to assist in the diagnosis. Cardiac myocytes and endothelial tissues manufacture and secrete a family of structurally related peptide hormones termed natriuretic peptides. Atrial natriuretic peptides (ANPs) are secreted in response to the atrial stretch that occurs in heart failure due to increased hydrostatic pressure within the atria. These peptides have diuretic, vasodilating, and kaliuretic (potassium-wasting) effects. B-type natriuretic peptide (BNP) is abundant in the heart and rapidly rises in the bloodstream in the presence of heart failure. A blood test can show elevated BNP within 15 minutes. In patients with the symptom of dyspnea, which can be either cardiac or pulmonary in origin, the BNP blood test can be used to rule out heart failure (Level I; Jessup et al, 2009). BNP is a cardiac marker that can be used in combination with other more definitive tests and is not solely relied on to diagnose heart failure. BNP can be elevated in pulmonary edema, COPD, pulmonary embolism, renal disease, and other conditions. However, a BNP level that is greater than 500 pg/mL is highly indicative of heart failure. In the Breathing Not Properly study, a BNP cutoff of 100 pg/mL alone had a sensitivity of 90% and a specificity of 73% to diagnose heart failure in the emergency department and had a diagnostic accuracy of 81.2% compared with 74% for clinical judgment alone. After instituting treatment for heart failure, the clinician can rely on BNP levels to monitor therapeutic effectiveness. In addition, there is a pharmacological form of BNP, nesiritide, that is used to treat heart failure. However, once nesiritide is initiated, BNP levels would not be of clinical use.

An echocardiogram is the diagnostic test used after demonstrable elevation of BNP. Echocardiography is the single best test to confirm a diagnosis of heart failure. Abnormalities of systolic and diastolic function are easily visualized, and ejection fraction can be estimated. An echocardiogram can also visualize different etiologies of heart failure and diseases of the pericardium, myocardium, and heart valves.

A CBC may show severe anemia associated with high-output heart failure. A urinalysis that shows proteinuria may indicate nephrotic syndrome, and red blood cells or cellular casts may indicate glomerulonephritis. A serum albumin elevation may indicate volume overload caused by renal failure. An ESR should be ordered because the ESR is typically decreased secondary to impaired fibrinogen synthesis and decreased fibrinogen concentration in patients with heart failure. Electrolytes may show hyponatremia, which may be either genuine (secondary to prolonged sodium restriction and diuretic therapy) or dilutional (secondary to expansion of extracellular volume). Hyponatremia may also signal pronounced activation of the renin-angiotensin system. Hypokalemia may be secondary to diuretic therapy or activation of the renin-angiotensin-aldosterone axis. Hyperkalemia may be secondary to renal failure as a result of the heart failure, especially if ACE inhibitors have been used. The blood urea nitrogen and creatinine may be elevated secondary to decreased renal blood flow. Liver function tests may show abnormalities as a result of hepatic congestion. There is also a decreased hepatic blood flow; therefore, drugs metabolized by the liver should be appropriately dosed. An arterial blood gas study may also be ordered for further acid–base evaluation. Finally, the thyroxine (T_4) and thyroid-stimulating hormone levels may indicate that the heart failure is aggravated by hypothyroidism or hyperthyroidism.

The clinician may also order the following diagnostic procedures to gather information in the diagnosis of heart failure. Although there is no specific ECG pattern for heart failure, an ECG may help diagnose the underlying cause, such as an MI. A chest x-ray film will show an alteration in cardiac silhouette as evidenced by a change in cardiac size and shape, a change in cardiothoracic ratio (cardiothoracic ratio more than 0.50 is considered cardiomegaly), and specific chamber enlargement. A chest x-ray film may also show pulmonary venous congestion as evidenced by distention of the pulmonary veins upward from the hila. Normally in the upright position, larger vessels are seen in the bases; however, with increasing capillary pressures, there is compression of the vessels to the lower lobes and dilation of upper lobe vessels. This might present on x-ray studies as an equalization of upper and lower lobe vessel size; loss of definition of pulmonary vascular markings, which is usually caused by perivascular edema; haziness of hilar shadows; and thickness of interlobular septa (Kerley B lines). Kerley B lines usually result from distended lymphatic vessels. As pulmonary capillary wedge pressure exceeds 25 mm Hg, alveolar edema is indicated by diffuse haziness, usually extending downward toward both lung fields (butterfly pattern). An echocardiogram can be used to identify underlying structural defects such as valvular defects, systolic dysfunction, and abnormal cardiac wall thickness. A radionuclide angiocardiography uses technetium-99m (multigated acquisition scan). This multigated blood pool imaging technique is useful in measuring the EF and wall-motion abnormalities, and right-heart catheterization is useful for determining response to therapy; it can be used in a monitored intensive care unit.

Left-heart catheterization is not usually indicated in heart failure; however, once the condition is stabilized, catheterization can be useful in identifying the underlying causes of the failure. Left-heart catheterization may be performed by the cardiologist if sudden murmurs are auscultated, including severe mitral regurgitation that may be caused by ruptured chordae tendineae, severe aortic regurgitation that may be caused by bacterial endocarditis, or perforation of the interventricular septum or papillary muscle rupture.

Differential Diagnosis

The symptoms of heart failure can be vague and progress slowly, or they can be sudden and overwhelming. In either event, the symptoms and findings of what appears to be heart failure may have other causes such as anxiety neurosis, lung disease, venous insufficiency, nephrotic syndrome, hepatic cirrhosis, superior vena cava syndrome, constrictive pericarditis, or pericardial effusion.

Management

The principles of management include identifying and treating precipitating or aggravating conditions, recognizing and treating underlying cardiac disease, and managing the cardiac failure.

When managing heart failure, the clinician must consider treatments that will decrease the cardiac workload, decrease the clinical volume overload, optimize LV function, reduce mortality, and control atrial fibrillation. To decrease the cardiac workload, the clinician must order rest until the patient's "dry weight" (non–heart failure weight) is achieved, order vasodilators, encourage weight loss if appropriate, and control HTN. Analysis of data acquired from the Systolic Hypertension in the Elderly Program indicates a marked effect in preventing development of heart failure in older patients with isolated systolic hypertension when diuretic therapy was instituted.

To reduce mortality, the health-care provider should order ACE inhibitors, which are indicated for all patients with LV systolic dysfunction unless there are specific contraindications, such as history of intolerance or adverse reactions to these agents, serum potassium greater than 5.5 mEq, or symptomatic hypotension.

ACE inhibitors may be the sole therapy for a patient with fatigue and mild dyspnea on exertion. They are referred to as the "cornerstone of heart failure therapy." ACE inhibitors have been demonstrated to counteract many of the neurohumoral changes in heart failure and, therefore, decrease mortality. For patients who cannot tolerate ACE inhibitors, angiotensin receptor blockers (ARBs) can be used. Vasodilators and nitrates can also be used in those who cannot tolerate ACE inhibitors. Diuretics should be added to this therapy if symptoms persist or volume overload becomes obvious.

To decrease clinical volume overload, diuretics should be initiated at the first signs of volume overload (stage C), e.g., orthopnea, paroxysmal nocturnal dyspnea; however, the clinician should avoid overdiuresis, which will lead to hypotension or renal insufficiency and may interfere with other medications. For mild heart failure, thiazide diuretics are used, and for severe failure, loop diuretics, such as furosemide (Lasix) or bumetanide (Bumex), should be ordered. Doses of these agents can be increased during acute heart failure exacerbations to counteract fluid overload. All patients should be on a sodium-restricted diet.

As a compensatory mechanism in heart failure, the sympathetic nervous system is stimulated. Sympathetic stimulation causes arterial vasoconstriction and increased heart rate, which have detrimental effects on the weakened heart. For this reason, beta-adrenergic blockers, such as carvedilol, have been recommended as part of the drug treatment regimen. Carvedilol is also an alpha-1 antagonist, and along with the beta-adrenergic blockade, slows heart rate, decreasing the work of the heart, and limits peripheral arterial vasoconstriction, decreasing afterload against the ventricles. Bisoprolol and sustained-release metoprolol are the other beta blockers shown to reduce mortality (Level I; Jessup et al, 2009).

Once heart failure has progressed to stage C, spironolactone, an aldosterone antagonist, has been shown to be of benefit in carefully selected patients. Refer to the latest AHA updates for heart failure to review criteria for stage C therapy. In addition, in stage C, the patient should be evaluated for biventricular pacing and an implantable defibrillator (Level I; Jessup et al, 2009). Heart failure often causes ventricular remodeling and arrhythmias such as left bundle branch block (LBBB). These conditions lead to unsynchronized ventricular contractions. Cardiac resynchronization therapy (CRT) has been shown to improve cardiac mechanics by inducing concordant contraction of the two ventricles. CRT involves implantation of a biventricular pacing device, and if necessary, an implantable cardioverter-defibrillator. Implantation of an internal cardiac automated defibrillator may be considered for primary prevention in chronic heart failure patients (NYHA functional class II or III and ACC/AHA stage C) with ischemic or nonischemic cardiomyopathy or with a patient with an EF less than or equal to 35%, given the patient's increased

risk of sudden cardiac death due to an increased risk of sustained ventricular tachycardia and ventricular fibrillation. CRT may also be used for patients with NYHA class III or IV heart failure with persistent symptoms who are already receiving optimal medical therapy. Heart transplantation may be considered for patients who have exhausted all other treatment recommendations with poor effect (ACC/AHA stage D). Psychological support is essential; patient support groups have been shown to be very effective in helping patients cope with their conditions and follow the prescribed regimen.

Historically, digoxin has been used to treat heart failure; however, with the establishment of ACE inhibitors and ARBs along with beta blockers and diuretics as the front-line treatment options, use of digoxin has declined. Digoxin may still be used in conjunction with other medications in patients with severe heart failure (ACC/AHA stage C). It may not be necessary in patients who become asymptomatic after treatment with ACE inhibitors and diuretics. Intravenous inotropic agents that may be ordered in a monitored setting for end-stage cardiac failure (stage D) include dopamine (Intropin), dobutamine (Dobutrex), and milrinone (Primacor).

Controlling and, when possible, eliminating atrial fibrillation is essential in treating heart failure. Atrial fibrillation in patients with asymptomatic or symptomatic left ventricular systolic dysfunction is associated with an increased risk of progression of the dysfunction and mortality. Because of this, anticoagulation treatment is instituted in heart failure to decrease the formation of thrombi in the dysfunctional heart chambers, thus preventing embolic cerebral stroke. Long-term oral anticoagulation with warfarin (Coumadin) is usually recommended.

CRT is an option for patients who present with a left ventricular EF less than or equal to 35%, a QRS greater than 120 ms, or who are NYHA class III of IV or who otherwise are not optimized.

Ventricular assist devices (VADs) are becoming more frequently considered in the management of end-stage heart failure than ever before. VADs can be a bridge to transplant or a destination therapy. With the implementation of a VAD program, a designated interprofessional team is implemented to optimize outcomes.

Once drug therapy is initiated, the clinician may manage the patient. Increasingly around the United States, heart failure clinics are becoming popular referral resources.

Other treatments include the following:

- Regular exercise should be encouraged for all patients with stable heart failure, because it improves functional status and decreases symptoms.
- Cardiac rehabilitation programs, although not specifically indicated for patients with heart failure, might benefit patients who are anxious about

exercising on their own or those who have low cardiac output.

- Dietary sodium is restricted to 2 g/day or less.
- Limitation of fluid intake should be advised for each patient based on his or her status.
- Alcohol consumption should be discouraged. A patient should drink no more than one glass of beer or wine or a mixed drink with no more than 1 ounce of alcohol per day.
- The patient should record his or her weight daily and notify the clinician of a weight gain of 3 pounds in 24 hours or 5 pounds or more within 1 week.
- Immunization with influenza and pneumococcal vaccines may reduce the risk of a respiratory infection.
- All barriers to adherence must be removed to assist the patient with management of the disease. Some barriers include the cost of medications, adverse effects, and the complexity of the medical regimen.
- The patient must be counseled concerning the prognosis, so that he or she may have the benefit of understanding the rationale for decisions made about care. This must be done while maintaining hope. The clinician should explain that good quality of life is still possible with cooperation in the treatment regimen. The patient must be given information regarding the prognosis so that plans can be made for the future.
- The patient should be encouraged to complete advance directives.

Follow-up and Referral

Referral to a cardiologist is recommended on onset of symptoms of heart failure; however, initial treatment should begin immediately in the clinician's office, with a phone referral made directly to the cardiologist. Patients in acute failure may be hospitalized. The clinician and the cardiologist will establish a plan of care with the patient and will decide who will manage the patient on an ongoing basis. It must be clear to all involved what the plan of care is to be. The Joint Commission has mandated that specific Core Measures of care be met before discharge. For the patient with heart failure, there must be an assessment of left ventricular function documenting an EF. If the EF is below 40%, the clinician must prescribe an ACE inhibitor or ARB. If the patient has had an allergic reaction to either of these drugs and cannot tolerate the drugs, this must be documented in the medical record. Additional Core Measures are advice/counseling on smoking cessation (other tobacco use should be discouraged) and discharge instructions that include reconciliation of medication regimen. For further information pertaining to Core Measures, the clinician is advised to review the Joint Commission's latest recommendations at www.jointcommission.org.

Patients in chronic cardiac failure may be treated on an outpatient basis. After a complete and detailed baseline history and physical exam, subsequent visits for the patient in chronic failure should assess the patient's cardiac status thoroughly. Questions regarding the patient's health-related quality of life (e.g., sleep, sexual function, mental health or outlook on life, appetite, and social activities) should also be asked. After the patient, family, and caregiver have been educated on the condition, they should be encouraged to communicate all signs, symptoms, fears, and concerns with the clinician. Patients are likely to experience changes in symptoms before there is evidence of deterioration on physical examination.

Frequency of follow-up should depend on the underlying cause of heart failure. Generally, the patient is seen by the clinician at least every 3 months. Intensive home-care surveillance has been shown to decrease the need for hospitalization and improve the functional status of older adult patients with heart failure.

Patient Education

Successful management of patients with heart failure requires an active partnership between the patient and all health-care providers. One of the most critical points in decreasing the possibility of the patient becoming "crippled" by the disease process is a thorough education regarding the condition and encouragement to take responsibility for personal care. The clinician should encourage and assist the patient to do the following:

- Keep a record of daily weights and notify the clinician of a 3-pound weight gain in 24 hours or a 5-pound or more weight gain in 1 week or less.
- Advise the clinician of symptoms or concerns.
- Exercise regularly.
- Rest with elevation of lower extremities.
- Use elastic stockings to reduce the risk of venous thrombosis and PE.
- Ensure emotional rest.
- Maintain an optimum body weight.
- Discuss with the clinician changes made in self-care. The clinician should explain to the patient that some things can be changed, and that by discussing what he or she wants to change with the clinician, before making changes, an "informed" change can be made.

In working closely with the patient and possibly the family to plan the patient's care, the clinician should never lose sight of the high esteem with which his or her opinions and directions are taken. In discussing the plan of care with the patient and family, the clinician should keep in mind that the family, who fears losing their loved one, will attempt to ensure that the plan is followed to the letter; therefore, the clinician should remember to "build in," and teach the patient and family how to "build in," some humane adaptations to the plan of care. For instance, as the clinician stresses that the diuretic must be taken every morning, he or she must realize that if the patient has an important family function one morning and chooses to take the diuretic later in the day, the mandate may cause needless stress and guilt. The patient may be frightened of getting into distress if he or she does not follow the orders. The family may "harass" the patient for deliberately not following the plan of care, or the patient may feel that participation in events that take place in the morning is forbidden. Any or all of these perceived restrictions compromise the quality of the patient's life and are unnecessary. It is critical that the clinician ensure that the patient understands the rationale for decisions about his or her care.

With the increasing incidence of heart failure, researchers have begun to look at areas of patient involvement in self-care and the impact on outcome. Exercise training is now being recommended for most individuals with moderate-to-severe heart failure. Activity intolerance associated with chronic heart failure has been studied from the perspective of physiological variables; however, very little research has been conducted on the outcomes of exercise training based on subjective data. A research study examined the perception of vigor as a subjective measure of personal health. In this study of person–environment interaction in patients with heart failure, the researcher found that an astute evaluation of the patient's environment, including his or her physical and social milieu, is warranted when assessment of energy level is undertaken. Purposeful activity and exercise should be encouraged and supported. During interviews with patients with heart failure, the researcher noted the hopeful and life-loving attitudes of the participants involved in exercise training in her study, which suggested coping strategies not often attributed to a population experiencing terminal illness. Conclusions were that reinforcement of these attitudes may be a key intervention in reversing the energy-draining sequelae of illness patterns experienced by the individual with a failing heart.

Coaching and encouraging a terminally ill patient in self-care is time consuming and can be draining. The clinician will need to have authentic presence and respond to calls for care that are often not timed with the patient's regularly scheduled appointment; however, the time invested in each patient cannot be charged appropriately on a ledger or justified to other patients who may be late for their visit with the clinician. Nonetheless, to patients with lifelong terminal illness, the importance of life and the significance of the effects of their illness are directly related to their perceptions of the attention and care they perceive being given.

■ ARRHYTHMIAS

Arrhythmias the clinician may encounter in primary-care practice include the atrial arrhythmias of atrial fibrillation, premature atrial contractions (PACs), atrial tachycardia, atrial flutter, and supraventricular tachycardia (SVT). Ventricular arrhythmias encountered include premature ventricular contractions (PVCs) and ventricular

tachycardia (VT). First-, second-, and third-degree heart blocks and arrhythmias associated with digitalis toxicity are other arrhythmias commonly encountered.

Atrial Arrhythmias
Atrial Fibrillation

Atrial fibrillation is one of the most common arrhythmias that clinicians will encounter in clinical practice. In most cases, atrial fibrillation initially will be associated with a rapid ventricular response, and most patients will have some type of underlying heart disease. In these patients, the loss of atrial contribution to left ventricular blood volume (atrial "kick"), along with a rapid ventricular rate, can have serious hemodynamic effects caused by diminished cardiac output. These effects may be seen in the form of hypotension, diaphoresis, dizziness, and syncopal episodes.

The loss of mechanically effective atrial contractions in atrial fibrillation leads to stasis of blood in the left atrium that predisposes an individual to formation of embolic atrial thrombi. Thrombi that form in the left atrium then have a propensity to travel into the left ventricle and into the aorta where they are propelled into the arterial circulation. A common route for the thrombus from the aorta is to the brachiocephalic artery, carotid artery, and then into the cerebral circulation. This pathway makes atrial fibrillation a risk factor for ischemic stroke because an embolus may lodge in a branch of the middle cerebral artery. All persons in atrial fibrillation should be evaluated for the risk of stroke and given recommendations for anticoagulant therapy using the most current version of the CHADS2 scoring tool. The CHADS2 risk score is calculated using 1 point each for **C**HF; **H**TN; **A**ge greater than 75 years; **D**iabetes; and 2 points for **S**troke or TIA (Levine, 2014). The clinician is encouraged to periodically review the latest criteria of this scoring method in the literature for current recommendations. All atrial fibrillation candidates for anticoagulant therapy need to be evaluated with regard to their individual circumstances and using the best available evidence.

Premature Atrial Contractions

PACs are very common, yet in most cases have no clinical significance. PACs are usually a benign arrhythmia that does not require pharmacological intervention unless there are underlying causes that can be corrected. This arrhythmia is commonly seen in young, healthy individuals. Cardiac stimulants such as caffeine, nicotine, alcohol, or over-the-counter medications sometimes induce PACs. They are rarely, if ever, symptomatic and are frequently seen in patients with obstructive lung disease and heart failure.

Supraventricular Tachycardia

Supraventricular tachycardia (SVT) is often described as a "catch-all" term that encompasses rapid arrhythmias above the ventricles. There continues to be confusion over specific terminology of these SVTs. Some experts feel that the confusion arises from failure to understand the mechanism and inability to differentiate true atrial tachycardias or atrial flutters from paroxysmal supraventricular tachycardias (PSVTs) that use reentry circuits. The use of the term *paroxysmal atrial tachycardia* (PAT) further confounds the terminology issue. This term is often incorrectly used for all SVTs (whether paroxysmal or not) that are not atrial flutter or atrial fibrillation.

Research has shown that the two most common forms of PSVT are atrioventricular node reentry tachycardia (AVNRT) and orthodromic circus movement tachycardia (CMT). For purposes of this discussion, the condition SVT is subdivided into PSVT, which includes AVNRT and CMT, and non-PSVT, which includes atrial tachycardia of nonreentry origin and atrial flutter. Although atrial fibrillation can also be classified as an SVT, this rhythm is discussed separately. Current Advanced Cardiac Life Support (ACLS) treatment standards require that the clinician be able to differentiate the aforementioned atrial tachycardias that are included under the term *SVT*.

The atrial rate differentiates atrial tachycardia from atrial flutter. This rate difference is particularly pertinent when the clinician is attempting to discern if the arrhythmia is an atrial tachycardia with block (seen in digitalis toxicity) or an atrial flutter. Both rhythms can present with more than one observable P wave before the QRS. An atrial tachycardia rate (140–250) is slower than an atrial flutter rate (250–350). Atrial flutter is less common than atrial fibrillation and most commonly occurs in older adults. Atrial flutter must be referred to a cardiologist and managed in an acute-care setting. These patients typically have some form of organic heart disease.

Ventricular Arrhythmias
Premature Ventricular Contractions

PVCs are usually a benign arrhythmia that does not require pharmacological intervention unless the rhythm progresses to VT. VT may be associated with any form of heart disease. It may be sustained or nonsustained. In patients who have had an MI, nonsustained VT is a risk factor for sudden cardiac death.

Heart Blocks

Atrioventricular (AV) blocks are classified as to the degree of severity of the disturbance of the impulse going through the electrical conduction system between the atria and ventricles. Heart blocks may be permanent or transient and are classified as first, second, or third degree. A *first-degree AV block* is observed with a regular rhythm and only a prolonged P-R interval. *Second-degree AV block* may be classified further as type I (Mobitz I or Wenckebach) and type II (Mobitz II). For purposes of this discussion, the terms "type" and "Mobitz" are combined as Mobitz type I and Mobitz type II. Mobitz type I occurs in the AV nodal area with progressive lengthening of the P-R interval until a QRS complex (ventricular contraction) is dropped. Mobitz type II occurs within or below the bundle of His, with a normal or lengthened PR interval and a periodic drop of a QRS complex in a set ratio of atrial to ventricular contractions. A *third-degree AV block* occurs when the atria beat regularly and at a normal rate but no excitation is transmitted from the atria to the ventricles. In turn, the atria and ventricles contract independently at their own intrinsic rates. This complete lack of coordination between the chambers of the heart severely compromises cardiac output and can prove fatal.

Third-degree heart block is classified as third degree at the junctional level or third degree at the ventricular level. A second-degree Mobitz type I block does not progress to Mobitz type II; rather, a Mobitz type I block typically progresses to a third-degree block with an idiojunctional response. In contrast, a second-degree Mobitz type II block progresses to third-degree heart block with an idioventricular response that carries a more ominous prognosis. If a rhythm presents with two P waves with a normal rate to every two R waves (referred to as 2:1 conduction), the origin of nodal or subnodal pathology must be determined. This rhythm is often referred to as second-degree AV block undifferentiated. If the QRS complex is narrow (0.04–0.10), it can be deduced that the location of the block is from the junctional area and Mobitz type I in origin.

Arrhythmias Associated With Digitalis

Historically, one of the most common agents used in the treatment of heart failure and supraventricular tachyarrhythmias has been digitalis. Although digitalis is not seen as often nowadays, it is still prescribed by many clinicians and merits discussion. It is a common cause of various degrees of AV block. There is a narrow therapeutic range for this drug; signs of toxicity can occur before acute symptoms are recognized. Digitalis toxicity can produce virtually any arrhythmia. Those arrhythmias most commonly seen in digitalis toxicity are atrial tachycardia with AV nodal block, accelerated junctional rhythms, atrial fibrillation with a slow or regular ventricular response, second-degree heart block or Mobitz type I (Wenckebach), and ventricular dysrhythmias. The serum digitalis levels may not reflect the amount of digitalis bound to the myocardial membrane, where it cannot be measured. A finding of a normal digitalis level should not be the determining factor in assessing digitalis toxicity. The onset of atrial tachydysrhythmias, noncardiac subjective symptoms (particularly altered visual color perception), and pertinent medication history should make the clinician highly suspicious of digitalis toxicity. ECGs representing these rhythms are shown in Figure 10.4.

Common Arrhythmias
ATRIAL ARRHYTHMIAS

Figure 10.4a Atrial fibrillation. Fibrillatory waves distort the baseline, and the R-R interval is characteristically irregular. The ventricular rate is approximately 100 beats/min.

Figure 10.4b Premature atrial contraction (PACs) or atrial premature contractions (APCs). A single complex occurs earlier than the next expected sinus complex. After the PAC, sinus rhythm usually resumes.

Figure 10.4c Atrial tachycardia with a rate of 180 beats/min.

Figure 10.4d Paroxysmal supraventricular tachycardia (PSVT) or paroxysmal atrial tachycardia (PAT). Sinus rhythm which changes into atrial tachycardia at a rate of 230 beats/min.

Figure 10.4e Atrial flutter. A characteristic sawtooth pattern at the baseline. Atrial flutter with a 4:1 conduction. The R-R interval is regular.

Figure 10.4f Atrial flutter with a 2:1 conduction. Initiation of carotid sinus massage temporarily slows the ventricular rate enough to unmask the flutter waves.

VENTRICULAR ARRHYTHMIAS

Figure 10.4g Premature ventricular contractions (PVCs). The ectopic QRS complex (the PVC) is wide, abnormally shaped, and appears earlier than expected. The length of the compensatory pause following a PVC indicates that sinus node discharge was undisturbed. A nonconducted sinus P wave distorts the T wave (the P wave appears on time).

Figure 10.4h PVC couplets. Pairs of uniform PVCs originating from the same ectopic site.

Figure 10.4i PVC bigeminy. A uniform PVC occurring from the same ectopic site; occurs every other beat.

Figure 10.4j Multifocal PVCs. PVCs coming from two ectopic foci.

Figure 10.4k Ventricular tachycardia. The ventricular rate is approximately 160 beats/min. The QRS complexes are wide, they look alike, and the R-R interval is regular.

Figure 10.4l Torsade de pointes. Polymorphic ventricular tachycardia, congenital or drug induced.

Figure 10.4m Ventricular fibrillation. Chaotic electrical activity with no ventricular contraction.

Figure 10.4n Atrioventricular (AV) blocks: First-degree AV block. The P-R interval is consistently prolonged at 0.20 second or longer. The underlying rhythm is sinus.

SECOND-DEGREE AV BLOCKS

Figure 10.4o Type I (Mobitz I or Wenckeback). The P-R interval lengthens until a beat is dropped. The QRS complexes are narrow. The nonconducted P waves are easily visible.

Figure 10.4p Type II (Mobitz II). The P-R interval remains fixed. The QRS complexes are wider than normal. The nonconducted P waves are visible. The conduction ratio (P waves to QRS complexes) is commonly 2:1, 3:1, or 4:1.

Figure 10.4q Third-degree AV block: There is no relationship between the P wave and the QRS complex. This is a third-degree AV block with a ventricular escape pacemaker.

Figure 10.4r Bundle branch block (BBB). Either the left or the right ventricle will depolarize late, creating a "notched" QRS complex.

Epidemiology and Causes
Atrial Arrhythmias

Most patients with atrial fibrillation have some form of heart disease. The most common form is CAD associated with heart failure, followed by hypertension and rheumatic heart disease. Frequently, the precipitating event is an acute illness, electrolyte imbalance, or major cardiac surgery. Atrial fibrillation is seen in 60% of patients after valvular surgery and in 33% to 42% of patients with mitral valve stenosis. Other causes of atrial fibrillation include abrupt discontinuation of beta blockers, alcohol ingestion (sometimes called "holiday heart"), hyperthyroidism, acute MI, and cor pulmonale. A danger of untreated atrial fibrillation, with or without rapid ventricular response, is the significant increased risk of embolic stroke. The risk of stroke is increased in untreated atrial fibrillation after 48 to 72 hours; therefore, it is important to diagnose and treat this arrhythmia in an expeditious manner. A beta blocker or calcium channel blocker should be given to slow AV conduction and control the ventricular rate of atrial fibrillation.

PACs typically have no clinical significance. In a normal patient, tobacco, caffeine, alcohol, or emotional stress may cause PACs. PACs may also result from stretch of the myocardium as a warning of developing CHF. In patients with organic heart disease, common causes of PACs are mitral valve stenosis and cor pulmonale secondary to atrial enlargement. Occasionally in patients with organic heart disease, PACs may precipitate PSVT, atrial flutter, and atrial fibrillation. Remember that the most common cause of a pause on the ECG is a blocked PAC. To differentiate this from heart block, assess if the P wave is early or on time. If the P wave is early, it is a premature atrial ectopic beat. If the P wave is on time, heart block should be considered.

Ventricular Arrhythmias

Frequent PVCs are seen in patients with cardiomyopathies of differing etiologies and arteriosclerotic heart disease. These patients are rarely symptomatic and in general do not need to be treated. In patients with frequent PVCs, it is worthwhile to rule out acute underlying causes of ventricular ectopy such as hypokalemia, hypomagnesemia, hypoxia, myocardial ischemia, or digitalis toxicity. Other common causes are stress and stimulants such as alcohol and nicotine. Sustained ventricular tachycardia is associated with a prior MI or CAD, electrolyte disturbances, and digitalis toxicity.

Heart Blocks

A first-degree heart block (P-R interval greater that 0.20 milliseconds) may be seen as a result of drugs that slow AV conduction or in persons with CAD and digitalis toxicity. A transient second-degree AV block type I may be associated with an acute inferior MI. It may also be associated with CHF or digitalis toxicity. A Mobitz type II AV block is a less common second-degree heart block; it is marked by an intermittent blocked impulse that can occur at the bundle of His or the right or left bundle branches. This type of block may occur as the result of an anterior wall MI. As this block progresses, complete heart block with an idioventricular response may follow. Insertion of a temporary pacemaker as soon as a Mobitz type II block is discovered is the standard of care. Other causes of AV block at this level are acute infections, valvular heart disease, and digitalis toxicity. This is not commonly a transient arrhythmia and can progress to third-degree AV block at the ventricular level; therefore, it must be monitored and treated appropriately.

Pathophysiology

The mechanism of atrial fibrillation remains controversial. Cardiac disease associated with atrial enlargement is the primary cause of the rapid firing (400–700 beats per minute) of the ectopic foci throughout the atrium.

Although electrical atrial activity is very rapid, only a small islet of myocardium is depolarized rather than the entire atrium. Because the atrium does not contract as a whole, there is no P wave. The chaotic atrial activity is seen as a wavy line between the QRS complex and is referred to as fibrillatory waves. These impulses are transmitted in variable fashion from the atria to the ventricles. The ventricular response rate to atrial fibrillation may be fast or slow, depending on the refractory nature of the AV node and the degree of AV nodal heart block or conduction delay within the AV node. In turn, therapy is usually geared toward rate control with AV nodal slowing agents, rather than toward complete resolution of the arrhythmia with antiarrhythmic medications.

Normally, electrical impulses from the sinoatrial node within the atria are conducted down the AV node to the His-Purkinje conduction system, disseminating throughout the two ventricles, thereby leading to subsequent contraction. However, in addition to the AV node, in some individuals a fast conducting accessory pathway exists between the atria and ventricles that bypasses the AV node. The tissue in these pathways depolarizes at a faster rate owing to the presence of faster inward sodium transport channels. One of the most common and well-characterized examples of these bypass tracts is the bundle of Kent accessory tract, which is seen in individuals with Wolff-Parkinson-White (WPW) syndrome. Because conduction down this bypass pathway directly transmits a depolarizing impulse to the ventricles faster than impulses sent down the AV node, this has been termed a "preexcitation" syndrome. ECG patterns in these patients demonstrate QRS fusion beats with a characteristic shape produced by the overlap of QRS complexes transmitted via each pathway in temporal proximity, hence creating a fusion complex. The first portion of the upswing in the R wave in this complex has a characteristic slanted appearance with a less steep angle than the remainder of the upward deflection, termed a *delta wave*. Figure 10.5 shows a delta wave present in WPW syndrome.

The most common mechanisms of PSVT observed in symptomatic patients are CMT (40% of cases) and

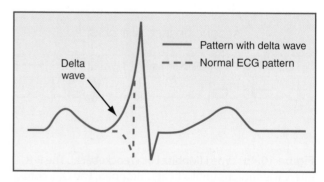

Figure 10.5 Delta wave present in Wolff-Parkinson-White syndrome.

AVNRT (50% of cases). CMT is distinguished by the dependence of the circular, reentrant impulse on an accessory conduction pathway, separate from the AV node itself. Thus, the fast bypass tract found in WPW syndrome is a perfect setup for CMT. Normal physiology dictates that cardiac conducting tissue become refractory (i.e., resistant to depolarization and electrical conduction) for a brief period of time following transmission of an electrical impulse. Bypass pathways such as that seen in WPW syndrome typically have shorter refractory periods than the AV node. Once depolarizing impulses are transmitted down the AV node to the ventricles, the refractory nature of the AV node prevents retrograde conduction back up this pathway. However, the same impulse may be conducted in retrograde fashion from the ventricles back up the accessory bypass tract to the atria. In turn, this impulse may then be conducted back down the AV node, which will have recovered from its refractory state by this time, only to circle back around once again to the atria via the fast accessory pathway. This type of circular, orthodromic conduction accounts for 90% of CMT cases, with a P wave occurring immediately after the QRS complex, rather than before it. The remaining 10% of CMT cases are considered antidromic, with the depolarizing impulse initially conducted down the fast accessory tract, only to circle back up the slower AV nodal pathway to the atria to complete the circular movement.

In AVNRT, PSVT typically results from an interplay of two conducting pathways within the AV node itself—one fast and one slow. The key aspect of this type of PSVT is that reentry of the impulse is dependent on an AV nodal pathway, as opposed to an accessory bypass pathway. In AVNRT, the fast AV nodal conducting pathway has a refractory period that lasts longer than that of the slow AV nodal pathway. Thus, if an electrical impulse enters both pathways of the AV node simultaneously, the fast pathway will remain refractory longer. In turn, if an early PAC then enters the AV node while the fast accessory pathway is still refractory, it can depolarize the ventricles only via transmission down the slower AV nodal pathway. By the time the impulse has traveled down this open slow pathway, the fast pathway is no longer refractory, and the impulse may travel in retrograde fashion back up to the atria via the fast pathway, and then back down again to the ventricles via the slow pathway. This mechanism activates the atria and the ventricles nearly simultaneously, which places the P wave within the QRS complex, distorting its terminal portion.

PVCs and VT may be the results of enhanced normal automaticity from catecholamines within the His-Purkinje system or abnormal automaticity anywhere in the ventricles from ischemia, injury, or electrolyte imbalances. Another mechanism for these arrhythmias is reentry through slowly conducting tissue within the His-Purkinje system or the ventricular myocardium related to catecholamines or digitalis excess.

Digitalis toxicity may cause delayed after-depolarizations that are oscillations in transmembrane potential that follow full repolarization of the membrane. These oscillations are caused by interference of the sodium-potassium pump by digitalis. Digitalis competes with potassium for a binding site on the cellular membrane wall, which disables the sodium-potassium adenosine triphosphatase (ATPase) pump. The less potassium there is to bind to receptors, the greater amount of receptors available for digitalis; thus, hypokalemia potentiates digitalis toxicity. Triggered activity is also another important mechanism in the pathophysiology of digitalis toxicity.

The mechanism of AV block is delayed conduction or nonconduction of an atrial impulse when the AV junction is not physiologically refractory. In first-degree AV block, there is not an actual block but rather a prolongation of conduction. In second-degree block, there is nonconduction of some of the atrial impulses. The pathology is either in the AV node itself or within or below the bundle of His. The QRS complex duration assists the clinician in localizing the level of block. A narrow QRS complex is seen if the ventricular response is initiated at the level of AV node and conducted down both bundle branches simultaneously, as seen in Mobitz type I block. A wider QRS complex indicates that the block is located further down the conduction system at the bundle of His or within the bundle branches. These criteria may not be helpful if the patient has a preexisting right or left bundle branch block, however. Such a patient could present with a prolonged P-R interval with a broad QRS complex, and the pathology could be either in the AV node or within or below the bundle of His. The clinician would then need to assess the P-R interval carefully for varying lengths and Wenckebach conduction patterns. If the patient is in a two P waves for every wide QRS complex (2:1 conduction) pattern, the origin of pathology is difficult to determine from the ECG.

Clinical Presentation
Subjective

A patient presenting with atrial fibrillation may complain of shortness of breath, palpitations, angina, changing level of consciousness, and syncope. If the patient is aware of palpitations, the clinician should have him or her "tap" out the rhythm in the palm of the hand. The irregular tapping at irregular intervals can differentiate this rhythm from the regular patterns of other arrhythmias.

A patient experiencing SVT will complain of dizziness, shortness of breath, and chest pain. As part of taking the patient's history, the clinician should ask about polyuria that is associated with SVT. Polyuria is present in 20% to 50% of patients with PSVT or atrial fibrillation. It is thought to be related to the cardiac secretion of atrial natriuretic factor released by changes in rhythm and atrial pressure.

A patient presenting with nonsustained VT may complain of palpitations or may present with symptoms similar to those of patients with sustained VT. Usually patients with sustained VT will have complaints compatible with a loss of cardiac output, such as decreased levels of mentation and hypotension.

If the patient is taking digitalis, the clinician should question him or her about anorexia, nausea, and vomiting. In addition, the patient should be asked about changes in the quality of color vision, especially red and green color distortions. These changes may be subtle; patients often do not volunteer them unless asked. Scotomas and flickering halos, although advanced signs, may also be present. Neurological symptoms such as headache, malaise, memory lapses, and insomnia may also be reported.

A patient experiencing first-degree heart block will be asymptomatic. With a third-degree AV block, the patient may exhibit signs of symptomatic bradycardia. The origin of the block may determine the degree of symptomatology. Patients with second-degree AV Mobitz type I that progresses into a third-degree block with an idiojunctional response may or may not exhibit overt signs or report symptoms of a bradycardia. The hemodynamic symptom present will depend on the rate of the junctional response (anywhere from 40–60 beats per minute), the status of the patient's left ventricular ejection fraction, and the loss of atrial kick (up to 20%–30% of the cardiac output). A patient whose Mobitz type II heart block progresses to third degree with a ventricular response of 20 to 40 beats per minute will almost always exhibit signs and symptoms of a severe bradycardia such as profound changes in level of consciousness and hypotension, which will prohibit reports of subjective data.

Objective

Atrial Fibrillation Physical examination of the patient with atrial fibrillation will yield an irregularly irregular heart rhythm. In most cases the rate is rapid (100–180 beats per minute). Some patients with a diseased AV node present with a slow or normal ventricular rate. Patients can be asymptomatic, although most cases present with some symptoms such as palpitations, dizziness, a decrease in BP, or are mildly symptomatic with new-onset activity intolerance. In a few cases, a stroke can be the presenting manifestation of atrial fibrillation as a result of emboli flowing from clot formation in the dysfunctional atrium into the cerebral vasculature. *Cannon waves,* which are unpredictable expansions of the jugular pulse caused when the atria contract against closed AV valves, causing a reflux of blood into the jugular

vein, may be seen. When present, Cannon waves signify AV dissociation as a result of the atrial fibrillation. The ECG strip will show fibrillatory waves representing (although unmeasurable) an atrial rate of 350 to 600 beats per minute, with a ventricular rate of 100 to 180 beats per minute. The rhythm is irregular. There are no discernible P waves, and a coarse or fine fibrillatory wave (f wave) is present. It is the hallmark of this arrhythmia and represents chaotic atrial activity. The P-R interval cannot be measured, and the QRS wave is usually normal.

Premature Atrial Contractions PACs may be found on a routine ECG. The rate is usually 60 to 100 beats per minute with a regular rhythm except when the premature beats are present. The premature beats have a different P wave configuration because of origination outside the sinus node. The PAC P-R interval may be different from the sinus P-R interval, and the QRS complex may be normal, aberrant (wide, different QRS complex), or absent.

The most common cause of a pause on an ECG rhythm strip is a blocked or nonconducted PAC. This occurs when the PAC comes so early that it falls in the T wave. If the AV node is still refractory, the early P wave does not conduct, and a pause is seen on the rhythm strip. If the clinician looks closely at the T wave and compares it to the patient's other T waves, the early nonconducted P wave can be seen distorting that specific T wave. If the nonconducted PACs present in a bigeminal pattern, the rhythm may be mistaken for profound sinus bradycardia or sinoatrial (SA) block. The clinician should always assess for nonconducted P waves within preceding T waves in any pauses observed on the ECG.

Observation of the neck veins may help the clinician rapidly distinguish between PSVT and VT. During PSVT, the atria contract against closed AV valves, resulting in a rapid, regular expansion of the neck veins (the same mechanism as Cannon waves). This physical finding has been called the "frog sign" because the rapid, regular expansion of the neck veins resembles the puffing motion of a frog. The patient's family may have noticed the frog sign of PSVT.

Supraventricular Tachycardia The ECG of a patient in SVT will show a regular rhythm with a rate of 150 to 250 beats per minute. The P waves are ectopic and distorted and may be initiated by a PAC. The P-R interval is shortened, and the QRS complex may be normal or distorted. If the patient is in atrial flutter, the atrial rate will be regular at 250 to 350 beats per minute, and the ventricular rate may be regular or slightly irregular. The P waves are discernible and "march out" (can be mapped out with a caliper) consistently throughout the strip. The P-R interval cannot be calculated, and the QRS complex has a variable conduction.

Premature Ventricular Contractions The ECG of a patient with PVCs will usually show a rate of 60 to

100 beats per minute. The rhythm will be irregular secondary to the premature ventricular beat. The PVC usually obscures the P waves; however, P waves may be visible if the PVC is late in diastole. These P waves are not related to the ectopic beat and occur at the same regular rate of the preceding sinus P waves. The P-R interval is not measurable on the PVC. The QRS complex for the PVC is wide and bizarre. It may be observed in patterns of ventricular bigeminy, trigeminy, or couplets. In the setting of an acute ischemic event, PVCs that occur close to the preceding T wave (R on T phenomena) may precipitate ventricular fibrillation.

Ventricular Tachycardia   VT can be categorized as monomorphic or polymorphic. The ECG of a patient with monomorphic VT will show a rate greater than 100 beats per minute with a regular rhythm; the P waves will be buried in the QRS complex or discernible after the QRS complex because of retrograde conduction. The P-R interval is not measurable, and the QRS complex is wide and bizarre. The ECG of a patient with polymorphic VT will show a "flipping" of the ventricular axis. For example, torsades de pointe is a form of polymorphic VT whose QT interval demonstrates prolongation before the onset of the dysrhythmia. It is essential to differentiate torsades from non–torsades polymorphic VT to optimize treatment.

Heart Blocks   In first-degree AV block, the pulse will usually be 60 to 100 beats per minute. The ECG rhythm is usually regular, with a P wave preceding each QRS complex and a prolonged P-R interval longer than 0.20 milliseconds. QRS complexes follow every P wave and are usually a normal width.

A patient with second-degree AV block Mobitz type I will have a ventricular rate of 50 to 70 beats per minute, although it may vary. The atrial rate is regular, whereas the ventricular rate is irregular. P waves precede each QRS complex, and the P-R interval progressively lengthens. The QRS complex is usually normal in width, unless a preexisting bundle branch block is present. As the P-R interval progresses, eventually the QRS complex disappears for a beat. In contrast, in a Mobitz type II AV block, the P-R interval may be prolonged or normal, but it remains constant, unlike the progressively lengthening P-R of a type I. The blocked P wave may occur in patterns of 2:1, 3:1, or 4:1. The width of the QRS complex indicates where the block is located. The wider the complex, the lower the block is located below the AV node. The P wave is regular and the P-R interval constant, with a wide QRS following every P wave until the QRS complex is not conducted.

With a third-degree block, the AV node (if the block is of a Mobitz I origin) or the ventricles (if the block is a Mobitz II in origin) set up an autonomous rhythm with a ventricular rate of 25 to 60 beats per minute. The atrial rate is 60 to 100 beats per minute. P waves are present and regular, but there is no relationship to the QRS complex. The P-R interval cannot be calculated,

and the QRS complex is wider and longer than 0.12 milliseconds if the block is at the ventricles; it is normal if the block is at the nodal/junctional level.

Diagnostic Reasoning
Diagnostic Tests
An ECG is the routine diagnostic test to determine the type of arrhythmia so as to direct treatment appropriately. The most definitive diagnostics are confirmed by electrical physiology studies. Electrophysiological testing using intracardiac electrocardiographic recordings and programmed atrial and/or ventricular stimulation is used in the diagnosis and management of complex dysrhythmias. Electrophysiological testing can evaluate recurrent syncope of possible cardiac origin and differentiate supraventricular from ventricular dysrhythmias.

Tilt-table testing, or autonomic testing, is useful in patients with arrhythmias when syncope may be due to a vasovagal response. The patient is tilted to approximately 70 degrees in conjunction with isoproterenol infusion. Syncope due to bradycardia and/or hypotension will occur in about one-third of patients with recurrent syncope.

Transesophageal echocardiography (TEE) is a diagnostic procedure used to visualize and rule out the presence of thrombi in the left atrium before cardioversion in atrial fibrillation. The presence of clots in the left atrium is a contraindication to cardioversion.

Differential Diagnosis
The differential diagnoses should consider conditions that could mimic the symptoms of dysrhythmia, such as panic attack, anxiety, valvular disorders, and syncopal episodes either neurogenic or cardiac in origin.

Management
Management of these patients by a clinician depends on the expertise of the clinician. If the clinician is at all unsure of the management of an arrhythmia, he or she should consult with the collaborating physician or a cardiovascular specialist.

Atrial Fibrillation
The initial goal of treatment in atrial fibrillation is to control the ventricular response and then convert the patient back to normal sinus rhythm (NSR) by using medications or electrical synchronized cardioversion.

Some patients with afib after cardioversion revert to a NSR. However, many patients with atrial fibrillation after cardioversion return to afib within a short period of time. This is seen particularly in patients with long-standing atrial fibrillation or in patients with advanced heart disease and a very large left atrium. Patients with new-onset atrial fibrillation or chronic atrial fibrillation with a very rapid ventricular response should be admitted to a unit where telemetry is available so that the response to treatment can be carefully monitored. Drugs that may convert atrial fibrillation to sinus rhythm are amiodarone and disopyramide. Digoxin is effective only for rate control at rest and should be used only as a second-line agent. This drug has been used less frequently with the advent of newer alternatives. Elective synchronized cardioversion is recommended if acute ischemic heart disease is present along with a rapid ventricular rate (120–200 beats per minute) or if the patient is in clinical distress. Always evaluate the patient for risk of atrial emboli before electrical shock.

Before cardioversion, the patient should undergo TEE to assess for the presence of mural thrombi. Successful cardioversion (in the absence of mural thrombi) and prevention of recurrence of atrial fibrillation depends on atrial size and the length of time in atrial fibrillation. In addition, valvular function should be assessed for further therapeutic interventions. Before electrical or pharmacological cardioversion is attempted, anticoagulants should be considered. Anticoagulation therapy should be initiated in all patients who remain in atrial fibrillation longer than 48 hours or who experience atrial fibrillation of unknown duration. Patients may be placed on IV heparin for rapid anticoagulation and started on warfarin (Coumadin), which takes approximately 5 days to achieve its full anticoagulant effect. A prothrombin time (PT) with international normalized ratio (INR) is drawn and the patient started on warfarin at 5 mg/day, with the dose adjusted according to the patient's INR. The target INR is between 2 and 3, and most patients require a maintenance dose of 2 to 7.5 mg/day. The PT should be checked at regular intervals to make sure the INR remains within the appropriate range. If the patient is hospitalized, these levels are usually monitored daily, but typically take 2 to 3 days to equilibrate in response to dosing changes. Once the patient is discharged, levels should be checked every week with the dosage adjusted accordingly, until the clinician has established the patient's individual response and optimal dose. Once a constant appropriate INR range has been established, PTs should be monitored monthly. Alternatives to warfarin may include dabigatran (Pradaxa), rivaroxaban (Xarelto), or apixaban (Eliquis). These agents are for the management of the patient with nonvalvular atrial fibrillation. Commonalities of these agents are shorter half-lives, fewer drug–drug interactions, and earlier peak blood levels compared with warfarin. Additionally, these newer agents do not necessitate dose titration or lab monitoring. Comparative studies suggest that with these agents, there is a 10% reduction in mortality, fewer strokes, and fewer systemic emboli. However, a disadvantage for these drugs is that there is not an established antidote for reversal. The clinician should try to maintain patients in chronic atrial fibrillation who are difficult to convert with a controlled ventricular rate and to keep them on anticoagulant therapy indefinitely. (See Table 10.9 for antithrombotic treatment options for stroke prevention in nonavalvular atrial fibrillation.) For patients refractory to the above therapies, ablation therapy is an option.

Premature Atrial Contractions

Treatment of PACs is not indicated unless patients are symptomatic or there are underlying causes that can be

Table 10.9 Antithrombotic Treatment Options for Stroke Prevention in Nonvalvular Atrial Fibrillation

Agent	Dosing	Implications for Nurse Practitioner Practice
Warfarin* (Coumadin)	Starting dose: 2–5 mg daily in the evening	Goal INR 2.0–3.0. Higher in mechanical valve patients. Antidote: Vitamin K
Dabigatran† (Pradaxa)	150 mg 2 times daily CrCl > 30 mg/mL 75 mg 2 times daily CrCl 15–30 Contraindicated if CrCl <15	Requires no lab monitoring. Do not cut, crush, or open pill. Antidote: None
Rivaroxaban† (Xarelto)	20 mg daily for CRCl > 50 mg/mL 5 mg daily for CrCl 15–49 mg/mL No dosing information if CrCl <15 mL/min	Requires no lab monitoring. If unable to swallow, pill may be crushed. No dosing if patient on dialysis Antidote: None
Apixaban† (Eliquis)	5 mg 2 times daily 2.5 mg 2 times daily with at least two of the following: age >80; body weight less than 60 kg; or creatinine >1.5 Contraindicated if CrCl <25 mL/min	Requires no lab monitoring. Antidote: None

*Pregnant women (with the exception of those who have mechanical heart valves) should not receive warfarin.
†These drugs should not be administered to those patients with prosthetic heart valves, hemodynamically significant valvular heart disease, severe kidney failure, and/or advanced liver disease.

corrected. Simple measures such as stopping tobacco use, reducing caffeine intake, and improving electrolyte imbalance may reduce the incidence of PACs. If symptoms persist, Holter monitoring may be indicated, and the patient should be instructed to maintain a diary of activities. The patient should be monitored for the first 3 months to establish whether this is an acute or a chronic condition. A cardiologist should follow the patient.

Supraventricular Tachycardia

The initial treatment for stable SVT consists of vagal maneuvers, such as carotid sinus pressure. Vagal maneuvers increase parasympathetic tone and slow conduction through the AV node. These techniques include coughing, lying on the floor while elevating legs against the wall, or squatting. If the clinician has the experience and knowledge of carotid sinus massage, this maneuver is usually effective. The vagal maneuver of carotid sinus massage is contraindicated in patients with carotid artery stenosis, bruits, or a history of transient ischemic attacks, or in patients older than age 65 years who may have an exacerbated parasympathetic response to carotid pressure. Facial immersion in cold water (dive reflex) is another method that has been used. The clinician must never use eyeball pressure as a vagal maneuver because it may cause retinal detachment and is unpleasant for the patient.

In the case of PSVT, adenosine is the treatment of choice; 6 mg in a peripheral IV is given rapidly. If treatment is unsuccessful, the dosage is increased to 12 mg and may be repeated once. Adenosine blocks the AV node and has an extremely short half-life of less than 10 seconds. Because of this short half-life, it is critical that this drug be delivered to the heart by a rapid IV push followed by a rapid saline flush. Adenosine does not usually cause a drop in BP and has replaced verapamil in the emergency treatment of PSVT. Verapamil hydrochlorate (verapamil HCl) may be used to treat tachyatrial arrhythmias and is given as a 2.5 to 5 mg IV bolus over 1 to 2 minutes; a second dose of 5 to 10 mg may be given IV 15 to 30 minutes after the first dose.

If the patient is symptomatic with atrial flutter, is hypotensive, has ischemic pain, or has severe CHF, synchronized cardioversion is usually recommended. Pharmacological intervention may involve beta blockers and calcium channel blockers along with digitalis. Patients who have recurrent symptomatic and refractory PSVT will need to see an electrophysiologist for possible radiofrequency ablation of the accessory pathway. Ablation therapy is often chosen over a lifetime course of prophylactic drugs.

Premature Ventricular Contractions

Treatment for PVCs is not usually needed in healthy adults because many adults experience PVCs with no untoward effects. If the patient is having PVCs related to an MI, however, it must be determined whether the PVCs are caused by a problem with oxygenation, hypotension, electrolyte or acid–base imbalance, other medications, or by an increased catecholamine state from unrelieved ischemic pain or anxiety. Typically, therapy in this case involves treating the underlying cause, such as the hypoxia, pain, electrolyte imbalance, or the alteration in hemodynamics with nitroglycerin, oxygen, pain medications, and beta blockers.

Heart Blocks

Treatment for a first-degree AV block is not advised because it is an asymptomatic arrhythmia. However, the clinician should assess and take note of the types of drugs that are being used that prolong AV conduction. For a Mobitz type I AV block, treatment is observational. If symptomatic bradycardia develops, a temporary or transcutaneous pacemaker may be needed, whereas a permanent pacemaker may be required for a Mobitz type II AV block. For third-degree heart block, the underlying pathological sites must be determined to prevent complications. The ability to determine whether this block has an idiojunctional response versus an idioventricular response is necessary for determining appropriate interventions. Third-degree heart block is considered an emergent and potentially life-threatening condition.

■ PREMATURE VENTRICULAR CONTRACTIONS AND VENTRICULAR TACHYCARDIA

Implantable cardioverter-defibrillator (ICD) devices are multiprogrammable antiarrhythmic devices capable of treating bradydysrhythmias, ventricular fibrillation, and ventricular tachycardia. These devices offer antitachycardia pacing as well as low- and high-energy shocks in multiple ranges of tachycardia rates. These devices are placed under the skin in the left chest. Patients need close follow up with a cardiologist and extensive patient education. Patients should carry a device identification card at all times. The American College of Cardiology/American Heart Association/North American Society of Pacing and Electrophysiology (ACC/AHA/NASPE) guidelines delineate indications for ICD therapy (http://content. onlinejacc.org/article.aspx?articleid=1357576).

Follow-up and Referral

A cardiologist should be consulted to establish the plan of care. The cardiologist may order a Holter monitor to establish if there is a routine pattern to the rhythm. Electrophysiological studies may be indicated to evaluate the patient for ablation therapy for PSVTs, such as WPW syndrome.

Patient Education

The education of a patient for atrial fibrillation should include a list of foods and prescription and OTC drugs that interfere with warfarin (Table 10.10). The patient on warfarin is at risk for bleeding; therefore, the clinician should provide literature on medical alert identification jewelry and instruct the patient how to assess for signs of bleeding, such as bruising and dark stools and to use electric razors and night lights. Patients should be taught to check their pulse rate. If the pulse rate is decreased (below 60 beats per minute) or the patient notices bursts in the rate, it should be reported to the clinician.

For patients being admitted to hospice care or on a withdrawal protocol, the clinician should consider de-activating the ICD/pacer.

■ VALVULAR DISORDERS AND MURMURS

Mitral and aortic valve disorders are the most common of the heart valve disorders. These disorders may be congenital or acquired and may be symptomatic or asymptomatic. Many are detected during heart auscultation when alterations in the normal heart rhythm, presence of extrasystoles, murmurs, and abnormal heart sounds are heard.

Heart murmurs are the sound of turbulent blood flow. Blood traveling through the chambers and great vessels is normally a silent event. When turbulence exists in the wall of the heart or a great vessel, a murmur occurs.

Murmurs may be benign, in that the clinician simply hears the blood flowing through the heart, but no cardiac structural abnormality exists. Certain cardiac structural problems, however, such as valvular and myocardial disorders, can contribute to the development of a murmur.

Benign systolic ejection murmurs such as physiological murmurs are found in the absence of cardiac pathology. The term implies that the reason for the murmur is something other than obstruction to flow and is present with a normal gradient across the valve. This murmur may be heard in up to 80% of thin adults or children if the cardiac exam is performed in a soundproof room; it is best heard at the left sternal border. It occurs in early to midsystole, leaving the two heart sounds intact. In addition, the patient with a benign systolic ejection murmur denies cardiac symptomatology and has an otherwise normal cardiac exam, including an appropriately located point of maximal impulse (PMI) and full pulses. No cardiac pathology is present with a

Table 10.10 Drugs and Foods That Interact With Warfarin (Coumadin)	
Increased Anticoagulant Effect	**Decreased Anticoagulant Effect**
Drugs	*Drugs*
acetaminophen (Tylenol)	carbamazepine (Tegretol)
allopurinol (Zyloprim)	cholestyramine (Questran)
amiodarone (Cordarone)	griseofulvin (Grifulvin)
cisapride (Propulsid)	oral contraceptives (Ortho TriCyclen, Loestrin)
cephalosporins (Keflex)	rifampin (Rifadin)
disulfiram (Antabuse)	spironolactone (Aldactone)
erythromycin (E-Mycin)	sucralfate (Carafate)
fluoroquinolones (Cipro, Levaquin)	
gemfibrozil (Lopid)	*Foods*
H_2-blockers (Pepcid, Zantac)	Chronic alcohol abuse
fluconazole (Diflucan)	
metronidazole (Flagyl)	
NSAIDs (Advil, Motrin)	
penicillins (Pen VK)	
propranolol (Inderal)	
quinidine (Quinaglute)	
selective serotonin reuptake inhibitors (SSRIs: sertraline [Zoloft], fluoxetine [Prozac])	
sulfonylureas (Glucotrol, Amaryl)	
tetracycline (Achromycin)	
trimethoprim-sulfamethoxazole (Bactrim)	
valproate (Depakene)	
Foods	
Excessive alcohol	
Vitamins A, C, E	

physiological murmur, so no endocarditis prophylaxis is needed.

A *hemic murmur* is heard in hyperkinetic or high-volume states such as anemia, fever, or response to exercise. The murmur is crescendo–decrescendo and harsh, and both heart sounds are preserved. Because there is no cardiac pathology associated with this condition, it resolves when its underlying cause is gone. As with a physiological murmur, no structural cardiac abnormality is present, and no endocarditis prophylaxis is needed.

An *aortic sclerosis murmur* is also called the 50/50 murmur because it is present in about 50% of adults older than age 50 years. Its etiology is likely fibrotic and/or calcific changes in the aortic valve. The valve can open enough to prevent a significant gradient but is restricted enough to cause the murmur. It differs from an aortic stenosis murmur in having an early peak and resolution, as well as lack of hemodynamic significance.

Types of Valvular Disorders

Aortic stenosis is the inability of the aortic valves to open to optimum orifice. The aortic valve normally opens to 3 cm^2; aortic stenosis usually does not cause significant symptoms until the valvular orifice is limited to 0.8 cm^2. The disease is characterized by a long symptom-free period, with rapid clinical deterioration at the onset of symptoms, including dyspnea, syncope, chest pain, and congestive heart failure. The clinician should look for a narrow pulse pressure on BP, a characteristic of severe aortic stenosis.

The murmur of *mitral regurgitation* (also referred to as mitral insufficiency) arises from mitral valve incompetency or the inability of the mitral valve to close properly. This allows a retrograde, "regurgant" flow from a high-pressure area (left ventricle) to an area of lower pressure (left atrium). Mitral regurgitation is most often caused by the degeneration of the mitral valve, most commonly by rheumatic fever, endocarditis, calcific annulus, rheumatic heart disease, ruptured chordae tendonae, or papillary muscle dysfunction. In mitral regurgitation from rheumatic heart disease, there is usually also some stenosis. Once the person is symptomatic, the disease progresses in a downhill course of heart failure over the next 10 years.

Mitral valve prolapse (MVP) is the most common valvular heart problem, with an incidence of 2.4% in the general population based on two-dimensional echocardiographic criteria. In most cases, MVP is a benign condition. However, MVP with mitral regurgitation may predispose the individual to thrombi and endocarditis. In the past, the prevalence of MVP was overestimated owing to lack of the availability of specific diagnostic procedures. Patients given this diagnosis more than 10 years ago may not have the disorder at all and should be reevaluated with two-dimensional echocardiography. (Table 10.11 presents the common valvular disorders.)

Epidemiology and Causes

Bacterial endocarditis, rheumatic heart disease, and aortic calcification are common etiologies of valvular disorders that cause heart murmurs. Bacterial endocarditis is most often due to septicemia caused by *Staphylococcus aureus* or *Streptococcus viridans* (alpha-hemolytic) infection. Valvular deformities are among a spectrum of abnormalities associated with endocarditis. IV drug abusers and patients with indwelling IV catheters are at risk for bacterial septicemia that can lead to endocarditis. Patients with prosthetic heart valves, heart murmurs, or valvular damage require prophylactic antibiotics to prevent endocarditis before any invasive procedures such as dental or surgical interventions.

Rheumatic heart disease is another cause of heart valve injury. Rheumatic heart disease is a result of rheumatic fever, an infection caused by group A beta-hemolytic *Streptococcus* infection. The pathological mechanism involves antibodies developed by the body against the bacteria. Antistreptococcal antibodies are thought to cross-react with the body's own tissues and "mistakenly" attack the heart valves in susceptible individuals. Because of the wide availability of antibiotics, rheumatic fever has become a less common etiology of valvular disease.

Calcification of the aortic valve is a common finding in elderly patients who present with the systolic murmur of aortic stenosis. A calcified aortic valve is often a result of long-standing arteriosclerosis. This calcification causes narrowing of the aortic valve resulting in an audible disturbance in blood flow through the valve.

In children and younger adults, aortic stenosis may also be present; it is usually caused by a congenital bicuspid (rather than tricuspid) valve or by a three-cusp valve with leaflet fusion. This defect is most often found in males and is commonly accompanied by a long-standing history of becoming excessively short of breath with increased activity such as running. The physical exam is usually normal except for the associated cardiac findings.

Mitral valve prolapse occurs in about 2% to 4% of the population and is usually detected in young adulthood. It is more common in women younger than age 20; the incidence is equal in men and women after age 20.

Pathophysiology

Normal heart valves allow one-way, unimpeded forward blood flow through the heart. The entire stroke output is able to pass freely during one phase of the cardiac cycle, and there is no backflow of blood. When a heart valve fails to open to its normal orifice, it is stenotic. When it fails to close appropriately, the valve is incompetent, causing regurgitation of blood to the previous

Table 10.11   Common Valvular Disorders

Disorder	Murmur Characteristics	Physical Exam	Diagnostic Findings
Aortic stenosis	Grade: 1–4/6, harsh systolic usually crescendo-decrescendo pattern. Heard best: Second right intercostal space (RICS), apex. Radiation: To carotids. Other: Softens with standing.	Cardiac: May have diminished S_2, slow-filling carotid pulse, narrow pulse pressure, loud S_4, heaving PMI. Other: Anxiety, difficulty breathing, compromised mental status, cyanosis, peripheral edema, hair loss, shiny skin over shins, cool extremities, decreased SBP, pulmonary edema.	Chest x-ray: Aortic valve calcification, left ventricle (LV) enlargement, prominent ascending aorta. ECG: LVH, sinus tachycardia, atrial fibrillation, AV conduction delay, left or right bundle branch block (LBBB, RBBB). Echocardiogram: Limited aortic valve movement, thickened left ventricular wall. Cardiac catheterization: Increased pressure gradient in systole across aortic valve, decreased size of aortic orifice, increased left ventricular end-diastolic pressure.
Aortic regurgitation	Grade: 1–3/4 high-pitched blowing diastolic murmur. Heard best: Third left intercostal space (LICS). Other: May be enhanced by forced expiration, leaning forward.	Cardiac: Usually with S_3 wide pulse pressure, sustained thrusting apical impulse, palpitations, dyspnea, orthopnea, paroxysmal nocturnal dyspnea (PND), syncope, signs of LV failure, peripheral edema, flushed skin, cardiomegaly. Other: More common in men, usually from rheumatic heart disease; occasionally caused by third-degree syphilis, fatigue, weakness, anxiety, compromised mental state. 16- next column is left ventricular end diastolic pressure	Chest x-ray: Aortic valve calcification, LV enlargement, dilation of ascending aorta. ECG: LVH, sinus tachycardia, PVCs. Echocardiogram: Dilated and hyperdynamic LV, enlargement of aortic root and LA, early closure of mitral valve, diastolic fluttering of aortic valve. Cardiac catheterization: Decreased aortic diastolic pressure, increased LVEDP, decreased regurgitant flow, reflux through aortic valve.
Aortic sclerosis	Grade: 2–3/6 systolic ejection murmur. Heard best: Second RIC. Other: "50 over 50" murmur (found in 50% of those over age 50). Grade: 1–3/4 low-pitched late diastolic murmur. Heard best: Apex. Radiation: Localized. Other: Short crescendo-decrescendo rumble, often with opening snap; enhanced by left lateral decubitus position, squat, cough; also immediately post–Valsalva maneuver.	Cardiac: Full carotid upstroke, no S_4. Cardiac: Accentuated S_1 in mitral area, atrial fibrillation, dyspnea, orthopnea, PND. Other: History of rheumatic fever; protracted latency period, then gradual decrease in exercise tolerance, fatigue, hoarseness, ruddy cheeks, peripheral edema, anorexia, enlarged liver, crackles, bloody productive cough.	Echocardiogram: Benign thickening and/or calcification of aortic valve leaflets. Cardiac catheterization: No change in valve pressure gradient. Chest x-ray: LA and RV enlargement, pulmonary venous congestion ECG: LAH, RVH, P-mitrale, prolonged notched P waves, atrial fibrillation. Echocardiogram: Thickened mitral valve with diminished movement of leaflets, left atrium (LA) and right ventricle (RV) enlargement. Cardiac catheterization: Increased pressure gradient across mitral valve, increased left atrium

Table 10.11	Common Valvular Disorders—cont'd		
Disorder	Murmur Characteristics	Physical Exam	Diagnostic Findings
			pressure (LAP) and pulmonary vascular resistance, increased LVEDP, increased PAWP, decreased CO.
Mitral stenosis	Grade: 1–4/6 high-pitched blowing systolic murmur, often extending beyond S_2. Heard best: Right lower sternal border (RLSB). Radiation: Radiates to axilla, often with laterally displaced PMI. Other: Sounds like a loon— "haa," "hoo." Decreased with standing Valsalva maneuver; increased by squat, hand grip.	Cardiac: History of ischemic heart disease, endocarditis, RHD (rheumatic heart disease), other valve abnormalities, dyspnea, orthopnea, PND, diaphoresis, cyanosis, jugular venous distention, peripheral edema. Other: Weakness, fatigue, anxiety, abdominal respirations, enlarged liver, crackles.	ECG: Atrial fibrillation, P mitrale (if patient is in sinus rhythm). Doppler echocardiogram: Detects and quantifies mitral regurgitation.
Mitral regurgitation	Grade: 1–3/6 late systolic crescendo murmur with honking quality. Heard best: Apex. Other: Follows midsystolic click; with Valsalva or standing, click moves forward into earlier systole resulting in a longer sounding murmur; with hand grasp, squat, click moves back further into systole, resulting in a shorter murmur.	Cardiac: Recurrent chest pain in the precordium and substernal areas, dyspnea, syncope. Other: Often seen with minor thoracic deformities (e.g., pectus excavatum, strait back, shallow anteroposterior diameter) or high arched palate, fatigue, light-headedness, migraine headache, exercise intolerance, anxiety, panic attacks; arm span often greater than height.	Chest x-ray: Normal. ECG: Normal. Two-dimensional echocardiogram: Demonstrates MVP.
Mitral valve prolapse	Grade: 1–3/6 ejection murmur. Heard best: Pulmonic area.	Cardiac: Widely split S_2 RV heave. Other: CHF, exertional dyspnea.	Auscultation: A split S_2 may be heard.
Atrial septal defect (uncorrected)	Grade: 1–3/6 ejection murmur. Heard best: Pulmonic area.	Cardiac: Widely split S_2 RV heave. Other: CHF, exertional dyspnea.	Auscultation: A split S_2 may be heard.

chamber or vessel. Both of these events place the patient at significant risk for embolic disease.

Clinical Presentation
Subjective

The patient may be asymptomatic or, depending on the specific problem, may complain of dyspnea, orthopnea, paroxysmal nocturnal dyspnea, fatigue, hoarseness, palpitations, weakness, chest pain, heart failure, vertigo, syncope, and peripheral edema. The patient may or may not know whether or not he or she has a heart murmur. (Table 10.11 lists the signs and symptoms of specific valvular disorders.)

Objective

When evaluating an adult with a cardiac murmur, the clinician should ask about major symptoms of heart disease, including chest pain, heart failure symptoms, palpitations, syncope, and activity intolerance. The bell of the stethoscope is most helpful for auscultating lower-pitched sounds, whereas the diaphragm is best used for hearing higher-pitched sounds. Systolic murmurs are graded on a 1 to 6 scale, from barely audible to audible with stethoscope off the chest (grades IV to VI must have a palpable thrill). Diastolic murmurs are usually graded on the same scale but are graded from 1 to 4 because these murmurs are not loud enough to reach grades 5 and 6. Advanced Assessment 10.3 gives more information about the cardiac examination, including assessing heart murmurs.

Diagnostic Reasoning
Diagnostic Tests

Initially, the clinician may discover a murmur on physical exam. Depending on the associated symptoms, the clinician may refer the patient for subsequent testing or may refer the patient directly to a cardiologist for more invasive testing. Two-dimensional echocardiography is the definitive procedure to diagnose heart valve disorders.

Various diagnostic tests used to detect valvular lesions or structural heart changes include echocardiography, ECG, chest x-ray film, and cardiac catheterization. The clinician usually should order an echocardiogram, ECG, and chest x-ray to confirm a definitive diagnosis of a murmur and then refer the patient to a cardiologist unless the clinician and patient agree on an initial course of therapy as a trial, such as in MVP. The ECG can reveal left ventricular hypertrophy (LVH). The chest x-ray may show an enlarged cardiac silhouette, left ventricular prominence, calcification of the aortic valve, and dilation and calcification of the ascending aorta. An echocardiogram is useful in demonstrating the underlying pathological process, whether the lesion involves the aortic root, or if valvular disease is present. Cardiac catheterizations can provide an accurate assessment of regurgitation and stenosis, along with left ventricular function and pulmonary artery pressures. Coronary angiography is often indicated to determine the presence of coronary artery disease before valve surgery.

Differential Diagnosis

The differential diagnoses for MVP include hypertrophic cardiomyopathies, papillary dysfunction, coronary artery spasm and/or disease, anxiety disorders, and congenital cardiac anomalies.

The differential diagnoses for mitral stenosis include atrial myxoma or vegetation caused by endocarditis,

---

Advanced Assessment 10.3 The Cardiac Exam and Assessment of Heart Murmurs

Area of Examination	Assess	Possible Clinical Correlation
Skin temperature	Variations from normal	Cool, moist skin may indicate a decrease in cardiac output Cool, dry skin may reflect environmental temperature or use of vasoconstricting substances such as sympathomimetics (caffeine, nicotine)
Skin color	Central cyanosis Peripheral cyanosis Palmar erythema Pallor	Poor blood oxygenation Excessive removal of oxygen from the blood Suggests liver impairment May be present in severe anemia (hemoglobin [Hgb] <8 g)
Pulse	Rate Rhythm Character and volume	Note presence of bradycardia, tachycardia Regular, irregular, regularly irregular (extrasystoles), irregularly irregular (likely atrial fibrillation) Normally full and rapidly filling
Blood pressure (BP)	Pulse pressure	Narrow pulse pressure may be found in volume depletion, aortic stenosis Wide pulse pressure may be found in aortic regurgitation
Point of maximum impulse (PMI)	Location	Normally located at fifth intercostal space (ICS) at midclavicular line With hypertrophy, PMI shifts laterally and may cover more than one ICS
Apical impulse	Sensation	Normally a gentle tapping sensation Forceful, thrusting seen with ventricular overload Diffuse, weak seen in cardiac hypertrophy Sustained in poorly controlled hypertension, aortic stenosis Double apex impulse in ventricular aneurysm

Advanced Assessment 10.3 The Cardiac Exam and Assessment of Heart Murmurs—cont'd

Area of Examination	Assess	Possible Clinical Correlation
Heart sounds	S$_1$ (normal heart sound)	Marks onset of systole, heard just before palpation of carotid artery High-pitched, click-like sound
	Variations from normal S$_1$	Unusually loud: mitral stenosis Unusually soft: In mitral stenosis, S$_1$ becomes softer as the valve calcifies and becomes more rigid and less mobile (mitral stenosis, mitral regurgitation) Abnormally wide split: delay in closure of tricuspid valve (RBBB)
	S$_2$ (normal heart sound)	Marks end of systole; vibration of aortic and pulmonic valve after closure
	Physiological split S$_2$	Occurs at end of systole Widest split at peak inspiration; may disappear with sitting, standing Normal finding in younger adult; usually disappears by middle-age
	Fixed split S$_2$	Occurs at end of systole No closure of split with position change; does not increase with inspiration Occurs with atrial septal defect, pulmonary stenosis
	Paradoxical split S$_2$ S$_3$ (third heart sound, ventricular gallop, protodiastolic gallop)	Occurs with coarctation of the aorta Likely produced by the rapidly filling ventricles at a point where ventricular filling slows or by a recoil of the heart as it is pushed against the chest Occurs in early diastole Heard best by the diaphragm; no change with respiration, although occasionally inspiration or expiration will increase its sound Found in disorders of systolic emptying, CHF, valvular heart disease, ischemic heart disease, hypertrophic cardiomyopathy
	S$_4$ (fourth heart sound, atrial gallop, presystolic gallop, S$_4$ gallop)	May be caused by the tug of the chordae and papillary muscles in the state of poor ventricular compliance Found in disorders of diastolic filling; poorly controlled hypertension, angina, ischemic heart disease

anemia, and thyrotoxicosis. For mitral regurgitation, the differential diagnoses include rheumatic or ischemic heart disease, MVP, infective endocarditis, mitral annular dilation or calcification, congenital valve deformities, cardiac trauma, and prosthetic mitral valve malfunction.

Management

The principle of management is to help the patient maintain a normal cardiac output, thus preventing manifestations of heart failure, venous congestion, and inadequate tissue perfusion. For an asymptomatic patient, no treatment is indicated. In recent years the recommendations for use of antibiotic prophylaxis before dental work has undergone revision and is more selective. For current guidelines pertaining to the use of prophylactic antibiotic therapy, the clinician is advised to refer to the ACC/AHA guidelines for the prevention of infective endocarditis (cited at end of Treatment Standards/Guidelines 10.1).

Mitral Valve Disorders

Mitral Valve Prolapse There is no medical treatment to correct MVP. Symptomatic management includes lifestyle changes, such as beginning a mild exercise program to reduce plasma catecholamines, lower the heart rate, decrease stress, and increase the cardiac output and blood volume. Beta blockers may be prescribed for patients with MVP to help control palpitations; however, because fatigue is a problem with this disorder, it may be exacerbated by beta blockers.

The clinician is referred to the most current guidelines available from the ACC/AHA regarding the use of antibiotic prophylaxis. Anticoagulation with aspirin

Treatment Standards/Guidelines 10.1   Infective Endocarditis Prophylaxis

The following are recommendations from the American Heart Association's guidelines regarding infective endocarditis (IE) antibiotic prophylaxis.

Only the people at greatest risk for or negative outcomes from IE should receive preventive antibiotics before routine dental or medical procedures, particularly if involving the gingival tissues or periapical region of a tooth and for those procedures that perforate the oral mucosa.

Antibiotic prophylaxis is recommended for high-risk patients with any of the following:

• Prosthetic heart valves
• Previous history of IE
• Complex cyanotic congenital heart disease (unrepaired or repaired)
• Cardiac valvulopathy in a transplanted heart
• Echocardiographic evidence of substantial leaflet pathology and regurgitation

Antibiotic prophylaxis is no longer indicated for common valvular lesions; however, clinicians should exercise judgment in selecting the dose and duration of antibiotics in individual cases or special circumstances.

Good oral hygiene is considered to be an important factor in preventing IE.

Endocarditis Prophylaxis (30–60 minutes before dental procedure)

If no penicillin allergy: Amoxicillin oral: Adults 2 g; children 50 mg/kg
Unable to take oral: Ampicillin IM or IV: Adults 2 g; children 50 mg/kg
OR
Cefazolin or ceftriaxone IM or IV: Adults 1 g; children 50 mg/kg
If penicillin/ampicillin allergic:
Cephalexin* oral: Adults 2 g; children 50 mg/kg
OR
Clindamycin oral: Adults 600 mg; children 20 mg/kg
OR
Azithromycin or clarithromycin oral: Adults 500 mg; children 15 mg/kg
If penicillin/ampicillin allergic and unable to take oral medication:
Cefazolin or ceftriaxone IM or IV: Adults 1 g; children 50 mg/kg
OR
Clindamycin IM or IV: Adults 600 mg; children 20 mg/kg

*Cephalosporins should not be used in persons with a history of anaphylaxis, angioedema, or urticaria with penicillins or ampicillin.
    Source: Allen, U. Infective endocarditis: Updated guidelines. *Can J Infect Dis Med Microbiol* 21(2):74–77, 2010.

(81–325 mg/day) is prescribed for some individuals with MVP who also have had a history of TIA, ischemic stroke, or atrial fibrillation.

Persons with MVP and severe mitral regurgitation should be followed with stress echocardiography periodically. Surgical intervention is indicated for MVP with severe mitral valve regurgitation.

Mitral Stenosis   For symptomatic mitral stenosis, diuretics and sodium restriction should be initiated to reduce the blood volume and pulmonary and systemic venous pressures, along with anticoagulation therapy with warfarin if there is a history of systemic embolism, atrial fibrillation, or a large left atrium. If the patient is in atrial fibrillation, the antiarrhythmic amiodarone or the calcium channel blocker diltiazem may be prescribed and are replacing the use of digitalis. Surgical intervention may be required for some patients; it may include mitral commissurotomy, balloon valvuloplasty, or mitral valve replacement.

Mitral Regurgitation   For a symptomatic patient with mitral regurgitation, vasodilators should be initiated to reduce ventricular filling volume and to decrease systemic vascular resistance. Diltiazem and anticoagulants should be prescribed to control the ventricular rate and decrease the embolic complications if the patient has atrial fibrillation. Sodium restriction and diuretics will relieve symptoms of heart failure if they are present in patients with mitral regurgitation. A mitral valve replacement may be required.

Aortic Valve Disorders

Aortic Stenosis   Aortic valve replacement or aortic commissurotomy may be required for aortic stenosis.
Aortic Regurgitation   For the patient with symptomatic aortic regurgitation, digitalis and diuretics can be used to treat the symptoms of heart failure; arterial vasodilators will reduce the left ventricular afterload. Aortic valve replacement may be required.

Follow-up and Referral

The clinician should follow the patient at regular intervals for close monitoring, as well as whenever a new drug has been added or a dosage changed. The patient should be referred to the collaborating physician or cardiologist when the diagnosis is unconfirmed or when the symptoms are not well managed with medical therapy.

Patient Education

Valvular heart disorders require lifelong management. Patients may benefit from maintaining a diary to monitor the effectiveness of lifestyle changes and compliance with drug therapy in controlling symptoms of the disorder. Patients with MVP should be instructed to begin a gradual program of exercise and to avoid caffeine, decongestants, and products containing ephedrine, alcohol, chocolate, and cheeses. They should be encouraged to drink at least eight glasses of water a day to prevent dehydration. Patients with aortic stenosis often require activity restrictions. The patient should understand how to pace activity, note an improvement in fatigue, and accept the activity restrictions.

A critical part of the evaluation of a person with a heart murmur is the decision to offer antimicrobial prophylaxis. No prophylaxis is needed with benign murmurs. Treatment Standards/Guidelines 10.1 presents the treatment guidelines for bacterial endocarditis prophylaxis.

■ PERIPHERAL ARTERY DISEASE

Peripheral artery disease (PAD) is an occlusive disorder of the arteries, which most commonly affects the lower extremities. PAD is most commonly the result of occlusive atherosclerotic plaques that impede blood flow to the peripheral vasculature. The resulting arterial insufficiency most commonly manifests itself in the form of lower extremity *claudication*—cramping pain triggered or exacerbated by exertion and relieved by rest. Although atherosclerosis is the most common etiology of arterial insufficiency, several other disorders may precipitate lower extremity ischemia, including vasculitis, radiation exposure, dissection, and aneurysm.

Epidemiology and Causes

Peripheral artery disease is caused by atherosclerosis, blood clots, trauma, spasms of smooth muscles in the arterial walls, and congenital structural defects in the arteries. Approximately 8 million people have PAD, and its most common symptom is intermittent claudication. In patients older than age 70, 20% suffer from PAD. The 5-year mortality rate for PAD approaches 30% as patients die from comorbid conditions of CAD and cerebrovascular disease. PAD is more common in men than women and nine times more common in smokers. (See Risk Factors Box 10.2.)

Pathophysiology

Atherosclerosis is the most common cause of arterial insufficiency of the lower extremity, also referred to as PAD. Arteriosclerotic plaque obstructs optimal arterial blood flow to the muscles of the lower extremity. With increased muscle activity, there is an increased need for arterial blood flow. For this reason, during ambulation or exercise, limitations of arterial blood flow cause muscle pain due to ischemia. This cramping muscle pain is referred to as *intermittent claudication* because in the initial stages of PAD, ischemia occurs periodically.

Risk Factors 10.2   Risk Factors for Peripheral Vascular Disease (PVD)

Peripheral Vascular Disease	
Arterial Risk Factors (Peripheral Arterial Disease)	Smoking: Vasoconstriction/spasm-decreased circulation Obesity: Increased cardiac workload Inactivity: Decreased circulation Hypertension: Increased fibrous tissue, which decreases stretch of arterial walls, which increases peripheral vascular resistance High cholesterol: Atherosclerotic plaque, which increases hyperlipidemia Diabetes: Increase in atherosclerosis of smaller vessels
Venous Risk Factors	Coagulation abnormalities Abdominal/pelvic surgery: Venous pooling/stasis Estrogen/oral contraceptives Pregnancy: Venous congestion Obesity: Increased cardiac workload, venous pooling Heart disease: Venous stasis Advanced neoplasm: Coagulation abnormalities; interference with venous blood flow

Muscle activity of the lower extremity requires increased circulation and arterial vasodilation. PAD causes lack of arterial vasodilatory ability. Thus, as PAD worsens, arterial circulation diminishes, and less muscle activity causes pain due to worsening ischemia. Eventually pain at rest occurs, which is a sign of severe PAD. In general, the clinical manifestations of PAD are extremity pain (claudication), weak pulse, pallor, paresthesias, and palpable coolness of the lower extremity. Long-standing PAD causes muscle atrophy, diminished hair growth, and discolored, hardened toenails of the extremity. All of these signs and symptoms are due to lack of arterial blood supply to the lower extremities. Early recognition of the signs of PAD and treatment are critical because severe ischemia can lead to the need for amputation.

Arteriosclerotic plaque formation within the lower extremities is accelerated by the presence of diabetes mellitus; therefore, PAD is more common in persons with diabetes. Hyperglycemia in diabetes causes endothelial injury, damaging arterial vessels. Clinical manifestations of arterial insufficiency are apparent in the lower extremities of individuals with diabetes. Many suffer the complications of diminished circulation of the legs, which include poor wound healing and peripheral neuropathy. The smaller caliber arterial vessels of the most distal regions of the lower extremity are initially affected. Therefore, careful periodic physical assessment of the feet and lower extremities is recommended in persons with diabetes, inspecting for poor wound healing and diminished peripheral pulses.

Aneurysms, another manifestation of arterial PVD, result from weakening in arterial walls, which renders them susceptible to rupture. The most common cause of this weakening is arteriosclerosis. Aneurysms appear as bulges in the arterial wall and are classified according to location. The aorta and cerebral arteries are the most common sites of aneurysms. In the aorta, a dissecting aneurysm, which is an incomplete tear in the vascular wall, may occur when elevated blood pressure (BP) leads to separation of the layers of aortic tissue.

Arteritis, a form of vasculitis, involves inflammation of arterial blood vessels. Inflammation decreases the vasodilatory capacity of arteries and may cause spasm of the arteries. This condition is often associated with autoimmune disease. *Raynaud's phenomenon* is a result of cold-induced vasospasm of the small blood vessels in the fingers and toes, causing a characteristic blanching that sometimes extends to the hands or feet. A tricolor change may also be stimulated, which appears first as blanching of the finger tips and toes, followed by cyanosis and rubor (redness).

Clinical Presentation

Subjective

The patient with PAD will usually present with intermittent leg pain (intermittent claudication) that increases in severity with exertion. The location of the lower extremity pain depends on where the occlusion is located. Aortoiliac occlusions typically produce claudication of the thigh and buttock, whereas occlusions of the femoral artery produce pain in the upper calf. The pain is described as severe, "grabbing," and cramplike. The pain lasts minutes (at most) and is relieved by rest and does not reoccur until the patient walks the same distance again. Pain at rest frequently signifies severe PAD. The patient usually denies swelling, pain at night, or color or temperature changes. The patient may also complain of thick toenails with corn-like material under the nails. Eventually, the lower legs and ankles may assume a purple-black color characteristic of cyanosis and gangrene.

Objective

Taking a thorough history distinguishes the cause of leg pain in more than 90% of patients. Assessing the risk factors assists in the diagnosis. The next step should be to determine the rapidity of onset of symptoms. PAD must be differentiated from a limb-threatened state that may need immediate treatment. If the onset of claudication has been gradual, this is more consistent with the progressive obliteration of the lower extremity vessels and the formation of collateral circulation, as seen with PAD, rather than an acute event such as an embolus from the heart or a proximal abdominal aortic aneurysm.

The clinician should evaluate the cervical, radial, ulnar, brachial, femoral, popliteal, dorsalis pedis, and posterior tibial pulses bilaterally. A consistent grading system should be used. Usually 0 refers to an absent pulse, 1+ a diminished pulse, 2+ normal, and 3+ bounding. The clinician should keep in mind that about 10% of the population has absent pedal pulses. Because a bruit indicates turbulence and possible atherosclerotic narrowing, the following pulse sites should be assessed using the diaphragm of a stethoscope: cervical, supraclavicular, abdominal, flank, and inguinal areas.

To differentiate chronic venous insufficiency from PAD, the clinician should raise the patient's legs for several minutes. When the legs are dependent again, the patient with PAD will have pale, dusky red (rubor) extremities and the patient with chronic venous insufficiency will have improved color in the extremities. Circulatory checks should be done to assess for acute arterial ischemia. The six P's of PAD are pain, pulselessness, paresthesia, paralysis, poikilothermia (coolness), and pallor. The clinician should do a sensory examination to rule out peripheral neuropathy associated with ischemia in patients with diabetes.

With PAD, the clinician may observe decreased or absent peripheral extremity pulses. The affected leg may be smaller in size as a result of muscular atrophy. The clinician will note thinning of the skin, loss of hair over the affected area, and possible leg ulcers. The extremity may be cool and pale, and the toenails will be thickened.

The patient will have a history of delayed wound healing. When the extremity is dependent, it will appear reddish blue in color.

Diagnostic Reasoning
Diagnostic Tests

If arterial insufficiency is suspected and the pulses are absent, a Doppler flow study should be performed, which can quantify the degree of the ischemia. Part of the Doppler flow study includes calculating an ankle-brachial index (ABI), which involves a comparison of arm BP to the ankle pressures, using a BP cuff and a Doppler. The normal ratio of ankle to brachial pressure is more than 0.9. An ABI reading of 0.6 to 0.9 indicates moderate level of disease, and levels less than 0.5 indicate severe ischemia. Although an arteriogram is not usually ordered as a diagnostic tool, it should be obtained preoperatively, after the patient has been assessed by a vascular surgeon.

Additional assessment tools and diagnostic procedures for PAD also include a walking impairment questionnaire (WIQ), treadmill exercise testing, lipid profile, and magnetic resonance angiogram. The WIQ is used to assess the ability of patients to walk defined distances at certain speeds and to climb stairs.

Differential Diagnosis

Differential diagnoses for PAD may include chronic venous insufficiency, thrombosis, phlebitis, polycythemia, anemia, Raynaud's disease, vasculitis such as Buerger's disease, aneurysms, and peripheral neuropathy.

Management

Treatment for PAD is aimed at improving blood flow by removing or lessening the cause of impaired circulation. Because the condition is usually chronic and irreversible, treatment involves education and lifestyle changes.

Patients with PAD should be counseled about modification of risk factors, and hypertension and diabetes should be aggressively managed. The clinician should encourage the patient to walk at least 30 minutes three to four times per week. Any ulcers or traumatic lesions to the extremities will need immediate care. The patient should be encouraged to keep the legs dependent (below the level of the heart) to improve blood flow and, therefore, oxygenation in the extremities. Tight bandages and stockings should be avoided.

Although drug therapy is not a substitute for exercise, some medications have been helpful in extending ambulation distances for more than 25% of patients.

Patients with PAD should be started on antiplatelet therapy with aspirin, or if they cannot tolerate aspirin, clopidogrel. These antiplatelet agents do not provide a measurable improvement in symptoms of claudication but are prescribed to reduce the risk of concomitant atherosclerotic disease such myocardial infarction and stroke. Current ACC/AHA guidelines recommend pentoxifylline as a second-line drug to cilostazol for the treatment of claudication. Cilostazol is a phosphodiesterase-3 inhibitor that causes vasodilation and in addition inhibits platelet aggregation. Cilostazol may be ordered specifically to treat leg pain and cramping due to the blockages from atherosclerosis in the leg arteries. Head-to-head trials have demonstrated that cilostazol is more effective at reducing symptoms of claudication compared with pentoxifylline because the former lengthens the pain-free walking distance for patients with claudication. Cilostazol should not be prescribed in the presence of any degree of heart failure because this is a contraindication to its use.

Most patients with moderate PAD can be effectively managed with medical therapy and risk modification alone. Surgical intervention and angioplasty are used selectively in patients with severe PAD. Indications for surgical or percutaneous revascularization include profound functional and occupational limitation due to claudication, disease refractory to pharmacological therapy, and limb-threatening critical ischemia. Patients must be able to demonstrate improvement in their symptoms on revascularization and not be severely disabled by other comorbid conditions (e.g., severe pulmonary disease, heart failure, coronary artery disease) that may render revascularization futile.

Follow-up and Referral

All patients with peripheral artery disease should be followed at least every 3 months to assess the effectiveness of lifestyle changes, skin care, and management of ulcers. If ulcers are present, the patient may need to be seen on a weekly basis. Patients with PAD may be referred to a vascular surgeon for evaluation and potential surgery, including a balloon angioplasty in the distal extremity or an arterial graft using a section of the great saphenous vein or a synthetic graft.

Patient Education

Patients who have been diagnosed with PAD should be counseled about the modification of risk factors. They should totally abstain from nicotine. It is essential to control hypertension and diabetes if present. Dietary control must include limitation of fat and salt intake. Patients must be taught to do meticulous daily foot care that includes inspecting feet daily for sores, ulcers, and abrasions, including the use of a mirror to check the soles of the feet. Patients should not walk barefoot and should wear well-fitting supportive shoes. They should not soak their feet and should be careful trimming their nails. All patients should be taught to watch for the signs and symptoms that might indicate progressive ischemia, such as increased pain, increased pallor or cyanosis, and rest pain.

Patients with PAD should be encouraged to perform Buerger-Allen exercises three to four times per day. The clinician should teach the patient to raise and lower the extremities, with each of five repetitions taking about 2 minutes. The legs should be raised to a 45-degree angle, and then lowered again to the supine position. The changes in position cause the veins of the legs to refill by gravity.

Additionally, exercise therapy is recommended for peripheral artery disease because it stimulates collateral vessel growth in the lower extremities. Patients should be encouraged to walk distances until moderate pain occurs, stop until pain subsides, and then resume walking. A supervised treadmill walking program three times a week over a 6-month period is part of cardiovascular rehabilitation. Treadmill grade and speed are gradually increased over time as the patient improves.

DEEP VEIN THROMBOSIS/ CHRONIC VENOUS INSUFFICIENCY

Deep vein thrombosis (DVT) is a disorder of the venous system characterized by clot formation in the deep vessels of the venous vasculature. DVT primarily results as a complication associated with Virchow's triad—venous stasis, endothelial injury, and hypercoagulable state. The resulting thrombus formation may lead to a variety of complications including chronic venous insufficiency and, most notably, pulmonary embolism (PE). Pulmonary embolism is a potentially life-threatening complication of DVT in which venous thrombi propagate to the pulmonary vasculature resulting in respiratory compromise. Chronic venous insufficiency is a disorder characterized by valvular incompetence, which manifests as lower extremity edema, skin discoloration, and ulceration as a result of poor antegrade venous flow. Although the condition is commonly a complication of DVT, it may be the result of inflammatory conditions such as phlebitis or anatomical disturbances.

Epidemiology and Causes

Chronic venous insufficiency and varicose veins usually result from venous incompetence secondary to valvular dysfunction. More than 20% of the population is affected with chronic venous insufficiency; the incidence increases with age with no evident ethnic predisposition. Chronic venous insufficiency is more common in women than men. DVT and PE are complications encountered during the treatment of medical and surgical patients. Risk Factors Box 10.3 presents risk factors for DVT. Approximately 300,000 to 600,000 hospitalizations can be associated with DVT and PE each year. Up to 50,000 deaths occur annually because of PE. It is estimated that there are more than 2 million cases per year of DVT. The actual number of cases is often underdiagnosed due to the silent nature of the problem.

Patients undergoing various types of surgical procedures, such as orthopedic, gynecological-obstetric,

Risk Factors 10.3 Risk Factors for Deep Vein Thrombosis (DVT)

Virchow's Triad	Clinical Risk Factors for DVT
Venous Stasis	Immobility
	Venous insufficiency
	Prolonged sedentary position
	Post-stroke
	Post–myocardial infarction
	Heart failure
Vessel Injury	Trauma
	Surgery (especially orthopedic)
	Indwelling IV catheters
Hypercoagulability	High estrogen states (oral contraceptives or hormone replacement therapy)
	Pregnancy/postpartum period
	Cancer
	Inherited coagulation abnormalities

Source: Teri Capriotti, DO, MSN, CRNP.

urological, neurosurgical, and general surgical procedures, are at high risk for developing DVT and PE. Of these groups, orthopedic patients appear to be especially prone to thrombosis, particularly patients with hip fracture. All elective orthopedic surgical patients undergoing lower extremity surgery are at risk for DVT. The risk is greatest for patients undergoing hip surgery and knee reconstruction, for which DVT rates range from 45% to 70%.

Patients with various types of medical diseases, usually chronic, are also at a high risk for venous thrombotic events. The risk of DVT in pregnancy has been reported to be five times higher than in nonpregnant patients in the same age-group and may be increased postpartum. A silent DVT may cause a postphlebitic syndrome. The postphlebitic syndrome is characterized by swelling and pain in an extremity that was previously affected by thrombophlebitis. A frequent complication of DVT is PE, which can obstruct blood flow to the lungs and cause significant morbidity. The mortality of PE is estimated to be approximately 30%, although with the availability of newer diagnostic tools such as computed tomography angiogram, which can detect smaller peripheral emboli, it is estimated that the actual mortality rate of PE is about 10%. More than 80% of patients who died from a pulmonary embolism showed DVT on autopsy.

Pathophysiology

Clots can originate anywhere in the venous system, but the majority begin in the deep veins of the pelvis and lower extremities, with a significant number at or above the popliteal vein. Clots that originate in the proximal veins are potentially more dangerous because they are larger in size and result in more clinically significant thromboembolic events.

The causative factors in the formation of blood clots are referred to as *Virchow's triad* (see Risk Factors Box 10.3). Clots are likely to form when two of the three factors in the triad—stasis, vessel wall damage, and coagulation changes—are altered. Stasis of blood may result from immobility, edema, or anesthesia; blood tends to coagulate in and around the valve cusps of the veins, thus increasing the likelihood of clot formation. Vessel wall damage may result from trauma, surgical incision, laceration, venous wall distention from immobility or anesthesia, or a previous DVT. Coagulation changes leading to activated coagulation factors as a result of damaged endothelium may be the result of surgery, trauma, injury, disease states (such as sepsis, infection, or cancer), pregnancy, or foreign substance invasion via IV lines or catheters. The damaged endothelium causes the local activation of coagulation factors as platelets come in contact with the exposed collagen found in connective tissue, including skin, bone, ligaments, and cartilage. The platelets release substances that cause vasoconstriction and accelerate clotting.

Once formed, a DVT can propagate, embolize, or lyse. When the clot propagates, it extends proximally and becomes larger and thus more dangerous, by obstructing blood flow, which causes the vein to dilate and the vessel wall to be damaged. When a clot embolizes, it travels; it may lodge itself in the arteries of the lungs, resulting in PE. When a clot lyses, it breaks down. Even if a clot lyses, it can still cause irreversible valve damage by allowing blood to reflux in the veins. The damage sets up a cycle of pooling and hypertension known as the postphlebitic syndrome. Patients with this syndrome experience chronic pain, swelling, and venous ulcers.

Deep venous thrombophlebitis/thromboembolism is a critical disorder of the veins of the lower extremity. The presence of a thrombus within a deep vein with an accompanying inflammatory response is termed *deep venous thrombophlebitis or deep venous thrombosis*. If the thrombus breaks away from the wall of the vein and travels upward toward the heart, it is termed a *venous thromboembolism*. Common causes of hypercoagulability are estrogen use, pregnancy, and neoplasms. Venous stasis occurs most often as a result of immobility. Vascular injury can be due to surgery or trauma. Orthopedic surgery is a major risk factor for DVT, and there is a high incidence of concurrent DVT in persons with cancer of the pancreas, lungs, breast, genitourinary tract, and stomach.

The signs of DVT may be subtle. Overt signs of DVT may include tenderness and a palpable cord along the course of a vein, although more often than not the only sign is a unilateral swelling of an extremity with or without signs of inflammation. The most common complaint is calf pain. Although used in the past, a positive *Homans' sign* (pain on dorsiflexion of the foot) is now considered an unreliable diagnostic indicator.

PE is a potential complication of DVT. The venous thrombus may break free from the venous wall and travel from the lower extremity to the inferior vena cava and up to the right atrium, right ventricle, and into the pulmonary arterial circulation. This may cut off blood flow to an entire lung segment, resulting in potentially fatal ventilation/perfusion (VQ) mismatch. In addition, any abnormal communication between the right and left chambers of the heart (e.g., atrial septal defect, patent foramen ovale, ventricular septal defect) creates the potential for cerebral thromboembolism (i.e., cerebrovascular accident or stroke).

It is critical to diagnose DVT early because the complication of PE can be life-threatening. A PE is a thrombus that obstructs circulation within the lungs, causing lack of oxygenation of blood. Signs of pulmonary embolism can be subtle or severe depending on the size of the embolus. Sudden death can result from pulmonary embolism and may not be heralded by clearly observable signs of DVT.

Chronic venous insufficiency is a disorder of the valves within the deep veins of the lower extremities. Valves within veins assist venous blood to flow upward toward the heart, regulating unidirectional flow by preventing retrograde flow of venous blood away from the heart. Weakened venous valves do not form tight closures, failing to prevent retrograde blood flow. The appearance of superficial varicose veins may be associated with chronic venous insufficiency. Superficial varicose veins are benign in most cases and are treatable with conservative measures. However, under more severe circumstances, venous stasis results, as excess pressure builds up in the legs, causing distention of the veins, thinning and scaling of the skin with dusky discoloration (stasis dermatitis), and eventually large venous ulcers. In addition, dependent edema and poor wound healing result.

Clinical Presentation

Subjective

Although many lower extremity thrombi are silent, the patient may present with a complaint of pain in the calf muscle, slight swelling, or muscle tenderness.

The patient with chronic venous insufficiency will complain of dependent edema, venous engorgement (varicose veins), and localized pain. The patient may complain of a darkened color in the lower extremities, along with dryness and scaling of the skin.

Objective

In patients with DVT, the clinician may note slight swelling, muscle tenderness, and pain in the calf muscle. The clinician may assess for warmth or heat of the affected extremity and note distention of the superficial veins. A slight fever and tachycardia may also be present. An acute DVT in the femoral or iliac veins may show symptoms of tenderness over the veins, swelling, and a slightly bluish skin color.

In patients with chronic venous insufficiency, the clinician may note a brownish hyperpigmentation of the extremities, edema, subcutaneous fibrosis, and possibly leg ulcers. When the clinician elevates the extremity, the sharp, deep muscle pain may be lessened. The peripheral pulses may be normal or diminished. There may be superficial ulcers around the medial malleolus.

Diagnostic Reasoning

Diagnostic Tests

If a diagnosis of DVT is suspected, the clinician should first assess the clinical pretest probability of thrombosis. This may be done using a clinical probability assessment model such as the Well's criteria. Further diagnostic work-up is contingent on the patient's clinical likelihood of DVT. If the patient is determined to have a low clinical probability of DVT, a D-dimer level may be ordered. In patients with an intermediate or high clinical probability of DVT, a Doppler ultrasound of the lower extremity should be obtained in order to confirm the diagnosis.

If the results of the ultrasound are inconclusive and the clinical suspicion for DVT is high, an ascending venogram may confirm the diagnosis. The ascending venogram has long been considered the "gold standard" for diagnosis of venous thromboembolism, although if an ultrasound confirms the diagnosis, usually no further testing is done. An ascending venogram is performed by injecting a contrast material into a vein in the foot. Sequential x-ray films are taken that may show abnormalities such as vein-filling defect, formation of collateral veins, or abrupt termination of the contrast material along the vein. One risk of the ascending venogram, however, is an actual DVT because the invasive nature of the procedure may actually cause the thrombus to release.

Magnetic resonance imaging (MRI) is an alternative to a venogram. MRI is expensive and should be reserved for those who cannot tolerate the IV dye needed for a venogram. Venous ultrasound and venogram are more cost effective. If pulmonary embolus is suspected, a VQ scan or a spiral CT of the pulmonary artery would be indicated.

The D-dimer assay can be helpful in ruling out, but not definitively confirming, the diagnosis of DVT. D-dimer is a breakdown product of fibrin and is positive in venous thrombosis and PE. However, the D-dimer assay has low specificity and cannot be solely relied on for diagnosis. If a D-dimer is present, it does not prove a DVT exists, because many conditions cause a positive result. However, if the D-dimer is negative, it effectively rules out the presence of DVT.

To confirm venous insufficiency if the history and physical exam are inconclusive, a venogram may be performed. This is a radiological test in which the vein is injected with a radiopaque dye. Sequential films will show the engorged and tortuous veins. In addition, plethysmography may be done to determine the changes in the fluid volume of the extremities. The air-cuff plethysmography measures the changes in the circumference of a limb by recording the changes in pressure in an air-filled cuff surrounding the extremity. This test is rarely done because the history, physical exam, and other tests are usually adequate to confirm the diagnosis.

Differential Diagnosis

Patients with chronic venous insufficiency may exhibit some of the symptoms of DVT. Patients who suffer from chronic venous insufficiency have swelling and dilated superficial veins. They may also complain of aching or fatigue in the legs while standing or walking. Other differential diagnoses for DVT include cellulitis, lymphedema, and a strained muscle.

Management

Chronic Venous Insufficiency

For the patient with chronic venous insufficiency, conservative treatment is effective in alleviating symptoms in 85% of patients. The dependent edema can be a guide to the effectiveness of therapy. The clinician should order light exercise, support or compression stockings, and weight loss and should stress the need to elevate the legs several times each day for approximately 30 minutes. Subsequent management involves aggressively treating any ulcers and reducing factors that cause atherosclerosis.

Deep Vein Thrombosis

Pharmaceutical modalities prevent coagulation changes in the blood that result in clot formation or prevent extension of the clot. Low-dose fractionated or unfractionated heparin, administered subcutaneously, is considered the mainstay of therapy for DVT. Some potential complications of low-dose heparin therapy include bleeding, wound hematoma, and thrombocytopenia. Low-dose heparin therapy is contraindicated for neurosurgical procedures, especially intracranial procedures.

Patients with DVT can be treated in an inpatient or outpatient setting (for an otherwise healthy patient with no significant comorbidities). In the hospital, patients are treated aggressively with anticoagulant therapy, IV unfractionated heparin, or low molecular weight heparin (LMWH) and monitored for signs of further thrombosis or iatrogenic bleeding. An initial IV bolus of heparin (5,000–10,000 units IV) should be followed by a continuous infusion at 1,000 units per hour. The dosage of heparin should be adjusted according to the partial thromboplastin time (PTT). The goal is to achieve a PTT of two times the control value. Alternatively, LMWH can be used as inpatient or outpatient management of DVT until warfarin is at a therapeutic level. Candidates for outpatient heparin therapy must have a supportive environment, be hemodynamically stable, be without renal failure, and not be at high risk for bleeding. Enoxaparin (Lovenox), dalteparin (Fragmin), and tinzaparin (Innohep) are examples of types of LMWH. LMWH can be administered subcutaneously once or twice daily. Lovenox may be used at 1 mg/kg injected subcutaneously every 12 hours. In this case, PTT need not be followed, although factor Xa levels may be measured to assess for therapeutic response to confirm the appropriateness of the dose. The side effect of thrombocytopenia is less likely, and less laboratory testing is required. Simultaneous initiation of warfarin and LMWH has not shown any adverse effects.

Only unfractionated heparin is readily reversible after several hours, once the IV drip is turned off. Subcutaneously injected LMWHs, on the other hand, will exert their effect for at least 12 hours after each dose. Warfarin therapy should be initiated after the patient has been on heparin for 1 to 5 days although the trend now is to start warfarin soon after heparin. Warfarin should be started at 5 to 10 mg orally daily, with the dose adjusted to the PT and INR, as stated previously.

If anticoagulant therapy is contraindicated, filtering devices such as a vena-cava filter may be used to trap emboli before they reach the lungs and cause a PE. Inferior vena caval filters are mechanical barriers that are inserted in the large vena cava under percutaneous radiological guidance. Although they do not prevent clot formation, they prevent clot migration from the legs to the lungs.

High-risk patients should also have nonpharmacological prophylaxis with intermittent pneumatic compression for at least the first 5 days of therapy. External pneumatic compression and gradient compression stockings are effective alternatives for decreasing lower leg thrombosis if lower extremity trauma does not preclude their use. Patients should also elevate the affected limb, apply heat, and limit activity.

Thrombolysis is not indicated for DVT except in cases of massive ileofemoral thrombus. Thrombolytic agents are indicated for patients with massive PE and associated hemodynamic instability. The role of thrombolysis in patients with lesser size PEs is controversial.

Follow-up and Referral

Most patients with acute DVT are hospitalized for about 1 week. Follow-up therapy for these patients includes anticoagulant therapy for 6 months after an initial episode of DVT and for 1 year after each subsequent episode. The clinician will follow the patient after he or she is released from the hospital. The patient on warfarin must be seen daily until the target INR range is achieved (usually in the hospital), then on a monthly basis thereafter.

Patient Education

Patients should be educated about DVT and treated prophylactically, depending on the number of risk factors exhibited and the resulting need for hospitalization or surgery. To prevent DVT, prophylactic modalities should be used for all patients at risk, including pharmacological, physical or mechanical, or a combination of the two.

Physical modalities that prevent DVT by reducing stasis include leg elevation, passive leg exercises, and early ambulation. Although these techniques are somewhat effective, each has some drawbacks and should be combined with other physical measures such as graduated elastic compression or external pneumatic compression devices. Graduated compression stockings provide safe, simple, and inexpensive prophylaxis. Besides preventing stasis, they also prevent venous distention, which potentially initiates vessel wall damage. Pneumatic compression devices are more effective at emptying the veins, sustaining femoral blood flow velocity, and expelling the blood from behind the valve cusps in the femoral vein, thus stimulating fibrinolysis.

Education for patients recovering from DVT includes teaching about the need to avoid trauma to the affected veins. The clinician should be educated regarding potential adverse effects of the anticoagulant medication, including signs and symptoms of bleeding, and when to seek medical care. The patient must avoid food fads and crash diets and should not drink alcohol or take vitamin E, cold medicines, antibiotics, aspirin, cimetidine (Tagamet), thyroid hormones, or NSAIDs without first consulting the clinician. Immobility should be discouraged. Patients must know when to return for a follow-up PT if they are on warfarin.

Davis*Plus* | For additional resources please visit http://davisplus.fadavis.com

References

Evidence-Based Practice

Brar, SS, et al. Long-term outcomes by clopidogrel duration and stent type in a diabetic population with de novo coronary artery lesions. *J Am Coll Cardiol* 51:2220–2227, 2008.

Calhoun, DA, et al. Resistant hypertension: Diagnosis, evaluation, and treatment. A scientific statement from the AHA. *Hypertension* 51:1403–1419, 2008. Retrieved from http://hyper.ahajournals.org/content/51/6/1403

Heart Rhythm Society. Syncope. Updated May 22, 2013. Retrieved from www.hrsonline.org/PatientInfo/SymptomsDiagnosis/Fainting/index.cfm

Institute for Clinical Systems Improvement. Diagnosis and treatment of chest pain and acute coronary syndrome (ACS). Updated November 2012. Retrieved from www.guidelines.gov/summary/summary.aspx?doc_id=134808nbr=006889& string=dyspnea

Jessup, M, et al. 2009 focused update: ACC/AHA guidelines for the diagnosis and management of heart failure in adults. *Circ J AHA* 119:1177–2016, 2009.

Levine, E. CHADS2 score for stroke risk assessment in atrial fibrillation. Medscape. Updated May 20, 2014. Retrieved from http://emedicine.medscape.com/article/2172597-overview

Michigan Quality Improvement Consortium. Medical management of adults with hypertension. Revised August 2011. Retrieved from www.guidelines.gov/summary/summary.aspx?doc_id=11549&nbr =005980&string

O'Gara, PT, et al. 2013 ACCF/AHA guideline for the management of ST-elevation myocardial infarction: A report of the American College of Cardiology Foundation/American Heart Association

Task Force on Practice Guidelines. *J Am Coll Cardiol* 61(4): e78–e140, 2013. Retrieved from http://content.onlinejacc.org/article.aspx?articleid=1486115

Page, MR. The new lipid guidelines: An in-depth look. *Pharmacy Times,* November 19, 2013. Retrieved from www.pharmacytimes.com/news/The-New-Lipid-Guidelines-An-In-Depth-Look

Bibliography

Arrhythmias

Camm, AJ, et al. The Task Force for the Management of Atrial Fibrillation of the European Society of Cardiology (ESC). Guidelines for the management of atrial fibrillation. *Eur Heart J* 31:2369–2429, 2010. Retrieved from www.escardio.org/guidelines-surveys/esc-guidelines/GuidelinesDocuments/guidelines-afib-FT.pdf

Thompson, D. Hospitalization rates soar for irregular heartbeat. Health-Day, November 18, 2013. Retrieved from http://consumer.health-day.com/senior-citizen-information-31/misc-aging-news-10/afib-hospitalization-rates-soaring-682259.html

Heart Failure

Anderson, KM. Clinical uses of brain natriuretic peptide in diagnosing and managing heart failure. *J Acad Nurse Pract* 20:305–310, 2008.

Dogar, M, et al. Chronic heart failure: When to consider device therapy. *Consultant* 49(5), 2009.

Gray, A, and Hendrix, C. Cross communication: Avoiding device interference in pacemakers and ICD's. *Adv Nurse Pract* 17(2):57–58, 2009.

Jessup, M, et al. 2009 focused update: ACC/AHA guidelines for the diagnosis and management of heart failure in adults. *Circ J AHA* 119:1177–2016, 2009.

Jurgens, C, et al. Why do elders delay responding to heart failure symptoms? *Nurs Res* 58(4):274–282, 2009.

Klapholz, M. B-blocker use for the stages of heart failure. *Mayo Clin Proc* 84(8):718–729, 2009.

Newsline. Heart failure strikes young black men hardest. *Clin Advis* 12(6), 2009.

Coronary Artery Disease

Allen, U. Infective endocarditis: Updated guidelines. *Can J Infect Dis Med Microbiol* 21(2):76–77, 2010. Retrieved from www.ncbi.nim.nih.gov/pmc/articles/pmc2912107

Cassar, A, et al. Chronic coronary artery disease: Diagnosis and management. *Mayo Clin Proc* 84(12):1130–1146, 2009.

Goff, DC, et al. 2013 ACC/AHA guideline on the assessment of cardiovascular risk: A report of the American College of Cardiology/American Heart Association Task Force on Practice Guidelines. *J Am Coll Cardiol,* November 12, 2013. Retrieved from www.cardiosource.org/science-and-quality/journal-scan/2013/11/2013-acc-aha-guideline-on-the-assessment-of-cv-risk.aspx

Keefe, JH, et al. Primary and secondary prevention of cardiovascular disease: A practical evidence-based approach. *Mayo Clin Proc* 84(8):741–757, 2009.

Keller, KB, and Lemberg, L. Electrocardiographic artifacts. *Am J Crit Care* 16(1):90–92, 2007.

Keller, KB, and Lemberg, L. Torsade. *Am J Crit Care* 17(1):77–80, 2008.

Kumar, A, and Cannon, CP. Acute coronary syndromes: Diagnosis and management, part II. *Mayo Clin Proc* 84(11):1021–1036, 2009.

O'Riordan, M. New cholesterol guidelines abandon LDL targets. Medscape, November 14, 2013. Retrieved from www.medscape.com/viewarticle/814152

Page, MR. The new lipid guidelines: An in-depth look. *Pharmacy Times,* November 19, 2013. Retrieved from www.pharmacytimes.com/news/The-New-Lipid-Guidelines-An-In-Depth-Look

Turris, SA. Women's decisions to seek treatment for the symptoms of potential cardiac illness. *J Nurs Scholar* 41(1):5–12, 2009.

Zoler, ML. Guideline authors, AHA-ACC leaders confident in risk calculator. *Family Practice News,* November 19, 2013. Retrieved from www.familypracticenews.com/single-view/guideline-authors-aha-acc-leaders-confident-in-risk-calculator/ae4a045d138f0a9580de194c2ef20957.html

Hypertension

AGS Beers criteria for potentially inappropriate medication use in older adults: The American Geriatrics Society. Retrieved from www.american geriatrics.com

Angeli, F, et al. Masked hypertension: Evaluation, prognosis, and treatment. *Am J Hypertens* 23:941–948, 2010.

Aronow, WS. Hypertension: How to treat the elderly in elders. *Consultant* 53(9), September 2013. Retrieved from www.consultant360.com/articles/hypertension-how-treat-elderly

Centers for Disease Control and Prevention National Analytic Guidelines. Center for Health Statistics Division of Health and Nutrition Examination Surveys, September 30, 2013.

Hickner, J. New CVD guidelines put focus in the right place. *J Fam Pract* 63(2):66, 2014.

James, PA, et al. Evidence-based guideline for the management of high blood pressure in adults: Report from the panel members appointed to the Eighth Joint National Committee (JNC 8). *J Am Med Assoc,* December 18, 2014 [e-pub ahead of print].

Kidney Disease: Improving Global Outcomes (KDIGO) Blood Pressure Work Group. KDIGO clinical practice guidelines for the management of blood pressure in chronic kidney disease. *Kidney Int* 2(suppl):337–414, 2012.

Michigan Quality Improvement Consortium. Medical management of adults with hypertension. 2005. Updated August 2011. Retrieved from www.guidelines.gov/summary/summary.aspx?doc_id=11549&nbr=005980&string

National Health and Nutrition Examination Survey:, 2011–2012.

National Institutes of Health, National Heart, Lung, and Blood Institute. The seventh report of the Joint National Committee on prevention, detection, evaluation, and treatment of high blood pressure (the JNC 7 report). *J Am Med Assoc* 289(19):2560–2572, 2003.

Page, MR. The JNC8 hypertension guidelines: An in-depth guide. 2014. Retrieved from www.ajmc.com/publications/evidence-based-diabetes-management/2014/jan-feb2014

Pierson, C, et al. The importance of managing cardiovascular risk in the treatment of hypertension: The role of ACE inhibitors and ARBs. *J Am Acad Nurse Pract* 20:529–538, 2008.

Polly, DM, et al. Management of hypertensive emergency and urgency. *Adv Emerg Nurse J* 33(2):127–136, 2011. doi:10.109/TME.06013e318217a564

Roberts, ME, and Epstein, BJ. Optimizing management of hypertension with combination therapy: Considerations for the nurse practitioner. *J Cardiovasc Nurs* 24(5):380–389, 2009.

Shimbo, D, et al. Masked hypertension and prehypertension: Diagnostic overlap and interrelationships with left ventricular mass: The Masked Hypertension Study. *Am J Hypertens* 25(6):664–671, 2012.

2013 ESH/ESC guidelines for the management of arterial hypertension: The task force for the management of arterial hypertension of the European Society of Hypertension (ESH) and of the European Society of Cardiology (ESC). *Eur Heart J* 34(28):2159–2219, 2013. doi:10.1093/eurheartj/eht151

Weber, MA, et al. Clinical practice guidelines for the management of hypertension in the community: A statement by the American Society of Hypertension and the International Society of Hypertension. *J Clin Hypertens (Greenwich)*.

Thrombosis

Creager, MA, and Loscalzo, J. Vascular diseases of the extremities. In Longo, D, et al, *Harrison's principles of internal medicine,* ed 18. McGraw-Hill, New York, 2012.

O'Gara, PT, and Loscalzo, J. Valvular heart disease. In Longo, D, et al, *Harrison's principles of internal medicine,* ed 18. McGraw-Hill, New York, 2012.

Resources

American College of Cardiology
www.acc.org
2014 Evidence-Based Guidelines for the Management of HTN in Adults
http://jama.jamanetwork.com/article.aspx?articleid=1791497
American Heart Association
www.americanheart.org
(Contact AHA for local state affiliate)
American Medical Association (AMA)
www.ama-assn.org

Cardiovascular Risk Calculator
http:myamericanheart.org/cvriskcalculator
Nova Online Cardiac Resources
www.pbs.org/wgbh/eheart/resources.html
Website for *Healthy People 2020*
www.healthypeople.gov/hp2020/objectives/topicarea

Chapter 11

Abdominal Problems

Debera J. Thomas, DNS, RN, FNP/ANP •
Dorothy J. Dunn, PhD, RNP, FNP-BC, AHN-BC

COMMON COMPLAINTS

■ ABDOMINAL PAIN

Abdominal pain is one of the most common complaints for which people seek medical attention. According to the 2010 National Ambulatory Medical Care Survey, abdominal pain is one of the top 20 leading principal reasons for office visits. Colorectal cancer is the fourth most common cancer and the third most common cause of cancer deaths. The *National Vital Statistics Reports* (Centers for Disease Control and Prevention, 2012) revealed that chronic liver disease and cirrhosis continues to rank twelfth in the leading causes of death. The causes of abdominal pain are numerous; a few are serious enough to require surgical intervention. Conditions associated with an acute abdomen can be inflammatory, metabolic, or structural; therefore, any acute abdominal pain must be evaluated quickly and precisely. Abdominal pain that occurs without any other signs or symptoms is rarely a serious problem. In instances when the exact cause of pain is not immediately evident, an empiric trial of therapy or test selection may help suggest the underlying pathophysiology, narrow the differential diagnoses, and guide further assessment and treatment. It is important to keep in mind that extra-abdominal etiologies such as ovarian cancer, ectopic pregnancy (see Chapter 14), or myocardial ischemia (see Chapter 10) may present as abdominal pain.

Half of patients who complain of abdominal pain do not receive an accurate diagnosis. The source of the abdominal pain may be from one of a triad of vascular emergencies: mesenteric ischemia, abdominal aortic aneurysm, or myocardial infarction. Conditions in this triad can cause severe pain and should not be excluded from the differential diagnosis.

Differential Diagnosis

Total patient presentation must be considered when evaluating abdominal pain. A careful history is the key to determining the severity of the condition. The onset, location, duration, characteristics, any associated/aggravating factors, relieving factors, temporal factors, and severity, as well as what the pain means to the patient, are useful in the diagnostic reasoning. The presence or absence of bowel sounds is also an important diagnostic factor. Tachycardia, tachypnea, and hypertension often indicate the intensity of the pain. Many nonsurgical conditions can present with classic acute "surgical" abdomen symptoms such as intense pain, rebound tenderness, and guarding. All patients with abdominal pain should undergo rectal, genital, and pelvic evaluations. Blood found in the stool or intense pain on examination may indicate more serious conditions.

The mechanism responsible for the abdominal pain is what gives certain characteristics to the pain. For example, pain that originates from pain receptors located in the viscera (organs) produces pain that is poorly localized and is described as dull. This is known as *visceral pain* and is caused by distention or spasm of a hollow viscus. Distention of an organ capsule, such as Glisson's capsule around the liver; vascular compromise; and mucosal irritations cause pain that is visceral in nature. Conversely, *parietal pain,* described as sharp and well localized, is caused by irritation of the peritoneum. Appendicitis often causes this type of pain as the peritoneum becomes involved. *Abdominal pain* described as colicky, which simply means that it comes and goes, may result from gallstones or renal stones. *Burning pain,* caused by irritation of the gastric mucosa by gastric contents, is associated with peptic ulcers and esophagitis.

A thorough history and physical examination are essential to narrow the list of differential diagnoses of patients with abdominal pain. First, the nature of the pain should be elicited in order to provide clues to the mechanism of the pain. Location of the pain is valuable information, but it is important to remember that abdominal pain can be referred from areas outside of the abdomen. Timing of the pain (onset, duration, frequency, and relationship to associated symptoms) can help eliminate some causes. The palliative and provocative aspects of the pain can give clues about the cause of the pain. For example, does moving, eating certain foods, assuming different positions, or taking medications make the pain better or worse? Associated symptoms will further narrow the list of diagnostic possibilities. Some causes of abdominal pain will necessitate a surgical referral. Any time the pain is very severe and associated with a rigid abdomen, referral to a physician is essential. Abdominal pain can be the presenting symptom of many different pathophysiological processes, ranging from very mild gastritis to more serious forms of abdominal pain associated with bowel obstruction or appendicitis.

A complete blood count, serum chemistries, liver function tests, urinalysis, pregnancy test, and abdominal films will help determine the acuity of the problem. Differential Diagnosis Flowchart 11.1 presents selected causes of abdominal pain and their characteristics. Treatment of abdominal pain depends on the cause.

Differential Diagnosis Flowchart 11.1

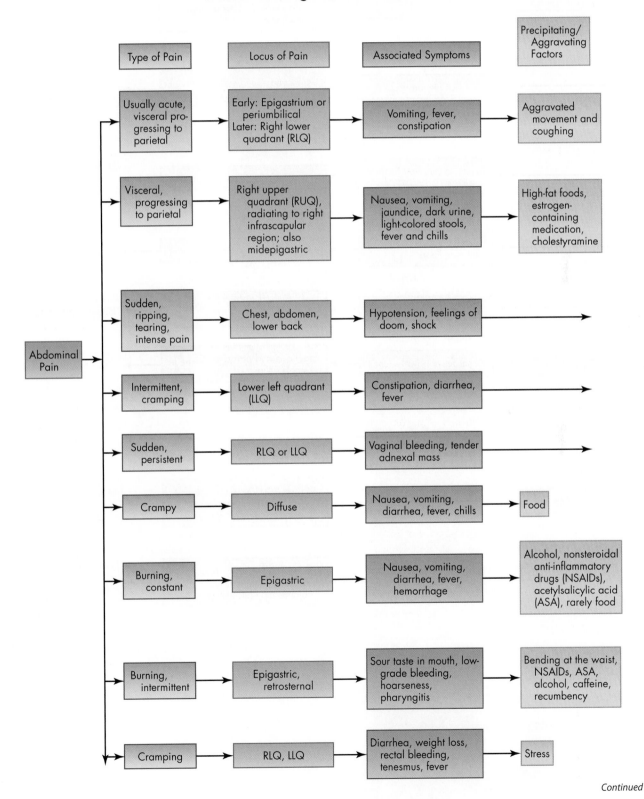

Continued

Differential Diagnosis Flowchart 11.1 (continued)

Relieving Factors	Physical Findings	Diagnostic Studies	Cause
Lying still	RLQ: Guarding and rebound tenderness	Complete blood count (CBC) with differential, ultrasound, computerized sonography (CT) scan	Appendicitis
	RUQ tenderness	Ultrasound, CBC with differential, liver function tests, amylase	Cholecystitis/ Cholelithiasis
	Shock, diminished femoral pulses	Radiography, CT scan	Dissection or Rupture of Aortic Aneurysm
	LLQ mass, mild tenderness in left iliac fossa	Laparoscopy, other labs are normal	Diverticulitis
	Tender adnexa	Human chorionic gonadotropin (hCG)	Ectopic Pregnancy
Relief with vomiting or defecation	Hyperactive bowel sounds	Stool ova and parasites (O & P), stool culture	Gastroenteritis
			Gastritis
Antacids		Barium swallow, upper gastro-intestinal (GI), esophageal endoscopy with biopsy	Gastroesophageal Reflux Disease (GERD)
	Tenderness in RLQ, LLQ	CBC with differential, small bowel follow-through (Crohn's), colonoscopy (ulcerative colitis)	Inflammatory Bowel Disease (Crohn's disease, ulcerative colitis)

Differential Diagnosis Flowchart 11.1 (continued)

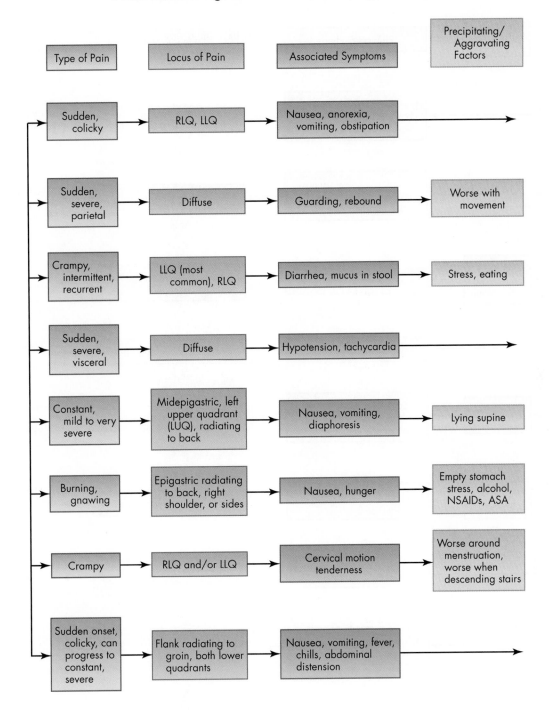

Continued

Differential Diagnosis Flowchart 11.1 (continued)

Relieving Factors	Physical Findings	Diagnostic Studies	Cause
	Hyperactive, high-pitched bowel sounds or hypoactive bowel sounds	Abdominal x-ray	Intestinal Obstruction
Lying still	Decreased bowel sounds, guarding, rebound tenderness	Abdominal x-ray	Intestinal Perforation
Pain often relieved by defecation	Colon tender to palpation	Small bowel follow-through to rule out other causes	Irritable Bowel
	Diminished bowel sounds	Abdominal arteriograms	Mesenteric Infarction
Leaning forward	Abdominal distension, diminished bowel sound, diffuse rebound tenderness	Amylase, ultrasound	Pancreatitis
Food, antacids	Epigastric tenderness to palpation	Endoscopy, barium swallow	Peptic Ulcer Disease (PUD)
	Tender adnexa and cervix	Ultrasound, CT scan, human chorionic gonadotropin	Salpingitis
	Costovertebral angle (CVA) tenderness, hematuria	Urinalysis, intravenous pyelogram (IVP), ultrasound	Urinary Stones

■ CONSTIPATION

Constipation is a common symptom in Western society and is the most common gastrointestinal (GI) disorder in the United States, particularly in older adults and sedentary individuals. There is no single definition of constipation, although it is often defined as a change in a person's normal bowel pattern, either a decrease in frequency or an increase in difficulty of defecation. The clinician and the patient must have a similar operational definition of constipation and what a normal bowel pattern is for that patient.

The most common cause of constipation in the United States is a lack of dietary fiber; the recommended amount is 30 grams daily for optimal bowel health. The average American consumes only about 10 grams per day. Other common causes of constipation are habitual use of laxatives, irritable bowel syndrome (IBS), decreased physical activity, a change in environment or travel, use of medications with constipating potential, suppression of the urge to defecate, and painful defecation caused by anorectal problems. Other less common but serious causes of constipation include bowel tumors and metabolic disorders such as hypothyroidism, diabetes, hypercalcemia, and depression.

Generally, there are three categories of constipation: simple constipation, disordered motility, and secondary constipation. *Simple constipation* results from a diet that is low in fiber and high in simple carbohydrates and meat. A sedentary lifestyle is also a common contributor to constipation. In addition, some people have difficulty defecating in an environment other than their own home; they frequently suppress the urge to defecate, thereby promoting simple constipation. The next most common category of constipation is *disordered motility,* which is seen most often in older adults and is caused by slowed transit time. Megacolon and megarectum are also common disorders of motility, but they most frequently occur in children with conditions such as Hirschsprung disease. Other conditions that cause disordered motility and constipation include IBS and diverticular disease. *Secondary constipation* often is a result of medications such as codeine, morphine, analgesics, calcium channel blockers, antidepressants, antiparkinsonian drugs, cough medicine, and aluminum antacids. Table 11.1 presents a list of constipating drugs. Other common causes of secondary constipation are chronic laxative use, prolonged immobilization, and organic diseases of the lower GI system, such as colorectal cancer.

Chronic constipation rarely results from a serious condition, and the patient can usually be treated symptomatically by increasing dietary fiber. Those whose constipation developed with a recent disability, a change in diet, recent depressive illness, or the ingestion of a constipating medication can also be treated symptomatically. Patients who develop constipation that cannot be explained, have abdominal pain, report blood or mucus

Table 11.1	Medications That Commonly Cause Constipation	
Aluminum-containing antacids	Antiparkinsonian drugs	
Anticholinergics	Antipsychotics	
Anticonvulsants	Bismuth-containing products	
• Phenobarbital	• bismuth subsalicylate (Pepto-Bismol)	
• Phenytoin	Iron preparations	
• Carbamazepine	NSAIDs	
Antidepressants	Opiates	
• Amitriptyline	• Codeine	
• Doxepin	• Morphine	
• Imipramine	• Heroin	
• Nortriptyline	• Fentanyl	
• Protriptyline	• Methadone	
Antihistamines	• Propxyphene	
Antihypertensives	Sympathomimetics	
• Calcium channel blockers		
• Clonidine		

in their stool, or require a substantial increase in their laxative use require more investigation. Constipation occurs in fewer than 30% of patients with colon cancer.

Differential Diagnosis

An accurate description of the feces can give clues to the cause of the constipation. For example, ribbon-like stools often indicate a motility disorder but can also be caused by an organic narrowing of the distal or sigmoid colon. If the patient complains of a progressive decrease in the diameter of the stools, this suggests an organic lesion. If steatorrhea and greenish-yellow stools are associated with the constipation, the practitioner should look for a small bowel or pancreatic lesion. Constipation alternating with diarrhea is often a result of IBS.

The cause of constipation is multifactorial, which can make the differential diagnosis difficult. Differential Diagnosis Flowchart 11.2 presents various causes of constipation.

Treatment

The management of simple constipation is straightforward. Most patients respond well to education about bowel habits, activity, and dietary intervention. Some patients may require pharmacological intervention as well. Patients should be instructed to slowly increase the amount of dietary fiber to 25 to 35 grams per day, with at least 12 to 15 grams at breakfast. Mild exercise after the morning meal is often helpful in stimulating peristalsis and promoting defecation. Uninterrupted toilet time in the morning is also helpful. Adequate hydration is essential in the prevention of constipation; patients should be encouraged to drink at least 64 ounces of fluids daily.

Differential Diagnosis Flowchart 11.2

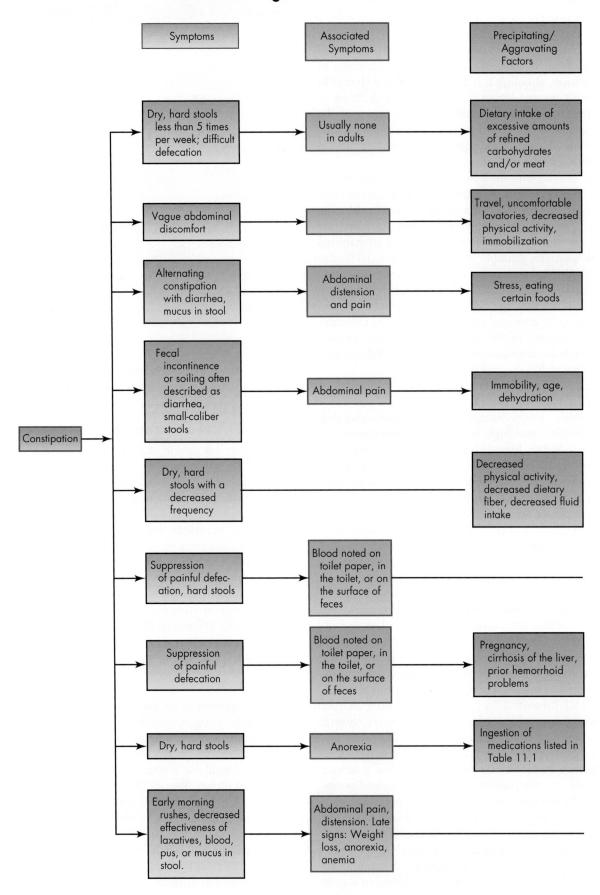

Differential Diagnosis Flowchart 11.2 (continued)

Treatment with a pharmacological agent may be needed for patients who do not respond to increases in fiber, fluids, and exercise. Most drugs should be used for a short time only, and most are available without a prescription. Because these agents are available without a prescription, patients may have self-medicated for some time; and by the time they seek medical attention, they may either have overused laxatives or may have a more serious underlying pathology. The only agents that are appropriate for long-term use are the bulking agents. The different agents used in the treatment of constipation are listed in Drugs Commonly Prescribed 11.1.

■ DIARRHEA

Just as with constipation, there is no single definition of diarrhea, but it is generally defined as an increase in the frequency, volume, or fluid content of bowel movements over what is normal for the individual. Because dietary intake of fiber in the United States is low, the average daily stool for each individual weighs about 200 grams. For most individuals, if the daily stool is more than 200 grams or the frequency of bowel movements is more than three times a day, the patient's condition can be considered diarrhea. Diarrhea is one of the most common presenting complaints in primary-care practice.

There are several types of diarrhea. The first is *osmotic diarrhea,* which is seen in patients with injury to the small intestine that results in malabsorption or maldigestion of nutrients, as in patients with short bowel syndrome. Lactase deficiency or disaccharidase deficiency can also cause osmotic diarrhea, as can ingestion of poorly absorbed solutes such as magnesium sulfate, laxatives, and sorbitol. Osmotic diarrhea usually responds to fasting. Celiac disease is described as a malabsorption syndrome related to immune reaction to gluten in the diet. It is most common

in women, and the peak incidence is in women aged 40 to 50 years. Gluten is found in food products that contain wheat, barley, and rye. The effects on the intestinal mucosa cause the villi to become flat, the crypts to hypertrophy, and an increased number of intraepithelial lymphocytes and plasma cells to appear. Complications such as collagenous sprue and intestinal ulcers, nutritional complications, and malignancy are possible. The patient will have a history of chronic diarrhea, foul-smelling stools, abdominal bloating, weakness, and fatigue. A presumptive diagnosis is based on a combination of clinical presentation and positive serology. Distal duodenal biopsy is needed to confirm the diagnosis. Treatment includes a lifelong gluten-free diet and treatment of nutritional deficiencies such as iron, folate, and vitamin B_{12}.

Another type is *secretory diarrhea,* which produces voluminous watery stools but is unresponsive to fasting. Secretory diarrhea is primarily the result of bacterial enterotoxins (most notably from cholera and strains of *Escherichia coli*). But it can also be caused by laxative abuse; bile salt malabsorption, which stimulates colonic secretion; and endocrine tumors that stimulate pancreatic or intestinal secretion.

Diarrhea is associated with *morphological changes* within the mucosa of the intestinal wall that occur with inflammatory conditions of the intestines, and these changes can result in acute or chronic diarrhea. Both Crohn's disease and ulcerative colitis cause inflammation of the mucosa of the intestinal lumen, resulting in diarrhea.

Diarrhea can also result from *altered intestinal motility* secondary to diabetic neuropathy, dumping syndrome, or irritable bowel syndrome (IBS). Some medications, such as antibiotics, can induce diarrhea by disrupting the normal balance of bacteria. Probiotics have been studied in the treatment of diarrhea. A systematic review

Drugs Commonly Prescribed 11.1   Pharmacological Agents Used to Treat Constipation

Drug	Indication	Adverse Reactions and Prescribing Considerations
Bulking agents Psyllium preparations Methylcellulose preparations	IBS Chronic constipation Diverticulitis	Causes flatulence, bloating and requires adequate fluid intake.
Stool softeners Docusate sodium	Frequently used for prevention of constipation, but not effective.	Hepatotoxic if combined with irritant laxatives.
Saline laxatives Magnesium hydroxide	Intermittent use in chronic constipation and bowel prep.	Can cause dehydration and electrolyte imbalance.
Stimulant/irritant laxatives Bisacodyl Senna Cascara	Acute constipation; should not be used for chronic constipation.	Patient can become dependent. Also causes dehydration and electrolyte imbalance.
Lubricants Mineral oil	Intermittent use in chronic constipation.	Can cause lipid pneumonia if aspirated.

of 63 probiotic studies of adults and children revealed that the duration of antibiotic-associated diarrhea was shortened by a mean of 25 hours with probiotics and hydration therapy. In another systematic review, acute infectious diarrhea of children with rotovirus concluded a decrease of between 17 and 30 hours in diarrhea duration with probiotics (Level II; Piascik & Sanders, 2012). Probiotic use for travelers' diarrhea, *Clostridium difficile*, and inflammatory bowel disease (IBD) has not proved efficacious. Pathogenic bacteria also cause increases in gastrointestinal motility and intestinal secretions. There have been promising results with the use of fecal microbiota transplantation (stool transplant) for the treatment of *C difficile* diarrhea. This procedure involves taking fecal bacteria from a healthy person and infusing this via enema into the person with the *C difficile* infection.

Differential Diagnosis

Differential diagnosis of diarrhea is aided by separating acute diarrhea from chronic diarrhea. *Acute diarrhea* usually has an abrupt onset and lasts for less than 1 week. Nausea, vomiting, or fever may be associated with acute types of diarrhea. On the other hand, *chronic diarrhea* lasts for more than 2 weeks or recurs over months or years. When diarrhea occurs suddenly in an otherwise healthy patient without signs or symptoms of other organ involvement, the most likely cause is an infectious agent, most often viral. The most frequent causes of chronic diarrhea are IBS, medications, dietary factors, IBD, and colon cancer.

A thorough history and comprehensive review of systems can elicit information that the patient may not think is important but that can facilitate diagnosis. For example, recent travel is particularly important because viral, bacterial, and protozoan causes are endemic in many areas. Hikers and campers in the United States who drink unfiltered water are at a high risk for giardiasis. Focus on History 11.1 presents important information to obtain from the patient's history.

Acute viral gastroenteritis is the most common cause of diarrhea. (Gastroenteritis is discussed in detail later in this chapter.) Other common causes of diarrhea the practitioner should consider are IBS, IBD, ingestion of magnesium-containing antacids, lactose intolerance, antibiotic therapy, laxative abuse, and AIDS. Differential Diagnosis Flowchart 11.3 presents the differential diagnosis of diarrhea.

■ DYSPEPSIA AND HEARTBURN

The frequency with which patients present with dyspepsia and heartburn as their chief complaint has been diminishing, probably because of the availability of over-the-counter histamine-2–receptor blockers and proton pump inhibitors. Aggressive advertising of these products by pharmaceutical companies over the last decade has led to the increase in self-medication for what could be a serious illness that the individual mistakes as simple heartburn.

Focus on History 11.1 Diarrhea

Characteristics of Feces
- Frequency
- Amount and fluidity
- Color and characteristics: Bloody, tarry, black, steatorrheaic, mucus

Other History
- Diet history: Intolerance to lactose or certain foods
- Recent travel
- Source of drinking water: Well or city water supply
- Medication use: Magnesium-containing antacids, antibiotics, chemotherapy, immunosuppressive agents
- Medical/surgical history: Diabetes mellitus, hyperthyroid, human immunodeficiency virus (HIV), organ transplant, GI surgery
- Sexual practices: Frequency of anal intercourse, number and sex of partners
- Social history: Living conditions
- Family history: Colon cancer, inflammatory bowel disease

Dimensions of the Problem
- Associated symptoms: Abdominal pain, fever, vomiting, neurological symptoms, headache, malaise, myalgia, muscle weakness
- Exacerbating or alleviating factors

Differential Diagnosis

Dyspepsia and heartburn are two different entities. *Heartburn* is occasionally described as extreme pain, and this makes it difficult to distinguish heartburn pain from that of angina pectoris. Patients with heartburn sometimes describe the pain as radiating to the back, arms, or jaw, which further complicates the diagnosis. Symptoms of *dyspepsia* include epigastric discomfort, postprandial fullness, early satiety, anorexia, belching, nausea, heartburn, vomiting, bloating, borborygmi, dysphagia, and abdominal burning. These symptoms most often have functional or organic causes. The possibility of an organic cause for dyspepsia increases as a person ages. Patients who ingest alcohol in significant amounts or take drugs such as salicylates, corticosteroids, NSAIDs, erythromycin (E-Mycin), or theophylline (Theo-Dur, Theo-24) often have dyspepsia as a result of medication-induced gastritis. Giardiasis can cause dyspepsia with only occasional bouts of diarrhea. Nonulcer dyspepsia caused by *Helicobacter pylori* causes vague abdominal pain, a sense of fullness, nausea, and bloating, which are worse after eating. If the symptoms of dyspepsia are continuous and associated with anorexia and weight loss, gastric cancer may be the cause.

Heartburn, a retrosternal burning sensation, is common in the general population, with 7% complaining of daily symptoms, 14% having weekly episodes, and

Differential Diagnosis Flowchart 11.3

Differential Diagnosis Flowchart 11.3 (continued)

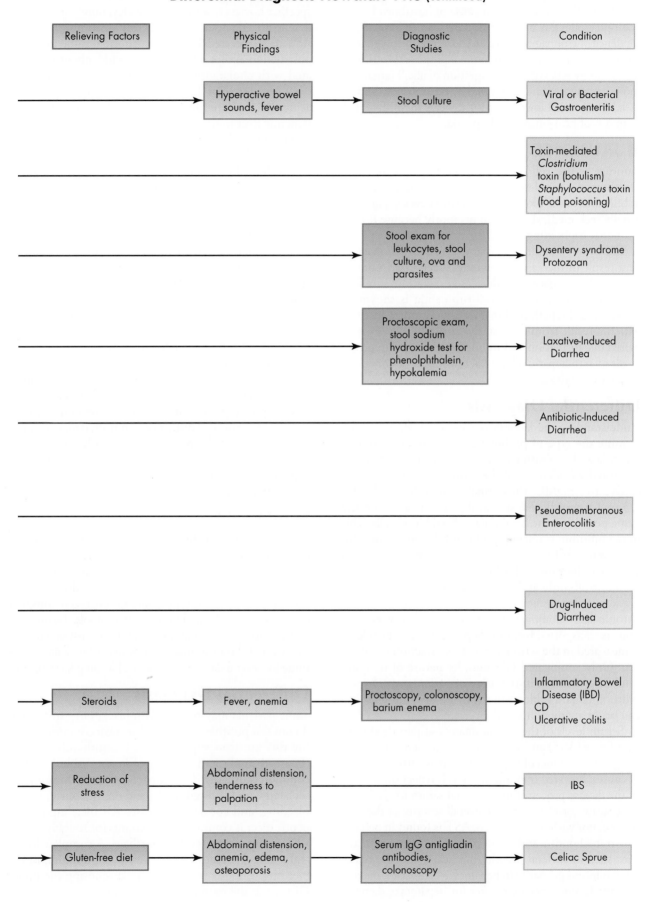

36% experiencing heartburn at some time or other in their lives. The most common cause of heartburn is gastroesophageal reflux disease. Pregnant women have a high incidence of esophagitis, most often later in the pregnancy because of increased intra-abdominal pressure. Heartburn is commonly relieved by the ingestion of alkali (antacids) and is precipitated and aggravated by recumbency. Differential Diagnosis Flowchart 11.4 reviews the differential diagnosis of heartburn and dyspepsia.

■ JAUNDICE

Jaundice is the yellow coloring of the skin, mucous membranes, and sclera resulting from an accumulation of bilirubin in the blood. Patients who develop jaundice usually seek medical attention promptly because it is so dramatic, frightening, and difficult to ignore.

The hyperbilirubinemia that causes the jaundice can be a result of increased production, decreased uptake, decreased conjugation, or decreased excretion of bilirubin. The etiology of hyperbilirubinemia is shown in Table 11.2. Hyperbilirubinemia and jaundice in most patients result from cholestasis, either because of impaired bile formation and/or bile flow, which can be the result of extrahepatic biliary tract obstruction or hepatic parenchymal disease.

Differential Diagnosis

Understanding the laboratory values is essential to determine the type of problem causing the hyperbilirubinemia and establish a differential diagnosis. Icterus is not usually evident until the serum bilirubin level exceeds 2 to 3 mg/dL. The normal serum bilirubin level is 0.3 to 1.0 mg/dL. Most bilirubin is formed from the heme portion of the breakdown of red blood cells. This initial bilirubin is unconjugated and therefore not soluble in water. When measured in the serum, it is reported as indirect bilirubin. This form of bilirubin is reversibly bound to albumin and transported to the liver, where it is taken up by the hepatocyte and conjugated with glucuronic acid. Conjugated bilirubin, which is water soluble, is transported from the hepatocyte into the bile. It is measured in the serum as the direct fraction of bilirubin. Only conjugated bilirubin, by nature of its water solubility, is found in the urine of patients with hyperbilirubinemia. Problems in the metabolism of bilirubin can occur at any point of the cycle.

Serum levels of the transaminases—aspartate aminotransferase (AST) and alanine aminotransferase (ALT)—are good indicators of hepatocyte damage from a variety of causes. Elevated transaminase levels reflect the activity of the disease process, but the actual serum levels do not necessarily correlate with the overall severity of the liver disease, nor with the prognosis. AST is found in hepatocyte mitochondria and cytoplasm and in nonhepatic tissues such as skeletal muscle, the heart, and the brain. ALT is found primarily in hepatocyte cytoplasm, making it a much more specific marker for hepatocyte damage.

Levels of AST and ALT that are below 300 U/L are nonspecific; however, some extreme elevations can be quite diagnostic. For example, it is very uncommon for the AST to be elevated 15 times the normal value in biliary obstruction except when it occurs suddenly or is associated with cholangitis. Striking elevations of ALT and AST (greater than 1,000 U/L) occur in patients with acute viral hepatitis, toxin- or drug-induced hepatitis, and ischemic liver injury. If the ratio of AST to ALT is high, it generally indicates severe hepatic necrosis, most often caused by alcoholic hepatitis.

Alkaline phosphatase is found in the biliary canalicular membranes and is useful in assessing cholestasis. Cholestasis is also characteristically accompanied by an increase in the serum gamma-glutamyl transpeptidase (GGT) and 5(-nucleotidase. Extreme elevations in alkaline phosphatase (greater than three times normal) in conjunction with elevation of the GGT indicate a mechanical obstruction of the biliary system by a tumor, stricture, or stone. Because alkaline phosphatase is also found in bone, an isolated elevation of that enzyme without elevation of the GGT is indicative of a bone disorder rather than a cholestatic process.

A patient who presents with jaundice often has complaints of pruritis, anorexia, nausea, vomiting, fever, light-colored stools, weight loss, and fatigue. Examination may reveal right upper quadrant pain and tenderness, dark urine, and abdominal distention. Pruritus, dark urine, and light-colored stools in conjunction with the jaundice are indicative of cholestasis, either intrahepatic or extrahepatic, such as cholelithiasis, cirrhosis, or other biliary obstruction.

■ MELENA

Melena is defined as black, tarry stools that test positive for occult blood. The most common cause of melena is upper gastrointestinal (GI) bleeding, but bleeding in the small bowel or the right colon can also produce melena. It is the action of gastric acid and intestinal secretions that reduces bright red blood to black, tarry stools. To produce melena, about 100 to 200 mL of blood must be present. Because of GI transit time, it is possible for melena to continue for several days after the acute bleeding has stopped.

Differential Diagnosis

Some patients may present with black, tarry stools that do not test positive for blood. The most common causes for this are iron supplements, bismuth subsalicylate (Pepto-Bismol), and a variety of foods. Table 11.3 lists common causes of GI bleeding. Signs and symptoms associated with GI bleeding depend on the source, rate of bleeding, and coexistent diseases. GI bleeding from a peptic ulcer is common and accounts for roughly half of all episodes of upper GI hemorrhage. A complete blood count can give clues to the severity and duration of the bleeding. Endoscopy is useful in diagnosing the upper GI tract as the source of the bleeding.

Differential Diagnosis Flowchart 11.4

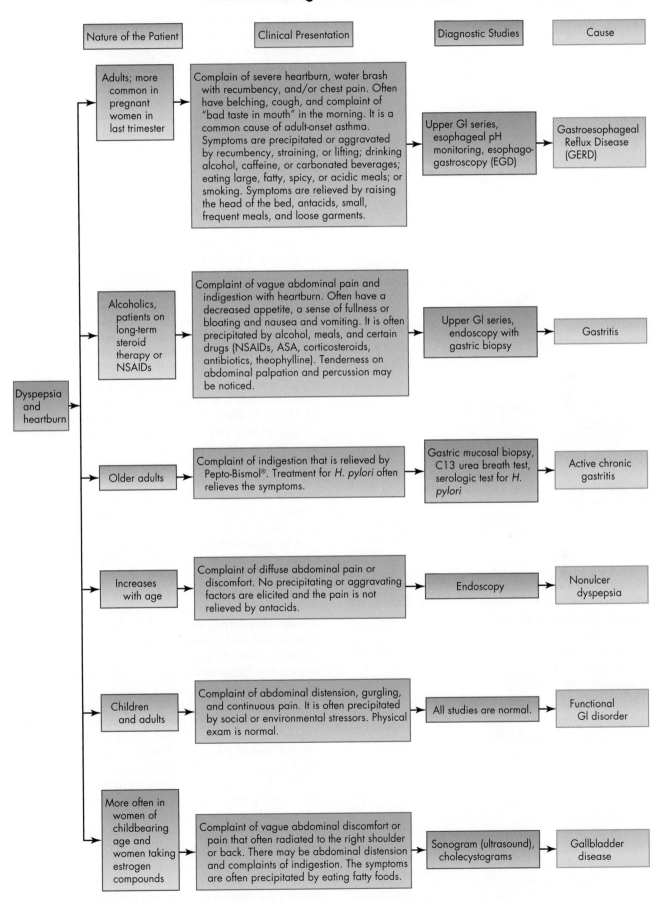

Table 11.2	Etiology: Hyperbilirubinemia

Increased Production

Hemolysis, resorption of hematomas, ineffective erythropoiesis
- Megaloblastic anemia, iron-deficiency anemia, sideroblastic anemia
- Thalassemia minor
- Polycythemia vera
- Lead poisoning

Decreased Clearance

Inherited disorder of bilirubin metabolism
- Gilbert's syndrome, Crigler-Najjar syndrome, Dubin-Johnson syndrome, Rotor's syndrome

Cholestasis
- Hepatocellular disease: Viral, drug-induced, or alcoholic hepatitis
- Biliary tract obstruction: Choledocholithiasis, tumor, sclerosing cholangitis, chronic pancreatitis, pancreatic cancer, primary biliary cirrhosis

Drugs
- Antibiotics (erythromycin, trimethoprim/sulfamethoxazole, amoxicillin/clavulanic acid, nitrofurantoin, griseofulvin)
- Analgesics (propoxyphene, sulindac, diflunisal)
- Allopurinol
- Warfarin
- Steroids (contraceptive and anabolic)
- Phenytoin
- Thiazide diuretics
- Phenothiazines
- Tricyclic antidepressants
- Haloperidol
- Parenteral gold
- Oral hypoglycemics (chlorpropamide, tolbutamide)

Table 11.3	Common Causes of Gastrointestinal Bleeding

Upper Gastrointestinal Tract

Peptic ulcer
- Gastric ulcer
- Duodenal ulcer

Gastric erosions
Erosive esophagitis
Esophageal varices

Lower Gastrointestinal Tract

Diverticular disease
Colon cancer
Intestinal polyps
Inflammatory bowel disease
Ulcerative colitis
Crohn's disease
Infectious colitis
Meckel's diverticulum
Small bowel neoplasm

■ NAUSEA AND VOMITING

Nausea is an unpleasant sensation in the stomach that is difficult to define because it is a sensory experience. It is often accompanied by diaphoresis, increased salivation, and the vasovagal signs of hypotension and bradycardia. Nausea can occur alone or precede vomiting. Vomiting is the forceful expulsion of gastric contents; it is a reflex response to stimulation of receptor sites in the mucosa of the upper gastrointestinal (GI) tract, the labyrinthine apparatus in the inner ear, higher cortical centers in response to emotional stimuli, or the chemoreceptor trigger zone of the medulla oblongata. Afferent nerve fibers carry these impulses to the vomiting center, where efferent fibers then send impulses to relax the gastric fundus and the gastroesophageal sphincter, to contract the pylorus, and to cause reverse peristalsis in the esophagus. The abdominal muscles and diaphragm contract, increasing the intra-abdominal pressure, which forces the gastric contents out through the mouth.

Differential Diagnosis

Gastroenteritis is the most common cause of nausea and vomiting in adults and children. Contaminated food should be considered in cases of acute nausea and vomiting, especially when more than one person is affected. Gastritis, usually associated with alcohol consumption or drugs (aspirin, NSAIDs, antibiotics, and illicit drugs), is also a very common cause of acute nausea and vomiting in adults. Nausea and vomiting are listed as adverse effects of a large number of medications; they are also common presenting symptoms for many disease entities such as hepatitis, myocardial infarction, and peptic ulcer. Table 11.4 provides common causes of nausea and vomiting.

A bit of detective work is necessary to determine the cause of the nausea and vomiting. The circumstances surrounding the episode or episodes give clues to the cause. Vomiting following a meal can occur with gastritis and in digitalis toxicity. If the vomiting occurs 1 to 2 hours after eating, diseases of the biliary tract or pancreas should be suspected. Projectile vomiting without nausea is classically a sign of a neurological source, such as increased intracranial pressure. If the nausea and vomiting occur in the early morning, the cause may be uremia, pregnancy, or chronic alcohol ingestion. The duration of the nausea and vomiting depends on the cause. Infectious agents in the GI tract usually cause nausea and vomiting only for 24 hours or less. On the other hand, nausea as a result of pregnancy can last for weeks.

The characteristics of the vomitus are important in determining the cause. For example, repeated vomiting without bile staining is indicative of pyloric obstruction, which can be caused by scars from an ulcer or a tumor, whereas vomiting of undigested food could indicate an esophageal obstruction. The odor of the vomitus is important information to elicit from the patient in determining the cause. Odorless vomitus indicates a lack of

Table 11.4	Common Causes of Nausea and Vomiting

Gastrointestinal Disorders and Problems

Gastroenteritis
Acute gastrointestinal infections
Food poisoning
Gastritis, including alcoholic
Peptic ulcer disease
Hepatitis
Food intolerance
Celiac sprue
Lactase deficiency
Ingestion of fatty foods
Intestinal obstruction
Appendicitis
Cholecystitis
Peritonitis
Diabetic gastric atony

CNS Disorders and Problems

Increased intracranial pressure
Migraine headache
Meningitis
Acute labyrinthitis
Ménière's disease
Altitude sickness

Other Disorders and Problems

Motion sickness
Uremia
Bulimia nervosa
Diabetic ketoacidosis
Adrenal insufficiency
Acute myocardial infarction
Congestive heart failure
Gastroparesis
Postinfectious gastroparesis

Acute Systemic Infections Accompanied by Fever
Pregnancy
Adverse Effect of Drugs and Chemicals

Antibiotics (erythromycin, metronidazole)
Opiates
Estrogen
Ipecac
Digitalis
Chemotherapy
Theophylline

gastric acid, possibly from esophageal stricture or achalasia. Fecal odor, on the other hand, indicates a bowel obstruction or gastrocolic fistula.

In the continued search for the cause of nausea and vomiting, associated symptoms can further narrow the field of possibilities. Ménière's disease or middle ear disturbances should be suspected if the patient complains of vertigo, tinnitus, or hearing loss. Nausea and vomiting often accompany migraine headaches, which are usually unilateral. Nausea and vomiting with diarrhea and abdominal pain are often caused by gastroenteritis. Differential Diagnosis Flowchart 11.5 delineates the differential diagnosis of nausea and vomiting.

Treatment

Management of nausea and vomiting is aimed at the underlying cause, which is covered in detail under the specific diagnoses in this chapter and in other chapters of this book. Symptomatic relief, however, is useful for the comfort of the patient and in preventing complications such as dehydration and electrolyte imbalance. Drugs Commonly Prescribed 11.2 presents a list of medications commonly used for the control of nausea and vomiting. Complementary Therapies 11.1 lists the uses of vitamins, minerals, and herbs for GI problems.

■ DYSPHAGIA

Dysphagia is defined as difficulty swallowing that may or may not have a component of *odynophagia*, or painful swallowing. Although dysphagia may accompany odynophagia, classic dysphagia is not usually painful. The prevalence increases with age and is common in older adults.

The process of swallowing is quite complex and involves 50 pairs of muscles and many nerves. Swallowing has three phases: (1) The *oral phase* involves movement of the tongue and jaw allowing for mastication and preparation of food into a bolus and making it ready for swallowing; (2) the *pharyngeal phase* includes the reflexive passage of the bolus from the oral cavity through the pharynx and into the upper esophagus; and (3) the *esophageal phase* is the reflexive passage of the bolus through the esophagus and into the stomach. There is often a combination of underlying factors that cause dysphagia.

Differential Diagnosis

Dysphagia can be caused by mechanical obstruction or be from a functional problem that impairs motility. Mechanical obstruction can be either intrinsic (strictures, tumors, diverticular outpouchings) or extrinsic (something outside the esophagus that presses inward compressing the esophageal wall with tumor being the most common). Functional dysphagia can have a neurological or muscular cause. Neurological conditions that interfere with voluntary swallowing or peristalsis are cerebrovascular accidents, Parkinson's disease, multiple sclerosis, amyotrophic lateral sclerosis, and achalasia. Eighty percent of oral phase and pharyngeal phase abnormalities have a neurological origin. Dermatomyositis is a muscular disease that causes functional problems in the upper esophagus leading to dysphagia. Dysphagia may be the first sign of such an underlying disorder. Psychological conditions may also cause the symptoms; the term *globus hystericus* refers to a manifestation of acute anxiety disorders and panic attacks. Dysphagia may also be associated with underlying depressive disorder.

Differential Diagnosis Flowchart 11.5

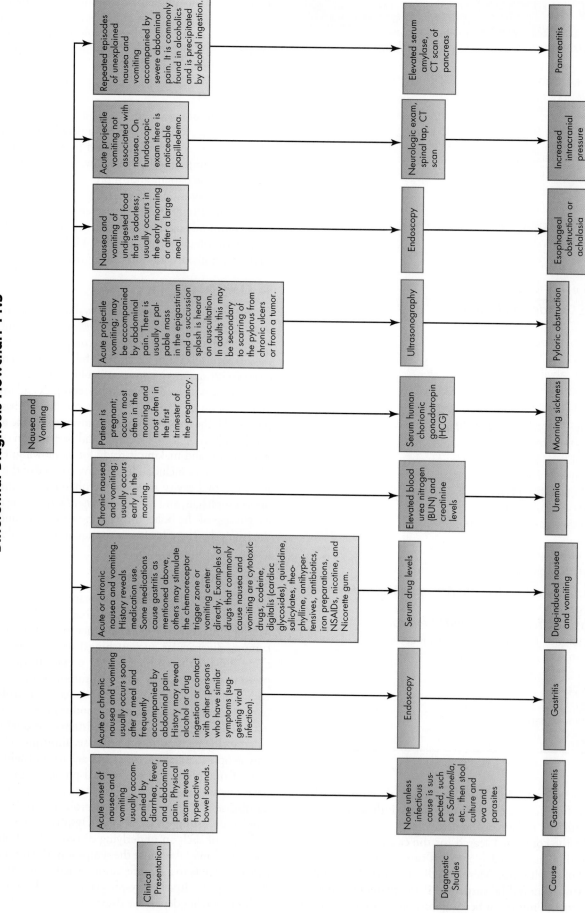

Drugs Commonly Prescribed 11.2 Medications for the Control of Nausea and Vomiting

Drug	Indication	Adverse Reactions and Prescribing Considerations
Antihistamines Dimenhydrinate Promethazine Hydroxyzine Meclizine	Motion sickness Drug-induced nausea Postoperative During labor	Sedation, dry mouth, blurred vision, headache
Antidopaminergics Prochlorperazine	Chemotherapy- and radiation-induced nausea and vomiting Postoperative	Sedation, dry mouth, urinary retention, constipation, extrapyramidal effects
Antidopaminergics and cholinergics Metoclopramide	Postoperative Diabetic gastroparesis	Restlessness, drowsiness, fatigue, extrapyramidal effects
Cholinergic antagonists Scopolamine	Motion sickness	Dry mouth, blurred vision, tachycardia, constipation, sedation
Serotonin receptor antagonists Ondansetron Granisetron	Chemotherapy- and radiation-induced nausea and vomiting	Anxiety, euphoria, depression, headache, insomnia, restlessness, weakness

Complementary Therapies 11.1 Complementary Therapies For Gastrointestinal Problems

Agent	Indication	Adverse Reactions and Prescribing Considerations
Senna (*Cassia senna*)	Constipation	1–2 tsp dried leaves per 8 oz water taken as a tea once daily (not to be taken for longer than a few days)
Milk thistle (*Silybum marianum*)	Hepatitis and liver toxicity	140 mg three times per day (oral)
Acupuncture	Heartburn/GERD IBD IBS	8–12 treatments
Licorice root	Peptic ulcer disease	5–15 mg three times per day Can cause high blood pressure
Ginger	Nausea and motion sickness	250 mg daily

Alterations of the swallowing process may manifest differently depending on the underlying pathology. For example, if there is a problem in the oral phase, dribbling, spillage, pocketing of food in the mouth, or aspiration may be present. The pharyngeal phase is the first reflexive, or involuntary, phase; problems during this phase are characterized by nasal regurgitation, aspiration, and/or altered voice. This is the phase where aspiration most commonly occurs during swallowing. Esophageal phase problems are characterized by neck pain, heartburn, and the sensation of food becoming "stuck" below the sternum.

A videofluoroscopic swallow study is considered the gold standard for evaluating swallowing. This imaging technique videotapes the entire swallowing process and shows an outline of the structures from the oral cavity to the stomach, as well as assessing the velocity and movement of oral and hypopharyngeal structures and their temporal relationship to each other. Through observation of the ingestion of various food consistencies, such as thin liquids, thick liquids, semisolids, and solids, the safest plan for oral intake can be determined.

Treatment

There are a number of approaches to treating dysphagia depending on the cause. One approach involves muscle strengthening exercises of the facial muscles to improve the coordination of swallowing. Most approaches involve instructing the patient and family members in ways to improve safe food intake, including positioning (usually sitting upright, with the head tilted slightly forward and downward) and food-consistency modification (no thin liquids, mechanical soft diet) during food intake. However, if the risk of aspiration is severe, the clinician may have to consider elimination of oral intake. For these patients, enteral feeding is the next choice.

COMMON PROBLEMS

■ GASTROESOPHAGEAL REFLUX DISEASE

Esophageal reflux is the backward flow of stomach or duodenal contents into the esophagus without associated retching or vomiting. It can occur in otherwise healthy people. If symptoms become severe or frequent or are associated with esophageal mucosal damage, the potential for serious clinical consequences becomes more likely, and the esophageal reflux is considered a disease. Gastroesophageal reflux disease (GERD) is a syndrome that results from esophageal reflux; the characteristic symptoms are caused by repeated exposure of the esophageal mucosa to the deleterious effects of gastrointestinal contents and the gradual breakdown of the mucosal barrier. See the Iceberg of GERD.

The Iceberg of GERD

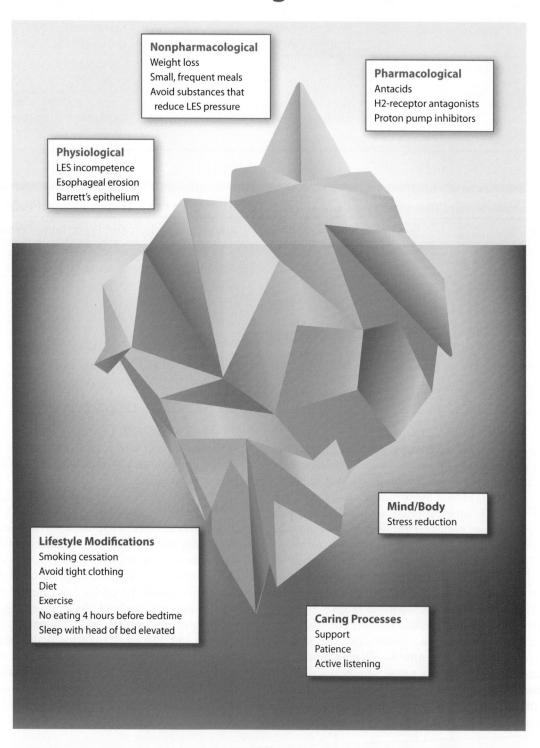

Nonpharmacological
Weight loss
Small, frequent meals
Avoid substances that
   reduce LES pressure

Pharmacological
Antacids
H2-receptor antagonists
Proton pump inhibitors

Physiological
LES incompetence
Esophageal erosion
Barrett's epithelium

Lifestyle Modifications
Smoking cessation
Avoid tight clothing
Diet
Exercise
No eating 4 hours before bedtime
Sleep with head of bed elevated

Mind/Body
Stress reduction

Caring Processes
Support
Patience
Active listening

Epidemiology and Causes

GERD can occur at any age. Some research indicates that it increases with age and then decreases after age 69. The prevalence of GERD is equal across gender, ethnic, and cultural groups in the United States; it is a common condition. There are higher rates of GERD in individuals who are overweight or obese and have a body mass index over 25. The prevalence rate for GERD in the United States is around 20%. The prevalence rate in other countries is less, ranging from 0.1% to 5% in China to 10% to 15% in the United Kingdom. Thirty-five percent to 45% of the adult population complain of heartburn at least once a month, and 10% of the adult population complain of symptoms daily. These figures may be significantly underestimated because many people with mild symptoms use over-the-counter (OTC) H_2-receptor antagonists (H_2-RAs) or antacids. Many individuals also believe that it is normal to have symptoms from time to time and attribute them to stress or dietary indiscretion.

The primary cause of GERD is the inappropriate, spontaneous, transient relaxation of the lower esophageal sphincter (LES) to an unknown stimulus. In most patients, the resting or baseline LES pressure is normal (10–30 mm Hg). In patients who have more severe disease, the LES is incompetent, with a resting pressure of less than 10 mm Hg. The incompetent LES results in free reflux during abdominal straining, lifting, bending, and recumbency. Gastric contents are acidic, and it is this low pH (less than 3.9) that causes injury to the esophageal mucosa in the majority of patients with GERD. Normally, refluxate is neutralized by swallowing salivary bicarbonate and cleared by esophageal peristalsis. Decreased swallowing (by two-thirds) during sleep, coupled with recumbency, significantly increase the duration of exposure of the mucosa to acid at night.

Historically, the presence of a hiatal hernia, which displaces the LES into the thorax, was believed to be the major cause of GERD. This is now disputed because, although most patients with hiatal hernias do experience reflux, not all patients who have reflux have hiatal hernias. The two conditions are related but separate. Delayed gastric emptying, which often worsens as people age, causes increased intra-abdominal pressure and may contribute to reflux. Obesity is also a risk factor for GERD. A number of foods and pharmacological agents are known to lower LES pressure. Table 11.5 lists the common substances that reduce LES pressure or cause direct gastric mucosal irritation.

Pathophysiology

Physiologically, gastric acid is prevented from refluxing into the esophagus by the presence of two areas of high pressure in the distal esophagus. The upper esophageal sphincter is a 3-cm segment at the proximal end of the esophagus. The LES is a 2- to 4-cm segment of the esophagus just proximal to the gastroesophageal junction

Table 11.5	Substances That Reduce Lower Esophageal Sphincter Pressure or Irritate the Gastric Mucosa

Food Substances

Alcohol

Caffeinated beverages (cola, tea, coffee)

Chocolate

Citrus fruits

Decaffeinated coffee

Fatty foods, fats (butter, margarine, shortening), and oils

Onions

Peppermint and spearmint

Tomatoes and tomato-based products (ketchup, cocktail sauce, tomato sauce, tomato paste)

Nonfood Substances

Anticholinergic drugs

Beta-adrenergic blocking agents

Calcium channel blockers

Diazepam

Estrogen and progesterone

Nicotine, including secondhand smoke

Theophylline

that prevents the reflux of gastric contents. These areas of the esophagus are under muscular, hormonal, and neural control. The anatomical placement of the LES within the abdomen supports its function, as does the acute angle (angle of His) that is formed as the esophagus enters the stomach.

Esophageal reflux occurs when the gastric volume (e.g., a large meal) or the intra-abdominal pressure is elevated (e.g., in pregnancy). It can also occur when the sphincter tone of the LES is decreased (e.g., by caffeine) or when the LES undergoes inappropriate relaxation. Gravity, saliva, and peristalsis combine to return refluxed contents to the stomach. As the esophagus becomes inflamed with repeated exposure to gastric acid, it cannot eliminate the refluxed material as quickly or efficiently, prolonging the duration of the contact with each subsequent exposure.

Because gastric contents are so irritating to the esophageal mucosa, an inflammatory response is established. With repeated exposure, the inflammation becomes chronic. In response to chronic inflammation, there is increased blood flow to the area, and erosion occurs. Frank bleeding is unusual, but minor capillary bleeding is common. As the erosion heals, the body replaces the normal squamous epithelium with metaplastic columnar epithelium (Barrett's epithelium) containing goblet and columnar cells. This new epithelium is more resistant to acid and, therefore, supports esophageal healing. Barrett's epithelium is a premalignant tissue, however, and presents a 40-fold increased risk for the development of esophageal adenocarcinoma. Fibrosis and scarring also accompany the healing process, leading to esophageal strictures.

Clinical Presentation

Subjective

The most typical symptom of GERD is heartburn, ranging in degree from mild to severe. It is usually associated with other symptoms, including regurgitation, water brash (reflex salivation), dysphagia, sour taste in the mouth in the morning, odynophagia, belching, coughing, hoarseness, or wheezing, usually at night. Substernal or retrosternal chest pain may also be present, but additional questioning can determine if the pain is activity induced, leading to the conclusion that the pain may be cardiac in origin. Factors that precipitate or make the symptoms worse, such as reclining after eating; eating a large meal; ingesting alcohol, chocolate, caffeine, fatty or spicy foods, or nicotine; wearing constrictive clothing; or working in an occupation in which heavy lifting, straining, or working in a bent-over position is involved also help establish the diagnosis of GERD. It is equally important to ask what the patient does that makes the symptoms better, such as taking antacids, sitting upright after a meal, or eating small meals.

Patients with chronic GERD may present with dysphagia as their chief complaint. The dysphagia is usually present only with the first swallow of every meal and is not progressive. Should the patient complain of progressive or persistent dysphagia, adenocarcinoma or the development of a stricture should be suspected.

Objective

The physical exam of the patient with GERD is usually normal. The only physical sign may be a stool positive for occult blood on rectal exam resulting from microhemorrhages in the irritated esophageal epithelium.

Diagnostic Reasoning

Diagnostic Tests

Diagnosis of GERD is usually made by history alone and has a sensitivity of 80%. The severity of the symptoms does not correlate well with the severity of the disease; some patients with the most severe disease have virtually no symptoms. GERD may also manifest with atypical symptoms such as adult-onset asthma, chronic cough, or sore throat.

When the diagnosis of GERD is unclear or when the patient fails to respond to 4 weeks of empiric therapy, the most accurate method of diagnosing the disease is by ambulatory esophageal pH monitoring, which involves placing pH probes 5 cm above the LES. If the pH is less than 4 above the LES and correlates with the occurrence of symptoms, the test is definitive for GERD. Esophageal manometry is indicated to determine the location of the LES before placement of the pH-monitoring probe. To prevent the overuse of upper endoscopy, the American

College of Physicians published best practice advice in 2012 for esophagogastroduodenoscopy (EGD) in adults with GERD symptoms. It recommended EGD for patients with heartburn and dysphagia, bleeding, anemia, weight loss, or recurrent vomiting. Upper endoscopy with a biopsy is the test of choice to document the type and extent of tissue damage (e.g., Barrett's esophagus) in the esophagus. It is also recommended for surveillance evaluation in anyone with Barrett's esophagus every 3 to 5 years and more frequently if there is Barrett's esophagus with dysplasia.

Differential Diagnosis

The symptoms of GERD are similar to those of peptic ulcer disease (PUD), and the two conditions often co-exist. Unlike GERD, however, PUD usually produces epigastric pain and tenderness on palpation. One pattern that can help differentiate GERD from PUD is that heartburn from PUD is usually relieved by food. This is not the case in GERD; instead, the symptoms are worse shortly after eating. Another possible differential diagnosis is gallbladder disease, which usually presents with epigastric or right subcostal pain. Nausea and possibly vomiting are usually associated with cholelithiasis and cholecystis; this is not the case in gastric reflux. There may be a strong association between the ingestion of a high-fat meal and the development of the symptoms of cholelithiasis. Occasionally, GERD may present with chest pain. In these patients, the practitioner must differentiate between symptoms of cardiac origin and those of GERD. If the pain is of cardiac origin (e.g., angina), the patient's history usually reveals that the pain is associated with exercise and is relieved by rest and nitrates. Patients with angina are often treated with medications (calcium channel blockers, beta-adrenergic blockers, nitrates) that decrease the LES pressure and produce a coexistent esophageal reflux, which complicates the differential diagnosis further.

Management

The goal of the management of GERD is to rapidly eliminate or reduce symptoms; to prevent meal- or exercise-related symptoms; and to prevent the complications of esophageal stricture, esophageal ulcer, Barrett's esophagus, pulmonary aspiration, and esophageal hemorrhage all in the most cost-effective way. The focus of management is patient education coupled with pharmacological intervention. The guidelines for treatment from the Agency for Healthcare Research and Quality include a "step-up" and a "step-down" approach. For all patients with GERD, lifestyle modifications are the first line of treatment. These include elevating the head of the bed 6 to 8 inches; smoking cessation; and avoiding high-fat meals, large meals, and certain foods such as chocolate, alcohol, peppermint, caffeine, onions, garlic, citrus, and tomatoes. The patient should be instructed to avoid recumbency or sleeping for 3 to 4 hours after a meal and avoid bedtime snacks. Some medications also should be avoided because they affect the LES pressure; these include calcium channel blockers, beta blockers, alpha-adrenergic agonists, theophylline, nitrates, and some sedatives. Weight loss should be encouraged in those patients who are overweight or obese.

If diet and lifestyle modifications are ineffective in controlling symptoms, the treatment is "stepped up" to medications. For patients with mild to moderate symptoms but nonerosion reflux disease, the first step-up is to H$_2$-RAs. These include cimetidine (Tagamet), ranitidine (Zantac), famotidine (Pepcid), and nizatidine (Axid). These are available OTC, as well as in prescription dosages. If there is no improvement, proton pump inhibitors (PPIs) are used in a dosage that effectively eliminates symptoms. Another alternative is to begin treatment with PPIs at higher doses and "step down" treatment to the lowest dose that effectively suppresses acid secretion. The most cost-effective approach is the patient-directed or "on demand" approach where the patient takes medication as needed.

Troublesome Symptoms

Initial Therapy Patients who have severe symptoms and have endoscopically documented erosive esophagitis or Barrett's esophagus are treated with PPIs such as omeprazole, rabeprazole, pantoprazole, or lansoprazole once a day 30 minutes before breakfast. An 8-week course of once-a-day treatment usually provides adequate control of heartburn in 80% to 90% of the cases and healing of erosive esophagitis in 80%, whereas twice-a-day dosing heals 95% of cases. If twice-daily dosing provides inadequate symptom relief, the patient should be evaluated with upper endoscopy. Chronic maintenance therapy with PPIs may be necessary for severe erosive esophagitis.

Long-term Therapy Patients with severe erosive esophagitis, Barrett's esophagus, peptic stricture, or who required twice-daily PPI therapy for initial symptom control should be maintained on long-term therapy. Over 80% of patients who achieved good symptom control with initial therapy and discontinue treatment will relapse. These patients may require intermittent 2- to 4-week courses of PPI therapy.

Evidence suggests that PPIs are more effective than H$_2$-RAs in all cases of GERD. These agents should not be used in combination, especially with older adults. The PPIs should be taken 30 to 60 minutes before breakfast to maximize effectiveness. If the patient requires a twice-a-day dosing, the second dose should be taken 30 to 60 minutes before dinner as well. H$_2$-RAs are considerably less expensive than PPIs but are ineffective in healing esophagitis in more severe cases. Patients on long-term therapy should have their symptoms reevaluated every 6 months in an effort to avoid potential adverse effects such as PPI-associated pneumonia, *Clostridium difficile*, osteoporosis, and vitamin B$_{12}$ deficiency.

Unresponsive Disease

The 5% to 20% of patients who do not respond to any of the above treatments may require surgical intervention. These patients are referred for laparoscopic Nissen fundoplication. Other minimally invasive procedures are also being used. These include the Endocinch procedure that endoscopically places a stitch at the junction between the esophagus and stomach that narrows the opening, thereby preventing reflux. The Stretta procedure is used to destroy the nerves at the LES, causing scar tissue and some stenosis that prevents reflux. Before referring a patient for surgical intervention, other causes of refractory GERD, such as gastrinoma, proton pump resistance, pill-induced esophagitis, or patient noncompliance, should be investigated.

Treatment Standards/Guidelines 11.1 outlines the step-up and step-down approach to the treatment of GERD and includes medications, dose, and dosing schedule.

Treatment Standards/Guidelines 11.1
Step-up/Step-down Treatment for GERD

Mild, intermittent symptoms	Trial for 4 weeks; if symptoms persist, step-up • Dietary and lifestyle modification • Pharmacological therapy • Antacids—may improve symptoms • OTC H$_2$-RA
Step-up	• Continue with diet and lifestyle modifications • Pharmacological therapy • H$_2$-RA at prescription doses (cimetidine 800 mg twice a day or 400 mg four times a day, or ranitidine 150 mg twice a day, nizatidine 150 mg twice a day, famotidine 20 mg twice a day) **OR** • PPI (omerprazole 20 mg, rabeprazole 20 mg, lansoprazole 30 mg, esomeprazole 20 mg, or pantoprazole 40 mg daily)
Troublesome Symptoms	Trial for 8 weeks; if symptoms persist, move to next step. • Dietary and lifestyle modification • Pharmacological therapy • PPI (omerprazole 40 mg, esomeprazole 40 mg daily)
Unresponsive Disease	• Dietary and lifestyle modifications • Surgical intervention (fundoplication)

Follow-up and Referral

GERD is a lifelong condition, and patients must be reevaluated on a regular basis to minimize the development of severe complications. Patients with mild-to-moderate symptoms should be instructed in the appropriate lifestyle modifications and treated with antacids or OTC H_2-RAs for a period of about 4 weeks. If on the 4-week follow-up visit there is no improvement in the symptoms, the patient can be advanced to step 2 treatment for 6 weeks. If this regimen is ineffective, the patient should be referred to a gastroenterologist. Patients who have self-medicated for a length of time may have developed erosive esophagitis or Barrett's esophagus and need aggressive treatment.

Patient Education

Education for patients with GERD includes instructing them on appropriate lifestyle modifications. Patients who are obese should be referred to a dietitian for counseling about weight loss. Dietary modifications are the keystone for lifestyle change; they include reducing the ingestion of foods that are irritating to the gastric mucosa and those that reduce LES pressure. Factors that increase intra-abdominal pressure should be avoided, such as large meals, tight or restrictive clothing, and bending or straining. It is most helpful for patients to eat small, frequent meals, with the main meal at midday. Eating less than 4 hours before bedtime, including snacks, should be avoided because this increases the chance of reflux. Patients should be instructed to sleep with the head of the bed elevated, which can be accomplished by placing blocks or bricks under the legs of the head of the bed. Sleeping with more pillows does not have the same effect as raising the head of the bed. With the head elevated, gravity helps in preventing reflux at night, when the swallowing reflex is reduced. Patients should be given assistance in smoking cessation, but the use of supplemental nicotine should be avoided because it reduces LES pressure. Programs for stress management have not been found to be helpful in reducing the symptoms of GERD.

■ GASTROENTERITIS

Gastroenteritis, also known as enteritis or gastroenterocolitis, is defined as an inflammation of the stomach and intestine that manifests as anorexia, nausea, vomiting, and diarrhea. Gastroenteritis can be acute or chronic and can be caused by bacteria, viruses, parasites, injury to the bowel mucosa, inorganic poisons (sodium nitrate), organic poisons (mushrooms or shellfish), and drugs. Chronic causes include food allergies and intolerance, stress, and lactase deficiency. Gastroenteritis caused by bacterial toxins in food is often referred to as food poisoning; it should be suspected when groups of individuals present with the same symptoms.

The symptoms and subsequent electrolyte imbalances are usually self-limiting in the healthy adult but can have serious consequences for older adults and immunocompromised or pediatric patients. The severity of the illness is indicated by the presence of dehydration secondary to profuse watery diarrhea, fever greater than 101°F (38.3°C), vomiting, or dysentery (frequent small stools containing blood and mucus). A careful history and physical exam provides clues about the causative agent and the suspected vector of transmission. Travel, dining locations, and antibiotic history should be included as part of the assessment.

Epidemiology and Causes

Acute gastroenteritis results most often from an infectious agent. Although it is one of the most frequent diagnoses in primary-care practice (about 30% of patients seen each year), the exact number of individuals affected is not known because acute gastroenteritis presents with a group of nonspecific symptoms that often go unreported or the etiology cannot be determined. Estimates are that the annual rate for gastroenteritis is approximately one episode per adult per year in the United States and Western Europe. Food- and water-borne outbreaks are of particular importance and gain the attention of the news media in an effort to identify and treat all the individuals who may have been exposed to the potentially harmful pathogen.

The most common mode of transmission for acute infectious gastroenteritis is the fecal–oral route from contaminated food or water. Person-to-person transfer of the disease is more common within the hospital setting and within day-care centers where there are larger groups of people capable of transmitting the disease. Groups considered at high risk for developing gastroenteritis include anyone traveling to a developing country, immunocompromised patients, anyone engaging in anal intercourse, residents of institutions or nursing homes, infants and children attending day-care centers, and individuals consuming raw shellfish and seafood.

Bacterial pathogens account for 30% to 80% of acute gastroenteritis cases and are an important cause of morbidity in tropical areas and in travelers to areas of high risk for the pathogens (traveler's diarrhea). Areas considered high risk for developing traveler's diarrhea include Africa, Southeast Asia, and developing countries in the Middle East or Latin America. Table 11.6 presents the most common bacterial, viral, and parasitic causes of gastroenteritis.

Gastroenteritis can also be caused by dietary factors such as coffee, tea, and sodas containing caffeine, medications (primarily antacids and antibiotics), and metabolic factors, including diabetes mellitus, hyperthyroidism, and adrenal insufficiency.

Pathophysiology

Pathophysiological causes of gastroenteritis are numerous; however, bacterial, viral, and parasitic infections are among the most common. Almost all forms of enteric

(Text continued on page 534)

Table 11.6 Organisms Causing Gastroenteritis

Pathogen	Pathogenesis	Duration/Onset	Clinical Findings	Diagnosis and Treatment
Bacterial Pathogens				
Bacillus cereus	Type of food poisoning from formation of enterotoxins within food or gut; two forms, differing in duration of illness.	Duration is normally less than 24 hours. Onset is within 1–8 hours after exposure.	Illness begins with vomiting and proceeds to diarrhea; no fever. Commonly occurs in rice dishes; the spores are heat resistant and not affected by cooking.	No antibiotic treatment is required; oral hydration and supportive care.
Campylobacter jejuni	Found primarily in eggs and poultry but may be found in domestic animals. Organism invades the intestinal mucosa and produces a cholera-like toxin. Organism grows within ileum and jejunum.	Duration of illness is 2–6 days. Onset of symptoms approximately 48 hours after ingestion of pathogen.	Common cause of traveler's diarrhea from ingestion of contaminated water. Symptoms include fever, bloody diarrhea, and abdominal pain. Stool is positive for polymorphonuclear neutrophils.	Normally self-limiting. Erythromycin ethylsuccinate (EES) can be used in severe cases. Rapid antibiotic resistance is common. Stool culture requires special media. Quinoline antibiotics have been effective in increasing recovery.
Clostridium botulinum	Anaerobic gram-positive bacillus that produces seven distinct toxins. In the food-borne type the toxin is ingested with contaminated food. Once absorbed, the toxin blocks the release of acetylcholine from peripheral nerve endings. Canned foods are the primary source.	Duration of illness depends on diagnosis and treatment. Mortality rate is high. Onset is abrupt, although incubation can be as long as 4–8 days.	GI symptoms often precede neurological findings, which are bilateral, are symmetrical, and occur in a descending fashion. Initial neurological symptoms include dry mouth, diplopia, and loss of pupillary reflex. Dysphagia and dysarthria can lead to aspiration pneumonia. Progression of neurological insult leads to paralysis of the diaphragm and death if mechanical ventilation is not employed.	Diagnosis is made by isolation of organism in suspected food, the serum, or feces. Symptoms are often confused with Guillain-Barré. Treatment is to first eliminate any unabsorbed food (toxin) by inducing vomiting or by gastric lavage, then administration of trivalent antitoxin (A, B, or E) from the Centers for Disease Control and Prevention (CDC). The antitoxin does not reverse the existing neurological symptoms but prevents progression. Little benefit if given after 72 hours. Toxin may cause serum sickness or anaphylaxis. Mechanical ventilation must be considered in an emergency.

Continued

Table 11.6 Organisms Causing Gastroenteritis—cont'd

Pathogen	Pathogenesis	Duration/Onset	Clinical Findings	Diagnosis and Treatment
Clostridium difficile	Gram-positive anaerobe maintained in spore form. It colonizes bowel when normal bowel flora are suppressed by antibiotics. It produces two toxins: toxin A, an enterotoxin, and toxin B, a cytotoxin causing pseudomembranous colitis and necrosis.	Duration and intensity of disease vary. Onset normally is in a hospitalized patient who has had recent antibiotic treatment.	Symptoms range from none to acute abdomen secondary to toxic megacolon with perforation; symptoms usually begin after initiation of antibiotics. Profuse, watery, or mucoid diarrhea, which may be blood tinged, accompanied by fever, abdominal cramping and distention, WBCs greater than 20,000, and ascites. Metabolic acidosis indicates severe colitis or toxic megacolon. Common cause of nosocomial infections in hospitals.	Diagnosis is confirmed with isolation of toxin A or B in the stool. Culture alone is no longer diagnostic because of the number of patients who are asymptomatic carriers. Flexible sigmoidoscopy may reveal pseudomembranous colitis. It is associated with recent abdominal surgery. It is treated with oral metronidazole (Flagyl) 250 mg four times daily for 10 days, vancomycin (Vancocin) 125 mg four times daily for 10 days. Relapse (20%) is treated with second course of above. Patients with multiple relapses may require 30 days of antibiotic treatment. Avoid antimotility agents.
Clostridium perfringens	Found in soil, feces, air, water. Outbreaks caused most often by contaminated meat. Type A enterotoxin causes mild to moderate gastroenteritis. Type C enterotoxin can be fatal.	Duration of illness is similar to mild gastritis, lasting 1–4 days without medical intervention. Fatal cases are less common. Onset is usually within 12 hours of ingestion of contaminated food.	Abrupt onset of diarrhea without fever. If fatal, cases have severe diarrhea with abdominal pain and distention.	Diagnosis is made by isolating organism in food or feces. Cultures usually show many clostridia in food or feces. No treatment is necessary for mild forms other than supportive care. Penicillin may be useful in severe cases.
Escherichia coli (E coli)	Five identified strains classified by pathogenesis of diarrhea. All are gram-negative rods.	Dependent on strain; epidemics are due to ingestion of contaminated meat or dairy products.		

Enterohemorrhagic *E coli* (EHEC). Most serious; produces a hemorrhagic infection; O157:H7 strain produces two toxins, which inhibit protein synthesis in intestinal cells.	Duration typically 1–8 days. Onset is 24 hours after ingestion of contaminated food.	Acute onset of dysentery with 12–24 hours of abdominal cramps, watery diarrhea, and fever is followed by bloody stools. Can cause hemorrhagic infection of colon and can be fatal. Complications include hemolytic-uremic syndrome (HUS) or thrombolytic thrombocytopenic purpura (TTP). WBCs are greater than 20,000; azotemia; dehydration. Infants and older adults are most prone to adverse effects.	Diagnosis is by isolation of *E coli* O157:H7 in stools. Look for the source of undercooked meat. It can be transmitted in feces and dirty diapers. Treatment is supportive. Antibiotics have not proved effective.
Enterotoxigenic *E coli* (ETEC). Adheres to the mucosa of small bowel releasing toxins, which cause diarrhea.	Duration 2–4 days. Incubation period is 24–36 hours.	Most common cause of traveler's diarrhea from contaminated food or water. Mild fever, abdominal cramps, watery stool, nausea, and vomiting are common.	Usually self-limiting, requiring no treatment other than supportive care. It is common in developing countries.
Enteropathogenic *E coli* (EPEC).	Duration is 1–3 days; 12- to 36-hour incubation period.	Profuse, watery, foul-smelling diarrhea. It is of special concern to infants and older adults who are prone to dehydration.	Usually self-limiting. Infants and older adults may require hospitalization. It is rare in the United States.
Enteroinvasive *E coli* (EIEC) causes invasion and proliferation within enterocytes, much like *Shigella* infection.	Duration is 4–10 days; 12- to 72-hour incubation period.	It is an uncommon cause of food-borne dysentery in the United States. Patients have fever, anorexia, cramps, and watery diarrhea. Stools may be mucoid or bloody. Clinical presentation is much like that of *Shigella* infection.	May isolate leukocytes in stool. Diarrhea is self-limiting. Food poisoning of this kind is rare in the United States.
Enteroadherent *E coli* (EAEC) is rare and adheres to liver cells.		Mild, nonbloody diarrhea; strain is uncommon.	No leukocytes in stool.

Continued

Table 11.6   Organisms Causing Gastroenteritis—cont'd

Pathogen	Pathogenesis	Duration/Onset	Clinical Findings	Diagnosis and Treatment
Vibrio cholerae	Commonly found in areas with poor sanitation; food and water contaminated with feces. Enterotoxin causes hypersecretion in small intestine. Rarely found in the United States but may be endemic along the Gulf Coast.	Incubation is 1–3 days. Duration is 1–2 weeks.	Most cases in the United States are hemolytic and are transported here from contaminated foods. Diarrhea can be severe, causing septicemia, especially in immunocompromised patients, children, or older adults. Diarrhea is profuse, "rice water" and can be life-threatening. There is no abdominal cramping or fever. Patients may stool at the rate of 1 L/hr.	To diagnose *V cholerae* a special *Vibrio*-selective medium must be used in the stool culture. Diarrhea requires prompt replacement of fluids and electrolytes. Antibiotic: tetracycline 500 mg PO every 6 hours for 2 days or Bactrim DS every 12 hours for 2 days.
Vibrio parahaemolyticus	Pathogen found in seafood. Produces toxins in the gut or invades intestinal mucosa. Outbreaks frequent in summer; usually associated with improperly cooked seafood.	Incubation period 8–24 hours. Duration is 1–3 days.	Patient presents with abdominal cramping, headache, fever. Usually associated with explosive, noninflammatory, watery diarrhea, which may be bloody depending on the degree of mucosal destruction.	Stool is positive for *Vibrio*. Often diagnosed when a group of people become sick after consuming seafood. Food cultures are positive.
Yersinia enterocolitica	Primarily transmitted via fecal-oral route; food borne. It is rare in the United States; more common in northern Europe and Canada. Organism forms an enterotoxin and invades the intestinal epithelium.	Onset and incubation are unknown. Duration usually resolves in 1–3 weeks.	Symptoms include fever, abdominal pain, and bloody diarrhea. Older children may develop mesenteric adenitis, which presents with fever, right lower quadrant pain, and leukocytosis; similar to symptoms of appendicitis. Adults may present with polyarthritis, Reiter's syndrome, and erythema nodosum. *Yersinia* can cause bacteremia.	Diagnosis is made by isolation of organism in the stool. Stool also tests positive for fecal leukocytes. Treatment for severe cases is tetracycline 250–500 mg every 6 hours for 7–10 days; ciprofloxin 500 mg PO twice daily; tobramycin 3–5 mg/kg per day every 8 hours.
Salmonella	One of the major causes of diarrhea worldwide. Three species: *S typhi, S choleraesuis,* and *S enteritidis.* Found	Duration is 2–5 days; onset is 8–48 hours after ingestion. Patients may become "chronic carriers," defined as	Peak incidence is in summer and fall. Symptoms begin with nausea and vomiting, followed by colicky abdominal pain and	Diagnosis is made by isolation of organism in stool. No treatment is necessary unless associated with fever

Organism				
	primarily in chicken, eggs, and livestock, causing 85% of community-acquired *Salmonella* outbreaks. Individuals must ingest 10,000–1 million organisms to become infected.	individuals with positive stool cultures 1 year after initial disease.	bloody or mucoid diarrhea. Enteric fever results from organisms entering the bloodstream via the bowel lymphatics, causing bacteremia, headache, and myalgias. Tissue abscesses may develop. Stools may be foul smelling.	and systemic disease. Treatment includes trimethoprim-sulfamethoxazole (Bactrim DS) or a quinoline, norfloxin 400 mg or ofloxin 400 mg PO twice daily for 7–10 days. Stress proper handling of food, thorough cooking, and good hand washing.
Shigella	One of the most common causes of bacillary dysentery. Several species: *S sonnei* is isolated in 75% of cases in the United States. Because of poor hygiene and overcrowding, it is spread via the fecal–oral route and requires only a small number of organisms to produce disease. Organism causes epithelial invasion of intestinal mucosa.	Duration usually 4–7 days and is self-limiting. Incubation period of 1–2 days after exposure or ingestion of pathogen.	Initially patients present with watery diarrhea and high fever. Later colitis-type symptoms develop: Abdominal cramps, tenesmus, urgency, frequent small stools with blood and mucus. Low-grade fever may persist for 2–20 days. Complications can include hemolytic-uremic syndrome (HUS) and colitis.	Diagnosis is made by isolation of organism in stool or rectal swab. In severe cases sigmoidoscopy shows mucosal hyperemia, friability, and ulceration. Treat with Bactrim DS twice daily for 3 days if infection was acquired in the United States.
Staphylococcus	Common cause of food poisoning. Caused by ingestion of enterotoxin found in improperly handled or stored foods. Enterotoxins produced by *Staphylococcus* act on receptors in the gut, which then transmit impulses to medullary centers.	Abrupt onset 1–8 hours after ingestion of contaminated food. Duration is usually less than 24 hours.	Abrupt onset of nausea, vomiting, colicky abdominal cramps, profuse watery diarrhea.	Definitive diagnosis is made only if contaminated food source is tested; otherwise, diagnosis is made based on short incubation and duration of symptoms.

Continued

Table 11.6 Organisms Causing Gastroenteritis—cont'd

Pathogen	Pathogenesis	Duration/Onset	Clinical Findings	Diagnosis and Treatment
Viral Pathogens				
Rotavirus	Very common cause of gastroenteritis in industrialized areas. Organism most often implicated in deaths from diarrhea. Frequently involves small bowel. A disaccharidase deficiency is common after rotavirus infections. Rotavirus is an RNA virus with four antigenic serotypes.	Incubation period 24–36 hours. Duration is 4–6 days.	Common in children younger than age 3. Peak incidence at age 6–24 months. Uncommon in adults because most have developed immunity. Symptoms include low-grade fever and copious watery diarrhea. Outbreaks are more common in winter months.	Diagnosis is made by electron microscopy. Serological enzyme-linked immunosorbent assay (ELISA) tests are available. No leukocytes found in stool.
Norwalk virus	Cube-shaped virus with seven known antigenic variants. It can cause large epidemics spread by contaminated water. It is transmitted by the fecal-oral route. It is a common cause of absenteeism due to "viral gastroenteritis."	Incubation is 18–48 hours. Duration is 48–72 hours.	Illness can be very debilitating to some patients. Symptoms are mild and brief and include vomiting, frequent watery diarrhea, diffuse myalgias, chills, and sometimes fever. Often causes family outbreaks.	No known antiviral therapy is available. Fluid and electrolyte replacement is the treatment of choice. Virus can be isolated with electron microscopy but is costly and the disease is self-limiting.
Protozoal Pathogens				
Giardia lamblia	Approximately 4% of healthy U.S. citizens harbor *G lamblia* in their intestines and are asymptomatic. *G lamblia* is a protozoon that attaches to the mucosa of the small bowel. Patients with hypogamma globulinemia and achlorhydria are predisposed to giardiasis. It is transmitted via oral–anal intercourse and is a common cause of traveler's diarrhea and diarrhea in children who attend day-care centers.	Incubation is 1–4 weeks. Duration usually 1–6 weeks.	Symptoms range from nonspecific complaints of bloating, flatulence, nausea, and watery, noninflammatory diarrhea to chronic diarrhea with weight loss, anorexia, and malabsorption.	Diagnosis can be made by examination of stool but is most often made by duodenal aspirate or small bowel biopsy. Stool exam is positive for trophozoites in about 50% of confirmed cases. Treatment with quinacrine hydrochloride (Atabrine) 100 mg three times daily after meals for 5–7 days or metronidazole (Flagyl) 250 mg three times daily for 5–7 days.

Entamoeba histolytica (amebiasis)	Transmitted via contaminated food and water, primarily in tropical areas with poor sanitation. Common in Mexican migrant workers and military personnel returning from the Far East. Human host becomes a reservoir after ingesting cysts from source and can transmit disease via fecal–oral route. Venereal transmission is common in the male homosexual population.	Most common clinical variant is the asymptomatic cyst carrier who can be a reservoir for an undetermined length of time. Duration can be weeks to months.	Symptoms include abdominal cramps, abdominal pain, and weight loss. Diarrhea contains blood and mucus. Patients may have hepatomegaly and pain over the cecum and ascending colon. Some patients may have fever, tenesmus, and acute dysentery illness. Complications can include peritonitis, toxic megacolon, and hepatic abscess. The encysted ameba is passed into the environment, where it can survive for up to 10 days.	Diagnosis is important to distinguish amebiasis from ulcerative colitis because treatment with glucocorticoids can accelerate amebic colitis and enhance systemic invasion. Sigmoidoscopy reveals discrete rectosigmoid ulcers with normal intervening mucosa. Indirect hemagglutination test is effective in detecting invasive amebic disease but remains positive long after treatment. Treat with metronidazole (Flagyl) 750 mg three times daily for 7–10 days.
Cryptosporidium	Enteric protozoan parasite that invades the small bowel located just below the basement membrane. Causes two distinct syndromes—one in immunocompetent and one in immunosuppressed individuals. Common cause of water-borne outbreaks from inadequate filtration. Parasite produces an exotoxin.	Incubation is 1–3 weeks. Usually self-limiting but can last 1–2 weeks in immunocompromised patients.	Outbreaks can occur after ingestion of water contaminated with livestock waste. Also common in day-care centers and patients with AIDS. Immunocompromised patients develop severe cholera-like diarrhea, which can last for months and cause daily fluid losses of 5–10 L/day.	Diagnosis by isolation of parasite in stool. Commercially available immunofluorescent antibody test can also assist diagnosis. Leukocytes not present in stool. Intestinal mucosa not inflamed but with ulcerations. Suggested treatment includes paromomycin (Humatin) 500 mg PO four times daily with food for 14–28 days, then 500 mg twice daily indefinitely. If treatment fails: azithromycin (Zithromax) 2.4 g PO on day 1, 1.2 g PO for 27 days, and then 600 mg/day for maintenance indefinitely.

infection manifest with diarrhea. Diarrheal diseases cause an increase in the frequency of stools, less well formed feces, and an increase in the fecal water content. The definition of diarrhea is dependent on each patient's normal bowel habits. Diarrhea is not considered a medical emergency unless it affects children or older adults who are less able to regulate their fluid intake. Diarrhea is a major cause of infant mortality in developing nations.

The gastrointestinal (GI) tract has several defenses against the development of infection. When bacterial or viral pathogens can overcome these barriers, they proliferate, causing varying degrees of gastroenteritis. The acidity of the stomach is normally maintained at a pH of 2, which creates a hostile environment for most microorganisms. This acidic barrier protects the small bowel and colon from ingested pathogens. If the organism is resistant to the acid environment or the patient has taken medications that alter the pH, the organism may thrive and cause illness.

Another host defense mechanism is the constant peristalsis of the small bowel, which prevents the colonization of pathogens within the lumen. Patients who have small bowel stasis as a result of obstruction, diverticuli, or blind loop syndrome frequently develop an overgrowth of bacteria within the stagnant segment, causing gastroenteritis resulting from the increased number of bacteria in the small bowel. In contrast, the colon is relatively stagnant; it typically harbors about 1 billion bacteria per gram of intestinal contents. Normal feces are composed primarily of water and bacteria. These beneficial bacteria protect against potential pathogens by consuming available nutrients and by producing by-products that create a hostile environment to the invading pathogens.

The GI tract also produces specific immunoglobulins that protect against invading organisms. After exposure to certain organisms, immunoglobulins may even protect against future invasions by the same organism, much like an antigen–antibody response. IgA, a secretory immunoglobulin, may help defend against many of the bacteria that cause gastroenteritis by invading the intestinal mucosa.

Ingestion of contaminated food can result in clinical symptoms of gastroenteritis, depending on the number and virulence of the organisms in the food. Almost all bacteria are capable of producing mild diarrhea if ingested in large enough quantities. Other organisms (e.g., *Shigella, Salmonella, Campylobacter, Cryptosporidium*) have such a high virulence that only a small inoculum can produce symptoms.

Often, the incubation time of the pathogen, coupled with the presenting symptoms, will give specific clues for establishing a diagnosis. Infectious processes of the small intestine often result in watery, secretory, or a malabsorptive type of diarrhea; infections of the large intestine tend to produce bloody diarrhea and abdominal pain. Gastroenteritis with an onset of nausea and vomiting within 6 hours after exposure to the pathogen suggests food poisoning resulting from the ingestion of a preformed toxin such as that of *Bacillus cereus*. Incubation periods greater than 14 hours and the initial symptom of vomiting are highly suggestive of viral infections.

Clinical Presentation
Subjective

Patients with gastroenteritis present with varying degrees of nausea, vomiting, diarrhea, fever, and abdominal pain and cramping. Symptoms depend on the underlying cause but can also include fatigue, malaise, anorexia, tenesmus, and borborygmus. Individuals with profuse diarrhea may complain of rectal burning and hematochezia from rectal abrasion and bleeding. Patients may complain of symptoms that suggest dysentery, including passage of numerous small-volume stools containing blood and mucus. Reports of voluminous stools are suggestive of a source in the small bowel or proximal colon; small stools accompanied by a sense of urgency suggest a source in the left colon or rectum. Bloody stools suggest mucosal damage and an inflammatory process secondary to invasive pathogens. Frothy stools and flatus suggest a malabsorption problem.

Objective

The physical exam is usually normal except for the aforementioned GI problems. Depending on the degree of dehydration, the skin turgor may be poor, and mucous membranes may be dry. Vital signs may reflect dehydration, such as a fever with an increase in temperature and heart rate. Older and very young patients with gastroenteritis may show signs of severe dehydration such as orthostatic hypotension and dizziness. Patients who have had prolonged illness and are malnourished may present with edema resulting from hypoalbuminemia.

Diagnostic Reasoning
Diagnostic Tests

Evaluation of the history is of vital importance to the appropriate diagnosis and management of the patient with gastroenteritis. The patient must be questioned thoroughly about the temporal association of symptoms with the suspected pathogen. Patient history should include a thorough drug history, including over-the-counter drugs, antibiotics, antacids, laxatives, alcohol, and sugar substitutes. It is important to know the patient's travel history, surgical history, and sexual orientation and practices. The duration of the illness is important in the differential diagnosis because acute diarrhea is usually caused by infectious agents or toxins, whereas chronic diarrhea usually has a noninfectious etiology.

Laboratory diagnosis of acute gastroenteritis is not always necessary in patients with nonbloody diarrhea and no evidence of systemic toxicity. In the average, otherwise healthy adult, the disease will normally run its course without incident, and there is no need for costly evaluation. Selection of the most appropriate tests is based on information received from the history and physical exam. In patients with severe diarrhea and dehydration, stools should be examined for consistency, blood, and fecal leukocytes. Numerous fecal leukocytes in patients with acute diarrhea is indicative of diffuse colonic inflammation and is highly suggestive of an invasive pathogen such as *Shigella, Salmonella,* or *Campylobacter.* Other causes of leukocyte-positive stools include *Clostridium difficile, Yersinia, Vibrio parahaemolyticus,* and *Escherichia coli.* In patients with chronic diarrhea, fecal leukocytes suggest inflammatory bowel disease (IBD) or ischemia.

A stool culture should be done on any patient who has severe diarrhea, a fever of 101.3°F (38.5°C) or higher, the presence of bloody stools, or stools that test positive for leukocytes, lactoferrin, or occult blood because these findings are indications of a bacterial pathogen. Routine stool culture will identify the presence of *Shigella, Salmonella, Campylobacter, Aeromonas,* and *Yersinia.* In diarrheal illnesses that are suspected to be caused by eating contaminated hamburger meat, stools can be cultured for *E coli.*

Blood cultures should be obtained from patients who show clinical signs of typhoid or enteric fever or from any hospitalized patient who has an intestinal illness with high fever. It is essential that the blood cultures be obtained before initiation of antibiotic therapy.

Stools should be examined for ova and parasites in cases of persistent diarrhea, especially if the symptoms began after travel to Russia, Nepal, the Rocky Mountains, or other mountainous regions, or after exposure to infants in a day-care center. Parasites should also be considered in homosexual males or any patient with HIV/AIDS who presents with diarrhea, as well as in a patient with diarrhea who lives in a community where a water-borne outbreak has occurred. If a patient has diarrhea that has lasted longer than 2 weeks and the stool is negative for fecal leukocytes, a stool exam for parasites should be considered. Patients with intestinal amebiasis usually have no leukocytes in their stool because of the noninflamed areas of intestinal mucosa between the areas of ulceration, as well as the lytic effects of the exotoxins produced by the parasite. If parasitic infection is highly suspected but the stool culture is negative, a small bowel biopsy is indicated to identify the causative agent. Immunofluorescent antibody tests and diagnostic enzyme-linked immunosorbent assay (ELISA) tests are more sensitive than microscopic studies for identifying *Giardia* and *Cryptosporidium.*

In patients with epidemiological evidence, stool samples should be sent to the laboratory for specific enteropathogen studies that are not normally detected with routine stool culture, such as enterohemorrhagic colitis (*E coli* O157:H7), *Vibrio cholerae,* other noncholera vibrios, and other Shiga toxin–producing *E coli.* Routine stool culture identifies certain strains of *Yersinia* and *E coli* O157:H7; however, some strains can be detected only by research laboratories. Any patient who develops diarrhea after initiation or completion of antibiotic therapy should have tissue culture assay or an ELISA test for *C difficile* toxin.

Viral gastroenteritis should be suspected in patients who present with vomiting as the major symptom and in cases where food- or water-borne contamination is suspected and the incubation period is greater than 12 hours. Although there are commercially available test kits that identify rotaviruses, their application is limited because there is no known treatment for viral causes of illness.

Flexible sigmoidoscopy is usually reserved for patients with colitis that is unresponsive to antibiotic therapy and for patients with persistent diarrhea undiagnosed by laboratory evaluation. Tissue biopsy can help identify the offending pathogen, as well as differentiate infection from chronic inflammatory changes consistent with IBDs or celiac disease.

Differential Diagnosis

The differential diagnosis of gastroenteritis, particularly in patients with persistent or chronic diarrhea and severe abdominal pain, should include inflammatory bowel syndrome, IBD, ischemic bowel disease (especially in patients with peripheral vascular disease), partial bowel obstruction, and pelvic abscess. Other considerations for diagnosis should include ruling out complications from diabetes mellitus, small bowel diverticulosis, Whipple's disease, chronic pancreatitis, and any surgical alteration of the GI tract that might interfere with normal absorption.

Management

All patients who present with diarrhea require fluid and electrolyte management, particularly children, older adults, and immunosuppressed patients. Patients who are dehydrated and able to tolerate oral fluid replacement should be instructed to drink fluids with a sodium content of 45 to 75 mEq/L (Pedialyte or Gatorade) or be provided with oral rehydration salts. In patients who are severely dehydrated or those who have chronic diseases and are hypotensive, hospitalization for IV hydration may be indicated. In otherwise healthy adult patients who are not dehydrated, sports drinks, diluted fruit juices, and broths or soups are usually adequate for fluid and sodium replacement.

Patients with diarrhea require a diet that includes calories that come from boiled starches and cereals (potatoes, pasta, rice, wheat, and oats), which will facilitate enterocyte renewal, with the addition of salt for the duration of illness. Once stools have started to become formed, the diet can be advanced as tolerated. Some authors advise avoiding dairy products; however, this is not necessary unless there is clinical evidence of lactose intolerance.

Nonspecific symptomatic treatment of acute diarrhea can decrease the occurrence by 50% and is most effective against secretory diarrhea. Antimotility drugs are the most frequently prescribed and most effective drugs for the treatment of symptomatic gastroenteritis. These agents work by slowing intraluminal peristalsis, thereby slowing the passage of fluids through the lumen, which facilitates absorption. Patients with febrile dysentery should not receive antimotility medications because slowing the intraluminal time may prolong the duration of the disease. Drugs Commonly Prescribed 11.3 lists medications commonly recommended for the symptomatic treatment of acute diarrhea.

Empiric antimicrobial therapy is recommended for patients with severe diarrhea, especially those with fever or stool positive for leukocytes. Traveler's diarrhea is treated empirically with trimethoprim-sulfamethoxazole (Bactrim DS), one double-strength tablet twice daily for 3 days. Other antibiotics that are effective for milder forms of illness include a single dose of ciprofloxacin (Cipro) 500 mg, norfloxacin (Noroxin) 400 mg, or ofloxacin (Floxin) 300 mg. Antibiotic prophylaxis, which has a 90% effectiveness rate, for people traveling in high-risk areas includes the antibiotics mentioned above in daily doses continuing for 2 days after returning home. Nonantibiotic preventive therapy includes bismuth subsalicylate (Pepto-Bismol), two tablets before each meal and at bedtime for a total of eight tablets/day for the entire trip. This remedy has an approximately 60% effectiveness rate.

Follow-up and Referral

Follow-up is not usually required except in those patients suffering from the chronic forms of infectious diarrhea such as from *C difficile*. Often, patients with serious infectious diarrhea will require home administration of IV antibiotics. Patients who require sigmoidoscopy for biopsy of intestinal mucosa for identification of the pathogen should be referred to a gastroenterologist.

Patient Education

The aim of patient education is prevention of the spread of disease from patients with infectious diarrhea to other individuals. Teaching includes good hand washing and safe disposal of waste products. Any infant or child with infectious diarrhea should not attend day care until the diarrhea has stopped or the child has completed the prescribed course of antibiotics. Good hand washing technique is imperative to prevent household outbreaks of the disease.

Patients traveling in high-risk areas should be instructed to consume only safe foods and beverages there and on the airplane leaving the area. "Safe" foods include acidic foods such as unpeeled citrus fruits; dry foods such as breads and cereals; steamed foods and beverages such as coffee, tea, and cooked vegetables; foods containing high amounts of sugar such as syrups, jellies, and jams; and bottled carbonated drinks such as soda and beer. It is generally not considered safe to drink bottled water (unless bottled from a safe source) or to eat raw, uncooked vegetables, including salad. Patients with known HIV infection and any other individuals with a known debilitating illness who may not tolerate any degree of gastroenteritis should be encouraged to take antibiotic prophylaxis.

■ PEPTIC ULCER DISEASE

Peptic ulcer disease (PUD) is a generic name for both gastric ulcers and duodenal ulcers. A peptic ulcer is a break in the surface mucosa of the stomach or duodenum, which results when there is disruption of the normal mucosal defenses and the tissue is exposed to the damaging effects of acid and pepsin. By definition, a peptic ulcer penetrates the muscularis mucosa and is

Drugs Commonly Prescribed 11.3 Symptomatic Treatment of Acute Diarrhea		
Drug	Indication	Adverse Reactions and Prescribing Considerations
bismuth subsalicylate (Pepto-Bismol)	Acute diarrhea	Not as effective as loperamide in acute diarrhea. May potentiate the effects of antidiabetic medications. Do not use with antibiotics in patients with HIV infection.
loperamide (Imodium)	Acute diarrhea	Drug of choice for afebrile, nondysenteric cases of acute diarrhea. Minimal central opiate effect.
diphenoxylate with atropine (Lomotil)	Acute diarrhea	Prescription only. For use in afebrile, nondysentery cases of acute diarrhea. Has central opiate effects. Overdose possible. Atropine has adverse effects that may limit use.

usually larger than 5 mm in diameter. Peptic ulcers occur when there is an imbalance between the protective factors of the mucosa and aggressive factors as acid and pepsin. The initial damage to the mucosa is usually a result of infection by *Helicobacter pylori* or medications, particularly NSAIDs.

Epidemiology and Causes

A person's lifetime risk of developing a peptic ulcer is from 5% to 10%. Approximately 500,000 new cases are diagnosed each year in the United States. Men and women are almost equally affected by peptic ulcers, with the incidence in men slightly higher. Most duodenal ulcers occur in patients between age 30 and 55, but gastric ulcers are more prevalent between age 55 and 70.

A variety of conditions are considered to be risk factors for the development of PUD, but the three major causes are infection with *H pylori,* chronic ingestion of aspirin and other NSAIDs, and acid hypersecretion such as in Zollinger-Ellison syndrome. Genetics, blood type, personality type, and cigarette smoking may also play a role in the development of PUD. Patients with chronic obstructive pulmonary disease, cirrhosis, renal failure, and renal transplant have a higher incidence of PUD than the general public, but the mechanism is not known. Dietary factors such as caffeine, alcohol, and spicy foods are no longer considered to be ulcerogenic.

Pathophysiology

The majority of ulcers are located in the duodenum and approximately 90% occur within 3 cm of the pylorus. Almost all patients with gastric ulcers have normal or subnormal amounts of gastric acid secretion. Only about 35% of patients with duodenal ulcers have demonstrated above-average rates of acid secretion but have impaired duodenal bicarbonate secretion that is *H pylori* dependent. The breakdown of the local mucosal defenses appears to play a larger role in the pathogenesis of ulcer formation. Mucosal defense is supported by surface mucus and bicarbonate, which form a thin alkaline gel coating mucosal cells, and by prostaglandin-enhanced mucosal blood flow and cell renewal.

A variety of factors can affect the development of ulcers. Cigarette smoking facilitates ulcer formation, which is proportional to the amount smoked. The mechanism by which cigarette smoking causes ulcer formation is unclear. Aspirin and other NSAIDs decrease the mucosal defense mechanisms by inhibiting prostaglandin synthesis, leaving the area vulnerable to the effects of gastric hydrochloric acid and pepsin. Many infectious agents have been detected in patients with ulcer disease, but *H pylori* is the most important. As many as 75% of patients with duodenal ulcers are infected with *H pylori,* and the bacterium is present in the majority of gastric ulcer patients although the association with gastric ulcers is less. Not everyone with *H pylori* infection, however, develops PUD.

Clinical Presentation
Subjective

The hallmark of PUD is a complaint of a burning or gnawing (hunger) sensation or pain (dyspepsia) in the epigastrium, which is often relieved by food or antacids. These complaints, however, are not specific or sensitive enough to be diagnostic of ulcer disease. Patients with PUD usually describe an episodic pattern of complaints in which the pain tends to cluster and last for minutes, with the episodes separated by periods of no symptoms. It is this alternating pattern that is more predictive of ulcer disease than the nature of the symptoms themselves. Almost half the patients with NSAID-induced ulcers are asymptomatic.

Nocturnal pain is present in two-thirds of patients with duodenal ulcers and one-third of those with gastric ulcers. This corresponds to the circadian stimulation of acid secretion. Nausea and anorexia sometimes occur in patients with gastric ulcer, whereas vomiting and weight loss are indications of more serious complications such as gastric malignancy or pyloric obstruction. Patients with duodenal ulcers may report a reduction in pain after eating; patients with gastric ulcers tend to experience more intense pain after eating, which is a result of secretion of gastric acids.

Objective

The physical exam is not useful in differentiating PUD from other types of upper gastrointestinal (GI) disorders. Patients with duodenal ulcers often demonstrate epigastric tenderness 2.5 cm to the right of the midline, but this may also be present with cholecystitis, pancreatitis, nonulcer dyspepsia, and other GI disorders. Reports of melena or coffee-ground–like emesis usually indicate a bleeding ulcer, and a perforated ulcer may present with abdominal rigidity.

Diagnostic Reasoning
Diagnostic Tests

Most routine laboratory tests are normal in patients with ulcer disease unless there is significant bleeding or vomiting, in which case the results show anemia and fluid and electrolyte disturbances. When a patient is actively bleeding, a complete blood count to evaluate hemoglobin levels is paramount. There is controversy in the literature regarding the hemoglobin level that would require transfusion. Most patients with upper GI bleeding should have *restrictive strategy,* defined as transfusing when hemoglobin levels fall below 7 g/dL. The diagnostic standard for PUD is upper GI endoscopy. It is much more accurate in diagnosing ulcer disease than the previously used upper GI radiographic series. Endoscopy also does not involve exposure to radiation, which is a concern, particularly in pregnant patients.

Research has implicated *H pylori* gastritis in 90% to 95% of both duodenal and gastric ulcers that are not associated with NSAIDs. *H pylori* infection increases with age, and in the United States more than 50% of asymptomatic persons older than 60 years show evidence of active or past infection. Worldwide, at least 30% to 50% of the population is colonized with this bacterium, but the rate is declining. The mode of transmission is unknown. In response to *H pylori*, the stomach produces more gastrin, which in turn leads to an increase in the amount of acid secreted by the parietal cells. The excess acid and pepsin on the stomach lining can cause the lining to erode and leads to the development of an ulcer. A simple serology test for *H pylori* can be done. *H pylori* can also be diagnosed by direct bacteriological analysis via an esophagogastroduodenoscopy (EGD) biopsy. EGD is an expensive, invasive procedure with possible complications; therefore, it is ordered for examination of individuals who have failed the standard triple-drug therapy for *H pylori* (see Drugs Commonly Prescribed 11.4) or for those who require direct visualization of the gastric mucosa for acute bleeding. There are a number of other ways to diagnose *H pylori*. A serological antibody (enzyme-linked immunosorbent assay) test can be used to detect infection with *H pylori*, but the test does not distinguish between active or past (treated) infection and is expensive. Urease is plentiful in patients with *H pylori* infection. Breath tests for *H pylori* are based on the production of ammonia from the metabolism of urea by urease. These breath tests indicate active infection and are a noninvasive way of diagnosing *H pylori* infection, although negative tests have a poor predictive value because false-negative results are more likely than truly negative findings.

In patients for whom an increase in gastric acid secretion is suspected, a fasting serum gastrin level should be drawn. Levels higher than 200 pg/mL should be confirmed on repeat testing and followed by basal and peak acid-output measurements. Zollinger-Ellison syndrome should be suspected in patients whose fasting serum gastrin level is above 600 pg/mL and who have a basal acid output of more than 15 mmol/hr.

Differential Diagnosis

PUD must be distinguished from other causes of epigastric distress, which can be problematic because a variety of thoracic and upper abdominal disorders can cause similar pain. Diseases to be considered in the differential diagnosis should include nonulcer dyspepsia, cholecystitis, pancreatitis, irritable bowel syndrome, gastroesophageal reflux disease, gastric cancer, myocardial ischemia, gastritis, and gastroenteritis. If the pain does not respond to food or antacids and there is severe pain and rebound tenderness, the cause is not likely to be an uncomplicated peptic ulcer. If the patient presents with weight loss, anemia, or exacerbation of the pain when eating, gastric cancer should be suspected.

Management

The principal aim of management for patients with PUD is to relieve pain, heal the ulcer, and prevent complications

---

Drugs Commonly Prescribed 11.4   Peptic Ulcer Disease

Drug	Indication	Adverse Reactions and Prescribing Considerations
First-line Therapy Antacids—only for symptom relief Mylanta II 2–4 tsp between meals and at bedtime Sucralfate 1 g four times per day for 4–8 weeks Proton pump inhibitors (PPIs)—all should be administered 30 minutes before breakfast Omeprazole 20 mg Lansoprazole 30 mg Esomeprazole 40 mg Rabeprazole 20 mg Pantoprazole 40 mg	Peptic ulcer disease	These medications should be used only as long as the patient is symptomatic and as needed.
Second-line Therapy PPIs as above PLUS Metronidazole 250 mg 4 times per day or Metronidazole 500 mg 3 times per day PLUS Tetracycline 500 mg 4 times per day PLUS Bismuth subsalicylate 2 tablets 4 times per day	When first-line therapy fails	These medication may inhibit absorption of digoxin, tetracycline antibiotics, and quinolone antibiotics. This regimen should be used for 10–14 days. Long-term use of PPIs is not advised. This drug may potentiate the effects of antidiabetic medications causing hypoglycemia.

or recurrences. Pharmacological therapy is the foundation of management for PUD, but nonpharmacological measures, such as smoking cessation, should be used as well. Cigarette smoking increases the risk for PUD; in patients with documented ulcers, smoking impairs healing, promotes recurrence, and increases the morbidity and mortality. There are no firm dietary measures for patients with PUD other than instructions to avoid foods that precipitate dyspepsia. Pharmacological intervention for PUD consists of H_2-receptor antagonists (H_2-RAs), proton pump inhibitors (PPIs), and agents that enhance the mucosal defenses, such as antacids, sucralfate (Carafate), bismuth subsalicylate (Pepto-Bismol), and prostaglandin analogs (misoprostol), as well as antibiotics.

Proton Pump Inhibitors

The PPIs are now the drugs of choice for treating PUD because they are more effective than H_2-RAs and are easier to use. The duration of action of the PPIs is more than 24 hours, whereas H_2-RAs inhibit only 65% of acid secretion over 24 hours. Another advantage of PPIs over H_2-RAs is that the PPIs are given on a once-a-day dosage schedule whereas H_2-RAs require at least twice-daily dosing. The usual dosage is either omeprazole 20 mg, rabeprazole 20 mg, lansoprazole 30 mg, esomeprazole 40 mg, or pantoprazole 40 mg. All of the PPIs inhibit parietal cell hydrogen-potassium adenosine triphosphatase (ATPase), which mediates hydrogen ion secretion. PPIs heal 90% of duodenal ulcers in 4 weeks of therapy and 90% of gastric ulcers after 8 weeks. Long-term use of these drugs is associated with slightly decreased absorption of vitamin B_{12} and iron.

H_2-Receptor Antagonists

If a patient has mild symptoms and no indicators of complications or a more serious disease, empiric therapy with an H_2-RA should be instituted for 2 weeks. After the initial treatment period, if symptoms persist or worsen, upper endoscopy should be considered for a more definitive diagnosis. When H_2-RAs are used for peptic ulcer treatment, the standard treatment is to administer an H_2-RA once a day at bedtime or half the daily dose twice a day for 8 weeks. More than 80% of ulcers are healed by the completion of this regimen. H_2-RAs effectively reduce basal and food-stimulated secretion of gastric acid and thus facilitate healing; they are generally well tolerated. Cimetidine (Tagamet), however, inhibits the hepatic cytochrome P-450 system and can increase levels of other medications that are metabolized by these enzymes, including warfarin (Coumadin), theophylline (Theo-Dur), and phenytoin (Dilantin). The other H_2-RAs have fewer adverse effects.

Other Pharmacological Agents

Antacids were traditionally the mainstay of ulcer treatment for decades and are still useful today. They neutralize acid rapidly, are generally well tolerated, and are inexpensive. One of the major disadvantages is that they require frequent (1- to 3-hour) dosing, which can contribute to patient nonadherence. They should be used with caution in patients with renal failure because of the risk of aluminum and magnesium toxicity. Antacids that contain calcium should not be used in patients with PUD because calcium causes rebound acid secretion.

Sucralfate is an aluminum hydroxide salt of sucrose that enhances the mucosal defenses and is used in healing duodenal ulcers and in the long-term treatment to prevent recurrence. Sucralfate works by forming a protective barrier to the action of acid and pepsin in the ulcer base. It also stimulates mucus, bicarbonate secretion, and prostaglandin production and binds fibroblast growth factor. Studies have shown that sucralfate 1 g four times daily heals duodenal ulcers as well as H_2-RAs do.

Bismuth preparations promote ulcer healing by stimulating mucosal bicarbonate and prostaglandin production. Bismuth also has antimicrobial action against *H pylori* and has been shown to eradicate the organism in up to 33% of cases. The two types of bismuth preparation available in the United States are bismuth subsalicylate and ranitidine bismuth citrate. Bismuth causes feces to darken or turn black. Patients should be warned of this effect to lessen their anxiety when it occurs. Bismuth subsalicylate also potentiates the effects of antidiabetic medications, so patients should be warned about the possibility of hypoglycemia.

Misoprostol (Cytotec), a prostaglandin analog, stimulates ulcer healing by promoting mucus and bicarbonate secretion. It is indicated for use only as a prophylactic measure to prevent gastric ulcer formation in patients who require treatment with NSAIDs for other conditions. It is ineffective in preventing duodenal ulcers caused by NSAID use. Misoprostol should not be used in pregnancy because it can cause abortion, premature birth, or birth defects.

There are a number of regimens used to eradicate *H pylori,* enhance ulcer healing, and prevent ulcer recurrence. Comparatively speaking, it is more cost effective to employ a regimen to eradicate *H pylori* than it is to maintain a patient on long-term therapy. Despite a number of randomized clinical trials, no optimal regimen has been identified. Most regimens use a combination of several drugs, including bismuth, amoxicillin, tetracycline, clarithromycin, metronidazole, H_2-RAs, and PPIs for a period of 2 weeks. Triple-drug therapy combining two antibiotics (clarithromycin and either amoxicillin or metronidazole) with a PPI has been shown to be very effective in the eradication of *H pylori* (75%–90%) (Level I; Chey and Wong, 2007). Amoxicillin is preferred over metronidazole because there are resistant strains of *H pylori,* and the adverse effects of metronidazole hamper patient adherence. Eradication of *H pylori* has also been demonstrated by combining bismuth subsalicylate and two antibiotics, but the dosing schedule is four times daily and has a higher incidence of adverse effects. Drugs Commonly Prescribed 11.4 presents the drugs used for PUD.

Follow-up and Referral

In patients empirically treated for ulcers, follow-up is necessary only if symptoms recur. If after 2 weeks the patient has seen no improvement or symptoms have progressed, referral to a gastroenterologist for upper endoscopy is indicated. Any time a gastric ulcer is suspected rather than a duodenal ulcer, the patient should be referred to a gastroenterologist because the incidence of gastric cancer in these patients is increased. In patients treated with an *H pylori* eradication regimen, retesting for *H pylori* is necessary only if symptoms recur. Follow-up is necessary for any patient who does not respond to therapy or who experiences worsening symptoms.

Patient Education

The most important aspect of patient education is to stress the importance of following the treatment regimen prescribed. The patient's anxiety can be eased by informing him or her of possible bothersome side effects of any medications, such as a change in fecal color when taking bismuth preparations. If the patient is taking sucralfate in conjunction with an antacid, PPI, or H_2-RA, it should be stressed that the sucralfate cannot be taken at the same time as the other medications or at the same time as digoxin, ciprofloxacin, or phenytoin because sucralfate binds to all of these medications. Dispelling myths about ulcers is also an important part of patient education.

■ CHOLECYSTITIS

Cholecystitis is an acute inflammation of the gallbladder wall, which is usually the result of an impacted calculus within the cystic duct, causing inflammation proximal to the obstruction. Cholelithiasis is found in 90% to 95% of patients presenting with cholecystitis. Cholecystitis without gallstones, acalculous cholecystitis, is a very serious disease with high morbidity and mortality rates. It usually occurs in patients who are already critically ill because of trauma, burns, surgery, or sepsis and who have had no oral intake or have been supplemented with hyperalimentation. Patients present with severe pain and tenderness in the epigastrium or right upper quadrant (RUQ) of the abdomen accompanied by nausea, vomiting, fever, and leukocytosis.

Epidemiology and Causes

Cholecystitis/cholelithiasis is prevalent in Western societies. Researchers estimate that the disease affects approximately 20 million Americans, the majority of whom are not aware they have cholelithiasis. About 50% of these asymptomatic patients never require treatment. Gallstones form in people as early as their 30s. In fact,

75% of American Indian women over age 25 have gallstones. The risk of requiring a cholecystectomy increases with age as a consequence of complications secondary to the lithiasis. By age 65, about 20% of women and 10% of men have symptoms related to gallstones that require medical attention. As many as 5,000 to 6,000 deaths each year are attributed to gallstone-related disease.

Cholesterol stones are the most common form and account for 75% of all gallstones. The remaining 25% are pigmented stones, which are categorized as black or brown depending on their chemical composition. Cholesterol stones contain between 50% and 90% cholesterol; the remainder of the stone is made of calcium salts from bilirubin pigment, carbonate, bile acids, phospholipids, fatty acids, and proteins. Risk Factors 11.1 describes the risk factors associated with cholelithiasis.

The well-known mnemonic regarding the typical cholelithiasis patient is the "six Fs": fat, female, forty, flatulent, fertile, and fat intolerant. After age 50, the gender distribution is equal. Pregnancy also predisposes women to cholelithiasis, presumably because of the increased abdominal pressure and increased cholesterol levels during the third trimester. Any condition that increases the development of cholelithiasis increases the chance of developing cholecystitis.

Pathophysiology

From 90% to 95% of cholecystitis cases are associated with cholelithiasis. Cholesterol stones are the most common form of gallstones. Cholesterol is insoluble in water; it is made soluble though interaction with bile salts and phospholipids, allowing it to be carried within the bile. There are two known transport systems for cholesterol within the bile, vesicular and micellar, both of which exist in the bile to maintain equilibrium. When this

Risk Factors 11.1   Risk Factors Associated With Cholelithiasis

Cholesterol Stones	Pigmented Stones
Female gender	Hemolytic diseases
Obesity	Increasing age
Pregnancy	Hyperalimentation
Increased age	Cirrhosis
Drug-induced (oral contraceptives, clofibrates)	Biliary stasis
	Chronic biliary infections
Cystic fibrosis	
Rapid weight loss	
Spinal cord injury	
Ileal disease with extensive resection	
Diabetes mellitus	
Sickle cell anemia	

equilibrium is disturbed and the bile contains more cholesterol than can be maintained, crystallization of the cholesterol, referred to as nucleation, occurs. Gradual deposition of cholesterol on these crystals leads to the development of a cholesterol gallstone. Although this process seems to contribute to the formation of gallstones, not all people with cholesterol-saturated bile form stones. Thus, there is more to the process of lithogenesis than is known.

The gallbladder is of primary importance in the development of gallstones because it provides an arena for bile stasis and allows time for the slow crystallization of cholesterol, which may also be enhanced by yet unknown proteins or other materials within the bile. Biliary cholesterol is increased by ingestion of estrogen and oral contraceptives, multiparity, and inflammatory terminal ileal disease, which decreases the bile acid pool. Bile stasis, which can contribute to gallstone formation, is increased by strictures within the ductal system, parenteral hyperalimentation, fasting, and mechanical obstruction secondary to tumor or cyst formation.

The pathogenesis of pigmented stones is less well understood but seems to be directly related to elevation in levels of unconjugated bilirubin. Any disease state that increases the amount of bilirubin increases the risk for pigmented lithogenesis. Black pigmented stones are formed within the gallbladder and are commonly associated with hemolytic diseases and in patients with cirrhosis and those who require long-term parenteral hyperalimentation. Black pigmented stones are more fragile and seem to crush more easily than cholesterol stones.

Brown pigmented stones are composed of alternating layers of calcium bilirubinate and calcium fatty acids. Chronic bacterial infections are believed to be partly responsible for the formation of brown pigmented stones because the enzymes the bacteria produce predispose the patient to this type of stone formation. Brown stones are typically found within the intrahepatic ducts and are rarely found within the gallbladder.

The pathophysiological changes occurring within the gallbladder before the diagnosis of acute cholecystitis are directly related to the amount of time the duct has been obstructed and the degree of inflammation that has taken place. The earliest pathological findings are erythema, edema, and a fibrinosuppurative exudate. Tissue examination reveals inflammatory infiltration, hemorrhage, and edema resulting in ulceration of the mucosa within a short period of time. The result is the development of gangrene, with abscess formation. As the acute process resolves, collagen deposits develop, usually within 1 to 2 weeks. The gallbladder eventually contracts and becomes scarred, causing thickening of the wall. Often the gallbladder becomes filled with pus preceding the development of gangrene. Perforation may occur, most often at the fundus, but it can occur anywhere there is erosion of an impacted stone. Perforation of the gallbladder allows bile to spill into the peritoneal cavity, causing bile peritonitis, abscess, and fistula formation.

Clinical Presentation

Subjective

Acute cholecystitis causes various symptoms, ranging from generalized gastrointestinal complaints to intractable pain. Most patients complain of indigestion, nausea, and vomiting, especially after consuming a meal high in fat. Acute cholecystitis usually begins with acute, colicky-type pain. About 80% of patients report that they have experienced this type of pain before. However, the pain associated with acute cholecystitis persists, and as the inflammation progresses, the pain localizes over the RUQ. Patients may complain of referred pain that radiates to the middle of the back, to the infrascapular area, or to the right shoulder. The pain is increased by any movement, including respiration. If the inflammation extends to the peritoneal area, the pain worsens, the abdominal muscles become rigid, and a fever is usually evident.

Objective

Physical findings are dependent on the degree of inflammation present. As the pain over the RUQ becomes severe, there is often involuntary guarding of the abdominal muscles over the right side. A positive Murphy's sign is elicited when the right subcostal region is so tender that there is painful splinting with deep inspiration or when palpation over the RUQ area causes transient inspiratory arrest. The gallbladder is palpable in fewer than 50% of the patients. Fever is usually low grade, 99° to 101°F (38.3°C); high fever suggests sepsis. Patients may develop mild jaundice from edema of the common bile duct. Hyperbilirubinemia should raise the suspicion of choledocholithiasis. Bowel sounds may be diminished.

In most cases, acute cholecystitis subsides spontaneously, with improvement in the first few days and no symptoms after about 4 days. If symptoms persist or become more severe, the potential for perforation, gangrene, empyema, and septic shock increases. Rebound tenderness, shaking chills, or increased fever should raise suspicion that perforation has occurred. Surgical referral is indicated early in the disease process.

Diagnostic Reasoning

Diagnostic Testing

During the acute presentation of cholecystitis, there is usually mild elevation of the white blood cell count, to 15,000/mL. Serum transaminases can be elevated up to four times the normal amount; aspartate aminotransferase and alanine aminotransferase can be elevated to 300 U/L. Alkaline phosphatase is elevated two to four times above normal levels, and bilirubin can be as high as 4 mg/dL. Profound elevation of the alkaline phosphatase and bilirubin is highly suggestive of chole-docholithiasis. An elevation in amylase can be the result of passage of a stone through the common bile duct but may also indicate gallstone pancreatitis.

Abdominal x-ray films may reveal gallstones, enlarged gallbladder, or air within the biliary system or peritoneal cavity. The gold standard for diagnosis of acute chole-cystitis is ultrasound; it is a quick, noninvasive, reliable, and cost-effective means of identifying the presence of cholelithiasis. Radionuclide scanning following admin-istration of technetium-99m (99m-Tc) is the most ac-curate means of confirming the clinical diagnosis of cholecystitis with cystic duct obstruction. If the gallblad-der fills with the isotope, the diagnosis of cholecystitis is highly unlikely; however, if the bile duct is visualized and the gallbladder is not, this is highly suggestive of cholecystitis. Oral cholangiograms are of no benefit in the acutely ill patient.

Differential Diagnosis

The differential diagnosis of acute cholecystitis in the presence of RUQ pain, nausea, vomiting, and fever in-cludes pancreatitis, myocardial infarction, appendicitis, peptic ulcer, pneumonia, and hepatitis. Most of these potential diagnoses can be effectively ruled out via stan-dard laboratory tests and ultrasound. Electrocardiogram can rule out myocardial infarction and is necessary as part of preoperative studies.

Management

Treatment of cholelithiasis depends on many variables, including age; presenting symptoms; past medical history; and size, type, and number of gallstones involved. Patients with symptomatic cholelithiasis can often be safely managed on an outpatient basis. Pa-tients must be advised to avoid foods high in fat, which can provoke an attack. Nonsurgical options for the treatment of gallstones include dissolution of the stone by oral ingestion of ursodeoxycholic acid (ursodiol) or direct dissolution by percutaneous instillation of methyl-tertiary-butyl ether. Both types of dissolution therapies are of limited value and can be used only with cholesterol stones. Recurrence rates with these treat-ments are almost 100%, and the length of treatment may be as long as 2 years.

Patients who are deemed poor surgical risks can also undergo extracorporeal shock wave lithotripsy along with chemical dissolution in an attempt to reduce the size of the stone. Patients who continue to have biliary colic or who have developed other complications should be hospitalized for further treatment, with prompt referral to a gastroenterologist and/or a surgeon.

Initial Management

Initial treatment begins with definitive diagnosis. For many, the diagnosis of gallstones is made as an incidental finding during medical treatment for another problem.

These patients are often asymptomatic and require no further treatment except awareness of the signs and symptoms of a "gallbladder attack." Patients who are considered a poor surgical risk can be treated nonsurgi-cally with dissolution therapy or lithotripsy. Those who remain symptomatic despite treatment or have devel-oped other complications should be hospitalized in an attempt to reduce the risk of a life-threatening event such as perforation or septic shock.

Management of acute cholecystitis includes rehy-dration with IV fluids and replenishing electrolytes as indicated by laboratory results. Patients are not allowed anything by mouth, and if vomiting is persist-ent, a nasogastric tube is inserted. Pain is managed with intramuscular analgesic agents. A third generation cephalosporin is started once the diagnosis is made. If sepsis is suspected, an aminoglycoside is added to the antibiotic coverage.

The treatment of choice for acute cholecystitis is early surgical intervention. Patients in the acute phase of the disease are usually stabilized before a cholecystectomy is scheduled. Patients who are considered a poor surgical risk may benefit from cholecystotomy, either opera-tively or percutaneously. Emergency decompression with cholecystotomy may be necessary to remove stones and purulent material before a cholecystectomy, which should be deferred for 6 to 8 weeks.

The mortality rate associated with acute cholecystitis is 5% to 10% and is usually associated with patients older than age 60 with comorbid conditions and those with septic complications. Approximately 50% of patients who do not choose to undergo cholecystectomy have a recurrence within 5 years, and complications are common.

Subsequent Management

The most common complications of acute cholecystitis are empyema and perforation. Perforation into the abdominal cavity can occur early in the disease process and is associated with a 30% mortality rate. Perforation may also occur into another hollow viscus or into the colon, causing draining fistulas, which may relieve the symptoms associated with cholecystitis. Surgical removal of the gallbladder with fistula repair is indicated when the patient is medically stable for surgery.

Follow-up and Referral

Patients with acute cholecystitis require referral to a general surgeon for removal of the gallbladder. Referral should be made after diagnosis of acute cholecystitis. Follow-up includes routine postoperative visits according to the surgeon. Patients who have persistent symptoms after the removal of the gallbladder (postcholecystectomy syndrome) may have a mistaken diagnosis, a functional bowel disorder, retained or recurrent common bile duct stones, or spasm of the sphincter of Oddi. Patients with incidental findings of asymptomatic gallstones should be referred to a surgeon and given the option for elective surgery, medical dissolution therapy, lithotripsy, or contact solvent dissolution.

Patient Education

Patient education for individuals declining surgical intervention should include the risks and benefits of each therapy. Dietary counseling should include weight loss for those patients who are obese and the avoidance of fatty foods that provoke attacks. Patients taking oral contraceptives should be given information about alternative forms of birth control, and menopausal women taking estrogen should be counseled about alternative sources of phytoestrogens, such as soy products.

■ ACUTE PANCREATITIS

Acute pancreatitis is defined as an acute inflammation of the pancreas and the surrounding tissues resulting from the release of pancreatic enzymes into these tissues. These enzymes cause a chemical burn in the retroperitoneal spaces, which leads to systemic toxicity. The degree to which the microcirculation within the pancreas is preserved determines the histological classification of pancreatitis. If the microcirculation remains intact, the process is defined as acute interstitial pancreatitis, but if the microcirculation is disrupted, necrotizing pancreatitis results. Acute pancreatitis normally resolves both clinically and histologically.

Epidemiology and Causes

Although there are many causes of acute pancreatitis, approximately 80% of all hospital admissions for acute pancreatitis are the result of biliary tract disease (passing of a gallstone) and alcoholism. The remaining 20% are caused by infection (mumps), hyperlipidemia (particularly types I, IV, and V), metabolic disorders (hyperparathyroidism, hypercalcemia), drugs (furosemide, valproic acid, sulfonamides, thiazides), endoscopic retrograde cholangiopancreatography (ERCP), structural abnormalities of the pancreatic duct (stricture, carcinoma, pancreatic divisum), structural abnormalities of the common bile duct and ampullary region, surgery (particularly of the stomach and biliary tract), vascular disease (atherosclerosis, severe hypotension), or trauma.

Acute pancreatitis is usually the result of some other process, such as passing of a gallstone, excessive alcohol intake, or some other biliary tract disease. Clinical pancreatitis is seen in up to 9.5% of alcoholic patients, and histological evidence is found in 17% to 45% of this group. Cholelithiasis is present in 60% of nonalcoholic patients with pancreatitis.

Pathophysiology

Pathological changes associated with pancreatitis range from acute edema and cellular infiltration to necrosis and hemorrhage. Although the exact pathogenesis is not known, temporary impaction of the sphincter of Oddi by a gallstone before its passage into the duodenum may cause edema or obstruction of the ampulla of Vater, with subsequent reflux of bile into the pancreatic ducts and injury to the acinar cells. This cascade of events causes an autodigestive process within the pancreas that can progress to shock and death without appropriate intervention. Inflammation is confined to the pancreas in edematous pancreatitis, and the mortality rate is less than 5%.

When inflammation and tissue necrosis extends beyond the pancreas, the associated mortality rate is 10% to 50%. Pancreatic exudate containing toxins and activated enzymes permeates the retroperitoneum and causes a chemical burn that increases the permeability of the blood vessels within the peritoneal cavity. As a result, large amounts of protein-rich fluid from the circulation are sequestered in these third spaces, producing hypovolemia and shock. As these toxins and enzymes enter the systemic circulation, they can further reduce vascular tone and, thus, the ability to correct the hypotension and shock.

Acute pancreatitis can be classified as either mild or severe. Mild acute pancreatitis normally improves within 48 to 72 hours and does not involve other organ systems. There is minimal interstitial edema, with only occasional microscopic acinar cell necrosis. Severe, acute pancreatitis is often associated with complications and multisystem organ failure. It can be a life-threatening condition, and the patient may require monitoring in the intensive care unit (ICU).

Complications during the first few days of diagnosis are associated with hemodynamic instability: shock, renal failure, respiratory compromise secondary to adult respiratory distress syndrome (ARDS), and hypoxemia. Pancreatic necrosis with secondary gram-negative sepsis has an associated 100% mortality rate unless there is extensive surgical debridement of the infected tissue. Up to 25% of patients diagnosed with acute pancreatitis develop some degree of fluid collection within a few days of diagnosis that resolves spontaneously half of the time. Those that do not resolve spontaneously form pseudocysts, abscesses, and other necrotic collections.

Pancreatic pseudocysts take at least 4 weeks to form and resolve spontaneously after about 6 weeks in 40% of the cases. If the pseudocyst does not resolve within 12 weeks after acute pancreatitis, the risk of complications in symptomatic patients (infection, bleeding, rupture) are as high as 60%, but there is little associated risk in asymptomatic patients. The decision for invasive intervention will depend on the progression of symptoms and cyst size.

Clinical Presentation
Subjective

The patient with acute pancreatitis usually presents with abrupt onset of deep epigastric pain that persists for hours to days and may radiate straight through to the back. The pain is intense and often refractory to large doses of parenteral narcotics. It is aggravated by any vigorous activity, such as coughing, and by lying supine; it improves when the patient is seated and leaning forward. The patient appears acutely ill, often with intractable nausea and vomiting. In some cases, depending on the severity, the patient may experience sweating, weakness, and anxiety. The patient may report a history of ingestion of alcohol or a big meal before onset of symptoms or mild biliary colic preceding the episode.

Objective

On physical exam, there is severe abdominal tenderness, particularly over the epigastric area, which may be accompanied by guarding but without rigidity or rebound tenderness, and there may be milder pain in the lower abdomen without guarding or rigidity. Abdominal distention is present in approximately 20% of the patients. Bowel sounds can be hypoactive or absent if associated with paralytic ileus. The rectal exam is normal, and the stool is usually negative for occult blood.

The patient is tachycardic (100–140 beats/min) with rapid, shallow respiration. Inspiratory effort is poor because deep inspiration causes pain. Blood pressure may be high secondary to pain or low if shock is imminent. The patient's temperature may initially be normal or subnormal but increases to 100.4° to 102.2°F (38° to 39°C) within a few hours. Mild jaundice and scleral icterus may be present. The patient's skin may be pale, cool, and clammy if shock is present.

Uncommon findings that can result from the pancreatic inflammatory process include left-sided pleural effusion, bluish discoloration over the flanks (Grey Turner's sign) or around the umbilicus (Cullen's sign), jaundice caused by impingement on the common bile duct, and epigastric mass secondary to pseudocyst development.

Diagnostic Reasoning
Diagnostic Tests

The diagnosis of pancreatitis is strongly suggested through the history and physical exam; however, because many other diseases present with similar symptoms, further testing is necessary. The gold standard for diagnosis is an elevated serum amylase (up to three times the normal level); however, in one-third of patients with alcoholic pancreatitis, the serum amylase level may be normal. The diagnosis of pancreatitis is supported by a concurrent elevation of the serum lipase. Serum amylase and lipase levels are increased on the first day of acute symptoms and return to normal in 3 to 7 days. These levels remain normal if there has been repeated prior damage to the acinar cells, rendering them incapable

of further enzyme secretion. The level of elevation of amylase and lipase is not indicative of the severity of the disease.

The white blood cell (WBC) count is usually between 12,000 and 20,000 cells/mL. The hematocrit can be as high as 50% to 55% because of hemoconcentration resulting from sequestered fluids in the third spaces.

A decrease in serum calcium may indicate saponification and is indicative of the severity of the pancreatitis. Calcium levels below 7 mg/dL (with normal serum albumin) can cause tetany and are associated with poor prognosis. Elevated C-reactive protein is correlated with pancreatic necrosis. The risk of infection is positively correlated with pancreatic necrosis and accounts for most of the deaths. Pancreatic necrosis requires surgical intervention; computed tomography (CT)–guided aspiration of the necrotic tissue for Gram stain and culture is indicated.

Patients presenting with biliary pancreatitis have an elevation of the liver enzymes. When alanine aminotransferase is up to three times the normal limit, the positive predictive value is 95% that the pancreatitis is caused by biliary disease (gallstones). Concomitant rises in the aspartate aminotransferase, alkaline phosphatase, and bilirubin suggest gallbladder disease.

Diagnostic imaging, especially CT of the abdomen, can provide fast and accurate information for the definitive diagnosis of acute pancreatitis. Although the CT scan can be normal in 15% to 30% of patients with mild acute pancreatitis, it is the most efficient means of discerning acute pancreatitis from other potentially fatal intra-abdominal processes. CT is also helpful in monitoring the progression or resolution of pancreatic pseudocysts.

Ultrasonography (US) is the gold standard for identification and location of gallstones and is considered mandatory because studies have shown that the morbidity associated with gallstone pancreatitis is dramatically reduced once the stone is removed. US can also detect dilation of the common bile duct, indicating obstruction. ERCP with sphincterotomy and stone extraction can be performed and has been proved to decrease morbidity and mortality.

If there is evidence that the pancreatitis is severe, additional testing with IV contrast is recommended; the necrotic pancreas has damage to its microcirculation and, thus, is not enhanced with IV contrast. If the microcirculation remains intact, there is uniform enhancement of the pancreas. Pancreatic necrosis is associated with much higher morbidity, mortality, and infection rates.

Pancreatic infection is a complication that requires immediate diagnosis and intervention. Infection should be suspected when the patient has persistently elevated WBC counts and fever. The patient normally looks very sick. Positive blood cultures and visualization of gas bubbles within the retroperitoneum on CT support the diagnosis.

Ranson's criteria are the most widely accepted and utilized system for assessing the severity of acute pancreatitis. Identification of early prognostic signs may provide the best indication of a serious outcome and can alert the practitioner that the patient may require transfer to the ICU. Listed within Table 11.7 are the 11 objective signs used to classify the severity of pancreatitis. Mortality rates correlate directly with the number of diagnostic criteria present. Pancreatitis is classified as severe when three or more of Ranson's criteria are met.

Differential Diagnosis

Differential diagnosis of acute pancreatitis is made by history and physical exam and supported by laboratory data and imaging studies. The gold standard for diagnosis is serum amylase; however, in cases in which the level is normal or mildly elevated, diagnosis can be confirmed by CT scan. CT scan is useful in differentiating other intra-abdominal processes from acute pancreatitis. However, it is less helpful in identifying gallstones as a potential cause. Laboratory data are helpful in differentiating other causes of acute abdominal pain with associated hyperamylasemia. Table 11.8 differentiates hyperamylasemia resulting from pancreatic and nonpancreatic causes.

Table 11.8	Hyperamylasemia: Pancreatic and Nonpancreatic Causes
Pancreatic Hyperamylasemia	Nonpancreatic Hyperamylasemia
Pancreatic pseudocyst	Salivary adenitis (secondary to mumps)
Perforated duodenal ulcer	Ruptured ectopic pregnancy
Small bowel perforation Mesenteric infarction Mesenteric vascular thrombus	Postabdominal surgery Lactic acidosis
Opiate administration Post-ERCP	Leaking aortic aneurysm Renal insufficiency

Table 11.7	Ranson's Criteria for Assessing the Severity of Pancreatitis

At admission or at time of diagnosis:
1. Age older than 55 years
2. White blood cell (WBC) count greater than 16,000/mcL
3. Blood glucose greater than 200 mg/dL
4. Base deficit greater than 4 mEq/L
5. Serum lactate dehydrogenase (LDH) greater than 350 IU/L
6. AST greater than 250 U/L

During the initial 48 hours:
1. Hematocrit (Hct) drop of more than 10 percentage points
2. Blood urea nitrogen (BUN) rise of greater than 5 mg/dL
3. Arterial PO_2 of less than 60
4. Serum calcium (Ca) of less than 8 mg/dL
5. Estimated fluid sequestration of greater than 6 L

Number of Diagnostic Criteria	Mortality Rate (%)
0–2	1
3–4	16
5–6	40
7–8	100

Adapted from Ranson, JH, et al. Prognostic signs and the role of operative management in acute pancreatitis. *Surg Gynecol Obstet* 139(1):69–81, 1974.

Management

Treatment of acute pancreatitis is aimed at limiting the severity of pancreatic inflammation, preventing further complications by interrupting the pathological processes, and managing the symptoms as they arise. Mild acute pancreatitis usually resolves spontaneously in a few days, so these patients can be managed conservatively as outpatients. Fasting is necessary until the symptoms of acute inflammation have subsided.

Treatment includes maintaining fluid status with parenteral fluids to prevent hypovolemia and hypotension. Traditionally, pain is controlled with meperidine (Demerol) rather than with other opiates, to prevent increased pressure within the sphincter of Oddi, although research indicates that morphine causes no more spasms in the sphincter of Oddi than meperidine. The patient is allowed nothing by mouth, and nasogastric (NG) tube insertion should be considered when there is persistent nausea, vomiting, or evidence of ileus. The use of empiric antibiotics, H_2-receptor antagonists, and pancreatic enzyme inhibitors have not been proven effective and are not recommended.

Judicious introduction of clear liquids can be instituted once the patient is pain free, the amylase and lipase have returned to normal range, and bowel sounds have returned. The diet may be advanced to regular low fat as the patient tolerates.

Patients with more severe pancreatitis tend to have sequestered larger amounts of fluid as a result of the "chemical burn" sustained by the tissues within the retroperitoneal space. These patients are usually transferred to the ICU under the care of a gastroenterologist or surgeon. Aggressive volume replacement is necessary and may require invasive hemodynamic monitoring to maintain appropriate fluid balance. Fluid resuscitation is an important part of therapy and 6 to 8 L/day may be required. Some patients may require infusion of fresh frozen plasma or serum albumin or blood transfusions, which can increase the risk of the development of ARDS. Cardiac function and fluid status can be monitored with a central line or pulmonary artery catheter. Measurement of hourly urine output is also necessary. If hemodynamic stability is not achieved through volume replacement, vasopressors may be necessary.

Daily monitoring of serum calcium, magnesium, glucose, electrolytes, total protein, albumin, amylase, lipase, and complete blood count with subsequent correction of abnormalities is required. In febrile patients, cultures of blood, urine, and sputum should be obtained, as well as CT-guided needle aspiration of necrotic areas of the pancreas with initiation of appropriate broad-spectrum antibiotic coverage as necessary to prevent increased morbidity and mortality. Arterial blood gas readings should be obtained daily, and hypoxemia treated accordingly. The patient may require assisted ventilation if hypoxemia persists or ARDS develops.

Correction of serum glucose is done with caution and should not begin until levels are greater than 250 mg/dL. Hypocalcemia is often corrected with the administration of albumin-containing fluids. Neuromuscular irritability, if present, can be corrected with a 10% solution of calcium gluconate. If there is a coexisting hypomagnesemia, correction of the magnesium level will often restore the calcium to its normal level. In patients with renal impairment, magnesium must be replaced cautiously.

Patients with severe pancreatitis must be maintained in a fasting state for prolonged periods of time, often for 2 to 4 weeks. Administration of antacids through an NG tube can help to prevent stress ulceration. The nutritional needs of the patient can be maintained with total parenteral nutrition until the gut becomes functional; enteral feedings can then be started, using the distal jejunum to reduce pancreatic stimulation. Oral feedings should not be started until any and all complications have been treated, the patient is free from nausea and vomiting, and amylase and lipase levels have returned to normal.

Surgical intervention is normally reserved for a pancreatic pseudocyst that has persisted for more than 6 weeks with ongoing symptomatology, necrotizing pancreatitis, pancreatic abscess, or severe hemorrhagic pancreatitis. Despite surgical intervention, the mortality rate for necrotizing pancreatitis remains high.

For pancreatitis caused by cholelithiasis, surgical intervention is determined by the presenting course of events. If biliary decompression is necessary, it can often be accomplished with ERCP. If the pancreatitis is mild, a cholecystectomy can be performed at a later time.

Follow-up and Referral

Patients with severe acute pancreatitis or those who do not respond to conservative treatment should be referred to a gastroenterologist for management. Surgical referral

should be made once the diagnosis of pancreatitis is made. The patient who develops a pseudocyst requires long-term follow-up with serial CT scans to observe the resolution or growth of the cyst, which may require surgical intervention. The patient who has gallstone disease should have a cholecystectomy.

The prognosis of the patient with pancreatitis correlates directly with the severity of the inflammatory process. Patients with interstitial, or edematous, pancreatitis even with systemic complications have a mortality rate of 1% to 2%; however, patients with necrotizing pancreatitis have a mortality rate of 10% with sterile necrosis and up to 30% with infected necrosis.

In patients for whom no cause has been found, studies have suggested that half of these patients have occult gallstone disease (biliary sludge) or sphincter of Oddi dysfunction. These patients require repeated abdominal US exams to detect the development of biliary sludge. Patients with hereditary hypercholesterolemia are often missed because serum triglycerides are not obtained until after several days of fasting, at which time the triglyceride level may have fallen to within normal limits.

Patient Education

Patients with biliary disease as the cause of the pancreatitis should be informed of the need for a cholecystectomy, as well as the benefit of reducing their dietary intake of fat. If the etiology of pancreatitis is alcohol abuse, the patient should be encouraged to abstain. Patients with genetic hyperlipidemia require diet instruction and information on avoidance of precipitating factors such as alcohol, estrogens, and certain drugs. These patients may benefit from lipid-lowering medications and must be taught to control their diabetes if present. If a drug is the suspected cause of the pancreatitis, it should not be restarted.

■ CHRONIC PANCREATITIS

Chronic pancreatitis is defined as a slowly progressive inflammatory process that results in irreversible fibrosis of the pancreas with destruction and atrophy of the exocrine and endocrine glandular tissue. There are varying degrees of ductal dilation and fibrosis. There can be intraductal formation of protein plugs, which calcify and cause further dilation and obstruction. *Chronic relapsing pancreatitis* is defined as acute attacks that occur in the setting of chronic pancreatitis and are usually precipitated by a specific event such as binge drinking or the passage of a stone.

Epidemiology and Causes

There is little reliable information on the prevalence or incidence of chronic pancreatitis. Alcoholism may account for between 70% and 80% of the cases in industrialized countries. Although there is no threshold for alcohol consumption and the development of chronic pancreatitis, there is a statistically significant increase in individuals who consume 120 grams of ethanol per day (eight 12-ounce beers, 8 ounces of 100-proof whiskey, or 30 ounces of wine). Diets high in protein in combination with either high or low fat can further predispose patients to pancreatic injury from alcohol.

Other causes of chronic pancreatitis include autoimmune disease, genetic mutations, hereditary predisposition, hypertriglyceridemia, severe malnutrition (especially protein-calorie deficiency in developing countries), tropical pancreatitis, and obstruction of the main pancreatic duct caused by stenosis, stones, tumor, or cystic fibrosis. In 10% to 30% of persons with chronic pancreatitis, the cause is unknown, but patients are divided into two groups: (1) those who present with abdominal pain (usually between ages 15 and 30) and (2) older individuals (ages 50–70) who present, often without pain, with pancreatic calcifications, glandular insufficiency, and diabetes.

The tropical, or nutritional, form of chronic pancreatitis is almost exclusively found in tropical countries. In these countries, the disease begins in early childhood and results in death in early adulthood because of complications. This type of pancreatitis also involves large intraductal calculi and a high susceptibility to pancreatic cancer. Malnutrition has a significant role, but it is not the sole cause because many areas with comparable malnutrition do not have equal prevalence of the disease. Key features of tropical pancreatitis include abdominal pain, maldigestion leading to steatorrhea, and diabetes.

Pathophysiology

The pathogenesis of chronic pancreatitis is unclear. Two characteristic findings in chronic pancreatitis are hypersecretion of protein without a subsequent increase in ductal bicarbonate secretion and inflammation. Chronic pancreatitis results in irreversible structural damage with permanent functional impairment of the pancreatic gland. For individuals who have alcohol-related disease, ductal obstruction is thought to be caused by changes in the chemical composition of the pancreatic juice, leading to protein plugging, calcification, and subsequent pancreatic damage. Another theory postulates that continuous injury to the acinar cells causes inflammation, necrosis, and fibrosis. Analysis of pancreatic juice obtained from alcoholic patients revealed protein plugs but not always chronic pancreatitis. Proponents of the theory favoring repeated damage to the pancreatic acinar cells believe that ductal obstruction is a result of changes in the pancreatic juice that cause increased viscosity and damage to the gland itself. These changes in the enzymatic properties result in chronic inflammation and fibrosis of the gland. Biliary disease has not been identified as a causative factor in the development of chronic pancreatitis.

With the progressive inflammatory changes occurring with chronic pancreatitis, it is not uncommon to find a fibrotic common bile duct and jaundice secondary to the obstructed common bile duct. Upper gastrointestinal bleeding can result from the formation of gastric varices or the development of a pseudoaneurysm in an artery within the pancreatic area. Steatorrhea and diabetes mellitus result from destruction of the pancreatic gland with subsequent endocrine and exocrine insufficiency. Steatorrhea develops as lipase and protease secretion drops below 10% of normal. Islet cell destruction reduces insulin secretion, causing glucose intolerance and diabetes.

Clinical Presentation
Subjective

The most frequent presenting symptoms are intractable abdominal pain, weight loss, and diarrhea; but symptoms can be as mild as dyspepsia, nausea, and vomiting. Abdominal pain is usually epigastric or in the left upper quadrant, may radiate to the back or left lumbar region, and is described as dull and constant. Pain may be absent in 5% to 10% of the cases or may represent an exacerbation of acute or relapsing pancreatitis. Pain may precede the development of other symptoms of chronic pancreatitis by years. The pain is often precipitated or aggravated by food or alcohol intake. In some patients, the pain diminishes over time (5–15 years) and is associated with burnout or calcification of the gland. Between 10% and 20% of older adults with idiopathic chronic pancreatitis have no pain with the disease.

Weight loss may result from anorexia caused by pain and nausea, malabsorption secondary to pancreatic exocrine insufficiency, or poorly controlled diabetes mellitus. Diabetes mellitus is present in approximately 50% of patients and is often the presenting sign in individuals who have no pain associated with pancreatitis. Steatorrhea develops after the pancreas loses the ability to secrete digestive enzymes, which results in bulky, foul-smelling, fatty stools. Patients often complain of "oil leakage" from the rectum or an "oil slick" in the toilet bowl, which is indicative of pancreatic insufficiency.

Objective

Abdominal assessment in patients presenting with pain reveals mild to moderate epigastric tenderness with no rebound tenderness or guarding. A palpable abdominal mass is suggestive of a pancreatic pseudocyst. Bowel sounds may be absent in patients with paralytic ileus. Lung sounds may be diminished in the bases, which is indicative of pleural effusion.

Diagnostic Reasoning
Diagnostic Tests

Diagnosis of chronic pancreatitis is normally made through evaluation of pancreatic function and radiographic visualization of structural abnormalities such as pancreatic calcification or abnormalities in the size or consistency of the pancreatic tissue. The patient usually presents with chronic abdominal pain, weight loss, exocrine insufficiency (malabsorption), and diabetes mellitus.

Tests for pancreatic function include assessment of endocrine and exocrine function. A 2-hour postprandial blood sugar level greater than 200 mg/dL or fasting glucose greater than 120 mg/dL on two occasions is diagnostic for diabetes mellitus. Glucosuria may also be present. The serum amylase level may remain within normal limits because the pancreas has lost the ability to mount a response due to the chronicity of the disease. Malabsorption is documented by a 72-hour stool analysis for fecal fat content. Although helpful for diagnosis of exocrine function, steatorrhea is not diagnostic of chronic pancreatitis because patients do not develop steatorrhea until lipase falls below 10% of normal.

Pancreatic insufficiency can be confirmed by the bentiromide (nitroblue tetrazolium–*para*-aminobenzoic acid [NBT-PABA]) test, which measures urinary excretion of pancreatic chymotrypsin, or a secretin stimulation test, which is more sensitive but is unavailable in many places. The test involves placing a tube within the duodenum and collecting pancreatic secretions after IV stimulation with secretin. Collections that are of normal volume and low in bicarbonate (HCO_3^-) suggest chronic pancreatitis; collections low in volume and with normal HCO_3^- suggest pancreatic cancer. The detection of decreased fecal chymotrypsin or elastase helps to diagnose pancreatic insufficiency, but these tests do not have widespread availability.

Imaging studies include plain films of the abdomen, which may show intraductal stones or a calcified pancreas caused by pancreatolithiasis and mild ileus. Computed tomography (CT) scan and/or ultrasound of the abdomen may show an abnormal size or consistency of the pancreas, a pancreatic pseudocyst, or dilated pancreatic ducts. Endoscopic retrograde cholangiopancreatography (ERCP) may also show abnormality of the main pancreatic duct or its secondary branches. Although not available everywhere, magnetic resonance cholangiopancreatography is an excellent alternative to ERCP.

Differential Diagnosis

Differential diagnosis includes diseases that present with persistent abdominal pain such as peptic ulcer disease or mesenteric ischemia; diseases that result in weight loss and abdominal pain, including abdominal malignancies, especially cancer of the pancreas; and intestinal disorders that may present with steatorrhea. The diagnosis of chronic pancreatitis can be confirmed by visualization of the calcified pancreas on x-ray films, which will also rule out most other disease processes.

Management

The treatment of chronic pancreatitis is aimed at preventing further pancreatic damage, managing pain, and supplementing exocrine and endocrine function. The major cause of chronic pancreatitis is alcohol abuse;

therefore, complete abstinence is imperative. Pancreatic enzyme supplementation may relieve pain in some patients. Generally, narcotics are necessary to manage pain. Patients whose pain is not managed by analgesics or pancreatic enzyme therapy should be considered for operative treatment.

Malabsorption is managed with a low-fat diet (less than 50 g/day) and oral pancreatic enzyme supplementation. Oral supplementation should be administered 20 to 30 minutes before meals and snacks. The usual dose is 30,000 units of lipase. Non–enteric-coated pancrelipase formulations (Viokase or Cotazym) should be given with H_2-receptor antagonists to prevent degradation by gastric acids. Enteric-coated preparations of pancrelipase (Pancrease or Creon) or pancreatin (Donnazyme) are stable at an acid pH and should not be given with acid neutralizers because this will promote enzyme release within the stomach. Fat-soluble vitamin (A, D, E, and K) replacement may be required. Favorable outcomes are weight gain, decreased number of stools per day, decrease in oil seepage from the rectum, and subjective improvement in well-being.

Endocrine insufficiency is controlled with insulin supplementation. Extreme caution must be used with insulin supplementation, because there is a deficiency of glucagon secretion, which can lead to prolonged hypoglycemia. Serum glucose levels of 200 to 250 mg/dL are considered acceptable and do not require treatment. The principal step in the management of diabetes associated with chronic pancreatitis is the correction of poor nutritional habits, malabsorption and malnutrition, and the elimination of alcohol. Normal insulin requirements range from 5 to 15 units per day but may fluctuate up to 40 units per day. It is best to maintain these patients at a higher than normal glucose level to avoid hypoglycemia while avoiding significant glucosuria.

Surgical intervention may be required to drain unresolving pseudocysts, for relief of pain, or to treat other complications associated with chronic pancreatitis. The goal of surgical intervention is to alleviate biliary tract disease, establish the free flow of bile into the duodenum, and remove obstruction of the pancreatic duct. Distal pancreatectomy may be necessary if the disease is located at the tail of the pancreas, and the Whipple procedure is performed when the disease is most extensive at the head of the pancreas. These procedures relieve the pain for 60% to 80% of patients.

In patients with alcoholic pancreatitis, ERCP examination often reveals alternating stricture and dilation ("chain of lakes") of the pancreatic duct. Treatment for this is a modified Puestow procedure (lateral pancreaticojejunostomy), which is 70% to 80% effective for pain relief.

Follow-up and Referral

Follow-up of the patient with chronic pancreatitis will depend on the complications resulting from the disease and the medical and surgical interventions employed to remedy the disease. Patients who have developed pseudocysts that have not resolved spontaneously will require periodic CT scans to monitor resolution or evolution of the cysts. Cysts that are consistently larger than 6 cm and are expanding should be referred for invasive treatment.

A nutritionist may be helpful in managing any protein-calorie malnutrition. The pancreas is very nutrition sensitive, and an improper diet can lead to atrophy and fibrosis. Follow-up with the nutritionist is often necessary for control of diabetes mellitus as well.

Patient Education

Patients should be taught about the natural history of this chronic disease, the common complications, and what to expect in the long term. Patients with chronic pancreatitis can expect that after 5 to 10 years, the episodes of pancreatic pain diminish in frequency and may in fact disappear. Patients should fully understand their medicine regimen, including appropriate time of medication and adverse effects. Patients have a tendency to be more compliant when they understand that the goal of treatment is to control diarrhea and gain body weight. Patients can be provided with written instructions to assist with adherence.

Patients should be cautioned against long-term narcotic analgesic use because it can result in drug dependence. If long-term narcotic use is necessary, patients may benefit from referral to a pain control clinic to learn how to relieve pain using nonpharmacotherapeutic measures.

■ HEPATITIS

Hepatitis is a common problem throughout the world and has many causes, including infectious, drug, vascular, and metabolic etiologies. Many cases of hepatitis are subclinical. Symptoms may be "flu-like" and go unreported so that the true incidence of the disease may be underestimated. Table 11.9 lists some of the causes of acute hepatitis.

Acute viral hepatitis is a systemic infection that predominantly affects the liver and can lead to liver inflammation and necrosis. There are many viral agents that cause hepatitis, but the most common, and the ones that have public health concerns, are hepatitis A virus (HAV), hepatitis B virus (HBV), hepatitis C virus (HCV), hepatitis D virus (HDV), and hepatitis E virus (HEV). All are endemic to the United States except HEV, which is common in Southeast Asia, India, parts of Africa, and Mexico. The prevalence of acute hepatitis has been slowly rising for the past few years.

Epidemiology and Causes
Hepatitis A

HAV is a small, single-stranded RNA virus of the picornavirus family. There was a 92% decline in the incidence

Table 11.9	Causes of Acute Hepatitis
Viral	Cytomegalovirus; Epstein-Barr virus; hepatitis A, B, C, D, and E viruses; herpes virus; rubella; varicella-zoster virus; yellow-fever virus
Nonviral	Amebic abscess, bacterial abscess, Lyme disease, syphilis
Metabolic disorders	Alpha-1-antitrypsin deficiency, Wilson's disease
Vascular	Budd-Chiari syndrome, congestive heart disorders failure, ischemia (hypotension, shock)
Drugs	Acetaminophen, allopurinol, ASA (high doses), captopril, carbamazepine, isoniazid, ketoconazole, methyldopa, NSAIDs, procainamide, sulfonamides
Toxins	Alcohol (ethanol), carbon tetrachloride, herbs, mushrooms

of hepatitis A infections in the United States between 1995 and 2007. In 1995, there were 12 cases per 100,000; in 2007 that number dropped to 1 case in 100,000. A total of 1,670 HAV cases were reported in 2010. HAV is endemic in the United States, with periodic outbreaks occurring in certain populations: Native Americans, Alaskan natives, and some Hispanic populations. Because the symptoms of HAV are often mild and nonspecific, many cases are undetected. Many other cases are asymptomatic, making it almost impossible to quantify the number of infections annually. Risk factors include crowded conditions, such as prisons, nursing homes, and day-care centers, and poor sanitation. Contaminated food or water is a common source of HAV. HAV can cause fulminant liver failure on rare occasions, usually in combination with an underlying liver disease.

Transmission is by the fecal–oral route, but HAV has been detected in blood. People contract HAV by consuming contaminated water or ice; raw shellfish harvested from sewage-contaminated water; and fruits, vegetables, or other foods eaten uncooked that may have become contaminated in handling. But HAV is also contracted through transfusion of infected blood. The virus is killed by heating at 185°F for 1 minute. Adequate chlorination of water also kills the virus. According to the Centers for Disease Control and Prevention (CDC) Viral Hepatitis Surveillance Program, household or sexual contact with a person who has HAV is the most frequently reported source of infection, accounting for 24% of the cases. The incubation period is 30 days but can be as long as 6 weeks. Excretion of HAV in feces occurs up to 2 weeks before clinical illness. It is rarely found in feces after the first week of illness. Blood and stools are infectious throughout the incubation period and early illness until the aminotransferase levels peak. A person is most infectious about 2 weeks before and during the first week that symptoms appear.

Chronic HAV does not occur. There is no carrier state, and HAV usually causes no long-term damage. HAV may persist for up to 1 year with relapses before full recovery. The mortality rate is less than 0.2%.

Hepatitis B

HBV is a DNA hepadnavirus with eight different genotypes and replicates in the liver. The incidence of HBV has decreased 81% in the United States since 1990, with 1.5 cases per 100,000 in 2007. There were 2,168 confirmed cases of chronic HBV in 2010. However, the risk of chronic HBV is as high as 90% for infected infants. The frequency of infection and the mode of transmission vary in different parts of the world. According to the CDC, in the United States, Canada, Western Europe, Australia, and New Zealand, the infection is of low endemicity and occurs primarily in adolescents and adults; 5% to 8% of the total population have been infected, and 0.1% to 2.0% are HBV carriers. More than 1 million people in the United States have chronic HBV infection; and although the overall prevalence of HBV in the United States is only 2% to 3%, the prevalence in the native Alaskan population is 6.4% and 14% among African Americans. Between 2000 and 2010, the reported number of HBV cases in the United States declined.

High-risk groups include male homosexuals, IV drug abusers, first generation immigrants from endemic regions (Southeast Asia, China, and the Middle East), and people with multiple sex partners. Other high-risk groups include nurses, physicians, dentists, and personnel working in clinical and pathology labs and blood banks where direct needle-stick contamination may occur. The risk of infection from a contaminated needle is 10% to 30%. Patients and staff at hemodialysis centers are also at high risk. The risk of contracting HBV from a blood transfusion is now 1 in 600,000 units transfused in the United States.

Transmission is usually by direct contact with infected blood or blood products or by sexual contact. The highest concentrations of HBV are found in the blood; however, other body fluids such as semen, cervical secretions, saliva, and wound exudates contain lower concentrations of hepatitis B surface antigen (HBsAg). Parenteral exposure is the most efficient route of transmission, most often occurring in IV drug abusers sharing or using nonsterilized, contaminated needles and in health-care workers by accidental needle sticks. HBV can be transmitted from contact with contaminated inanimate objects because the virus is capable of living in the open environment for approximately 1 week. HBV is not transmitted via the fecal–oral route. The vast

majority (90%) of acute HBV infections occur in young adults, especially men. HBsAg-positive mothers may transmit HBV to their babies during childbirth. HBV is not spread through food, water, or casual contact. The average incubation period for HBV is 12 to 14 weeks but can be anywhere from 6 weeks to 6 months.

The mortality rate for acute HBV infection is 0.4% to 1% but is higher when hepatitis D is superimposed. About 10% of patients infected with HBV develop chronic hepatitis. The risk of chronic infection with HBV is inversely proportional to the age at which infection occurred. Patients with chronic hepatitis are at an increased risk for cirrhosis and hepatocellular cancer. Infection with HBV is also associated with arthritis, glomerulonephritis, and polyarteritis nodosa.

Hepatitis C

HCV was first identified in 1989 and was previously known as hepatitis non-A non-B. It is a single-stranded RNA virus with 6 genotypes and more than 50 subtypes. Genotype 1 is the most common type in the United States and Europe (60%–70%). The clinical significance of the genotype is unclear, but different genotypes and subtypes have different responses to interferon treatment. The incubation period of HCV is 6 to 7 weeks. Transmission is similar to the routes for HBV, and before 1990, HCV was responsible for 90% of cases of post-transfusion hepatitis, but now very few cases of HCV infection are attributable to blood transfusion. IV drug use accounts for about 50% of HCV cases today. In 2011 there were 1,229 reported cases of acute HCV, but the estimated number of actual new cases of HCV is 16,500. This was a 44% increase over the previous year. The estimated number of chronic cases of HCV is between 2.7 and 3.9 million.

There are about 3.2 million Americans who have chronic hepatitis C infection. The prevalence of this infection is greatest in those individuals born between 1945 and 1965. They were most likely infected in the 1970s and 1980s. Injection drug use is the strongest risk factor. Having sex with an injection drug user is also a risk factor, although less robust. There is a 5% risk of maternal–neonate transmission at the time of birth, which tends to be greatest in patients with high circulating levels of HCV RNA. Anti-HCV antibodies are more common in non-Hispanic black and Mexican American people. Low family income and a lifetime history of more than 20 sexual partners are also risk factors. Rates of HCV infection are higher for men than for women, possibly due to more risky behavior. Other possible transmission can be through body piercing and tattooing, although there is little evidence to date. For many patients infected with HCV, the source is never determined.

Fewer than 25% of people with HCV infection are symptomatic, making diagnosis and treatment difficult in the 75% who are HCV RNA positive. Most acute cases go undetected until they present with symptoms of chronic liver disease. Seventy percent to 90% of patients with HCV develop chronic hepatitis. Of this group, 20% progress to chronic liver disease, liver failure, or hepatocellular carcinoma. Alcohol consumption appears to increase the chances of chronic disease and serious complications.

Hepatitis D

HDV is a defective RNA virus that requires HBsAg for its replication. Only individuals with HBV are at risk for HDV. The major risk factor for HDV is IV drug use. Transmission is by the parenteral route and should be suspected in any HBsAg-positive person with acute or chronic hepatitis. New cases of HDV are uncommon in the United States today, probably because of widespread vaccination for HBV. Incubation is 1 to 6 months, and the mortality rate is 3%.

Hepatitis E

HEV, formerly called enterically transmitted or waterborne non-A non-B hepatitis, is a single-stranded RNA virus. It is similar to HAV but not as easily transmitted. It is transmitted through fecally contaminated water and is responsible for water-borne hepatitis outbreaks; it is endemic in Southeast Asia, India, North Africa, and Mexico. Large outbreaks have occurred in refugee camps in Sudan and Chad. There have been relatively few cases in the United States, and most have been associated with global travel. There have documented cases in Germany and Japan of HEV infection with consumption of meat from animals that are infected with the virus. Interestingly, the seroprevalence of HEV in the United States is 21%. The illness is self-limiting, and there is no carrier state. The incubation period is from 2 weeks to 2 months. The mortality rate is low except in pregnant women, in whom the mortality rate is 10% to 20%. Table 11.10 lists the features of hepatitis A, B, C, D, and E.

Hepatitis G

Hepatitis G virus, also known as HGV/GB virus-C (HGV/GBV-C), is a single-stranded RNA flavivirus that is transmitted percutaneously. The clinical significance is yet to be determined. Most patients (75%) who are positive for HGV have normal liver function tests. Co-infection with HCV, HBV, and HIV is common. In patients with HIV infection, co-infection with HGV improves the survival rate (Jacobson, 2002). There is no evidence at this point that HGV causes liver damage.

Chronic Hepatitis

Chronic hepatitis, characterized by elevated aminotransferase (aspartate aminotransferase [AST] and alanine aminotransferase [ALT]) levels for more than 6 months, occurs in 1% to 2% of immunocompromised adults with HBV and in as many as 90% of neonates and infants with HBV. Chronic hepatitis occurs in up to 90% of the people infected with HCV. Cirrhosis develops in 40% of patients with chronic HBV, and 20% of those with chronic HCV are at high risk for developing hepatocellular carcinoma as well.

Pathophysiology

Hepatitis is an inflammation of the liver. It can result from a variety of causes. Viral hepatitis usually presents in one of three clinical manifestations: anicteric, icteric, or cholestatic. Despite the presentation, the progression of the disease follows the same pattern, differing only in severity, enzymatic abnormality, and possible outcomes. The pathological lesions of hepatitis are similar to those caused by other viral infections. Regardless of the type of hepatitis causing the infection, all the liver acini cells are affected by patchy cell dropout, acidophilic hepatocellular necrosis, scarring, Kupffer cell hyperplasia, and mononuclear inflammatory infiltrate. The degree of cellular change is proportionate to the severity of infection. Hepatocellular injury is mediated by cell-mediated immune response. Cytotoxic T cells and natural killer cells play an important part by killing the infected cells and releasing inflammatory cytokines. An intense immune response can decrease the chance of chronic infection; however, it does foster development of hepatocellular necrosis. Histological examination of tissue from livers infected with hepatitis demonstrates that even early in the disease process liver regeneration has already started.

Normally, in patients infected with hepatitis, the underlying reticulin network is preserved, allowing for complete histological recovery. If extensive necrosis of the bridging acini occurs, however, the inflammatory process can damage and obstruct the bile canaliculi, causing cholestasis and obstructive jaundice. In most mild cases of hepatitis, the liver parenchyma is not damaged; HBV and HCV tend to be the more severe forms of hepatitis, with histological evidence of parenchymal inflammation and necrosis. Although the histological changes in the liver tissue are the same for each type of hepatitis, occasionally HBV can be diagnosed from the presence of "ground glass" hepatocytes caused by HBsAg-infiltrated cytoplasm and by using special staining techniques that detect certain viral components. These findings are most often associated with chronic HBV infection. The long-term, asymptomatic chronic-carrier state is thought to result from an immunological tolerance to the hepatitis virus. The virus is not totally cleared by the immune system, and the hepatocellular injury is minimal, leading to a lifelong asymptomatic carrier state. This carrier state is most common in infants, whose immune system is immature and may be unable to overcome the virus. This chronic-carrier state is associated with a 10- to 100-fold risk of hepatocellular carcinoma.

HCV causes hepatocellular injury through direct cytopathic invasion by the virus. The viral load is directly

Table 11.10 Key Features of Hepatitis A, B, C, D, and E

Features	Hepatitis A Virus (HAV)	Hepatitis B Virus (HBV)	Hepatitis C Virus (HCV)	Hepatitis D Virus (HDV)	Hepatitis E Virus (HEV)
Transmission	Fecal–oral, sewage, contaminated water, and possibly shellfish and possibly blood	Percutaneous, permucosal through infected blood and body fluids, sexual	Percutaneous, community, a large percentage have no known risk factors	Percutaneous, but must have co-infection with HBV	Fecal–oral
Incubation period (days)	15–50 (average 20–37)	25–160 (average 60–110)	42–49	Same as for HBV	10–56
Laboratory tests	Anti-HAV IgM (acute); anti-HAV IgG (resolving)	HBsAg (confirms), IgM anti-HBs (acute phase), IgG anti-HBs (resolving/immunity), HBeAg, anti-HBe, anti-HBc (persists in carriers)	Anti-HCV appears in 6–37 weeks	Anti-HDV appears late	Anti-HEV IgM detected within 26 days of jaundice; IgG antibody persists
Immunity/immunization	45% of United States population has antibodies against HAV; HAV vaccine available	5%–15% of U.S. population has anti-HBs; HBV vaccine available	Unknown; no vaccine available	People immune to HBV are also protected against HDV	Unknown
Prevalence	Increasing in adults	Decreasing in the United States	4% of post-transfusion hepatitis; 50% IV drug users	Common in IV drug abusers	Rare in United States; endemic in Southeast Asia, India, North Africa, Mexico
Course/mortality	Does not progress to chronic state; mortality is 0–0.2% with fulminant hepatitis	Chronic liver disease occurs in 1%–5% of adults and 80%–90% in children; mortality rate is 0.3%–1.5%	Chronic active hepatitis develops in 70%–90% of cases; 20% develop chronic liver disease; mortality rate is the same as for HBV	Chronic liver disease develops if present in chronic HBV; mortality rate is 2%–20% for acute icteric hepatitis	Does not progress to chronic liver disease; mortality rate is 1%–2% but as high as 10%–15% in pregnant women

proportionate to the histological inflammation seen on liver biopsy. HCV is capable of rapid mutation, which allows it to elude immunity by development of resistant strains to the existing antibodies. Autoimmune hepatitis is most commonly associated with HCV, lending itself to the multiple extrahepatic manifestations of the disease. These patients develop autoimmune responses leading to membranous glomerulonephritis, vasculitis, dermatitis, pulmonary fibrosis, and rheumatoid arthritis. Chronic HCV occurs in approximately 50% of cases, with inflammatory changes leading to cirrhosis within 20 years.

Different drugs can cause different histopathological abnormalities in the liver. For example, acetaminophen damages hepatocytes by producing toxic metabolites that damage the cellular and subcellular structures of the liver. Hepatic injury resulting from sepsis is caused by direct bacterial invasion of the parenchyma, circulating endotoxins, and hypoxia. Cytotoxic lymphocytes attack hepatocyte membrane antigens in autoimmune chronic active hepatitis. All of these agents result in varying degrees of hepatocyte injury.

Clinical Presentation

Subjective

The clinical presentation of viral hepatitis is extremely variable; it can range from asymptomatic infection without jaundice to a sudden severe infection and death in a few days. Table 11.11 displays the clinical findings and

corresponding laboratory values for the different phases of viral hepatitis.

Prodromal Phase During the prodromal phase, the onset may be abrupt or insidious with anorexia, nausea, vomiting, malaise, upper respiratory infection, or flu-like symptoms. The patient may also complain of myalgia, arthralgia, and easy fatigability. Many patients report an aversion for smoking if they are smokers. Nausea and vomiting occur frequently. Diarrhea or constipation may be reported. In the early stage of acute HBV, skin rashes and arthritis may be seen.

Fever is usually present but rarely exceeds 103°F (39.4°C), except in HAV, in which it may go higher. Chills may mark an acute onset. A decrease in fever often coincides with the onset of jaundice.

Abdominal pain is usually mild and constant in the right upper quadrant or epigastrium. The pain can be aggravated by jarring or exertion. It is occasionally severe enough to simulate cholecystitis or cholelithiasis.

Icteric Phase During the icteric phase, jaundice and dark urine appear, usually 5 to 10 days after the initial symptoms, although some patients do not experience jaundice. With the onset of jaundice, the prodromal symptoms worsen and are followed by progressive clinical improvement.

Convalescent Phase The convalescent phase is marked by an increased sense of well-being. The jaundice, abdominal pain and tenderness, and fatigability disappear and the appetite returns. Chronic HBV begins at this point in the case of chronic disease.

Table 11.11	Clinical Findings: Viral Hepatitis	
Stage	**Subjective and Objective Complaints**	**Laboratory Tests**
Incubation	None	HBsAg late in the stage HBeAg
Prodromal	Onset abrupt or insidious Anorexia, nausea, vomiting, malaise, upper respiratory infection (nasal discharge, pharyngitis), myalgia, arthralgia, easy fatigability, fever (HAV), abdominal pain	HBsAg in HBV
Icteric	Jaundice, dark urine, light-colored stools Continued prodromal complaints with gradual improvement	Anti-HBc Anti-HAV (IgG and IgM) Anti-HCV HBsAg becomes negative High urine bilirubin Markedly elevated ALT and AST Elevated LDH, bilirubin, alkaline phosphatase Markedly increased PT indicates increased mortality
Convalescent	Increased sense of well-being Appetite returns Jaundice, abdominal pain, and fatigability abate	Anti-HAV IgG Anti-HBs Decreased liver enzymes

The acute illness usually subsides over 2 to 3 weeks. Complete clinical and laboratory recovery occurs by the ninth week in HAV and after 16 weeks in HBV. Five percent to 10% of the cases may last longer, and fewer than 1% have an acute fulminant course. Hepatitis B and C may become chronic.

Hepatomegaly is present in 50% of patients with viral hepatitis, and splenomegaly is seen in 15% of cases. Lymphadenopathy, especially in the cervical and epitrochlear areas, is commonly present. Signs of general toxemia may vary from minimal to severe. The clinical features of all the types of viral hepatitis are similar, with the exception of onset. Hepatitis A and E usually have an abrupt onset, whereas hepatitis B, C, and D have a more insidious onset, and the liver enzyme levels are higher. HVC is often asymptomatic.

Diagnostic Reasoning
Diagnostic Tests

Laboratory tests are used to diagnose, identify the serological type, and determine the current status of the disease.

Hepatitis A Two types of antibodies to HAV can be detected by radioimmunoassay and enzyme-linked immunosorbent assay. The first type of antibody to HAV is the immunoglobulin M (IgM) antibody (IgM anti-HAV), which appears about 4 weeks after exposure, or just before hepatocellular enzyme elevation occurs, and disappears in 3 to 6 months. Detection of IgM is the diagnostic gold standard for acute hepatitis A. The second type of antibody, immunoglobulin G (IgG) anti-HAV, appears about 2 weeks after the IgM anti-HAV begins to increase and peaks after about 1 month of disease. The IgG antibody persists for more than 10 years and provides immunity. If the IgM is elevated in the absence of IgG, acute hepatitis is suspected. If IgG is elevated in the absence of IgM, this indicates previous exposure to HAV, noninfectivity, and immunity to recurring HAV infection.

Hepatitis B Acute and chronic HBV can be differentiated from other forms of viral hepatitis by serological markers representing the body's immunological response. The HBV is made up of an inner core surrounded by an outer capsule. The outer capsule contains HBsAg (hepatitis B *surface* antigen). The inner core contains the HBV *core* antigen (HBcAg). HBeAg (the *extracellular* form of HBcAg) is also found within the core. Antibodies to these antigens are called anti-HBs, anti-HBc, and anti-HBe.

Detection of HBsAg is diagnostic for HBV and is the first test to order when HBV is suspected. It will appear 1 to 10 weeks after exposure to the hepatitis B virus and will remain positive throughout the acute phase of the illness. If HBsAg persists longer, this may indicate chronic hepatitis. HBsAg rises before the onset of clinical symptoms, peaks during the first week of symptoms, and returns to normal by the time the jaundice subsides. HBsAg indicates acute infection and infectivity. Anti-HBs appears about 4 weeks after the disappearance of the surface antigen and signifies recovery from the infection and noninfectivity, as well as immunity.

There are no tests available to detect the HBV core antigen (HBcAg), but the IgM anti-HBc appears shortly after HBsAg is detected and can persist for 3 to 6 months. The anti-HBc level is elevated during the time lag between the disappearance of HBsAg and the appearance of anti-HBs; this interval is called the *core window*. During this window, anti-HBc is the only detectable marker of a recent hepatitis infection. Anti-HBs is composed of IgG and IgM antibodies. The IgM titer is diagnostic for acute hepatitis, whereas the IgG antibody is usually positive for life after infection.

HBeAg is generally not used for diagnostic purposes but rather as an index of viral replication and infectivity. The presence of HBeAg correlates with early and active disease and with high infectivity in patients with acute HBV infection. HBeAg appears during the incubation period shortly after the detection of HBsAg. The continued presence of HBeAg predicts the development of chronic HBV infection. Table 11.12 displays the serology testing and results for HBV infection.

Hepatitis C The diagnosis of HCV is based on enzyme immunoassays (EIA) that detect antibodies to HCV (anti-HCV). Limitations of the enzyme immunoassay include moderate sensitivity for the diagnosis of acute HCV (false-negative result) and low specificity (50%) in healthy blood donors and some people with elevated gamma-globulin levels (false-positive result). In these

Table 11.12 Serologic Testing for Hepatitis B					
Interpretation	HBsAg	Anti-HBs	HBeAg	Anti-HBe	Anti-HBc
Acute hepatitis (confirms diagnosis)	+	–	+	–	IgM
Acute hepatitis	–	–	+ or –	–	IgM
Recovery from hepatitis (immunity)	–	+	–	+ or –	IgG
Vaccination (immunity)	–	+	–	–	–
Chronic HBV with active viral replication	+	–	+	–	IgG
Chronic HBV with low viral replication	–	–	–	+	IgG

particular cases, a diagnosis of HCV may be confirmed by use of a polymerase chain reaction to detect HCV RNA. The risk of transfusion-associated HCV has decreased from 10% in the early 1990s to less than 0.1% today as a result of the testing of donated blood for HCV.

Hepatitis D Diagnosis of HDV is via detection of anti-HDV or HDV RNA in the presence of hepatitis B markers. Rising titers of anti-HDV indicate acute infection and are detectable early in the disease.

Hepatitis E HEV is diagnosed via history and exclusion of other causes. There are no commercially available tests in the United States at this time, although certain research laboratories can detect anti-HEV in serum and HEV genomes in blood and stool.

Additional Testing In any patient in whom hepatitis is suspected, liver enzyme levels should be checked for signs of injury. Elevated aminotransferase levels are the hallmark of all forms of acute hepatitis. AST is usually markedly elevated early in hepatitis. ALT is often very elevated early in hepatitis, as is lactate dehydrogenase. All of these hepatocellular enzymes are elevated during the acute and chronic active phases of hepatitis. AST and ALT levels fluctuate during the course of the disease for unknown reasons. Bilirubin and alkaline phosphatase are usually elevated and may remain elevated after the AST and ALT have normalized.

The white blood cell count is normal or low, especially in the preicteric phase. Large atypical lymphocytes may occasionally be seen and are similar to those found in infectious mononucleosis. Mild proteinuria is common, and there is bilirubinuria just preceding and during the icteric phase. The prothrombin time may be prolonged in severe hepatitis and signifies increased mortality risk. Liver biopsy is rarely indicated unless there is evidence of liver damage from a chronic state of hepatitis.

Differential Diagnosis

Differential diagnosis for hepatitis includes other viral diseases that affect the liver, such as infectious mononucleosis, cytomegalovirus infection, and herpes simplex virus. Drug- or toxin-induced liver damage should also be included in the differential diagnosis list, as well as conditions that cause jaundice.

Management

The principle of the management of hepatitis includes prevention of transmission and symptomatic relief. Vaccinations are available to prevent HAV and HBV. Vaccination against HAV is recommended for people living in or traveling to endemic areas and prevents infection for at least 20 years. Immune globulin is recommended for close contacts of people with HAV within 2 weeks of exposure because it may prevent or lessen the severity of the disease.

HBV vaccine is recommended for people with high-risk factors, such as health-care workers, day-care workers,

IV drug users, male homosexuals, household contacts of HBsAg carriers, heterosexual contacts of HBsAg carriers, people with anticipated multiple transfusions, and patients undergoing dialysis.

Treatment for hepatitis, no matter what the cause, is largely supportive. Patients rarely require hospitalization. Balanced nutrition with adequate calories and fluids is recommended, and avoidance of alcohol is stressed. Activity is generally restricted during the acute phase and during a relapse with gradual resumption of activity.

Treatment of chronic HBV is currently intramuscular pegylated interferon alfa-2a. Treatment with interferon alone is not sufficient to eradicate HBV in most patients, so it is used in combination with an antiviral agent such as lamivudine. Candidates include patients with compensated liver disease, persistent elevated ALT, detectable HBsAg and HBeAg, low concentrations of HBV DNA, and fibrosis seen on liver biopsy. The response rate after this expensive therapy, however, is only about 40%.

HCV causes chronic hepatitis and liver damage. The goal of treatment is to eradicate HCV RNA. Treatment with pegylated interferon and ribavirin in the acute phase decreases the risk of chronic hepatitis. This treatment has a high sustained viral response rate (SVR) for those infected with genotype 2 or 3, and a liver biopsy is not necessary. However, SVR is not as good in persons with genotypes 1a, 1b, and 4. Pegylated interferon is a slow-release, long-acting drug that, when given once a week in a dose of 180 mg for 48 weeks, has shown an SVR in 38% of patients who already have chronic hepatitis C. SVR in patients who have genotype 2 or 3 is about 80%. Ribavirin in combination with pegylated interferon has been shown to be more efficacious in clearing the viremia. Ribavirin is given in divided doses of 1,000 mg per day for those weighing less than 75 kg (165 lb) and 1,200 mg for those over 75 kg.

Response to therapy is judged by an ALT returning to normal by 12 weeks and negative viral markers (HCV RNA). After the ALT has returned to normal, treatment is slowly discontinued. Consuming alcohol increases the risk of these patients progressing to cirrhosis and liver failure, so abstinence from all forms of alcohol (including in medications) is especially important.

Hepatic transplantation is indicated for patients with advanced liver disease as a result of chronic HCV, and in fact it is the most common reason for liver transplantation in the United States.

Follow-up and Referral

Any patient diagnosed with HCV should be referred to a hepatologist for follow-up because the chance of developing chronicity is great with this type of hepatitis. Patients with HAV usually do not require follow-up. Patients with HBV should be seen in 1 month and should have blood drawn for HBsAg after 6 months. Persistent elevation of HBsAg indicates a chronic state, and these patients should be referred to a hepatologist.

Patient Education

Patients and their intimate contacts should be given careful instructions about the cause of hepatitis, the mode of transmission, and measures to prevent the transmission. It is recommended that household contacts and sexual contacts be given passive immunity (immunoglobulin) for HAV and HBV, as well as active immunization. Hand washing and personal hygiene can help prevent the spread of the disease. Patients should also be taught not to share personal items such as toothbrushes, razors, and eating utensils during the period of infectivity. Patients with chronic hepatitis or a carrier state should be instructed to practice safe sex.

Patients who develop chronic liver disease as a result of hepatitis can contact the American Liver Foundation at www.liverfoundation.org.

■ CIRRHOSIS AND LIVER FAILURE

Cirrhosis is the end result of hepatocellular injury involving the entire liver, resulting in fibrosis, nodular regeneration, and distorted hepatic architecture. Cirrhosis is considered permanent and irreversible. Fibrous bands are formed during nodular regeneration in an attempt by the liver to repair itself, and these bands give the liver a hobnailed appearance. The fibrotic changes that occur within the liver parenchyma cause disruption and compression of the vascular, biliary, and lymphatic vessels and result in many of the characteristic findings common to liver failure. *Cirrhosis* and *fibrosis* are not synonymous terms; fibrotic changes are characteristic findings of cirrhosis.

Epidemiology and Causes

In the Western Hemisphere, cirrhosis is a leading cause of death in individuals older than age 40. Although there are many causes of cirrhosis (Table 11.13), chronic alcohol abuse remains the leading pathological insult in the United States.

Alcoholic cirrhosis—also known as Laennec's, portal, fatty, or micronodular cirrhosis—is the most common type of cirrhosis in the United States. An estimated 18 million people in the United States abuse alcohol, but only 25% of alcoholics develop cirrhosis. It is estimated that more than 30,000 people in the United States alone die from liver disease caused by alcohol abuse each year. Men are affected three times more often than women.

Alcoholic cirrhosis is often associated with nutritional and vitamin deficiencies but occurs in well-nourished individuals as well as in alcoholics. Studies have found no safe amount of alcohol that can be ingested daily without causing cirrhosis, which supports the theory that there are additional factors (genetic, environmental, nutritional) that may influence the development of

Table 11.13	Causes of Cirrhosis
Alcohol	
Direct hepatotoxins	
• Carbon tetrachloride	
• Phosphorus	
Indirect hepatotoxins	
• Tetracycline	
• Methotrexate	
• Acetaminophen	
• Mushroom toxin—*Amanita phalloides*	
• Alkylated anabolic steroids	
• 6-Mercaptopurine	
HBV and HCV	
Autoimmune chronic active hepatitis	
Diabetes mellitus and insipidus	
Thyroiditis	
Ulcerative colitis	
Glomerulonephritis	
Biliary cirrhosis	
Primary biliary cirrhosis	
Primary sclerosing cholangitis	
Chronic pancreatitis	
Sclerosing cholangitis	
Vasculitis	
Cholelithiasis	
Cystic fibrosis	
Genetic diseases	
• Wilson's disease	
• Hemochromatosis	
• Galactosemia	
Vascular/congestive disorders of the liver	
• Budd-Chiari syndrome	
• Ischemic hepatitis/shock liver	
• Right-sided heart failure (chronic)	

alcoholic liver disease. Women tend to develop cirrhosis more quickly with less alcohol intake than men, which suggests that a smaller, leaner body mass and enhanced absorption are both factors in the development of alcoholic cirrhosis.

There are three consequences of alcohol abuse: fatty liver, alcoholic hepatitis, and alcoholic cirrhosis. Fatty liver is a reversible condition where large vacuoles of triglycerides accumulate in the hepatocytes. The accumulation of fat in the liver causes an inflammatory reaction in the liver called steatohepatitis. Alcoholic hepatitis results from moderate to severe alcohol abuse for years and can lead to alcoholic cirrhosis quickly even with abstinence, but it is not an obligatory phase in the development of cirrhosis.

Primary biliary cirrhosis (PBC) is a disease that almost exclusively affects women aged 40 to 60. It is an autoimmune disease that causes destruction of the intrahepatic bile ducts, resulting in cholestasis. Autoimmune disorders such as scleroderma, Raynaud's syndrome, autoimmune thyroid disease, celiac disease, and Sjögren's syndrome have been linked to the development of PBC.

Primary sclerosing cholangitis (PSC) is most common in men aged 20 to 40 and is associated with inflammatory bowel disease, as well as with the histocompatibility antigens HLA-B8, HLA-DR3, and HLA-DR4, suggesting a genetic link. It is characterized by diffuse inflammation and fibrosis throughout the biliary tree. Factors contributing to the development of PSC are anything that obstructs or inhibits the flow of bile through both the extrahepatic and intrahepatic bile ducts. Smoking is associated with a *decreased* risk of PSC.

Budd-Chiari syndrome (BCS) is a disorder resulting from hepatic vein thrombosis and outflow obstruction, which can occur anywhere from the hepatic veins to the inferior vena cava (IVC) or the right atrium. Other disease processes associated with this form of cirrhosis are coagulopathies, lymphoreticular malignancies, ischemic hepatitis resulting from profound hypotension associated with shock, and liver arteriovenous malformations characteristic of hemorrhagic telangiectasia. There are numerous causes for BCS, and definitive diagnosis is found in only approximately 65% to 75% of cases. In the Western Hemisphere, thrombosis of the hepatic veins is most often associated with myeloproliferative and coagulation disorders, as well as oral contraceptive use. Venous thrombosis is also an associated risk factor in the third trimester of pregnancy. Malignant tumors arising from within the liver or metastatic renal carcinoma can result in mechanical obstruction of the IVC, causing thrombosis within the hepatic veins and resulting in cirrhosis.

Wilson's disease and *hemochromatosis* are both autosomal recessive metabolic disorders that often present with hepatocellular dysfunction and can lead to cirrhosis if left untreated. The liver is the primary organ involved in the metabolism of both iron (hemochromatosis) and copper (Wilson's disease); overload of either metal can cause cirrhosis. Hemochromatosis is diagnosed primarily in middle-aged whites, whereas Wilson's disease is a disease of adolescents and young adults of all ethnicities.

Pathophysiology

Cirrhosis is the irreversible, end stage of liver injury caused by a variety of insults. Fibrotic scarring and hepatocellular changes result from chronic inflammation; obstruction; and toxic, metabolic, and congestive injuries. The morphological changes resulting from the injury are often classified according to the size of the regenerative nodules: Patients may have micronodular, macronodular, and mixed forms of cirrhosis. The liver can develop cirrhosis as a result of severe acute injury, as is seen with hepatitis; or subsequent to moderate damage sustained over months, as seen with obstructive biliary diseases; or from chronic continuous abuse, as seen in alcoholic cirrhosis.

With cirrhosis, the normal lobular liver architecture is replaced by diffuse disorganization, resulting in proliferation of bands of fibrous tissue and nodular regeneration of the surviving hepatocytes. The extent to which this occurs depends on the degree of injury, the length of exposure to the injury, and the liver's reaction to the insult. The end result is a decrease in the total liver cell mass because of the collagen formation or fibrosis. During the repair process, there is distortion of the microcirculation, resulting in an increased resistance to blood flow, thereby causing portal venous hypertension. As the liver attempts to repair itself, it develops a series of collateral vessels from the newly regenerated nodules to the existing portal vein and hepatic artery. These vessels, which are much less efficient than those of the normal circulation, cause portal hypertension.

Histological classification of cirrhosis is useful for describing the major anatomical changes that result from the various insults. This type of classification gives no etiological information other than narrowing the scope to the injurious agents resulting in this specific histological category of injury. Moreover, it is important to remember that at any point in the disease process, a patient may exhibit varying degrees of histological change.

Micronodular (Laennec's) cirrhosis is characterized by regenerative nodules that are 1 cm in diameter or less, no bigger than normal liver lobules. Histological examination fails to identify portal tracts and hepatic venules. Alcohol abuse often results in this type of cirrhosis; the theory is that continuous damage is being done to the liver, preventing it from regenerating. Initially the liver becomes enlarged and fatty as changes in lipid metabolism lead to fatty infiltrates. As the disease progresses, the liver atrophies and hardens. Fibrous tissue forms in thin, regularly spaced bands throughout the liver, which in time result in a decreased liver mass.

Macronodular cirrhosis is characterized by larger nodules (diameters of 5 cm), which may be multinodular with varying size nodules and may contain central veins. These nodules are surrounded by broad fibrous bands of varying thickness, which correspond to postnecrotic types of cirrhosis as seen following hepatitis. As the normal liver architecture collapses, the portal tracts converge between the fibrous scars, which is a key histological finding. *Mixed cirrhosis* has characteristics of both micronodular and macronodular cirrhosis.

Drug-induced liver disease can be the result of the drug's metabolism itself or a combination of several drugs together. The resultant liver toxicity may be caused by metabolism that is enhanced, altered, or the result of idiosyncratic processes such as hypersensitivity or certain genetics. Intrinsic hepatic injury is drug-dose dependent, whereas idiosyncratic drug reactions are more frequent and are not dose dependent. Patients who have hypersensitivity reactions to a drug develop hepatotoxicity secondary to the formation of drug metabolites, which are harmful to the liver.

PBC and PSC are both chronic cholestatic liver diseases that affect adults. There is an immunological component to both diseases that causes inflammation and fibrosis, which ultimately results in bile duct destruction. Liver biopsy in patients with PBC is of limited value because the disease varies from portal tract to portal tract; biopsy is, however, helpful to validate cirrhotic changes. The beginning stages of PSC are characterized by portal infiltration of lymphocytes, plasma cells, macrophages, and eosinophils. These inflammatory changes are followed by "ductular proliferation," which is characterized by the replacement of mature bile ducts with small, ineffective ones. The inflammatory changes lead to fibrosis, and as fibrotic changes ensue, increased signs of cholestasis appear. The end result of these changes is cirrhosis.

Primary sclerosing cholangitis can involve any part of the biliary tract from the ampulla of Vater to the small bile ducts within the liver. The lumens of these ductal systems can be narrowed or completely obstructed by fibrous scar tissue, resulting in the key functional abnormality, which is cholestasis. The biopsy results show fibrosis with inflammatory changes as described for PSC. Bacterial infections that often occur in the area above the strictures and in the presence of long-standing disease lead to biliary cirrhosis.

The pathophysiology of liver disease caused by hereditary factors is essentially the same for both Wilson's disease and hereditary hemochromatosis. Wilson's disease results from decreased hepatic excretion of copper and excessive absorption of copper from the small intestine. There is a gradual accumulation of copper within the tissues, resulting in hepatotoxicity. Initial presentation of Wilson's disease may vary from acute hepatitis or chronic hepatitis, neuropsychiatric disease, cirrhosis, or fulminant hepatic failure in young adults. Histological examination of the initial lesions reveals hepatic steatosis, with increased glycogen deposits. These lesions eventually progress to fibrosis and finally cirrhosis.

Hereditary hemochromatosis is characterized by increased intestinal absorption of iron. Liver biopsy reveals increased iron deposition, predominantly within the hepatocytes. When levels of iron exceed 20,000 mcg/g of liver tissue, fibrosis and cirrhosis usually ensue.

Vascular causes of liver disease, which include BCS and congestive hepatopathology, cause cirrhosis as the end result of necrosis. Liver biopsies show centrilobular congestion, hemorrhage, necrosis, and dilation. The resultant disruption of the hepatic circulation causes portal hypertension, fibrosis of the surrounding tissues, and ultimately cirrhosis.

Clinical Presentation

Cirrhosis is often an incidental finding on an annual exam, revealed either by an asymptomatically enlarged liver or an elevation of the liver enzymes. The clinical manifestations of cirrhosis are the result of hepatocellular damage and portal hypertension. The cumulative effect of these signs and symptoms is often referred to as "the stigmata of liver disease." The onset of symptoms is usually gradual, and patients with cirrhosis may appear well and remain asymptomatic for years.

Subjective

Initial complaints generally include weakness, anorexia, weight loss, and fatigue. Malnutrition is usually evident and can be the result of anorexia or the effect of reduced bile salt excretion, resulting in fat malabsorption and deficiency of fat-soluble vitamins.

As cirrhosis advances, patients may present with upper gastrointestinal (GI) bleeding from esophageal varices, which develop secondary to portal hypertension. As the liver continues to fail, patients may present with ascites and/or encephalopathy. Patients with cirrhosis may complain of abdominal pain that is caused by the enlargement of the liver and stretching of Glisson's capsule or by the ascites itself.

Menstrual abnormalities, loss of libido, impotence, sterility, and gynecomastia are manifestations of increased levels of estrogen that result from the liver's inability to inactivate hormones. These symptoms may prompt individuals to seek medical attention. Previously undiagnosed cirrhosis is often the underlying cause of symptoms in patients presenting with one of the aforementioned complaints.

Objective

The physical exam findings depend on the stage and severity of the disease process. Initial exam findings may reveal an enlarged, firm liver edge (which is the left lobe) palpable below the right costal margin; however, in patients with advanced disease, the liver may be small and difficult to palpate. Often, a firm smooth mass is palpable over the epigastric area, which is the right lobe of the liver (Riedel's lobe). Occasionally, nodular deformities may be palpable along the liver's edge. These areas of liver enlargement are dull to percussion and can aid in measuring the expanse of the liver.

Manifestations of cirrhosis that are nonspecific but suggestive of chronic liver disease include spider nevi, which are normally found over the anterior chest; pectoral alopecia; generalized muscle wasting; Dupuytren's (palmar) contractions; parotid gland enlargement; palmar erythema; hair loss; and testicular atrophy. Patients may have dilated cutaneous veins called *caput medusae* (Medusa's head) radiating out from around the umbilical area. These varicose veins are a result of the shunting of blood to the paraumbilical veins and are a manifestation of portal hypertension. Signs of vitamin and mineral disturbances are glossitis, cheilosis, and peripheral neuropathies. Fever may indicate complications such as peritonitis, cholangitis, or hepatitis.

Jaundiced sclera, skin, and mucous membranes usually develop in the later stages of cirrhosis. The hyperbilirubinemia is a consequence of the liver's inability to conjugate and excrete bilirubin. Patients with hereditary hemochromatosis may have slate-colored skin from increased levels of iron stored in the tissue. Pruritus, although nonspecific, is often the presenting symptom in several forms of cirrhosis and can develop as a result of bile salts accumulating in the skin. Disruption in the liver's ability to synthesize clotting factors may manifest with bruising and complaints of a tendency to bleed. Peripheral edema results because of the decreased plasma osmotic pressure caused by hypoalbuminemia.

Ascites is a direct result of portal hypertension, which is a consequence of increased portal vein pressure. As liver function fails and healthy hepatic cells are replaced with fibrous nodules, the blood flow through the liver is impaired, causing increased resistance and back pressure that result in the accumulation of serous fluid within the abdomen. An abdominal exam reveals a positive fluid wave and shifting dullness on percussion. Splenomegaly results from splenic vein congestion. Esophageal varices, another consequence of portal hypertension, may be discovered after bleeding causes hematemesis, hematochezia, and/or melena. Hemorrhoids, which result from portal hypertension, are also present and cause bright red bleeding from the rectum.

Hepatic encephalopathy can range from mild confusion to coma and is the result of increasing blood ammonia, which is toxic to the brain. Characteristics of encephalopathy include asterixis (liver flap), reversal of sleep–wake patterns, tremors, hyperactive deep-tendon reflexes, dysarthria, delirium, and drowsiness.

Patients who present with Wilson's disease may have golden brown rings of color—called Kayser-Fleischer rings—located within Descemet's membrane of the cornea. These rings are usually found in patients with central nervous system (CNS) involvement and are seen with a slit lamp.

Diagnostic Reasoning

Diagnostic Tests

Results of initial laboratory testing vary depending on the stage of the disease process. If cirrhosis is in the early stages, laboratory results may be normal; however, in other patients, elevation of liver enzymes may be the only indicator of liver disease. Laboratory testing may reveal abnormalities, but these are nonspecific unless correlated with the history and physical exam.

Alcoholic cirrhosis may manifest in different ways depending on other coexisting processes such as malnutrition or hepatitis. The complete blood count commonly shows a macrocytic anemia and, depending on the severity of the disease, pancytopenia from the overall suppression of the bone marrow. The mean corpuscular volume does not correct quickly with abstinence from alcohol and may be the only key to occult alcohol use. Anemia can represent suppression of erythropoiesis from folic acid deficiency, occult losses from the GI

tract, or a combination of the two. The white blood cell and platelet counts can vary depending on whether there is infection or splenic sequestration. As the liver continues to fail and liver cell mass decreases, the prothrombin time (PT) increases as the liver loses the ability to synthesize the proteins necessary to produce clotting factors.

The blood chemistry may show mild to moderate increases in alanine aminotransferase (ALT) and aspartate aminotransferase (AST) levels; if, however, the patient has a superimposed alcoholic hepatitis, the classic enzyme elevation of ALT/AST may be reversed, with an AST/ALT ratio ranging from 2:1 to 3:1. The levels of AST/ALT do not reflect the severity of the disease process. The gamma-glutamyl transpeptidase level is a good measurement of recent alcohol ingestion and declines rapidly with abstinence. Alkaline phosphatase levels may be markedly elevated when there is biliary obstruction. Serum bilirubin levels can be as high as 30 mg/dL. Hypoalbuminemia is common and contributes to the development of edema.

The diagnosis of alcoholic cirrhosis may be difficult to differentiate from alcoholic hepatitis, which is a reversible process, unless a liver biopsy is obtained. Histological examination reveals hepatocellular necrosis and evidence of Mallory bodies within the damaged cells. Depending on the stage of the disease, there is fatty infiltration and fibrosis. In early disease, there are micronodular changes, which over time develop into macronodular cirrhosis.

Abdominal ultrasound (US) is helpful in determining the size of the liver and any ascites or nodule formation. Doppler studies, in combination with US, are used to evaluate patency of the venous system that, if disrupted, can lead to portal hypertension. Any nodular findings that are suspicious for malignancy should be biopsied. If a patient presents with melena or hematemesis, an esophagogastroscopy should be performed to assess for esophageal varices or ulcerative processes.

Diagnosis of cholestatic liver disease, specifically PBC and PSC, may be made in conjunction with various autoimmune disease processes. The initial hepatic blood work-up usually shows an alkaline phosphatase level that is three to four times normal, with mild to moderate increases in the transaminases. The cholecystitic nature of both processes leads to prolonged PT.

Patients with PBC may also present with mild elevation of serum bilirubin and more often hypercholesterolemia. Serum IgM levels are elevated in 50% of cases. Antimitochondrial antibodies (AMAs) are found in 95% of the patients with PBC; titers can exceed 1:500. Definitive diagnosis is made via liver biopsy, which reveals granulomatous bile duct destruction and accumulation of inflammatory cells within the portal tracts with resultant segmental necrosis of the interlobular and septal bile ducts (chronic nonsuppurative destructive cholangitis). Ultrasound evaluation of the biliary tree is negative for biliary obstruction.

Laboratory studies of patients with PSC show the typical cholestatic profile; however, unlike with patients with PBC, the AMA is negative. Total cholesterol levels increase as the disease progresses. Endoscopic or transhepatic cholangiography reveals characteristic beading and stricturing of the intrahepatic and extrahepatic bile ducts. Liver biopsy is diagnostic for fibrous obliterative cholangitis, with the hepatic ductal system being replaced with fibrous cords of connective tissue. The end result for both PBC and PSC is biliary cirrhosis.

Diagnosis of cirrhosis caused by vascular disorders such as BCS and other veno-occlusive diseases is normally made through imaging studies because laboratory findings are nonspecific. Serum bilirubin, transaminases, and alkaline phosphatase can be elevated as much as four times normal. A computed tomography scan demonstrates failure of the hepatic veins to opacify, indicating an occlusive process. Pulsed Doppler studies illustrate absent hepatic flow; a normal pulsed Doppler effectively rules out BCS. Venographic studies also demonstrate narrowing and obstruction of the hepatic venous system. Histological exam reveals centrilobular congestion with associated hemorrhage and necrosis.

Wilson's disease and hemochromatosis are inherited metabolic liver diseases that result in cirrhosis if diagnosis and treatment are not made early. Diagnosis of Wilson's disease is suggested by elevated serum copper levels in conjunction with low serum ceruloplasmin levels. Once an abnormal ceruloplasmin level has been documented, a 24-hour urine check for copper should be completed. Definitive diagnosis is made through quantitative copper levels in the liver on biopsy. The majority of patients with Wilson's disease have histological findings consistent with hepatic steatosis, which in time progresses to fibrosis and cirrhosis.

Iron metabolism studies are used to diagnose hereditary hemochromatosis and should be collected with the patient in the fasting state. The presence of an elevated transferrin saturation level in combination with an elevated ferritin level is suggestive of hereditary hemochromatosis. Liver biopsy is necessary for definitive diagnosis. Histological studies with quantitative iron levels greater than 20,000 mcg/g are consistent with advanced disease and cirrhosis.

Differential Diagnosis

The patient who presents with cirrhosis can be a diagnostic challenge. The differential diagnosis of cirrhosis varies little between the different etiologies, so the challenge is determining the cause in an attempt to prevent further liver damage. The differential diagnosis of alcohol-induced liver disease includes biliary tract disease, idiopathic hemochromatosis, nonalcoholic fatty liver disease, drug toxicity, and/or viral hepatitis. US exam of the liver can often rule out an obstructive process. Alcoholics with chronic pancreatitis frequently develop jaundice secondary to stricturing of the common bile duct, which is differentiated through endoscopic retrograde cholangiopancreatography. A liver biopsy is often the only definitive test for differentiating many of the hepatobiliary diseases from each other. Thorough history and physical exam can suggest a diagnosis, but histological study is necessary to distinguish one process from another.

Alcoholic patients also have a high incidence of coinfection with hepatitis, the cause of which is often unclear; this can alter the typical serological findings. A hepatitis panel will reveal active or prior infection. Drug toxicity, specifically with acetaminophen, even in low doses, can alter transaminase levels and necessitates obtaining a careful drug history from each patient. Because of the preexisting liver injury, alcoholics who present with acetaminophen toxicity have significantly higher morbidity and mortality with relatively low doses of acetaminophen.

The differential diagnosis of cholestatic liver disease must include all other causes of chronic cholestasis, such as tumors, strictures, or obstructions resulting from stone formation. Autoimmune chronic active hepatitis can mimic the signs and symptoms of PBC; however, laboratory studies will show a low or negative titer for AMA. US exam may reveal biliary duct dilation, a process consistent with both PBC and PSC, thus making cholangiography the diagnostic test of choice.

Management

Treatment of cirrhosis is aimed at identifying and removing the causative agent and treating the symptoms.

Alcohol-Induced Liver Disease

In a patient with alcohol-induced liver disease, the most effective treatment remains abstinence. Patients who continue to ingest alcohol and present with ascites can increase their 2-year survival rate to 95% if they can completely abstain from alcohol. Those who continue to drink have a 2-year survival rate of less than 25%. The liver has a remarkable regenerative potential; and despite slow progress, the patient can become functional if he or she is motivated to remain abstinent. Nutritional assessment with dietary supplementation to ensure adequate caloric intake (25–35 kcal/kg body weight per day) is imperative because many patients with alcohol-induced liver disease are also malnourished. Protein intake should be increased to 1 to 1.5 grams per kilogram of body weight per day unless there is evidence of hepatic encephalopathy, which necessitates a reduction in protein intake. Daily vitamin and mineral supplementation is also indicated: Specifically, patients should receive a multivitamin, additional vitamin B_{12}, folate, thiamine, magnesium, and zinc supplementation if 100% of the daily requirement of these minerals is not contained in the multivitamin. Patients who continue to show clinical deterioration despite abstinence can be considered for liver transplantation, provided they have remained alcohol free for more than 6 months.

Treatment of Complications

Many of the complications of alcohol-induced liver disease are the direct result of the development of portal hypertension and include ascites, hepatic encephalopathy, anemia, hemorrhage, spontaneous bacterial peritonitis, hepatorenal syndrome, hepatopulmonary syndrome, and hepatocellular carcinoma. Table 11.14 presents the treatment of these complications. Portal hypertension is the result of disruption of the hepatocellular circulation

causing an increase in portal venous pressure. As the liver becomes progressively more cirrhotic, collateral venous circulation develops to overcome the increased resistance to blood flow. The collateral circulation that develops between the portal and systemic circulation, specifically the azygos vein, is a much weaker system and results in dilated, tortuous vessels commonly known as varices. Development of varices within the esophagus and submucosa of the gastric fundus predisposes patients to

---

Table 11.14 Complications of Alcohol-Induced Liver Disease

Portal Hypertension and Variceal Hemorrhage

Portal hypertension is the result of disruption of the hepatocellular circulation, causing an increase in portal venous pressure. As the liver becomes progressively more cirrhotic, there is development of collateral venous circulation to overcome the increased resistance to blood flow. The collateral circulation that develops between the portal and systemic circulation, specifically the azygos vein, is a much weaker system and results in dilated, tortuous vessels commonly known as varices. Development of varices within the esophagus and submucosa of the gastric fundus predisposes patients to hemorrhage when the portal pressure gradient is greater than 12 mm Hg.

The most common site of variceal hemorrhage is from within the esophagus and can be life-threatening, with a mortality rate of approximately 50%. Patients with a massive acute hemorrhage require immediate attention to prevent hemodynamic instability and shock. Endoscopic exam can help identify the site of the bleeding and allows for banding or sclerotherapy, the treatments of choice for acute variceal bleeding. Pharmacological intervention includes IV infusion of vasoconstricting agents that assist in decreasing portal pressures.

Octreotide causes reduced splanchnic and hepatic blood flow and is effective in reducing portal pressures. Octreotide (Sandostatin) can be infused at 50–250 mcg/hr. A combination of band ligation or sclerotherapy and octreotide is the most effective treatment for bleeding varices. Patients who have failed both endoscopic and pharmacological intervention require emergent insertion of a Sengstaken-Blakemore tube for balloon tamponade of the bleeding variceal site. The risk for aspiration, esophageal rupture, or rebleed is great, and patients normally require intensive care monitoring.

Some patients may benefit from surgical placement of a portacaval shunt or more recently placement of a transjugular intrahepatic portosystemic shunt (TIPS). Both procedures are performed to decrease portal hypertension but are associated with a high operative mortality rate especially if performed on an urgent basis. Portacaval shunts are effective in reducing esophageal bleeding but carry an associated risk of developing postshunt encephalopathy and hepatic failure of about 50% and eliminate the possibility for future hepatic transplantation.

The risk of rebleeding from esophageal varices is about 70%, so patients should be placed on preventive therapy. The most well-known pharmacological intervention is the initiation of a nonselective beta blocker such as propranolol (Inderal) or nadolol (Corgard) to reduce portal pressure. Dosages of propranolol can range from a starting dose of 40 mg twice daily up to a total daily dose of 200 mg. The goal of treatment is to reduce the resting heart rate by 25% but not below 60 beats/min. The usual contraindications to beta blocker therapy must be considered before initiation of therapy. Also, any patient with known alcohol-induced cirrhosis should have beta blocker therapy as tolerated to decrease the risk of initial variceal bleed.

Prevention of recurrent bleeding can also be accomplished using sclerotherapy or variceal banding. Although both procedures are equally effective, endoscopic banding is associated with lower complications from ulcers or strictures than sclerotherapy. Surgical decompression of the portal system by shunt insertion or TIPS procedure can also be performed to reduce the risk of future variceal bleeding. Complications resulting from these procedures include hepatic encephalopathy, infection, shunt stenosis, and shunt occlusion.

Ascites

Ascites, the excess accumulation of serous fluid within the peritoneal cavity, is associated with unfavorable outcomes. Abdominal paracentesis should be performed and the ascitic fluid analyzed for cell count, culture, and albumin level. The serum albumin level minus the ascitic albumin level equals the serum-ascites albumin gradient (SAAG). An SAAG level greater than 1.1 g/dL is highly suggestive of portal hypertension but offers no information regarding the cause of the ascites. Ascites results from a combination of increased hydrostatic pressure (portal hypertension), decreased oncotic pressure (hypoalbuminemia), peripheral vasodilation probably mediated by nitric oxide released from the splanchnic vasculature, volume expansion resulting from a disturbance in the renin-angiotensin system with subsequent sodium and water retention, and impaired activation of aldosterone by the liver.

Continued

Table 11.14   Complications of Alcohol-Induced Liver Disease—cont'd

Ascites can be clinically observed on physical exam when 1,000 mL or more of fluid has accumulated within the abdominal/peritoneal cavities; smaller amounts are detectable with the use of ultrasound. Shifting dullness to percussion and a positive fluid wave are two findings consistent with the diagnosis of ascites.

Treatment of ascites begins with sodium restriction of 400–800 mg/day. The goal of treatment for the patient with ascites and peripheral edema is a daily weight loss of approximately 1 pound; if fluid is mobilized too quickly, it can further impair renal function by causing a prerenal azotemia. Treatment of ascites includes daily monitoring of weight, serum electrolytes, and renal function. Patients who present with ascites and have hyponatremia (serum levels less than 125 mEq/L) need fluids restricted to 800–1,000 mL/day. Although some patients respond with sodium and water restriction, diuretic therapy is usually required. Spironolactone (Aldactone), a potassium-sparing, aldosterone antagonist, is started at 100 mg/day and increased by 100 mg/week until diuresis is achieved or a maximum dose of 400 mg/day is reached. Adverse effects include painful gynecomastia and hyperkalemia. If effective diuresis has not been achieved, a loop diuretic is added. Furosemide (Lasix) is started at 40 mg/day and is titrated up to 240 mg/day as necessary.

Approximately 10% of patients with cirrhosis are resistant to diuretic therapy despite spironolactone 400 mg/day and furosemide 160 mg/day. These patients have persistent tense ascites and may also develop azotemia with creatinine levels greater than 2.0 mL/dL as a result of the intense diuretic regimen. The treatment for this "intractable" ascites is a large-volume paracentesis, but the practitioner must first determine whether the patient is adhering to the medical regimen, especially sodium restriction. If a large-volume paracentesis is necessary, up to 4–6 L of fluid can be removed per procedure. Intravascular volume expanders can be infused simultaneously to prevent hemodynamic instability secondary to removal of large volumes of ascitic fluid. Large-volume paracentesis is often the treatment of choice because it requires a shorter hospital stay and has fewer complications in comparison to diuretic therapy with regard to electrolyte imbalance and renal insufficiency.

The procedure can be performed daily until ascites is resolved, and then the patient can be maintained on diuretic therapy. The two major complications of paracentesis are spontaneous bacterial peritonitis (SBP) and hepatorenal syndrome.

Spontaneous Bacterial Peritonitis

SBP is a common complication of cirrhosis that can be fatal. Patients may present with abdominal pain, increasing ascites, fever, and progressive encephalopathy. Definitive diagnosis is made by paracentesis. The gold standard for the diagnosis of SBP is a total white cell count of greater than 300 cell/mcL with a polymorphonuclear neutrophil cell count of greater than 250/mcL. The protein concentration is usually less than 1 g/dL. Gram-negative bacilli are the causative pathogen in 70% of SBP, with *Escherichia coli* being isolated in 50% of the cases. Gram-positive organisms are isolated in approximately 25% of the cases, and infection with anaerobic organisms is rare due to the high oxygen content of the ascitic fluid. Because the mortality rate for untreated SBP is 50%, initiation of treatment is suggested before culture results are obtained. Cefotaxime (Claforan) is a broad-spectrum, third generation cephalosporin and is considered the treatment of choice for SBP. The usual dose is 2 g IV every 8 hours for 5 days. Post-SBP prophylaxis can be accomplished with norfloxacin 400 mg/day.

Hepatorenal Syndrome

Hepatorenal syndrome is a terminal complication frequently associated with advanced liver damage and is almost always found in patients with advanced ascites. The syndrome is characterized by oliguria, hyponatremia, azotemia, low urine sodium (less than 10 mEq/L), and hypotension. The hallmark to diagnosis is a disproportionate rise in creatinine with respect to the blood urea nitrogen. Histologically, the kidneys are normal, and diagnosis is often one of exclusion. Individuals with decompensated cirrhosis and ascites can precipitate hepatorenal syndrome after large-volume paracentesis, aggressive diuresis aimed at decreasing ascites, or sepsis. Patients are often misdiagnosed with prerenal failure, and the only way to differentiate between the two is through insertion of a central venous catheter and assessment of venous pressures. Treatment includes restoring the intravascular volume and avoiding any procedures that will dramatically disturb the patient's volume status, such as large-volume paracentesis and aggressive diuresis. The definitive treatment of patients with hepatorenal syndrome is liver transplantation.

Hepatic Encephalopathy

Hepatic encephalopathy, also known as portosystemic encephalopathy, is a complex process involving a change in mental status resulting from the failure of the liver to detoxify elements of gut origin and shunting of this blood from the portal to the systemic circulation and then to the brain. Nitrogenous agents such as ammonia are believed to enter into the CNS by way of shunted blood resulting in disturbances in neurological function. Although ammonia is thought to be the sole toxin responsible for hepatic encephalopathy, the serum levels do not correlate with the degree or presence of encephalopathy.

Table 11.14 Complications of Alcohol-Induced Liver Disease—cont'd

The diagnosis of hepatic encephalopathy is made clinically and often follows an event such as increased dietary protein, GI bleeding, constipation, infection, deterioration in hepatic function, hypokalemia, azotemia, alkalosis, and hypovolemia. Physical exam findings include an altered mental status such as personality (mood) changes, decreased reaction time, and intellectual deterioration, as well as neuromuscular dysfunctions such as asterixis or metabolic flap, absence of fixed sensory or motor deficits, and hyperreflexia. Other findings include fetor hepaticus (garlic odor of the breath caused by exhalation of sulfur-containing mercaptans), hyperthermia, and hyperventilation. Obtaining a fasting arterial blood ammonia level or a spinal fluid glutamine level can be helpful in confirming the diagnosis of hepatic encephalopathy although they are not necessary.

Treatment of hepatic encephalopathy begins with identification and treatment of factors that precipitate encephalopathy in patients with liver disease.

- *GI Bleeding.* Increases production of ammonia and other nitrogenous toxins.
- *Increasing Dietary Intake of Protein.* Provides building substrate for formation of nitrogenous toxins in the intestine.
- *Diuretic-Induced Problems.* Overdiuresis causes increased circulation of urea and ammonia production. Hypovolemia resulting in hypokalemia and alkalosis enhances the transfer of ammonia across the blood–brain barrier.
- *Constipation.* Decreases transit time within the intestine, which enhances contact time with ammonia-forming bacteria in the colon.
- *Drugs Causing CNS Depression.* Impaired liver function causes alteration in degradation and may accumulate, causing further depressant effects.
- *Infection.* Increases catabolism and production of nitrogenous toxins.

For instance, GI bleeding and diets high in protein provide the basic elements for formation of ammonia and other nitrogenous compounds from the action of bacteria in the gut, which can induce or aggravate the symptoms of encephalopathy. Colonic bacteria responsible for the formation of ammonia and other nitrogenous compounds can be reduced by administering oral neomycin (Mycifradin Sulfate Oral, Neo-Tabs Oral) 0.5–1.0 g every 4–6 hours for 5–7 days. Lactulose (Cephulac, Heptalac) is a nonabsorbable synthetic disaccharide, that, when digested by intestinal bacteria, is fermented and causes acidification of the colon contents. The lower stool pH binds the ammonia in the colon, rendering it nonabsorbable. Lactulose also changes the bowel flora so that there are fewer ammonia-forming bacteria. The initial dose of lactulose is 30 mL three to four times daily and is titrated until the patient has two or three softly formed stools daily.

Iron-Deficiency Anemia

Iron-deficiency anemia is a common finding in alcoholics. It can be treated with ferrous sulfate taken three times daily after meals. To avoid the constipating effect of iron, a stool softener can be given as well. If there is evidence of a macrocytic anemia, the patient may benefit from 1 mg of folic acid daily.

Hepatopulmonary Syndrome

Hepatopulmonary syndrome is a recently recognized pulmonary complication of cirrhosis and portal hypertension, which manifests through abnormal arterial oxygenation. The diagnosis is made when there is intrapulmonary dilation in the absence of other morphological pathology. The results are reversible with liver transplantation.

hemorrhage when the portal pressure gradient is greater than 12 mm Hg.

Irreversible, Chronic Liver Disease

Liver transplantation is the treatment of choice for irreversible chronic liver disease. Cirrhosis, hepatitis C, primary biliary cirrhosis, primary sclerosing cholangitis, alcoholic liver disease, autoimmune hepatitis, and genetic disorders of the liver are diseases for which transplantation has been successful. Five-year survival rates are documented as high as 80% with advancements in surgical techniques and immunosuppressive agents such as cyclosporine and tacrolimus (FK506). Contraindications to transplantation include malignant hepatobiliary processes, sepsis, and advanced cardiopulmonary disease.

In cases of hepatitis B and C, the virus can infect the new liver.

Primary Biliary Cirrhosis

Treatment of PBC is symptomatic. Pruritus is often the most aggravating manifestation of PBC. Cholestyramine (Questran) or colestipol relieves itching in patients with cholestasis by lowering serum bile acids and increasing the intestinal secretion of bile by preventing its resorption. The usual dose is 4 g or 5 g, respectively, in water or juice three times daily until the pruritus has been controlled, and then the dosage is decreased to that which maintains control of the symptom. Rifampin (Rifadin) 150 to 300 mg twice daily has been beneficial in relieving pruritus in some cases; ondansetron, a

$5-HT_3$ serotonin receptor antagonist, shows promise as well.

Fat-soluble vitamin deficiency occurs with the onset of steatorrhea and can be made worse with the administration of cholestyramine (a bile acid sequestrant). Vitamins A, D, E, and K can be replaced orally. Laboratory studies will reveal vitamin K deficiency as a prolonged PT. The deficiency can be treated with 5 to 10 mg daily of vitamin K by mouth; subsequent monitoring of the PT will indicate whether therapy is adequate. Overdosage of vitamin A can cause hepatotoxicity, so the dosage must be individualized based on serum levels and response to treatment.

Patients with PBC often have associated osteoporosis, which has no known treatment. If patients have been diagnosed with PBC and have osteomalacia, calcium supplementation with 500 mg three times daily and vitamin D 400 to 800 IU/day is indicated. Patients should be instructed to eat foods rich in calcium and phosphorus and to increase their exposure to sunlight.

Several immunosuppressive agents including corticosteroids, methotrexate, and azathioprine and the antifibrinogenic colchicine have been effective in reducing elevated serum alkaline phosphatase and bilirubin levels. Ursodeoxycholic acid (ursodiol), a choleretic, acts by stimulating excretion of bile by the liver, is much less toxic than the other drugs mentioned above, and has been effective in reducing symptoms and improving long-term survival.

Surgical reconstruction of the biliary tract, choledochoduodenostomy, and choledochojejunostomy are palliative treatments that alleviate the symptoms of PBC. If there is notable stricturing within the biliary tree, patients often do well with stenting. Liver transplantation for advanced PBC is the treatment of choice.

Hemochromatosis and Wilson's Disease

Two important but treatable inherited metabolic causes of cirrhosis are hemochromatosis and Wilson's disease. Early diagnosis and treatment are key to the management of hereditary hemochromatosis (HHC) and begin with liver biopsy for definitive diagnosis. If treatment is initiated in the precirrhotic phase, the disease can be controlled with weekly phlebotomies of 1 unit (500 mL) of blood, which contains approximately 250 mg of iron. This process is continued until there is depletion of the iron stores (which can be 2 years or more). Every 2 to 3 months, iron metabolism studies monitor the patient's progress. Once the iron stores are depleted—when serum ferritin levels fall below 50 ng/mL and transferrin saturation is less than 50%— patients can be maintained with periodic phlebotomies. Patients who are exhibiting cardiac symptoms may require the use of iron-chelating agents such as deferoxamine. Administered intramuscularly, it increases the urinary excretion of iron up to 5 to 18 g annually. Phlebotomy decreases the cardiac conduction defects and lowers insulin requirements.

Patients should be instructed to consume a low-iron diet that eliminates foods such as red meat, and they should avoid alcohol, vitamin C, raw shellfish, and any supplement containing iron. Patients may require specific treatment of diabetes mellitus, heart disease, arthropathy, hypopituitarism, and portal hypertension, all complications due to HHC. Patients whose disease has progressed to cirrhosis must be monitored for hepatocellular carcinoma either by liver US or measurement of alpha-fetoprotein levels. Because the disease is inherited, screening of all first-degree relatives is necessary.

Wilson's disease is also an inherited disease the early diagnosis and treatment of which can prevent the development of neurological or hepatic damage. Treatment includes both dietary and medicinal components. Limiting dietary intake of copper (legumes, animal organs, and shellfish) should become a lifelong habit. The administration of oral penicillamine (Depen) 0.75 to 2 g/day in divided doses induces the urinary excretion of chelated copper. If GI upset or hypersensitivity prohibits the use of penicillamine, trientine (Syprine) 250 to 500 mg three times daily can be substituted. Oral administration of zinc 50 mg three times daily as maintenance therapy also promotes excretion of copper in the feces. Patients who are receiving penicillamine, an antimetabolite of vitamin B_6, should receive pyridoxine (supplemental vitamin B_6) 50 mg/week. Liver transplant is the treatment of choice for patients with cirrhosis or fulminant hepatitis. Siblings and family members should be screened for the disease.

Vascular or Congestive Liver Disorders

Management of patients who present with vascular or congestive liver disorders, such as those with BCS and other hepatic occlusive diseases, is essential. Because of the many causes of BCS, initial treatment must begin with finding and treating the cause of the hepatic congestion. Hepatic vein thrombus is difficult to manage and requires a multidisciplinary approach including a hematologist, surgeon, hepatologist, and gastroenterologist. Ascites is initially managed with sodium restriction and diuretics; however, over time this is usually ineffective, and most patients will require large-volume paracentesis or shunting for symptomatic relief.

If diagnosis of acute thrombus is made early, thrombolytic therapy can be instituted and long-term anticoagulation with warfarin (Coumadin) can help prevent further thrombus formation. Surgical decompression shunting for refractive ascites can delay development of hepatic failure or cirrhosis but often results in graft thrombus. Patients with associated myeloproliferative diseases and hypercoagulopathies may benefit from low-dose aspirin therapy and chemotherapy as directed by a hematologist.

Follow-up and Referral

Any patient with advanced liver disease should be referred to a hepatologist or gastroenterologist trained to treat the disease and its subsequent complications. All patients require referral for liver biopsy to establish a definitive diagnosis. It is the responsibility of the clinician to recognize the onset of the disease process and obtain all the necessary testing in order to provide the most complete information to the accepting consultant. Patients with end-stage liver disease should be referred to a liver transplant facility. Patient follow-up can be shared between the primary-care practitioner and the consulting physician. Patients with chronic or advanced liver disease will require indefinite monitoring of their liver function tests, as well as their fluid and electrolyte status. Maintaining good nutrition is an important component of treatment of any disease process. Patients with advanced liver disease may benefit from consultation with a registered dietitian, who can review dietary restrictions and help patients understand how to achieve a balanced diet.

Patient Education

Patients with hepatic failure should be taught to check their weight daily as a way to monitor increasing fluid retention and ascites, which may indicate a developing complication. Patients with cirrhosis have a life-threatening terminal disease; therefore, attention must be given to promoting psychological well-being. Patients should be provided with education regarding medications to avoid to prevent further hepatotoxicity, such as acetaminophen (Tylenol), vitamin A, cocaine, tetracycline (Sumycin), phenytoin (Dilantin), and ethyl alcohol. Patients with liver failure should always ask their health-care provider about the potential liver toxicity of each of their medications. Patients with hepatic encephalopathy should avoid CNS depressants, which might intensify their lethargy or fatigue. These patients may also require education about the need for self-administering enemas if they become constipated, in order to decrease the time for bowel absorption of nitrogen-based compounds. All patients with ascites must be informed of the signs and symptoms of infection, which may indicate developing spontaneous bacterial peritonitis.

■ ABDOMINAL HERNIAS

An abdominal hernia is the protrusion of a peritoneally lined sac through some defect or weakened area in the abdominal wall. A history of heavy physical labor or heavy lifting can elicit a hernia. There are several different types of hernias, which are usually classified by the anatomical location of the protrusion.

Epidemiology and Causes

It is estimated that up to 10% of the population has some form of hernia. *Groin hernias* are the most common type and are classified as *indirect inguinal hernias,* which are responsible for 50% of hernias treated; *direct inguinal hernias,* which represent 25% of hernias seen; and *femoral hernias,* which represent 10% of hernias.

Hernias occurring through the anterior abdominal wall are called *ventral hernias;* these account for only 15% of all hernias. Ventral hernias are further broken down into epigastric hernias (5%), incisional hernias (5%), and umbilical hernias (3%).

Groin hernias are by far the most common type of hernia and occur in both men and women. Indirect inguinal hernias are the most common and occur in both genders, although they are frequently seen in young men. Direct inguinal hernias are more common in men older than age 40 and are caused by a congenital abnormality. Femoral hernias occur more often in women than in men and are rare in children.

The recurrence rate of hernias in general is about 10%, with direct and indirect hernias having a recurrence rate that is approximately equal. The subsequent recurrence rate of recurrent hernias is much higher, at 35%.

Ventral hernias include all other hernias of the anterior abdominal wall. Epigastric hernias are much more common in men than in women and are multiple in 25% of the cases. The peak age of incidence is age 20 to 50. Umbilical hernias are considered a normal occurrence in newborn infants, with about 20% of infants being affected. These hernias are more common in males of all ages and in African Americans of either gender. The presence of an umbilical hernia is considered normal until the child reaches age 2. Incisional hernias are considered the only iatrogenic type of herniation. Approximately 2% to 11% of all patients undergoing abdominal surgery develop incisional hernias. Women are affected twice as often as men.

Hernias occur because there is sufficient pressure to force tissue out through a defect in the abdominal wall, as well as a potential space for that protrusion. The etiology of hernias is multifactorial, with biological, congenital, and environmental influences contributing to their development.

Pathophysiology

In general, for any type of groin hernia to occur, two of the body's protective mechanisms must be overcome. The first is called the *shutter mechanism,* whereby the internal oblique muscle and the transversus abdominis muscles contract to overlap, strengthening the posterior wall of the inguinal canal. Second, a *closure* or *sphincter-type mechanism* causes contraction of the musculature, displacing the transversalis fascia, which in effect decreases the diameter of the deep inguinal ring.

Indirect Inguinal Hernias

Indirect inguinal hernias result when tissue herniates through the internal inguinal ring, which in men extends the length of the spermatic cord. With continued pressure, the sac can actually reach the scrotum, where it is then palpable just proximal to Hesselbach's triangle. The pathophysiology of indirect inguinal hernias in most cases begins with the herniation of tissue through a still-patent vaginal process that remains after the descent of the testes. In women, the vaginal process exists within the canal of Nuck. Indirect inguinal herniation is caused by a combination of this congenital defect and a disruption in the functioning of the sphincter mechanism as a result of a variety of environmental conditions, including increased abdominal pressure and trauma to the area.

Direct Inguinal Hernias

Direct inguinal hernias occur when the transversus abdominis and internal oblique muscles are attached, forming a high arch on the inferior border that results in a faulty shutter mechanism. Any environmental factors that increase abdominal pressure enhance the chance of herniation. As with indirect inguinal hernias, the presence of this congenital defect does not explain why herniation is more common later in life.

Femoral Hernias

Femoral herniation occurs at the fossa ovalis where the femoral artery exits from the abdomen. It is presumed to be caused because women have a larger femoral canal and smaller iliopsoas muscles. Other factors that contribute to femoral herniation are femoral engorgement during pregnancy and the size of the female pelvis.

Epigastric Hernias

Epigastric hernias occur along the midline between the xiphoid process and the umbilicus. The fibers along the linea alba are brought together in a patchwork-type closure; the defect exists within this decussation. As these fibers weaken, the contents can herniate through the abdomen. Epigastric hernias are three times more likely to occur in men than in women. Peritoneal fat, bowel, and omentum are the most common abdominal contents to protrude through the wall.

Umbilical Hernias

Umbilical hernias that develop in adulthood occur through a weakening in the abdominal wall around the umbilical ring. The herniation of abdominal contents through this defect is also dependent on environmental factors that increase intra-abdominal pressure. Of particular importance when diagnosing an umbilical hernia is to look for underlying ascites secondary to liver disease.

Incisional Hernias

Incisional hernias can occur anywhere along a surgical incision into the abdomen. They are classified into those that cannot be controlled by surgical technique and those that can be controlled by surgical technique. Controllable factors include the type of incision chosen and choice of suture and surgical techniques. Factors that are considered uncontrollable include the prior medical history of the patient, age, steroid use, nutritional status, obesity, and complications of the surgery, especially wound sepsis.

Clinical Presentation
Subjective

In any patient presenting with an abdominal hernia, the provider must determine whether there is an abnormal increase in intra-abdominal pressure that has contributed to the herniation. A thorough history and physical exam, with special attention to the genitourinary, respiratory, and gastrointestinal systems, will provide clues. All male patients who present with an abdominal hernia, regardless of age, require a prostate exam to determine if there is any obstructive process inhibiting urinary output, which in effect increases intra-abdominal pressure. Patients should be evaluated for ascites, which also increases intra-abdominal pressure.

Patients who have respiratory difficulty, such as obstructive pulmonary disease processes, have an increased risk of hernia because of the increased abdominal pressure associated with coughing and the downward expansion of the diaphragm found with hyperinflated lungs.

Objective

The presentation of inguinal hernias is not always obvious and is quite often an incidental finding on routine exam. Patients may present with complaints of pain while straining or lifting heavy objects or a swelling in the groin area. In general, the physical exam for all groin hernias begins with visual inspection of both groins and the genitalia. With the male patient standing, the spermatic cord is located on both sides and is palpated for any swelling into the scrotum. Once the inguinal canal has been palpated, three additional areas must be examined. After invaginating the scrotal sac, the examining finger follows the spermatic cord up to the external inguinal ring and the fascia of the external oblique muscle. The posterior wall is inspected for weakness or bulging, and the inguinal ring is also palpated for structural soundness. Once these areas have been examined, the provider then withdraws the finger slightly and the patient is asked to cough, which increases the intra-abdominal pressure. If the provider feels the presence of a tissue-like sac tapping against the finger, hernia is present. Other findings indicative of herniation are feeling a rush of fluid (peritoneal) under the examining finger or a patient's report of pain. In a female patient, the femoral areas are palpated while the patient increases intra-abdominal pressure by performing the Valsalva maneuver. Any bulging in the area is considered a positive finding.

Once a groin hernia has been diagnosed, the practitioner must determine whether the hernia is incarcerated or strangulated, both of which require immediate surgical attention, or whether a more chronic situation is present, which can be cared for electively. Most often this can be determined by patient history, as well as the physical ability to reduce the hernia on examination. A strangulated hernia is a nonreducible herniation in which the blood supply to the herniated tissue is compromised. An incarcerated hernia is a hernia that has caused a bowel obstruction as a result of the protrusion.

An indirect inguinal hernia presents as a soft swelling within the internal ring, when either provoked or unprovoked, and often descends into the scrotum. A direct inguinal hernia presents as a bulge in the area of Hesselbach's triangle (Fig. 11.1). Direct inguinal hernias are usually painless and easily reducible. The hernia bulges anteriorly, pushing against the side of the examining finger. Femoral hernias are more common on the right side and may be accompanied by severe pain. There is a palpable bulge through the femoral ring, and the inguinal canal is empty. Normally, it is the intestine that has herniated through the abdominal wall.

Epigastric hernias are normally asymptomatic and present as a small bump or bulge along the midline above the umbilicus. There may be variation in size with increasing intra-abdominal pressure. Peritoneal fat, omentum, and bowel are usually the tissues that herniate through the abdomen. The smaller hernias tend to be more painful because they involve the herniation of the preperitoneal fat, which is irritating. Larger hernias must be examined for incarceration and obstruction.

Incisional hernias manifest along the incision line of a previous abdominal operation and can be painful. Patients with incisional hernias may also have signs and symptoms of bowel obstruction, which are discussed under Bowel Obstruction later in this chapter.

Diagnostic Reasoning
Diagnostic Tests
Hernias are diagnosed almost exclusively by physical exam findings, as described in the preceding text. On occasion, a radiographic study is necessary to determine if an obstructive process is taking place. Other studies, such as pulmonary function testing or evaluation of a mass or lesion within the abdomen, may be indicated to assess the cause and/or extent of increased intra-abdominal pressure.

Differential Diagnosis
The differential diagnosis list for hernia is limited. It includes hydrocele, psoas abscess, femoral adenopathy or inguinal adenopathy, and ectopic testis.

Management
When a hernia is detected, the patient should be referred to a surgeon. Despite the evolution of hernia repair over the last century, the underlying principles remain the same: reinforce the two natural defense mechanisms discussed previously; decrease the size of the inguinal ring; and strengthen the posterior wall of the canal. Repair of femoral hernias is accomplished by reducing the size of the canal, whereas repair of indirect hernia is accomplished by dissecting the hernial sac and reduction of the repaired tissue. Frequently, there is not sufficient tissue to reconstruct and strengthen the posterior wall of the canal and synthetic mesh materials are used. Laparoscopic surgery has decreased the recovery time and allowed for a single intervention for bilateral hernia repair. All ventral hernias should be repaired to decrease the possibility for incarceration.

Postoperatively, the patient may experience incisional pain, which is relieved by oral analgesics. Pain that persists for more than a few days suggests impending wound infection. Normally, there is slight postoperative swelling, ecchymosis, and erythema of the skin, up to the scrotal area in male patients. Hernia repair with significant scrotal involvement may result in increased scrotal edema, which can be relieved with ice packs, elevation, and wearing a scrotal support. In female patients, swelling is usually limited to the surgical site but may extend to the labia and vulva.

Follow-up and Referral
All patients with abdominal hernias require surgical consultation, whether emergently or electively, and appropriate referral should be made. The patient is usually seen in the surgeon's office 3 to 7 days after surgery.

Patient Education
After typical groin surgery, the patient is allowed to return to normal activities, including work, after about

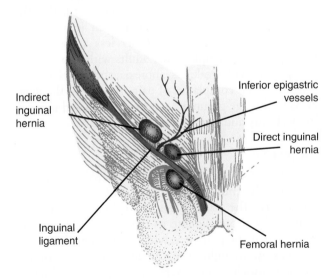

Figure 11.1 Locations of indirect and direct inguinal and femoral hernias. Anterior view of the groin, showing locations of indirect inguinal hernia, direct inguinal hernia, and femoral hernia, based on anatomical landmarks. *(Source: Kozol, AK, et al. When to call the surgeon: Decision making for primary care providers. FA Davis, Philadelphia, p 170. Reprinted with permission.)*

1 week but is instructed to avoid heavy lifting or contact sports for at least 4 to 6 weeks. Patients who have undergone laparoscopic repair of groin hernias are allowed to resume regular activities, including heavy lifting, as soon as 2 days postprocedure. Patients who have had a ventral hernia repair should follow routine postoperative instruction as directed by the surgeon.

■ APPENDICITIS

The appendix is a fingerlike projection located at the apex of the cecum just below the ileocecal valve. It has no known function in humans; however, it is thought to have some immunological function, based on the amount of lymphoid tissue it contains. The appendix fills with food, just as the cecum does, but because the lumen of the appendix is smaller, it has a tendency to become obstructed. Appendicitis is the inflammation of the vermiform appendix caused by an obstruction and/or infection. It is the most common cause of acute right lower quadrant (RLQ) abdominal pain requiring surgical intervention. Acute appendicitis results in more than 250,000 appendectomies annually in the United States and represents 1 million hospital day stays.

Epidemiology and Causes

Appendicitis can occur at any age; however, it is most common between ages 10 and 30 years. It is rare in infants and in older adults and is often associated with higher morbidity within these age-groups because of delayed diagnosis and intervention. During the peak incidence years, men are twice as likely to be diagnosed with appendicitis as are women, but the occurrence in both genders tends to equalize over the life span. It is estimated that appendicitis will affect 10 in 100,000 people in the United States, with an incidence of 1.1 cases per 1,000 people per year.

Appendicitis is more common in Western countries, where people have diets that are low in fiber, high in fat, and high in refined sugars and other carbohydrates. Obstruction of the appendix by a variety of pathological processes is the cause of the majority of appendicitis. Other contributing factors include intra-abdominal tumors and positive family history. Recent roundworm infestation or viral infection of the gastrointestinal (GI) tract have also been implicated.

Pathophysiology

Appendicitis typically begins with dilation of the appendix, followed by obstruction and subsequent bacterial infection. When the lumen of the appendix is obstructed by hardened feces (fecalith), inflammatory processes (including parasites, viruses, or bacteria), strictures, neoplasms, or foreign bodies (including vegetable or fruit seeds or barium), the mucosa of the appendix continues to secrete fluid, which further distends the lumen, impairing the venous blood flow and leading to tissue necrosis. Left untreated, this increased distention impedes arterial

inflow. Bacteria continue to proliferate and, in the absence of treatment, perforation of the appendix occurs. The incidence of perforation in patients with appendicitis is between 17% and 40%, with rates as high as 60% to 70% in older adults because of the nonspecific presenting symptoms. Gynecological disorders and gastroenteritis are the most common causes of misdiagnosis.

Clinical Presentation
Subjective

The diagnosis of acute appendicitis is made clinically and is based primarily on the patient's history and physical exam. The historical presentations of signs and symptoms are important keys to prompt diagnosis and treatment; therefore, it is important to obtain a thorough and accurate account of the events. The classic presentation of appendicitis begins with the acute onset of mild to severe colicky, epigastric, or periumbilical pain. The pain is often vague at first, but within 24 hours usually it shifts and localizes over the RLQ and is exacerbated by walking or coughing. In male patients, the pain may radiate into the testicles; pain (rigidity) also may be associated with abdominal muscle spasm in male or female patients. Most patients complain of nausea and anorexia after the onset of pain, which may or may not be associated with vomiting. If vomiting is present, the patient usually reports that abdominal pain was present before vomiting began. The sensation of constipation is typical, although diarrhea is present in some patients.

A mildly elevated temperature of 99° to 100°F is common. If the patient with RLQ pain presents with shaking chills (rigors), perforation of the appendix should be suspected. An important point to remember is that the very young and older adults may have an atypical presentation, which can mimic other less acute disease processes. For example, older adults with appendicitis may present with weakness, anorexia, abdominal distention, and mild complaints of pain. A delay in the diagnosis in this age-group has led to an associated increase in morbidity and mortality.

Objective

On physical examination, the patient may or may not look sick depending on the degree of pain and other symptoms. The patient may have hypertension and tachycardia proportionate to the degree of fever and pain. When the patient is lying recumbent, he or she may flex up the right knee to relieve the tension on the iliopsoas muscle, which overlies the appendix. Palpation of the abdomen early in the process may reveal diffuse tenderness over the umbilicus and midepigastric areas. As the process progresses, the tenderness localizes over the RLQ and may be accompanied by guarding. *Guarding* is defined as "the voluntary contraction of the abdominal muscles in anticipation of examination," as opposed to *rigidity,* which is caused by "the involuntary reflexive spasm of the muscles of the abdominal wall." Rebound tenderness is tested by placing the palmar aspect of the hand on the abdomen and pressing hard enough to depress the peritoneum. This may cause the patient pain, but the clinician should keep the abdomen depressed with constant pressure until the patient becomes accustomed to the pressure, and the pain decreases. Then, without warning, the clinician should remove the hand suddenly, preferably when the patient's attention is directed elsewhere. If positive for rebound tenderness, the patient will grimace in pain, which is a more reliable sign than a subjective complaint of pain. Asking the patient to cough helps to localize exactly the site from which the pain is coming. Advanced Assessment 11.1 outlines exam maneuvers that aid in the diagnosis of appendicitis.

A rectal exam can be performed, but it is open to greater subjective interpretation. Patients with appendicitis will normally perceive greater tenderness and fullness on the right than on the left during the rectal exam. The provider must keep in mind that both the bowel and the appendix are mobile organs; they can shift posteriorly or suprapubically, causing altered exam findings. Bowel sounds are a nonspecific finding—they may be present, absent, or decreased in patients with appendicitis.

Other physical exam findings can include alterations in vital signs consistent with increased pain, such as tachycardia or elevated blood pressure. Patients may be reluctant to take a deep breath for fear they will cause themselves pain.

If there is perforation of the appendix, there may be a sudden cessation of the pain, which is considered an emergency. Findings consistent with peritonitis include diffuse abdominal tenderness with rigidity. The patient may exhibit signs of septic shock, with marked leukocytosis, fever, and hemodynamic instability.

Diagnostic Reasoning

Diagnostic Tests

Laboratory findings are not diagnostic and are nonspecific, so they must be used in combination with data from the history and physical exam. The complete blood count usually reveals a mild to moderate leukocytosis (white blood cell count 10–20,000 mcg/L) with a left shift. Urinalysis shows microscopic hematuria or pyuria in 25% of patients. Women should have a urine human chorionic gonadotrophin test completed to rule out (ectopic) pregnancy. The lack of laboratory findings should not preclude the diagnosis of appendicitis.

No radiologic exam is of diagnostic importance early in appendicitis, but x-ray studies become more important as appendicitis progresses. A chest x-ray film rules out pneumonia as a source of abdominal pain and is necessary as part of the preoperative procedure in most hospitals. Plain x-ray films of the abdomen may show evidence of a fecalith, a gas-filled appendix, small bowel ileus, a deviation in the bowel gas pattern, or a loss of the right iliopsoas shadow. Any of these findings is suggestive of appendicitis when combined with a suspect history and physical exam.

A computed tomography scan of the abdomen is helpful in ruling out other diagnostic possibilities, as well as determining if there has been perforation of the appendix or development of a periappendiceal abscess. An abdominal ultrasound helps to visualize the inflamed appendix and is also useful in ruling out other potential diagnoses. Diagnostic laparoscopy may be considered in female patients to rule out ectopic pregnancy, tuboovarian processes, or pelvic inflammatory disease (PID).

Differential Diagnosis

The differential diagnoses of appendicitis include a host of problems, which include, but are not limited to,

Advanced Assessment 11.1	Physical Exam Maneuvers for Diagnosing Appendicitis	
Maneuver	Examination	Comments
Rovsing's sign	Deep palpation over the LLQ with sudden, unexpected release of pressure.	This causes tenderness over the RLQ and is considered a positive finding.
Psoas sign	The patient is instructed to try to lift the right leg against gentle pressure applied by the examiner or by placing the patient in the left lateral decubitus position and extending the patient's right leg at the hip.	An increase in pain is considered positive and is an indication of the inflamed appendix irritating the psoas muscle.
Obturator sign	With the right hip and knee flexed, the examiner slowly rotates the right leg internally, which stretches the obturator muscle.	Pain over the RLQ is considered a positive sign and indicates irritation of the muscle by the inflamed appendix.
McBurney's sign	Pressure is applied to McBurney's point, which is located halfway between the umbilicus and the anterior spine of the ilium.	Pain when pressure is applied to this area is considered a positive response.

urinary tract infection, ectopic pregnancy, ovarian cyst, pneumonia, gastroenteritis, Crohn's disease, diverticulitis, mesenteric adenitis, pancreatitis, PID, and cholelithiasis. If the diagnosis of appendicitis remains questionable after the history and physical exam have been completed and initial lab work has been obtained, radiographic studies are helpful in ruling out many of the processes found within the differential diagnoses. For women of childbearing age, the clinician should always obtain a pregnancy test before ordering any radiographic studies. In some cases, laparotomy or laparoscopy may be required to assist in definitive diagnosis.

Careful attention must be given to the sexual and menstrual history of all female patients because of the myriad of potential gynecological problems that present with the same signs and symptoms as appendicitis. A pelvic exam and a diagnostic laparotomy are often necessary for differential diagnosis.

Many GI disorders have symptoms that mimic those of appendicitis, and watchful waiting may be indicated in some cases. If appendicitis is at all a suspicion, however, the prudent practitioner will follow these patients closely until a diagnosis has been reached.

Management

The treatment of appendicitis is surgical; therefore, once a definitive diagnosis is made, prompt referral to a surgeon should follow. From 9% to 15% of appendectomies between 1998 and 2007 were considered unnecessary, or negative. This number is considered acceptable because of the morbidity and mortality associated with perforation. The incidence of appendiceal perforation ranges from 17% to 40% in patients with appendicitis; it is as high as 60% to 70% in older adults. With effective and timely treatment, the mortality rate is less than 1%; however, in the older adult population, mortality remains at 5% to 15%.

Preoperative management includes correction of fluid and electrolyte imbalances; bedrest; nothing by mouth, with placement of a nasogastric tube if indicated; and IV antibiotics. Narcotics should be avoided if possible because they mask any developing symptoms that might indicate a complication such as perforation. Laxatives are contraindicated in patients with appendicitis because they may cause the appendix to rupture. Stool softeners may be given if the patient is complaining about constipation and diarrhea is not present.

Third generation cephalosporins are the antibiotics of choice. If there has been perforation and peritonitis is suspected, antibiotic coverage for both gram-negative aerobic and anaerobic organisms is recommended. Some of the choices include ampicillin, gentamicin, clindamycin, metronidazole (Flagyl), ampicillin-sulbactam (Unasyn), and ticarcillin/clavulanate (Timentin).

Patients are normally discharged the same day as surgery unless there are complications. Early ambulation is encouraged, with progression to full activity as soon as possible. Diet is advanced when bowel sounds return. The patient is given standard postoperative guidelines for individuals who have had abdominal surgery.

Follow-up and Referral

The patient is normally followed by the surgeon, who will see the patient 5 to 7 days postoperatively to remove the sutures. If there was perforation of the appendix and the patient must remain hospitalized, the surgeon will follow the patient until discharge.

Patient Education

The patient will be given standard postoperative instructions from the surgeon, which should include advice to return to the hospital if anorexia, nausea, vomiting, abdominal pain, fever, or chills develop. Patients should understand that they are not to do any heavy lifting for at least 2 weeks.

■ INFLAMMATORY BOWEL DISEASE

Inflammatory bowel disease (IBD) is the term used to describe a chronic immunological disease that manifests in intestinal inflammation. The two most common IBDs are ulcerative colitis (UC) and Crohn's disease (CD). The disease is characterized by exacerbations and remissions that are experienced throughout an individual's lifetime and therefore result in significant disruption in the quality of life. The Patient's Voice 11.1 describes the impact of Crohn's disease on a 39-year-old woman with a 20-year history of the disease.

The Patient's Voice 11.1
Crohn's Disease
As a 39-year-old woman with a 20-year history of severe Crohn's disease (CD), I remain undecided as to which has been most difficult to deal with: the symptoms of the disease—uncontrolled diarrhea, bowel incontinence, malnutrition, pain, bloating, and flatulence, to name a few; the results of the symptoms—fatigue, malaise, anemia, anorexia, anxiety, embarrassment, guilt, fear, and shame; or the constant discipline necessary to incorporate lifestyle changes instrumental to the adaptation and management of this debilitating disorder—diet, stress elimination, exercise, rest, vitamin supplementation, and prescription compliance. Experience with CD has taught me that health and wellness is a personal choice and that whatever intestinal ailments or conditions one struggles with, incorporating the dietary changes necessary to promote wellness through nutrition, particularly raw, fresh fruit and vegetable juices, should be part of a comprehensive approach to achieving optimal health.

UC and CD are both IBDs that share similar characteristics and causes but are considered two separate diseases. UC involves only the mucosal surface of the colon, which ultimately results in friability, erosions, and bleeding. It occurs most often in the rectosigmoid area but can involve the entire colon. CD is also known as regional enteritis because of the characteristic segmental presentation of the diseased bowel, which is clearly separated by areas of normal mucosa, often referred to as "skipped lesions." CD can involve all or any layer of the bowel wall and any portion of the gastrointestinal (GI) tract from the mouth to the anus. Disease of the terminal ileus is present in about 80% of patients with CD, and in 20% of the cases only the colon is involved.

The peak age of onset is 15 to 30 years old, although it may occur at any age. UC is more common in males, and CD is more common in females. It is estimated that as many as 1.4 million people in the United States suffer from these diseases.

Epidemiology and Causes

The incidence and prevalence of these diseases vary widely, which supports a multifactorial theory in the development of the disease. Research supports a genetic predisposition for IBD, even though less than 15% of cases are familial. A gene on chromosome 16 that encodes the protein nucleotide-binding oligomerization domain 2 (NOD2) has variants that are found in about 62% of patients with CD. Genes associated with IBD have also been found on chromosomes 10 and 7 that encode for proteins that mediate epithelial cell–cell interactions and the transport of molecules into and out of cells. Another factor is the ability of bacteria in the gut to cause inflammation. Researchers believe that there is an exaggerated cell-mediated immune response to the bacteria. The intestinal epithelium plays an important role in the immune response, interacting with microbes and antigens and communicating with immune cells triggering the production and secretion of cytokines and chemokines.

The incidence of IBD is about equal in men and women. The highest prevalence for the disease is in Scandinavian and Northern European countries. The overall incidence and prevalence for both of these diseases is about equal worldwide, with incidence rates between 3 and 10 per 100,000 and a prevalence rate between 30 and 50 per 100,000. The age at onset is frequently in early adulthood but can be anywhere from age 10 to 40. Table 11.15 compares UC and CD.

Pathophysiology
Ulcerative Colitis

The inflammatory process of UC is confined to the mucosa of the colon and rectum and begins with neutrophil infiltration at the base of the crypt of Lieberkühn. The

Table 11.15	Comparison of Ulcerative Colitis and Crohn's Disease	
Feature	Ulcerative Colitis	Crohn's Disease
History		
Age at onset	Age 10–40	Age 15–25; age 50–80
Etiology	Unknown	Unknown
Genetic tendency	Familial tendency	Familial tendency
Nicotine use	Nonsmoker	Smoker
Assessment Findings		
Serological	+ (positive) for antineutrophil cytoplasmic antibodies (pANCA)	– pANCA
Fever/malaise	With severe disease	Common
Weight loss	Uncommon	Common
Rectal bleeding	Common	Dependent on location of lesion; occurs in about 50% of cases
Abdominal pain	Usually mild	Can be moderate to severe
Abdominal mass	Negative	May be present
Perianal lesions	Absent	May develop fissures, abscesses
Fistulas	Absent	Common
Strictures	Uncommon	Common
Common		
Rectal involvement	Always	50% of the cases
Distribution	Confined to colon; continuous	Any portion of GI tract; discontinuous, skipped lesions
Mucosa	Friable, granular	Cobblestone appearance
Ulceration	Crypt abscess development	Aphthous or linear ulcers
Inflammation	Surface involvement	Transmural involvement

disease most often occurs in the rectum and sigmoid colon. The mucosa in this area is thinner and has a dark red and velvety appearance in susceptible individuals. The cytokines released from the macrophages and neutrophils during the inflammatory response are responsible for tissue damage. Ulcers form in the eroded tissue, and abscesses form in the crypts. These abscesses become necrotic and ulcerate. The muscularis mucosa becomes edematous and thickened, narrowing the lumen of the colon. Bleeding, cramping pain, and the urge to defecate result from the mucosal destruction. The characteristic stool is diarrhea that contains blood and purulent mucus. There is also a loss of the absorptive surface leading to large volumes of watery diarrhea. Fecal leukocytes are always present with active colitis. Absence of these inflammatory changes within the deeper layers of the intestinal mucosa helps to differentiate UC from other inflammatory processes. Patients diagnosed with severe UC are at risk for a perforated colon. They require close observation and should have consultation with a surgeon.

Crohn's Disease

CD is an inflammatory process that begins in the submucosa of the intestine and gradually spreads to involve the mucosa and serosa. Any portion of the GI tract can be affected, but 80% of patients have small bowel involvement. There are abnormalities in the intestinal immune response where proinflammatory cytokines, interleukins, and tissue necrosis factor produce areas of tissue damage. Typically, some haustral segments are affected while others are not, creating a pattern called skip lesions. The ulcerations form longitudinal and transverse fissures, extending inflammation into Peyer's patches and the lymphoid tissue. The typical lesion is granulomatous with projections of inflamed tissue that is surrounded by scar tissue. It is described as a "cobblestone" appearance. With progression of the disease, fibrosis thickens the bowel wall, narrowing the lumen. Serosal inflammation causes bowel loops to adhere to one another, contributing to transmural inflammation, ulceration, and fibrosis, which can lead to obstruction, fistulas, and shortening of the bowel.

Individuals with IBD are at greater risk for developing colorectal cancer than the general population. Clinical findings suggest that carcinoma is less common in patients with CD than with UC and is attributed to the treatment of CD with colectomy.

Clinical Presentation

Subjective

Individuals with mild forms of UC commonly report four or fewer loose bowel movements per day associated with abdominal cramps that are relieved with defecation, small amounts of blood and mucus in the stool, and sometimes tenesmus. Usually there are no associated systemic symptoms. With moderate disease, patients have four to six loose stools a day containing more blood and mucus. They also have systemic symptoms such as tachycardia, mild fever, and weight loss and may have mild edema depending on the serum albumin level. Severe disease manifests with more frequent bloody bowel movements (6–10) per day; abdominal pain and tenderness; and symptoms of anemia, hypovolemia, and impaired nutrition.

The most common presenting symptoms of CD are abdominal cramping and tenderness, fever, anorexia, weight loss, spasm, flatulence, and right lower quadrant (RLQ) pain or mass. Individuals may report an increase in symptomatology during periods of stress or emotional upset or after meals consisting of poorly tolerated foods such as fatty or spicy foods or milk. Stools are soft or semiliquid. Observable blood is found in the stool intermittently; when present, it occurs in a larger amount than with UC. Because of the loss of healthy bowel mucosa, there may be insufficient resorption of bile salts, causing steatorrhea (foul-smelling, fatty stools). CD can involve the entire thickness of the bowel wall, causing microperforations and symptoms of acute localized peritonitis, which can mimic appendicitis or diverticulitis. If there is fistula formation, these symptoms may dominate the clinical picture.

Several patterns of symptom onset have been manifested—gradual, with vague abdominal discomfort, malaise, cramping, and bloody, mucopurulent stools; abrupt, with frequent periods of bloody diarrhea, anorexia, fever, and weight loss; and abrupt and fulminating, with sudden, violent diarrhea occurring nocturnally, high fever, intense abdominal cramping, signs of peritonitis, weight loss, and anorexia. Stools may contain blood, mucus, and/or pus. Typically, CD has a more insidious and gradual onset. Individuals often experience intermittent symptoms long before presenting for medical attention. The disease is characterized by periods of acute exacerbation alternating with complete remission.

If the UC is confined to the rectal or sigmoid area, the stools can be normal or hard and dry; however, the rectum will continue to dispel mucus containing both red and white blood cells. As the disease process moves proximally, the stools become looser. Patients may report eating less to decrease the frequency of bowel movements, which leads to more pronounced nutritional deficiencies.

Objective

On physical exam, there may be tenderness in the left lower quadrant or across the entire abdomen, often accompanied by guarding and abdominal distention. A digital rectal exam should be performed to assess for anal and perianal inflammation, rectal tenderness, and blood in the stool. Depending on the severity of the disease and the extent of potential complications, signs and symptoms of ileus and peritonitis may be found. Perirectal abscesses and fistulas are not associated with UC.

The physical exam may reveal abdominal tenderness with a tubular, tender mass in the RLQ. Fifty percent of individuals with CD have perianal involvement, including anal fissures, perianal fissures, and edematous, pale skin tags, which are often misdiagnosed as prolapsed hemorrhoids. Extraintestinal findings include episcleritis, erythema nodosum, nondeforming peripheral arthritis, and axial arthropathy, which may be more apparent than bowel symptoms and should prompt the practitioner to look for a diagnosis of CD.

CD tends to present in one of four patterns: (1) inflammation, RLQ abdominal pain, and tenderness, often presenting as appendicitis; (2) obstruction, fibrosis, and stenotic changes within the bowel, causing recurrent obstruction associated with severe colic, abdominal distention, constipation, and vomiting; (3) diffuse jejunoileitis involving the jejunum and ileum and characterized by both inflammation and obstruction, which can result in malnutrition and chronic debility; and (4) abdominal fistulas and abscesses, normally occurring late in the disease process and causing fever, generalized wasting, and abdominal masses. Although CD is uncommon among children, those with CD often present with extraintestinal symptoms, especially growth retardation, fever of unknown origin, and anemia.

Diagnostic Reasoning

Diagnostic Tests

Definitive diagnosis is made by correlating the symptoms with the history and physical exam. The results of diagnostic testing help to differentiate UC from CD. Stool analysis and cultures are obtained to rule out bacterial, fungal, or parasitic infection as the cause for diarrhea. The stool is also examined for mucus and blood, which are normally present with UC.

Patients with CD who have small intestine involvement may also require evaluation for malabsorption, which manifests as anemia secondary to bleeding and iron deficiency; for macrocytic anemia from inflammation of the terminal ileum and poor absorption of folate; and for hypocalcemia and vitamin D deficiency, hypoalbuminemia, and steatorrhea resulting from bile salt deficiency. Liver function tests may be helpful in screening for primary sclerosing cholangitis and other liver problems associated with IBD. Fluid and electrolyte disturbances are common in both diseases because of the extracellular fluid loss. CD may also present with an elevated white blood cell count and sedimentation rate, as well as a prolonged prothrombin time.

Imaging studies are necessary to confirm the diagnosis of IBD. Contrast radiography and endoscopy are the primary diagnostic tools. The diagnosis of UC should be supported with sigmoidoscopy, which defines the actual extent of the mucosal inflammation. Early in the disease, the mucous membrane is granular, friable, and edematous, with loss of the normal vascular pattern. In many patients, there may be scattered areas of hemorrhage that bleed with minor trauma. The resulting ulcerations develop after the mucosa breaks down, leaving the mucous membranes dotted with numerous bleeding and pus-oozing ulcers. Severe disease is characterized by copious amounts of purulent exudate. Colonoscopy should be avoided in individuals with severe colitis or deep ulcerations because of the risk of perforation or the development of toxic megacolon. Although there are periods of remission, sigmoidoscopy always shows some degree of friability and granulation in patients with UC. Biopsy results reveal chronic inflammation.

Plain films of the abdomen can help estimate the severity and proximal extent of the disease by demonstrating loss of haustration and the absence of formed stool within the diseased sections of bowel.

Every patient with UC requires a colonoscopy to determine the extent of the disease, but in order to avoid perforation, this is normally reserved for patients who have already begun treatment. Colonoscopy is preferred over barium enema (BE) because the former allows direct assessment of the colon and permits histological examination through biopsy. Ulcers suggestive of UC are shallow and confluent; they are erythematous, edematous, and friable, causing them to bleed easily. Individuals with UC usually have disease that begins in the rectum and extends proximally, without "skipped areas." Although BE is informative, it is contraindicated in individuals with moderate or severe disease because it can precipitate toxic megacolon.

Definitive diagnosis of CD is normally made via x-ray studies. The earliest manifestations of CD are aphthous and linear ulcers, which are best visualized with air contrast BE or small bowel follow-through, depending on the location of the lesions. BE may show reflux of barium into the terminal ileum. The ileum is stiff and nodular, and the lumen shows signs of thickening and narrowing. In advanced disease, the upper GI tract with small bowel follow-through may show the characteristic "string sign"—ileal strictures and evidence of bowel loop separation resulting from marked circumferential inflammation and fibrosis.

Colonoscopy reveals ulcers that are either minor erosions or deep longitudinal fissures. Segmental transverse fissuring creates the characteristic cobblestone appearance and is usually found above the rectum and rectosigmoid areas. Biopsies may be obtained to rule out pseudopolyposis, adenomatosis, or cancer. Computed tomography (CT) is often used in the evaluation of CD to identify bowel wall thickening or abscess formation.

If an abscess is found, CT may be useful for guided drainage of the abscess.

Differential Diagnosis

Differential diagnosis of UC must begin with the exclusion of an infectious cause for the colitis before treatment is initiated. Enteric infection is ruled out through fresh stool culture for ova and parasites. Infectious colitis caused by *Entamoeba histolytica, Campylobacter enteritidis,* and *Shigella* species and *Chlamydia* species can cause acute colitis, which is difficult to differentiate from UC both clinically and endoscopically. The distinction must be made because treatment with corticosteroids can be catastrophic. Obtaining a thorough travel, sexual, and antibiotic history is imperative. If the individual has had antibiotic exposure within the last 30 days, a stool sample to test for *Clostridium difficile* should be obtained. Homosexual men practicing anal intercourse should be screened for infectious proctitis as a cause of colitis. Individuals with HIV are susceptible to many opportunistic infections, which must also be considered as part of the differential diagnosis and treatment.

Older adults, patients with a history of coagulation disorders, and young women using oral contraceptives should be examined for ischemic colitis. Radiographic findings of "thumbprinting" and segmental distribution of lesions are typical of ischemic colitis. Although colon cancer rarely presents with fever and purulent diarrhea, it should be ruled out as a cause for bloody diarrhea.

As with UC, evaluation of CD must begin with ruling out infectious enteritis as the source of colitis. Enteric tuberculosis and fungal disease must also be considered in the differential diagnosis of CD. *Yersinia enterocolitica* enteritis, although a self-limiting infection, may require a 3-month follow-up examination because the initial clinical presentation is so similar to that of CD.

Although only 20% of patients with CD have disease that is limited to the colon, differentiation from UC must be made. CD is the more likely diagnosis when there is evidence of perianal disease and rectal bleeding. RLQ pain without a history of chronic bowel symptomatology may mimic appendicitis, pelvic inflammatory disease, ectopic pregnancy, ovarian cysts, or tumors; all of these must be ruled out in the differential diagnosis of CD. Both diverticular disease and ischemic colitis can present with the segmental involvement and luminal stricturing characteristic of CD.

Many drugs have been implicated in drug-induced colitis, the most common being NSAIDs and antibiotics. Many individuals who routinely take NSAIDs suffer damage to the GI tract characterized by bloody diarrhea and weight loss. Some antibiotics alter the bowel flora, allowing overgrowth of pathogens such as *C difficile,* which produces a toxin that is damaging to the bowel mucosa and can cause bloody diarrhea, abdominal pain, and weight loss. Although initial radiographic studies may be similar to those for CD, endoscopic examination reveals a more segmental distribution of lesions, and biopsy results are not supportive of inflammatory disease.

Colon cancers can cause bloody diarrhea; however, they usually do not have the associated fevers, leukocytosis, and purulent discharge. Diverticulitis can cause abdominal pain, fever, leukocytosis, obstruction, and diarrhea; however, endoscopic evaluation reveals the characteristic mucosal herniations in the bowel wall.

Management

There is no cure or definitive treatment for IBD. The initial therapy should depend on the severity of the presenting symptoms and must be individualized. Medical therapy is directed at reducing inflammation, correcting or maintaining fluid and electrolyte balance, and relieving the signs and symptoms of the disease.

Ulcerative Colitis

Initial treatment of UC includes nutrition counseling. Patients should avoid caffeine, raw fruits, vegetables, and other foods high in fiber, which can cause trauma to the already inflamed mucosal surface. Some patients may benefit from a lactose-free diet, but that is not recommended unless a trial produces symptomatic relief. A bland diet that is high in calories and protein yet low in fat can help to control diarrhea and flatulence and maintain nutrition and weight. Parenteral nutrition may be necessary in individuals with severe anorexia or uncontrollable diarrhea.

Antidiarrheal medications should be avoided in the acute phase but can be helpful for patients with mild symptoms. Patients with mild to moderate diarrhea may benefit from diphenoxylate with atropine (Lomotil) 2.5 to 5.0 mg by mouth twice daily up to four times per day, loperamide (Imodium) 2 mg after each bowel movement, or codeine 15 to 30 mg by mouth every 4 to 6 hours.

Disease that is limited to the rectosigmoid area can often be successfully treated with topical steroids or mesalamine (Drugs Commonly Prescribed 11.5). Steroid enemas and foams (e.g., hydrocortisone [Cortifoam] 100 mg) should be administered nightly for 2 weeks. If effective, this treatment will bring about remission in 70% of initial episodes of idiopathic UC. Patients may then taper the dose over the next week to prevent the side effects associated with rapid steroid withdrawal. Mesalamine (Rowasa), a form of 5-aminosalicylate (5-ASA), is more expensive; it is sometimes more effective than hydrocortisone for patients with refractory or left-sided colitis and is available in enema and suppository forms. Oral preparations of 5-ASA medications (e.g., Asacol) help to maintain remission after the enemas have been discontinued. 5-ASA preparations lack the sulfapyridine moiety (a by-product of the metabolism of sulfasalazine and responsible for most of the drug's toxicity), have

Drugs Commonly Prescribed 11.5   Inflammatory Bowel Disease

Drug	Indication	Adverse Reactions and Prescribing Considerations
5-Aminosalicylic acid agents mesalamine (Asacol)	None	Research indicated that these drugs are of little value in Crohn's disease. Continue to be used for ulcerative colitis.
Antidiarrheals loperamide (Imodium) diphenoxlate with atropine (Lomotil)	Diarrhea	Do not use in acute ulcerative colitis. Constipation may occur. Do not use if toxic megacolon occurs.
Corticosteroids prednisone budesonide (Entocort)	Moderate to severe disease	Drastically suppresses clinical symptoms. This preparation is ileal released and induces remission in 50%–70% of cases of Crohn's disease. Treatment is for 8–16 weeks followed by a 2–4 week taper in 3-mg increments.
Immunomodulating Drugs azathioprine mercaptopurine methotrexate	Moderate to severe disease that does not respond to corticosteroid therapy	This class of drugs can cause bone marrow suppression, and patients are at risk for life-threatening infections.
Anti-TNF therapies infliximab adalmumab certolizumub	Moderate to severe disease	This class of drugs causes bone marrow suppression and increase the risk for life-threatening infections.

fewer adverse effects, and are better tolerated for prolonged courses of treatment. Subsequent exacerbations of UC tend to show increasing resistance to therapy, requiring longer treatment regimens.

More advanced disease usually requires the addition of a systemic glucocorticoid in combination with sulfasalazine or 5-ASA therapy. Glucocorticoids are especially helpful in controlling the extracolonic manifestations of UC, which include peripheral arthritis, ankylosing spondylitis, erythema nodosum, anterior uveitis, and pyoderma gangrenosum. Peripheral arthritis and the skin lesions often parallel the course of the disease. Oral prednisone (Prelone), up to 40 to 60 mg in single or divided doses, must be tapered and not discontinued abruptly.

Severe or fulminant UC is manifested by 10 or more bloody stools per day, abdominal tenderness, fever, colon dilation, and tachycardia. Patients often require hospitalization for these symptoms. Patients with severe disease must be monitored closely for the development of toxic megacolon and colonic perforation. Any patient who does not show improvement after 7 to 10 days of maximized therapy should be considered for surgical intervention. Subtotal or total colectomy is often required to prevent perforation of the bowel and its complications. Some individuals may require restoration of their fluid volume and electrolytes, as well as blood transfusions, depending on the severity of the diarrhea and bleeding.

Immunosuppressive agents—azathioprine (Imuran), cyclosporine, and metabolite 6-mercaptopurine (6MP)—are used in cases of UC that are unresponsive to other

medical treatment and in patients who are not surgical candidates. The long-term use of immunosuppressive agents for relapse prevention must be balanced with the increased risk of developing a malignancy. Most commonly, these agents are used to allow patients to reduce the maintenance dosage of glucocorticoids. For disease that is unresponsive to other therapies, anti–tumor necrosis factor (anti-TNF) agents can be used. These include infliximab (Remicade) 5 mg/kg and adalimumab (Humira) administered subcutaneously 160 mg at week 1, 80 mg at week 2, and then maintenance of 40 mg every other week beginning at week 4.

Individuals who progress to fulminant disease are at risk for developing toxic megacolon—an atonic and distended, thin-walled colon. Approximately 1% to 2% of patients with UC develop this complication, which is characterized by fever, sepsis, electrolyte imbalances, hypoalbuminemia, and dehydration. Definitive diagnosis is made when radiographic measurement of the mid-transverse colon shows it to be dilated to greater than 6 cm. The patient is at risk for perforation until the dilation is reduced. If medical reversal is not accomplished within 48 hours, surgical intervention is indicated and consultation should be made early.

Patients with toxic megacolon should receive nothing by mouth, a nasogastric tube should be placed for intermittent suction, and all antidiarrheal medications should be discontinued. Fluid and electrolyte disturbances, particularly hypokalemia, should be corrected, and total parenteral nutrition may be required until the patient is able to tolerate oral food and fluids. Broad-spectrum antibiotics for peritonitis prophylaxis and parenteral administration of glucocorticoids are indicated. Patients must be monitored closely for signs and symptoms of perforation, which may be blunted because of the large doses of glucocorticoids. Loss of hepatic dullness on percussion may be the first sign of perforation. Daily abdominal x-ray films are necessary to assess colon distention and the presence of free air within the abdomen.

Over the long term, 25% of those with UC will require surgery. Emergent total colectomy is indicated for patients who do not respond to intensive medical therapy within 48 hours or who have massive hemorrhage or perforation. Surgical intervention is sometimes done in stages for patients who are severely ill. The most common procedure is the proctocolectomy with a Brooke ileostomy; it is a curative and functional procedure. Surgical intervention is also considered in patients who require large maintenance doses of glucocorticoids, are experiencing quality of life issues caused by severe diarrhea, or in children who are manifesting signs of growth retardation.

Crohn's Disease

Treatment of CD parallels that of UC including sulfasalazine (Azulfidine); however, 5-ASA medications have not been shown through research to be of any benefit. Glucocorticoids are used when initial treatment fails and for patients with moderate to severe disease. There is no curative therapy for CD; therefore, treatment is aimed at suppressing the inflammatory process and symptomatic relief of complications. The patient with CD has a much greater incidence of relapse once medications are discontinued; 70% of patients started on steroid therapy must remain on the therapy to prevent relapse. Oral prednisone 40 to 60 mg/day is used as initial outpatient treatment. Once maximal response has been achieved, the dose can be tapered over 2 to 4 months. Some patients may require a daily maintenance dose of 5 to 10 mg/day. As with UC, steroids are often helpful in managing the extraintestinal manifestations of the disease. Patients with disease within the rectum may benefit from enema preparations as well.

Sulfasalazine (Azulfidine) remains a common treatment for CD; however, new research is showing that it may have little value. There is a high incidence of intolerance, including nausea, anorexia, rash, and headache. When it is used, the initial dose of sulfasalazine for treatment of mild to moderate disease of the colon or ileocolon is 500 mg twice daily; the dose can be increased to 3 to 4 g/day. Clinical improvement is usually noted in 3 to 4 weeks, at which time the medication can be tapered to 2 to 3 g/day for 3 to 6 months. Sulfasalazine interferes with folic acid absorption, so patients should receive folic acid 1 mg/day while taking this medication.

The use of metronidazole has been effective in patients who are intolerant of sulfasalazine, although metronidazole's use is also limited by adverse effects, including nausea, anorexia, metallic taste, furry tongue, and paresthesias. Although the mechanism of action is not clear, metronidazole has been effective in the treatment of perianal disease and in controlling Crohn's colitis. There is a high rate of relapse, however, once the drug has been discontinued. Other antibiotics such as ciprofloxacin, ampicillin, and tetracycline have been effective in controlling Crohn's ileitis and ileocolitis.

The use of immunosuppressive medications has been shown to be effective in patients with CD that is unresponsive to other treatments, in individuals dependent on high-dose steroids, or in those with nonhealing fistulas. The clinical benefit of 6MP (the active metabolite of azathioprine [Imuran]) can take up to 3 months before being realized. These drugs can cause bone marrow suppression and pancreatitis; therefore, patients must be monitored frequently for leukopenia. The risk for developing malignancy is low but still must be considered. Patients remain on treatment for up to 2 years; in extremely refractory cases, treatment is continued indefinitely. Cyclosporine (Neoral, Sandimmune), an immunosuppressant drug typically used to prevent organ transplant rejection, is helpful in patients with steroid-resistant CD. Its use remains experimental, and it should be administered by practitioners who are experienced in caring for patients with complicated CD.

Other immunomodulating agents called TNF-α blockers such as infliximab (Remicade), adalimumab (Humira), and certolizumab are proving helpful in patients with moderate to severe CD. Rapid improvement is seen when infliximab is used initially. The regimen includes an initial dose of infliximab 5 mg/kg followed by repeat doses again at 2 weeks and 6 weeks, with maximal response seen in the first 2 weeks. Adalimumab (Humira) by subcutaneous injection is prescribed at 160 mg at week 1, 80 mg at week 2, and then maintenance of 40 mg every other week beginning at week 4. The side effects include infusion-related reactions and hypersensitivity reactions as a result of the development of antinuclear antibodies. This can be reduced by concomitant administration of other immunosuppressive medications. Serious infections may develop while patients are being treated with this medication.

Surgical intervention for CD is normally not indicated except for complications including intestinal obstruction, fistulas and abscess drainage, or perforation. Over the long term, up to 75% of patients with CD will require surgery. Patients with fistula formation (which may be enterocutaneous, enterovaginal, or enterovesicular) should be managed with bowel rest, parenteral nutrition, and antibiotic therapy before surgery is considered. Surgery is not curative and must be reserved for complications that are resistant to medical therapy. Intestinal obstruction caused by stricture formation is often successfully treated with strictureplasty, thus avoiding multiple colon resections and the risk of short bowel syndrome. Patients with symptoms of obstruction should avoid foods that contain nuts or seeds.

As with UC, the use of anticholinergic and antidiarrheal medications should be avoided in patients with severe disease because the drugs may precipitate toxic megacolon or ileus. Loperamide (Imodium), diphenoxylate (Lomotil), and codeine may be helpful in controlling chronic diarrhea in patients with mild Crohn's colitis.

Follow-up and Referral

UC and CD are both complex illnesses with periods of exacerbation and remission requiring lifelong intervention and follow-up. Adjustment of therapy is based on symptom analysis and examination. Confirmation of the diagnosis and uncontrolled exacerbations should be referred to the physician. Referral to a gastroenterologist is often necessary for endoscopic evaluation and tissue biopsy. Long-term use of steroids and immunosuppressive drugs dictates ongoing patient follow-up. Repeat evaluation may be indicated if symptoms of a major complication have developed. Routine colonoscopy for colon cancer surveillance is necessary in any patient with long-standing disease. Stool analysis for occult blood is not an effective means of surveillance. Individuals whose disease is not controlled with established medical therapy of low-dose prednisone should be referred to a gastroenterologist who is knowledgeable in the treatment of these chronic disease processes.

Patient Education

All patients need to be informed about the disease process, the treatment options, and the expected outcome of the treatment regimens. Patients must be a part of the treatment plan and must have the knowledge necessary to make informed decisions. Education about the disease, diagnostic and laboratory tests, and diet and lifestyle changes should be included in the education. Open, honest information is important in helping patients to develop realistic expectations with regard to treatment and outcomes.

The importance of adequate rest and stress reduction in an attempt to decrease bowel motility and promote healing is essential. Stress management techniques, such as guided imagery, should be taught, and patients can be referred for counseling if necessary. Patients should be provided with the information and addresses for national organizations such as the Crohn's and Colitis Foundation of America that have up-to-date information and local support groups.

Dietary concerns for patients with CD include a low-residue diet when obstructive symptoms are present. Patients on a low-residue diet should avoid all foods high in fiber, including whole grain breads and cereals, all fresh fruits and vegetables, and seeds and nuts. Patients are allowed to have canned fruits and vegetables and should have only white breads. If the patient is unresponsive to medical treatment or is exhibiting signs of growth retardation, oral elemental or parenteral nutrition may be necessary. Patients who are intolerant of lactose should be taught to avoid dairy foods. When patients are not in the middle of an acute attack, they can eat whatever they can tolerate.

Dietary instruction for patients with UC is the same as that for CD. If they are not having symptoms of an acute attack, patients may eat whatever they can tolerate. During an acute exacerbation, parenteral nutrition or oral supplementation for malnutrition may be necessary. Some patients will ask questions about the use of diet as a treatment. Studies to date show that diet is ineffective as a treatment or therapy for UC. Foods that can cause diarrhea and gas-producing foods should be avoided during acute attacks.

Female patients with IBD require special guidance and counseling before they attempt pregnancy. If pregnancy does occur, the patient must be followed closely by a gastroenterologist throughout her pregnancy.

■ IRRITABLE BOWEL SYNDROME

Irritable bowel syndrome (IBS) is a functional gastrointestinal (GI) disorder that is characterized by abdominal pain or discomfort. To be considered IBS, two of these features must be present: abdominal pain or discomfort that is relieved by defecation; change in frequency in stool; and a change in the appearance of the stool. Patients usually have other symptoms such as frequent stools (more than three per day) or fewer stools (less than three per week), passing mucus, feelings of straining, urgency or incomplete evacuation, flatulence, and abdominal distention. IBS is a common GI problem encountered in primary care. When patients present for medical attention, they have usually had the complex of symptoms for several weeks to several months.

Epidemiology

Traditionally, women have been affected more often than were men, at a rate of 3:1. Recent epidemiological studies, however, suggest that men and women are affected equally, but that men are underdiagnosed based on the current IBS diagnostic criteria. It is estimated that 9% to 20% of the general population is affected by symptoms that can be classified within the diagnosis of IBS, but fewer than one-third of those individuals seek medical attention. Typically, the symptoms first present in late adolescence and early adulthood but rarely in patients older than age 50.

Pathophysiology

The exact cause of IBS is unknown. IBS was once considered to have no organic cause, but several mechanisms have been identified. Normal bowel function is regulated by segmental contractions that limit the movement of bowel contents through the colon. An increase in these contractions causes constipation, and a decrease in the contractions results in frequent stooling or diarrhea. Myoelectric studies of colonic movement in individuals with IBS were inconclusive for diagnostic criteria, but the studies did demonstrate patterns of hypermotility, including high-amplitude pressure waves in patients, with pain as the predominant symptom during an acute IBS attack. Likewise, patients with diarrhea-predominant IBS had decreased and lower-amplitude pressure waves. Studies have confirmed alterations in colonic activity during periods of emotional stress, in which motility is decreased or inhibited with depression and increased with feelings of hostility and anger.

Another major investigative focus of IBS has centered on visceral hypersensitivity. Approximately 50% of the patients with IBS have perceptual abnormalities including heightened gut sensitivity, leading to a lower tolerance for abdominal pain and distention of the colon with gas and feces. Studies in which the rectums of IBS patients were distended by balloon dilation resulted in spastic contractions, leading to the characteristic symptoms seen with IBS. Patients with IBS are acutely aware of the intraluminal activities occurring with the digestive process. Sensations range from mild discomfort and tugging to frank pain. In summary, IBS patients do show evidence of abnormal colonic smooth muscle activity; however, the level at which the lesion originates is yet unknown.

Up to one-third of patients with IBS develop the disorder after bacterial gastroenteritis. It appears that patients with increased life stressors are more prone to developing IBS postinfection. Although the importance is unknown at this time, increased inflammatory cells have been found in all layers of the bowel in some patients with IBS.

The correlation between the symptoms of IBS and food intolerance is high. Careful diet history is necessary to distinguish between the two. The most common dietary triggers are lactose, fructose, sorbitol, and glutens. There is also a correlation between depression, anxiety, and somatization in patients who seek medical attention for their IBS symptoms.

Clinical Presentation
Subjective

Individuals with IBS typically present with symptoms that fall into two broad categories—those with abdominal pain and altered bowel habits, consisting of both diarrhea and constipation, and those with painless diarrhea.

Most patients with abdominal pain describe their pain as originating over some area of the colon, with the left lower quadrant (LLQ) being most often affected. The pain can be sharp and burning with cramping or a diffuse, dull ache. The description of the pain usually remains constant for the individual but can vary greatly among the patient population. Pain is often precipitated by eating or stress and can be relieved with a bowel movement or passing of flatus. The pain associated with IBS is usually not significant enough to interfere with sleeping, nor is it great enough to wake the patient from sleep.

More than 50% of patients with IBS describe an overly acute sensory ability with regard to the GI tract and the digestive process. This visceral hypersensitivity is manifested by frequent complaints of abdominal distention, gas, and belching. Many of these symptoms occur 2 hours after having a meal and are often thought to be food intolerances. Patients typically complain of urgency to defecate, abdominal pain, bloating, and gas. Some patients with IBS have upper GI complaints, including dyspepsia, pyrosis, nausea, and vomiting.

Patients who present with painless diarrhea usually report an urgent need to defecate immediately on awakening or after eating. Although diarrhea rarely occurs nocturnally, urgency is so great that it may cause incontinence.

Alteration in bowel habits is the most consistently reported symptom. The typical presentation is diarrhea alternating with constipation. Patients report that constipation that was once responsive to laxatives has become continuous and that the stool has become harder and is decreased in caliber. Many patients complain of a sense of incomplete evacuation and thus repeated attempts at defecation are necessary within a short period of time. Periods of predominant constipation can last for months, interrupted by periods of diarrhea and then back to constipation. Patients who have diarrhea as their predominant symptom complain of frequent, low-volume (less than 200 mL), loose stools. Diarrhea does not normally occur at night; however, it can be exacerbated by eating or stress. Many patients report the passage of large volumes of mucus within the stool. This differs from the mucus occurring with colitis because there is no associated inflammatory process nor is there any blood in the stool, other than if there is an incidental finding of hemorrhoids.

Patients diagnosed with IBS frequently have an associated psychiatric diagnosis, which presents in the form of anxiety, depression, and somatoform disorders. IBS symptoms are often precipitated by a recent stressful life event such as marital discord, death, or abuse.

Objective

As with any illness, a thorough and detailed patient history is the key to definitive diagnosis. The physical exam is usually normal except for tenderness in some area of the colon, most often the LLQ and over the umbilicus or epigastric area in those with small bowel involvement. Digital rectal exam is normal but may reveal tenderness and exacerbate symptoms in some individuals.

There is usually no associated weight loss or deterioration in health. History of psychosocial stressors can often be correlated with the onset of symptoms. Key to diagnosis is the lack of other systemic symptoms such as fever, leukocytosis, or bloody stools, which might suggest an organic cause for symptoms.

Diagnostic Reasoning

Diagnostic Tests

IBS is diagnosed based on a careful history and physical that reveals the characteristic increase in bowel symptoms with the onset of pain, relief of pain with defecation, heightened sensation of bowel activity, or sense of incomplete defecation. The criteria used for diagnosing IBS are provided in Advanced Assessment 11.2.

Initial laboratory testing should include complete blood count, erythrocyte sedimentation rate (ESR), chemistry panel including electrolytes and serum amylase, urinalysis, and stools for occult blood, ova and parasites, and cultures. Any abnormal lab value should prompt further investigation in the direction of the abnormal finding because most laboratory studies in the patient with IBS are normal and any diagnostic clue as to the cause is helpful. If white blood cells (WBCs) are found in the stool, it suggests an infectious or inflammatory process and not IBS.

Flexible proctosigmoidoscopy enables the provider to see up to 60 cm of the colon. No abnormalities are seen with IBS with the possible exception of an increased volume of mucus; however, increased tenderness and spasm may inhibit passage of the scope beyond 15 cm. Patients who present for initial treatment at age 40 or older should also be given an air contrast barium enema or colonoscopy.

Food intolerances should be ruled out, especially in patients who present with diarrhea and gas as predominant symptoms. Lactase deficiency can be identified with a hydrogen breath test or lactose tolerance test. Other intolerances are identified by removing the most common causative agents from the diet for 3 weeks and then slowly reintroducing them to the diet one at a time.

IBS is no longer a diagnosis of exclusion; thus, the practitioner must direct diagnostic testing as information is received and lends itself toward an organic cause of the symptoms. Patients should not be subjected to endless batteries of expensive and uncomfortable tests in search of an organic disease. Laboratory findings that support a cause other than IBS include elevated ESR, anemia, leukocytosis, blood or WBCs in the stool, or stool volumes greater than 300 mL.

Differential Diagnosis

The differential diagnosis of IBS can include any of the processes in Table 11.16, with emphasis on the organic GI disorders. Most of the disease processes can be ruled out with careful history and physical exam. Patients presenting with diarrhea as the dominant symptom should have thyroid function tests, 24-hour stool check for fecal fat, and stool weight and stool testing for laxative content. Patients who present with constipation as their predominant symptom may require referral to a specialist who can measure colonic transit time. A careful medication history is necessary for either presentation.

Patients with epigastric pain must have the pain differentiated from that produced by biliary tract pain, ulcerative disease, or malignancies of the stomach and pancreas.

Management

The initial step to successful management of IBS is making the diagnosis and then identifying the symptom pattern for each individual patient. Based on the symptom pattern of each patient, therapy may include diet, education, and pharmacological and supportive interventions. The patient with IBS requires reassurance and guidance throughout the course of the disease. There is evidence that a therapeutic relationship between the provider and the patient can reduce symptomatology (Level II; Kaptchuk et al, 2008). Patients must understand that there is no proven treatment and the therapy is often symptomatic. Much of the recent literature suggests that there is a high degree of placebo effect with varying treatments.

A careful diet history is important in identifying foods that may precipitate symptoms. IBS is often confused with lactose intolerance and can be evaluated by removing lactose from the diet for 2 weeks and monitoring the symptoms. Other foods that are frequently identified in producing IBS syndromes include caffeine, legumes (and other fermentable carbohydrates), and artificial sweeteners. If any foods are identified that provoke symptoms, they should be eliminated from the diet. Patients who

---

Advanced Assessment 11.2 Criteria for Diagnosing Irritable Bowel Syndrome

Abdominal pain or discomfort that is consistently relieved by defecation or has been associated with a change in the frequency or a change in the consistency of the stool for a period of 3 months either continuously or recurrently within that time frame
AND
Defecation with varying patterns of constipation and diarrhea 25% of the time
AND
Two or more of the following:

Altered stool frequency
Altered stool form including hard, loose, watery, mucoid
Altered sensory act of defecation including straining, urgency, tenesmus
Passage of mucus
Varied degrees of bloating and abdominal distention

Table 11.16	Differential Diagnosis of Irritable Bowel Syndrome

Food intolerance
- Lactase deficiencies
- Caffeine
- Fermentable carbohydrates
- Artificial sweeteners

Fat or bile acid intolerances

Pathogen-precipitated processes
- Intestinal parasites
- Bacterial overgrowth

Medication-induced alterations in bowel motility
- Laxative abuse
- Magnesium-based antacids
- Antibiotics
- Opiate analgesics

Functional upper GI disorders
- Dyspepsia
- Pyrosis
- Gastroesophageal reflux disease
- Peptic ulcer disease
- Cholelithiasis
- Biliary pain
- GI malignancy

Functional lower GI disorders
- Inflammatory bowel disease
- Crohn's disease
- Ulcerative colitis
- Diverticulitis
- Intestinal obstruction
- Hemorrhoids
- Lower GI malignancy
- Ascites

Endocrine disorders
- Hypothyroidism
- Hyperthyroidism
- Autonomic diabetic neuropathy

Psychological disorders
- Depression
- Anxiety

seem to suffer from postprandial discomfort may alleviate symptoms by eating a lower-fat diet that contains more protein. Dietary consultation can be helpful in assisting patients in developing a diet program that is palatable to them.

Diets high in fiber are beneficial regardless of predominant bowel habit. Patients are encouraged to increase their fiber intake to 20 to 30 grams per day. The hydrophilic properties of fiber or bulk-producing agents help to prevent excessive hydration or dehydration of stool; thus, fiber is indicated for both diarrhea and constipation symptom presentations. Foods high in fiber include whole grains, cereals, fruits, and vegetables; however, they must be introduced slowly for IBS patients in order to avoid

the sensation of bloating. Bulk-producing agents can be substituted for individuals who choose not to change their diet. Commercially prepared bulk-producing agents are started once a day and increased gradually to three to four times daily. Patients are encouraged to continue treatment for at least 2 months before termination in order to allow the bowel to adjust to the bulking agents. All patients should try to drink at least eight 8-ounce glasses of water per day. Individuals with constipation as their predominant symptom should be aware that fiber-bulking agents are not overnight laxatives, and they should not abandon this therapy because they did not get overnight results.

Pharmacological treatment is reserved for patients with moderate to severe symptoms and is directed at specific symptoms. Antidiarrheal medications are used only as a temporary measure. When the diarrhea is severe, episodic use of loperamide (Imodium) 2 mg or diphenoxylate (Lomotil) 2.5 to 5.0 mg every 6 hours can be used as needed. The use of codeine, tincture of opium, and paregoric should be avoided because of their addictive nature. Patients who anticipate stressful situations can use antidiarrheals prophylactically.

Patients with constipation who have not responded to a high-fiber diet, hydration, exercise, and bulking agents may benefit from intermittent use of stimulant laxatives such as lactulose or magnesium hydroxide. Long-term use of laxatives is discouraged.

Antispasmodic agents have been used successfully in controlling abdominal pain caused by intestinal spasm. Patients who suffer with postprandial pain not responsive to diet therapy can benefit from dicyclomine 10 to 20 mg three to four times a day by mouth or hyoscyamine 0.125 to 0.75 mg twice a day. Anticholinergics should be avoided in patients with glaucoma and benign prostatic hypertrophy because of the adverse effects and used with caution in the elderly.

Tricyclic antidepressants and selective serotonin reuptake inhibitors have been shown to relieve symptoms in some individuals. Individuals with IBS need reassurance and understanding that their disease is chronic. They often benefit from support groups and counseling. Psychiatric interventions that teach behavior modification and biofeedback or that can provide psychotherapy or hypnosis are helpful alternative measures for patients with refractory IBS.

Follow-up and Referral

The emotional support provided by regular follow-up appointments is important in the management of patients with IBS. A strong, honest relationship with the patient is necessary to allay fears and prevent unrealistic expectations of the patient regarding his or her disease. Follow-up is important to encourage preventive behaviors including high-fiber diet, regular exercise, and avoidance of foods that precipitate symptoms. Patients who are not responding to treatment should be referred to a gastroenterologist.

Patients who have IBS are often dissatisfied with treatment because no organic cause of their symptoms can be found. A second opinion is helpful in the management of these individuals; however, they must also be discouraged from continuing to search for organic causes for their symptoms. Referral for psychological intervention tends to be more helpful in patients with intermittent symptoms; those with chronic pain or intractable symptoms usually respond poorly.

Patient Education

Care of patients with IBS requires a positive and honest practitioner–patient relationship. Education is important in reducing the number of return visits for symptoms common to patients with IBS. The patients should understand that they have a real intestinal disorder, which is characterized by hypersensitivity to certain foods, hormonal changes, and stressors. Patients should be taught how to recognize these triggers and how to avoid or diminish their effects. Patients should understand that they have a chronic disease but that they do not have a shorter life expectancy because of it. A thorough understanding of the treatment regimen and setting realistic goals regarding treatment is the key to building a positive relationship with the patient. Patients must understand that the goal of treatment is to improve their symptoms, not cure the disease, and that improvement in symptoms can be a time-consuming process.

Dietary education is paramount to relief of the symptoms. Increasing fiber and water intake is an important component of the treatment. Teaching patients how to read nutrition labels will help them to quantify the amount of fiber they are consuming daily. Patients must be encouraged to take an active role in their treatment program and to understand that elimination of foods that trigger symptoms can be time consuming and requires their careful attention.

Establishing good bowel habits is also important in the treatment of IBS. A high-fiber diet and increasing water intake to eight 8-ounce glasses per day can help in maintaining a regular bowel program. Patients who suffer with constipation should avoid laxatives and instead practice bowel training. Allowing adequate time after breakfast to sit on the toilet without straining can help establish a daily schedule.

Helping patients recognize and understand environmental stressors that trigger symptoms should be included in patient education. Involving the patient's family is important in establishing a support system. A resource available to patients for both education and support is the International Foundation for Bowel Dysfunction.

■ BOWEL OBSTRUCTION

Bowel obstruction is the consequence of any condition that inhibits the normal flow of chyme through the intestinal lumen. It can be complete or partial and can involve any segment of the large or small bowel. Bowel obstruction is considered simple when it results from a mechanical blockage or functional (paralytic ileus) when there is a disruption in motility.

Epidemiology and Causes

Intestinal obstruction can be classified according to the onset. Acute obstruction is sudden and can be caused by torsion, herniation, or intussusception (the slipping of a proximal piece of intestine into the part below it). Chronic obstruction usually indicates a slow, gradual process often from tumor growth or strictures. Obstructions are also classed according to the degree of obstruction, either complete or partial, and the location of the obstructing lesion. Obstructions can develop within the lumen, as in the case of foreign bodies, tumors, or intraluminal fibrosis. This type of obstruction is considered intrinsic. Conversely, they can be extrinsic or from obstruction that arises outside the intestine. For example, intussusception, torsion (volvulus), fibrosis, and hernia can all cause intestinal obstructions from outside the bowel. Another aspect in the classification of intestinal obstruction is the effect it has on the intestinal wall. A simple obstruction indicates that there is no impairment of the blood supply to that portion of the intestine. A strangulated obstruction means that the lumen is obstructed and the blood supply is compromised. Bowel obstruction can be a complication of adhesions, which are fibrous bands of tissue that develop after a surgical procedure.

Pathophysiology

There are numerous physiological alterations resulting from an intestinal obstruction related to the onset, location of the obstruction, and the amount of intestine proximal to the obstruction. Immediately after the obstruction begins, there is distention of the intestine with sequestration of fluid and gas proximal to the obstruction. The gas is a result of bacterial fermentation and swallowed air. When the intestine begins to distend, its ability to absorb water and electrolytes decreases and more is left in the lumen adding to the distention. Sources of water and electrolytes include saliva, gastric juice, bile, and pancreatic juice, as well as intestinal secretions. Within 24 hours, as much as 8 liters can accumulate in the intestinal lumen, leading to vomiting. Because of the vomiting and sequestration of fluid and electrolytes in the intestinal lumen, profound fluid and electrolyte imbalances result, leading to dehydration, hemoconcentration, and ultimately hypovolemic shock. The increasing distention causes pressure on the diaphragm, thereby reducing the respiratory volume leading to atelectasis and pneumonia.

Depending on the location and stage of the intestinal obstruction, alkalosis or acidosis is possible. Alkalosis occurs early in intestinal obstruction or if the obstruction is in the proximal portion of the small bowel. This occurs because gastric juice, which is high in hydrogen ions, does not get absorbed through the intestinal lumen, resulting in loss of the ion. However, later in the course of obstruction, or if the obstruction is more distal, acidosis occurs because alkaline pancreatic secretions and bile cannot be reabsorbed. Potassium is sequestered in the intraluminal fluid, causing hypokalemia, which promotes acidosis and atony of the intestinal wall.

As pressure within the intestinal lumen increases, arterial blood flow may be compromised leading to ischemia, necrosis, perforation, and peritonitis. Metabolic acidosis is compounded by the buildup of lactic acid that results from the decreased arterial blood flow. Venous return is reduced leading to edema within the bowel wall. As the edema progresses, there is an increase in capillary permeability causing fluid to be lost into the peritoneum, contributing to the hypovolemia already present.

Clinical Presentation
Subjective

In general, patients with obstruction generally complain of a sudden onset of colicky abdominal pain accompanied by nausea and vomiting. The pain is usually intermittent and corresponds to peristaltic waves. Patients with obstruction at the jejunum or below may have emesis that has changed to a brownish, feculent type material. They may complain of initial bouts of diarrhea, but this is soon followed by constipation.

In the later stages of obstruction, patients may have constipation and lack of flatulence. It is important to obtain information regarding previous abdominal operations, which may help in the diagnosis of intestinal obstruction. The abdominal pain of small bowel obstruction is usually centered about the umbilicus or in the epigastric area, and vomiting usually occurs early in the disease process. If the arterial circulation to the bowel is compromised, the pain becomes more constant and severe. Perforation produces severe generalized abdominal pain, as well as the classic signs of peritonitis.

Objective

The physical exam should include careful inspection for abdominal scars and the presence of hernias. The patient may show signs of dehydration including poor skin turgor, dry mucous membranes, sunken eyeballs, and tachycardia. Blood pressure may be elevated depending on the degree of pain and if there is evidence of strangulation and subsequent ischemia. The degree of abdominal distention depends on the level of obstruction. The more distal the obstruction, the greater the length of proximal intestine producing greater distention. Also, if the obstruction is in the distal portion of the intestine, vomiting may occur only late in the course of the disease. The abdomen may be tender to palpation if strangulation is present. Bowel sounds are high pitched and

hyperactive; they may be accompanied by rushes, which coincide with the colicky abdominal pain. Patients with strangulation tend to have increased distention, abdominal tenderness, tympany to percussion, and hypoactive or absent bowel sounds. Sometimes a mass is palpable. If perforation has occurred, there may be a short period of pain relief, which is soon followed by increased pain, rebound tenderness, and fever, all suggestive of peritonitis.

Patients presenting with large bowel obstruction usually have a more gradual onset of symptoms, beginning with increasing constipation and abdominal distention. Large bowel obstruction is rare in patients younger than age 50. Lower abdominal cramps are unproductive of feces and are painful. Patients report a several-day history of no stools or flatus production. Vomiting occurs if there is an incompetent ileocecal valve or if there is a resultant superimposed, small bowel obstruction. The most common cause of large bowel obstruction is carcinoma of the sigmoid colon or diverticulosis.

Physical exam findings include a distended abdomen, particularly over the transverse and descending colon, with the presence of borborygmi. Patients are normally afebrile unless diverticulitis is suspected. There is usually no abdominal tenderness or guarding unless there are areas of ischemic bowel or associated small bowel obstruction with impending cecal perforation. A mass may be palpable over the area of obstruction. Rectal exam reveals an empty vault without tenderness unless there are obstructing rectal carcinomas. The systemic manifestations of large bowel obstructions are much less serious than those caused by small bowel obstruction.

Diagnostic Reasoning
Diagnostic Tests

Before diagnostic testing, patients must be thoroughly examined for any type of hernia that may be precipitating the obstruction. Diagnosis of small bowel obstruction is usually confirmed by supine and upright abdominal x-ray films that reveal a ladder-like distention of the small bowel. Upright films show multiple air-fluid levels within the loops of small bowel, which are the hallmark of small bowel obstruction. Findings indicative of other causes of small bowel obstruction are evidence of a foreign body or an actual mass suggestive of infarcted bowel. Oral contrast with small bowel follow-through can identify areas of partial obstruction. Oral barium studies are contraindicated and must be avoided unless large bowel obstruction has definitely been ruled out.

Laboratory studies include complete blood count and chemistry profile but are rarely useful for the diagnosis. Leukocytosis can indicate impending ischemia or strangulation of the bowel but is not diagnostic of such. Chemistry evaluation can help with proper fluid and electrolyte replacement. Serum amylase may be elevated and can lead to the erroneous diagnosis of pancreatitis. A finding of metabolic acidosis or an elevated lactic acid is highly suggestive of intestinal infarction.

Abdominal x-ray films of patients with large bowel obstruction usually show distention of the intestine down to the level of the obstruction. It is important to note the size of the cecum because as the diameter approaches 14 cm, the danger of perforation is imminent. If air is noted under the diaphragm, it is likely that perforation of the cecum or sigmoid colon has occurred.

Differential Diagnosis

Volvulus, a twisting of the bowel on itself, can happen suddenly, with loss of blood supply to the area and subsequent ischemia. Cecal volvulus presents as a large gas bubble within the midabdomen or left upper quadrant on abdominal x-ray film. A volvulus of the sigmoid colon usually occurs only in older adults. It typically appears as a "coffee bean" dilation arising from the pelvis. For both cecal and sigmoidal volvulus, a barium enema is done to reveal the precise location of the obstruction.

Colonoscopy and endoscopy are contraindicated in patients suspected of mechanical bowel obstruction because to visualize the intestine, air must be introduced into the colon and can increase the chance of perforation. The differential diagnosis of small and large bowel obstruction is presented in Table 11.17.

Management

All patients with suspected intestinal obstruction should be hospitalized and immediately referred to a surgeon. Therapy must be administered as definitive diagnosis is

Table 11.17	Differential Diagnosis of Bowel Obstruction

Pseudo-obstruction
Toxic megacolon
Twisting of a loop of bowel
 • Cecal volvulus
 • Sigmoid volvulus
Incarcerated or strangulated hernias
 • Abdominal
 • Femoral
 • Inguinal
Kinking of a loop of bowel
 • Adhesions secondary to previous abdominal surgery
Concentric narrowing of the lumen of the intestine
 • Neoplasms
 • Diverticulitis
 • Crohn's disease
Foreign body
 • Gallstones
 • Ingested objects
Intussusception
Paralytic ileus

being obtained. Most patients with a bowel obstruction will require placement of a nasogastric tube to decrease passage of secretions, aid in decompression, and ameliorate vomiting if present. Rehydration with IV fluids and replacement of electrolytes should be done as indicated by laboratory studies. Placement of an indwelling urinary catheter is necessary to monitor urine output accurately, which is recorded on a daily intake and output sheet.

Treatment of small bowel obstruction proceeds after the aforementioned therapies have been instituted and the patient is medically stabilized. Patients with upper small bowel obstruction are prone to alkalosis and hypokalemia caused by emesis; they must be monitored carefully and given IV fluid and electrolyte replacement as necessary. All medications that can decrease intestinal motility, including anticholinergics, narcotics, and calcium channel blockers, should be discontinued. If strangulation is suspected, the patient should be started on broad-spectrum antibiotic therapy, which provides coverage for anaerobic and gram-negative organisms. Laparotomy is indicated for all patients with complete bowel obstruction.

Patients with a large bowel obstruction are rehydrated and stabilized as previously described. If the patient has evidence suggestive of sigmoidal volvulus, an initial attempt to reduce the volvulus can be made with sigmoidoscopy, but surgery is required if that attempt is unsuccessful. Patients with Crohn's disease, intestinal lymphoma, or diverticulitis with subsequent concentric narrowing of the intestinal lumen may be given a trial of medical therapy specific to the disease process in an attempt to relieve the obstruction before surgical intervention.

Obstructing carcinomas can be treated with surgical resection and anastomosis. (Colon cancer is discussed later in this chapter.) If fecal impaction has been identified as the cause, it can often be removed digitally. If the impaction is barium and is located within the sigmoid colon, open laparotomy is required for removal. Adhesions can be relieved by surgical intervention; however, the chances are great that they will recur. Hernia reduction is indicated if this is the determined cause of obstruction. All patients who have undergone surgical intervention as definitive therapy must be monitored for paralytic ileus postoperatively.

Follow-up and Referral

All patients with suspected bowel obstruction must be referred to a surgeon, who will manage the patient's hospitalization and postoperative care. The prognosis of appropriately treated simple intestinal obstruction is good, with a mortality rate of less than 2%. If strangulation is suspected and intervention is delayed, the mortality rate can be as high as 25%.

Because patients are usually acutely ill, postoperative teaching should be delayed until the patient is more receptive to instruction. Initial follow-up visits should be with the consulting surgeon, who will direct the patient's care until the patient is released to his or her primary-care provider.

Patient Education

Follow-up of patients with bowel obstruction will be guided by the surgeon. Instructions on care of the incision, including dressing changes and signs and symptoms of infection, are provided before discharge from the hospital. Once the patient has been cleared by the collaborating surgeon, he or she will return to the primary-care setting. Patients should be instructed to report any recurrent abdominal pain with or without vomiting, fever, or problems regarding bowel function. Laxatives should not be taken without consulting the primary-care provider first. Stool softeners are prescribed as needed, and patients are encouraged to avoid foods that cause constipation. Patients should refrain from strenuous activity for at least 6 to 8 weeks.

■ DIVERTICULAR DISEASE

Diverticular disease is the term used to describe the inflammatory changes that occur within the diverticular mucosa of the intestine (diverticulitis), as well as the asymptomatic, uninflamed outpouchings called diverticulosis. Diverticula are pouchlike protrusions of the intestinal mucosa that occur most often within the descending and sigmoid segments of the colon. They decrease in frequency in the cecum and rarely are found in the rectum. Diverticula occur infrequently in the small bowel. There are two types, congenital and acquired. Congenital diverticula are situated on the antimesenteric margin of the bowel and consist of the intestinal wall layers. The acquired diverticula occur on the mesenteric margin of the bowel, where the blood vessels enter the bowel wall. A diverticulosis of the small bowel may cause malabsorption and steatorrhea. Diverticula tend to form at weakened areas of the intestinal wall, usually where arterial vessels perforate the colon. The inner layer of these pouchlike protrusions forms a narrow neck, which is continuous with the inner layer of the colon, and the sac herniates through the muscle wall. Most diverticula are asymptomatic and pose a problem only when they become inflamed or bleed. Most diverticula are found incidentally with endoscopy or barium enema (BE). Diverticula vary in size from 3 mm to 3 cm in diameter.

Epidemiology and Causes

Diverticula are uncommon in individuals younger than age 40, with the prevalence increasing steadily after that. More than one-third of the U.S. population is affected by age 60. Diverticular disease is more common in developed nations than in less-developed countries, with estimates as high as 40% to 50% in Western populations. The incidence is 2,200 to 3,000 per 100,000 people, occurring equally among men and woman. Diverticula are a rare finding in pediatric patients. Although they are common

in older adults, it may be difficult to diagnose diverticular disease in these patients because of their blunted immune response.

Although there is no known cause for diverticular disease, a low-fiber diet has been implicated because it causes increased intraluminal pressures within the colon, which lead to mucosal herniation through the weaker areas in the bowel wall. Other factors believed to contribute to the formation of diverticula include hypertrophy of the segments of the circular muscle of the colon, chronic constipation and straining, irregular and uncoordinated bowel contractions, obesity, and weakness of the bowel muscle brought on by aging. Risk factors are directly related to the suspected causes of the disease: older than age 40, low-fiber diet, previous diverticulitis, and the number of diverticula present within the colon. Diverticula occur most often in the left lower quadrant (LLQ); a right lower quadrant presentation is a rare condition, with a higher incidence in Asian populations.

Pathophysiology

The exact cause of diverticulosis is unknown; therefore, the pathophysiology is based on the speculative findings already mentioned. As a consequence of increased ingestion of refined foods and decreased fiber intake, the stool bulk is decreased and the colon transit time is increased, leading to the development of diverticula. Diverticula are thought to result from the increased pressure produced with the segmental contraction of the muscular portion of the wall of the colon. This increased pressure causes the herniation of the bowel wall through the weaker points in the muscle layer of the colon, normally occurring along the teniae at the penetration site of colonic vasculature. Inflammation occurring around the diverticular sac is often caused by the retention of undigested food and bacteria, which when formed into a hardened mass is called a *fecalith*. This mass in turn can disrupt the blood flow and lead to abscess formation. When the opening of this saclike projection becomes occluded and inflammation ensues, it can progress to the point of rupture. Acute diverticulitis is the result of this localized inflammation within the wall of the colon or peritoneum, causing the characteristic LLQ abdominal pain and tenderness. If the perforation is not localized, the patient can develop acute peritonitis and septic shock.

Fistula formation following acute diverticulitis is the result of a tract forming between the colon and other structures within the abdomen. These fistulas include colovesicular fistulas (urinary bladder), colovaginal fistulas (vagina), enteroenteric fistulas (loop of bowel), and colocutaneous fistulas (peritoneal tissue). Pericolitis is inflammation around the colon, which can result in fibrous strictures and obstruction.

Bleeding is a common complication of diverticulosis and is the most common cause of substantial lower gastrointestinal (GI) bleeding. Postbleeding examinations have discovered that most bleeding occurs from uninflamed rather than inflamed diverticuli.

Clinical Presentation
Subjective

Approximately 25% of patients with diverticular disease develop symptoms. Patients with diverticulosis characteristically present with pain in the LLQ of the abdomen. Some patients report that the pain is worse after eating, which may be a result of colonic distention, and that the pain is sometimes relieved with a bowel movement or passing flatus. Elimination patterns may alternate between diarrhea and constipation, and there may be associated abdominal distention and tenderness. Diverticulitis may present with bleeding, which can be massive and is not associated with pain or discomfort.

When the diverticula have become inflamed, there are the usual signs and symptoms of infection—fever, chills, and tachycardia. Patients typically present with localized pain and tenderness in the LLQ of the abdomen with associated anorexia, nausea, and vomiting. If there is fistula formation, there are symptoms associated with the particular organ involved. Patients may complain of dysuria, pneumaturia (passage of air in the urine), and/or fecaluria (passage of fecal matter in the urine) if there is fistula formation involving the bladder. Patients may be concerned about the development of hematochezia or frank bleeding from the rectum.

Objective

A physical exam reveals tenderness in the LLQ of the abdomen, and—if the patient can tolerate more vigorous examination—a firm, fixed mass may be identified in the area of the diverticuli. Patients may have rebound tenderness with involuntary guarding and rigidity. Bowel sounds may initially be hypoactive or can be hyperactive if an obstructive process has developed. Examination of the rectum may reveal tenderness, and the stool is usually positive for occult blood.

Diagnostic Reasoning
Diagnostic Tests

Initial laboratory testing can show mild to moderate leukocytosis, depending on whether the patient presents with diverticulitis or with a more advanced inflammatory process such as peritoneal abscess. The white blood cell (WBC) count is usually normal in patients with diverticulosis. Hemoglobin and hematocrit may be low if there is associated rectal bleeding. If there is fistula formation between the diverticula and the bladder, urinalysis may show elevated levels of both WBCs and red blood cells, and urine culture may be positive. Patients with signs suggestive of peritonitis should have a blood culture to assess for bacteremia.

Abdominal x-ray films should be obtained on all patients with suspected diverticulitis, especially if there are signs of perforation or peritonitis. Plain films of the abdomen can reveal free air (indicating perforation), ileus, or obstruction (small or large bowel). A BE outlines the lumen of the bowel clearly defining diverticula and is thus most helpful in the diagnosis of the disease process. If perforation is suspected, the study can be performed with Gastrographin, a water-soluble contrast medium. Barium studies help to identify sinus tracts, fistula formation, or obstructive processes. Diverticula are often an incidental finding on colonoscopy; however, colonoscopy is much less sensitive for the diagnosis of diverticular disease than BE. Colonoscopy may be helpful in ruling out cancer as the source of the symptomatology, as is cystoscopy in evaluation of colovesicular fistula.

Although diverticulitis can often be diagnosed clinically, a computed tomography (CT) scan with oral contrast is a much more sensitive and accurate test for cases in which confirmatory testing is necessary. CT scan can also determine if there is clinical deterioration by measuring the thickness of the bowel wall and assessing for the development of phlegmon over time using serial exams.

Patients who present with lower GI bleeding may require radioisotope scanning to locate the site of bleeding. Angiography is often nondiagnostic because the rate of bleeding is too slow or because bleeding has stopped.

Differential Diagnosis

The differential diagnosis of diverticular disease includes irritable bowel syndrome, carcinoma of the colon, inflammatory bowel disease, lactose intolerance, pelvic inflammatory disease, ovarian cyst, colitis (infectious or ischemic), appendicitis, and pyelonephritis. Most often the diagnosis can be made using the clinical findings and initial noninvasive ultrasonography. BE and colonoscopy are most helpful for definitive diagnosis of diverticulitis and colon surveillance for other colonic disease processes.

Management

With early detection and treatment of diverticulitis and the associated complications, the prognosis is good. An incidental finding of uncomplicated diverticulosis requires no further intervention and can be managed with a high-fiber diet or daily fiber supplementation with psyllium. Treatment of a patient presenting with mild symptoms can often be managed on an outpatient basis with rest, oral antibiotics, and a clear liquid diet. Initial antibiotic therapy varies with the extent of the inflammatory process and can include metronidazole (Flagyl) 500 mg by mouth three times daily with ciprofloxacin (Cipro) 500 mg by mouth twice daily, or trimethoprim/sulfamethoxazole (Bactrim DS) 160/800 mg by mouth twice daily for 7 to 10 days. The symptoms usually subside quickly; then the diet can be advanced to soft, low roughage and next to high fiber as tolerated. Pain due to spasms can be managed with antispasmodics such as hyoscyamine (Levsin) 0.125 mg every 4 hours, dicyclomine (Bentyl) 20 to 40 mg four times daily, buspirone (BuSpar) 15 to 30 mg/day, and/or meperidine (Demerol) 100 to 150 mg/day in divided doses.

Patients with more acute illness require hospitalization for intravenous antibiotics and hydration, analgesia, bowel rest, and possible nasogastric (NG) tube placement. If the patient requires analgesia, morphine sulfate should be avoided because it increases intraluminal pressures within the colon and causes or exacerbates the presenting symptoms or perforation. An NG tube should be placed if there is evidence of ileus or if there is intractable nausea and vomiting.

The choice of antibiotics will depend on the severity of the disease process and should cover both gram-negative bacteria and anaerobic organisms. If cultures are obtained from the diverticular abscess, antibiotic coverage can be altered according to the results of the culture. Use and dosage of aminoglycosides should depend on renal function as indicated by the creatine clearance. Patients who are immunocompromised will require broader antibiotic coverage, including an anti-*Pseudomonas* agent. IV antibiotic therapy is normally continued for 7 to 10 days and may be continued orally for an additional 7 to 10 days after discharge, depending on the severity of the illness.

Patients will usually experience relief in symptoms after 3 to 5 days of antibiotic therapy and may resume oral intake as tolerated. Once patients are able to maintain adequate nutrition and hydration, they can be discharged. A BE should be scheduled for 2 weeks after discharge to evaluate treatment.

Patients whose cases are complicated by bleeding that does not subside will require angiography to locate the site of bleeding; they may also require infusion of vasopressin (Pitressin) 0.2 to 0.3 units/min via an intra-arterial catheter placed during the radiographic procedure. If the patient shows signs and symptoms of acute blood loss, transfusion may be indicated. Twenty percent of patients who have experienced diverticular bleeding bleed again within a year.

If there is no improvement or if there is clinical deterioration after 72 hours of medical treatment, surgical intervention may be indicated. Approximately 20% to 30% of patients with the diagnosis of diverticulitis require surgical management. Surgery is usually required for patients who have had several episodes of diverticulitis within 2 years or for those who have had a single episode of diverticulitis with complications. Findings such as free peritonitis and large abscesses that do not respond to medical treatment are indications for emergent surgical intervention. The surgical procedure of choice is colon resection with a temporary colostomy. Once the inflammation and infection have resolved, the patient can undergo elective reanastomosis of the colon. Patients who have undergone the surgical procedure will require routine postoperative care, with emphasis on pain management, pulmonary hygiene, hydration, nutrition, and wound assessment.

Localized abscesses can be drained percutaneously with the assistance of the interventional radiologist. Once the inflammation and infection have resolved, the patient may require an elective single-stage colon anastomosis in which the affected portion of the colon is removed. Despite medical treatment, it is estimated that up to 40% of patients with diverticulitis continue to experience symptoms, and approximately half of these patients will need surgical intervention.

Follow-up and Referral

To evaluate or diagnose diverticular disease, all patients will require colonoscopy at some point during their disease process; therefore, referral to a gastroenterologist is indicated for symptoms that do not respond to treatment after 6 months. Early in the disease process, patients with diverticulitis should consult with a surgeon who can follow them and determine the necessity for emergent surgical intervention if complications should develop. If patients respond well to antibiotic therapy but suffer subsequent attacks of diverticulitis, they should be referred to a surgeon for elective removal of the affected portion of the bowel. Any patient who has had an acute attack of diverticulitis before age 40 will usually require surgical intervention and should be referred accordingly. Follow-up BEs can be repeated every 3 years if symptoms persist or after corrective surgery has been completed.

Patient Education

Patients diagnosed with diverticular disease will need to make modifications in their diets with an emphasis on increasing the amount of dietary fiber. Diet changes should be made slowly to avoid bloating, gas, and other GI problems that may discourage compliance. Fiber can be increased by eating bran, fresh fruits, vegetables, and whole grains. The goal of diet therapy is to avoid constipation and straining during bowel movements, which can further increase intraluminal pressures and cause complications.

Patients should also be instructed to drink at least ten 8-ounce glasses of water a day to have regular, soft bowel movements. If patients continue to have constipation despite increasing their fiber and fluid intake, a bulk-forming laxative such as psyllium (FiberCon, Metamucil) can be added.

Patients who have had a colostomy will need instruction regarding follow-up care, including how to assess the stoma and the skin (for skin breakdown); how to clean the stoma; and how to empty, reclose, and change the colostomy pouch. Diet instruction as previously discussed is important for patients with a colostomy to prevent constipation and promote bowel regularity.

Symptoms will recur in approximately one-third of all patients with diverticulitis who were initially treated with medical management. All patients with diverticular disease, therefore, should be instructed to return for follow-up if they develop signs and symptoms of infection or other associated complications of diverticulitis. Patients who present with another episode of diverticulitis warrant elective surgical resection. Patients should understand that despite adherence to diet and medication, they may have another attack.

■ COLORECTAL CANCER

Colorectal tumors are both curable and preventable; however, the systematic screening of such cancers is in its infancy. Colorectal tumor presentation can be either symptomatic or asymptomatic and is dependent on the location of the tumor. Polyps, the most benign form of tumors, are classified as hyperplastic (nonneoplastic), adenomatous (neoplastic), or submucosal (lipomas). Adenomatous polyps are believed to be the precursors to the malignant adenocarcinomas, which comprise more than 95% of all malignant tumors of the colon. Over the past 20 years, there has been a decline in the mortality rate associated with colorectal carcinoma, which has been attributed to improvement in screening, diagnosis, and treatment. Cure rates of colorectal carcinoma are estimated to be as high as 50%.

Epidemiology and Causes

Of cancers affecting both men and women, colorectal cancer is the second leading cancer killer in the United States. In 2009, 136,717 people were diagnosed with colorectal cancer and 51,848 people died from it; the incidence rate is 49.2 per 100,000 people, making colorectal cancer the third ranked incidence of top 10 cancer sites. Over a lifetime, colorectal cancer will affect 1 in 17 Americans. Approximately 148,810 individuals are diagnosed with colorectal cancer every year in the United States; the vast majority (108,070) have colon cancer, and the rest have rectal cancer.

Age is the most important risk factor for developing colorectal cancer in the United States. The risk increases steadily with age, especially after age 45, and is rare in individuals younger than age 35 unless they are predisposed to rare genetic diseases. The older adult population is at the greatest risk of developing colorectal carcinoma, with the median age at the time of diagnosis being 71 years. Colon cancer affects men and women equally; however, rectal cancers are more common in men. The overall survival rate of patients with colorectal cancer is approximately 50% to 55% and is attributed to early detection and treatment. African American males and members of low-income minority groups have, for unknown reasons, lower survival rates in comparison to national data for other groups. It is presumed—though not

proved—that the lower survival rates among minorities are in part a result of decreased accessibility to or underutilization of health care.

Seventh-Day Adventists are a religious group that subscribes to a vegetarian diet, and they also have a lower incidence of colorectal cancer. In the past, studies have shown that the Japanese have had a lower incidence of colorectal cancer; however, Japanese Americans who have adopted a diet high in fat and refined carbohydrates have a higher incidence of this type of cancer. In general, groups that migrate from areas of low to high incidence of colorectal cancer experience a change in cancer incidence that parallels that of the new region.

Other risk factors for colorectal cancer include a family history and a personal history of adenomatous polyps (multiple polyps or individual polyps greater than 1 cm in size) or colon cancer. Twenty-five percent of patients diagnosed with colon cancer have a family history of colon cancer. The risk of developing colon cancer is directly proportional to the number of first-degree relatives affected: For patients who have one first-degree relative with colon cancer, the risk increases twofold to threefold. Disorders involving increased colon mucosal cell turnover (such as inflammatory bowel disease and ulcerative colitis) have been implicated in greater risk for colon cancer. Familial adenomatous polyposis is an autosomal dominant condition that results in the development of thousands of adenomas within the colon but accounts for less than 1% of colon cancers. Other hereditary conditions that increase the chance of developing colorectal cancer include Peutz-Jeghers syndrome, Gardner's syndrome, and Turcot syndrome. Patients with a family history or personal history of gynecological (breast, ovarian, endometrial) cancers and individuals diagnosed with Barrett's esophagus also have an increased risk of developing colon carcinoma.

Although the etiology of colorectal cancer (adenomas) is unknown, both environmental and genetic factors have been implicated. Geographical variances and a positive correlation in the incidence of disease among migrant workers both suggest that environmental factors play a role. Diets high in fat, red meat, and refined carbohydrates and low in plant fiber have been correlated with the areas of highest incidence of colorectal cancer, whereas areas with the lowest incidence of colorectal cancer have diets high in fiber and rich in vegetables and fruits. It has been theorized that the excess fat interacts with colonic bacteria to form deconjugated bile acids, which have been associated with tumor-producing activity, increased deposition of fatty acids within the cell membranes, and increased synthesis of prostaglandins, which further stimulates cell proliferation. Ketosteroids are thought to be metabolic byproducts of cholesterol that induce genetic damage and have been found in higher concentrations among high-risk populations. Products of pyrolysis—decomposition of organic matter secondary to increases in temperature such as those resulting from char-broiling and frying—have also been implicated in carcinoma of the colon. Geographical areas with low levels of selenium also have higher incidence of colorectal cancer.

Conversely, diets high in fiber tend to reduce the transit time within the colon, thus decreasing exposure to potentially carcinogenic substances and altering the gut flora and decreasing fecal pH. (Populations with the highest incidence of colorectal cancer have an associated higher fecal pH.) When fecal contents take longer to transit the bowel, the deionized bile acids and free fatty acids stay in contact with the intestinal mucosa, which has been associated with development of colorectal cancer.

Pathophysiology

Adenocarcinomas account for more than 95% of colorectal malignancies. The evolution from adenoma to invasive carcinoma can take up to 10 years. *Adenomas* are benign neoplasms composed of granular epithelium that are not capable of metastasis or invasion of the muscularis mucosa. They are either sessile (attached by a broad base) or pedunculated (attached by a stalk). Most smaller adenomas (less than 1 cm in diameter) are of the tubular type, and less than 1% contain carcinoma. As the polyps increase in size (greater than 2 cm in diameter), they begin to show villous changes with increasing dysplasia; the chance of one of these polyps containing cancer is about 50%.

Most adenocarcinomas of the colon form hard, nodular areas that grow irregularly. Colon cancers are staged or classified according to histological changes in the infiltrative character of the tumor. The most common classifications used today are the Joint Committee Classification, Duke's staging system, and the tumor-node-metastasis system (Table 11.18). Histologically, colon cancers vary from well-differentiated cells that appear normal (grade 1) to highly anaplastic, poorly differentiated cells (grade 4). The accuracy of specimen collection is crucial. The most accurate method of evaluating a polyp is by removing the entire lesion for cytological examination. If the polyp is less than 7 mm in diameter, tissue for biopsy can be obtained while the polyp is destroyed through "hot" (fulguration) biopsy.

Metastatic progression of colon cancer usually involves spread by local invasion, lymphatic extension with

Table 11.18	Staging Classifications of Colorectal Cancer	
Tumor-Node-Metastasis (TNM) Class*	Description	Staging Groups
Tis	Carcinoma in situ	Stage 0
T1	Tumor invades submucosa. • Greater than 80% 5-year survival	• Tis N0M0 Stage I
T2	Tumor invades muscularis.	• T1N0M0 (Duke's classification Stage A) • T2N0M0 (Duke's classification Stage B1) Stage IIA
T3	Tumor penetrates through bowel wall. • 60%–80% 5-year survival	• T3N0M0 (Duke's classification Stage B2) Stage IIB • T4N0M0 (Duke's classification Stage B3)
T4	Tumor invades adjacent organ.	Stage IIIA
Any T	Any bowel wall perforation with lymph node involvement. • 20%–50% 5-year survival	• T1–2N1M0 (Duke's classification Stage C3) Stage IIIB
N0	No regional lymph node involvement.	• T3–4N1M0 (Duke's classification Stage C2–3)
N1	One to three pericolic or perirectal lymph nodes.	Stage IIIC
N2	Four or more pericolic or perirectal lymph nodes.	• Any T, N2M0 (Duke's classification Stage C1–3)
N3	Metastasis to lymph nodes along a vascular trunk.	Stage IV
M0	No metastasis.	• Any T, Any N, M1 (Duke's classification Stage D)
M1	Distant metastasis. • Less than 25% 5-year survival	

*American Joint Committee on Cancer.

spread to the mesenteric lymph nodes first, and then hematogenous spread through the portal system to the liver. In some patients, the cancer metastasizes throughout the peritoneal cavity and to the lungs. Rectal carcinoma spreads by direct extension through the perirectal fat to the lymph nodes and less often to the lungs and distant organs through hemorrhoidal circulation. Prognosis of colorectal carcinoma is a function of several factors, including poorly differentiated tissue histology, mucin production, aneuploidy (DNA abnormalities), tumor invasion to other organs, perforation, and venous involvement. The prognosis is not influenced by tumor size.

Colon cancers can develop as polyps within the lumen of the intestine or as a mass on the wall of the colon. Bulky polypoid tumors are more common within the right colon, whereas tumors that encircle the bowel, causing obstruction, are more common on the left side of the colon. Tumor growth is normally slow and, in most cases, is asymptomatic until the tumor becomes large. Diagnosis is usually made late in the course of the disease, often after metastasis, thereby making a surgical cure difficult. Colon cancers that produce intracellular mucin are called "signet ring"–type carcinomas; these tumors have a tendency to be more aggressive in their spread.

Several types of colon cancers have been linked to specific genetic defects. Hereditary nonpolyposis colorectal cancers include two autosomal dominant conditions that have been associated with a markedly increased risk for developing colon cancer. Although these patients have few or no adenomatous polyps, individuals diagnosed with Lynch syndrome I are at increased risk of developing colon cancer at an early age. This cancer has a propensity for the right side of the colon. Lynch syndrome II includes the features of Lynch syndrome I as well as an increased risk of developing tumors within the ovary, uterus, urinary tract, and stomach.

Clinical Presentation

Subjective

Signs and symptoms in patients with colorectal cancer will vary, depending on the tumor size, anatomical location, and associated complications, if any. There are very few early warning signs of colorectal carcinoma; in fact, most individuals are totally asymptomatic. Frequently, the cancer is found incidentally during abdominal surgery or during screening sigmoidoscopy.

Patients may present with melena or bright red bleeding from the rectum, depending on the location of the tumor. A change in bowel habits, including constipation alternating with diarrhea or a change in stool caliber (described as narrowed or ribbonlike), can be signs of colon cancer. Stools streaked with blood may be mistakenly dismissed as a sign of hemorrhoidal irritation. Abdominal pain is a rare presenting symptom but may

indicate obstruction resulting from tumors on the left side of the colon, which has a smaller diameter lumen, or from invasion of the bowel wall by a tumor. Patients rarely report colicky pain as a result of a right-sided colon cancer because of the larger diameter of the colon and the liquid consistency of the stool. Patients with rectal cancer may complain of tenesmus (spasm of the anal sphincter), urgency, and/or hematochezia. Patients with chronic occult blood loss from an undiagnosed tumor may experience weakness and fatigue caused by iron-deficiency anemia. Weight loss and anorexia are common with any malignant process but are usually manifested late in the disease process.

Objective

Physical exam may reveal a mass within the abdomen or an enlarged liver, which may be suggestive of metastasis. A digital rectal exam should be done even though most tumors are not palpable. The stool should be tested for occult blood, which, if positive, is pathognomonic for right-sided colon cancer. Approximately 50% of patients with a positive fecal occult blood test have either an adenoma (38%) or a neoplasm (12%). Conversely, fecal occult blood testing is positive in only 60% to 70% of patients with known large intestinal cancers; however, annual screening can reduce colorectal mortality rates by 33%.

Diagnostic Reasoning

Diagnostic Tests

Although there are no definitive laboratory tests for diagnosis of colorectal cancer, a complete blood count should be obtained to assess for iron-deficiency anemia or anemia of chronic blood loss, either of which can be a common finding in patients with colorectal cancer. Liver function tests may reveal an elevation of the liver enzymes, especially of alkaline phosphatase if there has been metastasis to the liver and/or bone. Usually, when there is liver metastasis, the bilirubin level tends to remain normal until late in the disease process.

The serum immune assay for carcinoembryonic antigen (CEA) was developed with the intent of providing an early means of detection for colon cancer; however, the test is too insensitive and nonspecific for screening. CEA levels have been poorly correlated with the stage of cancer; however, this test is useful for monitoring a patient's response to therapy, whether surgical or chemotherapeutic. CEA levels usually normalize after colon resection, and levels that remain elevated are associated with poor prognosis. A secondary spike in the CEA level after surgery is highly suggestive of recurrence and must be evaluated.

Colonoscopy with a biopsy and barium enema (BE) are used to establish definitive diagnosis of colorectal cancer. Air contrast BE enables the radiologist to detect small defects or lesions within the intestinal mucosa.

Colonoscopy is a more specific and sensitive test that can be used as follow-up to the findings of the BE; colonoscopy can also be used by itself to provide more definitive data through the biopsy of the suspect lesions. Colonoscopy establishes the diagnosis of colon cancer with almost 100% accuracy and is thus the diagnostic procedure of choice. Flexible sigmoidoscopy can be used for confirming lesions within the rectosigmoid area; however, full colon examination with colonoscopy is preferred. Computed tomography (CT) scan is used for evaluation of distant metastasis. Endoscopic ultrasound has been used to stage regional rectal cancers and is more accurate than CT scan in this particular area.

Patients with colonic polyps will require histological examination of the polyp. Polyps larger than 7 mm should be totally removed by snare cautery. Polyps that are less than 7 mm in size are usually not malignant and can be removed by "hot" biopsy, which destroys the polyp while obtaining the necessary tissue for cytological exam.

Differential Diagnosis

The symptoms of colorectal cancer are nonspecific; therefore, many disease processes can mimic the presenting symptoms of colon carcinoma and must be differentiated from it. Most of the inflammatory and irritable bowel disease processes can be confused with colon carcinoma. Ischemic colitis, diverticular disease, irritable bowel syndrome, inflammatory bowel disease, or infectious colitis can form strictures within the bowel that are indistinguishable from colon carcinoma. Colonoscopy with biopsy of the lesion is the diagnostic procedure of choice. Any patient older than age 50 who presents with iron-deficiency anemia, stool positive for occult blood, change in bowel habits, or hematochezia should have a thorough evaluation to rule out the possibility of neoplasm.

Management

The first step in the treatment of colon cancer is the staging of the disease. The staging of the cancer is of critical importance not only for the determination of the patient's long-term survival but also for determining which patients should receive adjuvant therapy. Staging of a neoplasm first involves understanding the characteristics used to describe the histological findings: tissue of origin (adenocarcinoma, sarcoma), origin of specimen (colon, breast), and the degree of tissue differentiation. Staging of the carcinoma includes both the primary site and the metastatic sites and allows for the development of the most optimal treatment plan based on those findings. More than half of all cancers are not curable using approved treatments available today. Many of the treatment regimens involve some form of experimental drugs or procedures; therefore, accurate staging is necessary to determine the efficacy of the treatment.

The only known cure for colon cancer is surgical resection. This is the treatment of choice for all patients who can tolerate the surgery. Even patients who have known metastasis can benefit from surgical intervention to reduce the chance of developing an intestinal obstruction or rectal hemorrhage later in the disease process. Most patients with colorectal cancer present with penetration of the mass through the bowel wall and with associated lymph node involvement. The surgeon will decide, based on the staging, what type of surgical resection is appropriate. The anatomical location of the tumor—left or right side of the colon—will dictate whether left or right hemicolectomy is performed. A wide margin of intestine (with careful ligation of the total arterial blood supply) will be resected to ensure that mesenteric and associated lymph node drainage is removed.

Lesions located within the rectosigmoid area are usually treated with anterior resection, which protects the rectal sphincter. (The rectum is the distal 8–11 cm of large bowel.) If the rectal lesions are small and are discovered early, they can sometimes be treated by local incision, laser photoablation, or cryosurgery. Larger lesions located within this lower portion of the large bowel usually require a combination of abdominal-perineal resection with a colostomy. Unresectable rectal cancers can be palliated with a diverting colostomy, or, if the patient is a poor surgical candidate, laser fulguration of the tumor mass can minimize the bleeding and maintain the patency of the rectum.

Adjuvant chemotherapy for colon cancer is based on the stage of the disease (see Table 11.18). From 6 months to 1 year of chemotherapy with 5-fluorouracil (5-FU) and levamisole continues to be the treatment of choice for carcinomas classified as stage III (node-positive) and, although it is not curative, it enhances the survival rate. Evaluation of the treatment is based on the initial response of the tumor to the therapy (e.g., shrinkage), as well as improvement in the 5-year survival rate.

Rectal carcinomas are typically treated with chemotherapy and radiation therapy. Radiation therapy for rectal cancer may involve both preoperative and postoperative radiation therapy. Depending on the size of the tumor, preoperative radiation therapy can help shrink the tumor, making it more amenable to resection. Postoperative combination therapy with 5-FU and radiation therapy has been effective in reducing both local and metastatic node occurrences.

Twenty percent of patients with colorectal cancer have known metastases at the time of diagnosis. Patients with known metastases to the liver may have improved survival rates with resection. Some patients with liver metastases have opted for infusions of 5-FU into the hepatic artery or portal vein, which has proved superior in the treatment of hepatic disease; however, this treatment has little effect on the overall survival rate for colorectal cancer and can be extremely toxic to the patient. Radiation therapy is often employed as a palliative measure for patients whose pain has been unresponsive to chemotherapy or other treatment modalities.

Although the oncologist will manage the patient's chemotherapy, the primary-care practitioner will continue to work closely with the patient to treat any of the numerous adverse effects caused by the chemotherapy and/or the radiation therapy. The potential toxic effects of adjuvant therapy for colorectal cancer are numerous and can range from nausea, vomiting, and weight loss to cystitis and radiation proctitis. Radiation therapy to the pelvic area can cause severe gastrointestinal disorders, including intractable diarrhea and even malabsorption syndromes.

Follow-up and Referral

Initial assessment and screening for colorectal carcinoma is the responsibility of every primary-care provider. Patients who are known to be at higher risk for the development of colorectal cancer, such as those who have a first-degree relative with the disease, a family history of adenomas, a personal history of adenomas or colorectal cancer, or a long-standing history of inflammatory bowel disease, will require a more in-depth screening by a practitioner who is well trained in this area. Screening for high-risk patients should include colonoscopy, which is best done by an experienced gastroenterologist. The recommended screening for average- and high-risk individuals is provided in Screening Recommendations/Guidelines 11.1.

Follow-up is vitally important in the treatment of colorectal cancer. In an effort to prevent recurrence, scheduled colon surveillance is required. Early detection and removal of adenomas can improve survival rates.

Close surveillance is necessary for patients who have undergone "curative resection" surgery. Recommendations include office visits every 3 months, which should include a CEA level, an annual CT of the abdomen and pelvis, and a chest x-ray film for the first 3 years postoperatively. A colonoscopy should be completed postoperatively; but, if the exam was not completed at that time, a colonoscopy should be scheduled for 3 months postoperatively and then again at 1 year, with special attention to anastomotic recurrences. If the results of the exam are within normal limits, patients may continue with follow-up exams every 3 years. Patients whose CEA levels normalize or stabilize after surgery and then spike suddenly require a thorough examination.

Patients who have undergone surgical resection for colon cancer and have a temporary or permanent colostomy may benefit from assistance from an enterostomal therapist. Consultation with a urologist for urological or sexual dysfunction resulting from surgical or radiation therapy may provide medical and social support. Patients suffering from metastatic disease can be referred to hospice service personnel, who are trained in providing comfort and support to both the family and the patient. They can give guidance regarding home and hospital care and are specially trained in providing appropriate analgesia for patients. Criteria for admission to the hospice program differ from one area to another; most require a physician statement that the patient has less than 6 months to live and is receiving only palliative or supportive treatments. Some hospice services require patients to have a "do not resuscitate" (DNR) order in place as a condition for admission.

Screening Recommendations/Guidelines 11.1 Colon Cancer Screening Recommended by the American Cancer Society

Risk	Screening Recommendations
Average risk	Annual fecal occult blood (FOB) test
	Flexible sigmoidoscopy every 5 years beginning at age 50 or colonoscopy every 10 years
High risk (general)	Annual FOB testing
	Double-contrast barium enema
	OR
	Colonoscopy every 3–5 years starting at age 40
Specific High-Risk Groups	
Prior colorectal cancer	Colonoscopy 1 year postfinding, then every 3 years
Hereditary nonpolyposis colorectal cancers	Colonoscopy screening must begin 10 years before the age at onset of the earliest affected family member
	OR
	Colonoscopy every 1–2 years beginning at age 20–25 and continuing until age 35 and then yearly
Inflammatory bowel disease	Annual colonoscopy beginning 8 years after onset of disease
First-degree family history	Colonoscopy every 3–5 years beginning 5 years before the age at onset of the youngest affected relative

Patient Education

Patient education should focus first on the prevention of colon cancer, stressing a diet that is low in fat and refined carbohydrates and high in fiber, fruits, vegetables, and complex carbohydrates. Some studies have shown favorable statistics when individuals supplement their diets with vitamins E and C and beta carotene and pursue a lifestyle that includes exercise. The risk/benefit/cost ratio makes these preventive measures worth suggesting.

■ HEMORRHOIDS

Hemorrhoids are defined as a mass of dilated and tortuous veins that represent prolapsed submucosal tissue. Hemorrhoids are classified as either internal or external, depending on their location. The primary cause of hemorrhoids is believed to be straining during defecation, which is further complicated by constipation, prolonged sitting, pregnancy, and anal infection. Some hemorrhoids are asymptomatic and require no treatment and typically resolve on their own within 3 weeks; others can result in profuse bleeding, requiring emergency ligation.

Epidemiology and Causes

Every year approximately 1 million people, or 5% of the American population, visit their medical provider for symptoms of hemorrhoids. Although hemorrhoids can occur at any age, their incidence increases with age.

Although the cause of hemorrhoids is not completely known or understood, they are common in countries where there is a known deficiency of dietary fiber. Thus, increased straining during defecation has been recognized as an important predisposing factor in the development of hemorrhoids. Heredity may also be a factor because 10% of the patients with hemorrhoids have a family history of the disease. Patients suffering from illnesses characterized by chronic diarrhea, such as inflammatory bowel disease, are also more likely to develop hemorrhoids.

Pathophysiology

External hemorrhoids are dilated varicose veins originating from the inferior hemorrhoidal plexus and are located below the anal-rectal line. Internal hemorrhoids are a dilation of the veins within the superior hemorrhoidal plexus and are located within the distal rectum and the anal canal.

The inferior hemorrhoidal plexus is prone to increased distention during defecation, which can result in rupture of a vessel and subsequent development of a perianal hematoma or thrombus within one of the vessels of the plexus. Patients who have a thrombosed hemorrhoid may present with a painful perianal lump.

Internal hemorrhoids are further classified by the degree of prolapse present. Table 11.19 describes the difference between each degree of prolapse.

Table 11.19	Classification of Internal Hemorrhoids
Severity	**Description of the Process**
First degree	Protrude into the lumen of the anal canal, usually without the sensation of protrusion.
Second degree	Protrude beyond the anal canal during defecation but spontaneously reduce when defecation is completed.
Third degree	Protrude beyond the anal canal during defecation but must be manually reduced after the completion of the bowel movement.
Fourth degree	Protrude beyond the anal canal and are permanently prolapsed despite attempts at manual reduction.

Clinical Presentation

Subjective

External hemorrhoids may present with an abrupt onset of pain that is associated with the development of a perianal lump. Many patients complain of more intense pain after defecation or other straining maneuvers, which result in further inflammation and engorgement. Mucus discharge from the anus can lead to poor hygiene and complaints of pruritus. The natural history of a resolved hemorrhoid is the formation of external skin tags, which are asymptomatic but may be irritating and interfere with daily hygiene.

Objective

On physical examination, external hemorrhoids may not be visible at rest but usually protrude on standing or with the Valsalva maneuver. Thrombosed hemorrhoids may appear as shiny, blue masses located at the anus. Evidence of hemorrhoidal skin tags may appear at the site of resolved hemorrhoids; these skin tags are fibrotic and painless.

Internal hemorrhoids most often present with rectal bleeding described as bright red streaks on the toilet paper. Patients may report that blood actually drips into the toilet after a bowel movement. Occasionally the bleeding is sufficient enough to cause anemia, which in any case merits further investigation.

Diagnostic Reasoning

Diagnostic Tests

Initial diagnosis is made by visual inspection of the anal area. Digital rectal examination is not considered an accurate means of diagnosis because most internal hemorrhoids are soft swellings that usually are not palpable, nor are they painful unless they have thrombosed or become infected, or unless a fissure has developed. External hemorrhoids can usually be diagnosed at physical exam, whereas internal hemorrhoids are visible on physical examination only if they have prolapsed.

Definitive diagnosis of internal hemorrhoids requires anoscopy for a proper inspection of the anal canal. With the anoscope in place, the patient is asked to strain as he or she would while having a bowel movement so that the degree of prolapse can be assessed. Patients may undergo proctosigmoidoscopy to effectively rule out any precipitating or coexisting diseases of the colon or rectum.

Differential Diagnosis

The differential diagnosis of hemorrhoids includes polyps, carcinoma of the anus, anorectal fistula, cryptitis, papillitis, or rectal prolapse. Proctosigmoidoscopy is an effective means of establishing the appropriate diagnosis.

Management

Initial treatment for symptomatic external hemorrhoids is focused on adequate pain relief with oral analgesia and sitz baths. If the hemorrhoids do not spontaneously regress, care is directed at decreasing straining with defecation and modification of toilet habits. Patients are encouraged to avoid sitting on the toilet for long periods of time, to use some form of bulk-forming laxative, and to increase their daily fiber intake slowly to 25 to 35 grams to establish regular, formed stools. Patients who suffer from diarrhea should be treated accordingly to control frequent loose stools. Individuals who suffer from pruritus should be instructed to maintain anal hygiene. Sitz baths, witch hazel, and application of topical hydrocortisone creams are all effective in controlling pruritus. If the external hemorrhoids continue to be painful or bothersome despite treatment, referral for surgical excision should be made.

Medical treatment of internal hemorrhoids follows the same principles previously outlined, with attention toward avoiding straining during defecation, modification of diet with the addition of fiber, increasing fluids, and the addition of bulking agents. If medical treatment is not effective, there are a number of nonsurgical treatments that may be employed. First-degree hemorrhoids can be treated by injection sclerotherapy or infrared coagulation. Infrared coagulation, much like electrocoagulation, uses high-intensity light to shrink the swelling. Second- and third-degree hemorrhoids are normally treated with rubber-band ligation, in which a rubber-banded ring is placed around the base of the hemorrhoid. This band acts a tourniquet, strangulating the tissue while fixing the mucosa proximal to the ligation into the muscularis. All of the nonsurgical techniques used to treat internal hemorrhoids are associated with some degree of pain and bleeding.

Large, advanced-degree hemorrhoids will most often require referral to a surgeon for a formal hemorrhoidectomy. Again, proper anal hygiene and correction of chronic constipation and diarrhea are essential to prevent the recurrence of hemorrhoids.

Follow-up and Referral

Excision of a single external hemorrhoid, evacuation of a thrombosed external hemorrhoid, and injection sclerotherapy of simple internal hemorrhoids can all be performed in the office by a trained provider. Band ligation and other specialized treatment of hemorrhoids will require referral to a gastroenterologist more familiar with these procedures. Follow-up will be based on the patient's postprocedure course. Most patients will require no further care except for instruction on proper anal hygiene and diet. The addition of a nonirritating laxative after the procedure will usually prevent the development of constipation and the associated fear of defecation.

Patient Education

Patient education for hemorrhoids is aimed at preventing the problem through increasing fiber in the diet. Fiber should be increased to 25 to 35 g/day, but this should be done slowly to prevent bloating and gas formation. Teaching patients to read the labels of their food can help them gain control over their nutrition. Often, patients associate salad and cereal with very high levels of fiber. This is not accurate information in many cases; for example, most breakfast cereals have only 1 to 3 g of fiber per serving, and iceberg lettuce has very little fiber as well. Over-the-counter bulking agents, such as psyllium (Metamucil), can be suggested to help eliminate constipation. It is important to teach patients the necessity of drinking no less than 64 ounces of water a day.

References

Evidence-Based Practice

Centers for Disease Control and Prevention. Deaths: Preliminary data for 2011. *Natl Vital Stat Rep* 61(6):1–5, 2012. Retrieved from www.cdc.gov/nchs/data/nvsr61/nvrs61_61_06.pdf

Chey, WD, and Wong, BCY. American College of Gastroenterology guideline on management of *Helicobacter pylori* infection. *Am J Gastroenterol* 102:1808–1825, 2007.

Jacobson, MA. The effect of hepatitis G coinfection on HIV disease progression. Presented at University of California–San Francisco, Positive Health Program at San Francisco General Hospital,

Journal Club, January 7, 2002. Retrieved from http://hivinsite .ucsf.edu/InSite?page=md-rr-01&ss=xsl/conf-sl&slide=2

Kaptchuk, TJ, et al. Components of placebo effect: Randomised controlled trial in patients with irritable bowel syndrome. *BMJ* 336(7651):999–1003, 2008.

Piascik, M, and Sanders, ME. Probiotic supplementation: What nurse practitioners need to know to recommend safe and effective formulations. Power-Pak C.E.: Continuing Education for Pharmacists and Pharmacy Technicians. Retrieved from http://powerpak.com/course/content/108730.

Bibliography

General

Bascom, A. *Incorporating herbal medicine into clinical practice.* FA Davis, Philadelphia, 2002.

Carey, WD. The prevalence and natural history of hepatitis B in the 21st century. *Cleve Clin J Medicine,* 2009, May; 76 Suppl 3:S2–5.

Centers for Disease Control and Prevention. *National ambulatory medical care survey: 2010 survey.* Retrieved from www.cdc.gov/nchs/data/ahcd/namcs_summary/2010_namcs_web_tables.pdf

Centers for Disease Control and Prevention. Deaths: Preliminary data for 2011. *Natl Vital Stat Rep* 61(6):1–5, 2012. Retrieved from www.cdc.gov/nchs/data/nvsr61/nvrs61_61_06.pdf

Dambro, MR. *Griffith's 5-minute clinical consult.* Lippincott Williams & Wilkins, Philadelphia, 2013.

Edmunds, MW, and Mayhew, MS. *Pharmacology for the primary care provider,* ed 4. Mosby/Elsevier, St. Louis, MO, 2013.

Fauci, AS, et al (Eds.). *Harrison's principles of internal medicine,* ed 18. McGraw-Hill, New York, 2011.

Huether, SE. Alterations in digestive function. In McCance, KL, and Huether, SE (Eds.), *Pathophysiology: The biologic basis for disease in adults and children,* ed 6. Mosby, St. Louis, MO, 2010, pp 1420–1515.

Kahrilas, PJ, et al. American Gastroenterological Association medical position statement on the management of gastroesophageal reflux disease. *Gastroenterology, 135*(4), 1383–1391, 2008.

Kee, JL. *Laboratory and diagnostic tests with nursing implications,* ed 8. Prentice-Hall, Upper Saddle River, NJ, 2010.

Papadakis, MA, and McPhee, SJ. *Current medical diagnosis and treatment,* ed 52. Lange/McGraw-Hill, New York, 2013.

Liver, Biliary, and Pancreatic Diseases

Afdhal, NZ. Epidemiology of and risk factors for gallstones. UpToDate Online. Retrieved from www.uptodate.com/online/content/topic.do?topicKey=biliaryt/5497&selectedTitle=4%7E150&source=search_result.

Bernadette Wilkie, J. Identifying and managing hepatitis C in the community. *Prim Health Care* 23(4):22–25, 2013.

Campos-Outcalt, D. Hepatitis C: New CDC screening recommendations. *J Fam Pract* 61(12):744–746, 2012.

Centers for Disease Control and Prevention. Updated CDC recommendations for the management of hepatitis B virus–infected health-care providers and students. *MMWR Recomme Rep* 61(RR-3):1–12, 2012.

Duke, RD. Demystifying the liver and its diseases. *Clin Advisor* 15(2):27–34, 2012.

Heliobacter pylori: Toward effective eradication. *Clin Advsor* 15(3), 20–26, 2012.

Krebbeks, VP, and Cunningham, VM. A DNP nurse-managed hepatitis C clinic, improving quality of life for those in a rural area. *Online J Rural Nurs Health Care* 13(1):127–148, 2013.

Lok, AS, and Pawlotshy, JM. Viral hepatitis at a crossroad. *Gastroenterology* 142(6):1261–1263, 2012.

Maasoumy, B, and Wedemeyer, H. Natural history of acute and chronic hepatitis C. *Best Pract Res Clin Gastroenterol* 26(4):401–412, 2012.

Medical Services Commission. *Abnormal liver chemistry—Evaluation and interpretation.* British Columbia Medical Services Commission, Victoria, BC, 2011.

National Guideline Clearinghouse. Hepatitis C. 2010. Retrieved from www.guideline.gov/content.aspx?id=24042

O'Brien, S. The clinical importance of hepatitis C genotyping in the United States. *MLO Med Lab Observer* 45(11):16–17, 2013.

Ranson, JH, et al. Prognostic signs and the role of operative management in acute pancreatitis. *Surg Gynecol Obstet* 139(1):69–81, 1974.

Sachs, CJ, and Kaku, S. Abdominal pain: A rational approach, part 1. *Consultant* 52(10):693–705, 2012.

Sacks-Davis, R, et al. Identifying newly acquired cases of hepatitis C using surveillance: A literature review. *Epidemiol Infect* 140(11):1925–1934, 2012.

Yu, ML, et al. Sustained hepatitis C virus clearance and increased hepatitis B surface antigen seroclearance in pathients with dual chronic hepatitis C and B during posttreatment follow-up. *Hepatology* 57(6):2135–2142, 2013.

Zheng, MH, et al. Interleukin-28B rs129860C/T and rs8099917T/G contribute to spontaneous clearance of hepatitis C virus in Caucasians. *Gene* 518(2):479–482, 2013.

Upper Gastrointestinal Diseases

Crosby, K, and Dexter, K. Clinical evaluation of peptic ulcer disease. *Clin Advisor* 16(6):42–103, 2013.

Crowe, SE. Treatment regimens for *Helicobacter pylori.* UpToDate Online. Retrieved from www.uptodate.com/online/content/topic.do?topicKey=acidpep/10778&selectedTitle=1%7E150&source=search_result

Evans, JA, et al; ASGE Standards of Practice Committee. The role of endoscopy in Barrett's esophagus and other premalignant conditions of the esophagus. *Gastrointest Endosc* 76(6):1087–1094, 2012.

Feldman, MJ. J. Edward Berk distinguished lecture: Gastric acid secretion still relevant? *Am J Gastroenterol* 108(3):347–352, 2013.

Kahrilas, PJ. Medical management of gastroesophageal reflux disease in adults. UpToDate. Online. Retrieved from www.uptodate.com/online/content/topic.do?topicKey=eso_dis/4448&selectedTitle=1%7E150&source=search_result

Katz, PO, et al. Guidelines for the diagnosis and management of gastroesophageal reflux disease. *Am J Gastroenterol* 108(3):308–328, 2013.

National Guideline Clearinghouse. ASGE guideline: The role of endoscopy in the surveillance of premalignant conditions of the upper GI tract. Retrieved from www.guideline.gove/summary/summary.aspx?doc_id=9306&nbr=004976&string=p

Ruttecki, GW. Less is more: A restrictive transfusion policy for acute GI bleeding. *Consultant* 53(2):89, 2013.

Shaheen, NJ, et al. Upper endoscopy for gastroesophageal reflux disease: Best practice advice from the clinical guidelines committee of the American College of Physicians. *Ann Intern Med* 157(11):808–816, 2012.

Soll, AH. Overview of the natural history and treatment of peptic ulcer disease. UpToDate Online. Retrieved from www.uptodate.com/online/content/topic.do?topicKey=acidpep/7085&selectedTitle=1%7E150&source=search_result

Thorn, AR. Not just another case of nausea and vomiting: A review of postinfectious gastroparesis. *J Am Acad Nurse Pract* 22(3):125–133, 2010.

Tsuboi, K, et al. Role of the lower esophageal sphincter on esophageal acid exposure—A review of over 2000 patients. *Tropic Gastroenterol* 33(2):107–111, 2012.

Wright, W. Diagnosis and treatment of heartburn: An update on therapies. *Adv Nurse Pract* 18(4):25–30, 2010.

Yuan, Y, and Hunt, RH. Evolving issues in the management of reflux disease? *Curr Opin Gastroenterol* 25(4):342–351, 2009.

Lower Gastrointestinal Diseases

Anastasi, JK, et al. Symptom management for irritable bowel syndrome: A pilot randomized controlled trial of acupuncture/moxibustion. *Gastroenterol Nurs* 32(4):243–255, 2009.

Ashktorab, H, et al. A 50-year review of colorectal cancer in African Americans: Implications for prevention and treatment. *Digest Dis Sci* 54(9):1985–1990, 2009.

Bakken, JS, et al. Treating *Clostridium difficile* infection with fecal microbiota transplantation. *Clin Gastroenterol Hepatol* 9(12):1044–1049, 2011.

Bautista, M, et al. Surgical outcomes in the elderly with inflammatory bowel disease are similar to those in the younger population. *Digestive Dis Sci* 58(10):2955–2962, 2013.

Ben-Horin, S, et al. Optimizing anti-TNF treatments in inflammatory bowel disease. *Autoimmunity Rev* 13(1):24–30, 2014.

Centers for Disease Control and Prevention. Age-adjusted invasive cancer incidence rates for the 10 primary sites with the highest rates within race and ethnic specific categories. 2009. Retrieved from www.cdc.gov/uscs/toptencancers.aspx

Kong, AP. Anorectal complaints: Office diagnosis and treatment, part 1. *Consultant* 52(8):567–570, 2012.

Leahy, Y. Inflammatory bowel disease: Patient education using Web-based resources. *Gastroenterol Nurs* 32(6):415–418, 2009.

National Guideline Clearinghouse. ASGE guideline: Colorectal cancer screening and surveillance. Retrieved from www.guideline.gov/summary/summary.aspx?ss=15&doc_id=10162&nbr=5347

Ng, SC, et al. Systematic review: The efficacy of herbal therapy in inflammatory bowel disease. *Alimentary Pharmacol Therapeutics* 38(8):854–863, 2013.

Panaccione, R, et al. Adalimumab maintains remission of Crohn's disease after up to 4 years of treatment: Data from CHARM and ADHERE. *Alimentary Pharmacol Therapeutics* 38(10):1236–1247, 2013.

Parikh, V. Jejunal diverticulosis. *Consultant* 53(4):283, 2013.

Peppercorn, MA. Definition of and risk factors for inflammatory bowel disease. UpToDate Online. Retrieved from www.uptodate.com/online/content/topic.do?topicKey=inflambd/4555&selectedTitle=19%7E150&source=search_result

Peppercorn, MA. Clinical manifestations, diagnosis and prognosis of Crohn's disease in adults. UpToDate Online. Retrieved from www.uptodate.com/online/content/topic.do?topicKey=inflambd/5518&selectedTitle=4%7E150&source=search_result

Randall, B. Celiac disease. *Clin Advisor* 14(12):103–106, 2011.

Rietdijk, ST, and D'Haens, GR. Recent developments in the treatment of inflammatory bowel disease. *J Digestive Dis* 14(6):282–287, 2013.

Richman, E, and Rhodes, JM. Review article: Evidence-based dietary advice for patients with inflammatory bowel disease. *Alimentary Pharmacol Therapeutics* 38(10):1156–1171, 2013.

Rubin, RN. Man with melena and epigastric pain. *Consultant* 52(11):747–748, 2012.

Shanahan, F. The microbiota in inflammatory bowel disease: Friend, bystander, and sometime-villain. *Nutr Rev* 79(S1):S31–S37, 2012.

Speight, RA, and Mansfield, JC. Drug advances in inflammatory bowel disease. *Clin Med* 13(4):378–382, 2013.

Stake-Nilsson, K, et al. A qualitative study of complementary and alternative medicine use in persons with uninvestigated dyspepsia. *Gastroenterol Nurs* 32(2):107–114, 2009.

Resources

American Liver Foundation
800-223-0179
www.liverfoundation.org
Crohn's and Colitis Foundation of America
386 Park Avenue, South, 17th Floor
New York, NY, 10016-8804
800-932-2423 ext. 12
www.ccfa.org

International Foundation for Bowel Disfunction
P.O. Box 17864
Milwaukee, WI 53217
414-241-9479

Renal Problems

Debbie J. Nogueras, PhD, MSN, ANP/FNP-BC • Debera J. Thomas, DNS, RN, FNP/ANP • Brian Oscar Porter, MD, PhD, MPH

Chapter 12

COMMON COMPLAINTS

■ DYSURIA

Dysuria is the subjective experience of pain or a burning sensation on urination and can include frequency, hesitancy, urgency, and strangury (slow, painful urination). Symptoms of dysuria can be secondary to several different medical conditions or certain medications; for example, a light burning sensation or discomfort can be normal when associated with concentrated acidic urine. Dysuria is most commonly associated with lower urinary system infection.

Differential Diagnosis

Dysuria is most often associated with a bladder problem and rarely with renal disease. Inflammatory lesions of the prostate, bladder, and urethra—including prostatitis in men, urethrotrigonitis in women, and bladder and urethral infections in men and women—are the most common causes of dysuria. When caused by bladder problems, frequency of urination usually occurs secondary to diminished bladder capacity or with pain when the bladder becomes distended. Urinary frequency may be a manifestation of urinary incontinence and can occur with prostatic hypertrophy or neurogenic bladder disorders.

Other conditions associated with dysuria are bladder tumors, chronic renal failure, nephrolithiasis, and occasionally diseases of the upper urinary system. Dysuria may also be associated with diseases outside the renal system such as sexually transmitted diseases, vaginitis, or prostatitis. For example, female patients may present with symptoms of dysuria or external irritation from the urine passing over the irritated labia. The dysuria may or may not be accompanied by vaginal discharge. Any woman who presents with dysuria should be questioned about an associated vaginal discharge or irritation. The symptoms of dysuria may lead to other diagnoses, including urethral strictures, prolapsed uterus, pelvic peritonitis, cancer of the cervix or prostate, dysmenorrhea, and conditions of the prostate. Prescribed medications such as opiates and those used to prevent motion sickness can also cause dysuria.

Urinalysis is the easiest, least invasive, and most economical way to identify urinary tract infections and other renal problems (Advanced Assessment 12.1). Once the underlying problem has been identified, appropriate treatment can be instituted.

Conditions associated with dysuria, such as bladder tumors, chronic renal failure, nephrolithiasis, and infections of the upper and lower urinary system, are discussed in the Common Problems section of this chapter. Problems associated with conditions of the prostate are discussed in Chapter 13 and those associated with dysmenorrhea in Chapter 14.

■ HEMATURIA

Hematuria is defined as blood in the urine and can be visible (gross) or occult (microscopic). It is characterized by more than three red blood cells (RBCs) per high-power microscopic field (hpf). Normal urinary excretion of RBCs is 2,000,000 per day, which corresponds to two or three RBCs per hpf. It actually takes very little blood to make the urine look very red. Urine will appear pink between 20 and 30 RBCs per hpf and becomes red at about 100 RBCs per hpf. There is a direct relationship between the quantity of blood found in the urine and the likelihood of pathology.

Transient hematuria occurs on one occasion whereas *persistent hematuria* occurs on two or more consecutive occasions. Both transient and persistent hematuria can be a sign of serious underlying disease. Urine color can vary widely from light pink to dark red and is sometimes characterized as "smoky." The color of urine is dependent on the amount of blood present, as well as on dietary intake, use of medications, and the dilution and pH of the urine. For example, the ingestion of beets can color the urine red to pink, and medications such as rifampin and phenazopyridine (Pyridium) can give urine a reddish-orange color. The presence of porphyrins, hemoglobin, or myoglobin can color the urine reddish-brown. Pus in the urine is indicative of bacterial infection, such as cystitis, urethritis, or prostatitis.

Rates of hematuria can be as high as 15% in the general population but are usually less than 1%. The age, gender, and activity level of the patient with hematuria should be considered on assessment. For example, long-distance runners and other athletes can have rates of hematuria as high as 18%. However, even transient hematuria in men older than age 50 may be an

Advanced Assessment 12.1   Urinalysis

Name	Abnormal Value	Common Differential Diagnosis
Appearance	Colorless	Diabetes insipidus, diuretic agents, fluid overload
	Dark	Hematuria, malignancy, stones, acidic urine
	Cloudy	UTI, hematuria, bilirubin, mucus
	Pink/red	Hematuria, hemoglobin, myoglobin, beets, food coloring
	Orange/yellow	Phenazopyridin, rifampin, bile pigments
	Brown/black	Myoglobin, bile pigments, melanin, cascara, iron preparation
	Green	Bile pigments, methylene blue, indigo carmine
	Foamy	Proteinuria, bile salts
Specific gravity	Increased	Dehydration, congestive heart failure, adrenal insufficiency, diabetes mellitus, nephrosis, antidiuretic hormone
	Decreased	Diabetes insipidus, pyelonephritis, glomerulonephritis, excess fluid intake
pH	Acidic	Diet, medications, acidosis, ketoacidosis, chronic obstructive pulmonary disease
	Alkaline	Diet, sodium bicarbonate, vomiting, metabolic alkalosis, UTI
Bilirubin	Positive	Jaundice, hepatitis
Blood	Positive	Kidney stones, tumors, kidney disease, trauma, infection, injury from instrumentation, coagulation problems, menses
Glucose	Positive	Diabetes mellitus, pancreatitis, Cushing's disease, shock, burns, steroids, renal disease, hyperthyroidism, cancer
Ketones	Positive	Starvation, diet, ketoacidosis, vomiting, diarrhea, pregnancy
Nitrate	Positive	Infection
Protein	Positive	Kidney disease, pregnancy, congestive heart failure, diabetes mellitus, cancer, benign cause
Leukocyte esterase	Positive	Infection
Reducing substance	Positive	Medications, glucose, fructose, galactose Liver disease, hyperthyroidism

indication of serious disease, with up to 2.4% of this population having urinary tract malignancies, typically a transitional cell carcinoma. In men older than age 60, this incidence of urinary tract malignancy increases to 9%. In older men with gross hematuria, the rate of associated malignancy is as high as 20%. In general, there is a higher correlation between underlying malignancy and gross hematuria as opposed to microscopic hematuria, especially in patients with a history of cigarette smoking.

Differential Diagnosis

A drug history is important because many drugs can cause hematuria. In addition, dietary substances such as caffeine, spices, tomatoes, chocolate, alcohol, citrus fruits, and soy sauce may act as bladder irritants. The patient's drug and food intake history should be assessed to rule out these substances as the causative agent. The drugs involved may be prescribed, over the counter, herbal, supplemental vitamins, or recreational in nature.

Some medications—beta-lactam antibiotics, sulfonamides, NSAIDs, rifampin, ciprofloxacin (Cipro), allopurinol (Zyloprim), cimetidine (Tagamet), and phenytoin (Dilantin)—can cause *nephritis*, which can result in destruction of nephrons and subsequently lead to impaired renal function and hematuria. Other conditions such as anticoagulation and papillary necrosis can result from the use of anticoagulants such as warfarin (Coumadin), heparin, aspirin, and NSAIDs. Glomerulonephritis can be caused by the use of hydralazine, hydrocarbons (including glue and paint sniffing), gold, penicillamine, amphetamines, NSAIDs, allopurinol, and Paraquat. Urolithiasis (discussed later in this chapter) can occur from the use of carbonic anhydrase inhibitors, triamterene, sulfonamides, and vitamin D metabolites and often presents with hematuria.

Menstrual history is always important in a female patient, as well as history of recent strenuous exercise, streptococcal infection (especially poststreptococcal glomerulonephritis), or nephrolithiasis; family history (e.g., of polycystic kidney disease); and recent travel (potential exposure to parasitic infections). Gross painless hematuria is a cardinal symptom of certain malignancies such as bladder cancer.

The physical exam may reveal costovertebral angle tenderness, which could indicate pyelonephritis, tumor, or glomerulonephritis. An abdominal mass may indicate a neoplasm (renal cell cancer) or polycystic kidney disease. Suprapubic tenderness is indicative of a bladder etiology, whereas urethral discharge indicates a urethritis. An enlarged prostate could indicate benign prostatic hypertrophy, whereas a tender prostate would more likely be suggestive of prostatitis; a prostate nodule may indicate a neoplasm. Skin lesions (e.g., ecchymosis) may indicate an underlying coagulopathy or vasculitis.

The most important diagnostic test in cases of hematuria is urinalysis. One major drawback of doing a urine dipstick test is that it detects the presence of heme (an iron-containing nonprotein portion of the hemoglobin molecule) in the urine but not RBCs. If the dipstick is positive for heme, but the number of RBCs on the microscopic exam is within normal limits, myoglobinuria and hemoglobinuria should be suspected. When hematuria of renal origin is suspected, laboratory tests should include antinuclear antibodies (ANAs); immunoglobulins; cryoglobulins; antiglomerular basement membrane antibodies; a full chemistry panel, including creatinine clearance and blood urea nitrogen; complete blood count and platelets; antistreptolysin O (ASO) titer; serum protein electrophoresis; and a Venereal Disease Research Laboratory (VDRL) test (to rule out syphilis). If these studies indicate a renal problem, the patient should be referred to a nephrologist. A urine culture and sensitivity should be done on all patients with hematuria, and if bacterial infection is found, treatment with appropriate antibiotics should be instituted with reevaluation for a persistent hematuria 2 weeks after completion of treatment.

Isolated asymptomatic hematuria is often found on a routine screening urinalysis with no apparent source determined by history and physical exam. The possibility of occult malignancy or other potentially serious etiology increases with age, and if the patient is older than age 40, he or she should be evaluated for urological tumor. Patients younger than age 40 should be monitored at least monthly for 3 months, and if the hematuria persists a more aggressive work-up is indicated.

Examination of the morphology of RBCs present in the urine using phase-contrast microscopy can provide clues as to the etiology of hematuria. Dysmorphic RBCs may indicate glomerular disease. A fresh urine sample is essential, because changes in morphology occur if the urine is allowed to sit. If the hematuria persists without evidence of infection, an intravenous pyelogram or renal ultrasound should be done to assess kidney structure. A computed tomography (CT) scan is the preferred imaging method for follow-up if a possible solid renal mass is found. Other tests that should

be done include a prothrombin time and partial thromboplastin time, a purified protein derivative test, erythrocyte sedimentation rate, an ANA test and complement level, antistreptococcal enzyme titers (ASO, anti-DNase B), cryoglobulin screen, and a urinalysis for cytology.

Cystoscopy is done to evaluate the upper urinary tract, and cytology can be done to evaluate the lower urinary tract. If the findings of these studies are negative and the patient continues to have gross hematuria, further investigation should include a CT scan, arteriogram, and/or ureteroscopy. The outcome of these studies will determine whether a referral for urologist or nephrologist follow-up is necessary.

The causes of hematuria are grouped according to anatomical site of the blood source. For example, *isolated hematuria* (no other abnormal urine components) may be from bleeding anywhere from the renal pelvis to the urethra, but is rarely caused by systemic disease. RBC casts usually indicate injury to the nephron and are diagnostic of hematuria of a renal origin. However, intact uniform RBCs with no casts suggests hematuria originating in the lower urinary tract. The presence of bacteria in the urine is diagnostic of a bacterial origin, as is fever. Acute cystitis and urethritis produce gross hematuria and are more common in women. The presence of both proteinuria and hematuria is suggestive of glomerular or interstitial nephritis. Hematuria accompanied by colicky flank pain suggests a ureteral stone. When bleeding occurs only at the beginning or end of urination, a prostatic or urethral source is likely. Hematuria accompanied by hypertension, edema, and a sore throat or a skin infection may be indicative of glomerulonephritis. Thirty percent of patients with gross hematuria are diagnosed with a malignancy of the prostate, urethra, bladder, kidney, or ureter. Differential Diagnosis 12.1 lists possible differential diagnoses of hematuria.

■ PROTEINURIA

The primary proteins found in urine are globulin and albumin. *Proteinuria* is usually indicative of a renal pathology, most often of glomerular origin. Proteinuria can be functional as a result of acute illness, emotional stress, or excessive exercise and is a benign process. It can also develop from overproduction of filterable plasma proteins, especially Bence Jones proteins associated with multiple myeloma. Abnormalities in the glomerular basement membrane produce glomerular proteinuria. Damage to the proximal tubule where filterable proteins are reabsorbed can result in tubular proteinuria.

Intermittent proteinuria is most often asymptomatic and discovered incidentally through urine dipstick testing and is associated with functional disorders. Continuous proteinuria is associated with renal pathology. The dipstick test does not detect Bence Jones proteins or light chain immunoglobulins and is most sensitive to albumin. A false-negative reading can occur because of a diluted urine

Differential Diagnosis 12.1   Hematuria

Problem	Differential Diagnoses
Urethra	Urethritis (gonococcal, nongonococcal)
	Stricture
	Calculus
	Trauma
Prostate/male genitourinary tract	Infection (prostatitis, epididymitis)
	Benign prostatic hypertrophy
	Tumor
Kidney	Infection (pyelonephritis)
	Nephrolithiasis
	Cancer (renal cell)
	Trauma
	Glomerular disease (vasculitis, idiopathic)
	Ischemia (embolism, thrombosis, papillary necrosis)
	Allergic interstitial nephritis (drug induced)
Ureters	Nephrolithiasis
	Tumor
	Endometriosis
Bladder	Infection (bacterial, parasitic)
	Calculus
	Tumor
	Endometriosis
	Drugs (hemorrhagic cystitis)
Pseudohematuria	Menstrual contamination
	Phenothiazines
	Red food dye
	Quinine
	Rifampin
	Hemoglobinuria
Systemic illness	Intense exercise
	Coagulopathies (thrombocytopenia, hemoglobinopathy, sickle cell)

sample, alkaline pH (normal 4.5–8 [usually 5.5–6.5]), or Bence Jones proteinuria. The most accurate way to quantify the amount of protein in the urine is a 24-hour urine collection; however, a spot urine albumin to urine creatinine ratio can be measured and is a close approximation of the 24-hour urine measurement. A 24-hour urine with more than 165 mg of protein is considered abnormal and a specimen with more than 3.5 g is indicative of a nephrotic problem. A urine albumin to urine creatinine ratio of less than 0.2 is normal and corresponds to an excretion of less than 200 mg/dL of protein.

Differential Diagnosis

Proteinuria may occur from "benign" causes. Causes of benign, or functional, proteinuria include orthostatic proteinuria, exercise, environmental conditions, fever, and acute illnesses. Orthostatic proteinuria occurs when the protein level is elevated only when the patient has been standing but not while he or she has been reclining. Exercise-induced proteinuria may occur in athletes such as runners or boxers; it may be accompanied by elevated catecholamines, hemoglobinuria, or hematuria. Proteinuria caused by environmental conditions such as emotional stress, exposure to cold, prolonged lordotic posture, and excess in the body's norepinephrine level will resolve spontaneously when the precipitating element is eliminated or removed. A mild, transient proteinuria may result from an albumin infusion or acute illnesses such as fever, congestive heart failure, acute pulmonary edema, head injury, or cerebrovascular accident; this type of proteinuria typically resolves as the medical condition improves.

When proteinuria is identified in a low-risk (nondiabetic or nonpregnant) patient, the urine should be tested for Bence Jones protein, the presence of which suggests multiple myeloma. In addition, a full chemistry panel should be done, including a fasting blood sugar, a lipid profile, urine culture and sensitivity, and a complete blood count with differential. If the patient's urine is positive for Bence Jones proteins, a serum protein electrophoresis should be done. Proteinuria associated with multiple myeloma, lymphosarcoma, Hodgkin's disease, and leukemia is called Bence Jones proteinuria. Bence Jones proteinuria is characterized as a free monoclonal light chain of protein.

Any persistent proteinuria that is not classified as functional proteinuria requires further work-up, beginning with a 24-hour measurement of urine protein and creatinine levels. If the excretion rate is above 3.0 to 3.5 g/day, the patient, by definition, has nephrotic syndrome and must be referred to a nephrologist. Nephrotic syndrome can lead to acute renal failure, hypertension, and end-stage renal failure.

If the excretion rate of protein is more than 2 g in 24 hours, a glomerular cause is most likely and further evaluation is warranted. If renal function is normal in a patient with an elevated urine protein, the patient should then be evaluated for orthostatic proteinuria. This involves having the patient collect a urine specimen on awakening but before assuming an upright position for longer than 1 minute. After the patient has been standing or walking for 2 hours, a second specimen is collected. If the patient has orthostatic proteinuria, the first specimen will be free of protein and the second will be positive for protein, and referral to a nephrologist is necessary. Although this condition is largely benign and self-limiting, orthostatic proteinuria is not well understood. Patients with nonorthostatic proteinuria and normal renal function in whom no Bence Jones proteins have been detected should also be referred to a renal specialist for renal biopsy. Proteinuria associated with a specific disease process involving the renal system is presented in Table 12.1.

Table 12.1 Proteinuria

Type of Proteinuria	Major Mechanism	Disease Process
Bence Jones proteinuria	Elevated plasma concentration	Multiple myeloma (lymphosarcoma, leukemia, Hodgkin's disease)
Tamm-Horsfall proteinuria	Increased tubular cell secretion	Normal mucoprotein in urine
Tubulointerstitial area involvement	Decreased tubular reabsorption of normal filtered protein	Pyelonephritis
Altered glomerular capillary permeability	Increase of filtered proteins	Glomerulonephritis, nephrotic syndrome
pH > 8.0	High-alkaline urines	False positive

Management of proteinuria depends on the underlying cause. Angiotensin-converting enzyme agents have been found to reduce proteinuria by decreasing interglomerular pressure. If hyperlipidemia and/or hypertension are present, they should be aggressively treated. Patients found to have chronic renal failure should also be aggressively managed to prevent or delay the onset of end-stage renal disease.

COMMON PROBLEMS

■ URINARY INCONTINENCE

Urinary incontinence (UI) is the involuntary loss of urine from the bladder. Incontinence is so frequent in women that many consider it normal. Incontinence is also common in older men as a result of an enlarging prostate. Incontinence can affect a person's quality of life and may be psychologically devastating. Ignoring the incontinence, or inadequate treatment of this condition, can lead to social isolation, body image problems, anxiety, or depression; therefore, prompt treatment is essential (see the Iceberg of Incontinence).

Epidemiology and Causes

The direct cost of treating and managing UI is reported to be more than $26 billion per year and affects more than 25 million Americans. Costs include diagnostic testing, medication, and adult incontinence products such as disposable pads and undergarments. One study estimates that more than 40% of American women are affected, and there seems to be a strong association between urinary incontinence and major depression. The prevalence of UI in the community population varies from 5% to 15% depending on age and gender, and more than 50% of the patients in long-term care facilities have incontinence. Women are more likely than men to have incontinence, and the incidence increases with age; in fact, the risk of UI increases 14% with each decade of life.

Transient UI is characterized by a sudden onset and can have several causes including delirium, infection, pharmacological agents, or underlying systemic illnesses such as diabetes, fecal impaction, and restricted mobility. Most new-onset incontinence that occurs in the hospital resolves with appropriate treatment, but this acute transient phase can become a chronic problem if left untreated. The basic types of persistent UI are categorized as stress, urge, overflow, and functional UI. A patient may present with mixed symptoms of urge and stress incontinence. Table 12.2 provides an overview of the types of urinary incontinence.

Pathophysiology

An understanding of incontinence requires knowledge of the physiology of micturition. Three major components are involved in urine storage and release: the central nervous system (CNS), the bladder, and the bladder outlet (urethral sphincters). Within the CNS, micturition is controlled by both the cortical (central) and brainstem (pontine) micturition centers. The cortical micturition center coordinates inhibitory stimuli from the frontal lobes and basal ganglia, permitting bladder relaxation and filling, as well as urethral sphincter closure to prevent urinary leakage, as the bladder increases in size. These efferent signals emanate from spinal levels T11 to L2 and are mediated by alpha-adrenergic receptors and cholinergic somatic stimulation. This maintains urethral pressure along the bladder outlet by both internal and external sphincters. Alpha-adrenergic stimulation causes muscle contraction of the internal sphincter, whereas the external sphincter is under voluntary control of striated muscle tissue (allowing patients to "hold their urine" for purposes of social appropriateness).

In contrast, bladder emptying is mediated by the parietal lobes and thalamus, which modulate afferent proprioceptive stimuli from the distended bladder wall detrusor muscle, sensing an increase in bladder pressure that is interpreted as bladder fullness. Once the patient has the urge to void, the inhibition by the cortical micturition center ceases. In turn, the brainstem micturition center sends impulses from the pons down the spinal cord to the sacral micturition center at S2 to S4,

The Iceberg of Incontinence

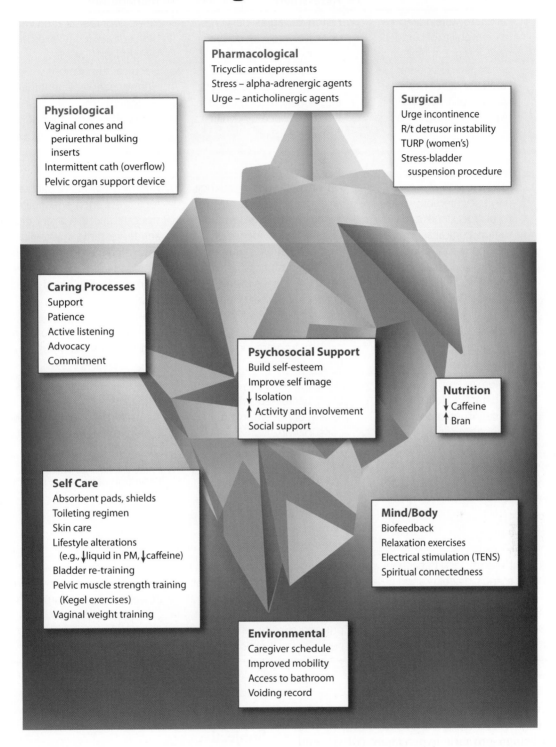

Pharmacological
Tricyclic antidepressants
Stress – alpha-adrenergic agents
Urge – anticholinergic agents

Physiological
Vaginal cones and
  periurethral bulking
  inserts
Intermittent cath (overflow)
Pelvic organ support device

Surgical
Urge incontinence
R/t detrusor instability
TURP (women's)
Stress-bladder
  suspension procedure

Caring Processes
Support
Patience
Active listening
Advocacy
Commitment

Psychosocial Support
Build self-esteem
Improve self image
↓ Isolation
↑ Activity and involvement
Social support

Nutrition
↓ Caffeine
↑ Bran

Self Care
Absorbent pads, shields
Toileting regimen
Skin care
Lifestyle alterations
  (e.g., ↓liquid in PM, ↓caffeine)
Bladder re-training
Pelvic muscle strength training
  (Kegel exercises)
Vaginal weight training

Mind/Body
Biofeedback
Relaxation exercises
Electrical stimulation (TENS)
Spiritual connectedness

Environmental
Caregiver schedule
Improved mobility
Access to bathroom
Voiding record

subsequently triggering the bladder detrusor muscle to contract via cholinergic stimulation of parasympathetic M2 and M3 type muscarinic receptors found within the smooth muscle of the bladder walls. This latter action is simulated by the pharmacological agent bethanechol (Urecholine), which is used to treat urinary retention from an atonic or poorly responsive bladder. In addition, preganglionic sympathetic inhibition relaxes the urethral sphincter, allowing for the egress of urine.

Age-related changes that may affect urological functioning are decreased bladder capacity, increased postvoid residual urine volume (greater than 50 mL), increased disinhibition of bladder contractions (i.e., overactive bladder), increased nocturnal sodium and

Table 12.2   Types of Urinary Incontinence

Type	Cause	Assessment	Management
Stress	Failure to store due to hypermobility of bladder neck, intrinsic sphincter deficiency, neurogenic sphincter deficiency Medications: Sedatives, hypnotics, antispasmodics	History of vaginal deliveries, urine leakage with cough or sneeze Evidence of urine loss Pelvic exam, pad test, stress test, urinalysis culture and sensitivity, video-urodynamics, cystometrogram	Pelvic floor reeducation with biofeedback (Kegel exercises) Weight loss, if obese Electrical stimulation Hormone replacement therapy (estrogen) Alpha-adrenergic agonist Surgical correction of hypermobile bladder neck Periurethral bulking injections
Urge	Failure to store due to urinary tract infection; vaginitis; bladder stones and tumors; cortical, subcortical, and suprasacral lesions; cerebrovascular accident; dementia; multiple sclerosis; Parkinson's disease; spinal cord transection Medications: Diuretics, narcotics	History of dysuria, frequency, urgency, hematuria, nocturia Evidence of a large amount of urine loss, evidence of unstable detrusor with decreased capacity Assess perineal hygiene Pelvic exam, smear, neurological exam, urinalysis, culture and sensitivity, cystometrogram, video-urodynamics	Antimicrobial agents, antiseptics, topical estrogen, anticholinergics, smooth muscle relaxers, tricyclic antidepressants, imipramine Pelvic floor reeducation with biofeedback (Kegel exercises) Prompted voiding and scheduled voiding Fluid intake management Removal of bladder stones, resection and/or tumor treatment
Overflow	Failure to empty due to underactive detrusor, outlet obstruction, diabetes mellitus Medications: Anticholinergics, disopyramide, antihistamines, calcium channel blockers	History of hesitancy, dribbling, decreased stream, feeling of not emptying, constipation Neurological exam, prostate exam (for males), prostate-specific antigen (for males), urinalysis, culture and sensitivity, serum creatinine, voiding cystometrogram, video-urodynamics	Scheduled toileting (Credé's maneuver) Treatment of underlying conditions Collection devices (intermittent or suprapubic) Alpha blockers Resection of prostate, balloon dilation
Functional	Delirium, fecal impaction, manual dexterity and immobility Medications: diuretics, hypnotics, alcohol, narcotics, decongestants	Fecal impaction Assess sleep patterns, mental state, hearing, vision, functional ability, intake and output, accessibility, infection, neurological function	Remove barriers Provide barrier-free environment Bowel and bladder program Collection devices Physical therapy Habit training

fluid excretion (nocturia), urinary overflow phenomena resulting from increased urethral resistance in men related to benign prostatic hypertrophy (BPH), and weakness of the pelvic muscle walls in women. Postmenopausal estrogen deficiency can result in decreased competence of the internal and external sphincters via atrophy of the urethral mucosal epithelium resulting in atrophic urethritis, loss of compliance, and a diminished urethral mucosal seal. It is important to note, however, that normal aging in and of itself does not cause urinary incontinence.

Clinical Presentation
Subjective

All assessments of the urinary system should begin with a detailed medical and surgical history, including the patient's voiding history. A voiding history includes the date of incontinence onset; number of times per day or night the patient voids; amount of urine voided each time; fluid-intake history, with types of fluids consumed; and the characteristics of the urinary incontinence, such as "occurs when sneezing," nocturia, frequency, urgency, or dysuria. Information regarding underlying medical conditions such as diabetes, cancer, acute illness, and neurological disease should be elicited.

Objective

The aim of the physical exam is to identify the underlying pathophysiological causes of incontinence, which can be multiple. The neurological assessment is important in differentiating diagnoses such as cerebrovascular accident (CVA) and Parkinson's disease and should include an assessment of the functional and cognitive ability. This provides information about limitations in mobility, self-care ability, mental status, and communication barriers, such as aphasia or language.

An abdominal exam should be done to rule out constipation, fecal impaction, masses, distended bladder, or cystitis, which can lead to incontinence. A pelvic exam will reveal the pelvic muscle strength, conditions such as uterine prolapse, and any problems associated with perineal structures. Inspection of the skin around the pelvic area is important. For example, in women, there may be atrophic vaginitis; in men, there may be abnormalities of the foreskin, penis, or perineum. A rectal exam should be done to determine the sphincter tone and the presence or absence of feces, to support causative complications such as fecal impaction. In men, a prostate exam is crucial in evaluating urinary tract complaints. The skin condition should be evaluated for breakdown or pressure areas during the pelvic exam because incontinence can lead to skin breakdown in the perineal area and buttocks which then can lead to decubitus ulcers. In female patients, particularly postmenopausal women, the perineum should be assessed for dryness and atrophy from decreased estrogenization of the vaginal mucosa.

During the physical exam, signs of congestive heart failure should be assessed; a cough stress test (which will allow direct observation of urine loss with a full bladder), bladder scan, or, if necessary, catheterization to determine postvoid residual volume should be done as well. The patient or caretaker should be instructed to keep a voiding record for 3 to 7 days. The voiding record includes the time of the incontinence episode, the amount of urine, whether there was an urge to void, and the patient's activity at the time of the voiding. This record also includes an hourly record of fluid intake. For patients with a questionable history of UI, a "pad test" can be done. This involves having the patient take oral phenazopyridine (Pyridium), which will color the urine orange, and then wear a sanitary pad that can be checked at intervals for staining.

Diagnostic Reasoning

Diagnostic Tests

A urinalysis and urine culture and sensitivity should be done, as well as measurements of serum electrolytes, blood urea nitrogen, creatinine, calcium (for polyuria in

the absence of diuretics), and glucose. Catheterization to assess postvoiding residual volume is important even on initial evaluation of the patient. Further testing will also depend on whether the onset of incontinence is acute, in which case testing related to other concurrent conditions may be warranted. The urinalysis is often normal but may show glycosuria (in patients with diabetes), proteinuria (in patients with glomerular disease), white blood cells (in patients with a bacterial infection), red blood cells (which may indicate the presence of a tumor), or bacteria (another sign of infection). A urine culture that is positive for bacteria also indicates infection; specific findings can be used to guide antibiotic therapy.

Other diagnostic options include urodynamic testing and cystometry, cystometrogram, video-urodynamics, and a postvoid residual catheterization to indicate the amount of retained urine. Reviewing the patient's use of medications for possible drug interaction, obtaining an accurate record of intake and output, and evaluating for other risk factors contributing to UI are also important. Patients who have indwelling catheters should be urodynamically evaluated for possible bladder retraining. Renal ultrasound may show renal pathology; a transrectal ultrasound can provide evidence of prostate disease; and a pelvic ultrasound may demonstrate pelvic pathology. A cystogram may show abnormal sphincter pressure or bladder pathology.

Differential Diagnosis

Many older patients may normally compensate for their incontinence, but any alteration—either physiologically or psychologically—such as a hospitalization can precipitate an acute onset of incontinence. The administration of IV hydration in an acutely ill or older adult may be sufficient to precipitate incontinence. Although the endpoint is the same for all types of incontinence (involuntary bladder emptying), the context in which this occurs may vary markedly. Thus, the primary goal of differential diagnosis is for the clinician to correctly identify the type and etiology of incontinence, which in turn drives management and treatment decisions.

In persistent UI, a number of factors must be evaluated. Normal micturition requires the coordination of both the central and peripheral nervous systems. The cerebral cortex exerts an overall inhibitory influence on the sacral spinal cord reflex. Delirium, dementia, parkinsonism, and stroke may all lead to urge incontinence without awareness. The brainstem, on the other hand, and the suprasacral spinal cord exert a predominantly facilitating and coordinating influence that may be overcome in disorders such as stroke and multiple sclerosis, leading to overflow incontinence without awareness. This is referred to as neurogenic or detrusor-sphincter dyssynergy. Local irritation and bladder or outflow obstructions may also lead to urge incontinence without awareness. Injuries to the sacral cord, which controls reflex bladder filling and emptying, persistent outlet obstruction, and diabetes mellitus may all lead to an acontractile bladder and overflow incontinence without awareness. Likewise, the bladder and lower genitourinary tract must perform their storage and emptying functions properly for normal micturition. Failure to store urine may be a result of a hyperactive or poorly compliant bladder (e.g., secondary to cystitis, stones, tumor, or diverticuli), leading to urge incontinence. Laxity of pelvic floor muscles, bladder outlet, or sphincter weakness all may cause diminished outflow tract resistance, leading to stress incontinence. The bladder may fail to empty completely if it is poorly contractile as a result of diabetes mellitus, thus resulting in overflow incontinence. Increased outflow obstruction may be caused by anatomical obstruction by the prostate, stricture, or cystocele, resulting in chronic urinary retention and overflow incontinence.

Mixed types of incontinence are the norm rather than the exception; many patients have an overlap of pathologies. Just as multiple etiological factors must be considered, a broad variety of interventions must be made available and are best approached through the *Circle of Caring.*

Management
Stress Incontinence

Stress incontinence is the involuntary loss of urine resulting from increased intra-abdominal pressure such as coughing, sneezing, and laughing. In this condition, the bladder is unable to retain urine because of hypermobility of the bladder neck, intrinsic sphincter deficiency, neurogenic sphincter deficiency, or use of medications such as sedatives, hypnotics, alpha blockers, and/or antispasmodics. Patients who present with stress incontinence report urine leakage with coughing or sneezing and typically have a history of vaginal deliveries and/or hysterectomy, as well as evidence of urine loss. A detailed history guides the diagnostic work-up, which will then include a pelvic exam, pad test to determine the amount and frequency of leakage, cough stress test, urinalysis with culture and sensitivity, video-urodynamics, and/or cystometrogram.

Once the diagnosis of stress incontinence has been made, treatment should be individualized and instituted to meet the patient's needs. Noninvasive treatments include pelvic floor reeducation (Kegel exercises) with biofeedback, weight loss (if the patient is obese), electrical stimulation, and medications such as alpha-adrenergic agonists, which improve the muscle tone of the urinary tract. Eliminating diuretics will also improve symptoms. Surgical options include correction of hypermobile bladder neck and periurethral bulking injections. See Drugs Commonly Prescribed 12.1 for a list of medications used for UI.

Urge Incontinence

Urge incontinence, also known as detrusor instability, is the involuntary leakage of urine resulting from inability to delay voiding. The patient has the sensation of a full

---

Drugs Commonly Prescribed 12.1   Urinary Incontinence

Drug	Indication	Adverse Reactions and Prescribing Considerations
Anticholinergic/Antispasmodic Agents		
tolterodine (Detrol LA) oxybutynin (Ditropan XL) solfenacin (Vesicare) darifenacin (Enablex) trospium chloride (Sanctura XR) transdermal oxybutynin (Gelnique) fesoterodine (Toviaz)	Urge incontinence Overactive bladder (OAB) Stress incontinence	**Contraindications:** Closed-angle glaucoma Myasthenia gravis Partial or complete gastric obstruction Severe colitis Urinary retention Gastric retention **Side effects:** Dry mouth Drowsiness Blurred vision Urinary hesitance Urinary retention Decreased GI motility Headache Constipation Vertigo/dizziness Abdominal pain

Drugs Commonly Prescribed 12.1 Urinary Incontinence—cont'd

Drug	Indication	Adverse Reactions and Prescribing Considerations
Topical Estrogen		
Premarin cream (conjugates estrogen) Estrace cream Estring	Stress incontinence Urge incontinence associated with atrophic vaginitis	**Contraindications:** Hypersensitivity Breast cancer Thromboembolic disorders Estrogen-dependent neoplasia Abnormal genital bleeding Pregnancy **Side effects:** Premenstrual syndrome–like syndrome Amenorrhea Nausea/vomiting Headache Dizziness Depression Changes in libido Dysmenorrhea Breakthrough bleeding Breast tenderness Photosensitivity Endometrial cystic hyperplasia
Alpha-1-Adrenergic Blocking Agents (Men)		
tamsulosin hydrochloride (Flomax) terazosin hydrochloride (Hytrin) doxazosin mesylate (Cardura)	BPH and related urinary symptoms	**Contraindications:** Hypersensitivity to tamsulosin terazosin, or doxazosin **Side effects:** Orthostatic hypotension Palpitations Dizziness Impotence GI upset Headache
Tricyclic Antidepressants		
imipramine (Tofranil) amitriptyline (Elavil)	OAB Urge incontinence	**Contraindications:** Hypersensitivity to tricyclic antidepressants Use of monoamine oxidase inhibitors **Side effects:** Dry mouth Urinary retention Blurred vision Orthostatic hypotension Sedation Confusion in the elderly Tachycardia Anxiety and nervousness Sexual dysfunction Constipation

bladder but is not able to store the urine long enough to reach the toilet. This failure can be caused by urinary tract infection; vaginitis; bladder stones; bladder tumors; cortical, subcortical, and suprasacral lesions; CVA; dementia; multiple sclerosis; Parkinson's disease; prostate problems; spinal cord transection; and medications such as diuretics and narcotics. The patient's history and physical exam may reveal evidence of dysuria, increased frequency or urgency, hematuria, large amounts of urine loss, and unstable detrusor muscle with decreased capacity, or nocturia. Assessment should include perineal hygiene, pelvic exam and a vaginal discharge smear, and a neurological exam including an assessment of mental status; a urinalysis with a culture and sensitivity should also be ordered. Invasive procedures that may be needed include cystometrogram and video-urodynamics.

Treatment begins conservatively, with pelvic floor reeducation and biofeedback, if the patient is capable. A prompted and/or scheduled voiding by a caregiver, with management of the patient's fluid intake, may be useful for patients who have cognitive impairments or are forgetful. Medications such as antimicrobial agents may be necessary to treat underlying conditions. Other medications may include topical estrogen, anticholinergics, smooth muscle relaxants, and tricyclic antidepressants to improve the neuromuscular function of the bladder and sphincter (see Drugs Commonly Prescribed 12.1). Surgical treatment may be indicated for the removal of bladder stones or tumors.

Overactive Bladder

The term *overactive bladder* (OAB) is often used interchangeably with the term *urge incontinence;* however, they are different conditions. OAB is a syndrome of symptoms that include urgency, frequency, and nocturia, all of which are associated with involuntary contractions of the detrusor muscle. Urge incontinence may or may not be a feature of this syndrome; about one-third have urge incontinence. OAB may occur as a component of other types of UI, such as with stress incontinence. The cause of OAB is multifactorial in that it can include disorders of the lower urinary tract, ingestion of alcohol and caffeine, use of a variety of prescribed drugs, or neurological conditions. This condition is most common in women and often results in anxiety and depression because of the restricted daily functioning. Sexual dysfunction can occur because of the fear of urine loss during sexual intercourse.

Treatment for OAB first begins with identifying women with the problem. It is estimated that only about 6% to 27% of women with this condition seek treatment. Nonpharmacological methods mentioned earlier are used to manage OAB as well, but pharmacotherapy plays an important role. Antimuscarinic agents are the most commonly used drugs and are effective because they block the parasympathetic stimulation of the detrusor muscle by blocking acetylcholine. See Drugs Commonly Prescribed 12.1 for a complete list of medications used for OAB.

Overflow Incontinence

Overflow incontinence is the involuntary leakage of small amounts of urine. This is caused by an overdistended bladder in a patient who does not feel the need to void because of an atonic detrusor muscle, outlet obstruction, BPH, diabetes mellitus, or use of medications such as anticholinergics, disopyramide (Norpace), antihistamines, diuretics, or calcium channel blockers. The history and physical exam may indicate hesitancy, dribbling, nocturia, decreased stream, feeling of not emptying the bladder, and/or constipation. A neurological exam, prostate exam, urinalysis with culture and sensitivity, serum creatinine, voiding cystometrogram, and/or video-urodynamics should be done.

Management of incontinence consists of treating the underlying condition; teaching scheduled toileting and Credé's maneuver; and the prescribing of medications such as alpha blockers (see Drugs Commonly Prescribed 12.1). It may be necessary to discontinue certain medications or to alter dosages to reduce the adverse effects causing overflow incontinence. Teaching scheduled toileting and Credé's maneuver to force the urine from the bladder may be helpful. Credé's maneuver involves applying pressure over the symphysis pubis and slowly pressing down. This is particularly helpful in patients who have a spinal cord injury or other neurological problems. Alternative collection devices may be indicated, including the use of external catheters; pads; and indwelling, intermittent, or suprapubic catheterization. In the case of outlet obstruction, a resection of the prostate may be necessary.

Functional Urinary Incontinence

Functional UI is incontinence that occurs in a normal functioning urinary system. The leakage of urine is caused by factors outside the lower urinary tract and can be transient in nature. The causes of functional incontinence may vary from delirium or fecal impaction to lack of manual dexterity and immobility problems. Medications such as diuretics, hypnotics, narcotics, and decongestants, as well as alcohol, may also play a role. Assessment for fecal impaction, sleep pattern disturbances, mental status, hearing and vision, functional ability, fluid intake, infection, and neurological function is essential.

Treatment for functional incontinence consists of removing barriers, providing education regarding a scheduled bowel and bladder program and the use of collection devices, referring patients for physical or occupational therapy, and habit training. Barriers to elimination may be identified when the patient cannot remove clothing or reach the toilet in sufficient time to avoid leakage. By identifying the barrier(s), interventions to resolve the problem can be developed. Some solutions include the use of hook-and-loop (Velcro) closures (which are easily managed by arthritic hands and fingers) instead of buttons and zippers, bedside commodes for nighttime use to eliminate the amount of time needed to get to the bathroom, or monitors for obtaining immediate assistance in getting out of bed and to the toilet.

A caregiver may be necessary to assist the patient in toileting; therefore, it is imperative to assess the caregiver's ability to provide care and determine his or her level of competency. Nursing research shows that caregivers want to give "good" care; however, the caregiver must be physically capable of providing the care through manual dexterity, strength, and cognition. Further, the caregiver must be able to comprehend and follow through with instructions that may be complex and require problem-solving ability.

Identifying patients who need physical or occupational therapy to improve their functional skills may be required. Initiation of a bowel and bladder program can decrease the incidence of constipation and fecal impaction; patients should also be encouraged to retrain the bladder to empty completely on a regular basis. For patients who cannot avoid UI, alternatives are available to keep them clean and dry. Condom catheters are effective in keeping male patients dry, and pads of various types are available for both males and females. Indwelling catheters, suprapubic catheters, and intermittent catheterization are options for urine collection in patients who cannot maintain bladder function or who have frequent or regular UI.

Medications used to treat incontinence are effective for patients who suffer from the inability to store urine. Pharmacological agents should be used in conjunction with other treatment modalities such as toileting and behavioral modification. Scheduled toileting along with regulation of fluid intake can have a positive effect on bladder control. Behavioral modification treatment such as pelvic floor reeducation is designed to increase pelvic floor muscular strength and endurance. Reeducation is accomplished through Kegel exercises of the targeted muscle group using biofeedback for a period of 4 to 6 weeks. Kegel exercises are the tightening and releasing of the pubococcygeal and levator ani muscles, accomplished by tightening the muscle group used to avoid defecation or urination. The patient may experience results within 2 weeks to several months of initiating the program. This treatment is noninvasive and, when appropriate, should be attempted before surgical intervention (Table 12.3).

Vaginal cones or rings may be used to retain the uterus in a more normal position. Cones can reduce the pressure on the bladder of the prolapsed uterine musculature.

Surgical intervention may be appropriate if all other measures have failed or in conjunction with the previous conservative approaches. Surgery may be indicated to correct anatomical abnormalities such as prolapsed uterus, hypermobile bladder neck, or obstructions such as enlarged prostate or tumors. Surgery should be used

Table 12.3	Kegel Exercises

Instructions for the patient:
- Locate the correct muscle. To do so, try stopping your urine flow by contracting the muscle. When the urine slows or stops, you are using the pubococcygeus (PC) muscle.
- Squeeze the muscle for 2 seconds. (Do not hold your breath or contract your abdomen, buttocks, or thighs.) Then relax for 10 seconds. This is one repetition. Do 10 repetitions twice a day.
- After you have mastered the technique, begin to lengthen the time you contract the muscle. Increase the time by 1 second every few days until you are able to contract the muscle for 10 seconds at a time (and relax for 10 seconds). Continue to do 10 repetitions twice a day.

as the last treatment option unless the causative agent is diagnosed as a tumor or severe obstruction.

Follow-up and Referral

Close follow-up is essential for patients with incontinence. This may be biweekly at first, while the patient is being taught the exercises and the medication dosage is being adjusted. Quarterly follow-up visits may be sufficient once incontinence is under control and medication dose has been stabilized. The patient should be monitored for adverse effects of medication and orthostatic hypotension. Periodic urinalysis should be done to detect any urinary tract infections early. Women should have regular pelvic exams to detect pelvic abnormalities early, and men should have regular rectal exams to pick up prostatic abnormalities.

Patient Education

Patient and family education is crucial in the treatment of UI. Environmental assessment should include recommendations about proximity of toilet facilities. An individualized toileting schedule should be geared to each patient's pattern of incontinence. Bladder training in the form of timed voiding, working up to 3-hour intervals, is an important intervention. Good general nutritional and exercise practices are important to the upkeep of overall health. Support and encouragement are essential. Interventions geared toward preventing social isolation, setting up necessary support services, and optimism in dealing with the problem are important interventions in the primary-care setting.

■ LOWER URINARY TRACT INFECTIONS

A lower urinary tract infection (UTI) occurs when the normally sterile environment of the urinary tract system is invaded by pathogenic bacteria. Infections of the lower urinary tract can occur in the urethra, bladder, and prostate. Infection of the urethra *(urethritis)* and infection of the urinary bladder *(cystitis)* usually occur together. Women may be diagnosed with chronic inflammation of the bladder wall *(interstitial cystitis [IC])*. Prostatitis is infection of the prostate gland.

Infections can be acute, chronic, recurrent, complicated, or uncomplicated. *Acute infections* are characterized by the onset of UTI in a previously symptom-free individual. Infections can become *chronic* when unresolved after the usual treatment is rendered. UTIs become chronic because of obstructions, antibiotic-resistant bacteria, or the presence of multiple strains of bacteria that are not susceptible to the antibiotic therapy prescribed. A UTI is considered *recurrent* when it recurs within 2 weeks of the original infection. A *complicated* UTI is either an acute or chronic infection that is accompanied by factors that complicate the infection, such as catheters (e.g., indwelling, suprapubic, or intermittent), underlying chronic disease, or pregnancy. An *uncomplicated* UTI is one that can be resolved without addressing such complicating factors.

Epidemiology and Causes

Lower UTI is a common problem that affects approximately 20% of women and 1% of men each year and accounts for more than 6 million visits to primary-care providers each year. UTI rarely occurs in men younger than age 50 and is usually caused by urinary catheters, anatomical abnormalities of the urinary tract, unprotected anal intercourse, or vaginal intercourse with a woman who has a bacterial infection. UTI may occur at all ages but is more prevalent in sexually active adults, very young children, or frail older adults. Other populations at risk include individuals with predisposing conditions such as a suppressed immune system, pregnancy, urinary obstruction, catheter dependency, neurogenic bladder, or diabetes mellitus.

Lower UTI may be the result of other conditions within the renal system. A urethral obstruction can create stasis of urine, providing a medium for bacterial growth. Other conditions that can contribute to UTI are a descending infection from the kidney, an anatomically short urethra (in female patients), and acute infections elsewhere in the body. UTI may also occur as a result of poor or nonsterile catheterization technique or reuse of disposable catheters, poor hygiene, unprotected anal intercourse, or simply from an indwelling catheter, which, as a foreign body, serves as a nidus of infection.

Interstitial cystitis (IC) is found primarily in women. Statistically, 3 to 8 million women and 1 to 4 million men seeking treatment for bladder pain are diagnosed with IC, also known as painful bladder disease. The cause of this condition is unknown at this time, but some researchers theorize that there is an abnormality in the bladder surface that allows potassium and urea to leak and absorb into the bladder interstitium. Other factors being investigated are lymphatic, infectious, neurological, psychological, autoimmune, and vasculitic. IC does not respond to antibiotics.

Pathophysiology

Lower UTIs usually occur as a result of contamination from the patient's own gastrointestinal tract. Bacteria may be introduced into the urinary tract from fecal contamination secondary to poor perineal hygiene, unprotected sexual intercourse, and/or an anatomically shortened urethra in women. The use of a spermicide during intercourse (especially with diaphragm forms of contraception) alters the vaginal microenvironment, predisposing to bacterial colonization. Immunosuppressed or medically compromised patients may have difficulty in suppressing bacterial growth as bacteria ascend the urethra. Patients who are dependent on catheters are at risk for introduction of bacteria into the urinary tract through contamination of the catheter. Alkaline urine is a common complication of diabetes mellitus. The elevated pH of the urine creates a medium in which bacteria can grow and proliferate. Renal stones can also create an environment that promotes bacterial growth, as the blockage causes stasis of urine or reflux. In turn, contamination can occur in the kidney when urine "backs up" in the kidney due to vesicoureteral reflux, in which the urine back-flows freely into one or both ureters, leading to urinary stasis.

In women, approximately 80% to 90% of cases of uncomplicated UTI are a result of the gram-negative rod bacterium *Escherichia coli.* The second most common cause (5%–20% of cases) of uncomplicated bacterial infection is the gram-positive coccus *Staphylococcus saprophyticus,* although this agent is rare in complicated UTI. Other gram-negative rods identified as causative pathogens in a smaller number of cases, but particularly in complicated UTI, are *Proteus mirabilis, Klebsiella, Enterobacter, Serratia,* and *Pseudomonas.* In addition, the gram-positive coccus *Enterococcus* has been identified. *Staphylococcus aureus* is a gram-positive coccus that can be introduced into the urinary tract system through instrumentation or as a complication of renal stones. Fungi, particularly *Candida* species, may also be causative agents in complicated UTI that fails to respond to antibiotic therapy, especially in the presence of an indwelling catheter. Candiduria may be asymptomatic, and fungal structures should be sought on urine microscopy, because fungal colonies may be more difficult to elaborate on standard urine culture, in turn leading to delays in treatment.

In up to 50% of all bacterial species associated with cystitis, genetic virulence determinants may be identified that contribute to the uropathogenicity of these organisms, such as adherence factors that allow for greater binding to the uroepithelium. Another is the urease gene, expressed by certain gram-negative bacteria such as *Proteus, Klebsiella, Ureaplasma, Providencia,* and

Pseudomonas species. This enzyme splits urea molecules within the urinary tract, creating ammonium and hydroxyl ions that produce an alkaline microenvironment. This higher pH facilitates survival of these bacteria, particularly when housed within triple phosphate (magnesium ammonium phosphate) stones, also known as struvite stones.

Cystitis is rare in men because the increased length and drier environment around the urethra contribute to less frequent bacterial colonization. In addition, prostatic fluid has inherent antibacterial properties, but when UTI does occur, it is often associated with abnormal urethral anatomy or inadequate treatment of prostatitis. Most antibiotic agents do not penetrate the prostatic tissue and, therefore, do not eliminate the infection. As a result, the bladder is reinfected from contaminated prostatic fluid.

Two well-documented phenomena related to classic UTI are asymptomatic bacteriuria and the dysuria–pyuria syndrome. As the name implies, in asymptomatic bacteriuria patients experience no obvious clinical symptoms or signs of UTI (including altered mental status in the elderly), yet urinalysis and culture yield findings consistent with bacteriuria. In contrast, the dysuria–pyuria syndrome (also called "acute urethral syndrome") is characterized by painful urination with white blood cells (WBCs) on microscopic urinalysis in the absence of a positive bacterial culture. Such a condition may be due to organisms such as *Chlamydia* that do not grow well on standard urinary culture. This condition may, however, be difficult to distinguish clinically from vaginitis due to sexually transmitted infection.

Clinical Presentation
Subjective

The presenting signs and symptoms of UTIs vary widely in intensity and occurrence. Women may present with urethritis and cystitis simultaneously. The most frequently reported symptoms in both males and females are dysuria, urinary frequency or urgency, nocturia, hematuria, low back or suprapubic pain, urinary incontinence, or cloudy, foul-smelling urine. These symptoms can occur in any combination. In elderly patients, altered mental status may be the sole manifestation of UTI and should create a high level of suspicion.

Urethritis in men is rare; if left untreated or treated inadequately, it can lead to complications such as urethral strictures, periurethral abscess, urethral diverticuli, and fissures. Vaginal discharge in women and urethral discharge in men may suggest sexually transmitted diseases (STDs). Purulent urethral discharge *(Neisseria gonorrhoeae)* or whitish-mucoid discharge *(Chlamydia trachomatis)* should be treated aggressively with the appropriate antibiotic therapy.

Objective

The physical exam should include a clean-catch, midstream urine sample for urinalysis. The urinalysis will reveal an infectious process in the urinary tract system and may exhibit any of the following: cloudy appearance, alkaline pH, hematuria, elevated levels of nitrites, leukocyte esterase (detecting pyuria of greater than 10 leukocytes per hpf), and urine sediments of red blood cells (RBCs), WBCs, mucus, and bacterial overgrowth. Of note, the *Enterobacteriaceae* convert urinary nitrates to nitrites, producing positive results on urine dipstick analysis if present in adequate numbers (greater than 100,000 organisms/mL). In contrast, however, staphylococci do not convert this substrate and are not detectable by this test. Moreover, false-positive urinary nitrite tests may result in the presence of the urinary tract analgesic phenazopyridine. A urine culture and sensitivity may be ordered to speciate and determine the sensitivity of the causative organism to specific antibiotic therapy.

Patients with IC may present with the need to urinate frequently because of reduced bladder capacity. This may occur up to 60 times per day in extreme cases. Other symptoms include pain or discomfort in the abdominal area that holds the bladder.

Diagnostic Reasoning
Diagnostic Tests

Diagnosis of lower UTI is made based on the subjective complaints of the patient and a clean-catch midstream urine sample showing the presence of bacteria, especially if more than 100,000 organisms/mL of the same morphology are present in a sample from a female patient. Traditionally, this concentration of bacteria (i.e., 100,000 cfu/mL on urine culture) has been used to define UTI, but UTI may result from far lower bacterial loads, UTI is currently defined as a urine sample with greater than 100 organisms/mL in the presence of characteristic clinical symptoms. The method of urine collection also influences interpretation of the urine culture, because the sterility of commonly performed "clean-catch" techniques is heavily dependent on the patient's ability to clean around the urethra before voiding. Sterile wipes containing iodine, chlorhexidine, or other acceptable cleaning agent must be used to wipe the urethral opening at least two to three times consecutively in a direction away from the perineum to minimize contamination by anorectal flora. Alcohol swabs are unacceptable cleaning agents. Straight catheterization samples obtained with sterile technique are the most reliable, whereas samples obtained from receptacles connected to indwelling catheters may prove unreliable owing to repeated manipulation of the collecting bag.

Although urine culture is considered the gold standard with the greatest sensitivity for laboratory confirmation of UTI, urinalysis with microscopy is also helpful and provides rapid results. Urinalysis also typically indicates pyuria (greater than 10 neutrophils per hpf on microscopic exam) and often the presence of RBCs. Hematuria is common in UTI but not with urethritis or vaginitis; however, blood in the urine is not a marker of complicated infection. UTIs may be treated with empiric antibiotic therapy based on knowledge of the most common bacterial etiologies. However, a urine culture and sensitivity testing will definitively identify the infecting microorganism and the appropriate antibiotic therapy. Although the diagnosis of UTI is made both clinically and by urinalysis, generally urine culture and sensitivities are indicated if complicated infection is suspected, if atypical symptoms are present, or if symptoms persist or recur within 1 month of the patient's receiving an empiric course of antibiotic therapy and a new regimen is desired.

Interstitial cystitis is mostly a diagnosis of exclusion. Although somewhat controversial, a useful diagnostic tool for this condition is the potassium sensitivity test. This test involves slow instillation of 40 mL of sterile water into the bladder and the patient is asked to grade the discomfort on a 0 to 5 scale, with 5 being the most severe. This establishes a baseline. Then the water is emptied and potassium chloride solution is instilled into the bladder and the discomfort graded as in the instillation of water. IC is suggested when there is a 2-point increase in the pain or urgency, indicating abnormal epithelial dysfunction.

Differential Diagnosis

The differential diagnosis of tumors, upper UTI (pyelonephritis), vaginitis, and STDs must be explored. Tumors of the renal system and upper UTI are discussed in this chapter. Vaginitis and STDs are discussed in Chapters 13 and 14. Patients with lower UTI differ from those with upper UTI in that they do not exhibit signs of sepsis such as fever and chills, have WBC casts in the urine (reflecting the passage of neutrophils through the renal tubules), or experience flank and costovertebral angle tenderness on exam.

Management

Pharmacological antimicrobial management is the mainstay of treatment. Drugs Commonly Prescribed 12.2 presents the oral agents typically used for the treatment

---

Drugs Commonly Prescribed 12.2 Urinary Tract Infections

Drug	Indication and Dosage	Adverse Reactions and Prescribing Considerations
Sulfonamides		
trimethoprim and sulfamethoxazole (TMP-SMX) Bactrim, Septra (80 mg TMP/400 mg SMZ) Bactrim DS (160 mg TMP/ 800 mg SMZ) [double strength]	Precoital or postcoital prophylaxis 100 mg trimethoprim after sexual intercourse Acute uncomplicated UTI 1 DS tablet 2 times daily × 3 days for uncomplicated UTI Complicated UTI 8–10 mg/kg/day IV in 2–4 equally divided doses every 6, 8, or 12 hours for up to 14 days For pyelonephritis 1 DS tablet every 12 hours for 7–14 days	**Contraindications:** Hypersensitivity to trimethoprim or sulfonamides Allergy to sulfa Folate deficiency megaloblastic anemia Pregnancy at term and lactation **Side effects:** Abdominal distress Nausea Rash Neutropenia **Special instructions:** Take with a full glass of water. Complete full course of therapy.
Fluoroquinolones		
ciprofloxacin (Cipro) (Cipro XR) [extended release] levofloxacin (Levaquin) ofloxacin (Floxin) norfloxacin (Noroxin)	Ciprofloxacin Uncomplicated UTI 250 mg 2 times daily × 3 days Complicated UTI 500 mg PO 2 times daily × 7–14 days Levofloxacin Uncomplicated 250 mg daily × 3 days Complicated 250 mg daily × 10 days or 750 mg daily × 5 days	**Contraindications:** Hypersensitivity to fluoroquinolones **Side effects:** Nausea Abdominal discomfort Diarrhea Photosensitivity Dizziness Superinfections

Drugs Commonly Prescribed 12.2   Urinary Tract Infections—cont'd

Drug	Indication and Dosage	Adverse Reactions and Prescribing Considerations
	Ofloxacin Uncomplicated 200 mg 2 times daily × 3 days Complicated 200 mg 2 times daily × 10 days Norfloxacin Uncomplicated 400 mg 2 times daily × 3 days Complicated 400 mg 2 times daily × 10–21 days	**Caution:** QTc prolongation, hyper- and hypoglycemia, tendinitis, and tendon rupture have all been associated with fluoroquinolones. Concomitant use with NSAIDs may increase risk of CNS stimulation and seizures. **Special instructions:** Complete the full course of therapy. Do not take at the same time as antacids, calcium, iron, or zinc preparations. Norfloxacin, ofloxacin should not be taken with food or milk.

Aminopenicillins

Drug	Indication and Dosage	Adverse Reactions and Prescribing Considerations
amoxicillin (Amoxil) amoxicillin and potassium clavulanate (Augmentin)	Amoxicillin Mild/moderate infections: 500 mg 2 times daily or 250 mg 3 times daily × 10 days Severe infections: 875 mg 2 times daily or 500 mg 3 times daily × 10 days Amoxicillin and potassium clavulanate Mild/moderate infections: 500 mg/ 125 mg 2 times daily or 250 mg/ 125 mg 3 times daily × 10 days Severe infections: 875 mg/125 mg 2 times daily or 500 mg/125 mg 3 times daily × 10 days	**Contraindications:** Penicillin allergy **Side effects:** Hypersensitivity reactions Urticarial rash Nausea Diarrhea Superinfections **Special instructions:** Complete full course of therapy. May decrease effectiveness of oral contraceptives. Augumentin should be given with food to decrease nausea.

Cephalosporins—Second Generation

Drug	Indication and Dosage	Adverse Reactions and Prescribing Considerations
cefaclor (Ceclor) cefuroxime (Ceftin)	Cefaclor 250–500 mg 3 times daily Cefuroxime (uncomplicated) 250 mg 2 times daily × 7–10 days	**Contraindications:** Allergy to cephalosporins **Side effects:** Pruritis Uticaria Erythema multiforme Rashes Arthritis/arthralgia (with or without fever) Diarrhea Nausea **Special instructions:** Renal dysfunction prolongs half-life. May be taken without regard to meals. Complete full course of therapy.

Cephalosporins—Third Generation

Drug	Indication and Dosage	Adverse Reactions and Prescribing Considerations
cefixime (Suprax) cefpodoxime (Vantin)	Cefixime 400 mg daily × 3–7 days Cefpodoxime 100 mg 2 times daily × 7 days	**Contraindications:** Allergy to cephalosporins **Side effects:** Diarrhea Abdominal pain Nausea

Continued

Drugs Commonly Prescribed 12.2   Urinary Tract Infections—cont'd

Drug	Indication and Dosage	Adverse Reactions and Prescribing Considerations
		Dyspepsia Flatulence **Special instructions:** Reduce dose of cefixime by 25% if renal dysfunction present. Cefpodoxime: avoid antacids 2 hours before and after dose. Complete full course of therapy.
Anti-infectives		
nitrofurantoin (Macrodantin, Furadantin)	UTI 100 mg 2 times daily × 7 days	**Contraindications:** Hypersensitivity to nitrofurantoin Renal function impairment Anuria or oliguria Pregnancy in third trimester, labor, or delivery **Side effects:** Nausea Vomiting Anorexia Abdominal discomfort **Special instructions:** Take with food. May cause urine to darken.
Urinary Analgesic		
phenazopyridine (Pyridium)	Relief of pain, burning, urgency, and frequency from UTI 200 mg 3 times daily after meals; maximum 2 days	**Contraindications:** Hypersensitivity to phenazopyridine **Side effects:** Headache Rash Itching **Special instructions:** Take after meals. May turn urine reddish-orange color and stain fabric.
Antispasmodic		
flavoxate (Urispas)	Relief of dysuria, urgency, frequency, and incontinence 100–200 mg 3–4 times a day	**Contraindications:** Use with caution in patients with glaucoma and older adults. **Side effects:** Nausea Vomiting Dry mouth Headache Drowsiness Blurred vision Vertigo

of lower UTI. Epidemiological surveillance has revealed increasing rates of resistance in *E coli* isolates to ampicillin and sulfonamides, including trimethoprim-sulfamethoxazole (TMP-SMX), but only a small percentage of these isolates were resistant to nitrofurantoin (Macrodantin, Macrobid), which is known to concentrate in the urine. Nitrofurantoin is also effective against many gram-positive cocci such as *Enterococcus faecalis,* whereas other key uropathogens such as *Proteus, Enterobacter,* and *Klebsiella* may be highly resistant. Thus, both TMP-SMX and nitrofurantoin may be used as empiric therapy for uncomplicated UTI only and, in fact, may prove to be inadequate. Indeed, one of the strongest risk factors predicting microbial resistance to TMP-SMX is the previous use of this or any other antimicrobial agent for any type of infection within the past 3 months.

The fluoroquinolones (e.g., ofloxacin, ciprofloxacin, levofloxacin), on the other hand, have widespread efficacy against most uropathogens, although their increasing use as first-line empiric therapy has clearly been associated with steadily rising rates of resistance, as well. Thus, for uncomplicated UTI, a 3-day regimen of TMP-SMX should be used empirically in patients with no history of sulfa drug allergy, previous hospitalization, or antibiotic use for any reason within the past 3 months (Level I; American College of Obstetricians and Gynecologists, 2008) in geographical areas where *E coli* resistance to this agent is known to be less than 20% (e.g., the Northeastern United States, as opposed to the Western United States). A 7-day course of nitrofurantoin should be used as an alternative in patients with documented sulfa allergies or in those with previous antibiotic use within the last 3 months.

The cost-effective 3-day treatment regimen for uncomplicated lower UTI reduces the risk of nonadherence and the development of *Candida* vaginitis due to clearance of normal urogenital flora. It is recommended for TMP-SMX or the fluoroquinolones, but not nitrofurantoin, which requires a longer course of therapy for maximum efficacy. Complicated UTI, on the other hand, requires at least 10 to 14 days of antibiotic therapy. The antimicrobial effects of these medications persist for several days after the final dose is administered. In particularly severe cases of UTI (especially in high-risk groups such as elderly or bed-bound patients) or in cases involving urinary tract instrumentation, hospitalization and broad-spectrum IV antibiotic coverage (e.g., ceftriaxone, piperacillin-tazobactam, or ampicillin plus gentamicin) may be required until symptoms wane and urine culture and antibiotic sensitivities confirm the most appropriate antibiotic choice. The same approach may be required for upper UTI (i.e., pyelonephritis).

Empiric treatment of UTI in men (by definition, a complicated UTI) should be extended to at least 7 days. Nitrofurantoin and beta-lactams should be avoided; fluoroquinolones are generally the antibiotics of choice, given their effectiveness in treating occult prostatic infection.

Treatment of UTI during pregnancy is especially important, because an established link exists between premature delivery and UTI (especially pyelonephritis). Empiric therapy may include ampicillin 500 mg PO four times daily, nitrofurantoin (Macrobid, Macrodantin) 100 mg PO two times daily, cephalexin (Keflex) 500 mg PO four times daily, or sulfisoxazole 1 g PO four times daily. Broader-spectrum regimens may include amoxicillin-clavulanate (Augmentin) 500 mg/125 mg PO two times daily or cefpodoxime (Vantin) 100 mg PO two times daily. Most clinicians will choose to treat UTI during pregnancy for 1 full week. Fluoroquinolones should be avoided, given concern for their effects on bone and cartilage formation in the developing fetus, and TMP-SMX should be avoided in the first and third trimesters of pregnancy. In women with a prior history of recurrent UTI, postcoital prophylaxis with a single oral dose of nitrofurantoin 50 mg or cephalexin 250 mg has been shown to be highly effective.

Fungal UTI due to *Candida* infection is typically associated with an indwelling urinary catheter, and nearly half of all cases resolve simply with removal of the catheter. However, reinsertion of a new catheter is associated with a high rate of relapse. Antifungal treatment is typically not required for asymptomatic colonization, but if indicated in the presence of dysuria, an appropriate regimen would be fluconazole (Diflucan) 200 mg PO (or IV for hospitalized patients) daily for 7 to 14 days.

The management of asymptomatic bacteriuria deserves special mention. This condition should be treated with antibiotics in pregnant women (Level II; Scottish Intercollegiate Guidelines Network, 2006), because it increases the risk of premature delivery. Although some studies suggest treatment in girls beyond preschool age is not warranted owing to the high rate of recurrent asymptomatic infection without obvious sequelae, general practice also calls for treating asymptomatic bacteriuria in young children. Treatment is also indicated in patients before they undergo a urological procedure to avoid operating on a contaminated field, after removal of a bladder catheter in place for less than 1 week, and in any patient with an underlying structural abnormality of the urinary tract, vesicoureteral reflux, or struvite stones. In contrast, treatment of this condition in adult men, nonpregnant women, the elderly, diabetic persons, and spinal cord patients with indwelling urinary catheters is not warranted. Although asymptomatic bacteriuria may be a harbinger of future UTI, antibiotic therapy has not been shown to persistently eradicate bacteriuria or urinary tract colonization in these populations.

After completion of antibiotic treatment, follow-up cultures may be obtained to ensure complete eradication of the pathogen in patients with a history of recurrent infection, during pregnancy, or in those prone to complicated UTI. Chronic or recurrent UTI may be prevented through prophylactic treatment either on a daily basis or after sexual intercourse, but this should be done only after all options to eliminate the causative factors of UTI have been explored. Strategies should be emphasized to decrease the incidence of infection through the guidelines outlined under Patient Education.

Although appropriate antibiotic treatment is often adequate to relieve dysuria, certain medications may also be prescribed for the first few days to decrease the pain and discomfort of UTI. Use of these agents should not be prolonged, however, given their significant side-effect profile. Effective treatment may involve anticholinergics, which produce an antispasmodic effect, including atropine (Donnatal), hyoscyamine (Levsin, Cystospaz), propantheline (Pro-Banthine), or oxybutynin (Ditropan). However, anticholinergics may also contribute to urinary retention (especially in the elderly), which is a clear risk factor for UTI, and should thus be used with caution. Analgesics may be prescribed such as phenazopyridine (Pyridium), but this alters the color of urine to orange and may cause urinary leakage secondary to anesthetization of the urethra and sphincter.

IC does not respond to antibiotics. However, this condition may be treated with pentosan polysulfate sodium (Elmiron), which tends to reduce the bladder wall inflammation. This drug has been shown to improve symptoms in 38% of patients with IC. IC is not curable, but it is controllable. If IC is left untreated, it becomes more difficult to treat and in severe cases can progress to the development of a fibrotic contracted bladder. Complementary therapies used for lower UTI are presented in Complementary Therapies 12.1.

Follow-up and Referral

Patients should follow up with a midstream, clean-catch urine sample for urinalysis to evaluate for the presence of WBCs or a culture and sensitivity for all recurrent infections. UTI that is secondary to other pathological conditions will not resolve until the primary causative factor is addressed. Indwelling urinary catheters should be changed every 4 to 6 weeks with new equipment using sterile technique. It is important to maintain adequate hydration and to monitor the urine output for signs of obstruction or renal failure. Urinary tract obstructions must be identified and removed to reduce the chances of chronic infection and renal damage leading to renal insufficiency and failure. It may be necessary to prescribe analgesics for the patient to reduce the pain associated with the UTI. Pain-relieving medications such as phenazopyridine (Pyridium) can be effective but should be prescribed for no more than 3 days.

Self-medication is usually adequate for female patients who have relatively few recurrences of UTI. If a diagnosis of recurrent bacterial UTI is confirmed, the patient should be given a supply of an antibiotic (preferably TMP-SMX or nitrofurantoin) and instructed to take it for 3 to 7 days whenever the symptoms recur. The patient should keep a diary of her infections and response to treatment and review it annually with a health professional so as to track medication-associated problems. The patient should also be advised to notify the clinician if symptoms such as flank pain, fever, hematuria, or lack of response to treatment occur.

If UTI recurs frequently (e.g., monthly), prophylactic therapy should be prescribed. After a course of 10 to 14 days of a suitable antibiotic (e.g., a fluoroquinolone), the patient should begin low-dose antimicrobial prophylaxis every other day at bedtime over a 4- to 6-month period. This regimen has proved as effective as daily dosing. Nighttime therapy is recommended because the patient generally does not void for a prolonged period, thus giving the bacteria the opportunity to adhere to the bladder wall. If this period of prophylaxis has been effective, the patient may switch to self-medication. If the frequency of recurrence increases at this point, however, prophylaxis should be extended to every other night indefinitely. However, all lifestyle issues should be investigated first. There is evidence that the use of cranberry products can reduce the frequency of UTI recurrence (Level I; Scottish Intercollegiate Guidelines Network, 2006).

Patient Education

Patient education should focus on teaching the patient to prevent recurrence of UTI. This is accomplished by advising the patient to follow these guidelines:

- Complete the full course of antibiotic therapy even if all symptoms subside (treatment may be anywhere from 3–14 days in duration).
- Increase fluid intake to eight 8-ounce glasses of water per day; this is most important to continue flushing out bacteria.

Complementary Therapies 12.1	Lower Urinary Tract Infections	
Therapy	Dosage	Comments
Herbs		
Cranberry	300–400 mg PO 2 times daily standardized cranberry extract capsules	Prevents the adherence of bacteria to the bladder wall (proanthocyanidins, active ingredient, inhibits adhesion of *Escherichia coli* to uroepithelial cells)

- Take cranberry supplement and drink cranberry juice to decrease the bacteria's ability to adhere to the epithelial cells that line the bladder.
- Self-medicate if symptomatic.
- Wear cotton underclothes rather than nylon to avoid moisture buildup and avoid wearing "thong" underpants.
- Avoid the use of harsh soaps or feminine hygiene products that can irritate the urethra.
- Use condoms to provide a barrier to infection from intercourse.
- Use proper techniques for self-catheterization to reduce the incidence of introducing bacteria.
- Empty the bladder frequently to avoid stasis of urine.
- Take showers instead of tub baths or bubble baths to avoid chemical irritation of the urethra.
- Keep a diary of urinary symptoms and review it annually if recurrent infections are a problem.
- Empty the bladder completely, possibly by double-voiding (i.e., completely emptying the bladder two times in 5 minutes), especially if recurrent infections are a problem.

The patient should also be educated regarding any potential adverse effects of medication, including urinary leakage associated with phenazopyridine (Pyridium) treatment or the subsequent development of vaginal yeast infections.

UPPER URINARY TRACT INFECTION: PYELONEPHRITIS

Pyelonephritis is an infection of the kidney that is characterized by infection within the renal pelvis, tubules, or interstitial tissue that may be unilateral or bilateral. The condition may be classified as either acute or chronic. The chronic condition leads to changes in the kidney that create atrophy and scarring of the kidney and calyceal deformity that may eventually lead to renal failure.

Epidemiology and Causes

Pyelonephritis occurs in both men and women, but it is more common in women. The occurrence is higher in older adults (especially if institutionalized or hospitalized), children, and immunocompromised patients. Community-acquired pyelonephritis is estimated to occur in approximately 15.7 persons per 100,000 per year. However, hospital-acquired pyelonephritis occurs in approximately 7.3 persons per 10,000 hospitalized persons. The incidence and risk of developing this disease is increased in patients with predisposing factors including anatomical abnormalities such as ureterovesical reflux, urinary obstruction, stress incontinence, multiple or recurrent urinary tract infections (UTIs), renal disease, kidney trauma, pregnancy, and metabolic disorders such as diabetes mellitus. Having an indwelling urinary catheter is always a prominent risk factor for pyelonephritis,

especially in hospitalized elderly women. An episode of acute pyelonephritis within the prior year also puts the patient at increased risk. Most of these risk factors alter the vaginal microenvironment and predispose individuals to lower UTI, as well.

In acute pyelonephritis, the actual insult to the kidney may be hematogenous seeding or urinary tract reflux, but most commonly it is an ascending infection from the bladder. It can often be attributed to untreated lower UTI that spreads to the upper urinary system or is introduced through instrumentation. Chronic pyelonephritis usually has no specific pathological explanation if anatomical abnormalities have been ruled out.

Pathophysiology

Pyelonephritis is typically caused by fecal flora that colonize the vaginal introitus and subsequently ascend along the urinary tract to the kidneys. It is unclear whether lower UTI always precedes pyelonephritis, because many patients present without clinical evidence of prior cystitis. However, bacteria are believed to enter through the urethral meatus and ascend upward from the lower urinary tract (urethra and bladder) to one or both kidneys via the ureters, the bloodstream (i.e., hematogenous spread), or the lymphatic system.

Escherichia coli (75%–95% of cases), *Proteus mirabilis, Klebsiella,* and *Pseudomonas* are the most common gram-negative causative agents. From 5% to 10% of cases are caused by gram-positive organisms, including *Enterococcus, Staphylococcus saprophyticus,* and *Staphylococcus aureus* (particularly in severe infection). *Ureaplasma urealyticum* and *Mycoplasma hominis* are rarer causative agents. In patients with normal urogenital systems, nearly all bacterial agents of pyelonephritis express virulence factors that contribute to their uropathogenicity (e.g., the *pap* and *sfa* operons and pathogenicity islands found in virulent *E coli* strains).

In acute pyelonephritis, swelling of the renal parenchyma occurs as a result of the patchy distribution of the acute infectious process throughout the kidney. In rare instances, scarring of the renal parenchyma leading to kidney atrophy, renal hypertension, and renal failure may occur if left untreated. When the infection is severe, abscesses may develop in the renal medulla leading to necrosis of the renal papillae. This infection can be potentially life-threatening in the elderly, in children, or in immunocompromised patients. In addition, diagnosis and treatment in pregnant women is particularly critical, because upper UTI has a clear association with premature delivery.

Chronic pyelonephritis is usually caused by a recurrent or chronic bacterial infection of the kidney, often related to the presence of instrumentation such as an indwelling catheter that serves as a nidus of infection. Patients often have other urological problems such as vesicoureteral reflux, neurogenic bladder, or urinary obstruction caused by renal tumors, stones, or prostatic hypertrophy. The persistent unresolved infection and inflammation cause fibrosis (scarring) of the tubulointerstitium, which may lead to hypertension as the body senses decreased renal blood flow or eventually chronic renal insufficiency.

Clinical Presentation

Subjective

The patient with acute pyelonephritis may present with a sudden onset of fever, persisting over a few hours or days and ranging up to 103°F (39.5°C). The patient may present with shaking, chills, nausea, and vomiting, as well as unilateral flank or localized back pain over the affected kidney (i.e., costovertebral angle tenderness), fatigue, diarrhea, or other symptoms resembling those of a gram-negative sepsis. Signs of urinary urgency or frequency and suprapubic discomfort may be present. In some cases, the presentation may mimic pelvic inflammatory disease. Otherwise, the patient may be largely asymptomatic and then progress to full-blown sepsis (i.e., urosepsis). In the elderly patient, altered mental status may be the initial manifestation of pyelonephritis.

Chronic pyelonephritis may present with the patient complaining of fatigue, nausea, decreased appetite with weight loss, nocturia, and/or polyuria. Patients may present with symptoms of renal failure resulting from asymptomatic chronic pyelonephritis that has persisted for several years. Symptoms of renal failure are discussed in detail later in this chapter.

Objective

The physical exam will elicit marked tenderness on deep abdominal palpation and/or percussion of the affected flank and back overlying the affected kidney (i.e., costovertebral angle tenderness). Patients may be hypertensive, and with severe pyelonephritis may remain symptomatic for several days, even if appropriate antibiotic therapy is administered.

Patients with chronic pyelonephritis may show minimal symptoms or symptoms similar to those of acute pyelonephritis. The early signs and symptoms may be vague; chronic pyelonephritis usually is first diagnosed when the patient presents with impaired renal function caused by damage to the kidneys.

Diagnostic Reasoning

Diagnostic Tests

The diagnosis of pyelonephritis is confirmed through urinalysis, which is positive for bacteria, proteinuria, leukocyte esterase, urinary nitrites, hematuria, pyuria, and specifically white blood cell (WBC) casts (reflecting the passage of neutrophils through the renal tubules), as well as urine culture, which typically demonstrates greater than 100,000 cfu/mL, allowing for identification of the causative organism. Any of these findings may be

altered, however, if the patient is already on antibiotic therapy, and colony counts may be as low as 10,000 cfu/mL in some cases. Blood cultures may also be positive in 10% to 20% of mild to moderate pyelonephritis, reflecting urosepsis.

Cystoscopy with ureteral catheterization, renal ultrasound (to reveal hydroureter and/or hydronephrosis), or intravenous pyelogram (IVP) may be indicated. However, the nuclear medicine–based dimercaptosuccinic acid (DMSA) scan is most sensitive for detecting pyelonephritis and renal scarring. Although rarely used, renal biopsy in acute pyelonephritis may reveal abscess formation with neutrophilic invasion. The area of the infection is wedge shaped, pointing toward the medulla, and the glomeruli are spared. Findings in chronic pyelonephritis will include fibrosis, scarring, and reduction of renal tissue, with calyceal clubbing, dilation, and distortion. A voiding cystourethrogram may reveal vesicoureteral reflux, which predisposes to both lower and upper UTI.

Differential Diagnosis

It can be difficult to differentiate pyelonephritis from cystitis; however, the presence of WBC casts is diagnostic for pyelonephritis. Hematuria is also often present in lower and upper UTI, but not in vaginitis or urethritis. Chronic pyelonephritis can sometimes be diagnosed through IVP, DMSA scan, and ultrasound, which may identify atrophied kidneys with "clubbing" of the affected calyces. A definitive diagnosis of chronic disease is made by identifying persistent pyuria and by positive urine cultures. Sometimes, chronic pyelonephritis is diagnosed only via kidney biopsy.

Management

Aggressive therapy is necessary to prevent permanent damage to the kidneys, a potential complication of upper versus lower UTI. Tissue penetration of antibiotics into the renal medulla appears more important than serum or urine levels. Oral antibiotics may be prescribed in mild cases of acute pyelonephritis, characterized by the absence of nausea and vomiting or signs of sepsis. First-line therapy includes ciprofloxacin (Cipro) 500 mg two times daily for 7 days, or ciprofloxacin extended-release (Cipro XR) 1,000 mg daily for 7 days, or levofloxacin (Levaquin) 750 mg daily for 5 days. In second-line therapy, trimethoprim-sulfamethoxazole (TMP-SMX) (Bactrim DS, Septra DS) taken orally for 14 days may be as effective as amoxicillin-clavulanate for 14 days in young women with their first pyelonephritis and without anatomical abnormalities. However, given the prevalence of sulfonamide and ampicillin resistance among common uropathogens, TMP-SMX and amoxicillin are likely to be ineffective in cases of recurrent or moderate to severe pyelonephritis (except in cases of *Enterococcus* infection, which calls for the addition of amoxicillin [Amoxil] 500 mg PO three times daily).

Nitrofurantoin should be avoided because it does not achieve adequate tissue levels. Other effective choices are third generation cephalosporins (e.g., cefixime, cefpodoxime, ceftriaxone), aminoglycosides (e.g., gentamicin, tobramycin), or aztreonam, with fluoroquinolones reserved for antibiotic-resistant organisms, hence the critical need for early urine culture to guide pharmacotherapy. Drugs Commonly Prescribed 11.2 presents the oral agents commonly prescribed for lower UTI and mild to moderate pyelonephritis (not requiring hospitalization or IV therapy).

Hospitalization may be indicated, depending on the patient's ability to maintain adequate fluid intake and to tolerate oral antibiotics, along with the severity of the symptoms and evidence of bacteremia. Hospitalization of patients who are pregnant, vomiting, or dehydrated should be strongly considered. Likewise, the patient's degree of systemic illness (bacteremia or urosepsis), age, history of chronic disease, or nonadherence to therapy may lead to the assessment that hospitalization is necessary. Ninety-five percent of patients demonstrate a good response within 48 hours to IV antibiotic treatment and may be discharged on appropriate oral medication, once urine culture and antibiotic sensitivity results are available and subsequent antimicrobial therapy may be narrowed in spectrum. Treatment courses should typically last for 7 to 10 days for mild to moderate cases, 14 days for severe cases, or 21 days in particularly slow responders. Ample evidence has demonstrated that once common 6-week regimens lead to increased adverse effects without improved treatment effectiveness. Selection of a regimen should be based on local resistance and susceptibility results.

Common choices for non-*Enterococcus* infection include ciprofloxacin (Cipro) 400 mg IV every 12 hours, or levofloxacin (Levaquin) 250 mg IV daily for 10 days or 750 mg IV daily for 5 days, except in pregnant patients, in whom fluoroquinolones are contraindicated, given the potential for adverse effects on bone and cartilage development in the developing fetus. Second-line therapy includes ceftriaxone 1 to 2 g IV daily, as well as other extended-spectrum cephalosporins or penicillins, carbapenems, monobactam (in penicillin allergy), and aminoglycosides (except in pregnant patients), such as gentamicin 3 to 5 mg/kg IV daily or tobramycin 3 to 5 mg/kg IV daily in three divided dosages. Fluoroquinolones are also appropriate choices, except in pregnant women, given concerns over their effects on bone and cartilage formation in the developing fetus. This class of antibiotics has virtually equivalent absorption when administered orally or intravenously at the same dose (see Drugs Commonly Prescribed 11.2). Thus, IV fluoroquinolone preparations should be used only for patients with active nausea and vomiting. When enterococcal infection is suspected, ampicillin 1 to 2 g IV every 6 hours should be combined with either gentamicin or tobramycin at 1 mg/kg IV every 8 hours added for synergy. Another option for empiric therapy is the broad-spectrum antibiotic piperacillin-tazobactam (Zosyn) 3.375 g IV every 6 hours given over 30 minutes. If the creatinine clearance is between 20 and 40 mL/min, the dose should be 2.25 g every 6 hours. If the creatinine clearance is less than 20 mL/min, the dose should be 2.25 g every 8 hours.

If the patient does not respond adequately within 48 hours, he or she should be reevaluated, the cultures reviewed, and an ultrasound, IVP, or DMSA scan performed. IV antibiotics may need to be administered for up to 7 to 10 days in severe cases. During treatment the patient must increase fluid intake, and an accurate intake and output record must be maintained for appropriate fluid management. Surgery may be indicated to remove or correct secondary causes of UTI such as urinary obstruction or anatomical abnormalities and neuropathic genitourinary tract lesions. Diagnostic studies requiring insertion of instruments should be delayed until the urine is sterile or free of bacteria and/or pus, to avoid the complications of bacteremia or septic shock. A urological anatomical evaluation should be performed for all men with pyelonephritis and women with recurrent pyelonephritis to elicit structural abnormalities that may be contributing to or causing the condition.

Follow-up and Referral

If undergoing outpatient treatment, the patient should be seen 48 hours later to assess responsiveness to therapy. Similarly, patients in the hospital should be evaluated in 48 hours for response to therapy and consideration of discharge. Follow-up urine cultures are not routinely recommended in asymptomatic patients. However, for those with recurrent pyelonephritis, reculturing at 2, 6, and 12 weeks after antibiotic therapy is initiated may be done to ensure complete and lasting eradication of infection. Further treatment decisions are based on clinical findings such as fever, pain, and culture of bacteria. When a diagnosis of chronic pyelonephritis is determined, the patient should be referred to a nephrologist because of the severe damage that can occur to the kidney. As discussed previously, a renal ultrasound, renal colic CT scan, or voiding cystourethrogram may detect structural abnormalities, renal stones, or vesicoureteral reflux—all of which predispose the patient to infection. Patients should also be monitored and treated for other conditions secondary to the pyelonephritis such as hypertension, chronic infection, renal insufficiency, or renal failure.

Patient Education

The focus should be on teaching the patient to prevent recurrence of lower UTI and pyelonephritis by following these instructions:

- Complete the antibiotic therapy even if symptoms subside.
- Prevent or reduce the incidence of lower UTIs by following the guidelines under Patient Education in the previous section.

- Increase fluid intake to eight 8-ounce glasses of water per day.
- Report any recurrence of UTI symptoms immediately.
- Take a cranberry supplement and drink cranberry juice to decrease the bacteria's ability to adhere to the epithelial cells that line the bladder.
- Control hypertension with medications, dietary regimen, and lifestyle changes as detailed in Chapter 10.

■ NEPHROLITHIASIS

Nephrolithiasis is a condition in which stones (renal calculi) originate in the kidney. The stones form from calcium salts (approximately 75%–85%), struvite (approximately 10%–15%), uric acid (approximately 7%), and cystine (1%–2%). These stone formations often cause acute episodes of urinary tract obstruction, infection, and severe pain in adults.

Epidemiology and Causes

The incidence of renal calculi occurs in people aged 20 to 60 years but peaks in those aged 20 to 30 years. It affects approximately 2% to 5% of individuals at some time during their lifetime, or about 70 to 210 per 100,000 of the population. Calcium oxalate stones occur more often in men, whereas struvite stones are more common in women. Formation of renal calculi is more prevalent in the Southeast, West, and Midwest. The patient may report a sedentary lifestyle or occupation that exposes him or her to high environmental temperatures. Renal stones can occur because of obstruction, urinary stasis, infection, dehydration and urine concentration, increased consumption of calcium or vitamin D, excessive excretion of uric acid, or vitamin A deficiency. Hereditary factors can also predispose the patient to kidney stone formation.

Calcium oxalate and calcium phosphate stones account for 65% to 85% of all cases of renal calculi. These types of stones are found predominantly in men and in individuals whose diet is high in salt, animal fat, animal protein, and oxalate from green leafy vegetables. Interestingly, a low-calcium diet is also a risk factor, as it leads to increased oxaluria because less oxalate is bound to calcium in the gastrointestinal tract. Vasectomy is a risk factor as well, and hypertension doubles the risk of stone formation for reasons that are as yet unclear. Patients with calcium oxalate or calcium phosphate stones typically do not have hypercalcemia except with certain disorders such as hyperparathyroidism, sarcoidosis, and hyperuricemia, which may lead to hypercalciuria or hyperuricosuria. Loop diuretics such as furosemide (Lasix) also promote calciuria, and hypocitraturia and hyperoxaluria similarly predispose to calcium stone formation, because an increased amount of calcium is available for complexing with oxalate or phosphate within the urinary tract. Inflammatory bowel disease is associated with marked hyperoxaluria. Medullary sponge kidney disease is found in 10% to 30% of persons with calcium stones.

Struvite stones are found predominantly in women; these stones are associated with urinary tract infections (UTIs). They occur when the urine is alkaline (pH greater than 7.0) and a urea-splitting organism such as *Proteus* or *Klebsiella* is present. Uric acid stones are formed from an increase in uric acid production or ineffective elimination of uric acid, as found in gout. This may result from dietary intake of foods high in uric acid, acidic urinary pH (e.g., type I renal tubular acidosis, significant bicarbonate loss associated with severe diarrhea), regional enteritis, hereditary factors (including a predisposition to gout), or ulcerative colitis. Uric acid stones account for approximately 15% to 20% of all cases of nephrolithiasis. Cystine stones are created because of a rare autosomal recessive disorder called cystinuria. These stones are formed when there is a metabolic error that causes a decrease in tubular reabsorption in the kidney, leading to urinary cystine concentrations greater than 250 mg/L. Cystine stones account for approximately 1% to 3% of all cases of renal stones.

Pathophysiology

Renal stone formation occurs when normally soluble mineral substances supersaturate the urine and deposit out of solution as crystals, which serve as nuclei for stone-forming substances such as calcium oxalate, calcium phosphate, triple-phosphate struvite (magnesium ammonium phosphate), uric acid, or cystine. Stone formation may also be facilitated by extremes in the urinary pH (alkaline or acid). This crystal combination becomes trapped within the renal system, where it continues to attract other crystals, causing the stone to increase in size. Stones are typically anchored at the ends of collecting ducts at sites of epithelial injury. The calculi vary in size and composition and typically grow within the renal tubules, calyces, renal pelvis, ureters, or bladder. Large stones are called staghorn calculi if they span more than one of the renal calyces. Although over the span of years their presence in the kidneys may lead to chronic renal failure, unless they fragment and pass through the urinary system, they are generally asymptomatic.

The four major types of stones and their characteristics, causes, etiology, diagnosis, and treatment are listed in Table 12.4. These forms are not mutually exclusive and share certain risk factors, and many patients have renal stones of a mixed etiology. Calcium stones are light in color; their crystals characteristically resemble red blood cells (RBCs) in shape and size or may be a larger "dumbbell" form. Formation of these stones may be secondary to hypercalcemia or they may be idiopathic. Hyperoxaluria and hyperuricosuria are more associated with calcium oxalate stones, whereas calcium phosphate stones are more associated with primary hyperparathyroidism. Struvite stones are flat and consist of hexagon-shaped crystals that are radiopaque. They often form secondary to UTI caused by *Proteus mirabilis*. Staghorn calculi are more likely to be struvite stones. Uric acid

Table 12.4   Renal Calculi

Type of Stone (percentage of all stones)	Characteristics	Causes	Management
Calcium (75%–80%)	Resembles RBCs in shape and size or large dumbbell form Light color	Idiopathic, hypercalcemia, or increased levels of uric acid	Thiazide diuretics Diet Cholestyramine or oral calcium Surgery
Struvite (15%)	Flat, hexagon shape Radiopaque	Alkaline urine, infection with urea-splitting organisms such as *Pseudomonas*	Antibiotic therapy Surgery
Uric acid (7%)	Teardrop-shaped or flat square plates Red-orange color	Increased uric acid production, high intake of uric acid, acidic urine, regional enteritis, ulcerative colitis, or idiopathic	Allopurinol Fluid replacement Diet Surgery
Cystine (<1%)	Lemon yellow and sparkle	Hereditary	Force fluids D-Penicillamine Tiopronin

stones are radiolucent and red-orange, with a teardrop or flat square shape. Formation of these stones may be associated with a hereditary etiology of gout or with idiopathic causes. Uric acid crystals may also serve as a nidus for calcium stone formation. Cystine stone crystals are lemon yellow, hexagonal, and sparkle under light microscopy. Finally, certain medications promote crystalluria and predispose the patient to renal stones; these medications include topiramate, triamterene, and sulfadiazine. The protease inhibitor indinavir (Crixivan) used to treat HIV-positive patients may actually precipitate within the renal collecting system, causing direct stone formation.

The incidence of recurrence of certain stones is approximately 40% to 50% within 5 years, with an estimated one-third of patients eventually losing a kidney if the condition is untreated or inadequately treated. Complications can occur when the stone obstructs the flow of urine. This can lead to urinary retention, accumulation of uremic wastes, end-stage renal failure, and/or electrolyte imbalances. Stones can predispose the patient to UTI and hematuria.

Clinical Presentation

Subjective

The patient with an acute episode of nephrolithiasis may present with a variety of signs and symptoms, depending on the location, size, and type of stone. Onset is usually sudden, with renal colic, which is a type of flank pain that is not relieved by changes in position or other measures. The pain may present with a referral pattern that originates in the flank or kidney area and radiates across

the abdomen down into the groin, perineal area, and inner thigh. This colicky pain occasionally progresses to constant pain at a level that can be excruciating and intractable. Other symptoms of renal calculi may include nausea, urinary frequency, vomiting, diaphoresis, dysuria, hematuria, and weakness. The patient may report a history of a recent or chronic UTI, previous diagnosis with nephrolithiasis, a dietary history consistent with stone formation, or alterations in voiding patterns.

Objective

The patient may present with abdominal distention and guarding on palpation, flank tenderness on percussion, and decreased or absent bowel sounds on auscultation. Fever may be present if there is acute infection related to obstruction. Blood pressure (as well as pulse rate and respiratory rate) may be elevated because of pain.

Diagnostic Reasoning
Diagnostic Tests

The diagnostic work-up should begin with a routine urinalysis, complete blood count, and blood chemistry profile. The urinalysis may be normal or it may show RBCs, WBCs, crystals, cast minerals, bacteria, pus, and an alkaline or acidic pH. Table 12.5 identifies the tests and the expected results that would lead to the suspicion of renal calculi. Either gross or microscopic hematuria is observed in the majority of cases but may be absent in up to 30% of cases, depending on the time of presentation. Identification of the type of stone formation is important for the appropriate treatment to be instituted. The results of these tests should lead the clinician to

Table 12.5	Tests for Renal Calculi
Test	Rationale
Urinalysis	Shows RBCs, WBCs, crystals, casts, minerals, bacteria, pus, abnormal pH.
24-hour urine	May show increased levels of creatinine, uric acid, calcium, phosphorus, oxylate or cystine.
Serum chemistry	May show increased levels of magnesium, calcium, uric acid, phosphorus, protein, and electrolytes.
Serum BUN and creatinine	Shows BUN elevated secondary to urinary tract obstruction; creatinine elevated secondary to damage to the kidney.
Complete blood count	May show infection or septicemia.
Kidney and upper bladder	Shows calculi and/or anatomical changes.
Intravenous pyelogram	Shows calculi and any abnormality in anatomic structures.
Cystoureteroscopy	May show calculi and/or abnormal structural defects.
CT scan	Identifies calculi and other masses in the renal system.

continue the diagnostic work-up with noninvasive tests to identify obstructions, masses, or anatomical abnormalities. Further diagnostic tests include the kidney, ureters, and bladder x-ray studies, abdominal or transvaginal ultrasonography (used for pregnant women and those of childbearing age in whom radiation must be avoided), or noncontrast helical computed tomography scan (contrast is avoided due to potential renal toxicity). Invasive procedures may be necessary to visualize or assist in removing the stone through IVP, cystourethroscopy, or other surgical procedures.

Differential Diagnosis

The differential diagnosis for renal calculi may include a variety of diseases, including appendicitis, diverticulitis, mesenteric adenitis, pancreatitis, ileus, peptic ulcer disease, abnormalities of the fallopian tubes and ovaries including ovarian cysts, ectopic pregnancy, gallbladder disease, and abdominal aneurysms. A tentative diagnosis of renal calculi is made from the history and the findings of the physical exam showing increased intensity of renal colic with flank pain or a pattern of referred pain, coupled with flank tenderness. Because hematuria may be the only presenting sign of stone formation, malignancy (renal cell carcinoma), which is typically painless, must also be considered. Diagnosis of renal stones is confirmed by urinalysis that is positive for blood and renal visualization by radiography or ultrasound.

Management

Treatment goals are to decrease the symptoms and complications arising from existing stones and prevent subsequent recurrence. It is important, therefore, to decrease the concentration of stone-forming substances in the urine. An intake of six to eight 8-ounce glasses of water a day is essential; this high fluid intake must continue indefinitely. Most stones smaller than 5 mm pass spontaneously; rates of spontaneous passage steadily decrease

for stones larger than this and is highly unlikely for stones larger than 10 mm.

Initially, pain management is the priority. Oral NSAIDs in doses of 600 to 800 mg 3 times daily or oral narcotics such as hydrocodone-acetaminophen (Vicodin, Lortab), acetaminophen-codeine (Tylenol #3), or oxycodone-acetaminophen (Percocet) are often necessary. In some cases, intramuscular or IV narcotic analgesics may be necessary, but most studies have demonstrated that NSAIDs are as effective as oral opiates, albeit slower acting. In addition, they have also been shown to relax ureteral smooth muscle, which may facilitate stone passage. Antispasmodics such as flavoxate or oxybutynin may also provide temporary relief, but the anticholinergic effects of these medications must be taken into account, because they may lead to urinary retention. Warm compresses to the lower back, focused breathing, imagery, and diversional activities may provide minimal relief.

Certain drugs help to reduce urinary excretion of stone-forming substances. Most notably, thiazide diuretics (e.g., hydrochlorothiazide) reduce calcium excretion; allopurinol reduces uric acid production by inhibiting xanthine oxidase; and D-penicillamine affects the excretion of cystine. Importantly, loop diuretics such as furosemide (Lasix) and triamterene increase calciuria and typically worsen renal stone formation.

Noninvasive or invasive surgical interventions may be necessary if the stone does not pass spontaneously; these are presented in Table 12.6. Noninvasive procedures to treat renal calculi are aggressive and have many of the same risks that occur with surgery. Extracorporeal shock wave lithotripsy (ESWL) sends shock waves throughout the outside of the body to disrupt proximal and midureteral calculi and is preferred for stones smaller than 10 mm. NSAIDs should be avoided at least 3 days before this therapy to minimize the risk of bleeding. The percutaneous ultrasonic lithotriptor (PUL) applies

Table 12.6	Surgical and Other Procedures for Renal Calculi Management		
Procedure	**Type of Procedure**	**Location of Calculi**	**Description**
Lithotripsy	Invasive	Bladder or urethra	Crushing of the calculi under direct visualization using a lithotriptoscope
Lithotony	Invasive	Renal system	Arthroscopic removal of the calculi
Lithonephrotomy	Invasive	Kidney	Incision of the kidney to remove the calculi
Lithotomy	Invasive	Bladder or urethra	Incision of the bladder or ureter to remove the calculi
Ureteral stent	Invasive	Kidney or ureter	Stent is placed in front of the calculi to facilitate elimination
Lithotrophic	Noninvasive	Renal system	Agent used to dissolve calculi
Percutaneous ultrasonic lithotriptor	Noninvasive	Renal system	Ultrasound waves are applied to the outside of the body to crush the calculi
Extracorporeal shock wave lithotripsy	Noninvasive	Renal system	Shock waves are applied to the outside of the body to crush the calculi

therapeutic ultrasound waves to the outside of the body to achieve the same results. A lithotriptic agent may also be used to dissolve the calculi stones.

Invasive procedures may be necessary to remove the stone because of the location of the stone or the failure of noninvasive procedures to destroy the stone. The procedure chosen is dependent on the location, size, and type of stone (e.g., struvite stones typically require ESWL or surgical intervention). First and second generation lithotriptors originally visualized stones via fluoroscopy or ultrasonography. However, advances in urethroscopy with flexible fiber-optic systems now allow for the direct visualization of stones virtually anywhere along the urinary tract from the urethra to the renal pelvis. Stones may be crushed via electrohydraulic or laser lithotripsy in conjunction with these visualization techniques. Flexible ureteroscopy combined with laser lithotripsy is now the preferred treatment for proximal ureteral stones larger than 10 mm. The patient is then able to eliminate the stones naturally after they are crushed into smaller pieces. *Lithotomy* is an incision into the bladder or ureter to remove calculi or place a ureteral stent, whereas *lithotony* specifically denotes arthroscopic extraction of a renal stone from the bladder. Ureteral stents may be placed within the ureters to facilitate the passage of stones through natural elimination. *Lithonephrotomy* is an incision into the kidney to remove a stone.

Preventive measures should be taken to reduce the incidence of recurrence. The incidence of calcium-based stones may be reduced by increasing fluid intake (greater than 2 L/day) and taking thiazide diuretics or allopurinol. In addition, an acidic diet higher in meat content actually promotes calcium excretion. Hypocitraturia and hyperuricosuria may both be treated with potassium citrate supplementation. However, this may alkalinize the urine, creating another risk factor for stone formation,

and care must be taken to stop this drug if urine pH is greater than 6.0. In similar fashion, appropriate treatment of UTI must be initiated to avoid recurrence of struvite stones, and the urease inhibitor acetohydroxamic acid (Lithostat) 250 mg PO three to four times daily may be given as adjunctive therapy to prevent urinary alkalinization, if infection with urease-producing organisms is confirmed.

Oxalate-containing stones should be prevented with a low-oxalate diet (see Patient Education). Struvite stone production may be decreased by preventing UTIs through patient education and self-care as previously discussed, maintenance of antibiotic therapy, or acidifying the urine with methenamine mandelate. Uric acid stones may be decreased through diet modification (see Patient Education) or medications that facilitate uric acid excretion, such as allopurinol. Recurrence of cystine stones may be reduced through maintenance doses of D-penicillamine, tiopronin, or captopril, which binds cystine via sulfhydryl moieties.

Follow-up and Referral

Most patients with renal calculi are treated and followed on an outpatient basis. The patient may need hospitalization for secondary complications that can occur, such as severe nausea and vomiting leading to dehydration, urinary obstruction, decreased renal function, severe bleeding, intractable pain, and significant infection. The patient should be referred to a urologist and/or nephrologist for stone removal under these circumstances or if stone formation is thought to be secondary to a metabolic abnormality.

Patient Education

The patient should be instructed to increase fluid intake to six to eight 8-ounce glasses per day unless prevented by cardiac complications, such as congestive heart failure. Increasing fluids will assist in the elimination of the stones. The patient should monitor intake and output and strain the urine for passed stones. Over-the-counter drugs that contain phosphorus or calcium, such as many antacids (e.g., Tums), and most vitamin supplements, especially vitamin D_3, should be avoided. The role of vitamin C supplementation is controversial. Although some promote high-dose vitamin C supplementation to acidify the urine and facilitate stone dissolution (especially the calcium phosphate type), excess vitamin C (1 g/day) is known to undergo chemical conversion to oxalate, which may promote oxaluria and calcium oxalate stone formation. In contrast, vitamin B_6 and magnesium are both known to decrease oxaluria by facilitating oxalate metabolism. Magnesium further competes with calcium, reducing calcium-containing stone formation. In turn, supplementation of vitamin B_6 and magnesium has been shown to reduce the incidence of oxalate stones, although the ideal doses have not been established.

The patient should be encouraged to increase his or her activity level as tolerated, because inactivity contributes to stone formation secondary to calcium shifts and urinary stasis. Dietary modification is also important. In general, caffeine, beer, and wine should be avoided. A low-oxalate diet is appropriate for calcium oxalate stones, which avoids oxalate-rich foods including beets, black tea, chocolate and cocoa, lamb, nuts, rhubarb, and spinach. A low-phosphorus diet for calcium phosphate or struvite stones would eliminate milk products and cola drinks. A low-purine diet is often effective in reducing stones formed from excess uric acid. This diet limits the intake of purine-rich foods, such as organ meats, red meats, seafood (especially sardines, anchovies, and scallops), poultry, legumes, whole grains, and alcohol (which decreases uric acid clearance).

■ RENAL TUMORS

Renal tumors (neoplasms) are characterized by abnormal tissue formations on or around the kidney that may cause or contribute to renal disease. They may be primary or secondary (resulting from malignant spread), although the latter are rarely clinically relevant and are typically found during postmortem examination. *Renal adenomas* (benign tumors) and adenocarcinomas are rare; these tumors usually create complications requiring surgical removal.

Epidemiology and Causes

Renal cell carcinomas originating in the renal cortex are the most common (85%) malignant renal tumors. These tumors occur most often in the parenchyma of the kidney, with ureteral and urethral tumors occurring rarely. Histologically, they are classified as clear cell (75%–85%), chromophilic or papillary (15%), chromophobic (5%), and the uncommon forms of oncocytic and collecting duct tumors. Transitional cell carcinomas

are the next most common, comprising 5% to 8% of all tumors; these typically affect the bladder and are discussed extensively in the next section.

Renal tumors are responsible for approximately 3% of all adult malignancies. The incidence is higher in men (although the difference in incidence has been decreasing over time), with onset between ages 55 and 70 years and rarely occurring in people younger than 35 years of age. These cancers are curable in more than 90% of patients if they are superficial and/or localized in the renal pelvis or ureter. Tumors that are invasive have a 10% to 15% chance of being cured. In children, nephroblastoma (Wilms' tumor) is common, comprising 5% of primary tumors, whereas sickle cell disease has a known, albeit rare, association with carcinoma of the renal medulla.

Obesity; exposure to asbestos, cadmium, and/or gasoline; the use of phenacetin- and aspirin-containing analgesics; and chronic hemodialysis for acquired polycystic kidney disease are all risk factors for renal cell carcinoma. Cigarette smoking has a 25% to 30% correlation with the development of renal cell carcinoma.

Pathophysiology

The urinary system is lined with transitional cell epithelium where tumors may form. The tumors often are asymptomatic and grow undetected until complications from the tumor present. The tumors are usually encapsulated and located near the cortex unilaterally. Renal neoplasms may be diagnosed as benign or malignant; they may be identified as either primary (originating in the kidney) or secondary (originating or spread from another source). Primary malignancies usually spread through the lymph nodes and blood vessels to the lungs, liver, and bone. Metastatic disease that spreads to the kidney, usually from the lung, is more common than primary renal neoplasms. Metastatic lesions to the ureter typically originate via hematogenous spread from breast or colorectal primary lesions. Direct extension into the ureter may also occur from cervical or colonic neoplasms, as well as pelvic retroperitoneal lymphoma. Benign renal neoplasms are rare but should be removed because of complications that may occur such as pain, bleeding, and obstruction.

Carcinogen exposure has been associated with specific gene mutations that appear to underlie the development of various forms of hereditary renal cell carcinoma, for example, the von Hippel–Lindau tumor suppressor gene on chromosome 3p25 to 26 (associated with both sporadic and hereditary clear cell carcinoma, i.e., von Hippel–Lindau disease), the fumarate hydratase gene, the Birt-Hogg-Dubé tumor suppressor gene on chromosome 17p, the c-*met* oncogene on chromosome 7 that codes the hepatocyte growth factor receptor (associated with hereditary papillary renal cell carcinoma), the *ras* gene family, and *p53* overexpression (implicated in cellular division). However, definitive causal relationships between these various mutational hot spots and renal cancer have not been proven.

Clear cell carcinomas consistently display mutations spanning the 3p14 to 3p26 chromosomal region. In contrast, chromophilic carcinomas lack these mutations but have been associated with various trisomies, including chromosomes 12, 16, and 20. Chromophobic carcinomas, which arise from the intercalated cells of the collecting duct system, typically display hypodiploidy with a wide variety of whole chromosomal deletions. The much less common oncocytic carcinomas have been associated with deletions in chromosome 11q13, but as with collecting duct tumors, no consistent chromosomal abnormalities have been identified.

Clinical Presentation

Subjective

Signs and symptoms vary depending on the size of the tumor. Early signs of tumor growth are silent: Approximately 60% of the time, patients present with gross hematuria as the only symptom. The patient complains of a dull, achy flank pain or abdominal mass in approximately 30% of cases. In 10% to 15% of patients, the triad of flank pain, hematuria, and abdominal mass is found, which is often a sign of advanced disease.

Objective

Examination of the patient may reveal other symptoms that may present alone or in combination with hematuria. General signs of advanced disease include weight loss and fatigue; more specific signs and symptoms of renal tumors include intermittent fever (not associated with infection), palpable abdominal mass, and nephralgia. Metastasis of renal cancer indicates a poor prognosis; it typically involves the lungs, lymph nodes, liver, bones, and contralateral kidney.

Diagnostic Reasoning

Diagnostic Tests

The diagnosis of a renal mass is initially confirmed by intravenous pyelogram (IVP) with nephrotomography; however, it is often impossible to determine if the mass is solid or cystic with this test. Generally speaking, a cancerous tumor splays, distorts, or occludes the visualization of the collecting system and prevents normal filling and draining of the renal system. Although hematuria is common, urine cytology is not consistently reliable for diagnosing these tumors. Ureteroscopy or ultrasonography with IVP can be used to differentiate a potentially neoplastic tissue from a cyst formation by direct or indirect visualization of the entire renal system. Once tissue biopsy samples are obtained, flow cytometric analysis is used to determine the ploidy (DNA content) of the tumor, and histological analysis determines morphology and tumor grade (degree of cellular differentiation).

Urine cytology samples often provide inadequate tissue for such analyses, however, and the mass must be biopsied directly. Treatment Flowchart 12.1 presents evaluation of treatment of a renal mass.

Magnetic resonance imaging and CT scan are useful in preoperative work-up and staging of the metastatic lesion. It is necessary to stage the advancement of the tumor to initiate appropriate treatment. Staging of the neoplasm is confirmed through surgical intervention. Staging identifies the tumor advancement and potential for survival.

- Stage I is defined as a tumor confined within the kidney capsule; it is treated by nephrectomy. The 5-year survival rate is 60% to 75%.
- Stage II is defined as the invasion of the renal capsule that is confined within the Gerota's fascia; it is treated by nephrectomy. The 5-year survival rate is 47% to 65%.
- Stage III is defined as involvement of the regional lymph nodes ipsilateral, renal vein, or vena cava. The 5-year survival rate is 5% to 15%.
- Stage IV is defined as distant metastasis, with a 5-year survival rate of less than 5%.

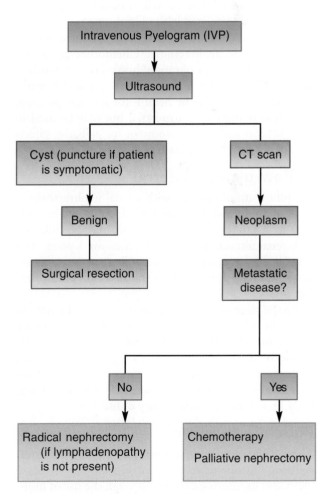

Treatment Flowchart 12.1 Evaluation of Treatment of a Renal Mass

Approximately 30% of patients with renal tumors have metastatic disease when diagnosis is made. The most common sites of metastasis are the lung (50%–60%), bone (30%–40%), regional nodes (15%–30%), brain (10%), and adjacent organs.

Differential Diagnosis

A renal cyst is differentiated from a renal tumor by biopsy. Renal calculi and renal infarction must be ruled out, as well as (rarely) renal tuberculosis. In addition, polycystic kidney disease and hydronephrosis must be considered and may be ruled out on biopsy.

Management

As with any cancer, treatment of renal tumors requires immediate specialist referral to a urologist or surgical oncologist, often with additional consultation by a medical oncologist or nephrologist, depending on the patient's renal function. Treatment for a renal neoplasm is primarily surgical with a partial or total nephrectomy, with or without regional lymphadenectomy if no metastatic disease is present. Less radical surgical interventions have been suggested by a minority of urologists, who stress the poor prognosis of advanced renal tumors, regardless of surgical intervention, as well as increased morbidity and mortality associated with radical surgery.

No universal standards have been accepted for the treatment after nephrectomy. Chemotherapy is not effective with this type of cancer; however, immunotherapy using lymphokine-activated killer cells with or without interleukin-2 may be helpful for selected patients. Radiation therapy is controversial but may be used in combination with nephrectomy or for palliative effects in patients with bone metastasis.

Follow-up and Referral

For follow-up of patients with a total nephrectomy, a CT scan of the abdomen and renal fossa should be done in 3 to 6 months; then the patient may be followed with renal ultrasound every 6 months for 3 years, then annually, unless symptoms occur. Chest x-ray studies are done quarterly for a year to monitor for pulmonary metastasis.

At the time of the neoplasm diagnosis, the patient should be referred to a urologist for a surgical evaluation and to an oncologist for cancer treatment. The patient should be seen by the primary-care provider as needed for problems not related to the cancer and to assist the patient with counseling regarding grief, death and dying, body image changes, and quality of life.

Patient Education

The patient needs preparation for the surgical intervention. Postoperatively, the focus is on pain management and promoting comfort through the use of moist heat, analgesic/narcotics, or positioning on the side with pillows and back support. Additional interventions include preventing pneumonia and atelectasis by encouraging the patient to do coughing and deep breathing exercises, incision care, and monitoring bowel and bladder function.

■ BLADDER TUMORS

Bladder tumors are abnormal tissue masses that occur in the bladder wall lining, which is composed of transitional cell epithelium, or "urothelium." These tumors commonly recur despite aggressive treatment.

Epidemiology and Causes

Bladder tumors are the most common cancer of the urinary system; they represent approximately 2% of all malignant tumors and result in 3% of cancer deaths per year. Bladder cancer is the fifth most common neoplasm in the United States; it occurs in men three times more often than in women, and most often in adults aged 60 to 70. It is also more common among non-Hispanic white men than in other ethnic or racial groups.

There is a significant correlation between bladder tumors and risk factors including cigarette smoking, presence of renal tumors, exposure to aromatic amine dyes known as arylamines (e.g., beta-naphthylamines, xenylamine, 4-nitrobiphenyl, and benzidine), arsenic, chronic use of phenacetin-containing analgesics, saccharin (in rodent studies), chronic lower urinary tract infection (UTI), schistosomiasis, and recurrent nephrolithiasis. Other predisposing factors include previous radiation treatment for cervical, ovarian, or prostate cancer and prior cyclophosphamide chemotherapy.

Pathophysiology

The second most common form of renal carcinomas arise from the transitional cell uroepithelium (urothelium), which lines the mucosal surfaces of the collecting tubules, renal calyces, renal pelvis, ureters, bladder, and urethra. Transitional cell carcinomas account for 90% of all tumors of renal pelvic or ureteral origin. Bladder tumors are primarily transitional cell carcinoma, which have the most favorable prognosis, but may also include squamous cell carcinoma and adenocarcinoma. Bladder tumors are described as papillary (90%) or nonpapillary (10%). Papillary bladder lesions form as a small protuberance attached to a stalk. Nonpapillary lesions are more invasive and have a poorer prognosis. Primary bladder cancer tends to metastasize to the lymph nodes, liver, bones, and lungs. Bladder cancer may be secondary to local extension and/or metastatic disease from adjacent organs such as the cervix in women and the prostate in men.

Genetic analyses of transitional cell carcinomas demonstrate a loss of heterozygosity at any one of multiple chromosomal locations, including 9q (most common), 5p, 8p, 10q, 11p, and 17p—all of which may represent sites of tumor suppressor genes. Genetic predispositions also appear to exist, based on allelic variants of the p450 cytochrome enzyme complex. For instance, smokers afflicted with bladder cancer express p450 enzyme variants that lead to increased activation of arylamine metabolites, a required step for their role in bladder carcinogenesis. Along this same line, allelic variants exist for the *N*-acetyltransferase gene *NAT2,* which (along with *NAT1*) serves as the primary pathway for the metabolism and detoxification of arylamines via *N*-acetylation. Individuals with *NAT2* variants conferring a "slow-acetylation" phenotype are up to 17 times more likely to develop bladder cancer than those with a "fast-acetylation" phenotype. A similar phenomenon exists regarding the glutathione-*S*-transferase M1 gene *(GSTM1),* which contributes to detoxification of carcinogenic compounds via conjugation to glutathione and the facilitation of excretion. In the United States, nearly 50% of white men display deletions in both alleles of this gene, effectively eliminating any enzymatic activity from the *GSTM1* gene product.

Transitional cell carcinomas often present multifocally along the urinary tract, spreading via intraluminal seeding or intraepithelial migration in a process known as "field cancerization." However, these multifocal tumors still display monoclonality along their entire distribution. Squamous cell carcinoma, a less common form of bladder cancer that also accounts for 7% of renal pelvis tumors, is typically associated with inflammatory processes, including chronic UTI and renal calculi. These tumors tend to be deeply invasive and carry a poor prognosis.

Clinical Presentation

Subjective

The patient with a bladder tumor frequently is asymptomatic until he or she has an episode of hematuria that varies in severity from microscopic to gross amounts and may be intermittent or continuous. Other presenting symptoms may include dysuria, frequency, chills, low-grade fever, weight loss, and urinary urgency. Patients with advanced disease may complain of pelvic pain and symptoms associated with urethral obstruction.

Objective

The physical exam may be positive for a palpable mass and/or metastatic manifestations. The urinalysis shows trace to gross hematuria, possibly with abnormalities in protein level, RBCs, or WBCs. The serum complete blood count may indicate that anemia is present.

Diagnostic Reasoning

Diagnostic Tests

The diagnosis of bladder tumor is confirmed by visualization of the lesion through cystoscopy and biopsy. A urine cytology positive for transitional cell cancer can confirm the diagnosis; however, negative results do not rule out the possibility of bladder cancer. Cystoscopic evaluation can be used to confirm the suspected

diagnosis, to determine the location of the tumor, and to aid in the staging of the tumor. The cystoscopy should include a bladder washing for cytology and a mucosal biopsy. An abdominal or pelvic CT scan, with or without IVP, may be useful for determining the metastatic progress of the disease.

In general, transitional cell carcinomas are staged from A to D, according to level of invasion: stage 0 tumors are confined to the mucosa; stage A tumors invade the lamina propria; stage B tumors invade the muscular layer; stage C tumors extend to the peripelvic fat or renal parenchyma; and stage D indicates metastatic disease. The tumor-node-metastasis (TNM) system of the American Joint Committee on Cancer may also be used, with nodal metastases reflecting stage IV cancer. When transitional cell carcinomas are looked at as a whole, in situ disease has a 5-year survival rate of 95%, localized disease nearly 90%, regional disease just over 60%, and distant disease only 17%.

Urine tumor marker tests can detect recurrent tumors. The *N*-benzoyl-L-tyrosyl-*p*-aminobenzoic acid (BTA) and nucleoside 5′-monophosphate (NMP22) tests are more sensitive for recurrent tumors than urine cytology.

Differential Diagnosis

Because this disease most often presents as painless hematuria, differential diagnoses such as stones, infections, trauma, other tumors such as renal cell carcinoma, arteriovenous malformations, and glomerulonephropathies should be ruled out. Differential diagnosis for bladder irritability includes inflammation, stones, neurological dysfunction, and foreign bodies. Biopsy is necessary for definitive diagnosis.

Management

Treatment is dependent on the type, size, and degree of invasion of the bladder tumor, which is classified as superficial, invasive, or metastatic. *Superficial tumors* involve the bladder mucosa and submucosa; they are treated by endoscopic resection or laser resection. These tumors tend to recur, and the patient must be reexamined every 6 months. *Invasive tumors* involve the muscle and/or perivesical fat around the bladder. These tumors are treated with radical cystectomy or with radiation and chemotherapy. The 5-year survival rate is 65% to 75% with treatment. Research indicates that neoadjuvant chemotherapy can improve the survival rate in cases of advanced urothelial cancer (Level I; Siefker-Radtke et al, 2013; International Collaboration of Trialists, 2011). *Metastatic tumors* involve the lymph nodes, bone, or viscera and are treated with radiation and/or chemotherapy. This stage of the disease has a 5-year survival rate of 10% to 15%.

For the majority of bladder tumors, surgical resection is the treatment of choice. Immediate referral to a urologist or surgical oncologist is critical, as well as follow-up with a medical oncologist and/or nephrologist, depending on functional renal status. Intravesical chemotherapy may prevent recurrence, but radiation therapy for bladder tumors is less effective than the other interventions. See Treatment Standards/Guidelines 12.1.

Follow-up and Referral

All patients diagnosed with bladder cancer should be referred to a urologist for evaluation and treatment. Obtain a urinalysis and cystoscopy every 3 to 6 months because of the increased risk of recurrence of bladder tumors. Patients who have been diagnosed with advanced metastatic disease should be referred to an oncologist. Home health or hospice care may be appropriate for patients who need skilled care and ongoing patient teaching; an ostomy nurse may be necessary for patients who have undergone an ileostomy or urostomy.

Patient Education

Teach the importance of ongoing follow-up care. For terminal patients, many issues must be addressed and discussed to give patients and their caretakers an improved quality of life. Some of these are fear and anxiety, grieving, anticipation, self-image issues (including loss of hair), nausea and vomiting, weight loss, anorexia, impotence, sterility, pain, fatigue, loss of job, loss of family member, and potential for infection. Ileostomy/urostomy teaching is indicated for patients whose bladders have been surgically removed. Preventive measures include not smoking and avoidance of other chemical carcinogens.

■ ACUTE KIDNEY INJURY

Acute kidney injury (AKI), also known as *acute renal failure,* is the sudden and rapid deterioration of renal function resulting in an inability to maintain acid-base, fluid, and electrolyte balance and an accumulation of nitrogenous wastes. AKI now has a universal definition and staging system to allow for earlier detection and management of disease. AKI is defined when one of the following criteria is met: serum creatinine rises 26 μmol/L or greater within 48 hours or 1.5-fold or greater from the reference value, which is known or presumed to have occurred within 1 week, or urine output is less than 0.5 mL/kg/hr for more

Treatment Standards/Guidelines 12.1 Bladder Tumors

Stage	Description	Treatment Options	Characteristics
Stage 0	Noninvasive papillary carcinoma (Ta). Has grown toward hollow center of bladder but not into connective tissue or muscle of bladder wall. Has not spread to lymph nodes or distant sites.	Endoscopic or laser resection intravesical immunotherapy OR intravesical chemotherapy	Recurrence is common; follow up every 6 months. Relative 5-year survival rate 98%
Stage I	Cancer has grown into the layer of connective tissue under the lining layer but has not reached the muscle layer in the bladder wall. Has not spread to lymph nodes or distant sites.	Simple or radical cystectomy, radiation, chemotherapy	Relative 5-year survival rate 88%
Stage II	Cancer has grown into thick muscle layer of bladder wall, but has not passed through the muscle to reach the fatty tissue surrounding the bladder. Has not spread to lymph nodes or distant sites.		Relative 5-year survival rate 63%
Stage III	Cancer has grown into the fatty tissue surrounding bladder. May have spread to prostate, uterus, or vagina, but not growing into pelvic or abdominal wall. Has not spread to lymph nodes or distant sites.		Relative 5-year survival rate 46%
Stage IV	Cancer has grown through the bladder wall and into pelvic or abdominal wall, may have spread to nearby or distant lymph nodes or to sites such as the bones, liver, or lungs.	Treatment is palliative only Systemic chemotherapy and/or radical cystectomy or external beam radiation therapy	Relative 5-year survival rate 15%

than 6 consecutive hours. The reference serum creatinine should be the lowest creatinine value recorded within 3 months of the event.

The most common causes of AKI are associated with intrarenal injury caused by renal hypoperfusion or nephrotoxins. The signs and symptoms vary with each patient and are most often due to uremia or its underlying cause. Persons with AKI usually do not experience the profound neurological and musculoskeletal disorders seen in patients with chronic renal failure (CRF). Although recovery from AKI may be rapid and complete, this disorder nonetheless has a high mortality rate, estimated at anywhere between 5% and 80%, depending on the patient's age, the cause of AKI, and the extent of multiorgan involvement.

Epidemiology and Causes

It is estimated that 5% of all hospitalized patients develop AKI; for patients in intensive care units, the rate is as high as 15%. Two percent to 7% of all post–open-heart surgery patients are estimated to develop AKI. Fifty percent of AKI that develops in hospitalized patients is considered iatrogenic. AKI affects all ages and both sexes equally.

Risk factors for AKI include surgery, especially for older patients or patients of any age with elevated creatinine levels. Community-based AKI occurs more frequently among vulnerable populations such as individuals with underlying renal disease, multiple myeloma, or diabetes. AKI is also one of the potential risks related to open-heart surgery and other cardiac procedures (e.g., cardiac catheterization) and use of IV contrast dyes. Any problem that causes decreased blood flow to the kidneys can lead to AKI: anaphylactic shock caused by drug or transfusion reactions, ingestion of nephrotoxic substances (aminoglycosides, angiotensin-converting enzyme [ACE] inhibitors in renal artery stenosis), malignancy, sepsis, cardiac problems, aneurysm, liver cirrhosis, trauma, dehydration, or shock.

AKI is classified into three major groups based on the anatomical nature of the lesion: prerenal azotemia, intrarenal azotemia, or postrenal azotemia. *Prerenal azotemia* is the name given to any condition that leads to an overall decrease in renal perfusion; etiologies in this group include hypovolemia, renovascular disease, decreased cardiac output, systemic vasodilation, renal vasoconstriction, and impairment of renal autoregulation of blood flow, which is often associated with drugs such as ACE inhibitors or NSAIDs. *Intrarenal* refers to disorders that affect the renal parenchyma itself, such as glomerulonephritis, acute tubular necrosis (often caused by ischemic insult or nephrotoxic drugs such as aminoglycosides), interstitial nephritis (often an allergic type of reaction to various drugs or transfusion reactions), and tubular obstruction. Immune-mediated phenomena may lead to AKI following acute bacterial infection, for example, thrombotic thrombocytopenic purpura (TTP) or hemolytic uremic syndrome (HUS) following *Escherichia coli* gastroenteritis. *Postrenal azotemia* refers to any etiology that might lead to an obstruction of flow of urine from the kidneys, including ureteral obstruction, bladder neck obstruction, or urethral obstruction. Major causes include benign prostatic hyperplasia/hypertrophy (BPH), prostate or bladder cancer, and metastatic disease affecting the urinary tract. An important consideration in the male patient with preexisting BPH is the use of over-the-counter sympathomimetic decongestants and other cold remedies, the alpha-agonist properties of which may lead to acute worsening of prostatic hypertrophy with resultant anuria.

Table 12.7 presents the major causes of AKI. Complications commonly seen as a result of AKI include intravascular volume overload, metabolic acidosis, anemia, hyperkalemia, and uremic syndrome, which is characterized by nausea, vomiting, anorexia, pericarditis, and both central and peripheral nervous system abnormalities including altered mental status, seizures, or coma. *Prerenal, intrarenal,* and *postrenal* mechanisms of AKI are not mutually exclusive, however, and many patients present with a combination of these pathologies.

Table 12.7   Major Causes of Acute Kidney Injury

Prerenal Acute Kidney Injury
- Fluid and electrolyte depletion
- Hemorrhage
- Septicemia
- Cardiac failure
- Liver failure
- Heat stroke
- Burns

Intrarenal Acute Kidney Injury
- Ischemia
- Toxins
- Radiocontrast agents
- Hemoglobinuria
- Myoglobinuria
- Acute glomerulonephritis
- Arterial or venous obstruction
- Tubulointerstitial nephritis
- Pyelonephritis
- Papillary necrosis
- Precipitation from hypercalcemia
- Urates
- Myeloma protein

Postrenal Acute Kidney Injury
- Prostatism
- Bladder tumor
- Pelvic tumor
- Retroperitoneal tumor
- Renal calculi

Pathophysiology

Prerenal Azotemia

Prerenal azotemia is caused by decreased blood flow to the kidneys, usually associated with poor systemic perfusion. Etiologies includes hypovolemia, altered peripheral vascular resistance, diminished cardiac output, congestive heart failure, renal artery disorders such as vasculitis, and to a lesser extent thromboembolic disease, as well as chronic liver diseases such as cirrhosis and the hepatorenal syndrome.

The kidney's compensatory mechanisms to hypoperfusion are autoregulation and activation of the renin-angiotensin-aldosterone axis via the release of renin. In the face of damage to select renal tissue, these mechanisms attempt to shunt blood to undamaged nephrons in a process called adaptive hyperfiltration. Autoregulation depends on the body's ability to control afferent arteriole dilation and efferent arteriole constriction in order to maintain normal glomerular filtration rate (GFR) and creatinine clearance. The release of renin activates the proenzyme angiotensinogen to the biologically inactive angiotensin I. In turn, ACE converts angiotensin I into angiotensin II, one of the most potent vasoconstricting agents in the body. Its production results in peripheral vasoconstriction and increased sodium reabsorption via increased aldosterone production. Antidiuretic hormone (ADH) is released in response to the increased plasma sodium concentration. ADH further enhances vasoconstriction and increases water reabsorption, thereby decreasing urinary output and increasing blood volume.

These mechanisms attempt to maintain systemic and renal perfusion. However, if the adaptive mechanisms of the kidneys fail, AKI develops because of hypoperfusion. As a result, glomerular filtration and the excretion of urea decrease, along with increased sodium and water reabsorption, resulting in an overall increase in blood urea nitrogen (BUN). Thus, although adaptive hyperfiltration is initially beneficial, allowing normal serum creatinine to be maintained in the face of mild renal insufficiency, prolonged activation of this compensatory mechanism leads to progressive renal failure.

Intrarenal (Parenchymal) Azotemia

Intrarenal azotemia results from injury to renal tissue; it is usually associated with intrarenal ischemia, toxins, or both. Accounting for up to 50% of all cases, intrinsic dysfunction is considered after prerenal and postrenal causes have been excluded. The sites of injury are the glomeruli, vasculature, interstitium, and tubules.

Acute tubular necrosis (ATN) is the most common cause of intrarenal azotemia and AKI in general. In ischemic ATN, the ischemic event refers to prolonged hypoperfusion and ischemia of the kidneys, with a sustained mean arterial pressure (MAP) in adults of less than 75 mm Hg. When renal autoregulation fails, the sympathetic nervous system (SNS) responds by initiating the renin-angiotensin system as the kidney attempts to redirect blood flow to the remaining healthy nephrons in a process called adaptive hyperfiltration, as explained in the preceding text. Again, however, this initial compensatory mechanism can eventually lead to progressive renal failure, because the SNS response and possibly endothelin production may lead to severe afferent renal arteriole constriction. As a result, overall glomerular hydrostatic pressure, glomerular blood flow, and GFR are decreased.

The length of the ischemic episode determines the amount and degree of renal cellular damage, which may continue after MAP and renal reperfusion are restored. Studies in animal models have demonstrated that a number of immunological mechanisms contribute to renal tubular injury, most notably early complement activation; intracellular adhesion molecule–1 (ICAM-1) expression, which may promote neutrophilic damage to the endothelium; T-cell–mediated cytotoxicity; macrophage activation; and pro-inflammatory cytokine expression (e.g., tumor necrosis factor–α, interleukin [IL]–6, IL-7, various chemokines).

Renal blood flow can be reduced by 50% after an ischemic episode; this is termed *no-reflow phenomenon*. The kidneys are unable to synthesize vasodilating prostaglandins, which usually exacerbates the ischemic injury. Blood flow is redistributed from the cortex to the medulla as a result of SNS stimulation and angiotensin II production. This further decreases glomerular capillary flow and worsens tubular ischemia because these structures are located primarily in the cortex.

With renal ischemia, the availability of nutrients and oxygen for basic cellular metabolism and the tubular transport system is diminished. There is a significant decrease in the production of adenosine triphosphate (ATP) by the mitochondria; and, with insufficient oxygen and ATP, metabolism shifts from aerobic to anaerobic. This shift corresponds with extracellular and intracellular acidosis that alters kidney function. Ischemia also causes a decrease in renal cellular potassium, magnesium, and inorganic phosphates and an increase in intracellular sodium, chloride, calcium, and reactive oxygen species. Sodium and calcium exchange is abnormal because of low ATP, altered Ca-ATPase activity, and increased intracellular sodium. This results in an increase in cellular calcium, which seems to increase cell injury. The formation of oxygen-free radicals further exacerbates cellular damage and apoptosis (programmed cell death) during reperfusion after a prolonged renal ischemic event, an event termed *reperfusion injury.*

The basement membrane is altered by tubular cellular edema and becomes necrotic because of prolonged tubular ischemia. Tubular obstruction occurs from sloughed necrotic cells and cast formation, which seems to be facilitated by a translocation of basement membrane cellular adhesion proteins called integrins to the luminal membrane. Tubular hydrostatic pressure and Bowman's capsule hydrostatic pressure, which opposes the glomerular hydrostatic pressure, increase as a result of tubular obstruction. This decreases GFR. Injury to the basement membrane increases tubular permeability, allowing tubular filtrate to leak back into the interstitium and peritubular capillaries, further decreasing tubular filtration.

Ischemic ATN is usually associated with oliguria (less than 500 mL/day in adults) because of extensive nephronal injury. Other clinical indications of ATN include decreased urea excretion and elevated BUN, decreased creatinine clearance and elevated serum creatinine, abnormal renal handling of sodium, and an inability to concentrate urine. Urinary osmolality may approximate plasma osmolality of 300 to 350 mOsm/L, a condition called *isosthenuria.*

Toxic ATN involves exposure to toxic by-products of microorganisms or to nephrotoxic agents. Renal toxic drugs often cause allergic interstitial nephritis, characterized by eosinophilic damage. Toxic ATN begins with an event that causes injury to tubular cells. Subsequent pathophysiology is similar to that of ischemic ATN because there is tubular cell necrosis, cast formation, tubular obstruction, and altered GFR. Unlike in ischemic ATN, the basement membrane is usually intact, however, and the injured necrotic areas are more localized. Other differences are nonoliguria, which occurs more often with toxic ATN than with ischemic ATN, as well as the extent of injury with toxic ATN, which may be less than with ischemic ATN. The healing process, therefore, can be more rapid in patients with toxic ATN.

There are several reasons why the kidney is so susceptible to toxic damage. Blood continuously circulates through the kidney, repeatedly exposing the kidney to all components in the blood. Also, the kidney is the major excretory organ for toxic substances, and, as these substances await transport within renal cells, they disrupt cellular function. If liver disease is present, substances that are usually detoxified by the liver can overload the kidney. The kidney also transforms many substances into metabolites that can be toxic to the kidney, and the countercurrent mechanism concentrates bodily substances and other substances that, in increased concentrations, can be toxic to the kidney.

Postrenal Azotemia

Bilateral (ureteral) or distal (bladder outlet or urethral) postrenal obstruction impedes urine flow and results in oliguria or frank anuria. Urine congestion increases pressure retrograde through the collecting system and nephron and slows the tubular fluid flow rate and GFR. There is increased reabsorption of sodium, water, and urea, which results in decreased urine sodium, increased urine osmolality, and increased BUN. The decreased GFR results in a decreased creatinine clearance and, therefore, in an increased serum creatinine level. If the postrenal obstruction is prolonged, the collecting system dilates and compresses parenchymal tissue. The nephron is injured, which results in dysfunction of the concentrating and diluting mechanism, causing the urine osmolality and sodium level to be similar to those of plasma. If the postrenal obstruction is temporary, there is little dilation of the collecting system and loss of renal tissue.

Clinical Presentation
Subjective

Symptoms of AKI are not usually present until the GFR falls to approximately 10% to 15% of normal. The most common symptoms, which are secondary to the accumulation of toxic metabolites such as urea, are fatigue, malaise, nausea, vomiting, pruritus, and mental status changes. Of note, the development of uremic syndrome symptoms bears no direct correlation to increases in BUN or serum creatinine, despite the critical role of hemodialysis in clearing the body of as yet unidentified uremic toxins. Oliguria or even anuria may also be a presenting symptom of AKI but is not present in every case; urine output depends largely on the stage of AKI, as well as the precipitating cause. In some cases, fluid overload may be present, resulting in dyspnea and orthopnea.

A detailed history can give clues to the etiology of AKI. The patient should be questioned about history of drug use, surgery, trauma, or infection as possible sources of renal insult. However, the actual diagnosis of AKI is often made by routine laboratory assessment.

There are multiple signs and symptoms of AKI and four identified stages: initiating, oliguric, diuretic, and recovery. The *initiating stage* begins when the kidney is injured; this stage is variable in length, from minutes to several days (e.g., damage caused by contrast dye occurs within 2 minutes). Decreased urine volume and other signs and symptoms of renal impairment may then become evident. These may include anorexia, lethargy, nausea, headache, muscle cramps, and fatigue. The cause of AKI must be determined, and the plan of treatment should be established in consultation with a nephrologist.

The *oliguric stage* usually lasts from 5 to 15 days but can persist for weeks, depending on the nature of renal damage. Renal repair begins as tubular cells regenerate. Destroyed basement membrane is replaced with fibrous scar tissue, and nephrons become obstructed with inflammatory products. Decreases in glomerular filtration, tubular transport of substances, urine formation, and renal clearance occur. When AKI persists for weeks or longer, renal endocrine functions such as the secretion of erythropoietin are altered. The longer this stage persists, the poorer the prognosis.

The next phase is the *diuretic stage,* defined as beginning when urine output is greater than 400 mL per day and when the BUN begins to fall. This stage is considered to last until the BUN is stabilized or is in the normal stage.

The fourth and final stage, referred to as the *recovery phase,* extends from the time the BUN is stable and the urine output normal to the day the patient returns to normal activity. The entire process may take 10 months, and some patients never recover but instead progress to CRF.

Objective

The objective manifestations of AKI depend on the stage of the disorder and may be extremely variable; however, these signs can provide an assessment of the degree of renal failure and provide clues as to the underlying etiology. Orthostatic vital signs, skin turgor, and distention of jugular veins should be assessed to obtain information on the patient's fluid balance. Signs of fluid depletion can point to a prerenal etiology, whereas signs of fluid overload suggest a greater degree of renal impairment. Severe proteinuria may lead to generalized edema (anasarca) due to the lack of intravascular oncotic pressure from hypoalbuminemia. Abdominal bruits can suggest renovascular disease. In cases of polycystic kidney disease or hydronephrosis, the kidneys may be palpable. A pelvic or renal exam may reveal causes of outflow obstruction such as an enlarged prostate or pelvic mass.

Diagnostic Reasoning
Diagnostic Tests

Elevated BUN and serum creatinine levels assist in establishing the diagnosis of AKI. GFR is difficult to measure directly and is most commonly estimated using a simplified formula for creatinine clearance (see Diagnostic Tests section under Chronic Renal Failure for complete discussion). However, because acute trends are most important in the diagnosis and follow-up of AKI, direct serum creatinine levels are often used as an estimate of renal function. However, it is critical to remember that these absolute values are heavily influenced by a patient's muscle mass, age, and gender, as well as the presence of any underlying renal disease. As such, serum creatinine levels may overestimate or underestimate renal function in certain populations (e.g., elderly or obese patients).

Serum electrolyte levels (sodium, potassium, chloride, bicarbonate, calcium, phosphate) should also be monitored for potentially life-threatening abnormalities that may develop secondary to impaired renal function. The presence of RBCs, either alone or as casts, may suggest a vascular or glomerular lesion, whereas WBCs and white blood cell casts are seen in interstitial nephritis and cases associated with infection. Eosinophiluria, in particular, is characteristic of allergic interstitial nephritis due to renal toxic drugs. "Muddy-brown" granular casts and epithelial cell casts are strongly associated with ATN but are not considered very specific. Moreover, their absence does not exclude intrinsic renal disease.

Urinary sodium tends to be less than 20 mEq/L in prerenal disease, whereas the kidneys "leak" or "spill" sodium by failing to reabsorb this electrolyte in ATN, resulting in urinary sodium values typically greater than 40 mEq/L. However, variations in water reabsorption also affect urinary sodium concentration. Thus, the fractional excretion of sodium (FENa) is easily remembered as the urinary clearance of sodium divided by the glomerular filtration rate:

$$FENa = 100 \times \frac{sodium\ (urinary) \times creatinine\ (plasma)}{sodium\ (plasma) \times creatinine\ (urinary)}$$

The FENa is more helpful in distinguishing prerenal azotemia from ATN. The FENa is generally less than 1% in prerenal disease related to hypoperfusion because the kidneys try to preserve intravascular volume by maximally conserving sodium. A FENa of greater than 2% reflects acute tubular necrosis, but values between 1% and 2% are considered inconclusive. Of note, FENa has little or no predictive value in the presence of diuretic therapy, because natriuresis is a mechanistic outcome of both thiazide and loop diuretics. Thus, increased urinary sodium may not exclude a prerenal etiology or implicate ATN. In addition, FENa is less helpful when ATN is superimposed on a chronic intravascularly depleted state, such as in hypoalbuminemic cirrhotic liver disease.

ATN is also characterized by an inability to concentrate urine; thus, urine osmolality is typically lower than 450 mOsm/L and in many cases lower than 350 mOsm/L. In contrast, the urine is highly concentrated in prerenal azotemia due to the secretion of ADH and intensified water reabsorption, producing urine osmolalities greater than 500 mOsm/L. As renal tubular function worsens under prerenal conditions, however, this distinction tends to blur, and concentrating ability may wane as ischemic damage sets in.

If a glomerular process is suspected, measurement of antinuclear antibody, antineutrophil cytoplasmic antibody (ANCA—seen in Wegener's granulomatosis), antiglomerular basement membrane (anti-GBM) antibodies, complement levels, and cryoglobulins can help the clinician determine whether immune-mediated disease is present (Level II; Lewington & Kanagasundaram, 2011).

A 24-hour urine test is the best way to measure proteinuria. A protein loss of more than 3.0 to 3.5 g every 24 hours indicates a glomerular lesion, whereas lesser amounts in the urine are more indicative of an interstitial disorder.

Renal ultrasound is commonly used to assess kidney size and rule out hydronephrosis. Ultrasound is used instead of intravenous pyelogram to avoid the risk of radiocontrast nephrotoxicity. If hydronephrosis indicative of obstruction is detected, the patient should be referred to a urologist. Computed tomography (CT) scan, retrograde pyelogram, and cystoscopy may all be useful in determining the exact location of the obstruction. Renal scan may be helpful in detecting unilateral renal artery stenosis but is less sensitive in detecting bilateral renal artery disease. Renal artery stenosis is better diagnosed via CT scan or magnetic resonance imaging/magnetic resonance angiography (MRI/MRA), although direct renal angiography is still considered the (albeit invasive) gold standard for diagnosis.

If the noninvasive work-up proves inconclusive, renal biopsy may be indicated in some cases. Most notably, biopsy is performed in cases of isolated glomerular hematuria with proteinuria to confirm acute nephritic syndrome, to better characterize nephrotic syndrome or suspected vasculitis, and to aid in the diagnosis of acute or subacute renal failure of unknown etiology. Percutaneous versus open biopsy techniques are chosen based on the propensity for bleeding diatheses and the difficulty in reaching the affected kidney as determined by renal imaging.

Differential Diagnosis

The main diagnostic challenge in AKI is to determine the underlying cause. This is often complicated by fluid and electrolyte alterations. Assessment of the patient involves taking a thorough history, physically assessing the patient, and ordering appropriate laboratory studies. When determining whether or not prerenal azotemia exists, the patient's history can provide information indicating poor renal and/or systemic perfusion. This information may include surgery, high fever, alterations in diet or fluid status (such as a patient receiving nothing by mouth and given bowel preparation repeatedly for diagnostic tests), a low-sodium diet with fluid restriction, use of diuretics and antihypertensives, anaphylactic drug or transfusion reaction, penetrating or nonpenetrating abdominal trauma, hemorrhage, burns, shock, excessive sweating and dehydration, peritonitis, malignancies, sepsis, neurogenic shock, drug overdose, acute myocardial infarction, congestive heart failure, cardiac tamponade, cardiac dysrhythmias, cardiac arrest survival, renal artery emboli, thrombi, stenosis, aneurysm, occlusion, trauma, and liver cirrhosis.

Physical assessment findings may vary depending on the etiology of AKI and need to be correlated with the patient's history and laboratory findings, such as fluid volume depletion or oliguria. Findings on physical exam consistent with a prerenal etiology may include dry mucous membranes, poor skin turgor, reduced jugular venous pressure, hypotension, oliguria, or weight loss. Significant laboratory findings are increased urine osmolality and specific gravity, decreased urine sodium and urea, increased BUN, increased BUN to plasma creatinine ratio (a ratio greater than 20:1 because plasma creatinine is usually normal), normal urinary sediment (in most cases), and oliguria.

Prolonged azotemia caused by a prerenal condition often leads to intrarenal failure. Nephrotoxic agents that may cause damage to the kidneys are drugs such as antineoplastics, anesthetics, antimicrobials, and anti-inflammatory agents; x-ray contrast media; biological substances (e.g., toxins, tumor products, and heme pigments from hemoglobin or myoglobin); environmental agents (e.g., pesticides and organic solvents); heavy metals (e.g., lead, mercury, and gold); and plant and animal substances (e.g., toxic mushrooms and snake venoms).

Other factors that may injure renal (parenchymal) tissue include inflammatory processes related to bacterial or viral infection and toxemia of pregnancy; immune processes, such as autoimmunity, hypersensitivity, and tissue or organ transplant rejection; trauma or radiation to the kidney; and obstruction (e.g., neoplasm, stones, and scar tissue). Intravascular hemolysis related to transfusion reaction and microangiopathic hemolytic anemia as seen in TTP and HUS also causes damage to renal tissue. In addition, systemic and vascular disorders, such as renal vein thrombosis, nephrotic syndrome, Wilson's disease, malaria, multiple myeloma (direct proteinaceous deposition of immunoglobulin light chains into the renal parenchyma), sickle cell disease, malignant hypertension, diabetes mellitus, and systemic lupus erythematosus all cause intrarenal injury. Pregnancy-related disorders, such as septic abortion, preeclampsia, abruptio placentae, intrauterine fetal death, and idiopathic postpartum renal failure, can also cause damage to the kidneys.

Data that identify an event, a series of events, an agent, or agents that may have caused renal injury, especially those related to ischemia or exposure to toxins, should be collected during the history. These may include nephrotoxins; radiological tests that require administration of a dye; hypersensitivity reaction to a drug or dye; recent infections, trauma, or sepsis; antineoplastics, with or without radiation therapy; multiple myeloma or pregnancy; and a history of cardiac, renal, or liver disease.

There is no one specific finding that pinpoints intrarenal azotemia during physical assessment. Findings on exam must be correlated with history and laboratory findings. Differentiating prerenal problems and actual ATN is a challenge. Because prerenal problems often correspond with the onset phase of ATN and because this is a reversible phase, it is essential for diagnosis and aggressive management to begin early. Laboratory plasma values, urinalysis, and microscopic examination of the urine provide important data that can help to differentiate prerenal azotemia from ATN.

Prerenal problems are indicated by high urinary specific gravity and osmolality, low urinary sodium caused by decreased renal blood flow, avid tubular sodium reabsorption, and decreased GFR. The kidneys interpret this as a state of dehydration and respond with aldosterone and ADH to maximize sodium and water reabsorption from the distal tubule and collecting duct into the peritubular capillary plasma. This results in a small amount of very concentrated urine with high specific gravity and high osmolality. Despite maximal sodium reabsorption, urine is concentrated because of urea or other solutes. Urinary and plasma creatinine levels often show wide variation in prerenal problems, with a slower rate of rise than in ATN and periodic decreases in serum creatinine.

ATN is characterized by altered renal ability to conserve sodium; clinically, ATN is seen as a urinary sodium level greater than 20 mEq/L. Depending on the state of hydration, the serum sodium levels vary in ATN. Oliguria is usually associated with postischemic ATN, whereas either oliguria or nonoliguria may be associated with nephrotoxic ATN. Creatinine clearance is severely decreased, and plasma creatinine rises about 0.5 to 1 mg/dL per day in ATN. BUN to serum creatinine ratio does not typically exceed 10:1 to 15:1 in ATN.

Response to therapy is another factor that distinguishes ATN from prerenal problems. The kidneys typically respond very quickly to therapy aimed at correcting an underlying prerenal problem in which no actual nephron damage has occurred; however, in ATN, response to treatment of the underlying cause may be minimal depending on the degree of *nephron damage*. Additional therapy for ATN should be aimed at correcting alterations related to inability of the kidneys to maintain their functions.

Postrenal azotemia results from interference with the flow of urine from the kidneys and is associated with obstruction or disruption of the urinary tract. Ureteral, bladder, bladder neck, or urethral obstruction may be the result of calculi, urinary tract or bladder neoplasms, or sloughed papillary tissue; strictures, trauma, or blood clots; congenital or developmental abnormalities; foreign objects or surgical ligation; prostatic hypertrophy; retroperitoneal fibrosis; abdominal and pelvic neoplasms; pregnancy; neurogenic bladder; bladder rupture; or use of drugs such as antihistamines and ganglionic blocking agents. The history should focus on collecting data that indicate obstruction or disruption of the urinary tract. Significant findings include change in urine volume, history of prostatic disease or abdominal neoplasms, history of urinary tract stones or nephralgia, pregnancy, recent abdominal surgery, and paralysis (e.g., quadriplegia).

Postrenal azotemia physical assessment findings also vary with etiology and need to be correlated with laboratory and history findings (e.g., nephralgia associated with moving urinary tract stones or rapidly developing hydronephrosis; or bladder distention associated with prostate, bladder neck, or urethral disorders). Laboratory findings include urine volume variations such as oliguria, polyuria, or abrupt anuria; urine osmolality variations (may be increased or similar to plasma osmolality); urine specific gravity variations; a decrease in urine sodium and urine urea; and a BUN to serum creatinine ratio that is normal to slightly increased. Microscopy of the urinary sediment is usually normal unless urinary tract infection (UTI) is present.

Management

Approximately 50% of patients with AKI are nonoliguric and have less severe signs and symptoms than oliguric patients. Because frequent causes of death are cardiac arrest resulting from hyperkalemia, gastrointestinal bleeding, and infection, the patient should be monitored very closely and treated appropriately on a day-to-day basis. The main goal is to keep the patient alive and to determine the underlying cause of the renal failure. The etiology of AKI will determine long-term management strategies.

In many cases of ATN, which is often caused by nephrotoxic agents, the removal of the offending agent will allow renal function to return gradually to normal. In the meantime, supportive measures should be provided, often in the form of peritoneal or hemodialysis. Prerenal azotemia secondary to absolute hypovolemia necessitates the restoration of intravascular volume. Replacement of fluids depends on the mechanism of loss. Gastrointestinal fluid loss is generally hypotonic and should be replaced accordingly; fluid loss as a result of hemorrhage usually indicates the need for administration of both saline and RBCs. In addition, fluid and electrolytes must be managed. Hyperkalemia in AKI can be life-threatening; emergent management is required in patients with extreme elevation of potassium levels (more than 6.5 mmol/L) or in any patient with electrocardiogram (ECG) abnormalities.

Certain diseases, such as glomerulonephritis or Wegener's granulomatosis, require immunosuppressive treatment with prednisone and cyclophosphamide to prevent irreversible renal damage. Postrenal azotemia involves identification of the level of obstruction followed by treatment to relieve the obstruction. If the obstruction is high, at the vesicoureteral junction or in the ureter or renal pelvis, percutaneous nephrotomy or ureteral stent placement by a urologist is necessary. For urethral obstruction, bladder catheterization or placement of a suprapubic tube may be sufficient to relieve the obstruction. Intermittent bladder catheterization four to five times a day poses less risk of UTI than an indwelling urinary catheter and is the preferred method for urinary outflow in cases of bladder atony and neuromuscular compromise such as with spinal cord injury. However, the presence of a bladder outlet or urethral obstruction, which is more likely to cause AKI, may necessitate placement of a long-term catheterization device until surgical intervention is possible.

In cases of intrarenal (intrinsic) failure, supportive methods are necessary while waiting for the kidneys to respond to reversal of the underlying problem. Several indications exist for temporary hemodialysis including, but not limited to, fluid overload unresponsive to diuretic therapy; hyperkalemia with symptoms or

ECG changes; uremic encephalopathy; severe metabolic acidosis; cardiorespiratory failure; and pleuritis, pericarditis, and other forms of inflammatory serositis. Forms of dialysis include traditional intermittent hemodialysis via large-bore venous and arterial catheters; peritoneal dialysis, which operates by osmotic diffusion via an indwelling dialysate within the peritoneal cavity; and continuous renal replacement therapy, which is a prolonged form of low-flow arteriovenous or venovenous hemofiltration appropriate for hemodynamically unstable patients.

Follow-up and Referral

After hospitalization, patient follow-up is necessary in about 1 week, then 1 month, 3 months, 6 months, and annually thereafter, providing there are no further complications. Blood chemistries, such as a basic metabolic profile and a complete blood count, should be checked at each follow-up visit. The patient should be assessed for signs and symptoms of fluid overload, such as crackles on lung auscultation, elevated blood pressure, shortness of breath, weight gain, jugular vein distention, and/or edema.

Patient Education

During the recovery stage there is no special form of treatment other than general healthy living. Lack of knowledge is a major problem with regard to acute episodes of renal failure. Patients require continual education throughout their clinical pathway and their treatment of AKI. Follow-up care, support, and prevention of another episode should be the teaching focus.

■ CHRONIC KIDNEY DISEASE

Chronic kidney disease (CKD) is characterized by a progressive loss of functioning nephrons, eventually leading to end-stage renal disease (ESRD). As the functional reserve of the kidneys is lost, signs and symptoms of renal failure appear. These signs may arise as sequelae of acute kidney injury (AKI), but most often CKD arises as a complication of chronic systemic disease, such as diabetes or hypertension. The time frame for the development of CKD is typically thought of as ranging from months to years, whereas AKI typically sets in over days to weeks (see previous section).

Epidemiology and Causes

According to the National Health and Nutrition Examination Survey (NHANES) (a large population-based representative health survey of the entire country done every 2 years), approximately 13% of the U.S. population suffers from CKD. The number of people with a chronic elevation of creatinine greater than 2.0 mg/dL is estimated to be 2.8 per 100,000. There are approximately 485,000 patients with ESRD, of whom 341,000 are on chronic dialysis. Older adults represent 33.8% of new patients, and diabetes mellitus and hypertension cause about 70% of ESRD cases. Compared with the

general population, African Americans are 3.9 times more likely to have ESRD and 6.7 times more likely to have hypertensive ESRD. It is estimated that HIV-associated nephropathy may soon be the third leading cause of ESRD (after diabetes mellitus and hypertension) in African Americans aged 20 to 64 years. Men are 1.3 to 1.4 times more likely than women to have ESRD. The peak age for onset of ESRD is between 65 and 75 years. Geriatric patients have the highest incidence and morbidity and mortality rates, because renal disease can result from many age-related illnesses. Some older patients tolerate dialysis quite well, however.

The major underlying conditions leading to ESRD are diabetes mellitus and primary hypertension (approximately 70%); glomerulonephritis, cystic diseases, and other urological diseases (approximately 15%); and assorted other causes (approximately 15%). Renal artery stenosis and chronic ischemic renovascular disease may cause up to 20% of CKD cases in persons older than 50 years. Analgesic overuse (e.g., NSAIDs), cigarette smoking, collagen vascular disease, AIDS-related nephropathies, cirrhosis, and multiple myeloma are examples of other risk factors for the development of CKD. Several hereditary renal diseases (e.g., polycystic kidney disease and Alport syndrome, which also causes congenital deafness) can lead to CKD in children and some adults.

Hypertension is present in at least 85% of patients with CKD. Hypertensive- and diabetic-related CKD is a form of microvascular end-organ damage caused by these cardiovascular risk factors. Thus, these patients must also be evaluated for other forms of end-organ damage related to atherosclerotic disease, because a significant correlation exists between microvascular CKD, peripheral vascular disease, coronary artery disease, and cerebrovascular disease.

Pathophysiology

The pathophysiology of renal failure is manifested somewhat differently depending on the underlying cause, although the end result is the same—a nonfunctional kidney. Diabetic nephropathy is the most common cause of ESRD and involves several mechanisms, including hyperglycemia, hormonal imbalances, and renal hemodynamic changes. Hyperglycemia leads to alterations in tubuloglomerular feedback, abnormalities in polyol (e.g., sorbitol) metabolism, and the formation of advanced glycosylation end products (AGEs) in tissues. Increases in circulating AGE peptides parallel the severity of renal dysfunction in diabetic nephropathy. Ultimately, defects in glomerular cellular metabolism lead to hemodynamic changes in the kidney.

Hormonal imbalances associated with diabetes and ESRD include decreased insulin, increased growth hormone and glucagon, and altered concentrations of or responsiveness to vasoactive hormones (angiotensin II, catecholamines, and prostaglandins). Growth hormones and glucagon (both elevated in poorly controlled diabetes) have been shown to produce glomerular hyperfiltration in the laboratory in recent studies.

Renal hemodynamic changes implicated in diabetes and ESRD involve glomerular hypertension and glomerular hyperfiltration. Changes in circulating levels of vasoactive hormones, or altered responsiveness to them, can result in hyperfiltration. Regardless of the inciting event, factors such as hyperglycemia-induced increases in extracellular fluid volume, renal hypertrophy, and/or altered glycoregulatory or vasoregulatory hormone action contribute to increased pressure and flow across the glomerular membrane, resulting in glomerular hypertension. This, in turn, along with associated renal vasodilation and hyperfiltration, increases transglomerular protein filtration. This leads to proteinuria and mesangial deposition of circulating proteins. As a result, mesangial expansion and glomerulosclerosis cause destruction of nephrons, and the glomerulus becomes a fibrinous scar that can no longer function. In addition, a positive feedback stimulus for compensatory hyperfiltration is initiated, with further increase in GFR and progressive renal injury. Ultimately, it is glomerular hypertension that mediates the progressive nephron destruction. Based on this glomerular hypertension–hyperfiltration hypothesis, therapies directed at lowering glomerular hypertension would protect the kidney from further progression of nephropathy.

Hypertensive nephropathy is the second most common cause of renal failure. The kidney is one of the major organs injured by hypertension. The resultant disease is termed *nephrosclerosis*. Benign nephrosclerosis is associated with chronic, mild, or moderate hypertension in which renal insufficiency develops slowly. The renal arterial vessels become thickened while the lumens become narrowed, resulting in decreased renal flow and autoregulation. Renal tubular changes correlate with the degree of reduction in renal blood flow. Signs and symptoms vary with the severity of renal injury; they include proteinuria, nocturia, casts, and azotemia. Patients with benign nephrosclerosis are very susceptible to AKI when a situation occurs that decreases blood flow to the kidney. Treatment is focused on control of hypertension.

Malignant nephrosclerosis is associated with marked hypertension, headache, congestive heart failure, and blurred vision. Unlike the progression of benign nephrosclerosis, renal failure develops rapidly. Renal arterioles and glomerular capillaries become thickened and necrotic, and tubules atrophy. Signs and symptoms are hematuria with red cell casts, proteinuria, and azotemia. Treatment includes immediate reduction of blood pressure (BP), which is necessary to prevent permanent renal loss and damage to other organs.

Renal artery stenosis occurs when the renal artery and the branches become thickened, stiff, and narrow because of atheromatous plaques (two-thirds of cases) or fibromuscular dysplasia (one-third of cases). As the body perceives the decreased blood flow (i.e., hypoperfusion) via the stenotic renal arteries as hypovolemia, the renin-angiotensin-aldosterone axis is activated, and mild to severe hypertension results from the retention of sodium and water. This condition becomes critical if both renal arteries are affected or if blood flow is compromised in patients with only a single kidney, either congenitally or after live organ donation of the other kidney. Other signs include a bruit auscultated in the flank or midabdominal region over the affected renal artery and an elevated blood renin level from the ipsilateral renal vein. The incidence of fibromuscular dysplasia is higher in women than in men, especially from 20 to 40 years of age. The treatment required is angioplasty or surgical repair to stent or reconstruct the stenotic vessels, along with medical therapy consisting of antihypertensives and diuretics.

Glomerulonephritis (GN) is the third most common cause of renal failure. GN is an inflammatory process that primarily affects the glomerular capillaries. It is also a major cause of ESRD. Approximately 25% of GN cases result from nonimmune mechanisms, whereas 60% to 75% stem from autoimmune mechanisms. Glomerular injury can be divided into two major categories based on pathology: *nephritis,* which is characterized by glomerular inflammation and/or necrosis; and *nephrosis,* which is characterized by abnormal permeability of the glomerular membrane. This allows macromolecules such as albumin to pass. These two forms of injury are not mutually exclusive. A single etiology can produce both forms of injury.

The immunological injury that characterizes glomerulonephritis functions in several different ways. Antiglomerular basement membrane (anti-GBM) disease is a result of direct glomerular injury occurring as a result of inflammation triggered by antibodies directed against components of the glomerular basement membrane. Linear deposits of immunoglobulin are seen via immunofluorescence (IF) microscopy of renal tissue. IF also reveals granular immunoglobulin deposits. Part of the inflammatory response that occurs is secondary to the glomerular deposition of immune complexes, composed of antibodies bound to a variety of circulating antigens. This is referred to as *immune complex disease.* Finally, pauci-immune ANCA disease is characterized by the presence of serum antibodies against the neutrophil cytoplasm that are associated with the multisystem disease. Minimal or no immunoglobulin is seen by IF, hence the name "pauci-immune." Nonetheless, the glomerular injury is still believed to be immune in nature.

The hallmark of nephrosis is increased permeability of the glomerular capillary wall to macromolecules, including serum proteins. Inflammatory changes are generally not seen but may be present. In classic forms of glomerulonephrosis, nephrotic syndrome develops, and various degrees of proteinuria may be present. In addition to hypertension, other characteristic findings include hypercholesterolemia with lipiduria and central edema from hypoalbuminemia due to albuminuria. In more than two-thirds of cases of glomerulonephrosis in adults, the cause is idiopathic; in the remainder, nephrosis is secondary to systemic disease such as diabetes, lupus, or amyloidosis.

Clinical Presentation
Subjective

Because of the significant functional reserve of the kidneys, symptoms do not generally appear until renal function (as measured by the GFR) declines to 10% to 15% of normal. At about 30% to 40% of normal GFR, biochemical evidence of renal failure may be apparent, but patients typically remain asymptomatic. Early prominent symptoms in renal failure include anorexia, lassitude, fatigability, and weakness.

The inability of the kidneys to perform their normal excretory, metabolic, and endocrine functions results in *uremia,* a complex syndrome that includes a variety of physiological and clinical abnormalities. Dermatological abnormalities may result in the patient complaining of pruritus and dry skin; gastrointestinal alterations may manifest themselves as complaints of anorexia, nausea, vomiting, and hiccupping. Neurological complaints may include emotional lability or depression, insomnia, fatigue (especially on exertion), confusion, headache, seizures, and coma. There may be a urine odor to the breath and perspiration, complaints of shortness of breath, a metallic taste in the mouth, impotence, nocturia, and muscle cramps. The patient may present with foot drop, infection, bleeding, or gout. Often the patient is being treated for a major systemic disease such as diabetes. It is, therefore, important to be alert to the potential for the onset of CKD.

Objective

The patient may appear pale, with a characteristic uremic frost appearance to the skin, or, conversely, hyperpigmentation may be apparent. There may be bruising and asterixis (i.e., hand-flapping on hyperextension of the wrists with complete forward extension of the upper extremities). Peripheral neuropathy and altered mental status may be present, along with peripheral edema and ascites from severe proteinuria and the resulting hypoalbuminemia, as well as auscultatory crackles and a pericardial rub. There may be an elevated BP and a hard, rapid pulse. Some abnormalities are the result of the accumulation of toxic metabolites; others are caused by underproduction (e.g., of vitamin D and erythropoietin) or overproduction (e.g., renin) of biochemically active substances produced by the kidney.

Diagnostic Reasoning
Diagnostic Tests

If a patient has a condition known to predispose the individual to the development of CKD, especially if that patient is in a high-risk population, biochemical monitoring (BUN, creatinine, and creatinine clearance) should be done to detect renal failure before it becomes clinically apparent. Serum creatinine can track the progression of CKD; however, the GFR (normally about 140–180 L/day) can fall to 40% to 50% of normal with only small changes in serum creatinine levels. Accurate measurement of the GFR itself is based on experimental calculations of renal inulin clearance. Inulin is a polymer of fructose secreted from the blood exclusively via the renal glomeruli and displaying no tubular reabsorption. Measurement of inulin clearance, however, requires a complex assay too cumbersome for daily clinical use and tends to be reserved solely for research purposes.

Alternatively, GFR can be estimated using the Cockcroft-Gault formula for creatinine clearance: (140 minus age × lean body weight in kilograms) divided by (72 stable serum creatinine in mg/dL). This value is multiplied by 0.85 (i.e., reduced by 15%) for women. It is important to realize that trends in GFR (as estimated by creatinine clearance or serum creatinine levels) are far more important in assessing renal function and stability of CKD than are the absolute values of these indices. A meta-analysis of 13 studies found that a lower GFR and a higher albuminuria independently predict mortality and ESRD in patients with CKD (Level I; Astor et al, 2011). This is especially true of direct serum creatinine measurements, whose interpretation must take into account a patient's muscle mass, age, and gender. Thus, creatinine clearance is a far more informative diagnostic tool as a measure of renal function.

Although no universally agreed on definition of chronic kidney disease exists, GFR and proteinuria are often used to stratify CKD patients by disease severity. The Third National Health and Nutrition Examination Survey defined **Stage 1** disease as persistent albuminuria with a normal GFR greater than 90 mL/min per 1.73 m^2 of body surface area (BSA); **Stage 2** disease has persistent albuminuria with a GFR between 60 and 89 mL/min per 1.73 m^2 of BSA; **Stage 3** disease is defined as a GFR between 30 and 59 mL/min per 1.73 m^2 of BSA; **Stage 4** disease is defined as a GFR between 15 and 29 mL/min/1.73 m^2 of BSA; and **Stage 5** disease is ESRD, defined as a GFR less than 15 mL/min/1.73 m^2 of BSA. Routine monitoring of the complete blood count (CBC) can detect anemia secondary to erythropoietin deficiency. Monitoring of urinalysis can detect increasing proteinuria. When renal function declines further, closer monitoring of routine laboratory tests to detect dangerous electrolyte imbalances (e.g., hyperkalemia) and acidosis is required.

Numerous laboratory alterations occur in patients who have developed ESRD. A CBC will usually reveal a normochromic, normocytic anemia; decreased hematocrit; increased bleeding time; capillary fragility; thrombocytopenia; and a decreased immune responsiveness. Blood chemistries typically reveal some of the following abnormalities: decreased active vitamin D; elevated ammonia, BUN and serum creatinine, uric acid, sulfate, potassium, phosphate, parathyroid hormone, and glucose levels, along with insulin resistance and a type IV hyperlipidemia. Urinalysis may reveal proteinuria (the greater the proteinuria, the quicker the progression of CKD) and coarse granular casts. Ketosis may artificially raise creatinine levels, and certain drugs (cimetidine, trimethoprim, cefazolin) may also alter diagnostic test results.

Twenty-four–hour urine studies (protein, creatinine clearance) may be done although samples often are difficult to obtain in ambulatory patients and have been largely replaced by spot urine checks. Complement levels, antinuclear antibody, and serum and urine protein electrophoresis may all provide data as to the underlying pathophysiology of CKD.

Renal ultrasound performed at least at baseline is indicated in all cases of CKD. Among other pathologies, sonography may reveal decreased kidney size (less than 11 cm), polycystic kidney disease, or an obstructed ureter or bladder outlet with hydroureter and/or hydronephrosis. Renal CT scan/CT angiography or MRI/MRA may detect and localize harder to visualize structural abnormalities, renal parenchymal disease, or renal artery stenosis. Duplex Doppler ultrasonography to assess renal vascular flow has a high sensitivity and specificity for arterial stenosis if conducted by an experienced ultrasonographer, but renal angiography remains the diagnostic

gold standard for this condition. However, unilaterally decreased kidney size on renal imaging is highly suggestive of vascular occlusive disease and may be quite helpful as a screening method. Renal biopsy is not utilized for CKD as much as for AKI, unless noninvasive modes of testing are unable to suggest a likely etiology.

Differential Diagnosis

The differential diagnosis of CKD is aimed at identifying the underlying etiology of renal failure, as discussed earlier. Although the terms *chronic kidney disease* and *chronic renal insufficiency* (CRI) are often used interchangeably, some authorities reserve the use of CKD to imply a dialysis-dependent state, whereas CRI denotes an earlier form of the condition not yet requiring dialysis or kidney transplantation, but that may clearly progress to CKD. The signs and symptoms and diagnostic test results commonly seen in the three stages of CKD (decreased renal reserve, renal insufficiency, and ESRD) are presented in Table 12.8.

Management

General principles of CKD management include (1) the determination and control of underlying etiology,

Table 12.8	Differentiating the Stages of Chronic Kidney Disease		
Stage	Glomerular Filtration Rate	Signs and Symptoms	Management
D1. Decreased renal reserve	Greater than 90 Normal kidney function	Asymptomatic Hypertension (mild)	Control blood pressure and observation
K2. Kidney Damage	60–89 Mildly reduced kidney function	Hypertension (mild) ↑ PTH Early bone disease ↑ BUN and serum creatinine	Observation Control blood pressure
3. Renal insufficiency 3a. 3b.	Moderately reduced kidney function 45–59 30–44	Hypertension Anemia due to ↓ erythropoietin ↑ BUN and serum creatinine Risk of cardiovascular events	Refer to specialist Evaluate serum creatinine, potassium, hemoglobin, urinary protein every 6 months Control blood pressure
4. Severe renal insufficiency	15–29 Severely reduced kidney function	Moderate hypertension Anemia Hyperphosphatemia ↑ Triglycerides Metabolic acidosis Hyperkalemia Water/salt retention ↑ BUN and serum creatinine	Refer to specialist Control hypertension Oral phosphate binders Cholesterol-lowering therapy Administration of erythropoietin drug (epoetins)
E5. End-stage kidney disease—kidney failure	<15 or on dialysis	Severe hypertension Anemia Hypophosphatemia Uremia	Refer to specialist Dialysis Transplant Same management as for Stage 4

Adapted from www.renal.org/whatwedo/InformationResources/CKDeGUIDE/CKDstages.aspx and www.kidney.org/PROFESSIONALS/kdoqi/guidelines_ckd/toc.htm

(2) monitoring changes in renal function, (3) conservative treatment of the physiological effects of CKD, and (4) instituting more aggressive treatment (dialysis and/or renal transplantation) when appropriate in later stages of treatment-refractory disease. Glucose levels and hypertension must be strictly controlled in diabetic patients, with a target hemoglobin A1C (HbA1c) less than 7%. For any patient with proteinuria of more than 1 g/day, the target BP is 125/75 mm Hg; for a patient with proteinuria of less than 1 g/day, the goal is a BP of 130/80 mm Hg. Given the importance of maintaining renal perfusion, systolic blood pressures lower than 110 mm Hg should be avoided. Angiotensin-converting enzyme (ACE) inhibitors or the newer class of angiotensin II receptor blockers (ARBs) should be used for BP control in patients with diabetes mellitus given their renoprotective effects. If monotherapy with one of these agents is insufficient to control BP, a diuretic should be added, followed by a calcium channel blocker (diltiazem or verapamil) or a beta blocker, as needed. If combination therapy using agents from these additional classes proves ineffective, an ACE inhibitor or ARB should be added (whichever class was not used initially).

Pharmacological BP management is equally as important for the medical treatment of renal artery stenosis. However, ACE inhibitors and ARBs are usually avoided in patients with bilateral renal artery stenosis, because their vasodilatory effects on the efferent renal arterioles effectively decrease GFR in the presence of reduced afferent blood flow from stenotic renal arteries. In turn, this may precipitate potentially devastating acute or chronic renal failure. Percutaneous angioplasty or surgical revascularization with arterial stenting should be considered for patients with severe hypertension refractory to pharmacotherapy, recurrent episodes of flash pulmonary edema due to CKD-related fluid overload, and progressive renal insufficiency that fails to improve despite effective BP control. Individuals with particularly severe CKD (serum creatinine greater than 4 mg/dL) or chronically atrophied kidneys (less than 7 cm) are unlikely to respond to such interventions, however. Revascularization is more likely to be effective in patients whose renal function rapidly declines, particularly after beginning ACE inhibitor or ARB therapy.

Dietary therapy is a cornerstone of conservative management of CKD. Restriction of fluid (limited to maintain a serum sodium concentration of 135–145 mEq/L) and sodium (especially if volume expanded) may decrease secondary hypertension or congestive heart failure, although volume depletion must be avoided given the potential for acute worsening due to renal hypoperfusion. Restricted protein intake is recommended (0.58 g/kg per day), although an adequate caloric intake (40–50 cal/kg per day) should be maintained, because malnutrition is a common complication of CKD. Consultation by a skilled nutritionist is

recommended at the time of diagnosis and periodically as the disease progresses and the patient's nutritional needs change. Foods rich in essential amino acids are the most effectively utilized source of nitrogen. Restriction of dietary phosphate (800 mg/day) and potassium may be necessary because of reduced excretion and the potential for hyperphosphatemia and hyperkalemia. Strict dietary restrictions may be unnecessary in older patients because they often have low protein and sodium intake, but treatment regimens must be individualized.

Low-dose sodium polystyrene sulfonate (Kayexalate) 5 mg PO daily to three times daily with meals may be used as a potassium binder for hyperkalemia. Oral phosphate binders such as calcium carbonate (2.5–20 g/day), calcium acetate (Phos-Lo; 1334 mg three times daily), or sevelamer (Renagel; 800 mg three times daily) are typically taken with meals when GFR falls below 30 mL/min. Sevelamer is used when CKD is complicated by iatrogenic hypercalcemia. Aluminum- and magnesium-containing salts should be avoided, owing to cumulative toxicity.

Given the kidneys' reduced ability to synthesize activated vitamin D in CKD and the propensity for subsequent hypocalcemia and renal osteodystrophy, oral 1,25-dihydroxyvitamin D (calcitriol 0.25 mg daily) and calcium carbonate (600 mg two times daily) supplements should be given, along with a renal-specific multivitamin (Nephrocaps). Importantly, however, this chronic treatment may result in hypercalcemia and worsen coronary artery calcification. Thus, close monitoring of serum calcium levels is critical. Vitamin E may also be helpful in treating muscle cramps.

Anemia should be treated with erythropoietin (80–120 units/kg subcutaneously per week), taking care not to induce polycythemia (goal Hgb = 11–12 g/dL) with its attendant risk of stroke. Dosing usually begins around 10,000 units per week but may be adjusted upward in frequency or dose, as needed. Darbepoetin alfa is an alternative erythropoietic agent with a longer half-life, allowing for less frequent dosing (0.45 mcg/kg subcutaneously per week). Patients with iron-deficiency anemia should take ferrous sulfate 325 mg PO daily to three times daily with meals, with lower doses in elderly patients being less likely to induce constipation. Gentle transfusion with packed red blood cells may be required in cases of extreme or acutely worsened anemia, but care must be taken not to induce high-output heart failure or fluid overload, because the heart typically adapts to the chronic anemia of CKD. In relation to this, bleeding diatheses due to uremic platelet dysfunction are not uncommon in both AKI and CKD. Active bleeding in these patients should be treated with desmopressin (DDAVP), cryoprecipitate, estrogen, or dialysis to remove uremic toxins believed to be qualitatively inhibiting platelet function.

Hypercholesterolemia should be treated with a statin drug with the low-density lipoprotein goal of less than 100, because CKD is considered a coronary artery disease equivalent. Recent evidence suggests this goal should be even lower to minimize the rate of disease progression due to atherosclerotic renovascular disease. Dietary modification to restrict cholesterol and saturated fats is also critical to adequately address hyperlipidemia, especially hypertriglyceridemia.

Both hypovolemia (renal hypoperfusion) and renal toxic drugs may exacerbate CKD and must always be considered when acute or chronic renal failure is observed. A judicious trial of isotonic fluid repletion may be appropriate in patients displaying the physical stigmata of dehydration, and careful attention must be paid to the dosing of all chronic and newly started medications. All nephrotoxic agents (e.g., NSAIDs, radiocontrast dye) should be avoided.

Other measures to relieve symptoms include skin moisturizers for dry skin, and menthol or phenol lotion, a trial of capsaicin cream, or diphenhydramine (Benadryl) may all be useful in treating pruritus. It may be necessary to give diuretics for edema, but dehydration must be avoided. Thiazide diuretics may be tried first, but they are far less effective at a GFR less than 20 to 30 mL/min (approximated by serum creatinine levels of greater than 2.5 mg/dL); however, they do provide an additive effect when used with a loop diuretic initiated for refractory edema. Potassium-sparing diuretics should be avoided, owing to the kidneys' reduced ability to excrete potassium.

As CKD progresses, the patient will have increased difficulties with fluid balance and may experience episodes of hyperkalemia, hypertension, acidosis, and severe uremia with altered mental status and qualitative platelet dysfunction with a tendency for bleeding diatheses. Metabolic acidosis should be treated with sodium bicarbonate 600 mg two times daily initially to titrate serum bicarbonate to the 16 to 20 mEq/L range. However, patients must display adequate respiratory function to avoid the accumulation of metabolized carbon dioxide and respiratory acidosis. The potassium and calcium levels should be monitored during treatment of acidosis, because both might fall. Hospitalization may be required for control of fluid overload, hypertension, hyperkalemia, or infection.

A GFR less than 10 mL/min per 1.73 m² of BSA, a serum creatinine level approaching 12 mg/dL, or BUN greater than 100 mg/dL all typically require more aggressive therapies to avoid life-threatening sequelae, including peritoneal or hemodialysis. Continuous venovenous or arteriovenous hemofiltration may be used in hemodynamically unstable patients, as an alternative to classic hemodialysis. Such therapies must be done only under the supervision of a nephrologist, however. Life-threatening indications for dialysis include pericarditis, diuretic-refractory fluid overload (e.g., pulmonary edema), medication-resistant or rapidly worsening hypertension, uremic syndrome with an attendant bleeding diathesis or neurological symptomatology, and persistent nausea and vomiting. In addition, protein malnutrition in the face of a creatinine clearance of less than 20 mL/min is considered an indication for early dialysis.

Follow-up and Referral

Patients with CKD should be referred to a nephrologist. The course of CKD is typically punctuated by periods of rapid deterioration, often precipitated by dehydration or infection. The rate of progression to kidney failure will depend in part on the underlying renal disease: It is usually more rapid in patients with diabetic nephropathy or severe hypertension and slower in patients with polycystic kidneys. In patients with advanced renal failure (creatinine levels greater than 10 mg/dL), however, mean survival time without intervention (e.g., dialysis or transplantation) is 100 to 150 days. Vascular access for hemodialysis (arteriovenous grafts or fistulae) must be obtained 2 to 3 months in advance to permit maturation of the fistulae and allow for potential revisions. Decisions regarding dialysis and transplantation require a team approach with the primary-care provider, nephrologist, patient, and family. Comprehensive evaluation of the patient's medical, psychological, and social situation is necessary for successful planning.

The patient may need to be hospitalized to control fluid overload, hypertension, hyperkalemia, or infection. In general, the multiplicity of metabolic demands on the patient with CKD will require careful and close follow-up and constant adjustments in treatment. The most important cornerstone of care is the monitoring and treatment of all underlying disorders known to lead to chronic renal failure. Successful therapy depends in good part on the maintenance of a strong relationship between the health-care provider and the patient and family. Nowhere is a *Circle of Caring* approach more important than in a chronic, progressive disorder such as CKD. Interventions should be geared toward minimizing the patient's dependence and social isolation. See Case Study 12.1.

CASE STUDY 12.1   Giving Up Hope

Hope began her life as a juvenile diabetic. She became sick early in life, but did not let that stop her from having a rewarding career as a teacher. Her favorite hobby was painting—a talent that proved to strengthen her throughout her illnesses.

When I met Hope, she was 47 years old, her kidneys were no longer functioning, and she had lost one leg below the knee. She also had recently been diagnosed with breast cancer and had chosen to undergo chemotherapy. No longer able to work, she began to paint and continued to fight her illness. Each complication drained her body more. She endured peritoneal dialysis and then hemodialysis after a bout with peritonitis. Finally, her breast cancer metastasized to the peritoneal cavity.

Hope returned from hemodialysis early one day. It would be for the last time. Her sixth dialysis shunt was no longer patent. I then realized why I had been drawn to Hope. She no longer needed medicine or therapy; she needed someone to help her die.

I'll never forget that day. Hope looked at me through her tears and said, "I don't want to die." Not knowing exactly what to say, I looked in her eyes and told her it was time. Her life was in someone else's hands now, not hers. She didn't have any more decisions to make, and she could try to find peace. Although her soul was strong, her body was not. By letting go, she wasn't giving up; she was saving herself.

I feel that we, as clinicians, touch life in the most profound way by giving certain patients permission to die. The true challenge lies in knowing when medicine is no longer what the patient needs.

Source: Astalos Chism, L. An unforgettable case. *Clin Advis* February 1998, p 12.

Patient Education

For care to be effective, the patient and family must have a good understanding of the chronic and progressive nature of CKD, of the importance of treating all underlying systemic diseases such as diabetes and hypertension, and of the specifics of the treatment plan. Avoidance of infection is important, as is maintaining a healthy diet as recommended. Patients should know when and how to report bleeding, fever, decreases in urine output, or episodes of nausea and vomiting.

 For additional resources please visit
http://davisplus.fadavis.com

References

Evidence-Based Practice

American College of Obstetricians and Gynecologists. *Treatment of urinary tract infections in nonpregnant women.* ACOG practice bulletin no 91. American College of Obstetrics and Gynecologists, Washington, DC, March 2008.

Astor, BC, et al. Lower estimated glomerular filtration rate and higher albuminuria are associated with mortality and end-stage renal disease. A collaborative meta-analysis of kidney disease population cohorts. *Kidney Int* 79:1331, 2011.

International Collaboration of Trialists. International phase III trial assessing neoadjuvant cisplatin, methotrexate, and vinblastine chemotherapy for muscle-invasive bladder cancer: Long-term results of the BA06 30894 trial. *J Clin Oncol* 29:2171–2177, 2011.

Lewington, A, and Kanagasundaram, S. Clinical practice guidelines: Acute kidney injury. The Renal Association. 2011. Retrieved from www.renal.org/Clinical/GuidelinesSection/AcuteKidneyInjury.aspx#downloads

Scottish Intercollegiate Guidelines Network (SIGN). *Management of suspected bacterial urinary tract infections in adults. A national clinical guideline.* SIGN publication no 88. SIGN, Edinburgh, Scotland, July 2006.

Siefker-Radtke, AO, et al. A phase 2 clinical trial of sequential neoadjuvant chemotherapy with ifosfamide, doxorubicin, and gemcitabine followed by cisplatin, gemcitabine, and ifosfamide in locally advanced urothelial cancer. *Cancer* 119(3): 540–547, 2013.

Bibliography

General

Dambro, MR. *Griffith's 5-minute clinical consult.* Lippincott Williams & Wilkins, Philadelphia, 2013.

Edmunds, MW, and Mayhew, MS. *Pharmacology for the primary care provider,* ed 4. Mosby/Elsevier, St. Louis, MO, 2013.

Fauci, AS, et al (Eds.). *Harrison's principles of internal medicine,* ed 18. McGraw-Hill, New York, 2011.

Kee, JL. *Laboratory and diagnostic tests with nursing implications,* ed 8. Prentice-Hall, Upper Saddle River, NJ, 2010.

Kumar, V, et al. *Robbins basic pathology,* ed 8. Saunders/Elsevier, St. Louis, MO, 2010.

McCance, KL, and Huether, SE. *Pathophysiology: The biologic basis for disease in adults and children,* ed 5. Elsevier Mosby, St. Louis, MO, 2012.

Papadakis, MA, and McPhee, SJ. *Current medical diagnosis and treatment,* ed 52. Lange/McGraw-Hill, New York, 2013.

Acute Kidney Injury

Berliner, AR, and Fine, DM. There's something fishy about this bleeding. *NDT Plus* 4:270, 2011.

Dirkes, S. Acute kidney injury: Not just acute renal failure anymore? *Crit Care Nurse* 31(1):37–49, 2011.

Grams, ME, et al. Fluid balance, diuretic use, and mortality in acute kidney injury. *Clin J Am Soc Nephrol* 6:966, 2011.

Ishani, A, et al. The magnitude of acute serum creatinine increase after cardiac surgery and the risk of chronic kidney disease, progression of kidney disease, and death. *Arch Intern Med* 171: 226–233, 2011.

KDIGO clinical practice guideline for acute kidney injury. *Kidney Int Suppl* 2:1, 2012. doi:10.1038/kisup.2012.1

Plantinga, L, et al. Nonsteroidal anti-inflammatory drug use among persons with chronic kidney disease in the United States. *Ann Fam Med* 9:423, 2011.

Bladder Tumors

American Joint Committee on Cancer. *AJCC cancer staging manual,* ed 7. Urinary bladder. Springer, New York, 2010, pp 497–502.

McDougal, WS, et al. Cancer of the bladder, ureter and renal pelvis. In DeVita, VT, et al (Eds.), *DeVita, Hellman, and Rosenberg's cancer: Principles and practice of oncology,* ed 9. Lippincott Williams & Wilkins, Philadelphia, 2011.

Moyer, VA. Screening for bladder cancer: US Preventive Services task force recommendation statement. *Ann Intern Med* 155(4): 246–251, 2011.

National Comprehensive Cancer Network. NCCN Clinical practice guidelines in oncology. Bladder cancer. V.2.2012. Retrieved from www.nccn.org/professionals/physician_gls/pdf/bladder.pdf

Silbert, JL, and Parsons, JK. Evidence-based principles of bladder cancer and diet. *Urology* 75(2):340–346, 2010.

Chronic Kidney Disease

Abboud, H, and Henrich, WL. Clinical practice. Stage IV chronic kidney disease. *N Engl J Med* 362:56, 2010.

Crews, DC, et al; Centers for Disease Control and Prevention Chronic Kidney Disease Surveillance Team. Prevalence of chronic kidney disease in persons with undiagnosed or prehypertension in the United States. *Hypertension* 55(5):1102–1109, 2010.

Gansevoort, RT, et al. Lower estimated GFR and higher albuminuria are associated with adverse kidney outcomes. A collaborative meta-analysis of general and high-risk population cohorts. *Kidney Int* 80: 93, 2011.

Glassock, RJ. Is the presence of microalbuminuria a relevant marker of kidney disease? *Curr Hypertens Rep* 12:364, 2010.

James, MT, et al. Early recognition and prevention of chronic kidney disease. *Lancet* 375:1296, 2010.

KDIGO. Chapter 1: Definition and classification of CKD. *Kidney Int Suppl* 3:19, 2013. Retrieved from www.kdigo.org/clinical_practice_guidelines/pdf/CKD/KDIGO_2012_CKD_GL.pdf

KDOQI clinical practice guideline for diabetes and CKD: 2012 update. *Am J Kidney Dis* 60(5):850–886, 2012.

Levey, AS, and Coresh, J. Chronic kidney disease. *Lancet* 379:165, 2012.

Plantinga, LC, et al; CDC CKD Surveillance Team. Prevalence of chronic kidney disease in U.S. adults with undiagnosed diabetes or prediabetes. *Clin J Am Soc Nephrol* 5(4):673_682, 2010.

United States Renal Data System. USRDS 2009 annual data report. U.S. Department of Health and Human Services. The National Institutes of Health, National Institute of Diabetes and Digestive and Kidney Diseases, Bethesda, MD. *Am J Kidney Dis* 55(Suppl 1): S1, 2010.

Wei, SY, et al. Chronic kidney disease care program improves quality of pre-end-stage renal disease care and reduces medical costs. *Nephrology* (Carlton) 15:108, 2010.

Nephrolithiasis

Baumgarten, DA, et al; American College of Radiology. ACR Appropriateness Criteria® acute onset flank pain—Suspicion of stone disease. National Guideline Clearinghouse. Retrieved from www.guideline.gov/content.aspx?id=32639

European Association of Urology. Guidelines on urolithiasis. National Guideline Clearinghouse. Retrieved from www.guidelines.gov/content.aspx?id=12528

Gücük, A, et al. Routine flexible nephroscopy for percutaneous nephrolithotomy in renal stones with low density: A prospective randomized study. *J Urol* 190(1), Jan 9, 2013.

Renal Tumors

Akdogan, B, et al. Prevalence and predictors of benign lesions in renal masses smaller than 7 cm presumed to be renal cell carcinoma. *Clin Genitourin Cancer* 10:121, 2012.

Millet, I, et al. Characterization of small solid renal lesions: Can benign and malignant tumors be differentiated with CT? *Am J Roentgenol* 197:887, 2011.

Smaldone, MC, et al. Small renal masses progressing to metastases under active surveillance: A systematic review and pooled analysis. *Cancer* 118:997, 2012.

Urinary Incontinence

Abrams, P, et al. Fourth International Consultation on Incontinence Recommendations of the International Scientific Committee: Evaluation and treatment of urinary incontinence, pelvic organ prolapse, and fecal incontinence. *Neurourol Urodyn* 29:213, 2010.

Huang, AJ. Nonsurgical treatments for urinary incontinence in women: Summary of primary findings and conclusions. *JAMA Intern Med* 173(15), 2013.

Loughlin, KR, and Prasad, MM. Post-prostatectomy urinary incontinence: A confluence of 3 factors. *J Urol* 183:871, 2010.

Nygaard, I. Clinical practice. Idiopathic urgency urinary incontinence. *N Engl J Med* 363:1156, 2010.

Ruby, CM, et al. The effect of medication use on urinary incontinence in community-dwelling elderly women. *J Am Geriatr Soc* 58: 1715, 2010.

Tennstedt, SL, et al. The effects of severity of urine leakage on quality of life in Hispanic, white, and black men and women: The Boston Community Health Survey. *Urology* 75:27, 2010.

Winters, JC, et al. Urodynamic studies in adults: AUA/SUFU guideline. *J Urol* 188:2464, 2012.

Urinary Tract Infections

Clark, CJ, et al. Pediatric urology urinary tract infection in children: When to worry. *Urol Clin North Am* 37(2):229–241, 2010.

Colgan, R, and Williams, M. Diagnosis and treatment of acute uncomplicated cystitis. *Am Fam Physician* 84(7):771–776, 2011.

Gupta, K, et al. International clinical practice guidelines for the treatment of acute uncomplicated cystitis and pyelonephritis in women: A 2010 update by the Infectious Diseases Society of America and the European Society for Microbiology and Infectious Diseases. *Clin Infect Dis* 52(5):e103–e120, 2011.

Gupta, K, and Trautner, B. In the clinic. Urinary tract infection. *Ann Intern Med* 156(5):ITC3-1–ITC3-15, 2012.

Little, P, et al. Presentation, pattern, and natural course of severe symptoms, and role of antibiotics and antibiotic resistance among patients presenting with suspected uncomplicated urinary tract infection in primary care: Observational study. *BMJ* 340:b5633, 2010. doi:10.1136/bmj.b5633

Litza, JA, and Brill, JR. Primary urology urinary tract infections. *Prim Care* 37(3):491–507, 2010.

Lumbiganon, P, et al. Screening and treating asymptomatic bacteriuria in pregnancy. *Curr Opin Obstet Gynecol* 22(2):95–99, 2010.

National Kidney and Urologic Diseases Information Clearinghouse (NKUDIC). Kidney and urologic diseases statistics for the United States. Retrieved from http://kidney.niddk.nih.gov/kudiseases/pubs/kustats/#urologic

Sandberg, T, et al. Ciprofloxacin for 7 days versus 14 days in women with acute pyelonephritis: A randomised, open-label and double-blind, placebo-controlled, non-inferiority trial. *Lancet* 380(9840): 484–490, 2012.

van Nieuwkoop, C, et al. Prospective cohort study of acute pyelonephritis in adults: Safety of triage towards home based oral antimicrobial treatment. *J Infect* 60(2):114–121, 2010.

Wang, CH, et al. Cranberry-containing products for prevention of urinary tract infections in susceptible populations: A systematic review and meta-analysis of randomized controlled trials. *Arch Intern Med* 172(13):988–996, 2012.

Resources

American Cancer Society
www.cancer.org
American Urological Association
www.auanet.org
Mayo Clinic
www.mayohealth.org
National Association for Continence
www.nafc.org

National Bladder Foundation
www.bladder.org
National Kidney Foundation
www.kidney.org
University of Pennsylvania Cancer Center
www.oncolink.upenn.edu

Chapter 13

Men's Health Problems

Debbie J. Nogueras, PhD, MSN, ANP/FNP-BC • *Debera J. Thomas, DNS, RN, FNP/ANP* • *Brian Oscar Porter, MD, PhD, MPH*

COMMON COMPLAINTS

■ NOCTURIA AND INCONTINENCE

Nocturia is currently defined by the International Continence Society as having to wake at night one or more times to void, each time being preceded and followed by sleep (Level I; Cornu et al, 2012). Recording the number of times a patient urinates at night and making a reasonable estimate of the amount voided is extremely important. The frequency of urination may vary from large volumes of urine (polyuria) voided infrequently to small quantities passed at frequent intervals. Adult men normally void five to six times during the day and once or not at all during the night. As men age, nocturia is usually a sign of a prostate problem, most often benign prostatic hyperplasia (BPH). Typically, 50% of men older than age 50 years have BPH, and the rate increases by 10% for every 10 years of age (i.e., to 60% of men older than age 60 years, to 70% of men older than age 70 years, and so on). BPH is discussed in more detail later in this chapter.

The occurrence of nocturia without discomfort may be due to diminished bladder capacity, overflow incontinence, or habit. In men with a normal bladder, the absence of nocturia while suffering from increased frequency of urination during the day suggests psychogenic origin. A rare finding might be a polyp or irritative lesion in the posterior urethra that is relieved by recumbence, so nocturia is not present.

Detrusor muscle instability may cause urinary incontinence as well as nocturia. Fifty percent of male patients in nursing homes are incontinent, whereas 15% to 30% of elderly men in the community have urinary incontinence, which may be caused by decreased bladder capacity, increased residual urine (from inability to empty the bladder), or involuntary bladder contractions. Moderate dribbling of urine may indicate overflow from a partially incompetent outlet and can be congenital or an acquired anomaly. Less common causes of incontinence are spinal cord disease, multiple sclerosis, tumors, trauma, syphilis, and diabetic neuropathy. Microorganisms that can cause nocturia and incontinence include *Klebsiella pneumoniae, Proteus mirabilis, Enterobacter, Staphylococcus,* enterococci (*Streptococcus* bacteria associated with the intestines), or *Pseudomonas.*

Medications, such as methyldopa, phenothiazines, diazepam, excessive vitamin D, and diuretics, may also cause nocturia, as well as precipitate or aggravate incontinence. Drugs that cause urinary retention include alpha-adrenergic agents, androgens, and sympathomimetic agents such as ephedrine and pseudoephedrine. Urinary retention can cause nocturia and incontinence.

Differential Diagnosis

Increased frequency may occur as a result of primary disease of the urinary tract or may result from metabolic disease such as diabetes mellitus or diabetes insipidus; it may also be associated with emotional tension. Documentation of the pattern of urination during a 24-hour period is vital to a diagnosis of nocturia. Although a patient may complain if he awakens frequently to urinate, the precipitating events and activities of the day may also give a hint to the cause. For example, alcohol intake before sleep may increase the number of times the patient urinates at night and may also increase urine volume.

Urgency, a desire to urinate, can be constant or intermittent. Urgency and frequency of urination often occur together. Urgency is frequently the result of prostatic disease or bladder infection. Hesitancy refers to difficulty in initiating a urine stream. *Oliguria* is a decrease in urinary output and can be caused by a decrease in the production of urine secondary to acute glomerulonephritis or other renal disease, as well as conditions that drastically decrease cardiac output. Dribbling can be symptomatic of disease; it may occur at night and during the day and usually indicates the presence of a urethral stricture or prostatic obstruction, but it may be caused by a neurological disorder.

Treatment

Treatment of nocturia depends on identifying the cause. A simple urinalysis is performed to rule out urinary tract infection. A prostate-specific antigen blood test and a digital rectal exam are done to rule out a prostate problem. The results may indicate a need for further testing.

Specific patient education is discussed under the particular disease causing the nocturia.

■ TESTICULAR PAIN

Testicular pain is probably the most urgent of patient complaints. Testicular pain as a single symptom is a fullness or heaviness of the scrotum, ranging from a dull ache to a sticking pain, and may occur in a wide variety of patients with no differentiation based on culture, race, or socioeconomic status.

The tunica vaginalis is a remnant of the processus vaginalis; a painful hernia can occur when an evagination of the peritoneal cavity is occluded by the adult spermatic cord. A patent processus vaginalis predisposes the patient to indirect or congenital hernias. Partial occlusion of the processus vaginalis can result in fluid accumulation, or hydrocele, that cannot be distinguished from a hernia or an incompletely descended testicle until surgery is performed. Anterior and lateral to the testes, the processus vaginalis remains patent, forming the tunica vaginalis, which represents the detached portion of the peritoneal cavity within the scrotum.

Differential Diagnoses

A cause of testicular pain may be swelling of the testis, the epididymis, or the spermatic cord or torsion of the testicle (the testicle may become twisted around the spermatic cord, causing acute pain; this condition is a urological emergency). Differential diagnoses for testicular pain include hydrocele, varicocele, epididymitis, and prostatitis. Pain from prostatitis usually occurs in the lower back and radiates to the testicles and is typically accompanied by fever. Cultures usually show *Escherichia coli,* with or without fistula formation. Hernias, hydroceles, and hematomas all must be excluded. A detailed history and physical exam will direct the assessment to exclude other diagnoses. A spermatocele may also cause testicular pain, although most spermatoceles are painless. A syphilitic gumma is a possibility, as is a varicocele; however, these conditions are usually not painful.

Because of the multiple possible diagnoses, specialized tests are performed. A scrotal ultrasound can identify any mass originating in the testicles and is noninvasive. An echo-texture pattern reveals the presence of a hypoechoic mass that is distinct from surrounding normal testicular tissue, spermatoceles, hydroceles, or varicoceles.

Treatment

Treatment of testicular pain is dependent on finding the underlying cause for the pain and treating it appropriately.

■ TESTOSTERONE DEFICIENCY (LOW T)

Testosterone levels peak during adolescence and early adulthood, and then gradually decline about 1% per year after age 30 years. As men age, there is a rise in follicle-stimulating hormone, which controls sperm production, and luteinizing hormone, which controls testosterone production; there is a simultaneous decline in testosterone. Normal testosterone levels are less than 300 ng/dL and are best assessed in the morning between 7:00 a.m. and 10:00 a.m. Testosterone decline may be a function of normal aging or may be due to hypogonadism. Other factors suppressing testosterone levels include stress, obesity, tobacco and alcohol use, obstructive sleep apnea, diabetes mellitus, and illness. Medications such as suramin (Germanin), ketoconazole (Nizoral), glucocorticoids, alkylating agents, and opiates used chronically may cause a decrease in serum testosterone.

Low testosterone (low T) affects multiple body systems. Cardiovascular effects include dyslipidemia and hypertension. Metabolic syndrome consists of these disorders, in addition to obesity and diabetes mellitus, which collectively increase the risk of cardiovascular disease. Low T is associated with type 2 diabetes mellitus, and men with the lowest levels of free testosterone are four times as likely to have diabetes. Osteopenia, osteoporosis, and fracture prevalence rates are greater in hypogonadal men, with 30% of fractures occurring in men with low T. Erectile dysfunction and decreased libido correspond with a decline in testosterone, which regulates nerve structure and function in areas of the spinal cord that are involved in erections. In addition, a decline in mental functioning has also been associated with low T.

First-line treatment for symptomatic men with low testosterone levels is testosterone replacement therapy. Testosterone gels and patches are the most prevalent hormone replacement formulations and can be found in the Drugs Commonly Prescribed 13.1. Testosterone therapy is contraindicated in men with breast or prostate cancer, palpable prostate nodules or induration, untreated obstructive sleep apnea, severe lower urinary tract symptoms with an International Prostate Symptom Score of greater than 19, and New York Heart Association Class III or IV heart failure.

COMMON PROBLEMS

■ BENIGN PROSTATIC HYPERPLASIA

Benign prostatic hyperplasia (also called benign prostatic hypertrophy) (BPH) is the common name for nodular hyperplasia of the prostate and is one of the most common conditions affecting men older than age 40 years. The prostate gland is a walnut-size gland positioned at the base of the bladder and in front of the rectum. The prostate gland, which starts enlarging in puberty and stops growing at around age 20 years, begins to enlarge again after age 50 years. The prostate has three distinct zones: the central zone, the peripheral zone, and the transition zone, which lies adjacent to the urethra (see Prostate Cancer later in this chapter for a more detailed description of prostatic anatomy). BPH develops primarily in the transition zone,

Drugs Commonly Prescribed 13.1   Erectile Dysfunction

Drug	Adverse Reactions	Prescribing Considerations
Hormone Replacement		
Parenteral agents: testosterone cypionate (Depo-Testosterone) testosterone enanthate (Delatestryl)	Sodium retention with dependent edema, increased risk of bleeding, pain at injection site, mild gynecomastia, mood swings, lipid abnormalities	Do not use in patients with serious liver, kidney, or cardiac disease, prostate or breast cancer, or in those with mercury allergy. The peak and trough effects that may lead to aggression, feelings of well-being, energy, and increased libido within 72 hours of injection. As the peak level falls, the patient may experience depressed mood and loss of libido.
Oral agents: fluoxymesterone (Halotestin) methyltestosterone (Android, Methitest, Testred, Virilon)	Same as for parenteral agents Not used much as transdermal or parenteral agents because of the difficulty in achieving adequate blood levels due to high first-pass loss in the liver.	Oral agents are not generally recommended because of the hepatotoxicity and unreliable androgenic effects.
Transdermal testosterone patch: Androderm Testoderm	Local irritation; burn-like blistering or irritation of skin where transdermal patch is worn.	NOT to be applied to the scrotum. Should be applied to the arm, back, abdomen, or thigh. May cause local irritation.
Transdermal testosterone topical gel or solution: AndroGel 1% (2.5- to 5-g packets) Testim 1% Gel (5- to 10-g packets) Axiron solution (60–120 mg)	Burn-like blistering or irritation of skin where gel is applied. Problems with urination.	Apply to the axilla, upper arm or shoulder, NOT the scrotum. May transfer to partner during close contact.
Testosterone implantable pellets: Testopel (150–450 mg)		Produces steady blood levels; must be implanted in subcutaneous tissue every 3–4 months.
Testosterone buccal system: Striant (30 mg)	Mouth or gum irritation Allergic reactions. Swelling of ankles or legs. Breathing disturbances, including those associated with sleep. Liver damage	Insertion twice a day, in the morning and in the evening, provides continuous systemic delivery of testosterone.
Vasoactive Therapy		
Oral agents: sildenafil (Viagra) vardenafil (Levitra) tadalafil (Cialis) avanafil (Stendra)	Headache, flushing, dyspepsia, nasal congestion, visual color changes, back, lower limb pain for all phosphodiesterase-5 inhibitors.	None of these agents should be used in patients taking nitrates or alpha blockers. Must wait 24 hours before giving a nitrate after sildenafil or vardenafil. The duration of action for tadalafil is 36 hours. Must wait 48 hours before giving a nitrate.
Injectables: alprostadil (Caverject)	Penile pain, prolonged erection, penile fibrosis, injection site hematoma, numbness, yeast infection, priapism. May also cause upper respiratory infection, headache, dizziness, hypotension.	Should not be used in patients with sickle cell anemia, penile fibrosis, coagulopathy, severe cardiovascular disease, myeloma, leukemia, penis deformity, morbid obesity, or penile implants. Can be used only once every 24 hours and a maximum of 3 times a week. Patient should be instructed to choose injection site along side of proximal third of the penis, alternate injection sites, and avoid visible veins.

Drugs Commonly Prescribed 13.1   Erectile Dysfunction—cont'd

Drug	Adverse Reactions	Prescribing Considerations
Vasoactive Therapy		
Transurethral suppositories: alprostadil (Muse)	May cause urethral irritation.	As above. Should not be used if partner is pregnant unless a condom is used. The suppository is inserted in the penis about 1 inch after the patient urinates. The button on the top of the applicator is pushed to release the suppository. A gentle rocking motion will separate the suppository from the applicator. After the applicator is removed, the patient should massage the penis firmly for about 10 seconds while standing. An erection begins in about 5–10 minutes.

whereas carcinoma of the prostate usually develops in the peripheral zone.

Epidemiology and Causes

The cause of BPH is not fully understood, but androgens play a key role. Aging is a primary risk factor, and BPH occurs in more than 50% of men older than age 50 years and 90% of men older than 80 years. Of these, 20% of men older than age 60 years have obstructive and irritative symptoms that are severe enough to require treatment. Genetic susceptibility to the disorder is also underscored by twin concordance and family history studies, with inherited forms predominating in men younger than 60 years of age.

Epidemiological studies of BPH have been hampered by inconsistencies in the definition and clinical criteria of this disorder. Most authorities consider not only prostate size (greater than 30 mL) but also decreased urinary flow rates (less than 15 mL/sec) and significant postvoid residual bladder volumes (greater than 50 mL).

BPH arises from a systemic hormonal alteration, which may or may not act in combination with growth factors that stimulate stromal or glandular hyperplasia. One risk factor for BPH is intact testes—more specifically, functioning Leydig cells. Castrated men or those with untreated hypogonadism before age 40 years rarely develop BPH. There has been no concrete evidence that dietary, environmental, or sexual practices are implicated in BPH, although obesity substantially increases the risk of BPH.

Pathophysiology

The prostate consists of two main sections. The inner section of the gland produces secretions needed to keep the lining of the urethra moist. The outer section contributes to seminal secretions. Prostatic secretions form part of the seminal fluid during ejaculation. The ejaculatory ducts from the seminal vesicles pass through the prostate gland and enter the urethra.

The importance of dihydrotestosterone (DHT) as a key androgenic hormone in the pathogenesis of BPH is well supported. Although concentrations of this pro-hormone (which is subsequently converted into testosterone) do not differ in men with or without BPH, prostatic receptors for this hormone have a much more heterogeneous distribution in men with BPH, whereas in normal controls, these receptors predominate within the epithelia. Thus, although necessary to the pathogenesis of BPH, androgen exposure alone is not sufficient to cause the disorder. Similarly, estrogen has been implicated as a necessary factor to maintain BPH in older men, but it is not sufficient to cause its pathogenesis alone. The data are conflicting, however. For instance, the concentration of estrogen receptors is actually lower in hyperplastic prostatic tissue, whereas the concentration of progesterone receptors does not differ in BPH versus the normal prostate.

The earliest histological signs of BPH usually appear in men in their 30s and 40s. The development of pathological BPH is similar in most cases. BPH usually presents as a predominance of stromal nodules (up to a fourfold increase), consisting primarily of smooth muscle and connective tissue, in the periurethral area of the transition zone. This may be followed by glandular hyperplasia (up to a twofold increase) with an increase in epithelial cells. Key growth factors include fibroblast growth factor, insulin-like growth factor–2, and transforming growth factor–b. In vitro data demonstrate a wider array of growth factors that stimulate prostatic epithelial cell growth. Anti-apoptotic factors such as bcl-2 are also upregulated in BPH tissue, and animal studies have implicated higher numbers of stem cells in hyperplastic prostatic tissue.

There are two documented mechanisms of obstruction—static and dynamic. *Static constriction* is caused by the buildup of prostatic tissue, with direct obstruction of the bladder neck. *Dynamic constriction* is an increase in prostatic muscle tone through adrenergic stimulation, leading to constriction of the bladder neck. A predominance of alpha-adrenergic receptors in the sympathetic nervous system controls stromal hyperplasia. If middle-lobe enlargement of the prostate predominates, the symptoms produced are similar to those of a ball-valve obstruction at the bladder neck.

Obstruction of the bladder outlet forces the bladder to generate higher pressures than normal to achieve micturition. Increased muscle mass in the bladder leads to reduced bladder elasticity and compliance, which manifests as a reduction in bladder capacity. If the bladder neck obstruction is not relieved, the bladder's smooth muscle begins to be replaced by connective tissue, leading to bladder failure.

Clinical Presentation
Subjective

Use of a standardized questionnaire such as the American Urological Association Symptom Index (AUASI) (shown in Focus on History 13.1), also known as the International Prostatic Symptom Score, is important in assessing the impact of BPH on the patient. This questionnaire is designed to uncover the degree of symptomatology in each patient. There are 7 items on the questionnaire that determine the severity of obstructive or irritative symptoms. Total symptom scores may range from 0 to 35. Obstructive voiding symptoms can be mild, with a score of 0 to 7. A score of 8 to 19 is considered moderate; 20 or higher indicates severe symptoms. Symptom scores are helpful to quantify the patient's symptoms. A score of 7 or higher on the AUASI, for example, can reinforce the need for further investigation of the cause of the symptoms. Although the scores alone are not diagnostic, they help to support the

---

Focus on History 13.1 AUA Symptom Score Index

Directions: Circle one number on each line.

Question to be answered	Not at all	Less than 1 time in 5	Less than half the time	About half the time	More than half the time	Almost always
1. Over the past month, how often have you had a sensation of not emptying your bladder completely after you finished urinating?	0	1	2	3	4	5
2. Over the past month, how often have you had to urinate again less than 2 hours after you finished urinating?	0	1	2	3	4	5
3. Over the past month, how often have you found you stopped and started again several times when you urinated?	0	1	2	3	4	5
4. Over the past month, how often have you found it difficult to postpone urination?	0	1	2	3	4	5
5. Over the past month, how often have you had a weak urinary stream?	0	1	2	3	4	5
6. Over the past month, how often have you had to push or strain to begin urination?	0	1	2	3	4	5

Focus on History 13.1 AUA Symptom Score Index—cont'd

Directions: Circle one number on each line.

Question to be answered	Not at all	Less than 1 time in 5	Less than half the time	About half the time	More than half the time	Almost always
7. Over the past month, how many times did you most typically get up to urinate from the time you went to bed at night until the time you got up in the morning?	0	1 time	2 times	3 times	4 times	5 times

Total sum of the 7 circled answers (AUA Symptom Score): _____

AUA Symptom Score Index

Score	Severity
0–7	Mild
8–19	Moderate
20–35	Severe

Source: Barry, MJ, et al. The American Urological Association symptom index for benign prostatic hyperplasia. *J Urol* 148(2): 1549–1557, 1992. Retrieved from www.ncbi.nlm.nih.gov/pubmed/1279218

diagnosis, as well as being useful in following a patient after initiating therapy to track the decrease in symptoms.

The symptoms of BPH vary and are dependent on the type of obstruction, but usually include a combination of obstructive and irritative voiding symptoms. Because the symptoms are not specific to BPH and may have other causes, a complete work-up is necessary. BPH is non–life-threatening, but it is a lifestyle-changing diagnosis.

Symptoms of obstructive BPH include decreased force of stream, hesitancy, postvoid dribbling, sensation of incomplete bladder emptying, overflow incontinence, inability to voluntarily stop the urinary stream, urinary retention, double-voiding (voiding a second time within 2 hours), and straining. Irritative symptoms of BPH include nocturia, urinary frequency, urgency, dysuria, and urge incontinence.

Objective

A digital rectal exam (DRE) is done to determine enlargement of the prostate gland. The prostate in BPH is usually diffusely smooth and enlarged. If the prostate is nodular and unusually firm, prostate cancer may be present. The size of the prostate does not correlate with the severity of the symptoms in men with BPH. Many men with palpably enlarged prostates are asymptomatic, whereas some patients with small prostates have irritative or obstructive symptoms.

Objective findings can include gross hematuria (in men older than 60 years of age), observation of a weak stream, distended bladder (to greater than 150 mL detected by percussion), increased postvoid residual volume (more than 100 mL), and prostate enlargement (to more than the normal "walnut" size, weighing 20 g or less).

Diagnostic Reasoning
Diagnostic Tests

Laboratory tests include a urinalysis, prostate-specific antigen (PSA), and the Prostate Health Index (phi). Urinalysis is done to exclude infection or hematuria. The American Urological Association (AUA) no longer recommends serum creatinine on the initial evaluation. PSA is done to assess for prostate cancer. There may be an elevation of the PSA in either prostate cancer or BPH; therefore, the PSA value alone is not diagnostic of cancer or BPH. Acute lower urinary retention or prostatitis will also elevate the PSA. The PSA in BPH is usually less than 10 ng/mL. PSA is a glycoprotein that aids in the liquefaction of the seminal coagulum. The phi blood test detects the [-2] proPSA isoform of prostate-specific antigen. This test may reduce the number of unneeded prostate biopsies, using a threshold of 27 when the total PSA is 4 to 10 ng/mL. An elevated pH results from the chronic residual urine. If an obstructive uropathy is present, the serum creatinine level will be elevated. Urine cultures are sometimes positive for bacteria because of the chronic residual urine. Urine cytology should be done to rule out carcinoma, particularly when hematuria is present. An intravenous pyelogram can identify an increased postvoid residual (PVR) volume of urine, a large prostatic impression on the bladder, trabeculated bladder, bladder diverticula, upper tract dilation, and/or bladder stones.

Subsequent testing should be done by a urologist if initial treatment does not relieve symptoms or if prostate cancer is suspected. Uroflow, for example, measures the amount of urine voided per unit of time. Flow of less than 10 mL/sec is indicative of obstruction. This test is accurate when the voided volume is greater than 200 mL. A cystometrogram measures bladder compliance and is usually reserved for patients with suspected neurological disease or whose prostate surgery was unsuccessful in relieving symptoms. A cystoscopy is usually done only to determine the best surgical approach for BPH.

Differential Diagnosis

The differential diagnoses that must be considered when evaluating a patient with suspected BPH are numerous and fall into three distinct categories: bladder outlet obstruction, nonobstructive etiologies, and irritative symptoms. Differential Diagnosis 13.1 presents the differential diagnosis for BPH.

When BPH is the presumptive diagnosis, other obstructive etiologies of the lower urinary tract (bladder calculi, bladder neck contracture, urethral stricture, and prostate cancer) should be explored. Careful history may

reveal previous urethral instrumentation, urethritis, or trauma as the source of the obstruction. Bladder calculi may present with pain and hematuria. Irritative etiologies (bladder cancer, lower urinary tract infection, prostatitis, or urethritis) may present with hematuria, urgency, and frequency. A history of diabetes mellitus, stroke, neurological diseases, or spinal cord injury can contribute to a neurogenic bladder, which has many of the same symptoms as BPH. Cancer of the prostate and BPH have many of the same symptoms. A PSA and DRE can help differentiate between these two disorders.

Management
Medical Management

Most patients with BPH can be treated as outpatients; the goal is to relieve the symptoms, specifically nocturia. The Patient's Voice 13.1 illustrates the patient's need for symptom relief. Inpatient treatment is required to manage fluid and electrolyte abnormalities of obstructive uropathy.

> ### The Patient's Voice 13.1
> #### Nocturia
> I had been getting up three or four times a night to urinate. It was getting to be a nuisance. At my annual exam, I was told I had mild BPH and that my PSA was normal. I told my primary-care provider that I was tired of getting up so often at night and that it made me tired the next day. The primary-care provider told me that if getting up several times a night was bothering me, that there were some medications I could try. I decided to give it a try. What relief! A simple pill and now I can sleep all night and wake up refreshed. I feel great. I am grateful that my primary-care provider took the time to listen to me.

Most urologists and primary-care providers have adopted a "watchful waiting" technique for BPH that has only mild symptoms. A patient with mild to moderate symptoms, minimal PVR, and no objective changes in the urinary tract may only require monitoring. The "watchful waiting" medical treatment is usually considered the most conservative and the most effective treatment for BPH, as long as more serious conditions have been ruled out. Watchful waiting is also the recommended treatment when BPH has little or no impact on the quality of life. As lifestyle changes do occur, however, or as the AUA score increases, several options may be offered to the patient. Avoidance of caffeine and alcohol, both known to be bladder irritants, is recommended. A patient with a high AUA symptom score, urinary retention, or complications of BPH, including a high PVR, renal insufficiency, hematuria, bladder stones, or anatomical urinary tract abnormalities, should not be treated with only watchful waiting, because these conditions require more vigorous treatment.

Once prostatic cancer has been ruled out, medications may be tried initially to treat the BPH symptoms. Medical

Differential Diagnosis 13.1   Benign Prostatic Hyperplasia

Bladder Outlet Obstruction
- Prostate cancer
- Urethral stricture due to trauma or sexually transmitted disease
- Bladder neck contracture (acquired or congenital)
- Anterior or posterior urethral valve failure
- Müllerian duct cysts
- Inability of bladder neck or external sphincter to relax during voiding

Nonobstructive Etiologies
- Neurogenic bladder (detrusor denervation)
- Myogenic cause (detrusor muscle failure)
- Diabetes mellitus
- Parkinson's disease
- Cerebrovascular accident
- Medications (parasympatholytics, sympathomimetics)
- Psychogenic stress–induced performance anxiety

Irritative Symptoms
- Neurogenic bladder (detrusor denervation)
- Neoplasm
- Bladder cancer
- Bladder calculi
- Prostatitis
- UTI
- Urethritis

management is used when no strong indication for surgery exists or when a patient refuses surgery or is a poor surgical candidate. Because the prostate and bladder contain alpha$_1$-adrenergic receptors that cause the prostate and bladder neck to contract when bound, alpha blockade decreases this effect and results in objective and subjective improvement in the manifestations of BPH. Most of the alpha blockers used in the treatment of BPH are selective alpha$_1$-adrenergic agonists. These include silodosin (Rapaflo) 4 or 8 mg daily or the longer-acting terazosin (Hytrin) 1 to 10 mg daily and doxazosin (Cardura) 1 to 8 mg daily. The subtype alpha$_{1a}$-adrenergic receptors have been identified in the bladder neck and prostate, with the subsequent development of medications that target these receptors, which include tamsulosin (Flomax) 0.4 or 0.8 mg daily and alfuzosin (UroXatral) 10 to 15 mg daily (immediately after the same meal each day).

The long-acting alpha$_1$-adrenergic blockers have the advantage of once-a-day dosing but still require a gradual dose titration. For example, doxazosin is usually started at 1 mg daily for 7 days and then increased by 1 mg per week until the dose is 4 mg daily. Terazosin is started at 1 mg daily for 3 days, then 2 mg daily for 11 days, then increased to 5 mg daily. The alpha$_{1a}$-adrenergic blockers (tamsulosin and alfuzosin) do not need to be titrated, but should be started at the lowest dose and increased if necessary. The dosage of silodosin is once daily with a meal. No dosage adjustment is required with mild renal impairment or mild or moderate hepatic impairment. In moderate renal impairment, the dose would be reduced to 4 mg daily. For those with severe hepatic or renal impairment, silodosin is contraindicated.

Another class of medications used to treat BPH are the 5-alpha-reductase inhibitors, which include finasteride (Proscar) and dutasteride (Avodart). These medications block the conversion of testosterone to DHT by inhibiting the enzyme 5-alpha-reductase. DHT is primarily responsible for the enlargement of the prostate gland. The maximum reduction in prostate size (20% reduction) may take 6 months of therapy. However, improvement in symptoms is seen only in men with very enlarged prostates (greater than 40 g). Finasteride is well tolerated in most patients, but adverse effects include decreased ejaculate volume, reduced libido, and erectile dysfunction in 3% to 5% of all patients. The adverse effects may decrease with time, however, and are reversible with the cessation of treatment. Finasteride also decreases the PSA concentration by almost 50%, which can complicate prostate cancer detection. Dutasteride (a second generation 5-alpha-reductase inhibitor) produces a more rapid reduction in DHT. For example, dutasteride 0.5 mg daily for 2 weeks reduced serum DHT concentrations by 90% and resulted in significant improvement in symptoms after 3 to 13 months of treatment. The side effects of dutasteride were similar to those of finasteride, but decreased over time and were only slightly higher than in men receiving placebo.

There is some evidence that combination therapy of terazosin and finasteride is superior to single-medication therapy (either alpha blockers or 5-alpha-reductase inhibitors) in long-term but not in short-term treatment. If a patient has reached the maximum dose of the alpha blockers and symptoms continue to progress, finasteride can be added at that point to improve prostate size and symptoms.

Complementary therapies may also be used to treat BPH. Complementary Therapies 13.1 presents herbal therapies, along with vitamin and mineral therapies, that may be used in the treatment of the symptoms of BPH and other men's health problems.

Invasive and Surgical Management

Urological surgery is another treatment option for BPH and in fact is the second most common surgery in men (cataract surgery is the first). Prostate surgery is indicated when there is urinary retention or when other symptoms are intractable because of the prostatic obstruction, as gauged by the AUA index (that is, in patients with a score of greater than 8). Obstructive uropathy, recurrent and persistent urinary tract infections (UTIs) resulting from the prostatic obstruction, or recurrent gross hematuria caused by the enlarged prostate also are indications for surgical resection.

Transurethral resection of the prostate (TURP) is the surgical treatment of choice for a patient with BPH. Candidates for surgical intervention include patients with severe symptoms, high PVRs, complications, upper urinary tract changes, and those who fail medical therapy. TURP is performed through a cystoscope, using a diathermy loop for resection of prostatic tissue. It usually is performed under spinal or general anesthesia, with a urethral catheter maintained in place for 36 to 48 hours postoperatively. Some patients may also need to be discharged from the hospital with a urinary catheter in place

Complementary Therapies 13.1 Benign Prostatic Hyperplasia			
Problem	Therapy	Dosage	Comments
BPH	Saw palmetto (*Serenoa serrulata sabal*)	60 mg 2 times daily	Saw palmetto inhibits 5-α-reductase activity and mimics the effects of finasteride (Proscar).
Urinary infection (cystitis, urethritis)	Cranberry	500 mg 2 times daily	(Level II; Vidlar et al, 2010)

for up to 2 weeks after surgery. Symptomatic improvement following a TURP occurs in 90% of the patients. Flow-stream rates are increased as much as 15 mL/sec. Unfortunately, a complication of TURP can be retrograde ejaculation, occurring in 65% of patients; another potential complication is erectile dysfunction, which occurs in up to 15% of patients. Less frequent problems include bleeding, UTI, and urethral stricture.

A transurethral incision of the prostate (TUIP) is limited to patients with moderate to severe symptoms and a small prostate who have an elevated bladder neck or posterior commissure hyperplasia. In this procedure, an instrument is passed through the urethra to make one or two cuts in the prostate and the prostate capsule, reducing urethral stricture. This procedure can be performed on an outpatient basis or during a 24-hour stay; TUIP has a lower complication rate than TURP.

Open prostatectomy is a surgical option reserved for prostate glands weighing more than 40 to 100 g. An open prostatectomy is the surgical removal of the inner portion of the prostate via a suprapubic or retropubic incision in the abdominal area. This procedure requires longer hospitalizations than the other two options and has far more complications. Nonetheless, this may be the only alternative for a patient who has failed medical treatment or when a carcinoma of the prostate is suspected.

Robotic simple prostatectomy is now being used with increasing frequency for the treatment of BPH. It is used for patients with very large prostates. During the procedure, the inner part of the prostate that is causing the obstruction is removed. This is a substitute for open prostatectomy and has drastically reduced blood loss, postoperative pain, and hospital length of stay. Although robotic prostatectomy has better outcomes with regard to sexual and urinary functioning than the open prostatectomy, most patients will experience some sexual dysfunction and urinary incontinence.

There are several minimally invasive procedures for BPH. Transurethral laser–induced prostatectomy (TULIP) is a type of coagulation necrosis and is done under transrectal ultrasound guidance. Other types of laser surgery (coagulation necrosis) are performed under direct visualization. In laser procedures, the ablated tissue sloughed in 3 weeks to 3 months. The main advantage of laser surgery is that it is minimally invasive and can be done in the outpatient setting. There is also minimal blood loss, and the occurrence of retrograde ejaculation and erectile dysfunction is reduced. Also, this procedure can be performed in patients who are taking anticoagulants.

Another procedure is transurethral electrovaporization of the prostate. This seems to provide results equivalent to those of laser ablation. In transurethral electrovaporization of the prostate, a grooved roller-blade electrode administers diathermic energy to the prostate, vaporizing the prostatic tissue. The procedure provides a patient with improved urinary flow through the urethra. Because this is a recent innovation, long-term studies are not yet available.

Transurethral microwave thermotherapy (TUMT) is another procedure that results in the ablation of prostatic tissue. In TUMT, microwave energy is applied to the prostate through a microwave antenna in a urethral catheter; temperature monitoring of the rectum and urethra is essential. Prostate tissue is heated to 55°C, resulting in necrosis of the tissue, causing obstruction. Urethral cooling prevents urethral necrosis and limits postoperative irritative symptoms. One of the adverse effects of TUMT postoperatively is urinary retention, requiring catheterization. Although symptom score and urine flow rates are improved, long-term studies are needed to assess the efficacy.

In transurethral needle ablation (TUNA), two radiofrequency energy waves are administered to prostatic tissue via needle electrodes applied through a cystoscope. Temperatures up to 120°F (48.9°C) destroy the prostatic tissue that had caused the urinary retention or obstruction while preserving prostatic urethral mucosa.

Another means of thermal tissue ablation is the high-intensity focused ultrasound. A rectal probe delivers a short burst of high-intensity focused ultrasound energy that heats the prostate tissue, resulting in coagulative necrosis. Clinical trials are ongoing and demonstrate symptom improvement, but long-term efficacy is not known yet.

Stents have been placed cystoscopically and may be effective in relieving severe urinary obstruction or retention without further surgical intervention. Within 4 to 6 weeks after placement, the stents become covered in urothelium. Stent placement is reserved for patients who are poor surgical risks or who have a limited life expectancy. Stent placement is being used less since the development of minimally invasive procedures such as the TUNA and TULIP.

Transurethral (balloon) dilation of the prostate involves the insertion of a catheter with a balloon at the end through the urethra and into the prostatic urethra. The balloon is then inflated to stretch the urethra at the stricture where it has been narrowed. Although this treatment has been associated with fewer complications, dilation is less effective than other methods. It may provide only a temporary solution, with symptoms recurring within 2 years, and is rarely used today.

Follow-up and Referral

Patient monitoring includes the use of the AUA symptom index, which should be monitored every 1 to 6 months; urodynamic testing, which should be done every 3 to 6 months; and DRE and PSA, which should be done yearly. In addition to the yearly PSA, urodynamic studies should be done every 3 to 6 months to evaluate flow rates and voiding pressures. Any patient with BPH who is suspected to have prostatic carcinoma should be referred to a urologist.

Patient Education

It is extremely important to stress to the patient with BPH that taking over-the-counter medications containing alpha agonists or anticholinergic agents can cause acute urinary retention that can result in acute renal failure. These patients may require an indwelling urinary catheter until the acute urinary retention is resolved. The most common offending medications are various cold and flu preparations. Patients should also be advised to avoid bladder irritants such as coffee, spicy foods, and alcohol. Patients should be instructed to void at least every 2 hours to help reduce the possibility of UTI.

■ ERECTILE DYSFUNCTION

Erectile dysfunction (ED), sometimes referred to as impotence, is the failure to consistently maintain a sufficiently rigid erect penis to allow for sexual intercourse and is considered a facet of male sexual dysfunction. ED can also manifest as a lack of sexual desire or inability to ejaculate. ED can result from many causes, including physiological, psychological, endocrine, vascular, and neurological.

The Iceberg of Erectile Dysfunction

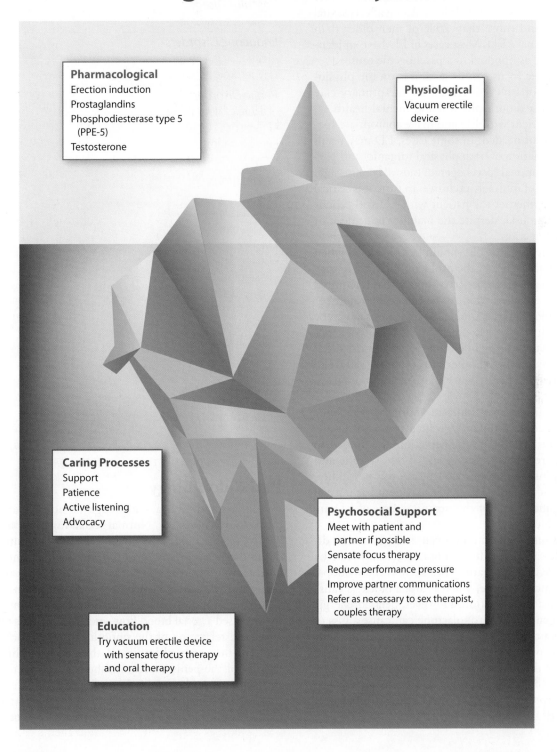

Epidemiology and Causes

ED is classified as mild if the patient fails to achieve a satisfactory erection in 2 out of 10 attempts. If all attempts at satisfactory erection fail, the ED is classed as severe. Moderate ED is somewhere in between mild and severe. It is difficult to estimate the number of men with ED because the definition is broad and some men may be reluctant to seek medical attention for the problem. Transient and limited episodes of impotence occur in about half of all adult men at one time or another in their lives and are not pathological. In the United States, between 15 and 30 million men are believed to suffer from ED at some time in their lives. Aging affects sexual functioning, and more than 25% of men older than 65 years of age have ED. Most cases of ED have an identifiable organic as opposed to a psychogenic cause.

Although the focus of this section is on the physiological causes of ED, it is critical for the primary-care clinician to assess both physical and mental health aspects in the patient with ED and make appropriate specialist referrals if needed. In some cases, ED may result from a combination of both physical (organic) and psychological/emotional (psychogenic) causes, because such etiologies are not mutually exclusive. In turn, it is critical to determine whether the patient with ED still experiences sexual arousal, despite the inability to achieve or maintain an erection.

Several categories of ED should be considered when determining the cause of the problem. First, there may be a failure to generate the nerve impulse that is required to initiate an erection. This can be caused by a number of endocrinological or neurological conditions or can be psychogenic in origin. ED can also be the result of a failure to adequately fill penile blood vessels, most often arteriogenic in origin. Another category is the failure to retain blood in the penis, which is usually veno-occlusive in origin.

A loss of libido may indicate androgen deficiency arising from either pituitary or testicular disease, resulting in a failure to initiate the nerve impulse needed to initiate an erection. Plasma levels of testosterone and gonadotropins are measured to rule out this possibility. Endocrine factors are unlikely if the patient has normal semen volume. Some of the organic causes of ED are listed in Table 13.1.

Medications are a common cause of ED, either directly or by adverse effects. Loss of erection can be caused by central sympatholytics such as methyldopa, clonidine, and reserpine, whereas alpha blockers cause few problems with erection. However, beta-adrenergic blocking agents and spironolactone can cause a loss of libido. Certain drugs, such as calcium channel blockers, can increase prolactin secretion and thereby cause ED. Some of the drugs of addiction can lower testosterone levels and lead to ED. In addition, zinc deficiency seen in malabsorption or malnourishment syndromes may also cause ED.

Table 13.1	Organic Causes of Erectile Dysfunction

Neurological Diseases
- Anterior temporal lobe lesions
- Disease of the spinal cord
- Loss of sensory input (secondary to diabetes mellitus, polyneuropathies), tabes dorsales (disease of dorsal root ganglia)
- Disease of nervi erigentes (secondary to complete prostatectomy, retrosigmoid operations, aortic bypass)

Vascular Disease
- Leriche syndrome

Endocrine Disorders
- Testicular failure (primary or secondary)
- Hyperprolactinemia

Penile Disorders
- Failure of detumescence
- Priapism
- Penile trauma
- Peyronie's disease

Medications
- Phenothiazines
- Thioridazine
- Imipramine
- Methyldopa
- Guanethidine
- Reserpine
- Spironolactone
- Alcohol
- Heroin
- Methadone
- Estrogen
- Beta blockers
- Antihypertensives
- Thiazide diuretics

Pathophysiology

To understand ED, a knowledge of normal erectile physiology is necessary. Normal sexual function in men has five phases: libido, erection, ejaculation, orgasm, and detumescence. For an erection to occur, there must be an intact autonomic and somatic nerve supply to the penis and the pudendal arteries. Erection begins with neurological and vascular stimulation and is maintained by increased arterial blood flow, increased venous resistance, and relaxation of the smooth muscle of the sinusoids in the corporal bodies of the penis. Additional rigidity of the penis is accomplished by contraction of the bulbocavernosus and ischiocavernosus muscles. The process is initiated by neurotransmitters, possibly nitric oxide, vasoactive intestinal peptide, acetylcholine, and prostaglandins, although the exact mechanism is unknown at this time.

In addition to the increase in arterial flow, the efflux of blood is reduced. As the erectile tissue expands, the peripheral veins are compressed against the enveloping tunica albuginea, which effectively impedes drainage of blood from the cavernous sinuses. The less turgid corpus spongiosum allows the urethra to dilate during ejaculation.

With continued sexual stimulation, the urethral meatus dilates and sperm move to the ejaculatory duct. Seminal fluid is added to the sperm cells by the seminal vesicles and prostate gland. At the time of vaginal penetration, the male secretions produced by the bulbourethral glands and the glands of the penile urethra combine with the female cervical secretions. The sperm cells move by emission into the prostatic urethra, where they become activated by seminal fluid and are motile. In the male, orgasm is concomitant with ejaculation, which is brought about by sympathetic activity transmitted along the hypogastric nerve and lateral pelvic plexus, and then through the prostatic and cavernous plexuses. Ejaculation is the strong rhythmic contraction of the vas deferens, seminal vesicles, epididymis, prostate, urethra, and penis. Retrograde ejaculation is prevented by partial bladder neck closure, mediated by sympathetic nerves. Orgasm is a sensory phenomenon in which the rhythmic contractions of the muscle are perceived as pleasurable.

Postcoital resolution, or detumescence, results from the sympathetic outflow to the genital areas; the periarterial muscle increases its tone, thereby reducing the flow to the erectile tissues of the penis. A refractory period of variable duration follows.

An understanding of vascular disease as a cause of ED is essential because continual high blood flow into the vascular system of the penis is necessary to maintain an erect state. Atherosclerosis can cause failure to fill; therefore, risk factors for this type of ED are heart disease, cigarette smoking, diabetes mellitus, aging, dyslipidemia, and hypertension. Trauma can also damage the pudendal and cavernous arteries, for example, from prolonged bicycling, and cause failure to fill. Leriche's syndrome, with impedance of the blood flow into the penis, occurs as the result of obstruction of the distal aorta at the bifurcation of the common iliac arteries. Presenting symptoms of this syndrome are claudication and ED, either separately or in combination.

Because resistance to the efflux of blood from the penis is necessary to maintain an erection, anything that impairs this ability is considered as a failure-to-store defect. It can result from insufficient relaxation or fibrosis of the corporeal smooth muscle. Adrenergic agonists and/or psychological stress can cause insufficient relaxation of the corporeal smooth muscle, whereas atherosclerosis and penile trauma can result in fibrosis. *Priapism,* persistent painful erection, is usually idiopathic but can be associated with sickle cell anemia, chronic granulocytic leukemia, or spinal cord injury. The persistent erection disrupts this vascular network and can lead to fibrosis and subsequent failure to store.

In addition to the inability to achieve or maintain an erection, ED may also involve abnormal functioning of several other sexual processes. Premature ejaculation seldom has an organic cause. It is usually related to anxiety about the sexual situation, performance-related fears, or an emotional disorder. Psychological disorders such as depression, bipolar disorder, anxiety disorders, and relationship dysfunction may all cause ED.

The absence of emission may be caused by three organic disorders: retrograde ejaculation, sympathetic denervation, or androgen deficiency. Retrograde ejaculation may occur after surgery on the bladder neck, or it may develop spontaneously in a male patient with diabetes. A postcoital urine sample can be analyzed to confirm the diagnosis. Smooth muscle contractions may not occur at the time of ejaculation as a result of the loss of the autonomic innervation of the prostate and seminal vesicles after sympathectomy. An androgen deficiency may lead to absence of secretions from the prostate and seminal vesicles. If libido and erectile function are normal, the absence of orgasm is almost always due to a psychiatric disorder.

Various penile diseases and anatomical abnormalities may also cause ED. Structural causes of ED include microphallus, Peyronie's disease, scarring of the corpora cavernosa, phimosis, hypospadias, and postsurgical sequelae. Peyronie's disease results from localized fibrotic thickening of the tissue around the corpora cavernosa. Plaque may be palpated along the penile shaft, usually on the dorsum, but plaque is sometimes present on any part of the corpora cavernosa. Inelasticity produces a curvature of the penile shaft on erection that may be very painful. There is a high correlation between Peyronie's disease and Dupuytren's contracture of the palmar fascia.

Clinical Presentation
Subjective
Because male sexual dysfunction can manifest in many ways and because the causes are numerous, a careful history is essential for the correct diagnosis and subsequent treatment. Impotence is a very personal complaint, and discussion requires a trusting relationship between patient and clinician and sufficient time during the visit for the patient to voice his concerns. He may complain of a loss of desire, an inability to obtain or maintain erection, premature ejaculation, or an absence of emission or inability to achieve orgasm. Frequently, the patient has a combination of these symptoms. It is essential to determine whether or not the patient has normal erections, most likely during sleep or early in the morning. If an erection does occur, an organic cause is most likely not the cause of the ED. In 25% of cases, medication use may be the cause of ED. The use of alcohol, tobacco, and recreational drugs increases the risk of sexual dysfunction.

Objective

A physical exam, including a thorough genital exam to rule out any abnormalities of the penis itself, is done. The testes should be palpated for size or abnormal masses. If the length is less than 4 cm, hypogonadism should be considered. Evidence of feminization such as gynecomastia and abnormal body hair distribution should be assessed. All pulses should be palpated, including the penile pulse, which can be felt by pressing both corpora between the thumb and forefinger and palpating to either side of the midline. If there is an indication of a vascular etiology from either the patient's history or physical exam, an aortogram may be indicated.

A neurological exam to evaluate the erectile reflex, including anal sphincter tone, perineal sensation, and the bulbocavernosus reflex, should be part of the physical exam. The reflex can be evaluated by squeezing the glans penis and noting the degree of anal sphincter constriction. An examination for signs of peripheral neuropathy, including distal muscle weakness and loss of tendon reflexes in the legs, is important, along with tests that will reveal any impairment of vibratory, position, tactile, and pain sensation.

Diagnostic Reasoning

Diagnostic Tests

Initially, laboratory tests that rule out causes of ED should be done. These tests include a fasting blood sugar to rule out diabetes mellitus, lipid profile to rule out dyslipidemia, thyroid-stimulating hormone (TSH), and a testosterone level. If the testosterone level is below 300 ng/dL, a serum prolactin level is warranted. Laboratory tests for patients with established ED should include a complete blood count, a blood chemistry profile (including fasting glucose or glycosylated hemoglobin levels), a TSH level, and a PSA in men as young as 40 years if they have a family history of prostate cancer. Most men older than age 55 years will have some abnormal laboratory findings or risk factors, but these may not necessarily be the cause of the ED. Several specialized tests can be done but usually only if the cause of the ED is not apparent from the more standard tests. The most useful of these tests is the nocturnal penile tumescence and rigidity (NPTR) test and color Doppler sonography of the penis.

NPTR testing is useful to assess the patient's physical ability to achieve an erection. Sensors are placed at the base and tip of the penis and record the circumference and rigidity of the penis during sleep. Typically, the test is done from one to three nights. Men usually have erections during rapid eye movement (REM) sleep. A physiological cause of ED is indicated if there is an absence or impairment of erections during sleep. This test is self-administered in the patient's home; however, it can be used in the clinical setting to determine erectile response to sexual stimuli.

There are, however, two medical conditions that cause ED in sexual situations yet still allow normal erectile activity during NPTR. The first is disruption of the afferent nerves that amplify the erectile response to external sexual stimuli but are bypassed in the nocturnal erectile activity. The second is called *pelvic steal syndrome,* which may occur in physiological states when the patient is awake, but not when he is asleep. This condition involves partial blockage of the iliac vessels and causes all erections to occur when the patient is at rest. Loss of erection ensues, however, with gluteal muscle activity during thrusting.

Color Doppler sonography is being used to assess vascular causes of ED. It measures the integrity of arterial influx in the cavernous artery during erection by measuring the peak systolic velocity in this artery.

Differential Diagnosis

Differential diagnosis of ED requires consideration of fibrosis secondary to trauma, severe urethritis, late-stage syphilitic lesions, penile infiltration with lymphogranuloma venereum, benign and malignant tumors, and congenital curvature. Urethral strictures produce an indurated area that may be identified by careful palpation along the penile urethra. A stricture can be identified more easily by the passage of a small urethral probe or catheter (urethral sound). Occasionally, strictures may be recognized by the presence of an indolent, firm, tender mass that may even involve the skin over the penile shaft. Restricted erections may cause ventral curvature of the penis, periurethral inflammations, and, at times, a purulent urethrocutaneous fistula.

Management

A number of options are available for the treatment of ED. If an organic cause cannot be found, these men will most likely benefit from behaviorally based sex therapy. Pharmacological treatments including hormone replacement are presented in Drugs Commonly Prescribed 13.1. Nonpharmacological interventions including vacuum constriction devices, vasoactive therapy, penile prostheses, and penile revascularization are discussed in the sections that follow.

Hormone Replacement

For men with documented testosterone deficiency who do not have prostate cancer, testosterone replacement is the treatment of choice. Testosterone replacement can be accomplished by several delivery methods that include injections, oral medication, topical patches, or topical gels.

Vacuum Constriction Devices

Most vacuum devices work in similar ways, using a process that takes about 2 minutes. The patient inserts his penis into the cylinder, then uses the pump to create a partial vacuum. This causes venous blood to enter the corpora cavernosa, initiating tumescence and rigidity. Once a sufficient erection is achieved, a latex constriction ring is placed around the base of the penis to help maintain the erection. This is a noninvasive procedure and complications are rare. Vacuum constriction devices are now available over the counter and cost between $300 and $500.

Vasoactive Therapy

The development of drugs that decrease the breakdown of 5-cyclic guanosine monophosphate (cGMP) has revolutionized ED treatment. cGMP is the intracellular second messenger of nitric oxide, which is the primary vasodilator and neurotransmitter involved in the erectile response. The first of these drugs was sildenafil citrate (Viagra). Sildenafil is an orally active cGMP-specific phosphodiesterase inhibitor. It results in an increased blood flow necessary for successful penile erection. The standard dose is sildenafil 50 mg taken orally at least 1 hour before sexual activity. Contraindications that can cause severe hypotensive effects are listed in Drugs Commonly Prescribed 13.1. Other medications in this class are vardenafil (Levitra), avanafil (Stendra), and tadalafil (Cialis). Phosphodiesterase-5 inhibitors do not affect libido and do not initiate an erection without sexual stimulation.

Vasoactive prostaglandins have been shown to be an effective treatment for ED. Alprostadil (Caverject) 5 to 40 mcg is injected directly into the base and lateral aspect of the penis using a tuberculin syringe. Erection occurs within 20 minutes and lasts for approximately 30 to 60 minutes. Prolonged erection (priapism) occurs rarely, but the patient should be instructed to seek medical attention if this does occur. Alprostadil is also available in a transurethral suppository in dosages of 125, 250, 500, or 1,000 mcg. Results have been good, with the suppositories producing an erection in about 5 to 10 minutes (see Drugs Commonly Prescribed 13.1 for instructions for use).

Penile Prostheses

Several prosthetic devices that can be surgically implanted into the penis are available in a variety of sizes and diameters. They are placed directly in the corporal bodies. Penile prostheses may be rigid, semifirm, hinged, or inflatable. The inflatable devices are more natural appearing; however, there is more opportunity for mechanical failure. Implantation of a prosthesis, which is a highly reliable but invasive form of therapy, may help men who have failed therapy with other methods; it is very expensive, however, ranging in cost from $9,000 to $20,000. Implantation may be covered by some insurance plans. Most patients desiring implants prefer spontaneity and therefore choose this invasive treatment. Significant problems associated with implants are infection, erosion, and occasional mechanical failure (in fewer than 5% of patients). The most common types of implants are nonhydraulic (using semirigid rods) and hydraulic (using inflatables). Both types of implants involve surgical placement of two cylinders inside the corpus cavernosum. Healing takes 4 to 6 weeks, after which the patient may have intercourse.

Penile Revascularization

The experience with penile revascularization is limited, and some patients fail to have a sufficient erection even after the procedure. Patients with arterial disorders may be candidates for the various procedures, which include endarterectomy and balloon dilation, or arterial bypass. For patients with venous disorders, ligation of the deep dorsal vein or emissary vein or ligation of the crura of the corpora cavernosus may be somewhat effective.

In younger men, several conditions may warrant penile revascularization surgery. Men younger than age 45 whose impotence is caused by severe pelvic trauma are the best candidates for this surgery. In patients with impotence of sudden onset, the possibility that trauma to the peritoneum or pelvis may have led to vascular injury should be considered. A congenital shunt should be ruled out in any patient who reports that he has never had a full erection.

Follow-up and Referral

Hormonal replacement therapies should be guided by a clinician experienced in the evaluation and monitoring of patients on hormonal replacement. For example, patients on testosterone replacement therapy should undergo monitoring prostate examinations and PSA screening tests, given the theoretical risks of BPH and prostate cancer associated with testosterone exposure. Blood levels of the hormone being supplemented (e.g., serum testosterone) and other regulatory hormones along the hypothalamic-pituitary-gonadal axis (e.g., luteinizing hormone, which stimulates testosterone secretion) should also be followed to prevent the risks of medication overexposure. However, interpretation of these levels requires expert knowledge of reproductive endocrinology and is influenced by both the timing of the hormonal treatments and the monitoring of blood draws.

Common psychogenic causes of ED include performance anxiety and relationship problems. Thus, referrals to sex therapy and/or marriage and couples counseling may be particularly helpful for some patients, especially in combination with other therapies. In addition, all of the invasive surgical interventions described above require appropriate referrals to a qualified urologist or pelvic surgeon.

Patient Education

The primary role of the provider in educating the patient with ED is to stress the importance of management of chronic conditions such as hypertension, diabetes mellitus, and stress. Guided imagery, regular exercise, and yoga may be recommended as a modality to reduce stress. Tight control of blood pressure and blood sugar should be encouraged as a way to limit further deterioration of erectile function. In addition, counseling for the psychogenic causes of ED is essential. Instructions regarding topical hormone replacement formulations should include warnings regarding the possibility of transfer to sexual partners during intimate contact, as well as the general risk to women and children from unintended exposure to medications affecting the hormonal axis.

PROSTATITIS

Prostatitis is one of several inflammatory and/or painful conditions affecting the prostate gland. Prostatitis accounts for about 25% of all office visits by men. Fifty percent of men will experience prostatitis in their lifetime. The classification of the type of prostatitis is important for both diagnostic and treatment purposes. Patients may present with acute bacterial prostatitis, chronic bacterial prostatitis, nonbacterial prostatitis, or prostatodynia (see Chronic Pelvic Pain Syndrome later in this chapter). Chronic nonbacterial prostatitis is the most common type; it is eight times more frequent than bacterial prostatitis.

In an effort to standardize this classification schema, the National Institutes of Health suggested that nonbacterial prostatitis and prostatodynia be grouped together as chronic prostatitis/chronic pelvic pain syndrome, which may be inflammatory or noninflammatory in nature. In addition, a final category of asymptomatic inflammatory prostatitis is used to denote persons with a significant inflammatory infiltrate in prostatic secretions but without overt pain or difficulty with urination.

Epidemiology and Causes

Acute bacterial prostatitis is always associated with a urinary tract infection (UTI) and has a characteristically abrupt onset. Chronic bacterial prostatitis is a major cause of recurrent bacteriuria. Nonbacterial prostatitis has findings similar to those associated with chronic bacterial prostatitis, but no evidence of bacterial infection will be present in a urine culture. Prostatodynia presents with signs and symptoms of prostatitis but without evidence of inflammation. Prostatitis occurs predominantly in sexually active men aged 30 to 50 years. Chronic bacterial prostatitis is more common in patients older than 50 years old. Athletes who run long distances—including cross-country runners and athletes who have vigorous exercise regimens—may be predisposed to prostatitis, although the etiology is not well documented at present.

Acute and chronic bacterial prostatitis are both caused by an infection that originates from the ascending urethral flexion or from the reflux of urine into the prostatic ducts. Infection may also spread directly to the prostatic ducts from the rectum. Infection may spread via the lymphatic system or bloodstream, with prostatic calculi serving as a nidus for infection. The most common aerobic gram-negative bacteria involved in prostatitis include *Klebsiella, Pseudomonas, Enterobacter, Escherichia coli, Proteus mirabilis,* and *Neisseria gonorrhoeae.* The causative gram-positive bacteria are *Streptococcus faecalis* and *Staphylococcus aureus.* Some organisms suspected but as yet unproven are *Staphylococcus epidermidis, Micrococcus,* non–group D *Streptococcus,* and diphtheroids. Rarely, fungi and *Mycobacteria tuberculosis* have been implicated in chronic prostatitis. The cause of nonbacterial prostatitis is currently under scrutiny;

however, *Ureaplasma, Trichomonas vaginalis,* and *Chlamydia trachomatis* may be involved. Risk factors for prostatitis are age (older than age 50 years), history of prostatic calculi, and history of a previously diagnosed UTI. Chronic prostatitis, in particular, is associated with a history of recurrent UTI, presumably due to repeated seeding of the urinary tract by the infected prostate.

Pathophysiology

The infectious processes resulting in acute or chronic bacterial prostatitis are a result of the organisms mentioned previously. Purulent prostatic discharge may or may not be evident in the absence of prostatic massage. Among patients who fall into the chronic prostatitis/chronic pelvic pain category, prostatic massage will effectively double the number of cases that are considered inflammatory, due to the presence of white blood cells (WBCs) in postmassage urine or seminal fluid.

The pathophysiology of nonbacterial prostatitis is less clear, but it may be related to a voiding dysfunction such as spasm of the bladder neck or urethra. The cause of prostatodynia is unclear, although it may be related to internal urethral sphincter problems or to abnormal tension of the pelvic floor musculature. Prostatodynia is also related to stress, anxiety, and depression.

Clinical Presentation

Subjective

The patient may present complaining of *tenesmus* (a spasmodic contraction of the anal sphincter), with pain and a persistent desire to empty the bowel or bladder accompanied by involuntary, ineffective straining efforts. Focus on History 13.2 presents common signs and symptoms of the different types of prostatitis. Obstructive symptoms, including weak urine stream, incomplete bladder emptying, and terminal dribbling, are common in both acute bacterial prostatitis and prostatodynia. Irritative symptoms are present in all of the classifications but are more common in chronic bacterial prostatitis and prostatodynia. In addition, the patient with prostatodynia typically does not have a history of recurrent UTIs.

Objective

The practitioner should assess the patient for the signs and symptoms listed in Focus on History 13.2. The rectal exam should be performed with care, because vigorous manipulation of the prostate can result in septicemia. In chronic prostatitis, the rectal exam may reveal a tender prostate, but it is usually not swollen or boggy.

Diagnostic Reasoning

Diagnostic Tests

A complete blood count will show leukocytosis and a shift to the left if the patient has acute bacterial prostatitis. A urinalysis is done to check for bacteriuria, which if found indicates the need for a fractional urine examination. In

Focus on History 13.2   Signs and Symptoms of Prostatitis

Type of Prostatitis	Common Signs and Symptoms
Acute bacterial prostatitis	General complaints: Fever, chills, low back pain; malaise, arthralgia, myalgia Urinary complaints: Frequency, urgency, dysuria, nocturia, bladder-outlet obstruction Physical exam: Warm, tense, boggy, very tender prostate
Chronic bacterial prostatitis	General complaints: Symptoms often absent, perineal pain, low back pain, lower abdominal pain, scrotal pain, penile pain, pain on ejaculation Urinary complaints: Dysuria, irritative voiding Physical exam: Normal, boggy, or focally indurated prostate
Nonbacterial prostatitis	Similar to chronic bacterial prostatitis Physical exam: Prostate tender on palpation
Prostatodynia	General complaints: Pelvic pain Urinary complaints: Irritative voiding, abnormal flow

this test, the first 10 mL of urine in a void (VB_1), 10 mL from midstream (VB_2), expressed prostatic secretions (EPS) obtained by prostate massage, and 10 mL of urine following massage (VB_3) are obtained, cultured, and microscopically examined. If VB_1 shows the highest number of WBCs and colonies on culture, urethritis is diagnosed. If VB_2 is highest, cystitis is probable. If EPS and/or VB_3 is highest, chronic bacterial prostatitis is confirmed. Some clinicians feel that vigorous prostatic massage can lead to bacteremia; therefore, the use of this test is left up to the individual clinician's discretion. Because this test is cumbersome to perform and studies have shown that prescribing patterns do not differ substantially between clinicians who do or do not perform this test, it is not necessarily done. A urine sample from a patient with nonbacterial prostatitis will show the presence of WBCs, but the urine culture will be negative. There are no abnormal laboratory findings associated with prostatodynia.

If a malignancy or abscess is suspected, computed tomography scanning or transrectal ultrasonography is indicated. A needle biopsy of the mass or aspiration of the abscess for culture may be done by the urologist.

Differential Diagnosis

The differential diagnosis for prostatitis includes cystitis, urethritis, pyelonephritis, epididymitis, prostatic abscess, malignancy, obstructive calculi, foreign bodies, and

acute urinary retention. Abscess is more common in men who are HIV positive. The manifestations of acute prostatitis can mimic those of acute diverticulitis, but history and laboratory tests usually differentiate between the two conditions. In the case of nonbacterial chronic prostatitis or chronic pelvic pain syndrome, the diagnosis is one of exclusion; other sources of perineal pain (hernias, testicular masses, and hemorrhoids) should be ruled out first. Asymptomatic inflammatory prostatitis is not yet fully understood, and guidelines as to its natural history and need for treatment are not yet established.

Management

The main principle of management for prostatitis is to treat the patient on an outpatient basis if he does not have a fever. Hospitalization may be necessary if the patient is toxic, is immunocompromised, has a proven or suspected abscess, or has signs of urosepsis.

An extremely ill patient with bacterial prostatitis should be treated in the hospital with ciprofloxacin (Cipro) 200 to 400 mg IV every 12 hours until he has been afebrile for 24 to 48 hours, then oral ciprofloxacin 500 mg PO every 12 hours or levofloxacin (Levaquin) 500 mg PO daily is used to complete 6 total weeks of treatment.

Men with bacterial prostatitis may be treated on an outpatient basis for 4 to 6 weeks with antibiotics such as ofloxacin (Floxin) 400 mg PO every 12 hours, ciprofloxacin 500 mg PO every 12 hours, or norfloxacin 400 mg PO every 12 hours. Alternatives to the quinolones are trimethoprim and sulfamethoxazole (TMP-SMX [160 mg/800 mg]: Bactrim, Septra, Cotrim) one double-strength (DS) tablet every 12 hours, or doxycycline (AK-Ramycin, AK-Ratabs, Doryx, Doxy-Caps, Doxychel Hyclate, Doxy-Lemmon, Vibramycin, Vibra-Tabs) 100 mg every 12 hours.

It is extremely important that the patient with acute bacterial prostatitis be kept well hydrated. IV fluids must be given if the patient is hospitalized and is unable to consume liquids orally. Urethral catheterization is contraindicated in patients with acute bacterial prostatitis, and percutaneous suprapubic catheterization is required if urinary retention develops.

The best cure rates in chronic bacterial prostatitis are associated with treatment with TMP-SMX, although other antibiotics such as carbenicillin, erythromycin, cephalexin, and the quinolones are effective as well. The patient with chronic infection is usually treated for 6 to 12 weeks.

The etiology of nonbacterial prostatitis is uncertain, but the patient may benefit from erythromycin 250 mg four times daily, TMP-SMX DS one tablet daily, or in combination with a fluoroquinolone. Other patients with nonbacterial prostatitis have responded to treatment with nitrofurantoin (Furadantin, Furalan, Furanite, Macrodantin, Nitrofan, Nitrofurantoin), 100 mg daily.

The irritative voiding symptoms associated with nonbacterial prostatitis may be treated with NSAIDs, muscle relaxants, anticholinergics, warm sitz baths, normal sexual activity, and regular mild exercise. Avoidance of spicy foods, caffeine, and alcohol may help some patients alleviate the irritative voiding symptoms. For patients with severe urinary retention, insertion of a suprapubic catheter may be necessary. Surgical resection for intractable chronic disease or to drain an abscess may also be performed.

Follow-up and Referral

Depending on the acute nature of the illness and the patient's response to treatment, referral to a urologist may be warranted. The patient with hematuria or significantly elevated prostate-specific antigen should prompt immediate urological referral. Patient monitoring for acute bacterial prostatitis should include a follow-up urinalysis and culture 30 days after beginning treatment. Chronic bacterial prostatitis requires urinalysis and culture every 30 days. Monitoring should continue until the patient no longer shows signs of infection. Suppression therapy with prophylactic antibiotics has also been tried if recurrent symptomatic infections occur.

Patient Education

The patient should be told that the prognosis for recovery from prostatitis is good, with a 55% to 97% cure rate. The cure rate depends on the population and the medications used. Prostatitis can, however, be difficult to cure and can last for a prolonged time. The National Kidney and Urologic Diseases Information Clearinghouse has printed information available for patient education.

■ CHRONIC PELVIC PAIN SYNDROME

As discussed in the section on prostatitis, the term *prostatodynia* is often used as a designation for unexplained chronic pelvic pain in men, which may be mistaken for inflammatory prostatitis. However, the nomenclature and conceptualization of prostatodynia has been expanded in modern clinical practice into a broader disorder called chronic pelvic pain syndrome (CPPS). This is considered predominantly a noninflammatory disorder that has many causes, including voiding dysfunction and pelvic floor dysfunction, but the prostate is normal.

Epidemiology and Causes

The term *prostatodynia* is not considered accurate nomenclature for CPPS, because it suggests that the condition stems from the prostate itself, despite the term being used historically to describe nonspecific groin pain of unclear etiology. No unifying cause of CPPS is known. CPPS affects mostly young and middle-aged men and is characterized by pain in the groin that may extend to the genitalia and perineum.

Pathophysiology

CPPS is considered by some clinicians to be equivalent to chronic nonbacterial prostatitis, although several lines of evidence point to nonprostatic causes. It may be considered an umbrella disorder of male patients with an array of chronic pelvic symptoms, consisting predominantly of groin pain that relates largely to anatomical structures in proximity to the prostate gland. Importantly, the symptoms of CPPS have no adequate treatment, cure, or objective explanation, although the disorder appears to relate to a combination of dysfunctional immune, endocrine, neurological, and psychological factors.

Clinical Presentation
Subjective

CPPS is often mistaken for chronic prostatitis because many of the symptoms and signs of these disorders are the same. The patient with prostatodynia may present with low back and perineal pain, urinary hesitancy, and interruption of urine flow. Unlike in chronic prostatitis, there is no history of urinary tract infections with CPPS.

Objective

On physical exam (including digital rectal exam), the prostate is normal, but there may be increased anal sphincter tone and periprostatic tenderness. The primary value of physical assessment is in ruling out identifiable diagnoses, such as prostatitis, urethritis, and prostate cancer.

Diagnostic Reasoning
Diagnostic Tests

There are no tests that specifically diagnose CPPS. Elevated prostate-specific antigen is not typically associated with classic prostatodynia and is more consistent with prostatitis. Urinalysis is normal without bacteriuria or pyuria, as are expressed prostatic secretions in most patients. Of note, some patients with CPPS have evidence of white blood cells (WBCs) in prostatic secretions, suggesting an inflammatory component, although this finding is not classically associated with prostatodynia. Moreover, significantly elevated WBCs in prostatic secretions should trigger the suspicion of acute or chronic infectious prostatitis.

There may be detrusor contraction without urethral relaxation, high urethral pressures, and spasms of the urinary sphincter on urodynamic testing. However, these tests are not performed unless the patient has no response after a trial of alpha blockers or anticholinergic medication, as described under Management.

Differential Diagnosis

The differential diagnoses for prostatodynia include acute and chronic prostatitis and nonbacterial prostatitis. Because the urinalysis is normal, acute infection can be ruled out. The normal expressed prostatic secretions distinguish prostatodynia from nonbacterial prostatitis. Of note, however, some clinicians may diagnose CPPS in patients, despite evidence of an inflammatory component to their condition, as reflected by WBCs in expressed prostatic secretions, suggesting heterogeneity of the diagnosis.

Management

The patient with CPPS is usually treated with alpha blockers to reduce bladder neck and urethral spasms. The most commonly used drugs are terazosin (Hytrin) 1 to 10 mg PO daily, doxazosin (Cardura) 1 to 8 mg PO daily, and tamsulosin (Flomax) 0.4 to 0.8 mg PO daily. Some patients benefit from myofascial release therapy and warm sitz baths, whereas others may experience relief using the muscle relaxant diazepam and biofeedback to relieve tension myalgia associated with pelvic floor muscle dysfunction. Psychotherapy is appropriate if sexual dysfunction accompanies CPPS. Antibiotics have no established role, given that CPPS is not infectious in origin, yet patients may be inappropriately prescribed antibiotics for prolonged periods of time, given the lack of a clear etiology.

Follow-up and Referral

Given that CPPS should only be diagnosed after thorough evaluation that rules out chronic prostatitis and other identifiable causes for persistent symptoms, referral to a urological specialist may be required for patients with intransigent symptoms.

Patient Education

Several patient education resources are available for patients with CPPS, including the Chronic Prostatitis/Chronic Pelvic Pain Syndrome Network, the Prostatitis Foundation, and the International Association for the Study of Pain interest group on Pain of Urogenital Origin.

■ EPIDIDYMITIS

Epididymitis is an inflammation of the epididymis, the coiled structure connecting the sperm-producing rete testis to the vas deferens, allowing for maturation and immunosurveillance of the sperm. This inflammation results in scrotal pain, swelling, and induration of the posterior-lying epididymis, with eventual scrotal wall edema and involvement of the adjacent testicle, possibly with reactive hydrocele formation. The inflammation of the testicle results in a unilateral painful testicle known as *epididymo-orchitis.*

Epidemiology and Causes

There is a predisposition to epididymitis when the patient has a history of unprotected intercourse, a new sexual partner, a history of urinary tract infection (UTI) with dysuria, or urethral discharge. Symptoms may also occur following heavy lifting or straining. Younger sexually active men or older men with UTI are the patients who most commonly present with epididymitis. It may also (but rarely) occur in prepubertal boys, which likely heralds a structural abnormality in the genitourinary tract.

The causes of epididymitis in males younger than 35 years are usually sexually transmitted diseases (STDs) such as *Chlamydia* or *Neisseria gonorrhoeae* infections. There is usually a difference in the type of discharge.

Chlamydia infection produces a serous urethral discharge, whereas gonorrhea produces a purulent discharge.

Causes of epididymitis in men 35 years of age and older include coliform bacteria (such as *Escherichia coli,* which is most common) and sometimes *Pseudomonas aeruginosa* or *Staphylococcus aureus.* Epididymitis is often associated with a distal urinary tract obstruction in men older than 35 years or with coliform infections in men engaging in insertive anal intercourse. Tuberculous epididymitis will present with sterile pyuria and nodularity of the vas deferens, as well as pain. Another cause of epididymitis is sterile urinary reflux following transurethral prostatectomy. A granulomatous reaction following bacille Calmette-Guérin intravesical therapy for superficial bladder cancer may also cause epididymitis.

Rare causes of epididymitis include syphilis, brucellosis, blastomycosis, coccidioidomycosis, and cryptococcosis. When nonbacterial epididymitis and epididymo-orchitis occur, the cause is not clear, but may be secondary to retrograde extravasation of urine.

Pathophysiology

UTIs, particularly prostatitis, predispose a patient to the development of epididymitis. Other risk factors include transmission of pathogens via indwelling urethral catheters or urinary instrumentation, or as a consequence of transurethral prostate surgery. A urethral stricture of any type may also be a risk factor. Epididymitis caused by STDs is transmitted through the urethra and may be accompanied by symptomatic or asymptomatic urethritis.

Other causes include immunosuppression, trauma, or reflux of urine from the urethra through the vas deferens, causing chemical inflammation and edema within the epididymis that leads to ductal obstruction. Predisposing factors for subacute presentations of epididymitis in otherwise healthy postpubertal male patients include heavy physical activity, prolonged bicycle or motorcycle riding, and sexual activity. These patients may have negative urinalyses and often do not experience dysuria.

Clinical Presentation
Subjective

The major complaint of patients with epididymitis is scrotal pain that often radiates along the spermatic cord or to the flank. The pain may appear relatively acute over several hours. Many experience pain at the tip of the penis and complain of urethral discharge or other symptoms of UTI, such as frequency of urination, dysuria, cloudy urine, or hematuria. Initially, only the lowermost tail section of the posterior-lying epididymis will be painful, tender, and indurated. Elevation of the testes and the epididymis will relieve the discomfort. Fever and chills occur with a severe infection and an abscess formation.

Objective

Physical exam reveals scrotal swelling, and the testis may be indistinguishable from the epididymis. The scrotum wall will be thick and indurated, and a reactive hydrocele may occur. In addition to nodularity of the vas deferens and tenderness of the epididymis, patients with the non-sexually transmitted variety of epididymitis will have pyuria. Rectal exam reveals a tender prostate.

Diagnostic Reasoning
Diagnostic Tests
Initially, a urinalysis will show pyuria and leukocytosis. A Gram stain of the urethral discharge may reveal gram-negative intracellular diplococci that are diagnostic of *N gonorrhoeae*. Culture of the penile discharge may be consistent with *Chlamydia* or gonorrhea infection. If no organisms are visible on the urethral smear, but white blood cells (WBCs) are evident, the diagnosis is usually nongonococcal urethritis and *Chlamydia* is the most likely pathogen. A complete blood count shows increased WBCs with a left shift. Interstitial congestion and fibrotic scarring may be present. An ultrasound of the scrotum can confirm the diagnosis of epididymitis.

Differential Diagnosis
The differential diagnoses for epididymitis include epididymal congestion following a vasectomy, testicular torsion, torsion of the appendix testis, mumps, orchitis, testicular tumor, and testicular trauma. An epididymal cyst, spermatocele, hydrocele, or varicocele should also be ruled out as part of the differential diagnosis. In epididymitis, the pain often improves when the scrotum is elevated above the level of the pubic symphysis (Prehn's sign).

Management
Initial treatment includes bedrest with scrotal elevation and ice packs, along with appropriate antibiotics; in severe cases, a spermatic cord block with local anesthetics may be necessary to relieve the pain. In men younger than age 35 with sexually transmitted epididymitis, treatment is a one-time dose of ceftriaxone 250 mg IM in addition to doxycycline (Vibramycin), 100 mg PO two times daily for 10 days. If the patient is allergic to cephalosporins or tetracyclines, a fluoroquinolone such as ofloxacin 300 mg PO two times daily or levofloxacin 500 mg PO daily can be given for 10 days. It is important to treat the sexual partner as well. Patients with nonsexually transmitted forms of epididymitis may be treated with ciprofloxacin 750 mg PO two times daily, ofloxacin 200 to 300 mg PO two times daily, or TMP-SMX (Bactrim, Septra) one DS tablet PO two times daily for 2 to 3 weeks. For patients with noninfectious epididymitis, treatment is with NSAIDs, rest, and scrotal support. Antibiotic therapy is for patients who are refractory to conservative treatment. Tylenol with codeine may be used for moderate to severe pain. For the septic or toxic hospitalized patient, ceftriaxone (Rocephin), 1 to 2 g given IV or IM every 24 hours, is the preferred treatment. An aminoglycoside (gentamicin) 1 mg/kg IV or IM every 8 hours (adjusted to the patient's renal function after a loading dose of 2 mg/kg) may also be administered.

Surgical procedures may be needed, depending on the severity of the case. An aspiration of the hydrocele may assist in examination of the scrotal contents and relieve discomfort. A vasostomy to drain the infected material may be done as well. Scrotal exploration should be done if there is uncertainty in differentiating epididymitis from testicular torsion. Drainage of abscesses, epididymectomy, or orchiectomy may be considered in severe cases that do not respond to antibiotics. The activity of the patient after these procedures is limited to bedrest for a minimum of 1 to 2 days.

Follow-up and Referral
Patient monitoring with office visits should continue until there are no signs of infection. Early treatment of prostatitis may prevent the development of epididymitis. Vigorous rectal examination of patients experiencing acute prostatitis should be avoided because this can lead to epididymitis. The prognosis is good if epididymitis is treated promptly. Pain improves in 1 to 3 days, but induration may last several weeks and take several months to resolve completely.

Complications of epididymitis include infertility or decreased fertility, recurrent epididymitis, abscess formation, or Fournier's gangrene (necrotizing synergistic infection), all possible when treatment is delayed or inadequate. Patients with sensory neuropathy as a result of diabetes may have little pain despite severe infections or abscesses; older adult patients may also present without significant pain.

Patient Education
The patient is instructed to limit activity and immobilize the scrotal contents, which will relieve the pain and aid in treating the infection. The patient will need to wear an athletic supporter and avoid sexual contact and physical activity as long as pain persists. Patient education includes stressing the need to complete the full course of all antibiotics, even after the patient becomes asymptomatic.

■ TESTICULAR TORSION
Testicular torsion is the twisting or rotation of the testes, resulting in acute ischemia. It is a urological emergency. The torsion may vary from 90 degrees to 360 degrees about the spermatic cord. An even more common phenomenon is torsion of the testicular appendix or appendiceal torsion, in which a small vestigial remnant of the Müllerian duct located on the anterosuperior portion of the testis twists about its base.

The testis is approximately 4.5 cm × 3 cm × 2.7 cm. Within the scrotum, each testis is surrounded by the tunica albuginea, a tough layer of connective tissue, as well as the tunica vaginalis, which is a potential space formed by a membranous sac covering the anterior two-thirds of the testicle. A cryptorchid testis that fails to descend into the scrotal sac is most prone to undergoing torsion.

Epidemiology and Causes

Testicular torsion can occur at any age, from the newborn to age 80 years; however, two-thirds of the cases occur between 10 and 20 years, with the peak at age 14 years. Testicular torsion is possible but rare in older men. Torsion of the appendix testis is more common in children aged 7 to 14 years.

The contributing factors of testicular torsion are usually idiopathic and spontaneous. There is a history of trauma in 20% of the cases, with one-third of the patients having had prior episodic testicular pain. One initiating factor of torsion appears to be the contraction of the cremaster muscle, which may occur during sleep in approximately 50% of patients. The contraction of the cremaster muscle may also be stimulated by trauma, exercise (most frequently in runners), extreme cold (torsion is more common in winter months), and sexual stimulation. Paraplegics are also at high risk for developing testicular torsion, probably as a result of constant pressure while sitting. Other factors contributing to testicular torsion are possible alterations in testosterone levels and cremasteric contractions during the nocturnal sex response cycle or a congenital abnormality of the tunica vaginalis or the spermatic cord.

Pathophysiology

If the base of the testis is inadequately fixed to the tunica vaginalis via the gubernaculum, the testis may twist around the spermatic cord under several of the conditions listed above. Arterial inflow becomes compromised and venous outflow is obstructed, resulting in ischemia of the testis. This is exquisitely painful and may lead to necrosis if it is not treated on an emergency basis. Irreversible cellular damage may result in as little as 6 to 12 hours. Even if the testis is salvaged, fertility may be permanently compromised owing to a disruption of the blood–testis immunological barrier. This exposes germ cell antigens to the systemic circulation, resulting in sperm-specific antibodies that lead to permanent destruction of spermatozoa.

Clinical Presentation

Subjective

The most common symptom of testicular torsion is acute onset of pain accompanied by swelling. Torsion of the appendices of the testis also presents with pain, but it may be more gradual in onset. The patient may have pain for several days before seeking medical attention.

Objective

The most common clinical sign of testicular torsion is the absence of the cremasteric reflex. The testicle may also be high in the scrotum, with a transverse, rather than longitudinal, lie known as a "bell-clapper" deformity. Elevation of the testis does not relieve testicular pain, as is sometimes observed in epididymitis (Prehn's sign). However, this physical finding is insufficiently specific to distinguish between these two disorders. Occasionally with torsion of the appendices of the testis there may be a small lump that is palpable on the superior pole of the testis. If the skin is pulled tautly over it, the lump may appear blue ("blue dot sign"). This "blue dot" results from infarction and necrosis of the appendix testis and is present in about one-fifth of cases.

Diagnostic Reasoning

Diagnostic Tests

Testicular torsion is diagnosed by the history and presenting manifestations. The only initial assessment required is a physical exam. Color Doppler ultrasonography or radionuclide scanning can be used to diagnose both testicular torsion and appendiceal torsion. Doppler ultrasound can detect an absent or reduced pulse with torsion and an increased flow with an inflammatory process (Doppler ultrasound is reliable only in the first 12 hours following torsion). A radionuclide testicular scintigraphy with technetium 99-m (99m-Tc) pertechnetate will show absent or decreased vascularity in patients with torsion; increased vascularity will be evident in patients with inflammatory processes, including torsion of appendix testes.

Differential Diagnosis

Differential diagnoses for testicular torsion include epididymo-orchitis, an incarcerated or strangulated inguinal hernia, an acute hydrocele, a traumatic hematoma, an idiopathic scrotal edema, a torsion appendix testis, an acute varicocele, a testicular tumor, or Henoch-Schönlein purpura. Scrotal abscesses and leukemic infiltrates are also important considerations in the differential diagnosis and must be ruled out.

Some pathological findings associated with testicular torsion include venous thrombosis, tissue edema, necrosis, and arterial thrombosis.

Management

Compression of the testicular vessels leads to ischemic necrosis of the testes within 6 hours. Failure to recognize the torsion and intervene immediately results in the loss of the testicle in 80% of the cases, with subsequent atrophy of the testis in 10% or more. Fertile resolution occurs in only 10% of patients.

On diagnosis, immediate referral of the patient to the emergency department is indicated. Testicular torsion is a urological emergency. In the emergency department, manual reduction may be successful. Manual reduction of the testis is classically done with gentle external rotation of the testis toward the thigh, because most cases of torsion occur with medial rotation away from the thigh. However, retrospective studies have demonstrated lateral testicular torsion in up to one-third of cases. Relief of pain, resolution of the "bell-clapper" deformity, and a restoration of arterial blood flow are used as the primary indications of effective reduction of testicular torsion. Reduction is followed by surgical exploration. Any testis that is not clearly viable (and obvious) is removed. Surgical exploration via scrotal approach—with detorsion, evaluation of testicular viability, orchidopexy of the viable testicle, and orchidodectomy of the nonviable testicle—is the preferred surgical intervention.

For a patient with torsion of the appendix, testis surgery may also be performed, but recovery is quicker, just several days. Conservative medical treatment may be initiated with rest, ice, and NSAIDs, but recovery is much slower and pain may persist from weeks to months. The dead appendiceal tissue is usually reabsorbed, though, and fertility is preserved.

Follow-up and Referral

Testicular salvage is directly related to the duration of torsion; the salvage rate is 85% to 90% if torsion has persisted for less than 6 hours. The salvage rate becomes less than 10% if the duration of the torsion is greater than 24 hours. Depressed spermatogenesis occurs in 80% to 94% of individuals and may be related to the duration of ischemic injury.

Patient Education

As many as two-thirds of testes salvaged may atrophy in the first 2 to 3 years post-torsion. The possibility of testicular atrophy in a salvaged testis, with depressed sperm counts, necessitates patient education and understanding. Patients should be taught to seek immediate care when experiencing testicular pain, to prevent permanent sequelae.

■ HYDROCELE

A *hydrocele* is a collection of peritoneal fluid within the scrotum around the testes, between the parietal and visceral (adjacent to the testis) layers of the tunica vaginalis—the two-layered sac that surrounds the testis and spermatic cord. A hydrocele forms when secretion of fluid into this potential space outweighs its reabsorption. These collections may range from only a few milliliters of fluid to enormous volumes measured in liters.

Epidemiology and Causes

The incidence rate of hydrocele is about 1% in adult men. Most hydroceles occur in men older than age 40 years. Causes of an acute hydrocele include nonspecific acute epididymitis, tuberculous epididymitis, trauma to the testes, tumor of the testes, or sequelae as complications of radiation therapy. Exstrophy of the bladder may increase the risk for hydrocele formation. Patients with Ehlers-Danlos syndrome have an increased risk for hydrocele, as do patients with a ventricular peritoneal shunt for dialysis or peritoneal dialysis.

Pathophysiology

A basic knowledge of scrotal anatomy is required to understand the pathogenesis of a hydrocele. The processus

vaginalis originates as a diverticulum of the peritoneal sac that lines the abdomen, just inferior to the testis. During development, as the testis descends into the scrotum, it brings this diverticulum down with it, eventually becoming engulfed by it. The sac surrounding the testis (now called the tunica vaginalis) remains connected to the peritoneal sac via the processus vaginalis. Typically, throughout infancy and childhood, the connecting portion of the sac between the tunica vaginalis and the processus vaginalis gradually closes, breaking communication with the peritoneal sac.

Hydroceles in infants typically result from a patent processus vaginalis that fails to close during in utero development, allowing for the free flow of fluid between the peritoneal sac and the tunica vaginalis. These hydroceles have been directly correlated with the risk of indirect inguinal herniation in which gut contents bulge through the patent processus vaginalis. A noncommunicating hydrocele results from complete closure of the processus vaginalis, trapping peritoneal fluid within the tunica vaginalis. This type of hydrocele may be self-limited in adults. A hydrocele of the spermatic cord forms when the distal processus vaginalis closes but the midportion surrounding the cord remains patent and filled with fluid. The proximal portion may be opened or closed.

Rapidly forming hydroceles may result from reactive inflammatory processes within the scrotum such as testicular or appendiceal torsion, epididymitis, and even testicular cancer. A chronic hydrocele may result from gradual fluid accumulation within the tunica vaginalis in young boys or men, caused by an imbalance in fluid secretion, conduction, and reabsorption.

Clinical Presentation
Subjective

Patients with hydrocele typically present with swelling in the scrotum or inguinal canal. If the size of the scrotum fluctuates, a communicating hydrocele could exist. Hydroceles are usually painless, although patients report a sense of heaviness in the scrotum. If pain is present, it may radiate to the lower back.

Objective

The scrotum is transilluminated with a penlight in a darkened room during the physical exam. The trapped fluid appears light pink, yellow, or red. The hydrocele can be illuminated to show the full size and shape, which assists in the diagnosis. The testes themselves do not transilluminate, nor do hematomas. Swelling may be noted in the groin or in the upper scrotum.

Diagnostic Reasoning
Diagnostic Tests

A detailed description of the events that precipitated finding the hydrocele should be obtained. Details of any trauma incurred will assist in the evaluation. If a hydrocele cannot be confirmed, the patient should be referred for an inguino-scrotal ultrasound, which can distinguish the presence or absence of bowel within the inguinal ring. A testicular nuclear scan is used to distinguish testicular torsion. Abdominal x-ray studies may be useful in distinguishing an incarcerated hernia from a hydrocele but are rarely needed.

Differential Diagnosis

The differential diagnoses for hydrocele include indirect inguinal hernias (because of the location of the hydrocele), orchitis (inflammation or infection of the testes) or epididymitis (an inflammatory process that can produce symptoms that mimic those of a hydrocele), or varicocele. Pain is more likely to be present with epididymitis. Traumatic injury to the testes must be ruled out by history and physical exam. Torsion of the testicle or torsion of the appendix of the testes must also be ruled out. Exploratory surgery is indicated for definitive diagnosis of a patent processus vaginalis in a communicating hydrocele. A mass of any type requires further evaluation for testicular or scrotal cancer.

Management

For adults, no treatment of a hydrocele is required unless complications are present or the clinician suspects a significant underlying cause, such as a tumor. If the hydrocele is painful, large, unsightly, or uncomfortable, however, several treatments are available. For example, a variety of outpatient surgical procedures are used to treat hydrocele. The Jaboulay-Winkelmann surgical procedure is for thick hydrocele sacs that form when the hydrocele has wrapped itself posteriorly around the cord structures. The Lord procedure is used for a thin hydrocele sac; the radial suture is used to gather the hydrocele sac posterior to the testis and the epididymis. The hydrocele can be surgically drained and the tunica vaginalis resected. Sclerotherapy (injection of a sclerotic irritant into the tunica vaginalis to induce scarring and adhesions between the adjacent layer of the tunica) and endoscopic procedures can also be performed to alleviate hydroceles. Aspiration of hydroceles is usually not done because the fluid rapidly reaccumulates; however, it may be done for a postoperative hydrocele.

Follow-up and Referral

Patient monitoring for a hydrocele should be at 3-month intervals until the decision is made for or against surgery. Postoperatively, patient monitoring should be in 2- to 3-week intervals, followed by 2- to 3-month intervals until there is resolution.

Postoperative traumatic hydroceles are common and usually resolve spontaneously. Other possible complications may be injury to the vas deferens spermatic vessels, suture granuloma, hematoma secondary to the surgery, or a wound infection.

Patient Education

For patients with a hydrocele, education regarding an explanation of the disease process and management plan is appropriate, along with reassurance of the overall benign nature of the condition (depending on the underlying cause).

■ VARICOCELE

A *varicocele* is an abnormal degree of venous dilation of the pampiniform plexus above the testes, which usually results in pain and engorgement of the testis.

Epidemiology and Causes

There is no ethnic predisposition or age differentiation among patients with varicoceles. The overall rate of incidence is 8% to 20%. In men evaluated for infertility, however, the rate of varicocele increases to 25% to 40%. A weak wall in the spermatic vein or excessive pressure are the leading causes of varicoceles.

Pathophysiology

The pathophysiology of a varicocele results from vascular engorgement of the internal spermatic vein. A varicocele almost always appears on the left or bilaterally, because the left spermatic (gonadal) vein empties into the left renal vein, whereas the right spermatic vein empties into the inferior vena cava. One of the longest veins in the body, the left spermatic vein, empties into the renal vein at a perpendicular angle. Compared with the right renal vein, the left renal vein has a higher intravascular pressure owing to its anatomical positioning between the aorta inferiorly and the superior mesenteric artery. In turn, if the valves of the left renal vein become incompetent because of this increased pressure, retrograde blood flow causes back-pressure to be transmitted to the pampiniform venous plexus, which overlies the testis. In contrast, a unilateral right-sided varicocele may result from serious pathology, causing increased pressure within the inferior vena cava, such as a tumor or thrombus.

Clinical Presentation
Subjective

The patient may present with pain and engorgement of the testes. The recognition of a varicocele is usually secondary to a problem with fertility, however. A patient with a varicocele often describes the sensation as feeling like a "bag of worms."

Objective

On physical exam, with the patient in an upright position, tortuous veins located posterior to and above the testis can be assessed. The engorged veins may extend up into the external inguinal ring, depending on development. Venous dilation can be increased by having the patient perform the Valsalva maneuver in a recumbent position. The reverse is also true: In the recumbent position, the venous distention will abate. Testicular atrophy with impaired circulation may be present.

Diagnostic Reasoning
Diagnostic Tests

A system of grading has been established to better define varicocele. A *grade 1* varicocele is one that is palpable only when the patient performs the Valsalva maneuver. A *grade 2* varicocele is palpable when the patient is standing. A *grade 3* varicocele may be assessed with light palpation and visual inspection.

Sperm counts and motility of the sperm are significantly decreased in patients with a varicocele approximately 65% to 75% of the time. There is evidence of a progressive decline in fertility in men with varicocele. Scrotal ultrasound, venography (shows testicular venous reflux from a varicocele), and thermography (shows increase in temperature at the varicocele) all help to confirm the diagnosis.

Differential Diagnosis

A differential diagnosis for varicocele must include a hydrocele, a spermatocele, testicular tumor, epididymal cyst, and a renal tumor. A diagnostic priority is questioning the patient. It is essential to note whether the onset of the varicocele has been rapid or has resulted from a gradual increase in the varices of the testicles. In an elderly patient, the development of a varicocele may be a late sign of a renal tumor.

Management

After a varicocele has been diagnosed, referral to a surgeon is indicated although most patients do not require surgery because most varicoceles are minor. Surgical treatment of a varicocele involves ligation of the internal spermatic vein, which usually results in decompression of the varicocele and improvement of the quality of semen, as well as decrease in the pain. The surgery can be laparoscopic, anteriorly via an inguinal or subinguinal approach; posteriorly, via a lumbar approach; or even microsurgical. Embolization with coils is a second-line approach, but appears to have a higher complication rate owing to migration of the coils. Testicular atrophy is a definite indication for treatment. Conservative treatment in older men with only minor pain or for whom fertility is no longer an issue or for men with normal fertility may consist of NSAIDs and scrotal support. Treatment has not consistently improved sperm count or fertility in controlled trials.

Follow-up and Referral

Complications of a varicocele (if not corrected) include infertility and testicular atrophy. A referral to a urologist is indicated and recommended for affirmation of the diagnosis and further explanation of treatment options. Any patient with a recent onset of varicocele, infertility, pain, or testicular atrophy should have a urology consultation.

Patient Education

Education for the patient should include an explanation of the disease process, signs, symptoms, and implications. The patient should be taught how to monitor growth and symptoms of the varicocele, especially if it is right sided. To relieve pain, the patient should be encouraged to wear a scrotal support; for some patients, wearing jockey shorts (briefs) rather than loose boxer shorts is sufficient to relieve discomfort.

■ PROSTATE CANCER

To properly understand the pathophysiology, diagnosis, and treatment of carcinoma of the prostate, a brief review of prostatic anatomy is warranted. The prostate is composed of acinar glands and their ducts, which are arranged in a radial fashion with the stroma containing blood vessels, lymph vessels, and nerves. Ninety-five percent of all prostate cancers are acinar adenocarcinomas. The prostate gland secretes 0.5 to 2 mL of fluid a day, and this constitutes 10% to 20% of the seminal fluid of the ejaculate. The prostatic fluid contains citric acid, prostaglandins, and fibrinogen. The epithelial cells of the prostate gland are the only source of the glycoprotein prostate-specific antigen (PSA).

The prostate lies between the base of the urinary bladder and the upper surface of the levator ani and deep transverse peritoneal muscles. The anterior surface is adjacent to the retropubic space; the posterior surface lies adjacent to the seminal vesicles and recto-vesicular (rectum–bladder) septum.

The prostate is palpable per rectum. The prostate gland is 2 to 3 cm across; at its midpoint, it is twice the breadth of the examining finger. A 20 g size is normal. A slightly enlarged gland is documented as +1 and is considered three finger-breadths across, with +2 being twice the normal breadth (or four finger-breadths across). Occasionally a +3 or +4 classification will present, which involves the anterior pelvic outlet with marked encroachment of the posterior lobe on the rectal wall, reducing the caliber of the rectal passage. A normal prostate posterior area can be palpated without moving the hand, but the clinician may need to move the hand side to side in order to palpate an enlarged prostate or nodular area.

The prostate gland is subdivided into five lobes, which include the left and right lateral lobes (which are extensive and make up what was formerly termed the anterior lobe), the left and right posterior lobes (which also include the apex of the gland), and the median lobe. Prostatic cancer is known to have a propensity for the gland's posterior and apical peripheral zone (thus palpable through the rectal wall), whereas benign prostatic hyperplasia (BPH) tends to affect the transition zone that surrounds the urethra.

Epidemiology and Causes

Prostate cancer is the most common cancer found in American men and ranks second in the number of cancer deaths (lung cancer is number one). In fact, more than 40% of men older than 50 years of age have been found to have prostate cancer on autopsy, and the prevalence increases with age. Clinical incidence of prostatic carcinoma is highest in North America and Europe and lowest in the Far East, suggesting that there may be environmental or dietary factors that increase prostate growth. In American men, those at highest risk for prostate cancer are African Americans; men with a family history of prostate cancer; and men with a diet high in fat, particularly animal fat.

Recently a major susceptibility focus for prostate cancer was found on chromosome 1 and is still under investigation. A man with a first-degree relative (a father or a brother) with prostate cancer is twice as likely to develop the disease and to do so at an earlier age. Occupational and environmental risks for development of prostate cancer include exposure to cadmium nitrates and heavy metals. As an occupational group, farmers are at the highest risk for development of prostate cancer. Further investigation continues on the subject of occupations as a risk factor.

Smoking has also been identified as a risk factor for prostate cancer; the risk appears to be proportional to the amount of smoking the patient does and may be related to the cadmium content of cigarettes. A patient's endogenous hormonal influences, characterized by increased levels of testosterone, have been shown to contribute to increased risk.

Pathophysiology

Prostate cancer is believed to result from a sequential accumulation of genetic abnormalities affecting the androgen receptors on prostatic tissue. These defects have been characterized as either genetic predispositions to disease that are seen to run in families (e.g., deletions in chromosome 1q); somatic mutations that activate prostatic oncogenes such as c-*myc*, *MKP-1*, *bcl-2*, and telomerase (e.g., mutations in the 7p and 8q regions); and somatic mutations that inactivate tumor suppressor genes such as *PTEN/MMAC-1*, *Mxi1*, *GSTP1*, *TGF-1*, and *Rb* (e.g., mutations in the 8p, 10q, 12q, 13q, and 17p regions). Such mutations accumulate over time, thus accounting for the strong correlation between age and disease prevalence.

The degree of malignancy may be graded according to several different scales. One method (Jewett system) utilizes the following stages:

A1–A2 and B1–B2 neoplasms are confined within the capsule.
C1 has extension of the carcinoma beyond the capsule.
C2 has malignancy that involves the seminal vesicles.
D1 involves metastatic disease in the regional lymph nodes.
D2 involves metastatic disease in bone or other organs.

The left and right posterior lobes of the prostate are most predisposed to malignant transformation. Extensive carcinoma may involve the capsule and the periprostatic tissues. Carcinomas of the prostate usually extend to the base of the bladder and the region of the seminal vesicles to form a shelf or a plateau. Usually, the periprostatic spread is limited by Denonvilliers' fascia, but once this area has been invaded, circumferential extension about the rectum occurs.

The lethality of malignant prostate cancers is a direct function of the heterogeneity in their cellular composition, which consists of both androgen-sensitive and androgen-insensitive cells. Anti-testosterone therapies work by suppressing androgen, which itself represses pro-apoptotic genes in cancer cells that would otherwise lead to cellular death. However, the apoptosis (nonnecrotic or programmed cell death) of androgen-insensitive cancer cells is not induced by anti-androgen therapies. Through progressive genetic mutations, the androgen receptors on cancerous prostatic tissue are increased in number, level of androgen-independent activity, and resistance to apoptotic death signals from tumor suppressor genes. This accounts for the progressive and inevitably increased androgen insensitivity of malignant prostatic tissue and, in turn, the persistent spread of disease.

Clinical Presentation
Subjective

Men with prostate cancer are usually asymptomatic early in the disease and may also be asymptomatic late in the disease. Latent symptoms include bone pain, weight loss, anemia, shortness of breath, lymphedema, and lymphadenopathy. Neurological symptoms (inability to perceive touch, pain, and temperature in the perineal or scrotal areas and a lack of sensation of bladder distention) occur with epidural metastasis and cord compression. Patient complaints also include bladder-outlet symptoms or acute urinary retention with very large or locally extensive tumors, but are most often due to BPH.

Objective

Rectal exam reveals a palpable hard prostate that may be localized or diffused; several hard areas may be present or the nodules may be limited to one hardened area. An induration of the prostate may also be noted. Hematuria and hemospermia are signs that appear late in the course of the disease; they are very rarely detected in early prostate cancer. Evaluation of the rectal sphincter, and the anal and bulbocavernosus reflex, directs attention to the possible lesion at the level of the conis.

Diagnostic Reasoning
Diagnostic Tests

PSA is prostate specific but not cancer specific (found only in the cytoplasm of benign and malignant prostate cells). The effectiveness of using PSA in screening programs for prostate cancer has been questioned because of the lack of evidence that routine screening for PSA can improve the quality and quantity of life for the overall population. The American Cancer Society (ACS) recommends that men with no symptoms of prostate cancer, who are in relatively good health and can expect to live at least 10 more years, should start screening at age 50 years. ACS recommends that African American men and men who have a father, brother, or son diagnosed with prostate cancer before age 65 years begin conversations about initiating screening at age 45 years. Men at higher risk should be screened beginning at age 40 years. The American Urological Association (AUA) recommends the use of PSA-based screening programs in conjunction with digital rectal exam (DRE) to detect prostate cancer in men aged 55 to 69 years who are at average risk and asymptomatic. The AUA guidelines state that PSA screening is not recommended for men younger than 40 years, for men 40 to 54 years who are at average risk, for men 70 years and older, or for men with a life expectancy of less than 10 to 15 years. The predominant age range for onset of prostate cancer is 50 to 60 years, which influences the recommendations for screening. Although approximately 67% of men 80 years of age have prostate cancer, only about 3% are expected to die from it.

Research continues on PSA levels as a viable means of identifying true prostate cancer, and the goal is to increase the specificity of the test. The strongest evidence of benefit for PSA screening is in the age-group of 55 to 69 years. In younger higher-risk men, screening should be individualized based on the uncertainty of benefit and associated harms of screening (false positives, unnecessary biopsies, etc.). Recent guidelines recommend 2-year PSA intervals, and for men over 60 years with PSA levels below 1.0 ng/mL, even longer PSA screening intervals (e.g., up to 4 years). There is no PSA level below which prostate cancer can be definitively ruled out; rather, the risk of prostate cancer increases as PSA level increases. Traditionally, a PSA level greater than 4.0 ng/mL is considered positive, and a level of 4.1 ng/mL has been considered a threshold for performing prostate biopsy. Serial PSAs are thought to be more accurate than a single test. Age-specific PSA norms have also been suggested as a method to increase the accuracy of the PSA test for the diagnosis of prostate cancer. However, the use of age-specific norms as biopsy decision points is controversial, given that they may potentially delay detection of prostate cancer in some patients.

Considering the current guidelines for PSA screening and the possible risks of biopsy (e.g., bleeding, infection, nerve damage), individualized informed decision making with the patient's active involvement is the best practice with regard to PSA testing and subsequent interventional diagnostic procedures. The ACS, the AUA, and the American College of Physicians all recommend that health-care providers have an open discussion with patients about the pros and cons of prostate cancer screening, as discussed in this section, and decide on a mutually agreeable course of action based on the patient's individual risk of developing prostate cancer and the implications of such a diagnosis (morbidity and mortality of both prostate cancer and its treatment). If screening is agreed to, it should begin at age 55 to 69 years for most men and at age 40 years for African American men or those with a family history of prostate cancer, especially in a father or brother. Screening may stop by age 75 years or in those with severe health problems, because prostate cancer is unlikely to be the cause of death for the large majority of these patients.

If prostate cancer is suspected (PSA greater than 10 ng/mL or laboratory-specific threshold), the patient should be referred to a urologist for a transrectal ultrasound (TRUS) and a transrectal biopsy of the prostate. The identification of any malignancies using TRUS-guided biopsy is not only a conclusive finding; this diagnostic procedure also provides information that is helpful in staging the disease and planning subsequent treatment, which may include radiation therapy and chemotherapy. Prostate screening using a combination of DRE, TRUS, and PSA with age-related values provides the most positive, predictive value of diagnosing prostate cancer. The potential complications of the TRUS-guided biopsy are hematospermia, hematuria, fever, hematochezia, or rectal bleeding. Biopsy may be repeated if initial results are negative and cancer is highly suspected. Free PSA levels in the bloodstream have also been tested as a screening tool and criteria for patients to have a follow-up TRUS. Free PSA occurs in greater concentrations in men without prostate cancer. Alternatively, the ratio of complex PSA to a total PSA is greater in individuals with prostate cancer. Complex PSA is PSA bound to the protease inhibitor alpha-1-antichymotrypsin, which is the form that is most elevated in prostate cancer. The predicted value is 24%, based on patients who underwent biopsies after having had the free PSA test.

Another group of researchers has been using the prostate-specific antigen density (PSAD) to screen for prostate cancer. PSAD can help differentiate BPH from prostate cancer because it is calculated by dividing the PSA by the volume of the prostate that is estimated via TRUS. Alkaline phosphatase is typically elevated in patients with metastases, but this finding is not specific for cancer of the prostate. Further studies that are done in patients with prostate cancer include a bone scan, which may show the presence of metastases. Computed tomography of the pelvic lymph nodes, ultrasound of the prostate, lymphoscintigraphy, and magnetic resonance imaging are alternate techniques that show metastases. On the horizon are molecular diagnostic tests on the urine postprostatic massage that detect highly specific genetic markers of prostate cancer, such as DNA hypermethylation (i.e., inactivation) of the genetic promoter for the tumor suppressor gene glutathione S-transferase (GSTP1).

Differential Diagnosis

BPH is the number one differential diagnosis in someone with suspected prostate cancer because the urinary outlet symptoms of nocturia, frequency, hesitancy, and weak urinary stream can be seen with both conditions but are far more commonly due to BPH. New-onset erectile dysfunction (ED), hematuria, or hematospermia are less common presentations of prostate cancer. Other differential diagnoses for prostate cancer include a benign nodule, prostate stones, nodular whorls, and seminal vesicle enlargement.

Management

Unfortunately, neither chemotherapy nor immunotherapy can cure prostate cancer once it has spread beyond the gland. If the findings are positive on both DRE and PSA, the patient should be referred to a urologist for a definitive diagnosis (biopsy) and staging.

Staging

Prostate tumors are classified according to the Gleason system in which first a "grade" is applied to the architectural pattern of the cancer in the largest segment of the specimen and then a second "grade" is given to the next largest area. The pathologist adds the two scores together to produce the Gleason score, which is on a scale of 1 to 10. Accurate staging provides an indication of the best treatment options.

Gleason score 1 to 4: Indicates a well-differentiated cancer that is likely to be slow growing.
Gleason score 5 to 7: Indicates a moderately differentiated cancer.
Gleason score 8 to 10: Indicates poorly differentiated cancer cells that are likely to be aggressive and rapid growing.

Prostate cancer is further staged according to the extent of the tumor, based on additional diagnostic studies or findings at the time of surgery. The most commonly used staging system is the American Joint Committee on Cancer tumor-node-metastasis (TNM) system, which grades tumors numerically within more detailed subcategories: "T" describes *tumors* according to their degree of differentiation; "N" describes the extent of *node* involvement; and "M" describes the degree of *metastasis*. For example, T1 tumors are microscopic, nonpalpable, and not visible by TRUS. Tumors classified as T2 are palpable but not beyond the prostate itself, and T3 tumors go beyond the capsule or into the seminal vesicles. T4 tumors are fixed and extend far beyond the prostate. Prostate cancer extending beyond the prostate itself is often fatal, and treatment is typically only palliative; however, localized disease is often curable by surgery, radiation therapy, and/or chemotherapy.

Patients Older Than Age 70 Years

Patients older than age 70 years are usually offered conservative treatment as an alternative to surgery. Radiation external beam therapy or brachytherapy with implants and total androgen ablation are the general measures that are used to treat prostate cancer in older men.

Patients Younger Than Age 70 Years

If the patient is younger than 70 years of age, surgery is often recommended for a prostate cancer cure. Surgical interventions may be used for Jewett stages A and B and selected C stages. If the patient is in agreement, an orchiectomy may be warranted to ablate endogenous hormonal effects.

The standard treatment options for prostate cancer include radical prostatectomy, radiation therapy, and watchful waiting. Treatment decisions are based more often on the adverse effects, long-term risks, and financial and emotional costs of different therapies, depending on the individual patient. Younger healthy patients are often encouraged to undergo the most radical treatment, whereas older patients are often directed to watchful waiting (observation) or radiotherapy. A relatively new surgical approach uses the da Vinci robotic system. For this surgery, a few small incisions are made rather than the typical large abdominal incision. The da Vinci system uses a magnified, three-dimensional, high-definition vision apparatus and mechanical wristed instruments that allow the physician to operate with enhanced vision, precision, dexterity, and control. The benefits of this surgical approach are a more precise removal of the prostate that causes less nerve injury, thereby improving sexual function and decreasing the chance of urinary incontinence. In addition, there is less blood loss during surgery and fewer postoperative complications.

Other treatments for prostate cancer include hormonal therapy to inhibit cancer growth by testosterone deprivation or administration of endogenous estrogen to block the release of luteinizing hormone (LH) from the hypothalamus. Unfortunately, estrogen therapy is associated with hypercoagulopathy, cardiomegaly, and gynecomastia. Newer hormonal preparations include leuprolide (Lupron), goserelin acetate (Zoladex), triptorelin (Trelstar), and histrelin (Vantas), which block the release of follicle-stimulating hormone (FSH) and LH. Luteinizing hormone–releasing hormone (LHRH) antagonists such as degarelix (Firmagon) reduce testosterone levels more quickly and are used to treat advanced prostate cancer. These agents are typically administered monthly. Adverse effects include loss of libido and hot flashes. Oral antiandrogens are also available, including asflutamide (Casodex), flutamide (Eulexin), and nilutamine (Nilandron), which inhibit the binding of testosterone to cancer cells. Finasteride (Proscar) is used to block the enzyme 5-alpha-reductase, which converts testosterone into DHT. A newer antiandrogen treatment is enzalutamide (Xtandi), which blocks signaling from the androgen receptor to the prostate cancer cell; abiraterone (Zytiga) blocks the CYP17A1 enzyme in the testosterone synthetic pathway and, in turn, reduces androgen production.

Cryosurgical ablation of the prostate is used to destroy cancer cells in patients who have had negative bone scans for metastatic prostate cancer. Cryosurgery destroys the prostate cancer cells through freezing. Unfortunately, the major adverse effects of this ablation technique include possible destruction of nerves and/or circulation, which can cause incontinence and ED.

Some research indicates that lifestyle modification in conjunction with "watchful waiting" improves the attitudes of men with early-stage prostate cancer. (See Nursing Research–Based Practice Box 13.1.)

Follow-up and Referral

Patient follow-up is determined by the radiation oncologist and urologist. Without fail, the patient should have a clinical examination every 3 months for a year. Chest x-ray studies and bone scans should be done every 6 months for a year and yearly thereafter. Potential complications of treatment may include cardiac failure, phlebitis, and pathological fractures secondary to the hormonal changes (testosterone suppression), as well as those mentioned in the previous section. With early diagnosis and treatment, the expected prognosis is good, and lesions should be curable, especially in young, healthy males.

Once prostate cancer has been diagnosed and treatment regimens have been chosen and implemented, the patient should be followed by the specialist and also seen by the primary-care clinician regularly for health maintenance, reassurance, positive outlook, and laboratory test follow-up.

Patient Education

Support groups and other advocacy organizations for prostate cancer patients are available, along with books on the subject, including reports from prostate cancer survivors. Churches are also being used as a forum for patient education, particularly those with older congregations. Given the widespread impact of prostate cancer, it is important for the clinician to be knowledgeable regarding the latest diagnostic and treatment options, as well as to remain attuned to patients' desires and fears regarding this diagnosis.

■ TESTICULAR CANCER

Primary testicular neoplasms may arise from any testicular or adnexal cell component. Each testis is covered externally by two layers of fascia: the outer layer, the tunica vaginalis; and the deeper albuginea layer, which extends internally and divides the testis into 250 to 300 lobules. Each lobule contains seminiferous tubules (the site of spermatogenesis) and the interstitial cells that produce androgens including testosterone. The epididymis lies along the external surface of each testis and is the site of sperm maturation and storage. Tumors of the germ cells

---

Nursing Research–Based Practice 13.1

Osei, DK, et al. Effects of an online support group for prostate cancer survivors: A randomized trial. *Urol Nurs* 33(3):123–133, 2013.

Prostate cancer is the most frequently diagnosed cancer in men. The American Cancer Society estimates for new diagnoses of prostate cancer in 2012 were at least 241,740 new cases and 28,170 deaths. The 5-year survival rate is close to 100%, and the 15-year survival rate is 91%. Thus, the number of prostate cancer survivors is significant, and although treatment options are highly successful, quality of life may be affected significantly.

The purpose of this study was to evaluate the effects of an online support intervention for patients with prostate cancer. This method of support is convenient, inexpensive, and anonymous. The sample consisted of 40 men between the ages of 53 and 87 years, with a diagnosis of prostate cancer within the previous 5 years, who were divided into two groups: those who participated in the online support group (treatment group) for 6 weeks and the control group who were given prostate cancer resource kits. Most participants were Caucasian (95% treatment, 75% control) with an education level of some college, college graduate, or graduate school (90%). This was a longitudinal, randomized, experimental study that collected data on quality of life and symptom manifestations using an online survey platform. Data were collected at 3 time points; baseline, 6 weeks, and 8 weeks. Quality of life was measured using 4 different tools, and the treatment group also completed a scale to measure their satisfaction with the online support group.

Multivariate analysis of variance was used to analyze differences across time and within groups, with outcomes on quality of life scales considered collectively. The results indicated the prostate cancer patients in the treatment group reported a statistically significant improvement in urinary irritation, sexual health, and hormonal health. Conversely, in the control group, quality of life declined with regard to perceived physical health, urinary irritation, sexual health, hormonal health, life satisfaction, and spouse negative characteristics at the 6-week time point. However, quality of life measures returned to baseline levels at the 8-week time point.

The researchers concluded that those patients who participated in the online support group had a positive improvement in their perception of quality of life. However, generalization of these findings is limited by the study's extremely low return rate using the online survey data collection platform. The researchers sent out 1,000 letters inviting potential subjects to participate, but received back only 51 responses (5%), with only 40 of those meeting the inclusion criteria.

and the seminiferous tubules are the most common testicular carcinomas.

Epidemiology and Causes

Although testicular malignancies comprise only 1% to 2% of all neoplasms in males, the psychologically and physically debilitating effects of testicular cancer affecting young men aged 15 to 35 years deserve mention, because testicular cancer is the most common solid malignancy in the age-group. Fortunately, it is also one of the most curable of solid cancers.

In the United States, there are five to six new cases of testicular cancer per year per 100,000 males. It is less common in African Americans, at 0.9 cases per 100,000 males. In adults, germ-cell types comprise 90% to 95% of testicular cancers, and in boys they represent 60% to 75%. The peak age at onset is between age 20 and 40 years. Smaller peaks occur between birth and 10 years of age and in men older than age 60 years.

No clear cause-and-effect relationships are identified for testicular cancer. Risk factors for testicular cancer include HIV infection and Caucasian race (especially Scandinavian background), with a much lower incidence among African Americans. Men who have experienced undescended or partially descended testes (cryptorchidism) are at a much higher risk for testicular cancer. Prior cryptorchidism is the only undisputed risk factor for this type of cancer, with 10% of testicular tumors associated with this condition. Importantly, a fourth of these tumors occur in the contralateral, descended testis.

Other possible risk factors that have been identified for testicular cancer include higher social status, being unmarried, or living in a rural area. Weak associations demonstrate that hormonal imbalances associated with in utero exposure to estrogen may increase the risk for testicular cancer later in life. One study of mothers who used diethylstilbestrol (DES) during the first trimester found a 2.5- to 5-fold increase of testicular cancer in the sons of exposed mothers.

Pathophysiology

Primary testicular neoplasm may arise from any testicular adnexal cell component. These are divided into germinal (90%–95%) and nongerminal (sex cord–stromal) tumors. For treatment purposes, the germinal tumors are further divided equally based on histology into seminomas and nonseminomas (i.e., embryonal carcinomas, teratomas, choriocarcinomas, and yolk sac tumors), which are epithelial in nature. In contrast, far rarer are the sex cord–stromal tumors, which consist primarily of Leydig cell variants that produce estrogen due to increased aromatase activity and Sertoli cell tumors, which may also present with estrogenic overload.

Only a small number of molecular markers have been consistently associated with testicular cancers, for example, an isochromosome of chromosome 12p, activating mutations in c-*kit,* increased p53 and telomerase expression. Abnormal DNA ploidy is also common in germ cell tumors. Although certain genetic alterations differ in germ cell tumors found in prepubertal males, all germ cell tumors are believed to arise from pluripotential primordial germ cells. One exception to this is the relatively rare spermatocytic seminoma, the pathogenesis of which appears to be fundamentally different based on unique molecular markers.

Except for spermatocytic seminomas, all germ cell tumors may be preceded by a premalignant condition known as intratubular germ cell neoplasia of unclassified type (ITGCNU) or testicular carcinoma in situ. It is found adjacent to 90% of germ cell tumors, implying that genetic mutations lead to gonadal dysfunction and subsequent malignancy over a large area of tissue—a phenomenon known as a field defect. At least half the cases of untreated ITGCNU will progress to invasive malignant disease within 5 years, predictably spreading to the retroperitoneal draining lymph nodes. Men with a history of cryptorchidism are recommended to have empiric testicular biopsy between ages 18 and 20 years to evaluate for ITGCNU.

Clinical Presentation
Subjective

Typically, the patient with testicular cancer presents with a hard lump or nodule on his testis that he felt while performing a testicular self-exam. He may also note scrotal swelling, heaviness in the scrotum that may be interpreted as pain, a sensation of fullness, or a previously small testis that has enlarged to the size of a normal testis or the contralateral testis. Generally, testicular cancer presents as a painless enlargement of the testis.

Objective

During routine physical exams (e.g., a sports physical), a scrotal nodule or swelling is most commonly detected in men with testicular cancer. A firm, nontender mass within the confines of the tunica albuginea is usual, palpable, and distinct from the spermatic cord structures. Acute or chronic epididymitis or epididymo-orchitis may result in delay of diagnosis of testicular cancer in about 10% of the cases. Gynecomastia may be present in 5% of patients with testicular malignancies. Hydroceles (seen in 5%–10% of patients) may be secondary to testicular cancer.

As many as 10% of patients with testicular cancer will be asymptomatic, and another 10% will present with manifestations of metastasis. Symptoms of metastases include respiratory symptoms (cough) due to lung metastases, low back pain and nerve root or psoas muscle irritation due to retroperitoneal metastasis, or lower extremity swelling from vena cava obstruction.

Diagnostic Reasoning
Diagnostic Tests

Several biochemical markers can aid in the diagnosis of testicular carcinoma, but their main use is in following disease progression or remission after treatment (looking at trends). These tests include human chorionic gonadotropin (hCG), alpha-fetoprotein (AFP), and lactate dehydrogenase (LDH). AFP levels are elevated by the pure embryonal carcinoma, teratocarcinoma, yolk sac tumor, or combinations of these three malignancies, but not by pure choriocarinoma or seminoma. However, AFP may be elevated in benign liver disease; telangiectasis; tyrosinemia; and malignancies of the liver, pancreas, stomach, and lung. Heavy marijuana smoking can also elevate levels of AFP. hCG levels are elevated by all choriocarcinomas and occasionally in seminomas; however, they are also elevated in liver, lung, pancreatic, and stomach malignancies, as well as by kidney, breast, and bladder tumors. Forty percent to 60% of patients with an embryonal carcinoma and 5% to 10% of patients with seminomas have detectable levels of hCG (usually under 500 ng/mL). Testing for LDH has fallen into disfavor because of the ubiquitous nature of the test. An elevated LDH level may be the sole biochemical abnormality in 10% of patients who have persistent or recurrent seminomatous tumors, and other liver function tests are elevated in the presence of hepatic metastases. In general, elevated AFP, hCG, or LDH is a poor prognostic sign, and prognosis worsens with the level of elevation. Elevated placental alkaline phosphatase (PLAP) may be the marker of choice for seminomas in 70% to 90% of patients. Patients with recurrent or disseminated seminomas have elevated PLAP levels. PLAP may also be elevated by heavy tobacco smoking.

Scrotal ultrasound is also a useful diagnostic tool for testicular cancer. The mass can be seen clearly originating within the testis. Using an echo-texture (hypoechoic) pattern, the mass will appear distinct from the surrounding normal testicular tissue on ultrasound. Uniformly cystic or fluid-filled masses are not likely to be testicular cancer, which is a solid tumor. However, ultrasound is not accurate for staging and should not replace orchiectomy as the procedure of choice. Magnetic resonance imaging is not usually more informative than scrotal ultrasound and pelvic/abdominal computed tomography (CT) for staging and identifying enlarged retroperitoneal lymph nodes, implying the need for lymph node dissection. Positron emission tomography scanning is usually used only to identify residual masses after treatment.

Chest x-ray studies, with both posterior-anterior and lateral views, are important for identification of metastasis and to rule out spread of malignancy above the diaphragm. A CT scan is able to define pelvic retroperitoneal and mediastinal lymphadenopathy, as well as to detect metastases to the abdominal viscera.

Differential Diagnosis

Definitive diagnosis of testicular cancer may be made with a transinguinal scrotal exploration and biopsy and/or radical orchiectomy (excision of the testicle and spermatic cord). Transscrotal open or cutaneous biopsy and transscrotal orchiectomy are contraindicated because of the potential for anatomical trespassing into the various lymphatic drainage systems. Testicular cancer is typically a painless mass in the testis, but the differential diagnosis should include epididymitis, hernia, hydrocele, hematoma, spermatocele, syphilitic gumma, and varicocele.

Management

The main principle of management for testicular cancer is a radical orchiectomy, which is also the major diagnostic tool, because the whole testis is removed for biopsy. Testicular cancer is very treatable, with fewer than 400 deaths per year in the United States at the present time. Treatment does, however, leave the patient with a high possibility of being infertile. Sperm-banking (semen cryopreservation) should be done before radiographic diagnostic studies, if desired. Many of these men have gonadal dysgenesis with baseline sperm count and morphology problems, but banking in general works well and future children do not have higher rates of congenital defects fathered by this banked sperm.

Staging

Testicular carcinoma is divided into two main categories when considering treatment. The first category, nonseminomas, includes embryonal cell carcinomas (20%), teratomas (5%), choriocarcinomas (less than 1%), and mixed cell types (40%). The second category is seminomas (35%). Staging depends on the type of tumor. See Table 13.2 for staging criteria.

The TNM classification of the American Joint Cancer Committee is also used for testicular cancer. The primary tumor (T) is classed from T0 (no evidence of primary tumor) to T4 (invades scrotum). Lymph node assessment (N) is from N0 (no regional lymph node metastasis) to N3 (metastasis in lymph node greater than 5 cm). Distant metastasis (M) is classified from M0 (no distant metastasis) to M1b (distant metastasis to sites other than nonregional lymph nodes or lungs).

Seventy-five percent of nonseminomas can be cured with orchiectomy alone, usually with modified retroperitoneal lymph node dissection. This is done to preserve

Table 13.2	Staging and Classification for Testicular Carcinoma
Nonseminoma Germ Cell Tumor Staging	
Stage A	Lesion confined to testis
Stage B	Regional lymph node involvement in retroperitoneum
Stage C	Distant metastasis
MD Anderson System for Seminomas	
Stage I	Lesion confined to testis
Stage II	Spread to retroperitoneal lymph nodes
Stage III	Supradiaphragmatic nodal or visceral involvement

the sympathetic innervation so the patient will still have ejaculatory function. The serum markers are monitored postorchiectomy, and those that return to normal have an excellent prognosis. For patients with nonseminomas that have metastasized or who have significant lymph node involvement (greater than 3 cm), combination chemotherapy is used following orchiectomy. Commonly used chemotherapeutic agents include cisplatin (Platinol) and etoposide (VePesid) and bleomycin (Blenoxane), or paclitaxel (Taxol). If the serum tumor markers do not normalize after chemotherapy, salvage chemotherapy is needed. Salvage chemotherapy includes cyclophosphamide (Cytoxan)– or ifosfamide (Ifex)–based protocols with mesna (Mesnex) to protect against hemorrhagic cystitis.

The 5-year survival rate for those with stage A nonseminomas is 96% to 100% after treatment. Patients with stage B nonseminomas have almost a 90% 5-year survival rate after treatment. For patients with stage C nonseminomas, the 5-year survival rate is between 55% and 80%.

Seminomas are chemosensitive and have good chemotherapeutic response and are also extremely sensitive to radiation therapy. All patients with seminomas will have radical orchiectomy surgery; and then, depending on the stage, irradiation and chemotherapy will be used. For patients with stage I and stage IIa (retroperitoneal disease less than 10 cm), surgery and radiation are the treatments of choice and are associated with a 5-year survival of 98% and 92% to 94%, respectively. More advanced stage II (retroperitoneal disease greater than 10 cm) and stage III seminomas received primary chemotherapy either with etoposide and cisplatin or a combination of cisplatin, etoposide, and bleomycin. If enlarged lymph nodes (more than 3 cm in diameter) persist after chemotherapy, a retroperitoneal lymph-node resection is done. In 40% of cases, there is residual carcinoma in these lymph nodes. Ninety-five percent of patients with stage III seminoma have a complete response to orchiectomy and chemotherapy. A viable tumor is present in more than 40% of cases. Primary chemotherapy is a last resort.

As with all chemotherapeutic agents, the precautions are specific for each. Cisplatin causes ototoxicity, nephrotoxicity, and neurotoxicity. Etoposide may cause thrombocytopenia. Cyclophosphamide and ifosfamide may cause hemorrhagic cystitis. Patients must be well hydrated to minimize the risk of hemorrhagic cystitis. Patients receiving ifosfamide should also receive mesna to reduce the risk of hemorrhagic cystitis. Bleomycin causes pulmonary fibrosis. One alternative drug may be carboplatin (Paraplatin), which can cause ototoxicity. Ondansetron (Zofran), dronabinol (Marinol), and metoclopramide (Reglan) and other medications may be used to control nausea. Follow-up is extremely important for patients with testicular malignancies.

Follow-up and Referral

For the first 2 years, tumor markers and chest x-ray films are assessed every month, and a physical exam emphasizing the lymph nodes should be performed monthly. After the first 2 years, tumor markers and chest x-ray films are checked every 2 months; the physical exam should be done every 2 to 4 months for another year. CT scans are usually done every 3 to 4 months for the initial 3 years. After year 3 with no further symptoms, the tumor markers, chest x-ray studies, and physical exams should be done every 6 to 12 months. If a patient had a diagnosis of teratoma, he will need to have a follow-up for at least 5 years, however, and a CT scan every year for 3 years. Radiation therapy can cause extreme fatigue and interfere with sperm production; it can also cause diarrhea, vomiting, and skin reaction at the treatment site. Adverse effects of chemotherapy include hair loss, immunosuppression, loss of appetite, and nausea and vomiting. Complications from retroperitoneal lymph node dissection include loss of seminal emission and/or hypoalbuminemia. Radiation treatment may cause nephritis or enteritis. Nonseminomatous tumors are more likely (50%–70%) to metastasize than seminomas (25%). Men who have been cured of testicular cancer in one testicle have a 2% to 4% chance of developing cancer in the remaining testicle. If cancer develops in the other testicle, it is almost always a new cancer, however, and not a metastasis from the first episode.

Patient Education

The question of life after testicular cancer becomes extremely important to the patient. The patient must be able to cope with the way testicular cancer affects his self-image. A low sperm count may occur after the loss of a testis. Patients who are concerned about their appearance after losing a testis can be educated about the availability of a prosthesis that simulates the weight and feel of a testicle. Although surgery to remove lymph nodes does not compromise a man's ability to have an erection or reach orgasm, it can interfere with ejaculation. Some men naturally regain the ability to ejaculate; others require medication. A patient should also be educated about sterility and hormone supplements. The option of sperm banking should be discussed with patients when the diagnosis of testicular cancer is first confirmed. Open discussions and reassurance are extremely important in patients diagnosed with testicular cancer.

The importance of a monthly testicular self-exam (TSE) cannot be stressed enough. Males aged 15 to 40 should be instructed on TSE at each primary care visit, and the technique should be demonstrated. Advanced Practice Nursing Interventions 13.1 presents information on how to teach the patient to perform a TSE.

Advanced Practice Nursing Interventions 13.1   Teaching the Patient to Perform a Testicular Self-Exam

Teach the patient the symptoms of testicular cancer. No symptoms may occur in the early stages. When symptoms do occur, they may include the following:

• Lumps on the testicle
• Slight enlargement of one of the testes
• Heavy sensation in the testicles or groin
• Dull ache in the lower abdomen or groin

Advise the patient that if hard lumps or nodules are found, or if any of the above symptoms occur, he should contact his health-care provider immediately.

Teach the patient when to perform the exam. The exam is best performed during or after a shower or warm bath, as the fingers glide more easily over the relaxed skin, making it easier to concentrate on the texture underneath. The heat causes the skin to relax, making the exam easier. The exam takes only about 3 minutes and should be performed once a month.

Teach the patient how to perform the exam:

1. Start by examining one of the testicles. Slowly roll the testicle between the thumb and fingers, applying slight pressure. Try to find any hard, painless lumps.
2. Now examine the epididymis. This comma-shaped cord is behind each testicle. It may be tender to the touch. It is also the location of the most noncancerous problems.
3. Continue by examining the vas (the sperm-carrying tube that runs up from the epididymis). The vas normally feels like a firm, moveable smooth tube.
4. Now repeat the exam on the other side.

SEXUALLY TRANSMITTED DISEASES

Sexually transmitted diseases (STDs) are on the rise. In response to that rise, the Centers for Disease Control and Prevention (CDC) has published Guidelines for Sexually Transmitted Diseases, which include information on prevention, diagnosis, and treatment for all known STDs. These guidelines are available online at www.cdc.gov.

STDs are a costly addition to the health-care burden in the United States, not only for the treatment of primary symptoms but also because of the increased risk of further complications from STDs. Open, frank discussions with patients about sexual practices is warranted from the early teenage years through old age. The primary-care clinician who is proactive and informative is the greatest resource that a patient can have. Pamphlets, posters, and patient education materials including videos and informational handouts are extremely helpful as a way to open a discussion on the topic.

Epidemiology and Causes

It is estimated that approximately one in five Americans is infected with a viral STD other than HIV. Perhaps even more alarming is that the United States, with the most educated population and highest standard of living, has the highest STD rates in the world. Increased

risks for STDs are associated with gender, marital status, race and ethnic background, level of education, number of sexual partners, and lack of availability of health care. The long-term effects of STDs can be devastating and, at times, lethal. Improved advances in treatment, screening tests, and diagnostic procedures aid in discussion of the patient's symptoms and treatment therapies.

Pathophysiology

STDs consist of a heterogeneous collection of causative infectious agents (see Table 13.3). However, the unifying principle of these disorders is their propensity for spread by intimate person-to-person sexual contact, particularly after exposure of the mucous membranes to infected bodily fluids. This typically occurs within the genitalia; however, the oral and anal mucosa are also highly susceptible entry points, as exemplified by the incidence of gonococcal pharyngitis after receptive oral intercourse.

Given the length of the male urethra and the relatively smaller area of exposed genital mucosa via the urethral meatus, men had traditionally been thought of as being less susceptible to STD infection. However, microabrasions in the outer skin of the penile shaft sustained during sexual intercourse have been well documented as another important entry site for sexually transmitted organisms to reach the subcutaneous tissue. Moreover, the presence of one STD increases the chances of becoming infected with another—especially HIV. This is likely due to compromise

(Text continued on page 677)

Table 13.3 Sexually Transmitted Infections

Infectious Agent	Clinical Presentation	Diagnostic Reasoning	Treatment as Recommended by the CDC
Bacterial Infections			
Chancroid (*Haemophilus ducreyi*)	Single painful ulcer (irregular, erythematous, and undermined edges) with a unilateral painful abscess. Painful lymphadenopathy.	Probable diagnosis is made if: patient has one or more painful genital ulcers; no evidence of syphilis on serological test performed at least 7 days after onset of ulcers; the clinical presentation is typical for chancroid; and test for HSV is negative.	azithromycin (Zithromax) 1 g PO × 1 OR ceftriaxone (Rocephin) 250 mg IM × 1 OR ciprofloxacin (Cipro) 500 mg PO 2 times daily for 3 days OR erythromycin (E-mycin) 500 mg PO 4 times daily for 7 days
Chlamydia (*Chlamydia trachomatis*)	Most commonly, no reported symptoms. Patient may note an increase in mucopurulent discharge and bleeding with intercourse.	Yellow, mucopurulent discharge. Wet mount: >10 WBCs per high-power field (hpf). DNA probe—concurrent testing for *Neisseria gonorrhoeae* can be done with the same probe. Direct chlamydia enzyme immunoassay.	azithromycin (Zithromax) 1 g PO × 1 OR doxycycline (Vibramycin) 100 mg PO 2 times daily for 7 days
Gonorrhea (*Neisseria gonorrhoeae*)	Usually asymptomatic; partner may have an infection. Purulent yellow/green discharge. Gonococcal pharyngitis manifests as any bacterial pharyngitis, but 60% are asymptomatic.	Gonococcal culture, DNA probe. Urine DNA (initial 15 mL of a urinary void). Urine will typically have WBCs or epithelial cells infected with *N gonorrhoeae*.	ceftriaxone (Rocephine) 125 mg IM in a single dose OR cefixime (Suprax) 400 mg PO × 1 PLUS azithromycin (Zithromax) 1 g orally in a single dose OR doxycycline (Vibramycin) 100 mg PO 2 times daily × 7 days
Granuloma inguinale (*Klebsiella granulomatis*)	Chronic, progressive papule that ulcerates to a beefy red, painless granular area with clean, sharp rolled edges; inguinal swelling; late painful abscesses (buboes).	History of travel and sexual contact in endemically infected area. Cannot be cultured; stained tissue sample may show Donovan bodies (bacteria-filled vacuoles).	doxycycline (Vibramycin) 100 mg PO 2 times daily for at least 3 weeks and until all lesions have completely healed OR azithromycin (Zithromax) 1 g PO every week for at least 3 weeks and until all lesions have completely healed OR ciprofloxacin (Cipro) 750 mg PO 2 times daily for at least 3 weeks and until all lesions have completely healed OR

Continued

Table 13.3 Sexually Transmitted Infections—cont'd

Infectious Agent	Clinical Presentation	Diagnostic Reasoning	Treatment as Recommended by the CDC
			erythromycin (E-mycin) 500 mg PO 4 times daily for at least 3 weeks and until lesions have completely healed.
Lymphogranuloma venereum [LGV] (*Chlamydia trachomatis*)	Lymphadenopathy, anorectal swelling, and fistula formation.	History of travel and sexual contact in endemically infected area. Serological LGV complement fixation test: suspect disease if titer is above 1:16; test is diagnostic if titer is above 1:64.	doxycycline (Vibramycin) 100 mg PO 2 times daily for 21 days
Nongonococcal urethritis [NGU] (*Chlamydia trachomatis*)	Dysuria and urethral discharge (40% of patients); sparse, mucoid penile discharge, usually only after "milking" penis.	Gram stain smear of urethral exudate; culture for sugar fermentation reaction for NGU. Chlamydial DNA probe.	azithromycin (Zithromax) 1 g PO × 1 OR doxycycline (Vibramycin) 100 mg PO 2 times daily for 7 days
Syphilis (*Treponema pallidum*)	**Primary:** Painless ulcer at initial site of contact (chancre), adenopathy **Secondary:** Maculopapular rash on palms and soles, condyloma lata/moist, flat wart-like lesions, adenopathy **Tertiary/late:** Cardiac, neurological, ophthalmic, auditory, and gummatous lesions	Dark-field microscopy: Positive for spirochetes. Direct microhemagglutination-treponema pallidum (MHA-TP): Antibody test. Fluorescent treponemal antibody absorption (FTA-ABS): Antibody test reported as positive. Venereal Disease Research Laboratory (VDRL) rapid plasma reagin (RPR): Reported as reactive with a titer; indicates degree of infection.	benzathine penicillin G 2.4 million units IM × 1 **Early latent:** benzathine penicillin G 2.4 million units IM in a single dose **Late latent or latent syphilis of unknown duration:** benzathine penicillin G 7.2 million units total, administered as three doses of 2.4 million units IM at 1-week intervals **Neurosyphilis (CSF) (infection confirmed):** Aqueous crystalline penicillin G 18–24 million units per day, administered as 3–4 million units IV every 4 hours or continuous infusion for 10–14 days

Table 13.3 Sexually Transmitted Infections—cont'd

Infectious Agent	Clinical Presentation	Diagnostic Reasoning	Treatment as Recommended by the CDC
Viral Infections Herpes simplex virus (HSV) infection	**First outbreak:** Flu-like symptoms with adenopathy, tingling of the site before outbreak, and very painful vesicular lesions. Ulcers form, with circumscribed erythematous edges and white exudate centrally; lesions may last up to 12 days. **Recurrent outbreaks:** Symptoms may be similar but are usually less severe and of shorter duration (4–5 days).	Viral culture of vesicle fluid most accurate if done within 48 hours of outbreak. Tzanck smear from the base of an early vesicle. DNA probe from lesion scraping.	**First outbreak:** acyclovir (Zovirax) 400 mg PO 3 times daily for 7–10 days OR acyclovir (Zovirax) 200 mg PO 5 times a day for 7–10 days OR famciclovir (Famvir) 250 mg PO 3 times daily for 7–10 days OR valacyclovir (Valtrex) 1 g PO 2 times daily for 7–10 days **Recurrent outbreaks:** acyclovir (Zovirax) 400 mg 3 times daily for 5 days OR acyclovir (Zovirax) 800 mg PO 2 times daily for 5 days OR acyclovir (Zovirax) 800 mg PO 3 times daily for 2 days OR famciclovir (Famvir) 125 mg PO 2 times daily for 5 days OR famciclovir (Famvir) 1,000 mg PO 2 times daily for 1 day OR famciclovir (Famvir) 500 mg PO once, followed by 250 mg 2 times daily for 2 days OR valacyclovir (Valtrex) 500 mg PO 2 times daily for 3 days OR valacyclovir (Valtrex) 1 g PO daily for 5 days **Suppressive:** acyclovir (Zovirax) 400 mg PO 2 times daily famciclovir (Famvir) 250 mg PO 2 times daily valacyclovir (Valtrex) 500 mg PO daily valacyclovir (Valtrex) 1 g PO daily

Continued

Table 13.3   Sexually Transmitted Infections—cont'd

Infectious Agent	Clinical Presentation	Diagnostic Reasoning	Treatment as Recommended by the CDC
Human immunodeficiency virus (HIV) infection (For more about HIV, see Chapter 17.)	Fever, malaise, adenopathy. Rash may occur in first few weeks after infection (acute retroviral syndrome). Bloody diarrhea. Opportunistic infections. Increased HPV infections.	Positive enzyme immunoassay (EIA). Positive Western blot (WB).	Treat infections as recommended by CDC. Refer to specialist. Long-term counseling and management. Highly active antiretroviral therapy (HAART) is key for the treatment of HIV. Initiation of therapy is a function of T-cell count, viral load, and concurrent symptoms. Treatment is heavily influenced by the ability to comply with various treatment regimens.
Human papillomavirus (HPV) infection	History of multiple partners or sexual abuse. Positive history of HPV. Itching, foul discharge. May be asymptomatic. Fleshy, soft, pale-colored keratinized growths.	Acetic acid test: lesions turn white with application of vinegar.	**Patient-applied treatments:** podofilox (Condylox) 0.5% applied thinly 2 times daily for 3 days, then rest for 4 days; may repeat up to 4 cycles OR imiquimod (Aldara cream) 5% applied once a day at bedtime, 3 times a week for up to 16 weeks. Wash treatment area with soap and water 6–10 hours after application. **Clinician-applied treatments:** Cryotherapy and liquid nitrogen treatments— repeat every 1–2 weeks. OR podophyllin resin (Podofin) 10%–25% in benzoin— apply thinly, allow to dry; patient should wash off in 1–4 hours. OR trichloroacetic acid and bichloroacetic acid (TCA/ BCA) (Tri-Chlor) 80%– 90% applied by clinician and repeated weekly as needed OR Surgical removal

Table 13.3	Sexually Transmitted Infections—cont'd		
Infectious Agent	Clinical Presentation	Diagnostic Reasoning	Treatment as Recommended by the CDC
Protozoa			
Trichomoniasis (*Trichomonas vaginalis*)	Heavy, odorous, yellow-green watery discharge. May have complaints of itching, swelling, and redness.	Discharge may be frothy. Wet mount: motile protozoa and WBCs.	metronidazole (Flagyl) 2 g PO × 1 OR tinidazole (Tindamaz) 2 g PO × 1

of mucosal and outer skin barriers, as well as interactions on the molecular level, for example, human papillomavirus (HPV) as a cofactor for HIV infection. Infectious organisms themselves may also express various genetic virulence factors that render them more susceptible to sexual transmission, including surface proteins that facilitate epithelial adherence to the urethral lining.

Clinical Presentation/Diagnostic Reasoning/Management

Table 13.3 presents the treatment of male reproductive system infections and STDs commonly seen by primary-care providers. STDs are typically distinguished from one another by their clinical presentation, although many STDs are asymptomatic in men or present with milder symptoms than in women. (Chapter 14 presents information on infections and STDs that are commonly seen in women.)

It is critical that all patients receiving treatment for one STD also be screened for syphilis with a serum rapid plasma reagin, as well as offered screening for HIV infection. In addition, given the frequently asymptomatic nature of *Chlamydia* infection in both men and women, all persons being treated for *Neisseria gonorrhoeae* should be concurrently treated for *Chlamydia trachomatis,* because these two STDs often occur concurrently.

It is a basic tenet of STD treatment that all sexual partners must be notified of their potential for infection (regardless of the original source of infection or index case) and the need for testing and/or empiric treatment with an appropriate regimen. Reporting of many STDs to public health authorities is mandatory, but these laws differ on a state-by-state basis.

There is some debate whether methicillin-resistant *Staphylococcus aureus* (MRSA) can be considered a sexually transmitted disease. It is transmitted primarily through skin-to-skin and other close contact. Although the use of barrier methods such as condoms minimizes the risk of contracting an STD, this method will have

no effect on MRSA transmission unless all infected skin surfaces are fully covered. Because at least 30% of the population is colonized with *S aureus* and at least 2% with MRSA, the likelihood of transmission with intimate contact is possible.

Follow-up and Referral

STDs have traditionally been treated in the primary-care outpatient setting unless clinical symptoms meet criteria for hospital admission, such as severe pelvic inflammatory disease in women or initial presentation of HIV infection with or without the presence of opportunistic infection. Advancement in public health practices gave rise to the development of specialized, high-volume STD clinics to serve urban areas with high STD prevalence rates. However, cases that are refractory to established treatment guidelines may be referred to an infectious disease specialist for further diagnostic testing and individually tailored therapeutic regimens. Regardless of the treatment setting, beginning in the early teenage years, patients need to be asked and/or advised at every visit about sexual practices, the consistent use of condoms, and the benefits of abstinence. Patients with previous STD infection or those practicing high-risk sexual practices should be screened on a regular basis for common STDs including HIV, syphilis, *Chlamydia,* and *Neisseria gonorrhoeae.*

Patient Education

A resurgence in public education about sexual health is probably the most effective and efficient way to decrease the risk of this contagion. The clinician, while providing direct treatments, must also accept the responsibility for educating the patient about the need to seek treatment as soon as any symptoms appear. Persons most at risk are those with multiple sexual contacts, adolescents, and individuals who need further education. Patients should understand that active STD infection increases the chance of becoming infected with HIV, as well.

References

Evidence-Based Practice

Cornu, J, et al. (2012). A contemporary assessment of nocturia: Definition, epidemiology, pathophysiology, and management—A systematic review and meta-analysis. *Eur Assoc Urol* 62:877–890, 2012.

Bibliography

General

Dambro, MR. *Griffith's 5-minute clinical consult.* Lippincott Williams & Wilkins, Philadelphia, 2013.

Edmunds, MW, and Mayhew, MS. *Pharmacology for the primary care provider,* ed 4. Mosby/Elsevier, St. Louis, MO, 2013.

Fauci, AS, et al (Eds.). *Harrison's principles of internal medicine,* ed 18. McGraw-Hill, New York, 2011.

Kee, JL. *Laboratory and diagnostic tests with nursing implications,* ed 8. Prentice-Hall, Upper Saddle River, NJ, 2010.

Kumar, V, et al. Robbins *basic pathology,* ed 8. Saunders/Elsevier, St. Louis, MO, 2010.

McCance, KL, and Huether, SE. *Pathophysiology: The biologic basis for disease in adults and children,* ed 6. Elsevier Mosby, St. Louis, MO, 2010.

Papadakis, MA, and McPhee, SJ. *Current medical diagnosis and treatment,* ed 52. Lange/McGraw-Hill, New York, 2013.

Prostate Cancer/Prostatitis/Benign Prostatic Hyperplasia

American Urological Association. Clinical guidelines: Management of BPH (revised 2010). Retrieved from www.auanet.org/education/guidelines/benign-prostatic-hyperplasia.cfm

American Urological Association. Detection of prostate cancer. Retrieved from www.auanet.org/education/guidelines/prostate-cancer-detection.cfm

American Urological Association. Phi blood test. 2013. Retrieved from www.auanet.org/advnews/press_releases/article.cfm?articleNo=316

Barry, MJ, et al. American Urological Association symptom index for benign prostatic hyperplasia. *J Urol* 148:1549–1557, 1992.

Carter, HB, et al. Early detection of prostate cancer: AUA guideline. American Urological Association, 2013. Retrieved from www.auanet.org/education/guidelines/prostate-cancer-detection.cfm

Grunfeld, EA, et al. Andropause syndrome in men treated for metastatic prostate cancer: A qualitative study of the impact of symptoms. *Cancer Nurs* 35(1):63–69, 2012.

Krader, DG. PSA screening reduces deaths by 29% in a large trial. *Urol Times* 40(9):1–42, 2012.

Harden, JK, et al. Partners' long-term appraisal of their caregiving experience, marital satisfaction, sexual satisfaction, and quality of life 2 years after prostate cancer treatment. *Cancer Nurs* 36(2):104–113, 2013.

Howrey, BT, et al. The impact of PSA screening on prostate cancer mortality and overdiagnosis of prostate cancer in the United States. *J Gerontol A Biol Sci Med Sci* 68(1):56–61, 2013.

Ladjevardi, S, et al. Treatment with curative intent and survival in men with high-risk prostate cancer. A population-based study of 11,380 men with serum PSA level 20-100 ng/mL. *BJU Int* 111(3):381–388, 2013.

McVary, KT, et al. Management of BPH. American Urological Association and Research, Inc., 2010.

National Comprehensive Cancer Network. NCCN clinical guidelines in oncology: Prostate cancer. Retrieved from www.nccn.org/professionals/physician_gls/f_guidelines.asp

Parsons, JK, et al. Obesity and benign prostatic hyperplasia: Clinical connections, emerging etiological paradigms and future directions. *J Urol* 189(1):S102–S106, 2013.

Watson, RA, et al. Chronic pelvic pain in men treatment and management. 2013. Retrieved from http://emedicine.medscape.com/article/437745-treatment#a1156

Impotence/Erectile Dysfunction

Burn, RM, and Evans, JD. Avanafil for treatment of erectile dysfunction: Review of its potential. *Vasc Health Risk Managem* 8:517–523, 2012.

Gupta, BP, et al. The effect of lifestyle modification and cardiovascular risk factor reduction on erectile dysfunction: A systematic review and meta-analysis. *Arch Intern Med* 171(20):1797–1803, 2011.

Harte, CB, and Meston, DM. Recreational use of erectile dysfunction medications and its adverse effects on erectile function in young healthy men: The mediating role of confidence in erectile ability. *J Sex Med* 9(7):1852–1859, 2012.

Jiminez-Pacheco, A, et al. Influence of endogenous hormones and testosterone in the prostate cancer. Endocrine Abstracts 29, p 1561. 15th International and 14th European Congress of Endocrinology. Florence, Italy, May 2012.

Ledet, EM, et al. Characterization of germline copy number variation in high-risk African American families with prostate cancer. *Prostate* 73(6):614–623, 2013.

Lolong-Muh, J, et al. Erectile dysfunction following retropubic prostatectomy. *Br J Nurs* 22(4):54, 57–59, 2013.

Margolis, ST. Advisor forum: Low testosterone in young and healthy men. *Clin Advisor* 14(12):97, 2011.

Salyer, SW. Symptoms and treatment of low testosterone in men. *Clin Advisor* 16(5):50–55, 2013.

Shamloul, R, and Ghamen, H. Erectile dysfunction. *Lancet* 381(9861):153–165, 2013.

Washington, SL, and Shindel, AW. A once-daily dose of tadalafil for erectile dysfunction: compliance and efficacy. *Drug Design Dev Ther* 4:159–171, 2010.

Testicular Cancer

Maule, M, et al. Age at puberty and risk of testicular cancer: A meta-analysis. *Int J Andrology* 35(6):828–834, 2012.

National Comprehensive Cancer Network. NCCN clinical guidelines in oncology: Testicular cancer. V.1.2013. Retrieved from www.nccn.org/professionals/physician_gls/pdf/testicular.pdf

U.S. Preventive Services Task Force. Screening for testicular cancer: U.S. Preventive Services Task Force reaffirmation recommendation statement. *Ann Intern Med* 154(7):483–486, 2011.

Vantori, M. Testicular cancer. *Semin Oncol Nurs* 28(3):180–189, 2012.

Sexually Transmitted Diseases

Centers for Disease Control and Prevention. 2010 STD treatment guidelines. Retrieved from www.cdc.gov/std/treatment/2010

Kaloczi, L, et al. Sexually transmitted infections. In McCance, KL, and Huether, SE (Eds.), *Pathophysiology: The biologic basis for disease in adults and children,* ed 6. Mosby, St. Louis, 2010, pp 923–951.

Vidlar, A, et al. The effectiveness of dried cranberries (Vaccinium macrocarpon) in men with lower urinary tract symptoms. *Br J Nutr* 104(8):1171–1189, 2010.

Women's Health Problems

Jill Johnson, DNP, APRN, FNP-BC •
Debera J. Thomas, DNS, RN, FNP/ANP •
Brian Oscar Porter, MD, PhD, MPH

Chapter **14**

COMMON COMPLAINTS

■ BREAST MASS

A breast mass is a lump in the breast, and discovering such a mass is one of the most anxiety-producing events a woman may encounter in her lifetime. Seventy percent of patients with breast cancer present with a lump in the breast; 90% of these breast masses are discovered by the woman herself. Benign breast disorders (e.g., fibroadenoma) are referred to as *fibrocystic disease* or *mammary dysplasia* and are the most frequent breast lesions. In benign breast disorders, the breast masses or lumps are tender and usually bilateral. There may be a rapid fluctuation in the size of benign masses compared with breast malignancies, which slowly increase in size. In premenopausal women, masses should be reassessed in 2 to 3 weeks during a different phase of the monthly cycle. Typically, the tenderness and size of the mass may increase before menses. Fibrocystic breast disease is most common in women aged 30 to 50 years or in postmenopausal women on hormone replacement therapy.

Differential Diagnosis

The symptoms that differentiate a breast cyst from breast cancer are the tenderness, the fluctuations in size, and the multiplicity of lesions. It is difficult to distinguish a breast cyst from cancer based on clinical findings alone; therefore, aggressive testing is warranted. The first step is to rule out benign causes of a breast mass such as infection (e.g., mastitis or cellulitis). A mammogram is usually the first test performed; however, the breast tissue in patients with fibrocystic breast disease may be too radiodense to provide a conclusive diagnosis. A breast ultrasound will differentiate a cystic mass from a solid mass. A definitive diagnosis is made via breast biopsy. Aspiration of a cystic lesion will relieve the pain and will assist in the diagnosis.

Treatment

Treatment of fibrocystic breast disease consists of avoiding trauma; wearing a firm bra day and night; eliminating coffee, tea, and chocolate from the diet; and taking 400 IU of vitamin E daily. Patients may be prescribed diuretics, oral contraceptives, NSAIDs, and supplemental progestin. For patients with severe pain, danazol (Danocrine) 100 to 200 mg two times daily has been found to be helpful. Danazol is an androgen derivative that suppresses pituitary gonadotropins. With its androgenic effects, such as acne, edema, and hirsutism, most women find that the treatment is worse than the condition itself and prefer to try milder forms of pain relief.

Patients with benign breast lumps tend to become complacent about examining their breasts because they know the lumps are there. Breast self-exam (BSE) is just as important with fibrocystic breast disease as it is for women without breast lumps and should be stressed along with instruction on how to perform BSE.

■ DYSFUNCTIONAL UTERINE BLEEDING

A change in the pattern or volume of menstrual blood flow is a common health concern of women from puberty to menopause. The literature suggests that 10% to 20% of women have abnormal uterine bleeding (AUB) at least once during their reproductive lives. Women may describe abnormal bleeding episodes as infrequent, prolonged in duration, occurring between regular menstrual periods, and/or excessive. Normal duration of menses averages 4 to 5 days. There may be no evidence of genital tract lesions. The causes of AUB are divided into two major categories: organic and dysfunctional (endocrine). The diagnosis of dysfunctional uterine bleeding (DUB) is considered only after organic, systemic, and iatrogenic causes are eliminated.

Abnormal vaginal bleeding is, therefore, considered DUB if it arises from the endometrium of the uterus with no demonstrable organic cause. It is frequently the result of an endocrine abnormality of anovulation or short ovulatory cycles in which estrogen stimulates the growth of the endometrium without the stabilizing effect of progesterone and is not the result of a normal menstruation. In adolescence, anovulatory DUB is commonly caused by an immature hypothalamic-pituitary system that does not respond to the positive feedback effect of estrogen. In contrast, perimenopausal women experience variable menstrual cycle durations and bleeding episodes secondary to a decrease in ovarian response to gonadotropin stimulation. In addition, DUB is commonly seen during the reproductive years of women who are experiencing stress, are participating in a strenuous exercise program, or have undergone a large weight change.

Differential Diagnosis

Anovulatory bleeding is the cause of DUB in approximately 95% of women younger than age 20 years and in 90% of perimenopausal women who experience DUB for 2 to 3 years before the onset of menopause. In contrast, ovulatory cycles are associated with certain features such as midcycle pain, specific vaginal mucus changes, dysmenorrhea, and premenstrual breast tenderness. Although approximately one-half of ovulating women experience midcycle spotting, it is self-limiting. Irregular endometrial shedding may occur with the prolonged production of progesterone with a persistent corpus luteum resulting in DUB; however, DUB is a diagnosis of exclusion. Emphasis on a thorough history, physical exam, and pelvic exam and selected laboratory tests usually will yield the appropriate diagnosis. One must inquire about the woman's age, date of last menstrual period, birth control method, frequency of menses, amount of menstrual blood flow (e.g., the estimated number of pads or tampons used daily), duration of menses, and if there is a menstrual pattern change. In women who report profuse acute bleeding episodes, the diagnosis of pregnancy (e.g., passing tissue, nausea, vomiting, breast tenderness) must be excluded. In an ectopic pregnancy, the woman may complain of abdominal pain. Complaints of fainting spells may be indicative of a ruptured ectopic pregnancy.

Up to 10% of patients who use oral contraceptives (OCs) report irregular bleeding episodes. Any woman who presents with AUB and is age 35 years or older should be evaluated for cervical and uterine cancer. Malignancy must also be excluded. Endometrial sampling is an office procedure to rule out unchecked proliferation of the endometrium that can lead to hyperplasia and potentially endometrial adenocarcinoma. Similarly, a colposcopy, cervical biopsy, and endocervical curettage are used to diagnose cervical cancer. Women with a history of an abnormal Papanicolaou (Pap) smear test or ulcerated or friable lesions on the cervix should be referred for colposcopy. In addition, benign neoplasms such as uterine leiomyomas (fibroids), endometrial polyps, and adenomyomas are commonly seen in patients aged 25 to 45 years. Trauma and foreign bodies are seen more commonly in children. A less common cause of uterine bleeding is blood dyscrasia, such as von Willebrand's disease or thrombocytopenia purpura.

Laboratory work-up is directed by the history and physical exam findings and usually consists of hematocrit, hemoglobin, platelet count, and Pap and pregnancy tests. In severe bleeding, partial thromboplastin time, prothrombin time, and bleeding time tests are indicated. Hysteroscopy may be performed immediately before a dilation and curettage to assist in diagnosis of polyps, exophytic endometrial cancer, or fibroids. Prolactin level and thyroid function tests are ordered to rule out hyperprolactinemia and hypothyroidism, respectively.

Treatment

Management of DUB is directed toward controlling bleeding and preventing a recurrence. For teenagers, management includes observation for those with mild cases and no anemia, medroxyprogesterone (if the patient is not sexually active), or OCs for sexually active teenagers. For women of reproductive age, treatment is based on the woman's desire for fertility or contraception. For women who cannot take OCs, medroxyprogesterone is offered. OCs containing ethinyl estradiol are used in acute bleeding episodes. For women with severe acute bleeding, but who remain hemodynamically stable, conjugated estrogen is used until bleeding stops.

■ DYSPAREUNIA

Dyspareunia is painful sexual intercourse that can occur as a result of either introduction of the penis into the vagina or deep penile penetration. Dyspareunia can also be experienced by lesbians with introduction of multiple fingers or sex toys. The pain a patient experiences can be a consequence of vaginal inflammation, structural (anatomical) abnormalities, vaginal atrophy or insufficient lubrication, pelvic pathology, or psychological issues.

Because patients tend not to report painful sexual intercourse, it is difficult to determine the incidence. A review of studies reporting the prevalence of chronic pelvic pain indicates that the rates of dyspareunia ranged from 1.3% to 45.7% in over 154 studies that included over 35,973 women. One study of 313 patients documented that more than 60% had experienced dyspareunia at some point in their lives. Risk factors include history of sexual trauma, history of sexually transmitted infections (STIs), recurrent candidiasis infection, poor hygiene, menopause, psychological issues, and difficulties in the relationship.

Differential Diagnosis

Obtaining a thorough history from the patient is essential in ascertaining the cause of dyspareunia. As noted earlier, pain may occur with initial or deep penetration and may occur with initial intercourse or after a long time of pain-free experience. The patient may complain of vaginal discharge or irritation. There may be a history of unrelated pelvic pain, recent pregnancy and childbirth, trauma, or surgery. The patient may, on questioning, reveal difficulty in using tampons or difficulty with prior pelvic exams.

On physical exam, the patient may present with signs of vulvar or vaginal mucosal irritation, inflammation, lesions, discharge, atrophy, hymenal remnants, Bartholin's cyst or abscess, or vestibulitis. *Vaginismus,* the involuntary contraction of perineal muscles, may occur during the speculum exam, impeding full visualization and examination of the vaginal vault and cervix. The clinician must proceed with sensitivity, allowing the patient control over the pelvic exam. The bimanual exam may reveal pelvic mass, cervical motion tenderness, uterine prolapse, rectocele, or cystocele.

The laboratory work-up is directed by findings from the history and physical exam and usually consists of urinalysis, wet mount of vaginal discharge, and cervical cultures. Urinalysis is useful in identifying any urinary tract conditions that may be a contributing factor to the source of the pain. The presence of white blood cells, red blood cells, or bacteria may indicate a urinary tract infection. Wet mount examination of vaginal discharge can reveal the presence of bacterial vaginosis *(Gardnerella vaginalis),* trichomoniasis, or candidiasis. Cervical cultures are useful in determining the presence of *Chlamydia* and gonorrhea.

Treatment

Management of dyspareunia depends on the symptoms and etiology. If the cause is atrophic vaginitis, estrogens, especially vaginal estrogens, may be helpful for postmenopausal women. Water-soluble lubricant (Astroglide, K-Y Jelly) can be used for vaginal lubrication and comfort. STIs are treated with appropriate antibiotic therapy. Progressive dilation and muscle awareness exercises such as Kegel exercises are recommended for treatment of vaginismus, hymenal strands, anatomically narrow introitus, and scar tissue. If psychological factors, such as sexual trauma, relationship conflicts, stress, and a restrictive sexual attitude, appear to be the cause, referral to a psychotherapist is indicated.

■ PELVIC PAIN

Pelvic pain is seen in 1% to 2% of patients in primary-care practice. Pelvic pain is categorized as acute, chronic, or recurrent and presents as both pelvic or lower abdominal pain. Genitourinary, gastrointestinal, or musculoskeletal system diseases or dysfunctions may cause sudden, acute pain in both areas. Chronic or recurrent pelvic pain is described as less urgent. Recurrent pain can be associated with menstruation or unrelated to menses. The origin of chronic pain can be related to benign or malignant neoplasms or characterized as psychogenic.

Differential Diagnosis

An acute onset of pelvic pain may be the result of pelvic disorders including pelvic inflammatory disease (PID); ruptured ovarian cyst; torsion of ovarian cyst, ovary, or fallopian tube; or ectopic pregnancy with rupture. PID accounts for about 20% of acute pelvic pain in women, ovarian cysts for up to 40%, and adnexal torsion for about 16%. Ten percent of women who report acute pelvic pain may have extrapelvic disease such as appendicitis.

Women reporting recurring pain with menstruation may have primary or secondary dysmenorrhea, endometriosis, adenomyosis, chronic PID, and/or pain related to intrauterine devices. Endometriosis is seen in up to 50% of women with chronic pelvic pain. Recurrent pain that is not associated with menses may have many causes, including Mittelschmerz (release of mature ovum from ovary), leaking ovarian cysts, incompletely treated or recurrent pelvic infections, or urinary tract infections. Nongynecological pathology includes adhesions, inflammatory bowel disease, and irritable bowel syndrome. However, for as many as 37% of women with chronic or recurrent pelvic pain, no physiological cause of the pain can be determined.

Treatment

Treatment for pelvic pain depends on the cause. Differential Diagnosis 14.1 outlines the differential diagnosis for pelvic pain and possible treatments.

■ VULVOVAGINITIS (VAGINAL ITCHING, BURNING, AND DISCHARGE)

Vulvovaginitis is defined as the simultaneous inflammation of the vulva and vagina. The patient complains of vaginal itching, burning, and vaginal discharge, which comprise the triad of vulvovaginitis symptoms and account for some of the most common reasons patients seek health care. Although frequently the result of infection, vulvovaginitis may also have noninfectious causes including allergic reactions, foreign body, atrophic vaginitis, traumatic vaginitis, or collagen vascular disease.

Differential Diagnosis

The delicate vaginal environment can be easily altered by numerous internal and external influences. In addition to the effects of normal changes in the body's hormonal condition, such as ovulatory midcycle mucus production, menstruation, or the atrophic mucosal changes that occur after menopause, the use of antibiotics, presence of diabetes mellitus or glycosuria, and stress can also cause symptoms of vulvovaginitis.

A thorough history should include time of symptom onset and a full description of the vaginal discharge and the relationship of the symptoms to the menstrual cycle, coitus, and use of medications (especially antibiotics). A detailed sexual history helps to identify whether the patient is at increased risk for the development of a sexually transmitted infection. It is important to determine whether the patient's partner has symptoms of infection (penile discharge or lesion) and if the woman has used spermicidal preparations, douches, bubble bath, or feminine hygiene deodorants and if she has done any self-treatment.

The most common cause of symptomatic complaints of abnormal vaginal discharge, itching, and burning is infection from bacteria, yeast, or parasites. Bacterial vaginosis caused primarily by *Gardnerella* accounts for almost 50% of all vaginal infections, followed closely by candidiasis (approximately 25%) and trichomoniasis (approximately 20%). Each infection is diagnosed based on the clinical presentation, which includes the type,

Differential Diagnosis 14.1 Pelvic Pain

Clinical Findings	Diagnosis	Treatment
Lower abdominal tenderness Cervical motion tenderness Adnexal tenderness	Pelvic inflammatory disease (PID)	Antibiotics (see CDC guidelines)
Oral temperature above 101°F (38.3°C) ↑ Erythrocyte sedimentation rate Abnormal cervical/vaginal discharge abscess or pregnancy. Evidence of *Chlamydia trachomatis* or *Neisseria* *gonorrhoeae* ↑ WBCs		Hospitalization may be required for uncertain diagnosis, pelvic abscess, or pregnancy.
Smooth mobile adnexal mass Percussive dullness on affected side Diffuse pain/pressure (if ruptured)	Ovarian cyst	Oral contraceptives may hasten cyst resolution. Cysts >6 cm require evaluation via laparoscopy and possible surgical removal.
Localized or diffuse colicky or dull pain Shoulder pain with hemoperitoneum Rebound tenderness/guarding (if ruptured) Abnormal vaginal bleeding Amenorrhea Quantitative serum hCG immunoassay positive (1 week after conception)	Ectopic pregnancy	Surgery
Dysmenorrhea Dyspareunia Pain on defecation Infertility	Endometriosis	Oral contraceptive if contraception is needed. NSAIDs if no contraception is needed. Possible laparoscopy to rule out pelvic pathology.
Flank pain, suprapubic pain, dysuria, frequency Fever, nausea, vomiting	Urinary tract infection	Antibiotics (see Chapter 12 for specific treatment for UTIs).
Acute, progressively severe pain Mass/tenderness on affected side on palpation Symptoms more impressive than exam	Adnexal torsion	Hospitalization/surgery
Initially: Epigastric to midabdominal pain and anorexia Later: Lower quadrant to suprapubic to flank pain and vomiting Rebound tenderness/guarding: tenderness over McBurney's point Psoas/obturator sign Low-grade fever	Appendicitis	Hospitalization and surgery
Palpable mass on uterus Back pain/pressure Dysmenorrhea/menorrhagia Anemia Frequency/constipation	Uterine fibroid (leiomyomas)	Hysterectomy Uterine artery embolectomy
Variable in intensity of pain lasting up to several hours	Mittelschmerz	No treatment. OCs may be offered to inhibit ovulation.

amount, color, odor, and pH of discharge. Physical exam includes visualization of the vulva and vagina for the presence of lesions, discharge, erythema, or atrophy. The cervix is examined for the presence of lesions, erosion, friability, or erythema. During the bimanual exam, the clinician should pay particular attention to the presence of cervical motion tenderness or the presence of adnexal and uterine tenderness or masses.

Laboratory work-up is directed by findings from the history and physical exam and usually consists of a saline wet mount of vaginal discharge to determine the presence of *Gardnerella, Trichomonas,* or atrophic vaginitis

and a potassium hydroxide wet mount to determine the presence of *Candida.* A Gram stain of vaginal discharge can reveal the presence of gonorrhea. In addition, a urinalysis should be performed to rule out the presence of a urinary tract infection.

Treatment

Differential Diagnosis 14.2 presents the differential diagnoses for vulvovaginitis. Treatment for vulvovaginitis depends on the cause. Drugs Commonly Prescribed 14.1 lists the treatments for the different causes of vulvovaginitis.

Differential Diagnosis 14.2   Vulvovaginitis

Clinical Findings	Diagnosis
Vaginal discharge, mild or none	Physiological leukorrhea
Vaginal pH: <4.5	
No amine odor	
KOH exam: negative	
Pruritus	Candidiasis
Dyspareunia	
Vulvar erythema and edema	
Thick white floccular nonadherent vaginal discharge	
Vaginal pH: <4.5	
No amine odor	
KOH exam: Pseudohyphae	
Saline microscopy: Pseudohyphae	
Malodorous, gray-yellow-green watery or thick adherent vaginal discharge	Bacterial vaginosis (*Gardnerella)*
Burning with urination	
No dyspareunia	
pH: >4.5	
Amine odor present	
KOH exam is positive	
Saline microscopy: Clue cells	
Homogeneous, malodorous purulent, green-yellow, thick, frothy vaginal discharge	Trichomoniasis
"Strawberry" cervix	
Vulvovaginal erythema	
Itching	
Burning on urination	
Dyspareunia	
pH: 5–6	
Amine odor is absent	
KOH exam is negative	
Saline microscopy: Motile trichomonads	
Dyspareunia	Atrophic vaginitis
Vaginal dryness	
Vestibular and vaginal thinning	
Vulvular and vaginal burning	
Bleeding	
Itching	
pH: >6	
Amine odor is present.	
KOH exam is negative.	

Drugs Commonly Prescribed 14.1   Vulvovaginitis

Drug	Indication	Adverse Reactions and Prescribing Considerations
butoconazole 2% (Gynazole-1 or Mycelex-3) cream 5 g intravaginally once at bedtime OR	Candidiasis	Adverse reactions include vulvovaginal burning, itching, irritation, swelling, cramping, abdominal pain, headache.
miconazole 2% cream (Monistat) 5 g intravaginally (1,200 mg at bedtime for 1 day; or 200 mg at bedtime for 3 days; or 100 mg at bedtime for 7 days) OR		Do not use contraceptive diaphragm or condoms within 3 days.
clotrimazole 1% (Lotrimin) cream 5 g intravaginally for 7–14 days OR clotrimazole 2% cream intravaginally for 3 days OR clotrimazole 100 mg vaginal tablet for 7 days OR tioconazole 6.5% (Vagistat-1) ointment 5 g intravaginally in a single application OR terconazole 0.4% cream 5 g intravaginally for 7 days OR		Do not use tampons, douches, or spermicides within 7 days.
terconazole 0.8% cream 5 g intravaginally for 3 days fluconazole (Diflucan) 150 mg PO ×1 for uncomplicated; if severe 150 mg every 72 hours ×2 doses; for recurrent 150 mg weekly ×6 months	Recurrent or chronic candidiasis	Adverse reactions include headache, nausea, abdominal pain, GI upset, dizziness, taste perversion, and hepatotoxicity. Use with caution in the elderly. Pregnancy Category C Not recommended for use with nursing mothers.
Metronidazole 500 mg PO 2 times daily ×7 days	Bacterial vaginosis (BV)	Avoid ingestion of alcohol with metronidazole and for 24 hours after treatment is complete.
OR metronidazole gel 0.75% one full applicator (5 g) intravaginally daily for 5 days OR clindamycin cream 2% one full applicator (5 g) intravaginally at bedtime ×3 or 7 days		Adverse reactions include GI upset, metallic taste, dysuria, cystitis, incontinence, *Candida* overgrowth, seizures, peripheral neuropathy, neutropenia. Pregnancy Category B during 2nd and 3rd trimesters. Preferred orally in pregnancy. Do not use in patients with a history of enteritis or colitis. Do not use contraceptive diaphragm or condom for 72 hours after treatment. Pregnancy Category B Not recommended for nursing mothers.
metronidazole 2 g PO single dose OR metronidazole 500 mg PO 2 times daily ×7 days for recurrent infection.	Trichomoniasis	Must treat partner. Avoid alcohol for 24 hours after treatment is completed.
estrogen cream (Premarin vaginal cream) 0.5 g twice-weekly continuous OR 21 days of therapy followed by 7 days off therapy.	Atrophic vaginitis	Decrease or eliminate based on symptoms.

■ FAMILY PLANNING

From menarche to menopause, a woman's health concerns may include controlling fertility. Women need to be able to prevent pregnancy, plan intervals between pregnancies, and find help if a desired pregnancy is not achieved. These decisions are related to one's values, professional role, friends, family, cultural and religious beliefs, self-perception, health status, economics, sexual lifestyle, options accessible, and partner status. Ideally, the birth control option should be affordable, easy to use, easy to obtain, 100% effective, safe, mutually acceptable, and reversible. The most popular birth control methods are oral contraceptives (OCs), the diaphragm, and condoms. Other popular choices include Depo-Provera injections and the copper intrauterine device.

Although preventing pregnancy is a major concern, some lifestyle behaviors may also cause concern for acquiring a sexually transmitted infection (STI). To control both pregnancy and disease, routine health care is important. The gynecological history and physical exam are essential to address both issues.

The gynecological history reviews risks for STIs, as well as past and current birth control methods, and identifies needs for health promotion. It also identifies sexual dysfunction or sexual concerns. Reviewing anatomy and physiology with the patient may help her understand her body and result in healthier lifestyle choices. Other items important in history taking include menstrual cycle information; age at menarche; use of tampons or pads; change in menses; number of sex partners in the past year and lifetime; age at initiation of coitus; dyspareunia; orgasms; history of STIs; medications used; results of previous Papanicolaou (Pap) smears and resolutions; and cigarette, drug, and/or alcohol use or abuse. It is important to obtain a basic health history as well to identify potential contraindications to new or previous birth control methods.

Wording questions in a nonjudgmental, supportive, accepting manner enables the patient to be open and honest in an area of great sensitivity and possible pain. The clinician addresses areas of concern, such as poor body image, depression, poor nutrition, emotional or physical problems, myths, abuse from others, smoking, obesity, alcohol or drug abuse, and family problems.

Physical exam includes blood pressure, weight, height, last menstrual period, breast cancer and breast self-exam (BSE) teaching, bimanual pelvic, a Pap smear, and culture for STIs and other infections as appropriate to the patient's risk factors and presenting information. During the initial examination, baseline lab studies should be done including a lipid profile and complete blood count (CBC). Other tests (dependent on presenting history) are thyroid profile, fasting blood sugar, or liver profile. In addition, after a 10-year period of OC use, a liver profile should be obtained.

Some facilities require signed consent for the birth control method selected that ensures that the patient has been given, in writing, full information on the use, risks, benefits, and follow-up needs of the method. Other facilities educate the patient at the time of the visit and give her the product insert and educational material to read at home. Ideally, both partners, if possible, need comprehensive information on birth control methods so that their choice is an educated decision based on their lifestyle and needs. The success or failure of any birth control method depends on the woman's motivation, adherence, partner support, consistency, and comfort. The main methods of birth control are listed in Table 14.1.

Barrier Methods

Barrier methods include male and female condoms, the diaphragm, and cervical cap. Some barrier methods have the dual advantage of preventing pregnancy and STIs. The most common STIs are caused by herpes simplex virus, human papillomavirus (HPV), HIV, *Neisseria gonorrhoeae,* and *Chlamydia.* Controlling HPV also reduces the risk of cervical cancer. Adverse effects of barrier methods are similar in some ways: messiness, handling of genitalia, precoital interruption of spontaneity, and allergy or contact dermatitis. The use of barrier methods requires motivation on the part of both partners.

Male Condom

The *male condom* is the most common barrier method and is most effective when combined with a spermicide such as nonoxynol-9. Condoms are available in various sizes, colors, flavors, strengths, and lubrication. They should not be applied tightly. The tip should extend one-half inch beyond the penis to collect ejaculate. Care must be taken during withdrawal of the penis to prevent the condom from coming off and spilling the semen. Other adverse effects include irritation, allergic reaction, unfavorable oral sex, and accidental splitting of the condom. Condoms are very effective, and when used with a spermicide the failure rate is equivalent to that of OCs. However, condoms may not be the best choice for the under-25-year-old group because of noncompliance, inconsistent use, and low motivation.

Female Condom

The *female condom* is a device that is disposable and made of seamless polyurethane. It fits loosely inside the vagina and covers the perineum. There are flexible rims on both ends. The inner rim sits on the closed end and is compressed for placement into the vagina over the cervix, which prevents contact between body secretions. The condom is soft, lubricated by spermicide, and inexpensive and may be purchased over the counter. Many patients state that it is difficult to handle, however. Adverse effects include irritation and allergic reaction. The

Table 14.1	Methods of Birth Control				
Method	**Type**	**Mode of Action**	**Duration**	**Rate (%)***	
Barrier Methods	Male condom	Prevents sperm from entering vagina.	Each use	3–12	
	Female condom	Prevents sperm from entering cervix.	Each use	5–21	
	Diaphragm	Prevents sperm from entering cervix.	Each use	2–20	
	Cervical cap	Prevents sperm from entering cervix.	48 hours	2–20	
	Vaginal contraceptive sponge	Prevents sperm from entering cervix.	24 hours	18–28	
	Spermicide nonoxynol-9	Immobilizes and kills sperm.	Each use	2–30	
Hormonal Methods	Combination oral contraceptives	Inhibits ovulation, hostile environment, slows tubal transport.	Continuous	0.1	
	Progestin-only pills	Inhibits ovulation, hostile environment, slows tubal transport.	Continuous	1–4	
	Depo-medroxyproges-terone (Depo-Provera)	Blunts LH, inhibits sperm penetration, endometrium unreceptive.	90 days	0.3	
Intrauterine Devices (IUDs)	Copper T-380A	Prevents fertilization and implantation.	10 years	0.8	
	Mirena	Prevents fertilization and implantation.	5 years		
Regulated Abstinence	Calendar calculation	Prevents fertilization.	Each cycle	9	
	Temperature and mucous changes	Prevents fertilization.	Each cycle	4	
Postcoital Controls	Chance	No protection.	N/A	85	
	Withdrawal	Prevents sperm from entering vagina.	Each use	18	
	Postcoitus douche	Flushes sperm from vagina.	N/A	—	
	Emergency contraception	Interferes with fertilization or implant.	Each use (Plan B)	2	
Sterilization	Female	Fallopian tubes cut/tied to prevent ovum moving to uterus or sperm entering tube.	Permanent	0.4	
	Male	Vas deferens cut to prevent sperm from leaving male.	Permanent	0.15	

*Percentage of women experiencing an accidental pregnancy in the first year of use.

failure rate of the female condom is 5% to 21% when used correctly and comparable to the efficacy of the diaphragm.

Diaphragm

A *diaphragm* is a latex hemisphere with a flexible rim that fits over the cervix. The failure rate is 2% to 20% when used with spermicidal jelly. This method allows the woman control and has no systemic side effects. The largest size that covers the cervix comfortably is best. Once the device has been fitted, the patient should insert and remove the diaphragm, then return for a recheck after 1 week of practice while using a backup contraceptive method. Before insertion, 1 teaspoon of spermicide is placed in the cup and a small amount is spread around the rim. The diaphragm must be left in place for 8 hours after intercourse; if additional intercourse is desired, additional spermicide is instilled in the vagina. The diaphragm should not be left in place for more than 12 to 18 hours. Once removed, the diaphragm is washed with a mild soap, dried, and stored. Before the diaphragm is

used again, it should be held up to the light to check for holes, tears, and breaks. The patient should be instructed to urinate before inserting and after removing the diaphragm to reduce the risk of urinary tract infections (UTIs). Under normal circumstances, the diaphragm is fitted during the annual gynecological visit; however, if the patient has pelvic surgery, pregnancy, or a weight change of 10 to 20 pounds, the diaphragm must be refitted.

Cervical Cap

The *cervical cap* is a cup-shaped plastic or rubber device that fits snugly around the cervix with a failure rate similar to that of the diaphragm. Like the diaphragm, the cap is used with a spermicide. Because the cap is smaller than the diaphragm, it may be more difficult to insert and remove. The advantage of the cervical cap is that it can be used in women who are unable to use a diaphragm because of a relaxed anterior vaginal wall or in those who have recurrent UTIs with the use of the diaphragm. The cervical cap should not be left in place for longer than 12 to 18 hours and should not be used during menstruation because of the slight risk of toxic shock syndrome (TSS). Only women with normal Pap smears should use the cap, and a repeat Pap smear should be obtained 3 months after its use is initiated. Adverse effects of the cervical cap are similar to those associated with the diaphragm: allergic reactions, irritation, and displacement.

Spermicidal Methods
Vaginal Contraceptive Sponge

A *vaginal contraceptive* sponge is a one-size-fits-all disposable sponge of polyurethane treated with nonoxynol-9, which protects against pregnancy but not against STIs. The sponge is placed under tap water and rinsed, then inserted into the vagina. Adverse effects include displacement, irritation, and a slight risk of TSS (1 per 2 million sponges). It should be left in place for 6 hours after intercourse, but not more than 24 to 30 hours (depending on product) to minimize the risk of TSS. It is not recommended for use during menses or puerperium to decrease risk of TSS.

Contraceptive Foam, Cream, Film, Jelly, and Suppository

Nonoxynol-9 is the spermicide contained in contraceptive foam, cream, film, jelly, and suppositories. These products have an overall failure rate of 2% to 30% when used correctly. The advantages to these forms of contraception are that they are available without a prescription, easy to use, readily available, and relatively inexpensive. Nonoxynol-9 may have some virucidal and bactericidal activity but does not offer any protection against HIV, as once thought. The disadvantage of these products is that they can cause irritation and allergic reactions.

Hormonal Methods

Hormonal methods include oral contraceptives—both combination and progestin-only pills and medroxyprogesterone (Depo-Provera) injections. The implantable progestin contraceptive levonorgestrel (Norplant) is no longer available in the United States.

Oral Contraceptives

Oral contraceptives (OCs) contain either a combination of estrogen and progestin or progestin only (commonly called the "mini-pill"). The most popular OCs are the 4-week cycle combination pills. These contain estrogen and progestin and are taken each day for 3 weeks, with inert (placebo) pills for the fourth week. The nonhormonal (fourth) week is the time when withdrawal uterine bleeding occurs. A recent introduction is the cycle of OCs that contain 84 active and 7 inert pills (Seasonale). This results in menses only every 3 months (4 times a year).

The estrogen-progestin OC prevents pregnancy by suppressing the hypothalamic releasing factor that inhibits the release of follicle-stimulating hormone and luteinizing hormone from the anterior pituitary, thereby preventing ovulation; estrogen in the pill inhibits implantation by changing normal uterine lining maturation, and the progestins slow ovum transport and uterine motility. Progestins also cause the cervical mucus to become thick and scanty, slowing sperm transport and capacitation. In addition, pH is altered, and the cervical and uterine environment becomes hostile to sperm. If taken as directed, OCs have a failure rate of less than 0.5%; however, the typical failure rate is 3%.

Ethinyl estradiol (EE) is currently the most popular estrogen used in OCs in the United States. The progestins used today include desogestrel (in Mircette, Cyclessa, Ortho-Cept, Desogen), levonorgestrel (in Alesse, Nordette, Seasonale, Trivora, Triphasil), norethindrone (in Estrostep, Norinyl 1/35, Ortho-Novum 1/35 and 7/7/7, Necon 1/35, Modicon, Ovcon 35, Loestrin 1.5/30, Tri-Norinyl), norgestimate (in Ortho-Cyclen, Ortho-Tri-Cyclen), drospirenone (in Yasmin), and *dl*-norgestrel (in Lo-Ovral, Low-Ogestrel).

All progestins, even in low doses, offer excellent cycle control and minimal metabolic changes. Progestins have variable estrogenic, androgenic, and progestational effects. The third generation progestins (desogestrel, drospirenone, norgestimate) are the least androgenic and are particularly good for women with acne or hirsutism. Progestins may also affect plasma levels of clotting factor, blood vessel disease, diabetes, lipids, and other changes discussed separately in the chapter.

The amounts of estrogen and progestin in OC pills have been greatly reduced since their inception. The lower the effective dose, the lower the adverse effects; the lowest acceptable dose is guided by the ability of the pill to prevent breakthrough bleeding. Breakthrough bleeding is an undesirable adverse effect. Estrogen content is usually 20 to 35 mcg of EE per tablet, with no more than 50 mcg available in the United States. Progestin content ranges from 0.1 to 1.5 mg. Both the estrogen and progestin doses may either be constant in a cycle pack (in monophasic contraceptives) or vary (in multiphasic contraceptives). The ratio of estrogen to progestin in combination pills can be 1:5 or 1:50; most commonly, it is 1:10 to 1:30. In the normal menses cycle, the ratio is 1:10 (early follicular), 1:5 (preovulation), and 1:30 (luteal phase). Multiphasic OCs are used in an attempt to emulate the menstrual cycle but may be associated with a higher incidence of breakthrough bleeding than monophasic pills.

To prevent ovulation, the OCs should be started either with the onset of menses (same-day start) or on the first Sunday of the week the menses starts (Sunday start). In a Sunday start, a backup method (e.g., condom or abstinence) should be used for at least 7 days.

The effectiveness of OCs is dependent on patient adherence. Each pill must be taken at the same hour, every day. Once the start date is established and the pack started, there is no waiting or menstrual impact to start the subsequent pack. As soon as the initial pack is completed, the next pack is started on the next day. Patients may need suggestions on how to take the pill on time and every day, whether it is when brushing teeth or at meal time or bedtime, as long as it is the same hour, every day. For women who experience nausea when taking OCs, taking them at bedtime can minimize this adverse effect.

The combination pills are provided in 28-day pill packs, color-coded by dose and time, and include the 21 active and 7 inert tablets. Some manufacturers include iron supplements in the 7 inert (placebo) pills; some eliminate the 7 inert pills and provide a 21-day pack. To keep a patient adherent and on time, it is usually best to recommend the habit of a pill a day and without stopping the last 7 days, to prevent forgetting when to restart again.

If the patient forgets to take one or more doses of the OC, the following guidelines are recommended:

- One dose missed at any time in the cycle: Take the missed dose as soon as remembered and the next dose at the usual time.
- Two doses missed during the first 2 weeks of the cycle: Take two doses daily for 2 days, then resume one dose a day. Use a backup form of birth control for the balance of the cycle.
- Two doses missed during the third week of the cycle: Take one dose daily until the last day (day 21), dispose of the remaining pills, and begin the new OC pack that day. Use a backup form of birth control for 7 days.
- Three or more doses missed at any time in the cycle: Take one dose daily until the last day (day 21), dispose of the remaining pills, and begin the new OC pack that day. Use a backup form of birth control for 7 days.

Some patients experience breakthrough bleeding with missed pills and doubling of pills. Some practitioners do not advocate using the methods outlined above but instead tell their patients to discontinue the pack, use a barrier method, and restart with a new pack when the regular menses begins. If menses does not occur as usual, a pregnancy test must be performed.

Patients need special instructions when starting OCs if they had a recent full-term delivery, are nursing, had a recent abortion or miscarriage, have infrequent or irregular menses, or are using other medications.

Many patients inquire about starting or restarting OCs postpartum. The Food and Drug Administration (FDA) package insert indicates that because the postpartum period lends itself to a higher risk of thromboembolism, OCs should be started no earlier than 4 to 6 weeks after delivery in nonnursing mothers. Ovulation rarely takes place before 4 weeks postpartum of a full-term pregnancy; however, if a patient is using drugs (such as bromocriptine [Parlodel]) to suppress lactation, ovulation may occur earlier, and the pill should be started by day 14 postpartum.

Similarly, many patients who are breastfeeding inquire about starting on OCs. Because estrogen decreases the amount and quality of breast milk, OCs are not recommended for lactating women. Conversely, progestins actually promote breast milk production, so that progestin-only OCs should be used in women who are breastfeeding and desiring contraception. Combination estrogen and progestin oral contraceptives should not be prescribed until at least 6 weeks postpartum.

Because ovulation is a possibility within 14 days after either a recent abortion or miscarriage, OCs should be started either immediately or no later than 7 days after a first-trimester (5–13 weeks) abortion. After a midtrimester abortion, the OC should be started the same way as after a full-term pregnancy.

If a patient is not pregnant (as confirmed by test), OCs may be started at any time, with backup contraception for the first cycle of pills. In women with amenorrhea or infrequent cycles, discontinuance of the OC may leave them anovulatory or fully amenorrheic if their history includes secondary amenorrhea, oligomenorrhea, or irregular cycles. These patients should, therefore, consider another method of birth control.

Ineffective contraception and breakthrough bleeding may occur as the result of an interaction between the OC and drugs taken simultaneously. Table 14.2 presents common drug interactions. The exact mechanism of action is not clear, but it may be the result of the alteration of the gastrointestinal tract's absorption ability or alteration of enzymatic action on medication (either accelerating or decelerating metabolism). It is often difficult to modify drug prescriptions in illness and far simpler and safer to consider another form of birth control.

The combination OC is the most effective reversible form of birth control, relatively inexpensive, and least invasive method of correcting painful and irregular cycles. Some of the other benefits include reduced blood loss, resulting in lower incidence of anemia; less risk of ectopic pregnancy and salpingitis; fewer ovarian cysts; reduction in dysmenorrhea; reduction in risk of ovarian and endometrial cancer; improvement in acne; decreased risk for developing myomas in long-term (greater than 4 years) users; and a beneficial effect on bone mass. In general, these benefits reduce the need for costly hospitalizations.

The benefits and safety of OCs are dependent on adherence, but are also affected by other factors such as smoking. There is an increased risk of cardiovascular disease and thromboembolic disease in women who are older than 35 years of age and who smoke while taking OCs. Women older than 40 years of age who are nonsmokers may safely continue low-dose OCs. OC use is safest throughout the menstrual life in women who are

Table 14.2	Oral Contraceptives: Drug Interactions	
Drug Interactions	Effectiveness	Drugs
Drug effect on OCs	Increased effectiveness Decreased effectiveness Possible decreased effectiveness	Carbamazepine
OC effect on drugs	Decreased effectiveness	Acetaminophen, benzodiazepines, guanethidine, methyldopa, oral anticoagulants, oral hypoglycemics
	Increased effectiveness	Alcohol, antidepressants, benzodiazepines, beta blockers, corticosteroids, theophylline

of normal weight, are nonsmokers, have normal blood pressure (BP) and cholesterol, have no diabetes, and have no family history of heart disease. Consequently, a full history, gynecological exam, Pap smear, infection checks, lipid profile, and CBC lab tests should be performed before an OC is prescribed. Evaluation of the history, physical exam, and lab results is necessary to prevent adverse effects.

OCs have a wide range of adverse effects, from simple to more serious. Primarily, the constant presence of low-level hormones creates a pregnancy-like environment in the body. Thyroid hormone and cortisol levels may be elevated. Progestins may alter the lipid profile. Estrogens decrease glucose tolerance, and women with diabetes should be monitored closely if using OCs. Estrogen-related increases in clotting factors result in an increased risk of thromboembolism. Women who will be undergoing surgery and postoperative bed confinement should discontinue OCs at least 4 weeks before surgery.

The risk of developing hypertension in OC users increases with the duration of use and also in older women. If a woman develops hypertension while taking OCs, the pills should be stopped and another form of contraception adopted. However, if a woman is younger than 40 years of age and has mild hypertension that is controlled with medication and does not smoke, OCs may be used as long as BP is closely monitored.

Other adverse effects of OC use are an increased risk of cervical dysplasia and cancer in long-term (greater than 3–4 years) users. There is some evidence that there is a higher incidence of liver (usually benign) tumors or gallstones, but this is usually associated with higher dosages, long-term use, and older age. The use of OCs can precipitate migraine or vascular headaches or make existing migraines worse. Another form of contraception should be used if headaches increase in severity or frequency. Other problems that have been reported with OC use are depression and fluid retention.

It is unclear whether OCs contribute to breast cancer. FDA packaging inserts imply an association related to duration of use and history. Fibrocystic breast discomfort has been found to be less in OC users. Breast swelling and tenderness are common premenstrual complaints. Low-dose OCs seem to decrease this complaint,

as does reducing caffeine intake, avoiding smoking, and reducing sodium intake.

Because the cervical mucus is affected by the progestin component and estrogen can cause cervical mucorrhea, it is not uncommon for OC users to experience mucus-causing irritation, including *Candida,* of the vagina and vulva. Antibiotic therapy may also cause this condition.

Patients who use OCs may have increased pigmentation of the face and forehead. Combination pill users find this in the areola and perineum as well. Weight gain may or may not be an OC effect; it may be simply overeating, lack of exercise, fluid retention, thyroid problems, or poor nutrition, but a gain of 2 to 5 pounds is not uncommon.

To metabolize OCs properly, certain vitamins are utilized and not necessarily stored. Women should be instructed to take a daily multivitamin and extra vitamin C while taking OCs to prevent deficiency of these nutrients.

When combination OCs are discontinued, 90% of women resume ovulation and menses within 3 months. A pregnancy test should be done to ensure the patient is not pregnant if normal cycles are not established after 3 months. If a woman does not wish to become pregnant, another form of contraception should be used when the OC is discontinued. If a woman becomes pregnant while using the OC, most studies show no increased incidence of congenital defects. However, it is best not to use OCs if a patient believes she is pregnant but to use another method until it is established whether or not she is pregnant.

The progestin-only pill, the "mini-pill," contains progestin only and has a reported failure rate of 1% to 4%, slightly higher than that of combined OCs. Progestin-only pills contain either 0.35 mg norethindrone (Ortho Micronor, Nor-QD) or 0.075 mg *dl*-norgestrel (Ovrette) and are taken continuously beginning on the first day of the menstrual cycle. The progestin inhibits ovulation inconsistently but does cause thickening of the cervical mucus (makes it hostile to sperm), alters ovum transport (higher risk of ectopic pregnancy), and inhibits implantation. The advantages of the mini-pill are that it is safe during lactation and may actually increase the flow of milk; it can be used in women older than 35 years of age; it can be used in women with sickle cell disease; and it can be used in women with myomas. The progestin-only pill is less likely to cause headache, high BP, depression, cramps, premenstrual syndrome, or glucose elevation than combination OCs.

Disadvantages of the mini-pill include contraceptive failure and ectopic pregnancy. Irregular bleeding (amenorrhea, breakthrough bleeding, prolonged flow) is common in progestin-only users and may necessitate frequent pregnancy tests. Absolute contraindications include pregnancy, current or past history of thromboembolic disorders, stroke or heart disease, breast cancer, liver mass, and undiagnosed abnormal vaginal bleeding.

If the woman taking OCs complains of any of the adverse effects typically associated with OCs (nausea, abdominal bloating, hair changes, weight gain, leg pain, cramps, swelling), often switching the patient to a pill with a lower estrogen dose or one with a less androgenic progestin will relieve the problem. For example, switching to an OC with less progestational activity relieves hypoglycemia. If the patient complains of abdominal bloating, a lower estrogen dose or different progestin may relieve this problem. Bowel irregularity can also cause bloating, so this should be evaluated. If a patient complains of nausea, she should be instructed to take the pill with food or at bedtime. If the nausea persists or worsens, the patient may need to consult a gastroenterologist.

Regarding hair changes, excessive facial and body hair is usually less obvious in OC users. Hair loss is not usually related to OC use and should be referred to a dermatologist for evaluation.

Progestin, especially at high androgenic activity levels, and estrogen may cause weight gain. The patient should be switched to an OC with lower progestin/androgenic activities and provided with a diet that is lower in calories. If weight gain is mainly in breasts, hips, and thighs; is cyclic; and causes bloating, a pill with lower estrogen content should be tried.

Leg pain, cramps, and swelling usually disappear after three cycle packs. A severe pain, especially unilateral pain, can indicate a thrombosis and requires immediate discontinuation of the OC and immediate medical evaluation.

Medroxyprogesterone Acetate Injections

Medroxyprogesterone acetate, or Depo-Provera injectable, consists of 150 mg of deep intramuscular (IM) injections given every 3 months and has an efficacy rate of 99.7%. The initial injection is given on day 5 of the menses, and once injected it may take 8 to 9 months for fertility to be restored. The mode of action, adverse effects, and contraindications are the same as those for progesterone-only OCs. After 5 years of use, bone density loss has been observed, and patients should be advised to have adequate calcium intake daily (1,200–1,500 mg) at

the onset of use. The thinning of the uterine lining tends to lend some protection against endometrial cancer but also makes it more difficult for the patient to conceive for up to a year after discontinuing the injection. Depo-Provera may be used for patients who smoke and who are not candidates for the oral combination pill. All patients, however, should stop smoking as soon as possible.

Intrauterine Device

The *intrauterine device* (IUD) is a highly effective method for most women, and contrary to previous thought, nulliparity is not a contraindication to IUD use. Available in the United States today are the Mirena IUD, which releases levonorgestrel slowly, and the Copper T-380A. The Mirena is effective for about 5 years, and the Copper T-380A is effective for about 10 years. The mechanism of action of an IUD is not totally understood, but it is believed to act either as a spermicide or to have inhibitory effects on sperm capacitation and transport. Clearly, however, the IUD is not an abortifacient.

The IUD is inserted by a clinician trained in the procedure and is done at midcycle to prevent implantation. A 6- to 8-week wait is customary postpartum before insertion. The IUD has two long, off-white monofilament tails that project from the cervix into the vagina. The patient should be instructed to check this string after each menstrual period to ensure the IUD is still in place. A Pap smear and cultures are done during pelvic exam before insertion to be sure there are no abnormalities or infections.

Adverse effects include heavier menstrual periods, bleeding between periods, and cramping, and women with these problems should seek an alternative form of contraception. In 10% to 20% of cases during the first year of use there is spontaneous expulsion of the IUD. During the first month after insertion, there is an increased risk of pelvic infection. There does not appear to be any greater risk for infection other than that for acquiring an STI. Fertility is not affected by the use of an IUD.

Absolute contraindications for the use of an IUD include pregnancy, acute pelvic inflammatory disease, and purulent cervicitis. An IUD should be used with caution in women with a history of pelvic inflammatory disease, menorrhagia or severe dysmenorrhea, cervical or uterine neoplasia, or an abnormal uterus.

Regulated Abstinence

Regulated abstinence is another form of birth control used for both preventing and achieving pregnancy. Abstaining from sexual intercourse during the days of the menstrual cycle when the ovum is most vulnerable to fertilization is one way of avoiding pregnancy. Likewise, if achieving pregnancy is the desired outcome, engaging in sexual intercourse at this time is desirable. There are several techniques used to predict the best time for abstinence. The *rhythm method* or *calendar method* is based on the assumptions that the ovum is viable 24 hours after ovulation, spermatozoa are viable 48 hours after coitus, and ovulation occurs 12 to 16 days before menses. The woman records the length of her cycle for several months and establishes her fertile period by deducting 18 days from her shortest cycle and 11 days from her previous longest cycle. Each subsequent cycle, abstinence occurs during this calculated fertile period. The patient must have regular cycles to use this method.

The *natural family planning method* is another technique used to predict the best time for abstinence. There are three types: the basal body temperature method, the cervical mucus method, and the symptothermal method. When used in combination, the period of abstinence can be reduced and the effectiveness is increased for both preventing pregnancy or achieving pregnancy (if this is the goal). In the *basal body temperature method*, the patient measures basal body temperature daily. Abstinence is observed from menses to 3 days of elevated temperature. The lengthy abstinence plus abstinence in anovulatory cycles make this an unfavorable method.

In the *cervical mucus method*, an interpretation and recognition is made of changes in the cervical mucus consistency, which occurs in response to the changes in estrogen and progesterone levels. Abstinence begins in menses (and every other day thereafter to reduce risk of confusing mucus with semen) until the first day of slippery, copious mucus. Abstinence is observed every day thereafter until 4 days after the last day that mucus is present, or the peak mucus day.

In the *symptothermal method*, the fertile period is determined by calendar calculation and cervical mucus changes to decide on the fertile period; changes in mucus and basal temperature are used to decide on the end of this period. This method is difficult to learn but is the most effective natural method to prevent pregnancy.

The greatest obstacle to acceptance of these techniques is the need to avoid sexual relations for many days each cycle. Some couples use the barrier method during fertile times for greater acceptance and reduced failure rate.

Recent developments have produced self-administered tests (ovulation prediction kits) for the detection of hormone changes, reducing abstinence to several days per cycle. Urine evaluation for hormones is another method of family planning.

Postcoital Controls

Postcoital controls are another method of birth control. There are three different types: withdrawal, postcoitus douche, and emergency contraception. The simplest, most practical method of preventing implantation after unprotected sex is the administration of emergency contraception. Several regimens are effective in preventing implantation if the ovum has been fertilized, and all have about the same failure rate, 1% to 3%. The first method is to give two doses 12 hours apart of levonorgestrel 0.75 mg (called Plan B in the United States). An alternative is levonorgestrel 1.5 mg in a single dose. Both of these methods must be instituted within 72 hours of intercourse. Another regimen is ethinyl estradiol 50 mcg with 0.5 mg of norgestrel and is prepackaged as Preven. Two tablets are given and then two more 12 hours later. A regimen that is comparable is to give two tablets now and two more 12 hours later of Lo/Ovral, Nordette, or Levlen. An alternative to this is to instruct the patient to take the yellow pills of either Triphasil or Tri-Levlen in the same regimen, two pills followed by two pills 12 hours later. The third regimen is for the patient to take ethinyl estradiol 2.5 mg 2 times daily for 5 days, but this method tends to cause more nausea, vomiting, and breast tenderness than the other regimens. It is good practice to check for pregnancy pretreatment in the event that the woman inadvertently became pregnant earlier in her cycle and then posttreatment because the effects on the fetus worsen as the treatment and pregnancy continue, although it is uncertain that birth defects are directly related to steroid exposure in early pregnancy. Again, careful menstrual history should be reviewed, and a consent form may be obtained before prescription. Some women elect to continue the pregnancy if the treatment fails, and 10% of such cases have been later diagnosed with ectopic pregnancies. Contraindications to emergency contraception are pregnancy and those as listed for OC pills.

Sterilization

The most permanent method of birth control is sterilization. After risks and benefits of sterilization are reviewed with the patient, consent is obtained. The presence of two witnesses is recommended for patients younger than age 25 or those who are childless and older than 40 years of age. One percent of 1,000 patients who undergo the procedure later request reversal of sterilization.

Male sterilization consists of vasectomy performed on an outpatient basis; the procedure typically takes 20 minutes under local anesthesia. The major complication is hematoma (5%), sperm granuloma, and spontaneous reanastomosis. After vasectomy, the man is not considered sterile until two sperm-free ejaculates have been produced. Semen analysis should be performed 1 to 2 months after the procedure. About 15 to 20 ejaculations are required postvasectomy for absolute sterility.

Female sterilization is performed under general anesthesia by transperitoneal incision for tubal ligation. If sterilization is performed postpartum, a small infraumbilical incision is made and a tubal ligation is performed in the delivery room immediately or in the operating room the next day. The failure rate is 1 per 1,000.

692 UNIT II Caring-Based Nursing: The Science

Complications are hemorrhage, puncture, and cautery of the bowel (0.6%).

Abortion

An elective abortion is one of the most common gynecological procedures in the United States and has been legal since 1973. In accordance with the landmark *Roe v. Wade* Supreme Court decision, the state may not interfere with the practice of abortion in the first trimester. To protect the health of the mother, a second-trimester abortion may be performed, and limiting restrictions have been declared unconstitutional. In fact, since legalized abortion in the United States, the maternal mortality rate has fallen considerably.

The primary method used for elective abortion in the first trimester is vacuum aspiration under local anesthesia. Dilation and evacuation can be used in the second trimester and is done under either local or general anesthesia. For pregnancy after 18 weeks, hypertonic saline solution is instilled into the amniotic cavity, or prostaglandins may also be used to induce labor. The prostaglandins used most often are E_2, as a vaginal suppository, and 15-methyl prostaglandin F_{2alpha}, as an IM injection. They are given at 2- to 3-hour intervals until evacuation. Both instillation of hypertonic saline and prostaglandin administration are difficult for the patient. Abortions are rarely performed after 20 weeks, because fetal viability is considered to be at 24 weeks.

Complications from abortions increase as gestation increases and include retained products of conception and unrecognized ectopic pregnancy. Currently, most abortions (90%) are performed before 12 weeks of gestation, and there is an overall mortality rate of 1:100,000. Patients should be counseled to obtain an abortion as early as possible if this is their choice.

In September 2000 the U.S. FDA approved mifepristone (RU486), a synthetic antiprogestational-antiglucocorticoid pill as an oral abortifacient. RU486 is used to induce abortion during the first 9 weeks of pregnancy. RU486 is given as a single dose of 200 mg and has a success rate of 85%, but if it is followed in 36 to 48 hours with a prostaglandin vaginal suppository the success rate in terminating pregnancy is 95%. Adverse effects include nausea, vomiting, bleeding, and abdominal pain.

Patient Teaching

Contraception is not just a method; it is part of a life decision and future plan. There is no ideal method for every woman, but because so many options are available today, contraception can be tailored for each person's lifestyle, motivation, and partner's participation. Research in reproductive biology may provide less invasive and more effective methods in the future. Maximum outcome still depends on consistent and accurate use—the human element.

Every heterosexual woman should consider contraception as part of her overall personal health maintenance just as every woman should include the following in her health regimen: an annual gynecological exam, BSE, balanced nutrition, smoking and alcohol cessation, weight control, mental health, exercise, and risk reduction. Fertility control and good health work hand in hand for the patient and her future plans.

COMMON PROBLEMS

■ BREAST CANCER

Cancer of the breast is the most common cancer in American women and accounts for approximately 30% of all cancers in women in the United States. Centers for Disease Control and Prevention (CDC) statistics indicate that 230,480 women were diagnosed with breast cancer in 2011, and in that same year, 39,520 women were expected to die from it (most recent statistics available). Breast cancer is second only to lung cancer as the leading cause of cancer death among women and is the main cause of death in women aged 40 to 44 years. During the 1980s, there were yearly increases in breast cancer incidence rates, probably as a result of an increase in screening; but this rise has slowed over the past few years. Mortality rates have been decreasing since 1990, most likely because of earlier detection and advances in treatment.

Epidemiology and Causes

In general, the lifetime risk of a woman getting breast cancer is 1 in 8, and the lifetime risk of dying from breast cancer is 1 in 28. In North America, the lifetime odds of a woman getting breast cancer are 1 in 6 for non-Hispanic white women, 1 in 14 for African American women, 1 in 21 for New Mexican Hispanics, and 1 in 40 for New Mexican American Indians. The risk increases with age: It is low in women in their 20s and 30s and continues to rise each decade, with the median age for breast cancer diagnosis at 64 years of age. Increasing age and other risk factors (see Risk Factors 14.1) have been associated with the development of breast cancer, but these factors explain only 50% of cases. All women have the potential for the development of breast cancer. Screening recommendations and guidelines are presented in Screening Recommendations/Guidelines 14.1.

Pathophysiology

Breast cancer is a disease of various cell populations, with different growth rates, cell surface markers, and tendencies to metastasize. It is often considered a systemic disease at the time of first diagnosis, because many patients with "early" breast cancer already have established but clinically occult micrometastases, reflecting the importance of adjuvant hormonal therapy (e.g., tamoxifen, anastrozole). Invasive breast cancer is often preceded by carcinoma in situ (CIS) lesions of either ductal or lobular

Risk Factors 14.1   Breast Cancer

Major Risk Factors

- Female gender
- Increasing age (>50 years)
- Personal history of breast cancer (in situ or invasive)
- Family history of breast cancer in a first-degree relative (parent, sibling, or child)
- Residing in North America or Northern Europe

Moderate Risk Factors

- Biopsy-confirmed atypical hyperplasia
- Early menarche (<age 12 years)
- Late menopause (>age 55 years)
- Nulliparity or first live-birth at a late age (>30 years)
- Long-term use of postmenopausal hormone therapy, especially unopposed estrogen
- Exposure to high-dose radiation
- History of ovarian or uterine fundus cancer
- Higher education and socioeconomic status

Possible Risk Factors

- High-fat diet and weight gain
- Alcohol consumption (two or more drinks/day)
- Physical inactivity
- Cigarette smoking, especially during adolescence
- Exposure to pesticides and other chemicals

Screening Recommendations/Guidelines 14.1 Breast Cancer

The American Cancer Society (ACS) recommends the following screening for the early detection of breast cancer in those who are asymptomatic (ACS does not specify an age at which screening should be terminated). Women age 20–39:

- Clinical breast exam performed by the practitioner every 3 years.
- BSE performed by the patient monthly.

Women age 40 and older*:

- Clinical breast exam performed by the practitioner annually. (This should be performed close to the scheduled mammogram.)
- Mammogram performed annually.
- BSE performed by the patient monthly.

The National Cancer Institute (NCI) recommends screening (mammogram and clinical breast exam) every 1–2 years for women in their 40s. A review of clinical trials by the NCI showed there to be insufficient data to evaluate the effectiveness of screening mammography in women age 70 and older.

*U.S. Preventive Services Task Force new recommendation is age 50; however, it has sparked much controversy.

distribution, as discussed under Prognosis. However, a malignant breast mass may be present for many years before the initial diagnosis, and it is not uncommon for invasive disease to be identified at the time of diagnosis, rather than a premalignant lesion. Breast cancers spread by contiguous, lymphatic, and/or vascular channels. The most common areas of metastasis are the regional lymph nodes, lung, skin, bone, liver, and brain.

The development of frank breast cancer may also be preceded by a variety of benign breast conditions characterized by multicentric proliferation of breast tissue. Several genetic mutations have been recognized in both precancerous and cancerous lesions, including genes affecting cellular proliferation, DNA mismatch repair, or the conversion of procarcinogens to carcinogenic compounds. Two of the most widely publicized breast cancer susceptibility genes are the tumor suppressor genes *BRCA1* and *BRCA2,* first cloned in the mid-1990s. These gene products are involved in the repair of double-stranded DNA breaks, and mutations predispose individuals not only to breast cancer in women and men, but also to cancers of the ovary, pancreas, and even prostate. However, *BRCA1/BRCA2* mutations are quite rare, accounting for only one-fifth of familial breast cancer cases.

The Knudsen hypothesis of malignant transformation is often credited with the pathogenesis of breast cancer. In this model, at least two sequential genetic "hits" or mutations that interfere with DNA repair are thought to underlie malignant transformation of normal breast tissue, which ultimately loses its capacity for programmed cell death (apoptosis). In familial cancers, the first of these hits is thought to be the inherited germline mutation, and the second mutation may be induced by an environmental carcinogen or related to one of many other predisposing risk factors.

Clinical Presentation
Subjective

History and risk assessment should include age, ethnicity, education and socioeconomic status; breast lump or area that feels denser (with or without pain), tenderness, dimpling, nipple retraction, nipple ulceration, erythema or *peau d'orange* ("orange peel"); change in breast shape, breast enlargement, and/or an alteration in the vein pattern of the breast tissue; nipple discharge; and one or more palpable enlarged axillary lymph nodes. The date of onset, location, and duration of any change in the patient's breast and if trauma occurred should also be elicited.

Assessment should also include any systemic symptoms, especially those that may indicate metastases to the skeleton (bone pain, fracture), spinal cord (localized and radicular back pain, lower extremity weakness, paresthesias, paralysis, bladder/bowel dysfunction), brain (headache, seizure, mental status changes, vision and speech defects, sensory loss/muscle weakness, ataxia, persistent nausea/vomiting), bladder or bowel (incontinence), lungs (chest pain, dyspnea on exertion, shortness of breath, cough), and liver (abdominal pain or distention, jaundice, weakness, fatigue, nausea, vomiting, appetite, weight loss, lower extremity edema).

The medical history should include illnesses, especially a previous breast cancer, a benign or preinvasive breast condition, or another cancer such as ovarian cancer; prior radiation exposure; medications; allergies; diet and other health habits (fat intake, alcohol consumption, cigarettes, weight gain, exercise); and past surgical history, especially breast biopsy and/or surgery. Questions should be asked regarding gynecological and obstetric history: age at menarche; age at menopause; last menstrual period; pregnancy history (age when first full-term pregnancy occurred, abortions, miscarriages); and use of hormone therapy, particularly unopposed estrogen. Frequency of mammograms and date of last mammogram; results of previous mammograms, noting any abnormalities; other related diagnostic tests and results; and frequency of clinical breast exams and breast self-exams should be determined. Family history questions should include information regarding a first-degree relative with a history of breast cancer (note age at diagnosis and bilaterality of disease) and a family history of ovarian cancer associated with breast cancer.

Objective

A thorough physical exam with a focus on the breasts and axillary and supraclavicular lymph nodes should be performed. Inspect for contour, symmetry, skin changes, and nipple changes. In premenopausal women, this assessment should be done during the follicular phase of the menstrual cycle, when hormone levels are low and less likely to affect the breast tissue. Examination of the breasts includes inspection and palpation in the upright and supine positions. The size, location, mobility, and consistency of any palpable breast mass or dense area and lymph nodes should be documented. Any breast changes noted on inspection and the characteristics of any nipple discharge are also recorded. Pain is present in fewer than 10% of patients with cancer.

Clinical manifestations of breast cancer include those stated above, but some patients may present only with an abnormality detected on a mammogram. The Patient's Voice 14.1 illustrates the individuality of symptoms.

The Patient's Voice 14.1
A Breast Mass
One Patient's Voice
It was on my 48th birthday that I noticed a slightly tender enlargement in my left breast. I had consistently checked my breasts for years during my period. I had no family history for breast cancer and never experienced breast tenderness or lumps on a regular basis. Even before my one pregnancy at age 34, I had never experienced significant breast soreness. My nurse practitioner saw me the next day and stated that she could feel something. She sent me for a mammogram. I had one 2 years ago, so I was sent to the same place. Two days later, I was told there are "changes" and I was referred to a surgeon. I did not know what that meant, except I knew it could be serious. I wanted to do everything they told me to do. I wanted to get better. I had a biopsy and then shortly after, a "lumpectomy." I was told I was very lucky because although the biopsy was positive for cancer, they said my "nodes" were cancer free. I was told I would need radiation therapy since I only had the lump removed. I experienced too much stress and fear at that time in my life. My yoga classes were very important to me then because they helped me relax and heal. I have been going for 7 years since the surgery and now teach yoga too. I know I was lucky and grateful that my nurse practitioner could see me the day after I felt the lump. Waiting is so stressful.

Another Patient's Voice
I went for my annual mammogram and later got the call; I was referred to a breast specialist and had a biopsy. On my 45th birthday, I got the news that I had bilateral breast cancer. I have had a bilateral mastectomy, and almost a year of treatment, first chemo and now radiation. I have a young son and husband. This will be the first Christmas since my diagnosis and I am grateful to be here. Having this diagnosis made me rethink the important things in life. I have slowed down and appreciate all the people in my life. I know people say this, but the diagnosis of breast cancer has really been a gift. I appreciate the small things, like a beautiful sunset, the gentle breeze in my face, and the love of family and friends. I don't take life for granted any more!

Diagnostic Reasoning
Diagnostic Tests

A diagnostic mammogram is necessary in any woman with a palpable breast mass, suspicious nipple discharge, or a suspicious area on a screening mammogram. A spot compression flattens and isolates a lesion. A diagnostic mammogram determines the needs for subsequent testing, and it determines if other suspicious nonpalpable areas are present in one or both breasts.

Suspicious areas on a mammogram include (1) asymmetry with definitive borders or discernible masses; (2) architectural distortion (a "pulling in" of breast structures) not resulting from previous surgery; (3) a nodule that is more radiodense, irregularly shaped, and has unclear margins; (4) calcifications that are irregularly shaped, clustered, and of varying sizes; (5) skin changes such as a thickening or retraction; (6) spiculations (needle-like); and (7) axillary lymph nodes more than

2 cm and/or intramammary lymph nodes more than 2 cm in diameter.

Additional studies that may be scheduled to further delineate the abnormality are ultrasound, ductal lavage, and galactography or ductography. An ultrasound, which differentiates solid from fluid-filled masses, may distinguish between benign and malignant disease. It may better visualize abnormalities in patients with dense breast tissue (women younger than age 30–35 years) and is used in place of mammography in pregnant patients. Genetic testing for the *BRCA1* and *BRCA2* gene is expensive and done only in women with a high suspicion of a familial breast–ovary cancer syndrome who have undergone extensive pretest (and posttest) counseling.

Mammography views, using the Eklund technique, are used in a patient with a breast implant to provide additional views behind the implant. Galactography or ductography is used in the presence of serous or bloody nipple discharge without a palpable mass to visualize an intraductal lesion; however, it cannot distinguish between benign and malignant disease.

A biopsy is performed next. Suspicious areas noted on a mammogram or ultrasound must be submitted for biopsy for a definitive tissue diagnosis. A mammogram may not always result in a visible lesion; therefore, all clinically suspicious palpable masses must be submitted for biopsy whether or not seen with mammography.

The patient should be referred to a surgeon for further evaluation at this point. One or more of the following biopsy techniques may be done in the outpatient setting, usually under local anesthesia:

- *Fine-needle aspiration* (FNA). FNA may be performed by a primary-care provider experienced in the procedure. A 21- or 22-gauge needle is used to aspirate a cyst or extract cells from a palpable solid lesion for analysis. It is easy to perform and provides rapid results with little trauma to the tissue. It is highly reliable when used as an adjunct to the clinical exam and mammogram. On the negative side, it requires an experienced cytopathologist, may yield false-negative results, and does not differentiate in situ from invasive cancer. A stereotactic or ultrasound-guided biopsy can be performed on nonpalpable lesions.
- *Core-needle biopsy.* A large-gauge cutting needle is used to provide a large core of tissue from the lesion for histological examination. The results of a core-needle biopsy are as accurate as those of a surgical biopsy, but the procedure is less invasive with better cosmetic results. A stereotactic or ultrasound-guided biopsy can be performed on nonpalpable lesions.
- *Incisional biopsy.* This procedure may be done when a mass is very large and cannot be removed without major surgery. A wedge of tissue is removed for histological examination.

- *Open surgical excisional biopsy (lumpectomy).* This procedure involves the entire removal of a palpable mass or a nonpalpable lesion (after stereotactic or ultrasound-guided biopsy or mammographic needle localization). To qualify as a lumpectomy, lesions suggestive of cancer should be removed with a margin of at least 1 cm of normal tissue. X-ray films of needle-localization specimens are obtained to confirm removal of mammographically detected abnormality. A postexcision mammogram should confirm complete excision. The open surgical excisional biopsy provides complete pathological assessment but may result in poor cosmesis.

If there is suspicion of inflammatory breast cancer or Paget's disease, a skin biopsy or nipple biopsy should be done at the time of the breast mass biopsy.

Prognosis Preinvasive breast cancers include ductal carcinoma in situ (DCIS) and lobular carcinoma in situ (LCIS). DCIS has malignant potential but infrequently disseminates; therefore, approximately 98% of patients are cured with local–regional therapy (total mastectomy or breast-conserving surgery and radiation therapy). The addition of tamoxifen (Nolvadex) decreases the incidence of subsequent invasive disease. LCIS has a propensity for bilaterality, multicentricity, and a 25% to 40% risk for development of subsequent invasive cancer. It is managed with close surveillance, a bilateral mastectomy, or chemoprevention (tamoxifen).

Invasive breast cancers have the potential to disseminate through lymphatic and vascular channels to other organs. Most of these cancers are adenocarcinomas. Approximately 80% are infiltrating ductal carcinomas, and 10% are invasive lobular carcinomas. Their prognosis is identical. Invasive lobular carcinoma differs in its slightly greater tendency toward bilaterality and metastasis to meningeal and serosal surfaces. Other histological subtypes are pure mucinous, tubular, medullary, and papillary carcinomas. These subtypes have a slight to somewhat better prognosis resulting from a smaller risk of dissemination. Paget's disease of the breast and inflammatory breast carcinoma are rare. Paget's disease of the breast, unilateral eczema of the nipple, is always associated with DCIS or invasive ductal carcinoma. Inflammatory breast carcinoma has the poorest prognosis of all breast cancers.

Prognostic factors, or tumor-related features, are biological measures done on the breast tissue specimen. They serve as guides for the oncologist in determining systemic adjuvant therapy for the breast cancer patient. In addition to the histological types of invasive breast cancer, lymph node status (0, 1–3, 4 or more, or 10 or more [range of good to poor prognosis]), tumor size (1 cm or less in diameter [good prognosis]), and histological differentiation (range of well differentiated [low grade] to poorly differentiated [high grade]) are the standard predictors of risk of recurrence and survival. High-grade tumors are poorly differentiated and carry a worse prognosis, whereas lower grade, well-differentiated tumors carry a more favorable prognosis. With reference to these factors, patients with breast cancer have an excellent prognosis if they have the following features: DCIS, negative lymph nodes with an invasive tumor size less than 1 cm in diameter, and special histological subtypes of breast cancer (e.g., pure tubular) less than 3 cm in diameter.

Patients who have potentially high recurrence rates and who would, therefore, greatly benefit from systemic therapy have the following features: positive regional lymph node(s) or invasive tumors more than 2 cm in diameter even with negative lymph nodes. Breast cancer patients who have a tumor that is poorly differentiated have an increased risk of recurrent disease, but they may also have a greater response to chemotherapy.

Hormone receptor status—for example, the presence or absence of estrogen and progesterone receptors—is another important prognostic factor especially in guiding the oncologist in the selection of hormonal therapy. More patients with breast cancer respond favorably if estrogen receptor levels are high and if both estrogen and progesterone receptors are positive. Also, a positive status of the pS2 protein (an estrogen-regulated secretory protein expressed mainly by estrogen receptor–positive tumors) is indicative of a better prognosis in women with both negative and positive lymph nodes.

Other prognostic factors such as those indicative of the proliferative capacity of the tumor (mitotic index, thymidine labeling index, S-phase fraction, ploidy, and Ki-67), nuclear grade, tumor necrosis, tumor microvessel density, peritumoral lymphatic vessel invasion, the protease cathepsin D, and proto-oncogenes (*ERBB2* [*HER-2/neu,* c-erbB-2] and c-myc), and p53 (a tumor-suppressor gene) expression may be helpful in predicting response to treatment. For example, the overexpression of c-erB-2 may predict that a breast cancer patient may be resistant to certain chemotherapy agents and possibly to hormonal therapy. It may also predict a shorter disease-free interval.

Reference to these additional prognostic factors, along with the standard ones, may be valuable in determining the need for systemic therapy in women who have an intermediate prognosis, such as node-negative patients with invasive tumors 1 to 2 cm in diameter.

Staging   After the diagnosis of breast cancer is confirmed, the stage of the disease is evaluated (Table 14.3). Certain laboratory tests may determine distant metastasis. A complete blood count may show an abnormality of white blood cells and platelets, and a low hematocrit may indicate bone marrow infiltration and occult metastatic disease. Liver enzymes and calcium and phosphorus abnormalities may indicate occult liver metastasis and/or bone metastasis. Tumor marker (e.g., CEA, Ca 27.29) abnormalities may indicate occult metastatic disease. If the tumor marker is abnormal, it will be useful in later assessing response to treatment (disease progression or recurrence). These radiology exams also determine distant metastasis: A chest x-ray abnormality may indicate lung metastasis, and a bone scan/skeletal survey or liver scan, if signs, symptoms, or laboratory tests warrant, may suggest an abnormality.

Differential Diagnoses

Several differential diagnoses should be considered. With breast cancer, a palpable mass is usually persistent, unilateral, solitary, discrete, firm, irregularly shaped, nontender, and may or may not be fixed to the skin or underlying tissue. Breast distortion and skin changes such as diffuse erythema, edema, *peau d'orange,* dimpling, nipple retraction, or nipple ulceration are also indicative of cancer. If present, nipple discharge is spontaneous, persistent, unilateral, localized to a single duct, watery or sticky, and clear, sanguineous, serosanguineous, or serous in color. Lymph nodes suggestive of a malignancy are large, firm, or fixed.

Fibrocystic changes (cystic breast disease, chronic cystic mastitis, or mammary dysplasia) may be difficult to distinguish from breast cancer by palpation alone. *Fibrocystic changes* are so common that they are considered a normal variant of breast tissue. However, if accompanied by significant pain, nipple discharge, or palpable physical exam findings that raise suspicion for breast cancer, the condition is termed *fibrocystic disease.* Cystic areas are unilateral or bilateral, somewhat more diffuse, 1 mm to many centimeters in diameter, soft, and mobile; they may also be tender and painful due to stromal edema, dilation of ducts, and accompanying inflammation. These cysts are hormonally regulated and may be worse premenstrually; this variation with menses usually distinguishes fibrocystic changes from fibroadenomas and breast cancer. Aspiration of clear fluid with complete disappearance of the cyst on follow-up examination or the appearance of a fluid-filled cavity on ultrasound confirms the diagnosis. These changes are most common in patients aged 30 to 55 years.

Fibroadenomas are benign, solid masses of fibrous and glandular tissue that are often confused with breast cancer. These masses may be isolated or multiple and are typically firm, nodular, usually well defined, freely mobile, and possibly tender. Growth of the tumor is hormonally stimulated; thus, it may grow rapidly during pregnancy, lactation, or hormonal manipulation. These are most common in younger patients and are not associated with an increased risk of breast cancer if in their simple form. However, *complex fibroadenomas* (i.e., containing cysts greater than 3 mm in size, calcification on mammography, or histological evidence of sclerosing adenosis or papillary apocrine changes) have been associated with a greater risk of breast cancer when accompanied by proliferation of surrounding glandular tissue.

Table 14.3	TNM Staging of Primary Breast Cancer	
Stage	TNM Staging	Description
	TX, NX, MX	Primary tumor (T), regional lymph nodes (N), or distant metastasis (M) respectively cannot be assessed (X)
0	Tis, N0, M0	Carcinoma in situ or Paget's disease of nipple with no tumor
I	T1, N0, M0	Tumor ≤2 cm; no regional lymph node metastasis; no distant metastasis
IIA	T0, N1, M0	No evidence of tumor, metastasis to moveable ipsilateral axillary lymph node(s); no distant metastasis
	T1, N1, M0	Tumor ≤2 cm; metastasis to moveable ipsilateral axillary lymph node(s); no distant metastasis
	T2, N0, M0	Tumor >2– ≤5 cm; no regional lymph node metastasis; no distant metastasis
IIB	T2, N1, M0	Tumor >2– ≤5 cm; metastasis to moveable ipsilateral axillary lymph node(s); no distant metastasis
	T3, N0, M0	Tumor >5 cm; no regional lymph node metastasis; no distant metastasis
IIIA	T0, N2, M0	No evidence of tumor, metastasis to ipsilateral axillary lymph node(s) fixed to one another or to other structure; no distant metastasis
	T1, N2, M0	Tumor ≤2 cm; metastasis to ipsilateral axillary lymph node(s) fixed to one another or to other structure; no distant metastasis
	T2, N2, M0	Tumor >2– ≤5 cm; metastasis to ipsilateral axillary lymph node(s) fixed to one another or to other structure; no distant metastasis
	T3, N1 or N2, M0	Tumor >5 cm; metastasis to ipsilateral axillary lymph node(s) fixed to one another or to other structure; no distant metastasis
IIIB	T4, any N, M0	Tumor of any size with direct extension to chest wall (excluding pectoral muscle) and/or edema (including *peau d'orange*) or ulceration of the skin or satellite skin nodules confined to the same breast, or inflammatory carcinoma; any nodal status as described above; no distant metastasis
IV	Any T, N3, M0	Any tumor status as described above; metastasis to ipsilateral internal mammary node(s); no distant metastasis
	Any T, Any N, M1	Any tumor or nodal status as described above; distant metastasis, including metastasis to ipsilateral supraclavicular lymph nodes

Hamartomas composed of stromal and epithelial tissue and *tubular adenomas* consisting of ductal tissue are less common benign tumors of the breast that may present similarly on physical exam but are not considered cancerous. Fat necrosis or *panniculitis* is another benign condition and is typically trauma induced. The mass is firm and possibly tender, often with calcification seen on mammography. *Diabetic mastopathy* results in a breast lump with a dense mammographic appearance but benign histology consisting of keloidal scar tissue and a lobular, lymphocytic inflammation. This is most often seen in women with type 1 diabetes mellitus who also suffer from additional end-organ microvascular damage such as retinopathy or neuropathy.

Intraductal papilloma is a benign condition with a small, usually solitary and nonpalpable mass in one mammary duct with an associated spontaneous sanguineous or serosanguineous nipple discharge. If large enough to palpate, the mass is most often close to or beneath the areola, soft, mobile, 1 to 3 cm in size, poorly delineated, nontender, and sometimes associated with skin dimpling. It is most common in patients aged 35 to 55 years. Solitary papillomas are not considered premalignant; however, diffuse papillomatosis characterized by the formation of multiple papillomas carries with it a greater risk of eventual breast cancer.

Duct ectasia is a benign condition involving inflammation of a subareolar duct, which may produce subareolar erythema and swelling, a mass with nipple retraction and/or dimpling, dull nipple pain, tenderness, burning, and itching. Nipple discharge is pasty and straw-colored, cream-colored, green, or brown. It is most common in perimenopausal or postmenopausal patients who have had children and have nursed.

Ductal hyperplasia without atypia is distinguished from ectasia, in that it is the most common benign breast lesion clearly associated with an increased risk of breast cancer. Epithelial cell proliferation along the basement membranes of the ducts, although benign histologically, varies in size and shape. *Atypical ductal hyperplasia* is associated with an even greater risk of breast cancer (up to sixfold in women with a strong family history of breast cancer), especially in premenopausal women. It is characterized by a loss of apical-basal cellular organization within ductal tissue. *Atypical lobular hyperplasia* is even more concerning because it is qualitatively (albeit not quantitatively) equivalent to LCIS, which is considered a precursor lesion to invasive breast cancer.

Sclerosing adenosis, most common in patients aged 35 to 45, is a benign proliferation of the breast epithelium with increased fibrous and glandular tissue, with hard, pea-sized nodules throughout the affected area. There is mild to moderate pain and swelling premenstrually. The presence of this condition has also been associated with an increased risk of breast cancer. *Radial scars* are another benign histological finding consisting of a fibroelastic core from which ducts and lobules radiate outward. If large, these lesions may appear similar to spiculated carcinoma on mammography and are indeed associated with an increased risk of breast cancer.

Mastitis, a benign infectious condition of the breast that may or may not include formation of an abscess, presents with redness, induration, pain, possible purulent nipple discharge, fever, chills, and myalgia. It is more common during lactation.

Management

The patient diagnosed with breast cancer is referred to oncology specialists, such as a surgeon, medical oncologist, and/or radiation oncologist for treatment of the disease (Table 14.4). The choice of treatment is influenced by such factors as tumor stage, estrogen and progesterone receptor levels and other prognostic factors, patient age, menopausal status, and the patient's general health. When detected in early stages, invasive breast cancer that is treatable with surgery, radiation therapy, chemotherapy, and/or hormonal therapy may be highly curable.

Surgical Management

The initial surgical management of stage I and stage II breast cancer includes one of several types of surgery. Breast-conserving surgery involves a partial mastectomy, lumpectomy, wide excision, segmental mastectomy, or quadrantectomy with a separate axillary node dissection and radiation therapy to the breast. A modified radical mastectomy is a total mastectomy with an axillary node dissection. Breast-conserving surgery removes a portion of the breast tissue, whereas a total mastectomy removes all but approximately 2% to 3% of the breast tissue. The survival rates for these two surgical treatment options are equivalent.

The type of initial surgery for a particular patient usually depends on the location and size of the tumor, breast size, characteristics of the disease on mammography,

patient age, and the patient's feelings regarding breast preservation. Breast-conserving surgery may not be an option if there is a tumor beneath the nipple; a large tumor-size-to-breast-size ratio; multicentricity; extensive intraductal carcinoma; diffuse malignant-appearing calcifications on the mammogram; or contraindications to radiation therapy such as pregnancy, collagen-vascular disease, or prior radiation therapy to the breast or chest wall.

After a mastectomy, the patient may choose immediate or delayed breast reconstruction with a submuscular saline implant or expander, a transverse rectus abdominis myocutaneous flap, or a latissimus dorsi flap. Depending on the type of breast surgery, the adverse effects may be wound infection, seroma, bleeding or hematoma, phantom breast syndrome (pain, numbness, or nipple itching), paresthesias, muscle atrophy, arm or shoulder weakness or stiffness, lymphedema, phlebitis, or a winged scapula (protruding scapula resulting from intraoperative injury to the long thoracic nerve). A new technique under investigation, lymphatic mapping and sentinel lymph node biopsy, may eliminate the need for an axillary lymph node dissection in some patients and thus prevent some of these adverse effects. The sentinel node (the first lymph node along a lymphatic drainage pathway) is identified after peritumoral injection with a radioisotope or vital blue dye. If the sentinel node is negative for metastatic disease, a complete axillary lymph node dissection is not indicated.

Radiation Therapy

Radiation therapy is indicated for local–regional control of the primary breast cancer or palliation of metastatic disease. After breast-conserving surgery, primary treatment includes external-beam radiation to the entire breast with or without a boost (interstitial radioactive implant or external-beam radiation) to the primary site. After a modified radical mastectomy, radiation therapy to the chest wall and regional lymph nodes is considered in women at high risk of local–regional recurrence, including those with known residual disease or four or more involved lymph nodes. Patients undergoing an axillary lymph node dissection generally do not require radiation therapy to the axilla. Internal mammary lymph nodes may be treated, and patients with four or more positive lymph nodes may require supraclavicular radiation therapy to reduce the risk of supraclavicular lymph node recurrence. A pregnant patient with breast cancer can begin radiation therapy after delivery. Potential adverse effects of radiation therapy include fatigue, edema, breast pain or tenderness, skin reactions, brachial plexopathy, radiation pneumonitis, and myocardial damage if the left breast is treated. Secondary malignancies, such as sarcomas, leukemias, and lung cancer, are rare, although smokers have an increased risk of lung cancer in the ipsilateral lung.

Table 14.4   Management of Invasive Breast Cancer

Stage	Surgery/Radiation Therapy	Adjuvant Therapy
I	Breast-conserving surgery with separate axillary node dissection and radiation therapy (RT) to the breast OR Modified radical mastectomy (MRM)	Suitable ER-negative patients: Adjuvant chemotherapy ER-positive patients: adjuvant chemotherapy or tamoxifen 20 mg daily
II	Breast-conserving surgery with separate axillary node dissection and RT to the breast OR MRM Consider RT to the chest wall and regional nodes for patients at high risk of local-regional recurrence, including those with known residual disease or four or more involved nodes	*Node-positive patients:* Premenopausal and postmenopausal (ER-negative) patients: adjuvant combination chemotherapy with or without tamoxifen Postmenopausal patients with positive hormone receptors: Tamoxifen alone *Node-negative patients:* ER-negative or ER-positive patients with large tumors: Adjuvant chemotherapy ER-positive patients: adjuvant chemotherapy or tamoxifen 20 mg daily
IIIA	*In operable cases:* MRM with or without RT or radical mastectomy (removal of breast tissue, all axillary lymph nodes, and underlying chest muscle) with or without RT RT should be given because of the high risk of local recurrence; postoperative external beam RT to chest wall with or without boost as necessary for positive or close margins	Combination chemotherapy with or without hormones Neoadjuvant therapy: chemotherapy may be given preoperatively if primary resection is not feasible or technically difficult
IIIB	Biopsy for diagnosis and estrogen/progesterone receptors (ER/PR) If good response to chemotherapy or hormonal therapy: Local therapy with surgery and/or RT If poor response to chemotherapy or hormonal therapy: Palliative RT	Chemotherapy/hormonal therapy: Combination chemotherapy with or without hormones OR tamoxifen (if ER/PR receptors positive)
IV	Biopsy for diagnosis and ER/PR receptors External beam RT or palliative mastectomy to control local disease	If visceral disease minimal or absent and ER/PR receptors positive: Hormonal therapy (as initial therapy) For premenopausal patients: Tamoxifen or oophorectomy For patients who relapse after a period of response or prolonged stability on initial hormone therapy: megestrol 40 mg 4 times daily or anastrozole 1 mg daily or letrozole 2.5 mg daily If visceral disease present or ER/PR receptors negative: Combination chemotherapy
Inflammatory Breast Cancer	Refer to options for stage IIIB or IV	Refer to options for stage IIIB or IV

Breast surgery or radiation therapy may make subsequent mammograms difficult to interpret. Masses (postoperative fluid collections and scarring), edema, skin thickening, and calcifications may be seen on these mammograms, especially during the first 6 months after treatment. During the next 6 to 12 months, slow resolution of these changes takes place and stability occurs within 2 years.

Chemotherapy

Antineoplastic chemotherapy as adjuvant therapy is indicated for the eradication of micrometastatic disease that may be present at the time of the original diagnosis. It should be initiated within 6 weeks (preferably less) of surgery (radiation therapy would follow the chemotherapy). Combination chemotherapy is the standard of care for the treatment of primary breast cancer because it most likely would overcome the potential for drug resistance. The most widely used regimens are CMF (cyclophosphamide [Cytoxan], methotrexate [amethopterin], and fluorouracil [Adrucil]), CAF (FAC) (cyclophosphamide, doxorubicin [Adriamycin], and fluorouracil), and AC (doxorubicin and cyclophosphamide) with or without sequential paclitaxel (Taxol). Other regimens are CMFVP (CMF and vincristine [Oncovin] and prednisone [Deltasone]), CFM (CNF, FNC) (cyclophosphamide, fluorouracil, mitoxantrone [Novantrone]), NFL (mitoxantrone, fluorouracil, leucovorin [Wellcovorin]), sequential Dox-CMF (doxorubicin followed by CMF), VATH (vinblastine, doxorubicin, thiotepa [Thioplex], and fluoxymesterone [Halotestin]), and vinorelbine (Navelbine) plus doxorubicin.

Second-line or later therapy, in the event of disease progression or recurrent disease, includes agents such as vinorelbine, paclitaxel, docetaxel (Taxotere), or gemcitabine (Gemzar). Some of the more common potential adverse effects of chemotherapy include myelosuppression, nausea and vomiting, anorexia, mucositis, alopecia, fatigue, and neurotoxicity. Less common toxicities include hemorrhagic cystitis (alkylating agents), cardiomyopathy (anthracyclines), thromboembolic events, and early menopause (in premenopausal patients). Paclitaxel and docetaxel may also produce myalgia and rare allergic reactions; docetaxel may cause cumulative fluid retention and symptomatic pleural effusions. A rare complication of antineoplastic chemotherapy may be the development of secondary leukemia. Hematopoietic growth factors (erythropoietin, granulocyte colony-stimulating factor [Neupogen], granulocyte-macrophage colony-stimulating factor [Leukine], and oprelvekin [Neumega]) and cytoprotective agents such as amifostine (Ethyol) and dexrazoxane (Zinecard) may help to prevent or reduce some of the chemotherapy-related complications. Pamidronate (Aredia), a second-generation amino-bisphosphonate, is used in cases of osteolytic bone metastases to prevent pathological fractures, cord compression, the need for radiation therapy or surgery to the bone, and hypercalcemia, and it significantly reduces bone pain. Pregnant breast cancer patients may receive antineoplastic chemotherapy during their third trimester or after delivery.

Monoclonal Antibodies

The newest treatment for metastatic breast cancer, trastuzumab (Herceptin), a recombinant DNA–derived humanized monoclonal antibody, is used as a single agent in second-line or later therapy for those patients with metastatic breast cancer whose tumors overexpress the HER2 protein. The combined regimen of trastuzumab and paclitaxel is used for the same patient populations who have not previously received chemotherapy for their metastatic disease. Potential adverse effects include cardiomyopathy, anemia and leukopenia, diarrhea, and infection.

Hormonal Therapy

Hormonal therapy includes the use of antiestrogens (tamoxifen), progestins (e.g., megestrol acetate), luteinizing hormone–releasing hormone (LHRH) agonists (e.g., leuprolide), or aromatase inhibitors (anastrozole and letrozole). Tamoxifen is the most prescribed of these agents, and the treatment period is 5 years. Because of its antiestrogenic effect, it is beneficial in breast cancer patients whose tumors have positive hormone receptors, with its greatest effect in those who have both estrogen-receptor (ER)–positive and progesterone-receptor (PR)–positive tumors. Tamoxifen also exhibits an estrogenic effect on the endometrium; therefore, it may increase the incidence of endometrial cancer. Potential adverse effects include mild nausea, hot flashes, menstrual irregularities, vaginal discharge, vaginal dryness and irritation, benign ovarian cysts, thromboembolic events, and ophthalmological toxicities.

Local Recurrent Disease

Local recurrent disease is usually indicative of widespread recurrence, especially in postmastectomy patients. Some patients initially treated with breast-conserving surgery and radiation therapy who later develop a local recurrence in the ipsilateral breast may be cured with surgery and/or radiation therapy. Prolonged survival is more likely if there is a chest wall recurrence less than 3 cm in diameter, axillary and internal mammary (not supraclavicular) lymph node recurrence, and a disease-free interval of more than 2 years after initial therapy. Treatment options for recurrent disease include surgery, radiation therapy, chemotherapy, and/or hormonal therapy. Surgery and/or radiation may be used for a local or visceral recurrence. In asymptomatic patients with a positive or unknown ER/PR status, and with absent or minimal visceral disease in one organ, tamoxifen in premenopausal and postmenopausal patients or oophorectomy (or LHRH agonists) in premenopausal patients may be the treatment option. In the event that a patient had an initial response to hormonal therapy but had a subsequent relapse, another type of hormonal therapy may be prescribed, such as tamoxifen, anastrozole, letrozole, Megace, androgens, LHRH agonists (for premenopausal patients), or aminoglutethimide. A subset of patients may respond to hormonal therapy withdrawal for approximately 10 months before switching to another form of hormonal therapy. Patients with positive visceral disease and a negative ER/PR status should receive chemotherapy. If a patient relapses a year or more after receiving adjuvant treatment with CMF, this same regimen may be readministered. If the patient relapses after treatment with an anthracycline-containing regimen, she may be retreated with other agents mentioned earlier. Recurrent breast cancer treatment may be palliative in nature, such as the use of radiation therapy to relieve the pain of bone metastases.

Clinical Trials

At any stage of breast cancer, patients may be eligible for clinical trials designed to improve survival or decrease the morbidity associated with current standard therapy. Some patients with stages II, III, or IV may be considered as candidates for clinical trials of high-dose chemotherapy with bone marrow transplantation or hematopoietic stem cell support.

Follow-up and Referral

Depending on the breast cancer patient's risk for both local and distant recurrence, a history and physical exam may be done according to the following schedule: every 3 to 6 months during the first 3 years (more frequently during adjuvant therapy), every 6 months for the next 2 years, and annually after the fifth year (more frequently for patients at very high risk for recurrence).

A baseline mammogram should be done 3 to 9 months after tumor excision and at the completion of all treatment. Thereafter, it should be done at least annually to detect a recurrence in the ipsilateral breast of patients who had breast-conserving surgery or to detect a second primary in the contralateral breast of most breast cancer patients. Further testing such as bone scans, chest x-ray films, computed tomography scans, and liver function tests are ordered for symptomatic patients as indicated. Patients treated with tamoxifen should have routine pelvic examinations. If abnormal uterine bleeding occurs, further evaluation is warranted.

The 5-year relative survival rate for patients with localized breast cancer is 98.4%, for regional spread it is 84.6%, and for distant metastases it is 24.3%. The 10-year survival for localized breast cancer declines to 82%, and 15-year survival declines to 75%.

Patient Education

The primary-care clinician may be involved at various phases of the patient's care, for example, prediagnosis, diagnosis, treatment, and posttreatment. Therefore, the clinician is in a valuable position to teach the patient and significant others regarding breast cancer prevention and detection and to reinforce information about a breast cancer diagnosis and treatment options (including benefits and potential complications).

The patient should be taught the breast self-exam technique, which can be found at www.breastcancer.org. Screening recommendations should also be reviewed. If diagnosed at an early stage, breast cancer may be curable with standard treatment.

The breast cancer patient needs to learn how to prevent potential postsurgical and/or radiation therapy complications such as lymphedema. In this situation, the patient should be taught range-of-motion exercises for the involved arm and shoulder. The need to avoid infections, injuries, strains, and constrictions of the arm is stressed. Antineoplastic chemotherapy and other forms of breast cancer treatment can be teratogenic; therefore, the patient must be advised to use effective contraception during treatment.

The breast cancer patient should be taught about the pharmacological and nonpharmacological management for the adverse effects of potential chemotherapy, radiation therapy, or hormonal therapy. For example, the patient may be instructed to take medications such as ondansetron (Zofran) and Decadron to prevent delayed chemotherapy-induced nausea and vomiting and to perform techniques such as relaxation with guided imagery to prevent or minimize these symptoms. The patient may also be directed in the purchase of a breast prosthesis, mastectomy bra, or wig.

The patient diagnosed with breast cancer may face many physical and psychosocial issues, such as an alteration in body image and sexuality, a role change, anxiety, denial, anger, and depression. The clinician is in a prime position to counsel and support the patient and significant others and to direct them to the many breast cancer resources available to the public that offer individual and group counseling, among other services.

There is confusion in the lay literature about the role of dietary soy intake and the risk for breast cancer in both women with no history of breast cancer and those who have had the disease. Some clinicians discourage their patients from consuming soy. (See Nursing Research–Based Practice 14.1.)

■ MASTITIS

Mastitis is a general term that refers to inflammation of the breast. The terminology for the various types of mastitis can be confusing. There are overlapping definitions and contradictions in the literature. For purposes of this discussion, there are three general categories: puerperal mastitis, nonpuerperal mastitis, and periductal mastitis. Each category is defined further by an explanation of the cause of the mastitis.

Puerperal mastitis is a cellulitis that develops in the lactating or nonlactating breast after parturition. Epidemic puerperal mastitis was a hospital-acquired infection most commonly seen in the preantibiotic era. The most common contagion for epidemic puerperal mastitis is *Staphylococcus aureus*. *S aureus* is spread by cross transmission from neonate to mother, as well as cross transmission in the nursery. There is multiple duct involvement, which results in inflammation of several nonadjacent lobes of the breast. With the progression of rooming-in and the introduction of antibiotics, epidemic puerperal mastitis has become a rare occurrence.

Nursing Research–Based Practice 14.1

Enderlin, CA, et al. Dietary soy intake and breast cancer risk. *Oncol Nurs Forum* 36(5):531–539, 2009.

Breast cancer affects about one in every eight women at some point in their lives. There have been confusing reports of soy foods. Soybeans and other soy products are high in phytoestrogens and isoflavones. The isoflavones are structurally similar to human estrogen and have estrogenic properties. Members of some cultures who consume large quantities of soy products also have lower prevalence rates for breast cancer.

The researchers conducted a metasynthesis of the literature of the relationship between dietary soy intake and breast cancer risk. They reviewed a total of 34 studies that represented samples from 12 countries and multiple races and ethnicities. The studies were published between 1997 and 2008. The analysis of these studies indicates that the dietary intake of naturally occurring soy foods is safe for women without breast cancer. The safety of soy supplements, however, is unclear.

Sporadic puerperal mastitis is an acute process that is far more common in women who breastfeed rather than in those who bottlefeed. It usually occurs in the second to sixth week postpartum; however, it has been reported in patients even after breastfeeding for 1 year. It is hypothesized that the higher occurrence of mastitis in the earlier postpartum period is due to the prevalence of nipple and feeding problems at this time, a risk factor for the disease. Feeding problems are more likely to occur in first-time breastfeeding mothers.

Nonpuerperal mastitis is a rare disease, which is usually found in patients who are immunocompromised, have undergone radiation therapy, or have had an autoimmune disorder. It can also occur in neonates. It is common in late adolescence or early adulthood. Nonpuerperal mastitis is a ductal abnormality or a local manifestation of a systemic problem. Several pathological pathways may be involved including squamous metaplasia of the lactational ducts, periareolar abscesses, and cellulitis. Squamous metaplasia is the most common nonpuerperal mastitis. Mastitis can also be caused by several obscure pathogens or by a substance in the breast such as silicone. This disease usually presents a clinical picture of a palpable mass and known infectious process such as tuberculosis (TB) or syphilis. Nonpuerperal mastitis must always be examined for the risk of carcinoma.

Periductal mastitis has been referred to and cross-referenced under several other names, such as mammary duct ectasia, mastitis obliterans, plasma cell mastitis, comedomastitis, and secretory disease of the breast. The term *duct ectasia* refers to the dilated

lactiferous ducts of the breast being filled with keratin and secretions. Periductal mastitis is the inflammatory process that occurs around these ducts. Some degree of duct dilation normally occurs with aging. Some researchers have suggested that periductal mastitis seen in younger patients represents a different disease from the more chronic clinical presentation seen in older women. The primary event of periductal mastitis is controversial. Some hypothesize that duct ectasia precedes the inflammatory process and vice versa. The disease is characterized by dilation of the subareolar ducts. The ducts become thick walled and surrounded by plasma cells. Inside the ducts there is a pasty, yellow-brown secretion, which is lipid-rich. The periductal regions become fibrotic and inflamed. This may be caused by rupture and leaking of the ducts themselves. Fat necrosis is often evident.

Epidemiology and Causes

The incidence of mastitis in breastfeeding women has been reported from 1% to 9%. One study found an incidence of 26% in a population of long-term breastfeeding mothers.

The causative organism of sporadic puerperal mastitis is *S aureus* in at least 50% of reported cases. *S aureus* is frequently found on skin and cultured from the neonate's mouth. Other organisms implicated in the infection are *Escherichia coli,* group A and group B *Streptococcus,* and *Mycobacterium tuberculosis.* TB mastitis occurs in populations in which TB is endemic.

There are a multitude of contributing factors for puerperal mastitis. Cracked, abraded, or otherwise damaged nipples provide a portal of entry for the microorganism. Patients who are having latch-on and positioning difficulty during feeding also increase their risk for both nipple skin disruption and milk stasis, which can lead to mastitis. Slow milk ejection reflex, engorgement, failure to empty the breast adequately, waiting too long between feedings, supplemental feedings, use of pacifiers, wearing a tight and restrictive bra, sleeping positions that constrict the breast, and weaning also contribute to a woman's risk of developing mastitis. Each of these situations can lead to blocked ducts and milk stasis. Unresolved milk stasis provides a medium for bacterial overgrowth.

Physiological and psychological stress are both significant risk factors for puerperal mastitis. Fatigue, improper nutrition, and life stress are predictors for breast infections. These situations lead to lower maternal immune defenses and an increased likelihood for the illness.

Periductal mastitis/mammary duct ectasia is seen primarily in perimenopausal and postmenopausal women. The peak incidence is between 40 and 49 years of age, but it can occur at any time after the menarche. The inflammatory process has been observed on microscopic exam in 30% to 40% of women older than age 50; however, clinical disease occurs much less frequently.

The actual incidence of the disease is unknown. Duct ectasia has a reported incidence of 5.5% to 25% as demonstrated on postmortem exams. A risk factor for periductal mastitis is cigarette smoking. The mechanism by which smoking increases the incidence of this disease is unknown, but there is a clear statistical link. Inverted nipples have been suggested to be a source of duct obstruction, which could lead to ectasia, but they have not been shown to be a risk factor.

The cause of periductal mastitis and ectasia is unknown. There may be an autoimmune explanation, but this has not been clarified. Infection by anaerobes and other bacteria may play a role, but this has not been verified either. Some patients with this mastitis do have bacteria in their nipple discharge.

Pathophysiology

The causative mechanism of the various forms of mastitis (puerperal, nonpuerperal, and periductal) has been discussed in the preceding text. However, the pathophysiology of the infectious process in the most common form, puerperal mastitis, is a classic example of a breakdown in the body's protective outer epithelial barriers. This results in entry of bacteria from the infant's mouth or mother's skin into her breast through cracked nipple skin or the nipple pores. With one or more lobes of the breast seeded, infection develops. Moreover, the symptoms of the disease, which include pain, tenderness, and maternal fatigue, contribute to further decreases in effective feeding practices and adequate emptying of the breast, thus worsening the infection. Milk of a mastitic breast has a higher than normal sodium and chloride content, and it is not unusual for an infant to refuse to nurse on that breast.

The infection of puerperal mastitis is primarily in the extraductal tissue, and thus breastfeeding through the infectious process generally poses no harm to the infant, provided skin breakdown has not resulted in frank bleeding from the nipples and there is no evidence of purulent nipple discharge. Purulent material may be present within the ducts, however. In addition, although bilateral infection is possible, mastitis is usually unilateral and localized to the upper outer quadrant of the affected breast. The incidence of mastitis progressing to a subareolar breast abscess has been reported to be as high as 4% to 11% in patients treated for the disease. It is much higher for those who do not seek treatment for mastitis.

Clinical Presentation

Subjective

The clinical presentation is acute in nature. The patient's first complaint is fatigue followed by the onset of flu-like symptoms and breast tenderness. The involved breast segments may be red and warm. Patients describe the affected area with a range of being tender to painful. A fever of at least 100.0°F (37.8°C) can be expected with myalgia, malaise, and chills. Nausea and vomiting can accompany these symptoms.

Many patients with periductal mastitis are asymptomatic. Others present with breast tenderness or pain, a breast mass, nipple discharge, nipple retraction, a nonpuerperal breast abscess, or a mammary fistula. The pain is usually subareolar and noncyclical. The nipple discharge varies in color and may contain occult blood. It is most frequently green and sticky and occurs spontaneously. The mastitis can be unilateral or bilateral. Nipple retraction and noninflammatory masses occur more commonly in older women. Pain and abscesses tend to occur in younger women. Periductal mastitis and ectasia account for 3% to 12% of benign breast lumps. The pain is usually focused behind the areola and tends to be more severe in younger patients.

Objective

On examination, there are varying degrees of erythema and edema of the affected breast. The erythema is most commonly in a V-shaped distribution and may or may not feel hard. Sometimes there is purulent nipple discharge. There may or may not be a palpable blocked duct.

Diagnostic Reasoning

Diagnostic Tests

Milk cultures are rarely done in first-occurrence cases of mastitis because they are costly and may delay treatment. They are warranted with a recurrence or failure of initial treatment. A breast milk culture can be obtained by manual expression of a midstream, clean-catch specimen. Washing the nipple with water and sterile gauze preps the breast. The first 2 to 3 mL of milk expressed should be discarded. The specimen needs to be fresh when sent to the lab. Breast milk is rarely found to be sterile and naturally contains leukocytes. A normal leukocyte count is 1,000 to 4,000/mL.

With patients symptomatic for mastitis, there are three diagnostic categories when cytology and cultures are performed on breast milk samples. Milk stasis is present with a white blood cell (WBC) count of less than 106/mL and a bacterial count of less than 103 colony-forming units (cfu)/mL. Noninfectious breast inflammation is considered with a WBC count of more than 106/mL and a bacterial count of less than 103 cfu/mL. A WBC count of more than 106/mL with a bacterial count of more than 103 cfu/mL is indicative of infectious mastitis. With the help of a milk culture and sensitivity, appropriate antibiotic treatment can be initiated. There are occasionally situations in which a patient develops a chronic puerperal mastitis. These patients may have anatomical strictures of some lactiferous ducts, which lead to chronic plugged ducts. Long-term antibiotic therapy and impeccable breastfeeding management can improve the outcome.

Ultrasound examination of the breast or mammogram may be helpful in making the diagnosis of periductal mastitis. The mammogram shows tubular dilated ducts. Calcification may be present in the lumen and walls of the affected ducts. Intense periductal mastitis may simulate carcinoma on the mammogram. Because carcinoma and mastitis can coexist, a biopsy may be warranted with such findings. In older patients, the mass from the ectasia can be hard to differentiate from carcinoma. Both masses can be hard, irregular, fixed or not to the surrounding tissue, and have skin or nipple retraction. When the nipple discharge is bilateral and multiple ducts are involved, the likelihood of malignancy is reported to be remote. Another diagnostic tool can be needle aspiration and culture of areas of inflammation. Fine-needle aspiration may show polymorphs, plasma cells, lymphocytes, and giant cells.

Differential Diagnosis

The first differential diagnosis to consider when presented with a patient symptomatic for puerperal mastitis is to identify that a condition of milk stasis or plugged ducts has led to an infectious process. The clinical presentation is invaluable in this judgment. There have been several cases of breast cancer in patients who are lactating or pregnant. Inflammatory breast cancer is a rare disease, but it can present with some of the same symptoms as a traditional puerperal mastitis. The patient with inflammatory breast cancer may have a red, swollen breast, and sometimes (but rarely) a fever. The patient commonly has no palpable breast mass and may or may not have *peau d'orange* (resembling orange peel). Reports differ on infants rejecting a breast later diagnosed with a cancerous disease. When inflammatory cancer is present, these symptoms do not respond to antibiotic treatment as mastitis generally does. With any suspicion of a cancerous process, the patient must be referred for biopsy and a definitive diagnosis.

Breast engorgement is often mistaken for mastitis but does not have the accompanying systemic symptoms of infection (e.g., fever, erythema, myalgia). If the infant has signs of poor "latch-on" during feeding (infant showing sunken cheeks, clicking sounds signifying breaking of suction, contact between the upper and lower lips at the corners of the mouth while feeding, etc.), this can also predispose the mother to mastitis. Galactoceles (milk retention cysts), which may result from plugged ducts, appear hard and red and may be quite painful (soreness, as opposed to the shooting pains of mastitis) but which lack the systemic signs of mastitis, should be considered as a possible diagnosis. Interestingly, hard, tender breasts with shooting pains but without redness or fever may be more associated with fungal infection of the breasts.

Management

The principle of management in puerperal mastitis is to decrease contributing factors and generally improve breastfeeding management.

Flu-like symptoms should always be treated as mastitis in postpartum patients unless proved otherwise. With a first occurrence, the diagnosis can be made by clinical symptoms alone. If there is no response to antibiotic treatment, or if there is recurrent mastitis, further diagnostics are indicated.

It is vital that the infant continue to breastfeed to avoid milk stasis. Because the infection is extraductal, there is no risk to the infant on continuing breastfeeding (except in HIV-infected mothers). Massage of the breasts during feeding helps to better drain the breast, and additional pumping may be needed, particularly if the infant is not nursing effectively on the affected side. Pumping breasts in addition to frequent infant feeding decreases the duration of symptoms (recommend every 6 hours feed or pump) and sequelae of the disease, notably breast abscess. Breastfeeding management should include correction of any latch-on or positioning difficulties and aggressive discovery and care of cracked or sore nipples.

Bedrest is imperative during the acute phase of the illness. The mother should be assisted with her household duties and rest in bed with her infant. Moist heat to the affected breast can be useful before feeding and pumping to increase milk expression. Cold application may be comfortable between feedings. Of course, stress management should be explored.

Antibiotic therapy is traditionally recommended to treat the infection. With no treatment at all, only 15% of patients recover without recurrent infection or breast abscess. Approximately 50% improve with pumping alone for treatment and more than 95% recover completely with combination therapy of pumping and antibiotics.

The best response is when antibiotics are started within the first 24 hours of symptom onset. A broad-spectrum antibiotic such as dicloxacillin or cloxacillin 500 mg PO every 6 hours is recommended for 10 to 14 days (for gram-negative organisms, use amoxicillin or cephalexin). If there is no response in the first 48 hours after initiation of antibiotic therapy, cephalexin or amoxicillin + clavulanate (Augmentin) is given for broader coverage. In addition, antibiotic sensitivity should be obtained from the milk culture. For those with a penicillin allergy, erythromycin (E-Mycin) (500 mg PO every 6 hours) can be prescribed. The patient must be instructed to continue her pharmacological therapy for the duration of the prescription to avoid a partially treated disease. Pain and other uncomfortable symptoms can be treated with nonsteroidal analgesics such as acetaminophen.

In the management of periductal mastitis, broad-spectrum antibiotics have been successful. They tend to treat the periareolar inflammation associated with this condition and reduce pain. If a mass is present, it must be biopsied to rule out carcinoma. If the nipple discharge is suspicious, a duct excision is necessary to confirm the diagnosis. Symptomatic treatment simply includes good nipple and areolar hygiene. Some have recommended no oral nipple stimulation.

The wound infection rate after breast biopsies where periductal mastitis and/or ectasia is present is high. The infection rate is 2% after biopsies with no evidence of this disease but 10.2% when it is present. This appears to be unrelated to trends in culture results.

Notable sequelae of this mastitis are breast abscesses and fistulas. Nonpuerperal breast abscesses are seen more frequently than those associated with lactation. The incidence of periareolar abscess is 10% in patients who are symptomatic with duct ectasia. The bacteria cultured are usually *S aureus* and anaerobes. Surgical excision and broad-spectrum antibiotic coverage is the treatment of choice. Needle aspiration may be performed if the risk of malignancy is low, but this treatment frequently needs to be done repetitively.

Abscess is one of the more common sequelae of puerperal mastitis. It can occur when the disease progresses either with or without treatment. The patient presents with worsening local symptoms and may or may not have systemic manifestations. A breast ultrasound can be useful to confirm the diagnosis. Most abscesses are surgically incised and drained under anesthesia. Biopsy of the cavity has been recommended to check for the presence of carcinoma. A drain is put in place, and broad-spectrum parenteral antibiotics should be started with anaerobic coverage pending culture results. A polymicrobial infection is common. The drain can be covered with a sterile gauze. It is not unusual for breast milk to leak around the drain because of severed lactiferous ducts. There are occasions when a breast abscess is treated with recurrent needle aspiration, but this is not currently the treatment of choice.

A recurrence of mastitis may occur for several reasons, including inadequate antibiotic therapy. When a recurrence is evident, a breast milk culture is indicated, as well as further exploration of the patient's breastfeeding management. Chronic mastitis may be treated with low doses of erythromycin (E-Mycin) 500 mg PO daily for the duration of lactation.

After antibiotic therapy, infection of the nipples with *Candida albicans* is not unusual. Topical treatment for the patient and concomitant oral nystatin for the infant is necessary. A fungal or *Candida* mastitis may develop, which is characterized by fiery pain shooting up the duct system. Oral antimycotic treatment would thus be indicated.

Follow-up and Referral

The patient may best be served by referral to an International Board–Certified Lactation Consultant for professional evaluation and assistance with infant feeding. The lactation consultant evaluates and corrects problems related to the infant's feeding, which may be causing or contributing to the occurrence of infection. If a patient's symptoms are not resolved after reasonable treatment attempts, or if there is no change in the size or condition of a breast lump presumed to be a plugged duct after 48 hours of care and treatment, the patient must be referred for further diagnostic evaluation.

Patient Education

Appropriate patient teaching and breastfeeding management in the early postpartum period can be the best prevention tool for puerperal mastitis. Early and frequent infant feedings with correct latch and positioning is necessary. No harsh substances such as soaps and lotions should be put on the nipples, and correct bra sizing, rest, and diet instruction can all help with disease prevention.

Patients with periductal mastitis and duct ectasia need much support. The fear of carcinoma in this age-group is high, and the patient must be reassured that this diagnosis has been considered and ruled out. Because of the prevalence of this condition, unclear cause, and uncertain absolute recovery, the patient only learns palliative and symptomatic treatment with a clear understanding of the disease process.

■ FERTILITY PROBLEMS

Fertility is the quality of being productive or fertile. Although science has begun to perfect some techniques that facilitate fertility, chance continues to play a large role in conception. *Infertility* is defined as lack of conception despite unprotected sexual intercourse for at least 12 months, because studies have shown a 93% cumulative probability of pregnancy in normal fertile couples after this period of time. Infertility occurs in 10% to 15% of couples in the United States. A woman younger than age 35 is considered infertile if no conception occurs after 1 year of unprotected intercourse. This time frame is shortened to 6 months in women aged 35 or older. A man is considered infertile if he does not produce and deliver enough quality sperm to initiate a pregnancy. Infertility is divided into two categories. *Primary infertility* refers to a woman who has never had a child, whereas *secondary infertility* applies to a woman who has delivered at least one child. *Sterility* is a term applied when there is an absolute factor preventing reproduction. Fecundability is the probability of successful pregnancy within one menstrual cycle.

Epidemiology and Causes

Approximately 10% of couples in the United States have difficulty conceiving a child after a year or more of trying. The American Society for Reproductive Medicine estimates that there are more than 6 million couples with infertility problems in the United States. Twenty-five percent of fertile couples conceive during 1 month of unprotected intercourse. Sixty percent conceive after 6 months, and 85% conceive after 12 months. These conception rates are averages and vary among couples. Primary infertility occurs in about 1 of 12 couples (8.3%). The incidence of infertility increases as the woman ages. For example, one in seven couples aged 30 to 34 are infertile, one in five aged 35 to 39, and one in four aged 40 to 44. These declines reflect the natural aging process and emphasize the need for rapid evaluation and treatment of infertility, especially in a patient older than 35 years of age.

Fertility patterns are dependent on many factors, including age, sex, and health. A major difference between male and female reproductive potential is that women have a finite reproductive life span (approximately 35 years), whereas men, after puberty, have the capacity to reproduce for the rest of their lives. However, fertility decreases in both men and women with aging. The causes of infertility are divided into categories. Male factors are responsible for a couple's infertility in 40% of cases. Testicular defects are a major cause with 10% to 20% from post-testicular defects (obstruction and disorders of sperm transport), 1% to 2% from hypothalamic-pituitary disease, and 40% to 50% from unidentifiable causes. Female causes are ovarian disease (failure to ovulate), 20%; tubal disease (obstruction), 25%; cervical factors (sperm cannot effectively pass the cervix), 5%; uterine abnormalities, less than 1%; and unexplained, 10%. In practical terms, infertility is caused by one of four conditions: the inability to produce healthy gametes (sperm or eggs); the failure of healthy gametes to come into close physical proximity, thus preventing fertilization; the inability of the fertilized egg to attach to the uterine lining successfully; and the inability to carry a pregnancy to term.

Infertility is a complex issue and is often caused by numerous factors. Couples should be referred for infertility evaluation if they have been unable to conceive after at least 1 year of attempting to achieve pregnancy. If the woman is older than 35 years of age, the couple should be referred after only 6 to 9 months of unprotected intercourse without conception. At age 25, the age at which couples are the most fertile, the average length of time needed to achieve conception is 5.3 months. The average 20- to 30-year-old American couple has intercourse one to three times a week, a frequency that should be sufficient to achieve pregnancy if all other factors are satisfactory. The number of women who give birth to their first child after age 30 continues to increase. Delaying parenthood appears to increase the possibility that one or more physiological processes necessary for conception will be adversely affected.

Even though infertility is defined as no pregnancy after 12 months of trying, evaluation should be initiated after 6 months in women between 35 and 40 years of age, and immediate evaluation is encouraged in women over 40 years, given the rapid increase in follicular atresia that occurs after age 37.

Pathophysiology

The following essential components must be present for normal fertility in women. The cervical mucus must be favorable to the survival of spermatozoa and allow passage to the upper genital tract. There must be clear passage between the cervix and the fallopian tubes. The fallopian tubes must be patent and have normal fimbria with peristaltic movements toward the uterus to facilitate normal transport and interaction of ovum and sperm. The ovaries must produce and release normal ova in a timely manner, and there must be no obstruction between the ovaries and fallopian tubes. Finally, the endometrium must be in a normal physiological state to allow implantation of the blastocyst and to sustain normal growth and development.

The most common cause of tubal infertility is antecedent pelvic inflammatory disease, caused most commonly by *Neisseria gonorrhoeae* and *Chlamydia trachomatis*. In addition, tubal endometriosis, pelvic tuberculosis, and adhesions from previous pelvic surgery or infection affecting any portion of the fallopian tubes may lead to obstruction. Hydrosalpinges, which are large, elongated typically fluid-filled cystic masses located anywhere along the adnexa, may form due to obstruction. These significantly interfere with the success of in vitro fertilization, thought to be due to components in the hydrosalpinx fluid that are toxic to developing embryos.

Uterine anatomical abnormalities have not been consistently identified as causal sources of infertility, because many women with abnormal uteri are able to conceive and carry pregnancies to term. However, septate uteri, synechiae (severe endometrial scarring), and polyps are all more common in infertile women. Similarly, uterine leiomyomata or fibroids (benign smooth muscle monoclonal tumors), which are the most common form of pelvic tumors in women, are observed in greater frequency in infertile women. However, it appears that only those with an intracavitary or submucosal component are associated with lower oocyte implantation and pregnancy rates.

Several other factors may affect the ability of the uterus to maintain a normal pregnancy. Endometriosis is more common in infertile women and, even when located outside the fallopian tubes, may contribute to infertility in a number of ways: pelvic adhesions affecting the reproductive tract; direct damage to ovarian tissue by endometrial implants or subsequent surgical removal; and cytokine and growth factor production by endometrial implants that interferes with ovulation, fertilization, or oocyte implantation. Cervical stenosis may occur congenitally, after trauma, or from infection and subsequent scarring. This, along with alterations in cervical mucus, may impair entry of sperm into the uterus. After implantation of the fertilized oocyte, impaired corpus luteum development may lead to inadequate progesterone production and delayed endometrial maturation, as demonstrated by endometrial biopsy. Likewise, in the presence of adequate progesterone, the endometrium may not be adequately responsive to this hormone. However, the importance of luteal phase defects as a direct cause of infertility is controversial.

Systemic factors also exist that affect the ability to initiate or maintain pregnancy. Hypercoagulable states, such as from antiphospholipid antibody syndrome, systemic lupus erythematosus, or other autoimmune and connective tissue disorders, are well known to be associated with early, first-trimester miscarriages—likely due to immunological rejection of the developing embryo or microthrombosis of placental vessels leading to placental insufficiency. Genetic anomalies in both women and men have been associated with infertility, the most common being Turner's syndrome (XO) in women and Klinefelter's syndrome (XXY) and fragile X syndrome in men. Defects in several genes capable of affecting fertility have been identified including *KAL1,* which leads to congenital hypothalamic hypopituitary hypogonadism (Kallmann's syndrome); the follicle-stimulating hormone (FSH) receptor, FMR1, which leads to fragile X syndrome; and *DAX1, FGFR1,* and *GPR54.*

For normal fertility to occur in men, the testes must produce an adequate number of morphologically normal, motile sperm. The male genital tract secretions from the seminal vesicles and prostate gland must be normal. The genital tract must not be obstructed, because sperm travel from the testis through the epididymis and vas deferens to the urethra. Finally, ejaculated spermatozoa must be deposited in the female genital tract in such a manner that they reach the cervix and enter the uterus where they may contact oocytes either within the uterus or more commonly within the fallopian tubes.

Primary hypogonadism is the most commonly identifiable cause of male infertility, resulting from congenital causes including chromosomal disorders (e.g., Klinefelter's and fragile X syndrome), azoospermia from cryptorchidism (i.e., failure of testicular descent from the abdominal cavity during in utero development), defects in androgen production (5-alpha-reductase deficiency) or receptor activity, as well as Y chromosome deletions, especially in the long arm at the Yq6 region. Acquired disorders such as testicular infection (e.g., viral orchitis from mumps paramyxovirus, echovirus, or arbovirus), drugs toxic to sperm (e.g., alkylating immunosuppressants such as cyclophosphamide, antiandrogens such as spironolactone and ketoconazole), radiation exposure, tobacco smoking, and hyperthermia have all been associated with decreased male fertility, as well as underlying systemic disease such as chronic renal insufficiency and cirrhosis. Antisperm antibodies have also been identified in some infertile men that presumably affect fertility, but it is not clear whether these form spontaneously or as a result of testicular injury that compromises the testicular–blood barrier.

In far fewer cases, defects exist higher up on the hypothalamic-pituitary-gonadal axis. A failure of hypothalamic gonadotropin-releasing hormone (GnRH) secretion and/or pituitary gonadotropin production may result from congenital defects (e.g., Kallmann's syndrome) or acquired conditions such as secreting or nonsecreting pituitary macroadenomas, prolactinomas, craniopharyngiomas, or infiltrative processes such as sarcoidosis, histiocytosis, or tuberculosis.

Sperm transport may be inhibited anywhere along the male reproductive tract. Intrauterine estrogen exposure may lead to epididymal defects, and infection (e.g., epididymitis caused by *N gonorrhoeae, C trachomatis,* or tuberculosis) and certain chemical toxins (e.g., chlorhydrin) may affect spermatozoal function within the epididymis. The vas deferens may similarly be affected by infection, intentional ligation as in surgical vasectomy, inspissation of thick mucoid secretions (Young's syndrome), or congenital absence due to defects in cAMP-regulated chloride ion channels, as in cystic fibrosis. Although secretions from the prostate and seminal vesicles contain several components (e.g., fructose) that contribute to sperm viability and motility, defects in glandular secretion have not been causally related to infertility. In addition, erectile dysfunction and ineffective ejaculation may result from spinal cord damage or disease, as well as defects in autonomic function from diabetes mellitus. Varicoceles (venous dilation of the pampiniform plexus proximal to the testicle) are also far more common in infertile men, but they may also be present in men with normal fertility. Although no definitive evidence exists, they are thought to impair spermatogenesis via increased testicular temperature, hypoxia, or vascular stasis with delayed clearance of toxic serum metabolites.

Clinical Presentation
Subjective
The patient presents with the complaint of inability to conceive and the desire to have a child.

Objective
Assessment of persons seeking evaluation and treatment of infertility should begin with a detailed comprehensive history. Before tests to determine the cause of infertility are made, a detailed medical, social, and family history must be obtained from both partners. Often the history uncovers important information. The history should elicit information about the duration of the infertility and whether it is primary or secondary; the frequency of sexual intercourse; the regularity, duration, and frequency of menstruation; and any premenstrual signs and symptoms. It should also include information on any vaginal discharge, cervicitis, pelvic infections, surgery, and trauma. General physical condition, illness, allergies, and drug intake (prescription and illicit) should be noted, as should any significant family history. Prior use of contraceptives, including type, duration, and complications, should be recorded. Information on maternal use of diethylstilbestrol (DES) should also be noted, because this can affect fertility.

Necessary information from the man includes any history of mumps, orchitis, trauma, diabetes mellitus, herniorrhaphy, or exposure to x-rays or toxic substances such as lead, iron, zinc, or copper. The male should also be questioned about exercise patterns, drug intake (prescription and illicit), exposure to heat (from the environment or from wearing tight underclothes), duration of infertility, whether the fertility is primary or secondary, frequency of coitus, and history of maternal use of DES (can affect a son's fertility). A complete physical exam of both partners is essential, particularly a thorough pelvic exam of the woman. The male examination should include testicular volume (below 15 mL is small) and testicular length (less than 3.6 cm is small). Certain laboratory tests, such as complete blood count, thyroid-stimulating hormone (TSH), T_4, and urinalysis, should also be included. If findings are negative, an infertility work-up is begun.

Diagnostic Reasoning
Diagnostic Tests

The easiest and least intrusive infertility testing should be used first. Extensive testing should be avoided until data confirm that the timing of intercourse and the length of coital exposure have been adequate. The couple should be informed of the most fertile times to have intercourse during the menstrual cycle. Teaching the couple the signs and timing of ovulation and the most effective times for intercourse within the cycle may solve the problem before extensive testing needs to be initiated. Primary assessment, including a comprehensive history and physical exam for any obvious causes of infertility, is done before a costly, time-consuming, and emotionally trying investigation is initiated. Because infertility is a couple's issue, it is important for both partners to be present. One basic test of ovulatory function is the basal body temperature (BBT) recording, which aids in identifying follicular, ovulatory, and luteal-phase abnormalities. With the additional documentation of coitus, serial BBT charts can be used to indicate retrospectively if, and approximately when, the woman is ovulating and if intercourse is occurring at the proper time to achieve conception. A proposed schedule for intercourse, based on serial BBT charts, might be to recommend sexual intercourse every other day in the period of time beginning 3 to 4 days before and continuing for 2 to 3 days after the expected time of ovulation.

Semen analysis is the single most important diagnostic study of the male and should be done early in the couple's evaluation and before invasive testing of the female. Semen analysis must be done within 1 day of donation, and normal sperm morphology may be as low as 15% to 20% with good results. Also, at least 25% of sperm should have rapid progressive mobility (not just moving in place). Sperm viability should be tested if

motility is insufficient. Semen pH is also important (low pH is correlated with decreased fertility). Cellular debris and agglutination are of concern for antibody-mediated autoimmune destruction of sperm. Antibodies may be detected and are considered concerning if they coat more than 50% of spermatozoa. The presence of immature germ cells may represent a maturation defect, and the presence of sperm leukocytes (greater than 1 million/mL) reflects infection within the reproductive tract. Semen culture is often sent, but this is usually not diagnostically useful. It is important to note that an absence of sperm may be due to spermatic duct obstruction, rather than a lack of sperm production by the testes. Patients lacking sperm in the semen should be referred to urology to rule out retrograde ejaculation, congenital absence of the vas deferens, or other forms of obstruction. A postejaculatory urine specimen will reflect retrograde ejaculation if sperm are present, whereas an absence of sperm may reflect obstruction or impaired spermatogenesis.

It is important to assess both partners because of the high incidence of multifactorial infertility. A thorough female evaluation includes assessment of the hypothalamic-pituitary axis in terms of ovulatory function. Progesterone levels are measured at different points along the luteal phase to confirm ovulation. In addition, LH levels can be measured in the serum and with home urine tests to help predict ovulation (as the surge occurs 1–2 days ahead of ovulation) to facilitate the timing of intercourse, but home urine tests are not as sensitive (85%) as serum tests done during formal fertility evaluation, because once-a-day testing can miss the surge because of variations in renal clearance of luteinizing hormone (LH). Examination of vaginal discharge for increased volume and clear, slippery mucus that stretches into strings (Spinnbarkeit) is a strong indicator of preovulatory estrogen effect. The progesterone challenge test, using medroxyprogesterone acetate 10 mg daily for 5 days and checking for induction of uterine bleeding in the week after treatment, confirms adequate production of estradiol (estrogen). An FSH level should be drawn on day 3 of the cycle to check for adequate ovarian reserve—a value less than 15 mIU/mL is suggestive of adequate reserve. Prolactin and TSH levels should also be checked to rule out hyperprolactinemia (which may be treated with a dopamine agonist such as bromocriptine, pergolide, or cabergoline), especially in women with galactorrhea, and thyroid disorders. Magnetic resonance imaging and hysterosalpingogram imaging are done to evaluate the structure and function of the cervix, uterus, fallopian tubes, and ovaries. Laparoscopy is more sensitive for detecting tubal abnormalities than hysterosalpingogram alone but may be unnecessary if the findings from the hysterosalpingogram are normal. Also, the performance of the hysterosalpingogram itself (flushing the tubes with oil-based contrast medium) increases the likelihood of pregnancy.

Evaluation of the man may include at least two semen analyses to confirm or rule out a seminal deficiency. Endocrine evaluation of men includes serum LH, FSH, and testosterone levels. If the LH and FSH are high and the testosterone level is low, this is consistent with primary hypogonadism, whereas a normal to low LH and FSH reflects secondary hypogonadism. In men with low testosterone and normal to low LH levels, prolactin should be measured to rule out prolactinomas.

If the results of both the male and female infertility work-ups are negative, a laparoscopic evaluation may be necessary. Table 14.5 outlines different fertility tests and favorable clinical findings that indicate that the couple is capable of conceiving.

Management

The principle of management is to assist the couple to achieve pregnancy before or during the natural age-related

Table 14.5		Fertility Tests and Favorable Clinical Findings	
Gender	**Test**	**How Obtained**	**Favorable Clinical Findings**
Male	Semen analysis	48–72 hr after abstinence from ejaculation	Normal amount of ejaculate (3–5 mL; range 1–7 mL).
	Karyotyping (in men with severe oligospermia or azoospermia)	Blood sample/bone marrow	No agglutination of sperm. (Agglutination suggests infection or autoimmunity.) Normal seminal fluid. Sperm count greater than 20,000,000 cells with at least 50% motility 2 hours after ejaculation and more than 60% normal-appearing cells. Chromosomal abnormalities can be detected.
Female	Basal body temperature (BBT) measurement	Oral temperature taken daily before arising throughout several menstrual cycles	Biphasic pattern with persistent temperature elevation for 12–14 days before menses.
	Postcoital test	Vaginal exam within 8 hours after intercourse, during time of presumed ovulation	Cervical mucus suggestive of ovulation. Microscopic ferning pattern present. Watery, slippery, abundant mucus. Spinnbarkeit is present (the act of pulling out a string of cervical mucus and measuring how far it can be stretched before breaking). Presence of normal live and motile sperm in cervical mucus.
	Serum progesterone measurement	Blood sample	3–4 ng/mL in early luteal phase. 10 ng/mL at midluteal phase.
	Serum LH (to predict ovulation)	Blood sample	6.17–17.2 IU/L at ovulation.
	Karyotyping (in women with ovarian failure or repeated spontaneous abortion)	Blood sample/bone marrow	
	Immunoassay tests	Semen and male/female serum	Absence of antibody reaction. Evidence of normal pelvic anatomy and tubal functioning.
	Hysterosalpingogram	Dye injected through cervix into uterus then fluoroscopic visualization of the spread of dye through fallopian tubes. Done during first half of menstrual cycle before ovulation	Patency of fallopian tubes and absence of abnormalities in uterine cavities and fallopian tubes.
	Laparoscopy	Direct visualization of pelvic structures through a small abdominal incision	Normal pelvic structures and absence of signs of infection, adhesions, endometriosis, or lesions.

decline in female fecundity. Several lifestyle changes can increase the chances that a couple will become pregnant. Women should limit caffeine intake to no more than 250 mg (2 cups of coffee) per day. Studies show that consumption of caffeine over 300 mg can delay conception and increase the risk for miscarriage and preterm labor. Caffeine intake in men does not seem to affect fertility. Likewise, alcohol affects fertility in women, and intake should be limited to no more than 4 drinks per week. Increasing sexual intercourse to 2 to 3 times a week is also advisable. These measures should be recommended before any other interventions. If the woman's body mass index is less than 20 or greater than 27, attempts should be made to get the body weight to a normal level. Loss of just 5% to 10% of body weight in obese anovulatory women with polycystic ovarian disease (PCOS) can restore ovulation within 6 months and should be a first-line therapy. For women with PCOS, in addition to weight loss, insulin sensitization with metformin has been shown to improve fertility.

A low percentage of body fat resulting from eating disorders (anorexia nervosa/bulimia) or from extreme exercise can lead to anovulation through GnRH or gonadotropin suppression and must be addressed. Pulsatile GnRH therapy may restore ovulation in these women, but this treatment is available only in Europe at this time.

If an ovulatory defect has been identified during fertility testing, the treatment depends on the specific cause of the problem. In the presence of normal ovaries, a normal prolactin level, and an intact pituitary gland (normogonadotropic normoestrogenic anovulation [World Health Organization class II anovulation], which is 70%–85% of cases), clomiphene citrate (Clomid), a selective estrogen receptor modulator (SERM) with both agonist and antagonist effects at the estrogen receptor level, is effective. Ovulation occurs in approximately 80% of properly selected women, and conception rates approach 40%. The risk of multiple gestation with clomiphene is 5% and is almost exclusively with twins. The woman takes a 50-mg dose of clomiphene each day from days 5 to 9 of the cycle. Ovulation can be expected to occur 5 to 10 days after the last dose. If ovulation is not achieved in the first cycle of therapy, the dose may be increased in 50-mg increments to a maximum of 200 to 250 mg daily for 5 days. After the first treatment cycle, a pelvic exam should be done to rule out ovarian enlargement or hyperstimulation. Ovarian enlargement and abdominal discomfort may result from follicular growth and the formation of multiple corpus lutea. Other adverse effects include hot flashes, nausea and vomiting, vision problems, headache, and dryness or loss of hair. Clomiphene citrate should not be used for more than six cycles, because it is unlikely to work after this many tries. Tamoxifen is another SERM that works with fewer antiestrogen effects, but it has no added fertility benefit over clomiphene citrate.

Aromatase inhibitors such as letrozole (Femara) and anastrozole (Arimidex) have a shorter half-life than the SERMs and fewer antiestrogen effects, producing fewer follicles and lower estradiol levels, reducing the risk of multiple gestations and miscarriage. These agents may be used for patients who do not respond to clomiphene.

Treatment with gonadotropins requires much closer monitoring, is more costly, and has a higher risk of multiple gestations but is considered the most effective medication used with intrauterine insemination for ovarian hyperstimulation. A laparoscopic technique called ovarian drilling may be used in which a laser is used to induce ovulation. This technique seems to work no better than gonadotropins, but it carries less risk of multiple gestations.

Cervical stenosis can be treated via catheter dilation for several days with concurrent antibiotic prophylaxis (doxycycline 100 mg PO 2 times daily). Women with systemic clotting disorders may also benefit from aspirin and heparin anticoagulation therapy to improve the likelihood of pregnancy.

Intrauterine insemination (IUI) just before ovulation (based on LH measurements) is often effective when other methods have failed. IUI may be tried before in vitro fertilization (IVF) because it is often effective and less expensive. IUI done high in the uterus is more effective than intracervical injection, which approximates normal intercourse. With high IUI, the probability of pregnancy is improved through concurrent treatment with clomiphene for three to six cycles, and if this fails, IUI with gonadotropin injections for at least three cycles can be tried.

The last resort for infertile couples is IVF and embryo transfer or, if the tubes are patent and normal, gamete intrafallopian transfer (GIFT). In some cases of tubal occlusion in which the rate of success with tubal repair is low (less than 30%), IVF appears to be preferable to surgery because of the more rapid conception rate. IVF has the highest pregnancy rate in the shortest amount of time, but it is also the costliest intervention, with a price tag of $50,000 to $100,000 per attempt. Intratubal transfer of embryos may improve the success rate over transcervical transfer, but this is unclear and may depend on how good the results are at the particular center with the regular IVF procedure.

The pregnancy rate with IVF has been highly variable from center to center, owing to the complexity of the techniques required, whereas the pregnancy rate with GIFT has been more consistent. The mean live delivery rates per retrieval with IVF and GIFT are approximately 21% and 28%, respectively. Ectopic pregnancy occurs in about 4% to 5% of these pregnancies, whereas the rate of fetal abnormalities is not increased. There are many ethical considerations associated with assisted reproductive technologies; some of these are presented in Table 14.6.

Table 14.6   Ethical Considerations and Assisted Reproductive Technologies

In vitro fertilization (IVF) has been a welcome solution for many couples who have been unable to conceive. Recently, advances in the application of IVF technology have spurred the emergence of even more new avenues of achieving pregnancy and parenting. With hormone replacement therapy (HRT) and donor egg embryos, women past menopause can achieve pregnancy. Other options include cryopreservation, fertilization of donor gametes (donor eggs, sperm, or both), IVF with the use of a gestational carrier, embryo adoption, and the use of surrogacy. All of these options are complicated by the introduction of a third party into the reproductive process and ethical concerns. Some of the issues raised in connection with these techniques include the following:

1. Is it a constitutional right for individuals or couples to be able to utilize donor gametes or to contract with a woman to carry their embryo to treat their infertility?
2. With a multiple pregnancy rate approaching 20% in couples undergoing IVF procedures, the potential (<3%) of having a grand multiple gestation forces some couples to consider embryo reduction (selective abortion) to avoid an adverse obstetric and/or fetal outcome.
3. If excess embryos are frozen and kept, how long can and should they be stored? What should be done in cases of death of one or both of the partners, divorce, or when couples choose not to claim their embryos?
4. Do providers have the right to decide who can participate in using donor gametes, embryos, gestational carriers, and surrogates? What about single women, lesbian couples, or crossing generational lines (daughter being a donor for mother)?
5. Does the use of assisted reproductive technologies take into consideration the best interests of the parties involved, including those of the resulting offspring? For example, what are the effects on a child of knowing or not knowing the identity of the donor?
6. How can the potential for consanguinity (having an ancestor in common) be controlled in the case of gamete and/or embryo donation?
7. Does the existence of new technologies make it more difficult to accept childlessness by increasing pressure on women to follow every avenue in an attempt to conceive?
8. To what extent should health insurance policies cover these modes of treating infertility at a time of growing health-care costs?

It is also possible to achieve pregnancy with IVF and embryo transfer using donor eggs, with a higher success rate than with regular IVF and embryo transfer (47% per retrieval). The eggs generally come from young fertile women (sisters or anonymous volunteers). The recipient's uterus can be prepared for optimal uterine receptivity by replacement doses of estradiol and progesterone.

Male infertility from hypogonadotropic hypogonadism may be treated with human chorionic gonadotropin (hCG) injections 1,500 to 2,000 IU subcutaneously or intramuscularly three times per week for at least 6 months. hCG acts similarly to LH. If this does not work, human menopausal gonadotropin 37.5 to 75 IU three times per week is added that contains FSH. Thus, this treatment can last more than a year. This combination therapy is typically needed for Kallmann's syndrome (congenital hypogonadotropic hypogonadism). Recombinant LH/FSH is also now available. Pulsatile GnRH treatment delivered via IV pump is also available for hypothalamic hypogonadotropic hypogonadism.

Sperm autoimmunity may be treated with high-dose steroids (prednisone 40–80 mg PO daily) for up to 6 months, but this regimen may be poorly tolerated. Thus, intracytoplasmic sperm injection (ICSI) is an important IVF alternative with a clinical pregnancy rate of

up to 20%. Retrograde ejaculation may be treated with IUI, traditional IVF, or ICSI as well. Repair of varicoceles is controversial and is usually recommended only with large defects or in younger men, because prolonged damage to the testes—indicated by testicular atrophy, epithelial damage, and severe oligospermia or azoospermia—is unlikely to be reversed by surgical ligation of the varicocele. Reversal of vasectomy can result in successful pregnancy in a female partner in up to 50% of cases. In cases of obstruction along the reproductive tract, sperm may be retrieved for ICSI via direct microsurgical aspiration from the epididymis or the seminiferous tubules of the testes. In all cases of congenital reproductive tract defects such as absent vas deferens, genetic counseling must take place before microsurgical aspiration and ICSI, given the risk of passing genetic defects, such as the cystic fibrosis gene, Klinefelter's, or deletions in the Y chromosome, onto these men's offspring.

Follow-up and Referral

After the initial exam and counseling regarding the frequency and timing of intercourse, if couples wish to proceed with testing and/or treatment, referral to a fertility clinic is indicated. Infertile couples need a great deal of support and advocacy, as well as education and help in decision making. The options must be presented in a nonjudgmental way to facilitate the couple's own decision making. Providing referral to other sources of assistance is another way in which the clinician supports the infertile person or couple. One important source of information is RESOLVE, a national organization composed of self-help groups that provide support and information about infertility. Providing anticipatory guidance for the battery of tests to which patients are subjected during infertility evaluation is important.

Patient Education

An important part of care for infertile persons is emphasizing and teaching self-care. Infertility is often experienced as being "out of control." Identifying and using successful coping strategies help the patient regain a sense of control. Stress-reduction techniques, such as exercise, relaxation techniques, and meditation, may be especially useful both for those with general concerns about fertility and for those concerned about specific diagnostic or treatment procedures. Infertility can become an all-encompassing concern, resulting in alterations in health and recreation patterns and a loss of interest in other aspects of life. It should be emphasized that one can be creative, productive, and successful in other areas even if unable to produce children. The emotional problems surrounding infertility illustrate the need for emphasis on family-centered care. Infertility is a highly emotional issue that has far-reaching implications for many family members.

◼ AMENORRHEA

Menarche usually occurs between ages 11 and 15 years, and the average age in the United States today is 12.7 years. Absence of menstruation is considered amenorrhea and can be primary or secondary. *Primary amenorrhea* is the failure to menstruate by age 14 in girls with no secondary sex characteristics (breast development) or failure to menstruate by age 16 years in girls who may or may not have developed secondary sexual characteristics. *Secondary amenorrhea* is the absence of menstruation for 3 or more consecutive months in a woman who has achieved menarche.

Epidemiology and Causes

Primary amenorrhea occurs in about 0.3% of women and may result from hypothalamic or pituitary failure, ovarian failure, or chromosomal or enzymatic abnormalities. Amenorrhea is a manifestation of a pathological process and is not a diagnosis itself. Causes of primary amenorrhea include congenital defects of gonadotropin production; genetic disorders (Turner's syndrome); congenital central nervous system (CNS) defects such as hydrocephalus; congenital anatomical malformations of the reproductive system (absence of vagina or uterus); abnormal outflow tract (vaginal aplasia or imperforate hymen); and acquired CNS lesions, including trauma, infection, and tumors. Females without a uterus or

vagina usually have normal ovarian function in which skeletal growth and secondary sex characteristics develop in the proper sequence, but menses does not occur. In cases of uterine hypoplasia, the uterus does not respond to hormonal stimulation during puberty.

If a woman is not pregnant (most common cause), secondary amenorrhea is usually associated with anovulation caused by neuroendocrine dysfunction. Secondary amenorrhea occurs in approximately 1% to 3% of women, with a higher incidence among college students (3%–5%) and athletes (5%–50%). Amenorrhea reflects a disruption in the normal physiological or anatomical function of the hypothalamus, pituitary gland, and ovary or outflow tract. Hormones produced by these structures play major roles in ovulation; any slight change in production may result in anovulation and absence of menstruation. Women taking anabolic steroids (weight lifters, body builders), elite athletes with low body fat, and those with anorexia nervosa may present with secondary amenorrhea.

Pathophysiology

The hypothalamic-pituitary-ovarian-uterine axis needs to function in a coordinated manner for menstruation to occur. The most frequent cause of primary amenorrhea is dysfunction of the ovaries resulting from gonadal dysgenesis. This may be caused by various chromosomal abnormalities that result in a depletion of oocytes and ovarian follicles, subsequently impairing the regulated cycle of menses. Turner syndrome, characterized by an XO (single X-chromosome) genotype, is one of the most common chromosomal disorders. In this condition, the ovaries are replaced by fibrous tissue (known as streak ovaries), which has a very limited or absent capacity for estrogen production. In addition, premature ovarian failure (menopause occurring before age 40 years), polycystic ovary syndrome (characterized by concurrent hyperandrogenism), and estrogen- or androgen-secreting tumors may all produce amenorrhea. Secondary amenorrhea is nearly universally a hormonal problem because, by definition, normal female sexual development has already occurred. By far, the most common cause of secondary amenorrhea is the normal hormonal changes associated with pregnancy, that is, increased progesterone production needed to maintain the pregnant uterus.

Under normal conditions, the hypothalamus produces gonadotropin-releasing hormone (GnRH) in a pulsatile fashion. In response to GnRH, the anterior pituitary gland produces the gonadotropins follicle-stimulating hormone (FSH) and luteinizing hormone (LH). In response to FSH and LH, the ovaries produce estrogen and progesterone, which subsequently drive secondary sexual development and cyclic menstruation. Factors such as stress, weight changes, nutritional deficiencies, strenuous exercise, or infiltrative CNS lesions including hypothalamic tumors (e.g., lymphoma, histiocytosis) or sarcoidosis may all disrupt the normal pulsatile release of GnRH. Pulsatile production of GnRH may also be affected by rare pituitary tumors including macroadenomas and microadenomas, which consist primarily of hyperprolactinomas and account for 20% of secondary amenorrhea cases. Amenorrhea may occur before or after the treatment of such tumors (i.e., surgical resection), depending on the underlying production of pituitary gonadotropins. Functional hypothalamic amenorrhea (which may be primary or secondary) is characterized by an absence of histological CNS pathology, despite an underproduction or overproduction of GnRH that leads to a decrease in gonadotropin surges and amenorrhea. In contrast, a complete absence of hypothalamic GnRH production may occur congenitally, inherited in an autosomal dominant, autosomal recessive, or X-linked fashion.

Whereas acquired endometrial scarring known as Asherman's syndrome is the only anatomical uterine etiology of secondary amenorrhea, nearly a quarter of primary amenorrhea cases are due to structural abnormalities that prevent menstrual outflow, including imperforate hymen, vaginal agenesis, absent or abnormal uterus, or the presence of a transvaginal septum between the hymen and the cervix. Such conditions may not be connected to any specific event or environmental exposure. However, some conditions may result from biochemical abnormalities in hormone receptor functioning, manifested on either an XX or XY genetic background. Thus, an advanced work-up of patients with primary amenorrhea should also include karyotyping to confirm that the patient is an XX genetic female.

Complete androgen insensitivity syndrome (testicular feminization syndrome) is the prototype for primary amenorrhea occurring in a genetic male who appears outwardly female on clinical exam. In this disorder, the external genitalia of XY males are unable to respond to testosterone because of a receptor defect and thus fail to undergo differentiation into a phenotypically male form, despite their XY karyotype. Internally, however, the testes do produce functional Müllerian inhibiting factor, causing the regression of all internal female reproductive organs, thus leading to primary amenorrhea. A congenital lack of 5-alpha-reductase enzymatic activity causes a similar phenomenon of external sexual ambiguity in which XY males do not undergo full secondary sexual development at puberty, because testosterone cannot be converted into its more potent metabolite dihydrotestosterone.

Clinical Presentation
Subjective

Amenorrhea is a symptom, so this is usually the reason the patient seeks health care. Other subjective data from the patient usually are obtained during the history. The detailed history must include a complete menstrual history including age at menarche, date of last menstrual period and last normal menses, cycle regularity, and flow; obstetrical history, including number of pregnancies, lactation, and birth control methods; developmental data, to evaluate for short stature or growth hormone or thyroid deficiency; nutritional history, including anorexia, diet, stress, and sports activities; family history, especially the mother's onset of menopause; symptoms that may arise from systemic disorders (diabetes, thyroid); the presence or absence of any secondary sex characteristics; and any medications being taken, such as hypertensive medications or oral contraceptive pills. Cyclic pelvic pain in a young teen or preteen could indicate Müllerian outflow tract obstruction.

Objective

The physical exam should include a neurological exam to assess for headaches and visual field abnormalities to rule out pituitary tumor; olfactory testing to screen for Kallmann's syndrome (hypothalamic or pituitary tumor); a pelvic and rectal exam (to assess for the presence of a vagina, condition of hymen, and presence of uterus); the existence of skin lesions, acne, needle marks, and skin darkening, to rule out adrenal insufficiency; and a breast exam, to observe for galactorrhea, which may be a sign of hyperprolactinemia.

Diagnostic Reasoning
Diagnostic Tests

A urine pregnancy test should be the first test performed in the patient with amenorrhea because it is inexpensive and easy. It should be done despite what the patient tells you about her sexual history. If the test is positive, a serum beta–human chorionic gonadotropin for approximate staging of pregnancy should be done. Other tests should include baseline blood chemistry profiles to evaluate for renal or hepatic disease; thyroid function tests; vaginal smears for estrogen effect; and FSH, LH, and prolactin levels.

Tests for secondary amenorrhea include androgen studies of total testosterone and dehydroepiandrosterone sulfate, which are specifically done in women who also have clinical signs of hyperandrogenism (acne, hirsutism, etc.); a progesterone challenge test; and the measurement of prolactin and FSH levels, which evaluate the hypothalamic-pituitary-ovarian axis.

A progestin (or progesterone) challenge indirectly provides information regarding outflow tract patency. This test, given once a negative pregnancy test is obtained, consists of giving medroxyprogesterone acetate 10 mg PO for 5 to 10 days or 200 mg IM once to induce withdrawal bleeding or spotting, which should occur within 14 days after the last dose. If withdrawal bleeding occurs, this indicates pituitary-gonadal function, and amenorrhea is probably the result of anovulation. The test is negative if no withdrawal bleeding occurs and suggests low levels of estrogen (premature ovarian failure or hypothalamic pituitary failure) or a nonpatent outflow tract.

Differential Diagnosis

Differential diagnoses include pregnancy (intrauterine or ectopic); menopause; premature ovarian failure; hyperprolactinemia related to tumor, stress, or thyroid dysfunction; and some genetic or chromosome-related problems. Outflow-tract abnormalities include Asherman's syndrome, which is characterized by endometrial adhesions and scarring as a result of aggressive dilation and curettage, uterovaginal malignancies, cervical stenosis, or imperforated hymen.

A genetic disorder of male pseudohermaphroditism may result in primary amenorrhea. The patient is male genetically but female morphologically. No male genitalia develop because androgen receptors are absent in undifferentiated target organs.

Management

The goal of management for amenorrhea is to initiate or restore menses while determining the cause. Treatment of amenorrhea is dependent on its etiology and the patient's wishes. For primary amenorrhea, estrogen therapy is indicated for patients to develop secondary sex characteristics and prevent osteoporosis.

For a patient with secondary amenorrhea whose progestin challenge test is negative, treatment consists of oral estrogen 1.25 to 2.5 mg daily for 21 to 25 days, along with oral progesterone 10 mg daily during the last 5 to 10 days of the estrogen doses. The patient should experience bleeding if the endometrium is normally responsive to estrogen and the outflow tract is patent.

For a patient with secondary amenorrhea who is anovulatory and has adequate endogenous estrogen, the common practice is to administer periodic or cyclic progesterone 10 mg PO daily for 10 days each month. These patients must experience withdrawal bleeding for at least 3 months to prevent endometrial hyperplasia or endometrial carcinoma related to unopposed estrogen. If the patient is anovulatory and wants to conceive, ovulation may be induced with clomiphene citrate (Clomid) 50 mg PO on days 5 to 9 of the cycle after induction of bleeding with progesterone.

If the patient wants contraception, oral contraceptives are beneficial for monthly cycle regulation. For patients with hyperprolactinemia, bromocriptine (Parlodel) is the drug of choice. Once hypothalamic failure is established, GnRH may be given in a pulsatile fashion. GnRH is given as a combination with estrogen and calcium because these patients are hypoestrogenic and at high risk for osteoporosis. In patients with thyroid dysfunction, replacement therapy should be initiated, and the amenorrhea should correct itself.

Surgical intervention is possible for women with endometrial scarring (Asherman's syndrome) from endometritis. Diagnosis and treatment are accomplished in the same way, through hysteroscopic inspection and lysis of adhesions. After this procedure, antibiotics are given, and a small Foley catheter is placed in the uterus and left for 1 week. When the catheter is removed, an intrauterine device is inserted and left in place for 2 months while the patient receives cyclic estrogen and progesterone to build the endometrial lining. This treatment usually restores normal menses and fertility, but complications of pregnancy are common, including spontaneous abortions.

Follow-up and Referral

A gynecologist and an endocrinologist should be consulted for further testing. If a CNS problem is detected, computed tomography scanning or magnetic resonance imaging should be performed to rule out pathology. The gynecologist may also consider an endometrial biopsy for patients who are at high risk (those with diabetes, hypertension, and obesity) for endometrial hyperplasia and adenocarcinoma before prescribing medications. Pelvic ultrasound may also be used to measure the endometrial strip and rule out ovarian masses.

Once the work-up is completed, the patient should be evaluated annually. Patients with primary amenorrhea should be referred to a gynecologist. Patients with secondary amenorrhea may need to be referred if initial treatment is unsuccessful.

Patient Education

Frequently, teenagers and their parents are apprehensive when menses do not start "on schedule," but reassurance and watchful waiting may be all that is needed. Patients should be taught about their medication regimen and the importance of taking medications exactly as prescribed. Patients must be aware of the need to notify their health-care provider if they take any new medications, because many drugs interact with others and have a potentiating effect as well as a negative effect on the action of some medications. Encourage patients to maintain a healthy diet and exercise regimen, because having less than adequate body fat can result in amenorrhea.

■ PREMENSTRUAL SYNDROME

Premenstrual syndrome (PMS) is a cyclic recurrence of a constellation of physical and psychological symptoms that arise during the second, or luteal, phase of the menstrual cycle, starting at day 14 after menses, immediately following ovulation and the midcycle luteinizing hormone (LH) and follicle-stimulating hormone (FSH) gonadotropin surge. The original term for these symptoms was *premenstrual tension syndrome* (PMT). Most women experience minor physical symptoms before their menstrual cycle; however, about 5% of women present with symptoms severe enough to disrupt their daily lives.

Epidemiology and Causes

Premenstrual dysphoric disorder (PMDD) is the term given to a severe form of PMS in the *Diagnostic and Statistical Manual of Mental Disorders, Fifth Edition* (DSM-V). Although PMS may affect up to 75% of women with regular menstrual cycles, only 3% to 8% of women suffer from true PMDD. To apply the DSM-V criteria for PMDD, women must chart symptoms daily for two cycles. Chief complaints must include 1 of the 4 core symptoms (irritability, tension, dysphoria, and lability of mood) and at least 5 of the 11 total symptoms that are listed under the subjective heading in the clinical presentation section later in this chapter. More than 150 distinct signs and symptoms have been ascribed to PMS within the medical literature (Table 14.7).

The psychiatric hypothesis regarding the etiology of PMDD centers around a woman's denial of her body and femininity, negative imprinting about menstruation, and poor coping skills. This associates PMS with other psychiatric disorders. There does not appear to be any difference in the prevalence of this disorder between racial or ethnic groups. PMS usually disappears at the time of menopause.

Many believe that PMS is a physical response to organic changes that occur during the luteal phase of the menstrual cycle and, therefore, is not a psychiatric diagnosis at all. Research has postulated that mood and anxiety disturbances arise from ovarian steroid hormones that affect the synthesis, release, and reuptake of neurotransmitters. Several neuroendocrine processes are also affected during this period that may affect mood. Other diseases that present with mood and mental status changes, such as thyroid disease and vitamin B_{12} deficiency, are not classified as psychiatric disorders, and many believe that PMS should likewise be considered a physical complaint.

Pathophysiology

PMS has no universally accepted definition. As discussed, the American Psychiatric Association has established diagnostic guidelines for PMDD, which are more stringent than criteria for PMS. PMS is a complex clinical somatic entity, and no specific list or number of symptoms has been established that would enable a definitive diagnosis of PMS to be made. However, certain basic facts have been agreed on. Although the medical literature states that PMS is a complex disorder linking ovarian steroid hormones and neurotransmitter release, some feminist authorities feel that PMS may be caused in part by the stressors on women within modern society and the need for women to masculinize their work lives to meet the standards of Western society.

The influence of cyclical ovarian hormones on various neurotransmitters has been cited, including the beta endorphins and gamma-aminobutyric acid (GABA). In fact, the progesterone metabolite allopregnanolone, which potentiates GABA receptor function, is lower in concentration in women experiencing PMS. However, the majority of evidence supports a deficiency in the tryptophan-derived neurotransmitter serotonin as the primary factor in the pathogenesis of PMS. Serum serotonin levels and serotonin uptake by platelets are both reduced during the luteal phase of the menstrual cycle in women with PMS. Moreover, the serotonin agonist fenfluramine and selective serotonin reuptake inhibitors (SSRIs) both improve PMS symptoms, whereas tryptophan depletion and the serotonin antagonist metergoline both worsen the syndrome.

Fluctuations in ovarian steroids are believed to underlie these abnormalities in neurotransmitter levels, as demonstrated by the efficacy of gonadotropin-releasing hormone (GnRH) treatments (e.g., leuprolide) that suppress ovarian hormones and relieve the symptoms of PMS. Interestingly, however, the concentrations of serum estrogen and progesterone do not differ between women experiencing PMS and controls; thus, it is the cyclical nature of the sex hormones that appears to be key.

Several subcategories of PMS have been suggested. PMT-A is categorized by the symptoms of anxiety, irritability, and nervous tension. PMT-B is categorized by fluid retention, abdominal bloating, mastalgia, and weight gain. PMT-C is categorized as premenstrual cravings for sweets, increased appetite, and food binges. PMT-D is categorized by depression, withdrawal,

Table 14.7 Common Symptoms of PMS

Core Symptoms
- Irritability
- Tension/anxiety
- Dysphoria/depression
- Lability of mood/mood swings

Other Symptoms
- Headache
- Food craving
- Anger
- Backaches
- Tender breasts
- Clumsiness
- Crying
- Dizziness
- Feeling faint
- Fatigue
- Fluid retention
- Forgetfulness
- Bloating
- Hostility
- Joint swelling
- Confusion
- Migraine

insomnia, forgetfulness, and confusion. These categories have some overlap.

Clinical Presentation
Subjective

Usual cognitive symptoms during the premenstrual period are crying spells, depression, hostility, anxiety, irritability, relationship conflict and feelings of inadequacy, increased or decreased libido, and inability to cope with ever-recurring symptoms. These symptoms often persist for years; women tend to seek help from a health-care professional only when adverse events are linked with these alterations in mood. A recent crisis or threat from a significant other may precipitate a perceived need for professional help. Often, women seek relief from a sense of desperation. The delay in seeking help could come from a fear of being labeled a hypochondriac or mentally unstable.

A variety of physical symptoms may accompany these alterations in mood, ranging from mild to severe, and may change from month to month. The following is a comprehensive list of symptoms by body system:

- Gastrointestinal: Abdominal bloating (most common [more than 90% of women]), nausea, vomiting, constipation, increased thirst
- Respiratory: Colds, hoarseness, rhinitis, asthma, sinusitis, sore throat
- Urological: Oliguria, urethritis, cystitis
- Ophthalmological: Conjunctivitis, visual changes, glaucoma, styes
- Mammalogical: Breast tenderness (more than 50% of women), swelling, heaviness
- Dermatological: Acne, boils, urticaria, spot bruising, recurrence of herpes
- Neurological: Headaches/migraines (more than 50% of women), aggravation of epilepsy, vertigo, syncope, fainting, paresthesias of hands or feet
- Miscellaneous: Fatigue (affecting more than 90%), backache, joint pain, edema of extremities, weight gain, palpitations, pelvic or low abdominal pain, cold sweats, hot flashes, food cravings, compulsive eating

Other changes perceived as "positive" have been reported by patients during the premenstrual period, including increased libido, more energy, more creative ideas, and increased ability to accomplish tasks. Although physical symptoms may be the presenting complaints when patients first seek medical treatment, mood alterations are the most incapacitating and distressing.

All of the symptoms that any one patient may exhibit and believe to be resulting from PMS will present in one of four cycle patterns:

1. Symptoms appear at midcycle, disappear, and reappear the week before menstruation.

2. Symptoms begin at midcycle, with subtle changes that gradually escalate until menses.

3. Symptoms appear the week before menses and intensify until menstruation ensues.

4. Symptoms appear in the first or second luteal weeks and do not disappear until the end of menstruation.

Objective

Increased age and parity are important indicators when assessing whether symptoms are genuinely PMS related, because both of these factors increase the possibility of PMS. A 3-month diary of symptoms, such as the one shown in Table 14.7, which includes the timing of symptoms in relation to menses and severity, should be obtained from the patient. This diary should also list treatments and what makes symptoms better or worse. The diary should also contain a description of the effect the symptoms have had on a patient's family and colleagues. The patient should be asked, after this diary has been compiled, about her expectations concerning evaluation and therapy.

Diagnostic Reasoning
Diagnostic Tests

The most commonly accepted method to diagnose PMS uses a diary during at least two menstrual cycles (three is preferred). If the intensity of whatever symptoms are present increases at least 30% in the 6 days before onset of menses (compared with days 5 through 10 of the cycle) and if the symptoms occur in 2 consecutive months, a diagnosis of PMS is made. This is a rather subjective method of diagnosis, because women are asked to assess the percentage of increase subjectively, and there is no objective means of comparison with other patients. Other questions relevant to this diagnosis include those asked during the sexual, reproductive, family, medical-surgical, and psychiatric histories. This enables the health-care professional to rule out other possible diagnoses. Dietary habits, drug and alcohol consumption, exercise, and social and occupational histories are also important. Once the diary of symptoms and impairment can be pinpointed to the luteal phase of the menstrual cycle, with abatement of symptoms during other parts of the cycle, a presumptive diagnosis of PMS can be made.

A complete physical exam including a gynecological exam is necessary to assess the health of women with PMS symptoms. This will enable the provider to rule out other possible causes for these symptoms. Diagnostic tests that may be useful to rule out other illnesses are a complete blood count, Pap smear, and urinalysis. Other blood tests can rule out thyroid abnormalities (thyroid-stimulating hormone, T_4), menopause (FSH), hypoglycemia or hyperglycemia (fasting blood sugar), and hyperprolactinemia (prolactin level).

Depression scales are also part of a complete work-up for PMS. These enable the practitioner to rule out depression during the follicular stage of the menstrual cycle and, therefore, to pinpoint the depression and its manifestations to the luteal phase of the menstrual cycle.

Differential Diagnosis

One of the most important assessment parameters in making a diagnosis of PMS is that symptoms occur only during the luteal phase of the menstrual cycle. If symptoms appear during the follicular phase, this may reflect a mood or anxiety disorder. It is important to note that there is a lifetime incidence of psychiatric disorders, especially depression, of nearly 80% in women diagnosed with PMS. Differential diagnoses that are possibly related to the symptoms of PMS are cyclothymic disorder; dysfunctional marital situation; depression; bipolar depression; perimenopausal status; poor diet; endocrine abnormalities, such as hypoglycemia, diabetes, hypothyroidism, hyperprolactinemia, and hyperandrogenism; alcoholism; drug abuse; and tumors of the brain, breast, and ovaries. These must all be ruled out before a definitive diagnosis of PMS can be made. Often it is easy to dismiss vague symptoms and use "PMS" as a catch-all term. This can lead to misdiagnosis, which could have serious consequences. The DSM-V criteria for diagnosing PMDD specify that a woman must have 5 of the 11 symptoms listed, and at least 1 symptom must be 1 of the first 4 on the list. In addition, to be considered as PMDD, the symptoms must occur during the week before menstruation and end a few days after onset of menses. The symptoms must interfere with work, school, usual activities, or relationships and not be merely an exacerbation of another disorder. This must be established for two consecutive menstrual cycles. The symptoms are as follows:

1. Depressed mood or dysphoria (a feeling of low mood, irritability, anxiety, and/or despair)
2. Anxiety or tension
3. Affective lability
4. Irritability
5. Decreased interest in usual activities
6. Concentration difficulties
7. Marked lack of energy
8. Marked change in appetite, overeating, or food cravings
9. Hypersomnia or insomnia
10. Feeling overwhelmed
11. Other physical symptoms (e.g., breast tenderness, bloating)

Management

The principle of management is to assist the patient in developing strategies to gain control over the symptoms, alleviate them as much as possible, and normalize life. Once an accurate diagnosis of PMS is made, appropriate interventions can be individualized. There are two principles to keep in mind when developing this plan. First, PMS is a chronic disorder that lasts until after menopause. This makes cost and adverse effects important issues when planning treatment. Second, patients have different degrees of severity of symptoms and different symptom profiles. Treatments should match both the symptoms and the severity of symptoms. Lifestyle changes should be recommended as first-line therapy.

Lifestyle Changes

Lifestyle changes include regularly scheduled meals that are relatively high in complex carbohydrates and low in salt, sugar, and caffeine; regular aerobic exercise (shown to decrease depression); and stress reduction techniques. Aerobic exercise can cause an increase in endorphin levels and thereby improve mood. Epidemiological studies comparing the severity of premenstrual symptoms in patients who exercise to those who do not have suggested that those who exercise have fewer symptoms. This is especially true for premenstrual depression. Moreover, it appears that the benefits are independent of the intensity of exercise; therefore, low levels of exercise intensity may be beneficial. An activity as simple as sitting quietly for 20 minutes twice a day and deep breathing while listening to relaxation music was shown to reduce mood symptoms of PMS twice as effectively as no active therapy.

Specific dietary interventions that are effective include a reduction in salt, sugar, alcohol, and caffeine intake and an increase in complex carbohydrates. It is hypothesized that carbohydrates are involved in the serotonergic pathway, and an increase in serotonergic activity caused by increased complex carbohydrate consumption may help to relieve symptoms. In one trial, patients were given a carbohydrate-rich beverage during the late luteal phase of the menstrual cycle. The control group was given an isocaloric control beverage. The patients who drank the carbohydrate-rich beverage reported lower adverse mood symptom scores, whereas the control group reported no effect on mood.

Calcium and magnesium supplements have been shown to help control the emotional and physical symptoms of PMS. In several large clinical trials, 1,000 mg of calcium per day decreased all PMS symptoms as well as any other medication or treatment. Women taking magnesium also experienced a reduction in total symptoms. This effect is thought to be due to the reversal of lower than average mononuclear blood cell magnesium concentrations in patients with PMS.

Other dietary supplements have also been tried for PMS, but the results are not conclusive. For example, micronutrients such as pyridoxine (vitamin B_6) 50 to 100 mg daily, folic acid 400 mcg daily, and tocopherol (vitamin E) have been used to treat PMS symptoms. Because the adverse effects of vitamins are minimal, a daily supplement may be helpful as long as the dosage does not exceed the recommended daily allowance. Vitamin E has been prescribed as a treatment for mastalgia (breast tenderness). Trials have demonstrated that vitamin E (at doses of 150, 300, or 600 IU daily) makes little difference in the mastalgia of patients with PMS but does help some women. Vitamin E can be toxic in high doses, so it is important to prescribe appropriate doses to patients with mastalgia; 400 IU is the most commonly available dose, which gives a minimum effect without danger of toxicity.

Medications

In addition to lifestyle changes, SSRIs such as fluoxetine (Prozac) 20 mg daily (most common) are effective in relieving tension, irritability, and dysphoria. Sertraline (Zoloft) may be used in doses up to 150 mg daily, paroxetine (Paxil) 20 to 30 mg daily, and citalopram (Celexa) 20 to 30 mg daily. These are relatively inexpensive and have limited adverse effects, which include nausea, headache, jitteriness, and decrease in libido. Lowering the dose of the SSRI may eliminate some of the adverse affects. If a therapeutic response is not reached within several cycles, the dose may be increased. Although SSRIs are generally administered daily, these drugs have been shown to be effective when administered only during the luteal phase. SSRIs can then be used advantageously from a cost and adverse effect aspect.

Other antidepressants that inhibit serotonin reuptake but are not selective have also been used. These include clomipramine (Anafranil), nefazodone (Serzone), and venlafaxine (Effexor) (50–200 mg daily), which inhibit both serotonin and norepinephrine reuptake. But they are definitely not first-line therapies, given their side-effect profiles. In fact, several studies have shown that antidepressants outside of the SSRI class are not consistently effective for PMS control.

Benzodiazepines (BZDs) such as alprazolam (Xanax) 0.25 mg three or four times daily are usually reserved for patients who fit the strict criteria of PMDD. Alprazolam is given starting on day 14 and continued through day 28. This will reduce the chances of developing BZD dependence. Thus, BZDs are considered only as a second-line therapy after SSRIs and only in patients with documented PMDD.

Patients who do not respond to the above measures are candidates for a trial of ovulation suppression therapy with danazol 200 to 800 mg daily. Danazol is a GnRH agonist, a nortestosterone hormone derivative with progestin-like effects that induces ovarian suppression. It works by continuously suppressing pituitary gonadotropin secretions (LH/FSH). It must be given continuously because pulsatile administration leads to FSH/LH secretion. When this therapy is used, "add back" therapy is also used to provide some of the hormones suppressed by the GnRH agonist. Estrogen and progestin are given in low doses. For patients on

GnRH agonist therapy, long-term alendronate is given to help prevent bone mineral density loss. Danazol has several undesirable adverse effects such as weight gain, increased facial hair, and acne.

Fluid retention is commonly reported during the luteal phase of the menstrual cycle and accounts for some of the physical symptoms of PMS. Spironolactone (Aldactone) 100 mg daily during the luteal phase has been shown to significantly reduce physical and psychological symptoms of PMS over placebo. With the use of spironolactone, participants reported improvement in irritability, depression, feeling of swelling, breast tenderness, and food cravings. Other forms of diuretics, such as thiazides, do not demonstrate effective reduction of the symptoms of PMS.

NSAIDs administered during the luteal phase significantly reduce physical symptoms of PMS. Naproxen sodium (Naprosyn) 500 mg 2 times daily, begun 1 week before the onset of menses and continued through the first few days of bleeding, is effective for both PMS symptoms and dysmenorrhea. This treatment is not recommended for anyone with renal impairment, gastrointestinal (GI) disorders, or inflammatory bowel disorders. As with any NSAID, GI distress and bleeding may occur. Although this is not first-line therapy for patients with PMDD, for patients with moderate symptoms, especially if associated with dysmenorrhea, headaches, or other musculoskeletal symptoms, NSAIDs may be beneficial. This is a relatively inexpensive and safe form of therapy for younger patients and may provide them with the help that they need to function normally during this period of the menstrual cycle.

Many folk remedies and complementary therapies have also been tried by women for centuries with varying degrees of success. Complementary Therapies 14.1 presents some of these measures.

Surgery (bilateral oophorectomy, usually with hysterectomy) is an option for women who respond only to GnRH agonist therapy for documented PMDD. This option should be reserved for women who no longer desire childbearing and is most appropriate for women who are not near menopause and will likely need therapy for several more years.

Follow-up and Referral

The first follow-up visit should be in 2 months to evaluate the data collected by the patient between visits to assess symptom patterns, enabling the diagnosis of PMS to be made and to begin treatment. Frequent visits may be required after that time to evaluate the effectiveness of treatments and to encourage patients to continue to examine and develop treatment plans. Eventually, once symptoms have been controlled, yearly visits should be sufficient.

Referrals to a specialist may be required, depending on findings from the diagnostic tests and physical exam. The diagnosis of PMDD requires referral to a

Complementary Therapies 14.1   Women's Health Problems

Problem	Therapy	Dosage	Comments
Premenstrual syndrome (PMS)	Evening primrose oil	250 mg PO up to 3 times daily 2–3 days before menses	Rare adverse effects: Headache, nausea, diarrhea
	Calcium	1,200–1,600 mg PO daily	Should be taken in divided doses and with optimal daily allowance of vitamin D (400 IU daily) for better absorption
	Vitamin B_6	150 mg PO daily	Those taking levodopa must consult their provider before taking
	Vitamin C	1,500–3,000 mg PO daily	Take in divided doses for better absorption and to avoid diarrhea
	Essential oils: Chamomile, basil, lavender, marjoram	Use as directed on label	Aromatherapy
Menopausal symptoms	Black cohosh	40–200 mg PO daily	Not recommended for more than 6 months
	Chaste tree berry	Extracts or tinctures to provide 20 mg of crude fruit or 30–40 mg of fruits decoction	Possible adverse GI effects; contraindicated in pregnancy
	Vitamin B complex	50 mg PO daily	High levels of estrogen related to hormone fluctuations can deplete vitamin B_6, resulting in anxiety, irritability, and depression
	Vitamin C	1,500–3,000 mg PO daily	Take in divided doses for better absorption and to avoid diarrhea
	Vitamin E	400–800 IU PO daily	Can interfere with anticoagulant therapy; consult with provider before taking or if taking warfarin (Coumadin) or heparin
Breast tenderness	Chaste tree berry	As above	
	Evening primrose oil	As above	
Candidiasis (yeast infection)	Vitamin C	3,000–6,000 mg PO daily	Take in divided doses for better absorption and to avoid diarrhea
Decreased sexual desire	Essential oils: Jasmine, neroli, rose, sandalwood, ylang-ylang, clary sage, patchouli	Use as directed on label	Aromatherapy; aphrodisiac

psychiatrist for treatment. The use of certain treatments for severe PMS, such as GnRH agents, is handled by a gynecologist.

Patient Education

It is important to listen to and evaluate the concerns of patients when they present with symptoms typically associated with PMS. PMS must not be identified with weakness on the part of the patient but rather recognized as a disease entity that must be investigated and treated. It may take time and energy to manage the symptoms and help the patient maintain a good quality of life. When a patient is able to reduce PMS symptoms, whether severe or mild, it helps her to function within

her societal role at a higher level and, therefore, benefits everyone.

■ DYSMENORRHEA

Dysmenorrhea is painful menses. It may be primary, with no pelvic pathology, or secondary, usually accompanied by pelvic pathology.

Epidemiology and Causes

Primary dysmenorrhea usually begins 1 to 2 years after the onset of menstruation, is associated with ovular cycles, and lasts 1 or 2 days each month. The menstrual pain associated with primary dysmenorrhea may lessen for some women as they age or after the birth of children or it can last until menopause. There is no associated pathology, and from 50% to 75% of women experience this at some time.

Secondary dysmenorrhea is caused by a physical condition. Women who experience this type tend to be older than those who have primary dysmenorrhea, sometimes beginning when a women is in her 30s or 40s. Menstrual pain is the predominant symptom, as in primary dysmenorrhea. Possible conditions responsible for secondary dysmenorrhea include endometriosis, pelvic inflammatory disease (PID), fibroids (uterine leiomyomas), adenomyosis, and endometrial polyps. Secondary dysmenorrhea is most common in women aged 40 to 50 years.

It is estimated that more than 140 million lost work hours are a result of dysmenorrhea. It is the most common gynecological complaint of women and the main cause of missed work, school, or other activities. An estimated 42 million women in the United States suffer from painful menstrual symptoms each month. Risk factors for primary dysmenorrhea include obesity, low body mass index, long menstrual cycles, menarche occurring before 12 years of age, nulliparity, cigarette smoking, and a positive family history for dysmenorrhea. Risk factors for secondary dysmenorrhea include pelvic infection, endometriosis, and sexually transmitted infections.

Pathophysiology

Dysmenorrhea is caused by the production of prostaglandins and leukotrienes, chemical substances that are released when uterine tissue breaks up and is sloughed off during menstruation. Prostaglandin F_2 (PGF_2) and prostaglandin E_2 (PGE_2) are two of the most important players. Elevated uterine levels of these arachidonic acid metabolites, and more specifically an increased ratio of PGF_2 to PGE_2, have been directly correlated with increases in subjective pain. Increased prostaglandin levels found in uterine tissue, but not in plasma, cause dysrhythmic uterine contractions and increased resting tone by stimulating smooth muscle tissue to contract, which compromises blood supply and oxygenation to uterine muscle, thus causing severe pelvic pain known as "cramps."

These uterine contractions may last for several minutes at a time, producing maximal pressures up to 400 mm Hg, with resting pressures as high as 80 mm Hg. In turn, if uterine muscle tone is consistently higher than systemic arterial pressure, uterine ischemia ensues, resulting in the production of anaerobic metabolites that stimulate small type C pain fibers. In turn, pain relief has been directly correlated with decreases in uterine contraction pressure. Because smooth muscle is found in the stomach, intestines, and blood vessels, as well as in the uterus, the excessive stimulation accounts for the nausea, diarrhea, and headache that often accompany dysmenorrhea. Cramps facilitate

the release of menstrual tissue, and because the cervical opening is usually widened after childbirth or years of menstruation, cramps may lessen in the older patient. In contrast, worsened cramps are associated with anovulatory menstrual cycles—a common phenomenon in young women, affecting up to half of adolescents within 2 to 4 years after the start of menses.

Clinical Presentation
Subjective

Description of the pain is an important factor. The type, severity, and duration of pain should be noted. A patient with dysmenorrhea may present with sharp stabbing pain and cramping, low back pain, nausea and sometimes vomiting, bowel changes, and fatigue. The pain with primary dysmenorrhea usually starts within 24 hours of menses and may last for 48 to 72 hours. Secondary dysmenorrhea may have the onset of pain a week or more before the onset of menses and continue after cessation of flow for a few days. The patient may state that she is immobilized by her period every month for the first day. Her pain may be so severe that at times she cannot do anything except stay in bed with a heating pad on her abdomen. She may lose her appetite and eat very little during this time. She may complain of pain during intercourse.

Diagnostic Reasoning
Diagnostic Tests

The physical exam (revealing no signs of pathology) and a history of consistent symptoms for 1 or 2 days each month will usually substantiate the diagnosis of primary dysmenorrhea, because the symptoms are fairly typical. Secondary dysmenorrhea may have a slightly varying description of symptoms; some menses are more painful than others, and the level of discomfort may be progressive. If the complaint of painful intercourse is present, a diagnosis of secondary dysmenorrhea, possibly related to endometriosis, should be explored.

Laboratory studies in the evaluation of dysmenorrhea are ordered to rule out potential causes of pelvic pain. They include quantitative human chorionic gonadotropin and complete blood count, urinalysis, erythrocyte sedimentation rate, and stool for occult blood. Serum CA-125 levels are known to be elevated in women with endometriosis (a common cause of dysmenorrhea), as well as ovarian pathology; however, this test is not sufficiently sensitive to serve as a reliable screening tool. Imaging studies are the choice for the initial evaluation of suspected pelvic disease. Gynecological consultation with visualization of pelvic organs via ultrasound is the definitive procedure of choice for evaluation of pelvic pathology. If such testing does not produce a definitive diagnosis, it may be followed up by laparoscopic exploration to directly visualize pathological conditions such as endometriosis.

Differential Diagnosis

The ultimate goal of the differential diagnosis of dysmenorrhea is to exclude underlying pelvic pathology to differentiate between primary and secondary dysmenorrhea. This includes diagnosing conditions that may produce or mimic dysmenorrhea such as endometriosis, ovarian cysts, ectopic pregnancy, urinary tract infection, vaginitis, dysfunctional uterine bleeding, uterine leiomyomas, appendicitis, lower back pain, trauma from sexual assault, and PID. Endometriosis is the most common cause of secondary dysmenorrhea.

Management

The principle of management for primary dysmenorrhea is to relieve the menstrual pain as much as possible. For secondary dysmenorrhea, the goal is to find a diagnosis.

Ordinary aspirin 325 mg two tablets (650 mg total) PO every 4 hours, started 1 or 2 days before menstruation, is helpful because of its antiprostaglandin activity as an inhibitor of the enzyme cyclo-oxygenase, which converts arachidonic acid into prostaglandin metabolites. Dietary changes such as the avoidance of caffeine during the first few days of menstruation have been shown to be helpful. Exercise may be of some benefit because it raises levels of beta endorphins, chemicals in the brain associated with pain relief. Cigarette smoking has been linked to increasing the duration of dysmenorrhea.

Interestingly, in clinical studies, placebo treatments have been shown to improve symptoms of dysmenorrhea, albeit often only transiently. But the NSAID ibuprofen (Advil, Motrin) 400 to 800 mg PO three to four times daily as needed remains the mainstay of dysmenorrhea therapy and is considered the most effective over-the-counter pain reliever for cramps. Several studies have demonstrated that if ibuprofen fails to relieve a patient's symptoms, it is appropriate to try an alternative NSAID agent such as naproxen sodium (Naprosyn 500 mg or Aleve 220 mg × 2 tablets PO 2 times daily as needed), indomethacin (Indocin), fenoprofen (Nalfon 300–600 mg PO 2–3 times daily as needed), or mefenamic acid (500 mg PO initially, followed by 250 mg 4 times daily for up to 3 days). The latter agent not only inhibits new prostaglandin formation but also inhibits the activity of preformed prostaglandins (Level II; Kaur Bajaj et al, 2012). In contrast, acetaminophen (Tylenol) appears to be less effective because it does not inhibit prostaglandin formation and is not considered an anti-inflammatory agent.

Application of a hot water bottle or heating pad to the abdomen or hot baths may help relieve discomfort and in some studies has been shown to be as effective as NSAID therapy. However, interestingly, the combination of heat therapy and NSAIDs together has been shown to be counterproductive. Acupuncture, transcutaneous electrical nerve stimulation therapy, and specific herbal teas (e.g., mint tea, certain ayurvedic preparations) have all been shown to decrease uterine spasms in small clinical trials. Relaxation or yoga-type exercises may also help to relieve pain. Dietary restriction of both caffeine and salt is also recommended, and vitamin E, vitamin B_1, vitamin B_6, magnesium, and vitamin D were found to reduce symptoms. There is some evidence that vitamin E therapy, 400 IU/day beginning 2 days before the onset of menstruation and for 5 days total for two cycles, decreases dysmenorrhea (Level II; Kashanian et al, 2013). Other research indicates that ingestion of a single high oral dose of vitamin D has a favorable effect on dysmenorrhea (Level II; Lasco et al, 2012).

For some women, even prescribed prostaglandin inhibitors are ineffective. Combined estrogen-progestin oral contraceptive (OC) agents may be considered for these patients because OCs relieve cramping by inhibiting arachidonic acid production and ovulation, in turn hindering high levels of prostaglandin production. These therapies may be given daily as 21-, 63-, or 105-day continuous courses, each followed by 7 days off medication, before repeating the cycle. Longer cycles of OC therapy decrease the frequency of menstruation occurring during the off-therapy week.

If no relief is achieved after NSAID and OC therapy, ultrasonography and even exploratory laparoscopy may be appropriate to rule out pelvic pathology. If endometriosis (the most common cause of secondary dysmenorrhea) is found, a gonadotropin-releasing hormone analog may be prescribed in continuous fashion to inhibit menses (see under Endometriosis).

Follow-up and Referral

Each patient with a case of pelvic pain should have follow-up care because treatment is ongoing and requires further evaluation of relief of symptoms or additional diagnostic evaluation for continued symptoms. Prognosis for primary dysmenorrhea is good with the use of antiprostaglandins, with a 70% to 80% relief of symptoms in some cases.

Patient Education

Advise the patient that ordinary aspirin, two tablets every 4 hours 1 to 2 days before menstruation begins, can significantly reduce prostaglandin levels. Education about changes in exercise and diet may also be useful. Dietary supplementation with omega-3 fatty acids has been shown to help provide relief in adolescents. Patients should be encouraged to stop smoking and decrease alcohol intake. Symptomatic treatment with a warm bath or locally applied heat may be helpful.

■ ENDOMETRIOSIS

Endometriosis is a painful, chronic disease, characterized by the presence and proliferation of abnormally placed endometrial tissue, which responds to hormone changes in the woman's body. Abnormally placed endometrial tissue has been found outside the uterus, usually in the abdomen, on the ovaries, fallopian tubes, and ligaments that support the uterus; in the area between the vagina and rectum; in the outer surface of the uterus; and in the lining of the pelvic cavity. Other sites for these endometrial growths may include the bladder, bowel, vagina, cervix, vulva, and in abdominal surgical scars. Rarely, endometrial tissue may be located in the lung, arm, thigh, brain, and other locations.

The Iceberg of Endometriosis

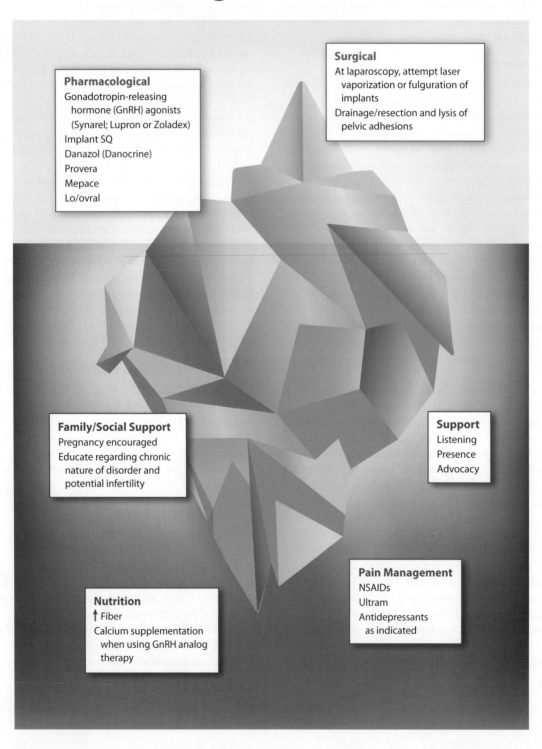

Pharmacological
Gonadotropin-releasing
   hormone (GnRH) agonists
   (Synarel; Lupron or Zoladex)
Implant SQ
Danazol (Danocrine)
Provera
Mepace
Lo/ovral

Surgical
At laparoscopy, attempt laser
   vaporization or fulguration of
   implants
Drainage/resection and lysis of
   pelvic adhesions

Family/Social Support
Pregnancy encouraged
Educate regarding chronic
   nature of disorder and
   potential infertility

Support
Listening
Presence
Advocacy

Nutrition
↑ Fiber
Calcium supplementation
   when using GnRH analog
   therapy

Pain Management
NSAIDs
Ultram
Antidepressants
   as indicated

This tissue reacts as correctly placed endometrial tissue would during the menstrual cycle. The bloody discharge produced by such tissue has no outlet. The presence of such discharge may cause severe pain with each menstrual cycle, either during ovulation, menstruation, or both. The accumulation of the discharge may form dense fibrous tissue, leading to adhesions, sterility, and destruction of ovarian tissue.

Epidemiology and Causes

Endometriosis affects an estimated 5.5 million women in the United States and Canada. Women at all levels of society and of all races may be affected. A study of 3,684 premenopausal women undergoing laparoscopy or laparotomy found a prevalence of endometriosis varying from 12% to 45%, depending on the indication for surgery. Delay in diagnosing endometriosis is common. Statistical analysis shows the highest level of occurrence reported in women 25 to 29 years of age and lowest incidence found in women over 44 years of age; however, the disease can be found at any age, including adolescents. Research conducted by the Endometriosis Association found that the recognition and diagnosis of endometriosis is still taking a combined average of 9 years (4.67-year delay in seeking medical help and 4.61-year delay in physicians' diagnoses). From the sample of 4,000 respondents, almost half said that they had to see a doctor five times or more before they were diagnosed, referred, or treated. Japanese women are twice as likely to have endometriosis as Caucasian women.

The cause of endometriosis is unknown. The retrograde menstruation and implantation theory suggests that during menses, some amount of menstrual tissue backs up through the fallopian tubes, implants in the abdomen, and proliferates in response to ovarian steroids. In turn, conditions that lead to genital tract obstruction and impede menstrual outflow contribute to reflux through the fallopian tubes. However, this theory has been found inadequate to explain all of the possible sites of endometriosis, and some experts believe that all women experience some menstrual tissue backup. Direct transplantation may account for endometriosis that develops in uterine surgical scars after a cesarean section or episiotomy. Another theory suggests that endometrial tissue is distributed from the uterus to other parts of the body through either the lymphatic or hematological circulatory systems. The coelomic (peritoneal) metaplasia theory suggests that undifferentiated cells lining the peritoneal cavity are triggered to differentiate into endometrial tissue by hormonal irregularities. There may also be a genetic predisposition to endometriosis; in addition, research by the Endometriosis Association has recently linked dioxin exposure to the development of endometriosis.

Pathophysiology

In addition to the etiological theories discussed in the preceding text, a link to immune system dysfunction and the pathogenesis of endometriosis has also been suggested. Reduced T-cell and natural killer cell function are thought to impair the ability of the body to recognize and destroy abnormally implanted endometrial tissue, that is, immunosurveillance. Interestingly, however, an increased number of peritoneal leukocytes and macrophages have been identified within ectopic endometrium. Increased levels of cytokines and chemokines produced by these cells have been identified, including interleukin-1 (IL-1), IL-6, IL-8, tumor necrosis factor, and RANTES (regulated upon activation normal T cell expressed and presumably secreted). These mediators act as growth factors for ectopic endometrium, and vascular endothelial growth factor stimulates capillary proliferation into this tissue. Interestingly, women with endometriosis are also more likely than controls to suffer from autoimmune inflammatory diseases.

Any pelvic organ may be a possible site of abnormal endometrial tissue known as endometriosis. The cyclical production of ovarian sex hormones allows for the proliferation and maintenance of these implants. Thus, endometriosis occurs primarily during a woman's active reproductive phase, rather than during premenstrual, immediately postmenarchal, or postmenopausal phases. This bleeding may cause severe pelvic pain and dyspareunia, infertility, and debilitation. In addition, inflammation of pelvic tissues may lead to adhesions and cyst development.

Endometriosis may be progressively staged from minimal (stage I: isolated implants without adhesions), mild (stage II: superficial implants less than 5 cm in aggregate without adhesions), moderate (stage III: multiple superficial and invasive implants with or without tubo-ovarian implants), to severe (stage IV: multiple superficial and invasive implants with large ovarian endometriomas and dense adhesions).

Clinical Presentation
Subjective

The primary symptom of endometriosis is recurrent abdominal and/or pelvic pain, which may range from very mild to completely incapacitating. The pain may be associated with menstruation (dysmenorrhea), or it may occur slightly before the menstrual period. Pain may be experienced as generalized abdominal or pelvic pain or pain associated with sexual intercourse (dyspareunia), urination, and defecation. Fatigue, diarrhea, constipation, or nausea may accompany the pain. The patient may complain only of premenstrual spotting.

A careful history of menstruation should be taken, with significant attention to any complaints of pain. A history of allergies, chemical sensitivities, and recurrent yeast (Candida) infections may be present. Infertility is associated with endometriosis; 30% to 40% of women diagnosed with endometriosis are infertile.

Objective

On physical exam, tenderness in the posterior fornix is the most common symptom. Lateral deviation of the cervix may be due to internal scarring, and bimanual examination may reveal palpable nodules on supporting ligaments and on affected ovaries. However, definitive diagnosis cannot be made via history and physical exam.

Diagnostic Reasoning

Diagnostic Tests

Direct visualization of endometrial implants through laparoscopy is the preferred diagnostic method, because most implants are located on the pelvic organs. A complete blood count may be done to diagnose anemia associated with blood loss resulting from endometriosis, and an elevated white blood cell count may also show evidence of an infection. This would tend to make endometriosis less likely, although it would not exclude abnormal endometrial tissue. Serum CA-125 levels are more likely to be elevated with advanced (stage III to IV) endometriosis, but this serum marker is not particularly sensitive and not a good screening tool.

Differential Diagnosis

The clinical manifestations of endometriosis are associated with many genitourinary disorders. The pain experienced is often discounted because it is a frequent (normal) accompaniment to menstruation. Pelvic and abdominal pain can be caused by gastroenteritis, appendicitis, ovarian cysts, fibroids, or ectopic pregnancy and these diagnoses must be ruled out. Specific differential diagnoses that must be considered are adenomyosis and endometrial polyps.

Adenomyosis is the presence of ectopic endometrial glands and stroma within the musculature of the uterus, which induces hypertrophy and hyperplasia of the myometrium in response to estrogen (and possibly progesterone); it may be microscopic or nodular on gross inspection, but endometrial biopsy is typically negative because of changes in the myometrium. Adenomyosis seems to be more associated with childbearing, but the pathogenesis is unknown. Although a third of women are asymptomatic, adenomyosis may present with abnormal uterine bleeding, dysmenorrhea, and menorrhagia—just as with endometriosis. Abdominal ultrasound may be able to identify these differential diagnoses, but laparoscopy is necessary to diagnose endometriosis.

Endometrial polyps are hyperplastic pedunculated/sessile growths of endometrial glands and stroma at the endometrial surface (millimeters to centimeters in size) and are common in middle-aged women. Metrorrhagia (irregular uterine bleeding) occurs in 50% of cases, and less frequently, menorrhagia, postmenopausal bleeding, prolapse through the cervical os, and breakthrough bleeding on hormonal treatments occur as symptoms.

Definitive diagnosis is made on microscopy (after dilation and curettage, biopsy, or hysterectomy), but sonohysterography (instillation of saline into uterus before ultrasound) is preferred to transvaginal ultrasound for noninvasive evaluation (but it cannot be diagnostic). Curettage via hysteroscopy, rather than blindly, is preferred for best detecting polyps.

Management

Currently, there is no cure for endometriosis. Management is linked to relieving or reducing pain, shrinking or slowing endometrial growths, preserving or restoring fertility, and preventing or delaying the recurrence of the disease. In women with mild disease or those who are perimenopausal and will soon stop ovarian cycling and the hormonal fluctuations that trigger bleeding endometriosis, expectant management (observation) is an important option.

Oral contraceptives are used with good results to provide adequate relief for women with mild disease. Studies indicate that low-dose drospirenone/ethinyl estradiol 3 mg/20 mcg, either continuous or cyclic oral contraceptives, are effective in reducing pelvic pain resulting from endometriosis (Level II; Harada et al, 2008; Mabrouk et al, 2012). In addition, pain relief is often achieved with NSAIDs and other prostaglandin inhibitors. Oral contraceptives (OCs) and NSAIDs are usually sufficient only for disease with minimal pain. Typically, the medications include ibuprofen (400–600 mg 4 times daily), naproxen sodium (220 mg 4 times daily), indomethacin, and mefenamic acid (Ponstel) (250 mg 4 times daily to 500 mg 3 times daily). Medication administration should begin with the onset of menstruation to avoid the possible influence of medications on pregnancy. Prescription pain medications may be necessary to control symptoms. Conservative management is to use the least powerful medications first. With consistent reevaluation of symptom reduction, the risks associated with medications can be minimized.

For women with moderate to severe disease, hormonal therapy may help relieve symptoms. Drugs such as nafarelin nasal spray (0.2–0.4 mg 2 times daily), long-acting leuprolide acetate (3.75 mg IM once a month), or goserelin (3.6 mg subcutaneously once a month) are gonadotropin-releasing hormone (GnRH) analogs and suppress ovulation by suppressing pituitary gonadotropin secretion and thus ovarian estrogen secretion. These drugs are used for 3 to 6 months, although the optimum length of therapy is unclear. Adverse effects of this medication are vasomotor symptoms (hot flashes), vaginal dryness, dyspareunia, decreased libido, insomnia, breast tenderness, headache, depression, and bone demineralization, which can be mediated by "add back" therapy with norethindrone, 5 to 15 mg daily.

Another hormonal treatment is danazol (200–400 mg 2 times daily), which is used for 6 to 9 months. Danazol is a testosterone derivative that acts like progesterone and suppresses menstruation. Adverse effects are androgenic and include weight gain, acne, hirsutism, muscle cramps, lower high-density lipoprotein, and decreased breast size.

Continuous combination OCs may also be given but are most effective in mild disease. Any of the combination OCs discussed earlier in this chapter can be used. Breakthrough bleeding may occur and is treated with conjugated estrogens 1.25 mg daily for 1 week or estradiol 2 mg daily for 1 week. Adverse effects are discussed earlier in the chapter.

Progesterone alone in the form of medroxyprogesterone acetate 100 mg IM every 2 weeks for four doses, then 100 mg every 4 weeks, can be given to inhibit endometrial tissue growth and initiate decidualization and atrophy of the endometrium. Oral therapy of medroxyprogesterone 10 mg three times daily or norethindrone 5 mg daily can also be used. These treatments provide 80% of women with complete or partial relief of symptoms. These treatments are used for 6 to 9 months. Oral estrogen can be added to control breakthrough bleeding.

Aromatase inhibitors, which decrease estrogen production, are still investigational. Regimens may be developed that combine these drugs with progestins or GnRH analogs.

Laparoscopy is used to ablate endometrial implants, which greatly reduces pain. Some women require removal of ovarian endometriomas along with ablation of implants, and this procedure improves fertility. For women who no longer desire to have children, a total abdominal hysterectomy and bilateral salpingo-oophorectomy (TAH-BSO) will treat the endometriosis definitively, but in women with deep implants, TAH-BSO may not be sufficient.

Medical treatment alone is inappropriate for moderate to severe disease, and in addition, in these women it does not improve fertility. Only surgical interventions are shown to improve fertility. For example, some reviews have shown that with observation alone, pregnancy rates in mild, moderate, and severe disease are 50%, less than 25%, and only 5%, respectively. With surgery, pregnancy rates rise to 50% and 39% in patients with moderate and severe disease, respectively. However, in vitro fertilization is usually needed postoperatively for women with severe disease in whom hysterectomy can be avoided. Infertile women who are trying to improve their chance of pregnancy typically benefit from laparoscopic ablation of endometrial implants.

Alternative therapies are gaining acceptance in the treatment of endometriosis. Visualization techniques, patterned breathing, massage therapy, and others may each have their place in the treatment of this disorder. Diet therapy and therapy to maximize the immune system may also be useful. Therapies must be evaluated for an appropriate match between patient and therapy.

Financial issues may be of concern. Hormonal therapies are significantly more expensive than dietary changes and massage therapy (see Complementary Therapies 14.1).

Follow-up and Referral

The signs and symptoms of endometriosis are related to the menstrual cycle. Follow-up visits should be timed to allow prescribed treatments to have affected the symptoms associated with the next menstrual cycle. The patient should be referred to a gynecologist experienced in laparoscopic diagnosis and treatment of endometriosis if the most conservative medical treatments are not sufficient to ameliorate the symptoms.

Patient Education

Each patient must receive appropriately formulated educational materials about endometriosis, including its signs and symptoms and the effects they may produce, because this is usually a lifelong condition. (See The Patient's Voice 14.2.)

The Patient's Voice 14.2
Endometriosis

I had a very painful menstruation from day 1. As long as I can remember, every month I was in bed doubled over in pain. Nothing seemed to relieve the intensity of the pain . . . even taking birth control pills. My periods were not heavy, but I always had pain and even a little spotting, especially after my period every month. About 1 year after the delivery of my third child, I began experiencing great discomfort with intercourse. My gynecologist suggested that since I was almost 40 years old, a surgical intervention was needed. He explained that laparoscopy or laparotomy and eventual hysterectomy was the usual treatment for women with severe pain. My first surgery did reveal that I had endometriosis . . . a small amount . . . but my surgeon said that some of the locations of the endometriosis made it even more painful. I had a difficult time with the hysterectomy . . . a lot of pain. But, since they removed my uterus, the pain I had for almost 27 years is finally gone. Why did it take so long for someone to give me relief?

◼ LEIOMYOMAS (UTERINE FIBROIDS)

Leiomyomas are most commonly called *uterine fibroids.* Fibroids are benign tumors (most common benign tumor of the uterus) and arise from the smooth muscle cells in the myometrium. Most are small and asymptomatic.

Epidemiology and Causes

Leiomyomas are extremely common, and the prevalence increases in women between 30 and 50 years of age. However, the prevalence decreases with menopause. By age 50 years, 50% of African American and Asian American women have leiomyomas and about 30% of white women have them.

The cause of leiomyomas is unknown, but clearly there is a hormonal link. Girls before menarche do not have leiomyomas, and they shrink after menopause, implicating estrogen. If a pregnant woman has a fibroid, it dramatically increases in size during pregnancy, but decreases after delivery. Risk factors for the development of leiomyomas include nulliparity, age between 30 and 50 years, obesity, and sedentary lifestyle. Interestingly, smoking seems to decrease the risk for developing fibroids.

Pathophysiology

Leiomyomas develop from a single neoplastic smooth muscle cell with abnormal chromosomal patterns. Leiomyomas are classified by location within the uterine wall and can be subserous, submucous, and/or intramural. Rarely, a leiomyoma can be intraligamentous, cervical, or parasitic (deriving its blood supply from an organ to which it becomes attached). Most uterine fibroids are surrounded by compressed (otherwise normal) myometrium. When leiomyomas outgrow their blood supply, they can become necrotic and ulcerate.

Clinical Presentation

Subjective

Most leiomyomas are asymptomatic. When symptoms are present, abnormal uterine bleeding is the most common symptom. The woman may also complain of pain, particularly with intercourse. If the fibroid is large enough, it can cause pressure on the bladder, resulting in urinary frequency, urgency, and possibly dysuria. The complaint of abdominal or genital heaviness is also common with large fibroids.

Objective

Pelvic exam will reveal one or more uterine masses. Leiomyomas are usually firm and nontender. If there are multiple fibroids (most of the time), the uterus will feel irregular and nodular in shape.

Diagnostic Reasoning

Diagnostic Tests

Because most women with leiomyomas have abnormal uterine bleeding, a complete blood count is ordered. The hemoglobin is decreased because of the increased amount and frequency of menstrual bleeding. Occasionally polycythemia may be present. A pregnancy test should be done to rule out intrauterine pregnancy. An endometrial biopsy may be done and will be normal, which helps rule out other diagnoses.

Pelvic ultrasound or magnetic resonance imaging will confirm the diagnosis of leiomyoma, but transvaginal ultrasound is used most often. Occasionally, hysterography or hysteroscopy is used to confirm cervical or submucous myomas.

Differential Diagnosis

Differential diagnoses should include other disorders that cause uterine enlargement and abnormal uterine bleeding, including pregnancy, adenomyosis (presence of endometrial glands and stroma in the myometrium), ovarian neoplasm, tubo-ovarian inflammatory mass, uterine cancer, and possibly diverticulitis.

Management

No treatment is necessary for women with asymptomatic or very small myomas. If the patient is severely anemic, measures should be undertaken to stop the prolonged, heavy menstrual periods and boost her hemoglobin. Medroxyprogesterone acetate 150 mg IM given every 28 days or Danazol 400 to 800 mg PO daily will usually slow or stop the bleeding. The woman should be instructed to take over-the-counter iron preparations (ferrous sulfate, ferrous gluconate, or ferrous fumarate 300 mg) daily. Folic acid 400 mcg PO daily will help boost red blood cell production as well.

The goal of conservative medical management is to shrink the leiomyomas. Oral contraceptives (OCs) may be effective for some women, but for others, the estrogen in the OC causes enlargement, so frequent monitoring is important. Gonadotropin-releasing hormone (GnRH) agonists are given to decrease the luteinizing hormone and follicle-stimulating hormone levels, thereby producing a hypoestrogenic effect that usually causes the leiomyomas to shrink. This is frequently used before surgery, because the risk of surgical complications is increased with large tumors. The GnRH agents that are used are leuprorelin (Lupron) depot injection of 3.75 mg every 28 days for 3 months or a single dose of 11.25 mg IM. Treatment lasts 8 to 12 weeks and is very costly. Because these drugs induce a menopausal state, the adverse effects reflect those of menopause (see under Menopause). These medications are contraindicated in women with undiagnosed abnormal uterine bleeding and in women who are breastfeeding. Insertion of the levonorgestrel intrauterine contraceptive device (Mirena) has been shown to significantly decrease bleeding with fibroids that are associated with menorrhagia. This device is removed after 5 years.

There are several surgical approaches for problematic leiomyomas. Myomectomy is removal of the myoma and is done when preservation of fertility is desired and the tumor is larger than 12-week gestational size. Hysterectomy (with or without removal of the ovaries) is the definitive treatment for very large fibroids, particularly when bleeding is very heavy and the patient is markedly anemic. Few adverse effects occur as a result of hysterectomy; infection, bleeding, and damage to surrounding organs are always possible with any surgical procedure. Other possible effects are depression, sexual dysfunction, and menopausal symptoms.

Uterine artery embolization is a relatively new alternative to surgery. The uterine arteries are embolized, producing end-organ ischemia and necrosis with subsequent shrinkage. This procedure is effective in reducing menorrhagia, pain, and uterine volume in 80% of patients. However, a large number of women report severe pelvic pain, fever, malaise, and nausea and vomiting resulting from the infarcted uterine tissue.

Follow-up and Referral

Any woman with severe bleeding, marked anemia, and palpable leiomyomas should be referred to a gynecologist for evaluation and treatment. Women with small uterine myomas should be reexamined at 3- to 6-month intervals or more often if symptoms increase. If menorrhagia is present, hemoglobin and hematocrit should be monitored frequently.

Patient Education

Women with leiomyomas should be reassured that this does not increase their chances of developing uterine cancer. If increased bleeding is a problem, the woman should be instructed to take an iron supplement daily and to increase iron-rich foods in her diet. She should report any shortness of breath, palpitations, or increase in fatigue or pain immediately.

■ ENDOMETRIAL CANCER

Endometrial cancer arises from the lining of the uterus, known as the endometrium. The majority are pure adenocarcinomas. Endometrial cancer accounts for at least 20% of cases of postmenopausal uterine bleeding.

Epidemiology and Causes

Cancer of the endometrium is the most common (50%) of all gynecological cancers. There are approximately 36,000 cases of endometrial cancer per year, with 6,000 annual deaths in the United States. The overall 5-year survival rate is 80% to 85% but is as high as 98% if the cancer is detected early and the depth of invasion is less than 66%. The 5-year survival rate drops to 78% if the depth of invasion is more than 66%. The average age at diagnosis is 60 years, and about 25% of all cases occur before menopause. African American women are at greater risk for most forms of endometrial cancer, and their stage-for-stage survival rates are also worse compared with those for Caucasian women. Oral contraceptive (OC) pills have been shown to have a protective mechanism against ovarian and endometrial cancer. Patients who use OCs have half the risk of developing these cancers. Women who use OCs for at least a year have this protective effect, which remains even after the OCs are discontinued. Risk factors for endometrial cancer include

unopposed estrogen, early menarche, advancing age, a high-fat diet, nulliparity, obesity, hypertension, and diabetes mellitus. Routine screening is neither cost-effective nor warranted, except in extremely high-risk women (40%–60% risk) with certain familial malignancy syndromes such as Lynch syndrome II (i.e., endometrial, ovarian, and colorectal cancers) who are at risk for hereditary nonpolyposis colorectal cancer. However, endometrial cancer screening has rarely been shown to be justified in asymptomatic women, even those on unopposed estrogen hormone replacement or the estrogen agonist tamoxifen.

Pathophysiology

The precursor of endometrial cancer is a hyperplastic state that may progress to invasive carcinoma. Endometrial hyperplasia of glandular tissue occurs when estrogen does not have progesterone as a counterbalance, resulting in a greater gland-to-stroma ratio. The mitogenic effect of estrogen on endometrial tissue appears to result from upregulation of the cell cycle protein cyclin D, as well as various proto-oncogenes and cellular growth factors and their receptors. These findings are also consistent with the protective effects of progestin-containing OCs or continuous progestin therapies. An unopposed estrogenic state may occur from multiple etiologies, including chronic anovulation such as in polycystic ovarian syndrome, an estrogen-secreting ovarian tumor, obesity that causes increased aromatization of androstenedione to estrone and testosterone to estradiol in peripheral adipose tissue with decreased levels of sex hormone–binding globulin, or iatrogenic estrogen exposure from older hormone replacement therapy regimens of estrogen monotherapy (10-fold increase in risk) or the selective estrogen receptor modifier tamoxifen (twofold to threefold increase in risk), which is used as adjuvant therapy for breast cancer. The potential for cytological atypia similarly increases with chronic unopposed estrogenic stimulation, creating a persistent proliferative phase within the endometrium, rather than the normal cycling of proliferative and progesterone-induced secretory phases.

This premalignant condition is characterized by either a simple (i.e., cystic dilation of the glands with occasional outpouching) or complex (more abundant and adjacent glands with outpouching and minimal stroma) architectural pattern of the endometrium, as well as the presence or absence of nuclear atypia and glandular mitoses. Simple hyperplasia without atypia is unlikely to develop into endometrial carcinoma (1% of cases), whereas complex architecture with atypia is most likely to progress to malignancy (30% of cases). Atypia is the key negative prognostic factor, because 25% of women with atypia on biopsy have coexistent malignancy on further evaluation. In fact, some pathologists group complex architecture with atypia together with differentiated adenocarcinoma under the common heading of endometrioid neoplasia. Indeed, 75% to 80% of all endometrial cancers are estrogen-dependent endometrioid carcinomas (type I).

Not all endometrial malignancy arises from hyperplastic tissue. For example, papillary serous endometrial tumors (5%–10% of cases) arise from atrophic rather than hyperplastic tissue and, as with clear cell (1%–5% of cases), mucinous, and squamous cell (fewer than 2% of cases) endometrial cancers, are estrogen independent (type II). These rarer forms of endometrial cancer tend to be more poorly differentiated (higher nuclear grade) than type I cancers, are highly aggressive with lymphatic invasion, and portend a worse prognosis. Uterine sarcoma is a rare form of cancer (5% of uterine malignancies), which may be completely nonepithelial in origin or of a mixed epithelial-nonepithelial phenotype. Most commonly arising from the uterine myometrium (e.g., mixed Müllerian carcinosarcomas of fibrous, vascular, or lymphatic tissue; leiomyosarcoma), uterine sarcoma may also arise from the endometrium and invade the myometrium (e.g., endometrial stromal sarcoma). These cancers are more aggressive than more common hyperplastic endometrial forms, are prone to metastasis to the retroperitoneal and intra-abdominal nodes and hematogenously to the lungs, and carry a poorer prognosis (e.g., 50% 5-year survival rate for stage I disease versus 90% for more common forms of endometrial cancer). They are more common in African American women (except the endometrial stromal form) and in women aged 40 to 60 years, and there appears to be a correlation with prior pelvic irradiation and, possibly, tamoxifen use.

Endometrial cancers may be mediated by mutations in a host of genes, such as the *p53* tumor suppressor gene, which is a late mutation in 20% of endometrioid carcinomas, an early mutation in 90% of serous adenocarcinomas, but rarely mutated in endometrial hyperplasia. Estrogen-dependent cancers also demonstrate mutations in *PTEN* (an early mutation seen in 80% of cases), microsatellite DNA (20%–30% of cases), and K-*ras* (a late mutation seen in 20% of cases). The cancerous cells lining the endometrium may extend directly into the cervix and through the uterine serosa. Both the pelvic (paravaginal) and para-aortic lymph nodes may become involved. Although endometrial cancer metastasizes slowly, malignant cells can be found in the peritoneal cavity.

Clinical Presentation
Subjective

The patient, usually postmenopausal, presents with abnormal bleeding in 80% of cases. Typically, this is the only patient complaint. Patients who are perimenopausal tend to have irregular periods of bleeding; however, irregular uterine bleeding must not be discounted in these women without further exploration.

Objective

The patient does not demonstrate any pain on the exam unless metastasis has already occurred and the pelvic organs are affected.

Diagnostic Reasoning
Diagnostic Tests

Any postmenopausal patient with abnormal uterine bleeding should be referred for endometrial biopsy. Eighty percent of cases of abnormal bleeding are from benign causes. A Pap test is not a reliable diagnostic indicator for endometrial cancer. Any atypical glandular cells reported on the Pap smear should be followed up by endometrial biopsy to rule out hyperplasia or carcinoma; the same may be done for women older than 40 years of age with normal endometrial cells on Pap smear, but this is more controversial. If endometrial biopsy reveals hyperplasia with atypia, a more extensive hysteroscopy with curettage should be done to rule out coexistent endometrial cancer. If abnormal bleeding persists after an otherwise normal endometrial biopsy (i.e., showing only atrophy, proliferative or secretory endometrium, or disordered/dyssynchronous endometrium reflecting irregular shedding of the endometrium seen with unopposed estrogen exposure and endometritis), further assessment should be done with transvaginal ultrasound (TVUS), hysteroscopy, and directed biopsy/curettage. TVUS is helpful in ruling out carcinoma in women not on hormone therapy (HT). A biopsy is done if the endometrial thickness is greater than 4 mm or in any woman with persistent uterine bleeding, regardless of endometrial thickness. However, TVUS cannot replace biopsy as a means of ruling out cancer. CA-125 should be checked to predict extent of extrauterine spread of the cancer. Depending on the results of the endometrial biopsy, the patient should be referred to a surgeon.

Differential Diagnoses

Differential diagnoses may include benign tumor (leiomyomas [fibroids]), ectopic pregnancy, intrauterine pregnancy, gastrointestinal masses, endometriosis, adenomyosis, and pelvic abscess or adhesions. Endometrial polyps should also be considered because they present mostly in middle-aged women, but account for 25% of cases of abnormal bleeding in premenopausal and postmenopausal women. They are hyperplastic pedunculated/sessile growths of endometrial glands and stroma at the endometrial surface (millimeters to centimeters in size). They are only rarely neoplastic (benign in 70%, hyperplasia without atypia in 25%, atypia in fewer than 5%, and cancer in fewer than 1%). Metrorrhagia (irregular uterine bleeding) occurs in 50% of cases of endometrial polyps; less frequently, menorrhagia, post-menopausal bleeding, prolapse through the cervical os, and breakthrough bleeding on hormonal treatments occur as symptoms. The only definitive diagnosis for endometrial polyps is microscopy (after dilation and curettage [D&C], biopsy, or hysterectomy), but sono-hysterography (instillation of saline into the uterus before ultrasound) is preferred to TVUS for noninvasive evaluation (but it cannot be diagnostic). Curettage via hysteroscopy, rather than blindly, is preferred for best detecting polyps.

Adenomyosis is the presence of ectopic endometrial glands and stroma within the musculature of the uterus, which induces hypertrophy and hyperplasia of the myometrium in response to estrogen (and possibly progesterone); may be microscopic or nodular on gross inspection, but endometrial biopsy is typically negative because of changes in the myometrium. It seems to be more associated with childbearing, but the pathogenesis is unknown (it is perhaps related to invagination of the endometrium, or it may arise de novo from Müllerian remnants). The uterus is large and boggy (as opposed to firm with fibroids). Adenomyosis is not related to endometriosis, although this is another form of ectopic endometrium. Although a third of women are asymptomatic, adenomyosis may present with abnormal uterine bleeding, dysmenorrhea, and menorrhagia.

Management

The primary principle of management is to obtain a correct diagnosis as early as possible, because the cure rate for endometrial cancer is very high if treated early.

Because primary prevention is the best management, women with chronic anovulation may benefit from the protective effects of progestin or progesterone-containing regimens (protects against hyperplasia and carcinoma [doses may be decreased from standard recommendations in women with significant side effects from this]). Women with hyperplasia without atypia can be given medroxyprogesterone acetate 10 mg daily for 12 to 14 days each month for 3 to 6 months, whereas women with atypia (premalignancy) need hysteroscopy with D&C and hysterectomy (preferred if childbearing is no longer an issue). If no cancer is found, women can receive megestrol acetate 10 to 80 mg four times daily continuously to suppress the hyperplasia or hysterectomy (if fertility is no longer an issue and the patient can tolerate the surgery). Obviously, any estrogen therapy should be stopped in these cases. In postmenopausal women not on HT who have hyperplasia without atypia, a hysteroscopy and D&C is done to find the source of the estrogen (such as a tumor or obesity). Women can be given medroxyprogesterone acetate 10 mg daily for 3 months, then reevaluated by biopsy as a guide for further management. If the woman is taking HT, it should be stopped immediately and a similar assessment done. In postmenopausal women with atypia, a hysteroscopy

with D&C is done to rule out carcinoma, and hysterectomy (preferred) is considered. As an alternative, megestrol acetate 40 mg two to four times daily can be given with a repeat biopsy in 3 months and hysterectomy done if atypia persists. Otherwise, if the atypia regresses, megestrol can be given and repeat biopsies done every 6 to 12 months for the rest of the woman's life.

Treatment of endometrial cancer is based on the International Federation of Gynecology and Obstetrics (FIGO) staging. Stage I is confined to the uterine corpus, stage II involves the cervix, stage III is regional spread to the pelvis, and stage IV is spread outside the pelvis (20%–25% 5-year survival). Node biopsy (lymphadenectomy) is done for clinically suspicious nodes and for anything beyond stage I disease—a tumor greater than 2 cm, type II endometrial cancer, or myometrial invasion beyond 50%—because all these indicate an increased risk of metastasis. Peritoneal cytology is also sent as a part of surgical staging, because a positive result with nonendometrioid tumors may indicate the need for postsurgical adjuvant chemotherapy. Bilateral salpingo-oophorectomy is done to check for adnexal micrometastases and to eliminate endogenous estrogen production.

In contrast to the treatment of early stage type I endometrial CA, uterine sarcoma is treated with total abdominal hysterectomy and bilateral salpingo-oophorectomy (TAH-BSO) with adjuvant radiotherapy (either external beam or brachytherapy). Although adjuvant chemotherapy has not been shown to be effective for uterine sarcoma, recurrent disease is treated with chemotherapy. Stage II or higher uterine adenocarcinoma is also treated with TAH-BSO, if the patient can tolerate surgery. Pelvic irradiation is an alternative to hysterectomy but entails significant comorbidities from fibrotic tissue damage that is progressive and nonreversible. Adjuvant postsurgical radiation may be used for women at intermediate to high risk of recurrent disease (grade 1 or 2 disease extending greater than 50% beyond the myometrium [stage IC] or stage II to IV disease) or reserved as salvage treatment for recurrent disease. Disease at high risk of recurrence (grade 2 disease extending to the cervix with greater than 50% myometrial involvement, grade 3 disease, involvement of the lymphatic or vascular system or other metastases) should be treated with surgery and adjuvant therapy—either chemotherapy or pelvic irradiation; the choice is individualized depending on potential side effects and patient tolerance. Recurrent or highly advanced disease is treated with a combination of chemotherapy and hormonal therapy, although the choice of regimen is controversial. Localized relapse may be treated with salvage surgery or pelvic irradiation.

Follow-up and Referral

If endometrial cancer is suspected in a postmenopausal patient with abnormal uterine bleeding, an immediate referral should be made to a gynecologist/oncologist for an endometrial biopsy.

Patient Education

The American Cancer Society recommends an endometrial biopsy at menopause for all patients and then occasionally for patients at risk. Healthy postmenopausal patients should be encouraged to seek care at the first sign of any abnormal bleeding. In addition, obese women should be encouraged to lose weight because it may prove protective and possibly therapeutic for women with chronic anovulation. The use of HT for any indication is controversial in women with prior endometrial cancer. All women should be encouraged to follow treatment regimens for any existing diseases such as hypertension and diabetes mellitus.

■ MENOPAUSE

Menopause has occurred when a patient has not menstruated for a period of 1 year. This takes place most often in women aged 48 to 55 years (average is 51.5 years), but the normal age range for the onset of menopause is wide—anywhere between ages 40 and 60 years. Menopause is not a disease state, but it portends a change in the hormonal, emotional, and reproductive lives of women. Many patients have an increased awareness of and respect for the wisdom of nature; they have philosophical and personal concerns about treating the symptoms and consequences of menopause not as a disease but as a normal part of their life cycle. Patients need to be aware of what is happening to their bodies so that they can make rational decisions about how to manage this stage of their lives.

The management of menopause and its symptoms has received a great deal of attention in recent years. As the life span for women lengthens—currently to an average of 84 years—menopause does not signal the end but rather another phase of life, with its own issues, challenges, and opportunities. Most women spend 30 years of their lives postmenopausal.

Epidemiology and Causes

Perimenopause is a triad of phases that include the climacteric, or menopausal, transition; menopause; and postmenopausal periods in a woman's reproductive life span. Throughout perimenopause, physical changes occur. The years immediately before and the decades after menopause are of much greater clinical significance than the cessation of menses, which identifies menopause itself.

The menopausal transition, or climacteric, is the phase that signals the nearing of menopause; it occurs approximately 10 years before the onset of menopause, usually between ages 38 and 42 years. The period of menopausal transition may have either an insidious or relatively abrupt onset. During this time, ovulation becomes less frequent, and the numbers of ovarian follicles are decreased and less likely to mature. Women note the beginnings of this phase usually with changes in the menstrual cycle, which can be a shortening of the menstrual cycle and an increase in menstrual bleeding.

Immediately before menopause, menstrual bleeding may occur after a short luteal phase or after an estradiol peak without ovulation. In approximately 70% of patients, menses then become lighter and farther apart until they stop. Another 10% of patients simply stop menstruating without any other symptoms.

The remaining 20% of patients experience heavier bleeding, which is often unpredictable. This group of patients is at risk for anemia and endometrial hyperplasia, a precursor for endometrial cancer. The diagnosis of endometrial hyperplasia is made by an endometrial biopsy. Other reasons for abnormal bleeding in this age-group can be endometrial cancer, endometrial polyps, uterine leiomyomas, and systemic clotting disorders. In the past, many patients were treated for increased menstrual bleeding with hysterectomies.

Premature ovarian failure is cessation of ovarian function before age 35 years. To determine true ovarian failure, two follicle-stimulating hormone (FSH) levels must be above the normal limit of 40 mIU/mL.

Pathophysiology

Menopause is the permanent cessation of menses and ovarian function in a woman. To understand menopause properly, however, knowledge of normal ovarian development is required. This is first characterized by germ cell differentiation (i.e., oocyte development) and primordial ovarian follicle formation, both of which begin during embryonic development, with a peak of 6 to 7 million oocytes present in a growing fetus at just 5 months in utero. FSH drives this process by stimulating granulosa cell formation in ovarian follicles and inducing luteinizing hormone (LH) receptor formation, which will eventually allow for ovulation to occur later in life in response to surges in LH at the time of menarche. In a sexually mature ovulatory female, follicular release of an oocyte leads to transformation of the follicle into a corpus luteum cyst, which produces less estrogen but increasing amounts of progesterone, capable of maintaining a pregnancy after fertilization and implantation of an oocyte into the uterine lining.

However, even during the fetal stages of development, follicular atresia and destruction of oocytes within the ovary itself are normal, continuous processes, which account for the reduction in oocyte number from its peak to 1 to 2 million at the time of birth and down to approximately 300,000 at the onset of puberty. Animal and human studies have shown this may be driven by reductions in FSH, decreased androgen production by ovarian thecal cells (reducing substrate for estrogen production via androgen aromatization), the upregulation of pro-apoptotic genes such as *Bax,* and the downregulation of anti-apoptotic genes such as *bcl-2* in both oocytes (primarily a fetal process) and follicular granulosa cells (primarily in adults).

Perimenopause, 2 to 8 years before and 1 year after the complete cessation of menses, is characterized by the waxing and waning of ovarian function, reflected in both ovulatory and anovulatory (estrogen-only) menstrual cycles of unpredictable duration and intensity, extended periods of estrogen deficiency, and heightened FSH/LH secretion with occasional follicular development and estradiol production. Over time, estrogen feedback to the hypothalamic-pituitary axis declines. In some women, estrogen positive feedback no longer leads to an LH surge capable of triggering ovulation, whereas in others, estrogen negative feedback fails to suppress LH production during the follicular phase. Moreover, the failure of corpus luteum cysts to form after ovulation leads to a decrease in progesterone and increased exposure to unopposed estrogen, which accounts for the increase in dysfunctional uterine bleeding (DUB) and endometrial hyperplasia observed during this period.

Although some degree of follicular atresia occurs continuously throughout a woman's reproductive lifetime and increases rapidly after age 37 years, the permanent cessation of both ovarian function and menses known as menopause is an event rather than a period of time. Occurring on average at age 51 years, factors that influence the timing of menopause have been the subject of much research. Whereas the age at menarche has steadily declined over recent decades (having been linked to nutritional status, environmental factors, and general health), the average age at menopause has remained remarkably constant since ancient times. Today, several factors have been well documented to lower the age at menopause, including smoking (which decreases the onset of menopause by 2 years on average), nulliparity, menstrual regularity and a shorter cycle length, a family history of early menopause, increased galactose intake, concurrent type 1 diabetes mellitus, and certain genetic variants in the estrogen receptor and galactose-1-phosphate uridyl transferase gene. Menopause occurring past age 55 years is defined as late menopause.

With the depletion of ovarian follicles that are able to respond to gonadotropins, both follicular development and cyclical estrogen production cease during menopause. FSH levels rise as the body tries unsuccessfully to stimulate follicular production of estrogen. FSH levels above 40 mIU/mL signal the approach of menopause, even though a patient may still experience occasional menstrual bleeding. LH concentration is also elevated, but menopausal levels are difficult to distinguish from LH elevations seen during preovulatory gonadotropin surges in the normal menstrual cycle. Persistently high LH levels lead to continued androgen production by ovarian thecal cells, namely androstenedione, contributing to some of the undesirable physical changes experienced by postmenopausal women such as increased facial hair. Biochemical studies have revealed that the gonadotropins in older women have a longer half-life (contributing to their increased serum levels)

but also contain higher levels of carbohydrate that tend to render them less biologically active. Moreover, although residual oocytes and differentiating follicles have been identified in postmenopausal women, the follicles are typically atretic and eventually become cystic in the absence of viable oocytes.

Without a follicular source, circulating levels of estrogen fall significantly during menopause—particularly the active form estradiol, produced from the aromatization of testosterone. High gonadotropin levels stimulate the ovarian stroma to produce the less potent hormone estrone, rather than estradiol, while androstenedione produced by the adrenal glands is converted to estrone by aromatization in the periphery, particularly within adipose tissue, which contains significant levels of the aromatase enzyme. In addition, serum levels of the hormone inhibin B also decline, closely correlating to the rise in FSH, implying an inhibitory action of inhibin B on FSH. Estrone and androstenedione levels remain relatively constant as the patient ages, whereas testosterone levels decline. Obese women, with larger amounts of adipose tissue, typically display higher levels of circulating estrogens; however, they are still subject to vasomotor symptoms triggered by estrogen deficiency. Patients who are thin tend to experience vaginal dryness and other symptoms associated with low estrogen levels, whereas obese patients are at greater risk of experiencing symptoms associated with unopposed estrogen, such as DUB, endometrial hyperplasia, and endometrial neoplasms. In turn, women who do not experience the vasomotor symptoms of estrogen deficiency during menopause (e.g., hot flashes) should be monitored yearly for endometrial pathology with vaginal ultrasound and biopsy as appropriate.

Clinical Presentation
Subjective

Many women do not seek medical attention while going through menopause; they simply stop monthly menstrual bleeding. Their first presentation may be for a yearly gynecological exam. If the patient has not menstruated for 12 months, she can be considered to be menopausal. Women should be counseled about the risks and benefits of hormone replacement therapy (HRT), calcium supplementation, and other steps necessary to remain healthy during the postmenopausal decades. If less than 12 months has passed, a reevaluation should occur at the next yearly gynecological exam.

Several factors have been identified that may alter menopause timing. Genetics and family history are factors that influence the age at which a woman experiences menopause. There is a similarity in menopausal age between mothers and daughters. Hysterectomy (removal of the uterus but not the ovaries) hastens the cessation of follicle stimulation and ovulation by 1 to 2 years. Women who smoke tend to have an earlier menopause.

Menopause can also be induced with chemotherapy and radiation treatments.

Most patients go through menopause without experiencing symptoms debilitating enough to make them seek medical attention. About 20% of patients seek attention for one or more symptoms related to menopause. The most common symptoms of menopause are the vasomotor symptoms of hot flashes, night sweats, and insomnia. Vasomotor symptoms are caused by thermoregulatory dysfunction in which inappropriate peripheral vasodilation, cutaneous blood flow, and perspiration lead to a rapid heat loss and a fall in core body temperature with chills/shivering as an involuntary reaction to increased body temperature; up to 75% of menopausal patients experience this symptom (more likely after surgical menopause). Hot flashes contribute to sleep disturbances commonly experienced by perimenopausal women; this has been linked to mood disorders including depression, irritability, and fatigue, although many studies have failed to show a direct connection between menopause and depression. It is postulated that menopause makes preexisting depression worse, rather than creating it de novo. Ten percent to 15% of all postmenopausal patients report frequent, severe episodes of symptoms that completely disrupt their lives.

Vaginal dryness or atrophy is a common complaint among menopausal women. Vaginal dryness results from decreased blood flow to the vaginal mucosa and vulva caused by estrogen deficiency contributing to the complaints of dyspareunia, or painful intercourse. Lack of estrogen also leads to thinning of the vaginal epithelial lining, decreased rugae, loss of elasticity, and decreased vaginal mucus. Atrophy can become so severe that a woman may complain of postmenopausal bleeding. Although an endometrial biopsy is needed to rule out hyperplasia, the bleeding may be a result of the vaginal dryness.

Five areas of change involving sexual relations have been described: diminished sexual responsiveness, dyspareunia, decreased sexual activity, decline in sexual desire, and a dysfunctional male partner. A decrease in estrogen influences peripheral blood flow responses to sensory stimulation, affecting the timing and degree of vasocongestive response during sexual activity.

Vaginal atrophy is a major contributor to both stress and urge incontinence in the menopausal woman, particularly atrophy of the urethral epithelium with atrophic urethritis, loss of compliance, and irritation interfering with adequate seal of the urethral meatus. Atrophy of the bladder trigone (outlet tract) and decreased responsiveness of alpha-adrenergic receptors at the bladder neck and urethral sphincter all impair continence as well. Detrusor instability is also a cause of urinary symptoms. Patients will report that they either leak urine when they laugh, cough, or sneeze or that when they feel the urge to urinate they cannot make it to the bathroom in time. This can be very disconcerting and uncomfortable and lead to urinary tract infection and urinary odor problems. Done correctly, Kegel exercises (described in Chapter 12) reduce incontinence in 50% to 90% of patients within a few months.

Objective

The only documented objective manifestation of menopause is bone demineralization and resultant osteoporosis. Postmenopausal osteoporosis is one of the most common and disabling diseases affecting North American patients today. During the climacteric, patients may lose 2% to 5% of bone mass per year. Predisposition to falling created by an unsteady gait and poor eyesight are significant factors equal to low bone density as cause for hip fractures in postmenopausal patients.

Until 2001, it was widely believed that hormone therapy would prevent heart disease in menopausal women. As a result of the Heart and Estrogen/Progestin Replacement Study (HERS) and the more recent Women's Health Initiative Randomized Control Study (WHI), it is fairly clear that hormone replacement does not prevent cardiovascular disease and in some cases can precipitate an adverse cardiac event, especially in the first 5 years of treatment. Critics of these studies argue that the women in the study were well past menopause when the study began. Clearly, hormone replacement had deleterious effects on older women, whereas the effect on younger women remains unclear. Current research on the relationship between menopause, hormone replacement, and cardiovascular disease remains controversial at best.

Diagnostic Reasoning

The diagnosis of menopause is based on a history of amenorrhea and the presence of associated symptoms including hot flashes, flushes, night sweats, and sleep disturbances in age-appropriate women. If these symptoms are present, laboratory testing is not necessary. Other causes of amenorrhea must be considered whenever the history is not consistent with estrogen deficiency. Such history would be amenorrhea without vasomotor symptoms. An FSH level above 40 mIU/mL with a history of prolonged amenorrhea is diagnostic.

Diagnostic Tests

The first test that should be done in a woman whose menses has ceased is a pregnancy test, because an elevated beta–human chorionic gonadotropin level could reflect pregnancy, molar pregnancy, ectopic pregnancy, or even certain germ cell tumors. It is simple and inexpensive.

Serum FSH and LH levels are elevated in menopause. FSH levels greater than 10 to 25 mIU/mL suggest relative ovarian resistance consistent with menopausal transition. FSH levels of greater than 40 mIU/mL are consistent with complete cessation of ovarian function. LH levels are less sensitive for hormonal and ovarian function. During the menopausal transition, LH levels begin to rise; however, LH may also be elevated during the midcycle surge and in cases of chronic anovulation.

In patients with amenorrhea who do not have menstrual bleeding after progestin withdrawal, measurement of a serum estradiol may be helpful. Normal estradiol levels range between 40 and 300 pg/mL. A level of greater than 30 pg/mL may indicate some degree of residual ovarian function. Levels less than 30 pg/mL indicate cessation of ovarian function.

Patients on combined oral contraceptives (OCs) should have levels drawn on days 5 to 7 of the placebo-pill week to get accurate FSH and estradiol levels. Patients on progestin-only contraceptive pills can have levels drawn at any time because these pills do not affect FSH and estradiol levels.

Menopausal status can also be determined by vaginal cytological examination. On microscopic examination, parabasal cells will predominate, indicating a lack of epithelial maturating resulting from low estrogen levels.

Differential Diagnosis

The differential diagnoses for patients presenting with menopausal symptoms are pregnancy, spontaneous abortion, anovulation, endometrial hyperplasia, carcinoma, infection, and abnormalities of the uterus such as fibroids or polyps, endometriosis, adenomyosis, injury, and ovarian abnormalities such as tumors or cysts.

Management

Management of menopause focuses on symptom management and includes lifestyle modifications and a variety of medications.

Lifestyle Modifications

Vasomotor Symptoms Lifestyle modification can assist in the management of vasomotor symptoms. These modifications include aerobic exercise, dietary, vitamin, and mineral therapies, and herbal therapies.

The North American Menopause Society (NAMS) recommends aerobic exercise, because physically active women have 50% fewer hot flashes than their sedentary counterparts. As with any strenuous activity, this may precipitate perspiration and hot flashes until the woman becomes physically fit or conditioned. The insomnia that often accompanies these vasomotor problems may be relieved with exercise. Physical conditioning also decreases cardiovascular risk.

In addition to aerobic activity, weight loss for women who are overweight may be beneficial. Women with a high body mass index (BMI) report having more hot flashes than those with a lower BMI. Weight loss, too, is beneficial for cardiac risk reduction.

Other lifestyle changes that can be helpful for hot flashes and night sweats include dressing in layers, avoiding becoming overheated, limiting intake of alcohol and caffeine, reducing stress, and smoking cessation.

Dietary habits are very personal and often very difficult to change. It is prudent to recommend a diet that is high in complex carbohydrates and fiber (25–30 g daily), low in fat (less than 30% of calories from fat), particularly animal fat, and high in antioxidants (fresh fruits and vegetables).

Herbal therapies include those that are similar to estrogen. Isoflavonoid phytoestrogens are contained within plant fibers and are functionally similar to estradiol. They produce estrogenic effects that may reduce vasomotor symptoms. This type of estrogen-like substance is found in soy products such as tofu and soy milk. An alternative herbal preparation that may alleviate vasomotor symptoms is black cohosh (40 mg PO daily) or red clover (40–160 mg PO daily), which has an estrogenic effect and reduces hot flashes. Selective serotonin reuptake inhibitors (SSRIs) and serotonin-norepinephrine (noradrenaline) reuptake inhibitors have been used with success in providing relief of hot flashes.

Vaginal Dryness For patients who complain of vaginal dryness, a Pap smear and urine analysis should be done to make sure the symptoms are a result of cellular changes and not infection. If positive for infection or cellular abnormalities (other than parabasal cells), these must be addressed and then symptoms must be reassessed. The most effective treatment for vaginal dryness or atrophic vaginitis is topical vaginal application of an estrogen product. The estradiol vaginal ring has little systemic absorption and is suitable for long-term use and is effective for vaginal atrophy and dryness. Progesterone therapy is not necessary with the ring because there is little systemic absorption of estradiol and therefore no need to protect the endometrium. Estrogen vaginal cream can be used for short-term therapy. Creams are inserted into the vagina daily for 4 to 6 weeks and can be continued for a few months if necessary to resolve symptoms. After initial therapy, use of 1 to 2 g of the cream twice a week will prevent recurrence. Because absorption is variable, the vaginal ring is preferable.

Water-soluble vaginal lubricants are alternatives to topical estrogen or may be used in conjunction with the estradiol ring or estrogen creams as needed. Lubricants (e.g., Astroglide, K-Y Jelly) used before intercourse to decrease dyspareunia do not alleviate the symptoms of vaginal atrophy. Other alternative therapies that may be useful for vaginal dryness include sitz baths, vinegar douches, and intercourse.

For the symptoms of urinary frequency and incontinence, Kegel exercises remain the first line of therapy. These exercises are a natural nonpharmacological therapy that improve the tone of the urethral sphincter in patients with stress incontinence.

Psychological Problems Many women experience emotional problems with menopause including depression, irritability, and anxiety. As previously stated, depression occurs more often in menopausal women who have experienced depression at other times in their lives. In addition to relieving symptoms of depression, many antidepressants also have a favorable effect on other symptoms such as hot flashes. For example, SSRIs may relieve hot flashes as well as hormone therapy can. Paroxetine (Paxil) 12.5 to 25 mg controlled released or venlafaxine (Effexor) 37.5 to 75 mg is given PO daily. The antiseizure medication clonidine 100 to 150 mcg daily can be given orally or transdermally to relieve hot flashes, but the adverse effects of dry mouth, drowsiness, and hypotension make is less desirable.

Regular aerobic exercise improves cognitive function, enhances mood, and promotes daytime alertness and nocturnal sleepiness. Recent studies have shown that a brisk daily walk enhances wellness and promotes a sense of well-being.

Hormone Replacement Therapy

Because of recent research, hormone replacement therapy is not a first-line treatment for menopausal symptoms and certainly is not prescribed to prevent heart disease. Hormone therapy (HT) can be estrogen therapy (ET) alone or estrogen plus progestin therapy (EPT). These are the new nomenclature promoted by NAMS to clarify different therapies. In mid-2001 the EPT arm of the Women's Health Initiative (WHI) was halted prematurely because of evidence that it increased women's risk for a cardiac event. However, the ET arm of the study is ongoing with no increase in cardiovascular disease noted. In the WHI, there was definitive evidence that EPT decreased the risk of postmenopausal osteoporotic fractures, but the ET did not show this. Also, these results are in postmenopausal women. Improvement in osteoporotic fracture rates for perimenopausal women has not been established in clinical trials. From these results, it is clear that HT is not a first-line treatment for osteoporosis; there are other nonhormonal therapies with proven efficacy in improving bone mineral density.

NAMS recommends HT only for women with moderate to severe menopausal symptoms, particularly hot flashes and sleep disturbances, but only for a short period, no longer than 5 years. In addition, NAMS clearly states that HT should not be used for prevention of heart disease or stroke or for prevention of dementia, but it does state that not all data apply to all women.

If, after reviewing the benefits and risks with the patient, the patient and clinician decide that HT would be the best option, factors such as frequency of dosage, mode of delivery, and convenience should be considered and the appropriate drug prescribed. See Drugs Commonly Prescribed 14.2 for different forms of HT and dosage. Different types of HT are as follows:

• Estrogen therapy (ET)—start with the lowest dose of estrogens (0.3 mg). Estradiol can be given in a transdermal skin patch (lowest dose 0.025 mg/day). The patch is changed once or twice a week. This is usually limited to women who no longer have a uterus.
• Estrogen plus progestin therapy (EPT) (used to be referred to as HRT)—this therapy can be delivered either continuous-sequential (CS-EPT) or continuous-combined (CC-EPT). In the case of CS-EPT, estrogen is given days 1 to 21 of each month, and a progestin is given on days 7 to 21. Hormones are withheld from days 22 to 30, causing endometrial sloughing and bleeding. Many women find this method unacceptable. In CC-EPT estrogen and a progestin are given every day continuously. There may be some spotting initially, but after a few months, the endometrium is atrophic and will not bleed.

Exogenous estrogen is contraindicated in patients with estrogen-dependent cancers, such as breast, endometrial,

Drugs Commonly Prescribed 14.2 Menopause	
Estrogen Therapy (ET) (oral)	Dosage available (use lowest possible dose to relieve symptoms for the shortest period of time)
Conjugated estrogen (Premarin)	0.3, 0.625, 0.9, 1.25 mg; can be given cyclic or continuous (0.625 mg usual if continuous)
Micronized estradiol (Estrace)	0.5, 1.0, 2.0 mg; can be given cyclic or continuous (1.0 mg usual if continuous)
Esterified estrogens (Estratab, Meneset)	0.3, 0.625, 1.25, 2.5 mg; used mostly for cyclic hormone therapy
Estropipate (Ogen, Ortho-Est)	0.75, 1.5, 3; ; given cyclic
Estrogen Therapy (ET) (topical)	Dosage and form
Transdermal estradiol	Released in mg/day
Climara	0.025, 0.0375, 0.05, 0.06, 0.075, 0.1 mg; change once weekly
Estraderm	0.025, 0.0375, 0.05, 0.06, 0.075, 0.1 mg change once weekly; may use 3 weeks on and 1 week off

Drugs Commonly Prescribed 14.2   Menopause—cont'd

Alora	0.25, 0.05, 0.075, 0.1 mg; change twice weekly
Vivelle	0.25, 0.0375, 0.05, 0.075, 0.1 mg; change twice weekly
Vaginal estrogen creams and tablets	
Estradiol	
Vagifem	25 mcg tablets; inserted vaginally daily for 2 weeks then 1 tablet twice weekly
Estrace	0.01 mg/g cream; given cyclically—3 weeks on, 1 week off
Estropipate	
Ogen	1.5 mg/g cream; given cyclically—3 weeks on, 1 week off
Conjugated estrogen	
Premarin	0.625 mg/g cream; given cyclically—3 weeks on, 1 week off
Estrogen ring	
Estring	2 mg with 7.5 mcg released per 24 hours; remains in place for 3 months
Estrogen plus Progestin Therapy (EPT)	Dosage available
Continuous-sequential (CS-EPT)	Estrogens given as above on days 1–21 of cycle
Estrogen	
See the ET above	
Progestins	
medroxyprogesterone acetate [MPA] (Amen, Cycrin, Provera)	2.5, 5.0, 10.0 mg; on days 14–25
norethindrone	2.5, 5.0 mg; on days 14–25
norethindrone acetate (Aygestin)	5.0, 10.0 mg; on days 14–25
Continuous combined (CC-EPT)	
Estrogen	
Conjugated estrogens	0.625 mg daily
Estropipate	0.625 mg daily
Micronized estradiol	1.0 mg daily
Progestins	
medroxyprogesterone acetate	2.5, 5.0 mg daily
norethindrone	0.35 mg daily
norethindrone acetate	1.0 mg daily
Micronized progesterone (Prometrium)	100, 200 mg daily
Combination Products	Dosage available
Premphase	Conjugated estrogens 0.625 mg for 14 days; conjugated estrogens 0.625 and MPA 5 mg for 14 days
Prempro	Conjugated estrogens 0.3 and MPA 1.5 mg OR conjugated estrogens 0.45 and MPA 1.5 mg; OR conjugated estrogens 0.625 and MPA 2.5 mg OR conjugated estrogens 0.625 and MPA 5.0 mg; continuously
Ortho-Prefest	Estradiol 1.0 mg and estradiol 1.0 mg with norgestimate 0.09 mg in alternating sequence of 3 tablets each
FemHRT 1/5	Ethinyl estradiol 5 mcg and norethindrone acetate 1.0 mg
Activella	Estradiol 1.0 mg and norethindrone acetate 0.5 mg

and ovarian cancer, or undiagnosed vaginal bleeding. Patients with liver disease, active thrombosis, or history of stroke should not take estrogen. Pregnancy is another absolute contraindication for estrogen or progestin therapy. Migraine headache is a relative contraindication for the use of estrogen because of the vasoactive properties of estrogen in some patients. Estrogen use has also been associated with a small increased risk of gallbladder disease. Recently, studies have demonstrated an association between estrogen therapy and adult-onset asthma. Increased risk for development of systemic lupus erythematosus exists when taking estrogen; however, the incidence is low.

There are many types of estrogen products. These include 17-beta estradiol, estrone, and estriol. Conjugated equine estrogens (Premarin) are commonly prescribed. Conjugated equine estrogen is derived from the urine of pregnant horses. It contains naturally occurring estrogens such as estradiol and estrone, as well as products not native to humans. Synthetic estrogens used for replacement therapy have a higher potency and increased deleterious effects on hepatic globulins.

Levels of androgens decrease slowly in patients who experience natural menopause and more rapidly in patients who have undergone oophorectomy because the majority of androgens are produced in the ovary. Androgens are also produced in skin, muscle, and bone tissue. A positive correlation may exist between reduced androgen production and decreased libido in postmenopausal patients. Androgens have been shown to decrease high-density lipoprotein levels, an undesirable effect; however, they have also been shown to decrease triglyceride levels, a factor in cardiovascular disease. Because the effects of androgen depletion on libido occur only in patients with testosterone levels of less than 20 to 60 ng/dL, a testosterone blood level is indicated before initiation of therapy. Androgens are available in synthetic form, either alone as methyltestosterone (Oreton, Android), or combined with estrogen. A natural micronized testosterone may be procured from a compounding pharmacy. The long-term effect of testosterone administration in postmenopausal patients is unknown.

Raloxifene HCl (Evista) is a selective estrogen receptor modulator and is a first-line therapy for prevention and treatment of postmenopausal osteoporosis. It protects patients from bone loss associated with decreased levels of estrogen. It does not affect breast or uterine tissue and, therefore, cannot cause breast tenderness, spotting, and other symptoms that can occur with the initiation of estrogen therapy. In initial studies, raloxifene did not demonstrate an increased risk for breast or uterine cancer. Raloxifene does not decrease hot flashes and may actually cause hot flashes in early treatment.

Bisphosphonates are a relatively new class of medications that are first-line therapies for the prevention and treatment of postmenopausal osteoporosis and include alendronate (Fosamax) and risedronate (Actonel). These drugs have been shown to increase spine and hip bone mineral density and decrease the risk of postmenopausal fracture. The patient should be instructed to take these drugs on an empty stomach in the morning and wait at least 30 minutes before eating or drinking. The patient must remain upright for 30 minutes after taking the medication. If heartburn or difficulty swallowing occurs, the patient should be instructed to stop the medication and seek medical attention.

Calcitonin can be used to decrease bone resorption in postmenopausal women. It can be used alone or in conjunction with hormone therapy. It is the drug of choice for women who cannot take HT, bisphosphonates, or raloxifene (Evista). The dose of calcitonin is 100 IU/day subcutaneously or 200 IU intranasally daily.

Bone mineral density can also be increased with teriparatide (Forteo, Parathar), which is an analog of parathyroid hormone. It is administered subcutaneously in 20 mg/day doses. A serious adverse effect is osteosarcoma when teriparatide is administered in high doses.

Vitamin D and calcium should be taken as supplements by most women. The recommendation is 1,200 to 1,600 mg of daily calcium and 400 to 1,000 IU of vitamin D to maintain bone health. The form of vitamin D should be ergocalciferol (vitamin D_2). Calcium supplements can be either calcium citrate or calcium carbonate. Some sources indicate that calcium citrate is better absorbed from the gastrointestinal tract.

Bioflavonoids are thought to have estrogenic activity. One study showed that grapefruit juice increased bioavailability of administered estradiol and estrone. Black cohosh, blue cohosh, ginseng, and wild yam have all demonstrated estrogenic effects. These compounds may result in endometrial hyperplasia, however, if unopposed with progesterone in patients with intact uteri.

Follow-up and Referral

When therapies recommended for the abatement of symptoms are followed without relief of symptoms, a referral to a gynecologist is recommended. Any patients with suspected abnormalities, especially carcinoma, should be referred to a gynecologist. Any perimenopausal or postmenopausal bleeding requires further evaluation with endometrial surveillance and biopsy to rule out endometrial hyperplasia or other pathology. Vaginal ultrasound may be used first, however, to avoid biopsy in women whose endometrial thickness is 4 mm or less. Estrogen-progestin therapy usually treats DUB, but intermittent ovulation may call for low-dose OCs as well. In smokers or women with contraindications to OCs (blood clots, breast or uterine cancer history) and no significant symptoms of estrogen deficiency, progestin therapy with medroxyprogesterone acetate 5 to 10 mg daily for 2 weeks a month can induce withdrawal bleeding and prevent endometrial hyperplasia. A depressed patient who does not respond to lifestyle changes and medications should be referred to a mental health specialist for counseling. Patients who are not responsive to therapy for insomnia may be referred to a sleep disorder clinic.

Patient Education

Pregnancy is still possible during perimenopause. When a patient presents with amenorrhea, it is important to perform a pregnancy test before assuming that the patient may be menopausal. Patients should be counseled about methods of birth control during this time so that undesired pregnancies do not occur.

The decision about the type of menopausal symptom treatment is made in conjunction with the patient. The following tests should be performed before a final decision to initiate therapy: Pap smear, blood chemistry, lipids, blood pressure, mammogram, endometrial biopsy in patients with breakthrough bleeding, and FSH and thyroid hormone levels.

Patients undergoing menopause may have deep feelings about what is happening. The clinician must assess and evaluate these feelings to understand better how to assist the patient. Studies show that fear, lack of knowledge about menopause, and the lack of an informed decision-making process are some of the factors leading to a woman's reluctance to seek treatment for menopausal symptoms. With much conflicting information in the media and among clinicians, patients may be especially interested in clarification of risks and benefits of all the treatments for menopausal symptom relief.

■ OVARIAN CANCER

Tumors of the ovary are common and most are benign. But malignant ovarian tumors are the leading cause of reproductive system death. *Ovarian cancer* has three main classifications: surface epithelial–stromal tumors, sex cord–stromal tumors, and germ cell tumors. The classifications are based on ovarian embryology and the differences in tissue origin.

Epidemiology and Causes

The cause of ovarian cancer is unknown. The risk factors for developing ovarian cancer include advancing age (more than half of the patients are older than 65 years of age); family history of a grandmother, mother, or sister with ovarian, breast, or colon cancer; father or brother with colon cancer (5%–10% are familial); nulliparity, early menarche, and late menopause ("incessant ovulation" increases possibility of ovarian epithelial damage and inactivation of tumor suppressor genes); lifestyle (high-fat diet, smoking history, lack of exercise); and a history of prolonged use of fertility drugs.

Ovarian cancer is quantitatively the rarest but most deadly of the gynecological cancers. In the United States, more than 25,000 cases of ovarian cancer are diagnosed annually, with approximately 14,500 deaths. It is the seventh most common woman's cancer in the world, with the greatest incidence in industrialized countries. It is most commonly diagnosed in white women with a northern European background and a strong family history. This familial predisposition may be strictly genetic or multifactorial, including environmental causes. The highest incidence occurs in the postmenopausal years, with a gradually rising incidence after age 45 years. Ovarian cancers have been associated with the number of ovulations in a woman's lifetime; therefore, nulliparity increases the number of ovulations and thereby the risk of a cell mutation occurring. Likewise, infertility drugs, which are known to hyperstimulate the ovaries, increase the chances of cancerous mutation.

Although the public is aware that early detection is crucial for cancer in general, no mass screening test has proved effective enough to be recommended at this time. For women who have risk factors for ovarian cancer, however, a pelvic exam, a cancer antigen 125 (CA-125) assay test, and a transvaginal pelvic ultrasound can be used at yearly intervals to increase the chance of early detection.

Pathophysiology

There are several distinct types of ovarian malignancies: epithelial cell, germ cell, and sex-cord stromal cell. By far the most common and life threatening are the malignancies of epithelial origin (80%–90% of ovarian tumors), which are derived from the epithelial layer of cells covering the surface of the ovary, continuous with the peritoneal mesothelium. These in turn are divided into several types, including papillary serous cystadenocarcinoma, which resembles the cells lining the fallopian tubes (75%); mucinous cystadenocarcinoma, which simulates the endocervical epithelium (10%); endometrioid tumors (10%), which are similar to endometrial cancers; and the much rarer clear cell, Brenner transitional cell, undifferentiated, and mixed cell–type tumors. Germ cell tumors comprise 20% to 25% of ovarian tumors, with fewer than 5% of these being malignant. Dysgerminomas are most common (30%–50%), followed by yolk sac (endodermal sinus) tumors and immature/mature teratomas—each of which accounts for approximately 20% of germ cell tumors. Much rarer forms of germ cell tumors include embryonal carcinoma, polyembryoma, choriocarcinoma, and carcinoid tumors.

Stromal cell tumors are less common, comprising only 5% to 8% of primary ovarian neoplasms. Neoplasms of stromal cells originate from the cells of the supporting structure of the ovary. These can be divided into gonadal support structures, which are the cells that support the ova or egg, and nongonadal stromal cells that are the nonspecialized support structures of the ovary. The gonadal cells are further divided into two specialized subgroups called the granulosa-theca and the

Sertoli-Leydig cells. Granulosa-theca cells surround the site on the ovary where the ovum is released and produce the female hormones. The second subgroup, the Sertoli-Leydig cells, is responsible for producing the male hormones. The nongonadal stromal cell tumors are derived from the smooth muscle and ligaments that give the ovary its basic structure and form.

Various germline mutations have been associated with epithelial ovarian tumors, such as *BRCA1*, *BRCA2*, and the hereditary nonpolyposis colorectal cancer gene, but only in a small minority of cases with serous ovarian adenocarcinomas predominating. These cancers, which appear to run in families, have an earlier age at onset than those in the general population. Mutations in well-characterized oncogenes including *HER-2/neu*, c-*myc*, *Akt*, and the tumor suppressor genes *p53*, *p16*, and *PTEN* have also been cited in noninherited forms of ovarian cancer. However, the precise pathogenetic mechanisms implicating these mutations, as well as most ovarian cancer risk factors, have yet to be determined.

A likely mechanism appears to be the increased frequency of genetic mutations associated with repeated injury and repair to the ovarian epithelium that occurs with cycled ovulation, thus explaining the correlation of ovarian cancer with nulliparity and early menses and the protective effect of oral contraceptives (OCs) that suppress ovulation. Hormonal stimulation of ovarian tissue by high estrogen and possibly also androgen levels has also been cited as a factor in malignant transformation, whereas progesterone has been shown to have protective effects. Interestingly, some case-controlled studies have demonstrated a connection between ovarian carcinogenesis and environmental agents believed to enter through the genitourinary tract that travel retrograde to the ovaries (e.g., perineal talc).

Clinical Presentation
Subjective

Symptoms can be vague or nonexistent in the early stages of the disease or seemingly unrelated to the ovaries. Such early symptoms include back pain, bloating, and constipation. As the tumor enlarges and the disease progresses, commonly expressed symptoms include a sense of pelvic pressure or discomfort; urinary frequency, pressure, and urgency; abdominal swelling and bloating; nausea and vomiting; gas and indigestion; rectal pressure; painful intercourse; diarrhea or constipation; abnormal vaginal bleeding; unexplained weight loss; and jaundice.

Objective

During the pelvic exam, a pelvic mass, decreased mobility of the cervix and uterus, fullness in the adnexal areas of cul-de-sac, and pain on palpation of the ovaries may be detected. A rectal exam may confirm a pelvic mass as well.

Diagnostic Reasoning
Diagnostic Tests

A comprehensive diagnostic work-up begins with a complete history and must include questions and discussions regarding the woman's current complaints, past health experiences, obstetric history, family history, and dietary habits. Further information that could be useful would be bowel and bladder habits and menstrual history.

If an ovarian neoplasm is suspected, a bimanual pelvic exam is the first step in the diagnostic work-up. Malignant ovarian tumors are usually large with irregular contour and decreased mobility, unlike benign tumors and cysts, which usually have smooth borders, are relatively small (less than 5 cm), and are mobile.

When a mass is palpated and suspicious of malignancy, subsequent diagnostic testing should include a pelvic ultrasound to evaluate the size, shape, and consistency of the mass. A serum CA-125 level is done. If the CA-125 is greater than 35 units, there is a greater likelihood that the ovarian mass is malignant, but the level may also be elevated in postmenopausal women with benign disease (e.g., endometriosis). CA-125, however, is most helpful for following the response to therapy and to help determine prognosis, but it is not an effective screening tool. A transvaginal ultrasound can help differentiate malignant ovarian masses from those that are benign. An intravenous pyelogram shows if the mass is impinging on the ureters or bladder. A barium enema determines involvement of the rectum or colon. In some cases a diagnostic laparoscopy can be used for direct visualization of the mass. Abdominal/pelvic computed tomography (CT) and magnetic resonance imaging are not useful to establish the diagnosis for pelvic masses, but these imaging tests are helpful in establishing the presence or degree of metastases from ovarian cancer or determining whether a primary cancer site exists outside the ovaries. A biopsy is not routinely recommended when an ovarian mass is present because this may cause the tumor cells to disseminate into the peritoneal cavity.

As part of a preoperative evaluation to further rule out other nonovarian primary cancer sites, a colonoscopy or barium enema should be done if the Hemoccult is positive or if the patient is obstructed. An upper gastrointestinal (GI) series is done if an upper GI site is suspected, bilateral mammography if any breast mass is present, and endometrial biopsy with curettage if uterine bleeding is present.

Differential Diagnosis

Differential diagnoses include ovarian cysts, benign tumors, ectopic pregnancy, hydrosalpinx, GI masses, pelvic kidney, endometriosis, tubo-ovarian abscess or adhesions, and intrauterine pregnancy. Other differentials include metastases to the ovaries from other primary sites, such as breast, uterus, or GI tract.

Management

The principle of management is early diagnosis and referral for treatment (surgery and oncological). Ovarian cancer is surgically staged, and the staging determines the specific treatment approach. Staging is done using the International Federation of Gynecology and Obstetrics (FIGO) staging, and this guides treatment. Stage I is confined to the ovaries. In stage II, there is extension to the pelvis, and stage III indicates spread beyond the pelvis to the peritoneal cavity or para-aortic/inguinal lymph nodes (but within the abdomen). Stage IV is distant metastasis. Seventy-five percent of women with epithelial disease present in stages III to IV, and 25% present in stages I and II. The 5-year survival rate for stage I ovarian cancer is 90%, but only 25% are diagnosed at this early stage. The 5-year survival rate declines rapidly as the stage increases. For example, 5-year survival for stage II is 40% to 60%, for stage III is 15% to 20%, and for stage IV is less than 5%.

Unlike other cancers, surgical resection for optimal cytoreduction is the standard of care for both early and advanced ovarian cancer. Therapy is based on appropriate surgical staging, unless there are clear contraindications to surgery. Surgery improves disease-related symptoms, improves response to chemotherapy (if cytoreduction leaves a tumor of less than 2 cm in the widest dimension), and decreases tumor-produced immunosuppressive cytokines. Surgical staging is done via laparotomy, checking for fluid in the cul-de-sac, as well as exploring the entire abdomen for disease. The para-aortic and pelvic lymph nodes are dissected as well, to look for microscopic extension into the nodes (stage III disease), which can occur in up to a third of cases that initially appear to be stage I.

Surgical removal usually includes hysterectomy and bilateral oophorectomy (because there is a large risk of contralateral disease) with appendectomy (which may be a site of isolated metastasis) and then additional resection of pelvic/abdominal structures as needed (especially the omentum). In very early stage disease, unilateral oophorectomy may be performed only if future fertility is desired, but endometrial biopsy should be done.

After surgical treatment, the patient is usually given a course of chemotherapy, with or without radiation. The amount and type of chemotherapy are based on the surgical finding and staging and subsequent pathological diagnosis and grading. Carboplatin plus paclitaxel is the standard of care for stage III to IV epithelial cancers. This same chemotherapy regimen may also be used for stage I to II epithelial cancers after surgery. It may suffice to just observe low-grade stage I disease after surgical resection, rather than treat with chemotherapy, as long as higher grade 2 or 3 disease is not noted. Chemotherapy

is started 4 to 6 weeks after surgery and continues for three to six cycles, depending on extent of disease and response to therapy (follow with physical exam/history, CA-125, imaging via CT scan, etc.). Most patients respond with first-line chemotherapy, but if recurrence occurs, chemotherapy may be used for palliative care. Patients with bulky residual disease survive a median of 26 months, whereas for those with small-volume residual disease, median survival is 60 months. Both maintenance chemotherapy (longer regimens of single or combination chemotherapeutic agents) and intraperitoneal (IP) chemotherapy are not current standards of care and are under investigation. IP chemotherapy has the advantage of direct contact with cancer cells, less systemic adverse effects, and less collateral damage to nonmalignant tissue. At present for stage III and IV disease, surgery followed by systemic chemotherapy is indicated, but a trial is currently ongoing to evaluate neoadjuvant (preoperative) chemotherapy. Currently, it is used for patients with poor performance status who would not tolerate surgery before treatment. Secondary cytoreduction after initial surgery and first-line systemic chemotherapy might be beneficial, however.

Diagnosis and treatment for ovarian cancer (and other gynecological cancers) is devastating. Several phenomenological studies have identified the themes of uncertainty, perceived lack of control, feelings of isolation, and hopelessness. These feelings can affect recovery and manifest in physical symptoms. Researchers at Yale University School of Nursing conducted a single-blind randomized clinical trial to determine if a specialized nursing intervention designed to help patients develop and maintain self-management skills and participate in decisions affecting their treatment would improve the quality of life (QOL) scores over those women who did not have the intervention. The women in the intervention group had less uncertainty, less symptom distress, and better scores on the QOL instrument than the control group (Level II; McCorkle et al, 2009).

Follow-up and Referral

When an adnexal mass is detected, the patient should be referred to a surgeon for prompt treatment. Patients who have been diagnosed with ovarian cancer and have undergone surgical and chemical treatment often are encouraged to have a second-look surgical procedure to assess the results of the prior treatments, both surgical and medical.

Patient Education

As mentioned previously, the number of ovulations in a patient's lifetime increases the risk of ovarian cancer; therefore, both pregnancy and use of OCs lower the risk of ovarian cancer. Patients should be aware of screening techniques, especially if they have any risk factors. Annual gynecological exams should be encouraged, and the importance of a low-fat diet and weight control should be stressed.

■ CERVICAL CANCER

Cervical intraepithelial neoplasia (CIN) has been explored and studied more than any other premalignant lesion of the genital tract. The accessible anatomical location of the upper vagina and cervix facilitates investigation. In addition, the development and use of colposcopy to identify sites of potential dysplasia and assist in directing biopsy have positively affected patient outcomes in the management of CIN. Several terms have been used to describe premalignant lesions of the cervix. These changes are described on a continuum from mildly atypical with a potential to progress to invasive carcinoma.

The grades of severity are CIN I (mild dysplasia), CIN II (moderate dysplasia), and CIN III (severe dysplasia to carcinoma in situ). Alternate nomenclature, as noted, is used to describe similar histological characteristics by using the term *dysplasia*. Hence, early premalignant changes in cervical epithelium are described as mild, moderate, or severe dysplasia. Mild involvement includes one-third of the cervical epithelium, moderate involvement includes two-thirds of the epithelium, and severe involvement includes the full thickness of the epithelium. Carcinoma in situ is considered the most advanced premalignant change.

Epidemiology and Causes

Cervical cancer is the 14th most common cancer in women in the United States and the most common cancer in women worldwide. With the prevalence of Papanicolaou (Pap) test screening in the United States, mortality rates have fallen by more than 45% since the 1970s. The American Cancer Society estimates that there will be 12,360 new cases of invasive cervical cancer and that more than 4,020 women will die of the disease in 2014. More than 20% of cases are found in women over age 65 years. Hispanic women in the United States have the highest incidence of cervical cancer followed by African American women. American Indians and Alaskan native women have the lowest risk.

Precancerous dysplasia, or CIN, occurs more often in younger women, with the incidence peaking in the early 30s. About 12% of women will have cervical dysplasia by age 20. However, the American College of Obstetricians and Gynecologists has issued new recommendations for cervical cancer screening. Screening should begin at age 21 years regardless of sexual history and is recommended every 2 years.

The cause of CIN remains unknown; however, studies implicate several factors that may be related to the development of CIN. In particular, the human papillomavirus (HPV) is believed to support the development of premalignant cervical lesions. Several different HPV types have been associated with various genital lesions. Three specific types have been associated with neoplasia

(higher grades of dysplasia and cervical cancer). Condom usage is promoted based more on general principles than on epidemiological data, and protection against HPV transmission is not 100% effective. HPV can be found in many genital areas (e.g., genital tract skin and mucous membranes). Hence, condoms do not protect the vulva from microscopic HPV particles on the skin. Although flat HPV cervical lesions are strongly associated with cellular transformation to CIN, most HPV infections are subclinical. Women may be unaware of their HPV status. In addition, women who have a history of early intercourse (age 14 or 15 years), begin to have children at an early age, and/or have a history of multiple sexual partners are at a greater risk for developing carcinoma of the cervix. A list of cofactors that may contribute to enhanced risk for cervical cancer is shown in Risk Factors 14.2.

Pathophysiology

A normal transformation zone includes columnar epithelium and squamous metaplasia. The squamocolumnar junction (SCJ) of the cervix is viewed via the colposcope, which magnifies the epithelium of the transformation zone. Colposcopic examination of this landmark site is important because this area is most vulnerable to neoplastic changes.

Risk Factors 14.2 Cervical Neoplasia

History

- Early intercourse
- Early marriage
- Multiple sex partners (more than two)
- Early childbearing
- Prostitution
- Immunosuppression
- Prior exposure to radiation
- Intrauterine DES exposure
- OC use
- Cigarette smoking
- Vitamin A, B, C, and folic acid deficiencies

Male Partner

- History of genital cancer, especially penile carcinoma; STIs, especially penile or urethral condylomas; CIN or cervical cancer in a previous partner; low socioeconomic status; multiple sex partners

Infections

- STIs (venereal infection)
- HPV infection (serotypes 16 and 18)
- HSV infection
- HIV infection
- *Chlamydia trachomatis*
- Cytomegalovirus infection

Examination of the exocervix reveals where the cervical glandular, grape-like in appearance, columnar epithelium meets the native squamous epithelium distal to the external os in young adult women. After childbirth this area may enlarge and move farther away from the os. The junction usually recedes after menopause into the endocervical canal. Throughout a woman's reproductive life, squamous metaplasia, a physiological process involving squamous tissue replacing columnar tissue, occurs. This process is most active during fetal development, adolescence, and pregnancy. The SCJ is first delineated in utero; however, metaplasia is an estrogen-dependent process that accelerates during puberty and pregnancy. As noted, SCJ cells are more vulnerable and especially prone to damage at these particular times in a woman's reproductive life. Abnormal colposcopic patterns that characterize an abnormal transformation zone are caused by neoplastic squamous epithelium, thus explaining why exophytic tumors are the most common presentation of cervical cancer.

HPV infection may also alter morphology of the cervical epithelium, leading to nuclear enlargement and multinucleation, hyperchromasia, and perinuclear cytoplasmic halos. Cellular findings of HPV infection on biopsy can be histologically similar to dysplasia, and misdiagnosis can occur. However, the diagnosis of HPV does not imply clinical disease. Thus, treatment is limited only to symptomatic patients (e.g., those with condylomas) or those with demonstrated evidence of neoplasia (e.g., positive colposcopy findings). There are two vaccines (Cervarix and Gardasil) for HPV infection prevention. Both of the vaccines protect against cervical cancer in women, but Gardasil also protects against genital warts and cancer of the anus, vagina, and vulva that are associated with HPV infection. Females should be vaccinated at age 11 but can be vaccinated up to age 26 years. Males should be vaccinated at age 11 but can be vaccinated through age 21 years. In some worldwide studies, the epitheliotropic HPV infection has been identified in greater than 99% of cervical neoplasias. Certain viral serotypes that undergo vegetative episomal replication without integrating into the host genome typically lead to condylomata acuminata or low-grade squamous intraepithelial lesion (LSIL; see discussion later in this section) (e.g., HPV-6, HPV-11), whereas more oncogenic forms of the virus (HPV-16, HPV-18, HPV-58, HPV-52, and HPV-31) that integrate into host DNA are more likely to contribute to malignant transformation—high-grade squamous intraepithelial lesion (HSIL; see discussion later in this section), invasive squamous cell carcinoma, or adenocarcinoma. The HPV E6 protein degrades the cell cycle inhibitory protein p53, and the HPV E7 protein interacts with the retinoblastoma protein Rb, causing dissociation of E2F, which also leads to dysregulated cell cycle progression. E7 protein also leads to upregulation of interleukin-6 (IL-6) and IL-8, both of which contribute to cervical

cancer progression. Importantly, HPV serotypes HPV-16 and HPV-18 most strongly correlate with invasive squamous cell carcinoma, with HPV-18 portending a worse prognosis. It is clear, however, that HPV infection alone is insufficient to lead to cervical neoplasia, and further insult by cigarette smoking, immunosuppression, or other risk factors appears necessary.

Although squamous cell carcinoma comprises 80% of all cervical cancers, at least 15% are attributed to adenocarcinomas, with another 3% to 5% being of a mixed adenosquamous phenotype. The incidence of adenocarcinoma of the cervix has steadily increased in women younger than 35 years since the 1970s, but this may be due to improved screening and early treatment of squamous cell disease. In addition, however, a greater association of adenocarcinoma with oral contraceptive use seems to imply the importance of underlying hormonal mechanisms in its pathogenesis. Far rarer forms include neuroendocrine tumors, small cell carcinomas, or rhabdomyosarcomas.

Clinical Presentation

Subjective

Patients with premalignant cervical lesions may present with one or more of the following: a history of one or more epidemiological risk factors associated with the development of cervical cancer; a concurrent vaginal infection with symptoms; a history of no recent gynecological care; and no Pap smear for a long time.

In contrast, women with invasive carcinoma may describe a brownish discharge or a history of abnormal vaginal bleeding occurring spontaneously or after intercourse. Women with a history of postcoital bleeding or irregular vaginal bleeding that cannot be explained should be referred to a gynecologist for further evaluation. Only with an extensive disease spread would other symptoms be manifested (e.g., weight loss, decreased appetite, and back pain).

Objective

Women with abnormal Pap smears are usually asymptomatic with normal cervical, vaginal, and abdominal findings on physical exam. Even if Pap smear findings are normal, any cervical or vaginal lesion that appears abnormal or is friable, is raised, or has the appearance of condyloma requires a referral for colposcopy. The location of the dysplasia directs the treatment.

The Pap smear report should include a statement on the adequacy of the specimen for examination, a general categorization, and the descriptive diagnosis. Pap smear results are described as follows:

- Satisfactory but limited (less than optimal; may be secondary to partially obscuring inflammation)
- Unsatisfactory (not acceptable for diagnostic evaluation and may require a repeat Pap or follow-up)
- Within normal limits

- Other (may require follow-up care; the report will have an additional notation if further action is required)

Protocol for triage of the patient with abnormal cytology is presented in Advanced Practice Nursing Interventions 14.1.

Diagnostic Reasoning

Diagnostic Tests

The American Cancer Society's (ACS's) Pap smear screening guidelines are supported by the American Medical Association, National Cancer Institute, American Nurses Association, American College of Obstetricians and Gynecologists, and American Academy of Family

Physicians. An issue that is the subject of ongoing debate concerns the mandated frequency for performing Pap smears. The ACS recommends that screening begin 3 years after the first vaginal intercourse or at age 21 years, whichever comes first. It also recommends that women older than age 30 be screened at longer intervals after three consecutive annual normal/negative Pap smear results, unless the woman has a history of diethylstilbestrol exposure in utero, is HIV positive, or is immunocompromised (organ transplant, chemotherapy, corticosteroid therapy). The ACS also recommends that screening be discontinued in women older than age 70 if they have had no abnormal Pap smears in the previous 10 years. If women have had a hysterectomy with removal of the cervix, they do not

Advanced Practice Nursing Interventions 14.1   Pap Smear Results: Treatment Protocols

Pap Smear Results	The Bethesda System (TBS) Category	Treatment Protocol
Sufficient number of cells were present to determine normalcy: Within normal limits.	Within normal limits	Repeat Pap test annually.
Sample was not prepared correctly or too few cells to be evaluated: Inadequate.	Less than optimal Unsatisfactory	Repeat Pap test in about 8 weeks.
Benign cellular change; may be caused by infectious agent such as *Trichomonas*, fungal organisms, *Gardnerella* and *Chlamydia*, or HSV.	Infection	Treat infections that present as symptoms or identified with Pap smear results, or do confirmatory study. Repeat Pap test after infection in 3–6 months; repeat annually if results are normal.
Benign cellular change secondary to inflammatory process and repair by body of injured tissue; may be caused by mechanical or chemical irritations (inflammation, atrophy, IUD use), trauma, or bacterial or viral infections.	Reactive/reparative	For inflammatory changes of unknown cause, repeat Pap test in 6–12 weeks. For repeated inflammatory changes on Pap test, refer to possible colposcopic examination. For Chlamydia or gonorrhea, treat as recommended and repeat Pap test in 1 year. For postmenopausal women with atrophic vaginitis and Pap test result of ASCUS or low-grade squamous intraepithelial lesion (LSIL), treat with topical estrogen cream for 4–6 weeks, then repeat Pap test.
Cellular changes from HPV or mild to moderate dysplasia.	Squamous epithelial cell abnormalities: Atypical squamous cells of undetermined significance (ASCUS) Squamous intraepithelial lesion: LSIL or high-grade squamous intraepithelial lesion (HSIL)	Refer for colposcopic examination.

Advanced Practice Nursing Interventions 14.1   Pap Smear Results: Treatment Protocols—cont'd

Pap Smear Results	The Bethesda System (TBS) Category	Treatment Protocol
Cellular changes from high-grade or squamous cell carcinoma.	Squamous cell carcinoma Adenocarcinoma	Refer to gynecologist.
Glandular cell findings–atypical glandular cells (AGC); considered less severe than adenocarcinoma but associated with a greater risk for cancer.	AGC	Refer to gynecologist.
Atypical glandular cells from endocervical, endometrial, or glandular not otherwise specified in origin (AGC-NOS); considered at lower risk for neoplasm than AGC women.	AGC–NOS	Refer to gynecologist.
Atypical glandular cells—favor neoplasm (AGC, favor neoplasm); high risk for high-grade CIN.	AGC–favor neoplasia	Refer to gynecologist.
Endocervical adenocarcinoma in situ (AIS); high risk for invasive cervical adenocarcinoma.	AIS	Refer to gynecologist.

need to be screened if the reason for the surgery was for a condition other than cancer or precancer.

It is important that the cytology laboratory comply with state and national regulations, utilize a sufficient number of reputable cytologists, maintain a quality assurance program, and support open, clear communication between health-care professionals and the laboratory.

Historically, several reporting systems have been developed to enhance communication between the cytopathologist and the clinician performing the Pap test. The oldest system was the class system that provided limited information and did not reflect the newer risk factors such as HPV infections. See Therapeutic Procedure 14.1 for specific techniques for obtaining a Pap smear.

Therapeutic Procedure 14.1   Pap Smear and Liquid-Based Cervical Cell Collection

Technique for Obtaining a Routine Pap Smear

1. Complete the cytology request form with all pertinent data.
2. Label the slide.
3. Insert the dry or water-lubricated speculum. Direct the speculum in a downward posterior direction.
4. Expose the cervix.
   - Avoid sampling if a vaginal infection is present.
   - Take the Pap smear sample before any other cervical sample.
5. Insert the cytobrush or cotton-tipped applicator in cervical os.
6. Use a vigorous rotary endocervical technique (clockwise fashion).
7. Use a paintbrush motion to place the sample on the glass slide.
8. Scrape the external os area with the cytology spatula.
9. Note the individual topography of the squamocolumnar juncture.
10. Obtain a vaginal specimen if needed (e.g., DES exposure, hormone evaluation, history of hysterectomy).
11. Smear the slide and fix immediately.

Technique for Obtaining a Liquid-Based Cervical Cell Collection

1. Complete the cytology request form with all pertinent data.
2. Label the container.
3. Insert the dry or water-lubricated speculum. Direct the speculum in a downward posterior direction.
4. Expose the cervix.
5. Insert cervical broom with central portion into the cervical os.
6. Rotate one-quarter turn only.
7. Place broom in fixative container and vigorously move about to dispel all particles into solution.

The Bethesda System (TBS) currently uses only two terms to describe the wide spectrum of squamous cell precursors: *low-grade squamous intraepithelial lesion* (LSIL) and *high-grade squamous intraepithelial lesion* (HSIL). TBS has also established a category called *atypical squamous cells* (ASC) and this is further qualified into two categories: *atypical squamous cells of undetermined significance* (ASC-US) and *atypical squamous cells; cannot exclude high-grade SIL* (ASC-H). TBS has also developed a classification for *atypical glandular cells* (AGC) that may be endocervical, endometrial, or glandular cells. There is *atypical glandular cells not otherwise specified* in origin (AGC-NOS), and these women are at lower risk for neoplasia than women with AGC. If the Pap smear shows AGC, this favors neoplasia. More worrisome is endocervical adenocarcinoma in situ (AIS) or true adenocarcinoma. These glandular findings are associated with a high rate of premalignancy, or true neoplasia, and thus these women should be referred for colposcopy; women older than 35 years of age and those with significant anovulatory unexplained bleeding should also get endometrial biopsy. If all cells are endometrial in origin only, colposcopy may be avoided in favor of initial endometrial biopsy.

LSIL is a combination of cytological changes consistent with HPV without evidence of dysplasia and changes consistent with mild dysplasia (CIN I). ASC-US is delimited to epithelial abnormalities of uncertain significance and usually represents about 5% of the smears in most populations screened. When cells are described as atypical, further evaluation is necessary.

(Table 14.8 presents a comparison of cytopathology reporting systems.)

Obtaining endocervical cells becomes more difficult as the patient ages and the SCJ migrates inwardly with age. An optimal smear contains squamous cells, endocervical cells, and potentially metaplastic cells. Absence of endocervical cells may indicate an inadequate sample and needs to be repeated. Table 14.9 presents factors affecting Pap smear results.

■ VULVOVAGINAL INFECTIONS AND SEXUALLY TRANSMITTED INFECTIONS

Several different sexually transmitted infections (STIs) affect the female reproductive tract and genitalia. STIs are transmitted through sexual intercourse between heterosexual or homosexual persons by intimate contact with the genitalia, mouth, or anus. STIs, called venereal diseases in the past, include infection by herpes simplex virus (HSV), *Chlamydia trachomatis, Neisseria gonorrhoeae, Treponema pallidum* (syphilis), human papillomavirus (HPV), trichomonads, and human immunodeficiency virus (HIV). Other vulvar lesions include chancroid, lymphogranuloma venereum (LGV), granuloma inguinale, and molluscum contagiosum lesions. Cervical infection known as mucopurulent cervicitis is also largely caused by community-acquired sexually transmitted agents, namely *C trachomatis* and *N gonorrhoeae.*

In contrast, vulvovaginal infections affecting the female genitalia that are not officially considered STIs include both vulvar disorders and selected vaginal and

Table 14.8   Comparison of Cytology Reporting Systems for Pap Smears

Class System	World Health Organization (WHO) System	Cervical Intraepithelial Neoplasia (CIN) System	The Bethesda System (TBS)
I	Normal	Normal	Within normal limits
II	Inflammation	Normal	Other: Infection, reactive and reparative
III	Dysplasia		Squamous epithelial cell abnormalities Atypical squamous cells of undetermined significance Squamous intraepithelial lesion Low grade (includes cellular changes associated with HPV)
	Mild	CIN-1	
	Moderate	CIN-2	High grade
	Severe		High grade
IV	Carcinoma in situ	CIN-3	High grade
V	Invasive squamous cell carcinoma Adenocarcinoma	Invasive squamous cell carcinoma Adenocarcinoma	Squamous cell carcinoma Adenocarcinoma Nonepithelial malignant neoplasma

Table 14.9 Factors Affecting Pap Smear Results

Patient History
- Previous treatment and/or surgery of reproductive tract
- Previous abnormal Pap test
- Diethylstilbestrol (DES) exposure in utero
- Current or recent vaginal or cervical infection and PID
- Any medications, especially hormones
- Bleeding abnormalities
- History of any malignancy
- Pregnancy suspected or current
- Partner history of genital or urological problems (e.g., discharge, infection, or bumps on penis or scrotum)

Patient Factors
- Intercourse
- Douching
- Birth control methods
- Menses
- Infection
- Accurate history

False-Negatives
- Rate for properly performed cytology smears is 1%–80%
- Rate of sample error (diagnostic cells not on the slide) is 60%; 40% for screening error (cells present on slide but missed by cytotechnologist)
- False or less than optimal reports are caused by clinician, patient, or cytopathologist factors

False-Positives
- Rate is <1%.

cervical infections. Painful vaginal disorders (vulvodynia) go by several names, including vulvar pain syndrome, chronic vulvar pain, vestibulitis, focal vulvitis, vestibular adenitis, and burning vulva syndrome. These may be caused by candidiasis (yeast infection), bacterial vaginosis (BV), atrophic vaginitis, allergic vaginitis, and irritation from foreign bodies or chemicals found in soaps, shampoos, or lotions.

Epidemiology and Causes

STIs are the most prevalent communicable diseases in the United States, with the exception of upper respiratory infections. STIs affect more than 12 million patients annually in the United States alone, with 25% being adolescents. Although STIs disproportionately affect adolescents and young adults (largely because of increased sexual encounters and risk-taking behaviors), no age-group is considered "safe." It is estimated that approximately one American out of five is infected with a viral STI other than HIV. Perhaps even more alarming is that the United States has the highest STI rates in the world despite being one of the most educated populations in the world and having the highest standard of living.

The causative agents of the most common vulvovaginal infections and STIs, as well as the clinical presentation, diagnostic reasoning, and recommended management, are presented in Table 14.10. Inadequately treated STIs have far-reaching implications for future health, including long-term fertility. Mucopurulent cervicitis may extend retrograde through the uterus and out the fallopian tubes to the ovaries and throughout the pelvic cavity, causing widespread inflammation, scarring, and adhesions. Known as pelvic inflammatory disease (PID), this condition may occur in up to 15% of mucopurulent cervicitis cases, requiring hospitalization and IV antibiotics in its most serious form and leading to obstruction anywhere along the reproductive tract. PID is the most common cause of tubal infertility (see section on infertility earlier in this chapter). Untreated syphilis may lead to a tertiary form of infection with serious central nervous system (CNS) insult (general paresis and dorsal motor column defects known as tabes dorsalis); aortitis; and nodular, granulomatous lesions on the skin, bone, and solid organs known as gummas. Untreated HIV infection progresses to clinical AIDS over 2 to 10 years, destroying the immune system and leading to increasing numbers of opportunistic infections of the lungs, genitourinary tract, and CNS, which eventually prove fatal. Even BV has been shown to be a risk factor in pregnant women for preterm delivery of low-birth-weight infants.

Pathophysiology

The female reproductive tract is normally protected from infection by several mechanisms, including a low, acidic pH resulting from vaginal secretions and the presence of commensal, nonpathogenic microbial flora, namely hydrogen peroxide–producing *Lactobacillus*. The normal flora environmentally compete and protect against the overgrowth of potentially pathogenic anaerobic and gram-negative bacteria. Disruptions of the mucosal surface either by trauma or preexistent infectious lesion predispose the reproductive tract to infection. In addition, although BV is not considered sexually transmitted (because it is caused by overgrowth of pathogenic vaginal flora), vaginal intercourse may raise intravaginal pH and predispose the woman to the development of BV. Ascending cervical infections, as seen in PID, also appear to be more common in the week following menses, possibly owing to the absence of endometrial sloughing mechanisms that protect against retrograde infection.

Although the pathogenesis of some vulvar and vaginal pain syndromes has not been fully elucidated, STIs are known to stem from a heterogeneous collection of causative infectious agents (see Table 14.10). However, the unifying principle of these disorders is their propensity for spread by intimate person-to-person sexual contact, particularly after exposure of the mucous membranes to infected bodily fluids. This typically occurs within the genitalia. However, the oral and anal mucosa are also

(Text continued on page 751)

Table 14.10 Vulvovaginal Infections and Sexually Transmitted Diseases

Problem	Clinical Presentation	Diagnostic Reasoning	Treatment: as Recommended by CDC
Vulvar Lesions • Chancroid (*Haemophilus ducreyi*)	Single painful ulcer (irregular, erythematous, and undermined edges) with a unilateral bubo If vaginal lesion, may be asymptomatic Painful lymphadenopathy	Risk factors: coinfection with HIV, HSV, and syphilis	azithromycin (Zithromax) 1 g PO × 1 OR ceftriaxone (Rocephin) 250 mg IM × 1 OR ciprofloxacin (Cipro) 500 mg PO 2 times daily for 3 days OR erythromycin (E-mycin) 500 mg PO 4 times daily for 7 days
• Lymphogranuloma venereum (LGV) (*Chlamydia trachomatis*)	Lymphadenopathy, anorectal swelling, and fistula formation	History of travel and sexual contact in endemically infected area Serological LGV complement fixation test; suspect if titer above 1:16; diagnostic if above 1:64	doxycycline (Vibramycin) 100 mg PO 2 times daily for 21 days OR erythromycin (E-mycin) 500 mg PO 4 times daily for 21 days OR azithromycin (Zithromax) 1 gram per week for 3 weeks; no recommended dosage from CDC
• Granuloma inguinale (granuloma venereum, Donovanosis) (*Klebsiella granulomatis*)	Chronic, progressive papule that ulcerates to a beefy red, painless granular area with clean, sharp rolled edges; inguinal swelling; late painful abscesses (buboes)	History of travel and sexual contact in endemically infected area Cannot be cultured; stained tissue sample may show Donovan bodies	doxycycline (Vibramycin) 100 mg PO 2 times daily for 3 weeks OR azithromycin 1 g PO once a week for 3 weeks OR trimethoprim 160 mg plus sulfamethoxazole 800 mg (Bactrim) 1 tablet PO 2 times daily for 3 weeks OR erythromycin (E-mycin) 500 mg PO 2 times daily for 4 weeks (during pregnancy) OR ciprofloxacin 750 mg PO 2 times daily for at least 3 weeks
• Molluscum contagiosum (large DNA virus from the Poxviridae family)	Pearly, raised, painless lesions with umbilicated center; diffuse or singular; may be self-limiting	Based on characteristic lesions	No treatment. Lesions may last months to years and often heal spontaneously. Once healed, the person has a lifetime immunity to the virus.
Vaginal Disorders • Vulvodynia	Burning and itching of vulva; tenderness at vaginal opening; dry and swollen vulva; associated with inflamed and painful	Diagnosis of elimination Changes in touch test Vulvar biopsy for inflammation	Treat symptomatically Mild pain: Topical lidocaine (Xylocaine) Antidepressants such as amitriptyline (Elavil) 50–100 mg

Table 14.10 Vulvovaginal Infections and Sexually Transmitted Diseases—cont'd

Problem	Clinical Presentation	Diagnostic Reasoning	Treatment: as Recommended by CDC
	Bartholin's, vestibular, and Skene's glands	Colposcopy for microfissures	PO at bedtime or fluoxetine (Prozac) 20 mg PO every morning or 20 mg PO every morning and noon Surgery (50% success rate)
• Candidiasis	Pruritus, redness, swelling, "curdy" (white, thick) vaginal discharge; occasional burning with urination, vaginal wall redness	Risk factors: previous antibiotic therapy, chronic vulva moisture, diabetes, HIV infection, immunosuppression Wet prep with saline, KOH, pH 4–5	fluconazole (Diflucan) 150 mg PO × 1 OR butoconazole 2% cream 5 g intravaginally at bedtime × 3 days OR miconazole 2% cream 5 g intravaginally at bedtime × 7 days OR clotrimazole 1% cream 5 g intravaginally for 7–14 days OR clotrimazole 100 mg vaginal tablet for 7 days OR tioconazole 6.5% ointment 5 g intravaginally in a single application OR terconazole 0.4% cream 5 g intravaginally for 7 days OR terconazole 0.8% cream 5 g intravaginally for 3 days
• Bacterial vaginosis (BV)	Thin discharge, malodorous, increased odor after intercourse, pruritus, edema, erythema	Based on symptoms, including homogenous white discharge with "fishy" odor, pH >4.5, clue cells on microscopic exam and a positive amine test (KOH applied to discharge releases fishy odor—"whiff" test)	metronidazole 500 mg PO 2 times daily × 7 days OR metronidazole gel 0.75% one full applicator (5 g) intravaginally daily × 5 days OR clindamycin cream 2% one full applicator (5 g) intravaginally at bedtime × 7 days
• Atrophic vaginitis	Dry, thin vaginal tissue; dyspareunia	History of perimenopause or menopause, pH 6.5–7, wet prep: negative for pathogens	Treat symptoms Vaginal lubricants Estradiol vaginal ring—50–100 mcg/24 hr; change every 3 months Estrogen vaginal cream—0.625 mg/g: Insert 0.5–2 g into the vagina once daily at night for 1–2 weeks. After initial therapy, use of 1–2 g of the cream twice a week will prevent recurrence.

Continued

Table 14.10 Vulvovaginal Infections and Sexually Transmitted Diseases—cont'd

Problem	Clinical Presentation	Diagnostic Reasoning	Treatment: as Recommended by CDC
• Allergic vaginitis	Excessive or malodorous vaginal discharge, pruritus, external dysuria	Obtain accurate history, pH normal (3.8–4.2)	Avoid offending substance Sitz baths Hormone-free vaginal creams and gels to restore vaginal pH and increase vaginal moisture
Cervical Disorders • Mucopurulent cervicitis (MPC)	Yellow mucous discharge, possible bleeding with intercourse, cervical tenderness, "beefy red" friable cervix	Wet prep: increase in WBCs	azithromycin (Zithromax) 1 g PO × 1 OR doxycycline (Vibramycin) 100 mg PO 2 times daily for 7 days OR erythromycin (E-mycin) 500 mg PO 4 times daily for 7 days OR erythromycin ethylsuccinate (EES) 800 mg PO 4 times daily for 7 days OR ofloxacin (Floxin) 300 mg PO 2 times daily for 7 days OR levofloxacin 500 mg PO daily for 7 days
STIs • HSV Infection	**First outbreak:** Flu-like symptoms with adenopathy, tingling of the site before outbreak, and very painful vesicular lesions Ulcers form with circumscribed erythematous edges and white exudate centrally; may last 12 days **Recurrent outbreaks:** Symptoms may be similar, usually less severe and shorter length (4–5 days)	Viral culture of vesicle fluid most accurate if within 48 hours of outbreak Tzanck smear from the base of an early vesicle DNA probe from lesion scraping	**First outbreak:** acyclovir (Zovirax) 400 mg PO 3 times daily for 7–10 days OR 200 mg PO 5 times a day for 7–10 days OR famciclovir (Famvir) 250 mg PO 3 times daily for 7–10 days OR valacyclovir (Valtrex) 1 g PO 2 times daily for 7–10 days. **Recurrent outbreaks:** famciclovir: 125 mg every 12 hours for 5 days OR famciclovir 1,000 mg PO 2 times daily ×1 day valacyclovir: 500 mg PO every 12 hours for 3 days OR valacyclovir 1 g PO daily for 5 days **Suppressive:** acyclovir 400 mg PO 2 times daily famciclovir 250 mg PO 2 times daily

Table 14.10   Vulvovaginal Infections and Sexually Transmitted Diseases—cont'd

Problem	Clinical Presentation	Diagnostic Reasoning	Treatment: as Recommended by CDC
			valacyclovir 1 g PO daily Evaluate after 1 year for recurrent episodes.
• *Chlamydia*	Most commonly no reported symptoms. Patient may have an increase in mucopurulent discharge and bleeding with intercourse.	Yellow mucopurulent discharge on cervix Cervix friable and inflamed May or may not have cervical motion tenderness Wet mount: >10 WBCs per high-power field (hpf) DNA probe (cervical swab)	azithromycin (Zithromax) 1 g PO × 1 OR doxycycline (Vibramycin) 100 mg PO 2 times daily for 7 days OR erythromycin base (E-mycin) 500 mg PO 4 times daily for 7 days OR ofloxacin (Floxin) 300 mg PO 2 times daily for 7 days
• *Syphilis*	Primary: Painless ulcer at initial site of contact (chancre), adenopathy Secondary: Maculopapular rash on palms and soles, condylomata/moist flat wartlike lesions, adenopathy Tertiary/late: Cardiac, neurological, ophthalmic, auditory, and gummatous lesions	Dark-field microscopy: positive for spirochetes Direct microhemagglutination–*Treponema pallidum* (MHA-TP): Antibody test Fluorescent treponemal antibody absorption (FTA-ABS): antibody test reported as positive Venereal Disease Research Laboratory (VDRL), syphilis test, rapid plasma reagin (RPR): with titer indicating degree of infection	**Early (less than 1 year duration):** benzathine penicillin G 2.4 million units IM × 1 OR doxycycline 100 mg 2 times daily for 14 days **Latent or late (duration longer than 1 year or unknown length):** benzathine penicillin G 2.4 million units IM once a week for 3 weeks **Neurosyphilis (CSF) (infection confirmed):** aqueous crystalline penicillin G 3–4 million units IV every 4 hours for 10–14 days Penicillin-allergic patients: doxycycline 100 mg PO 2 times daily for 2 weeks OR tetracycline 500 mg PO 4 times daily for 2 weeks
• *Gonorrhea*	Usually asymptomatic; partner may have an infection Purulent yellow/green discharge May have Skene's and Bartholin's gland inflammation	Gonococcal culture, DNA probe (cervical swab)	ceftriaxone (Rocephin) 250 mg IM × 1 OR cefixime (Suprax) 400 mg PO × 1 PLUS azithromycin (Zithromax) 1 g PO × 1 OR

Continued

Table 14.10   Vulvovaginal Infections and Sexually Transmitted Diseases—cont'd

Problem	Clinical Presentation	Diagnostic Reasoning	Treatment: as Recommended by CDC
			doxycycline 100 mg PO 2 times daily for 7 days Follow CDC guidelines for complicated or refractory gonorrhea.
• HPV	History of multiple partners or sexual abuse Positive history of HPV Itching, foul discharge May be asymptomatic Fleshy, soft, pale-colored keratinized growths on the vagina, cervix, vulva, or perianal area	Acetic acid test: Lesions turn white with vinegar application.	**Patient-applied treatments:** podofilox (Condylox) 0.5% applied thinly 2 times daily for 3 days, then rest for 4 days; may repeat up to 4 cycles OR imiquimod (Aldara cream) 5% applied 3 times a week for up to 16 weeks. **Clinician-applied treatments:** Cryotherapy and liquid nitrogen treatments—repeat every 1–2 weeks. podophyllin resin (Podofin) 10%–25% in benzoin—apply thinly, allow to dry; patient should wash off in 1–4 hours. TCA/BCA (trichloroacetic acid and bichloracetic acid, Tri-Chlor) 80%–90% applied by clinician every 4–7 days. Other therapies: Laser therapy, surgery, interferon lesion injections.
• *Trichomoniasis*	Heavy, odorous, yellow-green watery discharge May have complaints of itching, swelling, and redness on the vulva	Discharge may be frothy, with occasional characteristic "strawberry cervix" pH >5 Wet mount: motile protozoa and WBCs	metronidazole (Flagyl) 2 g PO ×1 OR metronidazole 500 mg PO 2 times daily for 7 days if pregnant OR clindamycin 300 mg PO 2 times daily for 7 days
• HIV infection	Fever, malaise, adenopathy, rash may occur in first weeks after infection (acute retroviral syndrome) Bloody diarrhea Opportunistic infections Frequent vaginal infections Increased HPV infections	Positive enzyme immunoassay Positive Western blot	Treat infections as recommended by CDC. Refer to specialist. Offer long-term counseling and management. Highly active antiretroviral therapy (HAART) is key for the treatment of HIV. Initiation of therapy is a function of T-cell count, viral load, and concurrent symptoms. Treatment is heavily influenced by the ability to comply with various treatment regimens.

susceptible entry points, as exemplified by the incidence of gonococcal pharyngitis after receptive oral intercourse.

Given the length of the vaginal canal and the relatively larger area of exposed genital mucosa, women appear to be more susceptible to STIs. They are also more likely to display symptoms of infection. The presence of one STI increases the chances of becoming infected with another—especially HIV. This is likely due to compromise of mucosal and outer skin barriers, as well as interactions on the molecular level, for example, HPV as a cofactor for HIV infection. Infectious organisms themselves may also express various genetic virulence factors that render them more susceptible to sexual transmission, including surface proteins that facilitate epithelial adherence to the vaginal or cervical mucosa.

Clinical Presentation

Subjective

The patient with a vulvar lesion may present with a complaint of a painful lymph node. With vaginal disorders, the patient typically complains of burning and itching of the vulva, along with tenderness at the vaginal opening. Usually there is a long-standing history of complaints with little or no response to treatment. There is increased pain with tight clothing such as jeans and panty hose, sitting, and external pressure. The discomfort can be so great that it interferes with or stops intercourse. Patients frequently describe "shards of glass" or "pins and needles" on the vulva and at the introitus and may complain of vulvar soreness for days after intercourse.

From 60% to 80% of STIs are asymptomatic; therefore, most are detected on routine exam. Other patients present with burning, itching, and a vaginal discharge that may range from clear to yellowish-green. Table 14.10 presents specific symptoms.

Objective

The primary lesions of some STIs may be painless and blisterlike, or the patient may have severe pain. All lesions of an ulcerative or wartlike nature should be serologically tested for syphilis. Any ulcer may become secondarily infected and may confuse the diagnosis. Manifestation of vaginal infections may include a slightly dry and swollen vulva with small splits present. There may be chronic inflammation, with possible glandular involvement. Bartholin's, vestibular, and Skene's glands may be inflamed and painful, with reddened areas. Scarring and muscle contracture may be present.

Diagnostic Reasoning

Diagnostic Tests

Diagnostic testing for some vulvovaginal infections is not available; therefore, the diagnosis is made by exclusion. Diagnosis of vaginal infections is made by eliminating other diseases as the cause and homing in on the patient's symptoms. Frequently there will be a history of treatment

for chronic yeast infections. Table 14.10 presents specific diagnostic tests.

If initial treatment is ineffective, an incorrect diagnosis may have been made initially. The vaginal exam should be repeated and any tests repeated to confirm the diagnosis. For vulvodynia, vulvar biopsy for inflammation, colposcopy for microfissures, and assessing for uneven hips caused by muscle contraction may confirm the diagnosis. Vulvodynia is not sexually transmitted, nor is it a condyloma. External events or irritants can trigger vulvodynia, so a comprehensive history should be obtained.

Differential Diagnosis

Differential diagnosis should include evaluation for chronic dermatitis, bacterial vaginosis, precancerous changes of the vulva, urinary tract infection (UTI), and vaginitis, along with assessing for any STI. The patient should be evaluated for allergies, urinary calcium oxalate, and increased sensitivity to touch, which may indicate a vaginal infection.

Management

The principle of management is to make the correct diagnosis, prescribe the correct treatment, and sufficiently educate the patient and partner so that there will not be a repeat occurrence. In response to the progressive rise in incidence of STIs, the Centers for Disease Control and Prevention (CDC, 2010) published treatment guidelines for sexually transmitted infections, which include information on prevention, diagnosis, and treatment for all known STIs. Table 14.10 presents the specific management of vulvovaginal infections and STIs.

All of the patient's sexual contacts from the 10 days before the onset of symptoms (30 days for STIs) should be treated. A recheck of symptoms is recommended in 3 to 7 days after the start of treatment. Improvement of objective symptoms is usually evident in 3 days and physical improvement within 7 days after treatment. The patient should be advised to apply warm compresses to promote healing of vulvovaginal infections. Treatment of LGV may include needle-aspirating enlarged lymph nodes to prevent rupture.

The use of the touch test is helpful for patients with vulvodynia to assess concretely the success of their treatment. To perform the touch test, the clinician lightly touches the vulvar area with a saline-moistened, cotton-tipped applicator and asks the patient to rate the pain on a scale from 0 to 5 (5 being the worst pain). A record should be kept of the pain scale and changes noted. Treatment should focus on eliminating the cause and reducing patient discomfort. Evaluate the patient for suicide risk secondary to the severe pain. Educate patients about long-term therapy and resources available, such as the Vulvar Pain Foundation.

If there is no improvement after treating vulvar lesions, the following questions should be considered: Is the patient HIV infected? Does the patient have a coexisting infection? Was the medication taken correctly? Is the diagnosis correct? Inform the patient that scarring may occur even with adequate treatment. Incision and draining of many lesions will increase scarring and is generally not recommended.

Diagnosis with any genital ulcer can be difficult. With chancroid *(Haemophilus ducreyi),* screening for HSV and syphilis is negative. Dark-field microscopy of bubo aspirate may be positive for the chains of gram-negative bacilli. Cultures are expensive and limited in availability. Polymerase chain reaction testing may be available soon. Preventing long-term sequelae and promoting the patient's optimum health depends on the patient's understanding and adequate treatment. Developing a trusting, compassionate relationship can make all the difference to a patient who may have a problem diagnosis.

Follow-up and Referral

Follow-up and referral depend on the specific diagnosis, cause, and management.

Patient Education

Treatment options have improved and simplified over the last few years, and some treatments are now available over the counter, which may lead to patient self-treatment that can confuse the diagnosis. Education is, therefore, most important.

Lesions of the vulva can be both painful and embarrassing for the patient. Frequently the patient may not realize that a lump or sore can be contagious, as well as evidence of a more serious disease. Another problem exists in the fact that the patient may not perform genital self-exam regularly, if at all. The first line of defense is prevention, which is best done through regular exams. Other preventive measures include patient education, abstinence, monogamy, use of condoms, and screening for infections. Education should include prevention of transmission and treatment of partners, along with medication use. Follow-up patient education can prevent transmission and promote adequate medication adherence for prevention of serious sequelae.

If the patient has HSV infection, long-term education, counseling, and compassion are indicated. Learning how to live with a lifelong disease is critical to decrease transmission of this STI. (See also discussion of HSV in Chapter 13.) The principal treatment for HSV focuses on the immune system, preventing outbreaks, and treating at the first sign of an eruption. Further study on herbal immune system treatments may provide additional help for a patient with HSV.

Genital warts (HPV infection) need aggressive partner follow-up to help decrease the spread of HPV. The patient should be educated that this infection can cause Pap smear changes and (if the patient is pregnant) that HPV can be transmitted to a newborn if the virus is active at the time of delivery, but the incidence is low.

Patients with molluscum contagiosum should be cautioned that scratching and picking can spread the infection. This also increases the chance of secondary infection. Patient education focuses on treatment, including that of the partner. Follow-up in 1 month for evaluation of all lesions is indicated.

General patient teaching should include the following. The patient should use unscented, hypoallergenic care products and wear loose clothing that is made of all-natural fibers, such as cotton. Very mild soap (e.g., Basis), daily sitz baths with baking soda, and vitamin E skin oil can decrease the pain associated with vulvovaginal lesions. Topical lidocaine/benzocaine may help mild pain. Dietary management should include a low–calcium oxalate diet. Teach the patient to avoid nuts, soy beverages and cheese, cocoa, chocolate milk, dark beer, black tea, instant coffee, high-fiber cereal, whole wheat products, and berries and to take vitamins and calcium citrate (Citracal) supplements to decrease urinary burning. Other treatments have had less success and can be disfiguring. The patient should be advised before any surgery for vulvar lesions that historically surgery has less than a 50% success rate and a second opinion is advised. Patient considerations for all these diseases include cost, convenience, lifestyle, pregnancy, other disease conditions, and medication use. Follow-up and testing for HIV and diabetes should be encouraged for patients with recurrent candidiasis.

Considerations when treating pregnant women who have STIs, UTIs, and BV/candidiasis are planning treatment to prevent adverse effects (dosage should be decreased) and evaluating the partner, especially with repeated infection. For foreign bodies, patient education about toxic shock syndrome, and careful use of tampons should be included. Any infection may interfere with the accuracy of a patient's Pap smear, so the patient needs to know that the smear may have to be repeated. For mucopurulent cervicitis, follow-up in some practices is 3 to 4 weeks after treatment to evaluate cervical healing. The CDC recommends treating for the identified STI; however, the tests are frequently negative, and some *Chlamydia* tests are only 60% accurate. Patient education should discuss partner treatment, medication use, and sexual abstinence during treatment. At every visit, safer sex practices should be encouraged.

References

Evidence-Based Practice

Centers for Disease Control and Prevention (CDC). Sexually transmitted diseases treatment guidelines, 2010. *MMWR* 59(RR12):1–110, 2010. Retrieved from www.cdc.gov/mmwr/preview/mmwrhtml/rr5912a1.htm

Enderlin, CA, et al. Dietary soy intake and breast cancer risk. *Oncol Nurs Forum* 36(5):531–539, 2009.

Harada, T, et al. Low-dose oral contraceptive pill for dysmenorrhea associated with endometriosis: A placebo-controlled, double-blind, randomized trial. *Fertil Steril* 90(5):1583–1588, 2008. doi:10.1016/j.fertnstert.2007.08.051

Kashanian, M, et al. Evaluation of the effect of vitamin E on pelvic pain reduction in women suffering from primary dysmenorrhea. *J Reprod Med* 58(1-2):34–38, 2013.

Kaur Bajaj, J, et al. Clinical efficacy of pyridoxine and mefenamic acid alone and in combination in premenstrual syndrome. *Int J Med Clin Res* 3(2):115–117, 2012.

Lasco, A, et al. Improvement of primary dysmenorrhea caused by a single oral dose of vitamin D: Results of a randomized, double-blind, placebo-controlled study. *Arch Intern Med* 172(4):366–367, 2012. doi:10.1001/archinternmed.2011.715

Mabrouk, M, et al. A new oral contraceptive regimen for endometriosis management: Preliminary experience with 24/4-day drospirenone/ethinyl estradiol 3 mg/20 mcg. *Gynecol Endocrinol* 28(6):451–454, 2012.

McCorkle, R, et al. Effects of a nursing intervention on quality of life outcomes in post-surgical women with gynecological cancers. *Psycho-Oncology* 18(1):62–70, 2009.

Bibliography

General

American Cancer Society. Cancer facts and figures 2013. Retrieved from www.cancer.org

Anonymous. The effectiveness of a pelvic floor muscle exercise program on urinary incontinence following childbirth. *Best Practice Information Sheets—Joanna Briggs Institute* 9(2):1–6, 2013.

Bascom, A. *Incorporating herbal medicine into clinical practice.* FA Davis, Philadelphia, 2002.

Bertone-Johnson, ER, et al. Cigarette smoking and the development of premenstrual syndrome. *Am J Epidemiol* 168(8):938–945, 2008.

Carey, WD. *2013 current clinical medicine,* ed 2. Saunders-Elsevier, Philadelphia, 2013.

Centers for Disease Control and Prevention (CDC). Sexually transmitted diseases treatment guidelines, 2010. *MMWR* 59(RR12):1–110, 2010. Retrieved from www.cdc.gov/mmwr/preview/mmwrhtml/rr5912a1.htm

Dambro, MR. *Griffith's 5-minute clinical consult.* Lippincott Williams & Wilkins, Philadelphia, 2013.

Edmunds, MW, and Mayhew, MS. *Pharmacology for the primary care provider,* ed 4. Mosby/Elsevier, St. Louis, MO, 2013.

Fauci, AS, et al (Eds.). *Harrison's principles of internal medicine,* ed 18. McGraw-Hill, New York, 2012.

Grigorieva, V, et al. Use of a levonorgestrel-releasing intrauterine system to treat bleeding related to uterine leiomyomas. *Fertil Steril* 79:1194–1198, 2013.

Hsu, AL, et al. Invasive and noninvasive methods for the diagnosis of endometriosis. *Clin Obstet Gynecol* 53(2):413–419, 2010. doi:10.1097/GRF.0b013e3181db7ce8

Hudelist, G, et al. Diagnostic accuracy of transvaginal ultrasound for non-invasive diagnosis of bowel endometriosis: Systematic review and meta-analysis. *Ultrasound Obstet Gynecol* 37(3):257–263, 2011. doi:10.1002/uog.8858

Hughes, E, et al. Ovulation suppression for endometriosis. *Cochrane Database Syst Rev* 3:CD000155, 2007. Review. PubMed PMID: 17636607.

Kao, A, et al. Dyspareunia in postmenopausal women: a critical review. *Pain Res Manage* 13(3):243–254, 2008.

Kee, JL. *Laboratory and diagnostic tests with nursing implications,* ed 8. Prentice-Hall, Upper Saddle River, NJ, 2010.

Kumar, V, et al. *Robbins basic pathology,* ed 8. Saunders/Elsevier, St. Louis, MO, 2010.

Latthe, P, et al. WHO systematic review of prevalence of chronic pelvic pain: A neglected reproductive health morbidity. *BMC Public Health* 6:177, 2006.

Liu, Z, et al. A systematic review evaluating health-related quality of life, work impairment, and health-care costs and utilization in abnormal uterine bleeding. *Value Health* 10(3):183–194, 2007.

McCance, KL, and Huether, SE. *Pathophysiology: The biologic basis for disease in adults and children,* ed 6. Mosby, St. Louis, 2010.

Newman, L, et al. Update on the management of gonorrhea in adults in the United States. *Clin Infect Dis* 44:s3, S84–S101, 2007.

Papadakis, MA, and McPhee, SJ. *Current medical diagnosis and treatment,* ed 52. Lange/McGraw-Hill, New York, 2013.

Tropeano, G, et al. Non-surgical management of uterine fibroids. *Hum Reprod Update* 14:259–274, 2008.

Woo, P, and McEneaney, MJ. New strategies to treat primary dysmenorrhea. *Clin Advisor,* November 5, 2010.

Breast Cancer

Adkins, BW. Maximizing exercise in breast cancer survivors. *Clin J Oncol Nurs* 13(6):695–700, 2009.

Boucher, BA, et al. Soy formula and breast cancer risk. *Epidemilogy* 19(1):165–166, 2008.

Breast cancer fast facts. Susan G. Komen, 2013. Retrieved from www.komenpugetsound.org/understanding-breast-cancer/about-breast-cancer/breast-cancer-fast-facts.html

Ciatto, S, et al. Integration of 3D digital mammography with tomosynthesis for population breast-cancer screening (STORM): A prospective comparison study. *Lancet Oncol* 14(7):583–589, 2013.

Howlader, N, et al (Eds.). *SEER cancer statistics review, 1975–2010.* National Cancer Institute, Bethesda, MD, 2013. Retrieved from http://seer.cancer.gov/csr/1975_2010

National Cancer Institute. Surveillance, Epidemiology, and End Results program. SEER stat fact sheets: Breast cancer. 2013. Retrieved from http://seer.cancer.gov/statfacts/html/breast.html

Pataky, R, et al. Cost-effectiveness of MRI for breast cancer screening in BRCA1/2 mutation carriers. *BMC Cancer* 13(1):1–9, 2013.

Plescia, M, and White, MC. The National Prevention Strategy and breast cancer screening: Scientific evidence for public health action. *Am J Public Health* 103(9):1545–1548, 2013.

Saadatmand, S, et al. Cost-effectiveness of screening women with familial risk for breast cancer with magnetic resonance imaging. *J Natl Cancer Inst* 105(17):1314–1321, 2013.

Skaane, P. Molecular imaging: A potential new tool for early detection and monitoring of targeted breast cancer therapy. *Acta Radiol* 50(10):1092–1093, 2009.

U.S. Cancer Statistics Working Group. *United States cancer statistics: 1999–2009 incidence and mortality Web-based report.* Department of Health and Human Services, Centers for Disease Control and Prevention, and National Cancer Institute, Atlanta, 2013.

Ovarian Disorders

Katsumata, N, et al. Long-term results of dose-dense paclitaxel and carboplatin versus conventional paclitaxel and carboplatin for treatment of advanced epithelial ovarian, fallopian tube, or primary peritoneal cancer (JGOG 3012): A randomised, controlled, open-label trial. *Lancet Oncol* 14(10):1020–1026, 2013.

Rafique, S, et al. A new approach to primary ovarian insufficiency. *Obstet Gynecol Clin North Am* 39(4):567–586, 2012.

Rooth, C. Ovarian cancer: Risk factors, treatment and management. *Br J Nurs* 22(17):S23–S30, 2013.

Shamilova, NM, et al. The role of genetic and autoimmune factors in premature ovarian failure. *J Assist Reprod Genet* 30(5):617–622, 2013.

Uterine/Cervical Disorders

ACOG Practice Bulletin No. 131. Screening for cervical cancer. ACOG Committee on Practice Bulletins, 2012. Retrieved from www.guideline.gov/content.aspx?id=38572

Howlader, N, et al (Eds.). SEER cancer statistics review, 1975–2010. National Cancer Institute, Bethesda, MD, November 2012. Retrieved from http://seer.cancer.gov/csr/1975_2010

Jayasekara, R. Menstrual bleeding (heavy): Surgery vs medical therapy. Evidence Summaries—Joanna Briggs Institute. 2009. Retrieved from Evidence-Based Resources from the Joanna Briggs Institute (Document ID: 1880534011).

Resources

American Society for Reproductive Medicine
1209 Montgomery Highway
Birmingham, AL 35216
Phone: 205-978-5000
www.asrm.org
Centers for Disease Control and Prevention
www.cdc.gov
Fertilitext
www.fertilitext.org
International Council on Infertility Information Dissemination
(INCIID)
PO Box 91363
Tucson, AZ 85752
Phone: 520-554-9548
www.inciid.org
Internet Health Resources: Infertility Resources
www.ihr.com/infertility

RESOLVE
1310 Broadway
Somerville, MA 02144
Phone: 617-623-1156
Helpline: 617-623-0744
www.resolve.org

Musculoskeletal Problems

Michael Zycowicz, DNP, FNP-BC, FAANP, FAAN •
Terry South, MSN, APRN, NP-C, FNP • Lori Martin-Plank,
PhD, FNP-BC, GNP-BC, FAANP •
Lynne M. Dunphy, PhD, APRN, FAAN

Chapter **15**

■ OVERVIEW

Musculoskeletal pain and dysfunction are one of the most common reasons for visits to a primary-care provider. Because of the complex and ill-defined nature of these problems and the variable differential diagnoses involved, the actual number of people affected is difficult to ascertain with true accuracy. Musculoskeletal problems in general are known to be the most frequent cause of disability in workers, and population surveys show a greater than 50% prevalence of musculoskeletal disorders among older Americans. Musculoskeletal problems are usually classified as acute (less than 6 weeks' duration) or chronic (more than 6 weeks' duration). Examples of chronic, recurrent musculoskeletal problems include arthritis (osteoarthritis [OA] and rheumatoid arthritis [RA]), fibromyalgia, and gout. Gout, fibromyalgia, and RA are important considerations in making a diagnosis, but given the underlying systemic nature of these disorders, they are covered in detail elsewhere in this text. (See Chapter 16 for gout and Chapter 17 for RA and fibromyalgia.) Osteoarthritis is covered in this chapter.

Musculoskeletal complaints are generally self-limiting. However, some conditions, if left untreated, can lead to a cycle of progressive joint instability and a higher risk of subsequent injury if recovery is not complete. It is essential to rule out any musculoskeletal emergencies (see Table 15.1; see Chapter 19 for assessment of musculoskeletal emergencies).

Delayed recognition of certain diagnoses may lead to permanent disability or death. Once these diagnoses have been excluded, proceed with an orderly evaluation of other diagnostic possibilities.

Musculoskeletal complaints can be a diagnostic challenge for the primary-care provider. There are no routine tests that can be employed in clinical practice to determine the presence of inflammation or muscle spasm. Much of the diagnosis is dependent on patient self-reporting of symptoms. An accurate patient history and clinician knowledge of underlying anatomy and physiology of the musculoskeletal system are essential keys to a correct diagnosis. A useful approach to the initial patient encounter is to determine whether the musculoskeletal complaint is

- Acute or chronic in duration
- Articular or nonarticular in origin
- Inflammatory or noninflammatory in nature
- Localized or systemic in distribution

Many musculoskeletal disorders resemble each other at onset, and some may take time to evolve into an identifiable diagnosis. Differential diagnoses of musculoskeletal problems include trauma, infection, metabolic or circulatory disorders, tumors, synovial conditions, congenital or developmental problems, or degenerative disorders.

Identifying the anatomical location of the musculoskeletal complaint is important. First distinguish between articular and nonarticular structures (see Table 15.2). Articular structures include the synovium, synovial fluid, articular cartilage, intra-articular ligaments, joint capsule, and juxta-articular bone. Disorders of these structures are characterized by deep or diffuse pain, limited range of motion (ROM) on active and passive movement, swelling (caused by synovial proliferation, effusion, or bony enlargement), crepitation, instability, "locking," or deformity. Nonarticular (or periarticular) structures are identified as supportive extra-articular ligaments, tendons, bursae, muscle, fascia, bone, nerve, and overlying skin. Nonarticular disorders are characterized by painful active but not passive ROM, demonstrated point or focal tenderness in regions distinct from articular structures, and physical findings far from the joint capsule. It is unlikely to see crepitus, instability, or deformity associated with these disorders.

Inflammatory disorders may be infectious or idiopathic. These are identified by the presence of all or some of the four cardinal signs of inflammation (erythema, warmth, pain, or swelling); systemic symptoms (fatigue, weight loss, morning stiffness, fever); or laboratory evidence of inflammation (elevated erythrocyte

Table 15.1   Musculoskeletal Emergencies

Clinical Manifestations	Musculoskeletal Emergencies: Differential Diagnoses
History	
Significant trauma	Soft tissue injury, internal derangement, fracture
Constitutional signs and symptoms (fever, weight loss, malaise)	Infection, sepsis, systemic rheumatic disease
Hot, swollen, painful joint	Infection, systemic rheumatic disease, gout, pseudogout
Physical Exam	
Weakness Focal	Compartment syndrome, entrapment neuropathy, mononeuritis, motor neuron disease, radiculopathy
Diffuse	Myositis, metabolic myopathy, paraneoplastic syndrome, degenerative neuromuscular disorder, toxin, myelopathy, transverse myelitis
Neurogenic pain (burning, numbness, paresthesia) Asymmetrical	Radiculopathy, reflex sympathetic dystrophy, entrapment neuropathy
Symmetrical Claudication pain pattern	Myelopathy, peripheral neuropathy Peripheral vascular disease, giant cell arteritis (with jaw pain), lumbar spinal stenosis

Table 15.2   Comparison of Articular and Nonarticular Structures

Articular Structures	Nonarticular Structures
Synovium and synovial fluid	Supportive extra-articular ligaments
Articular cartilage, intra-articular ligaments	Bone
Joint capsule	Nerve, overlying skin
Juxta-articular bone	Muscle, tendons, fascia

sedimentation rate or C-reactive protein, anemia of chronic disease, hypoalbuminemia, or thrombocytosis). Noninflammatory disorders tend to be related to trauma (meniscus tear), ineffective repair (OA), neoplasm, or pain amplification (fibromyalgia). There may be pain without swelling or warmth, absence of inflammatory or systemic features, minimal or absent morning stiffness, and normal (for age) laboratory testing.

The differential diagnoses may be narrowed by the identification of the underlying pathological process and the exact site of the complaint. These help to determine whether there is need for immediate diagnostic or therapeutic intervention or for continued observation.

The clinical history should contain the patient profile, including age, sex, race, family history, occupational history, medications, and leisure activities. The chronology of the complaint gives important diagnostic clues and may be divided into onset (e.g., abrupt), evolution (chronic, intermittent, migratory), and duration. The number and distribution of involved articulations should be noted. Articular disorders are classified based on the

number of involved joints: Monoarticular (one joint), periarticular (two to four joints), or polyarticular (more than four joints). Nonarticular disorders are classified as either focal or widespread. Precipitating events such as trauma or drug ingestion must be documented, as well as antecedent or current illnesses that may contribute to the patient's complaint. If the problem is chronic, ask the patient why he or she is addressing it at this particular time. A review of systems may provide useful diagnostic information, eliciting systemic features of diseases such as fever (systemic lupus erythematosus [SLE], infection). Musculoskeletal complaints may be associated with other organ systems, for example, such as the nervous system (Lyme disease, vasculitis), eye (sarcoidosis, Reiter's syndrome), and gastrointestinal tract (scleroderma, inflammatory bowel disease), to name just a few. (See Focus on History 15.1.)

Guided by the history, the physical exam helps to distinguish between mechanical problems, soft tissue disease, and noninflammatory and inflammatory joint disease. A major goal of the physical exam is to detect warmth over a joint, joint effusion, and pain on joint motion. These are hallmarks of synovitis. Limitations in movement and instability are also important to assess and are of particular concern in knee and ankle pain. The medial and lateral collateral ligaments of the knee can be assessed by valgus and varus stress of the joint. Excess laxity of the knee on anterior drawer test or Lachman's test may indicate an anterior cruciate ligament tear.

Always begin the exam by inspecting the site, observing for side-to-side symmetry. The patient must be undressed and draped so that visual inspection can be done.

Focus on History 15.1 Musculoskeletal Problems

Questions to ask:

1. Have you injured yourself?
2. Describe exactly how your injury occurred:
   - When the injury occurred, did it make a noise or sound? If so, describe the sound.
3. Where does it hurt? Does the pain radiate, or is it localized, or diffuse?
4. Do you have numbness or tingling?
5. Is there loss of function?
6. Is there swelling?
7. When did the pain first occur?
   - What relieves it?
   - What exacerbates it?
   - What time of day does it occur?
   - Does the pain awaken you at night?
8. Is there joint stiffness?
   - Does activity make it worse or better?
9. Do you have any other symptoms (or systemic processes)?
   - Do you have a fever?
   - Do you have a rash?
   - Do you have general fatigue?
   - Have you recently been traveling or camping?
   - Have you recently been immunized?
   - Have you recently been treated with antibiotics?
   - Do you have a history of upper respiratory infection? Sexually transmitted disease? Chronic disease?
   - Were you ever treated with steroids?
10. Describe your daily activities—work, hobbies, home.

The uninvolved side should be examined initially and compared with the involved side. The painful part should be examined last. The patient should actively perform as much ROM as he or she can.

If the patient complains about a specific anatomical area, examine that area to recognize, for instance, a frozen shoulder or hip trochanteric bursitis with pain over the greater trochanter. If the patient reports a history of hand numbness that awakens him or her at night, this suggests carpal tunnel syndrome, even with no physical findings. Foot pain that begins the first thing in the morning when the patient puts his or her foot out of bed is suggestive of plantar fasciitis or early RA.

The combination of point tenderness, reduced active ROM, and preserved passive ROM suggests soft tissue disorders, including bursitis, tendinitis, or muscle injury. If both active and passive ROM is limited, soft tissue contracture, synovitis, or a structural abnormality of the joint is possible. Tendinitis may be suggested by tenderness to palpation along the course of the tendon or by pain or rub produced when the tendon is stretched or stressed during active ROM against resistance. Inability to actively abduct the shoulder fully is suggestive of a rotator cuff tear. Crepitus (joint noises or palpable grinding during joint motion) may be due to articular surface abnormalities or synovitis. Crepitus not associated with pain or limitation of motion is generally of no clinical significance.

After the target area, if any, has been examined—or if the patient reports diffuse generalized musculoskeletal pain—a simple evaluation may begin with gentle palpation of the hands. Bony enlargements of the distal interphalangeal joints or Heberden's nodes are indicative of OA, whereas soft tissue swelling may indicate RA; inflammation may also be indicated by swelling of the metacarpophalangeal joints. If symmetrical swelling has been present for longer than 6 months, a presumptive diagnosis of RA may be made, regardless of laboratory results. Limitations of flexion and/or extension of the wrist are a sign of prior inflammation and a clue to earlier chronic RA. (See Rheumatoid Arthritis in Chapter 17.)

The shoulders can be examined by asking the patient to raise his or her arms above the head, put hands behind the head, and hands behind the back. Tender points in the muscles of the neck, shoulders, and back—a characteristic sign of fibromyalgia—are easily recognized by an experienced examiner. (See Fibromyalgia in Chapter 17.) Ask the patient to rise from a chair without holding on. If the patient cannot do this, there is an abnormality of the joints, nerves, or muscles, which requires further examination, usually by a specialist. Ask the patient to walk a few steps across the room and back and observe the gait. This should be included in all evaluations.

Have the patient lie down to assess ROM of the hips, knees, ankles, and feet. It is important to recognize flexion contractures, which, if not congenital or due to injury (ask the patient), are a sign of prior inflammation. All maneuvers described should take less than 2 minutes and should be included in the "general" physical exam. Note any endocrinopathies (irregular heart rhythms, weight gain, and thyromegaly) and possible malignancy (severe pain, weight loss, or palpable masses). In addition, muscle strength and function should be systematically evaluated. (See Advanced Assessment 15.1.) On physical examination, evidence of tender points and trigger points, as well as the absence of inflammation or swollen joints, increases the likelihood of a soft tissue problem. Many clinicians use a body drawing and mark the affected parts.

Extra-articular abnormalities, such as oral/nasal ulcers; iritis; rash; nodules; pericardial or pulmonary rub; enlargement of liver, spleen, or lymph nodes; and neurological abnormalities, suggest a systemic disease.

An accurate diagnosis of injury and/or rheumatic diseases can best be accomplished with careful history

The Iceberg of Low Back Pain

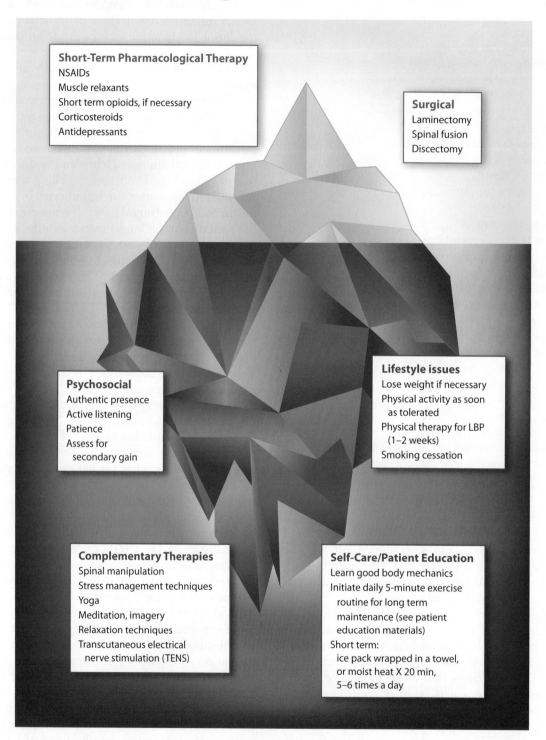

Short-Term Pharmacological Therapy
NSAIDs
Muscle relaxants
Short term opioids, if necessary
Corticosteroids
Antidepressants

Surgical
Laminectomy
Spinal fusion
Discectomy

Psychosocial
Authentic presence
Active listening
Patience
Assess for
  secondary gain

Lifestyle issues
Lose weight if necessary
Physical activity as soon
  as tolerated
Physical therapy for LBP
  (1–2 weeks)
Smoking cessation

Complementary Therapies
Spinal manipulation
Stress management techniques
Yoga
Meditation, imagery
Relaxation techniques
Transcutaneous electrical
  nerve stimulation (TENS)

Self-Care/Patient Education
Learn good body mechanics
Initiate daily 5-minute exercise
  routine for long term
  maintenance (see patient
  education materials)
Short term:
  ice pack wrapped in a towel,
  or moist heat X 20 min,
  5–6 times a day

and physical exam by an experienced clinician. At the same time, it should be recognized that in some patients—perhaps as many as 10%—a definitive diagnosis cannot be established, particularly at the first visit, and sometimes even over time. This is especially true in cases of chronic musculoskeletal pain. The diagnosis is not as important as the approach to treatment, which typically is similar for a range of diagnoses based on the presence or absence of inflammation (see Table 15.3).

Advanced Assessment 15.1 Grading of Manual Muscle Testing

Numerical Grade	Descriptive Grade	Description
5	Normal	Complete ROM against gravity with full or normal resistance
4	Good	Complete ROM against gravity with some resistance
3	Fair	Complete ROM against gravity
2	Poor	Complete ROM with gravity eliminated
1	Trace	Muscle contraction but no or very limited joint motion
0	Zero	No evidence of muscle function

ROM: range of motion.

Table 15.3 Examples of Disorders of Inflammation versus Noninflammation

Inflammatory Musculoskeletal Disorders	Noninflammatory Musculoskeletal Disorders
Infectious	Ineffective repair (osteoarthritis)
Crystal induced	Pain amplification (fibromyalgia)
Immune related (rheumatoid arthritis, systemic lupus erythematosus)	Trauma
Idiopathic	Neoplasm

Diagnostic Reasoning

Diagnostic Tests

Laboratory tests may be of limited use. One problem with using laboratory tests in the diagnosis is the fact that many people who have been told that they have SLE, gout, or Lyme disease do not have the disease at all, but simply an abnormal laboratory test such as a positive antinuclear antibody (ANA), elevated uric acid, or positive Lyme antibody test. These tests are abnormal in at least 5% of the general population, whereas the diseases identified are seen in less than 1%. Therefore, most individuals with positive laboratory tests do not have the associated disease. In contrast, many people with RA, for example, often have normal blood tests and x-ray findings, particularly in early disease, when aggressive treatment might be most effective. Some of these tests are useful to research laboratories in the identification and understanding of pathogenic mechanisms, but do not add anything to the meaningful diagnosis and management of the patient. A review of associated laboratory tests is presented here.

- Complete blood count—the presence of anemia may be a clue to inflammation, and leukopenia is seen in active SLE.

- Erythrocyte sedimentation rate (ESR) and C-reactive protein (CRP)—nonspecific indicators of inflammation. A highly elevated value indicates a likelihood of inflammatory rheumatic disease, infection, or malignancy. ESR increases with age, as does CRP, and some people (as many as 5%–10% of the general population) have elevated values with no explanation. Up to 40% of patients who present with RA have normal ESRs and CRPs. In patients with giant cell arteritis and polymyalgia rheumatica, the ESR is almost always markedly elevated, and therefore diagnostically useful.
- Rheumatoid factor (RF)—25% of patients with RA never have an elevated RF. It may also be elevated with other inflammatory conditions (e.g., SLE, subacute bacterial endocarditis, vasculitis, viral infection).
- Fluorescent ANA test—this test is positive in 99% of patients with SLE; however, it is also positive in 5% to 10% of normal blood donors, meaning only 1 in 100 people with a positive ANA has SLE. A positive ANA can also occur with certain drugs (procainamide, hydralazine); it may be transiently positive in people with a severe infection; and it is positive in a high percentage of people with other inflammatory rheumatic conditions, including RA (30%–50%), scleroderma (20%–50%), polymyositis (10%–30%), and idiopathic pulmonary fibrosis (10%–20%).
- Lyme borreliosis antibodies—Lyme disease is identified serologically by antibodies to the Lyme *Borrelia* organism. From 5% to 10% of normal individuals have a positive Lyme borreliosis titer, even in the best laboratories. A test for Lyme disease is not appropriate in patients with unexplained arthritis unless there are other risk factors such as living in an endemic area and frequent outdoor activities.
- Uric acid—uric acid measurement is often included in evaluation of patients with musculoskeletal symptoms, because elevated uric acid resulting from either overproduction or underexcretion is seen in more than 90% of people with gout. However, most people with elevated uric acid levels do not have

gout. A test for uric acid should be reserved for patients who have clinical evidence of episodic or atypical inflammatory arthritis. Alcohol and diuretics may cause moderately elevated uric acid levels. Asymptomatic hyperuricemia should not be treated. Further, some individuals with gout have normal serum acid levels, particularly at the time of the acute attack. A definitive diagnosis of gout requires identification of uric acid crystals in synovial fluid.

• Screening panels—these tests are available from all national laboratories and are marketed as "rheumatology screening panels" to rule out an inflammatory rheumatic disease. The simplest include rheumatoid factor, ANA, and uric acid, although more elaborate tests are available. These screens tend to be a major source of potential false-positive information in patient evaluations and are not advised for use by the general practitioner.

Imaging studies are indicated (1) when examination cannot localize the anatomical structure that is causing symptoms, (2) after a significant trauma, (3) when there is a loss of joint function (e.g., unable to bear weight), (4) when pain continues despite conservative management, (5) when a fracture or bone infection is suspected, or (6) when there is a history of malignancy. Clinicians who are unfamiliar with what views to order should contact the radiologist for guidance. Plain radiographs will be unrevealing (and are therefore not indicated) for most patients with acute and new symptoms of RA, SLE, gout, mechanical back pain, or tendinitis/bursitis.

Radiographs may confirm the diagnosis of OA and assess its severity, but normal findings on radiographs do not rule out the presence of OA. The earliest radiographic changes in RA are nonspecific and include soft tissue swelling and periarticular osteoporosis, but these features are often absent at the initial presentation. In established RA or long-standing gout, erosions may be diagnostic: Marginal erosions in the former and evidence of reparative process in the latter. Radiography (plain x-ray films) can reveal the following:

• Erosions
• Calcifications and cysts
• Osteopenia
• Narrowing of joint spaces
• Deformity of bones
• Separations (fractures, dislocations)

Repeat radiographs after 7 to 10 days are appropriate when a fracture is suspected despite an unrevealing initial examination because callus formation or abnormal alignment may be evident. Repeated imaging over time in patients with established rheumatic disease may be useful in assessing structural damage. For patients with typical acute mechanical low back pain, a plain radiograph adds little to the management decisions.

Ultrasonography may be useful in the detection of soft tissue abnormalities but has limited clinical value. The foremost application of ultrasound is in the diagnosis of synovial (Baker's) cysts although rotator cuff tears and various tendon injuries may be identified by ultrasound.

Computed tomography (CT) has proved most useful in the evaluation of the axial skeleton because of its ability to visualize in the axial plane. CT is useful in the diagnosis of low back pain syndromes (herniated intervertebral disc, spinal stenosis, spinal trauma), intra-articular osteochondral fragments, and advanced osteonecrosis. Helical or spiral CT can be useful in the detection of obscure fractures.

Magnetic resonance imaging (MRI) or radionuclide bone scanning is useful when specific disorders are suspected, and the management could be altered according to findings. Rotator cuff tear, spinal stenosis, avascular necrosis of bone, or mechanical derangement of the knee are some conditions that may be revealed with an MRI. A bone scan may be useful when osteomyelitis, stress fractures, or bony metastases are a concern. In general, MRI is useful for assessing soft tissue and spinal cord elements, whereas nuclear medicine studies are best for assessing bone turnover. MRI and bone scanning are expensive and the latter exposes patients to significant radiation. Rotator cuff degeneration and disc abnormalities are common in older patients. These studies should be reserved for patients in whom specific disorders are suspected, when the diagnosis cannot be made in a less costly manner, and only after a thorough history and physical exam.

Nerve conduction studies (electromyography) may be indicated when neurological abnormalities or paresthesias are present.

Differential Diagnosis

Joint symptoms of one and up to a few joints may be due to trauma, infection, crystal-induced inflammation (gout, pseudogout), or primary inflammatory arthritis (including spondyloarthropathies and atypical presentation of RA). In acute monoarthritis, it is essential that infection of a joint be diagnosed or excluded, and this can be done only via joint aspiration (see Therapeutic Procedure 15.1) and synovial fluid analysis and culture (see Advanced Assessment 15.2). Chronic monoarticular symptoms with little or no effusion are usually from OA. Tendinitis and bursitis generally involve one joint region, and physical exam is usually diagnostic. Common syndromes include de Quervain's tenosynovitis, olecranon bursitis, medial and lateral epicondylitis, bicipital and rotator cuff tendinitis, rotator cuff tear, trochanteric bursitis, patellar bursitis and prepatellar bursitis, anserine bursitis, plantar fasciitis, posterior tibial tendinitis, and Achilles tendinitis.

Polyarthritis has an extensive differential diagnosis. The presence of prolonged morning stiffness, systemic

Therapeutic Procedure 15.1   Arthrocentesis

Joint	Technique
Ankle	*Patient position:* Supine, with foot in plantar flexion *Needle size:* 20–22 gauge, 1-1/2 in. *Syringe size:* 10–30 mL and 2–5 mL *Procedure:* Locate the space between the medial malleolus and extensor hallucis tendon. Using an anteromedial approach, enter lateral to the medial malleolus, medial to the tendon, and aim the needle downward, laterally. Insert the needle 1-3/4 in. (3 cm).
Elbow	*Patient position:* Sitting, with elbow flexed to 90 degrees with the palm pronated on a table *Needle size:* 20–22 gauge, 1-½ in. *Syringe size:* 10–30 mL and 2–5 mL *Procedure:* Locate the space between the lateral epicondyle of the humerus and olecranon process (3/8 in. below the epicondyle). Using a posterolateral approach, insert the needle and direct it medially and slightly toward the hand. Insert the needle 5/8 in. (1.5 cm).
Knee	*Patient position:* Supine, with knee fully extended or bent slightly to 20 degrees over a rolled towel under the knee *Needle size:* 18–20 gauge, 1-1/2 in. *Syringe size:* 10–30 mL and 2–5 mL *Procedure:* Locate the joint space by moving medially from midpatella to a point halfway between the patella and underlying the femoral condyle. Using an anteromedial approach, aim the needle posteriorly (downward) and laterally. Insert the needle 3/8–5/8 in.
Knee (patient unable to extend knee)	*Patient position:* Sitting, with knee flexed 90 degrees over edge of examining table *Needle size:* 18–20 gauge, 1-1/2 in. *Syringe size:* 10–30 mL and 2–5 mL *Procedure:* Locate the triangle formed by the tendon and condyles. Using an anteromedial or lateral approach, enter distal to apex of patella medially or laterally to the tendon. Direct the needle slightly cephalad to a depth of 1-3/8–1-3/4 in.
Wrist	*Patient position:* Sitting, with palm pronated over a rolled towel, wrist flexed 20–30 degrees and with a slight ulnar turn *Needle size:* 24–26 gauge, 5/8 in. *Syringe size:* 10–30 mL and 2–5 mL *Procedure:* Locate the space between the bony processes of the radius and ulna and just lateral to the tendon. Using a dorsal approach, enter distal to the space and perpendicular to the skin. Insert the needle downward 3/8–3/4 in.

Advanced Assessment 15.2   Synovial Fluid Analysis

	Normal	Grade I: Noninflammatory	Grade II: Inflammatory	Grade III: Infectious
Visual analysis	Clear, straw-colored	Clear or slightly bloody and turbid	Turbid	Turbid, gray or yellow
Viscosity	Normal	Decreased	Decreased	Decreased
WBCs per mm^3	30–150	<2,500	2,500–25,000	>50,000
PMNs (%)	<20	20–50	50–70	70–90
Protein (g/dL)	1–4	1–5	3–6	3–7
Examples		OA, SLE, mechanical derangement	RA, gonococcal arthritis, rheumatic fever, gout, pseudogout, Reiter's syndrome	Septic arthritis, tuberculosis

OA: osteoarthritis; PMNs: polymorphonuclear leukocytes; RA: rheumatoid arthritis; SLE: systemic lupus erythematosus.

symptoms, Raynaud's phenomenon, rash, or sicca symptoms and manifestations of other organ involvement suggest a rheumatic disease. The specific evaluation is guided by the clinical manifestations and should screen organ symptoms that can be involved without overt signs, such as the lung, heart, liver, kidney, and bowel, for potential involvement. Precise diagnosis and management usually requires referral.

Arthralgia and/or myalgia without physical findings has an extensive differential diagnosis. Often, no definitive diagnosis is possible at the initial presentation. Common causes include fibromyalgia, viral infection, an overuse syndrome (tendon strain associated with repetitive motion injuries or muscle fatigue), a neuropathy, or hypothyroidism. If the history and physical exam do not provide a diagnosis, symptomatic management and reassessment over several weeks is more productive initially than is laboratory testing or diagnostic imaging.

After ruling out joint pain, trauma, overuse syndromes, and vascular components, primary differential diagnoses for muscle pain (myalgia) typically include infectious causes, such as viral syndromes, mononucleosis, Rocky Mountain spotted fever, or Lyme disease; systemic disorders such as fibromyalgia (FM) or polymyalgia rheumatica; or psychogenic causes. More than one syndrome may occur concomitantly. For example, bursitis may coexist with pain from FM. If the inflammation from the bursitis is overlooked, the patient may not receive the treatment indicated for the acute disorder (see Fig. 15.1).

COMMON COMPLAINTS

■ ACUTE MUSCULOSKELETAL INJURY

Acute musculoskeletal injury encompasses a number of common conditions characterized by acute pain and/or muscular spasm (persistent, painful, and reversible contracture of striated muscle). These symptoms may be caused by specific syndromes, such as low back pain and ankle sprain with well-documented and well-tested treatment guidelines; specific syndromes such as torticollis and "tennis elbow" with less-well-tested management guidelines; and a large group of disorders characterized by nonspecific musculoskeletal trauma, which results in tissue derangement that can lead to pain, limitations of movement, spasm, and the inability to perform activities of daily living. Sometimes a traumatic injury, such as from a car accident, or other significant precipitating factor, such as lifting a heavy object, may be identified as the initiating factor. In some cases a trivial movement such as bending over to tie a shoe or coughing may precipitate the injury. Acute musculoskeletal injury implies pain of less than 6 weeks' duration. (See Differential Diagnosis 15.1.)

The following are management principles in acute musculoskeletal pain/injury not requiring emergent treatment (see Chapter 19 for emergency care):

• The acronym RICE is commonly employed: *R*est the affected part, *A*pply ice for 48 hours, *C*ompression (Ace wrap), *E*levate it.
• Reassurance—most injuries are self-limiting and improvement should occur within approximately 2 weeks.
• Limitation of activity—immobilization of injury is appropriate during the diagnostic phase; if appropriate at all, bedrest should be limited to the most acute period (2 days or less) to control spasm and promote healing.
• Physical therapy—may include heat or cold application with the goal of returning the patient to full function as soon as possible with minimal limitation. Commonly cold/ice is recommended for 48 hours; then heat.
• Skeletal muscle relaxants—a 1- to 2-week course is valuable when injury is accompanied by spasm or tightness. Be aware of potential for sedation and abuse (see Drugs Commonly Prescribed 15.1: Skeletal Muscle Relaxants).
• NSAIDs/acetaminophen—first-line choices (see Drugs Commonly Prescribed 15.2: Pharmacological Treatment of Osteoarthritis).
• Opioids—useful for moderate or severe pain or if sedation desired—monitor adverse effects such as constipation, abuse potential.
• Referral—to orthopedic specialist if no relief with conventional methods.
• Imaging studies—radiograph, CT, MRI are usually *not* indicated for acute musculoskeletal injuries.

■ MUSCLE CRAMPS

Muscle cramps may be described as sudden, involuntary, painful contractions of a muscle or muscle part that last from seconds to several minutes. Cramps may occur spontaneously while at rest or may be precipitated by a brief muscle contraction. The cause is usually related to some hyperexcitability of the motor neurons supplying the muscles. In many cases, the reason for episodic, recurrent muscle cramps may remain unclear, even after complete diagnostic evaluation. Muscle cramps may also occur related to vigorous exercise and during sporting events. Monitor for dehydration.

Differential Diagnosis

The initial history should elicit whether the cramps occur with exercise or at rest. In pregnant women and children, leg cramps tend to occur at rest and are most often benign, requiring no treatment. Certain medications (e.g., some diuretics, some of the statin drugs, and clofibrate [Atromid-S]) may cause muscle cramping. Leg pain and cramps in adults that are precipitated by

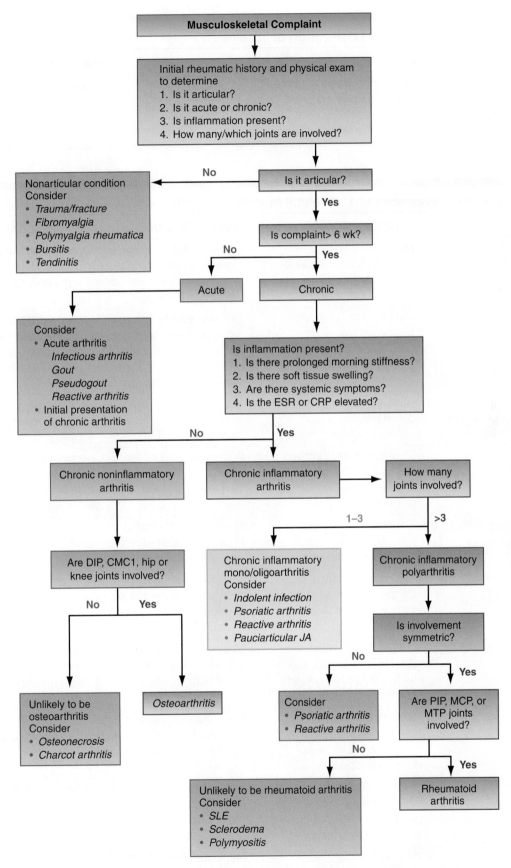

Figure 15.1 Diagnosis of musculoskeletal complaints. *(Source: Fauci, AS, et al (Eds.).* Harrison's principles of internal medicine, *ed 17. McGraw-Hill, New York, 2008.)*

Differential Diagnosis 15.1 Classification of Sprains

Grade	Degree of Injury	Treatment
Grade I	Partial tear; no instability or opening of the joint on stress maneuvers	Symptomatic only
Grade II	Partial tear with some instability indicated by partial opening of the joint on stress maneuvers	Immobilization to protect injured part, but full healing expected
Grade III	Complete tear with complete opening of joint on stress	Immobilization; possible repair

Drugs Commonly Prescribed 15.1 Skeletal Muscle Relaxants

Drug	Indications	Adverse Reactions and Prescribing Considerations
meprobamate (200 mg) and aspirin (325 mg) (Equagesic)	For short-term use only Adjunct for musculoskeletal pain, anxiety, tension	CNS depressant; driving and alertness precautions. Do not use with salicylate sensitivity. Caution in patients with depression, renal problems, or hepatic problems. Avoid with alcohol.
cyclobenzaprine HCl (Flexeril)	Maximum of 2–3 weeks Nonneurogenic acute muscle spasm, as adjunct to rest and physical therapy	CNS depressant; driving and alertness precautions. Same profile for toxicity as tricyclic antidepressants— arrhythmias, tachycardia, QT prolongation. Caution in glaucoma, hepatic impairment, urinary hesitancy, elderly. Avoid with MAO inhibitors, alcohol.
orphenadrine (Norflex) (anticholinergic muscle relaxant [central])	Painful musculoskeletal conditions	Potentiates anticholinergics, alcohol, other CNS depressants. CNS excitation, dizziness, blurred vision, dry mouth. Caution in elderly.
orphenadrine citrate 50 mg, aspirin 770 mg, caffeine 60 mg (Norgesic Forte)	Muscle relaxant; short-term use for acute conditions	Potentiates anticholinergics, alcohol, other CNS depressants. CNS excitation, dizziness, blurred vision, dry mouth. Increased risk of GI bleed; caution in elderly.
chlorzoxazone (Parafon Forte DSC)	Adjunct to PT and rest for short-term treatment of acute muscle spasm	May potentiate alcohol, other CNS depressants. Caution in cardiac, impaired renal or hepatic function, elderly. Dizziness, drowsiness.
methocarbamol (Robaxin)	Adjunct treatment of muscle spasm in conjunction with acute musculoskeletal condition	May potentiate alcohol, other CNS depressants. Dizziness, drowsiness, blurred vision, nasal congestion, hypotension. Caution in elderly.
metaxalone (Skelaxin)	Adjunct treatment of muscle spasm in conjunction with acute musculoskeletal condition	May potentiate alcohol, other CNS depressants. Caution with history of seizures, hepatic/renal impairment, elderly. Dry mouth, dizziness, blurred vision, nausea.
carisoprodol (Soma)	Used as adjunct to PT and rest in muscle spasm related to acute musculoskeletal condition	May potentiate alcohol, other CNS depressants. Caution in severe liver, kidney disease and in elderly. Dizziness, drowsiness, agitation, insomnia, irritability, syncope.
diazepam (Valium)	Skeletal muscle relaxant for short-term use in acute musculoskeletal conditions; also used for anxiety	Benzodiazepine; potential for dependence. May potentiate alcohol, other CNS depressants. Caution in hepatic, severe renal dysfunction and in elderly. Dizziness, drowsiness.
tizanidine HCl (Zanaflex)	Skeletal muscle relaxant for treatment of muscle spasticity	May potentiate alcohol, other CNS depressants. Avoid with severe renal, hepatic impairment; caution with elderly. Avoid with other CYP1A2 inhibitors. Visual hallucinations, sedation.

Drugs Commonly Prescribed 15.2   Pharmacological Treatment of Osteoarthritis

Drug/Usage	Indication	Adverse Reactions and Prescribing Considerations
acetaminophen (Tylenol)	Treatment of mild to moderate pain; fever; does not have anti-inflammatory properties	Monitor alcohol intake and limit to <3 drinks/day; hepatotoxicity may occur with chronic use or in doses >4 g/day. Low cost, easy availability, overall safety profile.
capsaicin cream	Topical for pain	Naturally occurring substance that seems to interfere with transmission of painful stimuli.
NSAIDs	Acute and chronic pain due to OA	Renal and/or platelet dysfunction; GI bleeding. Risk factors for GI bleed: Greater age, comorbidity, history of peptic ulcer, history of GI bleed, glucocorticoids, anticoagulation, combination NSAID therapy and increased dose.
tramadol HCl (Ultram; available in immediate and extended release); also available with acetaminophen (Ultracet)	Relief of moderate to moderately severe pain Opioid analgesic	Low abuse potential; nonscheduled; do not use with SSRIs, TCAs, MAO inhibitors to avoid serotonin syndrome. Do not use extended-release form with hepatic or renal disease. CNS depression, caution in elderly, use lowest dose initially.
codeine (Tylenol with Codeine)	Analgesic, opioid. Treatment of mild to moderate pain	Weak opioid; side-effect profile not good for older adults; also increased risk of hip fracture. Use with caution in head injury; constipation.
hyaluronic acid (Viscosupplement injection)—used as joint injection for pain relief for OA of knee only	Either three injections over 15 days or weekly injections for 5 weeks	Expensive; mild adverse effects include injection site inflammatory/allergic reaction, transient worsening of symptoms; systemic include occasional muscle cramps (not common); always risk of infection with intra-articular injection.
Corticosteroids—hydrocortisone (Cortisol)	Symptom relief for weeks to months; Intra-articular injection—dose depends on anatomical site and medication	Duration of relief may be short (1–2 weeks) in lower extremities, shoulder, or elbow; may be effective in hand for several months; always risk of infection with intra-articular injection; local reaction at injection site. Can increase blood glucose in diabetics.
prednisolone tebutate (Hydeltra)		
methylprednisolone acetate	No more than two injections should be given in any weight-bearing joint.	
(Depo-Medrol)		
triamcinolone acetonide (Kenalog)		
triamcinolone hexacetonide (Aristospan)		
betamethasone (Celestone)		

CNS: central nervous system; GI: gastrointestinal; MAO: monoamine oxidase; OA: osteoarthritis; SSRI: selective serotonin reuptake inhibitor; TCA: tricyclic antidepressant.

exercise and relieved by rest are usually caused by peripheral vascular disease. Blood chemistry tests may be necessary, including serum enzymes, to rule out causes such as dehydration (from diarrhea or sweating). (See Differential Diagnosis 15.2.)

■ PARESTHESIAS

Paresthesia is the sensation of numbness, prickling, or tingling experienced in central and peripheral nerve lesions. Frequently, the patient's understanding and use of the terms will differ from the clinician's; therefore, it is necessary to clearly establish the character of the patient's complaint. During the history, take time to differentiate between the lack of use of a limb from the sensation of tingling and numbness and the total loss of sensation. It is also important to ascertain if the loss or altered sensation ascends onto the abdomen or thorax.

The location of the paresthesia may be focal or generalized. It may also be nonspecific, as in multiple sclerosis, in which the initial presentation may be bilateral diminution of sensation or paresthesia in the upper or lower extremities, or unilateral, as in stroke or transient ischemic attack, in which unilateral extremity or face paresthesias may occur.

Paresthesias are also likely to be a result of anatomical or mechanical peripheral nerve injury, such as entrapment and compression neuropathies. These are most likely to occur at sites that are more susceptible to damage from an increase in pressure and mechanical forces, such as entrapment or compression of the medial nerve at the wrist (carpal tunnel syndrome), the ulnar nerve at the elbow, and the peroneal nerve at the knee.

Paresthesias also occur as a result of nerve-root injury, chlorinated hydrocarbon exposure, respiratory alkalosis, and the use of certain drugs, such as carbonic anhydrase inhibitors (which are used in the treatment of glaucoma).

The physical exam must determine if the sensory abnormality follows the distribution of a peripheral nerve or nerve root. Commonly affected nerves are cervical nerve roots 5 to 8 (C5–C8); ulnar and radial nerves of the hand; lumbar nerves 3, 4, 5, and S1; obturator, sciatic, and femoral nerves in the thigh; and peroneal and tibial nerves of the foot. (See Advanced Assessment 15.3.)

Differential Diagnosis
Cervical Radiculopathy

Cervical radiculopathy is commonly caused by compression of the cervical nerve roots, when the cervical discs place stress on the vertebral bodies. It usually is the result of age-related changes, cervical spondylosis, or a herniated disc. The most commonly involved nerve roots are C6 and C7, which produce paresthesias into the lower lateral arm, thumb, and middle finger.

Diagnostic tests include radiological assessment of the cervical spine, and if radicular pain is severe or if there is motor or sensory deficit or hyporeflexia, MRI is indicated. If only radiculopathy is present, a conservative trial of cervical traction as in the use of a soft cervical collar may be warranted. Newer findings on soft cervical collar usage discourage routine use, especially in cases where cervical radiculopathy is a chronic problem. Use of the soft cervical collar should be intermittent, meaning 1 to 3 hours on and then off for several hours. Usage should never be longer than a few days at most. In severe cases, a myelogram may be necessary to rule out neoplasm and to define the extent of compression. Surgery may be considered, but no long-term outcome studies have compared the benefits of surgery to nonoperative treatments such as heat and cold, ROM exercises, and limiting activity during acute outbreaks.

Brachial Plexus Neuritis or Radiculitis

Brachial plexus injuries include a broad array of neurological dysfunction ranging from momentary paresthesias to completely flail extremities. The mechanism of injury is equally diverse, from high-energy motor vehicle crashes, falls from a height, and gunshot wounds to lower-energy injuries such as most athletic injuries. "Burners" or "stingers" (transient brachial plexopathy)

Differential Diagnosis 15.2	Muscle Cramps
Symptom	**Possible Diagnosis**
Cramp-like symptoms	Intermittent claudication related to ischemia; drug induced (such as statin-induced myopathy)
Contracture	Thyroid disease, McArdle's disease
Tetany	Hypoglycemia, hypomagnesemia, respiratory alkalosis, hypokalemia
Dystonia	Occupational (such as writer's cramp)
	Drug-induced (antipsychotics, anti-parkinsonian) metabolic/neurological
True cramps	Ordinary (nocturnal), dehydration, drug-induced (nifedipine, beta agonists), lower motor neuron, hemodialysis (volume and electrolyte shifts), heat induced (volume depletion, hyponatremia)

Source: Adapted from McGee, SK. Muscle cramp. *Arch Intern Med* 150:571, 1990.

Advanced Assessment 15.3 Paresthesias and Affected Nerve Roots

Nerve Root	Paresthesia
C6 (6th cervical)	Thumb: Dorsal and lateral aspects
C7 (7th cervical)	Fingers: Index and middle
C8 (8th cervical)	Fingers: Fifth and ulnar half of fourth Hand: Ulnar side
L4 (4th lumbar)	Thigh: Anterior, just above knee
L5 (5th lumbar)	Foot: Dorsal aspect Great toe: Dorsal aspect
S1 (1st sacral)	Foot: Lateral aspect Small toe: Lateral aspect

are transient injuries to the upper trunk of the brachial plexus involving the C5 and C6 nerve roots. The most common mechanism of injury is a traction force when the shoulder is forcefully depressed and the head and neck are tilted toward the opposite side or the upper plexus is compressed between the shoulder pad and the scapula. These injuries are relatively common among college and professional athletes, especially in sports such as football and basketball.

Brachial plexus injuries involving axonal disruptions can be categorized further as occurring proximal to the dorsal root ganglion in the spinal foramen (preganglionic) or anywhere distal to the ganglion (postganglionic). This distinction is important because operative repair is impossible and the prognosis is poor for preganglionic root recovery.

The symptoms are severe—burning upper arm and shoulder pain that radiates down the arm, followed by weakness affecting C5 and T1 (thoracic) nerve root distributions. The patient is often seen holding the arm on the affected side, which hangs limply at the side.

A detailed neurological assessment is required, with examination of the neck and shoulder. Plain radiographs including the cervical spine should be obtained. If radiographs are abnormal, or if symptoms persist, progress to MRI. Cervical spine instability would be evident on radiograph. Depending on the location and severity of the brachial plexus injury, persistent pain, sensory loss, paresthesia, weakness, or paralysis is possible.

An athlete should not return to play while symptomatic. Athletes with prolonged or bilateral involvement should be referred. Treatment options vary from strengthening and stretching exercises to splinting to surgical intervention in some cases. Cervical spine precautions should be followed if cervical spine injury is suspected.

Thoracic Outlet Syndrome

Thoracic outlet syndrome is compression of the brachial plexus and/or subclavian vessels as they exit the narrow space between the superior shoulder girdle and the first rib. These structures can be affected individually or in combination. Women aged 20 to 50 years are most commonly affected. Etiology may be secondary to congenital abnormalities such as cervical rib or abnormally long transverse process of C7 or an anomalous fibromuscular band in the thoracic outlet. Post-traumatic fibrosis of the scalene muscles is also a possibility.

Symptoms may be vague and variable. Common symptoms are color changes in the hand along with sensory changes and weakness in the fourth and fifth fingers. Cervical spine (C-spine) films are necessary to document cervical rib placements, and electromyography (EMG) helps to delineate the specific nerve involvement. Ultrasound of the subclavian artery with the arm in different positions helps define the extent of compression.

Conservative treatment consists of shoulder exercises to improve posture. Orthopedic referral may be needed to evaluate for surgery to remove the offending bony structure.

Peripheral Polyneuropathy

Peripheral polyneuropathy is "stocking-glove" or distal sensorimotor paresthesia, with diminished or variable deep tendon reflexes. Diabetes mellitus is a frequent cause; early symptoms may respond to a regimen with tighter glucose control. A rapid onset of motor polyneuropathy is seen in Guillain-Barré syndrome, in which an ascending weakness occurs after a viral illness. Other etiologies include alcoholism, vitamin B deficiencies, vitamin B_6 excess, Sjögren's syndrome, AIDS, hypothyroidism, amyloidosis, and renal failure.

A complete history and physical exam to exclude muscle disease or weakness is necessary. Paresthesias result in weakness, sensory loss, and altered deep tendon reflexes, whereas primary muscle pathology produces only weakness. Complete blood count, erythrocyte sedimentation rate, blood glucose, liver function, blood urea nitrogen, creatinine, thyroid-stimulating hormone, and immunoelectrophoresis tests are indicated. A chest x-ray film and EMG will help confirm the diagnosis. A neurological consultation is indicated.

Sciatic Nerve Syndrome

Sciatic nerve syndrome is back pain that radiates into the buttocks and produces tingling in the posterior thigh and posterolateral calf to the lateral malleolus. Often the cause is a herniated disc, spinal stenosis, obturator neuritis, sciatic nerve irritation, direct trauma, or osteoarthritis. The pain may also be secondary to lumbar sacral strain but does not necessarily indicate disc herniation or prolapse. Sciatic nerve compression may result from tumors in the pelvis or from prolonged sitting or lying on the buttocks. The history may reveal twisting, bending, or heavy lifting.

The physical exam includes evaluating for point tenderness and ROM in the back. With the patient supine, perform straight-leg raising. A positive finding is radicular pain that occurs below the knee at less than 60 degrees of limb elevation, with pain in the buttock or posterior thigh. Treatment is usually conservative. Any change in bowel or bladder function (cauda equina syndrome) constitutes an emergency and needs immediate intervention.

Femoral Neuropathy

Arising from the second, third, and fourth lumbar nerve roots, the femoral nerve innervates the quadriceps and terminates as the saphenous nerve. Onset of femoral neuropathy is sudden and painful and is followed by wasting and weakness in the quadriceps, sensory impairment of the anteromedial thigh, and loss of the deep tendon reflex of the knee. Causes include nerve infarction due to diabetes mellitus, retroperitoneal compression by tumor, or hematoma from entrapment. Although improvement may occur, residual weakness is common.

■ NECK PAIN

Discomfort and limited ROM arising from the structures in the neck is a common complaint. The pain may originate from any of the musculoskeletal structures, including muscles, ligaments, tendons, cervical vertebrae, nerves, and vasculature. Pain referred to the neck from the temporomandibular joint, pleura, or mediastinum may also be seen. Causes of neck pain are generally structural in nature and most often are the result of trauma, degenerative changes, or muscle spasms. Stress, sedentary occupations, and improper biomechanics are frequently found to be contributing factors; questions regarding these factors should be asked during the history taking. The onset (rapid or insidious), location (arm, shoulder, head, or back), and character (sharp, dull, or aching) of the pain are essential in the differential diagnosis. Of particular note is pain (in the absence of trauma) that begins gradually and improves with rest, because infection and malignancy in the vertebrae do occur.

Physical exam of the neck begins with the evaluation of ROM, including flexion, extension, rotation, and side bending to determine limitations and the pain-producing movements. Spurling's maneuver should be used to assess nerve-root compression. (See Advanced Assessment 15.4.) This test is widely used in clinical practice; however, a review of studies assessing inter-rater reliability, sensitivity, and specificity revealed few methodologically sound studies and a need for more research on the usefulness of this test. Palpation of the neck must be done thoroughly, checking for tenderness, muscle spasm, and lymphadenopathy. Lymph nodes in the supraclavicular and axillary regions should be examined carefully; enlarged nodes in the absence of infection may indicate malignancy. Evaluate the vascular structures and the thyroid. The examination must also include a musculoskeletal and neurovascular assessment of the extremities, including assessments of the muscle strength of biceps, triceps, and handgrips. (See Advanced Assessment 15.4.) Abnormalities in sensation of any dermatome and altered deep tendon reflexes indicate cervical nerve-root compression.

Laboratory studies such as erythrocyte sedimentation rate, rheumatoid factor, or antinuclear antibody are necessary only if systemic or bone disease is suspected.

Differential Diagnosis
Torticollis

Often referred to as "wryneck," *torticollis* is a self-limiting condition that usually occurs after excessive exposure to the cold or activities that require unusual or prolonged rotation or twisting of the neck musculature. Torticollis most often occurs in young adults. Pain arises from acute muscle spasm and serves a protective function.

Questioning the patient about sleep positions and the number of pillows used may elucidate the cause of the condition. Physical examination findings in torticollis include limitation of neck flexion away from the affected side. Spasms of the sternocleidomastoid or trapezius areas are common.

Radiographic evaluation is not routinely needed, but x-ray studies may be useful if the symptoms continue past the time when improvement is expected.

Treatment involves decreased activity (which may be easiest to obtain with a soft cervical collar used intermittently for 2–3 hours at a time over the course of 2–3 days), moist heat, muscle relaxants, and any of the NSAIDs. Resolution is expected in 1 week.

Cervical Muscle Sprain/Strain and Spasm

Cervical muscle sprain/strain is a muscle injury in the neck, a common and largely self-limited condition. The soft tissue muscles of the neck are deeply buried and protected, and it is often difficult to differentiate injuries to the neck by either physical exam or more sophisticated imaging modalities. Thus, this term is also used to describe ligamentous injuries of the facet joints or intervertebral discs. After ruling out neurological dysfunction and unstable injuries, the treatments for a neck sprain or strain are similar.

Advanced Assessment 15.4   Spurling's Maneuver

To perform Spurling's maneuver (neck compression), follow this procedure:

1. With the patient's neck in extension, rotate the neck to the affected side.
2. Apply downward pressure on the head.
3. Assess for patient complaint of or accentuation of limb pain or paresthesia (a positive finding). Also observe for obvious atrophy in the neck.

"Whiplash" describes an acceleration–deceleration of the neck with rapid flexion–extension and is a common sequela of motor vehicle accidents. Despite no apparent instability, these injuries may cause prolonged disability, probably related to a combination of relatively severe ligamentous/muscle injury with nonorganic overlay.

Epidemiology and Causes

Cervical pain is common in both men and women and is usually described as lasting 2 weeks or longer. Mechanical disorders of the cervical spine are the most common cause of neck pain. Information on the prevalence and incidence of cervical pain is available from multiple sources but varies across a wide range. Consistent reporting of occurrence rates is also hampered by the lack of a reproducible definition of cervical pain across multiple studies. Terms such as *whiplash, acute neck sprain, neck spasm,* and *cervical strain* are frequently used to describe what seems to be a single condition. The prevalence of cervical pain in men and women is approximately 8% among persons aged 25 to 74 years. The highest prevalence (10%) is among persons aged 45 to 64 years. Rates are higher for whites than for blacks and other racial groups.

It has been estimated that 85% of all neck injuries presenting to primary-care providers result from automobile accidents. The National Safety Council estimates that 20% of all automobile accidents are rear-end impacts that can cause *whiplash*—an acceleration–deceleration injury related to cervical hyperextension, most commonly caused by a rear-end motor vehicle collision (MVC) occurring when the driver of a stationary car is struck from behind by another vehicle. The driver is usually relaxed and unaware of the impending collision. The sudden acceleration of the struck vehicle pushes the back of the car seat against the driver's torso. This force pushes the driver's torso and shoulders forward while the head remains static but moves posteriorly, causing hyperextension of the neck. This injury is most common in Western societies and metropolitan areas, where there are more automobiles. Approximately one-third of people will develop neck pain within 24 hours of the injury. The natural history of hyperextension cervical muscle strain and spasm injuries is that 60% get better within the first year, 32% get better within the next year, and 8% have permanent problems.

The relationship between occupational factors and cervical pain is difficult to study because exposure to those factors is usually difficult to quantify. Workers may be exposed to multiple risk factors both on the job and at home. The majority of work-related cervical injuries are diagnosed as a sprain or strain, and certain occupations appear to have a predisposition to cervical symptoms. Workers who do repetitive tasks with their upper extremities and prolonged sitting with their head in a flexed position are at risk of developing mechanical neck pain; these include machine operators, carpenters, office workers, dentists, and keyboard operators.

Pathophysiology

Cervical sprain is a clinical condition describing a nonradiating discomfort or pain in the neck area associated with a concomitant loss of neck motion and stiffness. The major biomechanical function of the cervical spine is to support the skull and provide movement in flexion, extension, and rotation. The supporting structures of the cervical spine are relatively unprotected; thus, injury to the muscles and ligaments that provide these motions can easily occur. Specific abnormalities in cervical strain can almost never be identified, except in traumatic injury to a specific structure.

Trauma to the cervical muscles that results in a strain may occur from elongation of muscle fibers with subsequent edema related to rupture of muscle tissue and secondary hemorrhage. The response of the muscle to injury is contraction, with reflex recruitment of surrounding muscles for protection (splinting) of the injured muscle. The contracted state may also occur because of poor posture, increases in muscle tension, or environmental trauma.

A *spasm* is caused by increased muscle tone that may be demonstrated by rigidity or spasticity. When a muscle cannot relax, it cannot recover from contracting. Muscle relaxation allows for restoration of internal blood flow, removal of metabolic by-products, and the influx of nutrients. Chronically contracted muscles develop subsequent ischemia and pain.

Normal posture should be effortless and painless. Abnormal forward posture of the head results in chronic strain on the posterior structures of the neck. A variety of daily activities may result in chronic abnormal posture, such as the prolonged use of a computer with a screen below eye level, a faulty sitting position, or the use of bifocal glasses.

Muscle tension is controlled by the interaction of spindle organs, Golgi's tendon organs, and extrafusal nerve fibers. A balance exists between these structures to coordinate muscular length, rate of contraction, and tension and relaxation of opposing muscles. A coordinating system in the spinal cord and the cerebral cortex influences the set point of this balance.

Muscle tone control is a multifactorial process, and the balance can be easily upset. In addition, a variety of factors extraneous to the muscles affect muscle tension, including fatigue, pain, anger, emotional stress, anxiety, and depression. Environmental trauma may lead to an acceleration–deceleration mechanism of energy transfer to the neck. The impact may result in bony or soft tissue injuries. The sternocleidomastoid, scalene, and longus coli muscles may be mildly or severely stretched or, worse, torn. In an MVC, the neck is subject to forced flexion, extension, and lateral flexion, as well as shear forces parallel to the direction of impact.

Clinical Presentation

Subjective

Pain is the most common presenting symptom although the associated complaint of a headache, usually occipital, which may persist for months, is not unusual. The pain is usually located in the middle to lower part of the posterior neck. The area of pain may be limited, or it may cover a large area. The pain may radiate toward the shoulders but usually will not radiate down into the arm. The pain associated with a cervical strain is most often a dull, aching pain that is exacerbated by neck motion and alleviated by rest or immobilization. The pain may follow a significant trauma or may be spontaneous in onset; pain following trauma often persists longer than sprains of spontaneous onset. Nonradicular, nonfocal neck pain is most common and may be noted anywhere from the base of the skull to the cervicothoracic junction. Pain is often worse with motion and may be accompanied by paraspinal spasm and discomfort in the region of the trapezius muscle. Pain may be accompanied by fatigue, sleep disturbance, irritability, and difficulty concentrating. Work tolerance may be impaired.

Cervical pain from an MVC usually does not appear for about 12 to 14 hours after the collision. The driver is often unaware at first of having been injured but later begins to feel stiffness in the neck. The pain at the base of the neck increases and is made worse by head and neck movement. Pain patterns should be evaluated carefully to differentiate muscular pain from radicular symptoms that typically radiate down the upper extremities.

Objective

Physical exam shows decreased neck ROM with poor quality of movement. With typical cervical muscle strain or spasm, Spurling's sign (radicular pain reproduced when the examiner exerts downward pressure on the vertex while tilting the head toward the symptomatic side) is usually negative.

Frequently, there is tenderness to palpation over both the anterior and posterior structures of the cervical spine, specifically the paraspinous muscles, spinous processes, interspinous ligaments, or medial border of the scapula. Pain is often noted at the extremes of motion. The neurological exam is normal in uncomplicated cases. The intensity of pain is variable and the loss of cervical motion correlates with intensity of pain. The presence of true spasm (continuous muscle contraction) is rare. Active motion of the cervical spine against any type of resistance causes an increase in pain. The shoulder exam, as well as the remainder of the physical exam, is typically normal.

Diagnostic Reasoning

Diagnostic Tests

Any evidence of neurological deficit merits further diagnostic testing (such as EMG or nerve conduction studies) to determine the cause. By definition,

hyperextension cervical injuries cause only soft tissue damage, but plain x-ray films of the cervical spine should be obtained in all instances. It is important to include radiographic studies so that unsuspected fractures or dislocations of the cervical spine, facet fractures, odontoid fractures, or spinous process fractures that might otherwise be missed in the neurologically intact patient can be identified or ruled out.

All seven cervical vertebrae must be seen. Anterior displacement of the pharyngeal air shadow indicates soft tissue swelling and possible disruption of the intervertebral disc or anterior longitudinal ligament and requires further evaluation. The width of the prevertebral soft tissue at the level of C3 should not exceed 7 mm in normal adults. The normal lordotic curve may be straightened or reversed with muscle spasm, but this limited finding is noted in approximately 10% of normal adults. Preexisting degenerative disease may be noted most frequently at C5 to C6 or C6 to C7 and is usually age related. In a patient with severe pain, the screening radiographs should be examined for signs of instability.

Differential Diagnosis

The diagnosis of cervical muscle strain is based on the history of localized neck pain and a compatible physical exam demonstrating localized pain, muscle spasm, and a normal neurological exam. Trauma to the cervical spine may result in major neural damage with paralysis; if the history reveals a significant trauma, a thorough evaluation with x-ray exam should be performed. Because of the significant consequences of potential damage to the spinal cord, referral to an orthopedic surgeon or neurosurgeon should be sought. Potential differential diagnoses include the following:

- Cervical disc herniation presents with associated radicular pain and neurological findings.
- Cervical spine tumor is accompanied by a history of night pain and weight loss.
- Cervical spine infection is accompanied by fever, sweats, and chills.
- Dislocation or subluxation of the spine would be evident on radiographs.
- Inflammatory conditions of the cervical spine (rheumatoid arthritis) would be accompanied by abnormal radiographs.
- Spinal fracture would also have abnormal radiographs.
- Malingering is accompanied by exaggerated symptomatology and evidence of secondary gain.

Management

Reassurance is a cornerstone of treatment in uncomplicated cases. The treatment of cervical muscle strain includes controlled physical activity and immobilization in a soft cervical collar, worn intermittently for 2 to 3 hours at a time for no more than 2 to 3 days. A decrease in activity allows the injured tissues to heal.

Nonnarcotic analgesics such as NSAIDs are helpful in making the patient more comfortable (see Drugs Commonly Prescribed 15.2). NSAIDs can be continued until symptoms have resolved. Long-term use of NSAIDs can lead to serious gastrointestinal disease, however, such as ulcers, gastritis, and hemorrhage. Thus, patients with gastrointestinal histories should use these drugs cautiously. Using the lowest possible effective dose can help to prevent this problem. It is particularly important to use caution in recommending doses for elderly patients who are more sensitive to the adverse effects of NSAIDs. This class of medicines affects renal and gastrointestinal prostaglandins and may cause fluid retention, edema, and increases in blood pressure; thus, patients should be monitored for weight gain. These problems may be very significant in elderly patients and in people with congestive heart failure.

Muscle relaxants may be helpful if palpable spasms are seen on physical examination, but the practitioner should use caution when prescribing them because they have a potential for addiction, and several studies have failed to show their efficacy beyond NSAIDs alone. Patients need to be aware that this class of drugs is for short-term use because the risk/benefit ratio for prolonged use of muscle relaxants is poorly established. Muscle relaxants cause drowsiness and dizziness, so patients need to avoid hazardous activities such as driving or operating machinery while using these medicines. Because these drugs are central nervous system (CNS) depressants, patients need to avoid taking them with alcohol or other CNS depressants to prevent additive effects. Dry mouth is another side effect of this anticholinergic class of drugs, so frequent mouth rinsing is recommended to prevent dental disease. Topical application of creams such as capsaicin may also help to relieve pain. Narcotic analgesics should be avoided if at all possible because very little research supports the use of narcotics in the treatment of soft tissue injuries.

Manipulation of the cervical spine is contraindicated in patients with osteoporosis, rheumatoid arthritis, carotid or vertebral atherosclerosis, or tumors. It is also contraindicated in the elderly, in patients with associated radiculopathy or myelopathy, and in those on anticoagulants.

Herbal preparations may also be used to treat the pain (see Complementary Therapies 15.1).

Neck pain and mobility are improved with physiotherapy. The goal of therapy is to maximize function of the cervical spine. Physical therapy modalities may take the form of cold (ice) initially or heat (warm bath) to help relieve pain and spasm. Activity should be encouraged as determined by the severity of the symptoms. Cervical traction may also be used to diminish pain and spasm if no improvement is seen with heat and medication. After 2 to 4 weeks of treatment with drugs and rest, if there is no significant improvement, a patient may benefit from an anesthetic injection, with or without the addition of corticosteroids. Administered only by experienced personnel, these injections can relieve pain and block reflex muscle spasms. Aerobic activity, such as walking, should be started as soon as possible. Once improvement is seen, a course of isometric exercises should begin. Encourage an early return to work and activities.

Follow-up and Referral

Usually the course of cervical muscle strain is one of progressive improvement with complete resolution of symptoms over several weeks. Recovery is usually complete without any lasting impairment; however, a small percentage of patients may continue to experience cervical spine pain despite treatment.

Complementary Therapies 15.1 Osteoarthritis and Musculoskeletal Problems

Acupuncture/Acupressure, Massage, and Bodywork Therapy

Acupuncture is used for treatment of osteoarthritis (OA) in Asia and is being used more frequently in other countries as a complementary modality for OA. Uncontrolled studies in which patients were treated with standard medical therapy and acupuncture have demonstrated significant improvement in functional status and pain relief. These findings have not been replicated in controlled studies using sham acupuncture; both groups in the controlled studies experienced marked improvement. Although further controlled studies on efficacy are needed, acupuncture can be used and is safe and well tolerated.

Acupressure is also used as an adjunct, as are various types of massage and bodywork therapy. Building on prior studies of spa therapy, a European randomized, controlled study used 3 weeks of spa therapy for older patients with OA of the lumbar spine, hip, or knee. Participants experienced significant improvement in function, decreased pain, and decreased use of analgesics and NSAIDs for 24 weeks after the final treatment. Tai-chi has also been studied as an intervention for OA.

Herbals may be used to treat the pain associated with cervical muscle sprain/strain and spasm. White willow is considered nature's aspirin and has been used in China since ancient times to relieve pain and inflammation. These herbs can be made into teas by using powder to brew. Care must be taken to follow directions regarding the amount needed and how often they are used, because renal and gastrointestinal side effects may occur. Massage may be especially helpful. Acupuncture or acupressure may also be considered as adjunctive therapy for patients with chronic cervical spine pain.

Continued

Complementary Therapies 15.1   Osteoarthritis and Musculoskeletal Problems—cont'd

The following table describes complementary therapies for different musculoskeletal problems:

Problem and Therapy	Indication	Adverse Reaction and Prescribing Consideration
Arthritis		
Turmeric	Used for anti-inflammatory and antioxidant properties	If allergic or hypersensitive to turmeric, curcumin, yellow food colorings, or plants belonging to the Zingiberaceae (ginger) family, do not use. Caution with a history of bleeding disorders, immune system deficiencies, liver disease, diabetes, hypoglycemia, or gallstones. Caution with blood thinners, such as warfarin and diabetes medications. Stop before surgery. May interfere with cancer chemotherapy agents.
Niacin (vitamin B$_3$; niacinamide)	Anti-inflammatory properties; decreases joint inflammation	Avoid with a history of liver disease or dysfunction, irregular heartbeats, heart disease, bleeding disorders, asthma, anxiety, panic attacks, thyroid disorders, stomach ulcers, gout, or diabetes.
S-adenosylmethionine (SAMe)	Pain reduction in arthritis; comparable to NSAIDs in efficacy in some studies	Avoid if allergic or hypersensitive to SAMe. Avoid with bipolar disorder. Use cautiously with diabetes, anxiety disorders, or during the third trimester of pregnancy. Avoid during the first trimester of pregnancy or if breastfeeding.
Selenium	Controls free radicals that may destroy cartilage	Avoid with history of nonmelanoma skin cancer; poor evidence of benefit.
Chondroitin	Pain reduction, increased function, and decreased use of anti-inflammatory drugs if used over a 6- to 24-month period	Avoid with prostate cancer or an increased risk of prostate cancer. Avoid if pregnant or breastfeeding. Use cautiously if allergic or hypersensitive to chondroitin sulfate products or with shellfish allergy. Use cautiously with bleeding disorders or if taking blood thinners such as warfarin.
Glucosamine	Pain relief in mild to moderate knee OA. Conflicting results in studies, one specific brand has been used	Avoid if allergic to shellfish or iodine; caution if diabetes or history of bleeding. Avoid in pregnancy.
Green tea	Reduce inflammation and slow cartilage breakdown	Contains caffeine.
Methylsulfonylmethane (MSM)	May inhibit transmission of pain impulses and has anti-inflammatory properties	Used alone or in combination with glucosamine for OA. The combination may provide pain relief and decrease inflammation; further studies needed.
Carpal Tunnel Syndrome		
Turmeric	See previous reference	
Muscle Cramps		
Magnesium	Necessary for muscle contraction and relaxation	
Musculoskeletal Pain		
White willow bark (Salix alba)	Has analgesic and anti-inflammatory properties; salicin is the active ingredient that the body converts to salicylic acid	Similar adverse effects as aspirin but not as pronounced; GI bleeding, abdominal pain, potential (rare) interference with platelet aggregation.
SAMe	See above.	
Sprains/Strains		
Arnica	Pain relief and healing; topical gel, cream, ointment	Do not use orally; toxic.
Glucosamine	Strengthen joints and accelerate healing	See above; further research needed.

If symptoms persist longer than 4 weeks after injury, further evaluation with CT scans or MRI is indicated. If these tests are normal, the patient can be assured that no compression of neural structures is present and can be strongly encouraged to increase activity. If imaging findings are abnormal, a referral to a neurologist, neurosurgeon, or orthopedic surgeon should be made for further evaluation.

If neck pain and restricted ROM are still present after patients have received analgesics and physical therapy and the findings on CT scan or MRI are normal, referrals for psychiatric support or vocational rehabilitation may be indicated to assist in recovery.

Patient Education

Knowing how a healthy neck works can help patients understand their cervical spine problems and how to care for them. It is important for patients to understand the concepts behind their treatments in order to receive the greatest benefits. They must also learn appropriate body mechanics to help protect the cervical spine from further damage by preventing its misuse or overuse. Stress from home or work can also lead to muscle tension and other symptoms, so the patient may need professional guidance in relieving or controlling these stressors.

Cervical Spondylosis

Cervical spondylosis (also known as *degenerative arthritis in the cervical vertebrae*) is a common cause of neck pain in older patients. Degenerative changes on radiography are found in 40% of the population at age 50 and in 70% of the population at age 65. These changes are usually asymptomatic, meaning that a finding on x-ray study does not necessarily account for the patient's pain. Progression of the osteoarthritis may result in subluxation, osteophyte formation, and disc protrusion.

Common symptoms are recurring neck stiffness and mild aching discomfort. There is pain and limited ROM with lateral rotation and lateral flexion of the neck toward the affected side. Paresthesias may also occur.

Radiographs will determine if subluxation and other osteoarthritic components are present, but an MRI will be necessary to identify disc herniation and soft tissue or spinal cord abnormalities.

Hallmarks of treatment are the use of NSAIDs, a conditioning program, and reeducation to result in better care of the neck.

When the secondary bony changes of cervical spondylosis encroach on the spinal cord, a pathological process called *myelopathy* develops. If this process involves both the nerve roots and spinal cord, it is called *myeloradiculopathy*. Regardless of its etiology, radiculopathy causes shoulder and/or arm pain, as well as numbness and/or tingling ("pins and needles"). Fewer than 5% of patients with cervical spondylosis develop myelopathy, and they are usually between ages 40 and 60. Acute myelopathy is most often the result of central soft-disc herniation that produces a high-grade block, which may be visualized on myelogram. This herniation may require surgical decompression and is a medical emergency. If pain is unremitting and cervical nerve-root compression is present, a neurosurgical consultation should be sought immediately.

■ MYOFASCIAL PAIN

Regional musculoskeletal pain or tender muscles are often the result of minor muscle tears following injury and are referred to as *myofascial pain,* meaning inflammation of a muscle and its fascia. Although the cause may not be readily identifiable, the pain is a result of local inflammation and produces a tender "trigger point" when a particular muscle group is palpated. The pain may radiate to surrounding structures. Even though this is a common cause of nonarticular rheumatic pain, it is often misdiagnosed. The trigger points are not visualized on routine imaging studies and cannot be objectively substantiated. There are commonalities between this disorder and fibromyalgia. (See Chapter 17.)

Treatment includes identifying and eliminating aggravating factors, injecting the trigger points with 1% procaine, and passive stretching of the muscle involved immediately after the local anesthetic has taken effect. Some patients achieve relief with a pharmacological regimen that includes NSAIDs and antidepressants, particularly amitriptyline, which appears to reduce pain and improve sleep. Some sources recommend sedatives such as clonazepam (Klonopin) to help relax muscles affected by myofascial pain syndrome. Sedatives must be used carefully because they can cause sleepiness and can be habit forming.

■ SHOULDER PAIN

Pain and dysfunction localizing in and around the shoulder girdle are common presenting musculoskeletal complaints. Shoulder pain affects patients of various ages and activity levels. Although shoulder pain can be referred from the neck, chest, or diaphragmatic region, it is most commonly caused by a local process. The shoulder joint includes three large bones (clavicle, scapula, and humerus) and four joints (sternoclavicular, acromioclavicular, glenohumeral, and thoracoscapular). The shoulder is a ball-and-socket joint, like the hip, but the two joints differ significantly in that the hip is a weight-bearing joint and the shoulder is a suspension joint, maximizing mobility. The two chief presenting complaints are usually related to pain and/or instability. Symptoms of decreased motion, power, or function can accompany complaints of pain or instability, but they are rarely the chief complaint.

Common conditions affecting the shoulder include acute injuries (less than 2 weeks' duration; common in younger patients), which include fractures, dislocations, and acute tendon rupture; chronic or repetitive injuries (impingement syndromes, most rotator cuff tears and biceps tendon ruptures); and degenerative, inflammatory, or idiopathic conditions (glenohumeral and acromio-clavicular arthritis, frozen shoulder). Although there have been many technological advances in diagnostic aids, most shoulder disorders can be diagnosed with careful history, clinical exam, and plain radiographs.

In the history, inquire about any precipitating injury and onset of pain. Obtain specific information about the location of the pain and the factors that aggravate or alleviate it. The relationship of the pain to the time of day, to active or passive movement, and to body position is significant. The patient's age, occupation, activities, medical history, and social factors will also be important in making a diagnosis. Patients with acute symptoms (less than 2 weeks' duration) usually have an injury, such as a fracture, dislocation, or rotator cuff tear. For patients with chronic shoulder pain, evaluate the activities related to the onset of symptoms.

Instability, another common complaint, can be classified by the frequency of symptomatic episodes, as well as the direction and degree of instability. Acute injuries may be a first-time dislocation or a recurrent episode. The instability episode may be partial (subluxation) with spontaneous reduction or may be complete (dislocation). The instability may be anterior, posterior, inferior, or multidirectional. Most traumatic dislocations are anterior. Multidirectional instability should be considered in patients who present with recurrent episodes of subluxations or dislocations and no history of significant trauma.

Determine if there is a discrepancy between active and passive motion. Disuse can cause some passive ROM loss; equal losses of active and passive ROM can be secondary to soft tissue contracture, as in frozen shoulder, or the result of joint incongruity from trauma or arthritis.

Muscle strength should be assessed and compared with the opposite shoulder. Pain can affect the accuracy of muscle testing. Tears of rotator cuffs and neurological injury can produce weakness. Assess functional status, although this may be affected by motivation and ability to adapt to impairment. The level of functional disability will depend on the normal intensity of activities that the patient performs.

A concise differential diagnosis is often obtained by evaluating the patient's chief complaint in the context of its chronicity and the patient's age. Patients younger than 30 years of age, for example, commonly present with traumatic injuries or instability such as gleno-humeral dislocations and acromioclavicular (AC) joint separation. Impingement syndromes and rotator cuff tears are more commonly seen in middle-aged patients. These must be distinguished from frozen shoulder, which produces a global loss of passive and active ROM. Glenohumeral dislocations are much less common and

must be treated with a high index of suspicion for a concomitant rotator cuff tear (50% of patients older than 40 years of age will have an acute tear). Older patients (over 55) are more likely to have rotator cuff tears or degenerative arthritis. Fractures and dislocations related to falls also occur in this age group.

The physical exam of the shoulder should begin with inspection of the shoulder for swelling, color, edema, and symmetry, followed by palpation for tender areas, crepitus, temperature, and deformity. The shoulder should be inspected anteriorly and posteriorly, particularly to observe scapular winging. Both active and passive ROM movements should be tested while comparing the painful shoulder to the unaffected side.

The most common ROM movements tested include the following:

- The Apley scratch test: This measures abduction and external rotation by having the patient reach behind the head and touch the superior aspect of the opposite scapula. Conversely, internal rotation and adduction of the shoulder are tested by having the patient reach behind the back and touch the inferior aspect of the opposite scapula. External rotation should be measured with the patient's arms at the side and elbows flexed to 90 degrees.
- Internal/external in flexion: With the patient's elbow flexed at the side, thumb pointing up, internally and externally rotate the elbow, taking care to keep the elbow against the body.
- Internal/external in abduction: Abduct the patient's shoulder to 90 degrees, keeping the elbow flexed at 90 degrees, and then have the patient lower his or her forearm from the horizontal plane, then raise the forearm, keeping the upper arm parallel to the ground.

Pain with abduction from 45 to 120 degrees (painful arc) indicates supraspinatus tendinitis or subacromial bursitis, which are early rotator cuff injuries. Muscle and bursae involvement produces pain only on active motion, whereas pain with passive ROM may involve tendons, bursae, or restricted joint movement and is generally indicative of more pathology. Resistive muscle testing, reflex testing, and an assessment of the neurosensory and neurovascular status complete the exam.

Specific findings can include inability to shrug the shoulders, which indicates trapezius muscle weakness, and weakness of forward flexion, which is associated with rotator cuff impingement. Because shoulder pain can be referred from other areas, the patient should be evaluated for cardiac, pulmonary, and abdominal causes, as well as neurological disease or injury. Pain caused by bony malignancy is usually gnawing, constant, and unrelated to movement. Malignant tumor is usually evident by a lytic lesion in the bone on x-ray film.

Plain x-ray films, including the anteroposterior (AP) projection and an axillary lateral view, are sufficient to reveal most fractures and dislocations. Additional views may include a transthoracic lateral, which images the glenohumeral joint at a 45-degree posterior oblique, or a 60-degree anterior oblique (Y view). A new view—the apical oblique—is suggested to reveal shoulder instability. This view is simple to obtain and painless for the patient. In addition to the standard x-ray studies, other diagnostic tests used in diagnosing shoulder pain include MRI, arthrography, and (if nerve involvement is suspected) EMG. Although the standard x-ray studies will often be normal, they should be done to rule out structural abnormalities, especially if there is history of trauma or if the problem is persistent. C-spine films and chest films may also be necessary if involvement in those areas is suspected. Laboratory studies should be done in accordance with the patient's history.

Differential Diagnosis

Shoulder disorders may be separated into acute versus chronic and traumatic versus nontraumatic. Problems in young adults are frequently the result of instability and traumatic injuries and tendinitis. The mature adult usually suffers with degenerative conditions of the tendons and joints.

Adhesive Capsulitis

Often referred to as a "frozen shoulder," adhesive capsulitis is defined as idiopathic loss of both active and passive ROM, with no clear predisposition based on gender, arm dominance, or occupation. Patients aged 40 to 60 years are more likely to be affected; diabetes mellitus (especially type 1) is the most common risk factor. Patients with diabetes tend to be refractory to treatment, and 40% to 50% will have bilateral involvement. Other underlying conditions related to frozen shoulder include hypothyroidism, Dupuytren disease, cervical disc herniation, Parkinson's disease, stroke, and tumors. In a short period of time, immobility will result in a tight, painful shoulder joint that has limited active ROM (a "freezing" phase of pain) and then typically progresses to a "thawing" phase of decreasing discomfort associated with a steady improvement in function. This process may take anywhere from 6 months to 2 years. Although adhesive capsulitis may result from any condition that produces pain and immobility, in older patients and individuals without predisposing factors, the possibility of underlying organic or neoplastic disease should be considered.

Physical exam typically reveals a 50% or more reduction in both active and passive ROM. Pain and tenderness are common with motion and at the deltoid insertion. Diffuse tenderness about the shoulder may also be present. AP and axillary radiographs of the shoulder are indicated to ensure that smooth, concentric joint surfaces with an intact cartilage space are present and to rule out other pathology such as osteophytes, loose bodies, calcium deposits, or tumors. Other studies, such

as arthrography, CT, or MRI, are rarely indicated if radiographs are normal.

Adhesive capsulitis is differentiated from chronic posterior shoulder dislocation, tumor, and osteoarthritis (OA) on radiograph. Post-traumatic shoulder stiffness is, obviously, related to a history of trauma. Rotator cuff tear is differentiated because of the presence of normal passive ROM.

Treatment consists of the application of moist heat, use of analgesics (NSAIDs and nonnarcotic analgesics), followed by a gentle stretching program, performed at home three to four times a day (should not cause significant pain). Advise the patient of lengthy recovery time and potential for chronic stiffness and residual pain.

Rotator Cuff Syndrome

Rotator cuff syndrome may include impingement problems, calcific tendinitis, and subacromial bursitis (shoulder bursitis). The term *impingement syndrome* refers to pathological changes that result when the subacromial bursa and/or rotator cuff become inflamed as a result of compression under the acromion or "roof" of the shoulder joint (rotator cuff tendinitis). It is the leading cause of shoulder pain, ranging from bursitis to rotator cuff tendinitis and, eventually, degenerative tears of the rotator cuff. In addition, the biceps tendon may be impinged (in bicipital tendinitis).

The rotator cuff covers the anterior, superior, and posterior aspects of the humoral head and is formed by the coming together of four muscles. These muscles assist in the elevation of the arm. Inflammation of the subacromial bursa and underlying rotator cuff tendons is a common cause of shoulder pain in middle-aged patients. Rotator cuff pathology presents a continuum from edema and hemorrhage to chronic inflammation and fibrosis to microscopic tendon fiber failure progressing to full-thickness rotator cuff tears. The etiology is multifactorial. A loss of microvascular blood supply to the tendon and repeated mechanical insults as the tendon passes under the coracoacromial arch combine to cause damage over time.

The history is usually one of gradual onset of anterior and lateral shoulder pain exacerbated by overhead activity. Night pain and difficulty sleeping on the affected side are also common. Atrophy of the muscles about the top and back of the shoulder may be apparent if the patient has had problems over a period of several months, although this may also indicate a full-blown rotator cuff tear.

On physical exam, palpation over the greater tuberosity and subacromial bursa commonly elicits tenderness and crepitus with shoulder motion. Pain will be elicited by having the patient slowly lower the abducted arm against downward resistance. Neer and Hawkins signs are generally positive. Impingement testing involves locally anesthetizing the shoulder. If the patient is then stronger and without pain after subacromial injection, pain inhibition from inflammation and fibrosis is likely rather than full-blown tear. AP and axillary radiographs are usually negative; narrowing of the space between the head of the humerus and the undersurface of the acromion suggests a long-standing rotator cuff tear.

Frozen shoulder is ruled out if active and passive ROM loss is not present; a rotator cuff tear will not improve with subacromial injection of local anesthetic; glenohumeral arthritis is evident on radiograph and there is pain on motion; acromioclavicular (AC) arthritis presents with tenderness over the AC joint.

Treatment includes resting from the offending activity and NSAIDs. The patient should begin a stretching program with emphasis on posterior capsule stretching. If home therapy of three to four times a day over a period of 6 weeks does not result in improvement, a subacromial corticosteroid injection can be administered, followed by continued stretching. Steroid injections should not be repeated if the previous injection does not produce significant and sustained (more than 2 months) relief. Significant rotator cuff weakness or failure to improve after 2 to 3 months of rehabilitation (with or without subacromial steroid injection) is an indication for further evaluation and operative consideration.

Calcific Tendinitis

Calcific tendinitis is a degenerative process accompanied by a local deposit of calcium that develops in the rotator cuff. The calcified material often creates inflammatory changes in the subdeltoid bursa and is frequently asymptomatic until an acute event or overuse exacerbates the condition. The symptom of calcific tendinitis is severe, localized pain that occurs with any movement of the shoulder. With the arm in a dependent position, the pain is absent or minimal. The shoulder is acutely tender and can be warm to the touch or swollen. X-ray films usually demonstrate the deposit. A transaxillary view is necessary if the deposit is anterior or posterior to the joint in the subscapularis muscle.

Minor or mild cases of calcific tendinitis rarely need invasive treatment. Anti-inflammatory medications, ultrasound, physical therapy, and rest are usually effective in ameliorating the pain. Some deposits appear soft, fluffy, or irregular on x-ray examination. Aspiration to remove some of the material while concurrently injecting an anesthetic with corticosteroid preparation can provide immediate relief. In more severe cases or those that fail to respond to conservative treatment, consider injection of corticosteroid.

Rotator Cuff Tear

Rotator cuff tear may occur secondary to trauma or from degenerative, calcific changes, chronic mechanical impingement, and altered blood supply to the tendons over time. The rotator cuff muscles insert into the tuberosities of the humerus and tightly hold the ball-and-socket joint of the shoulder together. Rotator cuff injuries are considered to be more serious than other soft tissue injuries

of the shoulder. Most full-thickness rotator cuff tears occur spontaneously in patients older than 50 years of age, presumably as a result of age-related changes in vascularity and tissue degeneration. The supraspinatus tendon is most often affected. Older people with rotator cuff tear may have only mild, disabling symptoms, or may even be asymptomatic. This injury can occur in individuals younger than 40 years of age, usually as a result of aggressive physical injury and repeated trauma from contact sports (e.g., football).

The patient will usually report a lateral deltoid pain, and weakness may be present. There may be a history of reaching overhead and feeling "something give" in the shoulder and then noting that the ipsilateral arm drops to the side. Thereafter it is difficult and very painful to abduct the arm. The pain is often worse at night, and the patient may report difficulty sleeping. To reach behind to scratch his or her back causes extreme pain.

The "empty can" test also isolates the mechanism of the rotator cuff. The patient's affected arm is abducted to 90 degrees, in neutral rotation (the thumb is pointed toward the ground). The patient is instructed to turn his or her arm and hand forward as if emptying a can. The examiner places his or her fingers on the outstretched arm near the hand and applies pressure, seeing if the patient can maintain position against resistance.

A suspected rotator cuff tear can be confirmed by performing the "drop arm" test. The examiner abducts the patient's shoulder to 90 degrees and instructs the patient to lower his or her arm slowly. If the arm drops to the side rapidly, the test is considered positive. Most tears are relatively small, however, and the patient is often able to maintain some control. It is clinically very difficult to differentiate tendinitis from a tear. The back of the shoulder may appear sunken, indicating atrophy of the supraspinatus and infraspinatus muscles following a long-standing cuff tear.

Soft tissue injuries do not show up on plain x-rays; therefore, findings are usually reported as within normal limits even though the films may demonstrate calcification from previous or chronic injuries. There may be spurring of the acromion process or calcium deposits in the soft tissue, as well as bony deformities from previous dislocations. Lytic lesions indicating metastatic disease can also show up on radiography. More aggressive diagnostic testing such as MRI, ultrasonography, or arthrography may be indicated in patients with a history of acute trauma or if there is no response to conservative treatment.

Nonoperative treatment includes icing the shoulder (most commonly in cases of acute injury), NSAIDs, physical therapy with stretching and strengthening exercises, and avoiding overhead activities. Ice the entire shoulder for 15 to 20 minutes twice daily. Corticosteroid injections should be used judiciously. Over time, steroid injections further weaken the tendon and can actually accelerate propagation of the rotator cuff tear. Patients should never receive more than three subacromial injections. Patients with significant failure and failed rehabilitation should be considered candidates for surgery. The exception to this rule is the patient younger than age 60 who has an acute traumatic cuff tear, in whom recovery is best accomplished within 6 weeks of the injury.

Degenerative Arthritis

Arthritis of the glenohumeral or AC joints can occur, but it generally is not isolated to the shoulders unless there is a history of old injury such as a dislocation or fracture. The common complaint is diffuse or deep-seated pain, aggravated by any strenuous activity. As the disease progresses any movement can cause the shoulder pain, and rest and night pain become prominent complaints. ROM may become progressively limited. As a result, activities of daily living, such as dressing, combing hair, and reaching overhead, are increasingly difficult. OA typically involves a single joint in an older patient, and generally there is no apparent relationship between the development of OA in the shoulder and the patient's previous activity level. Physical exam may reveal atrophy of the shoulder muscles; palpation elicits tenderness over the front and back of the shoulder. Crepitus is commonly present with rotation or flexion; ROM is usually decreased.

AP and lateral radiographs are indicated. The axillary view will demonstrate joint space narrowing that is indicative of cartilage destruction; there may be flattening of the humeral head, an inferior osteophyte, and posterior erosion of the glenoid. Treatment includes NSAIDs and application of heat and/or ice to relieve symptoms, and gentle stretching exercises to preserve motion. A trial of glucosamine and/or chondroitin sulfate can be considered, although their efficacy needs further evaluation. Activity modifications are beneficial in reducing pain. For advanced arthritis, total shoulder replacement may offer a very satisfactory solution.

Shoulder Dislocations

Shoulder dislocations are a common injury, occurring most frequently in younger adults. The mechanism of injury may be direct or indirect, usually with the arm in extension. There is often an obvious fullness of the anterior capsule on exam and a positive sulcus sign (space under the acromion). In an acute anterior dislocation, pain is severe and ROM is limited. The patient will usually hold the arm slightly abducted and externally rotated. There may be associated neurovascular and/or neurosensory trauma; therefore, the clinician should check the distal pulses and sensation, especially over the deltoid. Posterior dislocations are less common (2%) and less apparent. Deformity is minimal, but any motion of the extremity will cause severe pain. Recurrent dislocations can occur and do not require as severe a force as the initial injury. Reduction is usually the treatment of choice; occasionally, surgery is necessary.

Shoulder Fractures

Fractures of the humerus, clavicle, or acromion are common. Fracture of the clavicle typically occurs from a moderate fall (such as from a bicycle or down stairs) or from blows during a contact sport. Patients complain of sharp shoulder pain and are reluctant to move the upper extremity. It is important to verify that no neck pain or upper extremity paresthesias are present. These fractures usually best heal spontaneously after proper immobilization; they rarely require surgery.

Shoulder Sprains

Acromioclavicular joint (ACJ) sprain is classified as first, second, or third degree, depending on severity. These shoulder sprains often occur in young men, and are typically associated with a fall while the arm was adducted, causing trauma to the ACJ, although the injury may occur as a result of indirect trauma also. The patient will present with pain, especially on adduction or abduction past 90 degrees, point tenderness over the ACJ, swelling, and possible deformity. First-degree sprains involve a partial tear of the ACJ, whereas second-degree sprains involve a complete tear of the AC ligament and a partial disruption of the coracoclavicular ligament. In a third-degree ACJ sprain, both the AC and coracoclavicular ligaments are torn, and there is obvious displacement of the distal clavicle. X-ray confirmation can be sought. Treatment includes ice, NSAIDs, and a sling or figure-8 splint for 2 to 4 weeks, with daily gentle assisted ROM exercises. Patients with third-degree sprains should be referred to an orthopedic specialist.

Shoulder–Hand Syndrome

Shoulder–hand syndrome, also referred to as *reflex sympathetic dystrophy,* occurs as a complication of minor or major trauma, hemiplegia, myocardial infarction, pneumonia, or peripheral neuropathy. It is more common in elderly patients and is manifested by pain and stiffness in the affected hand. The pain is described as burning and is worsened by light touch and improved with application of cool moisture. The hand or shoulder is often mildly swollen and discolored, and abnormal diaphoresis of the affected areas may be noted. Treatment is early active and passive mobilization and use of NSAIDs. If necessary, a brief course of corticosteroids can be considered.

A summary of common differential diagnoses for shoulder pain is provided in Differential Diagnosis 15.3.

ARM (ELBOW, WRIST, AND HAND) PAIN

Pain in the upper extremity can be caused by problems in the elbow, wrist, or hand. These can be caused by trauma, nerve impairment, joint, muscle, bursa, or

Differential Diagnosis 15.3   Shoulder Pain

Musculoskeletal problems	Adhesive capsulitis (frozen shoulder)
	Rotator cuff syndrome
	Impingement
	Calcific tendinitis
	Subacromial bursitis
	Degenerative arthritis: glenohumeral, acromio-clavicular
Trauma	Fractures: Humerus, clavicle, acromion
	Acromioclavicular joint sprains
	Rotator cuff tear
	Dislocation: Glenohumeral
	Nerve injuries: Compression
Neurovascular problems	Reflex sympathetic dystrophy (shoulder–hand syndrome)
	Thoracic outlet syndrome
	Cervical root compression
	Brachial plexus injury
Systemic disease	Inflammatory disease
	Cancer

tendon disruption or inflammation. Infection is always a possibility, and gout (which can sometimes affect the elbow) is another consideration.

■ ELBOW PROBLEMS

Usually, elbow complaints in the adult occur as a result of overuse. The most commonly seen complaint is lateral epicondylitis of the humerus. Although this condition is often called "tennis elbow," it occurs frequently in patients who do not play tennis. It is associated with repeated extension of the wrist and pronation and supination of the forearm, particularly against resistance, which occurs in movements such as opening jars, hammering, and turning doorknobs. The common complaint is pain in the elbow that radiates into the forearm. There is pain and weakness with gripping objects ("coffee cup" sign). Tenderness is present over the lateral epicondyle, and wrist extension against resistance produces the pain. Rest, ice, NSAIDs, and physical therapy are generally effective; corticosteroid injections and wrist splinting may be considered in some cases and have been shown to be effective for short-term relief of lateral epicondylitis. Physical therapy is more efficacious than steroid injection if symptoms persist longer than 6 weeks (Stephens et al, 2008).

Medial epicondylitis is less common; this condition is often referred to as "golfer's elbow." It is a result of overuse or strain of the muscle group arising from the medial epicondyle, which is used in wrist flexion. Tenderness and pain is over the medial epicondyle and is exacerbated by wrist flexion. Diagnosis is by clinical exam only, and treatment is the same as for lateral epicondylitis.

Bursitis of the olecranon is often the cause of pain and swelling in the posterior aspect of the elbow. This may occur with forced extension of the elbow joint. Range of motion is generally normal, but caution is needed to rule out a septic bursitis. Monitor for fever, redness, heat, and warmth at the site. Synovial fluid aspiration can provide evidence of infection. Radiography is indicated to exclude bone infection.

Treatment may include ice for 15 to 20 minutes several times a day and rest. Assessment of position of computer keyboards or other workstation corrections may be helpful. NSAIDs are useful, and splinting with an elbow strap may ease pain by exerting counterpressure on the soft tissue below the lateral epicondyle, or short-term use of a wrist splint may reduce pain from lateral epicondylitis. An anterior elbow splint may be useful for medial epicondylitis management. Corticosteroid injection may be necessary. Refer to physical and/or occupational therapy. These measures are effective in 80% of cases. If the patient is still symptomatic, referral to a specialist is warranted. Surgical procedures are a last resort.

■ WRIST PROBLEMS

Wrist and hand problems may be assessed using Allen's test, Phalen's maneuver, the percussion test for Tinel's sign, and/or Finkelstein's test (see Advanced Assessment 15.5).

Wrist Injuries

Wrist injuries are common after falling on an outstretched hand. Patients present after trauma with pain and swelling in the distal forearm or wrist. Numbness may be present if the medial nerve is affected. The mechanism of injury will often provide important clues to the diagnosis. The exam begins with gentle palpation to locate the area of point tenderness and includes a thorough neurovascular assessment. A radiograph of the wrist (including an oblique view) will be necessary to rule out fracture. Common fractures are the Colles' fracture of the distal radius and the navicular (scaphoid) fracture of the anatomical snuffbox. It is not unusual to have a navicular fracture missed on radiography, so an orthopedic referral should be provided when the presenting complaint is pain and trauma to the soft tissue area of the anatomical snuffbox.

A common wrist ligamental injury is an ulnar collateral ligament tear at the base of the thumb. Often seen with ski-pole injury, this condition is related to repetitive gripping, and surgery is necessary to repair a tear in this area. Therefore, when the presenting complaint is pain and trauma to the proximal thumb, an orthopedic referral for stress testing is appropriate even if the x-ray result is negative.

Advanced Assessment 15.5 Tests for Wrist and Hand Problems

Test	Comments
Allen's test	*Purpose:* Assesses patency of radial and ulnar arteries and the arterial arch. *Procedure:* Compress the radial artery at the wrist. Have patient rapidly open and close his or her hand several times. Then have the patient open the hand. (Hand should be pale or white.) Release pressure from the artery. The hand should flush, indicating patency.
Phalen's test	*Purpose:* Assesses for median nerve compression. *Procedure:* Have the patient maintain forced flexion of the wrist for 1 minute or more, with the dorsal surface of each hand pressed together. If the patient complains of numbness and paresthesias in fingers, the test is considered positive.
Tinel's sign	*Purpose:* Assesses for compression neuropathy. *Procedure:* Percuss the median nerve at the wrist. If the patient complains of tingling in the digits (positive Tinel's sign), compression at the site of percussion is likely.
Finkelstein's test	*Purpose:* Assesses for de Quervain's disease. *Procedure:* Have patient touch thumb into palm and make a fist. Test is positive if moving the wrist into ulnar deviation causes pain.

Ganglion

A *ganglion* is a cyst that develops on or in a tendon sheath. It is filled with a thick, gel-like material that leaks from the joint into the weakened tendon sheath and forms a cyst sac. A ganglionic cyst is usually caused by frequent strains and contusions, resulting in joint inflammation. The most common sites are on the dorsum of the wrist over the radiocarpal joint or on the volar surface of the wrist near the flexor carpi radialis tendon. The ganglion can be asymptomatic, or it may be associated with dull aching and weakness. It can be distinguished from a tumor by its soft consistency and transillumination. Treatment includes aspiration or surgical removal, although a conservative approach is appropriate because spontaneous disappearance may occur.

Carpal Tunnel Syndrome

Carpal tunnel syndrome (CTS) is the most common entrapment neuropathy, affecting approximately 3% to 6% of adults. Symptoms are related to compression of the median nerve, which results in pain, paresthesias, numbness and tingling, and associated weakness in the hand and wrist that radiate to the thumb, index finger, middle finger, and radial half of the ring finger. (See full discussion of CTS later in this chapter.)

Hand Problems

When assessing and/or treating a patient with an injured hand, have the patient remove all rings as soon as possible. Inflammation secondary to most injuries will precipitate edema, making removal of rings difficult. A tight-fitting ring may cause arterial compression and ischemia if not removed. Usually soap or lubricant jelly will be sufficient to remove the ring. If this does not work, several other techniques may be used. (See Therapeutic Procedure 15.2.)

Osteoarthritis and Rheumatoid Arthritis

Although both osteoarthritis and rheumatoid arthritis affect the phalanges, the different types of arthritis occur in different locations. *Rheumatoid arthritis* usually presents as bilateral pain, swelling, and stiffness of the metacarpophalangeal and proximal interphalangeal (PIP) joints with characteristic deformities. Generally, other systemic complaints will occur, and joints other than just those in the hand will be affected as well. (See Chapter 17 for a full discussion of rheumatoid arthritis.) *Osteoarthritis* affects the distal interphalangeal joints (Heberden's nodes) and PIP joints (Bouchard's nodes) and presents with swelling, stiffness, pain, and deformity.

■ LOW BACK PAIN

Low back pain (LBP), also referred to as low back sprain or lumbar sprain, is, strictly speaking, an injury to the paravertebral spinal muscles. The term is also used to describe ligamentous injuries to the facet joints or anulus fibrosus. The disc may not herniate into the spinal canal, but substances can leak from the nucleus pulposus that induce inflammation and cause irritation of the lumbosacral nerve roots. Owing to the deep location of the lumbar soft tissues, localizing an injury to a specific structure is very difficult if not impossible. Whether muscle or ligamentous structures are involved, the treatment is similar.

LBP is also defined as activity intolerance because of lower back or back-related leg symptoms of less than 3 months' duration. LBP occurs in almost 70% of adults at some point in their lives. About 90% of patients with

Therapeutic Procedure 15.2   Removing Rings

Equipment: 2–0 or 3–0 nylon suture (string technique), rubber tourniquet (tourniquet technique), lubricant (tourniquet technique), mechanical ring cutter (ring cutter technique)

String Technique

1. In a distal direction, wrap 2–0 or 3–0 nylon suture tightly around the finger just distal to the ring.

2. Slip the proximal end of the string under the ring.
3. Pull the proximal end of the suture over the ring and firmly retract it distally over the axis of the finger. As each coil of the suture unwinds, it pulls the ring slightly over the coiled suture until it is free.

Tourniquet Technique

1. Carefully wrap the finger with a rubber tourniquet, starting at the fingertip and working up to the edge of the ring.
2. Have the patient lie supine on the exam table, with his or her arm pointed straight upward at the ceiling for about 5 minutes.
3. As soon as the patient lowers his arm, remove the tourniquet, apply copious amounts of lubricant, and slide the ring off.

Mechanical Ring Cutter Technique

1. Advise patient that the ring will be cut and obtain his or her consent.

2. Follow the manufacturer's directions.
Postprocedure: Give ring to patient, or secure as per institution policy and document.

acute LBP will spontaneously recover activity tolerance within 1 month. However, back pain associated with a neurological deficit, decreased or absent pulses, or bowel and bladder dysfunction is potentially life threatening and warrants immediate referral. Acute low back pain (ALBP) is pain that persists for less than 3 to 6 weeks. Chronic low back pain (CLBP) is defined as pain lasting longer than 3 months; symptoms are typically recurrent and episodic, but may be unremitting.

Epidemiology and Causes

LBP occurs in almost 70% of adults at some point in their lives. LBP is one of the most frequent reasons that patients visit primary-care providers and is the most common reason for loss of work time and disability in adults younger than 45 years. Most symptoms are of limited duration, with 85% of patients demonstrating significant improvement and returning to work within the month. The 4% of patients whose symptoms persist longer than 6 months generate 85% to 90% of the costs to society for treating LBP. Repetitive episodes, however, are common. Back pain is second only to headache as the reason for a complaint of pain. At any given time, 31 million Americans will be experiencing some sort of ALBP. ALBP occurs most frequently in adults between their 20s and 40s; CLBP typically is seen between the third and sixth decades of life, or even older for women.

The overall incidence of LBP is equal in men and women, but women report more LBP after age 60, most likely due to osteoporosis; these women are at risk for vertebral compression fracture. In addition, a woman's likelihood of experiencing LBP is increased after two or more pregnancies. Approximately 2% of patients with ALBP have lumbar radiculopathy, or "sciatica" and/or disc herniation (see next section on herniated disc).

There are two categories of risk factors that influence LBP: The first group of risk factors is occupational, and the second is patient related. Occupations that require hard labor and heavy exertion have been associated with increased risk of LBP. Lifting, pulling and pushing, twisting, slipping, sitting for an extended period, and exposure to prolonged vibration (such as driving or riding in a motor vehicle for long periods of time, as truck drivers do) have been attributed to the development of LBP. In addition, patients who view their occupations as boring, repetitious, or dissatisfying have been associated with a higher rate of LBP. LBP is the most frequent cause of lost workdays in the United States.

There is a higher risk of LBP in obese persons and in tall persons. No studies have proven posture as a definite risk factor for LBP, but spine pain from scoliosis is well known and is the basis of this risk factor. Many studies have shown decreased strength of abdominal and spinal muscles in patients with LBP. Physical fitness and conditioning have been found to have a preventive effect on low back injuries. Smoking has been shown to increase one's risk of LBP. Aging increases the risk for CLBP.

Psychosocial factors such as depression, anxiety, and alcoholism, among others, have been reported with higher frequency in patients with chronic LBP.

The cause of back pain is not always clear, but it may be related to ligamentous or muscular strain resulting from either a specific traumatic episode or an incompetence of the soft tissue structure (ALBP). Degeneration of the intervertebral disc, a physiological event of aging, modified by such factors as injury, repetitive trauma, infection, heredity, and tobacco use, may lead to CLBP. As the hydrophilic properties of the nucleus pulposus degrade, the disc loses height and formerly tight ligaments become loose. Motions such as sliding and twisting create tears in the annulus fibrosus. Osteoarthritis and CLBP may develop.

Pathophysiology

The lumbosacral spine supports the upper body in a balanced, upright position while allowing locomotion. In a static, upright position, maintenance of erect posture is achieved through a balance among the expansile pressure of the intervertebral discs, the stretch placed on the anterior and posterior longitudinal and facet joint ligaments, and the sustained involuntary tone generated by the surrounding lumbosacral and abdominal muscles. The balance of the spine is also related to the reciprocal physiological curves in the cervical, thoracic, and lumbosacral areas of the vertebral column. The balance in curvature results in an individual's posture. Proper alignment is also influenced by structures in the pelvis and lower extremities. Movement of the lumbar spine is associated with a lumbar pelvic rhythm that results in the simultaneous reversal of the lumbar lordosis and rotation of the hips. During flexion and extension of the lumbar spine, tension is produced in the paraspinous, hamstring, and gluteal muscles, the fasciae that surround the muscles, and the ligaments that support the vertebral bodies and discs. In addition to the normal stresses placed on these structures with lowering and raising of the torso, the stresses on these anatomical structures are increased to an even greater degree when an individual is required to lift a heavy object.

LBP that is associated with back strain may be related to anatomical structures that are tonically contracted in the resting position. LBP may also occur during motion if the stress is greater than the supporting structures can sustain or if the components of the lumbosacral spine are abnormal. Although the precise pathophysiology of uncomplicated lumbar strain (back strain) is not well characterized, damage may occur in lumbosacral spinal structures if the amount of force generated exceeds the stress capacity of the spine for an individual patient. If the lumbosacral spine is in a mechanically disadvantaged position (e.g., rotated or flexed) the force may not need to be that great to cause a disruption of annular fibers. These fibers may tear when stressed, which in turn causes degeneration of the disc. An annular tear is associated with the production of pain and may account for the frequent episodes of LBP in patients who eventually rupture a nucleus pulposus. Protruding or bulging intervertebral disc material may then impinge on a spinal nerve root, imparting specific radiculopathic symptoms depending on the spinal level affected. Disc herniation (herniated nucleus pulposus) is discussed as a separate entity in the next section of this chapter.

Several other less common spinal conditions exist that produce LBP. Spinal stenosis results in nerve impingement with back and lower extremity (calf) pain on extension of the spine owing to the narrowed spinal canal, because this maneuver lengthens and further narrows the canal. Osteoarthritis typically produces erosion with irregular bony deposition known as osteophytes at the articular sites of the vertebrae that may also result in nerve impingement and pain as a result of degeneration of the joint. Significant scoliosis can predispose a person to osteoarthritis and may result in chronic LBP resulting from a fundamental derangement of vertebral biomechanics, that is, the ability of the axial musculoskeletal system to appropriately distribute mechanical loads placed on the spine. Spondylolisthesis is a slipping (displacement) of one vertebral body either anteriorly or posteriorly relative to another and may be a congenital or acquired condition. Spinal hyperextension often causes increased or repeated stress on the bilateral pars interarticularis, the posterior bony plate connecting the superior and inferior articular facets of an intervertebral joint. A lesion or fracture of the pars interarticularis that causes the facet to separate without actual anterior or posterior slippage of a vertebral body is known as spondylolysis. Either of these conditions may result in nerve impingement with lower back and extremity pain. Although spondylolysis may be asymptomatic, this condition may progress to spondylolisthesis.

Clinical Presentation

Subjective

An acute onset of LBP often follows a lifting episode or may be precipitated by something as minor as a sneeze or cough. Patients may have difficulty standing erect and often change position frequently for comfort. The pain often radiates into the buttocks and posterior thigh. The condition often occurs for the first time during the young adult years. There may be associated grimacing and generalized hypersensitivity to light touch. Initial assessment of a patient with activity intolerance resulting from LBP consists of a focused medical history, including a history of the present illness and past medical, family, occupational, and social history. A review of systems, especially description of any injury, is essential and may alert the provider to possible "red flags" warranting immediate attention. A history of recent trauma, recent lumbar puncture, concurrent infection, or chronic use of high-dose corticosteroids is significant. (See Focus on History 15.2.) Some questions to consider while evaluating the patient's responses include the following:

• Is there a serious systemic disease causing the pain?
• Is there neurological compromise that might require surgical evaluation?

Focus on History 15.2   Low Back Pain

For the patient who complains of low back pain, focus the history by asking questions that will obtain the following information:

1. Mode of onset (abrupt or insidious?)
2. Characteristics:
   • Provoking factors
   • Aggravating factors
   • Relieving factors
3. Effects of activities
   • Posture
   • Coughing, sneezing, straining
   • Exercise, exertion, rest
   • Sleep
4. History:
   • Similar or different pains
   • Course (progressive, decreasing, increasing, fluctuating, episodic?)
   • Associated limb and/or neurological symptoms (pain, paresthesias, numbness, weakness, atrophy, cramps, fasciculations?)
5. Associated symptoms:
   • Urinary problems (frequency, urgency, retention, incontinence?)
   • Bowel problems (incontinence or constipation?)
6. Previous back pain history and treatment (medications, types of surgery, nonpharmacological management, lifestyle and work modifications, litigation or compensation issues?)

• Is there social or psychological distress that may amplify or prolong pain?

The hallmark symptom of CLBP is recurrent low back pain that often radiates to one or both buttocks. The pain may be described as "mechanical" in that it is aggravated by activities such as bending, stooping, or twisting. There may be stiffness and a history of intermittent sciatica (i.e., pain radiating down the back of the leg), but discomfort in the lower back remains the predominant symptom. This may be relieved with lying down or a good night's sleep, although if the pain is severe enough it may awaken the patient at night. Psychosocial indicators should be assessed because they can be barriers to recovery in all cases of LBP, both acute and chronic. Consider factors such as fear, financial problems, anger, depression, job dissatisfaction, family problems, or stress that can contribute to prolonged disability.

Objective

There is often diffuse tenderness to the lower back. ROM of the lumbar spine, particularly flexion, is typically reduced and elicits pain. Patients may exhibit a side or forward list from muscle spasm. The degree of lumbar flexion and the ease with which the patient can extend the spine are helpful parameters by which to evaluate progress. Though not characteristic, nonorganic findings, such as widespread sensitivity to light touch, nonanatomical localization of symptoms, inappropriate grimacing, inconsistent actions, and exaggerated pain behaviors, may be seen. In most cases of uncomplicated LBP, the motor and sensory functions of the lumbosacral nerve roots and reflexes of the lower extremities are normal. Negative straight-leg raise rules out surgically significant disc herniation in 95% of cases. (See Advanced Assessment 15.6.)

Diagnostic Reasoning

Diagnostic Tests

In cases of CLBP, anteroposterior and lateral radiographs often show age-appropriate changes, such as anterior osteophytes and reduced height of intervertebral discs on the lateral view. ALBP does not warrant radiographs except in the following circumstances:

- Unrelenting night pain or pain at rest
- Fever above 38°C (100.4°F) for greater than 48 hours
- Progressive neuromotor deficit
- Pain with distal numbness or leg weakness
- Loss of bowel or bladder control (retention or incontinence)
- Significant trauma
- History of suspicion of cancer
- Osteoporosis
- Chronic oral steroid use
- Immunosuppressed or immunosuppressive medication

- Drug or alcohol abuse
- Clinical suspicion of ankylosing spondylitis

Consider a complete blood count and erythrocyte sedimentation rate (ESR) if there is suspicion of cancer or infection. Routine imaging is not indicated in diagnosis of patients with nonspecific LBP (Chou et al, 2007, 2009).

Differential Diagnosis

LBP is a diagnosis of exclusion. The diagnosis of back strain is based on the history of localized LBP and a compatible physical exam demonstrating localized pain, muscle spasm, and a normal neurological exam. CLBP is recurrent and has lasted for a longer period of time, and the patient may also demonstrate mildly restricted straight-leg raising and spinal motion. (See Advanced Assessment 15.6.) Differential diagnoses for ALBP/CLBP include the following:

- Ankylosing spondylitis (family history, morning stiffness, limited mobility of the lumbar spine)
- Drug-seeking behavior (exaggerated symptoms, inconsistent and nonphysiological exam)
- Extraspinal causes (ovarian cyst, nephrolithiasis, pancreatitis, ulcer disease, abdominal aortic aneurysm)
- Fracture of the vertebral body (major trauma or minimal trauma with osteoporosis)
- Herniated nucleus pulposus or ruptured disc (unilateral radicular pain symptoms that extend below the knee and are equal to or greater than the back pain)
- Infection (fever, chills, sweats, elevated ESR)
- Myeloma (night sweats, men older than 50)

Advanced Assessment 15.6	Assessing the Lower Back—Special Tests
Test	Comments
Straight-leg raising—places the L5 and S1 nerve roots and the sciatic nerve under tension.	With the patient supine and relaxed, elevate the leg until either the leg begins to bend or the patient reports severe pain in buttock or back. Record degree of elevation at which pain occurs. It is considered positive when the pain is elicited below the level of the knee when the leg is raised less than 60 degrees. Next, dorsiflex the ankle to determine whether this motion increased pain (further stretch of the L5 and S1 nerve roots). Plantar flexion of the ankle relieves sciatic tension. Increased back pain with this maneuver is probably nonorganic. The straight-leg raising test is very sensitive, but not very specific. To increase specificity, raise the leg until pain is felt below the knee, then lower the leg about 5 degrees, which should eliminate the pain. Then, have patient dorsiflex the ipsilateral foot while the leg is raised. This should cause more traction on the sciatic nerve and reproduce the symptoms.
Reverse straight-leg raising—places the L1–L4 nerve roots under tension.	With the patient prone, lift the hip into extension while keeping the knee straight. Increased pain suggests compression of the upper lumbar nerve roots.
Prone rectus femoris test—places the L1–L4 nerve roots under tension.	With the patient prone, maintain the hip in a neutral position while flexing the knee. Increased pain suggests compression of the upper lumbar nerve roots.

Differential diagnoses for CLBP that are different than ALBP include the following:

- Depression (abnormal Beck Depression Inventory, sleep disturbances)
- Illness behavior (multiple surgeries, multiple illnesses)
- Inflammatory arthritides (morning stiffness for more than 30 minutes, positive human leukocyte antigen–B27, increased ESR)
- Intervertebral disc infection or vertebral osteomyelitis (history of excruciating pain, recent IV drug use, fever, recent infection/hospitalization, open wound)
- Metastatic tumors, myeloma, lymphoma (pathological fractures, severe night pain, weight loss, fatigue)
- Osteoporosis with compression fractures (female gender, previous fracture)
- Spinal tuberculosis (lower socioeconomic groups, history of AIDS)
- Workplace dissatisfaction (discontent with boss, job)
  See Differential Diagnosis 15.4.

Management

Reassure the patient that most episodes of ALBP are mild and self-limited; almost 90% are resolved within 1 to 6 weeks. Symptom control is considered an adjunct to helping the patient to overcome specific activity intolerance. The management of the patient with LBP, especially if pain is recurrent and/or chronic, requires a *Circle of Caring* by the practitioner. Multiple approaches are required to address the "iceberg" of LBP and the ways that it can interfere with the lives of patients and families.

Pharmacological Management

The oral medications used to control the discomfort of LBP primarily include acetaminophen, NSAIDs, muscle relaxants, and opioids. There is fair to good evidence that NSAIDs are effective for reducing pain in patients with LBP. Acetaminophen has also been found to be comparable in efficacy to NSAIDs for treating LBP, with fewer adverse effects. Health-care providers need to be aware that the long-term use of NSAIDs can lead to serious gastrointestinal (GI) disease such as ulcers and hemorrhage; thus, patients with GI histories should use this drug cautiously. Using the lowest possible effective dose can help to prevent this problem. Older adults are more sensitive to the adverse effects of NSAIDs, so it is important to use caution when prescribing NSAIDs for this age group. NSAIDs affect the renal prostaglandins and may cause fluid retention and edema, so it is also important for patients to monitor for weight gain. The risk of fluid retention and edema may be very significant in elderly patients and in those with congestive heart failure. In addition, there is the potential for nephrotoxicity.

There is moderate research evidence showing that muscle relaxants are more effective than placebo but no evidence that they are better than NSAIDs in relieving symptoms of acute LBP. Multiple trials found skeletal muscle relaxants moderately superior to placebo for short-term relief of LBP (duration less than 1 week) (American Pain Society/American Association of Pain Medicine, 2009). Patients need to be aware that this class of drugs is for short-term use because the risk/benefit ratio for prolonged use of muscle relaxants is not known. Muscle relaxants cause drowsiness and dizziness, so patients need to avoid hazardous activities when

Differential Diagnosis 15.4   Low Back Pain

Diagnosis	Spondylolisthesis	Muscle Strain	Scoliosis	Herniated Nucleus Pulposus	Osteoarthritis	Spinal Stenosis
Age	20	20–40	30	30–50	>50	>60
Pain location	Back	Back (unilateral)	Back	Back (unilateral)	Back (bilateral)	Leg (bilateral)
Pain onset	Insidious	Acute	Insidious	Acute (prior episodes)	Insidious	Insidious
Pain increases	When standing, bending	When standing, bending	When standing, bending	When sitting, bending	When standing	When standing
Pain decreases	When sitting	When sitting	When sitting	When standing	When sitting, bending	When sitting, bending
Straight-leg raising	Negative	Negative	Negative	Positive	Negative	Positive (stress)
X-ray (plain film)	Positive	Negative	Positive	Negative	Positive	Positive

taking them. This class of drug is a central nervous system (CNS) depressant, so patients need to avoid taking muscle relaxants with alcohol or other CNS depressants because the combined use will cause additive effects. Dry mouth is another side effect from this antimuscarinic class of drugs, so frequent mouth rinsing is recommended to prevent dental disease.

Research has shown that opioid analgesics did not enhance patients' ability to return to full activity sooner than that of patients taking NSAIDs or acetaminophen. In addition, the adverse effects of opioid analgesics were found to be substantial, including the risk for physical dependence.

Activity

It should be stressed that rest has been proven to have little to no effect on the resolution of LBP. Patients should do whatever activities are tolerable. Weight loss, physical activities, and exercise for 30 minutes a day (walking or biking with lumbar flexion and/or extension exercises) are also important. Deconditioning is a real phenomenon that occurs increasingly quickly with increasing age. Lack of activity, leading to deconditioning, becomes a vicious cycle. Reassurance is always appropriate after ruling out more serious causes of back pain. Avoid labeling patients as "disabled." Actively promote smoking cessation if the patient smokes.

Follow-up and Referral

The course of patients with back strain is one of gradual improvement, usually over a 1- to 2-week period. The recovery is usually complete, without any lasting impairment. The small percentage of patients who do not make a complete recovery may continue to experience LBP associated with muscle strain. Pain may continue for months or years. These patients are experiencing CLBP, which must be evaluated and treated in a manner that takes into account the special difficulties of individuals with chronic pain. Patients with more severe symptoms can have limited vocational and avocational activities, recreation, and sleep disturbances. Mood, sexuality, and concentration can be adversely affected. Deconditioning can be the result of reduced activities, making both symptoms and any occupational dysfunction worse. Suggest a modified work schedule and more recreational activities that improve general conditioning. Narcotic abuse and dependency can be a problem for patients with chronic pain; refer the patient to a pain management center where a variety of evaluation and treatment modalities are available.

In all patients, preventing recurrence of back pain is another important consideration. The first episode of back pain is usually the briefest and least severe. The vast majority of individuals with an episode of back pain are at risk of developing another episode of back pain that will be more severe and of greater duration. Patients with recurrence are usually resistant to therapies that are

beneficial in management of acute back pain, and therefore they may require chronic pain assessment and management strategies (including the use of complementary therapies such as acupuncture or acupressure). Consistent evidence from multiple trials demonstrates that acupuncture is moderately effective for short-term pain relief compared with no treatment or sham transcutaneous electrical nerve stimulation in patients with chronic low back pain. There was no difference in effect between acupuncture and sham acupuncture (American Pain Society/American Association of Pain Medicine, 2009).

Referral to a specialist (e.g., neurosurgeon, orthopedic surgeon) is recommended for any patient who has a neurological deficit or if the patient has a trauma history with x-ray exam revealing instability or fracture that could cause damage to neural elements.

Patient Education

Instruct the patient to carefully introduce activities back into his or her day as he or she begins to recover from the worst of the back pain episode. Gradual stretches and regular walking are good activities. Ice or heat, whichever provides more comfort, will help decrease the inflammation. Over-the-counter anti-inflammatory medications (e.g., aspirin, NSAIDs) or Tylenol may be used. Provide information on safe back exercises such as modified sit-ups and low back stretches. Encourage patients to make them a regular part of their lifestyle. Emphasize the need to relax. Patients should call if symptoms persist, worsen, or progress; significant pain persists beyond 1 week; or there is no improvement with home management. There is consistent evidence that application of heat for acute/subacute low back pain is superior to placebo for back functional status and short-term pain relief. There is insufficient evidence to evaluate ice therapy.

Agency for Healthcare Research and Quality guidelines suggest teaching the patient self-application of heat or cold but found insufficient evidence to endorse application of heat or cold products or justify their cost (American Pain Society/American Association of Pain Medicine, 2009).

■ HIP PAIN

Hip pain is discomfort within or around the hip. The largest joint in the body, the hip is subject to stress from ambulation and weight-bearing; it may suffer trauma and chronic mechanical stress. Possible causes are processes in the hip joint, the surrounding muscles, the soft tissues, or the neurovascular system. Diagnosis needs to consider the patient's age because certain problems are more prevalent in different age-groups. In adults, common problems include OA, RA, fractures, referred pain, bursitis, meralgia paresthetica, avascular necrosis, and malignancy.

Pain in and around the hip can often be felt in the groin or the buttock, or it can be referred to the thigh or knee. Conversely, pain may be referred to the hip if irritation to the femoral, sciatic, or obturator nerve roots occurs. These may be the result of herniation of lumbar disc, spinal stenosis, retroperitoneal tumor, or femoral hernia. Vascular insufficiency of the aortoiliac area may result in hip and buttock pain as well. The history should ascertain if pain is focal, as in bursitis, or diffuse, as in synovitis. The presence of stiffness should raise the suspicion of degenerative disease. Inquire about trauma, involvement of other joints, infection, fever, and relation of pain to activity.

Physical examination of the hip must first assess position at rest because fracture of the femoral head results in external rotation and flexion, and an internally rotated shortened leg may be a posterior dislocation. These patients should not have the hip moved until radiographic studies have ruled out fracture or dislocation. Performing palpation of the joint allows recognition of focal tenderness and swelling.

The ROM examination begins with assessment of gait, if possible. Next, the extremity should be put through passive ROM to detect crepitus, limitation of movement, muscle spasm, flexion contracture, or guarding. Flexion and extension need to be performed with the knee straight as well as flexed. Abduction, adduction, and internal and external rotation are assessed. Femoral and pedal pulses are auscultated for strength and bruits. Neurological testing for sensation and deep tendon reflexes concludes the exam. Diagnostic testing should include hip x-ray films. Other x-ray studies, such as spine or sacroiliac films or weight-bearing films, may be indicated in special circumstances. MRI, ultrasonography, and joint aspiration are other diagnostic techniques to be considered in special circumstances.

Differential Diagnosis

Osteoarthritis

OA usually causes stiffness or pain with use that is felt in the morning and improves during the day. Pain referred to the groin, thigh, knee, and lateral side of the leg may occur. Often pain or stiffness affects other joints as well. For more information, see the section on osteoarthritis that follows later in this chapter.

Trochanteric Bursitis

The hip area contains multiple bursae. The incidence of trochanteric bursitis peaks between the fourth and sixth decades of life; it is more common in women than in men. It is commonly associated with pain and limited ROM. Onset may be acute or insidious. Bursitis can be associated with trauma or overuse and may be inflammatory, hemorrhagic, infectious, or calcific. Inflammatory bursitis of the hip is the most common type. Trochanteric bursitis is often associated with lumbar spondylosis, degenerative arthritis of the hip, and lower limb–length discrepancy. It is characterized by chronic, intermittent, aching pain over the lateral aspect of the hip, and some patients report numbness in the upper thigh. Pain will increase with movement, especially external rotation and abduction, and can be triggered by prolonged standing or lying on the affected side. Other signs and symptoms include pain on forced hip abduction, distinct tenderness around the greater trochanter, and pain extending down the lateral aspect of the thigh. Trochanteric bursitis is treated with NSAID therapy (e.g., naproxen [Naprosyn] 375–500 mg PO 2 times daily for 1–2 weeks). Persistent cases may require corticosteroid injections.

Rheumatoid Disease

With rheumatoid disease, the hip pain is bilateral, and characteristics include morning stiffness and limited ROM that does not resolve with activity. The hip is generally not the first joint affected. During an acute phase there is tenderness and fullness or thickening seen in the joint.

Proximal Femoral (Hip) Fracture

Hip fractures are one of the most common of all adult fractures, accounting for at least half of all hospital days related to fracture care in the United States. The two primary types of hip fractures are *femoral neck* (intracapsular) and *intertrochanteric,* both of which occur most frequently in older adults who have sustained a fall at home or similar low-energy trauma. The incidence of hip fractures doubles for each decade of life after age 50 years, with women affected twice as often as men are.

Risks for hip fractures include physical activity, previous fracture, visual impairment, institutionalization, and osteoporosis. Pain in the hip area after trauma, such as a fall or motor vehicle collision, especially in patients older than age 50, should give rise to the suggestion of fractures. Neither a lack of trauma nor a long-standing history of hip pain rules out a fracture. In some cases, a fracture may occur as a pathological fracture secondary to an underlying neoplasm or chronic corticosteroid usage. The patient should be admitted to the hospital.

Obtain a history of how the injury occurred and whether the fall was witnessed by anyone other than the patient. A loss of consciousness for any period would necessitate a cardiac and neurological referral, as well as referral for orthopedic care. Determine the patient's mental status, and try to obtain a realistic assessment of the preinjury functional status.

Physical exam typically reveals an externally rotated and shortened injured leg. Any motion to this extremity will produce severe pain centered around the affected groin. Examine the pelvic bony prominences for tenderness because pubis ramus fractures may also be present or may be confused with the hip injury. It is important to check for lower-extremity pulses and neurological function. The entire limb should be assessed for points of tenderness or deformity that may indicate the presence of other fractures at sites such as the femur, tibia, or ankle. An anteroposterior view of the pelvis and "shoot-through" lateral views of the affected hip can provide definitive radiographic evidence to confirm the diagnosis. In most cases, surgical repair of the fracture is the treatment of choice.

Meralgia Paresthetica

Caused by compression of the lateral femoral cutaneous nerve, meralgia paresthetica is commonly seen in overweight middle-aged men. Symptoms include pain or paresthesias over the anterior superior iliac spine and the anterior lateral thigh, with decreased touch and pinprick sensation. Treatment includes analgesics and avoiding tight clothing around the waist.

Avascular Necrosis

Avascular necrosis appears as abrupt hip pain followed by progressive, intermittent episodes. Pain is worsened with motion and activity and often is worse at night. A limp, along with limited abduction and internal rotation, is present. MRI is needed for diagnosis, and an orthopedic referral is indicated. It often occurs as a serious complication of hip trauma, but it may occur unrelated to trauma.

Malignancy

Initially no signs may be present with malignancy; however, tenderness and palpable swelling may develop later over bony prominences. Night pain, systemic symptoms, and fractures may be seen.

■ KNEE PAIN

The knee is a complex, modified hinge joint consisting of three bones, three articulations, five major tendons, four major ligaments, and two menisci. The lateral and medial articulations are between the femoral and tibial condyles. The intermediate articulation exists between the patella and the femur. The knee is a relatively weak joint that gains its strength from the strong ligaments that attach the femur to the tibia. There are five intrinsic ligaments that assist in strengthening the articular capsule. The cruciate ligaments connect the femur and tibia within the articular capsule, crossing each other in the form of an X.

As a major weight-bearing joint, the knee is susceptible to many injuries. Torsion is limited in the joint, and any motion that extends beyond the defined range results in a ligamentous injury. Because the knee joint depends on the integrity of the ligaments to provide it with stability, an injury to the knee may be a calamitous event.

The arrangement of three articulations allows a combination of rolling, gliding, and rotation, in addition to flexion and extension. Although it is attached to the lateral tibia, the fibula does not articulate with the knee joint. The anatomy of the knee includes bony structures, ligaments, tendons, bursae, and cartilage. The femoral condyles and the tibial plateaus are capped by the patella and cushioned by the menisci, whereas the ligaments, muscles, tendons, and bursae provide stability.

The knee joint is a common site for discomfort due to trauma (24% of all activity-related musculoskeletal injuries in men, the highest of all sites), degenerative disease, and/or rheumatological conditions. Acute pain in the knee may be related to any of the following:

- Fractures
- Meniscal injuries
- Ligamentous injuries
- Musculotendinous strains
- Extensor mechanism injuries
- Contusions

Many knee complaints by adults are the result of overzealous exercise and sports activity. Fractures can involve the distal femur, patella, proximal tibia, and fibula. Inspect for swelling and deformity, palpate for tenderness in the bone itself, and obtain appropriate radiographs. Patellar fractures can result from indirect forces, such as falls, but fractures of the tibia and femur at the knee usually result from major trauma. Patellar dislocations are often reduced at the scene of injury when the knee is extended for transport.

Obtaining a history of the mechanism of injury is key in diagnosing meniscal tears. A history of a twisting injury sustained with the foot planted on the ground and locking (inability to extend the knee completely) with localized pain and tenderness along the joint are indicative of meniscal pathology. Some patients report that manipulating or pushing on the knee enabled them to "unlock it." Ask the patient if he or she heard or felt a "pop" when the injury occurred.

Patients with ligamentous injuries have acute pain, swelling, and instability. Strains of various musculotendinous structures around the knee also cause acute pain and swelling, but most do not result in instability. Patients with an injury to the extensor mechanism report a fall with a sudden weakness or collapse. Contusions are from direct blows and cause localized pain and tenderness.

Knee complaints are categorized as *injury* (trauma) or *overuse* and are either acute or chronic. Often chronic knee pain cannot be related to any recognized injury or overuse. Conditions that cause chronic knee pain include the following:

- Arthritis
- Tumors
- Sepsis
- Overuse syndromes (including bursitis/tendinitis and anterior knee pain)

Tumors are characterized by night pain and often can be palpated or identified on radiograph. Sepsis in the knee joint is rare; it is more commonly located in the prepatellar bursa. Inspection and palpation of the involved area easily determine the location of the infection. Bursitis/tendinitis and anterior knee pain have similar characteristics: both usually are chronic, often secondary to overuse, and often bilateral. The pain typically is worse with rising or walking after sitting, at night, and with prolonged exercise or use.

The physical exam of the knee begins with the patient standing. Inspect both knees anteriorly and posteriorly. Observe the gait. Inspect the knees for swelling, ecchymosis, erythema, abrasions, puncture wounds, and active range of motion (ROM). Assess the popliteal space for swelling that may occur with popliteal aneurysm, Baker's cyst, and tumors. It is important to assess movement in both the standing and supine positions and to note any limping, pain, locking, or giving way of the knee. As the patient lies supine, palpate the joint line, muscles, tendons, ligaments, and bones in an attempt to localize tenderness. An effusion may be demonstrated by eliciting the *bulge sign:* As the patient lies supine, massage the medial knee toward the head, then stroke the lateral aspect of the knee toward the medial aspect. A bulge sign or effusion is indicated if fluctuance occurs over the medial aspect. Palpation for crepitus while the knee is passively flexed and extended helps to determine if meniscal injury is present. Do muscle testing of the quadriceps and hamstrings.

A complete physical exam is also important to rule out the presence of systemic disease associated with knee pathology.

There are a number of specialized assessment techniques. Most are specific and technique driven, requiring practice to master them. The Lachman test should be done on most patients with knee pain; it is 94% specific and is helpful in diagnosing anterior cruciate ligament (ACL) injury. The McMurray and Apley tests are indicated in diagnosing meniscal tears. The anterior drawer test has a low sensitivity and high specificity for confirming ACL pathology, so a positive test strongly suggests a problem but a negative test does not rule out an ACL tear. The posterior drawer test is used to diagnose posterior cruciate ligament (PCL) injury. The collateral ligament stress test, also known as the valgus and varus stress tests, evaluates the intact function of the medial collateral ligament (MCL) and the lateral collateral ligament (LCL), respectively. The Fairbank test, also known as the Apprehension test, can identify dislocation of the patella. (See Advanced Assessment 15.7.)

Contusions are injuries to the leg by a direct blow. Disability may be minor; however, contusions can be quite painful, with significant swelling and tenderness. There may be ecchymosis, and active and passive stress will be painful.

Diagnostic testing includes the use of radiographs if mechanical injury or trauma is suspected. Specific weight-bearing views and sunrise or skyline views can be performed. MRI is helpful in diagnosing a torn meniscus or cruciate ligament injury. Arthrography is used for diagnosis of a Baker's cyst, and effusions can be aspirated for diagnostic purposes.

Differential Diagnosis
Inflammatory Arthritis

Knee arthritis, which may cause an inflammatory effusion, may be a primary manifestation in a number of conditions. It is one of the most common manifestations

---

Advanced Assessment 15.7   Assessing the Meniscus and the Patella—Special Tests

Test	Comments
McMurray circumduction test—to test for meniscal tear	Flex the knee to the maximum pain-free position. Hold that position while externally rotating the foot, and then gradually extend the knee while maintaining the tibia in external rotation. This maneuver stresses the medial meniscus and often elicits a localized medial compartment click and/or pain in patients with a posterior tear. The same maneuver performed while rotating the foot internally will stress the lateral meniscus. Pain-free flexion beyond 90 degrees is necessary for this test to be useful.
Apprehension sign—to test patellar instability	Have the patient seated with the quadriceps relaxed. Place the knee in extension. Displace the patella laterally and then flex the knee to 30 degrees. With instability, this maneuver displaces the patella to an abnormal position on the lateral femoral condyle. The patient often perceives pain and demonstrates apprehension.
Bulge sign—to assess for effusion	Apply lateral pressure to the area adjacent to the patella. Medial bulge will appear if fluid is in the knee joint.
Inspect/palpate—to assess for effusion	First, inspect the suprapatellar region. A large knee effusion will be visible. Subtle knee effusions can be demonstrated by "milking down" the joint fluid from the suprapatellar pouch. Hold the fluid wave in place with one hand and ballot the patella. Excessive fluid will create a spongy feeling as the patella is pushed down.

of osteoarthritis (OA). Often more than one joint is affected, and there is recurrence or chronicity. Gout, pseudogout, Lyme disease, septic arthritis, and avascular necrosis can also be responsible for the inflammatory response. It may be necessary to aspirate the joint and culture the synovial fluid to rule out infection. Treatment will depend on the underlying condition.

Fracture

A fracture is most likely to occur with direct trauma and result in acute onset of pain. Fractures of the knee and leg include those of the patella, tibial plateau, fibular head and shaft, and tibial pilon. Most, but not all, knee fractures are the result of fairly significant trauma; fractures of the knee are often present in conjunction with injury to associated structures. Most fractures around the knee are associated with a large effusion. If the joint is tapped, the presence of hemarthrosis with fat globules is clinically indicative of a fracture. Swelling and significant pain on movement will be present. It is important to ensure that no neurovascular compromise is present in the lower leg. Radiography should be obtained, and immediate referral is indicated.

Patellar fractures are usually the result of a direct blow from a blunt object or can be attributed to a fall or motor vehicle collision (MVC). The patient with a patellar fracture is usually unable to flex the knee. Marked joint effusion is usually present.

Stress Fractures

Stress fractures are common in patients who experience bone pain after initiating or increasing high-impact activity. Stress fractures are a result of repeated subtle bone trauma over a period of time that causes a gradual loss of bony substance. New bone is fragile until it calcifies. The cortex, temporarily weakened, is then susceptible to fracture. Common sites for stress fractures are the legs and feet.

There is point tenderness over the bone on physical exam. There may be ecchymosis and soft tissue swelling. Often the patient has altered his or her gait, causing pain to the knee. Resistive motion of the joint is painless. Radiographs may reveal a periosteal reaction or a hairline radiolucency but are usually negative until 2 to 3 weeks after the injury has occurred. Bone scans may be helpful.

Rest is the best treatment for a stress fracture. Once the patient is pain free, gradually resume activity. The best treatment of stress fractures is prevention. Exercise programs should begin slowly, and the patient should avoid the "weekend warrior" syndrome.

Runner's Injuries

Lateral knee pain frequently plagues runners, whether they are novices or seasoned athletes. When there is an inability to "run through the pain," runners will often seek care. Sometimes the pain occurs when the average running time or distance has been increased.

"Runner's knee," or *iliotibial band tendinitis,* may be related to improper footwear, uneven and bumpy paths, running on very hard surfaces, and lack of warm-up. The pain is based at the lateral edge of the patella, at the point where the iliotibial band crosses over the anterior aspect of the joint. Most runners with this condition have feet that supinate, meaning that they do not get a good push-off. Pain during a run suggests injury; pain after a run suggests an overuse problem.

Treatment includes rest, ice packs or ice massage, and NSAIDs. For runners with foot problems, orthotics may be indicated. Alternative low-impact activities should be encouraged (e.g., swimming, biking, or running in water). The symptoms should resolve in 10 to 14 days; at that time the individual may resume running at half the distance that he or she was running before. After 3 weeks, if the runner is pain free, the distance may be increased.

Collateral Ligament Sprains

Knee sprain or ligament tears often occur as a result of athletic injuries. Joint laxity will be present to a varying degree, depending on the injury. The two collateral ligaments, the MCL and the LCL, provide lateral stability to the knee. The MCL attaches to the medial condyle of the femur and the tibia. The LCL attaches to the lateral femoral condyle and extends to the lateral tibial plateau. The MCL and the LCL are injured when the valgus (MCL) or varus (LCL) stress to the joint extends beyond the defined range. MCL injuries are more common than LCL tears and often include an injury to the medial meniscus. Football players and skiers are more prone to ligamentous injuries, but they may occur just as easily on the dance floor or in the bathroom.

Wrenching the knee with the foot firmly planted causes injury to the MCL. In these injuries, the knee is in flexion and in a slight internal rotation. LCL injuries occur when the varus stress applied to the knee causes a "bend" toward the outside. The knee is painful and often swollen and may be ecchymotic over the body of the ligament. Some patients will report the feeling that the knee is "bent the wrong way." The knee swells within 20 to 30 minutes; more rapid swelling is an ominous sign and should be considered a "red flag."

Examining the knee immediately after the injury is easier and helps to ascertain the severity of the injury. The exam is more difficult once the joint swells. In a suspected collateral ligament sprain, there is tenderness along the body of the ligament, and point tenderness at the attachment sites is frequently present. In the MCL injury, there may be tenderness at the medial joint because the MCL attaches to the medial meniscus. Pain at the lateral joint line is equivalent to a joint injury.

Varus or valgus stress on the knee joint will determine joint laxity. The practitioner should always examine the unaffected knee first to establish the baseline and to allay anxiety about the evaluation.

Obtain plain radiographs to rule out fractures and dislocations. More extensive radiological exams such as stress films, CT scans, and MRI scans are obtained in consultation with an orthopedist. In an acutely swollen joint, MRI is often inconclusive. As in all musculoskeletal injuries, it is important to include fractures, dislocations, and tumors in the differential diagnoses.

Isolated first- and second-degree sprains can be managed with *r*est, *i*ce, *c*ompression (or immobilization), and *e*levation (RICE). The unstable knee requires an external knee immobilizer. No weight-bearing should be allowed on an acutely swollen or painful knee. Once the injury is past the acute stage, the patient should begin adductor-strengthening exercises with physical therapy referral. Once the swelling and pain subside, a more progressive rehabilitation program should begin.

All severe strains and fractures should be referred to an orthopedic specialist. Referral to a physical therapist to assist in complete rehabilitation should also be considered. An incompletely rehabilitated knee will be weak and potentially unstable. Without accurate diagnosis and treatment, the injury can become more extensive, jeopardizing joint stability and other structures. Traumatic arthritis can be the sequela to any joint injury.

Adherence to the rehabilitation process is imperative. In some instances, a knee support is necessary for sports. Pain and swelling are indicators that the knee is being overstressed or reinjured.

Cruciate Ligament Injuries

The two cruciate ligaments—the ACL and the PCL—provide rotational stability to the knee. The ACL attaches to the anterior part of the intercondylar area of the tibia, posterior to the medial meniscus. It rises superiorly, posteriorly, and laterally to attach to the posterior section of the medial side of the lateral condyle of the femur. The ACL restrains the anterior to the posterior translation of the knee, keeping the proper relationship of the femur to the tibia. It is loose when the knee is in flexion and tight when it is fully extended. It is the weaker of the two cruciate ligaments. The ACL is the most commonly involved structure in severe knee injuries. In 70% of the patients presenting with acute, traumatic hemarthrosis, the ACL is the injured structure. The ACL injury frequently occurs in combination with ruptures of the MCL and the medial meniscus. Once the ligament is torn, the knee is unstable. Swelling occurs rapidly in ACL or PCL injuries because of bleeding of the ligament tear.

The PCL originates in the posterior part of the intercondylar area of the tibia. It crosses superiorly and anteriorly on the medial side of the ACL and attaches to the anterior portion of the lateral surface of the medial femoral condyle. The PCL is tight in flexion. The PCL is injured less frequently than the ACL. It is usually injured by trauma to the anterior surface of the proximal tibia, as in hitting the dashboard in an MVC.

With either ACL or PCL injuries, the patient often reports hearing a "pop" or feeling the knee "snap." An instantaneous sensation of something being "terribly wrong" is also commonly reported. Pain from the injury prevents a return to activity. The patient may report a "distrust" of the knee during activities—the knee may give out, especially during exertion.

On examination, the knee is swollen, and the patient is unable to fully flex or extend the knee. There are four standard tests to perform to ascertain the integrity of the ligaments: the valgus and varus stress tests (collateral ligament stress tests), the Lachman test, and the thumb sign (see Advanced Assessment 15.8). Hamstring spasms and the posterior horn of the meniscus can stabilize the knee, so it is important for the patient to relax throughout the exam. Examine the normal knee first to allay anxiety and to establish a baseline because most people have some degree of laxity in the ligaments.

Obtain radiographs of the knee. Plain films will demonstrate effusions, loose bodies, and avulsion fractures. The Segond fracture—an avulsion off the lateral aspect of the tibial plateau—is pathognomonic of an ACL tear. The ligaments can be definitively evaluated by MRI.

Any trauma to the knee can cause fractures as well as cartilage, meniscus, ligament, and muscle damage. The clinician should consider all these injuries when evaluating the knee. The degree of the tear and presence of instability should direct the treatment plan. Partial tears and tears without concurrent fracture or meniscus tear can often be managed conservatively. Immobilize the acutely injured knee to decrease swelling and pain. The patient should avoid weight-bearing on the knee. The quadriceps muscle begins to atrophy with inactivity, so it is important to begin strengthening exercises as quickly as tolerable. The quadriceps muscles are adjunct stabilizers to the ACL, and rehabilitation should stress regaining full ROM and strength.

All patients who have sustained an injury to the cruciate ligaments require an evaluation by an orthopedic surgeon. An unstable knee is in jeopardy of fracture, worsening the initial injury, or falls as a result of the instability, resulting in other injuries. A knee that has sustained severe trauma is susceptible to developing arthritis. It is important that the patient understand that despite reconstruction and rehabilitation, the knee will never be perfectly normal. Nonetheless, it can be functional although it may require the use of a custom-made brace.

Cartilaginous Injuries or Meniscal Tears

Cartilaginous injuries or meniscal tears present with acute or subacute pain. The patient may complain of the knee "locking" or "giving way." Conservative therapy of rest, application of ice, and use of NSAIDs should be the initial treatment. If no improvement occurs, diagnostic evaluation of x-ray films (to rule out

Advanced Assessment 15.8   Assessing Knee Ligaments—Special Tests

Test	Comments
Valgus stress test—assess the medial collateral ligament (MCL) stability.	Support thigh to relax the quadriceps muscle. Apply stress initially with the knee extended and then flexed to 25 degrees. With the thigh supported and the knee extended, place one hand on the lateral side of the knee, grasp the medial distal tibia with one hand on the lateral side of the knee, grasp the medial distal tibia with the other hand, and abduct the knee. If the knee opens up in a valgus direction more than the opposite knee, the patient has either a complete or partial tear of the MCL.
Varus stress test—assess the lateral collateral ligament (LCL) stability	Assess LCL stability with the knee in extension and 25 degree flexion by reversing the stress pattern used for the MCL. If the knee opens up more than the opposite knee in a varus direction, the patient has either a complete or partial tear of the LCL.
Lachman test—anterior cruciate ligament (ACL)	With the patient supine and the knee flexed 15–20 degrees, grasp the calf, wrapping your hand around the leg, with your thumb on the tibial tubercle. With your other hand, stabilize the distal femur, pressing your thumb through the quadriceps tendon while the rest of your hand encircles the thigh above the patella. The knee should be relaxed so that you feel the full weight of it. Simultaneously apply pressure to the tibia posteriorly, attempting to move it forward while pushing backward on the femur, feeling for any anterior excursion of the tibia. The normal response is no forward translation of the tibia. With an ACL tear, there is anterior excursion of the tibia.
Thumb sign—posterior cruciate ligament (PCL)	With the patient supine, flex the knee to 90 degrees with the foot supported. Normally, the anterior tibial plateaus sit 1 cm anterior to the femoral condyles, and you may place your thumbs on top of the medial and lateral tibial plateaus. If the PCL is injured, the proximal tibia falls back and the area available to your thumbs decreases. When the tibial plateaus are flush with the femoral condyles, there is 10 mm or more of posterior laxity, consistent with a complete tear of the PCL.

fractures and OA), MRI, and orthopedic referral are indicated. (See Advanced Assessment 15.8.)

Meniscal Tears

Knee injuries are the most frequent sports-related injury. The knee is an inherently unstable joint held together by ligaments, cushioned by the menisci, and covered by muscles. The menisci are crescent-shaped fibrocartilaginous structures on the articular surface of the tibia. They act as shock absorbers for the knee and help to control normal knee motion. The medial meniscus is injured or torn more frequently than the lateral meniscus because of its more rigid structure, decreased mobility, and more vulnerable sites of attachment, which render it subject to greater stress. Meniscal tears ("torn cartilage" or "locked knee") can occur alone or in combination with ligament injuries such as cruciate ligament disruptions and/or collateral ligament tears. Meniscal tears disrupt the mechanics of the knee, leading to varying degrees of symptoms and predisposing the knee to degenerative arthritis.

Epidemiology and Causes

Meniscal and ligament tears affect two groups of patients primarily—young, athletic adults with a history of trauma and middle-aged or elderly patients with OA.

Several case series have indicated that meniscal tears are the most common of all knee injuries, accounting for an estimated 52,000 knees damaged by football injuries alone. Moreover, an estimated 1.7 million people undergo meniscal surgery each year. Traumatic tears may not always involve contact injury; however, most commonly, they are due to sports-related activities, particularly soccer, football, and basketball. In contrast to traumatic tears, degenerative tears result from the progressive weakening of the menisci and articular cartilage associated with aging.

Pathophysiology

The menisci are C-shaped fibrocartilaginous partial rings of tissue that line the surfaces of opposing bones within the mobile knee joint, maintaining the distance between the involved bones—the tibia and the femur. The medial and lateral menisci lie on the tibial plateau, with their curved portions facing outward. They consist of two phases: a liquid interstitial phase and a solid, extracellular collagenous (predominantly type I) matrix phase that is secreted by meniscal fibrochondrocytes. This dense viscoelastic structure allows them to provide nutrition and lubrication to the articular cartilage, as well as to serve a cushioning and stabilizing function, given their cup-like form. As the knee is fully extended from a flexed position, the distal end of the femur normally rotates slightly medially, with its bilateral bony prominences (femoral condyles) coming to rest within the cupped forms of the two menisci, essentially screwing into place when in the highly stable, fully extended position. When extended, the menisci support 50% of the load placed on the knee joint; when the knee is fully flexed, they support up to 85% of the load.

The menisci of the knee joint are particularly prone to injury when the knee is twisted while in the flexed position, as the femur compresses against the tibia and grinds against the meniscus. This grinding motion tears the meniscus because the force exceeds the strength of the fibrocartilage. The adult meniscus is poorly vascular, except for the peripheral 10% to 25%; thus, it is particularly slow to heal once torn.

Menisci tear either as a direct result of injury or indirectly because of the normal wear and tear on the knee. Traumatic tears are most commonly vertical, longitudinal tears (called bucket-handle tears when displaced), but transverse (radial) tears are also common. They are often associated with ACL or, less commonly, PCL tears. The second type of meniscal tear is known as a degenerative tear, which usually occurs in persons aged 40 years and older and is not preceded by trauma. Horizontal cleavage tears and flap tears are most common. These injuries have particularly poor healing capacity.

Microtears in the menisci heal via the formation of a fibrin clot, containing fibronectin, chemotactic growth factors, and mitogenic growth factors (e.g., platelet-derived growth factor) that cause undifferentiated mesenchymal cells to migrate into the tear, producing a meniscal scar that eventually transforms into fibrocartilage over the course of years. Meniscal chondrocytes act in concert with the scaffolding fibrin clot to contribute to this healing process. Articular damage from the meniscal tear may lead to osteoarthritis with progressive degeneration of the involved joint. Further, because the menisci stabilize the knee, loss of their integrity can lead to more extensive joint injuries.

Clinical Presentation

Subjective Patients with knee problems usually report pain, instability, stiffness, swelling, locking, or weakness. The patient with traumatic tears typically reports a "twisting injury" to the knee. Older patients with a degenerative tear may report a history of minimal or no trauma—they may simply stand from a different position or walk on an uneven surface. The patient may experience the knee "giving way," as well as a painful popping or locking. Typically patients can ambulate after an acute injury and may continue to participate in athletics.

In acute knee pain, obtaining a history of the mechanism of injury is essential to proper diagnosis.

Traumatic tears are typically followed by the insidious onset of knee swelling and stiffness over 2 to 3 days. Mechanical symptoms such as locking, catching, and

popping may continue. Patients usually experience pain on the medial or lateral side of the knee, particularly with twisting or squatting activities. Motion is often limited by a feeling of "tightness" secondary to effusion. In some cases, large fragments of meniscal tissue can become incarcerated in the knee joint, leading to a "locked knee." The mechanical symptoms and degree of pain tend to wax and wane.

Objective The most common finding on physical examination is tenderness over the medial or lateral joint line. Young patients who have traumatic tears that disrupt the peripheral blood supply typically present with a large effusion or hemarthrosis. In degenerative tears or tears that involve the avascular central body of the meniscus, effusions are typically small or absent. Knee motion may be limited secondary to pain or effusion in either instance. During provocative testing such as forced flexion and circumduction (internal and external rotation of the foot), pain is frequently elicited on the side of the knee with the meniscal tear. The McMurray test is positive when the flexion-circumduction maneuver is associated with a positive click.

Diagnostic Tests

Anteroposterior (AP), lateral, tunnel, and axial views are indicated for patients with a history of trauma or effusion. For patients with chronic conditions, the AP and lateral views should be weight-bearing. The definitive diagnostic test for a meniscal or ligamentous tear is MRI, which should be done only if the diagnosis is in doubt or if surgery is anticipated. MRI has also effectively supplanted invasive knee arthrography with intra-articular contrast media, except in contraindicated circumstances (e.g., preexisting metallic clips, severe claustrophobia). Aspiration generally yields noninflammatory fluid that may be bloody, depending on the extent of the tear.

Differential Diagnosis

In cases of acute knee pain, the following are diagnostic considerations:

- Fractures (distal femur, patella, proximal tibia, and fibula) may be ruled out on radiograph.
- Meniscal injuries are preceded in most cases by a twisting injury and "locking," inability to extend the knee completely, and localized pain and tenderness along the joint line.
- Ligamentous injuries show acute pain, swelling, and instability.
- Musculotendinitis strains demonstrate acute pain and swelling but rarely instability.
- Extensor mechanism injuries may cause a fall or collapse related to a sudden weakness.
- Contusions present with a history of a direct blow, localized pain, and tenderness.

Conditions that cause chronic knee pain include arthritis, tumors, sepsis, and overuse syndromes (including bursitis/tendinitis and anterior knee pain). Arthritis is relatively easy to diagnose because symptoms localize to the joint line and are associated with loss of motion and radiographic changes. Tumors are characterized by night pain (relentless and causing sleeplessness), often can be palpated, and should be identifiable on radiographs. Sepsis in the knee is rare in adults; it is more commonly located in the prepatellar bursa. Inspection and palpation of the involved area should determine the location of the infection. Bursitis/tendinitis and anterior knee pain have similar characteristics: Both usually are chronic, often secondary to overuse, and often bilateral. The pain typically is worse with rising or walking after sitting, at night, and with prolonged exercise or use.

Management

In the absence of mechanical symptoms and particularly when a degenerative tear is present, initial therapy should be conservative. RICE and the use of crutches help quiet the acute phase. A short course of oral analgesics, such as acetaminophen or NSAIDs, can facilitate return to normal activities. Rehabilitation to improve the strength of the quadriceps muscle is imperative. Straight-leg raises with the knee extended, but not locked, can be started immediately. Gradually increase weight-bearing, although non–weight-bearing activities such as swimming and riding a stationary bicycle are excellent for increasing ROM and strength.

Traumatic tears on younger patients should be treated aggressively. Sports activity should be restricted until MRI evaluation is made or symptoms resolve. Surgical repair is indicated in younger patients with significant tears in the vascular area (where healing can potentially occur). Other treatments that are being used but are too new to have evidence of long-term effectiveness are meniscal replacement with allogenic or artificial material in younger patients with prior total meniscectomy. For middle-aged or older adults there is no consensus on which treatments yield optimal outcomes. The dilemma is to decide if the meniscal tear will lead to OA or if the degenerative meniscal lesion was caused by OA. Even if the meniscal tear is surgically removed, OA can continue to progress if that was the underlying problem. Current best evidence indicates that medical treatment and planned exercise programs are as efficacious as arthroscopic surgery for middle-aged to older adults. There is a strong need for more research and randomized controlled trials in the area of management of meniscal tears and OA.

Follow-up and Referral

A patient with traumatic effusion, mechanical symptoms, or ligamentous instability requires further evaluation. Patients who do not respond to nonoperative treatment and have persistent joint tenderness or effusion may require further evaluation. Recurrent episodes of locking and damage to adjacent articular cartilage with subsequent OA are possible sequelae. With the exception of the outer rim, the blood supply to the meniscus is poor. Although small peripheral tears can heal, most tears are more central and cannot heal. Patients with recurrent stiffness, locking, or pain have a mechanically significant tear, which suggests ongoing internal damage. Failure to recognize and treat a traumatic tear can lead to progressive damage and a lost opportunity for surgical repair.

Patient Education

Maintaining quadriceps strength is key to minimizing disabilities from this injury. These include "closed-chain" exercises in which the bottoms of the feet are stabilized as they push directly against resistance (e.g., squats, stationary bicycle riding, leg presses). Although the knee will not return to 100% of baseline after healing, participation in sports with proper warm-up exercises and protective equipment can still be enjoyed. Achiness and swelling after a particularly strenuous workout may occur, reflecting the need for increased quadriceps strengthening, as well as the need to return to RICE therapy. Ice and NSAIDs will help control the symptoms but will not address the underlying pathology. Persistent swelling, pain, or episodes of instability should be evaluated further (see Advanced Assessment 15.8).

Patellofemoral Dysfunction

Patellofemoral dysfunction encompasses a continuum of disorders, including chondromalacia patellae and patellofemoral arthralgia. It is an overuse syndrome. Pain typically occurs when climbing stairs or when standing up after a period of sitting. Pain is often reproduced by direct pressure on the patella when the patient is supine with knee extended. X-ray films may reveal irregularity of the patella. Management is conservative; NSAIDs and quadriceps-strengthening exercises, such as tensing of quadriceps and straight-leg raising, are indicated.

Bursitis

Overuse may cause *anserine bursitis,* which produces pain over the inferomedial aspect of the patella, or *prepatellar bursitis,* which is usually a result of direct pressure and produces pain, swelling, erythema, and limited flexion. Initial treatment is the application of ice for 24 hours (then heat), rest, and use of NSAIDs. It is important to rule out infection with fluid aspiration and culture if infection is suspected.

Synovial Growths and Tumors

Pigmented villonodular synovitis is a benign neoplastic disorder, most often affecting young adults. Inflammation of the synovium, which lines the joints, bursae, and tendon sheaths, occurs causing recurrent unilateral pain, erythema, tenderness, and swelling, with intermittent knee locking. An orthopedic referral is necessary for diagnosis.

ANKLE PAIN

Most ankle pain is the result of ankle injury that results in ligamental damage (a *sprain*). A sprain occurs when the ankle is positioned in an unstable way, causing the ligaments to overstretch. A *first-degree sprain* involves stretching of ligamentous fibers; a *second-degree sprain* involves a tear of part of the ligament, with pain and swelling; and a *third-degree sprain* results in complete ligamentous separation (see Table 15.4). The inversion injury is most common, causing damage to the lateral ligaments of the ankle. By contrast, the medial ligaments are very tight and allow for much less motion than the lateral ligaments.

Initiate the history by asking an open-ended question about how the injury happened. Ask what happened after the injury: Was the patient able to get up and walk and continue activity? If so, a serious ligamental injury or fracture is less likely. If the ankle became swollen and discolored within minutes after injury, a severe soft tissue injury or even a fracture can be suspected.

The physical exam should include inspection and palpation. Look for swelling in the area of the internal and external malleoli and compare the landmarks with those of the opposite foot. The location of a deformity helps to localize the injury, and the degree of discoloration is associated with the extent of the injury. The ankle and foot should be palpated to localize the tenderness. It is also helpful to compare the passive ROM in one leg with the opposite extremity. It is important to note crepitus because it is often a sign of fracture. The anterior drawer test should be performed to test the stability of the anterior talofibular ligament, and the varus stress test should be performed to test the stability of the calcaneofibular ligament. (See Advanced Assessment 15.9.)

Radiographic examination of the injured ankle is necessary only in the following cases:

- The patient is not able to bear weight immediately after the injury.
- The ankle develops marked swelling and discoloration soon after the injury.

Table 15.4   Ankle Pain: Sprains

Classification	First Degree	Second Degree	Third Degree
Type of Pain	Stretching, minor tearing of ligament fibers	Partial tearing of ligament fibers	Complete tear of ligament
Clinical Manifestations			
Pain	Minimal	Mild to moderate	Severe
Swelling	Mild	Moderate	Significant; occurs rapidly, usually within the first 30 minutes
Ecchymosis	Mild	Moderate	Severe; occurs rapidly, usually within the first 30 minutes
ROM	Full, nonpainful	Slightly limited, painful	Limited; loss of function
Point tenderness	Mild	Point tenderness	Severe
Joint stability	Stable	Mild joint laxity	Abnormal
Weight-bearing	Able to bear weight	Painful or inability to bear weight	Inability to bear weight
Management	RICE Active ROM Partial weight-bearing activity Return to sports in 2–3 weeks with ankle support	RICE Active ROM Non–weight-bearing activity as tolerated Gradual return to sports with Aircast or taping	Refer to orthopedic specialist; surgery may be required Cast for 4–6 weeks No weight-bearing; rehabilitation Return to sports in 4–8 weeks with support
Complications	Recurrent sprains within 1 month if not fully rehabilitated	Recurrent sprains Joint instability Traumatic arthritis	Persistent instability Traumatic arthritis

RICE: rest, ice, compression, elevation; ROM: range of motion.

Advanced Assessment 15.9   Assessing Ankle Ligaments—Special Tests

Test	Comments
Anterior drawer test—to test stability of anterior talofibular ligament; place the ankle in approximately 20 degrees of plantar flexion	Stabilize the tibia, grasp the hindfoot, and pull forward. Asymmetrical or excessive motion will occur with chronic ankle laxity and severe ankle sprains.
Varus stress test—to test the stability of the calcaneofibular ligament	With the tibia stabilized and the ankle in neutral, grasp the calcaneus and invert the hindfoot. Excessive or asymmetrical motion will occur with chronic laxity of the calcaneofibular ligament.

- Pain occurs with ROM and manipulation of the areas most likely to be stressed in a particular injury.
- Crepitation occurs with palpation or movement of the ankle.
- There is a high risk for litigation.

Management includes application of ice or immersion in an ice water bath immediately after injury and every few hours for 48 hours after the injury, an elastic bandage or splint to stabilize the ankle against inversion and eversion stresses, limited activity until the pain and swelling subside, elevation of the affected foot, and the use of NSAIDs. Strenuous exercise should not be resumed until 2 weeks after the pain and swelling have ceased.

Differential Diagnosis

Nerve Entrapment

Nerve entrapment may occur secondary to ankle fracture, dislocation, or traction injury. If the tibial nerve is affected, there would be a loss of ankle plantar flexion, toe flexion, and weak ankle inversion.

Posterior Impingement Syndrome

Posterior impingement syndrome is most commonly seen in ballet dancers. It manifests with pain and swelling of the posterior ankle and worsens with plantar flexion or dorsiflexion of the great toe. Os trigonum is present on lateral x-ray film.

Referred Pain

Ankle pain may be referred pain secondary to disc herniation at the level of L5 to S1. Signs and symptoms include a sensory deficit over the malleolus, weak eversion, and a decreased Achilles reflex.

Peroneal Tendon Subluxation

Peroneal tendon subluxation may occur secondary to trauma; it will present with pain and a "snapping" over the posterior distal fibula. Pain will increase with active eversion of the dorsiflexed foot, and there may be palpable/visible movement of tendons.

Tendon Rupture

Achilles tendon rupture causes pain and inability to walk normally. Closed tendon ruptures usually result from a sudden excessive load applied to the musculotendinous unit, with failure occurring either within the tendon's substance (torn fibers) or at its insertion into the bone. A tendon rupture can occasionally occur spontaneously in healthy individuals from relatively minor trauma. Achilles tendon rupture is also an uncommon but potential side effect of fluoroquinolones.

Physical exam will usually reveal swelling, tenderness, and often bruising over the site of rupture. Test the tendon's continuity by performing Thompson's test. To do so, (1) have the patient lie prone, (2) bend the knee so that the leg is vertical, and (3) squeeze the calf. The test is positive if squeezing the calf does not produce plantar flexion of the ankle. This means the tendon is ruptured. Treatment is either surgical repair or immobilization with cast with the foot plantar-flexed.

Bursitis

Inflammation of the bursae of the ankle most commonly affects the retrocalcaneal bursa. There will be pain anterior to the Achilles tendon, just above its insertion into the calcaneus; the pain is aggravated by squeezing the area anterior to the tendon, as well as by dorsiflexion of the ankle. This injury is related to repetitive trauma.

Chronic Ligamentous Laxity

Chronic ligamentous laxity may produce few symptoms other than an aching and tenderness over ligaments after prolonged activity. Rest and NSAIDs are the treatment of choice.

Fracture

There will be pain, swelling, or inability to bear weight, decreased ROM, and obvious bony disruption on x-ray film. Stress fractures of the ankle may occur.

■ FOOT PAIN

The foot contains 26 bones, 33 joints, and more than 100 ligaments. Foot pain is usually related to an inflammatory process resulting from trauma (13% of activity-related musculoskeletal injuries in men), a deformity, or a foot–shoe incompatibility. The feet are subjected to numerous forces: For example, when an individual is standing, forces exerted on the foot are equivalent to four times the individual's body weight. Any alteration in ability to use the feet for any reason, such as pain secondary to hammer toe or corns and calluses, will have a significant effect on the health and well-being of the patient.

General treatment measures for foot pain include the use of footwear with roomy toes, supportive arches, and low heels. Heel lifts, cushioned inner soles, and arch supports can provide significant relief when used appropriately. Referral to a podiatrist may be necessary.

Differential Diagnosis

Forefoot Problems

Common problems in the forefoot are calluses, corns, plantar warts, bunions, neuromas, and stress fractures. The history in patients with calluses, corns, and warts would reveal discomfort related to pressure, whereas stress fractures cause pain of acute onset involving the metatarsals. An interdigital neuroma causes tenderness in the third and fourth intermetatarsal space with radiation into the toes. Physical exam findings in patients with stress fractures include point tenderness and swelling over the involved bone. The hyperkeratotic lesions of calluses and corns may be indistinguishable from each other, but plantar warts can be distinguished by the punctate bleeding associated with the wart. Interdigital neuromas may sometimes produce a tender nodule in the intermetatarsal space. A *bunion* or *hallus valgus* is the deformity of the first metatarsophalangeal (MTP) joint associated with the lateral drift of the toe. This presents as a painful swelling on the dorsomedial aspect of the first metatarsal head. Foot–shoe incompatibility may produce physical findings such as the toe deformities of hammer toe and mallet toe.

Midfoot Problems

Midfoot problems are generally the result of pes planus, or flat foot. This is likely to produce pain and stiffness in the midfoot region, often associated with degenerative arthritis or laxity of the posterior tibial tendon. Tenderness to palpation usually occurs along the medial plantar border of the sole with flat foot. Flattening of the medial longitudinal arch of the foot and often a valgus deflection of the heel are indicative of this condition.

Hindfoot Problems

Common hindfoot conditions include plantar fasciitis, infracalcaneal bursitis, and posterior heel problems such as Achilles tendinitis and posterior bursitis. The history of individuals with plantar fasciitis includes subcalcaneal pain that sometimes radiates to the arch of the foot while the person is running or walking. The pain is worse in the morning. Infracalcaneal bursitis produces an aching sensation in the midplantar region of the calcaneus that becomes worse the longer the heel is weight-bearing. The pain associated with Achilles tendinitis is at or proximal to the insertion of the Achilles tendon onto the calcaneus. In this condition, the physical exam reveals swelling and erythema. The pain is increased with dorsiflexion of the ankle, and crepitus may be palpated. Infracalcaneal bursitis produces pain and tenderness to palpation in the midplantar aspect of the calcaneus. Plantar fasciitis findings typically include tenderness along the medial plantar aspect of the calcaneus, with forced dorsiflexion of the digits increasing the pain. Differential Diagnosis 15.5 presents common differential diagnoses and their treatment.

COMMON PROBLEMS

■ ARTHRITIS

Osteoarthritis

Osteoarthritis (OA), also known as *degenerative joint disease* (DJD) or "wear and tear" arthritis, is the most common articular disease in adults older than age 45. It is the most widespread form of arthritis and is a significant cause of functional impairment, chronic pain, and disability in the older population.

OA is a gradual and progressive joint disease typically found in middle-aged to elderly patients. OA is the most common form of joint disease and is the leading cause of disability in the older adult. Although symptoms of OA occur earlier in women, the prevalence among men and women is equal. In addition to age, risk factors include genetics, female sex, joint injury, past trauma, advancing age, obesity, and mechanical stress (Rakel and Rakel, 2011). OA is a joint condition in which loss of articular cartilage and degeneration occur, which leads to pain and often deformity.

Often, OA is classified as "primary" or idiopathic, resulting from one or more of the following:

- Advancing age
- Obesity
- Occupational overloading of joints
- Familial type II collagen gene polymorphisms

This is contrasted to "secondary" OA, which may develop at varying intervals after trauma, infection, osteonecrosis, congenital malalignment, or in the setting of inflammatory arthritis or metabolic disease. In reality, both primary and secondary OA may coexist.

OA actually encompasses a group of subtypes with different etiological factors but a common response pattern in joint tissues. This type of arthritis is primarily noninflammatory and involves a combination of

Differential Diagnosis 15.5   Foot Pain

Differential Diagnosis	Management
Forefoot	
Hallus valgus or bunion	Avoid pressure on the tender bunion, NSAIDs, protective shields, orthotic devices, appropriate footware; if no relief, consider surgery.
Enlarged bone on the medial side of the first metatarsal	
Corns and calluses with keratinized skin	Moleskin protection, gentle rubbing with pumice, separating toes with cushions or orthotics; if unrelieved, consider surgery.
Sesamoid disorders	Protect the injured part by limiting weight-bearing, wearing protective padding or strapping, and NSAIDs.
Localized pain and swelling over first MTP joint	
Neuromas	Shoe modification: wide toe box, metatarsal bar, and soft inner soles; NSAIDs; and in severe cases, corticosteroid injections to reduce inflammation.
Stress fractures	Rest and efforts to disperse weight-bearing away from the fracture such as stiff-soled shoe, metatarsal bar, walking cast.
Infection	Treatment as appropriate.
Flat feet	Orthotics.
Bunion	Pad; surgery.
Peripheral neuritis	Investigate cause.
Midfoot	
Pes planus	No treatment if asymptomatic; if symptomatic: flexible arch support, heel-cord stretching, and toe exercises such as picking up objects with toes and spreading toes.
Hindfoot	
Achilles tendinitis	Initial treatment: Rest, ice and use of NSAIDs, and immobilization. Heel lifts and heel-cord stretching exercises. Corticosteroids are contraindicated.
Plantar fasciitis	Heel lifts, padded heel cups, and orthotic devices. Acute treatment is rest, ice, NSAIDs, and local corticosteroid injections. Heel-cord stretching exercises and use of a night-time dorsal splint to maintain ankle dorsiflexion and toe extension may be beneficial; surgical release of the plantar fascia is the measure of last resort.
Infracalcaneal bursitis	

MTP: metatarsophalangeal.

biomechanical stresses and biochemical changes in articular cartilage and synovial membrane. There is erosion and fibrillation of cartilage, with joint space narrowing and osteophyte formation. Principal sites for OA are the distal interphalangeal (DIP) joints, the proximal interphalangeal (PIP) joints, and the carpometacarpal (CMC) joint of the thumb in the hand; the first metatarsophalangeal or great toe joint; and the hips, knees, and cervical and lumbar spine. Although hand joints associated with the pincer grasp and lower-extremity weight-bearing joints are affected, the ankle, wrist, shoulder, and elbow are usually not, unless the cause of the arthritis is traumatic or occupational.

Epidemiology and Risk Factors

OA affects approximately 60 million Americans. Radiographic evidence of OA is present in about 33% to almost 90% of people older than age 65. Gender differences are not apparent before age 45. After age 50, however, women are more likely to have OA, with women representing 74% of cases, according to the Arthritis Foundation. The actual numbers are probably grossly underreported because many older adults are asymptomatic or do not report symptoms, which they mistakenly believe to be an inevitable consequence of aging, or for which they believe there is no treatment. Also, the definition of OA may differ among various authorities, leading to variations in reporting prevalence and incidence. Some health-care providers consider symptomatology alone, whereas others use radiographic (x-ray) evidence without symptoms; some include both. Studies stemming from autopsy analyses establish degenerative joint changes occurring as early as the second decade of life. Another confounding factor in interpreting prevalence and incidence is the fact that some sources list breakdowns by anatomical site, whereas others do not.

There is conflicting information on racial differences in rates of OA in African Americans and white Americans. Asian counterparts have a very low prevalence of hip OA, although hand OA is equally prevalent in Hong Kong Chinese and Europeans. Age is a risk factor, with a sharp increase in the middle to late years of life. The

Framingham Osteoarthritis Study and the English twin study have identified a genetic component in hand arthritis in women.

Genetic research on families with a preponderance of arthritis has demonstrated mutations of the *col2A1* gene, the precursor to type II collagen. Other genetic influences also have been identified, but the current approach to the study of genetics and OA is fraught with inconsistencies in defining the disease. Patients who have parents who developed OA at middle age or earlier or parents with polyarticular disease are considered at high risk for developing the disease themselves.

Obesity is a risk factor for arthritis of the knee and, to a lesser extent, the hip. Exercise, including recreational jogging, has not been shown to increase the risk of OA. Muscle weakness around the joints, abnormal gait pattern or weight-bearing, local joint injury, and repetitive occupational joint use are contributing factors. Cruciate ligament damage or meniscal tears, particularly when accompanied by partial or total meniscectomy, increase the risk of knee OA. Low levels of vitamin C and/or vitamin D have also been implicated as a risk factor for OA. Estrogen replacement therapy is associated with a reduced risk of knee and hip OA; it was also shown to have a moderately protective but not statistically significant effect against worsening of radiographic knee OA in a group of white American women enrolled in the Framingham study. Although all of these factors have been cited as having a role in OA, the definitive cause of the disease is not known. In general, biomechanical, biochemical, inflammatory, and immunological factors are all implicated in the pathogenesis of OA.

Pathophysiology

The exact pathophysiology of OA is still under study, with many promising developments on the horizon. Normal cartilage derives its viscoelastic and compressive characteristics from cellular and matrix components. Chondrocytes synthesize type II collagen and glycosaminoglycans to maintain the integrity of the extracellular matrix. These chondrocytes are also responsible for balancing cartilage degradation and repair. In contrast to the autoreactive inflammatory pathology associated with rheumatoid arthritis, systemic lupus erythematosus, and other inflammatory arthritides, in OA articular cartilage is thought to be initially damaged due to repetitive microtrauma or a single inciting macrotraumatic event. Bone and joint malalignment, ligamentous laxity, weakness in muscle groups that provide counterforce against the involved joint (e.g., quadriceps for the knee joint), and any type of underlying structural defect may magnify the damage imparted by this repetitive physical trauma. Proprioception is also impaired in affected knee joints. This diminishes muscular reflexes that normally provide compensatory mechanical mechanisms to counter destructive load-bearing forces on arthritic joints. In addition, underlying genetic defects in cartilage formation (e.g., type II collagen defects, ochronotic cartilage with abnormal pigment deposition) may lead to tissue damage from normal wear and tear in the absence of inciting physical trauma.

Mechanical loading of the joint has been shown to increase macromolecule formation by the chondrocyte within the extracellular matrix as a function of both load intensity and frequency of load-bearing, affecting not only the concentration of matrix proteoglycans but also the integrity of the collagen meshwork. The act of mechanical forces triggering biochemical reactions has been termed *mechanotransduction* and is only now beginning to be characterized within the chondrocyte. Although much of this pathogenesis is poorly understood and stems from preclinical animal studies, we know that cartilage matrix degradation predominates in OA, with greater fluid loss from joint cartilage in response to mechanical loading. In turn, attempts at repair by chondrocytes are ineffectual.

Current focus centers on the role of matrix metalloproteinases (MMPs) in mediating cartilage degradation. This family of proteolytic enzymes includes collagenase-1 (MMP-1), collagenase-2 (MMP-8), collagenase-3 (MMP-13), stromelysin (MMP-3), and gelatinase-A (MMP-2). They are secreted by chondrocytes and synovial cells and are regulated by plasmin, nitric oxide, interleukin-1 (IL-1), and other cytokines such as IL-6 and possibly tumor necrosis factor–alpha (TNF-α). Normally, these substances are tightly controlled by counterregulatory substances including tissue inhibitors of MMPs (TIMPs). However, in OA, pro-inflammatory cytokines, namely IL-1, stimulate MMPs and suppress cartilage self-repair by interfering with chondrocyte proliferation, collagen production, TIMP formation, and MMP inactivation. These processes are normally mediated by transforming growth factor–beta (TGF-β), which is found in decreased levels in OA patients. Dysregulated levels of anabolic cartilaginous growth factors including insulin-like growth factor–1 (IGF-1) and IGF-1 binding protein are also evident, as some studies have revealed lower levels of these factors in OA patients, as well. All these processes result in increased production of type 1 fibrous cartilage, rather than type 2 articular cartilage.

In addition, the disease process of OA includes sclerosis of underlying subchondral bone and abnormalities in the juxta-articular bone marrow. Abnormal bone deposition within the degenerating joint, which impinges on the joint space, is known as osteophyte formation. These osteophytes may give the impression of external bulging within the joint space, which may sometimes be mistaken for the inflammatory joint pathology of rheumatoid arthritis. However, if spinal osteophytes impinge on nerve roots, they may produce radicular symptoms, similar to those seen in intervertebral disc herniation.

Crystal deposition into the synovial fluid of osteoarthritic joints, particularly calcium pyrophosphate dihydrate and basic calcium phosphate crystals, also correlates with worsening degrees of radiographic joint pathology and cartilaginous fissuring. Although evidence for the pathophysiological nature of these crystals is primarily circumstantial, these crystals appear to initiate an inflammatory synovitis, MMP secretion, and synovial proliferation with subsequent cartilaginous destruction. Moreover, patients with an inherited predisposition to calcium pyrophosphate dihydrate deposition also develop severely degenerative OA.

Clinical Presentation

Subjective

Patients typically present with slowly developing, localized pain in the affected joint or joints that interferes with their usual activities. The onset is subtle, and the pain may be ignored initially. Patients with OA in the weight-bearing joints may have early morning stiffness or stiffness after inactivity, which subsides after 30 minutes, also referred to as the "gel phenomenon." Pain and stiffness are also present in hand OA, often accompanied by bony deformities such as Heberden's nodes, which affect the DIP joints, and Bouchard's nodes, which affect the PIP joints. Internal derangement in weight-bearing joints may cause them to "lock" or "buckle," increasing the risk for falls; patients often report that their knee "gave way" or "wouldn't bend." In the later stages of OA, pain may be also present at rest. OA may present as monoarticular or polyarticular.

The history should include information on the onset, location, and duration of pain; any self-care measures the patient has taken to alleviate pain and the effectiveness of these measures; and associated symptoms such as joint stiffness, swelling, or deformity. Does the pain interfere with sleep or awaken the patient at night? Inquire if there is a family history of OA. An occupational history should be explored for evidence of overuse; any trauma or surgery to the joint should be noted. Elicit a history of activity/exercise patterns, any changes in activities of daily living (ADLs) or instrumental ADLs, and weight changes, especially a gain in weight. Socioeconomic factors and vocational issues should be explored. It is also important to obtain a past or present history of any systemic illness or chronic disease state, along with a list of current medications, including over-the-counter (OTC) preparations, herbal remedies, and nutraceuticals. OA of the wrists, ankles, and shoulder is usually related to trauma or other secondary causes.

Objective

Typical clinical findings of OA include minimal or no swelling of affected joints, tenderness on direct palpation, crepitus, and reduced passive and active ROM. Crepitus is a common, although late, finding and a sensitive criterion for OA. There may be effusions in the large joints.

Physical exam findings include the following:

- Hands: Enlargement of the DIP and/or PIP joints. The CMC joint of the thumb may also be enlarged and in general there may be pain on motion.
- Feet: Swelling (bunion) of the big toe and DIP joints.
- Knees and hips: Possible pain and crepitus on passive ROM. There may be tenderness to palpation along the joint line, and some muscle atrophy may be present. Hard swelling, if present, is usually a result of bone spurs, whereas soft swelling is related to effusion. There may be significantly decreased ROM, both active and passive. Carefully examine the hip of any patient who complains of knee pain; pain referred to the knee may be the only symptom of hip OA.
- Spine: Degenerative changes are common. There may be limited motion and stiffness of the neck and/or lower back. Bony spurs at the facet joints may produce pain and compression of spinal root nerves.

The physical exam should include a functional status evaluation in the older adult. Gait abnormalities such as a limp are significant. Evaluation for spinal and hip alignment and leg-length discrepancy is helpful initially to detect contributing factors. Affected joints should be examined for tenderness, bony deformities, swelling, redness, warmth, and ROM. Tenderness along the joint line, crepitus, and limited ROM are typical but nonspecific findings. Knee joint effusion may also be seen, as well as Baker's cysts in the posterior popliteal area. Muscle strength, especially that of the quadriceps muscles, and joint stability should be assessed. The presence of fever or weight loss, especially when accompanied by fatigue and poor appetite, is suggestive of a systemic problem rather than OA; these symptoms need further investigation.

The most common symptom of OA is joint pain. OA pain tends to worsen with activity, more often following a period of rest. OA can also cause morning stiffness and generally lasts less than 30 minutes, unlike rheumatoid arthritis, which can cause stiffness for 45 minutes or longer (Rakel and Rakel, 2011). Frequently, the patient may report joint locking or joint instability. These symptoms result in loss of function, with patients limiting their ADLs due to the pain and stiffness. Early in the disease process, the joints may appear normal. However, the patient's gait may be antalgic if weight-bearing joints are involved.

The joints most commonly affected are the hands, knees, hips, and spine, but any joint can be involved. OA is often asymmetrical. Pain on ROM and limitation of ROM are common to all forms of OA. Table 15.5 explains the unique physical exam findings for common joints.

Table 15.5   Signs and Symptoms of Osteoarthritis

Hand	Spine
Pain on range of motion	Pain on range of motion
Hypertrophic changes at DIP and PIP joints	Limitation of range of motion
(Heberden nodes and Bouchard nodes)	Lower extremity sensory loss, reflex loss, motor weakness
Tenderness over carpometacarpal joint of thumb	caused by nerve root impingement
	Pseudoclaudication caused by spinal stenosis
Shoulder	**Hip**
Pain on range of motion	Pain on range of motion
Limitation of range of motion, especially external	Pain in buttock
rotation	Limitation of range of motion, especially internal rotation
Crepitus on range of motion	
Knee	**Foot**
Pain on range of motion	Pain on ambulation, especially at first metatarsophalangeal
Joint effusion	joint
Crepitus on range of motion	Limited range of motion of first metatarsophalangeal joint,
Presence of popliteal cyst (Baker cyst)	hallux rigidus
Lateral instability	Hallux valgus deformity (bunion)
Valgus or varus deformity	

DIP: distal interphalangeal; PIP: proximal interphalangeal.

Diagnostic Reasoning

Diagnostic Tests

Clinicians can make the diagnosis of OA based on the history and physical exam because OA is primarily a clinical diagnosis. Plain radiographs can be helpful in confirming the diagnosis and in ruling out other conditions (Fracture Management for Primary Care Expert Consult, M. Patrice Eiff and Robert Hatch, 2011). No laboratory tests are required to make the diagnosis.

Radiographic testing may be useful in the following situations:

* To establish diagnosis at the hip
* To assess disease severity at other joints
* To screen for other types of bone and joint pathology if pain is severe enough and disrupts sleep
* To determine baseline status to assess change over time

Early changes often do not appear, but as the disease progresses, x-ray findings include asymmetrical joint space narrowing, bony cysts and osteophytes, and subchondral sclerosis. Radiographic findings are poorly correlated to symptomatology. Further x-ray studies may be ordered to document progression of the disease if symptoms increase markedly, ADL levels change dramatically, or the patient is being evaluated for surgical intervention. MRI and CT scans may be ordered for patients with suspected spinal stenosis.

Laboratory testing is helpful in ruling out other conditions such as rheumatoid arthritis (RA), gout, lupus, sepsis, or polymyalgia rheumatica, but has little place in establishing a diagnosis of OA. Complete blood count (CBC), C-reactive protein, and erythrocyte sedimentation rate (ESR) are usually normal; the ESR in older patients is more likely to be elevated. Rheumatoid factor, antinuclear antibody, serum uric acid, or 24-hour urinary uric acid levels may be ordered to rule out RA, lupus, or gout, depending on the clinical presentation, but again may yield significant false-positive results. Synovial fluid analyses may be useful in ruling out inflammatory and/or infectious arthritis. (See Differential Diagnosis 15.6.)

Differential Diagnosis 15.6   Osteoarthritis

* Rheumatoid arthritis
* Crystalline arthropathies (i.e., gout and pseudogout)
* Inflammatory arthritis
* Seronegative spondyloarthropathies (e.g., psoriatic arthritis and reactive arthritis)
* Septic arthritis or postinfectious arthropathy
* Fibromyalgia
* Tendinitis
* Ankylosing spondylitis
* Avascular necrosis
* Patellofemoral arthritis
* Bursitis
* Lupus erythematosus
* Lyme disease
* Neuropathy
* Neuromuscular disease
* Parkinson's disease
* Osteopenia or osteoporosis
* Paget's disease
* Bone malignancy

The American College of Rheumatology (ACR) has identified criteria for the diagnosis of OA of the hand, knee, and hip.

Treatment

The goals of OA treatment include alleviation of pain and improvement of functional status. Optimally, patients should receive a combination of nonpharmacological and pharmacological treatment.

Nonpharmacological interventions, which are the cornerstones of OA therapy, include the following:

- Patient education
- Heat and cold
- Weight loss
- Exercise
- Physical therapy
- Occupational therapy
- Unloading in certain joints (e.g., knee, hip)

Four main categories of treatment choices are nonpharmacological, pharmacological, complementary and alternative, and surgical. In general, treatment should begin with the safest and least invasive therapies before proceeding to more invasive therapies. All patients with OA should receive treatment from the first two categories. Surgical management should be reserved for those who do not improve with behavioral and pharmacological therapy and who have intractable pain and loss of function (Sinusas, 2012).

Nonpharmacological therapy includes exercise and physical therapy that includes strengthening exercises and ROM exercises. The clinician should encourage regular exercise throughout the course of treatment and encourage weight loss for those patients who are overweight or obese. Consider physical therapy referral for supervised exercise and also bracing and splinting to help support painful or unstable joints. Therapeutic ultrasound is a physical therapy modality that is also used in OA treatment.

Pharmacological treatment should include acetaminophen for mild OA. If and when acetaminophen begins to fail in controlling symptoms or if symptoms are moderate to severe, NSAID therapy is recommended. NSAIDs are superior to acetaminophen for treatment of OA. Patients who take NSAIDs should be cautioned about the adverse effects, which may include gastrointestinal (GI) bleeding, renal dysfunction, and blood pressure elevation. COX-2 inhibitors (Celebrex) have an improved safety profile for adverse GI effects; however, they increase cardiovascular risks (Brown, 2012).

Opioids are used often in the treatment of OA pain; however, due to their potential for abuse, opioids should be an option only if the patient has not had a positive response to acetaminophen or NSAID therapy. Opioids should only be prescribed at low dosages and then slowly increased as needed, and the patient should be carefully monitored for potential dependence.

The ACR has issued guidelines for pharmacological treatment of OA of the hand, hip, and knee. For *hand* osteoarthritis, the ACR conditionally recommends using one or more of the following:

- Topical capsaicin
- Topical NSAIDs
- Oral NSAIDs
- Tramadol

The ACR conditionally recommends against using intra-articular therapies or opioid analgesics for hand OA. For patients 75 years and older, the ACR conditionally recommends the use of topical, rather than oral, NSAIDs.

For *knee* osteoarthritis, the ACR conditionally recommends using one of the following:

- Acetaminophen
- Oral NSAIDs
- Topical NSAIDs
- Tramadol
- Intra-articular corticosteroid injections

The ACR conditionally recommends against using chondroitin sulfate, glucosamine, or topical capsaicin for knee OA.

For *hip* osteoarthritis, the ACR conditionally recommends using one or more of the following for initial management:

- Acetaminophen
- Oral NSAIDs
- Tramadol
- Intra-articular corticosteroid injections

The ACR conditionally recommends against using chondroitin sulfate or glucosamine for hip OA.

The Agency for Healthcare Research and Quality (AHRQ) comparison found that acetaminophen was modestly inferior to NSAIDs in reducing osteoarthritic pain but was associated with a lower risk of adverse GI effects. On the other hand, acetaminophen poses a higher risk of liver injury. The AHRQ also noted that topical diclofenac was found to have efficacy similar to that of oral NSAIDs in patients with localized OA.

Management

The principles of management of OA are to control pain and other symptoms, to maximize functional independence and mobility, to minimize disability, and to preserve quality of life. A variety of modalities are utilized to achieve this, including patient education and self-care strategies, nonpharmacological and pharmacological interventions, and surgical management (see Table 15.6).

Pharmacological Management

Acetaminophen The goal of pharmacological management is pain control, with acetaminophen (Tylenol) as the first-line agent. Tylenol two tablets—regular strength

Table 15.6	Management of Osteoarthritis
General Management Pharmacological	Nonnarcotic analgesics Topical agents (e.g., capsaicin) Nonacetylated salicylates NSAIDs Intra-articular corticosteroids
Nonpharmacological	Activity modifications Exercise (biking, walking, swimming) Physical therapy Application of heat/cold Psychosocial support Pain management Self-help programs Surgical
Specific Management OA of the hand	Pharmacological: Analgesics Nonpharmacological: Occupational therapy
OA of the hip	Pharmacological: Analgesics, NSAIDs (at analgesic or anti-inflammatory doses) Nonpharmacological: Occupational therapy, physical therapy Surgical
OA of the knee	Pharmacological: Analgesics, NSAIDs (at analgesic or anti-inflammatory doses), intra-articular corticosteroids (intermittent) Nonpharmacological: Occupational therapy, physical therapy Surgical

(325 mg) or extra strength (500 mg)—may be taken every 4 to 6 hours as needed, or Tylenol Arthritis Extended Relief Caplets (650 mg) two tablets may be taken every 8 hours as needed, not to exceed 4,000 mg in 24 hours. The maximum daily dose of acetaminophen in patients receiving warfarin therapy should not exceed 2,500 mg PO. Several controlled studies have established the efficacy of acetaminophen, although other studies demonstrate that NSAIDs are more effective. However, recommendations begin therapy with acetaminophen, because this is a viable strategy for a long-term treatment plan. Patients should be cautioned about using alcohol with acetaminophen. Hepatotoxicity is a serious potential adverse effect. Patients should also be educated to read the label on OTC cold and sinus preparations because some of them contain acetaminophen. The acetaminophen in these preparations counts toward the daily maximum of 4,000 mg.

Nonsteroidal Anti-Inflammatory Drugs NSAIDs actually comprise several categories of pharmacological agents, all sharing comparable anti-inflammatory properties. Although each class acts in an individual manner, all inhibit the production of prostaglandins, which are inflammatory mediators. Cyclooxygenase (COX), or prostaglandin endoperoxide synthase, is the first enzyme in the prostaglandin synthesis pathway. This enzyme transforms arachidonic acid to other prostaglandin breakdown products. Two forms of COX are present: COX-1 is normally present in blood vessels, stomach, and kidney and promotes the normal functioning of those systems; COX-2 is generated in inflammatory settings by cytokines and inflammatory mediators. Aspirin and NSAIDs inhibit cyclooxygenase enzyme and prostaglandin production, but they have no effect on the arachidonic–lipoxygenase pathway resulting in the formation of leukotrienes. NSAIDs are nonselective COX inhibitors. All possess antipyretic, analgesic, and anti-inflammatory properties. Inhibition of COX-1 is largely responsible for the adverse effects associated with NSAID therapy, including GI bleeding, ulcerogenic activity, fluid retention, and blockade of platelet aggregation. Patients on NSAIDs are four to five times more likely to suffer GI bleeding than individuals who are not taking the drugs. The risk of bleeding is increased during the first month of treatment and with increased dosages of the NSAID; older age and polypharmacy are also risk factors. It was hoped that the use of the COX-2 inhibitors would be equally effective for pain while curbing GI side effects or platelets; however, subsequent data regarding the increased risk of vascular events such as myocardial infarction (MI) or transient ischemic attack (TIA)/stroke have resulted in withdrawal of several of these agents from the market. NSAIDs also interact with several other classes of medication. In addition, NSAIDs are well known to cause fluid retention, as well as having the potential to cause nephrotoxicity.

When initiating NSAID therapy, it is best to begin with the lowest dose possible and increase as needed. It is important to question the patient about use of OTC medications because many patients with OA take ibuprofen (e.g., Advil, Nuprin, Motrin IB) in a nonprescription strength for headache, fever, or other minor discomforts and do not associate the OTC form with prescribed medication. If the patient is intolerant of one medication in a specific class, another one in the same class may prove to be satisfactory. Individualization of therapy is the key to successful management.

Because of emerging data indicating that the COX-2 inhibitor celecoxib may be associated with increased risk of serious cardiovascular events (MI, TIA), especially when used for long periods of time or in very high-risk settings (such as after surgery), the U.S. Food and Drug

Administration (FDA) has issued a recommendation that prescribers consider this emerging information when weighing risks versus benefits for individual patients. According to the FDA, patients who are at high risk of GI bleed, have a history of intolerance to nonselective NSAIDs, or are not doing well on nonselective NSAIDs may be appropriate candidates for COX-2 inhibitor therapy; also, individual patient risk for cardiovascular events and other risks commonly associated with NSAIDs should be considered. There is considerable variability among patients in both effectiveness and tolerance of NSAIDs. If one particular drug proves ineffective or unacceptable, benefit may be obtained by changing to a drug of a different class. The doses of these drugs should be individualized. The addition of a proton pump inhibitor, histamine-2 blocker (H_2 blocker), or the prostaglandin analog misoprostol to NSAID therapy helps protect against gastroduodenal ulceration. In addition, meloxicam (Mobic) is a preferential inhibitor of COX-2, but it is not a true COX-2 inhibitor according to FDA criteria. It seems to be well tolerated with few side effects of drug–drug interaction. The American Academy of Family Practice Physicians has issued the following recommendations regarding NSAID use:

- Initiate therapy with acetaminophen, and if NSAIDs are needed, use the lowest dose for the shortest duration possible.
- Avoid NSAIDs in patients with preexisting renal disease, congestive heart failure, or cirrhosis.
- Avoid NSAIDs and aspirin in patients taking anticoagulants.
- Creatinine should be monitored for patients on angiotensin-converting enzyme inhibitors or angiotensin receptor blockers who are prescribed NSAIDs on a regular basis.

Recommendations from other medical experts emphasize that conservative treatments such as physical therapy and exercise should be first-line management. If NSAIDs must be used, those with the highest COX-1 selectivity should be tried initially (ibuprofen, aspirin, naproxen).

Additional Pain Relievers Tramadol hydrochloride (Ultram) is a nonopioid pain reliever that is indicated for moderate to moderately severe pain. It is available as a combination drug with acetaminophen that works synergistically; it can also be taken with NSAIDs. It is contraindicated with alcohol, hypnotics, and narcotics, and should be used with caution in patients with the potential to abuse it. There is no evidence that this medication is any more effective than NSAIDs. Likewise, although there are times when the prescription of opioids might be appropriate, no evidence exists that these medications provide any more relief than NSAIDs; given the side effects and abuse potential, they should be used only in selected situations. There is no clear evidence that muscle relaxants or benzodiazepines are helpful adjuncts,

although some clinicians continue to prescribe them because actual spasms of the paraspinous muscles are elicited on physical exam in the case of vertebral OA.

Other medications such as gabapentin (Neurontin), selective serotonin reuptake inhibitors, and tricyclic antidepressants have also proven effective in the management of patients with OA who have chronic pain.

Glucosamine with or without chondroitin, a dietary supplement not regulated by the FDA, is currently not recommended by the American Academy of Orthopaedic Surgeons (AAOS) for knee OA (Level I; AAOS, 2008).

Topical agents such as capsaicin (Zostrix) cream, applied three to four times daily to the painful areas, either alone or in concert with oral pharmacotherapy, may be helpful. The patient should be cautioned to avoid rubbing the cream in the eyes and to wash hands carefully after using capsaicin to avoid irritation. Some redness and burning at the site of application is normal initially, but it should disappear after 3 to 5 days. If irritation persists, the medication should be discontinued. Other topical agents, such as Ben Gay, Icy Hot, and similar preparations, are menthol based and have a temporary, local effect. Topical preparations also give the patient a sense of control over his or her own treatment. (See Drugs Commonly Prescribed 15.2: Pharmacological Treatment of Osteoarthritis.)

Intra-articular Injections Two groups of drugs are injected intra-articularly, particularly in arthritis of the knee. Intra-articular steroids have been used for some time in the treatment of OA of the knee. Several controlled studies document their efficacy for up to 4 weeks although some patients report a response for up to 6 months after injection. Agents include triamcinolone hexacetonide, triamcinolone acetonide, and methylprednisolone (Solu-Medrol). A 1% lidocaine solution is usually mixed with the steroid before injection. Patients are instructed to rest the joint for a day and to limit physical activity for 48 to 72 hours after the injection. The hip may also be injected. Joint injection is also used in these and other joints for bursitis or tendinitis.

The use of intra-articular injections of corticosteroids should be judicious: No more than three to four injections should be done per year and up to a maximum of 12 injections per joint, and they should be used only in episodes of acute flare-up. If steroid injections are administered excessively, they can accelerate joint deterioration. There is consistent evidence that intra-articular corticosteroid injections of the knee are effective for short-term pain relief (Stephens et al, 2008).

After the introduction of the needle into the joint and before steroid administration, aspiration of as much synovial fluid as possible should be attempted. Aspiration often provides symptomatic relief for the patient and allows laboratory evaluation of the fluid, if necessary. Infected joint fluid and bacteremia are contraindications to steroid injection.

In patients with osteoarthritic knee pain, steroid injections generally result in clinically and statistically significant pain reduction as soon as 1 week after injection. The effect may last, on average, anywhere from 4 to 8 weeks per injection, but the benefit is unlikely to continue beyond that time frame. Corticosteroid injections are effective for hip OA, with benefits often lasting as long as 3 months. Repeat injections are possible in the same joint, but usual practice is limited to four injections yearly.

Viscosupplementation Viscosupplementation with intra-articular hyaluronic acid is also used for treatment of knee OA. Hyaluronic acid is a naturally occurring component of synovial fluid; its purpose is to lubricate the joint for low-impact activities and potentially to prevent mechanical joint damage during high-impact activities. In patients with OA, the viscosity and elasticity of synovial fluid are decreased; there may be a lower concentration and limited distribution of hyaluronic acid. Consequently, all of the rheological features of synovial fluid, such as shock absorption, lubrication, and protection, may be decreased. This further increases damage to synovial tissue and the articular cartilage surface. Hyaluronan (Hyalgan), hylan G-F 20 (Synvisc), and hyaluronic acid (Orthovisc, a highly purified, high molecular weight form of hyaluronic acid, approved for use in the United States only fairly recently) are intended to restore all of the protective functions found in normal synovial fluid. They are indicated for pain relief of knee OA that has failed to respond to conservative measures. Intra-articular injections of hyaluronic acid are marketed as medical devices, not medications, and may be used in conjunction with NSAIDs. Hyaluronic acid is injected once a week for 3 to 5 weeks depending on the preparation, and it may provide benefit for 6 months or longer. Both hyaluronan and hyalin are produced from chicken combs, so patients should be screened for any allergy to avian proteins, feathers, and egg products before injection of hyaluronic acid. Other contraindications for intra-articular injections include knee joint infections, skin diseases, or skin infections at the injection site. If there is joint effusion, aspiration of synovial fluid before injection is advised. Adverse effects of hyaluronic acid injections include transient, localized pain, burning, and swelling at the injection site. Several studies have demonstrated the efficacy of viscosupplementation as equal to or better than continuous NSAID therapy, with significant improvement in pain at night or at rest as well as improvement of pain on motion, including walking pain. Duration of benefit was 8 to 12 months. Intra-articular injection has not been shown to be 100% effective; some studies suggested that the benefit was confined to patients with mild degenerative arthritis. Other conflicting information about viscosupplementation indicates the need for more studies and more rigorous methodology. The AAOS does not recommend for or against viscosupplementation at this time due to inconclusive results. Viscosupplementation is costly and is often not used unless the patient has insurance that will cover this cost.

Surgical Intervention

If nonsurgical strategies fail to provide sufficient pain relief and maintenance of function, referral to a rheumatologist or an orthopedic surgeon for surgical evaluation is indicated. Arthroscopic procedures can include joint lavage, partial medial or lateral meniscectomy or chondroplasty as indicated, lateral patellar retinacular release, fracture drilling of full-thickness defects, or chondral grafts. The AAOS does not currently recommend joint lavage or debridement; partial meniscectomy is advised only when there is strong evidence of a torn meniscus in addition to the OA. Large or open surgical procedures could include osteotomy and partial or total joint arthroplasty. For maximum success, ongoing communication among patients, medical and surgical providers, and physical therapists is essential in identifying appropriate candidates for surgery, treating comorbidities, and establishing rehabilitation goals. Outcomes following total hip and knee replacement demonstrated a higher level of postoperative function and better quality of life in candidates who had surgery earlier rather than waiting until the pain was intolerable and functional abilities had declined. It is also known that psychosocial factors such as motivation and emotional and social functioning (measured at baseline) are strong predictors of postoperative recovery. Annual radiographs to evaluate the position and fixation of the prosthetic components may also be recommended.

Surgery should be reserved for patients whose symptoms have not responded to other treatments. Indication for surgery is continued pain and disability despite conservative treatment. Arthroplasty consists of the surgical removal of joint surface and the insertion of a metal and plastic prosthesis. The prosthesis is held in place by cement or by bone ingrowth into a porous coating on the prosthesis. The use of cement results in faster pain relief, but bone ingrowth may provide a more durable bond; accordingly, prostheses with a porous coating are used in younger patients. Arthroplasty is performed if all other modalities are ineffective and osteotomy is not appropriate or if a patient cannot perform ADLs despite maximal therapy. The most effective surgical intervention is total joint replacement, with excellent patient outcomes following total joint replacement of the hip, knee, and shoulder. Most current joint prostheses function well for 15 to 20 years. After joint replacement, patients require partial weight-bearing, which progresses to full weight-bearing in 1 to 3 months; ROM and strengthening exercises are started within a few days after joint-replacement surgery and continued until the patient has good ROM and strength.

Long-Term Pain Management

For patients who are not candidates for surgery and who have intractable pain, long-term pain management is necessary. Goals of long-term pain management are to maximize quality of life and minimize pain and functional loss. Consultation with a pain management specialist for collaborative management may be beneficial; the use of alternative treatments, including massage therapy, acupuncture, or acupressure, can further enhance pain management and promote a feeling of relaxation and well-being. Pharmacological management should be individualized; it should take into consideration comorbidities, other medications, age, and functional abilities.

New technologies continue to be developed for this disabling disorder. Newer medications, complementary therapies, different prosthetic joint components, osteochondral replacement procedures, and gene therapy for rare hereditary forms of OA are some promising new directions. (See Nursing Research–Based Practice Box 15.1.)

Nonpharmacological Management

Self-Care Strategies   Initial management of OA includes patient education about the nature of the disease, the role of the patient in self-management, and sources of information and support for the patient. The Arthritis Foundation is an excellent resource and offers information sheets, local support groups, and an arthritis self-help course that includes exercise, joint protection, and relaxation techniques, along with information on medications that are typically used to manage symptoms. Weight loss is often an important component of the plan of care (see Table 15.7).

Involvement of the patient's spouse or significant other in the education and support of the individual with arthritis, specifically in helping him or her to develop coping skills, has proven superior to working with the patient alone. In a recent study of patients with OA, an informal network of social support appeared to be effective in mitigating the depression and functional limitations imposed by the disease and significantly enhancing quality of life. Trials of regular monthly phone calls by trained lay personnel to patients, discussing issues such as pain, medication, and treatment adherence, access to medical services, and functional concerns, were also effective. Patients experienced improvement in pain status and function with specific counseling; medical costs were negligible. (See Nursing Research–Based Practice Box 15.2.)

Physical Therapy   Nonpharmacological management strategies include weight loss (when appropriate) and physical therapy for muscle strengthening, particularly quadriceps strengthening for patients with knee OA. The physical therapist also evaluates mobility and the need for assistive devices such as canes or walkers to reduce load-bearing on the arthritic joint. The physical therapist may recommend environmental modifications to maximize functional independence and safety. Other orthotic devices, such as shoe lifts, splints, or bracing, may be prescribed to improve biomechanics. Heat, ice, or ultrasound may be applied locally to decrease pain. Whenever feasible, a supervised exercise program incorporating aerobic and resistive components should be instituted. Several significant studies of arthritis patients utilizing comparison groups attest to the safety and efficacy of fitness training programs versus ROM and health education alone. Participants in the fitness program experienced better task performance and reported less physical disability, less pain, and improved psychological functioning. Aquatic exercise programs are also excellent, particularly those that are tailored to the needs of arthritic patients.

Nursing Research–Based Practice 15.1

McCaffrey, R. The effect of music on acute confusion in older adults after hip or knee surgery. *Appl Nurs Res* 22:107–112, 2006.

McCaffrey (2006) used a randomized controlled design to test the effectiveness of music listening as a tool for decreasing acute confusion and maintaining cognitive function in older adults after hip or knee surgery. Twenty-two older adults undergoing hip or knee surgery were randomized into either a control group that received standard postoperative care or an experimental group that received standard care with the addition of the music intervention. Levels of cognitive function were found to be similar preoperatively in both groups when measured by the Mini–Mental State Exam (MMSE). All members of the experimental (music) group listened to lullaby music on transfer to the orthopedic floor from recovery. When alert, participants were asked to choose their own music from a preselected sample. The cognitive function and acute confusion of the control and experimental groups were then compared using the MMSE and NEECHAM Acute Confusion Scale, respectively, on days 1, 2, and 3 postoperatively. McCaffrey (2006) found that older adults who listened to music postoperatively had increased levels of cognitive functioning in comparison to the control group on postoperative days 1 and 2, with no significant difference on day 3. In addition, the music listening group achieved higher scores on NEECHAM on all three postoperative days, indicating decreased levels of acute confusion in comparison to the control group. Although the study was limited by its small sample size, the findings have implications for improving the nursing care of older adults after hip or knee surgery. "Music is a safe, inexpensive, easy-to-use intervention that can be used by nurses to improve cognition and episodes of acute confusion, thereby improving recovery in older adults after hip or knee surgery" (p. 111).

Table 15.7 Nonpharmacological Therapies for Osteoarthritis

Nonpharmacological Therapies	Comments
Continued reassurance and support	Simply telephoning patients periodically can be helpful; support group.
Patient education	Provide materials.
Protection from overuse	Educate.
Exercise: Only 24% of patients with OA report a level of activity consistent with health; >75% sedentary	Gentle, regular joint exercise helps maintain function and manage pain; water exercise especially effective; other non–weight-bearing, bicycling, for example, preserve muscle support; isometric exercises to maintain strength; moderate to vigorous exercise three times a week can lead to dramatic improvements.
Weight loss—BMI should be 25 or lower	Especially important for patients with lower extremity problems; needed after joint replacement also to preserve joint implant.
Surgery—indicated if patient has pain at rest, at night, unable to sleep, unacceptable loss of joint function	Joint replacement (hip and knee replacement especially effective in pain and function); patients who have undergone earlier preemptive procedure such as arthroscopic joint debridement or osteotomy may eventually require joint replacement.
Heat/ice	Application of heat to the OA joint effective—hot shower, bath; ice occasionally.
Shoe inserts, patellar taping, bracing (knee), gait aids (cane)	A variety of mechanical aids useful for support; patellar taping is recommended by the American Academy of Orthopedic Surgeons; shoe inserts and bracing are not recommended (Level II).

BMI: body mass index; OA: osteoarthritis.

Nursing Research–Based Practice 15.2

Davis, GC, and White, TL. A goal attainment pain management program for older adults with arthritis. *Pain Manage Nurs* 9(4):171–179, 2008.

The purpose of this study was to test the effectiveness of the Goal Attainment Pain Management Program (GAPMAP) for promoting the self-efficacy of older adults in managing chronic musculoskeletal pain associated with rheumatic disease. Seventeen older adults living in independent-living residential settings were included in the study, with an average age of 79.29 years. The GAPMAP intervention took place over a 3-month period and initially involved small group meetings to discuss pain management strategies and potential barriers to pain management. Participants then met with the nurse researchers individually to set personalized pain management goals. Attainment of these goals was assessed at the end of the 3 months. Participants received follow-up phone calls at weeks 1, 4, and 8 to assess progress and allow for discussion.

A significant finding of this study was that 13 of the 17 participants either met or exceeded their expected goals, examples of which include "pain reduction, pacing activities, walking, weight loss, performing selected exercises, and community participation" (p. 176). Additionally, participants were more likely to use "exercise" and "a heated pool, tub, or shower" as pain management strategies after the intervention. "Exercise and distraction" were found to be more helpful for participants after intervention, and there was a significant improvement in both the "experience of living with persistent pain" and "expected outcomes of pain management" (p. 177). The results of this study, although preliminary, highlight goal setting as a tool that nurses can use to help older adults take greater control over their own pain management. Supporting older adults to maintain their autonomy and participate in their own care through programs such as GAPMAP is an important part of nursing practice. More research with a larger sample size would be important for assessing the generalizability of these findings when applied to other aspects of the care of older adults.

Transcutaneous electrical nerve stimulation is sometimes used for arthritic pain, but studies to date have not established its effectiveness. Use of pulsed electric and electromagnetic fields (PEMF), more commonly used for the treatment of nonunion fractures, has shown some promise in preliminary studies of patients with knee OA, but further studies are needed before PEMF can be recommended as adjunctive treatment for OA.

Occupational Therapy Short-term occupational therapy to maximize ADL abilities and evaluate the need for adaptive devices is often overlooked, but it can be very valuable to the patient with arthritis. Devices such as a raised toilet seat, toilet side rails, elastic shoelaces, reachers, and various kitchen accessories can enhance functional capacity and independence.

Complementary Therapy   Acupuncture and nutritional therapy (including vitamin supplementation) are other therapies used for the management of OA and other musculoskeletal problems. (See Complementary Therapies 15.1.) Although some studies suggest that acupuncture may be beneficial as adjunctive treatment for OA, results are inconclusive. The AAOS does not recommend for or against acupuncture in OA of the knee due to conflicting evidence. Methylsulfonylmethane and *S*-adenosyl methionine are other dietary supplements some patients find beneficial, although at present no evidence exists to support this. Therapeutic magnets also appear helpful to some patients anecdotally.

Follow-up and Referral

Patients with OA may be referred to a rheumatologist or orthopedic surgeon for collaborative management. When conservative measures fail, the patient's quality of life can be markedly diminished. Frequent or constant disabling pain, especially pain at rest, and functionally limiting symptoms are the most important criteria for orthopedic referral. Patients may also be referred to physical therapy or occupational therapy for functional evaluation, education in joint preservation, and recommendations for environmental modifications to maximize function. Other options include referral to a pain management specialist, a professional massage therapist, or a licensed acupuncturist. Referral to the Arthritis Foundation for patient education and support is also valuable. The patient should be seen for follow-up at 3- to 6-month intervals and should be instructed to contact his or her primary health-care provider if pain increases or functional status declines. ROM and functional status should be assessed at each visit. There are a number of scales, such as the Arthritis Impact Measurement Scale–2, that allow the clinician to monitor the patient's perception of his or her progress with greater accuracy. This scale can be viewed at www.proqolid.org/instruments/arthritis_impact_measurement_scales_aims2. A short version of this scale is available also. A variety of other scales measure function and disability, such as the Pain Disability Index available at www.chronicpainnetwork.com/pdf/Pain_Disability_Index.pdf and the Stanford Health Assessment Questionnaire available at http://aramis.stanford.edu/HAQ.html. It is important to monitor all patients on aspirin or NSAID therapy for GI blood loss and cardiac, renal, and mental status. Practitioners should order periodic CBC, renal function tests, and tests for occult blood in stool.

Patient Education

Education of the patient and support persons is essential to successful management of OA. The Arthritis Foundation is an excellent resource for patient education, as well as a variety of services that are provided at the local and national level. In addition, courses such as the Arthritis Self-Help Course (ASHC) and People with Arthritis Can Exercise are available. Research has shown that patients who complete the ASHC show a decrease in pain and physician visits, even with increased physical disability. The improvements, sustained over a 4-year period, are attributed to these patients' feelings of enhanced self-efficacy.

Exercise programs should be individualized, with protection of the weight-bearing joints. Swimming or water exercise (which minimizes impact on joints) is especially recommended. Rest after exercise is also important.

The patient with OA needs to be aware of potential adverse effects of medications and drug interactions. Key areas for education include acceptance of the chronic nature of OA and lifestyle management to maximize function and minimize pain and the preservation of joint function. Vocational rehabilitation may also be necessary.

■ GOUT

Gouty arthritis accounts for approximately 3.9 million outpatient visits (Eggebeen, 2007). Gout is a disorder related to hyperuricemia. Urate crystals are deposited in certain joints, causing acute pain and edema. It typically occurs in the first metatarsophalangeal joint of the foot (podagra), but it may affect the wrist, elbow, or finger. Usually only a single joint is involved, with erythema, swelling, heat, and exquisite pain, but 10% to 15% of the patients with gout present with polyarticular symptoms. Attacks spontaneously resolve in 1 week but will recur with more frequency and severity. Diagnosis is made by joint aspiration; clinical symptoms are also used to diagnose. Acute episodes respond to oral ibuprofen; oral or IV colchicines may also be used initially, although GI side effects are a limiting factor. Lifestyle counseling regarding obesity, avoidance of high-purine foods, and alcohol moderation is indicated. Further testing is indicated if episodes recur despite lifestyle medications. Hyperuricemic agents such as allopurinol or febuxostat (Uloric) may be indicated for regular use. Urolithiasis is more common in patients with gout. (See Chapter 16 for a complete discussion of gout.)

■ OSTEOPOROSIS

Osteoporosis is a generalized skeletal disorder characterized by normal bone mineralization but low bone mass (bone mineral *density*) and disruption of the bony architecture, both of which result in an increased risk of fragility fractures. Its chief clinical manifestations are vertebral and hip fractures, although fractures can occur at any skeletal site. This is contrasted with *osteopenia,* which is a less severe form of decreased bone mineral density, and *osteomalacia,* which denotes a decrease in actual bone mineralization. Osteoporosis is now recognized as a significant public health concern with potentially devastating consequences in both human and economic terms. Increasing attention to women's health issues, the application of epidemiological research in prioritizing public health problems, and the need to minimize health-care expenditures have all contributed to recent efforts aimed at the prevention, identification, and effective treatment of this condition to avoid fractures. Fractures associated with osteoporosis are not only a physical stress to the individual and a burden for the health-care system; they also inflict great strain on the psychosocial well-being of individuals who suffer fractures and on the family or friends who take on the role of caregiver.

Epidemiology and Causes

Osteoporosis is characterized by microarchitectural deterioration of bone tissue, which leads to low bone mineral density (BMD) and fragility and a consequent susceptibility to fractures. Epidemiological studies in Europe, Japan, and the United States reveal that an estimated 75 million people are affected by osteoporosis. Roughly 4 out of 10 white women older than age 50 in the United States will experience a hip, spine, or wrist fracture during the remainder of their lives. Looking ahead, the lifetime risk of fractures will increase for all ethnic groups as people live longer. Approximately 10 million individuals older than age 50 in the United States have osteoporosis of the hip. An additional 33.6 million individuals older than age 50 have low bone mass, or osteopenia, of the hip and thus are at risk of developing osteoporosis and its potential complications later in life. Common consequences of osteoporosis are vertebral fractures and fracture of the hip and distal radius. In addition, a diagnosis of osteoporosis can lead to depression, a change in role, loss of independence, body deformities, and a real fear of initial or subsequent osteoporotic fractures.

As a result of both the aging of the population and the rise in the age-specific incidence of osteoporosis, the number of osteoporotic fractures has been increasing annually. Approximately 1.5 million osteoporotic fractures of the vertebral body, proximal femur, or distal radius occur each year in the United States. In 2005, osteoporotic fractures accounted for an estimated annual cost in excess of $19 billion per year. Proximal femur fractures, associated with the greatest health-care costs, are accompanied by a 20% risk of dying within 1 year of the fracture and impair the ability to perform ADLs in up to 75% of patients who survive. Women are more likely to have osteoporosis, but men also suffer from this condition. White women are more susceptible than black women; the prevalence of osteoporosis in Hispanic and Asian women is similar to that of white women.

Unless comprehensive prevention, screening, and treatment programs are initiated, as the average age of the American population continues to increase over the next 30 years, costs related to bone fragility could more than double. Women have two to four times greater lifetime risk of sustaining an osteoporotic fracture than men do as a result of the loss of BMD following the cessation of ovarian function at menopause. Bone loss after menopause is caused predominantly by estrogen deficiency and is most rapid (up to 7% per year) in the first decade after menopause. Postmenopausal osteoporosis is more prevalent in white and Asian women than in women of other races, with the majority of white women developing osteoporosis by the end of the first postmenopausal decade. By age 65, one-third of women will have had a vertebral fracture, and by the ninth decade of life, one in three will have had a hip fracture. The incidence, prevalence, and pathogenesis of bone loss in men are incompletely understood, and more research is called for in this area. Fractures of any type from osteoporosis are associated with a significantly higher likelihood of both physical and functional limitations. Patients who have already sustained a fracture from osteoporosis have a more than a fivefold increase in the risk of sustaining another fragility fracture.

The cause of osteoporosis is multifactorial. Although genetic factors are important determinants of bone density, other lifestyle, disease-related, and medication-related factors also contribute to an individual's risk for having osteoporosis, as shown in Risk Factors 15.1.

Risk Factors 15.1	Osteoporosis
Lifestyle	Low body weight
	Cigarette smoking
	Excessive alcohol intake
	Low dietary calcium intake
	Vitamin D deficiency
Disease-related risk factors	Thyrotoxicosis
	Hyperparathyroidism
	Cushing's disease
	Hypogonadism
	Rheumatoid arthritis
	Inflammatory bowel disease
	Chronic renal insufficiency
	Malabsorptive diseases
	Secondary estrogen deficiency resulting from anorexia or overexercise
Medication-related risk factors	Glucocorticoids
	Excessive thyroxine
	Long-term use of phenytoin
Other risk factors	Advanced age
	Family history of osteoporosis
	Postmenopausal
	Genetic predisposition

Although genetic factors may account for up to 70% of the variance in peak bone mass, many lifestyle factors play a significant role, and most are amenable to interventions aimed at primary and secondary prevention and treatment of osteoporosis. Regular exercise has been shown to preserve BMD, whereas a sedentary lifestyle probably contributes to osteopenia. Weight-bearing exercise, such as walking, is considered the best form of activity and is associated with higher bone density. There is increasing evidence that muscle strength training may prevent further loss of BMD in postmenopausal women. Further, the improved mobility, agility, and muscle strength that occur in people who engage in regular exercise may help to prevent falls and associated fractures.

The primary dietary risk factor for osteoporosis is lack of adequate calcium intake throughout the life cycle. The majority of cross-sectional studies support the supposition that long-term inadequate dietary calcium has a deleterious effect on skeletal mass. The importance of adequate calcium, phosphorus, and vitamin D intake for children, adolescents, and young adults should not be underestimated, because studies have indicated that women begin losing bone mass (albeit at a rate of less than 1% a year) in their early 30s. There is increasing evidence that vitamin D deficiency is more prevalent than previously thought, particularly among individuals at increased risk, such as the elderly; those living in northern latitudes; and in individuals with poor nutrition, malabsorption, or chronic liver or renal disease. Modest vitamin D deficiency can lead to a compensatory, secondary hyperparathyroidism and is an important risk factor for osteoporosis and fractures.

Cigarette smoking is an established risk factor for loss of bone density, with the proposed mechanism of action being a reduction in circulating estrogen levels, as well as toxic effects on osteoblasts.

Genetics are important determinants of the risk for developing osteoporosis. Although the specific genes that determine bone mass remain largely unknown, some investigators claim that polymorphisms in the vitamin D receptor gene may be associated with up to 75% of the variance in bone density.

A variety of disease-related conditions may be associated with an increased risk for osteoporosis. GI diseases such as inflammatory bowel disease, among others, that lead to malabsorption of minerals and/or vitamin D are associated with low BMD. Other generalized inflammatory diseases that elevate levels of cytokines—substances believed to induce bone resorption—have also been associated with lower bone density. Younger women with eating disorders and women athletes who have altered menstrual function secondary to a hypoestrogenic state are at increased risk for lower bone densities earlier in life and should be targeted for primary prevention interventions as early as possible, as well as treatment of the underlying disease when indicated. Finally, chronic renal impairment with parathyroid dysfunction and vitamin D metabolism abnormalities can lead to bone loss.

Among the medications associated with the development of osteoporosis, long-term use of glucocorticoids (steroids) has been shown to cause bone loss both rapidly and dramatically. Patients who take 7.5 mg or more of prednisone per day for more than 1 month have been identified as being at particular risk. Long-term excessive thyroid hormone may also potentiate bone loss, reinforcing the need to routinely monitor thyroid-stimulating hormone (TSH) levels in patients who require thyroid hormone replacement. Cyclosporine, cytotoxic drugs, anticonvulsants, excessive alcohol intake, heparin, and lithium are medications that have potentially detrimental effects on the skeleton. Long-term use of proton pump inhibitors for gastroesophageal reflux disease has recently been implicated in contributing to osteoporosis by inducing hypochlorhydria that interferes with calcium absorption.

In men, testosterone deficiency from primary or secondary hypogonadism is a common cause of osteoporosis, although few large-scale studies have been done in this area. One small cross-sectional study found that men who had undergone orchiectomy for prostate cancer had significantly higher rates of severe osteoporosis, some of which developed before castration. Research identifying the causes of and treatment for osteoporosis in men is both increasing and necessary, because preliminary data have shown a higher mortality rate in men with hip fractures compared with women. Measurement parameters for osteoporosis and osteopenia in men are different than women and controversy exists regarding the most accurate measurement factors. There is general agreement that osteoporosis in men occurs a decade or so after that in women.

Pathophysiology

Normal bone contains an abundance of intracellular mineral salts (calcium phosphate and calcium carbonate) referred to as *hydroxyapatites*. As hydroxyapatites are deposited in collagenous fibers within immature bone cells (osteoblasts), the tissue becomes hardened, or ossified. Essentially, two types of bone are formed—cancellous or dense. Cancellous bone tissue is spongy, containing many open spaces filled with marrow. It consists of an irregular latticework of thin plates of bone called *trabeculae* and provides some skeletal support. Overlying spongy bone is dense bone that is much more compact, providing substantial skeletal support.

There is a continual remodeling process of bone tissue throughout life, in which osteoclasts release proteolytic enzymes that are responsible for breaking down osseous tissue, and new bone tissue is formed in its place by osteoblasts. At menopause, the remodeling process becomes less homeostatic, and osteoclastic activity begins to predominate while the rate of bone turnover increases. Bony spicules are reduced in number and size, and horizontal spicules acting as struts do not fully extend to contralateral supporting structures from their sites of origin, thus drastically reducing structural support. This leads to a decrease in cortical thickness and both the number and size of trabeculae in cancellous bone, leading to a decrease in bone density.

Osteoporosis is likely to be a multifactorial process, relating to increased bone resorption, decreased bone formation, and an overall decrease in peak bone mass at baseline (largely determined by genetic predisposition). Each of these physiological processes may predominate to a different extent in different osteoporotic individuals. Studies exploring the genetic basis for osteoporosis have not yet proved definitive, but polymorphisms in the genes of several proteins have been implicated, including collagen, bone morphogenetic protein–2, apolipoprotein E, transforming growth factor–beta (TGF-β), and the estrogen receptor. Normal estrogen function is important in preventing osteoporosis in both men and women because it has been shown to inhibit osteoclastogenesis, induce osteoclast apoptosis, and decrease the erosive activity of osteoclasts. These activities are likely mediated through estrogen's inhibition of macrophages and osteoclasts to secrete tumor necrosis factor–beta (TNF-β), interleukin-1 (IL-1), and their binding proteins. New bone formation also appears to be impaired in estrogen-deficient states because estrogen has been shown to mediate TGF-β secretion by osteoblasts. Interestingly, androgen (e.g., testosterone) deficiency similarly results in increased bone turnover and can predispose an individual to osteoporosis as well.

Because serum hormone levels often do not differ between osteoporotic individuals and age-matched controls, changes in bone resorption and formation appear to be mediated largely by local factors, including mechanical loads on the bones themselves, as well as changes in the concentrations of local growth factors and their receptor proteins. Excesses in both exogenous (therapeutic) and endogenous (stress- or disease-related) glucocorticoids are well-known causes of osteoporosis, but unlike the role of sex hormones, glucocorticoids appear to be most involved in the regulation of new bone formation by osteoblasts. This growth effect is mediated largely by the inhibition of local growth factors including insulin-like growth factor and its cognate receptor binding proteins, as well as prostaglandins.

Research on the effects of prostaglandins and NSAIDs on osteoporosis is not definitive. It appears as though excess prostaglandin (PG) production (especially that of PGE_2) may increase bone resorption, whereas significant inhibition of prostaglandins may lead to reduced bone formation in response to mechanical weight-bearing. IL-6 produced by osteoblasts and other marrow-derived cells has been shown to increase osteoclastogenesis via a prostaglandin-dependent mechanism, leading to increased bone resorption in osteoporotic individuals. In contrast, IL-4 and IL-13 appear to inhibit bone resorption by

decreasing prostaglandin synthesis, whereas IL-7 may contribute to bone loss. Finally, excess production of parathyroid hormone (PTH) (as seen in primary hyperparathyroidism) and PTH-related protein (produced by bone and cartilage cells and the mammary gland in lactating women) both lead to increased bone resorption via their effects on downstream growth factors, possibly including fibroblast growth factor. Importantly, however, this complex set of interactions by secreted growth factors on bone resorption and formation has yet to be fully characterized, and the importance of the aforementioned cytokines and growth factors can only be suggested by the current literature.

Clinical Presentation
Subjective

Most often, there are no clinical symptoms with the onset of osteoporosis until a fracture occurs. The only "early" symptom that may be noticed is the gradual development of upper or midthoracic back pain associated with activity or long periods of sitting or standing, which is relieved with rest in the recumbent position. To emphasize the importance of taking a comprehensive history, a strong predictor for future osteoporosis-related fractures is a history of previous fractures, notably those occurring from minimal trauma.

Objective

Acute vertebral compression fractures generally occur in the thoracic or high lumbar region, with the patient experiencing a more sudden, severe onset of pain. With acute compression fractures, point tenderness in the specific area of the fracture can be elicited during the physical exam. As bone density decreases, microfractures of the anterior vertebral bodies in the thoracic spine are likely to accumulate over time, leading to the characteristic dorsal kyphosis (or "dowager's hump"). The resultant exaggerated kyphosis produces a loss of height, which is generally not a "complaint," per se, but may be only casually mentioned by a patient during the course of a health-care visit. This may be the only verbal cue the practitioner receives to help identify that patient as being at risk for having osteoporosis. As the kyphosis worsens over time, impairment of rib mobility, a decrease in lung volumes, and an increase in respiratory complaints may develop.

Diagnostic Reasoning
Diagnostic Tests

Although it is important for identifying patients who may be at particular risk for developing osteoporosis, clinical assessment alone cannot accurately identify patients who do or do not have this condition. For the practitioner, assessing a patient's risk for osteoporosis and signs of the disease based on the physical exam can provide support for the decision to proceed with further diagnostic testing. Risk assessment tools are currently available and may be used by clinicians as a quantitative means to support the need for additional diagnostic testing. The Simple Calculated Osteoporosis Risk Estimation (SCORE) instrument, for example, is estimated to have 90% sensitivity and approximately 40% specificity for identifying individuals with low BMD at the hip.

The American Association of Clinical Endocrinologists (AACE) recommends BMD testing in all perimenopausal or postmenopausal women who are willing to accept interventions should a low BMD be found. In the current health-care environment, insurance companies are increasingly requiring quantitative justification (e.g., in the form of risk assessments and/or other physical findings) from practitioners before paying for further diagnostic BMD testing. Standard radiographs are considered extremely insensitive for detecting bone loss, with films typically indicating bone loss only when it exceeds 30% or more. No biochemical marker currently exists that is used to detect bone loss; however, preliminary evidence from clinical trials suggests that such markers may be used in the future to evaluate early response to therapy.

The physiological process of bone turnover may be assessed with a variety of serum or urinary markers, allowing the monitoring of bone loss and reformation, although these markers do not provide bone mass density, which is considered the definitive test for diagnosis. However, these markers are useful in monitoring treatment and can serve as useful adjuncts in the original diagnosis of osteoporosis. In general, serum markers provide information about bone formation, whereas urinary markers supply evidence of bone resorption.

Bone alkaline phosphatase (BAP) is the most commonly available serum indicator of osteoblastic activity. These levels should be obtained before the initiation of therapy and then at 3- to 6-month intervals to monitor response. BAP levels that drop significantly may indicate lack of compliance with treatment. Urinary N-telopeptide is the most specific and newest urinary bone resorption marker available. This assay, which measures the urinary excretion of cross-linked N-telopeptide of type I collagen, is useful in identifying individuals with osteoporosis who have high rates of bone resorption and who might be good candidates for antiresorption therapy.

BMD measurement by densitometry is currently considered the gold standard diagnostic test for definitively diagnosing either osteopenia or osteoporosis. *Osteopenia* is the diagnostic term used when BMD is found to be less than normal but not severe enough to be considered osteoporotic. BMD densitometry is noninvasive and can be completed in 5 to 15 minutes. A number of BMD measurement technologies are available, including dual-energy x-ray absorptiometry (DEXA)—the "gold standard" for documenting osteoporosis of the proximal femur and lumbar spine; single-energy x-ray absorptiometry and peripheral DEXA for the radius and calcaneus

(heel); ultrasonography for the heel, fingers, and tibia; and quantitative computed tomography (QCT), including peripheral QCT for the spine, hip, and radius.

These technologies use a variety of anatomical sites from which to measure BMD and emit very low radiation doses (less than or equal to a standard chest x-ray study). Although all methods are considered accurate, the DEXA method is most widely accepted because prospective epidemiological studies have found it to be most precise for reproducibility in both the short and long term, making it an excellent method for monitoring responses to interventions over time. DEXA densitometry measures BMD at the central skeletal sites of the lumbar spine and hip (including both the femoral neck and greater trochanter).

BMD measurement reports are interpreted by using the calculated *Z*-scores and *T*-scores. Both use a normally distributed bell curve in determining how any one individual compares to a reference population, with *Z*-scores representing age- and sex-matched distributions and *T*-scores representing mean peak bone mass of a young adult distribution. The *T*-score is the most clinically relevant value on the BMD report and is used to confirm the presence of osteoporosis and to determine fracture risk. For every standard deviation below the young-adult matched mean, there is a significant increase in fracture risk.

Medicare-approved indications for BMD testing include (1) estrogen-deficient women at risk for osteoporosis, (2) patients with vertebral abnormalities, (3) patients receiving or needing to be on long-term glucocorticoids, (4) patients with primary parathyroidism, and (5) patients being monitored for response or efficacy of an approved osteoporosis drug therapy.

Secondary causes of osteoporosis should be considered in all patients with low BMD. The following routine laboratory tests are considered appropriate by the AACE for excluding secondary causes of osteoporosis: CBC, serum chemistry panel (calcium, phosphate, liver enzymes, total alkaline phosphatase, creatinine, electrolytes), and urinalysis, including pH.

Also based on AACE guidelines, additional laboratory analysis may be warranted if there are abnormalities in the aforementioned tests or if there is sufficient other evidence to suspect specific secondary causes for bone loss. These include sensitive TSH, 24-hour urinary calcium excretion, ESR, parathyroid hormone concentration, 25-hydroxyvitamin D concentration, dexamethasone suppression and other tests for hyperadrenocorticism, acid–base studies, serum or urine protein electrophoresis, and bone marrow examination or bone biopsy.

The World Health Organization's diagnostic criteria for osteoporosis are presented in Table 15.8.

Differential Diagnosis

If a fracture has occurred, it is important to distinguish the underlying cause. Was it related to trauma, or was

Table 15.8	World Health Organization Diagnostic Criteria for Osteoporosis
Diagnosis	Diagnostic Findings
Normal	BMD within 1 SD of young adult reference mean
Osteopenia	BMD >1 SD below young adult reference mean (21)
Osteoporosis	BMD >2.5 SD below young adult reference mean (22.5)
Osteoporosis (severe)	BMD >2.5 SD below young adult reference mean (22.5) *and* presence of osteoporotic fractures

BMD: bone mineral density; SD: standard deviation.

there an underlying pathological condition such as osteoporosis or neoplasm? Similarly, skeletal changes could result from a variety of underlying conditions, including a neoplasm, such as multiple myeloma or other neoplasias; osteomalacia; osteogenesis imperfecta tarda (type I); skeletal hyperparathyroidism (primary and secondary); and hyperthyroidism.

Management

The goals for either the prevention or treatment of osteoporosis are to prevent fractures, stabilize or improve bone mass, maximize physical functioning, relieve symptoms of fractures and resulting skeletal deformity, and maximize psychosocial functioning and coping.

The ability to meet these goals is dependent on both the patient and the practitioner's dedication to work as a team, first in determining what therapeutic regimen will be most beneficial and acceptable to the patient. Following this is the long-term commitment to continuing treatment, evaluating the therapeutic response, and assessing for the need to redirect the management plan based on the response. An algorithm outlining prevention, detection, and management strategies for osteoporosis is presented in Treatment Flowchart 15.1.

In addition to the physical and functional limitations that can be quantified, practitioners must also address the human and emotional aspects of being diagnosed with osteoporosis. Although not often the direct cause of death, and often identified as a "silent disease" until the patient sustains a fracture, for many individuals a fracture can lead to a downward spiral in physical and mental health and well-being. There may be an abrupt descent into disease, disability, and deformity. From an individual's perspective, osteoporosis can have a devastating effect on patients and their families, and can dramatically affect functional status, leaving the patient feeling vulnerable, isolated, and uncertain of the future. (See Treatment Flowchart 15.1.)

Lifestyle Management

For both the prevention and treatment of osteoporosis, smoking cessation, moderation of alcohol use, weight-bearing exercise, and adequate calcium and vitamin D intake are advised. In addition, avoidance of falls by eliminating hazards in the home and gait training or other exercises that improve strength and agility through physical therapy are important considerations. Nursing research has found that women with osteoporosis seek interventions that promote the ability to better care for themselves, reduce stress and isolation, and prevent further disability. Weight training and walking are effective interventions for prevention and/or treatment. An active lifestyle, including safe and appropriate exercise, should be actively encouraged by the provider. Protective pads worn around the outer thigh, which cover the trochanteric region of the hip, can prevent hip fractures in elderly residents in nursing homes. Patients with pain from osteoporotic fractures may find therapies such as massage, music, or acupuncture helpful.

Pharmacological Management
Calcium and Vitamin D Supplements

Optimal calcium intake varies according to age, sex, and other conditions. The recommended daily calcium intake as based on the Office of Dietary Supplements, National Institutes of Health, is as follows:

- Children: 800 to 1,300 mg/day
- Adolescents: 1,300 mg/day, including pregnant/lactating
- Adults aged 19 to 50: 1,000 mg/day, including pregnant/lactating
- Adults older than age 50: 1,200 mg/day
- Adults older than age 50 with low bone mass: 1,500 mg/day

An adequate calcium intake of 1,000 to 1,500 mg/day and sufficient amounts of vitamin D are necessary for both the prevention and treatment of osteoporosis. Supplementation is advised when dietary intake does not consistently meet the recommended amount. Fracture reduction in women aged 75 years and older who use only calcium and vitamin D supplementation has been previously demonstrated. There are many available forms, and patients may be confused about which type or brand is best. In general, the majority of commercially available supplements contain similar amounts of elemental calcium per calcium weight in milligrams (mg), and patient choice should be dependent on affordability, number of tablets per day necessary, and whether it is convenient for the patient to take them with food or not. Calcium carbonate is less expensive and more easily absorbed with meals. Individuals with hypochlorhydria can absorb calcium citrate more efficiently, and it can be taken with or without food. Inadequate levels of vitamin D interfere with the body's absorption of calcium. Recent

Treatment Flowchart 15.1 Osteoporosis

studies have indicated that the 400 IU/day of vitamin D previously recommended were not sufficient. The National Osteoporosis Foundation has updated its recommendations as follows:

- Adults younger than age 50: 400 to 800 IU of vitamin D daily
- Adults older than age 50: 800 to 1,000 IU of vitamin D daily

Estrogen Replacement Therapy Estrogen was the mainstay of treatment for osteoporosis for many years, until the Women's Health Initiative showed increased risk of cardiovascular disease and breast cancer from hormone replacement therapy (HRT). Despite a risk/ benefit ratio that is not favorable according to recent, large-scale clinical trials, women may still choose to take estrogen based on their own risk-factor profile.

Selective Estrogen-Receptor Modulators One of the most recent developments in osteoporosis prevention has been the introduction of a selective estrogen-receptor modulator (SERM; e.g., Evista). The approval of this drug by the FDA represents a new class of drugs that are nonhormonal but that modulate selective estrogen-receptor sites in skeletal tissue that decrease resorption of bone that occurs after menopause. The advantage of an SERM over traditional HRT is that it does not stimulate estrogen receptors found in the breast or uterus and therefore does not increase the risk for breast or uterine cancer associated with estrogen use (over 39 months of trials). Although SERMs do not adversely affect lipid profiles, whether they provide any cardiovascular benefit is under investigation. SERMs are currently approved for use in postmenopausal women only for the prevention of osteoporosis but not its treatment. For many women, the addition of this class of drug into the market may provide an appealing alternative. Tamoxifen is another SERM that, although not FDA approved for osteoporosis, has shown promise in some research.

Bisphosphonates Alendronate sodium (Fosamax), a third generation bisphosphonate, has been approved by the FDA for the prevention and treatment of osteoporosis. It is an aminobisphosphonate that binds to bone hydroxyapatite and specifically inhibits the activity of osteoclasts, thus reducing bone turnover. Treatment with alendronate sodium has been shown to increase BMD of the vertebrae, femoral neck, and femoral trochanter by 5% to 10% and to reduce hip, vertebral, and wrist fractures by approximately 50% over a 3-year study period, making it an effective alternative to HRT for treating osteoporosis in women who either cannot or will not take estrogen therapy. It is also available with vitamin D.

Like other bisphosphonates, alendronate sodium has the potential to irritate upper GI mucosa and is contraindicated in patients who have abnormalities of the esophagus that delay esophageal emptying or in patients who are unable to take the medication exactly as directed. Because of the very specific manner in which alendronate sodium needs to be taken, some individuals initially perceive it as an inconvenience they would rather avoid; with careful patient teaching and the willingness to try this medication, however, many patients find no difficulty incorporating it into their daily routine. Risedronate (Actonel) is another drug in this category, also available in weekly dosing, as is ibandronate (Boniva), which is available in monthly dosing. Only bisphosphonates have been demonstrated in large clinical trials to reduce the risk of fractures in patients being treated with glucocorticoid therapy. Risedronate (Actonel) prevents bone loss and reduces vertebral fracture risk by about 70%. Similar effects have been noted in alendronate (Fosamax) and etidronate disodium (Didronel). Zoledronic acid (Reclast, Zometa) is an IV third generation bisphosphonate. A once-yearly dosage of zoledronic acid (Reclast) 5 mg IV has been noted to reduce the incidence of bone fracture in the hip, spine, and other sites in postmenopausal women with osteoporosis. Adequate calcium and vitamin D must be maintained before, during, and after treatment. Zoledronic acid is approved for prevention and treatment of postmenopausal osteoporosis and glucocorticoid osteoporosis, as well as treatment of osteoporosis in men and treatment of Paget's disease. Concerns about osteonecrosis of the jaw are exaggerated; this complication is most likely when the drug is used in patients with malignancies.

Few studies have examined the effectiveness of bisphosphonates for fracture reduction in men although they have been shown to increase BMD. Currently, few well-designed trials have examined the effects of pharmacological therapy on BMD in men.

Calcitonin Calcitonin is another antiresorptive agent approved for the treatment of osteoporosis. It may be used for women who cannot or will not take estrogens or a bisphosphonate. Although it produces small increases in bone mass, there are conflicting data regarding whether calcitonin reduces fractures, because the quality of bone formed is in question and currently under further investigation. Calcitonin is available for subcutaneous or intramuscular (IM) injection and in a nasal spray preparation. Studies evaluating nasal spray calcitonin have documented an increased lumbar vertebral BMD after 1 year, but no difference from the placebo in BMD at the forearm or hip. Calcitonin has also been found to produce an analgesic effect in the treatment of bone pain and may be useful during the immediate post-fracture period. (See Drugs Commonly Prescribed 15.3: Osteoporosis, Paget's Disease.)

Androgen Supplementation Few studies have examined pharmacological therapy effectiveness in osteoporotic men. Preliminary data from one study showed an increase in BMD in men with idiopathic primary osteoporosis when treated with testosterone IM over 6 months. Although no adverse cardiovascular events were found in the treatment group, studies of longer duration are indicated in this area to better estimate the risks versus benefits of testosterone supplementation in men.

Fluoride Oral sodium fluoride has been used extensively in Europe for the treatment of osteoporosis and has been found to significantly increase vertebral bone density by increasing the number of osteoblasts. Large, prospective studies have not shown a concurrent reduction in fractures, however; and until future research shows otherwise, it is believed the quality of bone produced by fluoride is more brittle than that formed by antiresorptive agents. Therefore, in the United States sodium fluoride is currently not approved for the prevention or treatment of osteoporosis by the FDA.

Follow-up and Referral

Perhaps the most important part of managing the treatment of osteoporosis is improving adherence to treatment by individualizing the plan of care according to what is most effective in terms of increasing BMD and preventing fractures and what is most acceptable to the patient. There are currently no well-accepted guidelines for monitoring treatment of osteoporosis. Repeat BMD testing to monitor treatment response in osteoporotic patients should be limited to at least 2-year intervals. For patients with less-than-normal BMD (but who are not osteoporotic) or normal baseline BMD, repeat measurement every 2 to 3 years is indicated to monitor for either stabilization or progression of the disease. Referral to an endocrinologist is warranted any time secondary causes of osteoporosis cannot be excluded or if the response to treatment is less than expected for the type of therapy instituted.

Drugs Commonly Prescribed 15.3   Osteoporosis, Paget's Disease

Drug	Indication	Adverse Reactions and Prescribing Considerations
Bisphosphonates		
risedronate (Actonel) Available in daily, weekly, twice-monthly, and once-monthly dosage forms	Prevention and treatment of postmenopausal osteoporosis, to increase bone mass in men with osteoporosis, treatment of Paget's disease	Swallow whole; take in the morning with a full glass of water before other food or drink; remain in upright position for at least 30 minutes; caution with other GI irritants such as aspirin. Abdominal pain, atrial fibrillation, esophageal ulceration. Hypocalcemia is an absolute contraindication for all bisphosphonates.
alendronate (Fosamax) Also available with vitamin D; daily or once-weekly dosage	Prevention and treatment of postmenopausal osteoporosis and osteoporosis in men	Take on an empty stomach at least 30 minutes before a meal; drink full glass of water and remain upright for at least 30 minutes. Can increase toxic effects of aspirin; can decrease absorption of calcium supplements and vitamin D. See adverse effects above.
ibandronate (Boniva) Available in oral daily or monthly preparations and IV preparation for every-3-month dosing	Prevention and treatment of postmenopausal osteoporosis, osteoporosis in women with breast cancer on specific therapy, Paget's disease treatment, and treatment of hypercalcemia in malignancy	Swallow oral whole; take in the morning with full glass of water; remain upright and eat or drink nothing additional for 60 minutes; take on same day each month. See adverse effects above. Bone pain, arthralgia, and atrial fibrillation can occur in IV form.
zoledronic acid (Reclast)	Treatment of Paget's disease; prevention and treatment of osteoporosis in postmenopausal women and to increase bone mass in men with osteoporosis; hypercalcemia of malignancy	Obtain baseline renal function parameters within 10 days before initial dose. Avoid in renal disease. Adequate hydration is important, also concomitant administration of calcium and vitamin D before, during, and after drug administration. Osteonecrosis of the jaw has been seen; also arthralgia, atrial fibrillation, and bone pain can occur.
Diphosphonate		
etidronate disodium (Didronel)	Treatment of moderate to severe Paget's disease	Give daily (preferred) or in divided doses at least 2 hours before or after food; ensure adequate calcium and vitamin D. Bone pain, GI upset, arthralgias.
Calcitonin		
calcitonin-salmon (Miacalcin) nasal spray	Treatment of osteoporosis	Alternate nostrils—1 spray in 1 nostril daily. Must receive 1.5 g calcium + 400 IU vitamin D daily. Adverse effect of rhinitis in 12% of those treated.
Selective Estrogen Receptor Modulators (SERMs)		
raloxifene (Evista)	Prevention and treatment of postmenopausal osteoporosis Has not been shown to decrease hip fractures	May be taken any time of day, regardless of meals. Decreased effects of warfarin. Thromboembolic disease is a contraindication, as is breast cancer. Adverse reactions include flatulence, abdominal pain, hot flashes, increased risk of thromboembolism. Discontinue 72 hours before immobilization.
Parathyroid Hormone		
teriparatide (Forteo)	Treatment of osteoporosis in postmenopausal women at high risk for fracture (prior fracture and T score < −3)	Stimulates bone formation more than bone resorption. Contraindicated in hyperparathyroidism. Adverse reactions include dizziness, orthostatic hypotension, arthralgia, injection site reaction, secondary malignancy.

Continued

Drugs Commonly Prescribed 15.3   Osteoporosis, Paget's Disease—cont'd

Drug	Indication	Adverse Reactions and Prescribing Considerations
Hormone Replacement Therapy		
	Use as second-line therapy only	
Monoclonal Antibody		
denosumab (Prolia)	Treatment of osteoporosis in postmenopausal women at high risk for fracture, prior fracture, or failure on other therapy	Contraindicated in hypocalcemia. Increased risk of serious infection. Subcutaneous injection.

Patient Education

A number of informative patient education materials are available from a variety of sources, including pharmaceutical companies. Extensive, individualized education should be given to individuals when BMD results are available. This is particularly true for patients who are found to be osteoporotic and who have an array of interventions available to them. The amount of information about osteoporosis required for teaching can be overwhelming for patients; therefore, written information is essential. In addition, a number of resources are available to patients through both federal and national organizations. (See the Resources listed at the end of this chapter.)

Reviewing potential hazards that may lead to falls and reinforcing the importance of maintaining agility are equally important in the ongoing care and management of patients who are at increased risk for fractures. Referral to a physical therapist and/or a home-care nursing evaluation is often of value in this area. Referral to local support groups, national osteoporosis education groups, and mental health counseling may also be of benefit for patients who seek further assistance in either learning about their condition or coping with their situation. Active exercise, such as weight training and/or walking, should be encouraged and supported.

■ CARPAL TUNNEL SYNDROME

Carpal tunnel syndrome (CTS) is the most common cause of peripheral nerve compression. Pain and/or numbness affects some part of the median nerve distribution of the hand and in some cases may radiate into the arm. Symptoms tend to affect the dominant hand, but more than half the patients experience bilateral symptoms. Women are three times more likely than men are to be diagnosed with CTS.

Epidemiology and Causes

CTS is the most common entrapment neuropathy. It is most common in persons aged 40 to 60 years and affects females significantly more frequently than males, most commonly middle-aged and pregnant women. Roughly 80% of patients are older than age 40 years. Any condition that reduces the size or space of the carpal tunnel can cause compression of the medial nerve. Any movement that causes the wrist to repeatedly flex or extend out of the neutral position or that places pressure on the median nerve may contribute to the development of CTS. Direct compression may result from neoplasms, a misaligned fracture, or trauma to the carpal tunnel. The greatest risk is found in occupations that require repeated flexion or extension of the wrist, use of hand tools that require forceful gripping, or use of hand tools that vibrate. CTS has been reported to occur spontaneously, most often during conditions that affect hormone balance (e.g., pregnancy, menopause, myxedematous hypothyroidism, diabetes mellitus) or in patients with other underlying musculoskeletal disorders (e.g., gout, rheumatoid arthritis, acute injury, acromegaly). Although the mechanism is unclear, it is thought that the generalized fluid increase or deposition of matrix substances (e.g., myxedema, amyloidosis) in the body tissues causes impingement on the median nerve within the carpal tunnel. This is also likely to underlie the association of CTS with fluid overload in end-stage renal disease and chronic dialysis.

Past history of wrist trauma or Colles' fracture, degenerative (and inflammatory) joint disease, ganglionic cysts, obesity, fibromyalgia, and scleroderma are other risk factors for this disorder. There is no universal agreement that CTS is work related. Although no genetic mutations have been identified other than a rare chromosome 17 deletion that leads to an autosomal dominant neuropathic disorder prone to pressure-related nerve palsies, CTS is well known to occur in families. In fact, up to half the risk of developing CTS is thought to be attributable to genetic factors.

Pathophysiology

The anatomy of the wrist extends from the distal radius and ulna to the carpometacarpal joint. The eight small carpal bones of the wrist, arranged in two rows, account for numerous articulations and enable the wrist to perform a wide range of motion (ROM). The wrist is the second most mobile joint in the body, allowing for the exceptional mobility of the hand. Radial ligaments and the triangular fibrocartilage complex maintain the stability of the carpal bones. The carpal tunnel is formed by the arrangement of the wrist bones and the inelastic flexor retinaculum ligament. Through this tunnel run the finger flexor tendons and the median nerve. Any source of inflammation or pressure within this canal can result in symptoms of CTS.

Patients with CTS are exquisitely prone to developing increases in pressure within the carpal tunnel during wrist flexion and extension. In turn, this may lead to edema within the nerve tissue. Some studies have also demonstrated increased connective tissue proximal to the median nerve with a notable reduction in nerve fiber caliber following nerve impingement. These mechanisms may also result in venous congestion and stasis, compression of the median nerve, and resultant ischemia, leading to the pain and paresthesias associated with CTS.

Clinical Presentation
Subjective

Typically, the patient will present with an aching sensation that radiates into the thenar area; it may also be perceived in the proximal forearm, and occasionally the pain can extend to the shoulder. Paresthesias and numbness in the median distribution (thumb and index, long, and radial half of ring fingers, or some combination thereof) typically accompany the pain. Patients often report that they frequently drop objects and that they cannot open jars or twist off lids. Repetitive motions of the hand or stationary tasks with the wrist held flexed or extended for a period of time (such as when driving) worsen pain and numbness. A hallmark symptom is nighttime awakening with pain and numbness. Patients report that they must rub or shake the hand to "get the circulation" going. Persistent numbness and thenar atrophy can occur when the compression is severe and/or long-standing.

Objective

Examination of the patient with suspected CTS should include inspection of the wrist and hand for swelling, redness, nodules, deformity, and muscle atrophy. The thenar eminence (at the base of the thumb) is the best location to assess for atrophy. If the thenar eminence is atrophied or flattened, chronic CTS should be suspected. Palpation of the hand and wrist should be done to check for swelling, bogginess, or tenderness. Each distal interphalangeal (DIP), proximal interphalangeal (PIP), and metacarpophalangeal (MCP) joint should be palpated, as well as the wrist bones. Capillary refill time should be determined, and the radial and ulnar arteries should be assessed for patency. Allen's test should be performed to determine individual patency of both the radial and ulnar arteries.

ROM of the fingers and wrists should be assessed as follows:

- Have the patient make a fist with the thumb across the knuckles.
- Have the patient extend and widely spread the fingers.
- Have the patient touch each finger with the thumb of the same hand.
- With the palms facing down, passively move the fingers laterally and medially.
- Have the patient flex and extend the hands, with and without resistance.

Assessment may also include the following:

- Phalen's maneuver: Have the patient acutely flex the wrists by pressing the backs of the hands together for 60 seconds. An abnormal or positive Phalen's maneuver is present when the patient reports numbness and tingling in the thumb or first two digits.
- Tinel's sign: Lightly percuss the palmar surface of the wrist with a percussion hammer. An abnormal or positive Tinel's sign occurs when the patient reports tingling or a shocklike sensation that travels across the palm into the thumb and first two digits, a sign of nerve compression. There is broad variability in reported sensitivity and specificity of Tinel's sign in the literature, and it should not be relied on as a primary diagnostic modality.
- Carpal compression test: Place the thumbs over the flexor retinaculum and apply even pressure over the area of the median nerve for 30 to 60 seconds. A positive test is indicated by the occurrence of paresthesia in the hand or first three digits.
- Have the patient draw the pattern of numbness and tingling in his or her hand or indicate it on a preprinted picture of the hand and wrist.

The performance of sensory testing to aid in the diagnosis is of little clinical value. Many patients who do not have CTS have diminished ability to differentiate sharp and dull sensations on the fingers and therefore yield a high false-positive rate for this testing. Also remember that occupation and handedness may affect the muscular symmetry of the hands and wrists in the absence of a musculoskeletal condition.

Diagnostic Reasoning
Diagnostic Tests

Radiographs should be done if the patient has limited wrist movement; however, the most useful diagnostic test is a median nerve conduction velocity study. By measuring the velocity of sensory conduction, nerve entrapment may be conclusively validated. It is important to remember that this is an invasive test and that it is considerably more expensive than other diagnostic methods. In addition, a patient may have an abnormal nerve conduction velocity study but have no clinical symptoms; conversely, 5% to 10% of patients with CTS have normal test results.

Differential Diagnosis

The following is a list of differential diagnoses:

- Arthritis of the carpometacarpal joint of the thumb (painful motion)
- Cervical radiculopathy affecting the C6 nerve root (neck pain, numbness in the thumb and index finger only)
- Diabetes mellitus with paresthesias (determine on history)
- Median nerve compression at the elbow (tenderness at the proximal forearm)
- Wrist arthritis (limited motion, evident on radiograph)

Management

Conservative treatment is recommended for patients who present with acute symptoms. It has been reported that 50% to 75% of conservatively treated patients will attain symptom relief. The goal of treatment is to prevent the flexion and extension movements of the wrist. This is best accomplished through use of a splint that allows free movement of the fingers and the thumb while maintaining the wrist in the neutral position. Recommendations for wearing of the splint vary from constantly (day and night) to nighttime only. Some providers recommend using the splints day and night for 3 weeks, then nightly only for 3 more weeks. Splinting can be a cost-effective method for symptom control. Maximum results from splinting are attained if it is instituted within the first 3 months of symptom onset.

Oral NSAIDs are another conservative measure that can be used in conjunction with splinting. These drugs are often prescribed for patients who experience pain as part of the syndrome, but they may have some general usefulness in controlling edema in the carpal tunnel.

Corticosteroid injections, although used by some providers, are discouraged for treatment of CTS. Although the injections provide temporary relief, there is a concern that the median nerve could sustain damage and scarring or that infection may occur.

The use of vitamin B_6 (pyridoxine) in CTS has been reported in the literature over the past several years. Although there are no conclusive studies on the utility of this medication in treating or preventing carpal tunnel syndrome, use of this vitamin is becoming more prevalent. Care should be taken with dosing, because larger doses may result in neuropathies. It is also important to determine whether the patient is on any other medications that may be affected by pyridoxine; for example, serum concentrations of phenytoin and phenobarbital may be decreased with pyridoxine.

Management of concurrent disease (e.g., hypothyroidism, diabetes mellitus) is an important aspect of the conservative treatment of CTS. Treatment that diminishes fluid retention, when used with other conservative methods, will produce better results in relieving the symptoms of CTS.

CTS that occurs during pregnancy usually resolves when the pregnancy is over. Treatment consists of splinting and other nonoperative measures such as corticosteroid injections. CTS that is work related may respond to ergonomic modifications.

Follow-up and Referral

The presence of thenar atrophy or unremitting symptoms with conservative treatment warrant referral for surgical evaluation. Carpal tunnel release is one of the most commonly performed hand surgeries; it is usually done under local anesthesia on an outpatient basis. The surgery may be performed by a hand specialist, plastic surgeon, or neurosurgeon. Although small incisions are being used more frequently, some surgeons state that visual inspection of the entire carpal space is necessary. The use of a longitudinal incision must be weighed against the risks of wound infection, scarring, and diminished motor abilities.

Postoperatively, patients can expect to have the hand splinted for 8 to 14 days while the sutures remain in place. Depending on the type of surgical intervention, healing will occur within 4 to 10 weeks. Passive and active ROM exercises are encouraged to promote healing. Patients should be cautioned that subjecting themselves to the same risks that caused the CTS may curtail healing and cause the problem to return. Modification of the work environment may be necessary to reduce this possibility.

Patient Education

Workers who are exposed to occupational risks for CTS should be educated on the causes and prevention of CTS. The work environment should be assessed for ergonomic risks to workers; often an ergonomic specialist is needed to perform these assessments. *Ergonomics* means fitting the job to the worker, as opposed to the worker accommodating to the workspace. Special attention should be paid to jobs with a known ability to produce extreme or repeated flexion of the wrist. Ergonomic evaluations and recommendations include the following:

- Evaluating the workstations of computer keyboard workers in regard to the height of the keyboard, chair, and monitor.
- Teaching lifting techniques and reviewing them annually.
- Rotating jobs for workers who perform repetitive tasks.
- Resting frequently or wearing specially designed hand wear; for example, workers who use vibrating tools should wear antivibration gloves or should be given frequent, short rest breaks.

Outside of workplace risks, patients should be educated to consider the stress on the wrist during everyday activities such as gardening and cleaning. Knitting, sewing, and playing musical instruments may put tension on the wrist. Patients should be advised to avoid carrying heavy briefcases, packages, or purses with the hands. Bags with shoulder straps, backpacks, or bags with wheels should be recommended to patients with risk factors for CTS.

■ DUPUYTREN'S CONTRACTURE

Sometimes referred to as "Viking disease," or palmar fibromatosis, this condition affects the palmar tissue between the skin and the distal palm and fingers, most often in the fourth and fifth fingers but also in the thumb–index finger web space. Visible, palpable fibrous bands, reminiscent of tendons, can extend from the palm to the proximal interphalangeal joint of Dupuytren-affected fingers. It is a progressive condition that results in flexor contracture while not affecting the flexor tendons. As the contractures increase, patients have trouble grasping objects, pulling on gloves, and putting hands in pockets. Sensation in the affected fingers usually is normal. It occurs most frequently in persons aged 40 to 60 years and is a familial disorder, most commonly affecting males of northern European ancestry. It is dysfunctional and disfiguring but does not cause pain. Surgery is the only therapeutic option; recurrence is not uncommon.

■ BOUTONNIÈRE DEFORMITY

Another term for *boutonnière deformity* is "jammed finger" or "central slip extensor tendon injury." This deformity is caused by a rupture of the central portion of the extensor tendon at its insertion into the middle phalanx. The patient typically reports a history of trauma; the finger is held partially flexed at the PIP joint and extended or hyperextended at the DIP joint. With a recent injury, the PIP joint is painful and tender. Boutonnière deformity may not be apparent initially but can develop in 7 to 21 days as the intact lateral bands of the extensor tendon slip inferiorly. Ask the patient to extend the injured finger and observe the position of the DIP and PIP joints. The PIP joint will be flexed more than 30 degrees, and the DIP joint will be extended or hyperextended. A radiograph can rule out fracture. Flexion contracture of the PIP joint and extension contracture of the DIP joint are possible.

Splint the PIP joint in extension for 6 weeks in a young patient and for 3 weeks in an elderly patient. The DIP joint is left free. Initiate active and passive ROM at the DIP joint. If the injury is already 1 to 2 weeks old, this may not be possible.

■ HERNIATED LUMBAR DISC (HERNIATED NUCLEUS PULPOSUS)

The most common cause of radicular pain to the lower extremities is a herniated lumbar intervertebral disc. Over time, the lumbar discs are subjected to repeated deformations and large loads with physiological motion of the spine. In some individuals, fragmentation of the disc may result, followed by annular rupture, and finally a herniation of the nucleus pulposus into the lumbar canal. The resultant herniated disc syndrome (commonly called "sciatica" or "lumbar radiculopathy") may cause pain and/or numbness and/or weakness in one or both lower extremities. The pain results in part from direct mechanical compression of the nerve root and in part from chemical irritation of the nerve root by substances in the nucleus pulposus.

Epidemiology and Causes

Low back pain affects a significant portion of the population at some time in their lives, most commonly in persons aged 30 to 50 years. The lifetime incidence of low back pain is between 60% and 90%. Among patients with acute back pain, approximately 2% have nerve-root symptoms, but only 10% to 25% of those patients have symptoms that persist for longer than 6 weeks. Because fewer than 10% have symptoms after 3 months, only a limited number of patients require surgical treatment. Disc herniation occurs most commonly at the L4 to L5 or L5 to S1 levels with subsequent irritation of the L5 and S1 nerve root. Herniations at more proximal intervertebral levels constitute only 5% of all lumbar disc herniations. Fewer than 2% of patients with low back pain have infections, neoplasms, or inflammatory spondyloarthropathies. Spinal stenosis is more likely to be the etiology of radicular pain in patients older than age 55 years. Disc disease affects males and females equally.

Risk factors are normal aging (often difficult to distinguish between normal aging of the spine and pathological changes), cigarette smoking, a narrowed lumbar vertebral canal, obesity, osteoporosis, stress, and muscle tension. Causes include trauma (sudden or over time), frequent lifting without proper utilization of body mechanics, and vibration, such as driving and/or riding in a motor vehicle for prolonged periods of time.

Pathophysiology

An intervertebral disc is located between each vertebra and is connected to the vertebral body. The discs have a strong outer layer, the *annulus fibrosus,* and the inner *nucleus pulposus,* which is a jelly-like material that moves in the center of the annulus and redistributes itself as different stresses are placed on the disc, acting like a shock absorber. Disc anomalies begin when there is injury or degeneration of the annulus fibrosus—the outer portion of the disc. Bulging is an initial indication that the disc is showing signs of wear and tear.

The size of the individual's spinal canal becomes an important consideration when diagnosing a disc problem. A small canal will tolerate less disc material that is bulging or herniated, ruptured, or extruded. A small herniated disc in one patient will not be a problem; in another, the same size disc may cause significant compression of the neural structures. When a disc herniates, the nucleus pulposus pushes through a tear in the annulus fibrosis. The location and amount of disc material in the canal will determine the symptoms. A small amount of nucleus pulposus in a congenitally small canal can cause significant symptoms. Most discs will rupture more to one side than the other, producing more symptoms in the affected side via compression of a unilateral nerve root. Significant herniations may also bulge bilaterally, producing symptoms on both sides of the body. Thus, the nature of the symptoms is determined by the vertebral level of disc herniation.

In turn, radicular symptoms are the hallmark of disc herniation, and their absence makes this diagnosis highly unlikely. Lesions involving the L5 nerve root produce symptoms extending to the dorsum of the foot with weakened dorsiflexion of the large toe and weakened heel walking. Lesions involving both L5 and S1 nerve roots manifest with symptoms in the lateral and posterior calf, with S1 nerve root lesions extending to the heel, as well as gastrocnemius weakness, impaired toe walking, and a reduced or absent ankle reflex. Less common lesions affecting the L4 and L3 nerve roots include a diminished patellar reflex with symptoms extending to the anterior shin and thigh, with quadriceps weakness and difficulty rising from a squatted position.

The *cauda equina* is a continuation of the spinal cord below the first lumbar level in the adult. The "horse's tail" consists of an array of nerves that exit the conus of the spinal cord and continue down the lumbar spine, exiting at different lumbar and sacral levels through foramina. These nerves are responsible for specific sensory and motor functions, including perineal sensation and both bladder and anal sphincter function. In some instances, an acute herniation of the disc at the L5 to S1 level may cause acute cauda equina compression characterized by bilateral lower extremity weakness, anesthesia, or paresthesia of the perineum and buttocks (saddle anesthesia) and bowel or bladder retention and/or incontinence. This is a medical emergency and requires immediate decompression.

Clinical Presentation
Subjective

The onset of symptoms may be abrupt but is more likely to be insidious. Unilateral radiculopathy is frequently accompanied by low back pain. Some patients report that preexisting back pain disappears when leg pain begins signaling the herniation. The pain is often severe and exaggerated by sitting, walking, standing, coughing, and sneezing. Most often, the pain radiates down from the buttock to the posterior or posterolateral leg to the ankle or foot. These patients typically cannot find a position of comfort. Lying on their side in a fetal position or on their back with a pillow under the knees may afford some relief. Upper or midlumbar radiculopathy

(L1–L4 nerve root compression) refers pain to the anterior aspect of the thigh and often does not radiate below the knee.

Compression of the root may also cause paresthesias, loss of deep tendon reflex, and weakness of specific muscle groups. A herniated nucleus pulposus is most commonly seen in patients aged 20 to 50 years.

Objective

Most disc ruptures are posterolateral and press on a lumbar nerve root, which produces radiating pain. There may be paraspinal muscle spasm and lumbar scoliosis, with the trunk tilted away from the affected side. Look for a list with the patient standing. With the patient sitting, look for pain and spinal extension (leaning back) when the leg is raised (flip sign). When coupled with reproduced back pain with supine straight-leg raising limited to less than 45 degrees of leg elevation, these signs are highly reliable for herniated disc.

Evaluate motor and sensory function of the lumbosacral nerve roots and the deep tendon reflexes. Evaluate straight-leg raising on both the involved and uninvolved limbs with the patient in the supine position. This test places stress on the L5 and S1 nerve roots. Ipsilateral restriction on straight-leg raising is common with a variety of lumbar spine problems, but a positive crossed straight-leg raising test (pain in the involved leg or buttock that occurs when lifting the uninvolved leg) is highly specific for nerve root entrapment. To stretch the upper lumbar nerve roots, perform a reverse straight-leg raising test. With the patient prone, either extend the hip or do the prone rectus femoris test. With the patient in the prone position, flex the knee. Limited knee flexion in this position compared with supine flexion indicates tightness of the rectus femoris portion of the quadriceps muscle. With severe tightness, the pelvis will elevate as the hip moves into flexion. (See Advanced Assessment 15.10.)

Diagnostic Reasoning
Diagnostic Tests

Age-appropriate changes are usually demonstrated on radiograph. MRI might be useful if there is an unclear diagnosis or if the patient is being readied for surgery but otherwise is not indicated.

The majority of patients who present with low back pain do not require any imaging studies; however, there are several exceptions that warrant further diagnostic testing and immediate treatment. Patients who have recently experienced a trauma should be considered for radiographic evaluation. Imaging studies are used to evaluate the extent of ligamentous, neural, osseous, and soft tissue injuries. Patients suspected of having an infection or tumor should be initially screen with plain radiographs followed by MRI. Immediate imaging is also necessary for a patient who is suspected of having

Advanced Assessment 15.10	Classic Findings of Disc Herniation
Nerve Root	**Findings**
L3–L4 (L4 nerve root)	Weakness in the anterior tibialis, numbness in the shin, thigh pain, and an asymmetrical knee reflex (5% of all herniations)
L4–L5 (L5 nerve root)	Weakness in the great toe extension, numbness top of the foot and first web space, and posterolateral thigh and calf pain
L5–S1 (S1 nerve root)	Weakness in the great toe flexor and gastrocsoleus with inability to sustain tiptoe walking, numbness in the lateral foot, posterior calf pain and ache, and an asymmetrical ankle reflex

cauda equina syndrome. Cauda equina syndrome is most commonly seen in patients aged 30 to 40 years following an acute disc herniation. The physical exam reveals low back pain with bilateral weakness of the lower extremities, saddle anesthesia, and bladder and bowel incontinence. These patients should undergo immediate MRI and be referred to a surgeon.

In cases of neurological deficit, CT and/or MRI should be obtained in order to depict the spinal cord and surrounding tissue. The superiority of CT at capturing details of osseous structures allows for thorough assessment of fractures. CT is generally used to complement information obtained from other diagnostic imaging studies such as myelography, MRI, and radiographs. The value of the CT is its ability to demonstrate the osseous structures of the lumbar spine and their relationship to the neural canal. CT is helpful in the diagnosis of tumors, fractures, partial or complete dislocations, and spondylolisthesis. CT is not as useful as MRI in visualizing conditions of soft tissue structure.

Differential Diagnosis

The following is a list of differential diagnoses:

- Cauda equina syndrome (perianal numbness, urinary overflow incontinence or retention, reduced anal sphincter tone, bilateral involvement), which can lead to permanent motor loss if not immediately treated
- Demyelinating conditions (clonus)
- Extraspinous nerve entrapment (abdominal or pelvic masses)
- Hip or knee arthritis (decreased internal rotation of hip, knee deformity or effusion)
- Lateral femoral cutaneous nerve entrapment (sensory only, lateral thigh)
- Spinal stenosis (older population)
- Thoracic cord compression (clonus, spasticity, high sensory pattern, abdominal reflexes)
- Trochanteric bursitis (no tension signs, pain down lateral thigh and leg, exquisite tenderness over trochanter)
- Vascular insufficiency (absent posterior tibial pulse, claudication, trophic changes)

Management

Control of symptoms, relief of pain, and improved mobility are all goals of management. Most episodes improve with conservative treatment.

NSAIDs should be given for pain with 1 to 3 days of bedrest. If the pain is severe in the acute phase, which it can be, consider muscle relaxants and/or narcotics but for no longer than 7 to 10 days. The patient should be taught to limit sitting, prolonged standing, or walking and to take frequent rest breaks when resuming activity. Reassure patients that most disc herniations resolve without residual problems. Even ruptures with a significant inflammatory component should improve within 3 to 6 weeks. Refer if the problem persists longer than that, if pain increases, or if there is evidence of any "red flags." A short course of oral steroids (5 days) or an epidural injection may reduce leg pain within the first 2 weeks after herniation, although some recent studies have indicated that epidural steroids do not significantly alter pain that has persisted for more than 2 weeks or influence the outcome of the syndrome. Persistent numbness, progression of neurological deficits, and weakness can occur despite treatment.

Surgical options may need to be considered if symptoms persist for more than 3 months and other underlying causes are ruled out. Intolerable pain, multiple episodes of radiculopathy, severe postural tilt, and persistent dysfunctional pain are all indications for surgery. If cauda equina compression is confirmed, surgical lumbar decompression is the treatment of choice to halt neurological deterioration unless surgery is contraindicated for other medical reasons.

Follow-up and Referral

The patient should return in about 10 days for evaluation of pain and function. Monitor the patient every 2 weeks until he or she is fully functional. A progressive walking program should be initiated after pain is controlled (usually within 7–10 days). It is best to start with short walks initially, up to four times per day, lengthening the walks as tolerated. The patient should return to full activity as soon as possible but avoid high-risk activities such as heavy lifting and long car rides.

Most cases of acute back pain (90%) and/or radiculopathy (60%–80%) recover with conservative treatment; the same is true of most cases of chronic back pain and radiculopathy.

Progression of any neurological deficits, such as loss of ankle jerk; bladder and rectal sphincter weakness with retention or incontinence; foot drop with weakness of the anterior tibial, posterior tibial, or peroneal muscles; narcotic addiction in cases of chronic pain; limitation of movement; and restricted activity all warrant referral for further evaluation and treatment.

Patient Education

Cessation of smoking, weight reduction, good posture and body mechanics, and adherence to an exercise regimen are all ways to improve health and prevent recurrence. (See Patient Education 15.1 for exercises to recommend.) Modification of work environment may be necessary. Manipulation (chiropractic) and/or physical therapy may prove helpful.

■ LUMBAR SPINAL STENOSIS

Lumbar spinal stenosis is narrowing of one or more levels of the lumbar spinal canal and subsequent compression of the nerve roots. In the order of descending likelihood, L4 to L5, L3 to L4, and L1 to L2 are the levels most commonly involved. At L1 to S1, the stenosis is usually not central but foraminal, involving the same root (L5) as central canal stenosis at the L4 to L5 level. Typically, the stenosis must be severe before symptoms occur.

Epidemiology and Causes

Anatomically, as many as 30% of the population may have spinal stenosis after age 60, yet only a portion of this population has symptoms. Obesity is a predisposing factor, as is osteoporosis.

Pathophysiology

Lumbar spinal stenosis is defined as narrowing of the spinal canal with compression of the nerve roots. It may be congenital or acquired. It most frequently results from enlarging osteophytes at the facet joints, hypertrophy of the ligamentum flavum, and protrusion or bulging of the intervertebral discs. Lumbar spinal stenosis may produce symptoms by directly compressing nerve roots or by compressing nutrient arterioles that supply the nerve roots.

Clinical Presentation

Subjective

Onset of symptoms may follow a lifting incident or minor trauma or may gradually emerge. Often there is pseudoclaudication causing radicular complaints (with or without associated back pain) in the calves, buttocks, and upper thighs of one or both legs. Symptoms progress from a proximal to distal direction. Walking or prolonged standing causes pain and weakness in the legs and buttocks. In cases of vascular claudication, the pain stops when the patient stops walking, but pseudoclaudication does not immediately subside when walking stops. The patient may obtain short-term relief by leaning forward (manifested as "stooping"); when grocery shopping, the patient will be leaning on the cart. Relief after sitting is variable, depending on the degree of neural compression. Patients who sleep on their backs, meaning with the spine extended, might awaken after several hours with back and leg pain. Lumbosacral pain is associated with walking and standing. A vague aching in the legs or leg weakness may also be present. Spondylolisthesis (degenerative or spondylolytic), vascular insufficiency, and osteoarthritis of the hips are often associated with spinal stenosis, as well as obesity.

Objective

Muscle weakness of the legs is a subtle phenomenon. This may be best elicited after walking on a treadmill. Proprioception can be impaired; there may be a positive Romberg test. There may be sensory changes, and these are usually segmental and may involve more than one spinal level. Reflexes are often diminished. Some patients will have a lumbar scoliosis. With bowel or bladder symptoms, sphincter tone may be decreased. However, because many elderly patients have concomitant prostate problems or urinary incontinence, genitourinary evaluation may be necessary to differentiate these processes.

Diagnostic Reasoning

Diagnostic Testing

Radiographs may provide some evidence of spinal stenosis. AP and lateral view radiographs (up to L10 in the lateral view) may show significant narrowing of the intervertebral disc or spondylolisthesis. There may be osteopenia or an old burst fracture of the vertebral body.

Differential Diagnosis

The following is a list of differential diagnoses:

- Abdominal aortic aneurysm (palpable pulsatile mass)
- Arterial insufficiency (distance to claudication constant, recovery after rest, absent or diminished pulses)
- Diabetes mellitus (abnormal glucose metabolism, nonsegmental numbness, skin changes)
- Folic acid or vitamin B_{12} deficiency (confirmed by laboratory tests, anemia)
- Infection (fever, elevated ESR, intervertebral disc narrowing)
- Tumor (patchy neurological deficit, bone destruction, severe night pain)

Management

Any neurological deficit, gait disturbance, or bowel and bladder dysfunction should be evaluated further. These changes may not be reversed following surgery for decompression; thus the goal of the treatment is to prevent progression.

Intermittent use of NSAIDs may be helpful, as well as folic acid or vitamin B_{12} supplementation in some cases depending on results of laboratory tests. However, most management revolves around physical therapy or an exercise program that focuses on flexing the spine. Flexion of the spine increases intraspinal volume. Bicycling is one exercise that is done with the spine in flexion. Improving abdominal muscle tone lifts the pelvis anteriorly and flexes the lumbar spine. Reduction of intra-abdominal fat is critical to achieving the objective. Thus, weight loss may be pivotal. Lumbar flexion exercises increase spinal canal volume. Examples include exercise on all fours, arching the back, or in the fetal position. Exercises that extend the spine should be avoided (swayback).

Lumbar epidural corticosteroid injection may provide some immediate relief for approximately 50% of patients and more sustained relief for approximately 25%. When disabling symptoms persist, decompression laminectomy provides at least short-term relief in some patients but does not always rehabilitate lost function.

Follow-up and Referral

The rate of progression is variable from rapid to none. Many patients never develop any neurological deficits and tolerate the condition well. Pain and limited function, however, can become severe and lead to a secondary depression. Standing erect may become impossible, and the patient may be forced to adopt a stooped posture. Claudication may develop after walking only a few feet. Cauda equina syndrome develops in some patients, leading to loss of bowel and bladder function.

If nonoperative treatment is ineffective, specialty consultation is warranted. Night pain that disturbs sleep tends to be a sign of advancing disease and also indicates a need to refer and/or consult. Prolonged use of NSAIDs can cause renal failure, hepatotoxicity, and gastrointestinal ulcer disease and can exacerbate existing cardiac disease.

Patient Education

Educate the patient and family as to any potentially serious symptoms such as changes in bowel and bladder function, change in neurological status, and gait disturbance. Educate as to side effects of NSAIDs or narcotic usage. Support weight loss if necessary with dietary instructions and clear guidelines for activity and exercise. Because many of these patients are older adults, they may need a range of services arranged to accomplish these goals.

Common differential diagnoses for back pain include the following:

- Ankylosing spondylitis: Back pain and stiffness over several months; relief with exercise; reduced mobility of spine; painful or ankylosed sacroiliac joints; reduced chest wall expansion.
- Cauda equina syndrome: Acute urinary or rectal incontinence, with or without paraplegia.
- Dissecting aortic aneurysm: Sudden onset of severe low back pain in older adults; pain that is not relieved with rest; pallor, diaphoresis, and confusion may be present; possible asymmetrical pulses and blood pressure in extremities.
- Gallstones: Pain follows ingestion of a fatty meal and radiates around trunk to right scapula; belching, bloating, and stomach acid are present, along with right upper quadrant pain.
- Gynecological disorders: Vaginal discharge; pain worse around menstruation or ovulation.
- Herniated disc: Often preceded by years of recurrent episodes of localized back pain; leg pain overshadows back pain.
- Infection: Unremitting or progressive pain at rest; tender spinous process at level of involvement; fever; history of drug use; diabetes; immunosuppression or suspected systemic infection; previous genitourinary or spinal surgery.
- Musculoskeletal strain: Often no precipitating event; pain is over lower back and muscles without sciatica; aggravated by sitting, standing, and certain movements; alleviated with rest. Palpation localizes pain and muscle spasms may be seen. Insidious onset; progressive improvement.
- Prostatitis: Constant low back pain; urinary hesitancy; change in sexual frequency.
- Pyelonephritis: Ill-appearing patient with nausea and vomiting; back and flank pain excruciating with direct percussion.
- Sciatica: Pain radiating into the buttocks, thighs, and/or below the knees as the result of L5 or S1 nerve-root irritation, compression, or disc prolapse.
- Spinal fracture: Pain felt near the site of injury; history of major trauma to the back or (in older adults) a history of strenuous lifting or a minor fall.
- Spinal stenosis: Gradual onset in older adults; often mimics intermittent claudication, except pain is usually in buttocks, thigh, or calf, worsens with exertion and back extension (leaning backward or walking downhill), and is relieved with sitting, walking uphill, or leaning forward; weakness and/or bowel and bladder dysfunction may be present.
- Spondylolisthesis: Systemic inflammatory condition of the vertebral column and sacroiliac joints; most frequently affects men aged 20 to 30; chronic low back pain, worse in morning; excessive thoracic kyphosis is present.
- Tumor: Unremitting or progressive pain at rest, night pain; tender spinous process at level of involvement; variable neurological findings; weight loss, fever, or other systemic symptoms; known or suspected malignancy.

OVERUSE SYNDROME (REPETITIVE MOTION SYNDROME)

Overuse syndrome describes a constellation of cumulative soft tissue trauma disorders that develop in the absence of acute injury. All major tissues in the musculoskeletal system are subject to overuse injuries. Overuse syndromes may be referred to as *repetitive strain injury, chronic microtrauma, cumulative trauma disorders, soft tissue rheumatism,* and *work-related pain disorder;* all of these terms refer to syndromes that result in chronic localized pain and dysfunction. It may manifest itself as well-defined pathology of a single periarticular site or a regional myofascial pain syndrome. Examples of single-site periarticular pain generators include bursitis, tendinitis, or fasciitis (e.g., plantar fasciitis). Finding several pain generators in the absence of articular involvement suggests a chronic, low-grade, repetitive trauma disorder or an acute overexertion syndrome that one may find in "weekend warrior" athletes.

Proper diagnosis of overuse syndromes may be difficult because they often involve more than one type of tissue. Overuse problems usually develop in the muscles and tendons. Although it is common to divide the muscles and tendons for ease of presentation, it is important to remember that they function together as a unit—the musculotendinous unit. Other soft tissues, including the bursa, fascia, synovium, and nerves, may also be affected by overuse. *Muscle overuse injuries* may be divided into muscle strains and muscle soreness (acute and delayed); there are overuse injuries of the tendons and bursa; any joint that is subject to abnormal loads, ranges of motion, or activity may develop a reactive synovitis. Chronic compartment syndromes may occur related to entrapment of fluid in the fascial sheath. Common anatomical sites and types of overuse syndromes are described in Table 15.9.

Epidemiology and Causes

Overuse injuries are common in both athletes and nonathletes. It is difficult to determine the true incidence because frequently overuse injuries are not brought to the attention of a health-care provider. Despite this, such injuries account for more than 50% of the injuries seen in a primary-care setting and are the most frequently encountered athletic injury. Whereas individuals seem aware of the benefits of exercise, they do not always seem aware that these same activities can also bring problems with injury. Overuse injuries of soft tissue include damage to tendons, muscles, bursa, fascia, and nerves. They include impingement and snapping syndromes and compartment syndromes.

Given that repetitive stress can traumatize tissue, the potential for injury is enhanced by a wide variety of predisposing factors. Female sex, youth and old age, pregnancy, smoking, menopause, diabetes, poor physical

Table 15.9	Common Anatomical Sites: Overuse Syndrome
Anatomical Site	**Overuse Syndrome**
Shoulder	Rotator cuff tendinitis Thoracic outlet syndrome
Forearm	Lateral epicondylitis Medial epicondylitis Ulnar nerve entrapments
Hand and wrist	Carpal tunnel syndrome de Quervain's syndrome "Trigger finger"
Leg and foot	Chondromalacia patellae Iliotibial band syndrome Shin splints Achilles tendinitis Plantar fasciitis Stress fracture

conditioning, underlying anatomical imperfections aggravated by exercise or repeated motions, and obesity have all been identified as risk factors. In addition, poor cardiovascular or musculoskeletal conditioning, underlying cardiovascular disease, arthritis (osteoarthritis or rheumatoid arthritis), gout, and stress may all contribute to the development of overuse syndrome. In athletes, overtraining, running on uneven surfaces, poor equipment, inadequate footwear, and leg-length discrepancy may all contribute; in workers, unhealthy work environments both physically and emotionally are thought to contribute. Repeatedly performing arm and hand movements with a very short repetitive cycle of less than 30 seconds in the course of one's daily job is a risk factor. Repeatedly performing the same task over and over in a short period of time in a factory can impose the same level of risk. Dancers, musicians, grocery clerks, computer keyboard operators, and dental hygienists are all particularly susceptible. Vibration, cold environment, and use of some specific hand tools also are considered risk factors. (See Risk Factors 15.2.)

Sitting all day in an awkward body position may lead to muscle fatigue, for example. This may lead to generalized muscle inflammation and nerve compression throughout the upper extremities. Poor neck and shoulder posture places skeletal bone pressure on the nerve and blood supply to the arms, wrists, and hands, thereby diminishing circulation and nerve conduction to these areas. Fresh nutrient blood supply is diminished, thereby slowing recovery from microtrauma. Independent of whether muscle, tendon, cartilage, or hard tissue is involved, injury results from a simple mismatch between stress on a given tissue and the ability of that tissue to withstand the stress. There are two basic mechanisms behind tissue trauma: single-impact macrotrauma and

---

Risk Factors 15.2 Overuse Syndrome

- Arthritis (osteoarthritis and rheumatoid arthritis)
- Congenital defects
- Diabetes mellitus
- Ganglia
- Gout
- Hobbies (knitting, musical instruments, electronic games)
- Hormonal factors (pregnancy, oral contraceptive use, menopause, thyroid disorders, hysterectomy with bilateral oophorectomy)
- Hypertension
- Impaired circulation
- Inflammation of tendons and tendon sheath
- Obesity
- Occupational activities (computer usage, cash registers)
- Paget's disease
- Raynaud's phenomenon
- Renal disease
- Sports (racquet sports, golf, softball, running)
- Underlying anatomical abnormalities

---

repetitive microtrauma (damage at the microscopic or molecular level). Overuse injuries therefore can be defined as the level of repetitive microtrauma sufficient to overwhelm the tissue's ability to adapt or heal.

Pathophysiology

Overuse syndrome results from repetitive microtrauma to bones, ligaments, and musculotendinous units. This repetitive microtrauma causes a local inflammatory process, leading to pain and loss of function. In vitro studies have demonstrated that tendinous fibroblasts produce elevated concentrations of prostaglandin E_2 and leukotriene B_4 in response to repetitive stretch maneuvers. Thus, repetitive microtrauma is believed to lead to repeated cycles of inflammation and tissue regeneration, characterized by fibroblast proliferation, collagen production, and resultant tissue contraction.

Overuse syndrome most commonly involves the musculotendinous unit, resulting in tendinitis or tenosynovitis. Repetitive mechanical trauma to a joint may result in synovitis or arthritis, and repetitive overuse stress on bones can result in periostitis or stress fractures. Bone has the ability to constantly remodel and repair itself. However, if the degree of repetitive microtrauma exceeds the bone's capacity for repair, an overuse injury in the form of a stress fracture may occur. Stress fractures occur most commonly in the weight-bearing bones of the lower extremities, such as the tibia and metatarsals, but are sometimes seen in the upper extremities of athletes who throw (e.g., baseball pitchers).

Histopathological studies of muscle biopsies have also revealed differences in limbs affected by overuse syndrome. These include an increased number of type 1 muscle fibers (smaller, slow-twitch or red fibers) with a decreased number of hypertrophied type 2 fibers (larger, fast-twitch or white fibers). Muscle fibers affected by overuse syndrome also display mitochondrial changes with an increased number of muscle cell nuclei. These changes become increasingly evident at higher grades of overuse syndrome. Decreased blood flow to affected muscles has also been noted in some studies.

Clinical Presentation

Subjective

In general, overuse injuries are insidious in onset. Typical complaints include pain, fatigue, numbness, or any combination of the same. Patients often have difficulty localizing the pain and may report swelling and sensation not apparent on physical exam.

Often, the symptoms have existed for some time; it is when the symptoms occur more frequently or have become more intense and last longer that they may begin to interfere with function. This is most likely the point at which the patient seeks help.

Objective

Specific findings will vary depending on the joints and body area involved. However, in general, overuse syndrome may be categorized by grade. (See Advanced Assessment 15.11.)

Diagnostic Reasoning

Diagnostic Tests

The diagnostic tests indicated will vary depending on the body part involved. Radiographs are necessary with a history of trauma. A bone scan may be necessary to rule out stress fractures. Likewise, nerve conduction velocity studies can be ordered to rule out carpal tunnel syndrome or ulnar nerve entrapment at the elbow, but the results are usually negative. X-ray results are usually negative. MRI may help to visualize soft tissue injury.

Differential Diagnosis

The differential diagnoses will vary, depending on the joints and body area involved. Possible diagnoses include the following:

- Angina with referred arm pain (abnormal electrocardiogram)
- Claudication (decreased peripheral pulses)
- Deep vein thrombosis (abnormal venogram)
- Fibromyalgia (11 of 18 pressure points in four body quadrants)
- Herniated cervical or lumbar disc (abnormal spine radiograph, myelogram, and MRI)

Management

There are two primary goals in the management of overuse injuries: reducing inflammation and improving

Advanced Assessment 15.11   Grading Overuse Syndrome

Grade	1	2	3	4
Pain history	Hours after activity	Late, or just after activity	Early, or in middle of activity	At rest
Clinical manifestations	Tenderness (generalized)	Tenderness (localized)	Point tenderness Erythema Swelling	Point tenderness Erythema Swelling ROM decreased Function impaired
Management	Ice	Ice Decrease activity (25%)	Ice Decrease activity (50%)	Ice Rest NSAIDs

vascular blood flow. Overuse injuries can be very difficult to treat. Treatment should be initiated as early as possible because once chronic, they become even more difficult to treat both physically and psychologically. Exercise and physical therapy are the keys to successful recovery. Initial management should include *protection* from further injury, abstaining from the irritating activity, and, in some cases, splinting for immobilization; *rest; ice* applied for 10 to 30 minutes with an equal period without ice; *compression,* such as with an elastic bandage to provide support to injured tissue; and *elevation* to decrease swelling (*PRICE*). An individualized rehabilitation program should be designed and implemented as soon as possible. Flexibility, strength, proprioception, and endurance must be addressed and encouraged.

Pharmacological approaches may include NSAIDs during the acute phase and, in some cases, muscle relaxants; occasionally, antidepressant therapy may be used in chronic situations. Acupuncture is often effective, and some patients may benefit from the use of transcutaneous electrical nerve stimulation. Injured muscles, tendons, and nerves may require significant amounts of rest to allow healing to take place.

Follow-up and Referral

The degree of follow-up will depend on the location and severity of the injury. Once a diagnosis is made, treatment by a team of health-care professionals may be warranted. Considerable psychological sequelae may be involved. Better results are obtained when there is a specific, clearly identifiable syndrome such as carpal tunnel syndrome. Lack of job satisfaction and depression are also important predictors of recovery. Poor prognosis is associated with both long-standing disability (longer than 6 months) and litigation. With these disorders, patients often lose time from work and experience psychological changes. They may change occupations or never return to work.

Patient Education

The patient needs to be educated as to the precipitating activity and the need to refrain from that activity for a certain period of time. This can be especially difficult to reinforce with athletes. Patience and assistance in designing alternate activities will help so that the patient may remain active. If the cause is work related, monitor for chronicity and issues of secondary gain.

■ PAGET'S DISEASE

Paget's disease (osteitis deformans) of the bone, first diagnosed by Sir James Paget in 1877, is a disease of the osteoclast and is the most exaggerated example of disordered bone remodeling. It is characterized by excessive osteoclastic bone resorption followed by excessive bone formation from osteoblasts, resulting in bone that is architecturally unsound. This can lead to bone pain, bone deformity, and skeletal fragility and can involve a single bone or multiple bones.

Epidemiology and Causes

Prevalence of the disease is difficult to determine because it is often asymptomatic (70%–90% of cases). Older adults are most commonly affected; it is the second most common bone disorder after osteoporosis in older adults. It is estimated that the disease affects more than 10% of people older than 80 years of age. Ethnic and geographic clustering of cases has been well described for Paget's disease, and 40% of patients report a family history of the condition. This disease is common in England, with statistics indicating a prevalence as high as 5% of the general population in some areas. Australia, New Zealand, and Argentina are also high-prevalence areas. In the United States, the prevalence varies between 1% and 3%.

Although Paget himself felt the disease was caused by chronic inflammation, the etiology remains unknown to date. Bone biopsy data have identified various viral antigens, which suggests that a "slow virus" infection by a member of the paramyxovirus family (e.g., rubeola, which causes measles, respiratory syncytial virus, canine distemper) may be responsible for the disease.

Pathophysiology

The disease affects all aspects of bone metabolism and may be divided into three phases: lytic, mixed, and sclerotic. It begins with the lytic phase characterized by increased activity of multinucleate (up to 100 nuclei compared with 5–10 normally) osteoclasts, which leads to greatly increased resorption of bone (up to 20-fold). Hypercalcemia may manifest, particularly if the patient experiences prolonged immobilization. The mixed phase then follows, in which bone remodeling is abnormally increased, due to a greater number of osteoblasts of normal morphology. This leads to an abnormal, irregular deposition of collagen fibers. The final phase, known as the sclerotic phase, is notable for a predominance of abnormal bone formation. This is characterized by disorganized bone that takes on a mosaic pattern known as "woven bone," which is recognizable on x-ray exam. Eventually osteoblastic activity quiets, leaving sclerotic lesions. As the hypercellularity decreases, this bone becomes known as burned-out Paget's disease.

There are no Haversian systems within pagetic bone, and the bone marrow is eventually replaced by hypervascular fibrous tissue. Bones that are commonly affected with these sclerotic lesions include the cranium, long bones, and clavicles. These affected bones will change in shape, enlarge in size, and undergo changes in predominant direction of growth due to increased osteoid volume—all of which lead to considerable morbidity. Pagetic bone is weaker and less compact than normal adult lamellar bone, and bones affected by this change may be painful and, over time, may develop deformities, fractures, or nerve entrapment. Cytokines and growth factors that have been implicated, albeit inconclusively, in the pathophysiology of Paget's disease include IL-6, RANK-ligand (a member of the TNF-α superfamily), and macrophage-colony stimulating factor.

A rarer juvenile form of Paget's disease also exists. However, this form is fundamentally different from the adult form because it is typically polyostotic with widespread skeletal involvement. In addition, both histological and radiological findings differ from the adult form and may be readily distinguished.

Clinical Presentation

Subjective

The clinical presentation of Paget's disease is a function of the actual extent of disease, bones involved, and any complications present. Most (70%–90%) patients are asymptomatic. Although the affected bone may be larger than other bones, pagetic bones are weaker and more susceptible to fracture. The bones most commonly affected, in order of decreasing frequency, are the femur, sacrum, vertebrae, skull, tibia, and pelvis. Involvement of the tibia and humerus is less common, but the disease may occur at any site and may involve one (monostotic) or many (polyostotic) bones. Hands and feet are rarely involved.

The most typical complaint is one of pain at the involved site. The pain is usually dull or boring, but it can be shooting or knife-like, and often occurs at night. In some cases, a swelling or deformity of a long bone is noticed or the development of a change in gait. Back pain, with radiation to the buttocks or lower extremities, is another common complaint. Headache is a common complaint when the skull is involved.

Pagetic bone is of a highly vascular nature, and there may be increased warmth of the skin over the affected bones. The incidence of high-output cardiac failure may be tied to the increased vascularity of the involved bone, manifesting the classic symptoms of "dropsy" (generalized fluid overload). Though rare, this condition correlates with greater than 15% of skeletal involvement.

In patients with involvement of the ossicles of the inner ear or impingement of bone on the eighth cranial nerve, hearing loss may occur. Vertigo and tinnitus may also develop with skull involvement, as well as cranial nerve involvement resulting from compression by deformed bone. Spinal cord compression has also been observed with resultant cauda equina syndrome or paraplegia. Pathological fractures of vertebrae may also produce spinal cord lesions and pain. Articular complications, including asymptomatic hyperuricemia and classic gout, pseudogout, and degenerative arthritis, may occur. Fractures of the long bones occur most commonly in the femur, tibia, and humerus. Significant morbidity may result from heavy bleeding that may result from pathological fractures in these hypervascular bones.

Complications include cardiovascular problems, arthritic and osteoporotic problems, and neoplastic problems. When Paget's disease becomes widespread in the body, blood flow increases and may be associated with high cardiac output. The end result in this situation may be congestive heart failure. Arthritic changes in weight-bearing joints may result in pathological fractures. One dreaded complication is that of sarcoma. Incidence of sarcoma is approximately 1%; it may be in the femur, humerus, skull, facial bones, or pelvis. The extent of neoplastic involvement may be detected by CT and/or MRI.

Objective

Bowing of the long bones may be apparent, as well as enlargement of the skull (e.g., frontal bossing, maxillary enlargement). The sacrum, pelvis, and spine, particularly the lumbar spine, are the most common areas involved. Other less frequently involved sites include the femur (right more than left), cranium, sternum, and pelvis. Erythema and warmth is often noted over affected bone sites due to the increased hypervascularity.

Diagnostic Reasoning

Diagnostic Tests

Paget's disease is most commonly diagnosed through radiographs, radionuclide bone scanning, biochemical testing of bone resorption parameters, or biochemical testing of bone formation parameters. Biochemical tests reflecting osteoclast activity and resultant bone collagen resorption include measurements of urinary hydroxyproline/creatinine, as well as measurements of urinary and serum deoxypyridinoline, N-telopeptide, and C-telopeptide. Elevated 24-hour urinary deoxypyridinoline and type I collagen N-telopeptide excretion reflect bony destruction (resorption). As a marker of osteoblast activity, the measurement of serum alkaline phosphatase activity provides a general indication of bone turnover and disease activity in Paget's disease. Serum bone-specific alkaline phosphatase activity is helpful in patients who also have liver disease. At least one measurement of bone metabolic activity and x-ray films of affected bones are the minimum recommended level of evaluation to track and monitor the progression of treatment in Paget's disease.

Radiographs may illustrate three distinct stages of Paget's disease. In the earliest stage of the disease, an osteolytic lesion may be observed in the skull or a long bone. In the second stage of the disease, x-ray films reveal both osteolytic and sclerotic changes in the same bone. In the last stage of the disease, the sclerotic lesion dominates the bone and there may be an increase of the bone itself.

Although it is not a specific test, a radionuclide bone scan, using a radiolabeled bisphosphonate, is the most efficient means of detecting Paget's disease in a skeleton. The bisphosphonate is injected intravenously and is concentrated in areas of increased blood flow and high levels of bone formation, both common characteristics of Paget's disease. The test is used primarily to establish the full extent of skeletal involvement.

Diagnosis is often made when x-ray studies are performed or a high level of bone-specific alkaline phosphatase (a marker of bone formation) is found on routine screening. Immobilization in patients with Paget's disease is a primary risk factor for significantly elevated serum calcium and phosphorus, but immobilization alone will not necessarily result in hypercalcemia without underlying pathology. Occasionally, an associated hyperthyroidism can also lead to hypercalcemia. Quantitative histomorphometry of bone biopsies confirms the extent of remodeling present. Imaging studies to rule out malignancy should be performed whenever pathological fractures or elevated bone-specific alkaline phosphatase levels are detected.

Differential Diagnosis

When lesions are noted on x-ray film, metastatic cancer should be considered. Disseminated breast and prostate cancer are the cancers most likely to resemble Paget's disease radiographically and need to be ruled out. Occasionally, a hemangioma of bone may be sclerotic and mistaken for pagetic bone.

When making a diagnosis of Paget's disease, differential diagnoses such as osteoporosis, osteomalacia, hypercalcemia, and compensatory, secondary hyperparathyroidism should be considered. As with Paget's disease, osteoporosis involves the imbalance between bone formation and bone resorption. When bone formation exceeds resorption, the circulatory levels of parathyroid hormone may become increased, thus resulting in compensatory, secondary hyperparathyroidism.

Management

If Paget's disease is discovered incidentally and the patient is asymptomatic, no treatment may be necessary. However, there is an increasing trend to treat even if the patient is asymptomatic. This is based on evidence that failure to treat leads to further bone destruction, and that successful treatment is associated with restoration of normal patterns of new bone deposition. However, there is no direct evidence that aggressive treatment of Paget's disease is associated with prevention of progression or reduction in the risk of future complications.

There are four main approaches to treatment for a patient with Paget's disease:

- Nonpharmacological therapy, focusing mainly on physical therapy as a way to improve muscle strength
- Pharmacological therapy using either bisphosphonates or calcitonin
- Pain management using analgesics
- Surgery

Currently, bisphosphonates are approved by the FDA for the treatment of Paget's disease. Bone resorption is suppressed or reduced by bisphosphonates. They hinder the recruitment and function of osteoclasts, and they are thought to indirectly stimulate osteoblasts to produce an inhibitor of osteoclast formation. Alendronate, risedronate, tiludronate, and zoledronic acid are indicated for patients with Paget's disease of bone with alkaline phosphatase levels two times greater than normal, those who are symptomatic, or those at risk for future complications from their disease. Etidronate and pamidronate are designated for the management of moderate-to-severe disease. Ibandronate is not approved for Paget's disease treatment.

The bisphosphonates alendronate and risedronate have been shown to reduce biochemical indices for bone turnover into the normal range in many patients with a moderate to severe form of Paget's disease. Alendronate (Fosamax) is taken as a daily 40-mg tablet for 6 months;

risedronate (Actonel) is taken as a daily 30-mg tablet for 2 to 3 months. Calcium and vitamin D supplementation is also recommended for patients using either of these drugs. Etidronate (Didronel) is less potent than alendronate and risedronate but is recommended for treatment of symptomatic Paget's disease. It is given once daily (preferred) or in divided doses at least 2 hours before or after food, initially 5 to 10 mg/kg per day for a maximum of 6 months. Pamidronate (Aredia) is given by IV infusion, 30 mg/day for 3 successive days. Zoledronic acid (Reclast), 5 mg IV, is administered as a single infusion. IV treatments may require dosage adjustments in hepatic or renal impairment.

Subcutaneous injection of salmon calcitonin was the first widely used therapy for Paget's disease. Salmon calcitonin (Fortical, Miacalcin) has been shown to reduce elevated indices of bone turnover by 50%, decrease symptoms of bone pain, reduce warmth over affected bones, improve some neurological complications, and promote healing of lytic lesions. It is available in a nasal spray and an injectable (Miacalcin) form. The recommended dosage for the injectable form is 50 to 100 units per day or 3 times per week as subcutaneous or intramuscular injection. Its use today is primarily limited to patients who do not tolerate bisphosphonates. In the case of secondary resistance to salmon calcitonin, a switch to bisphosphonate therapy is necessary.

Pain directly attributable to Paget's disease is generally relieved through anti-osteoclast therapy as described earlier. Pain that is a result of bone deformity or arthritic or neurological complications may be treated additionally with acetaminophen, NSAIDs, and, depending on the circumstances, COX-2 inhibitors.

Surgical intervention is indicated in the face of significant bony deformities, nerve compression, or pathological fractures. Severe osteoarthritis of major joints such as the hip or knee may require artificial joint replacement with preoperative bisphosphonate therapy. Neurological sequelae from vertebral abnormalities may call for laminectomy for spinal decompression in lesions refractory to medical therapy. Osteosarcomas arising in pagetic bone may also require amputation to improve prognosis. In all these cases, extended physical therapy will follow.

Follow-up and Referral

Follow-up will depend on symptomatology, as will referral. Pain status needs to be monitored, as well as any laboratory abnormalities. If started on medication, the patient will need to be followed for therapeutic effects and any adverse effects that may occur secondary to therapy. Serum and urinary markers of disease activity should be followed 2 to 3 months after initiation of therapy and periodically thereafter. Any suspicion of malignancy warrants full evaluation and referral, because prognosis is particularly grim with the development of sarcoma with only a 1- to 3-year survival. Appropriate

referrals may include an orthopedic surgeon, neurosurgeon, physical therapist, and/or oncologist.

Patient Education

Patient education is important because so many people with Paget's disease are asymptomatic. The canine distemper virus has been postulated to be an etiological agent for Paget's disease; therefore, owners of unvaccinated dogs are at increased risk. Many of the medications prescribed for Paget's disease have significant adverse effects. Calcitonin analogs produced from other species may induce anaphylaxis and should be used with caution. Hypocalcemia may also result, and serum calcium should be monitored periodically. The bisphosphonates require ingestion on an empty stomach and the ability to stay in an upright position anywhere from 30 to 60 minutes. They can all cause gastrointestinal irritation, and other medications such as aspirin and NSAIDs should be used concurrently with caution. Adequate calcium and vitamin D intake must be maintained, because the bisphosphonates interfere with their absorption. These medications also interfere and interact with a wide variety of other drugs, blocking tetracycline, fluoroquinolone, and levothyroxine absorption. Warfarin must be monitored also.

■ COSTOCHONDRITIS

Costochondritis, also called *anterior chest wall syndrome,* is an inflammation of one or more costochondral junctions that manifests with chest wall pain. The pain may be sharp and acute or dull and persistent in nature. It is the most frequently occurring nontraumatic type of chest pain in adolescents and young adults. Pain is located over the costochondral and costosternal areas of the anterior chest.

Epidemiology and Causes

Costochondritis accounts for 10% of chest pain complaints in the United States. In the adolescent population, more than 20% of reported chest pain may be due to costochondritis. It is more common in women than in men, with a peak age range of 20 to 40 years. The cause of the problem is poorly understood, although trauma and overuse have been implicated in some cases. It is also sometimes seen in association with upper respiratory infection.

Pathophysiology

Costochondritis is an inflammation of the costochondral junctions manifesting only with pain in the absence of erythema, heat, or swelling. Repetitive minor trauma is currently believed to be the most likely etiology. However, epidemiological research has revealed an increasing incidence of costochondritis resulting from bacterial or fungal infections of the costochondral joints in injection drug users due to needle contamination or in people with postoperative thoracic wound infections.

When symptoms of costochondritis are accompanied by localized nonsuppurative swelling, this condition is termed *Tietze's syndrome,* which is characterized by a firm, palpable, tender fusiform swelling in the sternoclavicular joints or upper costal cartilages.

Clinical Presentation

Subjective

The patient presents with chest pain, which may be sharp and fleeting or intermittent. The patient may report previous episodes and may be concerned that there is something wrong with his or her heart. The onset of the pain is typically insidious and located at the costochondral junctions, most commonly involving the second to fifth costochondral joints. More than one site is involved in 90% of cases. There may be some radiation to the arm, but the pain is unrelated to position, respiration, or activity, although some patients report an increase in pain with trunk movements or deep breathing. The pain may persist for several months, causing the patient to return to the clinician for reassurance that nothing else is responsible for it. Chest tightness or localized muscle spasm may accompany the pain. There may be a history of recent upper respiratory infection, trauma, or unusual activity involving the chest or pectoral muscles.

Objective

In most cases, there are no objective physical findings other than sharply localized tenderness to palpation. These same sites may not be painful without direct palpation. In a few cases, inspection may reveal an area of redness, warmth, and nonsuppurative edema; however, this condition is more appropriately termed *Tietze's syndrome* and is seen most often in teenage girls. It is imperative in the examination of all patients with chest pain that the examiner apply pressure on the pectoralis muscles and each costochondral and costosternal junctions. This maneuver will reproduce the pain of costochondritis.

Diagnostic Reasoning

There are many causes of chest pain, ranging from life-threatening and acute to troublesome but benign etiologies. All of these must be considered in arriving at an accurate diagnosis.

Diagnostic Tests

The diagnosis of costochondritis is based on a thorough history and physical exam that reveal no red flags for more serious pathology. There are no specific diagnostic tests. However, testing may be initiated to rule out other conditions that manifest with chest pain and are part of the differential diagnosis. A chest radiograph is often helpful in this regard to evaluate for more serious lung, cardiac, or bony pathology. Erythrocyte sedimentation rate (ESR) is elevated in some instances of costochondritis, but inconsistently. Moreover, the lack of specificity of a positive ESR means that it cannot be used to exclude other conditions and rule in costochondritis. However, a nonelevated ESR may assist in ruling out more serious pathology.

Differential Diagnosis

Differential diagnosis includes cardiac-related chest pain such as the following:

- Mitral valve prolapse
- Myocarditis
- Pericarditis
- Left ventricular outflow obstruction
- Tachyarrhythmias
- Aortic aneurysm
- Acute coronary syndrome resulting from coronary artery disease or sympathomimetic drugs of abuse such as cocaine

Respiratory causes of chest pain include the following:

- Asthma
- Pneumonia
- Pleuritis
- Pneumothorax
- Pulmonary embolism
- Chronic cough

Gastrointestinal causes of chest pain include the following:

- Gastroesophageal reflux disease
- Esophagitis
- Gastritis
- Peptic ulcer disease (PUD)
- Esophageal spasm

Musculoskeletal causes of chest pain include the following:

- Muscle strain
- Trauma
- Hypersensitive xiphoid pain (xiphodynia or xiphoidalgia)
- Slipping rib syndrome (pain originating in the lower, floating ribs)
- Subacromial bursitis
- Fibromyalgia syndrome

Psychogenic disorders manifesting with chest pain include the following:

- Panic attacks
- Generalized anxiety disorder

Other diagnostic considerations with cutaneous pain include the following:

- Early herpes zoster (characterized by dermatomal clustered skin lesions)
- Pain related to chest wall tumors

Management

Management consists of reassurance and patient education regarding the benign and self-limited nature of the problem. Application of heat to the area may alleviate discomfort. NSAIDs may be prescribed for pain management, given the inflammatory nature of costochondritis. However, patients should be cautioned of the potential gastric and renal toxicities of NSAID overuse and contraindications should be stressed (e.g., PUD, gastritis, acute or chronic renal insufficiency). Drugs from these classes should be taken with food or milk. In addition, to avoid aggravating costochondritis, patients should be cautioned to avoid overuse or trauma.

Follow-up and Referral

The patient can be seen for reevaluation in 7 to 10 days or can be contacted by phone. The patient should be instructed to call the office if pain intensifies or other symptoms appear. One of the most important considerations when making the diagnosis of costochondritis is to rule out pathology of greater morbidity or potential mortality, as discussed earlier. A complete history and physical examination are the most important tools in guiding this evaluation; however, a complete work-up may require follow-up visitations to complete the diagnostic evaluation or assess changes in signs and symptoms over time.

Patient Education

The most critical point in many cases is convincing the patient that his or her condition is benign and self-limited despite the sharp nature of the pain. The patient is often fearful and requires reassurance. The clinician should educate the patient regarding the need to avoid overuse injury if any repetitive motion appears to be involved. It is important to stress the importance of avoiding any sudden, significant changes in activity.

■ TENDINITIS/TENOSYNOVITIS

Tendinitis is the inflammation of a tendon, which usually occurs at its point of insertion into bone or at the point of muscular origin. The term *tenosynovitis* refers to inflammation involving synovial sheaths surrounding the tendon in addition to the tendons. Common tenosynovitis syndromes, also referred to as "overuse" syndromes, include supraspinatus tendinitis, lateral epicondylitis or "tennis elbow," bicipital tendinitis, de Quervain's tenosynovitis (inflammation of the abductor pollicis longus and extensor pollicis longus and brevis tendons), "trigger finger" (volar flexor tenosynovitis), patellar tendinitis (patellar tendinosis or "basketball player's knee"), and Achilles tendinitis (see section on overuse syndrome in this chapter).

Epidemiology and Causes

This problem occurs commonly, with a slightly increased frequency in males, most likely related to sports. It occurs at all ages. Professional athletes and manual laborers are especially prone to tendinitis as a result of repetitive use. Painful areas of tendon are often labeled *tendinitis,* implying an inflammatory nature of the lesion; however, it is unclear whether inflammation is truly present in all forms of the pathology, especially in more chronic situations, which tend to have a more degenerative component. Some sources advocate the use of the term *tendinosis* for this reason. *Tenosynovitis* may result from inflammatory arthropathies such as rheumatoid arthritis or from gout. Tenosynovitis from amyloidosis is also common in renal dialysis patients. It also may occur for no discernible reason. Adults who overuse a joint with repeated motion are most likely to develop a *tendinitis.* Some classifications are based on degree of function and whether there is a partial or complete rupture of the tendon.

Pathophysiology

Exact pathophysiological entities involved with tendinitis and tenosynovitis have not been clearly established. It is understood that tenosynovitis involves inflammation of the synovial-lined sheath around one or more tendons, whereas tendinitis involves inflammation of the tendinous tissue itself. Because flexor tendons typically run in tight fibro-osseous tunnels, thickening of the surrounding sheath caused by inflammatory changes may in turn limit movement and cause pain as the trapped tendon attempts to glide within the thickened, tight sheath. The parietal and visceral layers of the synovium that surround flexor tendons typically provide nutrition and stability to the tendons, and they also allow for smooth movement of these connective tissues without extensive friction. However, infection may spread to these areas from nearby mucosal tissues, by direct extension from the skin through a puncture wound, or even hematogenously (as is the case with gonococcal tenosynovitis, which complicates 1%–3% of patients with mucosal infection of the pharynx or genitalia), because these synovial compartments normally offer little resistance. Tenosynovitis may also be associated with an inflammatory, infectious arthritis of large joints resulting from similar spread of infectious organisms (especially bacteria).

Tendinitis is usually associated with some degenerative changes in the tendon, including cell atrophy along with the presence of fibrinoid, mucoid, or hyaline degeneration of the connective tissue, which is visible under microscopic examination. Peritendinous scarring is not unusual, because tendons are relatively avascular and particularly sensitive to increased pressure within their synovial sheaths. Calcium deposits may also be noted along the length of the tendon, known as calcific tendinitis; this is especially common in the shoulder joint. These tendons tend to stiffen without treatment. Loss of function often follows, because they become progressively weaker and may eventually rupture.

Clinical Presentation

Subjective

Patients typically complain of pain and swelling over a localized area of tendon, usually in a region where the tendon passes through a tunnel. Pain is usually worse with motion, especially motion that stretches the involved tendon. A squeaking or rubbing and sometimes a triggering or catching sensation will be described by patients who have significant tenosynovitis. Tenosynovitis around the finger flexor tendon in the carpal tunnel region can have the associated symptoms of fingertip numbness from median nerve compression, as noted previously. A thorough history is essential, including all extracurricular activities.

Objective

The diagnosis of tendinitis is clinically driven. Early imaging is usually of minimal benefit. Perform a thorough physical exam that includes palpating any tender areas and ruling out any articular involvement of pain. One may see minimal swelling in tendinitis, although it can be impressive in cases of infection or with inflammatory causes of tenosynovitis. Examination may reveal localized pain, swelling, and tenderness. The pain will be worsened with certain motions, such as stretching the involved tendon, or with active work or activity that involves use of the tendon, especially against a resisting force. Crepitus and sometimes triggering can be palpated if a significant tenosynovitis has developed. These signs vary depending on the anatomical site of the tendinitis.

For example, tendinitis of the shoulder includes the bicep tendon and the tendons of the rotator cuff. This is similar to impingement syndrome. When patients have shoulder tendinitis, one will note tenderness with palpation of the subacromial space. These patients will have tenderness when one palpates the long head of the biceps tendon in the bicipital notch. To do this, have the patient keep his or her elbow at the affected side and externally rotate the shoulder to palpate the bicipital notch anteriorly and medially in the humeral head. When examining these patients, one can also elicit pain with resisted supination or flexion of the forearm. There is often an overlap of impingement syndrome with tendinitis of the shoulder.

If an inflammatory disease is present, associated redness, soft tissue swelling, and warmth may be present. Inflammatory processes of the tendon sheaths most commonly involve the dorsum of the hands, feet, and ankle and may cause marked soft tissue swelling. The ROM of contiguous joints may be limited by pain.

Diagnostic Reasoning

Diagnostic Tests

Diagnostics involve a thorough history and complete physical exam. Plain films may be useful to rule out other potential causes of pain in areas in question, but they will not show a tendinitis. MRI will show any significant tenosynovitis and tender nodules that sometimes develop. However, the diagnosis can almost always be made clinically without the need for MRI. Other options may include arthrography and MRI. In cases of tenosynovitis, there may be an associated anemia or elevation of the ESR.

Differential Diagnosis

Differential diagnoses to rule out include fracture, avulsion of the tendon, inflammatory arthritis, rheumatoid arthritis, and compartment syndrome. In the case of Achilles tendinitis, one must also consider a gastrocnemius strain, soleus strain, or tarsal tunnel syndrome. Tendinitis can be practically impossible to differentiate from bursitis, and the two conditions commonly occur together. The pain in tendinitis is localized to the side of the joint where tendon insertion occurs. Infectious tenosynovitis occurs primarily in the hand. In addition, the tenderness and swelling are located along the synovial lines proximally instead of at the insertion site and the pain is more marked, as are swelling and erythema. The ESR and white blood cell (WBC) count are more likely to be elevated in the case of infection.

Essentially, definitive diagnosis of tenosynovitis requires careful musculoskeletal examination, confirming the tendon source of the symptoms and excluding pathology from other contiguous musculoskeletal structures, including joints, bursae, and nerves. However, an inflammatory tenosynovitis of the dorsum of the hand or foot may require aspiration of synovial fluid, examination, and culture to confirm the diagnosis.

Management

Specific treatment requires an exact diagnosis to prevent further injury. An aggressive exercise program, for example, would be inappropriate for a compartment syndrome, complete tendon rupture, or nerve entrapment. Treatment will also depend on the stage of healing of the damaged tissue of the musculoskeletal system. There are essentially three phases of healing: (1) inflammation, (2) proliferation of new collagen and ground substance, and (3) scar remodeling and maturation.

Initial management should include protection, rest, ice, compression, and elevation (PRICE). The injury should be protected and rehabilitated in parallel with the healing process. The injured tissue needs to be stressed in order to activate collagen remodeling and realignment but also protected from overstress, which will cause reinjury and incite a further inflammatory response. Taping and bracing can both be helpful in providing protection. Ice is useful for treating pain, hemorrhage, and edema. It induces vasoconstriction, which results in a decrease in local blood flow. Ice acts as a topical anesthetic agent to control pain and decreases reflex muscle spasms by reducing the conduction velocity in peripheral nerves. Ice bags, compared with cold gel packs, elicit the greater decrease in tissue temperature over a longer period of time, and application for 15 to 20 minutes is recommended. Treatment may be repeated every 1 to 2 hours in acute cases. In lowering the temperature, ice decreases metabolism and enzymatic function; further, it slows down the inflammatory process. It is useful during the first 48 hours in acute cases, and in chronic cases it can be applied after activity for 30 to 50 minutes.

Compression in concert with cold therapy helps to reduce the swelling. Elevation decreases edema by aiding lymphatic and venous return. In acute ankle sprains, for example, elevation has been shown to be the most effective method of reducing swelling. The objective is to treat the initial symptoms with these techniques to prevent prolonged inflammation and avoid new tissue disruption. In addition, measures of relative rest are used to protect the tissue from further injury. In some cases, specifically carpal tunnel syndrome, for example, splinting may be effective. Ideally, the splint should be custom-made and fitted for the individual patient; an occupational therapist may assist with this.

In stage 2 of the healing process, the objective is to gradually introduce stress and apply modalities to increase collagen production, size, cross-linking, and alignment. The rate of collagen fiber formation is directly related to the functional state of the affected area. The collagen fibers reorient themselves in line with the tensile force applied to the tissue. In stage 3, the objective is to make the collagen as elastic as possible and decrease formation of scar tissue. Progressive stress is placed on tissue to promote an increase in collagen fibril size and to increase cross-linking in tissues. Flexibility training is needed to decrease cross-linking in the joint capsule.

Immobilization may be counterproductive, and absolute rest should be limited to 1 to 2 days at most until the inflammation response has settled or in the most severe, chronic cases of tendinitis after active rest has failed. *Active rest* means that the injured area can be used, but it should be protected from significant stress, which may cause further damage. The frequency and intensity of an activity may be decreased or altered, for example, but all activity should not be completely eliminated. Physical therapy is a cornerstone of treatment and can aid in the development of an individualized plan for the patient. Ice plays an important role once exercise and activity are resumed. It should be applied at the end of every exercise session to help prevent recurrence of inflammation and swelling.

Heat is effective after 48 hours in the acute phase and in the chronic phase. After the acute phase of the healing process, heat is useful in improving blood flow, relieving muscle spasm, and decreasing tissue stiffness, allowing greater ease of deformation. The most beneficial form of deep heat is ultrasound because the high-frequency waves render the tissues less stiff and more susceptible to remodeling by applied tensile forces. Ultrasound also increases local circulation and has been shown to speed

wound healing. Lasers are another modality that has positive effects on wound healing, but unlike ultrasound, they also decrease inflammation.

Two types of electrical stimulation may be used in treatment. Transcutaneous electrical nerve stimulation is used for pain relief and can be a useful adjunctive modality. High-voltage galvanic stimulation not only produces heat in the tissue but also has been reported to be effective in retarding the formation of edema. Deep friction massage is a modality used by physiotherapists to prevent the formation of adherent scars early in healing and later to break down scar tissue. It should be avoided in the first few days after injury because it can produce microtrauma, induce inflammation, and have a deleterious effect on healing.

NSAIDs are useful in the treatment of acute overuse injury, especially if used early, when they can decrease the production of arachidonic acid derivatives in the inflammatory pathway. They are probably best prescribed at maximum dose for 10 to 14 days. If no benefit is noted in the first 3 days, it is unlikely further benefit will be gained. They probably do not have a major anti-inflammatory role in the treatment of chronic injuries because there is scant histological evidence of true inflammatory response. Although widely prescribed, they have not been shown to effectively shorten recovery time; they may be useful in their analgesic effect in supporting a patient's compliance with physical therapy.

Corticosteroids are occasionally indicated in cases of chronic overuse syndromes. They should never be injected directly into a tendon, because this can lead to rupture. In addition, activity needs to be decreased for 5 to 10 days after injection. Tendon sheath injections, by contrast, are quite effective in treating tenosynovitis of the ankle or wrist. Steroid injections can also be given intra-articulately when there is significant reactive synovitis with effusion.

Follow-up and Referral

As noted in the section on overuse syndromes in general, soft tissue injuries cause considerable pain, discomfort, and potential dysfunction. A comprehensive, team approach, structured in a Circle of Caring model, is what is needed for these patients to avoid significant sequelae. As noted in the section on management, interventions need to be geared toward the stage of healing to be effective. The balance between rest and healing and the danger of erring in either direction can be great without thoughtful consideration by a team of providers, as well as maximum hearing of the patient's voice. Athletes may be overanxious and overdo; unhappy employees might have more of a psychogenic component to their pathology.

Referral to physical therapy is essential, as is referral to an orthopedic specialist if there is any question as to nature of pathology. Treatment must be individualized, and the patient must be a chief architect in the plan of care. Patients requiring corticosteroid injections should be referred. Occupational therapists can assist with fitting of splints if necessary. Adequate sleep is essential to the overall treatment plan and may also require follow-up. Aggressive intervention will potentially offset the possibility of the development of chronic pain syndrome.

Patient Education

It is important that patients understand the nature of their injury and be involved in the plan of care. In the case of athletes, careful evaluation of training schedules and circumstances surrounding the injury is essential so that appropriate preventive measures can be put in place to support healing and avoid future injury. In the case of a work-related repetitive motion injury, evaluation of the workplace may be necessary.

All risk factors should be assessed. In the case of a patient with obesity, nutritional counseling may be necessary. A diabetic patient may need additional assistance in controlling his or her disease and likewise with a patient with hypertension and cardiovascular disease. Managing household chores may be a challenge for individuals with tendinitis. Carrying groceries in a paper bag rather than a plastic bag, driving a car with an automatic transmission, placing hands properly on the steering wheel (at 9 o'clock and 3 o'clock), and using electric kitchen appliances such as a food processor or electric can opener can dramatically reduce strain on injured muscles and nerves. Some hobbies, such as quilting, knitting, gardening, playing certain musical instruments, computer games, frequent Internet usage, and needlepoint may have to be altered during the healing process and in some cases permanently. For many patients, stress management techniques such as yoga or meditation may be effective in promoting relaxation of injured, inflamed, and tense muscles.

In cases in which the patient's job is the source of repetitive strain injury, restrictions on work activity may be necessary. A careful and thorough occupational history can help make determinations about the contributing factors in the patient's job environment. A comprehensive ergonomic worksite evaluation may be conducted by a physical or occupational therapist in identifying specific problems. Ultimately, however, patients with severe forms of repetitive strain injury may be forced to change occupations.

Likewise, a severe tendinitis can potentially spell the end of a promising athletic career. From this vantage point, hearing the patient's voice—his or her concerns and feelings—is critical.

■ DE QUERVAIN'S TENOSYNOVITIS

De Quervain's tenosynovitis (stenosing tenosynovitis) is characterized by pain at the base of the thumb or at the radial styloid process on abduction and extension of the thumb. Within the wrist, there are six dorsal tunnels that transport the extensor tendons. The first tunnel transports the abductor pollicis longus (APL) and the extensor pollicis brevis (EPB) tendons. These tendons

form the radial border of the anatomical snuffbox. De Quervain's tenosynovitis occurs when the synovial lining of the tunnel becomes inflamed, thus narrowing the opening of the tunnel. This results in pain when the tendons move. The APL and EPB tendons are responsible for thumb flexion and extension and for establishing a grip. This condition is seen in patients who perform pinch-grip activities such as using hand tools with extreme pressure, carrying trays with a pinch grip, assembly work, and sewing/cutting activities. It is more common in middle-aged women and is often precipitated by repetitive use of the thumb.

De Quervain's tenosynovitis presents with pain at the radial side of the wrist, usually with lifting. This pain is aggravated by attempts to move the thumb or make a fist. Patients may complain of pain while turning a key or a doorknob or while attempting to open a jar. Often the condition occurs as the result of lifting infants with the second metacarpals (web between the thumb and the index finger) under the baby's axillae. Chronic pain, loss of strength, and loss of thumb motion can occur.

The history and physical exam should proceed as described for carpal tunnel syndrome. In addition, assess for crepitation over the radial styloid. On palpation, the tendon sheath may feel thickened. Allen's test, Phalen's maneuver, and Tinel's sign (see Advanced Assessment 15-5) should be negative. The confirmation test for de Quervain's tenosynovitis is Finkelstein's test. To perform this test, have the patient grasp the thumb in the palm while you deviate the wrist to the ulnar side. If this motion is painful, the test is considered positive. There is usually no need for additional diagnostic testing. Wrist x-ray studies are indicated only if there is a history of trauma. Calcification associated with tendinitis occasionally can be seen on radiographs.

Ask the patient to bring any work tools to the office visit to better evaluate risky hand and wrist positions. Observe if the patient has attempted to modify the tool (wrapping the handle in duct tape, adding a sleeve of rubbery material) to try to reduce the pressure on the hand surfaces. If there is a possible relationship to the patient's occupation/hobby, ask about the specifics of these activities.

The differential diagnoses include carpal tunnel syndrome, carpometacarpal joint arthrosis of the thumb, scaphoid fractures, and arthritis of the thumb and/or wrist.

Noninvasive treatment includes rest, splinting, and NSAIDs. Splints that are used are either a radial gutter splint or a customized long opponens splint. The splint should immobilize both the wrist and the thumb. Splinting is used for 3 to 6 weeks. A 2-week course of NSAIDs is usually helpful (see Drugs Commonly Prescribed 15.2).

Invasive treatments include corticosteroid injections into the tendon sheath. If the symptoms are not relieved with two to three injections, referral should be made for surgical release of the tendon sheath. Patients with unremitting symptoms after 6 to 8 weeks of conservative treatment should be referred for tendon release.

Patients should be educated regarding the cause of de Quervain's tenosynovitis. Modifications to hand tools or the work environment should be made. For example, hand tools may be retrofitted with a larger grip surface, so that pressure is more evenly distributed over the palmar surface of the hand. Avoidance of the precipitating factor is often enough to permanently resolve early symptoms.

■ TRIGGER FINGER

"Trigger finger" or "locked finger" is a common name for *stenosing tenosynovitis of the flexor tendons.* This problem can be painful and functionally limiting. Any digit can be affected, although it most commonly affects the ring or middle finger. Inflammation at the metacarpophalangeal (MCP) joint pulley causes a size discrepancy between the tendon and the pulley. Because the tendon no longer slides freely through the pulley, there is a snapping or locking phenomenon. The digit remains flexed or extended until the tendon pops through the pulley, causing severe pain. Tenderness with palpation of the flexor tendon over the MCP joint is noted. There is a higher prevalence of trigger finger in patients with carpal tunnel syndrome and de Quervain stenosing tenosynovitis.

Trigger finger may be idiopathic (more common in middle-aged women) or associated with rheumatoid arthritis (RA) or diabetes. Patients typically report pain and catching when they flex the finger and may describe the finger as going "out of joint." They may awaken with the finger locked in the palm although the finger gradually unlocks during the day. Physical exam reveals tenderness in the palm at the level of the distal palmar crease, usually overlying the MCP joint. A nodule may also be palpable. The nodule moves, and the finger may lock when the patient flexes and extends the affected finger. This movement is almost always painful. Full flexion of the finger may not be possible.

The most effective therapy for this problem is local anesthetic and corticosteroid injection into the tendon sheath, plus a modification of activities for about a month. A small number of patients require surgical release of the tendon. Splinting and NSAIDs have not proven effective.

■ BURSITIS

Bursitis, which is inflammation of a bursa, is a common cause of painful musculoskeletal syndromes. Bursae are sacs filled with synovial fluid, located between muscles, tendons, and bony prominences. Bursae cushion bony prominences from overlying muscles (deep bursae) or surface skin (superficial bursae); they may or may not communicate with the adjacent joint space. The bursa provides lubrication for movement of tendons over bones and can be affected by trauma, as in overuse, and by infection, inflammation, and neoplasms. The total number of bursae varies from person to person, but on average, this figure approaches 160. Some cases of bursitis may result from rheumatic afflictions and others

from a pathological condition of adjoining tissues. It may be acute or chronic.

Epidemiology and Causes

Bursitis is a common complaint, seen most often in patients who are skeletally mature. It is more common in males and tends to be more commonly associated with trauma (including overuse syndrome) in patients younger than 35 years of age. Interestingly, up to 85% of septic bursitis cases are in men. It is one of the most common reasons for visits to the primary-care setting; the incidence is clearly related to increasing age. The incidence of bursitis of the lower extremities is increased by obesity.

Bursitis commonly develops in the subdeltoid and subacromial bursa of the shoulder, the olecranon bursa of the elbow, the greater trochanteric bursa that is lateral to the hip, the ischial bursa, the prepatellar bursa of the knee, the anserine bursa, and the heel. The anserine bursa lies between the pes anserine tendons, which insert into the sartorius, gracilis, and semitendinosus muscles, and the medial collateral ligament, which lies over the medial aspect of the tibia.

Trauma in the form of repetitive motion injury is probably the most common cause of bursitis, as a result of constant friction between a bursa and musculoskeletal tissues surrounding it. Friction in turn causes irritation, edema, and, over time, inflammation and subsequent degeneration. The end result is an engorged bursal sac with surrounding tissue that has become tender and painful. Movement around the bursa may result in increased pain and pressure. In turn, flexion and extension of the closest joint may be limited by the affected bursa. Aging connective tissues are at a higher risk for microtears with bursitis.

Pathophysiology

Bursitis is an inflammatory process that may be acute or chronic; the exact etiology is often unknown. Bursitis may be caused by an infectious process, trauma (more common in patients under age 35 years), repetitive movement disorders, pseudogout, gout, or neoplastic disease. Less often, it may be attributed to rheumatoid disease (especially with nodular or bilateral bursitis) or infection by *Mycobacterium tuberculosis* or *Candida* fungal infection. Far more commonly, however, septic bursitis is due to bacterial infection.

Up to 80% of septic bursitis cases are due to infection by *Staphylococcus aureus,* with 5% to 20% due to *Streptococcus* and other gram-positive skin flora, which are typically introduced via direct trauma that compromises the protective skin barrier. Immunocompromised conditions such as diabetes mellitus, HIV infection, chronic steroid use, or autoimmune conditions such as RA may all predispose the individual to septic bursitis, and causative trauma to the overlying skin surface may even be microscopic in nature.

Bursitis is essentially a soft tissue problem rather than a joint problem such as arthritis, and often coexists with tendinitis or tenosynovitis. Overuse injury is characterized by repeated cycles of degeneration and regeneration with new collagen deposition. Synovial cells increase in thickness, and the normal bursal lining may be replaced by granulation tissue before eventual fibrosis. In turn, the bursa may become filled with transudative fluid with a high concentration of fibrin. At the conclusion of this inflammatory process, calcium deposition may occur proximal to the affected bursa.

Clinical Presentation

Subjective

The presenting symptoms are usually pain and sometimes swelling over the known locations of bursal sacs, which may be accompanied by swelling and warmth over the involved bursa. When the subcutaneous bursal sacs (olecranon and prepatellar) are inflamed by systemic illnesses such as RA, gout, or infection, additional clues to diagnosis may include fever, chills, and arthralgias. The prepatellar and olecranon bursae frequently present with local redness, swelling, and warmth that must be distinguished from septic arthritis. Patients who develop subcutaneous bursitis may have a family history of articular problems. An occupational history may provide a clue to diagnosis. Some examples include "weaver's bottom" (ischial-gluteal bursitis), "miner's elbow" (olecranon bursitis), and "housemaid's knee" (prepatellar bursitis). Bursitis of a deep bursa is manifested by pain over the bursa with activity or direct pressure. The pain may radiate some distance, as in the case of gluteal bursitis, in which the patient may complain of pain in a sciatic distribution.

Objective

Pain may be referred to other musculoskeletal structures contiguous to the bursa; therefore, careful examination is necessary to identify the source of the pain. Clinical signs and symptoms include induration, erythema, and effusion over the olecranon and prepatellar bursae. Gross distention of the bursal sac may be apparent. If there is significant limitation of ROM or pain on flexion, a co-incident arthritis must be suspected. Bursitis may also develop from repeated microtrauma, leading to effusion and thickening of the bursal sac. When irritation and inflammation continue, the bursa is at risk for calcification and development of adhesions around the bursa, thereby limiting tendon movement.

Diagnostic Reasoning

Diagnostic Tests

Laboratory findings will usually be normal. The ESR may be elevated by gout, RA, or infection. In cases of gout, uric acid levels would be elevated. In infectious leukocytosis, the WBC count may be elevated.

Differential Diagnosis

When formulating a diagnosis, RA, gout or pseudogout, and septic arthritis must be ruled out. A diagnosis is generally determined from an x-ray film showing the involved joint or bursa, with or without calcified deposits. Further diagnosis is determined from the aspiration of fluid in the affected joint. The fluid is cultured, and a WBC count done to assess the presence of bacterial infection. An elevated red blood cell count is associated with trauma.

Management

Medical management and treatment of bursitis includes avoidance of activities that can lead to constant irritation of the bursa and application of moist heat or ice to the affected area every 4 hours for 20 to 30 minutes. The use of moist heat versus ice is an individual preference. Immobilization of the affected area to reduce edema and provide support is recommended, along with ROM exercises to prevent loss of mobility and to help maintain motion. It has also been recommended in certain cases that an NSAID along with ultrasound therapy be used. If symptoms recur and fluid reaccumulates, an injection of a long-acting corticosteroid (triamcinolone 2–10 mg, hydrocortisone 25–37.5 mg, methylprednisolone 20–40 mg, or dexamethasone 4–16 mg, each mixed with an equal volume of lidocaine hydrochloride 1%) into the affected bursa is recommended, followed by application of ice for 10 to 20 minutes. Injections should not be repeated more than every 6 to 8 weeks, and most clinicians limit the number of intrabursal injections to two to the same site before referral for more invasive interventions, such as surgery, is initiated. In severe cases, surgery may be performed to excise the inflamed portion of bursa and calcified deposits and to aspirate bursal fluid.

Follow-up and Referral

Follow-up is determined by the response to therapeutic interventions.

Patient Education

Patient education is vital to ensure a rapid recovery. Encouraging a patient to decrease certain activities will speed up recovery. Encourage preliminary stretching and warm-up exercises before activities to maintain flexibility and strength. If medications are a part of the treatment regimen, reinforcement of proper administration and a discussion of their side effects are recommended.

References

American Academy of Orthopaedic Surgeons: Treatment of osteoarthritis of the knee (non-arthroplasty), 2013. Retrieved from www.aaos.org/Research/guidelines/OAKguideline.pdf

American Pain Society/American Association of Pain Medicine. Guideline for the evaluation and management of low back pain: Evidence review. 2009. Glenview, IL: American Pain Society Publisher.

Chou, R, et al. Diagnosis and treatment of low back pain: A joint clinical practice guideline from the American College of Physicians and the American Pain Society. *Ann Intern Med* 147(7):478–491, 2009.

Chou, R, et al. Imaging strategies for low-back pain: Systematic review and meta-analysis. *Lancet* 373:463–472, 2009.

Rakel, RE, and Rakel, DP. Textbook of family medicine, 8th ed. Elsevier Saunders, Philadephia, 2011.

Sinusas, K. Osteoarthritis: Diagnosis and treatment. *Am Fam Physician* 85:49–55, 2012.

Stephens, MB, et al. Musculoskeletal injections: A review of the evidence. *Am Fam Physician* 78(8):971–976, 2008.

Zhang, W, et al. OARSI recommendations for the management of hip and knee osteoarthritis, part II: OARSI evidence-based, expert consensus guidelines. *Osteoarthritis Cartilage* 16(2): 137–162, 2008.

Bibliography

Allen, RJ, and Wilson AM. Physical therapy agents. In Fishman, SM, et al (Eds.), *Bonica's management of pain,* ed 4. Lippincott Williams & Wilkins, Philadelphia, 2012

American Academy of Family Physicians. Acupuncture for pain relief. September 2009. Retrieved from www.aafp.org/afp

American Academy of Orthopaedic Surgeons. Treatment of osteoarthritis of the knee (non-arthroplasty), 2008. Retrieved from www.aaos.org/Research/guidelines/OAKguideline.pdf

American Pain Society/American Association of Pain Medicine: Guideline for the Evaluation and Management of Low Back Pain: Evidence Review, 2009.

American Society of Anesthesiologists Task Force on Chronic Pain Management. Practice guidelines for chronic pain management: An updated report by the American Society of Anesthesiologists Task Force on Chronic Pain Management and the American Society of Regional Anesthesia and Pain Medicine. *Anesthesiology* 112:810–833, 2012.

Avenell, A, et al. Cochrane Bone, Joint, Muscle Trauma Group. Vitamin D and vitamin D analogues for preventing fractures associated with involutional and post-menopausal osteoporosis. *Cochrane Database of Systematic Reviews* 4, 2009.

Barclay, C. Recommendations for prescribing NSAIDs in the primary care setting. *Am Fam Physician* 80:1371–1378, 2009.

Barnes, PM, et al. CDC National Health Statistics Report #12. *Complementary and alternative medicine use among adults and children: United States, 2007.* December 10, 2008. Retrieved from http://nccam.nih.gov/news/camstats

Benjamin, HJ, and Hang, BT. Common acute upper extremity injuries in sports. *Clin Pediatr Emerg Med* 8:15–30, 2007.

Bhatt, DL, et al. ACCF/ACG/AHA 2008 expert consensus document on reducing the gastrointestinal risks of antiplatelet therapy and NSAID use: A report of the American College of Cardiology Foundation Task Force on Clinical Expert Consensus Documents. *J Am Coll Cardiol* 52(18):1502–1517, 2008.

Boswell, MV, et al. Interventional techniques: Evidence-based practice guidelines in the management of chronic spinal pain. *Pain Physician* 10:7–11, 2007. Retrieved from www.painphysicianjournal.com/2007/january/2007;10;7–111.pdf

Buescher, JJ. Carbamazepine for acute and chronic pain. *Am Fam Physician* 73(9):1549–1550, 2006. Retrieved from www.aafp.org/afp/2006/0501/p1549.html

Burbank, KM, et al. Chronic shoulder pain: Part I. Evaluation and diagnosis. *Am Fam Physician* 77(4):453–460, 2008.

Burbank, KM, et al. Chronic shoulder pain: Part II. Treatment. *Am Fam Physician* 77(4):493–497, 2008.

Cameron, MH. Physical Agents in Rehabilitation: From Research to Practice, 4th ed. St. Louis, Missouri: Elsevier, 2012.

Chambers, RG. Corticosteroid injections for trigger finger. *Am Fam Physician* 80(5):454, 2009. Retrieved from www.aafp.org/afp/2009/0901/p454.html

Chen Gatti, J. Glucosamine treatment for osteoarthritis. *Am Fam Physician* 73(7), 2006. Retrieved from www.aafp.org/afp/2006/0401/p1245.html

Chou, R, et al. Clinical guidelines for the use of chronic opioid therapy in chronic noncancer pain. *J Pain* 10(2):113–130, 2009.

Clinical guidelines for best practice management of acute and chronic whiplash associated disorders. Clinical resource guide. TRACaa: Trauma and Injury Recovery, South Australia Adelaide. 2008.

Retrieved from www.mac.sa.gov.au/xstd_files/Whiplash-Clinical-Guidelines.pdf

Dachs, R. Exercise is an effective intervention in overweight and obese patients. *Am Fam Physician* 75(9):1333–1335, 2007. Retrieved from www.aafp.org/afp/2007/0501/p1333.html

Dahmer, S, and Schiller, RM. Glucosamine. *Am Fam Physician* 78(4):471–476, 2008.

Derry, MP, et al. Cochrane Pain, Palliative and Supportive Care Group. Topical rubefacients for acute and chronic pain in adults. *Cochrane Database of Systematic Reviews* 4, 2009.

Devereaux, M. Neck pain. *Med Clin North Am* 93:273–284, 2009.

Dixit, S, et al. Management of patellofemoral pain syndrome. *Am Fam Physician* 75:194–202, 204, 2007.

Dommerholt, J, and Shah, JP. Myofascial pain syndrome. In Fishman, SM, et al (Eds.), *Bonica's management of pain,* ed 4. Lippincott Williams & Wilkins, Philadelphia, 2009, pp. 450–471.

Ebbert, JO, and Tangalos, EG. Mindful practice: PPIs to prevent NSAID induced GI ulceration. *Dig Dis Sci* 53:2059–2065, 2008.

Elkins, G, et al. Hypnotherapy for the management of chronic pain. *Int J Clin Exp Hypn* 55(3):275–287, 2007.

Englund, M, et al. The meniscus in knee osteoarthritis. *Rheum Dis Clin North Am* 35:579–590, 2009.

Gennari, L, and Bilezikian, JK. Osteoporosis in men. *Endocrinol Metab Clin North Am* 36:399–419, 2007.

Gislason, GH. NSAIDs and cardiovascular risk. *Am Fam Physician* 80(12):1367–1368, 2009.

Govind, J, and Bogduck, N. Neurolytic blockade for noncancer pain. In Fishman, SM, et al (Eds.), *Bonica's management of pain,* ed 4. Lippincott Williams & Wilkins, Philadelphia, 2009, pp 1467–1485.

Goytia, RN, et al. Bisphosphonates and osteonecrosis: Potential treatment or serious complication. *Orthop Clin North Am* 40:223–234, 2009.

Graylee, JR, and Van Durme, DJ. Braces and splints for musculoskeletal conditions. *Am Fam Physician* 75(3):342–348, 2007.

Gregory, PJ, et al. Dietary supplements for osteoarthritis. *Am Fam Physician* 77(2):177–184, 2008.

Harrold, LR, et al. The dynamics of chronic gout treatment: Medication gaps and return to therapy. *Am J Med* 123:54–59, 2010.

Hitzeman, N, and Masley, C. Arthroscopic surgery for knee osteoarthritis. *Am Fam Physician* 78(3):331–332, 2008. Retrieved from www.aafp.org/afp/2008/0801/p331.html

Hoffman, BM, et al. Meta-analysis of psychological interventions for chronic low back pain. *Health Psychol* 26(1):1–9, 2007.

Holder, KK, and Kerley, SS. Alendronate for fracture prevention in postmenopause. *Am Fam Physician* 78(5):579–581, 2008. Retrieved from www.aafp.org/afp/2008/0901/p579.html

Hoppenfeld, S. *Physical examination of the spine and extremities.* Appleton & Lange, Norwalk, 1976.

Hunter, DJ, and Lo, GH. The management of osteoarthritis: An overview and call to appropriate conservative treatment. *Med Clin North Am* 93(1):127–143, 2009.

Jensen, ME, et al. Position statement on percutaneous verbal augmentation: A consensus statement developed by the American Society of Interventional and Therapeutic Neuroradiology, Society of Interventional Radiology, American Association of Neurological Surgeons/Congress of Neurological Surgeons, and American Society of Spine Radiology. *Journal of Vascular and Interventional Radiology* 20(7 suppl):S326–S331, 2009. Retrieved from www.jvir.org/article/S1051–0443(09)00319–4/fulltext

Karjalainen, KA, et al. Cochrane Back Group. Multidisciplinary biopsychosocial rehabilitation for subacute low-back pain among working age adults. *Cochrane Database of Systematic Reviews* 4, 2009.

Kassis, A. Antidepressants to treat nonspecific low back pain. *Am Fam Physician* 78(1), 2008. Retrieved from www.aafp.org/afp/2008/0701/p51.html

Keith, MP, and Gilliland, WR. Updates in the management of gout. *Am J Med* 120:221–224, 2007.

Kelly, RB. Acupuncture for pain. *Am Fam Physician* 80(5):481–484, 506, 2009.

Kkosla, S, and Riggs, BL. Pathophysiology of age-related bone loss and osteoporosis. *Endocrinol Metab Clin North Am* 34:1015–1030, 2005.

Koski, BL, et al. Daily activity patterns of an adult experiencing lower back pain undergoing electro-acupuncture: A case study. *Pain Management Nurs* 10(4):188–196, 2009.

Kuhlman, GS, and Domb, BG. Hip impingement: Identifying and treating a common cause of hip pain. *Am Fam Physician* 80(12):1429–1434, 1439–1440, 2009.

Lanza, FL, et al. Guidelines for the prevention of NSAID-related ulcer complications. *Am J Gastroenterol* 104:728–738, 2009. Retrieved from www.gi.org/physicians/pdfs/NSAIDJournal PublicationFebruary2009.pdf

Lash, RW, et al. Diagnosis and management of osteoporosis. *Prim Care Clin Office Pract* 36:181–198, 2009.

Last, AR, and Hulbert, K. Chronic low back pain: Evaluation and management. *Am Fam Physician* 79(12):1067–1074, 2009.

Liebson, C. Functional Training Handbook. Wolters-Kluwer Health, 2014.

Lim, LS, et al. Screening for osteoporosis in the adult US population: ACPM position statement on preventative practice. *Am J Prev Med* 36(4):366–375, 2009.

Malanga, GA, and Nadler, SF. *Musculoskeletal physical examination: An evidence-based approach.* Mosby/Elsevier, St. Louis, 2006.

McGee, S. *Evidence based physical diagnosis,* ed 2. Saunders/Elsevier, St. Louis, 2007.

Melton, S, and Liu, SS. Regional anesthesia techniques for acute pain management. In Fishman, SM, et al (Eds.), *Bonica's management of pain,* ed 4. Lippincott Williams & Wilkins, Philadelphia, 2010, pp. 723–754.

Meriwether, RA, et al. Physical activity counseling. *Am Fam Physician* 77(8):1029–1136, 1138, 2008.

Millett, PJ, et al. Shoulder osteoarthritis: Diagnosis and management. *Am Fam Physician* 78(5):605–611, 612, 2008.

National Osteoporosis Foundation. Clinician's guide to prevention and treatment of osteoporosis: 2008. Retrieved from www.nof .org/professionals/NOF_Clinicians_Guide.pdf

National Osteoporosis Foundation. National Osteoporosis Foundation's updated recommendations for calcium and vitamin D intake: 2008. Retrieved from www.nof.org/prevention/calcium_and_ VitaminD.html

National Osteoporosis Guidelines Group (NOGG). Diagnosis and management of osteoporosis in postmenopausal women and older men in the UK: National Osteoporosis Guidelines Group (NOGG) Update 2013. Retrieved from http://dx.doi.org/10.1016/j.maturitas.2013.05.013.

North American Menopause Society. Management of osteoporosis in postmenopausal women: 2006 position statement of the North American Menopause Society. *J North Am Menopause Soc* 13(3): 340–367, 2006.

Papaloannou, A, et al. *Review:* 2010 clinical practice guidelines for the diagnosis and management of osteoporosis in Canada: summary. *Canadian Medical Association Journal, Vol 182,* 17:1864–1873, 2010.

Pasternak, GW. Molecular insights into mu opioid pharmacology: From the clinic to the bench. *Clin J Pain* 26(suppl 10):S3–S9, 2010.

Pelland, L, et al. Cochrane Musculoskeletal Group. Electrical stimulation for the treatment of rheumatoid arthritis. *Cochrane Database of Systematic Reviews* 4, 2009.

Pujol, LM, and Herbert, B. Integrative approaches to the management of chronic pain. In Monti, DA, and Beitman, BD (Eds.), *Integrative psychiatry.* Oxford University Press, New York, 2010, pp 240–267.

Qaseem, A, et al. Pharmacologic treatment of low bone density or osteoporosis to prevent fractures: A clinical practice guideline from the American College of Physicians. *Ann Intern Med* 149(6): 404–415, 2008.

Qaseem, A, et al. Screening for osteoporosis in men: A clinical practice guideline from the American College of Physicians. *Ann Intern Med* 149(8):680–684, 2008.

Raj, PP, and Erdine, S. Pain-Relieving Procedures: The Illustrated Guide. Wiley-Blackwell, 2012.

Rand, SE, et al. The physical therapy prescription. *Am Fam Physician* 76:1661–1666, 2007.

Rathmell, JP. A 50-year-old man with chronic low back pain. *JAMA* 299(17):2066–2077, 2008.

Risser, A, et al. NSAID prescribing precautions. *Am Fam Physician* 80(12):1371–1378, 2009.

Robb, K, et al. A Cochran systematic review of transcutaneous electrical nerve stimulation for cancer pain. *J Pain Symptom Manage* 37(4):746–753, 2009.

Robinson, JP, and Tait, RC. Disability evaluation in painful conditions. In Fishman, SM, et al (Eds.), *Bonica's management of pain,* ed 4. Lippincott Williams & Wilkins, Philadelphia, 2010, pp 279–288.

Roskos, SE. Intra-articular corticosteroid for treating osteoarthritis of the knee. *Am Fam Physician* 72(7):1222–1223, 2005. Retrieved from www.aafp.org/afp/2005/1001/p1222.html

Simel, DL, and Drummond, R. *The rational clinical examination: Evidence-based clinical diagnosis.* McGraw-Hill, New York, 2009.

Simpson, MR, and Howard, TM. Tendinopathies of the foot and ankle. *Am Fam Physician* 80(10):1107–1114, 2009.

Staud, R. Mechanisms of acupuncture analgesia: Effective therapy for musculoskeletal pain? *Curr Rheumatol Rep* 9(6):473–481, 2007.

Sweet, MG. Diagnosis and treatment of osteoporosis. *Am Fam Physician* 79(3):193–200, 2009.

Trinh, K, et al. Cochrane Back Group. Acupuncture for neck disorders. *Cochrane Database of Systematic Reviews* 4, 2009.

van Tulder, MW, et al. Cochrane Back Group. Muscle relaxants for non-specific low-back pain. *Cochrane Database of Systematic Reviews* 4, 2009.

Wailoo, K. *Pain: A Political History.* Baltimore, MD: Johns Hopkins Press, 2014.

Wasserman, AM. Diagnosis and management of rheumatoid arthritis. *Am Fam Physician* 84:1245–1252, 2012.

Wells, GA, et al. Cochrane Musculoskeletal Group. Risedronate for the primary and secondary prevention of osteoporotic fractures in post menopausal women. *Cochrane Database of Systematic Reviews* 4, 2009.

Yang, J, and Monti, DA. Acupuncture and Chinese medicine. In Monti, DA, and Beitman, BD (Eds.), *Integrative psychiatry.* Oxford University Press, New York, 2010, pp 127–158.

Zoler, M. New axial spondyloarthritis criteria poised to broaden, hasten diagnosis. *Ann Rheum Dis* 68:777–783, 2009.

Resources

American Academy of Orthopaedic Surgeons
www.aaos.org
American Association of Clinical Endocrinologists (AACE)
www.aace.com
American Orthopedic Foot and Ankle Society
www.aofas.org
American Academy of Physical Medicine and Rehabilitation
www.aapmr.org
American Academy of Physical Therapy
www.aaptnet.org
Arthritis Foundation
www.arthritis.org

Arthritis Source
www.orthop.washington.edu/arthritis
Association of Hip and Knee Surgeons
www.aahks.org
California Center for Minimally Invasive Spine Surgery
www.spinecenter.com
Creighton University Osteoporosis Research Center
http://creighton.edu/org
Fitness Partner
www.primusweb.com/fitnesspartner
Mayo Health Oasis Back Care
www.mayohealth.org/ivi/mayo9401/htm/backcare.htm

National Institute of Arthritis and Musculoskeletal and Skin Diseases
www.nih.gov/niams
National Library of Medicine
www.nim.nih.gov/melineplus
National Osteoporosis Foundation
www.nof.org
National Women's Health Resource Center (NWHRC)
www.healthywomen.org
Natural Standard Databases for Complementary and Alternative
  Therapy
www.naturalstandard.com
Osteoporosis and Bone Disease
www.osteo.org
Osteoporosis and Related Bone Diseases National Resource Center
  (ORB-NRC)
www.osteo.org

Osteoporosis Society of Canada
www.osteoporosis.ca
A Patient's Guide to Low Back Pain
www.sechrest.com/mmg/back/backpain.html
Physical Therapy Association
www.apta.org
Physician and Sports Medicine
https://physsportsmed.org
Rehabilitation Foundation
www.rfi.org
Spine Center
www.spinenet.com
Virtual Hospital: Acute Low Back Problems in Adults
www.vh.org/providers/clinguide/backphysician/backphysician.html

Endocrine and Metabolic Problems

Chapter 16

Angela K. Golden, DNP, APRN, FNP-C, FAANP • Debera J. Thomas, DNS, RN, FNP/ANP • Brian Oscar Porter, MD, PhD, MPH

COMMON COMPLAINTS

■ CARPOPEDAL SPASM (HYPOCALCEMIA)

Carpopedal spasm is a violent, painful contraction of the hands or feet. It is one of the neuromuscular signs indicating hypocalcemia and is a significant sign of tetany. Neuromuscular signs and symptoms occur in the presence of hypocalcemia because calcium is an important mediator in neurotransmission and other intracellular biochemical activities. In response to hypocalcemia, there is an increased secretion of parathyroid hormone, which leads to immobilization of calcium stores from the bone and an increase in the absorption of calcium in the intestines.

Differential Diagnosis

Acute neuromuscular irritability producing carpopedal spasm occurs when the serum calcium drops abruptly by 2 to 3 mg/dL. Parathyroid hormone (PTH) deficiency disease or inadvertent damage to the parathyroid glands during neck surgery may cause acute severe hypocalcemia. Acute transient hypocalcemia may occur in burns, severe sepsis, pregnancy, extensive blood transfusions with citrated blood, acute pancreatitis, and acute renal failure.

Aggressive treatment of hypercalcemia with plicamycin (Mithracin), bisphosphonates, and calcitonin (Cibacalcin, Calcimar) may result in acute hypocalcemia. Other drugs that may produce hypocalcemia include radiographic contrast dyes that contain a calcium-chelating agent, EDTA, and foscarnet (Foscavir).

Chronic hypocalcemia is usually caused by the absence of PTH, ineffective PTH, vitamin D deficiency, chronic renal failure, hypomagnesemia, or hypoalbuminemia. Other potential causes of chronic hypocalcemia include alkalosis, malabsorption syndromes, chronic pancreatitis, laxative abuse, chronic liver failure, phosphate excess, and osteomalacia.

Patients with carpopedal spasm should be immediately assessed for hypocalcemia. Normal serum calcium values in adults range from 9 to 11 mg/dL. Immediate medical treatment is indicated in patients with marked hypocalcemia (less than 6.5 mg/dL).

A focused history, clinical exam, and subsequent laboratory tests may determine the cause of hypocalcemia. In absence of a clearly identifiable etiology such as a medication, chronic liver or renal disease, or an acute disease process, additional laboratory studies are needed. Further laboratory evaluation should begin with serum magnesium, serum phosphorus, and albumin levels. Depending on these findings, the practitioner should initiate treatment if indicated. A serum PTH level will assist in the diagnosis of parathyroid disease. A direct measure of serum vitamin D levels is the 25-hydroxycholecalciferol (25-[OH]D_3) assay.

Trousseau's sign (carpal spasm) is one of two neuromuscular signs indicative of hypocalcemia. It is often preceded by muscle cramps in the legs and feet. Carpal spasm consists of a flexed elbow and wrist, adducted thumb over the palm, flexed metacarpophalangeal joints, adduction of hyperextended fingers, and extended interphalangeal joints. The response is elicited by inflation of a blood pressure cuff to 20 mm Hg above the level of the systolic blood pressure. Inflation is maintained for 3 minutes to elicit the response, which is secondary to ulnar and median nerve ischemia. In severe hypocalcemia, spontaneous spasms may also occur in the lower extremities and feet. *Chvostek's sign* is the second neuromuscular sign associated with hypocalcemia. It is an abnormal unilateral spasm of the facial muscle when the facial nerve is tapped below the zygomatic arch anterior to the earlobe.

Patients exhibiting either Trousseau's sign or Chvostek's sign accompanied by respiratory distress (e.g., stridor, loud crowing noises, and cyanosis) require immediate referral for emergency care because the neuromuscular irritation produced by hypocalcemia may progress rapidly to laryngospasms, seizures, and dysrhythmias. If the serum calcium levels have gradually declined, symptoms are usually subtle.

Other symptoms of hypocalcemia include various neuropsychiatric disorders, including irritability, emotional instability, problems with memory, and psychosis. Complaints of paresthesias, fatigue, muscle cramps, or muscle weakness may be elicited on history. Gastrointestinal manifestations include dysphagia, nausea, vomiting, biliary colic, and abdominal pain or cramping. Patients may also complain of chronic constipation or diarrhea. Cardiovascular symptoms include hypotension, bradycardia, congestive heart failure, and dysrhythmias. Prolonged QT intervals may be seen on the electrocardiogram.

Chronic hypocalcemia may cause the skin to be coarse, dry, and scaly. Alopecia may present with thinning of the eyebrows and eyelashes. Nails are often rigid, brittle, and thin, with transverse grooves. Subcapsular cataracts, optic neuritis, intracranial calcification, papilledema, and parkinsonian-type movements may also be present in chronic hypocalcemia.

Management

Emergency treatment of hypocalcemia is IV replacement of calcium and is guided by severity of hypocalcemia paired with the patient's signs and symptoms. Patients with tetany, dysrhythmias, or seizures are treated with calcium gluconate (94 mg of elemental calcium) in bolus and maintenance infusion. Patients with hypomagnesemia also require IV magnesium replacement. During acute therapy and the initial therapy of chronic hypocalcemia, patients must be monitored closely for signs of hypercalcemia such as confusion, abdominal pain, dehydration, weakness, polydipsia, anorexia, nausea, vomiting, constipation, pancreatitis, peptic ulcer, polyuria, hypertension, and a shortened QT interval.

The goal of treatment of chronic hypocalcemia is to restore the serum calcium level to the low to normal range, and therapy includes calcium and vitamin D. Various preparations of calcium can be used, including calcium carbonate, calcium gluconate, calcium citrate, and calcium lactate. Calcium carbonate is the least expensive formulation; however, it may not be absorbed as well, especially in the elderly.

■ GYNECOMASTIA

Gynecomastia is the enlargement of glandular breast tissue in men, resulting in increased breast size. True gynecomastia involves enlargement of the stromal and ductal tissues; it may present unilaterally and progress to bilateral symmetrical or asymmetrical enlargement. Gynecomastia results from an imbalance of androgen and estrogen or an increase in prolactin. Growth hormones, estrogen, and corticosteroids stimulate ductal growth in the breasts. Progesterone and prolactin stimulate alveolar lobular growth of the breasts.

Gynecomastia is estimated to affect 12% to 40% of the male population in the United States and is present in 40% to 60% of men older than age 50 years. Transient gynecomastia occurs in male neonates and at puberty.

Differential Diagnosis

Asymptomatic gynecomastia may be an incidental finding on routine examination. It may also present as an acute unilateral or bilateral painful tender mass beneath the areola or as a progressive painless enlargement of breast tissue. The enlargement may be obvious by observation alone; however, less severe cases are noted only during palpation. Pain in the nipple or breast and tenderness often accompany gynecomastia. Gynecomastia lasting longer than 1 year is usually asymptomatic. Nipple discharge is rare (present in fewer than 5% of cases).

Gynecomastia associated with puberty has an age at onset of 12 to 14 years. The duration is approximately 6 months and then regression is expected. Gynecomastia that presents before or after puberty and cannot be associated with physiological aging, a drug, or chronic disease requires further investigation by an endocrinologist. Associated symptoms may assist in identifying the cause.

When gynecomastia is accompanied by other breast abnormalities, especially if they are unilateral, a mammogram is indicated to rule out a neoplasm. A disc that is greater than 4 cm in diameter should be evaluated via mammography.

True gynecomastia must be differentiated from pseudogynecomastia, which is fatty enlargement of the breast. The patient is examined in a supine position while the examiner grasps breast tissue between the thumb and forefinger and gently moves the two digits toward the nipple. A firm or rubbery, mobile, disclike mound of tissue at least 2 to 4 cm in diameter arising concentrically from beneath the nipple and areolar region confirms gynecomastia. The glandular enlargement of gynecomastia is usually resistive and ropy in texture. Severe cases present with more extensive enlargement. Lack of a disc of tissue suggests the enlargement is the result of adipose tissue deposition (pseudogynecomastia). Mammography will distinguish between the two if the clinical exam is inconclusive.

When true gynecomastia has been established, the patient is evaluated for physiological (developmental) or pathological causes. The most common causes of gynecomastia are puberty (25%), idiopathic (25%), drug related (15%), cirrhosis or malnutrition (10%), and testicular failure (10%). Other causes include renal failure, thyroid disease, neoplasms (including testicular cancer), hyperprolactinemia, Klinefelter's syndrome, and gonadotropin deficiency. Although physiological development of gynecomastia is the most common cause of gynecomastia, pathological causes should always be considered and ruled out via a thorough history and physical exam.

Medications that are implicated in gynecomastia are highly active antiviral therapy, calcium channel blockers, tricyclic antidepressants, and selective serotonin reuptake inhibitors. Less common medications are amiodarone, human growth hormone, amphetamines, and diazepam.

Malignant breast tumors (which represent about 3% of all cases of gynecomastia) in men are typically unilateral, firm, and immobile; grow rapidly; and are often painful. Nipple retraction and discharge, skin dimpling, and axillary lymphadenopathy also may accompany breast neoplasms. Mammography and fine-needle biopsy are essential for confirming the diagnosis.

Decreased libido and impotence may accompany gynecomastia and may indicate the presence of chronic pulmonary, renal, or liver disease; testicular failure; or endocrine pathology.

Management

Idiopathic and pubertal gynecomastia should resolve spontaneously within 1 to 2 years and require no medication. The patient should be followed every 3 to 6 months, and the size of the disc should be measured until it has resolved. Tamoxifen (Nolvadex) 10 mg twice daily may be useful in treating painful gynecomastia. It is generally used for up to 3 months and is an off-label use of tamoxifen. Cold compresses and analgesics may also relieve discomfort. Attention to any impact on body image, especially in adolescents, is important. Low-dose radiation or tamoxifen may prevent gynecomastia in men receiving estrogen or antiandrogen therapy for prostate cancer.

A referral to an endocrinologist is required for all cases in which gynecomastia appears before puberty, if gynecomastia does not resolve 2 years after puberty, if it occurs in the presence of abnormal serum levels of free testosterone and luteinizing hormones, or when gynecomastia is accompanied by the abnormal presence or the absence of secondary sex characteristics; undermasculinization; or small, asymmetrical testes. In a pubertal male, a referral is indicated at any time when physical findings are not consistent with normal growth and development.

The patient should be provided with information about gynecomastia and its cause. Reassurance is very important in a pubertal male. Patients should receive instruction on breast and testicular self-exam.

■ HIRSUTISM

Hirsutism is an increase in terminal hair growth on the face, chest, back, lower abdomen, pubic area, axilla, and inner thighs. It is present in approximately 5% of the female population in the United States. Almost 25% of these women have terminal hair growth on the face, especially on the upper lip. Hirsutism is caused by increased secretion of androgens by the ovary or adrenal glands or an increased sensitivity to androgens. It is often accompanied by menstrual irregularities.

There are two major types of hair: vellus and terminal. Vellus hair is found over most of the body and is fine, soft, and unpigmented. During puberty, vellus hair often changes to terminal hair in the presence of an increase in androgen. Terminal hairs are characteristically dark, coarse, pigmented, and thicker compared with vellus hair. Terminal hairs are found on the scalp, eyebrows, and the axillary and pubic areas after puberty. They are found in lesser abundance on the extremities.

Differential Diagnosis

The characteristic increase in terminal hair growth occurs in areas most sensitive to androgen: the upper lip, chin, chest, upper arms, upper abdomen, lower abdomen,

thighs, and upper and lower back. Accompanying signs of virilization, hoarseness of the voice, clitorimegaly, receding temporal hairline, acne, loss of body fat, and breast atrophy may be due to an ovarian or adrenal tumor. Markedly increased levels of plasma androgens often accompany virilization.

Although most cases (87%) of hirsutism are idiopathic or result from polycystic ovary syndrome (PCOS), more serious underlying disease entities must be ruled out. A targeted history with emphasis on when hirsutism was first recognized and how rapidly it has progressed, a detailed menstrual history, and a review of associated symptoms may provide some insight into the cause of hirsutism. The physical exam should focus on signs of adrenal disease and virilization that may further clarify possible causes.

Laboratory evaluation of hirsutism is indicated in women with menstrual irregularities, a history of sudden onset or rapid progression of hirsutism, associated symptoms of ovarian or adrenal pathology, and moderate to severe presentations. Evaluation of free testosterone levels, androstenedione, total testosterone, 17-hydroxyprogesterone, urine 17-hydroxycorticosteroids, thyroid-stimulating hormone, prolactin levels, luteinizing hormone (LH), follicle-stimulating hormone (FSH), and dehydroepiandrosterone sulfate (DHEA-S) will provide insights into possible causes or the need for further evaluation. Slightly elevated levels of serum androgens (free testosterone) are found in 40% of women with idiopathic hirsutism, whereas LH/FSH levels are increased in 75% of cases of PCOS. Testosterone levels greater than 200 ng/dL (in women) and/or DHEA-S levels above 700 ng/dL indicate the need for an ovarian and adrenal work-up, because these levels are rarely seen in idiopathic hirsutism or PCOS.

Androgen-dependent terminal hair growth may be caused by pathology in the adrenal glands or ovaries or by exogenous androgen administration. The age, associated symptoms, and rapidity of onset are critical factors in differentiating potential causes.

Idiopathic hirsutism in women is the result of excessive androgenic activity and begins during puberty. There is a gradual development over 2 to 3 years followed by a period of stability. There is a familial tendency toward hirsutism. Women of eastern European or Mediterranean descent are likely to have increased terminal hair growth. Idiopathic hirsutism usually occurs in women aged 15 to 25 years without symptoms of virilization. It is usually mild and not accompanied by menstrual irregularities. Hirsutism may present in pregnancy owing to production of androgens by the placenta and corpus luteum. Postmenopausal women experience an increase in androgen production, with 75% experiencing noticeable facial hair growth.

Management

When the cause of hirsutism is determined to be of adrenal or ovarian origin, the patient is referred to an endocrinologist for treatment. Discontinuing a drug that is determined to be the cause or substituting an alternative may stop the rapid progression of terminal hair growth.

Treatment of idiopathic hirsutism and hirsutism resulting from PCOS is dependent on the severity and treatment preferences of the patient. Hirsutism is often perceived as a loss of femininity and sexuality; women affected will need reassurance. Idiopathic hirsutism does not frequently interfere with fertility.

Weight reduction may assist patients. Obese women have increased androgen levels due to insulin-stimulated androgen production in thecal cells. Weight reduction may also improve menstrual function in these patients.

Mild cases of hirsutism can be managed by cosmetic therapy, including physical removal, chemical depilatories, and bleaching. Electrolysis and laser therapy are more permanent solutions but are costly. Androgen production may be reduced with weight loss if the woman is obese.

Pharmacological therapy may be indicated in women with more severe hirsutism, such as that caused by a tumor. After the tumor has been removed, oral contraceptives, either monophasic or triphasic, may be effective. Estrogen-dominant medications, such as the Ortho brands of contraceptives, are effective and will increase sex steroid–binding globulin. Progesterone-dominant medications, such as the Wyeth brands of contraceptives, will increase clearance of testosterone. Medroxyprogesterone (Depo-Provera) is also effective. Hormonal therapy will stop further hair growth but will not reverse the present hair growth, which must be treated cosmetically. It may take 6 to 24 months to see results of hormonal treatment, which may need to be lifelong. Spirolactone (Aldactone) has been studied and demonstrated to reduce hair growth (100 mg/day), but it may take 6 months of therapy to see a clinically significant effect. Eflornithine 13.9% (Vaniqa) cream has been approved by the U.S. Food and Drug Administration and has evidence of reducing hair growth on the upper lip, especially when combined with laser therapy (Level I; Wolf et al, 2007).

■ INCREASED NECK SIZE

The neck contains 75 lymph nodes, the trachea, larynx, pharynx, the submandibular and salivary glands, cervical vertebrae, and the parathyroid and thyroid glands. Pathology in one of these structures or in an area that is drained by one of the many lymph nodes may increase neck size.

A patient with increased neck size may present with complaints that shirt collars are tight. The patient should be evaluated immediately for difficulty swallowing or breathing problems. An immediate referral is indicated in the presence of either symptom. Some patients may complain of pain.

Differential Diagnosis

Increased neck size may be caused by a mass in any structure in the neck, including glands, lymph nodes, larynx, or pharynx. Cysts may also develop in the neck and increase the size of the neck. Blockage of the salivary glands produces neck enlargement. The most common cause of increased neck size is an enlarged thyroid gland. Other potential causes include trauma, masses, neoplasms, cysts, and lymph node enlargements.

The history can assist in diagnosing the cause of increased neck size. Patients reporting a recent fall, automobile accident, or injury may have sustained cervical trauma. History of a recent infection may cause lymph node enlargement. The patient should be questioned about a history of thyroid problems or recent surgeries, allergies, sinus problems, and any complaints of headaches. Symptoms of dysphagia, dyspnea, chest tenderness, cough, and hoarseness should be addressed. Complaints of pain should be investigated, including if the pain is aggravated by range-of-motion movements, breathing, swallowing, or chewing.

The physical exam should assess whether the swelling (enlargement) is focal or diffuse. One or more focal masses may be enlarged lymph nodes related to Hodgkin's disease, sarcoidosis, a thyroglossal cyst, thyroid adenoma, or carcinoma. If the swelling is diffuse, venous distention of congestive heart failure (CHF), Graves' disease, subacute thyroiditis, superior vena cava syndrome, or subcutaneous emphysema (which is usually accompanied by subcutaneous crepitus) is suspected. If the swelling is focal, it should be noted if the lesion is midline or lateral because midline masses can be indicative of thyroglossal cysts or adenoma of the thyroid; lateral masses are more likely related to Virchow's node, Hodgkin's lymphoma, bronchial cysts, a pharyngeal pouch, or a stone of Wharton's duct. Intermediate swelling suggests venous congestion of CHF, a bronchial cyst, a stone of Wharton's duct, or an aneurysm.

A technique for detecting thyromegaly is to have the patient sit upright for examination. During examination, the neck is exposed down to the sternal notch while the examiner stands directly in front of the patient with the thyroid gland at the examiner's eye level. The patient should take several sips of water while the examiner observes for an enlarged thyroid gland. After visual examination, the thyroid is palpated anteriorly and posteriorly.

Thyroid nodules can be palpated in about 5% of Americans. Women are more likely to have palpable thyroid nodules, and the frequency of nodules increases with age. Fewer than 10% of singular nodules are malignant. Thyroid-stimulating hormone and thyroxine (T_4) levels should be obtained on the patient with enlargement or any abnormalities in the thyroid.

A single enlarged lymph node is unlikely to result in a significant increase in neck size. Sudden complaints of a lymph node enlargement suggest an infectious process.

Patients who present with enlargement of a node over several months or multiple node involvement are more likely to have neoplastic disease. A hard, immobile mass is also suggestive of a neoplastic process. A referral is indicated for biopsy of the nodes. Laryngeal cancer produces cervical lymphadenopathy and increases neck size. Pain, dyspnea, dysphagia, hemoptysis, stridor, and hoarseness may also be present.

Management

Management of the patient with increased neck size due to endocrine (glandular) abnormalities is to treat the underlying cause.

■ POLYDIPSIA, POLYPHAGIA, AND POLYURIA

Polydipsia is excessive thirst; it is associated with several endocrine diseases and certain drugs. Polydipsia may accompany increased urine output (polyuria), which can be related to excessive loss of water and salt.

Polyphagia refers to excessive eating before satiety. This symptom can present as a persistent or intermittent condition, resulting from endocrine and psychological disorders. Certain drugs are also known to cause polyphagia. Elevated thyroxine (T_4) levels increase metabolism and thus the body's need for calories, often causing polyphagia.

Polyuria is a condition associated with increased urine production; it is defined as excretion of more than 3,000 mL (3 L) per day. Any condition that increases hyperosmolar states will increase urination as a consequence of osmotic diuresis. The patient with polyuria is at risk for fluid volume deficit that could result in hypovolemia.

Differential Diagnosis

Differential diagnoses for the patient with symptoms of polyuria, polydipsia, or polyphagia include diabetes mellitus (DM), diabetes insipidus, diuretic abuse, head trauma, and psychiatric disorders. See Differential Diagnosis Flowchart 16.1 for other cause of these symptoms.

The patient should be questioned about any history of head trauma, weight changes, thyroid disease, hypertension, and family history of diabetes. The patient should also be questioned about any history of psychiatric illnesses or changes in mental status, for example, alertness or memory, as well as symptoms of fatigue. A detailed 48-hour history of intake and output should be obtained, including the type of fluid intake over 48 hours, as well as the characteristics of the urine output. Urine output is often difficult for patients to estimate and objective measurement may be needed. A weight history should be obtained.

The patient should be assessed for signs of dehydration and malnutrition. Weight and vital signs are assessed. Initial laboratory testing includes urinalysis, urine specific gravity, serum electrolytes, blood urea nitrogen, serum creatinine, complete blood count, fasting serum glucose level, and glycosylated hemoglobin percentage (A1C).

Polydipsia, polyphagia, and polyuria are the classic symptoms of DM. Blood glucose levels should be evaluated in patients who experience these three symptoms. An A1C equal to or greater than 6.5%, a fasting (following

Differential Diagnosis Flowchart 16.1

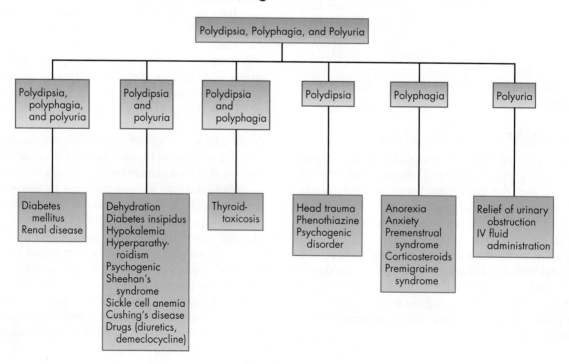

8 hours of no caloric intake) blood glucose level equal to or greater than 126 mg/dL, a 2-hour plasma glucose equal to or greater than 200 mg/dL following a 75-g oral glucose tolerance test (OGTT), or a random blood glucose level greater than 200 mg/dL in persons with classic symptoms of hyperglycemia (polyuria, polydipsia, polyphagia, weight loss) or hyperglycemic crisis confirm the diagnosis of DM. Additional symptoms indicating DM include weakness, fatigue, increased susceptibility to infections, and nocturia.

Management

Management of the patient with polydipsia, polyphagia, and/or polyuria is dependent on treating the underlying cause.

■ WEIGHT GAIN

Weight gain is a common complaint in clinical practice. It may be assessed as a risk factor, such as in coronary artery disease; as a symptom of another disorder, such as the edema seen with congestive heart failure (CHF); as a "sign of aging"; or it may indicate a problem such as hypothyroidism, Cushing's disease, or obesity.

Energy expenditure is composed of the resting energy expenditure, the thermic effect of food, and physical activity. Weight gain results from the ingestion of more calories than are expended. Most often, weight gain is a result of a combination of genetic and environmental factors. However, endocrine disorders, nephrotic syndromes, cardiovascular disease, and some drugs may be the cause of weight gain.

Differential Diagnosis

The history of weight gain, a 24- to 48-hour diet recall, and assessment of activity may provide insight into potential causes. Weight gain, when not associated with pathological disease, results from a complex combination of genetic and environmental factors. The incidence of weight gain increases with age. Several factors account for this weight gain, including a decrease in metabolic rate, decreasing muscle mass, and decreased physical activity. Weight gain results when there is no reduction in caloric intake.

Multiple complex factors interacting simultaneously within the individual usually lead to weight gain. These include biological, genetic, metabolic, psychological, environmental, and social factors. Americans tend to have high-fat diets and put taste and convenience ahead of nutritional content. A sedentary lifestyle and a variety of psychological factors, including depression, anxiety, guilt, and seasonal affective disorder, all contribute to weight gain.

The major differential diagnoses that present with weight gain include hypothyroidism, Cushing's syndrome, renal or hepatic disease, CHF, premenstrual syndrome, pregnancy, medication use, depression, and excessive caloric intake (see Differential Diagnosis Flowchart 16.2).

The patient's history may reveal a family history of obesity, recent weight changes, precipitating psychosocial factors, or a past dieting experience. Food intake (including alcohol) and exercise behaviors should be examined, as well as tobacco and drug use.

A complete physical exam may be needed to evaluate potential pathological causes for weight gain. The weight is recorded and abdominal girth measured, as well as vital

Differential Diagnosis Flowchart 16.2

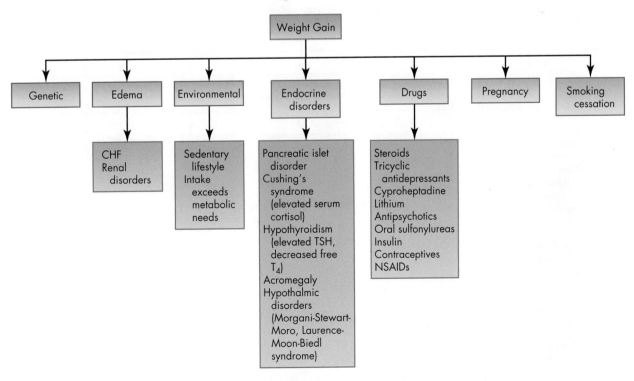

signs taken. Thyroid function tests (thyroid-stimulating hormone and thyroxine [T$_4$]), a serum blood glucose level, and a complete blood count are done in the initial evaluation of patients first presenting with weight gain. Serum cholesterol level, triglycerides, and a lipoprotein panel should be obtained to assess the patient's risk factors for cardiovascular disease.

In addition to the complaint of weight gain, patients may present with fatigue, inability to engage in physical activity, dyspnea on exertion, and pain in weight-bearing joints or in the spine. Patients may also present for the treatment of hypertension, diabetes, cholecystitis, or cardiovascular complaints.

Management

Treatment requires a variety of approaches and depends on the cause. Assessing the patient's motivation is crucial in assisting the patient to set realistic goals. The patient may require in-depth counseling and close follow-up. Many commercial and community programs exist to assist the individual with weight control. If an endocrine disorder is suspected, referral to an endocrinologist is indicated.

■ WEIGHT LOSS, UNINTENTIONAL

Unintentional weight loss of more than 5% of usual body weight within 6 to 12 months may reflect a physical or psychological illness, and a 10% loss of body weight in 1 to 2 months is predictive of a poor clinical outcome. Underweight is defined as being 15% to 20% or more below ideal body weight or a body mass index (BMI) of 18 kg/m^2 or less.

Unintentional weight loss is often a presenting symptom for many underlying pathologies. It may result from a decrease in intake, an increase in metabolic needs, or a combination of the two.

Differential Diagnosis

The history and physical exam may provide initial clues to the cause of the weight loss. The patient's height, weight, and BMI should be recorded, as well as the details about the onset and progression of the weight loss. Actual weight loss needs to be confirmed because it cannot be substantiated in up to 50% of all patients with this complaint. History should include a 3- to 5-day diet record; use of cigarettes, alcohol, or over-the-counter and street drug use; any active medical problems; prescribed medication use; and previous surgery.

Diagnostic testing should be based on the findings of the history and physical exam. Basic screening should include a complete blood count, comprehensive chemistry profile, thyroid function studies, urinalysis, chest x-ray film, and stool for occult blood.

A physical cause of weight loss can be found in about 65% of patients, psychiatric cause in 10%, and no identifiable cause in approximately 25% of cases. Physical causes of weight loss are almost always apparent after a brief evaluation or within 6 months of the first evaluation, even when the initial diagnosis is elusive. Many prescription medications, as well as poor dentition, oral lesions, irritation, and infection, have the potential to cause weight loss (see Differential Diagnosis Flowchart 16.3).

Differential Diagnosis Flowchart 16.3

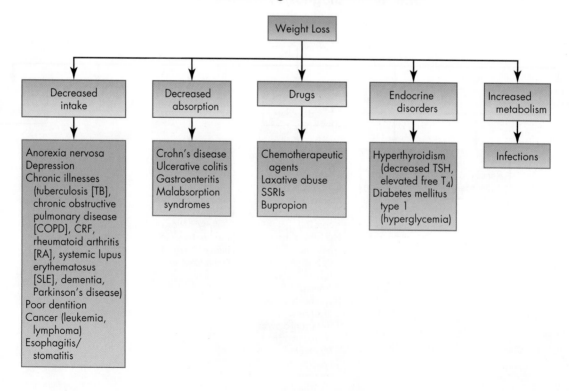

Management

The underlying medical or psychiatric causes of weight loss should be treated. Neurological causes may respond to medications or rehabilitation. Nutritional deficiencies must be corrected with oral or parenteral supplements; an additional 500 to 1,000 calories per day may be indicated.

Megestrol (Megace) 800 mg/day is used as an appetite stimulant in patients with anorexia associated with HIV/AIDS. Tricyclic antidepressants (amitriptyline [Elavil], imipramine [Tofranil], doxepin [Adapin, Sinequan]) are effective in patients with weight loss associated with depression and stimulate appetite.

Follow-up is determined by underlying cause and plan of management. If no cause is found, the clinician should reevaluate the patient thoroughly in 2 to 3 months. The patient should be referred for systemic medical problems or for psychiatric evaluation. Referral to a nutritionist, a dentist for oral problems, or a social worker may also be indicated. The patient needs to understand the nature of the problem and participate in the development of the treatment plan.

COMMON ENDOCRINE PROBLEMS

■ HYPERTHYROIDISM

Hyperthyroidism, a common clinical condition, includes a heterogeneous group of conditions characterized by the excessive secretion and synthesis of one or both of the thyroid hormones: thyroxine (T_4) and triiodothyronine (T_3). Although many clinicians use the terms interchangeably, *thyrotoxicosis* is a larger term that encompasses hyperthyroidism, as well as exogenous thyroid hormone intake and subacute thyroiditis, in which acute inflammation of the thyroid gland results in the rapid excretion (rather than overproduction) of stored thyroid hormones.

The clinical manifestations of hyperthyroidism result from the effects of excessive thyroid hormone on body tissue, resulting in alterations in growth, metabolism, and development. These manifestations are sometimes mistaken for signs of psychiatric illnesses. The long-term effects of inadequately treated overt hyperthyroidism are heart disease, osteoporosis (in postmenopausal women), mental illness, and infertility.

Epidemiology and Causes

Hyperthyroidism occurs in 1.2% of the U.S. population. It may occur at any age but peaks in persons aged 20 to 40 years. Only 10% to 15% of hyperthyroidism is diagnosed in older adults. The prevalence of hyperthyroidism is 2% in women older than 70 years and 4% in women aged 40 to 60 years, with an overall prevalence of 1% to 3%. Hyperthyroidism is much more common in women than men (8:1).

National organizations differ in their recommendations for routine screening in asymptomatic patients. In 2004 the U.S. Preventive Services Task Force (USPSTF) concluded that there was insufficient evidence for or against routine screening for thyroid disease in adults without symptoms, and the USPSTF has not updated this recommendation. If the patient is symptomatic or in a high-risk category, such as having a family history of thyroid disease or previous history of thyroid disease or autoimmune disorders, screening is appropriate.

Hyperthyroidism often occurs spontaneously and can result from the excessive intake of thyroid hormones. Graves' disease is by far the most common cause of spontaneous hyperthyroidism in the United States. An autoimmune disorder characterized by autoreactive, agonistic antibodies to the thyroid-stimulating hormone (TSH) receptor, Graves' disease accounts for 80% to 90% of hyperthyroid cases, peaking in young adults aged 20 to 40 years. It is also the most common form of hyperthyroidism occurring in pregnancy.

Subacute thyroiditis is the most common cause of thyrotoxicosis, accounting for 15% to 20% of cases. Characterized by glandular inflammation and follicular cell destruction, it is thought to be of viral etiology, frequently occurring following an acute viral infection. More common in middle-aged adults between 40 and 50 years, subacute thyroiditis is more likely to develop in women than in men. Silent thyroiditis is a form of subacute thyroiditis in which the thyroid gland is moderately enlarged and nontender. It usually occurs in adults between 30 and 40 years and is also more common in women.

Toxic multinodular goiter (Plummer disease) is as common as subacute thyroiditis, accounting for 15% to 20% of thyrotoxicosis cases. This type of goiter is more common in older adults and is a complication of chronic, inactive nodular goiter. This condition is more common in other parts of the world where dietary iodine deficiency is prevalent. A single, toxic thyroid adenoma is the next most common cause of thyrotoxicosis, accounting for 3% to 5% of all cases.

The inappropriate use of thyroid replacement or treatment errors may also produce symptoms of hyperthyroidism. Thyrotoxicosis factitia is a form of thyrotoxicosis in which a patient takes excessive amounts of either thyroxine (T_4) or triiodothyronine (T_3). This condition should be considered in a patient with access to hormone supplements or with a psychiatric problem. An excess of dietary iodine may also precipitate symptoms of hyperthyroidism.

A tumor of the pituitary gland causing hypersecretion of TSH (thyrotropin) is a rare cause of hyperthyroidism. Other uncommon causes include metastatic follicular thyroid carcinoma; ingestion of iodine-containing drugs (e.g., certain expectorants, amiodarone, seaweed-containing health food supplements) or iodinated radiocontrast media; choriocarcinoma or hydatidiform molar pregnancy producing high amounts of human chorionic gonadotropin (hCG), which is capable of weakly activating the receptor for TSH; struma ovarii (ectopic thyroid tissue), which is associated with dermoid tumors and ovarian teratomas; and testicular embryonal carcinoma (Table 16.1).

Pathophysiology

All types of hyperthyroidism are a result of overproduction and/or secretion of thyroid hormones, and the clinical manifestations of hyperthyroidism are a direct result of the effect of excessive thyroid hormones on essentially all organ systems and bodily tissues. Although thyroid hormones are required to regulate normal growth and development, excessive release of T_4 and T_3 from the thyroid into the circulation upregulates metabolism, leading to an increase in total body heat production, heart rate and contractility, and vasodilation. This explains the clinical manifestations of thyrotoxicosis, which include palpitations, diaphoresis, heat intolerance, and anxiety. T_3 is normally 20 to 100 times more biologically active than T_4, which is converted to T_3 in peripheral tissues. Interestingly, the degree of symptomatology does not consistently correlate with the extent of thyroid hormone overproduction. In general, younger patients tend to have symptoms more reflective of sympathetic activation (tremors, anxiety, and hyperactivity), whereas older patients manifest more cardiovascular symptoms, including atrial fibrillation and dyspnea, as well as weight loss.

Graves' disease is believed to result from an autoimmune response that may reflect a defect in suppressor T-cell function. Serum evaluation usually reveals the presence of antibodies to the thyroid-stimulating hormone receptor (TSH-R), known as thyroid-stimulating immunoglobulin (TSI). This antibody reacts with the TSH-R on thyroid follicular cells and allows release of thyroid hormones independent of the effects of pituitary TSH. Thyroid hormone levels are typically highest with this form of thyrotoxicosis. Excessive thyroid hormone

levels result in thyroid growth (hypertrophy), hypermetabolism, and sympathetic overactivity. Circulating antithyroperoxidase (anti-TPO) is another common finding. A diffusely enlarged goiter involving both thyroid lobes, hyperthyroid ophthalmopathy (periorbital edema, conjunctival edema and injection known as chemosis, proptosis, lid lag, and even diplopia), and excessive uptake of radioactive iodine on diagnostic testing are all common characteristics. Graves' disease has a higher prevalence in people with human leukocyte antigen (HLA)–DRw3 and HLA-B89. It also strongly correlates with other autoimmune conditions including vitiligo, type 1 diabetes mellitus (DM), pernicious anemia, myasthenia gravis, or adrenal insufficiency.

In contrast, subacute thyroiditis produces symptoms of thyrotoxicosis via the release of preformed thyroid hormones, in response to an inflammatory response after an acute viral infection. Thus, unlike other common causes of thyrotoxicosis including toxic multinodular goiter and an isolated toxic adenoma that involve increased production and hypersecretion of thyroid hormones, subacute thyroiditis demonstrates a very low uptake of radioactive iodine on diagnostic testing. Subacute painful or granulomatous thyroiditis is associated with HLA-Bw35.

Toxic multinodular goiter typically arises in areas on dietary iodine deficiency. As scattered portions of the thyroid gland increase in activity in an attempt to compensate for insufficient iodine, hormonal excess develops slowly over time. In fact, this condition may be asymptomatic at the time of diagnosis, especially in older individuals in whom the classic symptoms of hyperthyroidism may be blunted (a condition termed *apathetic hyperthyroidism*).

Nuclear scintigraphy demonstrates scattered areas of both increased and decreased iodine uptake, which reflect the increased thyroidal activity that manifests in the setting of adequate dietary iodine. In contrast, a single

Table 16.1	Hyperthyroidism: Common and Rare Causes	
	Disorder/Problem	**Etiology**
Common Causes	Graves' disease	Autoimmune disease
	Toxic nodular goiter	Unknown development of nodules that progress from nontoxic to toxic over time
	Subacute thyroiditis	Thought to be caused by viral infection
	Thyrotoxicosis factitia	Excessive ingestion of exogenous thyroid hormones
	Jod-Basedow phenomenon	Large intake of iodine in diet in a person with thyroid disease
Rare Causes	Pituitary adenoma	Rare tumor of the pituitary gland
	Struma ovarii	Rare secretion of thyroid hormones by thyroid tissue located in ovarian dermoid tumors
	Metastatic thyroid cancer	Very rare cause
	High-dose amiodarone	Excessive dosage of iodine-containing amiodarone
	Pregnancy and trophoblastic tumors	Very high serum levels of hCG

hyperfunctioning monoclonal follicular adenoma will demonstrate only a single focus of increased uptake on a radioactive thyroid scan. Such nodules tend to be functional only once they reach at least 2.5 cm in size. As pituitary TSH production is suppressed by the adenoma, the remaining glandular tissue becomes hypofunctional and actually demonstrates decreased uptake on nuclear scintigraphy.

Autoregulation of the thyroid normally prevents thyrotoxicosis in the face of dietary iodine excess, a phenomenon known as the Jod-Basedow effect. However, in the setting of a particularly concentrated iodine load (such as with iodinated radiocontrast media), patients with one or more autonomous thyroid nodules may lose this adaptive capability and be thrown into thyrotoxicosis (Jod-Basedow syndrome).

Clinical Presentation

The clinical presentation of hyperthyroidism depends on the duration and the amount of excessive thyroid hormone secretion. Symptoms are varied and depend on the cause and the multiple organ systems affected. Patients may be asymptomatic in the presence of mild elevations of thyroid hormones; they are more likely to remain asymptomatic at increasing levels if the increased secretion has been gradual.

Subjective

Because thyroid hormones have effects on most organ systems, a complete history and review of systems is indicated. Most patients with hyperthyroidism will complain of some combination of anxiety, nervousness, diaphoresis, fatigue, heat intolerance, palpitations, weight loss, and insomnia. In situations in which the thyroid tissue has become enlarged, the patient may complain of fullness or pressure in the neck. Additional symptoms include weakness, exercise intolerance, tremors, lower extremity edema, weight loss in the presence of an increased appetite, menstrual irregularities, frequent bowel movements or diarrhea, and exertional dyspnea.

Eye complaints include blurred vision, proptosis (downward displacement of the eyeball), photophobia, and double vision. Patients may also report that they are unable to concentrate, extremely irritable, and emotionally labile. Older patients may present with vague symptoms such as unexplained weight loss, apathy, worsening of angina, depression, change in bowel habits, and weakness. A summary of potential signs and symptoms of hyperthyroidism is presented in Table 16.2.

Patients should be questioned about current and prior endocrine diseases (in the patient and family), as well as a personal or family history of thyroid nodules, goiter, use of iodide-containing drugs, and thyroid neoplasms. Radiation to the head and neck increases the risk of thyroid cancer, which can produce hyperthyroidism. A weight history should be obtained, including recent and long-term weight patterns. If the patient is currently taking thyroid hormone replacement medication, how the medication is being taken should be assessed. Patients should also be questioned about any recent viral infections or the possibility of pregnancy, as well as use of other medications.

Objective

Signs of thyrotoxicosis on physical examination are associated with the various forms of hyperthyroidism and range from overt manifestations in young adults with an acute onset to a more subtle presentation in older adults. Often, an older adult will present with symptoms typically diagnosed as failure to thrive.

On physical examination, the thyroid may be enlarged, nodules may be palpable, and a bruit may be heard over the thyroid gland with the bell of a stethoscope. The neck should be examined for visual enlargement of the thyroid and palpated for lymphadenopathy. The thyroid must be palpated thoroughly, noting any nodules or enlargement, both anteriorly and posteriorly. Whereas the goiter of Graves' disease is often somewhat firm, the thyroid in toxic multinodular goiter may be softer, but with several palpable nodules. The neck should be moderately extended during examination, and water should be provided to the patient to aid swallowing. The thyroid gland moves with swallowing; however, a very large goiter or a large thyroid mass may prevent movement.

In subacute thyroiditis, the patient will present with a firm, painful, thyroid gland enlargement, fatigue, and possibly a low-grade fever. An enlarged painful thyroid gland is also consistent with degeneration or hemorrhage into a thyroid nodule, as well as either granulomatous or suppurative thyroiditis. In contrast, in silent thyroiditis or subacute lymphocytic thyroiditis, the gland is swollen but not usually tender.

Cardiovascular manifestations include tachycardia (resting heart rate greater than 90 beats per minute), irregular pulse, systolic murmurs, and widening of the pulse pressure. Although rare, an infiltrative dermopathy may be present in the lower extremities, which includes myxedema (deposition of glycosaminoglycan material in the dermis of the lower extremities causing nonpitting pretibial edema), erythema due to an inflammatory cell infiltrate, and skin thickening along the ankles and pretibial areas.

Visual acuity is tested, and the patient is assessed for lid lag. Lid lag is assessed by instructing the patient to slowly gaze up and down. As the patient gazes downward, the upper lid will lag behind the globe. Lid lag can also be detected by the globe lagging behind the lower lid as the patient gazes upward. Hyperthyroid ophthalmopathy occurs in 40% of patients with Graves' disease and is rare in patients with subacute thyroiditis. The conjunctiva may be inflamed, and visual acuity may be affected. Exophthalmos, excessive lacrimation, lid retraction, and lid lag may be present.

Table 16.2 Hyperthyroidism: Clinical Presentation

Body System	Subjective	Objective
General	Fatigue Weight loss Increased appetite	Muscle atrophy Tremors
Integumentary	Diaphoresis Heat intolerance	Warm, flushed, moist skin Onycholysis Hyperpigmentation Fine and silky hair Thinning hair Dermopathy of legs Pretibial myxedema urticaria Pruritus vitiligo
Gastrointestinal	Diarrhea Increased bowel movements Increased appetite	Increased liver function
Eye	Blurred vision Increased tearing Double vision Decreased visual acuity Photophobia Feelings of increased orbital pressure	Increased exophthalmos Lid lag and edema Corneal ulceration
Neurological	Tremors of hands	Hyperactive reflexes Tremor
Cardiopulmonary	Palpitations Exertional dyspnea	Sinus tachycardia Elevated blood pressure Symptoms of congestive heart failure Dysrhythmias (atrial fibrillation)
Genitourinary	Menstrual irregularities (decreased menstrual flow)	Gynecomastia
Head and neck	Pressure in neck Increased neck size	Enlarged thyroid gland
Psychosocial	Anxiety Nervousness Insomnia Irritability Emotional lability Restlessness	Increased pulse rate Increased respiratory rate Increased blood pressure
Musculoskeletal	Weakness	Proximal muscle weakness Loss of muscle tone Osteoporosis (postmenopausal women)
Hematological	Fatigue Breathlessness Palpitations	Normochromic normocytic anemia
Metabolic		Hypercalcemia Potassium wasting Increased alkaline phosphatase

The examiner should assess the skin for edema, general appearance, and signs of thinning hair. The skin may be moist and velvety to the touch, with increased pigmentation, spider angiomas, and vitiligo. Onycholysis (splitting and spooning of the nails) may be present.

Deep tendon reflexes may show a rapid relaxation of the reflex, and the most predominant hyperactive reflex is usually the Achilles tendon reflex. The patient may have decreased strength in the extremities and fine tremors, especially of the hands when the arms are fully outstretched. Lymphadenopathy and splenomegaly may also be present. A few patients may also have nonpitting pretibial edema.

Patients with long-standing hyperthyroidism may also have clubbing of the digits and signs of new bone growth in the hands, termed *thyroid acropachy*. Older adults with hyperthyroidism often appear apathetic. Physical examination may reveal atrial fibrillation (present in one-third of all older adults with hyperthyroidism), fine skin, brittle nails, and symptoms of congestive heart failure. The thyroid gland is often not enlarged in older adults.

Thyroid storm or crisis is a severe, sometimes fatal form of hyperthyroidism and requires immediate emergency medical care. Assessment, contributing factors, and treatment are listed in Table 16.3.

Diagnostic Reasoning
Diagnostic Tests

Initial Testing Laboratory examination is undertaken with the understanding that in many situations, levels of thyroid hormone often do not correlate reliably with the clinical presentation. The initial screening tests for suspected hyperthyroidism are measurement of the serum-sensitive TSH assay to detect suppressed levels in the setting of elevated thyroid hormones, T_4 and T_3. Laboratory protocols that add free thyroxine immunoassay (FT_4) and T_3 if the TSH is low can avoid additional blood draws and expense. If the protocol is not in place, an FT_4 and T_3 should be tested next. The sensitive TSH assay has a functional sensitivity of 0.02 mcg/dL or less, although units for this test are typically expressed as mIU/L or mcIU/mL.

In most cases of hyperthyroidism, a TSH level less than 0.35 mIU/L usually accompanies an elevated FT_4 measurement (above 12.5 mcg/dL). Measurement of

Table 16.3	Thyroid Storm/Crisis		
Contributing Factors	Acute infection		
	Trauma		
	Stress in patient with hyperthyroidism		
	Uncontrolled DM		
	Severe drug reaction		
	Following withdrawal of antithyroid medication or radioactive iodine therapy		
Symptoms: Initial	Fever (usually initial symptom), often >100.4°F (38°C)		
	Nausea, vomiting		
	Abdominal pain		
Symptoms: Progressive	Severe agitation, occasional psychosis		
	Elevated temperature		
	Diaphoresis		
	Tachycardia, heart failure		
	Dysrhythmia (atrial fibrillation of flutter)		
	Confusion		
	Cardiovascular collapse		
	Malignant exophthalmos		
	Elevated free thyroid hormone (T_4) levels but no more increased than hyperthyroidism; clinical diagnosis, not biochemical		
Management	Hospitalization and aggressive reversal of thyrotoxins		
	1. To block thyroid hormone synthesis, propylthiouracil (PTU) is given daily in two to four divided doses; methimazole is typically not used during thyroid storm because it does not prevent peripheral conversion of T_4 to T_3.		
	2. To alleviate the beta-adrenergic symptoms, beta blockers are given (propranolol [Inderal] IV).		
	3. To block conversion of T_4 to T_3, hydrocortisone is given IV.		
	4. If radioactive iodine is prescribed but not given for a few days, potassium iodide oral solution (SSKI) or telepaque may be given.		
	5. Supportive measures—decrease fever, treat underlying infection, give fluids and glucose.		

FT_4 is generally preferred over total T_4 because it measures the level of T_4 unbound to carrier proteins, which is, therefore, biologically active. In turn, a significant number of medications may alter the laboratory results due to alterations in protein binding. These include anabolic steroids, androgens, estrogens, heparin, iodine-containing compounds, phenytoin (Dilantin), rifampin (Rimactane, Rifadin), and salicylates. In addition, in the setting of a low TSH, T_3 levels should be obtained because about 5% of hyperthyroid patients have normal T_4 levels but elevated T_3 levels. Normal levels for T_3 range from 100 to 200 ng/dL.

Subsequent Testing In Graves' disease, antithyroglobulin and antimicrosomal antibodies are elevated. A TSH receptor antibody test is usually elevated in Graves' disease and is part of subsequent testing. The diagnosis of thyrotoxicosis is considered in cases of hyperthyroidism when TSH levels are depressed and measurements of T_4 are normal. Subacute thyroiditis may also have laboratory abnormalities of elevated erythrocyte sedimentation rate and C-reactive protein. Mild anemia is also common.

Nuclear scintigraphy with radiolabeled iodine (^{123}I) or technetium (^{99}Tc) helps in assessing the functional status of the thyroid gland. A 24-hour radioactive iodine uptake (RAIU) test can differentiate Graves' disease from subacute thyroiditis and toxic nodular goiters, thereby refining treatment recommendations. It identifies areas of increased and decreased thyroid function, often termed *hot* and *cold* spots, within the gland. Patients with toxic nodular goiter and Graves' disease have a high RAIU, whereas in subacute thyroiditis, iodine uptake is low. Importantly, however, toxic adenoma and toxic multinodular goiter both present with areas of decreased isotope uptake as well, because the hyperfunctioning nodules lead to suppression of TSH via negative hormonal feedback. A thyroid scan is critical to determining functionality of any dominant thyroid nodule in a patient presenting with thyrotoxicosis, because cold nodules are highly suspicious for concomitant malignancy and must be evaluated further.

An ultrasound of the thyroid will assist in differentiating a cyst from a nodule. A pure thyroid cyst is less likely to be malignant than a nodule. A fine-needle biopsy is the preferred initial diagnostic technique for evaluation of thyroid masses, particularly solid masses, to rule out malignancy. Magnetic resonance imaging is the preferred test to assess for ophthalmopathy resulting from Graves' disease. It is especially beneficial in ruling out an orbital tumor.

Differential Diagnosis

Thyrotoxicosis, with high levels of TSH, is seen in a rare pituitary tumor. Excessive exogenous thyroid administration will produce the same symptoms seen in thyrotoxicosis. Thyroid cancer must be considered when the thyroid gland is hard and enlarged or when nodules are palpated.

T_4 levels may be elevated in acute illnesses such as hepatitis, in the presence of elevated estrogen levels, acute psychiatric problems, hyperemesis, familial thyroid hormone binding abnormalities, and autoimmunity. Dopamine (Intropin, Dopastat) and high dosages of glucocorticoids may decrease TSH levels. Drugs that may increase T_4 levels are amiodarone (Cordarone), amphetamines, clofibrate (Atromid-S), glucocorticoids in high doses, heparin administered during dialysis, heroin, levothyroxine (Synthroid), methadone (Dolophine), and perphenazine (Trilafon).

Management

Treatment of hyperthyroidism differs depending on the cause and patient characteristics. A euthyroid state is the goal of treatment, while minimizing the adverse effects of treatment and decreasing the incidence of hypothyroidism.

Emergency treatment is necessary if the patient presents in thyroid storm (see Table 16.3). The patient should be hospitalized for oral and IV hydration, if needed, and immediately begin thyroid-blocking medications, beta-adrenergic blockers, and corticosteroids if signs of ophthalmopathy are present. Iodine blocks the release of stored thyroid hormones, and glucocorticosteroids block the conversion of T_4 to T_3. Patients intolerant of beta blockers (asthmatics, patients with chronic obstructive pulmonary disease [COPD]) may be treated with calcium channel blockers as an alternate therapy. Supportive measures include treating any underlying infection; managing fever with antipyretics, hydration, and cooling blankets; and correcting any fluid and electrolyte imbalances. In critically ill patients, utilization of plasma pheresis or dialysis may reduce the circulating levels of T_3 and T_4.

Multinodular and uninodular goiters should be referred to an endocrinologist for evaluation of possible malignancy. Nonmalignant thyroid nodular disease with laboratory evaluations indicating hyperthyroidism is most often treated with radioactive iodine.

Management of Graves' Disease

The three treatment options for Graves' disease are antithyroid drugs, radioactive iodine, or surgery. None of these treatments alters the underlying autoimmune process of Graves' disease. The most successful treatment in achieving a permanent euthyroid state is surgery; however, it is rarely the preferred method of treatment unless the thyroid gland is extremely enlarged and is pressing on other structures in the neck. Many patients treated with radioactive iodine will experience a relapse and require a second treatment. Radioactive iodine also may worsen ophthalmopathy if present. Currently the majority of endocrinologists use an ablative dosing of radioactive iodine. This allows the resolution of hyperthyroidism, although patients then become hypothyroid and require thyroid replacement therapy for life.

Pharmacological Therapy Patients experiencing tachycardia, palpitations, or tremor benefit from the introduction of a beta blocker during initiation of therapy. Beta blockers provide effective, short-term relief of hyperadrenergic symptoms. Use of a beta blocker is contraindicated in patients with COPD, bronchospasm, or uncompensated heart failure. It is used cautiously in patients who take insulin for DM because it may block symptoms of hypoglycemia. Beta-adrenergic blockers often require higher and more frequent dosing because of the frequent resistance to usual doses. Once ablative treatment is completed, beta blockers will be tapered and discontinued. As stated previously, calcium channel blockers are an option in patients for whom beta blockers are contraindicated; however, this class of drug should also be avoided in patients with uncompensated heart failure, given their propensity to decrease inotropy (cardiac contractility).

Antithyroid medications work by inhibiting thyroid hormone synthesis at multiple steps. They are used as a primary treatment to reduce the level of hormone on initiation of radioactive iodine therapy, as well as before and after thyroid surgery. These drugs take time to achieve their peak effect, however, and hormone levels may not be significantly decreased for up to 2 to 8 weeks. These medications are not used as primary or sole treatment in the majority of patients.

Two antithyroid drugs are being used at present—propylthiouracil (PTU) and methimazole (MMI). These drugs are the treatment of choice for pregnant women, especially PTU, because it is less likely to cross the placenta than MMI. As a pregnancy progresses, the dose of PTU often decreases and can frequently be discontinued before delivery. It is important to remember that antithyroid drugs do cross the placental barrier, and overtreatment can have adverse effects on a fetus, thus the importance of having a clinical endocrinologist consulting on a pregnant woman's care. They are often used in persons awaiting surgical intervention and in patients of childbearing age. Antithyroid drug treatment is often the preferred treatment in patients without significant thyroid gland enlargement. PTU has an added therapeutic effect of inhibiting T_3 activity and preventing peripheral conversion of T_4 into T_3—the more biologically active of the two main thyroid hormones. Thus, it is useful in cases of thyrotoxicosis to rapidly reduce hyperthyroid symptoms.

PTU is usually started at doses of 50 to 150 mg PO two or three times per day (150–300 mg per day). MMI (Tapazole) is given at an initial dosage 10 to 40 mg orally or rectally daily. The dosage is titrated every 3 to 4 weeks based on thyroxine levels and TSH levels. TSH and T_4 levels are evaluated every visit, and a targeted history and physical is performed to monitor therapeutic response. (See Drugs Commonly Prescribed 16.1: Hyperthyroidism.)

Because of the amount of thyroid hormone stored in the thyroid gland, it may take 2 to 8 weeks to see a therapeutic response to antithyroid medication. These drugs are not indicated for long-term use because more than one-half of patients on these drugs alone experience resumption of symptoms. Once the patient has achieved a euthyroid state, the frequency of follow-up visits is extended to every 4 to 6 weeks for a period of 3 to 4 months. If the TSH and free T_4 remain stable during this time, the follow-up is extended to every 3 to 4 months. In patients taking antithyroid medication, a serum FT_4 level should be evaluated with TSH levels, because the TSH level may remain suppressed due to chronic hyperthyroidism long after T_4 levels are decreased.

Common adverse reactions to antithyroid medications include rash, urticaria, and arthralgias, which may occur in 1% to 5% of patients. Rare but serious adverse reactions include agranulocytosis, aplastic anemia, and hepatitis, which may occur in up to 0.5% of patients taking antithyroid medications. Except for agranulocytosis, which is more common with MMI, these reactions are more likely to occur with PTU. Thus, patients taking these drugs should be instructed to report immediately any signs of infection, especially a fever, sore throat, malaise, or mouth sores. The antithyroid medication must be discontinued immediately if any of these symptoms are

Drugs Commonly Prescribed 16.1 Hyperthyroidism

Drug	Indications	Adverse Reactions and Prescribing Considerations
propylthiouracil (PTU)	Hyperthyroidism	Common: Pruritus, drowsiness, allergic dermatitis, nausea, vomiting, arthralgia Rare: Agranulocytosis Note: Onset of drug action is 1 week, peaking in 4–10 weeks with a duration of 1–4 weeks.
methimazole (MM) (Tapazole)	Hyperthyroidism	Common: Pruritus, drowsiness, allergic dermatitis, nausea, parotitis, arthralgia Rare: Agranulocytosis Note: Onset of drug action is 1 week, peaking in 4–10 weeks with a duration of 36–72 hours.

experienced. The patient is often changed to a regimen of radioactive iodine to produce a euthyroid state. Agranulocytosis may take up to 10 to 14 days to resolve fully after the medication is stopped and may require concomitant administration of granulocyte colony-stimulating factor (filgrastim).

Before initiation of antithyroid therapy, a baseline complete blood count and liver function tests including hepatic aminotransferases (aspartate aminotransferase, alanine aminotransferase) should be obtained. During therapy, the white blood cell count is checked every 2 weeks during the first month and then every 4 to 6 months thereafter. Liver enzymes should be evaluated every 3 to 6 months.

Antithyroid drugs (see Drugs Commonly Prescribed 16.1: Hyperthyroidism) are used for 6 to 24 months after achievement of a euthyroid state. The dosage is then gradually decreased until the drug is withdrawn. The patient is followed every 1 to 2 months initially after cessation of therapy for a possible relapse. Many patients will experience a permanent remission after a 1- to 2-year course of antithyroid medications.

Radioactive Iodine   Radioactive iodine–131 (^{131}I; Iodotope) is the treatment of choice for hyperthyroidism in the United States, especially in middle-aged or older adults. Typically, a 24-hour radioiodine uptake dose of 75 to 200 mcCi per gram of estimated thyroid tissue is administered orally, which concentrates in overactive thyroid cells, where it emits radiation, causing inflammation and the ultimate destruction of the pathological cells. It is less invasive than thyroidectomy, is a targeted therapy that is focused solely on the thyroid, and does not require hospitalization. Although response to this therapy is slower than with antithyroid drugs or surgical excision, radioablation is indicated in patients who have a poor response to antithyroid medication, as well as in cases of toxic multinodular goiter. Radioiodine is contraindicated in pregnancy and breastfeeding. The recurrence rates for hyperthyroidism are relatively low. For patients with Graves' disease, there is a 5% recurrence 1 year after treatment and that remains steady for 5 years as opposed to patients with uninodular or multinodular toxic goiter, which has a 6% to 7% recurrence rate and a 30% recurrence rate after 5 years (Level II; Bakos et al, 2013).

Women receiving radioactive iodine therapy should refrain from becoming pregnant for 4 months after therapy. T_4 levels need to be checked monthly for 3 months after the administration of radioactive iodine in patients receiving radioactive thyroid ablation therapy. Euthyroid patients should be assessed every 3 to 6 months for hypothyroidism by monitoring the FT_4 and sensitive TSH levels. Hypothyroidism may occur at any time, but is most likely to present during the first year. Some patients will fail treatment and require a second dose. First-time failure rates may be as high as 45%, but about 70% of patients receiving radioactive iodine therapy eventually develop hypothyroidism.

Hyperthyroid ophthalmopathy is often exacerbated with radioactive iodine treatment; however, research has found that the incidence of ophthalmopathy is reduced when prednisone (0.4 mg/kg) is given concurrently with radioactive iodine treatments. If ophthalmopathy occurs, the patient requires referral to an ophthalmologist. Treatment often includes diuretics and ophthalmic prednisone. Methylcellulose eyedrops (Tear Naturale) are useful to protect against excessive eye dryness.

A nonradioactive alternative to thyroid radioablation for severe Graves' disease or subacute thyroiditis involves administering a large quantity of concentrated iodine as a saturated solution of potassium iodide (SSKI, 35–50 mg iodide per drop, 1–2 gtts in water PO 2 times daily; Lugol solution, 8 mg iodide per drop, 3–5 gtts in water PO 3 times daily) or iopanoic acid (Telepaque, 1–3 g PO or 0.5 g PO 2 times daily). These concentrated iodine therapies effectively block the conversion of T_4 to T_3 and inhibit the release of thyroid hormones. SSKI and Lugol solution should not be used when autonomous thyroid nodules are present, however, such as in toxic multinodular goiter or toxic adenoma, because they may worsen thyrotoxicosis. In addition, these therapies are generally used only in severe cases of thyrotoxicosis because their use precludes definitive therapy with radioactive iodine for several months (the thyroid must first process out the iodine load).

Surgery   Surgery (subtotal or total thyroidectomy) is required for patients with compressive symptoms of the neck such as hoarseness (from compression of the recurrent laryngeal nerve) or respiratory stridor, which indicates displacement of the trachea. It may also be considered for cosmetic reasons, for patients who have failed other treatment options, and for patients with refractory amiodarone-induced hyperthyroidism. Surgery is often recommended in a patient with a large gland, multinodular goiter, or when thyroid cancer is suspected. It is also indicated in individuals who cannot tolerate antithyroid medication; however, an antithyroid medication may be administered during the initiation of therapy to prevent excessive release of stored thyroid hormones. In addition, propranolol is typically used to decrease the resting heart rate to below 80 beats per minute, and SSKI may be administered (1–2 gtts PO 2 times daily) for 2 weeks before surgical resection. Before the development of these preoperative pharmacotherapies, thyroidectomy was one of the most common causes of thyroid storm. Today, important complications of surgery include permanent hypothyroidism, which will require lifelong thyroid hormone replacement, and laryngeal paralysis via damage to the recurrent laryngeal nerve. Hypoparathyroidism may also result if one or more of the parathyroid glands are inadvertently resected during surgery.

Management of Subacute Thyroiditis

Subacute thyroiditis is a self-limiting condition treated with beta-adrenergic blocking medications and NSAIDs.

If patients have moderate to severe symptoms or do not respond to beta blockers and NSAIDs, they are candidates for treatment with corticosteroids. Subacute thyroiditis often follows a viral illness. After the thyroiditis, some patients may experience a transient hypothyroid state. These patients will need thyroid hormone until they return to a euthyroid state. For the patient with severe pain, an NSAID may help. Short-term use of oral prednisone (Deltasone) may be indicated for severe inflammation and pain. Doses of 40 mg daily for 1 to 2 weeks with a gradual taper over 2 to 4 weeks are usually effective.

Management of Subclinical Hyperthyroidism

Subclinical hyperthyroidism is characterized by undetectable TSH levels and normal levels of T_4 and T_3. Treatment is only recommended for patients over 65 years of age or patients with cardiac disease or some evidence of symptoms related to hyperthyroidism. There is an increased risk of atrial fibrillation in hyperthyroid patients over age 65 years who have a TSH level between 0.1 and 0.5 mIU/L. Consultation with an endocrinologist is indicated for these patients. If treatment is not initiated, the patient should be monitored every 6 months for overt hyperthyroidism.

Patients experiencing symptoms of infiltrative ophthalmopathy will need to be followed by an ophthalmologist. Glucocorticoids, diuretics, and methylcellulose eyedrops may provide symptomatic relief. Radiation or surgical decompression may be initiated by the ophthalmologist in severe cases.

Follow-up and Referral

The complex nature of thyrotoxicosis requires collaboration and referral to an endocrinologist for effective management and close follow-up. Importantly, up to half of all patients with Graves' disease who go into remission after starting antithyroid pharmacotherapy without definitive thyroid ablation with have a second attack of thyrotoxicosis within 1 year. In addition, all patients with Graves' disease should be referred to an ophthalmologist for full evaluation, because up to half of these patients have some form of ophthalmopathy, which may present subclinically. In contrast, Graves' disease ophthalmopathy may present before the patient develops symptoms of full-blown thyrotoxicosis.

Specific time frames for follow-up are dependent on the treatment and patient response. TSH, FT_4, and T_3 levels should be monitored at each follow-up visit, as well as measurements of blood pressure, pulse, weight, and character of the thyroid gland. General guidelines include the following:

1. Monitor thyroid function tests at least twice a year.
2. Initial treatment should be evaluated at 1 month and at 6 months or more frequently if the patient is symptomatic.
3. Therapy with antithyroid medications should continue for 3 to 24 months.
4. After radioiodine therapy, thyroid function tests should be performed at 4 to 6 weeks, 12 weeks, 6 months, and annually thereafter, if stable.

Patient Education

After diagnosis, the patient with hyperthyroidism must be provided with the various treatment options available. The risks and benefits of each treatment must be explained. The importance of strict adherence to provider guidelines for follow-up must be stressed to each patient. If the treatment regimen has produced a state of hypothyroidism, the patient is informed that thyroid replacement therapy must continue for life.

Patients must be instructed that it takes 4 to 6 weeks after medication begins to notice an improvement in symptoms because of the amount of stored hormone in the thyroid gland. Patients who are unaware of this phenomenon may not comply with the treatment regimen. Patients need written instructions for the signs and symptoms of thyroid storm, as well as signs of hypothyroidism once treatment is initiated. The patient should be informed of all potential adverse reactions of all medications, particularly those of antithyroid preparations, and to discontinue the medication and to call the primary-care provider if a fever, sore throat, or malaise develops.

Persons receiving radioactive iodine therapy should avoid contact with infants, children, and pregnant women for 7 days after ingestion. Women who receive this treatment postpartum must not breastfeed for at least 3 to 6 months, because radioactive iodine is excreted in breast milk and can ablate the infant's thyroid.

The need for adequate rest and exercise should be stressed. Patients will need adequate sleep, as well as relaxation time, and should be taught methods to promote relaxation, such as biofeedback, music, or guided imagery. Patients should be encouraged to express their concerns regarding psychosocial implications of their disease, and the physiological basis for their symptoms should be reinforced.

Patients who complain of heat intolerance may benefit from wearing or sleeping on natural fabrics during the summer months and should remain adequately hydrated. Patients who have experienced significant weight loss may benefit from a high-carbohydrate, high-calorie diet. A patient with Graves' disease may benefit from dividing food intake into six smaller meals daily. If diarrhea is a problem, discourage foods that increase peristalsis such as highly seasoned foods and bulky or fibrous foods. The patient should check his or her weight daily and report any weight loss of more than 4 pounds in 1 day immediately. A consistent weight loss of 1 to 2 pounds daily should also be reported. A supplemental multivitamin, particularly with vitamin B complex, is needed to prevent deficiencies in times of severe hyperthyroidism because of a high level of vitamin consumption during states of elevated thyroid hormone levels.

Once treatment is initiated and the patient is euthyroid, caloric needs decrease but the patient may still have an increased appetite. A sensible diet low in fat and sugar with adequate protein may avoid a significant unwanted weight gain during this period. The patient should be instructed to check his or her weight frequently and to adjust intake to maintain an ideal weight. Stimulants such as caffeine should be avoided. A multivitamin is often indicated for patients who have sustained thyrotoxicity. Patients suspected of having long-standing hyperthyroidism may benefit from vitamin D and calcium supplementation because osteoporosis is a complication of elevated thyroid hormones.

Some patients may experience depression as the levels of thyroid hormones change, and this should be explained. The patient should be instructed to report any worsening of symptoms of depression. If the patient presents with signs or symptoms of depression or anxiety, he or she should be evaluated for depression or anxiety. If reassurance does not relieve anxiety, temporary symptomatic treatment may be indicated.

Patients with exophthalmos should wear dark lenses outdoors during the day. The use of artificial tears may relieve feelings of dryness and provide some corneal protection. Glasses or eye protection should be worn during any activity that may introduce dust or dirt into the eyes. A sleeping mask should be worn at night if the patient cannot close the eyes adequately. Elevating the head of the bed at night and restricting sodium intake may relieve edema.

Patients taking antithyroid medications should wear a medical identification bracelet.

■ HYPOTHYROIDISM

Hypothyroidism is a common, treatable disorder in which there is a slow progression of thyroid hypofunction, followed by signs and symptoms indicating thyroid failure. It is a disease of various causes that lead to inadequate amounts of thyroid hormone being produced and/or secreted, resulting in a slowing of many body functions and metabolic processes. Because hypothyroidism has an insidious onset and progresses slowly, the clinical manifestations may go unrecognized.

Thyroid hormone deficiency present at birth was historically called *cretinism* but is now known by the less pejorative term *congenital hypothyroidism.* Affecting 1 in 4,000 newborns, the causes of congenital hypothyroidism include developmental abnormalities of the thyroid gland, enzymatic defects, iodine deficiency, maternal antibodies to thyroid hormones, and excessive intake of goitrogens by the mother. In such instances, the mother may also suffer from thyroid deficiency. Thyroid hormone deficiency beginning in early infancy and childhood is characterized by growth retardation, mental deficiency, and delayed dentition. Adolescents with primary hypothyroidism may manifest an enlarged sella turcica and, rarely, precocious puberty, in addition to growth retardation.

Growth retardation is treatable with hormone replacement therapy, but mental retardation persists.

Subclinical hypothyroidism is the presence of normal free thyroxine immunoassay (FT$_4$) with an elevated thyroid-stimulating hormone (TSH). As many as 15% of patients older than age 65 years have these levels, as do many other adults. However, few of these patients report symptoms, or their symptoms are nonspecific.

Epidemiology and Causes

The incidence of hypothyroidism varies with age, gender, and geographical and environmental factors. The incidence from numerous surveys ranges from 3 to 14 cases per 1,000 women, with significantly fewer cases reported in men. In fact, the incidence in women is 2 to 8 times greater than it is in men. It is estimated that as many as 4.6% of the U.S. population has an elevated TSH with a higher incidence in whites (5.1%) than in either Hispanics (4.1%) or African Americans (1.7%).

The most common worldwide cause of thyroid disorders is iodine deficiency, with a worldwide prevalence of 2% to 5%. In the United States, where iodine ingestion is usually adequate, autoimmune processes are the primary cause of thyroid disease. Hashimoto's thyroiditis, a type of primary hypothyroidism, is the most common form of autoimmune thyroid disease. This type of hypothyroidism occurs at least four times more often in women than in men, with the average age at onset from 30 to 60 years.

Iatrogenic hypothyroidism, which occurs after treatment with radioactive iodine (for hyperthyroidism) or surgery (for hyperthyroidism, thyroid nodules, or thyroid carcinoma), is the next most common cause of hypothyroidism, accounting for 30% to 40% of cases. Hypothyroidism also becomes increasingly common with age; in individuals older than age 50 years, up to 10% may have elevated TSH levels.

More than 95% of patients with hypothyroidism have primary or thyroidal hypothyroidism, involving dysfunction or atrophy of the thyroid gland. When the thyroid dysfunction is caused by failure of the pituitary gland, the hypothalamus, or both, it is known as central hypothyroidism. More specifically, secondary hypothyroidism refers to the failure of the pituitary gland to secrete adequate amounts of TSH. Tertiary hypothyroidism is a type of hypothyroidism resulting in inadequate secretion of thyrotropin-releasing hormone (TRH) by the hypothalamus or failure of TRH to activate its cognate receptors within the pituitary (peripheral resistance). Table 16.4 summarizes the causes of hypothyroidism.

Although one in five women will develop an alteration in thyroid function in her lifetime, recently published clinical guidelines do not recommend routine screening of asymptomatic women before age 50 years. Many clinicians, however, still use age 40 years as their criterion to begin screening. In 2004 the U.S. Preventive Services Task Force (USPSTF) found insufficient evidence to

Table 16.4	Causes of Hypothyroidism
Cause	**Etiology**
Loss of functional thyroid tissue	Idiopathic hypothyroidism: Atrophy (probably autoimmune), TSH receptor–blocking antibodies.
	Chronic autoimmune thyroiditis (Hashimoto's disease), subacute, postpartum, treatment with cytokines or amiodarone, external radiation.
	Status—post-radioiodine (^{131}I) treatment
	Status—post-thyroidectomy
	Infiltrating disorders: Malignancy, granulomatous disease
	Thyroid dysgenesis
Biosynthetic defects in thyroid hormone production	Inherited defects in hormone synthesis
	Iodine deficiency
	Antithyroid agents: Thioamides, lithium, iodide
Central hypothyroidism	TSH deficiency caused by pituitary disease: Postpartum infarction (Sheehan syndrome), tumors (e.g., craniopharyngioma, pituitary adenoma), granulomatous disease (sarcoidosis), irradiation, idiopathic
	TSH deficiency caused by hypothalamic disease: Tumors, irradiation, and transiently occurring nonthyroid illness
	Peripheral resistance to TSH by the pituitary
Transient hypothyroidism	Postpartum thyroiditis
	Subacute thyroiditis (usually viral)
	Withdrawal of thyroid hormone therapy in a euthyroid patient

recommend for or against routine screening for thyroid disease in adults. The American Thyroid Association recommends measuring thyroid function in all adults starting at age 35 years and then at least every 5 years. The American College of Physicians recommends TSH measurement in women older than 50 with one or more general symptoms that could be caused by thyroid disease. These organizations and many others have come to no clear recommendation for screening asymptomatic adults. All patients with a prior history of any medically or surgically treated thyroid disease should be screened with a serum TSH measurement yearly. In addition, patients with other autoimmune diseases and those with unexplained depression, diabetes mellitus (DM), cognitive dysfunction, prior external radiation to the head and neck, hypercholesterolemia, or other risk factors should be screened with TSH measurements. Women experiencing unexplained infertility should be screened for thyroid dysfunction, and postpartum women with vague complaints may benefit from screening.

Risk factors for thyroid failure include a family history of thyroid disease; personal history of thyroid disease; presence of antithyroid antibodies; radiation treatment to the head, neck, or chest; other autoimmune disease; old age; and use of lithium, amiodarone (Cordarone), or iodine.

Although production of T_4 decreases with age, serum T_4 and TSH levels remain stable, whereas T_3 levels may decrease in persons older than age 80 years. In many cases, hypothyroidism in the older adult is characterized by symptoms that may be subtle and similar to the normal signs of aging, thus making it easy to overlook. Common symptoms include hoarseness, deafness, confusion, frank psychosis, dementia, ataxia, depression, constipation, intolerance of cold temperatures, dry skin, or hair loss.

Pathophysiology

Normal thyroid function is required for every metabolic process in the human body. Growth and development, protein synthesis, and cell metabolism are all dependent on an adequate supply of thyroid hormone to the peripheral tissues. The thyroid plays an essential role in fetal development; oxygen consumption; heat production; sympathetic nervous system function; and cardiovascular, hematopoietic, pulmonary, and renal system function. Because of the multiple physiological effects of the thyroid gland, a deficiency of the T_4 hormone can lead to a complex array of clinical findings.

Localized thyroid disease is the most common cause of hypothyroidism in the United States, namely Hashimoto's autoimmune thyroiditis; worldwide, iodine deficiency is the primary etiology, because this element is a critical component of all thyroid hormones and incorporation of iodide molecules is a critical step in thyroid hormone synthesis. Under normal circumstances, the thyroid secretes 100 to 125 mcg of thyroxine (T_4) per day, but only minute amounts of triiodothyronine (T_3). T_4 is converted to T_3 in peripheral tissues, and T_3 is 20 to 100 times more biologically active than T_4.

When the production of T_4 is inadequate, the thyroid gland enlarges in response to increasing levels of pituitary TSH. This stimulates hypertrophy and hyperplasia of the thyroid gland, resulting in a *goiter*. In addition, deiodinase activity within the thyroid is increased, allowing for greater conversion of T_4 to T_3. Thus, the thyroid attempts to compensate by secreting increased amounts of T_3. However, in areas where the soil and water are deficient in iodine, inadequate substrate exists for these compensatory mechanisms, and endemic goiter results. Thus, a simple (nontoxic) goiter is the most common type of thyroid enlargement.

Hashimoto's thyroiditis is the most common etiology of hypothyroidism in the United States. This autoimmune form of hypothyroidism results when the body pathologically recognizes thyroid antigens as foreign, leading to a chronic immune response involving lymphocytic infiltration, vacuolization, and fibrosis of the parenchyma, which eventually leads to atrophy of the thyroid follicles. Autoantibodies may be undetectable early on in the disease process. However, over the course of the disease, up to 95% of these patients demonstrate serum antibodies to thyroid tissue, including antimicrosomal (antithyroperoxidase) antibodies (95% of patients) and antithyroglobulin antibodies (60% of patients). Over time, however, these autoantibodies usually become undetectable.

Inflammatory hypofunctioning thyroiditis may also result from other etiologies. Destructive thyroid inflammation may occur due to immune cross reactivity after viral infections, producing transient forms of hypothyroidism including de Quervain or painful thyroiditis, as well as subacute thyroiditis. In addition to a painful and tender thyroid gland, these patients are often significantly fatigued. Lymphocytic thyroiditis and transient hypothyroidism also occur in up to 10% of new mothers 2 to 10 months postpartum. This figure may rise as high as 25% in those with other autoimmune conditions such as type 1 DM. Although this condition is usually transient, lasting less than 4 months, and responds well to short courses of thyroid hormone replacement, postpartum thyroiditis predisposes these women to long-term hypothyroidism in the future.

Several iatrogenic causes of hypothyroidism have been recognized. Amiodarone (Cordarone), an iodine-containing antiarrhythmic, is one of the best known offenders because of its direct effects on the thyroid gland. However, both dopamine and lithium are associated with central (secondary or tertiary) hypothyroidism owing to their effects on the hypothalamic-pituitary axis and the secretion of TRH from the hypothalamus or TSH from the pituitary gland. Interferon-α, thalidomide, and the antiretroviral agent stavudine have also been associated with primary hypothyroidism.

Central hypothyroidism may also result from direct impingement by tumors on the pituitary gland (e.g., a pituitary adenoma that fails to produce TSH) or the hypothalamus. Brain irradiation has also been associated with subsequent defects along the hypothalamic-pituitary hormonal axis. However, by far the most common reason for iatrogenic hypothyroidism is the therapeutic result of previously treated hyperthyroidism (see previous section on hyperthyroidism in this chapter). Radioactive iodine treatment (^{131}I, Iodotope), concentrated iodine therapy (SSKI, Lugol solution), therapeutic surgical resection, or treatment for head and neck cancer involving external beam irradiation to the neck or surgical excision of a cancerous mass may all result in permanent hypothyroidism. Thus, these patients require close follow-up to detect clinical or biochemical evidence of hypothyroidism.

Low levels of thyroid hormones affect virtually every bodily system, resulting in an overall decrease in basal metabolic rate. An insufficient amount of thyroid hormone causes abnormalities in lipid metabolism, with an increase in total cholesterol, low-density lipoproteins, and triglycerides. These increases are associated with the development of atherosclerosis and cardiac disease in the hypothyroid patient. The gastrointestinal tract may be slowed in both gastric emptying and intestinal transit time, and gastric parietal cell dysfunction may result in achlorhydria and impaired digestion. Endocrine abnormalities of hypothyroidism include menstrual irregularities, infertility, delayed onset of puberty, and insulin resistance. Adequate amounts of thyroid hormone are also necessary for optimal erythropoiesis, and anemia is common in patients with hypothyroidism. Deficiencies in vitamin B_{12}, iron, and folate may also occur.

A characteristic pathophysiological change of hypothyroidism is the accumulation of hydrophilic proteoglycans within the interstitial space, which causes an increase in interstitial fluid. Pleural, cardiac, and peritoneal effusions are a common result of this process, as is the characteristic mucinous edema seen in long-standing hypothyroidism, known as myxedema. In a general sense, myxedema denotes infiltration of various bodily tissues with glycosaminoglycan substances, which may have widespread effects. In the heart, this infiltration decreases both chronotropy and inotropy, leading to cardiac hypertrophy as the body attempts to compensate for the decreased cardiac output.

Clinical Presentation
Subjective

The clinical presentation of the patient with hypothyroidism varies with the age at onset, duration of illness, and severity of disease. Regardless of the type or cause of hypothyroidism, the signs and symptoms are similar. Because this can be an insidious disease, the early symptoms are often subtle and nonspecific, increasing the risk of a missed diagnosis. The severity of symptoms may be related to the duration of hypothyroidism. A rapid onset of hypothyroidism is associated with more recognizable symptoms than is a gradual onset. The signs and symptoms are directly related to the inadequate amount of thyroid hormone at the peripheral tissue level.

Early classic symptoms include fatigue, dry skin, slight weight gain, cold intolerance, constipation, and heavy menses. Myalgia, muscle cramps, headaches, and weakness may also be present. Later symptoms include very dry skin, coarse hair, loss of lateral eyebrows, alopecia, hoarseness, continued weight gain, slight impairment in mental ability, depression, decreased libido, and hypersomnia. Many of the symptoms are common complaints, which are not specific by themselves but together make up the manifestations of clinical hypothyroidism. Subclinical disease may be even more subtle or asymptomatic.

A complete review of systems is needed because symptoms are often subtle and may involve every body system. The presence of pain and swelling or enlargement in the neck, a history of radiation to the neck, and previous endocrine problems in the past medical history or family history should be elicited. It is also important to obtain a complete medication history, and for women, a complete menstrual history is essential, including the most recent date, characteristics, and duration of last menstrual period. Some findings are more specific for Hashimoto's thyroiditis including painless thyroid enlargement, neck pain, sore throat, feeling of fullness in the throat, low-grade fever, and exhaustion.

Patients with hypothyroidism often experience decreased motility of the gastrointestinal (GI) system, and constipation may be present. Although the exact mechanism of the effect of thyroid hormone on the GI tract is not fully understood, many patients experience atrophic gastritis and pernicious anemia.

Objective

The physical exam should begin with observation of the overall appearance of the patient, noting slow movements and dull facies. The blood pressure, resting pulse, respiratory rate, and weight should be compared with previous exams.

The hair may become coarse and thin, and thinning of eyebrows may occur. Patients with hypothyroidism frequently have a thickened tongue, evident by the indentation of the teeth around the edges. The thyroid may be enlarged and tender or not palpable. The consistency, size of thyroid, and nodules (focal or diffuse) should be noted, as well as any scars present on the neck. A visible goiter may also be present.

The heart may be hypertrophic, which may be assessed by identifying the point of maximal impulse. The patient is usually bradycardic and may have a pericardial effusion.

The lung exam may reveal a pleural effusion. Abdominal exam usually reveals diminished or hypoactive bowel sounds. On neurological exam, the patient may be hypotonic and hyporeflexic with a prolonged relaxation phase and/or ataxic.

The patient with hypothyroidism may have facial puffiness; periorbital edema; dry, coarse, thick skin and hair; brittle nails; slow speech; bradykinesia; hoarseness; large tongue; bradycardia; mild diastolic hypertension; psychological disorders; and pitting edema of the lower extremities. Myxedematous changes occur in the later stage with thickened, scaly, and "doughy" skin, enlarged tongue, muscle weakness, joint complaints, hearing impairments, and ascites. Table 16.5 summarizes the clinical presentation of hypothyroidism.

Diagnostic Reasoning

Diagnostic Tests

Initial Testing   Although there are no universally accepted screening recommendations for hypothyroidism, the American Thyroid Association recommends a baseline screening at 35 years, with close attention to high-risk patients (pregnant women, women older than 60 years, persons with other autoimmune diseases). The American Association of Clinical Endocrinologists recommends checking the TSH in women of childbearing age even before pregnancy and then in the first trimester. The USPSTF does not recommend routine screening in adults without specific reasons. Congenital hypothyroidism is routinely screened for in neonates, as mandated in most states, because not treating hypothyroidism in this group has devastating effects (mental retardation). There is evidence to screen individuals with autoimmune disease, a first degree relative with autoimmune thyroid disease, pernicious anemia, a history of thyroid surgery or neck radiation, an abnormal thyroid exam, a psychiatric diagnosis, and patients taking amiodarone or lithium.

The diagnosis of hypothyroidism is made by measuring serum TSH. TSH and FT_4 should be used to follow treatment. When autoimmune thyroiditis is the suspected underlying cause, it is helpful to confirm this via antithyroid antibody titers, either antimicrosomal antibody (antithyroid peroxidase [TPO] antibody) or antithyroglobulin antibody. The antimicrosomal antibody test is more sensitive and specific. If the TSH is low, inappropriately normal, or insufficiently elevated in the presence of low T_4 values, central hypothyroidism caused by hypothalamic or pituitary disease should be excluded before starting thyroid replacement therapy.

The sensitive thyrotropin assay is the most specific test for diagnosing primary hypothyroidism. A rise in the TSH will precede any other abnormality of thyroid function as the first evidence of primary hypothyroidism. Hypothyroidism caused by primary thyroid failure can be confirmed by a concomitant finding of a decrease in serum FT_4. Patients in an early stage of hypothyroidism may present with an increase in serum TSH together with a normal or low-normal serum FT_4.

By radioimmunoassay, primary hypothyroidism is associated with low FT_4 with an elevated TSH level. The normal range of TSH is 0.35 to 2.5 mIU/L. However, an age adjustment may be needed, because the elderly may have normal values greater than 3 mIU/L. There is general

Table 16.5 Clinical Presentation: Hypothyroidism

Body System	Subjective	Objective
General	Fatigue Lethargy Mild weight gain Cold intolerance Mild depression Decreased libido Hypersomnia Muscle weakness and cramping	Slowing of mental processes Dull facial expression Periorbital puffiness Hypothermia Yellow skin (carotenemia) Facial pallor/swelling (myxedema)
Integumentary	Decreased sweating Hair loss Ankle swelling	Dry, cool, rough skin Alopecia Dry, coarse, thick hair Nonpitting edema
Gastrointestinal	Constipation Nausea	Hypoactive bowel sounds Large tongue Ascites
Neurological	Memory deficits Personality changes	Hyporeflexia Bradykinesia Delayed relaxation of reflexes Slowing of mental processes
Cardiopulmonary	Inability to exercise	Bradycardia Cardiac enlargement Pleural effusion
Genitourinary	Menorrhagia, irregular menses	Decrease in fertility
Head and neck	Enlargement of the neck	Enlarged tongue (late) Hoarseness

agreement that a TSH level above 10 mIU/L should be treated in patients with primary hypothyroidism. Levels of 4.5 to 10 mIU/L have varied recommendations. Absent cardiovascular disease, there are no outcome data to suggest that treatment for levels between 2.5 and 4.5 mIU/L is beneficial. An elevated TSH (up to 15–20 mIU/L) may be temporarily seen in euthyroid patients with a systemic illness. In this situation, the TSH and T_4 should be repeated in 2 to 3 weeks for confirmation. Patients with secondary or tertiary (central) hypothyroidism show a low, normal, or mildly elevated TSH level with low FT_4 and T_3 by radioimmunoassay. The laboratory values for patients with subclinical hypothyroidism show a mildly increased TSH (4.5–10 mIU/L) with a normal FT_4 level. Measurement of free T_4 is always preferred over total T_4, owing to alterations in hormone protein binding that may result in large fluctuations in total serum T_4 levels. Free thyroxine index (FTI), although not the test of choice, may be used because not all laboratories have the capacity to measure FT_4. FTI uses a T_3 resin uptake test to calculate the percentage of hormone binding sites available and multiplies this by the total T_4 level to give an estimation of the free T_4 level.

The antimicrosomal antibody (anti-TPO antibody) is diagnostic for Hashimoto's thyroiditis when found in high titers (1:400). The degree of elevation of this antibody correlates directly with clinical hypothyroidism. When hypothyroidism is present for a long period of time, the antibody titers fall. The antithyroglobulin antibody is also increased, but it is not as specific for Hashimoto's thyroiditis. If no antibodies are identified at the time of diagnosis, the condition is called *idiopathic hypothyroidism,* a form of autoimmune thyroiditis. The antimicrosomal antibody should also be evaluated in patients with repeat miscarriages.

Medications such as metoclopramide (Reglan) increase the TSH level. Dopamine (Intropin), glucocorticoids, NSAIDs, and somatostatin decrease the TSH level. Other medications, such as phenytoin (Dilantin), amiodarone (Cordarone), and lithium carbonate, can also affect thyroid function tests. Smoking (nicotine) can also affect thyroid hormone levels. There are many mechanisms by which medications affect thyroid function. The drug may bind with albumin and displace the thyroid hormones off the carrier proteins, or it may prevent albumin from binding with T_3 or T_4, in each case resulting in more active hormones in circulation. Some drugs may cause an upregulation in processing proteins (different cytochrome P oxidase isomers). These normally inactivate thyroid hormones, so the upregulation can lead to more rapid processing of thyroid hormones, in turn, affecting TSH levels.

Subsequent Testing Once a diagnosis of hypothyroidism is confirmed, additional testing may be necessary to determine the effect of the disease on other body systems. Because T_3 is nonspecific and not sensitive, it is not routinely used as an initial diagnostic tool. In the early stages of hypothyroidism, T_3 levels may be normal because of TSH-induced hyperstimulation. T_3 levels may not fall until late in the disease. Because the T_3 level correlates well with clinical status, the patient will not be as severely hypothyroid clinically until the T_3 falls to significantly low levels. In addition, the T_3 level may be below normal or elevated in patients with chronic disease.

Because anemia is a frequent complication of hypothyroidism, a complete blood count should be done. A complete blood chemistry profile should be done to assess for alterations in electrolytes, blood urea nitrogen, creatinine, serum osmolarity, and glucose, because a decreased glomerular filtration rate (affecting renal function) can occur. A complete urinalysis should also be performed, with specific attention to the presence of protein (indicating possible renal impairment). Changes in the chemistries may be an indication of deteriorating thyroid function leading to myxedema.

Patients with mild to moderate hypothyroidism have a tendency to develop hypertension (especially diastolic hypertension); therefore, the blood pressure should be monitored. Interestingly, patients with long-standing or severe hypothyroidism tend to be normotensive or hypotensive. Depression of the biosynthesis of cholesterol causes a decreased rate of cholesterol catabolism and leads to hypercholesterolemia. These patients tend to have elevated triglycerides and elevated low-density lipoprotein cholesterol. The combination of hypertension and hyperlipidemia increases the risk of atherosclerotic heart disease in a hypothyroid patient. Thus, an annual lipid profile and an electrocardiogram (ECG) should be done. As the cardiac system continues to deteriorate, the ECG may show nonspecific ST- and T-wave changes or low-voltage QRS complexes.

Unless there is reason to suspect a nodule or to confirm multinodular goiter, radioactive iodine scans and uptake are not usually necessary. As part of the complete examination, patients should have an annual chest x-ray exam to rule out the complications of hypothyroidism, including cardiomegaly, congestive heart failure, and pleural effusion.

Ultrasound studies of the thyroid may be useful if a nodular thyroid is detected or if infiltrative disease is suspected (amyloidosis, sarcoidosis, or tuberculosis). Fine-needle aspiration is indicated for suspicious nodules, which may be found in patients with hypothyroidism, hyperthyroidism, or euthyroidism. In fact, 5% to 6% of isolated nodules are malignant, especially larger ones, and ultrasound may reveal suspicious findings such as irregular margins or microcalcifications.

Differential Diagnosis

Marked variations in TSH may occur in the setting of an acute illness or psychiatric disorder when the body's metabolic demands are altered. TSH levels normally peak in the evening and are at their lowest in the afternoon. Nonthyroid illness is often associated with decreased TSH, T_3, and free T_4 levels without clinical hypothyroidism, with a reduction in the conversion of T_3 from T_4. In addition, usually the TSH level is normal or mildly increased during recovery from nonthyroid illness.

In euthyroid hypothyroxinemia, the patient is euthyroid with a decreased T_4 level due to increased thyroid-binding globulin concentration caused by nephrotic syndrome, exogenous testosterone, or high-dose steroids. Also, drugs that inhibit T_4 binding, such as phenytoin, phenobarbital, and salicylates, may decrease the total T_4 level.

Management

The goal of thyroid hormone replacement in primary hypothyroidism is to normalize, not suppress, the TSH. Suppressed TSH, particularly in postmenopausal women or individuals with levothyroxine overreplacement, causes decreased bone mineral density after several years, leading to osteoporosis. The replacement goal in central hypothyroidism is to normalize the FT_4 because the TSH is not reliable. Hypothyroidism is typically treated medically; however, surgery may be indicated for particularly large, nonfunctional goiters that impair tracheoesophageal functioning.

Management of Hypothyroidism

The treatment for hypothyroidism is the daily administration of thyroid hormone to restore the patient to a euthyroid state (see Drugs Commonly Prescribed 16.2: Hypothyroidism). The usual medication is levothyroxine (Synthroid, Levothroid, Levoxyl), a synthetic preparation of T_4, which has generally replaced a desiccated thyroid preparation. Levothyroxine preparations are manufactured in numerous dosages, allowing for specific, precise titration to meet individual patient requirements.

According to the medical guidelines developed by the American Association of Clinical Endocrinologists, the usual dose is 1.6 mcg/kg per day for full replacement. Healthy patients younger than age 60 years may receive 50 to 100 mcg daily (full replacement dose). Patients who are older or have coronary artery disease should begin with one-half of the expected replacement dose or 25 to 50 mcg/day PO, increasing the dose gradually by 25 mcg/day once every 4 to 6 weeks. The TSH level should be measured every 4 to 8 weeks after initiating therapy and before each dosage increase. The common dosage is 75 to 150 mcg/day. Dosing is best done in the morning to avoid nighttime insomnia. Many other medications and mineral supplements interfere with GI absorption, including iron, calcium carbonate, aluminum hydroxide, sucralfate, and tube feedings. Thus, these medications require separation

Drugs Commonly Prescribed 16.2   Hypothyroidism: Lifelong Pharmaceutical Treatment

Drug	Indications	Adverse Reactions and Prescribing Considerations
Synthetic L-thyroxine* T_4 (Levothroid, Levoxyl, Synthroid)	Patients with increased TSH level, usually three times the upper limit of the assay. Overt hypothyroidism, lifelong pharmaceutical treatment. Goal: To give enough thyroid supplement orally to result in normal free T_4 and TSH levels.	Monitor antihyperglycemics, oral anticoagulants, and potential sympathomimetics. Wait 4–5 hours after cholestyramine ingestion. Not to be prescribed for obesity. Use with caution in patients with cardiovascular disease, diabetes, adrenal insufficiency. Increased sensitivity in myxedema and severe hypothyroidism. Start with the lowest dose and increase by 0.025 mg/day every 3–6 weeks to a maximum of 0.3 mg per day. Older adults require a beginning dose slightly lower.

*Synthetic T_3 supplements (Cytomel) are not recommended as a drug of choice.

of dosing in time, whereas patients receiving continuous tube feedings require IV thyroxine dosing.

Replacement with T_3 preparations (liothyronine [Cytomel, Triostat]) is usually not indicated; however, anecdotal reports exist that indicated combination T_3/T_4 therapy may be helpful in patients who do not respond adequately to T_4 replacement alone. Although T_3 is better absorbed via the GI tract than T_4, the appropriate ratio of triiodothyronine preparations versus thyroxine in combination therapy has not been well established, and such treatment decisions require expert input from an endocrinologist.

Another treatment of historical importance that is still used today in some settings owing to its relative lower cost is desiccated bovine thyroid (Armour Thyroid). Obtained from pooled thyroid extracts from cows, these preparations contain multiple foreign antigens, and the specific levels of active hormone are difficult to control. Some manufacturers standardize preparations based on bioassays, whereas others use iodine content as a surrogate measure of activity. T_3 and T_4 are both present, usually in a 1:4 ratio. Although some older patients who have been treated for many years with desiccated thyroid are wary of changing medications after decades of replacement therapy at stable doses, few clinicians in the United States will start new patients on these preparations. They should not be used for patients with underlying cardiac disease given the varied concentrations of highly active T_3, which poses a greater risk of overreplacement and iatrogenic thyrotoxicosis.

Regardless of choice of replacement therapy, all patients should be monitored for signs of thyrotoxicity, especially angina pectoris and arrhythmias, because optimizing thyroid replacement dosing can be difficult and time consuming. If significant adverse symptoms occur during levothyroxine replacement, the dose should be decreased and the patient should be referred to an endocrinologist for evaluation before reattempting replacement therapy at the original higher dose.

Concurrent severe illness or major surgery may alter dosing requirements in either direction in the hypothyroid patient. Pregnancy is also well known to increase replacement therapy requirements. Some clinicians suggest increasing replacement dosing by 30% on confirmation of pregnancy with subsequent adjustments per TSH levels, because untreated hypothyroidism in pregnancy is associated with preeclampsia, postpartum cardiac dysfunction, anemia, miscarriage, and low birth weight. The levothyroxine dose should be returned to the prepregnancy dose after delivery, and a serum TSH level should be obtained 6 to 8 weeks postpartum.

Untreated hypothyroidism may progress steadily for 10 to 15 years before resulting in *myxedema coma*—a life-threatening state of multiorgan failure, characterized by progressive respiratory depression, decreased cardiac output, and fluid and electrolyte abnormalities (including hyponatremia)—or even death. Box 16.1 presents the assessment and management of patients with myxedema coma.

Management of Subclinical Hypothyroidism

Treatment for subclinical hypothyroidism has varied recommendations. The American Thyroid Association and the American Association of Clinical Endocrinologists recommend treating subclinical disease when there is presence of antithyroid antibodies, when evidence of atherosclerotic cardiovascular disease exists, when heart failure exists, or if the patient is symptomatic at this TSH level.

Box 16.1   Assessment and Management of Myxedema Coma

Untreated hypothyroidism may progress steadily for 10–15 years before resulting in myxedema coma (a life-threatening condition characterized by progressive respiratory depression, decreased cardiac output, and fluid and electrolyte abnormalities) or death. Myxedema coma is severe hypothyroidism, most commonly seen in older adult women, presenting with altered mental status (profound lethargy or coma), hypothermia, bradycardia, hypoventilation, hypoglycemia, and adrenal insufficiency. It is usually triggered by a precipitating factor such as noncompliance with levothyroxine therapy, ingestion of narcotics or analgesics, sepsis, cerebrovascular accident (stroke), myocardial infarction, trauma, or severe stress. The mortality rate can be greater than 50% despite emergency medical intervention.

Assessment
The patient is usually pale with periorbital edema, dry skin, decreased temperature, macroglossia, distant heart sounds, bradycardia, and delayed deep tendon reflexes. The patient may have hyponatremia, seizures, and hypotension, with secondary respiratory acidosis, hypoxia, retention of CO_2. Clinical diagnosis, not laboratory diagnosis, is required; T_4 is usually low, and TSH is high.

Management
Give ventilatory support if indicated, treat hypothermia, and give levothyroxine (Synthroid, Levothroid) IV 300–500 mcg over 15 minutes; then IV 100 mcg every 24 hours to bring thyroxine concentrations back to normal quickly. Glucocorticoids should also be administered until coexistent adrenal insufficiency can be ruled out. Hydrocortisone hemisuccinate 100 mg IV bolus is initially given, followed by 50 mg IV every 12 hours or 25 mg IV every 6 hours until plasma cortisol level is confirmed as normal. Administer IV hydration to correct hypotension and hypoglycemia (if present). Avoid overhydration because clearance of free water is impaired in these patients. Rule out and treat precipitating factors (if septic, treat with antibiotics). Patients with myxedema coma need emergency medical intervention and should be treated by an endocrinologist in an intensive care setting.

Some patients with subclinical hypothyroidism feel better when treated with levothyroxine. Medication therapy has potentially dangerous adverse effects but may improve subtle abnormalities, prevent goiterous growth, and prevent the development of frank hypothyroidism. Therapy is advisable especially if thyroid autoantibodies are positive, because overt hypothyroidism frequently develops.

In young patients or patients with goiter, consider initiating levothyroxine therapy. If the decision is made not to treat these patients, they should be evaluated at 6- to 12-month intervals for evidence of more severe clinical and biological loss of thyroid function. A lower dose (0.5–1.0 mcg/kg) could be given in the treatment of subclinical hypothyroidism. If the diagnosis of hypothyroidism is uncertain in a patient who is already on levothyroxine, the dose can be reduced by one-half, and the FT_4 and TSH levels can be reassessed in 6 to 8 weeks. If the TSH level is increasing, the patient should resume the previous dose. If the TSH is normal, the patient should discontinue the levothyroxine, and the TSH level should be rechecked in 6 to 8 weeks for any increase.

Follow-up and Referral

After therapy has been initiated with levothyroxine, the practitioner should check the patient's levothyroxine levels in 4 to 8 weeks by evaluating the TSH level to determine whether adjustment of the levothyroxine dose is necessary. The target TSH level is 0.3 to 2.4 mIU/L. Increasing the levothyroxine dose more often than at 6-week intervals will probably lead to overreplacement.

Once a stable dose of levothyroxine has been established, the TSH level in primary hypothyroidism or the FT_4 level in central hypothyroidism can be checked biannually or annually.

The patient should be examined annually for manifestations of thyrotoxicity (e.g., tachycardia, nervousness, or tremor) before increasing dosages. Laboratory values (FT_4 and TSH levels) within normal limits and a satisfactory clinical exam suggest that treatment is adequate. For maintenance treatment, the medication should be titrated to the lowest dosage required to maintain euthyroidism, with a normal TSH and a normal or slightly elevated T_4.

Undetectable TSH levels suggest overtreatment; medication should be decreased in these patients. TSH levels greater than 10 mIU/L indicate undertreatment, and medication should be increased.

Referral to an endocrinologist is necessary if the patient has cardiac disease, symptoms of myxedema, or central (secondary or tertiary) hypothyroidism. After starting hormone replacement therapy, if signs or symptoms of myxedema, chest pain, or thyrotoxicosis occur, the endocrinologist should be consulted. These patients are at high risk for serious complications related to hypothyroidism or its treatment. Hypothyroid patients with severe illness or those who present with unusual or confusing laboratory findings should be referred to an endocrinologist. Referral to an endocrinologist is indicated in patients younger than age 18 years, when there is evidence of pituitary disease, in pregnant and postpartum patients, and in those taking lithium or amiodarone (Cordarone).

For asymptomatic patients with subclinical hypothyroidism who (after consultation) are not being treated with medication, a TSH should be performed yearly, along with a focused history and physical exam.

Patient Education

During the follow-up visits, emphasis should be placed on compliance with lifelong thyroid replacement therapy (if indicated), reviewing the symptoms of hypothyroidism and hyperthyroidism, and stressing the importance of follow-up.

Instructions should be simple and repeated frequently with written information in the patient's primary language. An older adult or patient with decreased mental status or depression with hypothyroidism may need additional emotional support, reinforcement, and follow-up teaching. Support in the home setting may be necessary until the symptoms of slowed mental processes and depression abate. Initially, a family member may be needed to remind the patient to take his or her daily dose of medication.

Patients should be encouraged to wear an extra layer of clothing if they have cold intolerance and should be warned not to use a heating pad. Patients with diminished mental status and slowed responses may be at risk for burns. If psychomotor symptoms are present, the patient should be cautioned against operating dangerous machinery or driving a motor vehicle until the symptoms have resolved.

Because heredity is implicated in hypothyroidism, patients with children should be instructed to advise their child's primary-care provider of their diagnosis.

Patients who are at high risk for hypothyroidism (those who have had thyroid surgery, radioactive iodine treatments, history of thyroiditis, and postpartum women) should be taught the common symptoms of hypothyroidism (lethargy, fatigue, cold intolerance, constipation, weight gain, dry skin). The patient and family should also be instructed that hypothyroidism is a chronic, sometimes progressive disease requiring monitoring every 6 to 12 months. Patients and their families should be reassured that as the treatment progresses, the symptoms will resolve.

Practitioners are encouraged to write prescriptions that do not allow substitution and use the same brand for the patient throughout treatment. The same brand of thyroid preparation is recommended because the bioavailability, stability, and content of the medication may vary with the different brands. Patients should be given the rationale for treatment, adverse effects, and dosage for their medication. Emphasis should be on the fact that medication use is lifelong. The patient needs to understand that as the body ages or there are changes in body weight, the dosage of medication may need to be adjusted.

The patient should be taught the signs of hyperthyroidism (thyrotoxicity) in the event of thyroid replacement overdosage—for example, nervousness, palpitations, insomnia, and tremor. It is important to explain that it will take 1 to 2 weeks for the medication to be effective. During this time, patients may experience an increase in urination and a decrease in periorbital puffiness.

The Patient's Voice 16.1
One Patient's Story

I had pretty much a normal life. I was working in an administrative job, was in a bad relationship, and was perimenopausal. I would get home from work and it was a struggle to make dinner and clean up. I was exhausted all the time. I had trouble getting out of bed in the morning even after going to bed at 7:00 p.m.! On the weekends I would sleep for 14 hours a night and still wake up tired. At meetings, where I had once been quick with suggestions, I couldn't seem to think and put two sentences together. I had trouble finding the right words. I thought I was getting early Alzheimer's.

I was 50 years old, and I felt like 100! I was constipated, cold all the time, and in a mental fog every day. I saw my primary-care provider. She told me I was probably depressed because of my life situation and being perimenopausal and prescribed an antidepressant. After taking that for more than a month, I was not feeling any better and saw a different provider. That provider did a bunch of tests and a thyroid-stimulating hormone (TSH) assay was one of them. The results were through the roof. My thyroid was almost entirely shut down. If someone had just done the test earlier, I could have been spared a few years of total exhaustion.

The absorption of levothyroxine from the GI tract may be slowed by concurrent use of certain drugs, such as ferrous sulfate, sucralfate (Carafate), or antacids. The dose of thyroid hormone should be taken 2 hours before or 4 hours after ingestion of these medications. Because levothyroxine supplements may increase blood glucose levels, patients with DM should carefully monitor their blood sugar levels; their dose of insulin or oral hypoglycemic agents may need to be adjusted. Thyroid hormones may also affect the levels of phenytoin (Dilantin), lithium, tricyclic antidepressants, estrogen, digitalis, anticoagulants, and indomethacin (Indocin). The appropriate blood tests and screenings should be performed, and patients should be instructed on the important adverse reactions to report should they occur.

Because of increased sensitivity to certain medications in hypothyroid patients, patients should be cautioned against the use of analgesics and sedatives. Even in small dosages, these medications can cause severe somnolence and respiratory depression. Infrequently, a patient with normal TSH levels may continue to feel fatigued but should be discouraged from increasing the dose of medication, which some patients may be tempted to do. This symptom warrants further investigation as to the underlying cause and should be discussed during a clinic visit. In cases where patient compliance may be a problem, weekly dosages can be given, because the half-life of T_4 is approximately 1 week.

Patients should be taught to follow a healthy diet, with an emphasis on low-fat, high-fiber foods. Some patients may need to follow a diet that promotes weight loss once medication has been started. Because many patients with hypothyroidism experience constipation, they should increase their intake of raw fruits and vegetables and bran or high-fiber cereals and breads, and add unprocessed bran (two tablespoons/day) to cereal or liquids. A bulk-forming laxative containing psyllium may be taken on a daily basis. Increasing water intake to six to eight glasses a day is often beneficial in reducing constipation, as is increasing physical activity. A low-fat diet is recommended because there is a high incidence of atherosclerotic heart disease in patients with hypothyroidism.

Once therapy with levothyroxine is initiated, the patient should be able to resume all previous activities. Initially, rest periods with a gradual increase in exercise and activity, as tolerated, may be indicated. The patient must be instructed that if he or she develops any signs or symptoms of cardiac or respiratory difficulty, it is essential to seek immediate medical attention.

■ THYROID CANCER

Thyroid cancer is classified as differentiated (papillary and follicular) and undifferentiated (medullary and anaplastic). Most thyroid cancers (60%) are papillary, 20% are follicular, and the remaining tumors are medullary or anaplastic. Medullary thyroid cancer is more likely to be familial. Anaplastic tumors are the fastest growing of all thyroid neoplasms; they are more common in older adults and are associated with a high mortality rate. A rare type of thyroid cancer is non-Hodgkin's lymphoma, which should be considered in persons with a rapidly growing goiter. Hürthle cell carcinoma is a rare type of thyroid malignancy (2%–3% of thyroid cancers) that is often considered a variant of follicular carcinoma. Consisting almost exclusively of Hürthle cells (also called oxyphilic or oncocytic cells) that contain abundant granular acidophilic cytoplasm, these malignancies are highly aggressive, metastasize in more than half of cases, and are difficult to follow because they do not respond to TSH or take up radioiodine.

Epidemiology and Causes

Thyroid cancer is the most common endocrine-related cancer. The incidence of thyroid cancer in the United States is small, with only 0.4% of the population diagnosed with this type of cancer; however, 13% of people in the United States are found to have thyroid cancer on autopsy. Most thyroid cancers are small and slow growing. Thyroid cancer accounts for 0.5% of all cancer deaths per year. The incidence increases with age, and it is more common in adults aged 20 to 54 years, but it can occur at any age.

Thyroid cancer is more common in women than in men (3:1). Thyroid nodules found in persons younger than 20 years of age or initially found in adults older than age 60 years are more likely to be cancerous. Nodules are often found on routine physical examinations, by the patient, or during imaging for other purposes.

The major risk factor for development of thyroid cancer is exposure to ionizing radiation. Several historical incidents resulting in high-dose radiation exposure have been linked to an increased incidence of thyroid papillary malignancies in children, including the atomic bombings of the Japanese cities of Hiroshima and Nagasaki, military atomic testing near the Marshall Islands, and the nuclear power plant meltdown in the Russian city of Chernobyl. Moreover, until the 1950s, radiation treatments were given to children for an enlarged thymus, enlarged tonsils, and acne. It is estimated that 1 to 2 million individuals were exposed to this risk factor. Studies have estimated that one-third of patients who received radiation therapy to the head and neck will develop a thyroid nodule, and one-third of these patients will later develop a malignancy. It may be advisable for patients who received head and neck irradiation as children to have an ultrasound for screening purposes.

Importantly, low-dose radiation exposure associated with routine radiographic imaging studies has not been shown to be tumorigenic. Interestingly, ^{131}I radioablation therapy for thyrotoxicosis and high-dose external beam radiotherapy have also not been associated with papillary thyroid carcinoma, presumably because of the greater amount of cellular apoptosis associated with these doses of radiation.

There is also an increased incidence of follicular and anaplastic thyroid carcinoma in areas where iodine deficiency and goiter are more prevalent. Thyroid cancer is also more common in persons with autoimmune disease. Medullary carcinoma is an inherited form of thyroid cancer, with 90% of those inheriting the autosomal dominant gene ultimately developing cancer.

Metastatic cancer of the thyroid is less common, but renal cancer, breast cancer, lung cancer, and malignant melanoma may metastasize to the thyroid gland.

Pathophysiology

Though thyroid carcinomas are relatively rare in the United States, benign thyroid disease is significantly more common. An estimated 4% to 7% of the general population develops thyroid nodules; although the vast majority of these represent benign disease, it is estimated that 5% to 6% of isolated nodules are malignant. Thus, distinguishing malignant from nonmalignant cases requires careful clinical evaluation.

As with all types of cancer, thyroid cancer is believed to develop from a series of mutational events producing a cell that is genetically different from its source. This explains the strong association of thyroid cancer with radiation exposure, which increases the incidence of DNA mutation and transformation of normal thyroid cells into malignant clones. Similarly, germline mutations in the RET proto-oncogene have been associated with the inherited cancer syndromes multiple endocrine neoplasia (MEN) 2A, MEN 2B, familial adenomatous polyposis, and familial medullary thyroid carcinoma (FMTC) syndrome—all of which are associated with medullary thyroid carcinoma.

Thyroid cancers range from those that are well differentiated and slow growing to those that are poorly differentiated and aggressive. As with other malignancies, poorly differentiated thyroid cancers have an unfavorable prognosis. Cancers of the thyroid gland are typically classified into primary and secondary (metastatic) tumors. Primary tumors include papillary (80% of cases), follicular (10% of cases), anaplastic (2% of cases), and medullary tumors (5%–10% of cases), and rarely primary thyroid lymphomas (2%–5% of cases) and sarcomas. Papillary, follicular, and anaplastic tumors derive from the endodermally derived thyroxine- and thyroglobulin-producing follicular epithelium, whereas medullary tumors arise from the neuroendocrine-derived parafollicular or C cells. Thyroid lymphomas arise from intrathyroid lymph tissue and are strongly associated with chronic lymphocytic thyroiditis (Hashimoto's autoimmune thyroiditis), whereas sarcomas are derived from the vascular and connective tissue interwoven throughout the thyroid gland.

Clinical Presentation

Subjective

The major symptom of thyroid cancer is a lump or nodule in the neck, which is usually painless. Patients may also complain of a tight or full feeling in the neck, difficulty breathing or swallowing, hoarseness, hemoptysis, and swollen lymph nodes. New onset of hoarseness with hemoptysis is strongly suggestive of a malignant growth. Progressive dysphagia and shortness of breath may indicate invasiveness. Pain in the neck is usually a late symptom. History may reveal exposure to radiation as a child.

Objective

From 4% to 7% of the U.S. population have a palpable thyroid nodule, making clinical examination of the thyroid an ineffective method of screening. Differentiated thyroid carcinomas most commonly present as a thyroid mass or nodule. Although malignant neoplasms are more likely to be fixed, nontender, firm, and irregular in shape, only a biopsy can rule in malignancy. The physical exam should include examination of the tongue, oropharynx, and cervical spine for swelling, nodules, or tenderness.

Diagnostic Reasoning

Although there are some typical presentations of benign versus malignant nodules of the thyroid, many malignant lesions have an atypical presentation. A biopsy is the only reliable method of differentiating a benign from a malignant lesion; therefore on palpation of a nodule, the patient should be referred for evaluation and probable biopsy. Early referral of patients with nodules to an endocrinologist for evaluation and treatment reduces costs, decreases patient hospital time, and increases the precision of the diagnosis.

Nodules that develop in men, in persons younger than age 20 years or older than age 60 years, in persons with a family history of thyroid cancer, or in those with a personal history of exposure to radiation are suggestive of malignancy. Malignant growths are more likely to be irregular in shape, fixed, firm, and nontender. Multiple nodules of the same consistency are more likely to be benign. Fewer than 5% of nodules are malignant. The prognosis is good for thyroid cancer that is found early, is less than 2 cm in diameter, is of a favorable histological type, and has not invaded locally or metastasized.

Diagnostic Tests

Initial Testing   High-resolution ultrasonography is beneficial in identifying thyroid nodules but is not reliable in differentiating a benign from a malignant lesion. It is indicated when there is suspicion of multinodular disease or when the thyroid is difficult to evaluate clinically.

Subsequent Testing   A fine-needle aspiration (FNA) biopsy is usually successful in differentiating a benign from cancerous lesion of the thyroid gland and has an 83% sensitivity and a 92% specificity. Thus, the FNA will not capture all cases, and repeat biopsy may be necessary. The sensitivity of FNA is increased when it is ultrasound guided. Nondiagnostic FNA biopsies may require surgical lobectomy to confirm that the nodule is not in fact malignant. Psammoma bodies are found in 50% of papillary carcinomas; they are circular, laminated bodies found in the stroma of the tumor.

Elevated serum calcitonin is a strong tumor marker of medullary thyroid carcinoma, but these cancers are somewhat rare overall, so this test is not usually used in the initial work-up. For the inherited cancer syndromes MEN 2A, MEN 2B, and FMTC, polymerase chain reaction assays are used to detect germline mutations in the *RET* oncogene. Radioiodine uptake testing is a means of determining functionality of a thyroid nodule.

Computed tomography and magnetic resonance imaging are used when the tumor is large or recurrent or when there is expected extrathyroidal extension of the tumor, but these are not helpful for evaluation of a simple, isolated nodule. However, they can be used to assess for distant metastases and regional lymph node involvement. Spread to lymph nodes is more common with papillary than with follicular carcinomas; if metastasis does occur, lung and bone are the most common sites. Interestingly, lymph node metastases are not an important prognostic factor, but distant metastasis is associated with a nearly 70-fold increase in death.

Thyroid neoplasms are often painless, and thyroid function tests may show levels within the normal range unless the patient has thyroiditis.

Differential Diagnosis

Differential diagnoses include lymphocytic thyroiditis, multinodular goiter, benign thyroid nodule, cystic nodules, and regional lymphadenopathy. Mass-related effects may be similar to those associated with laryngeal or other forms of neck cancer (e.g., dysphagia or hoarseness due to recurrent laryngeal nerve involvement with vocal cord paralysis, hemoptysis due to local invasion through the trachea).

If medullary thyroid carcinoma is diagnosed, it is critical to take a thorough family history to assess whether this presentation occurs as a component of several inherited cancer syndromes, including MEN 2A or Sipple syndrome (which may present with concurrent pheochromocytoma and hyperparathyroidism), MEN 2B (which may present with concurrent pheochromocytoma, tall and slender Marfanoid body habitus, and ganglioneuromas), and FMTC syndrome.

Management

Initial Management

Any swelling suggestive of malignancy should be referred for evaluation of the mass. A surgeon and an oncologist (possibly a radiation or medical oncologist) will be necessary for determination of the diagnosis and treatment plan. Thyroidectomy or near-total thyroidectomy is the treatment of choice. The decision is based on the type of tumor, the size, and whether the tumor is compressing other structures. A surgeon with expertise in thyroid surgery should perform the procedure because of the potential of damage to the laryngeal nerves and the parathyroid glands. For small, noninvasive tumors, some surgeons prefer to perform a lobectomy, a more conservative approach. However, if there is local invasion, there is a greater possibility of recurrence. Radical neck surgery may be indicated for tumors with extensive local invasion.

Subsequent Management

After a total thyroidectomy, patients are often treated with radioactive iodine therapy to ablate any remnant thyroid tissue. Thyroid replacement therapy is initiated to suppress TSH to a goal of 0.1 mIU/L, and patients are monitored closely for response to therapy. They are subsequently followed every 6 to 12 months by an endocrinologist. A thorough neck exam, a chest x-ray exam, and physical exam are performed with observations for thyrotoxicosis. Thyroglobulin levels may also be measured for well-differentiated carcinomas. The endocrinologist may perform a follow-up ^{131}I scan 6 to 12 months after a total thyroidectomy and may initiate further radioactive iodine ablation therapy if indicated. A follow-up ^{131}I scan is not useful in medullary cancer because medullary carcinoma does not take up the radioactive isotope.

Some forms of malignancy have unique treatments. In addition to thyroidectomy and postoperative radiation therapy, thyroid lymphomas may also require chemotherapy directed by a medical oncologist. Sarcomas are particularly aggressive and, after thyroidectomy, are poorly responsive to chemotherapy and carry a poor prognosis.

Long-term prognosis of thyroid malignancy depends on cell type of tumor, size of the primary growth, gender (men are twice as likely to die from thyroid cancer as women), age at diagnosis (death is more common in those diagnosed younger than 20 years or older than 40 years of age), and extent of metastasis at the time of excision. Fortunately, papillary thyroid cancer is rarely fatal.

Follow-up and Referral

Follow-up is directed by the knowledge that no single diagnostic tool is sufficient to evaluate for recurrent disease. The follow-up of patients who have been treated for thyroid cancer includes periodic clinical exams, serum thyroglobulin measurements, chest x-ray films, and ultrasound examination to assess for recurrence. The patient is followed more closely during the first 3 to 4 years after surgery because recurrence is more likely within this time.

The patient with a total thyroidectomy will require thyroid hormone replacement for life. See Management of Hypothyroidism for specific guidelines.

Patients with medullary carcinoma MEN2 should be offered RET (rearranged during transcription) proto-oncogene testing. Provided the mutation is identified, all first-degree relatives should be offered the RET mutation analysis as well.

Patient Education

Patients with a family history of thyroid cancer should be advised to perform a "neck check" monthly. Patients with a history of goiter or irradiation should also perform this screening technique. The check is performed at home with a glass of water and a handheld mirror. The patient should be instructed to hold the mirror to visualize the area between the Adam's apple and clavicle. Then the head should be tilted backward, enough to adequately visualize the area without producing coughing or choking. As a sip of water is taken and swallowed, the patient should observe the area for any bulging. The maneuver should be repeated several times. Any signs of bulging should be reported immediately. Free copies of the *Neck Check* can be obtained at www.thyca.org/download/document/287/NeckCheckCard.pdf.

■ CUSHING'S SYNDROME

Cushing's syndrome includes a myriad of symptoms and physical features produced by persistent inappropriate hypercortisolemia. The condition was named after Harvey Cushing, a physician who found pituitary adenomas in six of eight patients with symptoms of adrenocortical hyperfunctioning in 1932. Cushing's syndrome may be caused by cortisol hypersecretion by the adrenal cortex due to cortical hypertrophy or to a tumor of the adrenal gland. However, the prolonged administration of large doses of exogenous glucocorticoid hormones will also cause this cluster of signs and symptoms and simulate disordered adrenal function. The term *Cushing's disease* refers specifically to pituitary adrenocorticotropic hormone (ACTH) excess caused by a pituitary tumor (adenoma), which, in turn, causes oversecretion of cortisol by the adrenal gland and is a form of Cushing's syndrome.

Epidemiology and Causes

Cushing's syndrome may be classified mechanistically as ACTH-dependent or ACTH-independent hypercortisolemic states. The former mechanism results in adrenocortical hyperplasia and is most frequently due to an ACTH-secreting pituitary adenoma (70% of cases). Known as Cushing's disease, this condition occurs more commonly in women. The tumors are usually small (microadenomas) and may not be recognizable on pituitary imaging, with some patients demonstrating only hyperplasia of pituitary corticotrophs. Fewer than 10% of affected patients have a tumor greater than 10 mm in diameter. The tumors are not encapsulated and present in the anterior pituitary gland. Spontaneous cases of Cushing's syndrome are rare, occurring in 2.6 persons per 1,000,000 per year. Malignant pituitary tumors are, fortunately, rare.

Nonpituitary tumors account for ectopic ACTH secretion in 10% to 15% of ACTH-dependent cases of Cushing's syndrome. In contrast, excessive administration of exogenous ACTH and ectopic secretion of corticotropin-releasing hormone (CRH) by nonhypothalamic tumors each account for less than 1% of ACTH-hypersecretion cases.

The majority of ACTH-independent cases of Cushing's syndrome are due to iatrogenic administration of glucocorticoid hormones for therapeutic purposes. However, tumors of the adrenal cortex account for up to 20% of ACTH-independent cases, and both micronodular and macronodular dysplasia of the adrenal gland have been observed, although these etiologies are both quite rare, accounting for fewer than 1% of cases.

Pathophysiology

A basic knowledge of the hypothalamic-pituitary-adrenal neurohormonal axis is required to properly understand the pathophysiology of Cushing's syndrome. Ultimately regulated by the central nervous system, CRH is first produced by the hypothalamus and released into the hypophyseal portal circulation, where it stimulates the production of proopiomelanocortin (POMC) by corticotrophs in the anterior pituitary gland, from which ACTH (also called corticotropin) is derived as a cleavage product. ACTH then acts directly on the adrenal cortex to stimulate the production of cortisol and other adrenal hormones that act at peripheral tissue sites as intranuclear transcription factors for steroid-responsive genes. Cortisol is then metabolized by the liver and kidneys,

and its breakdown products are secreted in the urine as 17-hydroxycorticosteroids, 17-ketogenic steroids, and 17-ketosteroids.

A key regulatory mechanism of this neuroendocrine axis is the negative feedback exerted by each downstream product on its preceding hormone—namely, the inhibitory effects of ACTH on CRH secretion, as well as serum cortisol on the secretion of ACTH and CRH at the level of the pituitary and hypothalamus, respectively. The pituitary is also likely subject to other forms of positive feedback from additional secretagogues. For example, pituitary corticotrophs have been shown to express receptors for growth hormone–releasing peptide and increase ACTH production in response to GRP secretion.

The secretion of ACTH (and, hence, serum cortisol) is normally pulsatile in nature in terms of frequency and remains constant. However, with the extent of ACTH release with each pulse varies according to the body's circadian rhythms (sleep–wake cycles), which accounts for the variation in serum cortisol levels observed through serial measurements at different times of the day. Physical and emotional stressors that increase the body's metabolic demands also increase ACTH and cortisol secretion. In the normal diurnal sleep–wake cycle, levels are highest in the early morning on awakening and are lowest late in the evening and during the very early morning hours after midnight.

In patients with Cushing's disease, pituitary adenomas secrete excessive amounts of ACTH. The hypersecretion is random, is episodic, and does not follow the usual circadian rhythm of ACTH secretion in terms of amplitude and duration. ACTH stimulates the secretion of glucocorticoids, mineralocorticoids, and androgenic steroids from the adrenal cortex. As cortical hyperplasia increases, the adrenal glands secrete increasing amounts of cortisol in response to each incremental pulse of ACTH. Moreover, in the presence of an adenoma, the usual negative feedback mechanism of excessive glucocorticoid secretion does not suppress ACTH production to the same extent as in unaffected persons, possibly owing to a defect in the glucocorticoid receptor in adenomatous corticotrophs. In turn, these patients present with hypercortisolemia and elevated levels of ACTH—particularly those with macroadenomas.

Importantly, however, in contrast to the ACTH-producing cells of relatively rarer ectopic, nonpituitary adenomas that remain virtually unresponsive to negative feedback mechanisms, pituitary adenomatous corticotrophs appear to still retain a threshold level, albeit a higher one than in normal corticotrophs, for cortisol-mediated negative feedback. This allows a high-dose dexamethasone suppression test to differentiate between pituitary and nonpituitary sources of ACTH hypersecretion. With ectopic, nonpituitary ACTH secretion, both hypothalamic CRH secretion and pituitary ACTH secretion from normal corticotrophs are suppressed. A number of different tumor types have been implicated with ectopic ACTH hypersecretion, most commonly small oat-cell carcinoma of the lung and carcinoid tumors of the thymus or pancreas, all of which arise from neuroendocrine cell precursors. Interestingly, most of these tumors secrete a greater proportion of POMC precursors than ACTH itself.

In patients with Cushing's syndrome, cortisol measurements taken at various times during a 24-hour period will demonstrate prolonged elevations of cortisol levels, even though some readings may be within the normal range. The normally tight regulatory relationship between ACTH and cortisol secretion is lost, with late evening levels being particularly high. This excessive production of cortisol over the entire 24-hour sleep–wake cycle results in the clinical signs and symptoms of Cushing's syndrome.

The most frequent cause of Cushing's syndrome, however, is prolonged administration of exogenous glucocorticoid hormones—an iatrogenic etiology that is considered ACTH independent. Thus, any medical problem requiring the prolonged use of corticosteroids predisposes the patient to develop this syndrome. Examples include autoimmune disorders, reactive airway disease, and chronic obstructive pulmonary disease—all of which may involve long-term systemic steroid use as maintenance therapy or for recurrent exacerbations. Rarely, megestrol acetate (Megace), which has intrinsic glucocorticoid activity, may also lead to Cushing's syndrome. Exogenous steroid administration leads to suppression of CRH and ACTH excretion, as well as steroid production by native adrenal tissue. This results in bilateral adrenocortical atrophy and low salivary and urinary levels of 17-hydroxycorticosteroid and cortisol, unless cortisol itself is the steroid being administered.

Primary adrenocortical disease including cortical tumors and both micronodular and macronodular hyperplasia is much less common. Adrenal tumors may be benign adenomas or malignant carcinomas. Both types of tumors demonstrate altered expression of genes involved in apoptosis and telomeric function, which appears to underlie clonal immortalization. However, a number of significant differences exist between benign and malignant tumors. Adrenal adenomas produce cortisol from cholesterol backbones very efficiently, secreting relatively low levels of the cortisol precursors dehydroepiandrosterone (DHEA-S) and 17-ketosteroids. Adenomatous cells have also been shown to respond to beta-adrenergic agonists and multiple cytokines, including interleukin-1 (IL-1), gastric inhibitory peptide, vasopressin, and serotonin.

In contrast, adrenal carcinomas are far less efficient at producing cortisol, secreting cortisol precursors at disproportionately higher concentrations. Adrenal carcinomas are still capable of leading to Cushing's syndrome, however, owing to their size and secretory cell mass. They are also more likely than adrenal adenomas to produce elevated levels of the aldosterone precursor corticosterone

and its hydroxy and deoxy variants. Adrenal carcinomas also produce high levels of vascular endothelial growth factor–A (VEGF-A), insulin-like growth factor (IGF)–1, IGF-2, IGF-2 receptor, cell cyclins, cyclin-dependent kinase, and the chemokines IL-8 and epithelial neutrophil-activating protein–78. In contrast, levels of the antiangiogenic factor thrombospondin-1 are reduced.

With primary adrenocortical tumors, hypercortisolemia allows for negative feedback of both CRH and ACTH secretion. Thus, pituitary corticotrophs atrophy, as do the normal adrenal cells of the zona fasciculata and zona reticularis. In contrast, macronodular adrenal hyperplasia results in glands weighing 25 to 500 g or more, with multiple benign nodules greater than 5 mm in diameter and a hypertrophic (rather than atrophic) internodular cortex.

Clinical Presentation
Subjective
The clinical presentation of Cushing's disease is usually gradual, developing over months or years. Signs and symptoms of Cushing's disease are those of hypercortisolism and androgen excess.

The presentation of patients with Cushing's syndrome is similar. Common complaints include weight gain, back pain, headaches, skin changes (see later), and muscle weakness. Women may complain of menstrual irregularities and hirsutism, and men often report decreased libido and impotence. Patients may also complain of emotional lability, increased appetite and weight gain, increased irritability, anxiety, poor concentration and memory, and sleep disturbances.

Objective
Patients with Cushing's syndrome predominantly present with generalized or central obesity. In fact, obesity is the most common and often the first clinical manifestation of this disorder. Excessive accumulation of fat in the face leads to the typical "moon face" appearance. Facial plethora often accompanies the moon facies. The "buffalo hump" appearance is caused by excessive accumulation of fat in the supraclavicular and dorsocervical area.

Most patients will have readily recognizable skin changes. There is atrophy of the epidermis and connective tissue, producing a thinning of the skin and easy bruising. Additional skin changes include hirsutism, acne, and striae. Striae are typically red to purple and usually are present on the abdomen but may be present on the hips, buttocks, thighs, breast, and axilla. Hyperpigmentation, commonly found in some types of Cushing's syndrome, is rare in patients with Cushing's disease.

Fungal infections of the skin, nails, and oral mucosa are common. Skin wounds heal slowly in the presence of excessive cortisol.

Most patients have muscle weakness, which is more prominent proximally and in the lower extremities. The extremities are usually thin, with muscle wasting. Osteoporosis is common in patients with prolonged elevated cortisol levels, and pathological fractures may be evident on radiographic examination.

Other manifestations include glaucoma, leukocytosis, granulocytosis, lymphopenia, and psychiatric symptoms. Less common clinical findings include renal calculi and edema. Hypokalemic alkalosis is rare in Cushing's disease but is often seen in Cushing's syndrome.

Hypertension is often present secondary to sodium and water retention. Glucose intolerance and hyperglycemia result because cortisol interferes with the transfer of insulin across the cell membrane.

Diagnostic Reasoning

Cushing's syndrome and disease is diagnosed via a combination of laboratory testing and radiographic examinations.

Diagnostic Tests

Initial Testing The Endocrine Society released diagnostic guidelines recommending that one of four tests be used in the initial testing for Cushing's syndrome: urine free cortisol (at least two measurements), late-night salivary cortisol (two measurements), 1-mg overnight dexamethasone suppression test, or longer low-dose dexamethasone suppression test (DST; 2 mg/day for 48 hours). Additional laboratory tests should include a complete blood count, blood glucose levels, and comprehensive metabolic panel. Hypercortisolemia impairs glucose tolerance and often produces hypokalemia and leukocytosis.

Initial tests to assess cortisol levels include serum cortisol levels and urinary cortisol. The overnight DST assists in the confirmation of hypercortisolemia. To do the overnight DST, the patient takes 1 mg of dexamethasone (Decadron) orally at 11:00 p.m., and the plasma cortisol level is measured at 8 a.m. the next morning. A normal finding is a value below 1.8 mcg/dL, because an elevated morning cortisol level would indicate that the patient's endogenous cortisol secretion is insensitive to the negative feedback imparted by the exogenous dexamethasone dose. False-positive results may occur in patients who are obese, depressed, or under extreme stress. Medications that may also produce high cortisol levels are estrogens, antiseizure medications, and rifampin. Phenytoin (Dilantin), phenobarbital (Luminal), and primidone (Mysoline) accelerate the metabolism of dexamethasone and can also produce a false-positive dexamethasone test.

A nighttime (11:00 p.m.) salivary cortisol level is normally below 4.2 nmol/L and when obtained on two samples within this range excludes the diagnosis of Cushing's syndrome. Levels twice this high are suggestive of Cushing's syndrome. Although this is a relatively easy test to perform (samples are stable at room temperature), it requires special sample collection tubes and a nighttime collection schedule but has a sensitivity of 93% to 100%.

A urinary free cortisol 24-hour collection test requires the patient to collect urine for 24 hours, which is often not a practical expectation, unless the collection is done in an inpatient setting. The majority of patients with Cushing's syndrome will have an elevated level; if it is fourfold the upper limit of normal, this result is considered diagnostic for Cushing's syndrome. However, mild Cushing's syndrome may still have normal levels; thus, normal urinary free cortisol levels (less than 50 mcg/24 hr) do not rule out Cushing's syndrome entirely. If the test result is positive for Cushing's syndrome, the patient should be referred to an endocrinologist, who will conduct further testing to determine the cause and subtype of Cushing's syndrome. If symptoms of Cushing's syndrome are present but tests do not confirm the diagnosis of hypercortisolism, a low-dose DST should be performed.

Subsequent Testing The low-dose DST involves administration of dexamethasone 0.5 mg PO every 6 hours for 48 hours. Urine is collected on day 2 of the test. Urinary free cortisol above 20 mcg/dL or a 17-hydroxy-corticosteroid level above 4.5 mcg/dL confirms the diagnosis of hypercortisolism. Many medications, including corticosteroids, phenothiazines, phenytoin, diuretics, quinidine, penicillin G, oral contraceptives, lithium, acetylsalicylic acid, and monoamine oxidase inhibitors, may affect the accuracy of test results.

Baseline plasma ACTH levels should be assessed once hypercortisolism is confirmed. Levels are highest between 7:00 a.m. and 10:00 a.m (8–80 pg/mL) and lowest just before bedtime (less than 10 pg/mL). Generally, levels below 20 pg/mL indicate a possible adrenal tumor, and levels exceeding 20 pg/mL are indicative of a pituitary or ectopic secreting ACTH tumor.

After completion of hormonal studies, radiological studies are performed to localize the possible source of excess cortisol production. Most microadenomas of the pituitary gland are detected by imaging. An abdominal computed tomography (CT) scan of the adrenal glands is done to detect adrenal tumors. In Cushing's disease, the adrenal glands are enlarged. A CT scan of the chest and abdomen is also beneficial in detecting possible sites of ectopic secretion. Because the lung is the most likely source of ectopic secretion, special attention to the chest is indicated. If the source is determined to be the pituitary gland, magnetic resonance imaging is indicated.

Patients should also be assessed for other sequelae of Cushing's syndrome such as hypokalemia, anemia, metabolic alkalosis, hyperglycemia, and hypercholesterolemia. Except for initial testing, the diagnosis of Cushing's syndrome and the differentiation as to cause are best accomplished either by an endocrinologist or in collaboration with an endocrinologist.

Differential Diagnosis

Pregnancy, obesity, and excessive activity may produce elevated serum cortisol levels. Other conditions that may produce elevated cortisol levels are alcoholism, severe depression, obesity, hypertension, DM, glucocorticoid therapy, estrogen replacement therapy, and oral contraceptives. There are also various familial (genetic) predispositions to hypercortisolemia. Type 1 multiple endocrine neoplasia (MEN 1) syndrome presents with pituitary corticotroph adenomas in 2% of cases, whereas Carney's syndrome is a rare autosomal dominant complex consisting of bilateral micronodular dysplasia, pigmented lentigines, and blue nevi on the head and trunk, as well as multiple endocrine and nonendocrine neoplasms.

Management

The goals of treatment are to reduce the cortisol levels to normal and treat the underlying cause. The initial clinical management of patients with Cushing's syndrome should be handled by an endocrinologist. Despite successful treatment, some patients may relapse, so the patient must be evaluated for recurrence of hypercortisolemia.

Initial Management

Transsphenoidal pituitary microsurgery is the treatment of choice for pituitary adenoma causing Cushing's disease. If surgery is unsuccessful, irradiation of the pituitary may be considered. Complications from surgery include transient diabetes insipidus, visual disturbances, cerebrospinal rhinorrhea, and meningitis. After microsurgery, 75% of patients will experience dramatic decreases in cortisol and will require exogenous glucocorticoid therapy for 6 to 36 months after surgery. For patients who fail to respond or who have a recurrence, treatment may include stereotactic pituitary radiosurgery (gamma knife) or laparoscopic bilateral adrenalectomy. Conventional pituitary irradiation therapy has a 23% cure rate. Failure rates with both types of treatment increase over time. Diagnostic errors (depression and lack of a pituitary adenoma) increased failure rates of patients treated with surgery.

After a transsphenoidal pituitary microsurgery, 25% of patients have persistent signs and symptoms. This is more likely to occur if the tumor was not completely removed and in patients with corticotrophic hyperplasia. These patients require a second pituitary operation, radiotherapy, or bilateral total adrenalectomy.

In younger patients who are not surgical candidates, mitotane (Lysodren) or alternatively ketoconazole (Nizoral) 200 mg every 6 hours may be used alone or in combination to reduce cortisol overproduction. Older adults who are not surgical candidates may tolerate the use of ketoconazole; however, liver enzymes may be elevated with this treatment and need to be monitored by an endocrinologist.

Subsequent Management

After resection of a pituitary adenoma, normal corticotrophins are suppressed; temporary cortisone replacement therapy is indicated for 9 to 12 months, but may be as long as 36 months. The drugs of choice for replacement therapy are hydrocortisone (Cortef), prednisone (Deltasone), and fludrocortisone (Florinef). Dexamethasone (Decadron) is an alternative. The lowest dose effective in maintaining hormone levels is recommended. Complications of untreated or inadequate treatment of Cushing's disease are increased susceptibility to infections, nephrolithiasis, hypertension, and osteoporosis. Inadequate treatment may also lead to psychosis or uncontrolled DM.

Medications for corticosteroid replacement are listed in Drugs Commonly Prescribed 16.3: Corticosteroid Replacement Therapy.

Follow-up and Referral

The follow-up for each patient depends on the therapy. The patient should be followed monthly for the first year and checked for signs of adrenal hypofunction, and then every 6 to 12 months thereafter. Excessive corticosteroid treatment should be avoided as much as possible. The patient may need education to cope with lifelong symptomatology (specifically information on the importance of early interventions for infections), a prevention of emotional lability mechanism to cope with overwhelming stress, use of potassium supplements, and maintenance of a high-protein diet.

The disorder is usually chronic, characterized by periods of cyclic exacerbation and rare remissions. Complications are osteoporosis, increased susceptibility to infection, hirsutism, and metastases of malignant tumors (depending on causality).

Referrals are suggested for surgical intervention for the following conditions associated with Cushing's syndrome:

1. *Primary hypersecretion of ACTH.* Transsphenoidal microsurgery is recommended and is often followed by radiation and sometimes by medication (adrenocortical inhibitors).
2. *Adrenocortical tumors.* Surgery is recommended, but prognosis is still poor. Replacement therapy is used but usually for only 3 to 12 months. The patient may need treatment with adrenocortical inhibitors if not treated with surgery, which should be managed by an endocrinologist.
3. *Ectopic ACTH production.* Surgery is recommended for removal of neoplastic tissue to manage symptoms, although surgical cure is unlikely. Sometimes a bilateral adrenalectomy is performed. Follow-up for these patients would depend on causality and recommended treatment.

Patient Education

Although patients with Cushing's syndrome will be managed initially by an endocrinologist, the primary-care clinician often manages other aspects of the patient's health. It is important to work collaboratively with the patient in managing symptoms successfully.

Patients need a thorough understanding of their medications and the warning signs of undertreatment or

Drugs Commonly Prescribed 16.3   Corticosteroid Replacement Therapy

Drug	Indication	Adverse Reactions and Prescribing Considerations
prednisone (Deltasone, Meticorten) Supplied PO	Adrenalectomy Pituitary resection	Glucocorticoid activity: Moderate Mineralocorticoid activity: Weak Use the lowest effective dose to prevent side effects such as DM, psychosis, osteoporosis, infections.
prednisolone (Delta-Cortef, Prelone)	Adrenalectomy Pituitary resection	Glucocorticoid activity: Moderate Mineralocorticoid activity: Weak Use the lowest effective dose to prevent side effects such as DM, psychosis, osteoporosis, infections.
methylprednisolone (Medrol, PO) or Depo-Medrol IM or IV	Adrenalectomy Pituitary resection	Glucocorticoid activity: Moderate Mineralocorticoid activity: None Use the lowest effective dose to prevent side effects such as DM, psychosis, osteoporosis, infections.
hydrocortisone (Cortef, Hydrocortone) Supplied in PO, IM, IV, topical, ophthalmic	Adrenalectomy Pituitary resection	Glucocorticoid activity: High Mineralocorticoid activity: Yes Use the lowest effective dose to prevent side effects such as DM, psychosis, osteoporosis, infections.
cortisone acetate (Cortone) Supplied PO and IM	Adrenalectomy Pituitary resection	Glucocorticoid activity: High Mineralocorticoid activity: Yes Use the lowest effective dose to prevent side effects such as DM, psychosis, osteoporosis, infections.
dexamethasone (long-acting) (Decadron) Supplied PO, IM, IV	Adrenalectomy Pituitary resection	Glucocorticoid activity: Very high Mineralocorticoid activity: Weak Use the lowest effective dose to prevent side effects such as DM, psychosis, osteoporosis, infections.
fludrocortisone (Florinef) Supplied PO	Adrenalectomy Pituitary resection	Glucocorticoid activity: None Mineralocorticoid activity: High Use the lowest effective dose to prevent side effects such as sodium and water retention, edema, hypertension, hypokalemia.

DM: diabetes mellitus

overtreatment with cortisone. Cortisone preparations should be taken with food. Patients need to be told that they should consult with the primary care clinician when initiating additional medications, both prescription and over the counter. Patients on high doses should wear a medical identification bracelet. Because these patients are prone to infections, they should be instructed on how to avoid common infections, both bacterial and fungal. Patients cannot rely on elevated temperature to indicate the seriousness of any infection; therefore, they need to report any initial signs of infection.

Nutritional counseling may be indicated, including information on avoidance of excessive sodium and on a well-balanced, low-fat diet. Many patients are obese, and the importance of weight loss must be addressed.

Patients should monitor their glucose levels at least weekly. During periods of stress or medication adjustment, glucose levels will need to be tested more frequently.

Patients should assess their glucose levels daily during periods of medication adjustment. If levels are stable and within normal levels, they may continue testing glucose levels until at least 1 week after final dose adjustment. They should resume daily glucose testing in times of stress or if any signs of infection are present. If the morning glucose level at any time is above normal, more frequent testing is indicated. The patient should be given a log to record the glucose test results and instructed to bring the log to each primary-care visit.

Patients with Cushing's syndrome will need to have their blood pressure monitored weekly. As with glucose monitoring, the frequency will depend on their symptoms and coexisting cardiovascular disease. More frequent monitoring will be needed during times of stress. The patient should obtain a sphygmomanometer for home use and keep a log of his or her blood pressures so that the primary-care provider can see the pattern.

The patient should be instructed about fall prevention. Because of the potential for osteoporosis, the patient should avoid activities that are likely to cause falls. Simple environmental changes can be made in the home to increase safety, such as removing small rugs, placing rails around the bathtub, and using a shower chair.

Patients should also report any symptoms of gastrointestinal upset (nausea, bloating, vomiting) and monitor themselves for signs of gastrointestinal bleeding (vomiting blood, tarry stools, increasing fatigue).

Instructions on skin care are essential. Research indicates that older adults with a history of long-term corticosteroid use are more prone to pressure ulcers. Thin, easily traumatized skin must be protected. These individuals should avoid applying tape and adhesive bandages directly to their skin. They should wear protective clothing for outdoor activities such as gardening.

There is potential for failure of the surgical intervention. Instruct the patient to report any return of symptoms if he or she has been asymptomatic for a period after the operation.

■ ADRENAL INSUFFICIENCY

Low levels of cortisol secretion by the adrenal glands can result from inadequate stimulation of the adrenals by adrenocorticotropic hormone (ACTH) from the anterior pituitary or because the adrenals are unable to produce adrenocortical hormones. *Addison's disease,* also known as primary adrenal insufficiency, is relatively rare and results from a failure of the adrenals to produce hormones because of a problem in the gland rather than a problem with the pituitary (ACTH). Other types of adrenal insufficiency, or hypocortisolism, occur from secondary sources, such as a failure of the pituitary gland to produce adequate levels of the adrenal-stimulating hormone ACTH or the abrupt withdrawal of exogenously administered glucocorticoids, which previously suppressed endogenous adrenal hormone production.

Epidemiology and Causes

Addison's disease is primarily (80% of cases in the United States) caused by autoimmune destruction of the adrenal cortex. Although it can occur at any age, Addison's disease most often occurs in persons aged 30 to 60 years. Women are diagnosed slightly more often than men, with an overall incidence of 0.6 per 100,000 and a prevalence of 4 per 100,000. Risk factors for Addison's disease include having a first- or second-degree relative with the disease.

Other causes of (secondary) adrenal insufficiency are chronic corticosteroid use followed by a physiologically stressful event, such as severe infection, trauma, or surgical procedure, in which adrenal hormone levels are inadequate, due to the iatrogenic suppression of endogenous hormone production. TB infection is the most common infectious cause of adrenal insufficiency worldwide, whereas HIV is the most common infectious cause in the United States, resulting from direct effects on the adrenal glands themselves. Other causes include bilateral adrenal hemorrhage and infarction, tumors of the adrenal gland causing decreased function, drugs (ketoconazole [Nizoral], etomidate [Amidate]), sarcoidosis, hemochromatosis, amyloidosis, and congenital causes.

Pathophysiology

Idiopathic Addison's disease is an autoimmune disorder and can occur at any age. Adrenal-specific autoantibodies are present in 50% to 70% of cases and are more likely to be present in younger patients and those with other autoimmune diseases. These autoantibodies are specific for cells of the adrenal cortex and for the enzyme(s) responsible for the production of cortisol and aldosterone. A combination of autoantibodies and cell-mediated immune responses is responsible for this disease. Frequently, idiopathic Addison's disease appears with other autoimmune diseases, which are collectively termed *autoimmune polyendocrine syndrome* (APS). Type 1 APS is an inherited autosomal recessive disease and, along with Addison's disease, includes hypoparathyroidism and mucocutaneous candidiasis. Type 2 APS is the more common type, with a constellation of disorders that includes Addison's disease, diabetes mellitus, celiac disease, immune thyroid disease, and hypogonadism.

Secondary hypocortisolism is usually a result of low ACTH levels and subsequent adrenal atrophy. The resulting hypocortisolism causes clinical manifestations similar to Addison's disease. However, in this type of hypocortisolism, there is no hyperpigmentation, as typically seen in Addison's disease, and the renin-angiotensin system functions normally, resulting in normal aldosterone and potassium levels.

Clinical Presentation

Clinical manifestations of Addison's disease include fatigue, weakness, anorexia, weight loss, nausea, abdominal pain, diarrhea, hypoglycemia, and hypotension (particularly orthostatic hypotension), which are primarily the result of hypocortisolism and hypoaldosteronism. Patients with Addison's disease typically exhibit hyperpigmentation due to elevated levels of ACTH, which is derived from the precursor protein proopiomelanocortin (POMC) that also gives rise to melanocyte-stimulating hormone. In severe cases, when a patient has Addison's disease that is well managed but the patient subsequently experiences a physiological stressor of some kind (e.g., infection, surgery), the requirement for cortisol increases and the patient may experience an Addisonian crisis, manifesting as severe hypotension and vascular collapse. The decreased adrenal androgen secretion associated with Addison's disease results in the loss of secondary sex characteristics (loss of pubic and axillary hair) in women, but because the adrenals are not a major source of androgens in men, male patients do not experience any loss of secondary sex characteristics.

Diagnostic Reasoning

Diagnostic Tests

When Addison's disease or other forms of hypocortisolism are suspected, a plasma cortisol level should be obtained. A morning (8:00 a.m.) cortisol level of less than 3 mcg/dL is consistent with Addison's disease, especially if accompanied by a plasma ACTH level greater than 200 pg/mL. Diagnosis is confirmed by a cosyntropin stimulation test, in which a synthetic form of ACTH is given intramuscularly (IM) and a serum cortisol level is obtained 45 minutes later. In Addison's disease, the exogenous ACTH dose does not result in a corresponding increase in cortisol secretion, demonstrating primary failure of the adrenal glands to respond to ACTH. Small, noncalcified adrenal glands on CT scan are indicative of autoimmune Addison's disease.

Differential Diagnosis

Patients with Addison's disease generally have an elevated ACTH level, which is associated with hyperpigmentation of the skin. In contrast, if a patient has hypocortisolism that is a result of hypopituitarism resulting in a low ACTH level, he or she will have normal pigmentation. In any patient with unexplained hypotension, Addison's disease and other forms of hypocortisolism should be considered. Other nonspecific clinical manifestations that may be associated with Addison's disease but are also common in other conditions are nausea, unintentional weight loss, weakness, and anorexia. Hypocortisolism should be considered when other causes for the constitutional symptoms have been ruled out.

Management

Initial therapy for adrenal insufficiency consists of hydrocortisone 15 to 30 mg in two divided doses, with two-thirds of the dose given in the morning and one-third given in the early evening. Prednisone can be used if the patient does not respond well to hydrocortisone. The dose of prednisone is 2 to 4 mg in the morning and 1 to 2 mg in the evening. The dose is adjusted based on the clinical response.

Stress hormone supplementation is necessary for patients who experience significant physiological stressors, such as serious infection, trauma, or surgery. In cases of severe stress, hydrocortisone is given IV or IM every 6 hours at a maximum dose of 50 mg. Oral medication at lower doses can be prescribed if the stress is less severe and then reduced to normal when the stress subsides.

In addition to hydrocortisone (glucocorticoid), mineralocorticoids must be replaced, although not all patients require daily therapy. Fludrocortisone (Florinef) acetate is the drug of choice and has a potent sodium-retaining effect. The usual dosage is 0.05 to 0.2 mg PO daily, which should be determined in conjunction with an endocrinologist. Symptoms of fatigue, postural hypotension, hyponatremia, or hyperkalemia may indicate the need for a higher dosage. Of note, in contrast to glucocorticoid requirements, increased mineralocorticoid supplementation is not required during times of increased physiological stress.

Some patients require androgen therapy along with the medications mentioned above. Dehydroepiandrosterone (DHEA) 25 to 50 mg PO daily has been shown to improve sense of well-being, increase muscle mass, and reverse bone loss. When prescribed DHEA, older women should be monitored for masculinizing effects.

Follow-up and Referral

Patients with adrenal insufficiency require chronic glucocorticoid and mineralocorticoid supplementation and are prone to Addisonian crises, due to the inability to mount an appropriate stress hormone response with endogenous cortisol. Determination of an appropriate replacement dose and regimen requires periodic assessment for signs of both underdosing (weakness, dizziness, and headaches on waking) and overdosing (Cushingoid features).

Once chronic maintenance dosing is established in conjunction with an endocrinologist, the primary-care provider will be able to meet most of the patient's ongoing health-care needs but should also evaluate for iatrogenic complications of chronic corticosteroid use, including cataract formation (requiring annual ophthalmological examinations) and the development of osteopenia/osteoporosis (requiring periodic dual-energy x-ray absorptiometry [DEXA] scanning). Expert consultation with an endocrinologist should be sought if dose adjustments or a change in class of hormone replacement is indicated.

Patient Education

Any patient with Addison's disease or adrenal insufficiency needs to be well informed about this condition and the potential implications for Addisonian crisis if the patient should develop a serious infection or experience other physiological stressors. Given the significant risk from systemic illness, patients should be instructed to see their health-care provider during times of illness. In these instances, additional corticosteroid supplementation (stress hormones) may be required, for example, a doubling or tripling of the dose of hormone replacement therapy in the setting of an illness, surgery, or dental procedure. This may require parenteral (IM) dosing if oral supplementation is not possible (e.g., because of significant nausea and vomiting or diarrhea). Thus, if possible, patients should be trained to self-administer IM injections and may be given a reserve prescription for parenteral hydrocortisone or similar agent to be used in these situations.

DIABETES MELLITUS

Diabetes mellitus (DM) is a syndrome of disordered carbohydrate, fat, and protein metabolism and hyperglycemia resulting from deficits in insulin secretion, insulin action, or a combination of both. There are two distinct types of DM, type 1 and type 2 (each with a distinct epidemiology and etiology), but impaired fasting glucose (IFG) and impaired glucose tolerance (IGT) are used to describe a fasting glucose between 100 and 125 mg/dL or a 2-hour postglucose load blood glucose of 140 to 199 mg/dL. Some sources state that IGT and gestational diabetes are now considered under the IFG category.

DM is the most common endocrine disorder, affecting 25.8 million people in the United States, up to 7 million of whom may be undiagnosed. In 2011, DM affected 8.3% of the adult population in the United States. The complications of DM include cardiovascular and peripheral vascular disease, decreased immune system functioning, renal failure, and retinopathy. Diabetic nephropathy is now the leading cause of end-stage renal disease. DM also is the leading cause of acquired blindness in the United States. Tight control of blood glucose levels reduces the morbidity and mortality rates associated with DM, but control is not without its costs. The costs of long-term management of diabetes have serious implications on the quality of life of those affected and their families.

■ DIABETES MELLITUS TYPE 1

Diabetes mellitus type 1 is a metabolic disorder characterized by a severe insulin deficiency resulting from beta-cell destruction and producing hyperglycemia. The lack of insulin alters lipid, carbohydrate, and protein metabolism. Chronic hyperglycemia of DM results in damage to various body organs, especially the eyes, kidneys, nerves, heart, and both small and large blood vessels. Loss of vision, renal failure, loss of a lower extremity, and chronic foot ulcers caused by peripheral neuropathy are common sequelae of long-term hyperglycemia. Chronic hyperglycemia affects all body systems and places significant social, economic, and psychological demands on patients and their families.

Diabetic retinopathy remains the leading cause of new-onset blindness among adults aged 20 to 74 years. After 20 years of type 1 DM, nearly all patients have some retinopathy. Impairment of growth, an increased susceptibility to infection, and autonomic neuropathy, resulting in gastrointestinal, genitourinary, and cardiovascular symptoms including sexual dysfunction, also occur. Persons with DM have an increased incidence of atherosclerotic heart disease, peripheral vascular disease, and cerebrovascular disease. Diabetic ketoacidosis (DKA) and hyperosmolar hyperglycemic syndrome (HHS) are both life-threatening sequelae of hyperglycemia. HHS is more commonly seen in type 2 DM, however. Tables 16.6 and 16.7 provide more information on these conditions.

Table 16.6 Diabetic Ketoacidosis (DKA)

Overview	Clinical Presentation	Management
DKA is an acute decompensation in diabetes and requires immediate medical attention. The cardinal features of DKA: **Hyperglycemia**—blood glucose >359 mg/dL **Ketonemia**—plasma ketone level >5 mmol/L **Acidosis**—plasma bicarbonate level <9 mEq/L **Causes:** Lack of insulin Stress (physical or emotional), even with continued insulin therapy • As insulin levels drop, concentrations of glucagon rise, which increases glucose levels • Epinephrine inhibits glucose transport in peripheral tissues, thereby stimulating the production of glucose in the liver and noncarbohydrates are used to produces glucose in the liver. • Free fatty acids from adipose stores are oxidized in the liver for energy, and this causes a release of ketones and resultant acidosis.	DKA begins with: • Anorexia • Increased thirst • Nausea/vomiting • Abdominal cramping • Increased urine formation Later signs: • Kussmaul respiration • Signs of dehydration (usual fluid deficit is 3–5 L) • Oliguria • Altered consciousness Left untreated: • Coma • Vascular collapse • Renal shutdown • Blood glucose increases from 300–800 mg/dL. Diagnostic tests: • Serum glucose • Sodium potassium • Phosphate • Bicarbonate • Beta-hydroxybutyrate • Osmolarity • pH • Calculated anion gap	Goals: • Correct dehydration. • Normalize electrolytes. • Correct acidosis. First line of treatment is insulin. • Continuous-dose insulin infusion: 0.1–0.2 units/kg per hour Correct dehydration and electrolyte imbalance: • Rapid infusion of normal saline or Ringer's lactate IV: 1–2 L • Potassium replacement 3–4 hours after initiation of insulin and fluid therapy • Bicarbonate therapy if pH is 7.0 or below After recovery, causes for the DKA should be explored. Patient teaching about the need for more insulin during periods of illness and stress.

Table 16.7	Hyperosmolar Hyperglycemic Syndrome (HHS)	
Overview	Clinical Presentation	Management
HHS is characterized by: • Severe hyperglycemia—blood sugar >600 mg/dL • No ketosis • Hyperosmolality • Dehydration • High mortality rate Seen in: • Older diabetics who develop infection or other illness • Undiagnosed diabetics • Patients with diabetes diagnosed after a long period of hyperglycemia Precipitating factors: • Peritoneal dialysis • Hemodialysis • Tube feeding with high-protein formulas • Mannitol • Phenytoins (Dilantin) • Steroids • Immunosuppressive agents • Diuretics • Surgery • Myocardial infarction • Sepsis • Renal insufficiency • Congestive heart failure	Insidious onset with subtle initial symptoms. History may indicate decreased fluid intake. Patients may present with: • Polyuria • Polydipsia • Weakness • No ketoacidosis • Lethargy and confusion develop when serum osmolality >310 mOsm/kg • Coma Laboratory tests: • Severe hyperglycemia— blood glucose >600 mg/dL • Initial serum sodium is decreased. • Serum sodium increases as dehydration progresses. • Serum osmolality >400 mOsm/kg	Goals: • Correct dehydration. • Normalize electrolytes. Correct dehydration and electrolyte imbalance. • Rapid infusion of hypotonic saline (0.45% NaCl) • In cases of hypovolemia, then use normal saline • Fluid needs may be 4–6 L in 8–10 hours • Correct serum sodium with following equation: Corrected sodium = measured sodium + (0.8 × every 50 mg/dL increment of plasma glucose above 100 mg/dL). Once blood glucose is <250 mg/dL, fluid replacement should be 5% dextrose in 0.45% saline solution or normal saline. An important end point of fluid therapy is to return urine output to 50 mL/hr or more. Less potassium is needed than in DKA.

Epidemiology and Causes

Type 1 DM occurs in approximately 800,000 Americans and accounts for about 10% of all cases of diabetes mellitus in the Western world. It is more common in whites (1.5–2 times higher than in nonwhites), and 60% of patients are under age 18 years on first presentation. Although there is no gender predisposition, marked variations have been observed across ethnocultural groups, correlating with differential expression of human leukocyte antigen (HLA) haplotypes. Type 1 DM was previously known as insulin-dependent diabetes mellitus (IDDM) or juvenile-onset diabetes. However, cases may occur at any age with a fairly abrupt onset. It is uncommon in children younger than 1 year of age and in adults older than 30 years. In nonpediatric patients, this condition is sometimes known as latent autoimmune diabetes of adults (LADA; see later discussion).

Currently, the American Diabetes Association (ADA) does not recommend screening for type 1 DM in apparently healthy individuals who have no risk of type 1 DM. Current clinical trials are being conducted to evaluate prevention strategies to delay clinical disease, and the ADA is hopeful that effective preventive therapies will eventually be found.

Type 1 DM has two forms—immune-mediated DM and idiopathic DM. *Immune-mediated diabetes mellitus* accounts for 90% of type 1 DM and results from an autoimmune destruction of insulin-producing pancreatic beta islet cells. It typically occurs in childhood or adolescence but can arise at any age. Current thinking on the etiology of type 1 DM is that it results from an infection or toxic insult in persons with a genetic predisposition. It is believed that there is a cross-reactive autoimmune response against pancreatic beta-cell antigens, with the most commonly identified infectious agents being congenital rubella, cytomegalovirus, adenovirus, mumps virus, and coxsackie B4 virus. Sensitized immune cells may release destructive cytotoxins and antibodies that contribute to the development of type 1 DM. Patients with immune-mediated diabetes are rarely obese and are prone to other autoimmune diseases such as Graves' disease, Hashimoto's thyroiditis, Addison's disease, vitiligo, and pernicious anemia. *Idiopathic diabetes mellitus* has no known cause with no evidence of autoimmunity and accounts for less than 10% of type 1 DM cases. It is a rare form of DM, is inherited, and is more common in people of Asian or African origin. The need for insulin replacement therapy in these patients is variable.

Pathophysiology

Type 1 DM is characterized by a reduction or absence of functioning beta cells in the pancreatic islets of Langerhans. Although the exact process is not well understood, it is speculated that the sequence begins with a genetic susceptibility that has been mapped to the HLA region on chromosome 6p. Specifically, an increased risk of type 1 DM has been associated with polymorphisms in at least five genes (*HLA-DQα, HLA-DQβ, HLA-DR3, HLA-DR4, HLA-DR9*), as well as preproinsulin (the primary protein product of the insulin gene) and PTPN22 (a lymphocyte-specific tyrosine phosphatase involved in T-cell receptor signaling, which also confers susceptibility to other autoimmune disorders). Inheritance of type 1 DM appears to be polygenic, however, because expression of a particular HLA allele alone is insufficient to lead to autoimmune beta-cell destruction.

Although other genes located within major histocompatibility complex (MHC) genetic loci, as well as non-MHC genes such as cytotoxic T-lymphocyte–associated antigen 4 (*CTLA-4*), influence diabetes risk, class II HLA genes have the greatest effect. In fact, certain non-MHC genes confer an increased risk of type 1 DM only in the presence of particular HLA haplotypes, implying the importance of polygenic interactions.

Much of our understanding of the pathogenesis of autoimmune DM stems from studies in diabetogenic murine models, including nonobese diabetic (NOD) mice and biobreeding (BB) rats. Some triggering mechanism such as a viral infection or other environmental factor is believed to stimulate an inflammatory response and initiate autoimmune infiltration of the pancreatic beta cells within the islets of Langerhans—a process termed *insulitis*. Strongly associated with interleukin-18 (IL-18) (interferon-gamma–inducing factor [IGIF]) and IL-12 expression, as well as interferon-gamma–positive Th1 T cells in NOD mice, insulitis involves autologous beta cells being recognized as foreign by the body's immune system. Islet cell antigens are presented by macrophages and other antigen-presenting cells within the context of class II MHC proteins to autoreactive T cells that mediate much of the subsequent beta islet cell destruction. Alterations in just one or two amino acid positions within certain class II MHC proteins can markedly increase their capacity to present autoantigens to autoreactive T cells. In turn, more than 90% of patients with type 1 DM express *HLA-DR3, DQB1*0201* or *HLA-DR4, DQB1*0302,* and persons expressing both of these HLA haplotypes are most susceptible to developing this disease. By contrast, other HLA polymorphisms confer a protective effect against type 1 DM, presumably due to their decreased affinity for binding autoantigen.

It is known that type 1A DM is clearly associated with an increased incidence of other autoimmune disorders, including thyroid, adrenal, and gonadal insufficiency.

The coexistence of all these conditions has been termed *polyglandular autoimmune disease type 2.* Other rare autoimmune syndromes that involve insulitis shed further light on the importance of genetic pathogenic mechanisms. Autoimmune polyendocrine syndrome type 1 results from a mutation in the *AIRE* gene, an autoimmune regulatory gene that controls the subsequent expression of multiple peripheral autoantigens within the thymus (including insulin itself), which is believed to mediate T-cell self-tolerance. The IPEX syndrome involves mutations in *foxp3,* which is considered a master control gene for regulatory T cells. T suppressor cells are subsequently reduced in activity, allowing for the development of autoimmune disease in affected infants, including DM and fulminant enteritis, which is often fatal.

Both Th1 and Th2 cells are capable of inducing beta-cell destruction, underscoring the importance of both cell-mediated and humoral immune processes in the pathogenesis of type 1 DM. Indeed, the presence of functional autoreactive B lymphocytes and islet cell–specific autoantibodies has been shown both to increase the incidence and shorten the time to progression of type 1 DM. Interestingly, however, autoantibodies are not absolutely required for the development of type 1 DM, as demonstrated by documented cases of the disease occurring in humorally immunodeficient persons with X-linked (Bruton's) agammaglobulinemia.

Nonetheless, islet cell–specific antibodies may be identified in 70% to 80% of prediabetic and newly diagnosed type 1 diabetic patients. Multiple species of autoantibodies have been identified, including immunoglobulins specific for the islet cell enzyme glutamic acid decarboxylase (GAD), the tyrosine phosphatase insulinoma-associated protein 2 (IA-2), and the insulin molecule itself. It has not been fully determined whether these antibodies are themselves pathogenic or simply formed as a consequence of immunological upregulation. For example, although anti-GAD antibodies are found in 70% of human patients with type 1 DM, they do not play a significant role in the pathogenesis of diabetes in NOD mice.

However, even before GAD-specific immunoglobulins form, anti-insulin antibodies may be detected. Studies in NOD mice and humans have confirmed the role of both pathogenic CD8+ and CD4+ T-cell clones that recognize peptide epitopes of the insulin B chain. IA-2-specific immunoglobulin is typically detected after antibodies to insulin and GAD. Identification of two of these three classes of autoantibodies is strongly predictive of progression to type 1A DM in genetically predisposed individuals.

Research continues on the genetic predispositions of type 1 DM and individualized treatments based on genotype. For example, the single gene *SIRT1* was demonstrated using mouse models to be involved in the development of type 1 DM, because a mutation in the *SIRT1* gene was destructive to pancreatic beta cells. Genetic predisposition alone, however, does not fully account for disease pathogenesis. Identical (monozygotic) twin studies reveal only a 30% lifetime risk of developing type 1 DM in twin siblings of probands; however, this compares to only a 5% risk in nonidentical siblings. Moreover, twin studies also demonstrate that autoantibodies against beta islet cells may be present for years in the unaffected sibling of a proband before autoimmune diabetes develops in the second twin. Thus, destruction of a significant amount of beta-cell mass may take months to years but will eventually lead to a lack of insulin.

It is this lack of insulin that disturbs the regulatory mechanisms that control the metabolism of glucose in the body. Hyperglycemia typically develops once 80% to 90% of a patient's beta cells have been destroyed. However, there are animal (baboon) models of autoimmune DM that demonstrate insulin deficiency with as much as 50% of beta-cell mass still intact. Moreover, inflamed islet cells from NOD mice explanted to isolated cell cultures slowly regain their ability to secrete insulin after 1 week of incubation. Thus, external factors such as the inflammatory cytokine milieu are believed to play an important role in diabetic pathogenesis, despite the presence of adequate beta-cell mass. The treatment implication of this is that some patients with autoimmune DM may have a reversible component to their disease if the autoinflammatory process can be stopped early enough and an adequate number of beta cells salvaged. For example, insulin-like growth factor–1 (IGF-1) has been cited as a cytokine that plays an important role in preserving beta-cell function.

However, progressive beta-cell destruction with hyperglycemia remains the hallmark of type 1 DM. In turn, it is this hyperglycemia that leads to both microvascular and macrovascular complications, which underlie long-term diabetic damage. Vascular endothelial dysfunction and inflammation result in fibrosis and intimal thickening, leading to progressive narrowing of the vascular lumen. In turn, blood flow through the microvasculature is reduced, leading to tissue ischemia throughout the body, which results in functional impairment of multiple end organs. Several clinical trials have demonstrated that careful glycemic control reduces the development and delays the progression of microvascular manifestations of diabetes, including nephropathy and retinopathy. Thus, patients with type 1 DM universally require exogenous insulin to maintain glycemic homeostasis.

Identifying the triggering event or events that are capable of inducing the pathogenesis of autoimmune diabetes has been the subject of much research and debate. Molecular mimicry is often cited as the mechanism by which seemingly innocuous environmental (e.g., food-based epitopes) or infectious (e.g., viral) antigens that share homology with beta islet cell antigens initiate a destructive autoimmune process, with the development of cross-reactive antibodies (e.g., the association of coxsackie B viral infection with anti-GAD antibodies and

the shared homology between the FC2 protein of the coxsackievirus B4 virus and human GAD). Another proposed mechanism of pathogenesis observed in BB rats involves delayed expression of islet cell antigens, which is thought to eliminate self-tolerance mechanisms associated with thymic T-cell education early in development, that is, negative thymic selection of autoreactive T lymphocytes. How this mechanism may relate to autoimmune diabetes in humans is less clear, however.

Some research has identified certain perinatal factors as increasing the risk of type 1 DM (e.g., maternal age greater than 25 years, preeclampsia, neonatal respiratory disease, neonatal jaundice secondary to ABO incompatibility). However, the increase in risk noted in this study was small. One systematic review of 12 studies involving 2,398,150 persons demonstrated that high birth weight (greater than 4,000 g) and increased weight gain in the first year of life were associated with an increased risk of type 1 DM. In contrast, a significant body of research has established viral antigens and certain dietary influences as having the strongest impact on the development of autoimmune DM. Direct viral infection of pancreatic beta islet cells may play a role, but evidence for this mechanism is lacking. However, acute immunoglobulin M (IgM) titers to coxsackie B virus are known to be elevated in the mothers of children with type 1 DM. In addition, enteroviral infections are also more common in type 1 diabetics compared with their nondiabetic siblings. Congenital rubella syndrome has also been associated with the development of type 1 DM and other autoimmune syndromes up to 5 to 20 years later, especially in individuals with the HLA-DR3 haplotype.

Contrary evidence also exists, however, that appears to exonerate viral infection as a triggering mechanism. Human immunization with either viral or bacterial antigens has never been shown to increase the risk of developing autoimmune diabetes. Moreover, when NOD mice and BB rats are raised in pathogen-free conditions with no viral contact, they display an increased incidence of autoimmune DM. In fact, infection of either of these animal strains by the lymphocytic choriomeningitis virus early on in development actually protects against type 1 DM. The precise mechanism is poorly understood, however.

The impact of dietary influences on the development of type 1 DM has been heavily studied. Although food epitopes may not mimic beta-cell antigens directly, similar proteins from other animal species are thought to trigger autoimmune reactions leading to type 1 DM. Epidemiological research from at least 10 countries has implicated key protein components of cow's milk including bovine serum albumin and beta-casein as the most likely triggers of these autoimmune responses. However, cross-sectional and prospective studies have not confirmed these associations. In fact, some work has even suggested that vitamin D confers protection against autoimmune DM. In contrast, one epidemiological study indicated that the risk of developing type 1 DM was 30% higher in regions of the United Kingdom where drinking water contained high levels of nitrates (14.8 mg/L vs. 3.2 mg/L).

The timing of the introduction of gluten- and rice-containing cereals into an infant's diet has also been implicated in increasing type 1 DM risk, specifically, when cereals are introduced before 3 months or after 7 months of age. The early introduction of rice cereals before 3 months is also associated with the development of celiac disease. Fortunately, these parameters correspond with the current American Board of Pediatrics recommendation to begin rice cereals (ostensibly, for their iron content) at 4 to 6 months of age.

Finally, secondary causes of diabetes may mimic either type 1 or type 2 DM, depending on whether the primary disease mechanism is destruction of beta islet cells with subsequent insulin deficiency or, rather, peripheral insulin resistance in which the body still produces insulin but the peripheral tissues utilize it less efficiently. Nonimmune mechanisms of beta-cell destruction that produce a type 1B diabetes–like state include hemochromatosis, cystic fibrosis, and pancreatitis.

Clinical Presentation

Subjective

The manifestation of symptoms varies, but the majority of patients seek medical attention because of symptoms related to hyperglycemia. The diagnosis of DM type 1 is often made when a patient presents with DKA.

The classic symptoms of type 1 DM are polydipsia, polyuria, polyphagia, anorexia, and weight loss. Nocturnal enuresis is often a disturbing symptom reported by many patients. Visual changes, especially blurred vision, weakness, and fatigue, are frequently present.

Polyuria, or increased urination, results from osmotic diuresis secondary to sustained hyperglycemia. The loss of glucose, free water, and electrolytes induces a hyperosmolar state, which causes thirst (polydipsia). Blurred vision results from the lenses and retina being exposed to hyperosmolar fluids. There may be a decreased plasma volume, which causes dizziness. Weakness is due to the catabolism of muscle and potassium loss.

The patient may also complain of nausea or abdominal pain. Urinary tract infection and pyelonephritis should be ruled out, especially in patients with abdominal pain, because diabetics are more likely to experience serious complications of pyelonephritis including renal papillary necrosis, emphysematous (necrotizing) pyelonephritis, or progression to gram-negative sepsis.

Patients with DM have impaired immunity and may present with repeated infections, decreased wound healing, or infections that are uncommon in the general public, including staphylococcal and *Klebsiella pneumoniae* infections. Hyperglycemia worsens humoral immunity and leukocyte function. In fact, infections such as malignant (necrotizing) otitis externa (due to *Pseudomonas*

aeruginosa) and rhinocerebral mucormycosis occur almost exclusively in patients with DM. Patients may present with complaints of pruritus caused by an infection such as vulvovaginitis. Patients with poorly controlled DM may have chronic pyogenic infections of the skin. Necrobiosis lipoidica diabeticorum is rarely seen in any patient without DM and consists of plaques with demarcated borders and a shining yellow surface occurring on the anterior surfaces of the legs or dorsal aspect of the ankles. Because most patients with DM also have microvascular and macrovascular complications that decrease the blood flow to the tissues, pathogens are able to multiply rapidly because the increased glucose in body fluids is a good source of energy for them.

Diabetic foot ulcers result from a combination of factors including decreased circulation, infection, decreased immune response, and peripheral neuropathy. Occasionally, the patient may present with a complaint of paresthesia, which is related to a temporary dysfunction of peripheral sensory nerves. The patient with peripheral neuropathy presents with a stocking-glove distribution of anesthesia, leading to missed foot ulcers or burns on the hands (from cooking or smoking).

Objective

Weight loss despite normal or increased appetite occurs as water, glycogen, and triglyceride stores are depleted. There is a reduced muscle mass as amino acids are used by the liver for gluconeogenesis with resultant ketone bodies formed. Signs of dehydration such as poor skin turgor and dry mucous membranes may be present. Genital or urinary tract infections may be present as a result of the hyperglycemic state. Ketoacidosis is usually present and may be mild to severe. Hyperosmolar hyperglycemic nonketotic acidosis is a second complication of prolonged hyperglycemia.

Patients with long-standing DM frequently develop diabetic retinopathy, which is a result of retinal ischemia. Five stages of retinopathy are evident on physical exam: (1) dilation of retinal venules and retinal capillary microaneurysms; (2) increased vascular permeability; (3) retinal ischemia due to vascular occlusion; (4) angiogenesis with proliferation of new retinal surface blood vessels; and (5) retinal hemorrhage with fibrovascular proliferation and contraction, which may lead to retinal detachment. These patients must be referred to an ophthalmologist for evaluation.

Physical exam also requires a detailed neurological exam because DM can have neurological complications. For example, diabetics may have third cranial nerve palsy, or the sixth (abducens) and fourth (trochlear) cranial nerves can also be affected in cranial neuropathy.

Diagnostic Reasoning

Immediate testing in the clinic setting can be accomplished by utilizing a portable monitor to test capillary blood glucose level. This test is referred to as a random plasma glucose measurement and is given without regard to time of last meal. It is important to consider that certain drugs, including glucocorticoids, furosemide (Lasix), thiazide diuretics, estrogen-containing products, beta blockers, and nicotinic acid, can produce hyperglycemia. If the random plasma glucose level is elevated in the clinic, the urine should be tested for ketones and additional blood plasma glucose testing should be done.

Diagnostic Tests

Initial Testing Current guidelines for the diagnosis of diabetes include any one of the following:

- Glycosylated hemoglobin (A1C) of 6.5% or higher
- Symptoms of diabetes (e.g., polyuria, polydipsia, weight loss) plus a random plasma glucose level of 200 mg/dL or higher
- Fasting plasma glucose level of 126 mg/dL or higher (following 8 hours of no caloric intake)
- Two-hour plasma glucose level of 200 mg/dL or higher during an oral glucose tolerance test (OGTT) with a 75-g glucose load (not for routine use)

These criteria should be confirmed by repeat testing on a different day, except in the case of unequivocal hyperglycemia with acute metabolic decompensation.

Patients with latent autoimmune diabetes of adults (LADA) or patients at risk for developing type 1 DM can be tested for islet antibodies (IAs); however, this is not a current recommendation for all type 1 DM patients. This test will help differentiate type 2 DM from LADA. Instead of IAs, a clinical screening tool can be utilized first to assess for signs and symptoms of diabetes, and then the IA test may be performed, because patients with LADA will have positive serum IA. Another test that may be helpful in assessing beta-cell function in a patient with type 1 DM is the C-peptide level. Proinsulin is cleaved into insulin and C-peptide, the latter being biologically inactive. Therefore, C-peptide levels are found in amounts equal to endogenous insulin. However, exogenous insulin preparations do not include C-peptide. Thus, a patient with residual pancreatic beta-cell function will have decreased but nonetheless detectable levels of C-peptide, whereas if no insulin is being produced, the levels of C-peptide will be negligible (normal fasting level = 0.51–2.72 ng/mL or 0.17–0.90 mmol/L).

The International Expert Committee on Diabetes recommends that an A1C of 6.5% or greater can be used to diagnose diabetes with a repeat level for confirmation. The confirmation is not needed if a patient has the clinical symptoms of DM or the glucose level is greater than 200 mg/dL. This cannot be used for diagnosis in pregnancy, hemoglobinopathy, or abnormal erythrocyte turnover situations.

Subsequent Testing A1C determination gives valuable insight into the mean plasma glucose concentration over the preceding 2 to 3 months and is helpful in documenting the degree of glycemic control at the time of diagnosis and

as part of continuing care. The ADA recommends that the treatment goal should be A1C below 7.0%. The A1C level roughly correlates to the mean plasma glucose: 6% = glucose of 135 mg/dL; 7% = 170 mg/dL; 8% = 205 mg/dL; 9% = 240 mg/dL; 10% = 275 mg/dL; 11% = 310 mg/dL; and 12% = 345 mg/dL.

Additional laboratory tests that are appropriate to the evaluation of the patient's general medical condition should be performed. They include fasting lipid profile (total cholesterol, high-density lipoprotein [HDL], low-density lipoprotein [LDL], and triglyceride levels), urinalysis, microalbuminuria, thyroid function tests, liver enzymes, and serum creatinine if protein is present. Urine cultures are obtained if indicated. A 12-lead electrocardiogram (ECG) should also be included in the diagnostic for adults at onset of diagnosis. Screening for other autoimmune diseases (vitamin B_{12} deficiency, celiac disease, and hypothyroidism/hyperthyroidism) should be considered as well.

Differential Diagnosis

With the classic symptoms of DM confirmed by blood plasma glucose testing, a diagnosis of DM can be made; however, other potential causes of hyperglycemia should be considered. Hyperglycemia and glucosuria are present in patients with Cushing's disease, pheochromocytoma, or acromegaly. Extreme stress or trauma, such as that seen in extensive burns, may produce transient hyperglycemia. Renal tubular disease may produce glycosuria without concurrent hyperglycemia. Several pharmacological agents can cause hyperglycemia, including glucocorticoids, sympathomimetic agents, and niacin.

Management

Type 1 DM is a chronic illness that requires ongoing health care and education to prevent acute and chronic complications. The complexity and lifelong management regimens necessitate that the patient and clinician work as a team to develop and implement the treatment plan. The ADA recommends a team approach to care, including the primary-care provider, an endocrinologist periodically when indicated, a certified diabetes educator, a dietitian, the patient, and the patient's family. Essential to successful implementation of the treatment plan is the plan's fit with the patient's lifestyle to the extent possible. This is where a diabetes educator is of the most assistance. Children with type 1 DM will also need school personnel involved in the treatment team.

To be effective, the treatment program requires insulin regimens, frequent self-monitoring of blood glucose (SMBG), medical nutrition therapy, regular exercise, continuing education in the prevention and treatment of complications, and periodic assessment of treatment goals. The principles of assessment and management are summarized in Table 16.8.

A diagnosis of diabetes, as with any chronic illness, requires the incorporation of the diagnosis and ultimate

Table 16.8	Outpatient Assessment and Management of the Patient with Diabetes Mellitus Type 1	
Assessment	**Laboratory Monitoring**	**General Health Maintenance**
Every visit:	A1C every 3 months during the first	• Pneumococcal vaccine
• Symptoms of hypoglycemia and	year of initiation of insulin therapy	• Influenza vaccine annually
hyperglycemia	and during periods of insulin dosage	• Aspirin prophylaxis in
• Results of SMBG	adjustment	patients older than
• Any self-adjustments based on	In patients who have met treatment	40 years of age
SMBG or symptoms	goals, measure twice a year.	Patient education:
• Problems with adherence	Initially and annually:	• Preconceptive or contra-
• Symptoms of complications	• Lipid profile	ceptive counseling (initial
• Any other medical illnesses	• Urinalysis	and quarterly when
• Medications (prescription and	• Serum creatinine	applicable)
over the counter)	Microalbuminuria screening annually:	• Smoking cessation
• Height and weight	• Method 1: measurement of albumin-	recommendations if
• Blood pressure	to-creatinine ratio (can be performed	applicable
• Cardiovascular assessment	in clinic; first morning void is	
• Thyroid exam	preferred because of the diurnal	
• Ophthalmic exam (with an annual	variation in albumin excretion;	
dilated retinal eye exam)	>30 mcg/mg creatinine indicates	
• Peripheral vascular assessment	microalbuminuria)	
• Feet and skin assessment	• Method 2: 24-hour urine collection	
• Neurological assessment		
• Oral exam		

management into the patient's lifestyle. It may take a traumatic event or "turning point" in a patient's management to break the complacency of management to one that focuses on lifestyle changes.

Initial Management

Insulin Therapy The initial goal of treatment for type 1 DM is to normalize the blood glucose level. This is best accomplished by intensive insulin regimens to accomplish the following goals: plasma glucose levels at 80 to 120 mg/dL before meals, plasma glucose levels of 100 to 140 mg/dL at bedtime, and an A1C below 7%. The new type 1 diabetic patient often presents in crisis and requires hospitalization. These patients should be managed by or in close collaboration with an endocrinologist and a comprehensive health-care team. It is beyond the scope of primary care to manage this patient alone.

When patients present in acute hyperglycemia, it is essential not only to treat the hyperglycemia but also to determine its underlying cause (medication nonadherence, underlying infection [the most common cause of DKA], or dietary indiscretion). See Table 16.6 for the management of DKA.

The Diabetes Control and Complications Trial conclusively demonstrated that in patients with type 1 DM, the risk of development or progression of retinopathy, nephropathy, and neuropathy is reduced 50% to 75% by intensive insulin regimens compared with conventional treatment regimens. Individual treatment goals

should, however, take into account the patient's capacity to understand and carry out the treatment, the risk for severe hypoglycemia, and any other factors that increase risk or decrease benefit. Tight glycemic control increases the chance of hypoglycemic episodes and may not be appropriate for many elderly diabetics, patients with coronary artery disease who may be prone to hypoglycemia, or those with diabetic neuropathy who may lack the early neurological (adrenergic) warning signs of hypoglycemia.

Some patients may experience early morning hyperglycemia due to complete absorption of the evening insulin dose before the early morning hours (dawn phenomenon), particularly if an intermediate-acting form of insulin is used, such as neutral protamine Hagedorn (NPH), which has a peak effect at 6 to 10 hours and a duration of action of 10 to 16 hours. In addition, humans have an increased insulin requirement in the morning because of early morning secretion of growth hormone and cortisol. Thus, increasing nighttime insulin may just lead to late evening hypoglycemia, in the absence of an adequate insulin effect in the early morning hours. In turn, if NPH is being used, the evening dose should be given later. Alternatively, it may be more efficient to prevent early morning hyperglycemia by switching the regimen from NPH to a longer-acting form of insulin, such as glargine (Lantus) or detemir (Levemir).

The initiation of insulin therapy in newly diagnosed type 1 DM patients should be managed by or in close collaboration with an endocrinologist. The majority of insulin used today is made chemically identical to human insulin by recombinant DNA technology or by chemical modification of pork insulin; however, beef and pork insulins are still available. Insulin is available in rapid, short, intermediate, and long-acting forms. The optimum dosage is highly individual and can depend on site and depth of injection, skin temperature, and exercise. Human insulin is preferred for patients newly beginning insulin therapy, pregnant women, and persons with allergies.

In the United States, insulin is available in concentrations of 100 or 500 U/mL, but the higher-concentrated preparations are used only in rare cases of insulin resistance, when the patient requires large doses. The 2013 ADA Standards of Medical Care in Diabetes state that the majority of patients with type 1 DM should be treated with three to four injections of insulin per day (including an injection of long-acting [basal] insulin once daily and an injection of prandial fast-acting [regular or lispro] insulin before each meal) or a continuous subcutaneous insulin infusion pump. Both strategies require diligent and frequent blood glucose monitoring by the patient and should be chosen only if appropriate for the patient. Commercially mixed NPH and regular insulin preparations are available, or the patient can custom mix his or her own insulin. Dose amount and timing should be individualized for the patient according to his or her health needs and lifestyle (see Drugs Commonly Prescribed 16.4: Diabetes Mellitus Type 1).

Self-Monitoring of Blood Glucose Self-monitoring of blood glucose (SMBG) is the testing of capillary blood to determine the blood glucose level. Typically, plasma venous glucose measurements are within 15% of the results of whole blood capillary test results.

Drugs Commonly Prescribed 16.4 Diabetes Mellitus Type 1 Insulin Regimens

Single-Dose Therapy

Single Injection
• Intermediate or long-acting insulin with or without regular insulin in the morning OR Intermediate or long-acting insulin at bedtime
• Recommend minimal SMBG in the morning and at bedtime.

Conventional Split-Dose Therapy

Two Injections
• Mixture of NPH and regular insulin in the morning and evening
• Recommend minimal SMBG before each dosing and at bedtime.

Intensive Insulin Therapy

Three Injections
• NPH and regular insulin in the morning; regular insulin at dinner; NPH insulin at bedtime
• Monitor for increased risk of hypoglycemic episodes.

Four Injections
• Regular or lispro insulin before meals and long-acting insulin to maintain basal insulin levels
• Monitor for increased risk of hypoglycemic episodes.

Types of Insulin	Species	Onset, Peak, and Duration	Route
Lispro Insulin			
Humalog	Recombinant DNA technology (usually used in combination with other insulins)	>15 min, 30–60 min, 3–4 hr	SC
Regular Insulin			
Humulin R	Human	30–60 min, 2–6 hr, 6–8 hr	SC, IM, IV
Iletin II Regular	Pork	30–60 min, 2–6 hr, 6–8 hr	SC, IM, IV
Novolin R	Human	30–60 min, 2–6 hr, 6–8 hr	SC, IM, IV
Purified Pork Regular	Pork	30–60 min, 2–6 hr, 6–8 hr	SC, IM, IV
Velosulin	Human	30–60 min, 2–4 hr, 6–8 hr	SC, IM, IV

Drugs Commonly Prescribed 16.4   Diabetes Mellitus Type 1 Insulin Regimens—cont'd

Types of Insulin	Species	Onset, Peak, and Duration	Route
Insulin Isophane Suspension (NPH)			
Humulin N	Human	1–1.5 hr, 4–12 hr, 18–24 hr	SC
Iletin II NPH	Pork	1–1.5 hr, 4–12 hr, 18–24 hr	SC
Novolin N	Human	1–1.5 hr, 4–12 hr, 18–24 hr	SC
Purified Pork NPH	Pork	1–1.5 hr, 4–12 hr, 18–24 hr	SC
Insulin Isophane Suspension (NPH)/Regular Insulin			
Humulin 70/30	Human	30–60 min, 2–12 hr, 24 hr	SC
Humulin 50/50	Human	30–60 min, 3–5 hr, 24 hr	SC
Novolin 70/30	Human	30–60 min, 2–12 hr, 24 hr	SC
Insulin Glargine			
Lantus	Insulin analog	Slowly absorbed with gradual onset, peakless, lasting up to 24 hr	SC
Insulin Detemir			
Levemir	Insulin analog	Slowly absorbed with gradual onset, relative constant concentration with peak at 6–10 hr, lasting up to 24 hr	SC

SMBG: Self-monitoring of blood glucose

SMBG is recommended for patients with type 1 DM to evaluate the effectiveness of the insulin regimen, medical nutrition therapy, and exercise. Used properly, it is the most useful mechanism to maintain glucose levels as close to normal as possible and prevent the single most common complication of diabetes therapy, hypoglycemia.

The frequency and timing of monitoring are dependent on the needs and goals of the individual patient. Optimal monitoring for patients with type 1 DM is three to four times a day—before each meal and before bedtime. Barriers to frequent monitoring in all patients with type 1 DM are cost, inconvenience, and the discomfort produced by the finger pricks. The benefit versus cost ratio must be thoroughly explored with each patient as a treatment plan is developed and goals are established. Table 16.9 presents the goals of glucose management in the patient without symptoms of hypoglycemia.

Continuous Glucose Monitoring Continuous glucose monitoring (CGM) utilizes a device that measures interstitial glucose and can be utilized with intensive insulin therapy. This measurement correlates with SMBG. The device has been studied in adults older than 25 years of age and found to reduce the amount of time type 1 DM patients spent in hyperglycemic and hypoglycemic ranges. The measurement of CGM must be calibrated with SMBG, and SMBG should be utilized to make acute treatment decisions. Patients who have limited awareness of hypoglycemic episodes, or ones who have them frequently, may also benefit from CGM.

There are many different types of blood glucose meters, and one should be selected that best fits the needs and resources of the patient. Many of the meters have the ability to download records into personal computers, which allows the clinician to view the data. This can provide helpful information on trends of blood glucose control. The patient should, nevertheless, be instructed to keep a log of results along with insulin doses so that adjustments can be made to the treatment plan. There are more than 1,100 smartphone apps available for helping to manage diabetes. The glucose meter, as well as the individual patient's testing technique, should be assessed at each visit for accuracy while the patient's ideal dose is being adjusted and then annually once the patient is stabilized.

Management of Hypoglycemia Hypoglycemia (plasma glucose less than 70 mg/dL) is a common occurrence in patients with type 1 DM. It can occur for a variety of reasons: excessive exogenous insulin, missed meals or inadequate food intake, exercise, alcohol ingestion, drug interactions, and a decrease in liver or kidney function.

Table 16.9	Goals of Glucose Management*
Time	**Goal**
Before meals	80–120 mg/dL
Bedtime	100–140 mg/dL
Postprandial	<180 mg/dL

*Goals are for glucose management without symptoms of hypoglycemia.

Signs and symptoms include diaphoresis, tachycardia, hunger, shakiness, altered mentation (ranging from inability to concentrate to coma), slurred speech, and seizure. The signs and symptoms exhibited by the patient are highly individual and can vary from mild to severe.

The goal of treatment is to normalize the plasma glucose promptly. If the patient is conscious and able to swallow, this is best accomplished by the ingestion of 15 g of carbohydrate. Examples include one-half cup of any fruit juice (no additional sugar added), 6 ounces of regular soda (not diet), 1 cup of milk, or glucose tablets. Candy (no chocolate) can be used but is not recommended because the patient may eat it when it is not needed. Blood glucose should be checked 15 minutes after treatment, and additional carbohydrate should be given if the blood glucose results remain less than 60 mg/dL. For severe hypoglycemia and if the patient is unconscious or unable to swallow, 1 mg of glucagon can be given subcutaneously. Another treatment alternative is 50 mL of 50% dextrose solution given IV.

Nocturnal hypoglycemia can occur if the predinner, intermediate-acting insulin dose is too high or if the patient skips dinner or eats an inadequate amount. The patient may not awaken with symptoms but on arising may note an increased fasting glucose level. This is due to a compensatory mechanism in the liver, which responds in the event of sustained hypoglycemia. After hypoglycemia has been resolved, the possible causes should be reviewed with the patient and preventive measures discussed. The Somogyi effect, for example, is a unique combination of hypoglycemia during the night with rebound hyperglycemia in the morning. Although several studies failed to confirm the validity of this pathological process, many clinicians still feel the Somogyi effect exists and is most common in children with type 1 DM. This possibility should be investigated whenever fluctuations in blood sugar levels are serious.

Once the patient has been educated in insulin therapy, SMBG, and hypoglycemia, subsequent management should include education in meal planning and assistance in developing a regular exercise program. Most patients will benefit from a referral to a certified diabetic educator for a group program or individual counseling. A referral to a dietitian should be ordered for all patients.

Diet Meal planning or medical nutritional therapy is one of the most challenging aspects of diabetes management because achievement of treatment goals may require substantial lifestyle changes. The goals of nutritional therapy are to maintain normal blood glucose level, prevent hypoglycemia, maintain normal serum lipid levels, attain or maintain reasonable body weight, and promote healthy eating patterns. The meal plan should be based on the patient's food choices; exercise; medical history; weight; lifestyle; and cultural, ethnic, and financial factors. The first step of the nutritional consultation should be an initial assessment of the patient's nutritional status, including a diet history. Recommendations for change should not be made until the patient's current eating patterns are determined. Most patients with type 1 DM are lean, so weight loss is generally not a factor in meal planning. The following formulas can be used to determine the total number of kilocalories needed to maintain current weight:

For men: 66 + 13.7 (weight in kg) + 5 (height in cm) – 6.8 (age)

For women: 65 + 9.6 (weight in kg) + 1.7 (height in cm) – 4.7 (age)

Complementary Therapies 16.1

Problem and Therapy	Dosage	Comment
Diabetes Mellitus		
• Cinnamon (*Cinnamomum cassia*)	1–2 tsp daily	In one study, the ingestion of 1–6 g of cinnamon for 20 days reduced blood glucose, LDL cholesterol, triglycerides, and total cholesterol.
• Fenugreek (*Trigonella foenum-graecum*)	0.5 g of seeds in 150 mL of boiling water; steep for 3 hours and strain. Do not exceed 6 g/day.	Contains soluble fiber that decreases blood glucose. Has anti-inflammatory properties.
• Zinc	15 mg daily	May improve effectiveness of insulin.
• Niacin	500 mg 3 times daily	May slow the progression of type 1 diabetes mellitus and may prevent complications of the disease.
• Alpha-lipoic acid	200 mg 2 times daily	Used in Europe for decades for the treatment of diabetic neuropathy. Prevents nerve damage by toxic free radicals and may improve the action of insulin.
• Biofeedback-assisted relaxation for type 2 diabetes mellitus		Patients enrolled in a biofeedback relaxation therapy group were found to have significantly decreased blood glucose levels.

Multiply the result by 1.2 for a fairly active person and up to 1.5 for an ill person. Individuals on insulin should eat at consistent times that are synchronized with their insulin administration.

A nutritionally balanced meal plan is important for the patient with type 1 DM and should take into account the higher prevalence of atherosclerosis. The ADA guidelines recommend that the meal plan consists of the following:

- Protein: 10% to 20% of daily caloric intake from protein
- Fat: 10% to 20% of daily caloric intake from fat (less than 8%–9% saturated fat with no more than 300 mg of cholesterol)
- Carbohydrates: A minimum of 60% to 70% of daily caloric intake from carbohydrates (with 20–35 g of fiber)

Previously, it was a widely held belief that simple sugars should be avoided based on the assumption that sugars (simple carbohydrates) are more rapidly digested and absorbed than starches (complex carbohydrates) and can therefore aggravate hyperglycemia. There is very little scientific evidence to support this. Although various simple and complex carbohydrates do have different glycemic responses, the first priority should be given to the total amount of carbohydrate consumed rather than the source of the carbohydrate. This means that sucrose and sucrose-containing foods must be substituted for other carbohydrates gram for gram. Other nutritive sweeteners (such as fructose, dextrose, and maltose) and sugar alcohols (such as sorbitol, mannitol, and xylitol) do not have any significant advantage over sucrose in improving overall diabetes control, and sugar alcohols in excessive amounts may have a laxative effect. The calories and carbohydrate content of all these sweeteners should be taken into account in the meal plan. Nonnutritive sweeteners such as saccharin, aspartame, acesulfame potassium, sucralose, and the Latin American herb stevia are noncaloric and do not affect the blood glucose level. The majority of patients with type 1 DM can safely use them.

Although soluble fiber can inhibit the absorption of glucose from the small intestine, the amount contained in most foods will not have a significant effect on blood glucose levels. Fiber recommendations for individuals with diabetes, therefore, are the same as for the general population (20–35 g/day).

Vitamin and mineral supplementation is not generally recommended for persons whose dietary intake is adequate. Chromium replacements have no known benefit except for the patient who may be chromium deficient as a result of long-term parenteral nutrition. Magnesium and sodium replacement should be given only if medically warranted.

The same recommendations used for the general population concerning alcohol ingestion are appropriate for the patient with type 1 DM. Moderate consumption does not adversely affect blood glucose control if the patient has overall good control, but calories from alcohol should be included as part of the total calorie intake. Heavily sweetened drinks should be avoided, and alcohol should be taken with and in addition to the meal plan.

Exercise Before beginning an exercise program, the patient should be screened for the presence of macrovascular and microvascular complications that may be aggravated by exercise. These include coronary artery disease (CAD), peripheral arterial disease, retinopathy, nephropathy, and peripheral or autonomic neuropathy. The patient with type 1 DM can perform all levels of exercise as long as glycemic control is good and there is no evidence of the complications that would preclude exercise. The ADA recommends that patients with diagnosed CAD should undergo a supervised evaluation of exercise tolerance before beginning an exercise program.

Because the metabolic adjustments that occur to maintain blood glucose levels during exercise in a nondiabetic individual are absent in patients with type 1 DM, exercise can exacerbate hyperglycemia if the patient has too little insulin. Conversely, if there is too much insulin, hypoglycemia may occur. The patient must, therefore, use the following general guidelines regarding exercise to regulate the glycemic response:

- Check blood glucose before, every 30 to 60 minutes during, and after exercise.
- Avoid exercise if the fasting glucose is more than 250 mg/dL and ketosis is present or if the glucose level is more than 300 mg/dL, regardless of whether ketosis is present.
- Consume additional carbohydrate if the glucose is less than 100 mg/dL and as needed to avoid hypoglycemia.
- Identify when changes in insulin or food are necessary.

Any exercise prescription should be individualized to take into account the patient's interest, lifestyle, physical condition, and motivation. The program should include 150 minutes per week of moderate-intensity aerobic activity. Muscle-strengthening exercises can also be added. With careful instructions, the patient with type 1 DM can enjoy the benefits of an exercise program.

Urine Ketone Testing Urine ketone testing is recommended for patients with type 1 DM and should be performed when the patient is experiencing stress and when SMBG levels are greater than 300 mg/dL. During an acute illness, especially if the patient is nauseated and vomiting, urine ketones should be monitored. Because pregnancy is a stress on the diabetic patient, pregnant women should assess urine for ketones periodically. Ketonuria can reflect dehydration and the need for extra fluid, as well as an increased insulin requirement.

Follow-up and Referral

Continuing care is essential in the management of type 1 DM. Long-term surveillance for potential complications of DM demands almost as much daily attention of the patient and office time of the provider as do the daily regimens needed to manage this disease effectively.

The frequency of patient visits depends on the degree to which blood glucose levels are controlled, changes in therapy, and the presence and degree of complications or other medical conditions. If the patient is performing SMBG, telephone consultations instead of clinic visits may be possible. Once regulated, the patient should be seen at least quarterly. These visits should include a discussion on results of SMBG; adjustments to therapy made by the patient; symptoms of medical illnesses; problems with adherence to the treatment plan; changes in lifestyle; medications; and frequency, causes, and severity of hyperglycemia or hypoglycemia.

The National Institutes of Health (NIH) has set up a multicenter program called Trialnet that accepts referral of relatives of patients with type 1 DM for screening with islet cell antibody measurements. It offers treatment with various agents that are being investigated as potentially preventing the development of the disease. The Web site is www.diabetestrialnet.org.

Complications

Risks of type 1 DM complications (retinopathy, nephropathy, and neuropathy) are significantly reduced when A1C levels are maintained below 7%. A1C determination should be performed at least twice a year in patients with good control and quarterly in patients whose therapy has changed or who are not meeting glycemic goals. The physical exam should include a comprehensive foot exam and a funduscopic exam.

Referral to a specialist for the following complications may be indicated:

- *Retinopathy:* The ADA reports that after 20 years, almost all patients will have some degree of retinopathy, documenting the need for annual ophthalmic evaluations. Comprehensive dilated eye and visual exams should be performed annually by an ophthalmologist who is knowledgeable and experienced in the management of diabetic retinopathy for all patients age 10 years and older who have had diabetes for 3 to 5 years, all patients diagnosed after age 30 years, and any patient with visual symptoms or abnormalities.
- *Hyperlipidemia:* Adults with type 1 DM should be retested annually for lipid disorders with a complete fasting lipid profile, because there is an increased risk in these individuals for coronary artery disease.
- *Nephropathy:* A routine urinalysis should be performed annually in adults with type 1 DM to monitor for developing nephropathy. Screening for microalbuminuria should begin with puberty and after 5 years' duration of the disease. Persistent microalbuminuria (greater than 30 mg/24 hr) has been shown to be the earliest stage of diabetic nephropathy. Overt nephropathy

(albuminuria greater than or equal to 300 mg/24 hr) will develop over a period of 10 to 15 years in approximately 80% of patients who develop microalbuminuria, many of whom will also develop hypertension. Transient elevations of albumin excretion occur during acute febrile illnesses, marked hypertension, short-term hyperglycemia, exercise, urinary tract infections, and in heart failure. Angiotensin-converting enzyme (ACE) inhibitors have been found to postpone progression of microalbuminuria and ultimately nephropathy in patients. They have few adverse effects and are suggested as part of the initial therapy for diabetic patients with nephropathy. Their use is contraindicated in women who are pregnant, and they should be used with caution in women of childbearing age. ACE inhibitors may also exacerbate hyperkalemia in patients with advanced renal insufficiency or hyporeninemic hypoaldosteronism. Older adults with advanced renal disease and patients with renal artery stenosis may experience a decline in renal function with ACE inhibitors. If a patient does not tolerate the use of ACE inhibitors, angiotensin receptor blockers (ARBs) can be used. Some studies suggest that they be used together in all diabetic patients for the benefit in nephropathy, because the medications act by different mechanisms.

- *Hypertension:* In a patient with type 1 DM, hypertension is often a manifestation of nephropathy. Control of hypertension has been demonstrated to reduce the rate of progression of nephropathy and to reduce the complications of cardiovascular disease. ADA guidelines recommend that the goal for blood pressure control in nonpregnant adults is to maintain the systolic blood pressure less than 140 mm Hg and the diastolic less than 80 mm Hg. Studies have shown that the closer patients with DM get to the target blood pressure, the less likely they are to develop cardiac sequelae. The goal for patients with isolated systolic hypertension is the aforementioned target blood pressure, but a more realistic goal may be for a patient with a systolic blood pressure of 180 mm Hg or higher to decrease the systolic blood pressure to less than 140 to 160 mm Hg and for patients with isolated systolic blood pressure of 160 to 170 mm Hg to decrease by 20 to 30 mm Hg. Recommendations are that initial treatment for patients with hypertension should include lifestyle management and, if medication is required, an ACE inhibitor or ARB should be started, unless contraindicated. Patients with signs of congestive heart failure and a normal or higher than normal ejection fraction should be screened for diastolic dysfunction and treated to target accordingly.
- *Macrovascular disease:* Diabetic patients are at risk for developing macrovascular complications including stroke, peripheral vascular disease (PVD), and CAD/cardiovascular disease. Evidence of uncontrolled angina, carotid bruits, and ECG abnormalities may

require advanced intervention. Daily intake of aspirin has been shown to reduce cardiovascular events in patients with diabetes. Patients with disabling claudication or nonhealing ulcers require a vascular consultation for their PVD. All diabetic patients should be screened for these diseases, because symptoms may not be present until late in the course of the disease process.

- *Neuropathy:* Foot ulcers and related problems resulting from the decreased peripheral sensation in diabetic patients with significant neuropathy are a major cause of morbidity and mortality. Half of the patients with hyperglycemia extending over 15 years will develop some degree of neuropathy. Peripheral neuropathy may result in pain, loss of sensation, and muscle weakness. The feet and ankles are affected most often, but many patients also complain of pain in the knees and upper extremities. Severe pain from neuropathy can lead to sleep and mood disturbances. A thorough initial foot exam followed by annual foot exams are indicated in asymptomatic patients. A 10-g Semmes-Weinstein monofilament should be used to assess sensation at least annually. Abnormal findings indicate the need for a thorough vascular, neurological, musculoskeletal, and soft tissue evaluation. Many patients take several medications to control the pain or discomfort of neuropathy. Analgesics, narcotic analgesics, tricyclic antidepressants, antiarrhythmics, and local anesthetics are frequently prescribed. Tricyclic antidepressants are commonly prescribed for painful neuropathies and are often the first-line drug in patients for whom they are not contraindicated. Gabapentin (Neurontin) may be an alternative choice for patients who cannot take tricyclic antidepressants. Patients suffering from chronic pain syndromes may benefit from a referral to a chronic pain clinic. Patients with neuropathy require professional nail and callus care because most ulcers begin at the site of a callus. Supportive athletic shoes are recommended for all patients for walking. Extra-depth shoes and custom-molded shoe inserts are indicated for patients who are at high risk for foot ulcers.

  Patients at high risk include those with neuropathy; structural deformities of the feet, skin, or nails; or a history of previous ulcers. Charcot foot disorders occur in 9% of patients with neuropathy, and its symptoms may be confused with those of cellulitis. It leads to bony destruction, joint subluxation, and bony remodeling of the foot. Patients with abnormal findings on radiological exam should be referred to an orthopedist for initial evaluation.

- *Pregnancy:* Of the 10% of all pregnancies that are complicated by diabetes, 0.2% to 0.5% are women with type 1 DM. There is an increased risk for many complications such as preeclampsia, preterm delivery, intrauterine fetal demise, or cardiac and renal malformations, just to name a few. There should be preconception counseling and then frequent follow-up to stress the importance of extremely tight glucose control.

- *Other:* Autonomic involvement can affect gastrointestinal, cardiovascular, and genitourinary function. Sexual dysfunction, particularly impotence, may occur. The demands of glycemic control on lifestyle often lead to depression. Patients should be evaluated for depression initially and annually.

Patient Education

Insulin administration involves the use of subcutaneous syringes marked in insulin units. Regulations governing the purchase of syringes vary greatly from state to state. Although syringe manufacturers recommend that syringes be used only once, it appears safe and practical for the patient to reuse the syringe if needed, but it should be discarded if the needle integrity is compromised. Syringes should be recapped by the patient using a one-handed technique, and they should be discarded according to state requirements. Patients with visual or dexterity difficulties may benefit from prefilling syringes. Prefilled insulin syringes may be stored in a vertical position in the refrigerator for up to 30 days with the needle pointing upward.

Alternatives to syringes include jet injectors and penlike devices. Jet injectors are useful for patients who have needle phobias, but they are expensive. Penlike devices hold insulin cartridges and are useful if the patient is visually or neurologically impaired, and they help to increase the accuracy of insulin administration. Unlike older insulins, the new varieties do not require refrigeration, which makes them more convenient. Another alternative is the insulin pump, which is a small device (about the size of a pager) that is worn externally. Continuous subcutaneous insulin is delivered via tubing attached to the pump. Use of the insulin pump requires care by skilled professionals, careful selection of patients, frequent blood glucose monitoring, and comprehensive patient education.

Insulin should be injected at room temperature, and bottles not in use should be stored in the refrigerator. It should be injected into the subcutaneous tissue of the upper arm, anterior or lateral aspects of the thigh, the buttocks, or the abdomen. Rotation of the site within one area is recommended rather than rotating to a different site with each injection.

Foot care should be reviewed at each visit. Patients at high risk for foot ulcer development need continued education to follow through with professional foot care and daily foot hygiene. Patients at low risk should be encouraged to continue good hygiene; wear proper footwear; avoid trauma to the feet; stop smoking if they do; and report any blisters, macerated skin, or hemorrhage into a callus immediately and limit weight-bearing on the affected extremity.

Any illness maximizes stress, and this is especially true for diabetics. When ill, all diabetics must continue to take their insulin and increase blood glucose monitoring to every 2 hours. Supplemental dosages of regular insulin may be needed to control blood glucose levels. If blood sugar is higher than 240 mg/dL, the urine should be checked for ketones every 4 hours. A caloric intake of 50 g of carbohydrates every 4 hours should be maintained. A variety of clear fluids, including some with glucose, should be encouraged, as well as gelatin, ice pops, regular soda, soups, and toast, if tolerated. Patients should be encouraged to maintain an oral fluid intake of 6 to 9 oz/hr to avoid dehydration.

If vomiting or diarrhea persists over 2 hours, a fever of 101ºF (38.33ºC) or higher is present, or blood glucose is 240 mg/dL or higher and ketones continue to appear in the urine despite additional insulin, the patient should be instructed to seek medical attention immediately.

Signs of DKA to be alert for include extreme fatigue, abnormal cramping, and alterations in breathing pattern.

The Iceberg of Diabetes Mellitus

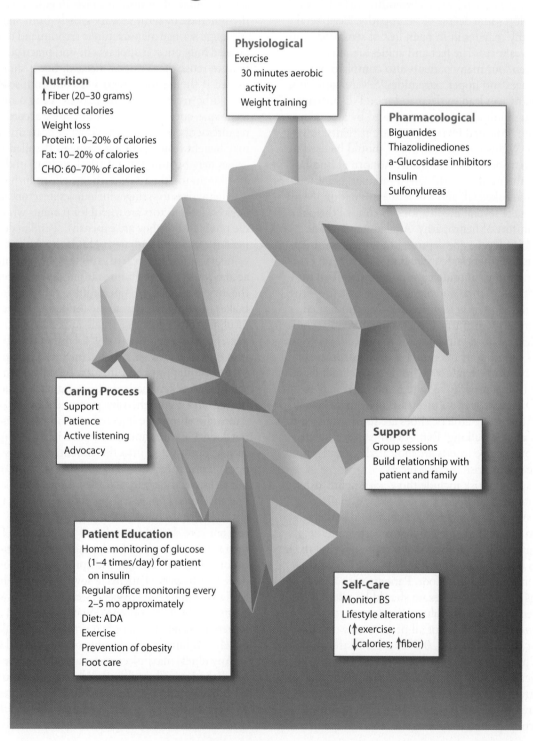

■ DIABETES MELLITUS TYPE 2

Type 2 DM is the fifth leading cause of death in the United States; however, it contributes to many other diseases, particularly heart disease, which is the leading cause of death. Type 2 DM is a group of heterogeneous forms characterized by insufficient circulating endogenous insulin, resistance to insulin action, and an inadequate compensatory insulin secretion response. Approximately 90% of all Americans diagnosed with diabetes have this type of DM. Type 2 DM reduces life expectancy because of complications, which are affected by the duration of diabetes, the degree of blood glucose control, and other cardiovascular risk factors such as smoking and hypertension.

Epidemiology and Causes

The prevalence of type 2 DM in the United States today is 6.6%. About 18 million Americans have type 2 DM, but nearly one-third of individuals are unaware that they have the disease. The disease is often asymptomatic in its early stages; as a result, individuals can remain undiagnosed for many years. The chronic hyperglycemia, however, is associated with long-term damage and dysfunction of various organs, including the kidneys, eyes, nerves, heart, and blood vessels. The comorbidities associated with type 2 DM are thus quite extensive, as reflected in the per capita health-care costs for diabetics in the United States, which are five times higher than those of nondiabetics.

Numerous risk factors are associated with the development of type 2 DM (see Risk Factors 16.1). At risk are those with a first-degree relative with type 2 DM, who demonstrate a 5- to 10-fold higher lifetime risk of developing the disease than age-matched controls with no family history. Moreover, nearly 40% of patients have at least one affected parent with the disease, and monozygotic twin studies further demonstrate between 60% and 90% concordance.

Risk Factors 16.1 Diabetes Mellitus Type 2

Family history (first-degree relative)
Age greater than 45 years
Impaired fasting glucose
Delivery of baby weighing more than 9 pounds
Hypertension
Hyperlipidemia (high-density lipoproteins <40 mg/dL in men and <50 mg/dL in women, triglycerides >250 mg/dL)
Obesity
Ethnicity/racial
• African American
• Hispanic American
• Native American
• Asian American
• Pacific Islander

Racial and ethnic variations also affect the prevalence of type 2 DM. A disproportionate number of African Americans, Hispanic Americans, Native Americans, Asian Americans, and Pacific Islanders have diabetes. The prevalence of type 2 DM in Native Americans and Alaskan natives is approximately two to six times that found in non-Hispanic whites. Pacific Islanders living traditionally have a prevalence of 2.9% whereas those who immigrate to the United States and adopt Western ways have a prevalence rate of 12%. Along with genetic differences, there are a host of factors that may underlie this disparity in disease prevalence, including socioeconomic factors, differential health-care practices, unequal access to health-care resources, and ethnocultural influences in diet and activity and the impact of institutionalized racism. However, the overall prevalence rate of type 2 DM appears to be increasing in the general population, as well as among specific ethnic minority groups.

The incidence of diabetes increases with age, especially in those 45 years of age and older. However, it is important to note that the condition may be diagnosed at any age. Paralleling the marked increase in childhood obesity over the last several decades, rates of newly diagnosed cases of type 2 DM among children are on the rise. Prevalence rates in adolescents and young adults are increasing faster than in any other age-group.

Those previously identified as having an elevated fasting glucose, impaired glucose tolerance, a history of gestational DM, or past delivery of an infant weighing more than 9 pounds are also at greater risk. Gestational DM is defined as any degree of pregnancy-associated glucose intolerance that affects 2% to 4% of all pregnancies in the United States. It is associated with significant fetal morbidity including macrosomia, congenital heart defects, hypoglycemia, hyperbilirubinemia, hypocalcemia, and sepsis. At the other end of the spectrum is polycystic ovary syndrome—a condition characterized by obesity, infertility, and insulin resistance in women, which is also a major risk factor for type 2 DM.

Several pharmacological agents are associated with iatrogenic hyperglycemia and the eventual development of overt DM. These include glucocorticoids, hormonal therapies such as oral contraceptives, the immunosuppressants tacrolimus and cyclosporine, nicotinic acid (niacin), antiviral HIV protease inhibitors (which also cause central fat redistribution known as lipodystrophy syndrome), several atypical antipsychotic agents including clozapine and olanzapine, and certain antihypertensives including beta blockers, calcium channel blockers, clonidine, and thiazide diuretics. In contrast, both angiotensin-converting enzyme (ACE) inhibitors and angiotensin II receptor blockers (ARBs) appear to improve insulin sensitivity and reduce the development of type 2 DM in hypertensive nondiabetics.

Increasing evidence points to linkages among CAD, hyperlipidemia, obesity, and DM, as discussed extensively under Pathophysiology. Because early detection and prompt treatment may reduce the complications of type 2 DM, screening for diabetes as part of routine medical care is appropriate under certain circumstances. Testing for diabetes should be considered in all individuals age 45 years and older and, if normal, should be repeated at 3-year intervals. Testing should be considered in younger individuals who are obese (more than 20% over desired body weight), have a first-degree relative with diabetes, are members of high-risk ethnic populations, have delivered a baby weighing more than 9 pounds, or have an impaired fasting glucose during pregnancy.

Pathophysiology

Type 2 DM is associated with two physiological abnormalities: insulin resistance and impaired insulin secretion. Insulin resistance is associated with acquired traits, such as obesity and aging.

Initially, as insulin resistance increases, insulin levels begin to rise, and the glucose level remains normal, causing a state of hyperinsulinemia. In turn, both fasting and postprandial hyperinsulinemia are predictors of future weight gain, which, in turn, predisposes the individual to hyperglycemia. Thus, this compensatory hyperinsulinemia fails to keep pace if blood glucose begins to rise as in a postprandial state. Moreover, hyperglycemia itself is toxic to pancreatic beta cells, possibly via decreased expression of the insulin gene. As a result, over time, this hyperinsulinemia actually progresses to relative hypoinsulinemia.

Unlike the pattern in type 1 DM, there is no autoimmune destruction of pancreatic beta cells. Rather, there is a decline in their endocrine function, with impaired insulin secretion in response to a glycemic load, which produces elevated plasma glucose levels. This appears to occur at the level of proinsulin, the secreted precursor form of insulin. In nondiabetic individuals, 10% to 15% of secreted insulin may be detected via immunoassays as proinsulin or one of its conversion intermediates. However, in diabetic patients, this value may be as high as 40%. Although the resultant hyperglycemia drives increased insulin secretion even further, obesity and insulin resistance alone do not appear to account for the increased fraction of proinsulin, thus implicating a potential defect in the conversion of proinsulin to insulin or the premature, dysregulated secretion of proinsulin.

Amylin, an islet cell–produced amyloid polypeptide, is also present in beta-cell secretory granules. Serum levels of amylin decrease in concert with those of insulin in type 2 diabetics, whereas pancreatic concentrations of the polypeptide are markedly increased in type 2 diabetics. These observations, along with amylin antagonist studies performed in rat models, have suggested that amylin may be a negative regulator of insulin secretion in type 2 DM; however, this hypothesis has yet to be confirmed in rigorous human studies.

Regardless, in conjunction with hyperinsulinemia, insulin resistance worsens, manifesting first as postprandial hyperglycemia and eventually as fasting hyperglycemia,

once hepatic gluconeogenesis increases. The sequence of impaired insulin secretion preceding worsening insulin resistance has been documented in prospective studies. However, several other studies have indicated that these two pathophysiological mechanisms are independent risk factors for the development of type 2 DM and, in fact, occur in concert with one another, rather than in a sequential manner. Indeed, double-knockout mouse models lacking activity in both the glucokinase (involved in insulin secretion) and insulin-receptor substrate–1 (IRS-1) (involved in insulin sensitivity) genes develop DM, whereas single-knockout mouse strains lacking only one of these genes do not. Although insufficient to cause DM alone, insulin resistance appears to be the strongest predictor of type 2 DM development, an observation that is reinforced by the importance of insulin resistance as a component of the insulin-resistant metabolic syndrome (syndrome X).

There is a strong non-Mendelian genetic component to type 2 DM. Only about 5% of type 2 DM cases can be attributed to single-gene mutations that decrease insulin secretion or function, for example, glucokinase (a probable beta-cell glucose sensor), insulin promoter factor–1 (an insulin gene transcription factor), and beta-3-adrenergic receptor (a regulator of lipolysis). However, several other genetic defects have been associated with insulin resistance, including mutations in the genes encoding the protein components of the insulin receptor, which is a tetramer consisting of two extracellular alpha subunits and two transmembrane/intracellular beta subunits with inherent tyrosine kinase activity that initiates intracellular signaling on binding of the insulin molecule. In addition, genes not directly involved in insulin secretion or function, such as the hepatocyte nuclear factors 1-alpha, 1-beta, and 4-alpha, have each been associated with different forms of maturity-onset diabetes of the young—a rare form of type 2 DM that may first manifest in a patient's early 20s.

However, the most common forms of type 2 DM likely involve insulin resistance that is due to postreceptor genetic defects. Candidate genes that may play an important role include those for glycogen synthase (needed for hepatic glucose stores), IRS-2 (a cell-signaling mediator downstream of the insulin receptor), calpain-10 (a cysteine protease particularly important in diabetic Mexican Americans), and peroxisome-proliferator–activated receptor (PPAR) γ-2 (the target molecule of the thiazolidinedione class of antihyperglycemic drugs, which plays an important role in adipocyte differentiation).

Obesity is a major modifiable risk factor for developing type 2 DM, affecting up to 90% of type 2 diabetics. Moreover, patients who are not obese but have an increased percentage of body weight distributed in the abdominal area rather than the hips (also known as central obesity, upper body obesity, or male-type obesity) are also at greater risk. Although this mechanism has not been fully elucidated, obesity is known to contribute to peripheral insulin resistance, both impairing glucose uptake and decreasing pancreatic beta-cell sensitivity to plasma glucose levels, thereby decreasing reactive insulin secretion. The aforementioned beta-3-adrenergic receptor and the c-Jun amino-terminal kinase (JNK) intracellular signaling pathways have both been implicated. Moreover, adipocyte-derived tumor necrosis factor–alpha (TNF-α) has been positively correlated with increasing insulin resistance, as has the adipocyte hormone resistin. In contrast, the adipocyte hormone adiponectin appears to be negatively correlated with insulin resistance. However, the bulk of the evidence for all these hormones comes primarily from rat and mouse studies, whereas human data are lacking. Whatever the case, physical exercise with a corresponding weight loss of just 10% to 20% of total body weight confers protection against the subsequent development of type 2 DM in overweight individuals, generating marked improvement in glucose tolerance.

Elevated plasma glucose levels may be well tolerated for many years by the diabetic patient, who may not seek treatment until chronic complications result. Eventually, however, insulin secretion will become insufficient to compensate for insulin resistance. Moreover, hyperinsulinemia and hyperglycemia increase lipid synthesis, raising the serum levels of fatty acids, triglycerides (greater than 150 mg/dL), and low-density lipoprotein (LDL) cholesterol, while lowering high-density lipoprotein (HDL) cholesterol. As a result, increased lipids are deposited on vessel walls more readily.

Hyperglycemia thus leads to both microvascular and macrovascular complications, which underlie long-term diabetic damage. Vascular endothelial dysfunction and inflammation result in fibrosis and intimal thickening, leading to progressive narrowing of the vascular lumen. In turn, blood flow through the microvasculature is reduced, leading to tissue ischemia throughout the body, which results in functional impairment of multiple end organs. This explains how DM can simultaneously reign as the leading cause of acquired blindness (due to retinopathy), end-stage renal disease (due to nephropathy), and nontraumatic lower extremity amputation (due to PVD and infection), as well as its major contribution to heart disease and stroke. In turn, several clinical trials have demonstrated that careful glycemic control reduces the development and delays the progression of microvascular manifestations of DM, including nephropathy and retinopathy.

Sympathetic tone and cardiac contractility are increased by hyperinsulinemia due to increases in the plasma catecholamines epinephrine and norepinephrine. With high levels of circulating glucose caused by cellular resistance to insulin, the distal nephron of the kidney absorbs increased amounts of sodium and water, expanding the intravascular volume and increasing the blood pressure. The triad of disturbed glucose metabolism, hypertension (greater than 140/90 mm Hg), and dyslipidemia with obesity is variably referred to as insulin resistance syndrome, syndrome X, obesity dyslipidemia syndrome, or the metabolic syndrome. This condition may exist in prediabetic, glucose-intolerant, or overtly diabetic states. Typically, this syndrome culminates in significant CAD and PVD and is strongly associated with the development of full-blown type 2 DM in prediabetics.

Clinical Presentation

Because the onset of diabetes may occur years before a diagnosis is made, individuals who are asymptomatic tend to be diagnosed during a routine physical exam or during treatment for another condition.

Subjective

Because the onset of type 2 DM is usually insidious, only a minority of patients are initially symptomatic. The patient may, however, present with pruritus or neuropathic complaints such as numbness and tingling. Some patients present with increased urination, nocturia, thirst, or polydipsia. In many cases, type 2 DM first presents as an infection, especially vaginitis (candidiasis) or a skin infection. Cardiovascular symptoms such as angina may prompt the patient to seek health care. The symptoms of type 1 and type 2 DM are basically the same. See the previous section on type 1 DM for a complete discussion.

Objective

There may be no dramatic change in objective findings, although the patient is often obese, with a history of dyslipidemia, hypertension, and CAD. Abnormal healing and an increased occurrence of infection, especially yeast infection, may be present.

Hyperosmolar hyperglycemic syndrome (HHS) is profound dehydration that results from prolonged hyperglycemia (see Table 16.7). Formerly known as hyperosmolar hyperglycemic nonketotic coma, HHS is associated with a high mortality rate and is seen in older adults who have developed an infection or other illness. It is commonly recognized in the older adult with pneumonia. Patients with undiagnosed DM may develop this condition because of prolonged hyperglycemia without treatment. Other risk factors for development include peritoneal dialysis; hemodialysis; tube feedings with high-protein formulas; and the use of mannitol, phenytoin, steroids, immunosuppressive agents, and diuretics. Symptoms are dramatic, including severe hyperglycemia (greater than 600 mg/dL), plasma or serum hyperosmolality (more than 340 mOsm), and profound dehydration. Ketosis may or may not be present, and neurological symptoms range from clouded sensorium to coma. The condition requires immediate referral for acute-care management.

Diagnostic Reasoning

Diagnostic Tests

Initial Testing Immediate testing in the clinical setting can be accomplished by using a portable monitor to test capillary blood glucose level. This test is referred to as a random capillary glucose measurement and is given without regard to time of last meal. A result of 200 mg/dL or more should be evaluated by screening for blood glucose with whole blood. It is important to consider that certain drugs, including glucocorticoids, furosemide (Lasix), thiazides, phenytoin (Dilantin), estrogen-containing products, beta blockers, and nicotinic acid, can produce hyperglycemia. If the random plasma glucose level is elevated, the urine should be tested for ketones and additional blood glucose testing should be done. There are four ways to diagnose diabetes:

1. A glycosylated hemoglobin (A1C) level greater than or equal to 6.5% on two occasions.
2. Symptoms of DM plus random plasma glucose of 200 mg/dL or higher on two occasions.
3. Fasting plasma glucose of 126 mg/dL or higher on two occasions. *Fasting* is defined as no caloric intake for at least 8 hours.
4. Two-hour postload plasma glucose of 200 mg/dL or higher during an oral glucose tolerance test (OGTT) on two occasions. The test should be performed using a glucose load containing the equivalent of 75 g of anhydrous glucose dissolved in water. This test is not recommended for routine clinical use or in pregnancy.

Subsequent Testing An A1C determination gives valuable insight into the mean glycemia over the preceding 2 to 3 months and is helpful in documenting the degree of glycemic control at the time of diagnosis and as part of continuing care. An A1C value less than 7% indicates good control; however, a value less than 6% has been shown to significantly decrease the occurrence of complications.

Additional laboratory tests that are appropriate to the evaluation of the patient's general medical condition should be performed at the time of diagnosis and at least annually thereafter. These include a fasting lipid profile, serum creatinine, and urine albumin.

Correct classification of patients with diabetes can be difficult. A determination of the C-peptide level may be helpful in determining the extent to which exogenous insulin is being produced. Proinsulin, a precursor of insulin, is produced in the pancreas and is split into insulin and C-peptide. Unlike insulin, C-peptide is not metabolized in the liver; its serum concentration thus reflects insulin secretion. If the basal (fasting) C-peptide level is more than 0.5 nmol/L (greater than 1 ng/dL), the patient most likely has type 2 DM. In type 1 DM, the basal C-peptide level is less than 0.2 nmol/L.

Differential Diagnosis

Differential diagnosis includes type 1 DM, impaired fasting glucose, genetic defects in insulin action, diseases of exocrine pancreas, drug- or chemical-induced DM, immune-mediated infections, and neurological disorders that mimic diabetic neuropathy.

Management

Type 2 DM is a chronic illness that requires ongoing health care and education to prevent acute and chronic complications. To be effective, the treatment program requires frequent self-monitoring of blood glucose (SMBG), medical nutritional therapy with weight reduction when indicated, use of oral glucose-lowering agents and/or insulin, regular exercise, continuing education in the prevention and treatment of complications, and periodic assessment of treatment goals. Careful attention should be given to the control of cardiovascular risk factors, such as hypertension, smoking, and dyslipidemia. The lifestyle behavioral changes needed to improve glycemic control are best accomplished with frequent and concise direction. Diet and exercise therapy must be addressed with specific instructions.

Research confirms the benefits of improved glycemic control in the improvement of work and disability outcomes, quality of life, decreased symptomatology, and health-care cost savings. However, studies have also shown that although tighter intensive glycemic control in type 2 DM reduces microvascular complications, it does not improve quality of life or decrease mortality.

Although the primary-care provider's focus is often on glycemic control, the patient's focus is on the need to fit control into an acceptable lifestyle. Research has identified that dietary modifications, the need for frequent blood glucose monitoring, and subsequent follow-up with health-care providers place a financial and psychological burden on patients and families.

Initial Management

Diet and Weight Loss Meal planning or nutritional therapy is one of the most fundamental and challenging components of diabetes management. The goal of nutritional therapy is to achieve and maintain blood glucose level, lipid, and blood pressure goals. Most patients with type 2 DM are overweight, so weight loss is generally a significant factor in meal planning. Although hypocaloric diets and weight loss usually improve blood glucose control, traditional dietary strategies have not been very effective in achieving long-term weight loss. As research continues to explore why weight loss and maintenance is so difficult, the emphasis should be on controlling glucose and promoting healthy eating patterns. The meal plan should be based on the patient's food choices, exercise, medical history, and weight, as well as lifestyle, cultural, ethnic, and financial factors.

If weight loss is indicated, a moderate caloric restriction (250–500 calories less than average daily intake as calculated from food history) and a nutritionally adequate meal plan with a reduction of total fat (especially saturated and trans fats) is recommended. A hypocaloric diet, independent of weight loss, is associated with increased sensitivity to insulin and improvement in blood glucose levels. Moderate weight loss, irrespective of starting weight, has significant benefits, especially in decreasing morbidity and mortality rates. In fact, weight loss is a primary intervention because it improves the serum lipid profile, reduces blood pressure, decreases insulin resistance, and ameliorates glucose intolerance.

Individuals on oral glucose-lowering agents and/or insulin should eat at consistent times that are synchronized with their medication administration. A nutritionally balanced meal plan is important for the patient with type 2 DM and should take into account the higher prevalence of atherosclerosis.

Specific diets for patients with diabetes are no longer recommended by the ADA; however, their recommendations for the composition of a healthy diet are 10% to 20% of daily intake from protein, 10% to 20% from fat (less than 7% being saturated fat), and 60% to 70% from carbohydrates.

Self-Monitoring of Blood Glucose   The optimal frequency of SMBG in patients with type 2 DM has not been clearly established. The frequency, however, is dependent on the attainment of blood glucose goals. SMBG may be useful for guiding treatment decisions or patient self-management when being treated with oral medications or insulin and in patients who have not consistently achieved blood glucose treatment goals. The patient should, nevertheless, be instructed to keep a log of results for periodic review by his or her primary-care provider.

Urine glucose testing provides only a rough estimate of blood glucose levels and is infrequently recommended; however, in patients who cannot or will not implement SMBG, urine glucose testing is an alternative. Urine glucose testing does not reflect blood glucose levels until the renal threshold of 180 mg/dL of blood glucose is exceeded.

Exercise   Exercise is an integral component of management of type 2 DM. Before beginning an exercise program, the patient should be screened for the presence of macrovascular and microvascular complications that may be worsened by exercise. These include coronary artery disease, peripheral arterial disease, retinopathy, nephropathy, and peripheral or autonomic neuropathy. The patient with type 2 DM can perform all levels of exercise as long as glycemic control is adequate and there is no evidence of complications that would preclude exercise. If the patient is taking oral antidiabetic agents or is on insulin, exercise can cause hypoglycemia. Thus, patients initiating an exercise regimen should be aware of the signs of hypoglycemia and be prepared to treat such an event.

Any exercise prescription should be individualized to take into account the patient's interest, lifestyle, physical condition, financial situation, and motivation. The program should include an aerobic activity, such as walking, for at least 150 minutes per week of moderately intense aerobic activity. Muscle-strengthening exercises can also be added. With careful instructions, the patient with type 2 DM can enjoy the benefits of an exercise program.

Subsequent Management

If fasting plasma glucose measurements are less than 200 mg/dL and presenting symptoms are not severe, a course of diet and exercise should be initiated to control hyperglycemia. The patient with type 2 DM will need frequent follow-up during the trial period. Symptomatic patients and patients with marked hyperglycemia (fasting plasma glucose 300 mg/dL or more) will show significant improvement in both with initiation of an oral agent.

Pharmacological Therapy   Pharmacological therapy for type 2 DM is required when dietary modification and exercise do not result in blood glucose control. Drug therapy should always be considered an adjunct therapy to diet and exercise and not as a substitute. Oral medication is initiated when 3 months of nutritional therapy and exercise have not achieved and maintained fasting plasma glucose levels less than 120 mg/dL and an A1C of less than 7%. There is some suggestion that an A1C of 9% or more at time of diagnosis should be treated with medication in conjunction with lifestyle changes at the onset of care.

Current therapy for type 2 DM includes drugs that alter insulin action, stimulate insulin secretion, affect the absorption of glucose, mimic the effects of incretin, act as an insulin secretagogue, or suppress postprandial glucagon release, as well as insulin itself.

Metformin (Glucophage) is a biguanide that works by suppressing excessive hepatic glucose production and by increasing glucose utilization in peripheral tissues. Metformin reduces fasting and postprandial hyperglycemia and reduces hepatic gluconeogenesis. It may also improve glucose levels by reducing intestinal glucose absorption. Metformin does not stimulate endogenous insulin secretion but does lower triglyceride and LDL cholesterol levels while increasing HDL cholesterol.

Metformin can be used as a monotherapy or in combination with sulfonylureas or insulin. Metformin is the first-line medication recommended by the ADA and the European Association for the Study of Diabetes. It is also beneficial in persons with type 2 DM who have been taking sulfonylureas and remain hyperglycemic despite treatment, as well as in patients who are obese, because it has a neutral effect on weight. Metformin should be used only in patients with adequate renal function (serum creatine less than 1.4 or creatinine clearance greater than 50 mL/min). Because metformin can cause fatal lactic acidosis, albeit rarely, it should not be used in patients with liver impairment, in alcoholic patients, or in patients who may develop hypoxia due to cardiopulmonary insufficiency. The risk for lactic acidosis increases if contrast dyes for radiological procedures (which decrease kidney function) are used in patients taking metformin. In this case, and in the case of any surgical procedure (which also decreases kidney function), metformin should be discontinued 24 to 48 hours before diagnostic and surgical procedures. Metformin administration should not be resumed for at least 6 hours after these procedures or until the patient is adequately hydrated. Initial dosing is 500 mg once or twice a day with breakfast and/or dinner (or 850 mg once per day) for 1 week, then twice daily with breakfast and dinner. The dosage should be titrated toward a maximum dose of 2,000 mg, although some studies have shown modest increased effectiveness up to 2,500 mg/day. Several weeks are needed to achieve the maximum effects of the dose. Common adverse reactions are diarrhea, nausea, anorexia, and abdominal discomfort, which usually resolve with a gradual increase of dosage. At the maximum dose, the monthly cost of metformin in the United States is about $4 on many generic formularies. A recent study examined the use of glimepiride (Amaryl) or canagliflozin (Invokana) as an add-on to metformin therapy in type 2 DM patients. The results indicated that canagliflozin reduced A1C and was better tolerated than glimepiride (Level I; Cafalu et al, 2013).

Sulfonylureas work by stimulating pancreatic insulin secretion, which then reduces hepatic glucose output and increases peripheral glucose metabolism. First generation sulfonylureas include acetohexamide (Dymelor),

chlorpropamide (Diabinese), tolazamide (Tolinase), and tolbutamide (Orinase). Second generation sulfonylureas include glimepiride (Amaryl), glipizide (Glucotrol), and glyburide (DiaBeta, Glynase, Micronase). The benefits of second generation sulfonylureas are that they are more potent, tend to produce fewer adverse effects, and have fewer interactions with other drugs.

Sulfonylureas are not recommended for use during pregnancy or for women who are planning a pregnancy. Sulfonylureas are metabolized in the liver, and their use should be avoided in persons with significant hepatic dysfunction. Patients with severe insulin resistance may respond better to metformin or thiazolidinedione (Actos, Avandia) therapy than to the use of sulfonylureas (see Drugs Commonly Prescribed 16.5: Diabetes Mellitus Type 2).

Therapy with sulfonylureas should be initiated at the lowest possible dose and usually begins with a once-daily dose before breakfast, although twice-daily dosing is an option. The dose can be increased every 2 weeks until the desired response is achieved, the maximum dose is reached, or the side effects preclude any further increase. Common adverse reactions are mild gastrointestinal upset and skin rashes. Numerous drugs can interfere with sulfonylureas and can alter their effects.

Drugs Commonly Prescribed 16.5 Diabetes Mellitus Type 2

Drug	Indication	Adverse Reactions and Prescribing Considerations
First Generation Sulfonylureas		
• chlorpropamide (Diabinese) • tolazamide (Tolinase) • tolbutamide (Orinase)	For use as adjunct to diet and exercise in type 2 DM Contraindicated in ketoacidosis	*Applicable for all first generation sulfonylureas:* Reduce dose in older adults; potentiated by NSAIDs, alcohol, salicylates, sulfonamides, probenecid, monoamine oxidase inhibitors, tricyclics, beta blockers. Antagonized by diuretics, steroids, phenothiazines. NIH precautions: Monitor urine and blood glucose; discontinue if jaundice or persistent rash occurs. Secondary failure may occur with prolonged usage. Sulfonylureas are contraindicated in pregnancy and lactation.
Second Generation Sulfonylureas		
• glyburide (DiaBeta, Micronase) • glipizide (Glucotrol) • glimepiride (Amaryl)	For use as an adjunct to diet and exercise in type 2 DM	*Applicable for all second generation sulfonylureas:* Same as for first generation sulfonylureas
Biguanides		
metformin (Glucophage)	Monotherapy; may be used as an adjunct to diet in type 2 DM or with a sulfonylurea or insulin	Contraindicated in renal disease; check renal function before starting prescription. Monitor for hypoglycemia, especially in older adults. Adverse reactions: GI disturbances, metallic taste.

Drugs Commonly Prescribed 16.5   Diabetes Mellitus Type 2—cont'd

Drug	Indication	Adverse Reactions and Prescribing Considerations
Thiazolidinediones		
• rosiglitazone (Avandia) • pioglitazone (Actos)	Adjunct to diet and exercise in type 2 DM; used as monotherapy or added to metformin Not for use with type 1 DM or in ketoacidosis	*Applicable for all thiazolidinediones:* Insulin resistance reducer. Do not give to patients with liver disease or if ALT is greater than 2.5 × upper limit of normal. Monitor transaminases—obtain baseline and check every 2 months for first 12 months, then periodically. Discontinue drug if levels increase or jaundice occurs. May cause resumption of ovulation in an anovulatory patient (and thus may result in an unintended pregnancy). Side effects: Swelling of legs, fluid retention, weight gain (upper respiratory tract infections, headaches, muscle aches, toothaches, sore throat in fewer than 1%)
Alpha-Glucosidase Inhibitors		
• acarbose (Precose) • miglitol (Glyset)	Adjunct to diet and exercise in type 2 DM; used as monotherapy or with insulin, metformin, or a sulfonylurea	*Applicable to all drugs in this class:* Adverse reactions: Asthma, dizziness, hepatic injury Do not use if serum creatinine is greater than 2 mg/dL. Use glucose, not fructose, to treat hypoglycemia. Monitor serum transaminases. Adverse reactions: Occasional diarrhea, flatulence, abdominal pain—advise patient to take with first bite of main meal.
Meglitinides		
• repaglinide (Prandin)	Adjunct to diet and exercise in type 2 DM; used as monotherapy or in combination with metformin	This class stimulates the release of insulin from islet cells. Use with caution in older adults and patients with renal or hepatic dysfunction. Interacts with many drugs. Adverse reactions: Hypoglycemia, upper respiratory infection, headache, diarrhea, arthralgia
Phenylalanines		
• nateglinide (Starlix)	Adjunct to diet and exercise in type 2 DM	Resembles sulfonylurea agents. This agent has fewer side effects than biguanides or alpha-glucosidase inhibitors.
Incretin Mimetics		
• exenatide (Byetta) • pramlintide acetate (Symlin) (synthetic hormone) • sitagliptin (Januvia) • saxagliptin (Onglyza) • liraglutide (Victoza)	For use as adjunct to diet and exercise in type 2 DM Can be used with insulin for type 1 and 2 DM	Adverse reactions include severe pancreatitis. Action is to mimic incretin: Slows gastric emptying and mimics glucose-dependent insulin secretion. Suppresses postprandial glucagon release, gastric emptying, and appetite, thereby lowering postprandial glucose. If using with insulin, the insulin dose should be decreased by 50%.

Acarbose (Precose) and miglitol (Glyset) are alpha-glucosidase inhibitors that slow down the breakdown of complex carbohydrates into monosaccharides. This causes a delay in the absorption of glucose and reduces postprandial blood glucose levels. They do not stimulate insulin secretion, and if used as single therapy, they usually do not produce hypoglycemia. However, if used with insulin or sulfonylureas, the potential for hypoglycemia is present. The recommended initial dose of acarbose is 50 mg/day; it should be titrated slowly up to the maintenance dose of 50 to 100 mg 3 times daily with meals. Miglitol also delays absorption of carbohydrates, thereby lowering the postprandial glucose. Therapy is initiated with the lowest effective dose of 25 mg 3 times daily, but the maintenance dose is 50 mg 3 times daily. Both drugs have similar adverse effects—flatulence and diarrhea—which are thought to be caused by the osmotic effect of undigested carbohydrates in the distal bowel. The cost of monthly therapy with these medications is between $79 and $84.

Two thiazolidinediones, pioglitazone (Actos) and rosiglitazone (Avandia), constitute a newer class of antihyperglycemic agents. They work by sensitizing peripheral tissues to insulin and can be used either alone or in combination with sulfonylureas, metformin, or insulin. Neither of these agents should be used in any patient with liver disease or if the alanine aminotransferase (ALT) level is greater than 2.5 times the upper limit of normal. Liver enzymes should be monitored every 2 months for the first year of therapy and then periodically thereafter to monitor for liver failure, which has occurred with drugs of this category. If the ALT level is 1 to 2.5 times the upper limit of normal, the patient should be monitored closely or the drug should be discontinued.

Other categories of drugs for type 2 DM are incretin mimetics (glucagon-like peptide–1 [GLP-1] and glucose-dependent insulinotropic polypeptide [GIP] analogs) and dipeptidyl peptidase–4 (DPP-4) inhibitors. Exenatide (Byetta) is an incretin mimetic and has the same effects as the human incretin hormone GLP-1. It enhances glucose-dependent insulin secretion and slows gastric emptying, possibly leading to decreased food intake. Exenatide is given initially in a dose of 5 mcg two times daily subcutaneously and can be increased to 10 mcg after 1 month. The approximate monthly cost in the United States for an incretin mimetic is $270. Pramlintide acetate (Symlin) is an amylin (hormone secreted by beta cells) analog that suppresses postprandial glucagon release, gastric emptying, and appetite, thereby lowering postprandial glucose levels when given before meals. It can be used in both type 1 and type 2 DM and is used in conjunction with insulin. Pramlintide is given at a dose of 60 mcg subcutaneously initially just before each meal and then titrated up to 120 mcg. It is important to note that the dose of insulin should be reduced by 50% when given with pramlintide. DPP-4 is an enzyme that enhances glucose metabolism. Sitagliptin (Januvia) inhibitors enhance the effects of GLP-1 and GIP,

thereby enhancing insulin secretion and suppressing glucagon secretion. DPP-4 inhibitors can be used as monotherapy but are more likely to be used in combination with metformin or thiazolidinediones. When used as monotherapy, the drug does not cause hypoglycemia and is weight neutral. The starting dose is also the maximal daily dose of 100 mg/day. Recently the FDA added a recommendation to monitor for acute pancreatitis for sitagliptin formulations with (Janumet) and without (Januvia) metformin. The approximate monthly cost in the United States for a DPP-4 inhibitor is $194.

The patient who fails to respond to the use of metformin or other agents should be evaluated for the possibility of type 1 DM. Although type 1 DM infrequently presents in older adults, it should be considered in patients with other autoimmune disorders, patients without a family history of type 2 DM, and patients of normal weight.

When nutritional therapy, exercise, and oral antidiabetic agents have failed to control blood glucose levels, the addition of insulin is recommended. The ADA recommends insulin as second-line therapy for type 2 DM or at the time of diagnosis in a newly identified patient with significant symptoms or high blood glucose or A1C levels. Relatively large doses of insulin may be required for type 2 DM patients, given their degree of insulin resistance, in comparison to patients with type 1 DM. Type 2 DM patients often require 1 U/kg or more. The recommendation is to start with bedtime intermediate-acting insulin or with a morning-dosed long-acting insulin and utilize SMBG to determine the amount of insulin dosing increases or decreases (see discussion in section on type 1 DM on insulin therapy). Metformin and thiazolidinediones can be used with insulin therapy, but sulfonylureas should be discontinued. Metformin and thiazolidinediones facilitate lower doses of insulin in maintaining glycemic control. Individual treatment goals should take into account the patient's capacity to understand and carry out the treatment, the risk for severe hypoglycemia, and any other factors that increase risk or decrease benefit.

Because several different types of oral antidiabetic agents can be used as monotherapy or in combination with each other or with insulin therapy treatment decisions can be complex. The following is a synopsis of treatment recommendations (each patient will require individualization dependent on starting A1C and specific lifestyle issues or comorbidities):

- Immediately on diagnosis of type 2 DM begin lifestyle therapy.
- If glycemic goals are not achieved within 3 months (or blood glucose levels and A1C are high), initiate monotherapy with metformin and/or consider basal insulin.
- If glycemic goals are still not met 3 months later, begin combined therapy with oral antidiabetic agents or consider intensive insulin therapy.

Monitoring for Hypoglycemia Hypoglycemia (plasma glucose less than 70 mg/dL) may occur in patients with type 2 DM for a variety of reasons: excessive exogenous insulin, excessive dosing of oral antidiabetic agents, missed meals or inadequate food intake, exercise, alcohol ingestion, drug interactions, and a decrease in liver or kidney function. When using two oral antidiabetic agents, the potential for hypoglycemic episodes is greater, and the patient and family should be aware of this. Signs and symptoms include diaphoresis, tachycardia, hunger, shakiness, altered mentation (ranging from an inability to concentrate to coma), slurred speech, and seizure. The signs and symptoms exhibited by the patient are highly individual and can vary from mild to severe. When the patient becomes ill, blood glucose will need closer monitoring; parenteral insulin may be necessary if oral agents cannot be tolerated.

Follow-up and Referral

On initial diagnosis, the patient should be referred to a dietitian and a certified diabetes educator. Because type 2 DM is a chronic disease, continuing care is essential, and the goal of treatment is to prevent or slow the chronic complications. The frequency of patient visits depends on the degree to which blood glucose levels are controlled, changes in therapy, and the presence and degree of complications or other medical conditions. If the patient is performing SMBG, telephone consultations may be possible instead of clinic visits. Once regulated, the patient should be seen at least quarterly. These visits should include a discussion on the results of SMBG; patient adjustments to therapy; symptoms of illnesses; problems with adherence to the treatment plan; changes in lifestyle; medications; and frequency, causes, and severity of hyperglycemia or hypoglycemia if the patient is on insulin or oral antidiabetic agents.

A1C determination should be performed at least twice a year in patients with good control and quarterly in patients whose therapy has changed or who are not meeting glycemic goals. The physical exam should include a comprehensive foot exam and a funduscopic exam.

Research indicates that patients are more successful in accomplishing lifestyle changes when there is regular contact with the health-care provider. This can be expensive and inconvenient. Community-based telemedicine programs can be helpful. (See Nursing Research–Based Practice Box 16.1.)

Complications

Referrals for the following complications are indicated:

- *Retinopathy:* Comprehensive dilated eye and visual exams should be performed annually by an ophthalmologist or optometrist who is knowledgeable and experienced in the management of diabetic retinopathy for all patients who are diagnosed with type 2 DM, because most individuals have had diabetes for several

Nursing Research–Based Practice 16.1

New, N. Teaching so they hear: Using a co-created diabetes self-management education approach. *J Am Acad Nurse Pract* 22(6):316–325, 2010.

Diabetes self-management programs have been shown to be effective in lifestyle changes, including diet and exercise, with results of better blood sugar control. The purpose of this pilot study was to determine if a co-created diabetes self-management education (DSME) program improved diabetes self-care activities when compared to a typical DSME program. This study used a quasi-experimental design which consisted of 3 phases with a group of adults with type 2 DM. The first phase used a qualitative design to develop and evaluate a co-created DSME intervention. The second phase involved the intervention that was developed as a result of the first phase. This quasi-experimental design included pre- and post-intervention data collection. The data collected was about diabetes knowledge, self-management activities, and adaptation. The control group received the usual DSME education while the experimental group received the new intervention. Phase 3 involved measures of satisfaction with the program for both groups. There were 20 participants in each group. Both groups had improvements in the dependent measures, but only the intervention group showed a statistically significant increase in the Diabetes Self-Care Activities score. The intervention based on patient-perceived problems and needs was a community-based self-management educational program and resulted in improvements in self-care activities.

years before they are diagnosed. Type 2 DM is the leading cause of acquired blindness in adults aged 20 to 74 years, and up to 25% of newly diagnosed patients may present with retinopathy at the time of diagnosis.

- *Hyperlipidemia:* Adults with type 2 DM should be retested annually for lipid disorders with a fasting lipid profile including serum cholesterol, triglyceride, HDL, and calculated LDL cholesterol measurements. ADA guidelines suggest that emphasis in clinical management should be directed toward lowering of the LDL, increasing the HDL, and lowering elevated triglyceride levels. Aggressive therapy is indicated because it is suggested that it will lower the risk of CAD. LDL levels should be less than 100 mg/dL in a patient with no overt cardiovascular disease (CVD) and less than 70 mg/dL with overt CVD. In patients with diabetes without a history of coronary vascular disease, behavioral therapy is indicated when the LDL is 100 mg/dL or more. If behavioral and medical nutritional therapy is unsuccessful, the use of statins (HMG CoA-reductase inhibitor) antihyperlipidemic therapy is indicated. Research indicates that intensive-dose statins increase the risk of diabetes compared with moderate-dose statin therapy (Level I; Preiss et al, 2011).

- *Nephropathy:* A routine serum creatinine and urinalysis should be performed annually for all patients. Screening for elevated serum creatinine and albuminuria in the patient with type 2 DM should begin at the time of diagnosis because it is not known how long the patient has had diabetes. Albuminuria is found in a high proportion of patients when first diagnosed with type 2 DM. The ADA recommends screening at the time of diagnosis of type 2 DM followed by annual screening because 20% to 40% of patients with type 2 DM will progress to overt hyperalbuminuria, and 15% to 20% will progress to renal disease. ACE inhibitors or ARBs are the recommended treatment for increased albuminuria.

Nephropathy has been associated with increased levels of plasma homocysteine. The Diabetic Intervention with Vitamins to Improve Nephropathy (DIVINe) trial was a randomized study examining the use of vitamin B therapy on adults with diabetic nephropathy. Although the therapy did reduce homocysteine levels, there was an increased risk of MI, stroke and all-cause mortality in addition to a detrimental effect on kidney function by reducing the mean glomerular filtration rate (Level II; House et al, 2010).

- *Hypertension:* In a patient with type 2 DM, hypertension is often a part of a syndrome that includes glucose intolerance, insulin resistance, obesity, dyslipidemia, and CAD. It is present in one-third of patients diagnosed with type 2 DM. Isolated systolic hypertension may occur with long duration of diabetes and is due in part to inelasticity of atherosclerotic large vessels. Control of hypertension has been demonstrated to reduce the rate of progression of nephropathy and to reduce the complications of cardiovascular disease. Systolic blood pressure should be less than 140 mm Hg and diastolic below 80 mm Hg. As with patients with type 1 DM, ACE inhibitors should be the initial treatment unless there are contraindications to their use.
- *Macrovascular disease.* Evidence of uncontrolled angina, carotid bruits, and electrocardiogram (ECG) abnormalities may require advanced intervention. An ECG is indicated in patients older than 40 years of age. Daily aspirin is recommended for cardiac prophylaxis in patients with a 10-year risk of CVD greater than 10% at a dose of 81 to 165 mg/day. Given the increased risk of bleeding due to its antiplatelet effects, aspirin is not recommended in low-risk patients with a 10-year CVD risk of less than 5%. Diabetic patients are at risk for developing macrovascular complications including stroke, PVD, and CAD/CVD. Patients with disabling claudication or nonhealing ulcers require a vascular

consultation for their PVD. All diabetic patients should be screened for these diseases, because symptoms may not be present until late in the course of the disease process. Type 2 DM is the leading cause of nontraumatic lower extremity amputation due to PVD and peripheral neuropathy. Problems involving the feet may require care by a podiatrist, orthopedic surgeon, vascular surgeon, or rehabilitation specialist. Assessment guidelines are addressed in the section on type 1 DM.

- *Neuropathy:* Peripheral neuropathy may result in pain, loss of sensation, and muscle weakness. Its incidence increases over time in patients with type 2 DM, and it is more prevalent in patients with low serum insulin concentrations and poor glycemic control. Autonomic involvement can affect gastrointestinal, cardiovascular, and genitourinary function. Patients with significant urinary symptoms or impotence should be referred to a urologist. All patients should be screened for neuropathic symptoms at the time of diagnosis and then at least annually.
- *Pregnancy:* To reduce the risk of fetal malformation and maternal and fetal complications, every pregnancy in a woman with type 2 DM should be planned in advance. Pregnancy is contraindicated in women taking oral antidiabetic agents, and, if receiving this treatment, the patient must switch to insulin. The pregnant woman with type 2 DM requires excellent blood glucose control and should be monitored closely by a multidisciplinary team, which includes the obstetrician or certified nurse midwife.
- *Psychosocial:* The complex management of DM places stress on the patient and family. Research has shown that obese women with type 2 DM reported increased stress, anxiety, and guilt. The complex self-management skills required to manage DM and its impact on well-being may affect the quality of life and contribute to depression. Patients should be monitored for problems with treatment adherence and for depression.

Patient Education

Successful diabetes management involves a team effort to achieve mutually agreed on treatment goals. To achieve these goals, it is crucial that the patient and family or significant other be educated in all aspects of the treatment plan. The following list is a synopsis of the salient topics for patient education:

- *Introduction:* Definition of type 2 DM, causes of diabetes, and function of the pancreas and insulin
- *Regulation of blood glucose:* Role of diet, exercise, insulin; signs and symptoms of hyperglycemia; causes, treatment, and prevention of hyperglycemia; signs and symptoms of hypoglycemia; causes, treatment, and prevention of hypoglycemia; when to contact the practitioner

- *Blood glucose monitoring and urine testing:* How to perform SMBG, how often to test, recording and reporting results, and urine ketone testing
- *Medication and insulin administration:* Actions and adverse reactions of oral antidiabetic agents; actions of insulin; types of insulin, effects on blood glucose; storage of supplies; drawing, mixing, and injecting insulin; site selection and rotation; and needle disposal
- *Meal planning:* Types of nutrients (carbohydrates, proteins, fats), timing of meals, portions, use of sweeteners, eating out, use of alcohol, and sick-day management
- *Exercise:* Benefits, types of exercise, effects on blood glucose, planning and measuring exercise, snacks
- *Prevention of long-term complications:* Importance of blood glucose control, vision exams, foot care, prevention of infection, and signs and symptoms of complications

■ HYPOGLYCEMIA

Hypoglycemia is a clinical syndrome of subnormal plasma glucose concentration that may affect infants through the elderly, although the primary etiology of the disorder differs markedly among various age groups. Hypoglycemia in patients with diabetes mellitus (DM) has been discussed previously in this chapter. In this section, hypoglycemia in patients without diabetes will be explored. Adult hypoglycemia is characterized by blood glucose levels of less than 55 mg/dL of blood, whereas neonatal hypoglycemia is typically defined as a level below 30 mg/dL in the first 24 hours of life. There is no universal agreement about these thresholds, however, with some research supporting a level of less than 50 mg/dL for men, 45 mg/dL for women, and 40 mg/dL for infants and children as indicative of hypoglycemia. Clinical hypoglycemia occurs when the blood glucose level is low enough to cause signs and/or symptoms.

Hypoglycemia with diabetes is the most commonly occurring endocrine emergency; however, it is not common in patients without diabetes. There are three types of hypoglycemia: fasting, reactive, and induced. Fasting hypoglycemia is a low blood sugar level more than 5 hours after eating; it can be subacute or chronic, but blood glucose does not return to normal without glucose ingestion or administration. Reactive or postprandial hypoglycemia is less common and is most often acute in nature. Reactive hypoglycemia usually produces symptoms 2 to 4 hours after a meal rich in carbohydrates, and symptoms rarely occur in a fasting state. Within 5 to 6 hours after a meal, the blood glucose level will return to normal. Induced hypoglycemia is the most common form. Medications and alcohol are the most frequent causes of induced hypoglycemia.

Another option for classifying hypoglycemia in adults is to use the patient's clinical presentation: ill or seemingly well. The Endocrine Society suggests this alternative to assist guiding diagnostics and also in situations where patients typically present with one type of hypoglycemia but may also experience a second classification of hypoglycemia. For instance, patients with insulinomas typically present with fasting hypoglycemia, but they also frequently experience postprandial hypoglycemia, making a classification of their hypoglycemia difficult.

Epidemiology and Causes

Hypoglycemia as a separate disease entity is most common in the elderly and is more prevalent in women overall. About 1% of the nondiabetic population is affected. Although endocrine disorders are the most frequent cause of hypoglycemia, bariatric surgery, insulinomas, non–islet cell neoplasms, liver disease, pregnancy, medications, and alcohol consumption are also causes. Hypoglycemia in neonates is a unique phenomenon, largely related to the immature developmental stage of the neonatal endocrine system, as discussed under Pathophysiology.

Classic hypoglycemia denotes a low plasma glucose level in the setting of insulin-dependent DM. Inconsistent subcutaneous absorption of insulin, decreased food intake, missed meals, and increased insulin secretion during exercise produce hypoglycemia in patients with DM. Moreover, physical and emotional stress may alter the body's reaction to insulin. Sulfonylureas also can produce hypoglycemia in patients with type 2 DM, but it occurs less commonly than with type 1 DM.

The symptoms of fasting hypoglycemia occur when the patient has not eaten for 5 or more hours. The possible causes of fasting hypoglycemia include pancreatic beta-cell tumors, extrapancreatic tumors, hypopituitarism, myxedema, glycogen storage diseases, ethanol-induced hypoglycemia, severe malnutrition, septicemia, pregnancy, and renal failure which results in decreased clearance of insulin from the body. The list of drugs that can cause fasting hypoglycemia is lengthy: insulin and sulfonylureas, fluoroquinolones, propanolol (Inderal), salicylates, quinidine, pentamidine (Pentam 300, NebuPent), coumarin, sulfonamides, tricyclic antidepressants, disopyramide (Norpace), didanosine, ritodrine, chlorpromazine, isoniazid (INH), selective serotonin reuptake inhibitors, clofibrate, thiazide diuretics, lithium, and ACE inhibitors. Poisoning with organophosphate and carbamate-based pesticides also results in hypoglycemia. Illegal sexual-enhancement drugs have also been associated with severe hypoglycemia. In adrenocortical insufficiency, there is a decreased production of cortisol which is required for gluconeogenesis, thus leading to hypoglycemia. Liver diseases, including hepatitis, cirrhosis, hepatomas, and hepatic congestion, interfere with the uptake and release of glycogen from the liver and ultimately may lead to hypoglycemia.

Postprandial hypoglycemia, or reactive hypoglycemia, may be caused by gastrointestinal surgery or any other alimentary tract disorder that affects absorption; congenital deficiency of enzymes necessary for carbohydrate metabolism; and late insulin release caused by B-cell dysfunction. It is an early manifestation of DM and has been seen with extreme exertion in untrained, physically unfit persons, as well as in patients with sepsis or heart failure. Idiopathic or functional postprandial hypoglycemia also exists that cannot be ascribed to any discrete cause.

Hypoglycemia may be factitious or self-induced by the excessive intake of sulfonylureas or insulin. Timing of these types of hypoglycemic events is not related to food intake. If this type is suspected in patients with known access to these drugs (health-care workers and caregivers of diabetic patients), serum and urine sulfonylurea levels should be obtained. A very low or nonexistent serum C-peptide level confirms that insulin is being injected exogenously.

Lifestyle patterns may contribute to hypoglycemia as well. The excessive consumption of simple sugars, an excessively refined and processed diet, excessive exercise, stress, irregular eating patterns, or missing meals may cause abnormal fluctuations of blood sugar levels. Nutrient deficiencies, food allergies, and poor digestion may also contribute to hypoglycemia. Cigarette smoking and high caffeine intake also produce instability in blood glucose levels. (Table 16.10 lists the causes of hypoglycemia.)

Table 16.10	Causes of Hypoglycemia
Type of Hypoglycemia	**Causes**
Fasting hypoglycemia	Renal failure (decreases rate at which insulin is secreted contributing to hypoglycemia)
	Hepatic disease
	Insulinomas
	Pancreatic tumors
	Autoimmune disease
	Hypopituitarism
	Extrapancreatic tumors
	Ethanol intake
	Septicemia
Reactive hypoglycemia	Postgastrectomy
	Gastric bypass surgery
	Hereditary fructose intolerance
	Congenital enzyme deficiency
	Pancreatic beta-cell dysfunction
	Meals high in carbohydrates
	Exercise
	Pregnancy
Drug-induced hypoglycemia	Exogenous insulin
	Sulfonylureas
	Propranolol
	Salicylates
	Quinine
	Pentamidine
	Disopyramide

Pathophysiology

To understand the clinical and biochemical phenomenon of hypoglycemia, it is important to grasp the mechanics behind the body's careful regulation of euglycemic plasma glucose levels between 80 and 90 mg/dL. After a carbohydrate-containing meal in which glucose is absorbed from the gut into the bloodstream, plasma glucose levels transiently increase to 120 to 140 mg/dL. Glucose subsequently enters pancreatic beta cells via the GLUT1 and GLUT2 cell membrane transporters, where the enzyme glucokinase phosphorylates it to glucose-6-phosphate, thereby acting as a glucose sensor and triggering the passive entry of calcium into beta cells, causing insulin secretion. Insulin lowers plasma glucose levels by decreasing hepatic glycolysis (glycogen breakdown) and gluconeogenesis (de novo glucose synthesis), driving glucose uptake by skeletal muscle and adipose tissue via the translocation of intracellular glucose transporter molecules to the cell membrane surface, and decreasing both proteolysis and lipolysis, which decreases the number of gluconeogenic precursors. In turn, plasma glucose levels typically return to normal within several hours after a carbohydrate-containing meal.

Hypoglycemia is sensed by central nervous system receptors in the hypothalamus as well as peripheral receptors that act via afferent nerves to trigger an appropriate hormonal response to maintain glucose homeostasis. The body counters glucose levels below 80 mg/dL by decreasing pancreatic insulin production, eventually secreting several counterregulatory hormones at levels below 70 mg/dL, including glucagon from pancreatic alpha cells, which acts directly on the liver, and epinephrine from the adrenal medulla, which acts similar to glucagon via hepatic beta-adrenergic receptors, as well as mediating the autonomic (sympathetic, adrenergic) symptoms of hypoglycemia (e.g., diaphoresis, anxiety). Epinephrine also directly inhibits insulin secretion via alpha-2-adrenergic receptors. If hypoglycemia is severe (less than 60 mg/dL) or persists for several hours, additional counterregulatory hormones are mobilized, including cortisol from the adrenal cortex and growth hormone from the pituitary gland.

These counterregulatory hormones increase hepatic glucose production via a number of mechanisms, including glycogen breakdown into individual glucose monomers (glycogenolysis) and, once intrahepatic glycogen stores are depleted, de novo glucose synthesis from amino acid, pyruvate, glycerol, and free fatty acid precursors (gluconeogenesis). In turn, the body also metabolically shifts away from glucose utilization toward alternate sources of fuel to maintain euglycemia, for example, proteins and ketone bodies converted from fats. Increased lipolysis is thus reflected in increased plasma free fatty acids, and increased protein breakdown is reflected in higher concentrations of the amino acids alanine and glutamine.

The brain utilizes glucose almost exclusively as its fuel source; however, it is not capable of synthesizing or storing it. Thus, the brain is particularly sensitive to dramatic changes in blood glucose concentration. Hypoglycemia, in which plasma glucose falls below 60 mg/dL, prevents the brain from receiving an adequate supply of blood glucose, thereby impairing function. Even asymptomatic hypoglycemia has been associated with neurocognitive impairment in infants and children. In adults, cognitive dysfunction can be detected in otherwise normal individuals at plasma glucose levels between 50 and 55 mg/dL; older men are particularly prone to this type of neurological impairment. At levels between 45 and 50 mg/dL, lethargy and obtundation follow, with coma occurring at levels below 30 mg/dL, followed by convulsions below 20 mg/dL and eventual death. Severe hypoglycemia has also been associated with cardiovascular dysfunction.

The histological structure of the pancreas is uniquely designed to prevent these events. Within the pancreas, each islet of Langerhans consists of several hundred cells, including a core of insulin-producing beta cells surrounded by glucagon-secreting alpha cells and an outer layer of somatostatin-producing delta cells and PP cells, which make pancreatic polypeptide. As arterial blood enters the islet core, the beta cells are the first to encounter plasma glucose concentrations. Thus, the function of alpha cells is determined largely by the normal activity of beta cells. For example, insulin directly inhibits glucagon secretion by pancreatic alpha cells.

In adults, reactive hypoglycemia occurs when these counterregulatory responses fail after the person consumes a carbohydrate load, causing blood glucose to fall 2 to 5 hours after eating. Patients with decreased glucagon and epinephrine responses to low blood glucose levels have up to a 25-fold greater risk of experiencing hypoglycemia, particularly during sleep, as sleep itself decreases counterregulatory hormonal responses.

Unfortunately, an initial hypoglycemic episode appears to contribute to a vicious cycle of hypoglycemia, as recurrent hypoglycemia has been associated with autonomic failure and a delay in the early warning signs associated with a subsequent hypoglycemic episode. This may relate to an increased production of cortisol, which decreases glucagon and epinephrine responses, as well as upregulation of glucose transport in the brain, which renders the central nervous system less sensitive to producing neuroglycopenic symptoms.

Hypoglycemia in infants has an extensive differential diagnosis of potential etiologies, because a number of congenital genetic defects exist that may initially present with neonatal hypoglycemia. These include disorders of glucose utilization related to hyperinsulinemic states (e.g., persistent hyperinsulinemic hypoglycemia of infancy, macrosomia associated with maternal diabetes, insulinoma), disorders of glucose metabolism (e.g., Krebs cycle or oxidative respiratory chain defects), genetic defects in the metabolism of alternate fuel sources (e.g., carnitine acyl transferase deficiency, long and medium chain acyl–coenzyme A dehydrogenase deficiency), and hypermetabolic states such as sepsis, severe burns, hyperthermia, polycythemia, or congenital hyperthyroidism. Persistent hyperinsulinemic hypoglycemia of infancy is the most common etiology of hyperinsulinemia during the first 3 months of life. This primary disorder of the pancreas is more commonly observed in infants who are small for gestational age and those born to mothers with toxemia (maternal sepsis).

Infants may also suffer from inadequate glucose stores (e.g., prematurity, malnutrition, intrauterine growth restriction), congenital hormonal deficiencies (e.g., growth hormone, cortisol, panhypopituitarism), or disordered gluconeogenesis (e.g., glucose-6-phosphatase deficiency, glycogen synthase deficiency, galactosemia, maple syrup urine disease, or any one of several glycogen storage diseases). Perinatal asphyxia potentiates hypoglycemia, worsening the resulting neurological impairment that is associated with sustained or recurrent hypoglycemia.

Clinical Presentation

The clinical presentation of hypoglycemia, especially subjective symptoms, varies depending on the physical status of the person. Older adults with neuropathy may lack awareness of its symptoms unless they are severe. In an accidental exposure to hypoglycemic agents, the symptoms are often not recognized or associated with this disease. Whipple's triad includes signs/symptoms, a low plasma glucose level, and resolution of the signs/symptoms after plasma glucose is back into the normal range.

Subjective

Symptoms of hypoglycemia may be present when the blood glucose level falls below 60 mg/dL. Brain function is often impaired when levels fall below 50 mg/dL. Some patients may exhibit symptoms with abnormal fluctuations of glucose and insulin. Symptoms vary from very mild to severe and are classified into adrenergic and neuroglycopenic.

Adrenergic symptoms include sweating, tremulousness, dizziness, confusion, anxiety, and palpitations. Neuroglycopenic symptoms include headaches, seizures, fatigue, weakness, drowsiness, syncope, diplopia and blurred vision, and personality changes. The neurological manifestations of hemiparesis, convulsions, confusion, and coma are more common in patients with DM. Symptoms are often relieved with ingestion of carbohydrates. Seizures and coma are severe complications.

The history should focus on eating habits, meal times, exercise habits, alcohol intake, and any history of liver or renal disease, as well as on family history of endocrine disorders, including DM and hypoglycemia.

Objective

Objective findings that accompany hypoglycemia may include tachycardia with or without premature ventricular contractions, diaphoresis, hypothermia or hyperthermia, coma, seizures, trembling, Babinski's sign, aphasia, and hemiparesis.

A physical exam with special attention to objective signs of endocrine disease is indicated initially. Assessment for an enlarged liver and neurological indications of chronic alcohol abuse should also be performed. In patients unable to provide an adequate history, the skin should be examined for needle marks, which may reflect possible insulin injections.

Infants prone to hypoglycemia have a unique physical presentation. Hyperinsulinemic babies (e.g., those born to diabetic mothers or babies with insulin-producing tumors) have large body size because of the growth effects of insulin. In contrast, those with decreased body fat are more likely to suffer from insufficient glucose stores. Poor linear growth reflects growth hormone deficiency, whereas midline craniofacial defects may indicate more global pituitary hormone defects. Hepatomegaly is a common sign of glycogen storage diseases. In more general terms, neonatal hypoglycemia may present with jitteriness, hypotonia, lethargy, poor feeding, cyanosis, apnea, or hypothermia.

Diagnostic Reasoning

Diagnostic Tests

Plasma blood glucose levels are used to diagnose hypoglycemia. Hypoglycemia is suspected if the plasma blood glucose level is between 45 and 60 mg/dL or if an overnight fasting glucose level is less than 60 mg/dL. Hypoglycemia is present if the plasma blood glucose level is 45 mg/dL or less. Evaluation of the etiology, when not attributed to treatment of DM, requires subsequent laboratory evaluations.

Initial Testing Initial testing includes a blood glucose level. The best time to obtain a blood glucose level is when the patient is experiencing symptoms. If hypoglycemia and symptoms occur concurrently and if both are relieved with eating, the diagnosis of postprandial hypoglycemia is confirmed. However, finger-stick monitors are not very accurate at extremes of high and low glucose concentrations. They are a helpful tool in detecting high and low blood glucose, but the number itself may not be accurate. An oral glucose tolerance test may be done; however, overinterpretation of the glucose tolerance test may lead to an overdiagnosis of hypoglycemia. More than one-third of normal patients have hypoglycemia with or without symptoms during a 4-hour fasting test. For definitive diagnosis, the patient should have (1) documented occurrences of blood glucose levels, (2) symptoms that occur when the blood glucose level is low, (3) evidence that symptoms are relieved by sugar or other foods, and (4) identification of the particular type of hypoglycemia. It is important to remember that whole blood glucose levels are 10% to 15% lower than serum glucose levels, because red blood cells consume glucose. The most reliable method of diagnosing hypoglycemia is

with a plasma glucose 72-hour fast. During this test, the patient is allowed calorie-free, caffeine-free fluids; and the patient fasts at least overnight, but it may be as long as 72 hours. Before and after the fast, a baseline serum glucose, insulin, proinsulin, and C-peptide measurement is obtained. Urine is tested for ketones throughout the test, and capillary glucose measurements are taken every 6 hours. The test is terminated when symptoms of hypoglycemia appear, and a blood glucose level is measured immediately. A positive test result for men is considered to be a blood glucose level less than 55 mg/dL and in women, less than 45 mg/dL. If after 72 hours of fasting and light exercise, hypoglycemia (less than 60 mg/dL) is not demonstrated, the test is negative. This test is performed in a hospital under close observation. Chronic hypoglycemia may be evident by a low glycohemoglobin level.

Subsequent Testing The following laboratory tests assist in the diagnostic reasoning during a hypoglycemic episode: plasma insulin level, insulin antibodies, plasma and urine sulfonylurea levels, and C-peptide. Other tests include a blood urea nitrogen, creatinine, alcohol levels, and liver function tests. To rule out endocrine pathology, if suspected as a possible cause, obtain cortisol and ACTH levels. The first void in the morning can be tested to detect ketones; a lack of them would imply a defect in the fatty acid oxidation pathway, because ketone bodies are not formed. In infants, urine may also be sent for organic acid analysis.

Fasting insulin levels range from 8.0 to 16.0 mcU/mL or 3.0 to 0.6 ng/mL. An abnormally elevated insulin level is seen in patients with insulinomas, exogenous insulin administration, insulin resistance syndrome, and reactive hypoglycemia in developing DM. An elevated insulin level in the absence of blood glucose variation is suggestive of insulinomas, exogenous insulin administration, insulin resistance syndrome, and reactive hypoglycemia in developing DM. Elevated insulin levels in response to glucose fluctuations suggests functional or reactive hypoglycemia.

C-peptide analysis is done with radioimmunoassay techniques and provides an index of beta cell function. Normal values range from 0.9 to 4.2 ng/mL. A low C-peptide level with an elevated insulin level confirms insulin administration. C-peptide levels are elevated in insulinomas. To differentiate insulinoma from factitious hypoglycemia, the ratio of insulin to C-peptide is determined. If the insulin:C-peptide ratio is less than 1.0, the hypoglycemia is a result of endogenous insulin secretion; if greater than 1.0, then exogenous insulin administration is confirmed.

Differential Diagnosis

Differential diagnoses include generalized anxiety disorder, panic attacks, hyperventilation, pheochromocytoma, drug or alcohol intoxication, transient ischemic attack, cerebrovascular accident, and psychosis. Causes of reactive hypoglycemia include meals high in refined carbohydrates; certain nutrients such as fructose and galactose cause a burst of insulin secretion. Drugs (e.g., sulfonylureas, salicylates) can cause excess glucose utilization or deficient glucose production. Oral diabetic medications are especially prone to causing reactive hypoglycemia when used in combination therapy. Insulinoma (adenoma of islets of Langerhans), although rare, should be considered in an otherwise healthy adult who is found to have fasting hypoglycemia.

Management

The goal in management of hypoglycemia is to normalize the blood glucose levels and treat the underlying cause. The patient with pathology is referred to an endocrinologist for further evaluation and treatment. In cases of functional and idiopathic hypoglycemia, the initial management plan may be developed in consultation with an endocrinologist.

Initial Management

Treatment of acute hypoglycemia for alert patients is 6 to 12 ounces of orange juice or another fruit juice without additional sugar. One cup (8 oz) of milk can be substituted if juice is not available. Glucose tablets, if available, can be used. In acute care settings, glucose is provided emergently as standardized IV bolus preparations of dextrose diluted to various concentrations in water (e.g., D25% or D50%), as opposed to the standardized hypotonic saline solutions with lower amounts of dextrose that are used primarily for maintenance glucose requirements (e.g., D5% 0.45% NaCl). The blood glucose level should be monitored closely after bolus IV administration of dextrose and then periodically while the patient is on a dextrose-containing continuous IV drip. Glucagon hydrochloride (0.03–0.1 mg/kg per dose; 1–2 mg in adults; 1 mg in children older than 5 years or weighing more than 20 kg; 0.5 mg in children younger than 5 years or weighing less than 20 kg) may be given IM, SC, or IV if the patient is unresponsive. Doses may be repeated as needed every few hours in adults and even more frequently in children (up to every 20–30 minutes initially).

Hypoglycemia is a medical emergency because of the seriousness of the potential sequelae (e.g., seizures, coma, cardiovascular dysfunction, death). Even if euglycemia is readily restored, patients must be evaluated for potential hospital admission for inpatient care and close observation if there is any concern for symptom recurrence. Patients requiring admission include those with hypoglycemia without an obvious cause or severe or persistent neurological deficits.

Subsequent Management

Long-term management of hypoglycemia includes treatment of underlying causes and dietary modifications. If hypoglycemia is a result of pancreatic or extrapancreatic

tumors, surgical excision is recommended. Although the treatment of choice for insulinoma is surgical resection, there is only an 85% success rate with an experienced surgeon. If the tumor is small, it may not be found on an exploratory laparotomy. When surgery is unsuccessful, an endocrinologist may initiate diazoxide (Hyperstat, Proglycem; 3–8 mg/kg per day PO in divided doses 3 times daily or 200 mg every 4 hours in adults) therapy to reduce insulin secretion. If hypoglycemia is caused by rapid gastric emptying following a gastrectomy, an anticholinergic drug may delay gastric emptying, decrease intestinal motility, and provide relief.

In patients with pseudohypoglycemia or idiopathic hypoglycemia, in which the cause cannot be identified, the treatment is primarily with dietary modifications. A high-protein, low-carbohydrate diet divided into six small daily feedings often relieves the symptoms. Caffeine, refined sugars, and alcohol should be restricted. If food allergies are suspected, allergy testing may be indicated to identify offending foods. If a medication is at fault, an alternative drug should be considered.

In a hyperinsulinemic infant, therapy may be only supportive with glucose infusions if the increased insulin levels are due primarily to maternal diabetes and are transient. However, if increased insulin levels are intrinsic to the infant, diazoxide is typically the first step in pharmacological treatment (15–20 mg/kg per day PO in divided doses 3 times daily). Octreotide (Sandostatin; 2–10 mcg/kg per day SC in divided doses every 4–6 hours), a long-acting analog of somatostatin, may be used as second-line therapy for short-term management of hypoglycemia. The dihydropyridine calcium channel blocker nifedipine (Adalat, Procardia; 10 mg PO 3 times daily initially and titrated up to 80 mg/day) has also been shown to be useful in hyperinsulinemic children, because it interferes with the calcium-dependent secretion of insulin (other calcium channel blockers have not been approved for this indication). There is no role for cortisol in acute treatment.

SMBG is the cornerstone of self-management. Patients may need to monitor blood glucose levels frequently during initiation of lifestyle changes to evaluate success. Monitoring glucose levels during exercise, eating at regularly scheduled intervals, and understanding the importance of SMBG may prevent severe hypoglycemic reactions. All patients with hypoglycemia will benefit from home blood glucose monitoring.

Infants younger than 3 months who have refractory hypoglycemia that cannot be treated pharmacologically may require pancreatic resection. Usually, a near-total resection of 85% to 90% of the pancreas is recommended, but development of diabetes is a subsequent risk. In infants between 3 and 6 months of age, frequent feedings may first be attempted for up to 1 month to see if this addresses a temporary phenomenon.

In patients with inoperable pancreatic tumors or patients in whom resection has been unsuccessful, small frequent feedings that are high in carbohydrates (every 2–3 hours) may be effective in preventing acute hypoglycemic episodes. In patients with renal failure, small frequent high-carbohydrate meals may prevent episodes.

Follow-up and Referral

Patients with a history of hypoglycemic events need frequent follow-up and evaluation. On each visit, the record of hypoglycemic events should be reviewed. More frequent SMBG may be indicated, especially 12 to 24 hours after a hypoglycemic event. Patients who continue to experience hypoglycemic episodes despite intervention should be referred to an endocrinologist.

Patient Education

The importance of dietary modifications must be stressed. Nondiabetic patients with reactive, functional, and fasting hypoglycemia should eat five or six small meals daily to steady the release of glucose into the blood. The meals should be balanced with carbohydrates, protein, and some fat. Instruct the patient who experiences symptoms after a meal high in refined sugar, but not after a regular meal, to restrict refined sugars in the diet. Patients who cannot eat small meals throughout the day should be encouraged to carry raw seeds and nuts mixed with dried fruits.

Patients with diabetes should be instructed to maintain their glycemic goals, report any episodes of hypoglycemia, and monitor their blood glucose at bedtime and before, during, and after exercise. Alcohol, cigarette smoking, and caffeine should be avoided.

COMMON METABOLIC PROBLEMS

■ METABOLIC SYNDROME

Metabolic syndrome is a constellation of risk factors. There is a body of evidence recognizing a metabolic origin for patients with cardiovascular risk *and* prediabetes. The metabolic origin of this syndrome is not well understood, although the involvement of insulin resistance may be the linking factor. However, the importance of these two disease processes and the increased risk for some patients cannot be overlooked. The American Diabetes Association (ADA) has published a statement with five other groups, and the Endocrine Society has a practice guideline stressing the importance of recognizing these at risk patients.

The cluster of factors for metabolic syndrome include hypertension, hyperlipidemia, and insulin resistance. Patients with these characteristics are at twice the risk for cardiovascular disease (CVD) over 5 years, compared with those without these comorbidities, and have a fivefold increase in risk of type 2 DM. Patients with this presentation should have intense lifestyle modification education as well as treatment to reduce the lifetime CVD risk, including decreasing blood pressure and hyperlipidemia and reducing the prothrombotic state. There is also evidence that patients may delay the onset of diabetes with aggressive lifestyle changes and possibly using metformin or a thiazolidinedione agent. Both medications have been shown to delay the conversion of prediabetes to diabetes.

Patients with the constellation of factors for metabolic syndrome are at increased risk of lifetime CVD and diabetes. Primary-care providers are obligated to assist these patients with the modification to prevent these lifelong risks by recognizing the factors and starting lifestyle treatment early. For more information about metabolic syndrome, see Chapter 10.

■ OBESITY

Obesity is an excess of adipose tissue (body fat) and is manifested by body mass index (BMI) of 30 kg/m² or higher for adults and a BMI at or above the 95th percentile for children and adolescents. Published clinical guidelines on the identification, evaluation, and treatment of overweight and obesity cite that the complex etiology of overeating makes this chronic illness poorly understood and often intractable to medical management. The two major types of obesity are upper body (apple-shape) and lower body (pear-shape) obesity. Patients with central or upper body obesity have excessive body fat in the abdomen and flank areas and are at a greater risk for type 2 DM, coronary artery disease, stroke, and early death than those with lower body obesity. Patients with lower body obesity have excessive adipose tissue in the buttocks and thighs.

The direct and indirect costs of obesity are more than $152 billion per year in the United States, including the direct medical costs and the cost attributable to lost wages. Americans spend more than $40 billion a year on diets and dietary products. The psychological cost of obesity in those affected includes stigmatization and discrimination.

Epidemiology and Causes

Overweight and obesity are epidemic in the United States today. Thirty-five percent of men and 36% of women are obese. Another 30% of Americans are overweight with a BMI between 25 and 29 kg/m². African American women are more likely to be obese than are white women. The incidence of obesity is higher in those of lower socioeconomic status regardless of race. Central and upper body obesity is more common in men, whereas lower body obesity is more common in women.

Worldwide, obesity is more prevalent in industrialized countries, and the prevalence is increasing worldwide, including in developing countries. The World Health Organization (WHO) classifies obesity as one of the world's most neglected public health problems.

The causes of obesity are categorized as essential and secondary. Essential obesity is the most prevalent type and is a result of the intake of more calories than are expended. This type of obesity results from the multiple interactions of genetic and environmental factors (cultural, metabolic, social, and psychological factors). Numerous genes have been identified that affect control of appetite, and mutations in these genes, along with environmental factors and behavior, result in obesity.

Secondary obesity is rare; possible causes include Cushing's disease, polycystic ovary syndrome (PCOS), hypothalamic disease, hypothyroidism, and insulinoma. Some medications associated with weight gain include glucocorticoids, tricyclic antidepressants, and phenothiazines.

Risk factors for development of obesity include diet, lifestyle, environment, and the interaction among the aforementioned causes. A diet high in fat contributes to obesity because dietary fat has more than twice the calories of carbohydrates or proteins. A sedentary lifestyle or a sudden decrease in physical activity without a reduction in caloric intake may cause obesity. An environment that supports sedentary lifestyles and facilitates access to fatty foods, processed foods, and refined sugars contributes to the incidence of obesity today.

Obesity affects almost every body system and is associated with an increased risk of multiple diseases. The consequences of obesity are listed in Table 16.11. The different types of obesity are related more closely to specific complications. Central trunk obesity is closely related to diabetes mellitus (DM), coronary heart disease, stroke, and early death. The health risks associated with obesity are directly correlated with the severity of obesity and include metabolic, structural, and psychosocial changes. Mortality risk increases as complications of obesity develop and approaches 50% when weight is 30% to 40% above the ideal. Reduction in body weight by 5% to 20% significantly decreases these comorbid risk factors in obese individuals.

Table 16.11   Consequences of Obesity
• Coronary heart disease/congestive heart failure
• Hypertension
• Dyslipidemia/hyperlipidemia
• Type 2 diabetes mellitus/metabolic syndrome/insulin resistance
• Sleep apnea
• Restrictive lung disease
• Asthma
• Varicose veins and venous insufficiency
• Gout and hyperuricemia
• Osteoarthritis
• Reflux esophagitis
• Gallbladder disease
• Thromboembolic disease
• Cancers: Endometrial, breast, prostate, colon

Obesity is also associated with an increased risk of colon, rectal, and prostate cancer in males. In obese females, uterine, gallbladder, biliary tract, breast, and ovarian cancer are more prevalent. Persons who are obese have an increased surgical and obstetrical risk. Psychosocial disability is also related to obesity. This is often a result of the societal stigma attached to obesity. Pickwickian syndrome is associated with severe or morbid obesity. This syndrome includes hypersomnolence, congestive heart failure, and hypertension.

Pathophysiology

Obesity results when one's intake of calories exceeds metabolic needs. The control of appetite and the mechanisms that govern food intake are complex and incompletely understood. The hypothalamus controls certain aspects of appetite and appears to have a role in an individual's food preferences. Other important central nervous system sites include the tractus solitarius of the hindbrain, the arcuate and paraventricular nuclei, and the amygdala. Mediated by several neurotransmitters including norepinephrine, dynorphin, hypocretin, serotonin, neuropeptide Y, and ghrelin, to name just a few, both the central and peripheral nervous systems produce and integrate a complex array of neural inputs that regulate diet and weight. In contrast, other hormones such as cholecystokinin, enterostatin, leptin, and the gut hormone peptide YY 3-36 have all been shown to suppress food intake through appetite suppression and inducing feelings of satiety. Whether obesity can be significantly attributed to dysregulation in one or more of these neuroendocrine regulatory mechanisms remains to be seen.

There is, however, a well-documented genetic predisposition to the development of obesity. Twin studies have revealed high correlations in obesity prevalence between siblings raised apart in separate households as well as together by the same set of parents, whereas the BMIs of adoptees correlate more closely with those of their biological rather than adopted parents. Secondary causes of obesity due to medical conditions are rare, however, and include various endocrine and neurological diseases.

In many individuals, obesity, overweight, and overeating appear intrinsically tied to a fragile emotional state, poor self-esteem, and dissatisfaction with life circumstances. The stressors and psychological demands that underlie a patient's poor dietary choices may be powerful influences that are capable of defying the counterbalancing knowledge that overeating and obesity lead to ill health. Thus, an addictive behavioral component to overeating appears to be a driving factor in many obese individuals. The complex psychology of obesity has been the subject of extensive study, and the most effective obesity treatment programs typically involve some sort of psychiatric analysis or counseling as primary or adjunctive therapy.

Whereas most individuals tend to underestimate their food intake by 10% to 20%, obese individuals underestimate caloric intake even further, by 30%. However, behavioral choices alone do not explain the entire pathophysiology of obesity.

The body is known to have neuroendocrine homeostatic feedback control mechanisms involving both the peripheral and central nervous systems, which seek to maintain nutrient intake and ideal weight. Examples include glycemic levels (hypoglycemia is a trigger to eat), serum leptin concentrations, glucocorticoids that act as appetite stimulants, sympathomimetic hormones that act as appetite suppressants, and the peptide ghrelin—a ligand for the growth hormone secretagogue receptor that increases appetite (ghrelin levels increase in anticipation of a meal and in response to diet-induced weight loss). Differences in fat-free body mass also correlate strongly with differences in energy expenditure among different individuals. In particular, weight gain is associated with increased metabolic demands and energy expenditure that retard further weight gain, whereas weight loss is associated with reductions in energy expenditure that counter further weight loss. Thus, a formerly obese individual who loses weight will experience a relative decrease in energy expenditure compared with a nonobese individual and will thus require 15% fewer calories to maintain his or her reduced weight. In turn, failing to reduce one's caloric intake appropriately may result in progressive weight gain.

On a molecular level, the bulk of our understanding of the pathophysiology and genetics of obesity stems from preclinical animal models—particularly that of the obese mouse, for which a number of genetically altered strains are available. Through genetically engineered knockout mice that lack one or more target genes, as well as transgenic models that overexpress either a functional or nonfunctional version of a target gene, researchers have identified several single gene defects that result in murine obesity. Some of these genetic findings have been further generalized to humans.

Expressed by adipose, intestinal, and placental cells, the leptin gene has been the subject of much controversy in human obesity. Serum leptin concentrations strongly correlate with body fat content, and leptin-deficient mice demonstrate insulin resistance, hyperinsulinemia, and hyperphagia. Leptin has been shown to reduce levels of neuropeptide Y, a potent stimulus for food intake produced in the brain's arcuate nucleus. Human obesity due to leptin deficiency has been identified in two consanguineous families, as has obesity due to leptin receptor deficiency. However, leptin overexpression has not been shown to reduce appetite or weight, and most obese patients express normal levels of this protein. Thus, decreased leptin levels appear to signal that fat stores are insufficient for growth and reproduction; however, the hormone itself is not a negative regulator of appetite or weight gain. Obese individuals appear to have decreased sensitivity to leptin.

Other single-gene defects associated with murine obesity include mutations in carboxypeptidase E, the enzyme responsible for the cleavage of proinsulin, and the *tub* gene, which is associated with neurological deficits, hypothalamic damage, and increased appetite. The *agouti* gene, which encodes an antagonist protein for the hypothalamic melanocortin-4 receptor, has also been associated with murine obesity and hyperphagia, as have deletions in the melanocortin-4 receptor. Mutations in multiple species of serotonin receptors are associated with murine obesity, a finding that appears to underlie the role of serotonergic pharmacotherapies that reduce appetite.

Mutations in prohormone convertase-I have been associated with human obesity in one family. In contrast, the role of the *agouti* gene in human obesity has not yet been confirmed. Other candidate genes involved in human obesity include the beta-3-adrenergic gene, which is involved in sympathetic autonomic responses that affect appetite, and peroxisome-proliferator–activated receptor (PPAR) γ-2, a gene involved in adipocyte differentiation. Genome scans have identified other potential DNA regulatory sites (e.g., chromosome 10p), but definitive gene products have yet to be identified.

Obesity is also a presenting feature of at least 24 different genetic syndromes, displaying an entire range of heritability patterns. These syndromes are relatively rare, but the most common are Prader-Willi syndrome, a neurodegenerative disorder resulting from genetic abnormalities in the long arm of chromosome 15q11 to 13, and the autosomal recessive Bardet-Biedl syndrome involving concurrent hypogenitalism, mental retardation, and renal abnormalities.

Clinical Presentation

Subjective

Patients will often present to their health-care provider with some or all of the following symptoms as a result of obesity: fatigue, decreased energy, weakness, joint pain, shortness of breath, increased daytime sleepiness, and depression. Most will seek help for another medical condition or present with one or more of the aforementioned complaints. When weight history is obtained, patients often report several attempts at weight loss.

Objective

The diagnosis of obesity is having a BMI of 30 kg/m^2 or greater (Table 16.12). In extremely muscular individuals, BMI is not an accurate gauge of obesity; in such cases, a body-fat analysis will yield more accurate information about body composition. In children, obesity is diagnosed as having a BMI in the 95th percentile or higher on age- and gender-specific pediatric growth charts.

Historically, ideal body weight was calculated by comparing actual body weight to population tables from the Metropolitan Life Insurance Company. Weights for the original and updated tables were calculated based on data from middle-class Americans seeking insurance, and

Table 16.12	Calculating Body Mass Index and Classifying Obesity

Calculating Body Mass Index

The most recent formula for calculating body mass index (BMI) was developed by a panel convened by the National Heart, Lung, and Blood Institute and the National Institute of Diabetes and Digestive and Kidney Diseases. The equation for BMI is weight (kg) divided by height (m) squared (kg/m^2).

Classifying Obesity

Classification	Relative Weight	BMI
Overweight	100%–120%	25–29.9 kg/m^2
Obesity	140%–200%	30–40 kg/m^2
Severe (morbid) obesity	>200%	>40 kg/m^2

as Americans grew heavier, the weights in the table increased.

Measurements of weight and height are used to calculate the BMI for the exact classification of obesity. BMI is calculated by taking the body weight in kilograms divided by the height in meters squared. Despite criticism, BMI remains the measurement most frequently used in research and clinical practice because it is easily calculated without laboratory equipment. In research, BMI correlates with percentage of body fat measurements taken with underwater weighing but is not as reliable in older adults.

Owing to differences in complications of different types of obesity, two methods can be used to assess for central obesity. The first is to do a waist measurement. Greater than 40 inches in men and greater than 35 inches in women signifies increased risk for central obesity. The second method is a waist-to-hip ratio, which is calculated using the following formula:

$$\text{Waist-to-hip ratio} = \frac{\text{Waist measurement at smallest part}}{\text{Hip measurement at largest circumference}}$$

A ratio of greater than 1.0 for males and greater than 0.8 for females indicates central truncal obesity.

Diagnostic Reasoning

Secondary causes of obesity must be ruled out before initiating a treatment plan with the patient. Cushing's syndrome, hypothalamic injury, and hypothyroidism should be considered as potential causes. A complete history and physical with anthropometric measurement are essential elements of the initial assessment. A comprehensive history includes a weight history and attempts at weight loss. Family history of obesity and cultural food preferences must be addressed in the assessment.

The amount of control the patient maintains in food purchasing and preparation should be considered.

The patient should be questioned about any periods of rapid weight gain and environmental or psychosocial changes in lifestyle during these periods explored. An exercise history should also be obtained, with special emphasis on the relationship of any weight gain or loss periods to exercise. Specific questions to assess current or past eating disorders are essential.

A past medical history and complete medication profile are necessary, especially the intake of corticosteroids, laxatives, diuretics, and appetite suppressants. Although rarely the cause of obesity, a personal or family history of thyroid disease should be explored.

The complete physical exam with a focus on signs of a possible cause of obesity (Cushing's syndrome or thyroid disease), as well as complications of obesity, should be done.

Diagnostic Tests

Initial assessment of the patient who is obese should include the following laboratory tests: thyroid-stimulating hormone (TSH), complete blood count, fasting glucose, liver function tests, and a lipid profile. An electrocardiogram (ECG) should also be obtained.

Differential Diagnosis

The diagnosis of obesity is usually straightforward. Acute or chronic fluid retention should be distinguished from increased adiposity, because edematous states and water balance must be considered. The differential diagnosis of obesity is geared toward determining the underlying cause. Although the vast majority of cases are due to nonnutritive dietary choices and sedentary lifestyle, certain medical conditions such as hypothyroidism should be ruled out with simple lab tests (e.g., TSH). But in general, an extensive laboratory work-up is not necessary. Patients should be evaluated for other risk factors associated with obesity, however, especially those implicated in coronary artery disease (CAD), such as hyperlipidemia and insulin resistance associated with type 2 DM.

Management

Whether weight gain is related to exogenous factors or endogenous factors is an important difference. Clinical management of obesity requires the balancing of energy intake and expenditure. All of the current clinical evidence suggests that successful management must include a combination of diet, exercise, and behavioral interventions. Multidisciplinary approaches to weight loss have a higher success rate. It also appears that continued close contact with a healthcare provider is more important for long-term success than any particular diet program. Because of the chronicity of obesity, the patient must learn long-term management skills. Cognitive therapy in conjunction with education is effective in increasing self-esteem, improving depression, and decreasing patients' dissatisfaction with their bodies.

The management plan should focus on reducing comorbidity and reducing visceral obesity, not solely on improving cosmetic outcomes. In fact, dietary instructions are essentially the same for the obese individual as for a healthy nonobese person: low-fat, high-fiber, high–complex carbohydrate eating plan with emphasis on portion control. A management plan that is realistic, that can fit into the patient's lifestyle, and that includes gradual changes in diet and activity is more likely to be accepted.

Assisting the patient to identify reasons for overeating may benefit the patient in managing his or her behavior. Being tired, anxious, and angry are major triggers for overeating. Remember the acronym HALT: hungry, angry, lonely, and tired.

Counseling of patients should include the benefits of weight loss: reduction in blood pressure, serum triglycerides, and blood glucose levels and an increase in HDL cholesterol. Patients with type 2 DM may experience a decreased A1C level. Management should be directed toward an initial goal of decreasing the patient's weight by 10% over 6 months. Subsequent goals are made after achievement of the initial goal. Treatment guidelines include measuring BMI at each patient encounter. If a patient has a BMI of 25 kg/m^2 or more or a waist circumference greater than 35 inches in females or greater than 40 inches males, care should be taken to assess for risk factors. All patients, regardless of their BMI, should be counseled about healthy lifestyle behaviors, including diet and exercise. The weight-loss goals and plan should be made in consultation with the patient to devise a program that is "doable" for the patient. If on repeated visits the patient has failed to lose weight, the provider should explore possibilities with the patient.

Management of the patient will depend on the patient's motivation and the cause of the obesity. Research has shown that attempts to lose weight almost always follow a major life transition such as an acute life-threatening illness, divorce, or death of a loved one. Other recent research with overweight women found incongruities in women's beliefs about the causes of their being overweight and how they planned to lose weight. Although many women identified stress as a major factor for overeating, they believed that dieting, not stress reduction, was the key to weight management.

Cultural and socioeconomic factors affect not only the prevalence of obesity but also attitudes as to acceptable weight and its implications. For example, some cultures view being overweight as a sign of good health and prosperity. In many Western cultures, obesity is seen more as a cosmetic problem than a major health problem.

Dietary Management

Before dietary modifications are initiated, a 3- to 7-day diet history should be evaluated. The patient should keep a diary, recording all oral intake, including water and drinks. It is often beneficial for evaluation to have the patient record daily activity along with food intake. Clues as to lifestyle patterns and behavioral eating patterns can be assessed more adequately with both sets of data.

The overall goal of weight loss depends on a calorie deficit. To calculate the energy requirements of patients, the following formula can be used: Multiply body weight by 10 for women and 12 for men. This will provide the amount of calories needed to maintain the current weight. A weight-loss goal of 1 pound per week can be achieved by reducing caloric intake by 500 kcal daily, because 1 pound of fat accounts for about 3,500 kcal. The National Institutes of Health guidelines suggest that the ideal weekly weight-loss goal is 1 to 1.5 pounds. More weight loss can be expected during the first week of a calorie-restricted diet because of excessive loss of water.

The diet should be balanced, and the patient should follow current guidelines for a healthy diet. Total calories eaten should consist of 30% or less from fat, 15% from protein, and 55% or more from complex carbohydrates. Saturated fats should be avoided. Besides restriction of fat intake, dietary recommendations must take into consideration minimum daily requirements, the patient's food preferences, and the patient's lifestyle.

Usual calorie restrictions range from 1,200 to 1,800 kcal daily. A restriction of 1,000 to 1,500 kcal per day is classified as a low-calorie diet (LCD). This level of restriction is indicated in patients who are at least 40% over the ideal weight.

A very low calorie diet (VLCD) includes 800 kcal daily, or 6 to 19 kcal/kg of body weight. VLCDs have short-term effectiveness and usually do not produce long-term results if used alone. A VLCD should be reserved for patients who are more than 40% over ideal body weight and at high risk for serious health consequences. VLCDs are contraindicated in older adults, pregnant and lactating women, and individuals with cardiovascular disease, gout, DM, cancer, severe renal or hepatic disease, and hypertension. Most VLCDs are liquid protein preparations. The major advantage of protein-formula liquid diets is that they remove the patient from the food environment.

Patients on VLCDs will need fluid, mineral, and nutritional supplements and frequent laboratory evaluations of potassium, magnesium, and uric acid levels. An initial ECG is done to rule out cardiac arrhythmias. Patients with this level of dietary restriction will need weekly evaluations by a specialist skilled in weight-loss management. Most patients will average a 1.5 to 2.5 kg per week weight loss on this restriction. Men are more likely to respond to a VLCD. VLCDs, although initially very successful, often are not effective in producing long-term maintenance of the weight loss. Fifty percent of patients will gain the weight back within 1 year.

The patient on a VLCD must be monitored for hypomagnesemia, hypokalemia, hyperuricemia, ECG changes, and cardiac arrhythmias. The overall long-term effectiveness of these diets remains controversial, and they should be reserved for patients who are extremely obese.

Exercise

Exercise is a significant part of a weight-loss and maintenance program. It is especially beneficial in the long-term management of weight loss, lowering blood pressure, increasing muscle mass, increasing insulin sensitivity, improving the lipid profile, and improving glucose metabolism. Unless specific contraindications exist, exercise should be prescribed for all patients. Including resistance exercises in the exercise prescription will help maintain lean body mass.

Slow, sustained exercise, 45 to 60 minutes daily, is more beneficial for weight loss than are high-impact exercise routines. Adults should engage in at least 30 minutes of moderate-intensity physical exercise on most days of the week. Moderately intense physical exertion is equal to a brisk walk of 3 to 4 miles per hour. Patients are more likely to continue low-intensity exercise than high-intensity exercise. A 20-minute walk is usually acceptable to most patients as a starting point.

Younger patients with obesity may begin an aerobic exercise program if physical examination results are within normal levels. Older, sedentary patients should begin with walking programs. Exercise tolerance testing may be indicated for older adults and adults at risk for CAD before beginning an exercise program.

Behavior Modification

Behavior modification is essential for initial weight loss and weight maintenance. Unless the patient can identify eating patterns and lifestyle patterns that have contributed to weight gain and change those within his or her control, long-term weight management will not be achieved.

Restrictive eating behavior control includes cognitive strategies for portion control and healthy food selections. The need to identify impulsive and binge eating is also important. Behavioral management is enhanced by avoiding high-risk environments or altering the environment to reduce triggers to overeating.

Stress has a significant impact on eating behavior. During times of stress, the patient may find it impossible to implement behavior modification techniques. Relaxation techniques can assist in managing stress. Relaxation techniques must be practiced frequently in times of low stress so they can be effectively used in times of excessive stress.

Pharmacological Management

Appetite suppressants are available over the counter (OTC) and by prescription and are classed as either catecholaminergic or serotonergic. Pharmacological therapy for obesity has received much press, especially because the combination of fenfluramine (Fen Phen) and dexfenfluramine (Redux) produced an increased incidence of cardiac valvular disease in some users. Both of these drugs were classed as serotonergic agents, and they have both been withdrawn from the market, raising significant concerns for this class of medications.

Catecholaminergic agents include amphetamines, but also non-amphetamine schedule IV appetite suppressants including phentermine (Fastin) and diethylpropion (Tenuate). These pharmacological agents typically reduce weight by 5% to 10% but must be administered continually or the weight is regained. The potential for adverse reactions, lack of evidence for long-term effectiveness, and potential for drug dependence make their use in the management of obesity debatable.

There are two other medications approved by the FDA for weight loss: orlistat (Alli and Xenical) and the combination of phentermine plus extended-release (ER) topiramate (Qsymia). Orlistat functions by blocking the absorption of fat in the gastrointestinal tract. Phentermine plus ER topiramate suppresses appetite and increases feelings of satiety.

Orlistat 60 mg is available OTC and is taken with each fat-containing meal and inhibits gastric and pancreatic lipases, reducing fat absorption. It is also available by prescription at a dose of 120 mg. Demonstrated results are a weight loss of 2 to 4 kg maintained for 2 years. Adverse effects of orlistat include diarrhea, gas, and abdominal cramping. Some studies suggest it may also inhibit the absorption of fat-soluble vitamins.

Phentermine plus ER topiramate has four dosing preparations to allow for titration of the medication when starting and stopping. The usual dose for weight loss is 7.5 mg/46 mg or 15 mg/92 mg. It is taken each morning to suppress the appetite (phentermine), increase satiety, decrease food appeal, and increase metabolic rate (topiramate). In studies, patients lost approximately 8% of their starting body weight using this combination medication. Adverse reactions include dry mouth, paresthesia, constipation, irritability, and seizures if abruptly discontinued.

Surgical Intervention

Surgical intervention for obesity should be reserved for those patients who have a BMI over 40 kg/m^2 or over 35 kg/m^2 with comorbid conditions. It is usually not considered until the obese patient has failed more conventional weight-loss methods. The incidence of bariatric surgery is booming in the United States today. The most common surgical procedures are the vertical-banded (Mason) gastroplasty and the roux-en-Y gastric bypass, which may both be done laparoscopically. Some studies have shown that surgery can produce up to a 50% loss of initial body weight. Complications may occur in up to 40% of patients after surgery and include peritonitis, abdominal wall hernia, dumping syndrome, infection, acute cholecystitis, hypoglycemia, pyloric outlet obstruction, chronic diarrhea, nausea, and vomiting. Patients should be counseled regarding these potential complications. They should also be informed of the possibility of regaining much of the lost weight if lifestyle changes are not also undertaken and sustained.

Follow-up and Referral

Most weight-loss programs require close follow-up. The severity of the problem and the nature of the interventions should govern how frequently the health-care provider sees the patient, but clearly, patients are more successful in maintaining weight loss with frequent follow-up visits. Many patients will benefit from frequent clinician visits that provide medical guidance, goal setting, and emotional support throughout the weight-loss process. In addition, the importance of clinical follow-up once weight-loss goals have been achieved should be emphasized, because recurrent weight gain following periods of significant weight loss is common. The patient should be seen for a weigh-in, blood pressure measurement, and discussion of progress at least monthly, but once a week is often most beneficial until the patient has developed habituated lifestyle changes.

Patient Education

Patient education includes instruction on how to maintain a balance between intake and energy expenditure. Exercise, a low-fat diet, and lifestyle changes should be emphasized. Patients may benefit from a referral to a dietitian. Many patients are unaware of techniques to reduce fat in their diet by cooking methods alone. One suggestion that may help is to use nonstick cookware so that there is no need to use fat or grease in the pan. Other suggestions are to bake, broil, and braise rather than fry foods. Patients with obesity must be educated about the importance of a combination of therapies. They must be guided to set realistic goals. Most obese persons skip breakfast and eat more in the late afternoon and evening, which is not helpful.

Sustaining weight loss requires behavioral changes. Patients should plan out their weight-loss strategy in writing. The plan should include diet modifications, exercise routine, and behavioral strategies. A calendar should be developed outlining the schedule. If lapses in the plan are experienced, the patient should explore the reasons for the lapse. Health-care providers should review this outline on each visit.

Some patients will benefit from support groups. Support groups for weight loss and overeating are listed in the Resources section at the end of this chapter. Patients who feel "sabotaged" by family members will need to explore methods for support outside of the family. Finding a walking partner or walking right after work before going home are some strategies to suggest.

Challenges in Caring for Obese Patients

The increasing number of obese and morbidly obese patients brings a challenge to primary-care providers. Caring for patients who are obese certainly includes treating the obesity, but many of these patients will have diseases and illnesses that will bring them to the provider's office. The National Institute of Diabetes and Digestive and Kidney Diseases Weight-control Information Network (WIN) offers suggestions for health-care providers in the care of these individuals separate from the need to treat the obesity. Providers and staff need to receive education related to respect for patients, appropriate equipment in the clinic, and providing the same level of care for obese patients as nonobese patients. Table 16.13 provides details to guide providers in creating an accessible and comfortable clinic environment, including medical equipment that can accurately assess patients who are obese and ways to reduce patient fears about their weight.

■ GOUT

Gout is a metabolic disease that produces an inflammatory arthritis. Gout was identified in the days of Hippocrates and was often referred to as "the disease of kings" because of its prevalence in the wealthy, who were able to afford the rich foods that typically trigger this

Table 16.13	Provider's Guide to Caring for Obese Patients

Create an accessible and comfortable clinic environment.
- Provide sturdy, armless chairs and high, firm sofas in waiting rooms.
- Provide sturdy, wide examination tables that are bolted to the floor to prevent tipping.
- Provide a sturdy stool or step with handles to help patients get on the examination table.
- Provide extra-large examination gowns.
- Install a split lavatory seat and provide a specimen collector with a handle.

Use medical equipment that can accurately assess patients who are obese.
- Use large adult blood pressure cuffs or thigh cuffs on patients with an upper-arm circumference greater than 34 cm.
- Have extra-long phlebotomy needles, tourniquets, and large vaginal speculae on hand.
- Have a weight scale with adequate capacity (greater than 350 pounds) for obese patients.

Reduce patient fears about weight.
- Weigh patients only when medically appropriate.
- Weigh patients in a private area.
- Record weight without comments.
- Ask patients if they wish to discuss their weight or health.
- Avoid using the term *obesity*. Your patients may be more comfortable with phrases such as "difficulties with weight" or "being overweight." You may wish to ask your patients what terms they prefer when discussing their weight.

disorder. Once a disabling chronic disease, current medical diagnostics and treatment modalities have decreased its disabling effects.

An overproduction or underexcretion (or both) of uric acid with tissue deposition of monosodium urate crystals causes the metabolic disease underlying gout. Most individuals with gout (90%) have a problem with underexcretion of uric acid. The arthritis produced by gout is characterized by recurrent, painful attacks of monoarticular joint inflammation caused by the phagocytosis of urate crystals, which deposit in joints, soft tissue, and cartilage.

Epidemiology and Causes

Gout occurs rarely in children, premenopausal women, or men younger than 30 years of age. Seventy percent of people with gout are men, with a peak incidence between 40 and 50 years. Gout is more prevalent in black men, possibly because of the increased prevalence of hypertension in this group. The increased incidence in older adults has been associated with the increased use of diuretics.

Twenty percent of patients who present with gout have a family history of the disease. Persons from the United States, the Pacific Islands, and countries with abundant lifestyles have an increased incidence of gout. Gout affects 8.3 million adults in the United States.

Hyperuricemia (uric acid levels exceeding 7 mg/dL in men and 6 mg/dL in women) occurs in 5% to 10% of the United States population. Most of these adults, however, are asymptomatic. One in five persons with hyperuricemia will develop urate deposits in a joint, soft tissue, or cartilage.

The risk factors and predisposing factors for development of gout are listed in Risk Factors 16.2. Causes of primary gout include the idiopathic inborn error of purine metabolism, decreased renal clearance of uric acid, and specific enzyme defects such as Lesch-Nyhan syndrome and glycogen storage disease. Secondary causes of gout include other disease processes and medications that produce an overproduction or underexcretion of uric acid.

Patients with gout may experience an acute attack with rapid fluctuations of serum urate levels. Surgery, dehydration, binge alcohol consumption, emotional stress, infection, diuretics, and uricosuric drugs can cause rapid fluctuations.

Pathophysiology

Gout is a direct result of hyperuricemia (high serum uric acid). Gout is characterized by an increased saturation of urate in the plasma and bodily fluids. Supersaturation of bodily fluids results in a precipitation of monosodium urate crystals out of body fluids into the joints, soft tissues, and cartilage. This leads to the symptoms and clinical findings of gout, because the deposition of urate in the joints and its crystallization trigger an inflammatory response. Several mechanisms may trigger an acute

Risk Factors 16.2   Gout

Primary Risk Factors
- Enzyme defects
- Decreased renal clearance of uric acid

Secondary Risk Factors
- Excessive daily intake of purine
- Obesity
- Starvation
- Alcohol abuse
- Medications: Thiazide diuretics, ethambutol, nicotinic acid, pyrazinamide, low-dose salicylates, cyclosporine
- Paget's disease
- Chronic hemolytic anemia
- Psoriasis
- Cytotoxic drugs
- Carcinoma and sarcoma
- Chronic renal disease
- Hypothyroidism
- Lead poisoning
- Hyperparathyroidism
- Diabetes insipidus
- Diabetic ketoacidosis

attack of gout, the most common being trauma or surgery. Gouty attacks may also be triggered by prophylactic or uricosuric agents, which are known to lower serum uric acid levels.

At the time of puberty, serum uric acid levels increase in men; however, most (90%–95%) remain asymptomatic throughout life. Estrogen is believed to protect women from hyperuricemia. Acute attacks are more likely to occur at lower serum uric acid levels in persons with alcoholism due to decreased urinary excretion. There is also an increased incidence of hypothyroidism in persons with confirmed crystal aspirates in synovial fluid. Although gout is frequently cited as a risk factor for the development of coronary artery disease, subsequent studies did not confirm previous findings of the Framingham Heart Study.

For unclear reasons, gouty arthritis has a predilection for the first metatarsophalangeal joint (the great toe)—a condition known as podagra. This may result from the relative coolness of this peripheral joint which allows for greater crystal deposition, the constant microtrauma to which this joint is subjected, and the differential impact weight-bearing alternating with recumbency has on the resorption of joint fluid and intra-articular urate. Gouty arthritis may extend to several joints and is classified into four stages based on timing and clinical presentation (Table 16.14).

In general, urate crystallization is more likely to occur at lower temperatures. Noninflamed synovial fluid in the knee is significantly cooler (90–91°F [32.2–32.78 °C]) than core body temperature. Thus, although a serum

Table 16.14	Stages of Gout		
Stage	Subjective Findings	Objective Findings	Diagnostic Findings
I. Asymptomatic	None	None	Microtophaceous deposits of urates in joints and bursae
II. Acute phase (inflammatory phase)	Extremely painful monoarticular or polyarticular attack Pruritus and desquamation of the skin surrounding the joint as the inflammation subsides	Affected joints are red, warm, swollen Early acute attack subsides within a few days; may last up to 2 weeks; inflammation gradually subsides 10% of patients experience only one acute attack during their life span	Elevated WBC count Elevated temperature Elevated serum uric acid or normouricemia
III. Intercritical (the interval between acute attacks)	None; patient is asymptomatic	Intervals between attacks decrease as the disease progresses. If a second acute attack occurs, it usually presents within the first year after the initial attack	
IV. Chronic (chronic tophaceous gout phase; occurs as a result of recurrent attacks with multiple sites of urate deposits [tophi] in articular and periarticular tissue)	May restrict movement of affected joints Chronic pain, stiffness, decreased joint function, joint derangement, secondary degeneration	More than 50% of patients progress to this stage within 20 years of the initial attack if not properly managed Occasionally, tophus ulceration and erosion with chalk-textured drainage Uric acid kidney stones (5%–10% of patients)	Tophi

uric acid concentration of 7 mg/dL appears to be the threshold level above which gout is more likely to develop, crystallization may be more likely to occur at lower concentrations intra-articularly. Hyperuricemia alone is insufficient to lead to crystallization, however. As part of the inflammatory process, urate-specific immunoglobulin (Ig) molecules coat monosodium urate crystals in gouty synovial fluid, likely serving as a promoter of nucleation for urate crystals.

As gout progresses, crystals are deposited into multiple bodily tissues. In severe cases with repeated attacks, monosodium urate monohydrate crystals form into a nodular deposit known as a *tophus,* surrounded by granulomatous inflammation consisting of monocytes and giant cells. In addition to the skin and joints, *tophaceous* swellings may be found in a number of bodily tissues, including the heart valves, kidneys, and larynx, capable of leading to significant pathology. Microtophi, consisting of collections of urate crystals surrounded only by a thin fibrocytic ring, may also be present in gouty synovial fluid. Some researchers have suggested that these microtophi release their urate crystals into the joint fluid after the initiation of synovial inflammation in the early stages of a gouty attack.

Urate crystals induce intra-articular inflammation via a number of mechanisms. Synovial lining cells, monocytes, and endothelial cells have all been shown to phagocytose urate crystals in vitro and subsequently increase their production of inflammatory mediators via transcriptional upregulation and mRNA stabilization, including interleukin (IL)–1, IL-6, IL-8, and tumor necrosis factor (TNF). Blockade of IL-8 and TNF activity has been further shown to counter urate-induced inflammation.

However, neutrophilic migration into affected joints and their subsequent phagocytosis of urate crystals appears to play a central role in the pathogenesis of gouty arthritis. Neutrophils undergo an oxidative burst during this process, releasing lysosomal enzymes, superoxide anions, leukotriene B4, and IL-1, among other mediators. In fact, the complexities of neutrophilic chemotaxis and function within gouty joints have been a central focus of gout research. Studies have indicated tyrosine kinases, phospholipases, adhesion molecules such as E-selectin, and several chemotactic factors play key roles in neutrophilic recruitment and activation by urate crystals. This explains the efficacy of colchicine in treating acute attacks, because it inhibits neutrophil tyrosine kinase activity in response to both gout and pseudogout crystals, as well as downregulates the activity of adhesion molecules on both neutrophils and endothelial cells.

A number of proteins interact with urate crystals to increase their pro-inflammatory properties. Immunoglobulins bound to urate crystals lead to a greater release of lysosomal and superoxide enzymes by neutrophils. In turn, neutrophil mediators have been shown to cleave Ig molecules from urate crystals to reduce their inflammatory nature. The inflammatory properties of tophaceous urate crystals are also reduced after protease treatment in vitro. In contrast, lipoproteins (specifically apolipoprotein B) reduce the inflammatory potential of urate crystals after binding, indicating that they may be involved in the self-limited resolution of acute attacks. The complement and kinin systems have also been implicated in urate crystal pathology, but they are not requisite for acute gouty inflammation.

The self-limited nature of an acute gouty attack involves several mechanisms. In addition to the deactivation and death of inflammatory cells and the inactivation of secreted pro-inflammatory mediators, leukocytes, monocytes, and macrophages have been shown in vitro to alter their cytokine transcriptional activity over time. In turn, they secrete several anti-inflammatory cytokines on resolution of an acute attack, including IL-1 receptor antagonist, transforming growth factor–β, and peroxisome-proliferator–activated receptor (PPAR) γ. Although acute attacks of gout typically resolve spontaneously within several weeks, if left untreated or if inadequately treated, gout leads to chronic arthritis and bony erosions within 5 to 10 years, producing joint deformities and ultimately restricting function.

Clinical Presentation
Subjective

A thorough evaluation of the onset, characteristics, and potential potentiating causes of the pain is completed on initial evaluation. The patient will present during an acute attack with pain, tenderness, erythema, and swelling. Usual presentation is monoarticular, and the joint most frequently affected is the first metatarsal joint; however, the midfoot, knees, fingers, wrists, and elbows may also be affected. The typical presentation is excruciating pain that awakens the patient at night. Patients often describe the pain as throbbing, crushing, and pulsating. The pain is not relieved by rest or position change. Pain prevents any weight-bearing on the affected limb. Often the patient cannot tolerate anything coming in contact with the affected part—even bed clothing touching the part is extremely painful. The patient may also report an episode of recent trauma to the affected joint, a recent drinking binge, or an eating binge before the acute attack. Patients may report a recent operation or severe illness, especially one producing a shift in fluid balance.

The patient's past medical history, including any joint or musculoskeletal trauma, should be reviewed, along with any family history of gout. Because gout is more prevalent in patients with hypertension, obesity, and hyperlipidemia, history taking should focus on these contributing factors. In addition, a drug history, specific for recent increased intake of aspirin or cyclosporine, should also be obtained.

Objective

Even though the patient initially presents with monoarticular complaints, a complete bilateral examination of all joints should be performed. Joints should be assessed for symmetry in appearance and range of motion. Asymmetrical presentation of joint inflammation, redness, tenderness, and limitations in range of motion are typical of gout.

The joint most frequently affected in the initial attack is the first metatarsophalangeal joint (podagra). Podagra is experienced by approximately 90% of patients with gout. Subsequent attacks may progress to include several joints (polyarticular). Other joints that are frequently affected include the instep of the ankle, the heels, knees, wrists, fingers, and elbows. Peripheral joints are more likely to be involved, because central joints are warmer and less conducive to crystal formations. In polyarticular episodes or if a large joint is involved, the patient may have an elevated temperature, tachycardia, anorexia, malaise, headache, and chills. On physical examination, the affected area is warm or hot to the touch. The patient will complain of pain on palpation, and range of motion will be limited. Skin overlying the affected area is often red and taut. Several days after an acute attack, desquamation over affected joints may be evident.

Patients who have progressed to the chronic tophaceous stage will have palpable tophi. *Tophi* are nodular deposits of monosodium urate monohydrate crystals that initiate an inflammatory process. Most tophi are firm and movable, whereas the overlying skin is thin and red. Tophi are most likely to develop on the pinnae, olecranon tips, and the distal joints of the hands and feet. Extensive tissue deposits of urate may also occur on the helix and antihelix of the ear, the eyelids, the sclera, and cornea.

Diagnostic Reasoning
Diagnostic Tests

Clinical presentation and history are often diagnostic of gout. Serum uric acid levels and radiographic imaging provide some confirmation; however, a definitive diagnosis is made only with identification of sodium urate crystals of aspirate.

Initial Testing Initial testing for gout includes a serum uric acid level. Most patients will have an elevated serum urate level in the absence of elevated blood urea nitrogen, because serum urate is above 7.5 mg/dL in up to

95% of persons with gout. However, some studies have suggested that serum urate levels may be normal in up to 15% of patients at the time of an acute gouty attack. In addition, elevated serum urate levels alone are not diagnostic of gout in the absence of characteristic joint signs and symptoms, and the clinician should look for other supportive laboratory findings. The erythrocyte sedimentation rate and white blood cell (WBC) count may also be elevated during an acute attack. The WBC count is typically greater than 10,000 cells/mcL, but values up to 100,000 cells/mcL may occasionally be observed.

The classic radiographic findings of gout are tophi, normal mineralization of bone, joint space preservation, asymmetrical polyarticular distribution, overhanging edge cortex, and punched-out erosions of bone. Radiographs of affected joints may show no changes in early stages. The only radiographic evidence in early stages may be asymmetrical soft tissue swelling. With recurrent attacks and progressive disease, however, radiolucent urate tophi and punched-out appearing areas are apparent in bone. Tophi appear as cloudlike increases in density, which may show signs of calcification. Urate crystals may also be seen in subcutaneous tissue, cartilage, joints, and other tissues. In the very late stages of gout, demineralization and loss of articular structures may be apparent on radiographic examination. Most changes are asymmetrical and occur predominantly in the feet, ankles, and knees. Patients with severe disease often have involvement of the hands and elbows.

Subsequent Testing   The definitive test to confirm the diagnosis of acute gout is urate crystals in joint fluid aspirate. The synovial fluid will be turbid during an acute attack. The crystals are identified by compensated polariscopic examination of wet smears of the aspirate and are noted to be negatively birefringent (a diagnostic finding). Aspiration and subsequent examination of the fluid should provide evidence for the diagnosis. Patients who present with gout and comorbid symptoms of abdominal pain, peripheral neuropathy, and proteinuria should be assessed for lead exposure.

Differential Diagnosis

Differential diagnoses include septic arthritis, cellulitis, rheumatoid arthritis, bursitis, fracture, acute trauma, and reactive arthritis (previously known as Reiter syndrome).

Septic arthritis should be considered when a patient presents with joint pain, swelling, and erythema. Septic arthritis occasionally coexists with gout. It should also be strongly considered when a patient does not respond to initial management for gout. Septic arthritis more commonly occurs in larger joints. Gram stains and cultures of synovial fluids are positive for bacteria in septic arthritis. Patients often present with fever and chills. Radiographic examinations often reveal joint-space narrowing and erosions within 1 to 2 weeks of the onset.

The rheumatoid factor titer may help rule out rheumatoid arthritis. Rheumatoid arthritis may resemble gout, but it typically has a symmetrical subjective presentation and radiographic presentation. Joint-space narrowing is also typical of rheumatoid joint disease.

Psoriatic arthritis may resemble gout in its early stages; however, the initial joints affected are frequently the hand, feet, sacroiliac joint, and spine. Fusiform soft tissue swelling is typical of psoriatic arthritis, and early joint-space narrowing is common.

The development of an inflamed joint in a young man or woman following a gastrointestinal (GI) (*Campylobacter, Salmonella, Shigella*) or genitourinary (*Chlamydia trachomatis*) infection would raise suspicion for reactive arthritis. In its typical presentation, this form of autoimmune joint inflammation is accompanied by conjunctivitis and noninfectious urethritis, comprising the classic triad of reactive arthritis.

Pseudogout presents with many similar characteristics to gout. However, polarized microscopic examination of joint fluid aspirate reveals calcium pyrophosphate dihydrate crystals, rather than the negatively birefringent uric acid crystals associated with gout. Pseudogout usually presents at a later age, and the symptoms are characteristically less acute and severe. Pseudogout is usually polyarticular (in approximately 75% of patients) and typically affects the knees and larger joints. Pseudogout is associated with hyperthyroidism and hypothyroidism, hypomagnesemia, amyloidosis, hypercalcemia, hypophosphatemia, and hemosiderosis.

Management

The goals of clinical management are to terminate an acute attack, prevent future attacks, normalize hyperuricemia, and prevent potential complications of urate deposits. Management of gout includes pharmacological treatment of acute attacks and long-term medical and pharmacological treatment of hyperuricemia. Acute management of gout includes generalized rest, elevation and immobilization of affected joints, and pharmacological treatment. Prevention of disability due to gout is a reality today because of advances in pharmacological treatment; however, the patient must become an active participant in the long-term treatment plan (Table 16.15).

Initial Management

Pharmacological treatment for an acute attack includes NSAIDs, colchicine (if onset is less than 36 hours), and corticosteroids.

Nonsteroidal Anti-inflammatory Drugs   The medication of choice initially is an NSAID. Traditionally, indomethacin (Indocin) has been the most commonly prescribed NSAID for an acute attack of gout, but the other NSAIDs are just as effective. Indomethacin 25 to 50 mg every 8 hours is given until symptoms subside, usually 5 to 10 days. A good alternative to indomethacin is naproxen (Naprosyn). The first dose of naproxen is 750 mg, followed by 250 mg every 8 hours for 5 to 10 days. NSAIDs are discontinued after the pain has dissipated. Contraindications

Table 16.15	Management of Gout
Acute attack	NSAIDs Colchicine Corticosteroids Rest
No further attacks	Avoid excessive alcohol Dietary modification to avoid purine-rich foods
Additional acute attack	NSAIDs Colchicine Corticosteroids Rest Avoid alcohol and binge eating Low-purine diet
Two or more additional attacks	Uric acid secretion <1,000 mg/24 hr: probenecid Uric acid secretion >1,000 mg/24 hr: allopurinol Dietary modification to avoid purine-rich foods Lifestyle modification Colchicine

to the use of NSAIDs are active peptic ulcer disease, impaired renal function, and allergic reactions to NSAIDs. Potential adverse reactions of NSAIDs include GI bleeding, nausea, rash, hypertension (especially in the elderly), hepatic impairment, fluid retention, and acute tubular necrosis with subsequent acute renal insufficiency (particularly at high doses or with chronic use).

Colchicine Colchicine is an effective medication to terminate an acute gout attack if administered within 36 hours of the initial onset of symptoms. If administered within this time frame, it is effective in 90% of all patients. Colchicine can be administered orally or IV. The IV route is rarely used due to its low benefit versus toxicity ratio. In acute attacks, administer 1 to 1.2 mg of oral colchicine at the first sign of attack, then 0.5 to 0.6 g every hour or 1 to 1.2 mg every 2 hours until pain is relieved. The cumulative dose of colchicine should not exceed 4 to 6 mg during one course of therapy for an acute attack.

Adverse reactions include nausea, vomiting, diarrhea, and abdominal pain and cramping. Colchicine usually provides relief within 18 hours; however, many patients will experience diarrhea or nausea within 24 hours of the first dose. In the past, colchicine was often intentionally dosed until patients experienced vomiting or diarrhea; however, this is no longer considered an appropriate gauge of dosing adequacy, because such GI complications are adverse (rather than expected) drug effects. In the Acute Gout Flare Receiving Colchicine Evaluation (AGREE) trial, patients were randomized to three groups: usual colchicine treatment, low-dose treatment (1.2 mg orally

followed by 0.6 mg 1 hour later), and placebo group. Researchers found that the low-dose group had a 50% pain reduction without rescue medication compared with the placebo group. They also found that the low-dose group had fewer adverse events compared with the traditional therapy (Level II; Terkeltaub et al, 2010). Colchicine is contraindicated in patients with a hypersensitivity to colchicine; severe cardiovascular, renal, or GI disease; or blood dyscrasias. Patients with renal or hepatic disease require a decreased total dose. In addition, colchicine must be used with caution in older adults.

Corticosteroids Corticosteroids can provide dramatic systematic relief and can be administered orally, intramuscularly, or intra-articularly. In most cases, corticosteroids are reserved for refractory cases or cases where the use of colchicine and NSAIDs is contraindicated. Corticosteroids are contraindicated in septic conditions; therefore, they should not be administered before analysis of the synovial aspirate. For polyarticular gout, prednisone, 40 to 60 mg PO daily, usually produces a good response. The dose should be tapered quickly over 5 to 7 days. Patients with monoarticular disease who cannot tolerate oral corticosteroids or NSAIDs benefit from intra-articular steroid injection. Intra-articular injection is with triamcinolone 10 to 40 mg and depends on the size of the joint.

Subsequent Management

The long-term management of gout includes pharmacological agents, dietary modifications, activity evaluation, and education regarding the prevention of gout.

Pharmacological Management Pharmacological prophylaxis should be initiated after the second or third attack. In patients with hyperuricemia and a history of only one acute attack, modification of lifestyle may prevent further attacks. Alternatives to thiazide diuretics should be addressed. Pharmacological prophylaxis, however, should be considered in patients with polyarticular gout and patients with consistent hyperuricemia greater than 8 mg/dL. Colchicine and NSAIDs may be continued in lower doses up to 12 months following an acute attack.

Colchicine is often used to prevent further acute attacks triggered by changes in uric acid levels. Colchicine does not correct the underlying causes of an acute attack, however. Adverse reactions to long-term use of colchicine are bone marrow depression, peripheral neuritis, and GI symptoms, especially diarrhea. The dosage of colchicine for long-term preventive management ranges from 0.5 to 1.2 mg daily. Colchicine is often used to prevent an acute attack with the initiation of probenecid or allopurinol, because they may precipitate an acute attack by rapidly decreasing the urate serum level. Before scheduled surgery, colchicine 0.5 to 0.6 mg PO three times daily for 3 days before and 3 days after surgery may prevent an acute attack of gout.

Three agents are currently available to lower uric acid levels—probenecid (Benemid) is a uricosuric agent that blocks tubular reabsorption of filtered urate; allopurinol

(Zyloprim) and febuxostat (Uloric) are xanthine oxidase inhibitors that lower plasma urate and urinary uric acid concentrations. They should not be started during or within 1 month after an acute attack. Before initiation, a 24-hour urinary uric acid excretion test is performed to differentiate between patients who are hypersecretors from those who are hyposecretors, because pharmacological management of the two conditions differs.

Before initiation of probenecid therapy, a 24-hour uric acid excretion test should be performed. Uric acid excretions greater than 1,000 mg in 24 hours are abnormal, and levels between 800 and 1,000 mg in 24 hours are considered to be borderline. Probenecid is indicated in patients whose excretion of uric acid is below 700 to 800 mg in 24 hours.

Probenecid is the drug of choice in persons younger than 60 years of age without a history of blood dyscrasias, renal failure, or kidney stones. An initial dosage of 500 mg is recommended, increasing gradually to 1 to 2 g after 1 week. Dosage is increased based on uric acid levels, with a maximum dose of 2 g daily. Major adverse reactions of this drug include skin rash, uric acid stones, and GI upset. It may also precipitate an exacerbation of gout if it produces rapid shifts in uric acid levels. Probenecid inhibits the excretion of penicillin, indomethacin (Indocin), and acetazolamide (Diamox). Allopurinol (Zyloprim) is used to decrease uric acid production in patients who are unable to take probenecid. It is indicated in patients whose 24-hour uric acid secretion is greater than 1,000 mg. Adverse reactions include GI upset, headache, rash, bone marrow suppression, fever, liver or kidney failure, vasculitis, lymphadenopathy, hepatitis, alopecia, and dermatitis. It is contraindicated in persons with idiopathic hemochromatosis and renal and hepatic disease. Serious hypersensitivity reactions to allopurinol may occur but are rare. However, patients should still be cautioned to discontinue use and immediately report any rash or fever that occurs after starting the drug. Twenty percent of patients on both allopurinol and ampicillin develop a rash. The safety of its use in pregnant or lactating women has not been established. The initial dose is 100 to 200 mg daily, with the average daily dose ranging from 200 to 300 mg. Dosages of 400 to 600 mg daily are indicated only in severe gout. The maximum daily dose is 800 mg. The goal of therapy is to decrease the serum uric acid levels below 6 mg/dL. Dosage should be adjusted based on serum uric acid levels every 2 to 6 months.

Febuxostat (Uloric) is also used to lower serum uric acid levels by blocking uric acid production. The dosage is 40 to 80 mg daily. Serious adverse reactions may occur including hypersensitivity rhabdomyolysis, interstitial nephritis, stroke, and myocardial infarction.

Dietary Modifications

Dietary modifications include avoiding high-purine–containing foods, maintaining adequate fluid intake, and

Table 16.16	Foods High in Purine

- All meats and seafoods (especially organ meats such as liver, kidneys, and sweetbreads)
- Meat extracts and gravies
- Yeast and yeast extracts (brewer's and baker's)
- Beer and alcoholic beverages
- Beans, peas, lentils, oatmeal, spinach, asparagus, cauliflower, and mushrooms

moderate alcohol intake. The complete restriction of purine in the diet has not proven effective; therefore, a moderation of purine in the diet is now recommended. Foods high in purine content are listed in Table 16.16. Fluid intake should be sufficient to maintain an output of 2,000 mL/day. Patients should force fluids to exceed 3,000 mL/day, especially if they are prescribed a uricosuric agent.

Lifestyle Modifications

Activity must be restricted during an acute attack, and bedrest should be maintained 24 hours following the acute attack. The joint should be immobilized; if a lower extremity is involved, no weight-bearing should be allowed during the acute attack. During intercritical periods, physical therapy may be indicated to maintain or improve function.

Hot compresses may promote comfort after an acute attack but should not be instituted until the acute pain subsides, usually 24 to 72 hours after initiation of therapy. Instruct the patient to apply heat for 20 minutes two to three times daily. Heat can be applied with moist heating pads, warm showers and baths, or moist towels heated in a microwave. Relief may also be obtained using ice packs during an acute attack. Patients should be instructed to apply packs only for 10 to 20 minutes sessions and to discontinue if pain is not relieved.

Long-term management includes dietary moderation (one to two servings of purine-rich foods per day), alcohol in moderation, weight maintenance, and maintenance of joint mobility.

Surgical Intervention

Patients with extensive or large tophi may benefit from surgical excision and should be referred to a surgeon.

Follow-up and Referral

The patient should be evaluated 1 to 2 weeks after an acute attack. If antihyperuricemia therapy is initiated, the patient needs to be followed every 4 to 6 weeks to adjust medications and review the goals of treatment.

Annual follow-up is recommended. Special attention is given to previously affected joints as to their range of motion and stability. Joints should be symmetrically evaluated for tophi. Annual serum uric acid levels are indicated in all patients, and evaluation of renal function is indicated for patients on prophylactic antihyperuricemic therapy. An evaluation of the patient's diet (including specific questions about alcohol intake) and exercise regimen should be conducted during the annual exam. Reinforcement of previous education is essential to increase adherence to medication and physical regimens during intercritical periods. Patients who are overweight will need continued reinforcement to lose weight and reduce stress on weight-bearing joints. Patients younger than age 35 years, premenopausal women, patients with frequent acute attacks despite prophylactic treatment, and patients with renal insufficiency should be referred to a rheumatologist for an initial evaluation.

Patient Education

Patients need instructions on avoidance of triggers for acute attacks. Excessive exercise, trauma, and alcohol or eating binges may precipitate an acute attack. Patients need explicit information on the adverse reactions of medication and measures to allay some preventable adverse reactions.

Fluid intake should exceed 2,000 mL daily to prevent formation of uric acid kidney stones. Patients should avoid dehydration because it may precipitate an acute attack. Diet modifications must be reviewed with patients in detail and written information provided. Because both wine and spirits in excessive amounts impair the kidney's ability to excrete uric acid, they should be used in moderation. Patients must be aware that binge drinking may provoke an acute attack. If the patient is obese, weight loss should be encouraged because loss of excess body fat may normalize serum uric acid without pharmacological intervention. Weight loss will also decrease stress on weight-bearing joints. Caution as to severe, rapid weight loss should be given because secondary hyperuricemia may result. A very low calorie diet may precipitate an acute attack.

Patients may need to take colchicine before having elective surgery if they are not already taking it regularly. They should be instructed to avoid aspirin.

Good posture and protection of weight-bearing joints are essential. Because the feet are most frequently affected, the patient should wear supportive and properly fitting shoes. Some patients may benefit from a physical therapist's exercise prescription or a visit to a podiatrist for an evaluation. At the first signs of an acute attack, the patient should limit all activity, limit weight-bearing if appropriate, and contact the primary-care provider.

 DavisPlus | For additional resources please visit http://davisplus.fadavis.com

References

Evidence-Based Practice

Bakos, B, et al. Long term efficacy of radioiodine treatment in hyperthyroidism. *Exp Clin Endocrinol Diabetes* 212(8):494–497, 2013.

Cafalu, WT, et al. Efficacy and safety of canagliflozin versus glimepiride in patients with type 2 diabetes inadequately controlled with metformin (CANTATA-SU): 52 week results from a randomised, double-blind, phase 3 non-inferiority trial. *Lancet* 382(9896), 941–950, 2013.

House, AA, et al. Effect of B-vitamin therapy on progression of diabetic nephropathy: A randomized controlled trial. *JAMA* 303(16):1603–1609, 2010.

Preiss, D, et al. Risk of incident diabetes with intensive-dose compared with moderate-dose statin therapy: A meta-analysis. *JAMA* 305(24): 2556–2564, 2011.

Terkeltaub, RA, et al. High versus low dosing of oral colchicine for early acute gout flare: Twenty-four-hour outcome of the first multicenter, randomized, double-blind, placebo-controlled, parallel-group, dose-comparison colchicine study. *Arthritis Rheum* 62(4):1060–1068, 2010.

Wolf, JE, et al. Randomized, double-blind clinical evaluation of the efficacy and safety of topical eflornithine HCl 13.9% cream in the treatment of women with facial hair. Int J Dermatol 46(1): 94-8, 2007.

Bibliography

General

Adler, GK. Cushing's syndrome. Retrieved from http://emedicine.medscape.com/article/117365-overview

American College of Rheumatology. 2012 Guidelines for management of gout. Part 1 & 2: Therapy and antiinflammatory prophylaxis of acute gouty arthritis. Retrieved from www.guideline.gov/content.aspx?id=38625

Ansstas, G, and Ansstas, M. Gynecomastia. 2013. Retrieved from http://emedicine.medscape.com/article/120858-overview

Buttaro, TM, et al. *Primary care: A collaborative practice*, ed 4. Mosby, St. Louis, 2012.

Cleary, J, and Webb, K. New strategies against comorbidities of obesity. *Clin Advisor* 14(9):33–48, 2011.

Cook, D. Creating an effective weight management plan. *Nurse Prescribing* 11(11):561–565, 2013.

Dambro, MR. *Griffith's 5-minute clinical consult*. Lippincott Williams & Wilkins, Philadelphia, 2013.

Edmunds, MW, and Mayhew, MS. *Pharmacology for the primary care provider*, ed 4. Mosby/Elsevier, St. Louis, 2013.

Fauci, AS, et al (Eds.). *Harrison's principles of internal medicine*, ed 18. McGraw-Hill, New York, 2011.

Goldman, L, and Schafer, AI. *Goldman's Cecil medicine*, ed 24. Elsevier, New York, 2011.

Griffing, GT. Hirsutism. 2012. Retrieved from http://emedicine.medscape.com/article/121038-overview

Harrison, S, et al. Update on the management of hirsutism. *Cleve Clin J Med* 77(6):388–398, 2010.

Institute for Clinical Systems Improvement (ICSI). Prevention and management of obesity (mature adolescents and adults). Retrieved from www.guideline.gov/content.aspx?id=32825&search=obesity

Kee, JL. *Laboratory and diagnostic tests with nursing implications*, ed 8. Prentice-Hall, Upper Saddle River, NJ, 2010.

Johnson, RE, and Murad, MH. Gynecomastia: Pathophysiology, evaluation and management. *Mayo Clin Proc* 84(11):1010–1015, 2009.

Masters, RK, et al. The impact of obesity on US mortality levels: The importance of age and cohort factors in population estimates. *Am J Public Health* 103(10):1895–1901, 2013.

McCance, KL, and Huether, SE. *Pathophysiology: The biologic basis for disease in adults and children*, ed 6. Mosby, St. Louis, 2010.

NIDDK. Medical care for patients with obesity. Retrieved from http://win.niddk.nih.gov/publications/medical.htm#optimal

Papadakis, MA, and McPhee, SJ. *Current medical diagnosis and treatment*, ed 52. Lange/McGraw-Hill, New York, 2013.

Adrenal Disorders

Ceccato, F, et al. Performance of salivary cortisol in diagnosis of Cushing's syndrome, adrenal incidentaloma, and adrenal insufficiency. *Eur J Endocrinol* 169(1):31–36, 2013.

Crawford, A, and Harris, H. Adrenal cortex disorders: Hormones out of kilter. *Nursing* 42(10):32–39, 2012.

Dekkers, OM, et al. Multisystem morbidity and mortality in Cushing's syndrome: A cohort study. *J Clin Endocrinol Metab* 98(6):2277–2284, 2013.

Falorni, A, et al. Therapy of adrenal insufficiency: An update. *Endocrine* 43(3):514–528, 2013.

Poullot, A, and Chevalier, N. New options in the treatment of Cushing's disease: A focus on pasireotide. *Res Rep Endocrinol Disord* 3:31–38, 2013.

Van Ryzin, C. Adrenal insufficiency: Causes of adrenal insufficiency and prevention of adrenal crisis. *J Pediatr Nurs* 28(2):206–207, 2013.

Diabetes Mellitus

American Diabetes Association. Standards of medical care in diabetes—2013. *Diabetes Care* 36(Suppl 1), 2013.

Balamurugan, A, et al. A pilot study of diabetes education via telemedicine in a rural underserved community—opportunities and challenges: A continuous quality improvement process. *Diabetes Educator* 35(1):147–154, 2009.

Carmichael, KA. What is a logical approach for choosing among new agents for patients with type 2 diabetes? *Consultant* 53(2):100–102, 2013.

Cherner, R. Diabetes: 12 treatment pitfalls—and how to avoid them. *Consultant* 52(11):735–743, 2012.

Debella, YT, et al. Chronic kidney disease as a coronary disease equivalent—comparison with diabetes over a decade. *Clin J Am Soc Nephrol* 6(6):1385–1392, 2011.

Dokken, BB. Optimizing technology for diabetes care. *Clin Advisor* 15(5):37–43, 2012.

Gitt, A, et al. Achievement of recommended glucose and blood pressure targets in patients with type 2 diabetes and hypertension in clinical practice—study rationale and protocol of DIALOGUE. *Cardiovasc Diabetol* 11(1):148–155, 2012.

International Expert Committee. International Expert Committee report on the role of the A1C assay in the diagnosis of diabetes. *Diabetes Care* 32(7):1327–1334, 2009.

Kapustin, J. Uncomplicating insulin therapy. *Adv NPs PAs* 3(2):20–30, 2012.

Markey, O, et al. Effect of cinnamon on gastric emptying, arterial stiffness, postprandial lipemia, glycemia, and appetite responses to high-fat breakfast. *Cardiovasc Diabetol* 19(78):1–9, 2011.

Mingrone, G, et al. Bariatric surgery versus conventional therapy for type 2 diabetes. *N Engl J Med* 366(17):1577–1585, 2012.

New, N. Teaching so they hear: Using a co-created diabetes self-management education approach. *J Am Acad Nurse Pract* 22(6):316–325, 2010.

Rendell, M. Diabetes: New drug options and old choices. *Consultant* 53(4):217–227, 2013.

Sherman, C. Exercise guidelines for patients with diabetes. *Clin Advisor* 13(9):46–51, 2010.

Smith, D. The dyslipidemia of type 2 diabetes: Treatment strategies. *Consultant* 53(3):137–144, 2013.

Waryasz, GR, and McDermott, AY. Exercise prescriptions and the patient with type 2 diabetes: A clinical approach to optimizing patient outcomes. *J Am Acad Nurse Pract* 22(4):217–227, 2010.

Thyroid Disorders

American Association of Clinical Endocrinologists and American Thyroid Association. Clinical practice guidelines for hypothyroidism in adults. Retrieved from www.thyroidguidelines.net/sites/thyroidguidelines .net/files/file/thy.2012.0205.pdf

Azizi, F, et al. Long-term continuous methimazole or radioiodine treatment for hyperthyroidism. *Arch Iran Med* 15(8):477–484, 2012.

Hyperthyroidism and other causes of thyrotoxicosis: Management guidelines of the American Thyroid Association and American Association of Clinical Endocrinologists. Retrieved from https://www.aace.com/files/hyper-guidelines-2011.pdf

Khandelwal, D, and Tandon, N. Overt and subclinical hypothyroidism. *Drugs* 72(1):17–33, 2012.

Pangaluri, R, et al. Prevalence of metabolic syndrome and its components in women with subclinical hypothyroidism. *Asian J Pharm Clin Res* 6(4):82–84, 2013.

Synder, S, et al. Total thyroidectomy as primary definitive treatment for Graves' hyperthyroidism. *Am Surg* 79(12):1283–1288, 2013.

Weedman, A. Current choice of treatment for hypo- and hyperthyroidism. *Prescriber* 24(13-16):22–33, 2013.

Yapar, AF, et al. Efficacy of radioiodine treatment in subclinical hyperthyroidism. *Acta Endocrinol* 8(1):77–86, 2012.

Resources

American Association of Clinical Endocrinologists
www.aace.com
American Cancer Society
www.cancer.org/search/index?QueryText=Endocrine+diseases
Centers for Disease Control and Prevention
www.cdc.gov/search.do?queryText=endocrine+diseases&searchButton.x=26 &searchButton.y=10&action=search
Dr. Andrew Weil (alternative health)
www.drweil.com
Endocrine Society
www.endo-society.org
Food and Drug Administration
http://google2.fda.gov/search?q=obesity&client=FDAgov&site=FDAgov&lr =&proxystylesheet=FDAgov&requiredfields=-archive%3AYes&out- put=xml_no_dtd&getfields= *
http://google2.fda.gov/search?q=endocrine+diseases&client=FDAgov&site= FDAgov&lr=&proxystylesheet=FDAgov&requiredfields=-archive% 3AYes&output=xml_no_dtd&getfields= *
National Institutes of Health
http://search.nih.gov/search?utf8=%E2%9C%93&affiliate=nih&query= endocrine+diseases
U.S. National Library of Medicine
www.nlm.nih.gov
RxList—The Internet Drug Index
www.rxlist.com

Thyroid Disorders

American Thyroid Association
www.thyroid.org

Diabetes Mellitus

American Association of Diabetes Educators
444 N. Michigan Ave., Suite 1240
Chicago, IL 60611
(800) 338-3633
www.diabeteseducator.org
American Diabetes Association
1660 Duke Street
Alexandria, VA 22314
(800) 232-3472
www.diabetes.org
American Dietetic Association
(800) 366-1655 (Spanish speaking assistance available)
(800) 745-0775
www.eatright.org
Centers for Disease Control and Prevention—Diabetes
www.cdc.gov/diabetes
Indian Health Services Diabetes Program
www.ihs.gov/MedicalPrograms/Diabetes
Juvenile Diabetes Foundation International
120 Wall Street, 19th Floor
New York, NY 10005
(800) 223-1138
National Diabetes Information Clearinghouse
1 Information Way
Bethesda, MD 20892
(301) 654-3327
http://diabetes.niddk.nih.gov

National Eye Institute
National Eye Health Education Program
Building 31, Room 6A32
31 Center Drive, MSC-25 IO
Bethesda, MD 20892
(800) 869-2020
www.nei.nih.gov
National Institute of Diabetes and Digestive and Kidney Diseases
www.niddk.nih.gov
Gout
Arthritis Foundation
PO Box 19000
Atlanta, GA 30325
(800) 283-7800
www.arthritis.org

National Institute of Arthritis and Musculoskeletal Disorders
Building 31, Room 4C05
Bethesda, MD 20892
(301) 496-8188
www.niams.nih.gov
Obesity
American Society of Bariatric Physicians
5600 S. Quebec Street, Suite 160-D
Englewood, CO 80111
(303) 779-4833
www.asbp.org
Overeaters Anonymous
www.oa.org
Obesity Society
www.obesity.org
Take Off Pounds Sensibly
www.tops.org

Chapter 17

Hematological and Immune Problems

Brian Oscar Porter, MD, PhD, MPH •
Jill E. Winland-Brown, EdD, APRN, FNP-BC

COMMON COMPLAINTS

■ BRUISING

A *bruise* (ecchymosis) is an integumentary manifestation of extravasated blood. Discoloration of the skin is attributed to a local interstitial pool of erythrocytes, which causes a light to dark blue skin color associated with red pigment. The bruise sets off a local inflammatory event that includes macrophage invasion and histamine release and may be associated with edema. Macrophages engulf red blood cells (RBCs) to clear the area.

Macrophages that contain the RBCs excrete hemosiderin and hematoidin. Hemosiderin is brown, and hematoidin is yellow. The release of these molecules from macrophages accounts for the characteristic color changes in bruises during their resolution. Hematomas (larger bruises) require lengthier periods of time to resolve than smaller bruises.

Bruising may result from blunt trauma or occur spontaneously in the absence of trauma. Thrombocytopenia (platelet counts below 50,000 cells/mL) predisposes an individual to bruise formation with minor trauma, given the integral role of platelets in the formation of blood clots. Spontaneous bruising may be seen with platelet counts below 30,000 cells/mL, particularly on the arms and legs. Spontaneous bruising may also be associated with the chronic use of corticosteroid or anticoagulant therapies. Steroids weaken the vascular walls, making them prone to release erythrocytes. Anticoagulants, when their levels exceed the therapeutic range, can permit microvascular ruptures to spill blood into interstitial spaces.

Anticoagulant therapy consists of warfarin (Coumadin) in oral dosages that are intended to keep the international normalized ratio (INR) between 2.0 and 3.0 for most disease-related prophylaxis, such as the prevention of valvular thrombus in atrial fibrillation. Initial dosing of warfarin is 2 to 5 mg per day for 3 days, followed by measurement of prothrombin time (PT) and INR. This initial loading dose starts the process of anticoagulation. Dosages thereafter range from 2 to 7.5 mg, on average, per day. Dosages can be higher than 10 mg if the INR dictates.

If the INR result is above the therapeutic range, several options can be followed depending on how far above range it is. First, the clinician should consider withholding one or more days of anticoagulant therapy. Second, therapy should be restarted at a lower dose after a hiatus of therapy. Finally, the PT and INR should be reevaluated within 3 to 5 days of the dosage adjustments.

Differential Diagnosis

The differential diagnoses of bruising include chronic use of steroid and anticoagulant therapies, thrombocytopenia, hemolytic anemia, domestic violence, self-inflicted injury or other blunt trauma, and hypersensitivity vasculitis. A thorough history and physical exam by the clinician should focus on the cause of the bruising.

■ FATIGUE

Fatigue presents as a complaint of tiredness that cannot be explained on the basis of exercise or other activity. It may be either acute or chronic, associated with a disease or independent of other pathophysiology.

Acute fatigue is most often associated with viral or bacterial infections and may serve as a harbinger of impending symptoms such as fever. Determining the etiology of chronic fatigue that may last for months is far more complex. A patient seeking relief from chronic fatigue may occupy the clinician's attention during many visits before the causes can be identified. The patient usually cannot explain the cause of chronic fatigue without the clinician asking appropriate assessment questions.

The clinical history of fatigue offers insights into the nature of the cause. Patient reports of fatigue that increases over the course of a day and abates after rest indicate an organic origin for fatigue. Functional fatigue, on the other hand, is characterized by fatigue on awakening that may actually improve after exercise. The close associations of depression and anxiety with fatigue make for a difficult task in distinguishing these functional causes of the fatigue from the fatigue itself. In addition, fatigue may reflect hematological abnormalities associated with other disease conditions, such as chronic anemia that results in decreased oxygen-carrying capacity, which makes the patient less tolerant of physical exertion and may contribute to persistent fatigue.

Differential Diagnosis

Fatigue by itself presents a complicated differential. Fortunately, it seldom presents without other comorbidity.

Acute fatigue is perhaps the simplest type to diagnose and treat. For example, acute fatigue typically appears in a clinical history that is positive for viral or bacterial exposure, combined with examination findings of fever and other systemic abnormalities.

Chronic fatigue has many causes, including chronic anxiety or stress reactions, lack of restorative sleep due to poor sleep hygiene or sleep apnea, depression, infectious mononucleosis, hepatitis, tuberculosis, anemia, heart disease, lung disease, electrolyte disturbances, rheumatoid diseases, and cancer. Thus, a detailed history and physical examination are key to distinguishing these underlying conditions. For instance, in the case of anemia, a detailed history may reveal fatigue worsened with exertion, and physical examination may demonstrate findings of pale nailbeds, gingivae, and tongue, along with sinus tachycardia.

■ FEVER

Fever is defined as a temperature elevation above normal baseline in which pathology can be identified as the cause. On average, most individuals maintain a body temperature close to 98.6°F (37°C), which may normally fluctuate up to ± 0.9°F (± 0.5°C) throughout the day. Physical exertion can elevate body temperature temporarily, followed by a return to baseline after the activity ends. A persistent elevation in temperature is clearly pathological, however.

Fever may be either acute or chronic. If acute, body temperature tends to be greater than 101.3°F (38.5°C). Acute fever is associated with upper respiratory infections (URIs) that are either bacterial or viral in nature, drug reactions, gastroenteritis, or urinary tract infections. Physiologically, fever is associated with the release of inflammatory immune mediators (e.g., interleukin-6, tumor necrosis factor–alpha) that act as pyrogens, presumably to create an environment within the body that is not conducive to microbial growth and replication. The ability of the body to elevate the temperature in the event of infection diminishes with advancing age; therefore, acute fever in an older adult might not be comparable to that in a younger patient.

Chronic fevers tend to be low-grade temperature elevations. Temperatures rise to 100.4°F (38°C) in cases of hepatitis, infectious mononucleosis (especially in the third and fourth weeks after the onset of symptoms), cancer, sinusitis, dental abscess, prostatitis, and tuberculosis (TB).

The origin of a fever may not be apparent from the patient's history, physical examination, or laboratory testing. If the cause is not evident after a thorough work-up, a persistent fever should be classified as a *fever of unknown*

origin (FUO). Specifically, FUO is defined as a fever of greater than 101.3°F (38.5°C) that occurs on at least three occasions over a 3-week period in an ambulatory patient. A hospitalized patient is diagnosed with FUO if the unexplainable fever persists for 1 week.

Differential Diagnosis

The magnitude of fever elevation may guide the clinician in differentiating its cause. Fevers can vary widely, however, based on the patient's age, history of pathogenic exposure, and many other factors. Fevers in excess of 104°F (40°C) tend to be associated with pancreatitis, pyelonephritis, and intracranial pathology. Fevers between 101.3°F (38.5°C) and 104°F (40°C) are associated with URIs and some acute viral syndromes. Fevers less than 101.3°F (38.5°C) are characteristic of hepatitis, some acute viral infections, and TB.

Differentiations in fever elevation guide the decision-making process of which laboratory evaluations to recommend. Correlated with history and physical examination findings, fever elevation determines the type of sampling of blood or other bodily fluids to be ordered. In addition, in the absence of definitive test results, knowledge of the categories of fever elevation may give the clinician more or less reason for alarm. For example, when a middle-aged woman with a 3-day fever of 102.2°F (39°C) presents with a nonproductive cough, chills, and inspiratory chest discomfort, and her lungs are clear but dull to percussion in the bases, the suspicion of a pulmonary consolidative process should cause the clinician to order a chest x-ray exam and complete blood count; however, the clinician may not order blood cultures because the fever is not high enough to suggest systemic infection, for which blood cultures would otherwise be indicated. Moreover, there are focal symptoms that explain the fever.

Environmental toxins may also cause fever. When this etiology is suspected, the history should focus on exposure to industrial chemicals, including pesticides and herbicides used in animal husbandry and agriculture. Fevers of environmental origin tend to follow an indolent course, often showing peaks and troughs. Physical signs may also be absent, thus adding to the indolence of the presentation.

■ LYMPHADENOPATHY

The term *lymphadenopathy* is used in clinical practice to designate any abnormality of lymph nodes and, in particular, enlarged lymph nodes. Perhaps the more exact term should be *lymphadenitis,* which suggests that inflammation is the cause of the lymph node enlargement. Lymph node enlargement may be regionally or systemically associated with inflammation. If the inflammation is regional, the lymph nodes that are proximal to a site of infection will show enlargement. If the disease process is systemic, lymph nodes in three or more sites that are dispersed across the body may become enlarged. An example of regional lymph node enlargement is cervical lymphadenopathy associated with pharyngitis. An example of systemic lymphadenopathy is HIV infection, in which there may be lymphadenopathy in three or more extrainguinal lymphatic chains.

Lymphadenopathy follows the course of the disease. Thus, nodes may be acutely or chronically enlarged depending on the duration of the disease. Acute infection often leaves the regional nodes tender to touch. Chronically enlarged nodes, on the other hand, may be nontender.

Differential Diagnosis

The differential diagnosis for lymphadenopathy depends on the location of involvement and associated findings. Neck masses, for example, involve a differential that is based on node location in the neck, age of the patient, and associated morbidities, such as tobacco use. The clinician should distinguish between slow growth in nodes and rapid or acute onset of lymphadenopathy. Acute onset is characteristic of inflammation and acute infection, whereas slow-growing nodes in the neck suggest neoplasm, such as lymphoma. However, there are exceptions. For example, a young patient with no history of tobacco or ethanol use may present with slow-growing cervical lymphadenopathy, but the possibility of neoplasm is minimal in a patient of this age and with this history. Nonetheless, an adult older than age 70 years with even a remote history of tobacco use is likely to be diagnosed with lymphoma if there is slow-growing neck lymphadenopathy. Thus, the patient's age is an important consideration in the differential diagnosis of neck lymphadenopathy.

HIV-associated lymphadenopathy presents challenges to the differential diagnosis. The average HIV-infected patient is younger than age 50, has a history of alcohol and/or tobacco use, and may also be antibody-positive to other sexually transmitted diseases. Lymphadenopathy could occupy the neck, axillae, inguinal region, breasts, and thorax. Reactive lymphadenopathy is characteristic of early and middle stages of the disease attributable to HIV infection itself; later disease findings contributing to lymphadenopathy may include lymphoma or infection with cytomegalovirus, human papillomavirus, toxoplasmosis, or *Mycobacterium avium* complex. Persistent slow-growth enlargement, therefore, is reason to consider lymph node aspiration and cytological evaluation in this setting.

COMMON HEMATOLOGICAL PROBLEMS

■ MICROCYTIC ANEMIA

Anemia can mean any of several problems that involve suboptimal red blood cell (RBC) number or function

(Table 17.1). The diagnosis suggests low hemoglobin (Hgb), low hematocrit (Hct), and/or a low number of RBCs. All of these problems involve a reduced amount of oxygen circulating in the body, because RBCs carry oxygen to tissues and cells. The World Health Organization (WHO) identifies *anemia* as an Hgb of less than 13.0 g/dL in men (less than 42% Hct) and less than 12.0 g/dL in women (less than 36% Hct). Slightly higher values of Hgb and Hct are considered standard in developed versus underdeveloped regions of the world.

As a rule of thumb, the estimated level of hematocrit is three times the value of the Hgb. For example, an Hgb value of 13.0 g/dL amounts to an estimated Hct of 39%.

Microcytic anemia is a category of anemia based on the small size (*micro-*) of the RBCs (*-cytic*). It has been linked to nutritional deficiencies, particularly a deficiency in dietary intake or uptake of iron. The small size of the RBCs is identified via one of the three indices of RBCs, the mean corpuscular volume (MCV). Microcytosis, therefore, is defined by an MCV value of less than 80 fL. In short, the clinician can make a diagnosis of microcytic anemia by identifying the presence of anemia combined with a low MCV.

Epidemiology and Causes

Microcytic anemia, as related to iron deficiency, is one of the most common anemias throughout the world. The incidence is high among women of childbearing age, with up to a third of pregnant women developing anemia in the third trimester. The ratio of incidence between women and men is 4:1. In the United States, 20% of adult women are affected by the condition compared with 3% of adult men. These statistics have remained constant for the past decade.

The causes of microcytic anemia include (1) an inadequate oral intake or gastrointestinal (GI) uptake of dietary iron, (2) anemia of chronic disease (ACD), (3) thalassemia, and (4) sideroblastic anemias.

The incidence of iron-deficiency anemia has been estimated to be 1:2.0 to 2.5 among pregnant women and 1:6 in persons older than age 75 years. Iron-deficiency anemia is often the easiest type to correct and remedy, unless it is caused by a GI malignancy. Iron deficiency is, therefore, less important in the differential even though it remains the most common cause of microcytic anemia.

Most adults in the United States ingest and absorb enough iron in their diets. It is estimated that the average dietary intake of iron in the United States is 10 to 15 mg per day, of which not more than 10% is absorbed in the stomach, duodenum, and jejunum. The average healthy adult, therefore, absorbs approximately 1 to 2 mg of iron per day. In addition, the same adult loses an amount of iron equal to that ingested and absorbed, thereby maintaining homeostasis.

ACD, unlike iron-deficiency anemia, presents a more complex diagnostic picture because of the many and

Table 17.1   Classification of Anemias

Anemia	Examples of Causes	Mean Corpuscular Volume (mm³)	Mean Corpuscular Hemoglobin (pg)	Mean Corpuscular Hemoglobin Concentration (%)
Microcytic, hypochromic	Iron deficiency, lead poisoning, thalassemia, rheumatoid arthritis	50–80	12–25	25–30
Microcytic, normochromic	Renal disease, infection, liver disease, malignancies	<80	20–25	27
Normocytic, normochromic	Sepsis, hemorrhage, hemolysis, drug-induced aplastic anemia, radiation, hereditary spherocytosis	82–92	25–30	32–36
Macrocytic, normochromic	Vitamin B_{12} and folic acid deficiency, some drugs, pernicious anemia	95–150	30–50	32–36

Indications for Hemoglobin Electrophoresis

- Suspected thalassemia, especially in individuals with positive family history for the disorder
- Differentiation among the types of thalassemias
- Evaluation of a positive Sickledex test to differentiate sickle cell trait (20%–40% Hgb S) from sickle cell disease (>70% Hgb S)
- Diagnosis of Hgb C or sickle cell anemia (hemoglobin SC disease)
- Identification of the numerous types of abnormal Hgb, most of which do not produce clinical disease

Hemoglobin Electrophoresis	Percentage of Hgb	Comments
Hgb A$_1$ Infants	>95 10–30	Low: Alpha- and beta-thalassemia major and minor
Hgb A$_2$ Cord blood Birth–6 months >6 months	2–5 0–1.8 0–3.5 1.5–3.5	Elevated: Beta-thalassemia major and minor up to 9%
Hgb F Neonates 1 month 2 months 3 months 6 months–1 year	<10 70–80 70 50 25 3	Elevated: Beta-thalassemia minor up to 9% Elevated: Thalassemia major and minor (after 6 months)
Hgb C	Absent	Usually asymptomatic, but can cause red blood cells to sickle due to osmotic fragility; occurs in 2%–3% of blacks
Hgb D Hgb E	Absent Absent	Hgb D and E rarely occur alone but worsen disease when in combination with sickle cell anemia or thalassemia
Hgb H	Absent	Unstable tetramer of beta hemoglobin chains; 30% of hemoglobin in severe alpha-thalassemia with 3 of 4 mutated alpha genes (hemoglobin H disease)
Hgb M	Absent	Any of several mutated forms of hemoglobin that cannot be reduced to an oxygen-carrying state, resulting in congenital methemoglobinemia
Hgb S	Absent	Elevated—sickle cell anemia: <40% in sickle cell trait; 85%–95% in sickle cell disease. Most common beta Hgb variant: if both beta chain genes affected, then sickle cell anemia (1% of population); if only one gene affected, then sickle cell trait (8%–10% of population)

varied causes of inflammatory disorders in chronic disease, which include rheumatoid arthritis, malignancies, and serious infections. Given its complex diagnostic picture, ACD must always be considered in the differential for microcytic anemia, although despite its importance, the incidence and prevalence of ACD are unknown.

The thalassemias are a group of inherited diseases of alpha- or beta-globin chains. Microcytic anemia is caused by hemolysis that results from the suboptimal synthesis of alpha- or beta-globin chains, hence the categories of thalassemia known as alpha- and beta-thalassemia. Beta-thalassemia is associated with descendants of groups of individuals who originated in areas around the Mediterranean Sea. Alpha-thalassemia is far more widespread, occurring in individuals with ancestry from the Asian continent, including China and Southeast Asia. Prevalence has also been noted among persons living along the western coast of Africa.

Sideroblastic anemia reflects a disorder of heme synthesis, resulting in abnormal hemoglobin and disordered RBC function. It may be caused by chronic alcoholism or lead poisoning or may be a stage in the evolution of a generalized bone marrow disorder that may progress to acute leukemia.

Pathophysiology
Normal Hemoglobin Formation

The predominant normal adult hemoglobin (hemoglobin A; $\alpha_2\beta_2$) comprises one pair of alpha-globin chains and one pair of beta-globin chains, accounting for 90% to 95% of total adult hemoglobin. Each of these globin chains is linked to an individual heme group, which consists of a protoporphyrin IX molecule bound to a ferrous (Fe^{2+}) reduced iron ion. It is this heme unit that reversibly binds oxygen, allowing for transport of oxygen by the hemoglobin tetramer to the bodily tissues.

Several other forms of hemoglobin are formed during human development. At least three distinct forms of hemoglobin consisting of different combinations of zeta (ζ), epsilon (ϵ), gamma (γ), and alpha (α) chains present themselves throughout embryonic development in the following order: hemoglobin Gower I ($\zeta_2\epsilon_2$), hemoglobin Portland ($\zeta_2\gamma_2$), and hemoglobin Gower II ($\alpha_2\epsilon_2$). In contrast, the predominant normal hemoglobin form in infancy is hemoglobin F or fetal hemoglobin (approximately 80%), which has two gamma-globin chains substituted for the beta-chains ($\alpha_2\gamma_2$). Hemoglobin F has a stronger affinity for oxygen than hemoglobin A does, allowing for oxygen transport across the placenta from the mother to the developing fetus. As a newborn ages, this form of hemoglobin slowly clears from the circulation, accounting for less than 1% of hemoglobin by 6 months of age, with a corresponding increase in hemoglobin A. Finally, an additional form of adult hemoglobin known as hemoglobin A_2 also exists, which is present in far smaller amounts than hemoglobin A (about 2% to 5% of total adult hemoglobin). With a slightly higher oxygen affinity than hemoglobin A, hemoglobin A_2 has two delta (σ)-globin chains substituted for the beta-globin chains ($\alpha_2\sigma_2$).

Iron-Deficiency Anemia

Because the reduced ferrous (Fe^{2+}) ion is a critical component of the heme moiety in hemoglobin, sufficient iron stores are critical for adequate erythropoiesis in the bone marrow. In low-iron states, the production of hemoglobin is severely reduced, resulting in marked microcytosis. Iron deficiency remains the most common cause of microcytic anemia in the United States. Because most adults receive enough iron in their diets to prevent microcytosis (other than strict vegan vegetarians), the clinician's attention should turn to malabsorption or occult loss of blood as the primary causes of iron-deficiency anemia.

The majority of iron uptake occurs in the duodenum and upper jejunum. Thus, malabsorption of iron is linked to underlying GI problems such as celiac sprue; surgical resections involving the stomach, duodenum, or jejunum; inflammatory bowel disease such as Crohn's disease; rapid GI motility; gastroenteritis; and selected drugs such as the histamine receptor 2 (H_2) antagonist cimetidine (Tagamet). Decreased levels of iron can also occur as the result of molecular bonds between plasma iron stores and certain drugs. These bonds develop during the distribution phase of pharmacokinetics, sequestering iron ions and decreasing the plasma pool available for integration into heme molecules. For example, sulfonamide drugs such as sulfamethoxazole-trimethoprim (co-trimoxazole, Bactrim, Septra) can cause decreased plasma levels of iron.

Iron deficiency resulting from acute or chronic (occult) blood loss is perhaps the most prevalent cause of microcytic anemia. A net loss of blood depletes iron stores and impairs the bone marrow's ability to synthesize new RBCs, due to progressively decreased heme synthesis. Thus, RBCs are decreased not only in number but also in size, producing a characteristic microcytic anemia. Common sites of bleeding (which may be either painless or painful) include the GI tract (e.g., upper tract lesions such as peptic ulcers or gastritis; lower tract lesions such as colon cancer, ulcerative colitis, Crohn's disease, diverticulosis, ruptured hemorrhoids) and the genitourinary (GU) tract (e.g., heavy endometrial bleeding known as menorrhagia, hematuria from bladder cancer). In fact, microcytic anemia may be the first laboratory finding that initiates a line of investigation identifying underlying malignancy. For example, heme-positive stools or melena are strong indications for colonoscopic cancer screening in men and women older than 50 years or in younger individuals with a strong family history.

Anemia of Chronic Disease

Anemia of chronic disease (ACD) may cause microcytic or normocytic anemia. ACD as a cause of microcytic anemia results from mechanisms that involve inflammation, infection, and/or underlying malignancy. Inflammation may lead to occult and progressive blood loss, because microvascular eruptions may result from histamine-release and immune complexes that physically invade the involved region. When these eruptions occur in the GI tract, occult blood escapes through the intestines. Thus, of particular concern is the relationship of occult blood in the stool to GI malignancy. Alternatively, chronic use of NSAIDs, such as ibuprofen (Motrin, Advil) and aspirin, for chronic pain conditions must also be considered as a cause of occult blood loss. NSAIDs and aspirin are used in the routine management of both rheumatoid arthritis and osteoarthritis. Blood loss results from erosion of the protective mucosal lining of the stomach, in particular, due to decreased production of prostaglandin formed by the enzymes cyclooxygenase-1 and cyclooxygenase-2—the molecular targets inhibited by NSAIDs.

Thalassemias

The pathology of thalassemia is related either to depletion or mutation in the genes that code for the subunits of the protein component of adult hemoglobin—the alpha- and beta-globin chains. Alpha-thalassemia is caused by gene depletion that, in turn, creates a reduction of alpha-globin chain synthesis. Because two copies of the alpha-globin chain gene are inherited from each parent on chromosome 16, mutations or deletions may exist in one or more of these four genes, producing distinct clinical manifestations. Mutations or deletions in all four genes results in alpha (O)–thalassemia or alpha-thalassemia major. No hemoglobin A, A_2, or F can form in this disorder, which is incompatible with extrauterine life. Rather, there is an excess of Bart's hemoglobin, which consists of gamma chain tetramers (γ_4). Bart's hemoglobin has an oxygen affinity at least 10-fold greater than that of hemoglobin A and, thus, cannot effectively release oxygen to fetal tissues. This causes severe anemia with resultant congestive heart failure, widespread capillary leak, and anasarca known as hydrops fetalis (widespread edema of all fetal tissues), typically resulting in fetal demise by the third trimester of pregnancy.

Mutations in three of the four alpha genes results in hemoglobin H disease, characterized by the widespread formation of hemoglobin H, which consists of a tetramer of four beta-globin chains (β_4). This results in moderate to severe lifelong hemolytic anemia, which typically requires repeated blood transfusions. Mutations in only two of the four alpha genes is called alpha-thalassemia minor or alpha-thalassemia-1 trait. This results in a mild anemia with only minor clinical manifestations. Mutation in only one of the four alpha-globin genes is a silent carrier state called alpha-thalassemia minima or alpha-thalassemia-2 trait and can be diagnosed only through DNA analysis because it has no clinical manifestations.

In contrast, only one gene for the beta-globin chain is inherited from each parent. Mutation or deletion of one of these genes results in beta-thalassemia minor or beta-thalassemia trait, characterized by a mild anemia that is typically asymptomatic. Deletions or severe mutations in both beta-globin genes result in beta-thalassemia major (Cooley's anemia), characterized by a severe transfusion-dependent, lifelong anemia with skeletal abnormalities due to bone marrow expansion in the body's attempt to increase hematopoiesis. An intermediate form of the disorder known as beta-thalassemia intermedia also exists in which a patient inherits two mutated, albeit expressed, beta-globin genes, each with a different type of mutation (a compound heterozygote) that results in varied levels of expression or functionality. Clinical manifestations may be worsened by acute illness or infection that impairs erythropoiesis and exacerbates the anemia.

Sideroblastic Anemias

Sideroblastosis and its resulting microcytic anemia are caused by a host of molecular defects that affect the biosynthesis of the heme moiety of hemoglobin. Heme is normally formed first by the creation of 5-aminolevulinic acid (ALA) from glycine and succinyl-coenzyme A by the erythroid isoform of the mitochondrial enzyme ALA synthase, which requires vitamin B_6 (pyridoxine) as a cofactor. Although the underlying genetic defects in many forms of hereditary sideroblastic anemia have not been characterized, known mutations occur most commonly in the genes for the erythroid form of ALA synthase (located on the X chromosome), the mitochondrial transporter ABC7, pyridoxal 5-phosphate (a reversible form of the disease responsive to pyridoxine therapy), ferrochelatase, the copper-dependent enzyme cytochrome oxidase, and pseudouridine synthase–1.

In most forms of sideroblastic anemia, elemental iron is typically delivered appropriately to erythrocyte precursors. However, underlying enzymatic mutations prevent or reduce the ability of heme to incorporate into protoporphyrin IX. A reduced number of RBCs form from ring sideroblast precursors (a diagnostic hallmark) found in the bone marrow, because peripheral reticulocytosis is markedly diminished. Despite an increase in the RBC growth factor erythropoietin, anemia results from the destruction of the abnormal erythroid precursors in the bone marrow via apoptosis and intramedullary hemolysis.

Sideroblastic mutations result in excessive iron deposition in the mitochondria of affected erythrocytes (erythropoietic hemochromatosis) which, nonetheless, are hypochromic and microcytic because this form of mitochondrial ferritin cannot be utilized for cytoplasmic maturation in the developing erythrocyte. Intestinal iron absorption is actually increased in sideroblastic anemia, owing to ineffective erythropoiesis, as is also observed in the thalassemias. Thus, iron overload occurs not only in erythroid cells but throughout the body, similar to genetic (familial) hemochromatosis, with predictable end-organ damage due to iron deposition (e.g., cirrhosis [liver], cardiomyopathy [heart], and endocrine defects [pancreas and adrenals]).

Acquired forms of sideroblastic anemia also exist. The most common causes include chronic alcoholism, which results in a multifactorial pathogenesis including many of the hypoproliferative mechanisms previously cited; iatrogenic associations with the antituberculous drug isoniazid and the antibiotic chloramphenicol; zinc toxicity, in which zinc ions preferentially bind to protoporphyrin in place of iron; and copper deficiency, which leads to decreased intestinal absorption of iron and diminished reduction of iron ions from the ferric (3+) state to the bioavailable ferrous (2+) form as a result of reduced cytochrome oxidase activity. Lead poisoning is also often cited as an acquired cause of sideroblastic anemia because lead inhibits ALA synthase. However, with lead toxicity true ring sideroblasts are typically not seen in the bone marrow, owing to the inhibitory effect of lead on the enzyme ferrochelatase, thereby preventing the integration of ferrous ions into heme. Idiopathic acquired sideroblastic anemia may also occur when a single erythroid progenitor cell develops a mutation affecting the heme synthesis pathway but is also conferred a survival advantage. As clonal proliferation of this precursor cell ensues, the bone marrow is largely replaced by this single sideroblastic lineage that is prone to apoptosis, which results in a myelodysplastic anemia.

Clinical Presentation
Subjective

Overall, patients with microcytic anemia present with subjective findings of tachycardia, fatigue, shortness of breath, dyspnea on exertion, palpitations, listlessness, poor concentration, anorexia, and dizziness or light-headedness. Because similar subjective findings are also associated with many additional diagnoses other than microcytic anemia, the history of patient complaints is unlikely to be conclusive.

Objective

As the Hgb drops below 10 g/dL (approximately 30% Hct), many patients present with a facial mask of fatigue, sallow-colored skin, pale mucous membranes, tachycardia, and tachypnea at rest. It is possible also to note a prolonged blanch response in the nailbeds (more than 3 seconds), although many patients may never present with this sign. Severe iron-deficiency anemia can cause progressive skin and mucosal changes, such as brittle nails, cheilosis (reddened appearance of lips with fissures formed at the angles of the mouth), and a smooth appearance to the tongue. In addition, pica is considered an objective finding associated with severe iron deficiency. *Pica* is identified as an eating disorder of craving for food substitutes, such as clay, dirt, ice chips, or cotton.

Diagnostic Reasoning
Diagnostic Tests

Initial diagnostic testing is focused on obtaining a complete blood count (CBC), from which an RBC count and RBC indices (MCV, mean corpuscular hemoglobin [MCH], and mean corpuscular hemoglobin concentration [MCHC]) are isolated. A low RBC count, Hgb level, and/or Hct identify anemia (see Table 17.1).

Secondary diagnostic testing for specific causes is described below.

Iron-Deficiency Anemia   The diagnostic tests for iron-deficiency anemia are relatively simple to perform and are readily available. Serum ferritin is a reliable test of low stores of iron, provided the patient does not have advanced liver disease. A serum ferritin value of less than 30 mg/L is considered pathological. As the ferritin level falls, the total iron-binding capacity (TIBC) rises above the normal range. If the drop in ferritin and rise in TIBC continue untreated, the serum iron level will also fall (to less than 30 mg/L), as will the transferrin saturation (to less than 15%). In addition, secondary testing should focus on results of RBC morphology from the CBC. Findings such as anisocytosis (variable RBC size), poikilocytosis (variable RBC shape), and hypochromasia (pale-colored RBCs) may be revealed when samples severely deficient in iron are evaluated under the microscope.

Anemia of Chronic Disease   Diagnostic tests for ACD focus on distinguishing ACD from iron-deficiency anemia. Unlike iron-deficiency anemia, ACD presents with a low serum iron level, along with a low TIBC. In addition, the serum transferrin level is either normal or increased in patients with ACD. Finally, the clinician should expect the transferrin saturation to be low, as it is in iron-deficiency anemia.

Thalassemias   The thalassemias, both alpha- and beta-thalassemia, require a CBC and Hgb electrophoresis for diagnosis. The CBC is essential to determine the diagnosis of microcytic anemia, and the MCV is low for each group of the thalassemias. In alpha-thalassemia trait, the Hgb electrophoresis reveals no increase in hemoglobin A_2 or hemoglobin F. In addition, no hemoglobin H is present. Plasma iron parameters remain normal. The anemia of alpha-thalassemia is modest, as evidenced by Hct level between 27% to 40%.

Beta-thalassemia minor patients also have a modest anemia. In these patients, unlike those with alpha-thalassemia trait, Hgb electrophoresis reveals an elevated hemoglobin A_2 level and, in some cases, an elevated hemoglobin F. Neither Hgb elevation will typically be greater than 9%, however.

Patients with beta-thalassemia major present very differently from patients with other forms of thalassemia. Their anemia is severe. Left untreated, their Hct levels will fall to less than 10%. Electrophoresis results show little or no hemoglobin A, with variable amounts of hemoglobin A_2 present. The clinician should expect hemoglobin F to be the primary hemoglobin that is detectable in these patients. As with all of the thalassemias, findings in patients with beta-thalassemia will include abnormal RBC morphology such as poikilocytosis and anisocytosis.

Sideroblastic Anemia   A diagnosis of sideroblastic anemia is confirmed by a Prussian blue stain of a bone marrow aspirate. The Prussian blue stain reveals tinged sideroblasts, which have iron deposits located in the mitochondria that surround the red blood cell's nucleus. In addition, erythroid hyperplasia is present in the aspirate from patients with sideroblastic anemia. A high level of serum iron and a high transferrin saturation should accompany these findings. Without a stain of the bone marrow aspirate, the laboratory profile could mimic iron-deficiency anemia, with a moderately low Hct of 20% to 30% and a low MCV.

Differential Diagnosis

The differential diagnosis depends on the blood work results. For microcytic anemia, it may be summarized by reference to its four predominant causes: iron-deficiency anemia, ACD, thalassemias, and sideroblastic anemia. The ultimate goal of the diagnostic evaluation is to identify the underlying cause of the microcytic anemia, such as GI malignancy, iron malabsorption, blood loss, menorrhagia, and so forth.

Management

The management of microcytic anemia focuses on treating and eradicating the cause of the anemia. If amelioration of the cause is not possible, symptomatic care is indicated.

The severity of the anemia will direct the intervention. The decision to transfuse a patient with red blood cells is a major clinical step that may be indicated if the Hct is 27% or less. The decision requires a thoughtful analysis of the overall clinical setting and hemodynamic status of the patient, which may not be severely compromised, even at low Hgb levels. Transfusing patients with comorbidities such as congestive heart failure (CHF) calls for great caution (given risks of fluid overload and high output heart failure). In addition, the risk of iron overload following repeated RBC transfusions must be carefully considered.

Iron-Deficiency Anemia

Iron-deficiency anemia is treated first with an increase in dietary iron and thereafter with supplemental iron. Foods rich in iron should be recommended, such as animal proteins, legumes, and dark green leafy vegetables, such as spinach. Diet alone may be sufficient in treating iron deficiency if the patient is either young or middle-aged or the cause of the anemia is short-lived. However, as the patient ages (particularly beyond age 65) and if the cause of the anemia is chronic, iron deficiency must be treated with either supplemental oral or parenteral iron.

Supplemental oral iron is best given as ferrous sulfate, 325 mg three times daily; 10 to 20 mg will be absorbed from the total daily regimen if the serum iron is moderately low. In more severe cases, however, the level of absorption will increase. The clinician should recheck the RBC indices and iron values 2 to 4 weeks after starting the regimen to ascertain the effectiveness of the oral regimen. The patient's adherence to the regimen could be complicated by the requirement that iron supplements be taken on an empty stomach to achieve maximal absorption. Therefore, if no measured improvement in anemia (Hct elevated by one-half of baseline), MCV, and iron stores appears after 1 month of therapy, the clinician should confirm adequate adherence to the regimen along with the underlying cause of the iron deficiency. The patient should continue to take supplemental iron for 3 to 6 months after normal levels in the blood and serum indices have been restored. Thereafter, the clinician should recheck laboratory values as indicated by the clinical assessment. If the patient does not respond to supplemental iron, then the clinician should doubt the initial diagnosis of iron-deficiency anemia. In particular, ACD should be suspected as the cause, or the clinician should reconsider whether the rate of GI blood loss might exceed stem-cell deployment from the bone marrow.

Supplemental iron by a parenteral route is indicated only when there is documented failure of therapy with oral iron supplements. The clinician should calculate the daily dose by subtracting the patient's measured MCV from the normal lower range value (which varies by age and gender). This value is considered the total number of milligrams of iron to add according to the MCV. In addition, the clinician must add 1,000 mg to the delivered dose to cover the storage of iron in the body. Overall, the daily dosage of supplemental parenteral iron is approximately 1,300 to 2,000 mg (1.3–2.0 g) of iron. The preferred route of administration is IV. Because anaphylaxis is possible with IV iron, the initial dose should be delivered over 4 to 6 hours to prevent adverse effects; some practitioners even advocate giving 50 mg over the first hour as a trial.

Anemia of Chronic Disease

ACD is treated symptomatically. Red blood cell transfusions may become necessary when the Hct falls below 27% to 30%. In most cases, however, the Hct will stay above 30%. Chronic ACD might require treatment with drugs that stimulate erythropoiesis given subcutaneously, including erythropoietin alfa and darbepoetin alfa. Typical ACD causes that require this are chronic renal failure and HIV infection or AIDS. The dosage varies according to patient tolerance and hematological requirements. Erythropoietin alfa (Epogen, Procrit) is given three times weekly, then adjusted. Darbepoetin alfa (Aranesp) may be given weekly initially and then adjusted to dosing every 2 weeks. These medications can be administered IV in the hospital or clinical setting. In addition, patients can learn to self-inject these medications subcutaneously, just as diabetic patients learn to self-inject insulin.

Thalassemia

The thalassemias often require no treatment other than vigilance by the clinician concerning hematological markers. If a clinician diagnoses microcytosis with mild anemia, the patient should not be subjected to further checks for iron deficiency if there is a distinct thalassemic etiology. Clinical vigilance may be all that is required for microcytosis with mild anemia.

Patients with severe anemia, however, such as that associated with beta-thalassemia major and hemoglobin H disease, require regular transfusion with RBCs. In addition, these patients require folate supplementation and possibly oral iron chelation therapy to prevent hemosiderosis and hemochromatosis resulting from multiple transfusions. Hemosiderosis of chronic standing may also require referral for a splenectomy.

Sideroblastic Anemia

There are few options for the treatment of sideroblastosis. Depending on the severity of anemia, RBC transfusions may be required. Large doses (200 mg/day) of vitamin B_6 (pyridoxine, e.g., Beesix) have benefited some patients. Erythropoietin alfa (Epogen) has proven to be of little aid in supporting these patients.

Follow-up and Referral

Iron-deficiency anemia that is mild necessitates follow-up every 4 to 6 months. There should be no need to retest iron stores after the first follow-up visit following the initial diagnosis, unless indicated by patient complaints or physical examination findings. Thus, typical follow-up testing may consist only of serial CBCs. A referral to an appropriate specialist may be necessary if a thorough work-up identifies serious pathology that could account for iron-deficiency anemia, such as GI malignancy or other type of occult blood loss. These patients may require upper and/or lower endoscopy or other type of work-up to exclude serious pathology. Anyone 50 years or older with heme-positive stools or evidence of iron-deficiency anemia should be referred for a colonoscopy unless the risks of colonoscopy outweigh the potential benefits of catching a GI cancer early—such as in elderly patients in whom the risk of perforation is greater and could prove fatal.

In general, the plan of referral for microcytic anemia should facilitate isolating the cause of the anemia, initiating treatment in the primary care setting, and involving specialty care referral as needed. The primary care clinician, therefore, has the responsibility to perform all screening tests and to seek to diagnose the underlying cause. In turn, referral to a specialist for iron-deficiency anemia is almost never required unless it is complicated by concurrent diagnoses, including other causes of microcytic anemia. For example, iron-deficiency anemia secondary to menorrhagia would necessitate appropriate gynecological referral if procedural interventions such as uterine ablation or hysterectomy are indicated.

ACD follow-up can be more complicated than follow-up of iron-deficiency anemia. If the patient requires erythropoietin injections, then he or she should be maintained on a 30-day follow-up schedule for the first 6 months after initiating therapy. In most cases, only a CBC will be required to determine the effectiveness of this therapy. It is exceptional for patients with ACD to require transfusions. The clinician should refer patients with ACD to gastroenterologists, hepatologists, oncologists, rheumatologists, hematologists, or other specialists depending on the suspected underlying pathology. For example, if the clinician were to detect occult blood in the stool of a patient with microcytic anemia and the history did not reveal a likely cause, referral to a gastroenterologist would be warranted.

Patients diagnosed with one of the thalassemias may or may not require referral to a hematologist. Although patients with the more aggressive thalassemias (such as beta-thalassemia major or hemoglobin H disease) must be referred promptly to a hematologist, who will be entrusted with managing the plan of care, patients with alpha- or beta-thalassemia minor may be managed by the primary care clinician following initial diagnosis. In these patients, it may only be necessary to monitor serial CBCs every 3 to 4 months. More frequent observation and intervention is required, however, for the other types of thalassemias, which require transfusion therapy, and the plan of care established by the hematologist will dictate the follow-up schedule.

Because sideroblastosis is diagnosed by examination of a bone marrow aspirate, early referral to a hematologist is required for suspected sideroblastic anemia. The hematologist may also perform tests to determine lead exposure and resultant damage from lead toxicity. Follow-up evaluation will become the responsibility of the primary care clinician, however, and the CBCs of these patients should be monitored every 2 to 3 months.

Patient Education

Education should focus on self-care and primary care management of the underlying cause of microcytic anemia. Self-care encompasses topics such as adherence to the medication regimen, dietary changes, level of activity, self-monitoring for signs and symptoms of anemia, and adjustment to the requirements of new health-related practices. For example, patients with iron-deficiency anemia must be educated to perform the following self-care behaviors: (1) take ferrous sulfate (supplemental iron) on an empty stomach or at the most with a small snack; (2) eat foods that are rich in iron, vitamin C, and B-complex vitamins, which are all necessary for RBC development; (3) remain as active as possible, and if fatigued, rest before resuming activity; (4) self-monitor for fatigue, shortness of breath, pale-colored stools (before initiating supplemental iron), and palpitations or tachycardia, which may all be associated with decreased oxygen-carrying capacity due to anemia; and (5) share information about iron deficiency so that friends and/or family can assist in adjustments that new health-related behaviors will require.

Additional patient education focuses on primary care management. Patients need to understand the importance of timely clinical laboratory evaluations, return visits, recognizing signs and symptoms of recurrent anemia that should be reported to the clinician, and proper techniques for administering or receiving drugs that must be delivered via a parenteral route, such as erythropoietin or IV iron supplements. Most important for patients with severe anemia is the necessity to remain vigilant in receiving blood transfusions and monitoring for the signs of potential iron overload, including liver dysfunction (nausea, loss of appetite, weight loss, yellowing of the skin, swelling of the lower legs).

■ NORMOCYTIC ANEMIA

Normocytic anemia is defined as an anemia associated with normally sized red blood cells (RBCs) (mean corpuscular volume [MCV] = 81–99 fL), although normal ranges vary with age. Many forms of normocytic anemia have normally shaped RBCs as well, although some conditions are recognized by typical abnormal morphological findings on peripheral blood smear. Most commonly, this type of anemia results from chronic disease states, but acute blood loss, hemolysis, and volume overload are other important etiologies of normocytic anemia.

Epidemiology and Causes

Normocytic anemias cover a broad range of diseases and conditions, each with its own epidemiology and prevalence rate. Nonetheless, it is possible to estimate the incidence of normocytic anemia of chronic disease (ACD) by recognizing that at least half of all patients with an underlying chronic disease will develop normocytic anemia over the course of their illness.

Pathophysiology

Most chronic diseases create mechanisms that reduce the life cycle of erythrocytes. In addition, chronic diseases may also be myelosuppressive. As discussed earlier, ACD may be microcytic. However, the combination of reduced cell life and impaired stem cell production (hypoproliferation) associated with chronic illness typically results in a normocytic, normochromic anemia. This may be related to a variety of different underlying conditions including infection, inflammation, autoimmune activation, malignancy (with or without marrow invasion), cardiac disease,

diabetes mellitus, endocrine disorders (e.g., hypothyroidism, hypoadrenalism, hypopituitarism, hypogonadism), acute renal insufficiency (due to the accumulation of uremic metabolites that decrease RBC life span), and chronic renal insufficiency (due to impaired erythropoietin synthesis by the kidneys). Severe trauma, surgery, or major acute disease states such as sepsis and myocardial infarction may also result in normocytic anemia, possibly due to the significant tissue damage and inflammatory response associated with these events.

Hypoproliferation appears to be the major contributing factor to normocytic ACD, resulting primarily from iron sequestration in bone marrow macrophages, which effectively decreases the plasma iron pool available for integration into newly synthesized hemoglobin molecules. In addition, patients with ACD are less capable of adequate erythropoietin upregulation in response to their anemic state, compared with patients with non–iron-sequestering anemias (e.g., iron-deficiency anemia). Moreover, although absolute erythropoietin levels may be increased in ACD compared with nonanemic normal values, the bone marrow demonstrates a decreased erythropoietic response to this growth factor. Animal studies have shown that certain inflammatory cytokines including tumor necrosis factor, interferon (IFN)–βeta, and IFN-γamma may underlie these mechanisms of hypoproliferation in normocytic ACD. In addition, expression of the acute phase reactant protein hepcidin is also increased in ACD. Upregulated by the pro-inflammatory cytokine interleukin-6 (IL-6), hepcidin has been shown in animal models to directly inhibit iron absorption by the gut, resulting in decreased plasma iron levels.

Acquired aplastic anemia also results in a normocytic anemia. This may be a primary condition affecting only the erythroid lineage or it may encompass more than one cell line (e.g., white blood cells [WBCs] or platelets), which would indicate a proliferative defect in an earlier common progenitor cell that gives rise to more than one bone marrow lineage. Aplastic anemia may also be associated with certain types of viral infections in high-risk individuals, such as parvovirus B19 infection in patients with sickle cell disease or hereditary spherocytosis. A failure of erythropoietin production by the kidneys, as is also observed in chronic renal insufficiency, will similarly result in reduced RBC production and decreased reticulocytosis.

Normocytic anemia may also be caused by a relative increase in plasma volume, such as that which occurs in pregnancy or iatrogenic parenteral overhydration. This results in a dilutional drop in plasma hemoglobin, which may be physiological, as in pregnancy, or which may be reversible via pharmacological diuresis, as in the case of fluid overload.

Increased blood loss, such as from acute bleeding or hemolysis, is another major cause of normocytic anemia. As bleeding progresses and the marrow undergoes reticulocytosis, MCV may be transiently increased due to the relatively larger size of reticulocytes. However, once plasma and bone marrow iron stores are exhausted, hemoglobin production decreases, and this anemia transitions to a normocytic state and then eventually into a microcytic anemia characteristic of iron-deficiency anemia.

If hemolysis occurs intravascularly, fragmented RBCs termed *schistocytes* are seen on peripheral blood smear. This type of anemia is most commonly associated with hemolytic uremic syndrome (HUS), thrombotic thrombocytopenic purpura (TTP), disseminated intravascular coagulation (DIC), or heart valve abnormalities that cause mechanical RBC shearing. Hemolysis may also occur extravascularly with clearance of RBCs by the reticuloendothelial system. This is characterized by rounded RBCs termed *spherocytes* on peripheral blood smear and occurs most commonly due to splenic removal of RBCs, as seen in hypersplenism or autoimmune hemolytic anemia (AIHA).

Immune-mediated hemolysis typically occurs when RBC-specific antibodies coat erythrocytes, rendering them prone to splenic removal or direct hemolysis by antibody-mediated complement fixation. RBC-specific antibodies may form as a consequence of antibody upregulation from viral infections such as mononucleosis, malignancies (especially chronic lymphocytic leukemia), or autoimmune disorders such as systemic lupus erythematosus. When these antibodies are primarily of the immunoglobulin G (IgG) class, they are known as warm agglutinins, because they result in RBC aggregation (agglutination) at warmer temperatures, due to the binding of two RBCs at a time (one to each of the IgG molecule's two antigen-binding sites). In contrast, IgM RBC-specific antibodies, such as those associated with *Mycoplasma* infection, are called cold agglutinins, because they are capable of causing RBC aggregation at relatively lower temperatures, by virtue of a greater number of antigen-binding and complement fixation sites that results from their tendency to cluster in pentamers (i.e., aggregates of 5 IgM molecules with a total of 10 antigen-specific binding sites).

Extravascular hemolysis may also result from a whole host of intrinsic RBC membrane defects, such as mutations in the membrane protein spectrin that cause hereditary spherocytosis. In addition, mutations in certain cytoplasmic enzymes render RBCs more prone to hemolysis. A prime example are disorders of glucose-6-phosphate dehydrogenase (G-6-PD), an enzyme critical to the production of glutathione, a powerful reducing agent and the RBC's main protective mechanism against highly oxidizing compounds such as naphthalene (the active chemical agent found in mothballs) or certain drugs such as trimethoprim-sulfamethoxazole (Bactrim), primaquine, and dapsone.

Clinical Presentation
Subjective

The patient presentation will depend on the severity of the anemia. Because normocytic anemia rarely presents with a moderate to severe anemia of less than 30% Hct, many patients with the diagnosis do not report subjective findings. On closer questioning, however, they might note malaise or fatigue.

Objective

The objective findings are the same as for microcytic anemia.

Diagnostic Reasoning
Diagnostic Tests

Initial testing begins with the CBC. The clinician should expect the finding of anemia not to be accompanied by an alteration in the RBC indices (MCV, mean corpuscular hemoglobin [MCH], mean corpuscular hemoglobin concentration [MCHC]), in order to establish a diagnosis of normocytic normochromic anemia, such as that associated with acute blood loss, sepsis, underlying malignancy, mechanical shearing from prosthetic heart valves, aplastic anemia, or ACD.

Subsequent testing begins with an absolute reticulocyte count (normal range for adults is 0.5%–2.5% of the total RBC count). Reticulocytes are the less mature type of RBCs. They acquire their name from their fine cytoplasmic network of ribosomal RNA used for hemoglobin synthesis, which is called a *reticulum;* this network appears when stained with certain dyes such as new methylene blue. The reticulum is lost as the RBC matures but is prominent in these less mature cells of the RBC lineage, which are larger than their mature RBC counterparts. Thus, the reticulocyte count is always higher than normal in any proliferative condition (proliferative normocytic anemia) and overall MCV may be elevated due to this abundance of immature reticulocytes. However, MCV may paradoxically be normal in a true microcytic anemia with a significant reticulocytosis, because the average (mean) RBC size may appear normal in the face of both small and large cells.

Proliferative microcytic anemia may be difficult to diagnose solely from laboratory testing. If the patient has a recent history of trauma, the diagnosis of proliferative microcytic anemia secondary to hemorrhage should be considered. However, when hemorrhage is not part of the clinical picture, attention should turn to evaluating the patient for hemolysis as a potential etiology.

Testing for hemolysis requires a peripheral smear, as RBC morphology is useful in determining the cause of the hemolysis. Possible morphological changes in RBC appearance include spherocytes, sickle cells, and schistocytes. Spherocytes are erythrocytes shaped like rounded spheres or globes, which are abnormal shapes for an erythrocyte. Sickle cells assume the shape of a quarter moon or the curved metal blade instrument known as a sickle, from which these erythrocytes take their name. Schistocytes, on the other hand, are classically called "fragmented" and appear as many varied shapes.

Further genetic testing may be required if these abnormal RBC morphologies are detected on the peripheral smear. The presence of sickle cells on the smear implies a sickle cell anemia diagnosis or one of its variants, such as sickle beta thalassemia, or sickle C disease. The presence of spherocytes necessitates obtaining a Coombs' test to detect anti-RBC antibodies, because a positive Coombs' test suggests hemolysis due to AIHA, whereas a negative test may suggest hereditary spherocytosis. Schistocytes require the clinician to order a prothrombin time (PT) and partial thromboplastin time (PTT), because elevated PT/PTT values may reflect disseminated intravascular coagulation (DIC) if there is also thrombocytopenia, given that platelet consumption from widespread thrombi/microthrombi is characteristic of this disorder. This results in bleeding and/or oozing, which may be refractory to treatment and ultimately prove fatal. Normal PT/PTT values in the presence of schistocytes suggests any one of several diagnoses, including severe hypertension; HUS/TTP; heart valve abnormalities (such as mitral valve stenosis); vasculitis; or hemolysis, elevated liver enzymes, and low platelet count (HELLP) syndrome. HELLP syndrome is typically associated with pregnancy, especially later-term pregnancies, and delivery of the baby is the primary intervention.

Although the peripheral smear typically reveals morphological changes in RBCs in the patient with hemolysis, RBC shape may be normal in some forms of hemolysis, such as with deficiency in the enzyme G-6-PD. A low level of G-6-PD in the absence of morphological changes in the peripheral blood smear of a patient with normocytic anemia strongly implicates the lack of this enzyme as the cause for the hemolysis. However, G-6-PD levels measured during an acute attack of hemolytic anemia may appear paradoxically elevated in patients with G-6-PD deficiency because of the relatively higher concentration of G-6-PD found in reticulocytes, which are upregulated during acute hemolysis as the bone marrow attempts to compensate for the increased hemolysis. Thus, serum levels are often normal during acute hemolytic attacks, and the diagnosis of G-6-PD deficiency must be confirmed by redrawing G-6-PD levels several weeks after the acute anemia has resolved.

Should the G-6-PD level be within normal limits in a patient who reports voiding dark red urine in the morning, then it is necessary to consider conducting the Ham acidified serum lysis test, as dark red urine raises suspicion that the diagnosis may be paroxysmal nocturnal hemoglobinuria (PNH). The traditional Ham acidified serum lysis test may provide a definitive diagnosis, although state-of-the-art diagnostic testing typically involves flow cytometric analysis, which directly evaluates RBCs for reduced or absent levels of the cell surface molecules CD55 and CD59 that result from the genetic defects underlying PNH.

In patients diagnosed with a hypoproliferative normocytic anemia with a normal MCV and low reticulocyte count, attention should turn to the white blood cell (WBC) count and platelet count. If both are low, the clinician should suspect pancytopenia affecting all the major bone marrow lineages. If the WBC and thrombocyte counts are high, however, then either ACD or renal disease is the likely cause of the normocytic anemia. Subsequent tests, therefore, involve renal function studies (e.g., blood urea nitrogen [BUN] and creatinine) and a careful review of the patient's medical history. Assessing endogenous erythropoietin levels is an important part of this work-up as well.

Differential Diagnosis

The differential for normocytic anemia includes mixed anemias of other classifications. Differentiation should be made between three major causative mechanisms: *deficiency* (iron, vitamin B_{12}, folic acid, pyridoxine [vitamin B_6]); *central*— caused by impaired bone marrow function (anemia of chronic disease, anemia of the elderly, malignant blood disorders); and *peripheral* (bleeding and hemolysis). Mixed anemias may appear normocytic because the MCV is within normal range even though iron-deficient RBCs may be small and vitamin B_{12}- or folate-deficient RBCs are megaloblastic. Moreover, because ACD is part of the differential for microcytic anemia as well as normocytic anemia, the clinician must distinguish between the RBC indices of the two in addition to focusing on the underlying chronic pathology.

Management

Management of normocytic anemia focuses on the cause of the disorder. Causes of normocytic anemia include ACD, renal disease, pancytopenia, hereditary spherocytosis, AIHA, sickle cell anemia, G-6-PD deficiency, paroxysmal nocturnal hemoglobinuria (PNH), DIC, heart valve abnormalities, HUS/TTP, vasculitis, severe hypertensive nephropathy, and HELLP syndrome. In the initial phase of management, treatment should be symptomatic, thereby alleviating the common downstream effects of anemia. Subsequent management consists of correcting, stabilizing, or preventing the cause for normocytic anemia. Correcting and/or stabilizing the underlying cause is limited to some cases of ACD, AIHA, heart valve abnormalities, vasculitis, severe hypertension, HELLP syndrome, and DIC.

Apart from appropriately treating the underlying disease pathology, management of ACD usually requires only watchful waiting; however, if the patient's Hct drops below 30%, the clinician may consider using erythropoietin alfa. Dosing with erythropoietin alfa for ACD is highly individualized and is dependent on the underlying causative disease pathology. In general, treatment should be targeted to increase hemoglobin to 11 to 12 g/dL, but not above 13 g/dL. Starting doses range from 50 to 150 U/kg SC three times per week, depending on the underlying pathology, and should only be initiated after carefully reviewing dosing guidelines in the specific product labeling. For the first 3 weeks of therapy, the clinician should check the Hct twice weekly until the dosage level is stabilized. Two to 6 weeks may pass before the Hct undergoes an appreciable elevation.

Endogenous erythropoietin levels do not aid in determining the starting dose of exogenous erythropoietin alfa therapy. Moreover, the clinician may increase the dosage and frequency of administration until the Hct rises to an appropriate level. As the dosage level rises, however, it is possible that polycythemia (Hct greater than 60%–65%) may develop as a side effect of exogenous erythropoietin usage. Thus, if hemoglobin rises above 12 to 13 g/dL or the patient becomes frankly polycythemic, the drug should be discontinued. Within a week of discontinuing therapy, the Hct should start to decline. Otherwise, in rare cases, it may be necessary to phlebotomize the patient, removing enough volume to cause a drop in the Hct. After the clinician achieves and maintains a normal Hct, the dosage level may be reduced and/or the frequency of administration changed. Thus, the management of dosing of exogenous RBC growth factors such as erythropoietin alfa (Epogen, Procrit) darbepoetin-alfa (Aranesp) requires expert consultation with a hematologist or other appropriate specialist, given the significant risks of overdosage associated with polycythemia, including thrombosis, stroke, and myocardial infarction.

First-line treatment of AIHA consists of oral or intravenous corticosteroid therapy, such as prednisone 1 to 2 mg/kg per day in divided doses. Thus, an adult who weighs 70 kg would receive between 70 and 140 mg of prednisone in two or three divided doses each day. After an initial response is documented, the prednisone dose is decreased to 20 to 30 mg/day within several weeks, followed by a slow taper over several months to prevent recurrence of the condition. As for other patients on chronic corticosteroid therapy, supplementation with calcium, vitamin D, and folic acid may be initiated, along with bisphosphonate therapy, as prophylaxis against osteoporosis. If transfusion is required for severe anemia, the clinician should be aware that the risk of transfusion reaction is very high owing to crossmatching difficulties for these patients, given their Coombs' test positivity. The clinician should expect that the transfused cells will survive no better than the patient's own erythrocytes if the underlying AIHA is left untreated.

Surgical consultation is required for possible splenectomy should prednisone become ineffective or too toxic from chronic administration. In emergency situations, short-term hemolytic control of 1 to 3 weeks may be achieved with IV immune globulin (500 mg/kg per day for 1–4 days). In addition, off-label use of rituximab (Rituxan), an anti-CD20 B-cell–depleting monoclonal antibody therapy, has been used as second-line therapy for AIHA.

Heart valve abnormalities require an individualized plan of care developed with referral to an interventional cardiologist, which may include surgical correction of the abnormality. Many patients with heart valve abnormalities will have already started taking warfarin sodium (Coumadin) to prevent embolism formation. They should not stop taking anticoagulant therapy unless their platelet counts fall along with the Hct or active bleeding is present. Anticoagulation should also be stopped in the face of a rapidly falling Hgb, even in the setting of a normal platelet count.

Treatment of vasculitis consists of high-dose prednisone, and it may be necessary to raise the prednisone dose to 60 mg daily. The clinician should slowly taper the steroid dose as the lesions of vasculitis heal, fever declines, and other symptoms abate. Additional immunosuppressive therapy may also be required to augment the prednisone. Cyclophosphamide (Cytoxan) in a dosage range of 1 to 2 mg/kg per day may be added to the prednisone regimen. These drugs should be taken either along with or following a meal to avoid GI upset. If the dosage of cyclophosphamide exceeds 100 mg, the clinician can anticipate that only 75% of the dose will be absorbed via the GI tract. Therefore, for doses that exceed 100 mg, the dose should be split. Weekly or biweekly monitoring of the patient's complete blood count (CBC), liver and renal function tests, and uric acid level are necessary, given the potential toxicities of these agents.

Severe hypertension (greater than 180 mm Hg systolic and 110 mm Hg diastolic) can be treated with one antihypertensive agent or a combination of agents. Hemolysis that is secondary to severe hypertension may present in a patient that is known to the clinician, in which case drug therapy should be adjusted according to the history of treatment for the individual patient. (See the section on management of hypertension in Chapter 10.)

HELLP syndrome typically occurs during the third trimester of pregnancy. Because of its late onset in pregnancy, delivery of the infant is the treatment of choice. Most hematological indices return to baseline within 2 to 3 days after delivery; however, thrombocytopenia may persist for a week or more.

DIC requires treatment with heparin and platelet transfusions (replacement therapy). Platelet transfusion parameters run as low as greater than 20,000/mcL to minimize the risk of spontaneous bleeding, greater than 50,000/mcL in the setting of active bleeding, or higher in the anticipation of invasive procedures. Platelet transfusions, however, are often futile because of severe consumptive coagulopathy that quickly extracts platelets from the circulation.

Although the role of heparin is controversial, especially before or after surgery, heparin is mandated if thrombus is diagnosed in DIC. In addition, fresh frozen plasma (FFP) is an important therapy in DIC. It is often used empirically, rather than waiting for tests that specifically confirm deficits in certain clotting factors. Before symptoms are present, anticoagulation in the form of low molecular weight heparin (LMWH) such as enoxaparin (Lovenox) is an accepted therapy for patients at risk of postoperative deep vein thrombosis, provided renal function is normal (because LMWH is renally cleared). There are also recombinant versions of certain human clotting factors such as factor VIII that are available for use in significant bleeding disorders.

Because patients who require heparin therapy for DIC require around-the-clock nursing care, they should be admitted to a hospital, where they can receive 500 to 750 U/hr of heparin, according to established weight-based dosing nomograms. Platelet transfusions should be used to maintain the thrombocyte count. In addition, cryoprecipitate should be given to raise the fibrinogen level to 150 mg/dL or more.

Prevention of hemolysis caused by low levels of G-6-PD by avoiding hemolytic triggers is preferred to treating hemolysis once an attack has initiated; however, the primary care clinician must understand both prevention and treatment strategies for hemolysis resulting from G-6-PD deficiency. Avoidance of oxidant drugs, such as dapsone (Avlosulfon), quinidine (Quinaglute Dura-tabs), and sulfonamide drugs (e.g., sulfamethoxazole/trimethoprim) and environmental triggers such as naphthalene (moth balls) is critical to prevent hemolysis in patients who are G-6-PD deficient. Treatment for acute hemolytic attacks consists of discontinuing all oxidant drugs, increasing oral and/or IV fluids, and administering RBC transfusions as indicated by the Hct level. Screening for G-6-PD among patients who may require one or more oxidant drugs has become standard in the management of patients with HIV/AIDS (sulfamethoxazole/trimethoprim treatment and prophylaxis for *Pneumocystis jiroveci* pneumonia) and patients such as elderly women who are susceptible to UTIs and may require frequent antibiotic treatment.

Follow-up and Referral

If normocytic anemia is not accompanied by an abnormal reticulocyte count, then follow-up every 6 months is sufficient for most patients. Follow-up should consist of a history and physical examination, along with obtaining a CBC and reticulocyte count. The patient's records should be constructed so that these values are readily retrievable. No referral is required for these patients.

If the peripheral smear is positive for spherocytes, sickle cells, or schistocytes, the clinician should refer the patient to a hematologist for further diagnostic evaluation and management. The hematologist will create a plan of care, which the primary care clinician can co-manage. Routine follow-up with the hematologist should occur every 3 to 6 months, depending on the severity and chronicity of the hemolysis.

If the reticulocyte count is low and the clinician discovers a low WBC and platelet count, the patient is diagnosed as being pancytopenic, and referral to a hematologist is indicated. If the evaluation of a bone marrow aspirate suggests the need for treatment, then the hematologist will determine the plan of care. Normal or high WBC and platelet counts suggest the need for referrals

to specialists who can treat the underlying causes of ACD or renal disease. These referrals may include gastroenterologists, hepatologists, rheumatologists, infectious disease specialists, nephrologists, and cardiologists.

Patient Education

Education should follow the pattern outlined in the section on microcytic anemia; thus, patient education should address self-care regimens and primary care management.

Self-care of normocytic anemia is similar to that for other anemias. The patient should be instructed to remain as active as possible, and, if he or she becomes fatigued, to rest. In addition, the patient must remain vigilant for the signs and symptoms of a declining Hct—malaise, fatigue, shortness of breath, tachycardia, and palpitations. If a deficiency in G-6-PD is diagnosed, the patient should be made aware of this and of all the potential oxidant drugs that could serve as triggers of hemolysis and should, therefore, be avoided.

Patient education concerning primary care management should address topics including their respective cause of normocytic anemia. Because of the chronicity of several of these causes, patients must be instructed at every visit to adhere to their treatment regimens and follow-up plan, including pertinent laboratory testing. For example, sickle cell disease patients require frequent follow-up, infectious disease prophylaxis, and assistance from their families during sickle crises. Establishing a plan for the management of sickle cell crises is an important preparatory step in anticipation of an event and is discussed in greater detail later in this chapter in the section on sickle cell anemia.

■ MACROCYTIC ANEMIA

Macrocytic anemia is defined as anemia with a mean corpuscular volume (MCV) equal to or greater than 100 fL. These anemic states are typically normochromic and may be normoblastic or megaloblastic with large erythroid precursors. Macrocytic anemias result most commonly from defects in DNA metabolism or changes in red blood cell (RBC) membrane structure. Macrocytic anemia has four general categories of causes: (1) vitamin B_{12} deficiency, (2) folate deficiency, (3) antimetabolite drugs such as methotrexate, and (4) miscellaneous etiologies.

Epidemiology and Causes

Both sexes are equally affected by macrocytic anemia. Prevalence is greatest among people of northern European lineage and Caucasians. Incidence increases past age 60 years, but it has been observed in all age-groups. The most common cause of megaloblastic anemia is a hereditary autoimmune disorder called pernicious anemia, which results in vitamin B_{12} deficiency, a critical component to the RBC maturation pathway and effective erythropoiesis. In contrast to other forms of macrocytic anemia, pernicious anemia affects women over men at a rate of 5:1, and onset occurs in midlife, often after age 40 years.

Pathophysiology
Vitamin B$_{12}$ Deficiency

Pernicious anemia is a macrocytic anemia caused by a hereditary autoimmune disorder in which destructive antibodies are directed against intrinsic factor, a 45-kDa protein produced by gastric parietal cells that binds to dietary vitamin B$_{12}$ (cobalamin) during the digestion and absorption of nutrients and is critical to DNA synthesis and RBC maturation.

Under normal conditions, dietary vitamin B$_{12}$ is cleaved from carrier proteins in the acidic environment of the stomach by the protease pepsin. However, it is then rapidly bound by cobalamin-binding factors known as R-proteins, which are found in gastric secretions and the saliva. As these complexes are not absorbable, they pass out of the stomach and into the duodenum. However, the alkaline environment produced by pancreatic proteases in the duodenum allows for the release of vitamin B$_{12}$ from R-factor and its subsequent rapid, high-affinity binding to intrinsic factor. This newly formed vitamin B$_{12}$–intrinsic factor complex then binds to specific receptors for this complex (e.g., cubilin) in the ileum, where absorption into ileal enterocytes is mediated primarily by transcobalaminase II (complexes bound to transcobalaminase I and transcobalaminase III are metabolically inert).

Vitamin B$_{12}$ is essential to the maturation of erythrocytes via the conversion of homocysteine into methionine and the demethylation of tetrahydrofolate. Demethylated tetrahydrofolate is a key component in the conversion of deoxyuridate to thymidylate and in purine synthesis involved in DNA metabolism. Anti-intrinsic factor antibodies are present in up to three-fourths of all patients with pernicious anemia and act either by blocking the binding of vitamin B$_{12}$ to intrinsic factor or by blocking the binding of the cobalamin-intrinsic factor complex to ileal enterocyte receptors. In addition, autoantibodies produced against gastric parietal cells and pathogenic CD4+ T cells act in concert to destroy gastric parietal cells, producing a morphological change in the stomach lining known as atrophic gastritis.

A subsequent decrease in gastric acid production compounds vitamin B$_{12}$ deficiency, as cobalamin cannot be freed from its carrier proteins in the less acidic stomach environment, thereby preventing its subsequent binding to intrinsic factor in the duodenum. Prolonged use of medications that counter gastric acid production such as histamine-2 blockers (e.g., ranitidine, famotidine, cimetidine) and proton pump inhibitors (e.g., esomeprazole, omeprazole, pantoprazole) have a similar effect. The widely used diabetic drug metformin (Glucophage) also decreases vitamin B$_{12}$ absorption in up to one-third of patients taking this medication.

Thus, insufficient levels of vitamin B$_{12}$ cause erythrocytes to expand in size compared with normal RBCs, thereby producing a characteristic megaloblastic anemia.

In turn, pernicious anemia is characterized by a macrocytic anemia, a low serum level of vitamin B$_{12}$, atrophic gastritis, achlorhydria secondary to gastric atrophy, and a greater probability of other autoimmune diseases, such as hypothyroidism and vitiligo.

Normally, the complex of vitamin B$_{12}$ and intrinsic factor is absorbed through the terminal ileum and then travels to the liver where it is stored. Studies have estimated that the liver may store up to 5000 mcg/day of vitamin B$_{12}$. Because the body requires no more than 10 mcg/day, liver stores of vitamin B$_{12}$ typically last for several years before anemia ensues. Therefore, megaloblastic anemia is insidious in onset. In patients with HIV disease and liver dysfunction, both the depletion of liver stores of vitamin B$_{12}$ and the destruction of storage sites within the liver have been identified as underlying causes of megaloblastic anemia.

Dietary deficiency of vitamin B$_{12}$ in the typical American diet is rare because of its rich supply in animal proteins. However, because meats and dairy products are the only dietary source, vegetarians and particularly vegans (who completely avoid all meat and dairy products) may consume inadequate amounts of vitamin B$_{12}$. Other reasons for poor absorption include a number of mechanical causes, such as those associated with surgical GI resections (e.g., partial or total gastrectomy, resections of the terminal jejunum or proximal ileum) and Crohn's disease, which can destroy sections of the small intestine where absorption of vitamin B$_{12}$ might otherwise occur.

Folic Acid Deficiency

Folic acid is a critical nutrient that acts in concert with vitamin B$_{12}$ to further nuclear maturation in erythrocytes. Folate deficiency leads to decreased levels of tetrahydrofolate, an important building block of DNA. As with vitamin B$_{12}$ deficiency, abnormal erythroid precursors deficient in folate are prone to intramedullary hemolysis within the bone marrow, leading to a characteristic anemia clinically indistinguishable from that of vitamin B$_{12}$ deficiency. Animal models have also demonstrated that RBC precursors in folate deficiency are more prone to apoptosis or programmed cell death, although human studies are less definitive. However, in contrast to vitamin B$_{12}$ deficiency, folic acid deficiency does not produce neurological sequelae.

Macrocytic anemia due to folate deficiency presents with a low serum folate level and a normal level of vitamin B$_{12}$. It is almost always related to inadequate dietary intake, although folic acid is found in citrus fruits, dark green leafy vegetables, and animal proteins. Adequate dietary intake is 50 to 100 mcg/day, except in pregnant women who need 800 mcg/day. Even in developed countries such as the United States, pregnant patients may not consume adequate amounts of folate in their diets, and folic acid deficiency increases in incidence in multigravid patients and with multigestational pregnancies.

Less common causes of folic acid deficiency are impaired metabolism and storage of folate. The liver typically stores enough folic acid as N^5-methyltetrahydrofolic acid (approximately 5,000 mcg) to serve the body's needs for several months, given the body's use of 50 to 100 mcg/day, as long as hemolysis and increased erythrocyte production are not issues, as in sickle cell anemia. There are many causes of impaired folate metabolism and hepatic storage, including chronic alcohol use resulting in decreased enterohepatic cycling and drugs such as phenytoin (Dilantin), sulfamethoxazole/trimethoprim (Bactrim), methotrexate, and oral contraceptives, which contribute to folic acid deficiency via a variety of mechanisms.

Impaired absorption of folic acid is another cause of folic acid deficiency. Tropical sprue, GI resections, Crohn's disease, and a few intestinal parasitic infections are the primary causes of impaired folic acid absorption. Unlike vitamin B_{12}, however, folic acid can be absorbed along the entire GI tract.

Antimetabolite Drugs

Any chemical that serves as a potential inhibitor of DNA or RNA synthesis is a potential cause of macrocytic anemia. Drugs such as hydroxyurea (an inhibitor of ribonucleotide reductase), the antiviral zidovudine, and the chemotherapies methotrexate, azathioprine, and 6-mercaptopurine can all cause macrocytosis, with methotrexate being best known for leading to anemia. Methotrexate interrupts purine metabolism in the liver by preventing molecular binding with dihydrofolate reductase, an enzyme required for the storage of folic acid. Thus, less folic acid can be stored, thereby leading to a reduction in serum folate levels.

Miscellaneous Etiologies

Various unrelated causes for macrocytic anemia include thiamine- or pyridoxine-responsive anemias and Lesch-Nyhan syndrome. Macrocytic anemia may also be caused by chronic alcoholism (ingestion of at least 80 g of alcohol per day), possibly via changes in RBC membranes caused by the alcohol breakdown product acetaldehyde. In addition, liver disease may lead to macrocytic anemia, possibly via increased lipid deposition in RBC membranes, and myelodysplasia, which causes a normoblastic (albeit macrocytic) anemia.

Clinical Presentation

Subjective

Patients with macrocytic anemia typically complain of stomatitis, glossitis, nausea and anorexia, diarrhea, peripheral neuropathies, and malaise if they are deficient in vitamin B_{12}. Macrocytic anemia caused by folate deficiency, drug toxicity, impaired folate storage in the liver, and miscellaneous etiologies will cause similar symptoms as vitamin B_{12} deficiency, with the exception of peripheral neuropathy, which does not occur in folate deficiency but is part of the symptom constellation associated with chronic vitamin B_{12} deficiency.

Objective

The clinician may note any of the following findings: pale or icteric mucosa, a dry and cracked oropharynx, a thickened and smooth-surfaced tongue, tachycardia, a systolic ejection murmur, tachypnea, and diffuse abdominal tenderness without organomegaly. Long-standing vitamin B_{12} deficiency may also result in a variety of neurological signs and pathological manifestations, including peripheral neuropathy in a glove and stocking distribution on the distal extremities, increased or decreased deep tendon reflexes, impaired position sense, diminished vibratory sensation in the lower extremities, a positive Romberg sign, a variable Babinski sign, and pronounced irritability or other mental status changes, including even frank dementia in severe cases. Of the megaloblastic anemias, neurological signs related to myelin defects in the dorsal and lateral spinal columns present only in vitamin B_{12} deficiency and not with isolated folic acid deficiency.

Diagnostic Reasoning

Diagnostic Tests

Initial testing involves confirmation of a megaloblastic macrocytic anemia on the peripheral blood smear. Expected findings include anemia and an elevated MCV (greater than 100 fL). The MCHC should be within normal limits, as the anemia is usually normocytic. It is important to note that the pathological processes that underlie macrocytic anemia may occur simultaneously with causes of microcytic or normocytic anemia, such as iron deficiency and thalassemia (microcytic) or anemia of chronic disease (normocytic). In these mixed anemias, MCV may actually be within a normal range, and the RBC indices are difficult to predict, typically requiring referral to a hematologist.

Reticulocytes may be either low or normal in number, depending on the cause of the anemia. If the cause of macrocytosis is a deficiency in vitamin B_{12}, then the serum level should be less than 0.1 mcg/mL and hypersegmented neutrophils will be present on the peripheral smear. Macroovalocytes will also be evident. In the case of folic acid deficiency, the serum folate level will typically be less than 3 ng/mL, although levels may vary in patients with chronic deficiency. Even one meal can normalize folate levels in a person with true deficiency. However, homocysteine and methylmalonic acid levels can distinguish between these two etiologies, with both values being elevated in vitamin B_{12} deficiency, whereas only homocysteine levels are elevated in folic acid deficiency. Common to both etiologies is a high serum iron level and findings consistent with mild hemolysis including low haptoglobin, elevated LDH, and mildly increased unconjugated bilirubinemia.

The Schilling test is rarely performed today but was classically used to diagnose GI malabsorption as a common etiology of vitamin B_{12} deficiency. The Schilling test uses orally administered radiolabeled vitamin B_{12} to measure the ability of the small intestine to absorb vitamin B_{12}, which is subsequently secreted in the urine. It involves a two-stage 24-hour urine collection that needs to be done before any radioactive scans are performed, as the material used in these scans may confound measurements of the radiolabeled vitamin B_{12}.

When diagnosing iatrogenic etiologies of macrocytic anemia, it is important to recognize that blood levels of specific drugs such as the antimetabolite methotrexate may vary according to individual laboratory standards. Additional tests may be indicated to assess for changes in liver function that may also be impaired by drugs, as reflected in elevations of hepatic transaminases (alanine aminotransferase [ALT] and aspartate aminotransferase [AST]), bilirubin, and lactate dehydrogenase (LDH). Urobilinogen may also be identified in the urinalysis.

Differential Diagnosis

The differential diagnoses for macrocytic anemia include all of the causes identified in this section: vitamin B_{12} deficiency, folate deficiency, antimetabolite drugs, and miscellaneous causes. In addition, the differential diagnosis includes anemia of chronic liver disease and myelodysplasia.

A thorough patient history often leads the clinician to the cause of the anemia even when diagnostic laboratory results might be equivocal. For example, if the patient is pregnant, then the clinician should suspect folate deficiency over vitamin B_{12} deficiency. In addition, megaloblastic anemia due to vitamin B_{12} or folate deficiency is also often characterized by thrombocytopenia and neutropenia due to defects in megakaryocyte and myeloid precursors. This same pancytopenia is also commonly seen in the various types of myelodysplasia.

Management

A general approach to the patient with macrocytic anemia should address the cause of the anemia, as well as the downstream effects of anemia itself. Thus, the goal is to correct or ameliorate the underlying cause while addressing clinically significant sequelae of the anemia. For example, it might be appropriate to deliver supplemental vitamin B_{12} or folate while providing RBC transfusions as needed. Transfusion is rarely indicated for macrocytic anemia, other than in severe cases, and the clinician must consider that these patients are often elderly and unable to handle large-volume transfusions, due to the risk of fluid overload.

If the cause of vitamin B_{12} deficiency anemia is not pernicious anemia (malabsorption), then the clinician may follow these guidelines for oral supplementation: prescribe up to 1,000 mcg/day of oral cobalamin until normal serum levels of vitamin B_{12} are achieved (usually 6–12 weeks after initiation of therapy). High doses such as these may even be effective in some cases of pernicious anemia, despite the lack of intrinsic factor, given the presence of an additional lower-efficiency GI absorption system that works independently of intrinsic factor and does not require a functional terminal ileum. Daily oral therapy, however, requires a high degree of patient commitment and compliance.

Thus, in most cases of pernicious anemia, and especially if neurological symptoms are present, more aggressive therapy is warranted. In these cases, the preferred route of administration is parenteral with 1,000 mcg of vitamin B_{12} intramuscularly (IM) daily for the first 7 days, then weekly for 1 month, followed by once monthly for life. Lower parenteral doses of 100 mcg have been advocated, although toxicity related to vitamin B_{12} overtreatment is not typically observed, as excess vitamin B_{12} is excreted in the urine. After depleted stores are replaced, patients may transition to oral, sublingual, or nasal preparations of vitamin B_{12} for ease of administration; however, serum levels of vitamin B_{12} and methylmalonic acid should still be followed periodically to ensure compliance with these medication regimens.

For folic acid deficiency, the clinician should prescribe 1 mg/day of supplemental folic acid. The effects of therapy should be reassessed after 2 to 3 months. It is critical to understand that treatment of folic acid deficiency will reverse many of the hematological defects shared with vitamin B_{12} deficiency; however, the neurological manifestations of cobalamin deficiency will progress and may be devastating if treated inappropriately with folic acid supplementation alone. Thus, it is important to rule out vitamin B_{12} deficiency before starting a folate replacement regimen, and if empiric therapy must be started before testing is available, patients should be treated with both folic acid and vitamin B_{12} supplements. Patients suspected of having either condition who do not respond with a significant reticulocytosis after 1 week of therapy should be evaluated further for a mixed anemic process originally masked by the megaloblastic manifestations.

It is also important to evaluate serum potassium levels in profoundly anemic patients once they start treatment, as increased erythropoiesis will markedly increase potassium utilization. As a result, as the anemia corrects, these patients may become significantly hypokalemic, requiring oral potassium repletion.

If the cause of the macrocytic anemia is an antimetabolite drug or other iatrogenic drug toxicity, the patient should discontinue all suspected drugs. Laboratory tests for elevated drug levels should be ordered; the liver transaminases (AST, ALT) should also be monitored for evidence of liver dysfunction, as well as coagulation times (PT/INR and PTT) as an indication of hepatic synthetic function. For patients with macrocytic anemia from miscellaneous causes, the individual etiologies and underlying disorders must be addressed.

Follow-up and Referral

Follow-up of the patient with vitamin B_{12} deficiency involves assessing the severity of the anemia. Serial CBCs and monitoring of vitamin B_{12} levels are required on a monthly basis after starting oral cobalamin therapy. If parenteral therapy is initiated, more frequent testing is required, such as once every 2 weeks. Additional testing includes liver function tests (LFTs). If LFTs reveal elevated transaminase levels before cobalamin replacement is started, then their course should be evaluated every 2 to 4 weeks. If liver enzyme levels rise after the start of therapy, more frequent testing might be required, as well as additional diagnostic testing for evolving hepatotoxicity.

Referral for vitamin B_{12} deficiency is often not required unless the diagnosis is pernicious anemia or the patient suffers from a particularly difficult to diagnose mixed anemic process. A hematologist and gastroenterologist should be consulted in the event of pernicious anemia, as these patients are at greater risk for gastric cancer, carcinoid tumors, and colorectal carcinoma. Thus, stool should be monitored periodically for occult blood as a trigger for colonoscopy. In addition, the hyperhomocysteinemia that accompanies vitamin B_{12} or folic acid deficiency is a risk factor for atherosclerosis and venous thromboembolism and should be addressed as an independent risk factor.

Follow-up of the patient with folic acid deficiency consists of a CBC and serum folate level drawn 2 to 3 months after starting therapy. The problem should be corrected by this point if the patient has adhered to the daily regimen of folic acid replacement. No referrals are indicated unless the anemia does not resolve.

Patient Education

Patients need to learn how to enrich their diets with folic acid and vitamin B_{12}. Increasing dark green leafy vegetables in one or two meals daily can support supplements and other therapies. In addition, patients should be educated about the basic signs and symptoms of macrocytic anemia so that they can self-monitor the effectiveness of therapy and possible recurrence of the anemia.

■ SICKLE CELL ANEMIA

Sickle cell anemia is an autosomal recessive disorder. The disease is caused by a point mutation in the DNA sequence of the gene for the beta-hemoglobin chain (termed the *hemoglobin S gene*), resulting in a marked hemoglobinopathy in which intracellular hemoglobin molecules form abnormal polymers that cause gross sickling of RBCs under hypoxic conditions. It is therefore diagnosed by the detection of sickled (scythe-shaped) cells on peripheral blood smear, a positive familial history, recurrent painful episodes of vaso-occlusive pain, and a pattern demonstrating mutated hemoglobin S on a hemoglobin gel electrophoresis profile.

Epidemiology and Causes

Sickle cell anemia and sickle cell trait are inherited conditions that occur most commonly in people of West African descent. The disease has also been identified in persons of European or Middle Eastern ancestry, although these cases are extremely rare. The disease is not prevalent among persons of Asian or Pacific Island descent.

Initial symptoms appear within the first year of life for those born with sickle cell anemia. Given the perinatal manifestations and associated comorbidities, prenatal screening is now available for at-risk couples, consisting of DNA analysis from fetal cells. The procedure should be offered to these couples as part of their prenatal counseling. If both the father and mother have sickle cell trait and each carry one copy of the mutated hemoglobin S gene, their offspring have a one in four chance of developing true homozygous sickle cell anemia. In more than 40 states, newborns undergo universal neonatal screening for hemoglobinopathies, including Hgb protein electrophoresis screening for sickle cell disease, the thalassemias, and other variant hemoglobinopathies.

Autosomal recessive genes for hemoglobin S are distributed equally between both sexes. Individuals who are homozygous for the hemoglobin S gene will develop sickle cell anemia and experience recurrent sickle cell crises throughout their lives. In addition, overall life expectancy is typically reduced to between 40 and 50 years of age. Those who are heterozygous for the hemoglobin S gene are said to carry the sickle cell trait, which is asymptomatic because hemoglobin A accounts for more than half of their hemoglobin. About 8% to 10% of persons of West African descent in the United States carry the sickle cell trait. One in 400 to 500 West African descendants suffers from sickle cell anemia, whereas up to 2% of all African Americans are affected.

Pathophysiology

The cause of sickle cell anemia is a point mutation in the genetic sequence of the beta chain gene of hemoglobin which results in the replacement of glutamic acid by valine at the N-terminal amino acid position 6 of this protein chain. The substitution of valine leads to the production of hemoglobin S, which is poorly soluble and prone to rigid polymerization when in its deoxygenated state. This typically occurs under conditions of physiological stress, such as physical overexertion, muscle tissue ischemia causing lactic acidosis, dehydration, infection, or exposure to cold environmental temperatures. However, the majority of acute sickling events have no identifiable cause.

Polymerized deoxyhemoglobin S takes on a rope-like form, aligning itself with other polymerized strands and transforming erythrocytes into a rigid, sickled, crescent-like shape. In turn, these sickled erythrocytes regularly become lodged in the microvasculature of various organs and bodily tissues, causing small but highly symptomatic infarcts throughout the body. Sickled cells adhere rigidly to the inner membranes lining small blood vessels, inducing intimal hyperplasia that contributes to the obstruction of free blood flow in the smaller capillaries, as well as inducing RBC hemolysis due to this adherence to the inner vessel wall. RBCs in patients with sickle cell disease have an average life span of 17 days, versus the normal length of 100 days.

Sickled cells become lodged in the microvasculature as small thrombi. Once the thrombi are situated against the vascular membrane, they attract plasma proteins, leukocytes, and platelets, creating an occlusion to blood flow. This inflammatory process escalates, as ischemia to the surrounding tissue unfolds. Ischemic injury and infarcts cause pain as perimeter tissue is increasingly starved for oxygen and other nutrients. The rate of sickling increases as tissues become more hypoxic and acidotic. Erythrocytes, with or without hemoglobin S, that are lodged in and around the microthrombi lose intracellular water, which results either in hemolysis occurring before RBC sickling or in escalated sickle cell formation and plasma hyperviscosity. As hypoxia and acidosis increase, more erythrocytes begin to sickle, and nearly all sickled cells in the area of the thrombus will eventually hemolyze.

The body attempts to compensate for this resultant anemia (which is typically normocytic, unless also associated with iron deficiency or a form of thalassemia) with expansion and upregulation of the bone marrow. This has several pathological implications. Chronically elevated white blood cell (WBC) counts result in the production of inflammatory cytokines, which further complicates vaso-occlusive crises. The additional blood flow also leads to cardiomegaly and eventual high-output congestive heart failure. This results in greater metabolic and caloric requirements as the affected individual ages, leading to stunted growth and lower than average adult weight if the condition is poorly controlled and nutritional requirements are not met with dietary supplements.

Anemia is also worsened by impaired production of the RBC growth factor erythropoietin (which is normally produced in the kidney), owing to the presence of progressive renal disease from microinfarction of the vasa recta capillaries in the renal medulla. Hemolysis results in hyperbilirubinemia, which predisposes to the development of pigmented cholelithiasis (gallstones). In turn, cholecystectomy is the most common surgical procedure in patients with sickle cell anemia.

The formation of microthrombi occurs in many parts of the body but is especially prone to occur in the chest, vertebrae, and long bones of the legs. In pediatric patients, swelling, tenderness, and inflammation of the hands and feet (especially the fingers and toes, termed *dactylitis*), known as hand–foot syndrome, is a common manifestation before age 2 years. Leg ulcers are also common, typically affecting the skin over the lateral and medial malleoli and subject to infection by *Staphylococcus aureus, Pseudomonas, Streptococcus* species, or *Bacteroides*. Bone manifestations also occur. As ischemia progresses

due to vaso-occlusion, the affected bone eventually infarcts and becomes susceptible to osteomyelitis by *Salmonella* species and, less commonly, *Staphylococcus aureus.* Severely debilitating noninfectious aseptic necrosis of the hip or shoulder joints may also occur due to vaso-occlusion of the arterial supply to the femoral or humeral heads, resulting in eventual loss of the entire joint.

Organs including the heart, liver, penis, and kidney also tend to be affected by vaso-occlusive crises, particularly during childhood and adolescent years. Priapism (painful and sustained penile erection often lasting several hours) is an emergent condition requiring inpatient treatment with hydration, transfusion, and in some cases surgical intervention to release engorged blood, as ischemia of the penis may lead to tissue necrosis. Retinopathy and its associated complications caused by microvascular ischemia increase in prevalence with age as well, including proliferative retinopathy, retinal hemorrhage and detachment, as well as retinal artery occlusion. Such changes may begin in childhood, and in turn, many patients with sickle cell anemia become blind before age 40 years.

Splenic sequestration results when large numbers of sickled erythrocytes become lodged in an engorged, functional spleen during early childhood, resulting in severe anemia and potentially fatal hypovolemic shock, carrying a mortality rate of 10% to 15%. Because this condition tends to be recurrent, splenectomy is often performed after the first episode. Later in adult life, vaso-occlusive episodes in the spleen lead to autoinfarction, with replacement of splenic parenchyma by fibrotic tissue, resulting in functional asplenia. Although this obviates the occurrence of splenic sequestration syndrome, splenic autoinfarction results in increased susceptibility to infection by encapsulated organisms, such as *Streptococcus pneumoniae* and *Haemophilus influenzae.*

In addition to splenic sequestration, severe anemia may also result from aplastic crises, in which patients experience extreme suppression of bone marrow erythropoiesis. This is often a postinfectious phenomenon that may follow infection with Epstein-Barr virus, *Streptococcus pneumoniae, Salmonella,* and especially parvovirus B19, seen classically in pediatric patients, which directly infects erythroid progenitors. The bone marrow is also susceptible to infarction, which may further exacerbate the chronic anemia.

Sickle cell disease patients are at risk for other life-threatening conditions, as well. In acute chest syndrome, bilateral pulmonary infiltrates occur with fever and significant pleuritic chest pain, resulting in a "splinting" pattern of respirations that consists of shallow breaths of suboptimal volume, which leads to progressive atelectasis and hypoxia. This condition may be triggered by vaso-occlusion, pulmonic infection, in situ thrombus formation with pulmonary infarction, or pulmonary emboli associated with bone marrow infarction (including fat emboli). Respiratory failure may eventually occur if the condition is not treated aggressively with IV hydration, RBC transfusion, pain management to relieve respiratory splinting, supplemental oxygen, and antibiotics for documented infection (e.g., community-acquired pneumonia or less commonly bacteremia).

Another serious complication of sickle cell disease is the tendency for cerebrovascular accidents (e.g., strokes, transient ischemic attacks). In fact, a significant percentage of these patients will experience strokes before reaching adulthood, some repeatedly, but with the first episode most commonly occurring between 2 and 8 years of age. Myocardial infarction may also occur in the presence or absence of documented coronary artery disease, believed to be due either to occlusion or to severe hypoxemia resulting from the reduced oxygen-carrying capacity of the blood.

Clinical Presentation
Subjective
Subjective findings are associated with the severity of the anemia and with pain. Pain is evident only when there is a crisis, but the subjective findings of anemia may be apparent without concurrent crisis. In brief, the subjective findings of sickle cell anemia are similar to those of other types of anemia.

The cardinal subjective symptom of a sickle cell crisis is pain. Pain appears suddenly in the back, chest, abdomen, or extremities, which patients typically characterize as excruciating. It may last for several hours or several days and is unrelieved by rest or change in body position. Massaging the site is of little value in relieving pain. Other subjective findings may include nausea, anorexia, light-headedness, significant anxiety or panic, heart palpitations, and shortness of breath.

Objective
The patient may present with a low-grade fever (less than 101.3°F [38.5°C]) during and preceding a sickle cell crisis. Additional symptoms may include point tenderness and guarding at the sites of pain, pinpoint pupils, inability to follow commands, photophobia, tachycardia and systolic murmur, tachypnea, diminished respiratory excursion, hepatomegaly, a nonpalpable spleen (due to infarction and fibrosis), and pretibial ulcers.

Outside of a sickle cell crisis, the clinician may note characteristic physical findings resulting from chronic bone marrow expansion including a lengthened tower-shaped skull, frontal bossing of the forehead, and fish-mouth deformities of the vertebrae. During the objective examination, the clinician may note chronic effects of hemolysis, such as jaundice or a sallow color to the skin. The patient may appear older than his or her stated years. Personality traits characteristic of patients who have lived with a chronic debilitating disease may also be present.

Diagnostic Reasoning
Diagnostic Tests
Initial testing involves a CBC and a peripheral blood smear. It should be clear, however, that adults with sickle

cell disease do not present de novo. They are typically diagnosed soon after birth and learn to cope with sickle cell crises even as they face delayed physical and psychological maturation. Postnatal infant screening in the United States, therefore, typically includes a CBC and peripheral blood smear.

Sickled cells will constitute 5% to 10% of the peripheral blood smear in most patients. The elevated reticulocyte count (greater than 10% of the total erythrocyte count) is characteristically accompanied by the presence of Howell-Jolly bodies, which are small remnants of nuclear material from hemolyzed erythrocytes that reflect hyposplenia from autoinfarction, and target cells, which are erythrocytes with a deeply stained core surrounded by a lighter-stained margin that resemble a target with a bull's eye. The clinician should also expect the WBC count to be elevated to 12,000 cells/mcL or greater, especially during and soon after a sickle cell crisis.

Further testing may include an indirect bilirubin level, which will be elevated after a sickle cell crisis due to hemolysis. Conversely, haptoglobin, a glycoprotein that binds free hemoglobin released from hemolyzed erythrocytes, will be significantly decreased, as it cannot be replaced quickly enough after a severe hemolytic episode.

Differential Diagnosis
The differential diagnosis for sickle cell anemia includes anemia resulting from other causes, sickle thalassemia, hemoglobin C disorders, nonspecific abdominal pain, UTI, poisoning, and diabetes mellitus. Each of these mimics some or all of the subjective and objective findings from the history and physical examination.

Sickle cell anemia is differentiated from sickle thalassemia by the MCV. The MCV should be low if there is any combination of sickle cell anemia and beta-thalassemia (a microcytic anemia) and normal if only sickle cell anemia is present. A combination of sickle cell anemia with alpha-thalassemia may cause a slower rate of sickling due to a reduced MCHC in the erythrocytes caused by the alpha-thalassemia. Therefore, the sickle cell crises in these patients are typically less damaging and possibly less painful than those in patients without this combination.

Hemoglobin C disorders are differentiated by a much milder onset and course of anemia than sickle cell anemia. Indeed, some patients with hemoglobin C disorders may pass their lives without any crises caused by the disorder. The underlying pathology is differentiated by the substitution of lysine for valine at amino acid position 6 of the beta-globin chain. Definitive differentiation between these disorders comes with a peripheral blood smear, which reveals rectangular crystals of hemoglobin C. With sickle cell/hemoglobin C disease (sickle C disease or SC disease), adult patients may still be prone to splenic sequestration crises, as their spleens typically do not autoinfarct and fibrose. Sickle beta-thalassemia may also be a milder, but nonetheless significantly morbid, condition compared with homozygous sickle cell disease. It is usually microcytic. If there is no other production from the other beta-globin gene (*sickle beta thal⁰*), these patients will be the most symptomatic. Alternatively, reduced production from the other beta chain gene (*sickle beta thal⁺*) gives a milder condition, as there is still some functional hemoglobin A present. There are also rarer forms of doubly heterozygous hemoglobinopathies when hemoglobin S is combined with hemoglobins A, G, or O.

Nonspecific abdominal pain that mimics sickle cell anemia will have none of the characteristic laboratory markers of sickle cell anemia, other than possibly an elevated WBC count or a low Hct. Sickle cell anemia in crisis usually also manifests with extra-abdominal pain.

Urinary tract infection is linked to sickle cell anemia as these patients experience UTIs more frequently than other individuals. A UTI can present with excruciating abdominal pain and referred pain to the back and chest. The WBC count is typically elevated, and there could be a low-grade fever with either frank or microscopic blood present in the urine. Thus, the distinguishing differences between isolated cases of UTI and those associated with sickle cell anemia include the history and laboratory markers of sickle cell anemia.

Poisoning with certain agents may present with hypoxemia and acidosis that are similar to what is observed in a sickle cell crisis. For example, ingestion of strong alkalines, such as those contained in household cleaning compounds, causes nausea, vomiting, acute abdominal pain, and dyspnea. The history and CBC should aid in the rapid and almost certain differentiation of poisoning from sickle cell anemia.

Finally, diabetes is in the differential because of the similarities in blood chemistries, such as renal and hepatic function tests, an acidic blood pH, urinalysis, and physical examination. Again, as is the case with the other differential diagnoses, the history, CBC, and peripheral blood smear should readily differentiate these etiologies, even in an emergent situation.

Management
Initial Management

Folic acid (Folvate) supplementation of 1 mg/day by mouth is indicated, along with a diet that is rich in the complex B vitamins and vitamin C. Significant rehydration is needed as a part of management and is a key to reversing sickle cell crises. It aids in keeping the blood pH normal, thereby preventing acidosis with the sequela of sickling. Hydroxyurea, a chemotherapeutic agent, is a common treatment to increase hemoglobin F levels, an infant hemoglobin form with a higher affinity for oxygen than hemoglobin A or S, which allows for less hypoxemia and less sickling of RBCs. In turn, it reduces the frequency of painful crises.

Although packed RBC transfusions may be indicated in sickle cell anemia treatment to decrease the fraction of hemoglobin S prone to polymerization, especially in children, they are less commonly used in adults and must always be weighed against the risks of infection (especially with hepatitis C), transfusion reactions, and iron overload. Anemia with Hgb of less than 7 has been associated with a greater risk of stroke, severe vaso-occlusive episodes, acute chest, and death in children. Chronic transfusions, however, lead to iron overload and iatrogenic hemochromatosis, which can destroy solid organs such as the liver and adrenal glands. Exchange transfusion may be used when the clinical manifestations of sickle cell anemia (e.g., acute chest, priapism) are severe and refractory to initial treatment, in order to decrease hemoglobin S to less that 50% of total hemoglobin. If osteomyelitis is confirmed with magnetic resonance imaging (MRI), which is the diagnostic imaging test of choice, then antibiotic therapy is required. *Salmonella* predominates in osteomyelitis of sickle cell patients over *Staphylococcus aureus,* which is seen more commonly in non–sickle cell patients. Dactylitis (painful swelling of the feet and hands during the first several years of life in children with sickle cell anemia) requires urgent treatment, as do aseptic necrosis of the hip and priapism.

Subsequent Management

Management of sickle cell crises often requires hospitalization. General goals include symptomatic control of pain with opioid-type drugs, IV rehydration, oxygen supplementation to reestablish normal or near-normal oxygen tension and to prevent or control acidosis, and vigilance against possible damage to vital organs such as the heart, liver, and kidneys.

Given the increased risk of infection by encapsulated organisms (*Streptococcus pneumoniae, Haemophilus influenzae*) in sickle cell anemia patients, prophylactic penicillin should be used in children 2 months to 5 years of age and lifelong in children who have had splenectomies secondary to splenic sequestration crises. In addition, patients should receive all age-appropriate immunizations, including antipneumococcal vaccines (7-, 13-, and 23-valent forms are available), Hib vaccine, influenza vaccine, and meningococcal vaccine. Parents or other family members should also be taught how to assess for splenic size so that they can recognize the early signs of splenic sequestration syndrome in affected individuals.

Given the chronicity of sickle cell anemia and the propensity for recurrent sickle cell crises, there is a phenomenon of learned helplessness, narcotic addiction, and drug-seeking behavior that may develop in sickle cell disease patients who are afflicted with chronic pain. These are critical conditions that must be considered when developing a treatment plan for the management of sickle cell anemia, because they can significantly affect the patient's capacity for effective self-care.

Follow-up and Referral

Follow-up visits with sickle cell anemia patients should occur every 3 months during periods of stability when they have not been in crisis for 6 months or more; however, the frequency and duration of crises may increase the required frequency of follow-up examinations with appropriate laboratory evaluations. Routine clinical markers to be assessed include a CBC, fasting blood sugar, electrolytes, renal and liver function studies, and urinalysis. Annual or biannual 12-lead electrocardiograms (ECGs) are also necessary to rule out cardiac pathology.

Every patient with sickle cell anemia should be evaluated at least twice per year by a hematologist. In addition, retinal examinations should be performed by an ophthalmologist on an annual basis. Retinal photographs may be required once retinopathies have been diagnosed. Other referrals become evident as organs start to fail; therefore, cardiologists, gastroenterologists, nephrologists, orthopedic surgeons, and general surgeons may be enlisted as necessary.

Patient Education

Education should focus on the patient's maturation and personality development, within the context of living with this chronic disease. Secondary gains (in the form of extra attention) that the patient received due to the illness early in life may result in the patient regressing to childish behaviors and coping mechanisms during sickle cell crises. In turn, these patients often present with poor coping skills. Patients who exhibit such regressive behaviors should understand that friends, acquaintances, and particularly prospective life partners and spouses may be offended by these behaviors. The patient, therefore, should be educated in ways that provide anticipatory guidance to others who witness such events.

Self-care behaviors that may prevent sickle cell crises should be reinforced regularly. These include adequate hydration, folic acid supplementation, avoidance of situations that tax the patient's physical and emotional stamina, and adequate sleep and rest as part of everyday activities. Additional self-care actions include participation in peer support groups, pregnancy prevention unless the patient is prepared for the possibility of additional sickle cell crises during pregnancy and lactation, involvement in prenatal counseling and testing of the fetus for DNA evidence of sickle cell disease, and avoidance of alcohol and adrenergic dietary elements, such as caffeine, that can cause diuresis and dehydrate the body.

Self-care also involves the patient's own spiritual practices. Spiritual beliefs and practices provide a unique contribution to the course of disease adaptation. In light of the early death of sickle cell anemia patients compared with the general population, spiritual practices may enhance personal acceptance of the disease. In addition, spiritual practices can marshal inner resources to resolve feelings of hopelessness and helplessness during sickle cell crises.

Because sickle cell disease is a lifelong condition, problems unique to children and adolescents with chronic disease are abundant. There is an important transition period in which the specialty care of these patients typically transitions from a pediatric to an internal medicine setting. Thus, these patients are often shocked to find that they are treated differently in an adult medicine setting, with more stringent requirements for adhering to a chronic treatment plan—especially regarding patient compliance and its relationship to the emergent treatment of chronic pain exacerbations. Peer support groups can be particularly helpful for these patients.

■ POLYCYTHEMIA

Polycythemia involves an increase in erythrocyte volume, which results in an increase in blood viscosity. The disorder may be either relative or absolute. A hematocrit (Hct) greater than 51% in women and 54% in men is characteristic. The term *polycythemia* is somewhat misleading. It means too many cell lines (*poly* = "many"; *cythemia* = "cell lines"), in general, and not just too many erythrocytes, in particular. Nevertheless, the name is associated with erythrocytes only.

Epidemiology and Causes

The incidence of polycythemia increases with age. It remains more prevalent in older men (older than age 70 years) than in women of similar age by a 2:1 ratio. On average, the incidence is 1.9:100,000. These statistics have remained stable for the past 60 years, according to three retrospective analyses. The incidence and prevalence of polycythemia increase among persons who reside at high altitudes, given the body's compensation for the relatively lower environmental oxygen tension through the upregulation of erythropoiesis.

Causes of relative polycythemia include decreased fluid intake, increased fluid loss, and extravasation of fluids. Absolute polycythemia, on the other hand, may be caused by either primary or secondary mechanisms. Primary polycythemia involves the proliferation of stem cells independent of erythropoietin and is termed *polycythemia vera*. In contrast, causes of secondary absolute polycythemia include Cushing's syndrome, erythropoietin-secreting tumors, and chronic hypoxia, such as that associated with residence at high altitudes and carboxyhemoglobinemia.

Pathophysiology
Relative Polycythemia

Relative polycythemia is a condition in which there is a decrease in plasma volume while the total number of circulating erythrocytes remains the same. The underlying pathology is almost always dehydration, which may be either acute or chronic. Acute dehydration is associated with vomiting, burns, crush-type injuries, and fevers, whereas chronic dehydration is an outcome of long-term use of diuretics, such as furosemide. Another chronic cause of dehydration is decreased oral fluid intake, a condition frequently encountered in older adults. Cigarette smoking, though an important cause of absolute polycythemia, is also known to decrease plasma volume. Interestingly, this reduction reverses on cessation of smoking (with a reduction in Hct of 4 or more percentage points in just a matter of days). Terms such as *pseudo-* or *spurious polycythemia, stress erythrocytosis,* and *Gaisböck's disease* have all been used to label chronic states in which plasma volume is reduced while Hct and hemoglobin (Hgb) are elevated.

Absolute Polycythemia

Absolute polycythemia is a condition in which the actual numbers of circulating erythrocytes are increased with a corresponding increase in measured red blood cell (RBC) mass. (One exception is *inapparent polycythemia* in which the increase in RBC numbers is counterbalanced by an increase in plasma volume, often masking the polycythemia on standard blood tests.)

Absolute polycythemia may be divided into primary and secondary categories. Many diagnosticians consider primary disease to be polycythemia vera, which is a chronic myeloproliferative disorder caused by an abnormally dividing pluripotential stem cell that leads to a clonal erythrocytosis that is erythropoietin independent, as well as a variable leukocytosis (increased myelocytes) and thrombocytosis. The molecular defect underlying polycythemia vera has yet to be fully characterized, but aberrant cell signaling pathways involving tyrosine kinases, tyrosine phosphatases, insulin-like growth factor–1, and transcriptional dysregulation have all been suggested. Interestingly, however, the defect does not appear to be in the erythropoietin–erythropoietin receptor pathway, because erythropoietin levels are typically low in these patients.

Physiologically, erythropoietin has many functions: (1) stimulating mitogenicity (cell division) of progenitor cells, (2) protecting progenitor cells from apoptosis, and (3) inducing specific proteins involved in the differentiation and terminal maturation of erythrocytes, such as ankyrin and spectrin (structural membrane proteins) and the oxygen-binding globin chains. In turn, primary polycythemia may result from congenital or acquired mutations in erythroid progenitor cells that affect the erythropoietin–erythropoietin receptor pathway. For example, primary familial and congenital polycythemia (PFCP or benign erythrocytosis) is an autosomal dominant disorder thought to result from mutations in the erythropoietin receptor that lead to increased responsiveness of erythrocytes to this growth factor. However, the specific molecular defect remains undefined in many patients.

There are several causes of secondary absolute polycythemia—chronic hypoxia, carboxyhemoglobinemia, Cushing's syndrome, chronic corticosteroid use, erythropoietin-secreting tumors, and cardiopulmonary diseases (the most common cause of secondary polycythemia),

which decrease oxygen saturation or diminish renal blood flow. Acquired forms include polycythemia due to the chronic hypoxia associated with prolonged high-altitude living, where the partial pressure of ambient oxygen is decreased. Carboxyhemoglobinemia is a condition associated with tobacco use, in which carbon monoxide–containing cigarette smoke increases carboxyhemoglobin (hemoglobin bound stably to carbon monoxide) levels, preventing the binding of oxygen to hemoglobin molecules and resulting in a leftward shift in the hemoglobin dissociation curve. This shift reflects a decrease in oxygen delivery to the tissues and, in turn, is compensated by polycythemia. Cushing's syndrome (abnormal corticosteroid production arising from the pituitary gland [ACTH overproduction], adrenals, or a hormonally active tumor [cortisol overproduction]) and chronic exogenous steroid use (either corticosteroids or anabolic steroids) are erythrogenic and, when left unchecked, may lead to polycythemia. In addition, the act of blood doping, in which RBC infusions are administered before sporting events by some athletes to increase oxygen-carrying capacity, is an important iatrogenic source of polycythemia. Finally, erythropoietin-secreting tumors tend to be located in the kidneys (e.g., renal cell carcinoma), liver (e.g., hepatocellular carcinoma, hepatoma), uterus (e.g., leiomyomata or fibroids), or central nervous system vasculature (e.g., hemangioblastoma).

Although these congenital forms are quite rare, secondary polycythemia may also be congenital, caused by inborn mutations that alter the oxygen affinity of hemoglobin, leading to decreased oxygen delivery to peripheral tissues with resultant hypoxemia. These include mutations in the alpha- and beta-globin genes that cause a marked increase in oxygen affinity with compensatory polycythemia, congenital methemoglobinemia in which the iron moiety in hemoglobin is trapped in the oxidized ferric form and therefore unable to bind oxygen (mutations in cytochrome b5 reductase prevent reduction of ferric ions back to the oxygen-binding ferrous form), and mutations that lower levels of 2,3-bisphosphoglycerate, a key molecule involved in oxygen delivery to peripheral tissues.

Several other erythroid growth factors have also been shown to exist. Stem cell factor (SCF), granulocyte-macrophage colony-stimulating factor (GM-CSF), and interleukin-3 (IL-3) are responsible for the growth of early pluripotent stem cells that give rise to the erythroid lineage. In addition, insulin-like growth factor–1 (IGF-1) also stimulates erythropoiesis in early progenitors and appears particularly important in patients with end-stage renal disease who no longer produce adequate amounts of erythropoietin due to parenchymal kidney damage. Type 1 receptors for angiotensin II have also been identified on erythroid progenitor cells, and both angiotensin-converting enzyme (ACE) inhibitors and angiotensin II receptor blockers (ARBs) have been shown to counteract erythrocytosis in renal transplant patients. Thus, secondary polycythemia may result from any number of mutations that affect these different growth factors, although these molecular lesions tend to be rare, many of which have only been identified in familial cohorts. Along this same line, iatrogenic polycythemia secondary to excessive use of exogenous RBC growth factors such as erythropoietin-alpha and darbepoetin alfa should always be considered in patients on medications of this class.

Clinical Presentation

Subjective

Many subjective complaints do not arise until the Hct is greater than 60%. Because cardiopulmonary disease is the most common cause of polycythemia, the clinician should elicit an effective history of pulmonary symptoms such as chronic cough, cyanosis, hypersomnolence, or shortness of breath and dyspnea on exertion.

Common complaints include headache, blurred vision, weakness, fatigue, irritability, dizziness, and, on occasion, tinnitus. Epistaxis, however, may be the complaint of clinical presentation. Epistaxis is due to mucosal engorgement in the nares and irregularities in clotting. After a warm bath or shower, patients may complain of generalized pruritus, which is caused by the release of histamine from basophils that become released from the vasculature or pool along dilated vascular walls.

Eliciting a detailed smoking history is also crucial. The constellation of symptoms that reflect chronic carbon monoxide exposure should also be assessed in patients with high-risk occupations, such as taxi and bus drivers, toll booth operators, and underground tunnel or parking garage attendants.

Objective

The clinician should assess for erythromelalgia (burning pain in the hands and feet pathognomonic for polycythemia vera), as well as the tendency toward venous and arterial thrombosis or hemorrhage in this condition due to hyperviscosity and thrombocytosis. Gastrointestinal manifestations are also common, including peptic ulcer disease and gastroduodenal erosions. These are believed to be from hyperviscosity and increased histamine release. On an ocular examination, the clinician may note new vessel growth on the retinae as well as vascular engorgement. Splenomegaly is almost always present. Tenderness may be elicited from palpation of both upper abdominal quadrants. The left quadrant may be tender because of gastric ulceration and the right quadrant because of duodenal ulcers or, infrequently, due to hepatomegaly.

The skin (especially on the face) and mucous membranes have a dark, flushed (plethoric) appearance. The skin appears purplish or cyanotic as a result of inadequate tissue oxygenation, and a ruddy cyanosis may be apparent on the fingers and toes. Finally, Cushingoid features may be present if Cushing's syndrome or chronic corticosteroid use is the cause of secondary absolute polycythemia.

Diagnostic Reasoning

Diagnostic Tests

Polycythemia tends to be suspected when Hct is greater than 48% or Hgb is greater than 16.5 g/dL in women or Hct is greater than 52% or Hgb is greater than 18.5 g/dL in men. These levels should always be age-adjusted. Thus, initial testing always includes a complete blood count (CBC), which starts the process of differentiating absolute from relative polycythemia. If the patient has polycythemia vera or one of the other absolute polycythemias, the Hct is typically greater than 55% for women and 60% for men. In fact, if the Hct is not greater than these percentages, Cushing's disease and overuse of steroids should be ruled out, as both cause milder degrees of polycythemia. By definition, there is an elevated RBC count in absolute polycythemia, but RBC morphology is classically normal on the peripheral blood smear.

In the absence of concurrent infection, the white blood cell (WBC) count in absolute polycythemia typically ranges between 10,000 and 20,000 cells/mcL. The differential is usually unremarkable except for occasional basophilia. The clinician should expect the platelet count to be elevated and to vary—at times exceeding 1 million cells/mcL.

Secondary tests aid in the differentiation of primary versus secondary causes of absolute polycythemia. Diagnosis of polycythemia vera is based on detecting splenomegaly in combination with an elevated Hct and platelet count. However, a definitive diagnosis of polycythemia vera may call for bone marrow biopsy if other biochemical studies are inconclusive. Erythropoietin levels are usually low in polycythemia vera, and a normal or elevated erythropoietin level necessitates a search for other causes.

Secondary testing is directed by the suspected underlying pathology. Pulse oximetry should be measured after minimal exertion as an important part of the diagnostic work-up. In addition, an arterial blood gas (ABG) drawn to measure the partial pressure of oxygen in arterial blood (PaO_2) and co-oximetry to assess for the effects of carbon monoxide exposure (carboxyhemoglobin) or oxygen-poor methemoglobin may be indicated. Carboxyhemoglobin levels greater than 5% suggest CO poisoning.

If the patient has relative polycythemia, the CBC will reveal an elevated RBC mass, but the Hct will often not be as high as 55% to 60%. Plasma volume may also be measured to help distinguish relative versus absolute polycythemia, but values are not always predictable. In addition, the WBC and platelet counts are lower for relative polycythemia compared with absolute polycythemia.

Differential Diagnosis

The differential diagnoses for polycythemia vera include chronic myeloid leukemia, myelofibrosis, and essential thrombocytosis. Chronic myeloid leukemia would have an extremely elevated WBC count (30,000/mcL). Myelofibrosis would have a normal or decreased Hct and abnormal RBC morphology. Essential thrombocytosis would have a normal Hct with a markedly elevated platelet count. Spurious polycythemia, in which there is a contracted plasma volume rather than a true increase in RBC mass, may be due to diuretic therapy.

Management

In general, the principles of polycythemia management concern the difference between relative and absolute causes. This section, therefore, presents management of polycythemia according to underlying pathology.

Initial Management

Relative Polycythemia Relative polycythemia is associated with dehydration; therefore, the clinician's objective is to rehydrate the patient. Rehydration in the primary care setting generally consists of oral hydration and medication adjustment if the cause of dehydration is related to a pharmaceutical agent, such as diuretics. Thus, the clinician must decide whether the patient is able to adhere to instructions regarding oral fluids and changes in drug regimens. Should IV rehydration be required, other factors must also be considered, such as the patient's age, associated comorbidities (e.g., cardiopulmonary disease such as congestive heart failure), ability to adhere to self-care instructions following discharge, and the availability of outpatient nursing care. Because of the complexity of care required for IV rehydration, acute-care or in-hospital nursing management is often the preferred setting for IV fluid therapy. Central to the decision to initiate oral versus IV hydration is the capacity of family or other caregivers to assist in the patient's rehydration.

Absolute Polycythemia Absolute polycythemia management begins with progressive phlebotomies if the Hct is greater than 55% to 60%. Phlebotomy is required to prevent thrombus formation, which can lead to a fatal embolic event, cerebrovascular accident, or myocardial infarction in a polycythemic patient. The goal of phlebotomy is to decrease Hct to 45% or lower. This goal can be achieved by the weekly removal of 500 mL of whole blood. For example, if the starting Hct is 65% and 3% to 4% Hct is lost with each 500 mL of blood, the goal of a 45% Hct can be reached after six phlebotomies. Maintenance of an Hct at or below 45% will require subsequent phlebotomies. Iron deficiency will develop after repeated phlebotomy.

Patients will report abatement of symptoms as the Hct falls. Should iron deficiency ensue, iron supplementation should not be started because supplements can stymie therapeutic gains achieved by phlebotomy. Despite potential iron deficiency, the fatigue associated with polycythemia should not recur once a Hct of 45% or less has been achieved.

Initial management of all absolute polycythemias follows the path of phlebotomy outlined above. Additional guidelines for initial management are specific to the underlying cause, for example, Cushing's disease, corticosteroid use, erythropoietin-secreting tumor, hypoxia, and carboxyhemoglobinemia. Surgical resection of the pituitary gland may be indicated for Cushing's syndrome depending on the source of the excess corticosteroids—the pituitary gland, the adrenal glands, and so forth. Tapering of steroids, if possible, is the management of steroid-induced polycythemia. Tumor excision or reduction is the management for erythropoietin-secreting tumors. Oxygen supplementation may be the initial management for chronic hypoxia (if PaO_2 is less than 60 mm Hg). Cessation of smoking is the management for carboxyhemoglobinemia due to tobacco use.

Given the significant risk of clot formation, hydroxyurea (Hydrea) is particularly useful in patients at risk for thrombosis, and low-dose aspirin should be started in all patients (especially those with thrombocytosis) unless contraindicated by another condition. IFN-α is useful in patients refractory to other treatments or in those with significant refractory pruritus although it may cause troublesome side effects, including flu-like symptoms and depression. Antihistamines may be helpful in treating the pruritus associated with polycythemia vera, although some patients may experience significant sedation with these medications. Anagrelide (Agrylin) is an antiplatelet agent that reduces platelet count and can be useful in patients with thrombocytosis although it should be used in caution in patients with coronary artery disease. Allopurinol should be used in patients with significantly elevated uric acid levels due to high RBC turnover, provided any acute gout attack has already been treated with colchicine, because allopurinol may precipitate uric acid deposition in the joints.

Subsequent Management

Subsequent management follows the steps taken in initial management. Patients with polycythemia vera will require repeated phlebotomies. Nonalkylating agents may be employed to suppress stem-cell formation, such as hydroxyurea (Hydrea) 60 to 80 mg/kg three times per week. Alkylating agents such as busulfan (Myleran) may also be used (1–3 mg/day as maintenance, with higher doses for induction), but these medications carrying a greater risk of long-term leukemia development. The risks of myelosuppression, such as systemic infection, must be considered with all of these agents, particularly if used at higher doses.

Secondary maintenance of patients with absolute polycythemia may also include antiplatelet aggregation therapy with aspirin although this treatment is controversial because the risk of thrombosis is also decreased with phlebotomy alone. If aspirin is used, a dose in the range of 81 to 325 mg/day should be sufficient although there is no consensus among hematologists and oncologists regarding the effectiveness of aspirin or the most appropriate dose in this population.

Follow-up and Referral
Relative Polycythemia

After dehydration has been treated, usually no long-term follow-up or referral is required, provided the underlying cause of the dehydration has been addressed. However, follow-up of patients who receive diuretics should be based on the need to monitor electrolytes and the therapeutic aims of diuretic therapy (e.g., follow-up of cardiac function). In turn, evaluating for normal potassium and sodium levels is an important goal of follow-up visits typically scheduled at 3-month intervals for patients maintained on chronic diuretic therapy.

Absolute Polycythemia

Because weekly phlebotomies are required to achieve and maintain an Hct of 45% or less, weekly assessments of the CBC and brief office visits are also necessitated. An initial referral to a hematologist is also required to confirm the diagnosis and establish the plan of care. If secondary management strategies such as myelosuppression are required, the clinician should rely on the hematologist for recommendations and comanagement. Specialty referral is also important because polycythemia vera carries a significant risk of transforming over time into myelofibrosis with myeloid metaplasia or acute myeloid leukemia.

Referrals to surgeons are required for tumor excision or pituitary resection, if indicated. A positive finding from computed tomography of the abdomen or magnetic resonance imaging of the brain should involve an immediate surgical consultation. A pulmonary referral may become necessary if the clinician does not detect lower carboxyhemoglobin levels as expected after a patient stops smoking.

Patient Education

Patients should learn that absolute polycythemia reduces life span. On average, patients live for less than 15 years after this diagnosis because of the risks of thrombosis. In spite of this grim prognosis, however, they should be reassured that active participation in their care may extend the quality of their lives and may increase longevity.

Increased quality of life is associated with improvement in the subjective presentation of the disease. Points to address in patient education include adherence to fluid intake requirements, drug regimens, exercise recommendations, laboratory evaluations, and adherence to follow-up visit schedules with the clinician and all specialty referrals.

Fluid intake requirements may fluctuate according to the stage and duration of treatment. As the disease progresses and phlebotomies occur repeatedly, the daily fluid intake should average 2 L for a 70-kg adult. Earlier in the treatment before blood volume is reduced, the necessary fluid intake is likely to be less—on average, 1 to 1.5 L/day. Drug regimen adherence may require learning how to self-medicate with a parenteral agent such as IFN-α. Therefore, teaching the patient and/or loved one how to deliver the drug is essential to the educational plan.

Instruction regarding exercise is dependent on the patient's level of tolerance for physical activity. The goal, however, should remain clear that increasing the level of activity can reduce thrombosis formation. Simplest among exercise plans for persons older than age 60 years is regular walking. The clinician should recommend that the patient walk with a friend in a safe place, such as an indoor shopping mall. An alternative is walking from side to side in a pool of waist-high water. This form of aquatic exercise can be helpful for patients with joint- and bone-related immobilities who otherwise experience increased pain when walking out of water.

Adherence to laboratory evaluations may diminish over time as the patient copes with this chronic and indolently fatal disease. Drawing the family and other loved ones into the circle of education and social support may enhance the patient's adherence to follow-up regimens. Call-back schedules for laboratory evaluations that fit with the individual's daily activities and provide rhythm to the patient's life are more likely to generate improved adherence.

Finally, visits to the clinician and specialists are times when patient education should be reinforced. Importantly, addressing and treating depression—an anticipated outcome of absolute polycythemia—can enhance adherence to all other elements of patient education. Therefore, teaching the patient and loved ones to recognize and report depression is a critical component of the educational plan.

■ LEUKEMIA

Leukemia is a neoplastic disease of malignant hematopoietic stem cells that differentiate and proliferate according to specific lineage trajectories that distinguish the types of leukemia as either acute or chronic. Further classification of leukemia specifies the stage of development and type of white blood cell (WBC) (immunophenotype) that is involved in the malignant transformation (see Table 17.2). The involved leukocytes proliferate and occupy space previously filled by nonmalignant cell lines. Thus, one significant outcome of the malignancy is the suppression of nonmalignant blood cells.

Epidemiology and Causes

The incidence of leukemias varies according to childhood and adult age groups. Overall, there is a slight predominance of male to female cases. Acute lymphoblastic leukemia (ALL) is the predominant form in children between 2 and 15 years of age, with higher prevalence seen among children younger than 5 years.

Other types of leukemia more commonly strike adults. Acute granulocytic leukemia (AGL) and acute myelocytic leukemia (AML) may be seen in adults of all ages, but their incidence increases after age 40 years. The

Table 17.2 Types of Leukemia and Treatment

	Age at Onset	Treatment—Combination Chemotherapy*	Treatment*—Other
Acute Leukemia			
Acute lymphocytic/ lymphoblastic leukemia (ALL)	2–15 years, rarely in adults	*Induction:* 4-drug regimen daunorubicin (Cerubidine) vincristine (Oncovin) prednisone (Deltasone) asparaginase (DVP L-asp) *Consolidation:* daunorubicin (Cerubidine) cytarabine (Ara-C) *Maintenance:* 4-drug regimen	CNS intrathecal methotrexate and cranial irradiation Allogeneic BMT in high-risk patients in first remission
Acute nonlymphocytic leukemia (ANLL) or acute myelogenous leukemia (AML) and acute granulocytic leukemia (AGL)	All adults but more prominent >40 years	daunorubicin (Cerubidine) OR idarubicin (Idamycin) OR mitoxantrone PLUS cytarabine (Ara-C)	Autologous or allogeneic BMT for high-risk patients in first remission
Chronic Leukemia			
Chronic granulocytic leukemia (CGL) or chronic myelogenous leukemia (CML)	All patients, but more prominent >60 years Median age 42 years	imatinib (Gleevec) PLUS hydroxyurea (Hydrea)	Allogeneic BMT in chronic phase (greater success in younger patients)
Chronic lymphocytic leukemia (CLL)	>60 years	cladribine OR fludarabine (Fludara) OR chlorambucil (Leukeran) PLUS cyclophosphamide May be used in combination with rituximab (Rituxan) or alemtuzumab (Campath)	Allogeneic BMT

*For all leukemias, the need for epoetin (Epogen, Procrit), darbepoetin (Aranesp), and/or pegfilgrastim (Neulasta) must be assessed.

incidence of acute lymphocytic leukemia increases in adults older than age 60 years. Chronic lymphocytic leukemia (CLL) and chronic granulocytic leukemia (CGL) are more prevalent among adults older than age 60 years; however, they may appear in persons of any age. CLL is the most common leukemia in developed Western countries, with a median age of onset of 70 years. Chronic myelocytic or myelogenous leukemia (CML) strikes middle-aged persons, with a median age of 42 years.

The etiology of leukemia is complex and not fully understood. Researchers have linked leukemia to environmental toxins such as chemical solvents, petroleum products, and insecticides, as well as heredity, although familial leukemias are rare. It is unclear whether the incidence of leukemia is higher among adult identical twins than among other adults; however, CLL in particular appears to have a familial predisposition.

The complications of mutagenic pharmacotherapies used to treat lymphoma, rheumatoid arthritis, or to maintain immunosuppression post-transplantation have provided insight into disease etiology. For example, alkylating agents, such as melphalan (Alkeran) and cisplatin (Platinol), have been implicated in a 5% to 10% increased incidence of leukemia among patients who have been receiving them for an extended period of time. Likewise, prolonged exposure to high doses of ionizing radiation is also associated with leukemia. In cases of prolonged toxin and radiation exposure, a latency of up to 20 years may pass before a leukemia diagnosis is established. Shorter latency periods are seen following exposure to chemotherapeutic agents that inhibit the

DNA-splicing enzyme topoisomerase II, such as etoposide, doxorubicin, or mitoxantrone.

Pathophysiology
Acute Nonlymphocytic Leukemia

By far, the largest number of adults with acute leukemia (as high as 80%) suffer from acute nonlymphocytic leukemia (ANLL). ANLL is a category that includes the leukemias formerly known as AML and AGL. ANLL presents after age 40 years and increases in incidence with each year thereafter. It originates in the malignant transformation of a single stem cell or a few select cells. At least 85% of all cases have been associated with defined clonal karyotypic abnormalities. Cells in the progenitor line are universally affected, thus providing a clue that the leukemia is intrinsic to the cell line following malignant transformation.

ANLL has been divided into eight distinct morphological classes (M0 to M7), according to the French-American-British (FAB) system, with classes M3 to M5 further subdivided into two subclasses each. Thus, the pathophysiology of ANLL is exceedingly complex. Each of these subtypes is characterized by one or more cytogenetic abnormalities that may be used to predict prognosis and guide treatment, as they can determine responsiveness to specific chemotherapies. For example, acute promyelocytic leukemia (AML class M3) is associated with a translocation between chromosomes 15 and 17 that juxtaposes the PML and retinoic acid receptor (RAR)–alpha genes, repressing the latter and preventing retinoic acid–induced differentiation of promyelocytes. Nonetheless, this mutation portends a favorable prognosis, as promyelocytic M3 cells are particularly sensitive to therapy with all-trans retinoic acid (ATRA).

In contrast, abnormalities that carry a particularly poor prognosis include mutations with monosomy (entire chromosomal deletion) of chromosomes 5 or 7 or trisomy of chromosome 8. The former monosomies are particularly associated with AML resulting from previous chemotherapy with alkalinizing agents or exposure to ionizing radiation. In contrast, AML associated with past exposure to topoisomerase II inhibiting agents is often associated with mutations in chromosome 11.

Acute myeloblastic leukemia (AML class M2) and acute myelomonocytic leukemia (AML class M4) have both been associated with a balanced translocation between chromosomes 8 and 21, which juxtaposes the transcription factor genes *AML1* and *ETO,* leading to dysregulated transcription of genes directly involved in myeloid cell division (e.g., granulocyte-monocyte colony stimulating factor, interleukin-3, and the antiapoptotic gene *BCL-2*). AML class M4 has also been associated with inversions or translocations in chromosome 16, creating a fusion of the genes *CBFB* and *MYH11,* which leads to repressed transcription of genes involved in myelocytic differentiation. Acute monoblastic leukemia (AML class M5) is associated with rearrangements of chromosome 11, whereas mutations in chromosome 3 appear to confer thrombocytosis in the setting of AML.

Acute Lymphoblastic Leukemia

ALL can appear among persons of all ages but is clearly a disease predominantly of early childhood, as noted earlier. B-cell lymphoblasts or, in far fewer cases, T-cell lymphoblasts increase in number after a single hematopoietic stem cell undergoes transformation (immortalization). Interestingly, the cytogenetics of ALL in children is far different from that in adults. For instance, the Philadelphia chromosome (a balanced translocation between chromosomes 9 and 22 that juxtaposes and activates the *BCR* and *ABL* oncogenes) is seen in only 5% of childhood cases, whereas this is the most common abnormality in adult ALL and may be found in up to 40% of cases. In contrast, hyperdiploidy (in which greater than 50 chromosomes are found in malignant clones) is seen in up to 30% of childhood cases but in no more than 5% of affected adults.

In contrast to CML (see next section), the presence of the Philadelphia chromosome is a poor prognostic indicator in ALL, contributing to dysregulated activation of the RAS intracellular signaling pathway that leads to uncontrolled cell division. These patients often have additional karyotypic abnormalities such as monosomy of chromosome 7. Studies have shown that ALL patients with the Philadelphia chromosome may be divided into two subsets that are distinguished by differing translocation breakpoints along the BCR gene—one in which this karyotypic abnormality appears restricted to a B lineage lymphoblastic cell clone and another in which the Philadelphia chromosome is further identified in myelogenous cell lines as well, indicating that these patients may actually have a indolent form of CML that underwent a B-lineage lymphoblastic crisis at the time of diagnosis.

As with AML, different forms of ALL have been distinguished on the basis of morphology, with certain cytogenetic profiles correlating with each. For instance, ALL of L3-type B-cell origin often shares a translocation of chromosomes 8 and 14 that is also seen in B-cell–derived Burkitt's lymphoma, suggesting that these cancers are varied manifestations of the same underlying malignant transformation event. Pre–B-cell ALL has been associated with translocations between chromosomes 1 and 19, which lead to a fusion protein between the highly active transcription factors *E2A* and *PBX1,* with subsequent immortalization of this early B-cell progenitor and a particularly poor prognosis. Infantile ALL has been associated in up to 80% of cases with translocations involving the mixed lineage leukemia (MLL) gene at chromosome 11q23, which is thought to regulate a number of downstream genes involved in lymphocyte differentiation, thereby resulting in extremely poor outcomes. A poor prognosis is also seen in ALL associated with translocations between chromosomes 4 and 11, a mutation that is commonly seen in AML class M5.

Translocation between chromosomes 12 and 21 that produces a fusion protein between the transcription factors *TEL* and *AML1* is the most common mutation seen in childhood ALL. Fortunately, this translocation confers a favorable prognosis in ALL, as does the presence of hyperdiploidy (a cellular complement of 50–60 chromosomes) with occasional structural abnormalities such as partial duplications and translocations. Multiple copies of chromosome 21 and the X chromosome are the most common findings in hyperdiploidy, but several other duplications have been noted as well (e.g., chromosomes 4, 6, 10, and 14). The high prevalence of these karyotypic abnormalities in childhood ALL underlies the generally favorable outcomes associated with this leukemia in children.

T-cell ALL is a less common entity that typically strikes young men. Related to T-cell lymphomas, these patients may present with particularly high WBC counts, invasion of malignant cells into the central nervous system (CNS) via the cerebrospinal fluid, and the presence of a mediastinal tumor. Well over half of these cancers are characterized by mutations in genes coding for the various protein components of the T-cell receptor—alpha, beta, gamma, or delta subunits. The T-cell receptor is a heterodimeric protein composed of either alpha–beta or gamma–delta subunits, expressed on the surface of the T cell, allowing for the recognition of specific antigens. Mutations commonly occur in chromosome 14, which encodes the alpha and delta receptor subunits, or chromosome 7, which encodes the genes for the beta and gamma chains. Translocations at these sites typically juxtapose these genes with various transcription factors that lead to dysregulated expression of the receptor subunit and proliferation of the T-cell clone. Mutations in the same chromosomes that do not involve these receptor subunits as well as others such as chromosomes 6 and 11 have also been identified in T-cell ALL. Interestingly, prognosis does not appear tied to these particular cytogenetics, and outcomes are generally favorable in both adults and children with T-cell ALL.

Chronic Myelogenous Leukemia

CML (chronic myelocytic leukemia, chronic myeloid leukemia) is most commonly associated with the development of the Philadelphia chromosome in a hematopoietic stem cell that commits to the myeloid lineage. Although differentiation is typically unaffected, the leukemic stem cell is self-renewing and produces a tremendous number of daughter cells, with the same leukemic clone dominating up to 90% of the bone marrow at the time of diagnosis. In this mutation, breaks occur in the DNA resulting in an equivalent exchange of genetic material between chromosomes 9 and 22. Oncogene activation occurs, as the reciprocal translocation [t(9;22)(q34;q11)] juxtaposes the *BCR* and c-*ABL* genes, creating a BCR–ABL fusion protein that confers a proliferative advantage to the leukemic clone, even in the absence of cellular growth factors.

The functions of the native BCR and ABL proteins are not fully elucidated, and neither gene alone is capable of malignant transformation; however, the fusion protein is oncogenic, giving rise to malignant clones through upregulated tyrosine kinase (phosphorylation) activity within a number of intracellular signaling pathways contributing to cell division (e.g., RAS, c-myc, and JAK/STAT molecular pathways). This explains the effectiveness of treatment with the tyrosine kinase inhibitor imatinib (Gleevec). Depending on the site of the chromosomal breaks, various types of the BCR-ABL fusion protein may be formed. In turn, cells transformed by these different species appear to respond differentially to specific therapies.

Although IL-3 and G-CSF mRNA transcripts are both upregulated in leukemic cell clones, the precise role of cytokines in the dysregulated growth of these cells remains unclear. As with other forms of leukemia, leukemic cell clones appear to arise from a self-renewing pool of mutated leukemic stem cells, which are typically less mature than the differentiated granulocytic leukemic clones themselves. In fact, the Philadelphia chromosome has been further identified in a number of cell lineages in CML, including granulocyte, macrophage, erythrocyte, megakaryocyte (platelet), and B-lymphocyte precursor cells, indicating that the mutation first occurs in an early, noncommitted, multilineage hematopoietic stem cell.

The creation of the Philadelphia chromosome may predate the onset of disease symptoms by many years, a pattern suggesting that the disease progresses through a latent or asymptomatic phase before becoming active. For example, the karyotypic abnormality may first arise in the third decade of life, with symptom onset as much as 10 to 20 years later. In fact, normal bone marrow function is characteristic of the disease trajectory in the early years after development of the Philadelphia chromosome. The pool of leukemic stem cells may not be expanded in number; however, leukemic daughter cells undergo clonal expansion and eventually crowd out normal bone marrow components. In addition, cell surface adhesion factors (e.g., beta-1 integrin) are downregulated, eliminating adhesion-dependent growth inhibition in which normal cells are triggered to stop proliferating after coming into contact with one another.

As with any chronic leukemia, a dreaded complication of CML is degeneration into a leukemic blast crisis, in which leukemic progenitor cells develop self-renewing properties as they undergo further mutations resulting in clonal proliferation of either myeloid or lymphoid (almost exclusively B lineage) blasts, given the widespread presence of the Philadelphia chromosome in multiple lineages. Most commonly, the additional mutations described include trisomies of chromosomes 8 or 19, duplication of the Philadelphia chromosome itself, or mutations in the *p53* tumor suppressor gene on chromosome 17. These blast cells may express many of the same proteins as hematopoietic stem cells, such as the transcription factor beta-catenin. Both leukemic stem cells and their progeny appear more resistant to apoptosis than wild-type (nonmutated) cells, but the significance of this to the pathogenesis of CML is not fully known. However, resistance to apoptosis appears to be important, because the life span of leukemic cell clones is not significantly greater than that of wild-type granulocytes and does not appear to account for their increase in number.

Finally, CML may also occur in the absence of the Philadelphia chromosome mutation, which is known as atypical CML. Up to 15% of CML patients may suffer from this condition, although some hematologist-oncologists have chosen to classify these patients as having a distinct myeloproliferative disease, rather than true CML. For reasons that are poorly understood, these patients have a worse prognosis with a poorer response to therapy and shorter survival times.

Chronic Lymphocytic Leukemia

CLL is a chronic lymphoproliferative disorder typically associated with increased numbers of small B lymphocytes. In fact, it is clinically indistinguishable from small lymphocytic B-cell lymphoma. After a malignant alteration occurs in a B-cell precursor, thus forming a malignant line, the clonal abnormality is passed on to slowly replicating progeny that are functionally incompetent.

The genetics of the malignant alteration in CLL are not as well established as they are for CML. Malignant B cell clones are known to be frozen in a state of differentiation somewhere between the pre-B and mature B-cell phase, with rates of proliferation and cell death varying widely among different individuals. These cells express very low levels of surface immunoglobulin, various B-cell–specific cell surface proteins (e.g., CD19, CD20, CD21), as well as CD5, which is primarily considered a T-cell marker. Variant forms exist that do not adhere to these criteria, although some hematologist-oncologists feel that a proliferation of non–CD5-expressing B cells represents a leukemic phase of non-Hodgkin's lymphoma, rather than true CLL.

The relative percentages of both T cells and natural killer (NK) cells are reduced in CLL, although absolute numbers of T lymphocytes may be increased, given the tremendous expansion of lymphocytes. Moreover, some CLL patients demonstrate unusual forms of T cells with low levels of surface CD4 and CD8 proteins. Such nonclassical T cells are also found in other autoimmune diseases. In addition, although hypogammaglobulinemia is common in patients with CLL, immunoglobulin receptors on leukemic cells may demonstrate autoimmune specificity, which may explain the increased frequency of AIHA, idiopathic thrombocytopenic purpura (ITP), and pure red cell aplasia in persons with CLL. Owing to their lack of protective antibodies, infection by gram-negative or encapsulated organisms is the most frequent cause of morbidity and mortality in persons with CLL.

Cytogenetic analysis of CLL cell clones has revealed chromosomal abnormalities in up to 70% of cases. The most frequent karyotypic abnormalities include trisomy of chromosome 12, partial deletions in chromosome 13 that affect the tumor suppressor retinoblastoma gene, and partial deletions in chromosomes 11 and 17 that are associated with a particularly poor prognosis and shorter survival. The *p53* tumor suppressor gene located on chromosome 17 is often affected, either by deletion or expression of a mutated, nonfunctional protein, with both conditions leading to unregulated cellular proliferation. In contrast, the overexpression of survival factors has also been identified in B lineage CLL, including the antiapoptotic molecules BCL-2 and inducible nitric oxide synthetase.

Clinical Presentation
Subjective

Patients with acute leukemia complain of bone and joint pain. Fevers, chills, palpitations, shortness of breath, and signs of infection typically constitute the initial subjective presentation. Patients may also have gingival bleeding associated with gingival hyperplasia. Skin eruptions, easy bruising, or prolonged bleeding time from simple wounds form a significant part of the subjective history.

Patients with chronic leukemia complain of fatigue, night sweats, and low-grade fevers. Although there is no clear differentiation in subjective findings between CML and CLL, CML may present with the symptoms of leukostasis associated with very high WBC counts (greater than 500,000 cells/mcL). The syndrome of leukostasis is characterized by blurred vision, respiratory distress, and occasionally priapism (prolonged and painful erection that lasts for several hours). Nausea and vomiting may be associated with organomegaly in both types of chronic leukemia. Bone and joint pain are typically limited to the myeloproliferative stages of CML.

Objective

The clinician will often note a high fever in patients with acute leukemia. Tachycardia and tachypnea are related findings. Patients appear pale and manifest eruptions such as petechiae and purpura. The patient's confusion—related to hypoxemia and fever—may be evident using standardized evaluation tools such as the Folstein Mini–Mental State Exam (MMSE).

In chronic leukemia patients, heart and lung sounds are typically within normal limits except during infection, in which case the lungs may reveal adventitious sounds. Splenomegaly may be evident and variably associated with hepatomegaly and/or lymph node enlargement. Temperature may not be elevated in chronic leukemia, as it often is in acute leukemia, unless the disease has progressed or there is a concurrent infection. In addition, the patient's skin color varies between pale and normal, and few, if any, skin eruptions are evident.

Diagnostic Reasoning

Diagnostic Tests

Initial testing for suspected acute leukemia includes a CBC with peripheral blood smear and platelet count. The WBC count may be significantly elevated (more than 300,000 cells/mcL). Granulocytes (polysegmented and banded forms) are typically diminished in number as will be platelets (often less than 50,000/mcL). A hematocrit of less than 30% is a common finding, especially if the WBC count is markedly elevated. The peripheral smear reveals a blastocystosis of greater than 25% in almost all cases.

Initial tests for suspected chronic leukemia are the same as for acute leukemia: CBC, peripheral blood smear, and platelet count. The WBC count should be elevated in CML and CLL, but typically more so in CML (elevations greater than 100,000 cells/mcL are common). Lymphocytosis, however, differentiates CLL from CML. Lymphocytes occupy as much as 90% of the peripheral smear in CLL. The peripheral smear of CML is characterized by a left-shifted myeloid series, with mature forms of myeloid cells predominant in the smear. Platelets may be elevated and are rarely diminished.

Subsequent testing for both acute and chronic leukemia includes a bone marrow aspirate. Results should parallel the peripheral blood smear, thus confirming the initial diagnosis with greater accuracy in quantitative and qualitative indices. In acute leukemia, the bone marrow aspirate reveals hypercellular components, which are dominated by blasts. At least 30% of the cells must be blasts to diagnose acute leukemia. Auer bodies are rod-shaped structures, present in the cytoplasm of myeloblasts, myelocytes, and monoblasts in leukemic patients. They predominate among myeloblasts in the bone marrow aspirates of patients with AML. Serum chemistry profiles are critical for secondary testing in acute leukemia patients because of rapid cell turnover in the WBC population, which liberates intracellular uric acid and leads to significant increases in serum concentration.

In CML, bone marrow evaluation typically reveals the Philadelphia chromosome along with a left-shifted myelopoiesis. Blasts occupy less than 5% of the aspirate sample. Subsequent testing of CML also includes measuring leukocyte alkaline phosphatase, which is usually low, thus reflecting the abnormal function of neutrophils. Additional testing includes measuring the vitamin B_{12} level and serum chemistries. The vitamin B_{12} level should be elevated, as should the uric acid level.

Subsequent CLL bone marrow results confirm the initial peripheral blood smear. Small, mature lymphocytes dominate the field. Surface immunoglobulin on the monoclonal malignant lymphocytes aids in distinguishing these small cells from their normal counterparts. Another secondary test, immuno-electrophoresis, further supports the diagnosis of CLL in about half of patients. The profile from the electrophoresis shows that the patient is hypogammaglobulinemic.

Molecular methods of cytogenetic analysis (fluorescent in situ hybridization [FISH], Southern blot, reverse transcriptase–polymerase chain reaction [RT-PCR]) to identify the Philadelphia chromosome and other karyotypic abnormalities are critical for predicting prognosis and determining the most effective treatment plan for each type of leukemia. These analyses have revolutionized leukemia treatment by facilitating the use of individualized, directed therapy.

Differential Diagnosis

Acute Leukemia The left-shifted (immature) bone marrow aspirate of acute leukemia must be distinguished from the left-shifted aspirates that are associated with recent exposure to toxic chemicals and radiation. The clinician should expect that the full recovery period after toxic exposure will be at least 6 weeks and may extend to 12 weeks. It is possible to rule out so-called false-positive left-shifted aspirates by repeating the procedure several days later. If the exposure to toxins and not monoclonal malignant mutations was the cause, then the subsequent test should reveal maturing cell lines.

Acute leukemias must be distinguished from their chronic counterparts and from similar myeloproliferative disorders, such as polycythemia. ALL resembles lymphoproliferative diseases, such as lymphomas and mononucleosis; therefore, a skilled pathologist is required to distinguish the lymphoproliferative disorders from particular acute leukemias.

Chronic Leukemia The Philadelphia chromosome of CML distinguishes this disease from myeloproliferative responses to infection, systemic inflammation, and other malignancies. Clinical wisdom will also help the practitioner distinguish the leukocytosis of CML from other reactive states. CML will likely present with more than 50,000 cells/mcL, but reactive states will not mount as great a response. In addition, CML is clearly different from other myeloproliferative diseases; the erythrocyte count, RBC indices, and hematocrit are generally normal in CML.

Microscopic evaluation of a bone marrow aspirate differentiates CLL from other lymphocytic disorders, such as viral infections. Unlike CLL, viral infections will present with flu-like symptoms, which include fever, chills, myalgias, and arthralgias. Thus, CLL is perhaps the easiest among the leukemias to distinguish.

Management

The probability of successful treatment and subsequent cure for acute leukemia decreases with increasing age. In addition, a cure for acute leukemia is less probable if the patient is diagnosed late in the disease trajectory, after several physiological systems have become involved. In general, treatment begins with combination chemotherapy to induce remission (i.e., induction phase), followed by a stage of chemotherapy called the consolidation phase, and finally a prolonged maintenance phase. Unlike the acute leukemias, the chronic leukemias usually follow an indolent course, which means that myelosuppressive chemotherapy may not be initiated until symptoms necessitate action. Symptoms, therefore, are managed as they appear.

Acute Leukemia

ANLL patients receive combination chemotherapy. (Medications are listed in Table 17.2.) The oncologist will set the dose ranges for at least two drugs—daunorubicin (Cerubidine) or idarubicin (Idamycin) plus cytarabine (Ara-C). The clinician is responsible for monitoring hepatic function throughout the course of combination therapy, which may run in 3- to 6-day cycles every 3 to 4 weeks for a total of 3 to 6 months, depending on successful remission and patient tolerance. Combination therapy produces bone marrow aplasia, which abates after 2 weeks following the conclusion of therapy. Aplastic patients, therefore, require supportive antibiotic prophylaxis, vigorous stoma care given severe denuding of mucosal surfaces, and possible RBC transfusions. The clinician's role is to comanage the adverse effects of the chemotherapy and to monitor serum chemistries, including liver function tests.

Adult patients with ALL may enter remission in initial management (albeit not as quickly or easily as children with ALL) without the aplastic disorders associated with the initial treatment of AML. Combination chemotherapy is the mainstay for initial management, including vincristine (Oncovin), daunorubicin (Cerubidine), and prednisone (Deltasone). Other combinations are under investigation. Comanagement with the oncologist is the same as for patients with ANLL, except that vigorous stoma care and associated weight reduction may not figure as prominently in ALL. Glucose intolerance may develop due to prednisone therapy, particularly in patients suffering from diabetes mellitus at baseline. Thus, the clinician is responsible for making adjustments to antidiabetic agents during chemotherapy.

After remission has been achieved for the patient with acute leukemia, a consolidation course of management is begun. Consolidation cycles differ for the acute leukemias. ANLL patients receive one complete chemotherapy consolidation cycle. Alternatively, they may receive a bone marrow transplantation (BMT) to consolidate the gains of earlier therapy. Transplantation may be autologous (an individual's own marrow saved before treatment), allogeneic (marrow donated by someone else), or syngeneic (marrow donated by an identical twin). Advanced Practice Nursing Interventions 17.1 presents information that should be provided to the patient who will be undergoing bone marrow transplantation.

Patients with ALL, on the other hand, face different challenges. They must receive CNS prophylaxis against malignant lymphocytes that may have crossed the blood–brain barrier to hide in meningeal crypts. CNS prophylaxis typically consists of intrathecal methotrexate and cranial irradiation.

Chronic Leukemia

Patients with CML are initially managed with watchful vigilance. Should treatment be required for extreme hyperleukocytosis–related symptoms, such as blurred vision and respiratory distress, leukophoresis may be initiated. In addition, depending on severity of symptoms, hydroxyurea (Hydrea) may be initiated at 2 to 4 g/day PO, followed by maintenance therapy of 0.5 to 2 g/day. The leukopenic goal of 5,000 to 10,000 WBCs/mcL requires frequent monitoring.

Symptom management and clinical vigilance are the initial therapies for patients with CLL. Symptoms that require intervention include thrombocytopenia (less than 50,000 platelets/mcL), anemia (less than 27% Hct), lymphadenopathy that impedes activities of daily living, and fatigue that reduces nutritional intake and immobilizes the patient. Whereas some sources cite a threshold of 50,000 platelets/mcL for thrombocytopenia requiring intervention, most oncologists tolerate much lower values before giving transfusions of platelets (even as low as 10,000/mcL, provided there is no active bleeding). If combination chemotherapy is utilized, the monitoring of platelet and erythrocyte counts is required because of myelosuppression secondary to chemotherapy.

Exogenous erythropoietin (Epogen, Procrit, or Aranesp) may assist in countering chemotherapy-induced anemia. In addition, the use of pegfilgrastim (Neulasta) and other granulocyte colony-stimulating factors may counter neutropenia.

Follow-up and Referral

When suspicion is elevated concerning a diagnosis of leukemia, the clinician should refer the patient to an oncologist. Pertinent laboratory results along with a clinical history should accompany the patient for the oncologist's appointment, although the oncologist typically requests and interprets bone marrow analyses.

For the patient with acute leukemia, comanagement of adverse effects from combination chemotherapy will require primary care follow-up monthly during the course of chemotherapy. The oncologist will direct treatment recommendations and adjustments and supervise laboratory analyses. The primary care clinician will provide oversight of the same laboratory results, along with recommendations for symptom management.

For the patient with chronic leukemia, if clinical vigilance is all that is required, the clinician should order laboratory evaluations including a CBC, platelet count, and peripheral blood smear every 6 weeks. Depending on symptom onset and severity, physical examinations may be done as infrequently as every 2 to 3 months, if the patient is otherwise stable. Once chemotherapy intervention begins, however, the oncologist will make treatment recommendations and alterations.

Advanced Practice Nursing Interventions 17.1   Bone Marrow Transplantation

The following information should be provided to patients undergoing bone marrow transplantation.

What It Is

A bone marrow transplantation (BMT) is the intravenous administration of 500–700 mL of bone marrow. The patient is "conditioned" to receive the bone marrow through a regimen of immunosuppressive therapy (chemotherapy or radiation). This conditioning eradicates malignant cells, provides immunosuppression, and creates a space for the bone marrow to engraft the transplanted marrow stem cells. The marrow is usually infused 48–72 hours after the patient's last dose of chemotherapy or radiation.

The bone marrow is "harvested" from a donor. It may be an autologous transplant (aspirated from the pelvic bones of the patient during a remission), an allogeneic transplant (from a compatible donor such as a parent or sibling with a similar tissue type), or a syngeneic transplant (from an identical twin). Peripheral stem cell transplants are currently the state of the art in bone marrow reconstitution, in which rare peripherally circulating stem cells are collected from the donor through an apheresis procedure, rather than harvesting whole marrow directly from the pelvic bones. This has greatly reduced the pain, discomfort, and complications associated with bone marrow (i.e., hematopoietic stem cell) donation.

What Will Happen Before the Procedure

• The health-care provider should provide complete information about the specific procedure (e.g., pretreatment, medication and activity restrictions), answer any questions, and provide emotional support.

• The patient should prepare for an extended hospital stay.
• The patient should prepare for side effects that are anticipated with immunosuppressant and cytoablative therapies (e.g., nausea, vomiting, cataracts, sterility, hair loss).

What Will Happen During the Procedure

• The nursing staff will do the following:
1. Monitor vital signs and for complications (e.g., allergic reactions, fluid overload, pulmonary embolism)
2. Provide support and reassurance

What Will Happen After the Procedure

• The nursing staff will monitor the following:
1. Routine vital signs
2. Signs and symptoms of infection (e.g., fever and chills)
3. Potential complications from chemotherapy given to prevent graft-versus-host disease
4. Signs and symptoms of graft-versus-host disease (e.g., rash, jaundice, joint pain, diarrhea, failure to engraft [pancytopenia])
• Mouth and skin care will be provided every 2 hours to help prevent infection
• IM injections will be avoided because they may lead to increased bleeding into the muscles

What To Do After Discharge

• Avoid infection by staying away from crowds and people with known infections
• Avoid sharp objects; for example, shave with an electric razor rather than an exposed razor blade

Patient Education

The patient may not be prepared for diseased-based education soon after receiving a clinical diagnosis of leukemia; therefore, it is important to involve not only the patient but also significant others in any education provided. Particular attention should be focused on treatment recommendations and their proposed impact on daily life and the patient's state of well-being. Treatment recommendations that include myelosuppressive therapies will require self-care activities that may not be in the patient's repertoire of capabilities. Thus, education should begin with an assessment of the patient's ability to monitor for infection, adverse effects of treatments, integrity of skin and mucous membranes, and fluid/nutritional status. Any deficits in the patient's ability to follow through with self-assessment should increase suspicion of complications from treatment yet to come; thus, resources that can aid the patient in self-assessment should be lined up before treatment is started.

In addition to self-assessment, the patient's education must address the anticipated burden on caregivers. Older patients and family members may not be able to adapt to the demands of treatment schedules, aplastic crises, and the like. A number of strategies can assist in this regard. The clinician should plan teaching sessions with the patient and caregivers present. The information should be repeated in subsequent sessions, and the patient should be asked to recall and repeat instructions provided in earlier sessions to confirm proper understanding. In addition, the clinician should monitor not only the patient but also caregivers for signs of strain and possible depression.

Patients need to be reassured that for all forms of leukemia, clinical vigilance is a form of treatment just as surely as is chemotherapy. Thus, if clinical vigilance is indicated, the patient and caregivers should learn the reasons to withhold pharmacological interventions while maintaining a watchful eye. Finally, patient education may require referral to support groups with other patients who have learned to live with cancer. Thus, referrals can include connections to other patients with leukemia within a primary care practice as well as support groups convened by local chapters of the American Cancer Society. The goal of support group referral is to advance the patient's connection with others who can share treatment-related information and advance coping strategies. Caregivers may require a separate support group where they can discuss issues that are unique to their role.

COMMON IMMUNE PROBLEMS

■ ALLERGIC REACTIONS

Allergy is defined as an immune-mediated reaction to a foreign environmental allergen. It is characterized by an inflammatory response to allergen exposure to the body. Typical sites for allergen exposure are the skin and respiratory tree, where local reactions may occur. Allergen exposure may also lead to a systemic response, however, whereby multiple organs and the circulatory system may become involved. Allergenic shock or anaphylaxis is an extreme example of this systemic response.

Atopy is a term used to characterize an IgE-mediated immune response that is exaggerated or out of character for exposure to what appear to be innocuous environmental allergens. Whereas allergic skin reactions are classically characterized by raised, erythematous wheal and flare reactions termed urticarial plaques, another common allergic skin condition, atopic dermatitis, has several different manifestations whose pathophysiology extends beyond IgE-mediated allergic processes (see Chapter 7).

Epidemiology and Causes

In contrast to autoimmune reactions, which tend to have a female predominance, allergic reactions are equally distributed between the sexes, affecting women as often as men, without regard to race. The incidence of allergies is greater in children than adults, perhaps because of the immaturity of immune responses in children and the tendency toward humorally mediated T helper cell–2 (Th2) type responses.

Seasonal allergies vary according to hemispheric geography, which means that pollen, mold, and fungal spores affect individuals according to seasonal patterns of exposure in the Northern and Southern hemispheres. In North America, pollens rise and fall in a May to September pattern, whereas molds follow a March through December pattern in outdoor environments; therefore, there are only 2 to 3 months of the year, in the late winter, when pollens and molds tend not affect the population. During cold weather, however, individuals remain indoors for longer periods of time, which can increase the risk of more frequent exposure to dust mites and other indoor allergens, including indoor mold species that tend to propagate in cool, dark interior environments, such as damp basements or bathrooms.

Causes of allergies include a wide array of environmental allergens and the corresponding intrinsic immune complexes formed by the body as it mounts a vigorous response to allergenic exposure. Environmental allergens include natural *inhalants* such as pollen, mold, and fungal spores, *ingestants* such as food and drug allergens, *injectants* such as animal or insect venoms, and *contactants* including dust mites and their feces, animal hair and dander, as well as chemical components in hair- and skin-care products. Regardless of the source, the allergen invades the body, either locally or systemically, eliciting a complex immune-regulated response that results in either local or systemic effects.

Pathophysiology

All allergens are foreign substances to the body. Cellular and humoral immune responses occur after initial exposure to a foreign substance. Immune responses result from a complex, coordinated set of events requiring several different cell types, cell surface signaling proteins, and secreted regulatory cytokines. Key cell types include histamine-containing mast cells and basophils, as well as highly granular eosinophils. Also important are antibody-secreting plasma cells that are specialized, differentiated B-lineage cells designed to produce monoclonal antibody of a single antigenic specificity. Also important are CD4+ T helper cells that are also antigen specific and produce an array of regulatory cytokines after their T-cell receptors come into contact with specific antigens. Helper T cells of the Th2 class produce cytokines (e.g., IL-4, IL-5, IL-13) that upregulate humoral antibody-mediated immune responses, whereas Th1 helper T cells produce a separate set of cytokines (e.g., IFN-γ, IL-12) that upregulate cell-mediated antibody-independent cytotoxic responses.

According to the Gell-Coombs classification system, there are four basic types of immune responses to allergens (termed *hypersensitivity responses* as a group), categorized by whether or not they are dependent on circulating antibodies (types 1 through 3) or only cellular immune components (type 4). Type 1 immune responses are considered classic allergic hypersensitivity reactions. However, type 3 immune responses often underlie what are termed *drug and food allergies,* whereas type 4 immune reactions mediate contact dermatitis, a pathological response to certain skin irritants, such as the allergens in poison ivy and poison oak.

Type 1: IgE-Mediated Immediate Hypersensitivity Response

In the first step of initial exposure to an allergen, the immune system must recognize that the allergen is foreign. Immunoglobulin E (IgE) is an immunoglobulin class present in relatively low concentration in the circulation. As with all immunoglobulins, IgE molecules are antigen specific in their variable arms, allowing for binding of more than one IgE molecule to a single circulating antigenic molecule. However, the constant portion of the IgE molecule (Fcε) allows for its binding to the surface of cells specifically expressing high-affinity receptors for the IgE molecule (FcεRIII). IgE molecules are bound to tissue-derived mast cells located primarily in the skin, respiratory system, and gastrointestinal (GI) tract, where allergens are most likely to contact or invade the body. In addition, circulating basophils are bound to allergen-specific IgE molecules.

Antibody cross-linking is the process by which two or more IgE molecules bound to the cell surface bind a common antigen, thereby triggering intracellular signaling and degranulation, with the release of cytokine mediators. Such responses do not typically occur on initial exposure to an allergen. On first exposure, specific IgE molecules are formed via class-switching of preformed antigen-specific B cells of the IgG or IgM classes to IgE, based on the constant portion of cell surface antibody molecules. These molecules then bind to mast cells and basophils, and upon reexposure to the same antigen when an allergen again binds to cell-bound antigen-specific IgE, a cascade of cellular events occurs, resulting in intracellular calcium shifts, which facilitate cyclic nucleotide signaling molecules to trigger leukocytic degranulation.

This leads to the excretion of preformed inflammatory mediators including histamine, heparin, tryptase, and other proteolytic enzymes, thromboxane, arachidonic acid, prostaglandins, superoxides, and several eosinophilic and neutrophilic chemotactic factors, as well as triggering the synthesis of newly formed inflammatory mediators including leukotrienes and key cytokines.

Inflammatory mediators cause venules, capillaries, and arterioles to dilate and become hyperpermeable. The mucous membranes are triggered to increase mucus excretion and the walls of hollow visceral structures to spasm as a result of smooth muscle contraction. Dehydration may result from a relative shift of fluid that follows intravascular proteins out of the vasculature and into the extravascular space, thus potentially lowering the blood pressure. Hypotension may also be aggravated by other environmental factors such as relative heat and humidity.

IgE activation and cellular excretion of inflammatory mediators may take place within seconds to minutes after antigenic exposure. Whereas the effects of initial inflammatory mediators may last for 30 minutes or less, repeated allergenic exposure can prolong the inflammatory cycle for hours. A prolonged and intractable inflammatory cycle produces the clinical picture of atopic (hypersensitivity) diseases characterized by type 1 allergic responses, such as allergic rhinitis and allergic asthma, which are heavily dependent on inflammatory cells including mast cells, eosinophils, and Th2 cells.

A second category of type 1 allergic reaction is *anaphylaxis*. Unlike atopic diseases, which are characterized by localized effects in the skin or respiratory tract, anaphylaxis is systemic in scope. All of the inflammatory processes of hypersensitivity become exaggerated, leading to life-threatening hypotension, bronchospasm, laryngospasm, angioedema, smooth muscle and visceral organ contractions, and raised inflammatory skin eruptions (generalized urticaria). Anaphylaxis may follow exposure in susceptible individuals to well known allergens, such as insect venom (bee or wasp stings) or certain drugs such as penicillin. However, these responses are not limited to individuals with a history of atopic disease and may occur unexpectedly in any individual. Therefore, a history of atopy does not predict anaphylaxis. If left untreated, anaphylaxis is typically fatal. Advanced Practice Nursing Interventions 17.2 describes a seven-step treatment algorithm for anaphylaxis.

Type 2: Antibody-Mediated Cellular Cytotoxicity Response

Type 2 antibody-mediated cellular cytotoxicity responses introduce an immune mechanism different from type 1

Advanced Practice Nursing Interventions 17.2
The Seven-Step Treatment For Anaphylaxis

- Step 1: Administer aqueous epinephrine 1:1,000 dilution 0.3–0.5 mg (0.3–0.5 mL) IM into the upper lateral thigh, in a supine position with head below heart level, if possible.
- Step 2: Repeat epinephrine every 5–15 minutes as required by clinical picture. If hypotensive, position the patient supine with feet elevated.
- Step 3: Support bronchodilation if patient is without laryngospasm by administering albuterol 3 mL (2.5 mg) inhalation via nebulizer.
- Step 4: If patient is in laryngospasm or pulmonary arrest, perform emergency endotracheal intubation and provide respiratory support.
- Step 5: Start IV fluids using normal saline or Ringer's lactate solution to maintain systolic blood pressure greater than 90 mm Hg. The rate of flow should be determined by the blood pressure reading but typically may be bolused.
- Step 6: If the patient is conscious and without laryngospasm, administer diphenhydramine (Benadryl) 25–50 mg to relieve cutaneous symptoms. H_2-blockers may also be added (particularly if GI symptoms are present) but have not been shown to be as effective as H_1-blockers.
- Step 7: Transfer the patient to an acute-care emergency center for continued support and observation. Add corticosteroids (IV or PO) to prevent late-phase anaphylactic reactions, which may be as severe as early-phase reactions.

See text regarding teaching about injectable epinephrine (EpiPen, Twinject).

immediate hypersensitivity responses. Type 2 responses involve the activation of antigen-specific IgM and IgG molecules. These humoral immune molecules bind to foreign antigens and activate serum immune complement. This leads to destruction of any cell to which an allergen-antibody complex is bound; thus, a type 2 immune response is cytotoxic. Examples of such type 2 responses include neonatal Rh-incompatibility hemolytic disease and immune-mediated hemolytic anemia. In addition, once antibodies bind to foreign antigens such as microbial cell surface proteins, these invading microbes become prone to phagocytosis and destruction by other immune cells, a process known as opsonization.

Type 3: Antibody–Allergen Immune Complex Response

The third category of immune responses also requires immunoglobulin M (IgM) and IgG activation, as is characteristic of a type 2 immune response. However, type 3 responses denote an immune complex that is formed between these immunoglobulins and the allergen. These complexes become deposited into the various tissues of the body, activating serum complement that in turn triggers various inflammatory mediators. These illnesses tend to be systemic, as immune complexes affect multiple organs and tissue types throughout the body. The reaction is not immediate, and in fact, may occur up to 2 to 3 weeks after antigenic exposure. Hypersensitivity-type pneumonitis secondary to inhaled allergen and serum sickness are two examples of type 3 immune responses. Delayed drug reactions are also classic examples of type 3 responses, with the most common offenders being the antiepileptic drugs phenytoin, phenobarbital, and carbamazepine, as well as various antibiotics.

Type 4: Delayed-Type Cellular Hypersensitivity Response

The fourth category of immune responses is defined as a cell-mediated delayed-type immune response that is unlike the three previous categories, which are all mediated by humoral factors (antibody-dependent). The other three categories directly involve few, if any, T lymphocytes. However, type 4 reactions are T-cell dependent and usually begin in the skin, where large numbers of T cells are found. Antigen contacting the skin is endocytosed (taken up) by antigen-presenting cells, which process and relocate small antigenic peptides on the cell surface, coupled to antigen-presenting proteins known as major histocompatibility complex (MHC) molecules.

Antigen-specific T-cell receptors recognize and bind to these antigenic peptide–MHC complexes, which leads to a series of inflammatory reactions including cellular lysis of the antigen-presenting cell and cytokine production. Because of this delay in cellular lysis, which may take up to 2 to 3 days after antigenic exposure, skin eruptions do not appear immediately. Contact dermatitis (e.g., poison ivy, chemical irritations, nickel metallic allergies) is the

classic example of a type 4 immune response. In addition, the wheal and flare response to *Mycobacterium tuberculosis* purified protein derivative (PPD) used in TB screening is also a type 4 immune response, when resulting positive in persons previously exposed to TB. This explains why the tuberculin skin test (TST) is read at 48 to 72 hours after placement.

Clinical Presentation

Subjective

Patients with classic atopic disease report fatigue and/or malaise, irritability, itchy and watery eyes, sneezing, rhinorrhea, nasal congestion, coughing without sputum production (unless a secondary bacterial infection accompanies the allergy), pruritus, and, in more severe cases, wheezing. Two elements are common to subjective complaints associated with allergies. First, an exposure to an allergen precedes the onset of symptoms. Thus, allergic rhinitis can be distinguished from perennial rhinitis because environmental seasonal allergen exposure precedes the former. Second, patients typically attempt to control their symptoms with self-care. For example, their subjective picture usually includes self-medication and may be somewhat controlled with over-the-counter (OTC) agents. A history of subjective allergic symptoms, therefore, requires accompanying inquiry concerning the use of OTC antihistamines and decongestants.

Objective

The sinuses may be tender to percussion if nasal congestion has predisposed a patient to sinusitis (due to impeded mucous drainage); otherwise, the sinuses are typically nontender in uncomplicated allergic rhinitis. The conjunctivae and mucous membranes in general will be injected. Nasal turbinates should be erythematous. Cervical nodes will feel shotty, with few greater than 1 cm in size. Postauricular nodes and thoracic nodes may not be involved. Tympanic membranes may appear dull to light but will be otherwise unremarkable.

Tachycardia typically accompanies OTC decongestant use, but fever does not contribute to the tachycardia because fever is almost always absent. Drowsiness is also typical with OTC antihistamine use (especially with first generation H_1-blocking agents). Lungs will be clear after several deep breaths and coughs unless allergic asthma causes wheezing to appear. Except in patients with anaphylaxis or allergenic invasion of the GI tract, the abdominal exam will prove unremarkable. In these exceptional cases, profound abdominal tenderness may inhibit deep palpation.

Skin eruptions will depend on the type of allergic reaction and may include urticarial (type 1 response), fissures, circumscribed papules, bullae, and petechiae. The clinician should expect no singular picture of skin eruptions that corresponds with the allergenic source; however, there are associations in skin presentation and history that lend themselves to diagnostic conclusions. For example, a history of exposure to poison ivy and multiple circumscribed papules in the anatomic place of exposure provides an association that is diagnostic of a specific exposure. Poison ivy, poison oak, and poison sumac all produce contact dermatitis by virtue of the oily irritant substance urushiol, which is contained in the leaves of these plants and acts as a contact allergen, leading to a delayed, cell-mediated (type 4) immune response.

If the patient's sensorium is affected, an objective mental status examination may reveal diminished problem-solving ability, impairment in recent recall, and unfocused attention. These signs are particularly evident in older adults and others who practice polypharmacy with combination OTC agents. Thus, it may be difficult to distinguish between the sedative effects of antiallergy medications (in particular, antihistaminic agents) versus the impact of a chronic atopic condition that is affecting the patient's sleep–wake cycle, such as severe allergic rhinitis or nighttime asthma.

Diagnostic Reasoning
Diagnostic Tests

Initial evaluation begins with the clinical history. The clinician should ask the patient to describe any changes in diet, skin-care products, or activities involving environmental exposures that preceded the onset of allergic symptoms. Suspicions raised by the history will often be confirmed or at least supported by subsequent diagnostic testing. Thus, particularly with regard to the evaluation of environmental exposures, a detailed history informed by the clinical presentation should largely drive diagnostic allergy testing.

Type 1 Response Initial testing continues with skin tests to diagnose the response to specific allergens. Skin tests involve first pricking the epidermis with a small amount of a liquid extract of the allergens of interest and later injecting the intradermal layers of the skin with these extracts, which is believed to be a more sensitive form of testing. (Patch testing, in which small amounts of emulsions of potential allergens are applied directly to the skin and left in place for 24–48 hours, is generally performed to diagnose contact dermatitis reactions and other manifestations of type IV hypersensitivity reactions.) Skin pricking testing is the first stage of allergen testing because of the very slight but potentially fatal risk that the applied allergen could cause a systemic allergic response (anaphylaxis). For every negative prick test, an intradermal injection may be placed as a more sensitive, albeit potentially higher risk, method of allergen testing.

The selection of antigens to be tested follows a pattern of reasoning based on the question: What are the most likely culprits? The exact composition of skin-test panels is determined by regional and patient-specific determinants. The allergist will expose the patient to small amounts of regional and suspected environmental allergens

in skin-test panels by prick or injection. If the test is positive, a wheal should appear in 15 to 20 minutes. The reliability and sensitivity of skin testing make it the preferred test for initial diagnosis. Skin tests are done with both positive (histamine) and negative (inert substances, such as saline) controls, and results must be judged against these controls as some individuals are sensitive to any kind of scratching or pricking of the skin, just by the nature of the insult to the skin, and not due to hypersensitivity to the antigen. However, given the sensitivity of allergen skin testing, a high false positive rate means that this testing should not be done indiscriminately or overinterpreted. In fact, many environmental and food allergens may test positive in up to half of the general population who otherwise demonstrate no other manifestations of hypersensitivity to these antigens. In turn, skin tests are far more useful in ruling out (i.e., excluding, rather than confirming) specific antigenic hypersensitivities, when reactions are negative.

Alternatives to allergen skin testing include in vitro serum-based testing methods, such as the radioallergosorbent test (RAST), the enzyme-linked immunosorbent assay (ELISA), and the fluorescent antibody staining technique (FAST). These serum tests reduce the risk of hypersensitivity-type reactions from allergens as seen in skin testing because they only measure antigen-specific IgE levels in the blood, rather than assess for functional hypersensitivity responses. Thus, skin tests are typically more sensitive than serum RAST tests in detecting true hypersensitivity responses because more atopic individuals will be positive on skin tests than will have elevated antigen-specific IgE serum levels. RAST tests are usually considered more specific than allergen skin testing as nonatopic individuals are unlikely to have high allergen-specific IgE levels, which must be balanced with their relatively decreased level of diagnostic sensitivity.

Consideration of sensitivity and specificity of allergy testing is particularly important for food challenge testing, which often utilizes skin prick testing as an initial screen, given its high sensitivity. Some clinicians also complement skin testing with RAST testing because although some food allergies may be type 3 immune complex responses, there certainly are anaphylactic food allergy reactions, which are IgE mediated and may be clinically severe. Definitive testing for such reactions may take place in an office setting by an allergy specialist (with ready access to endotracheal intubation supplies and injectable epinephrine) in the presence of physicians or other persons qualified to treat anaphylactic reactions. Set amounts of food are given to persons suspected of food allergy (typically children) in progressively increasing amounts, and individuals are subsequently monitored for several hours for any reaction. This is a highly specific test and is thus very effective in ruling out food allergies. Obviously, however, this testing method carries a great risk of anaphylaxis. Thus, RAST testing may be done instead of an observed food challenge to avoid needlessly subjecting individuals with high food-specific IgE levels to intentional exposure with that food trigger.

The most common form of asthma is an allergen-driven atopic disease characterized by type 1 immune responses to environmental allergens although it is distinct from systemic anaphylaxis. Atopic airway hyperreactivity may also be triggered by environmental irritants, such as tobacco smoke, which is not a true allergen. Thus, these individuals do not express true tobacco-specific IgE levels although smoke and other environmental pollutants may certainly trigger an asthma attack. Reactive airway disease (bronchial hyperresponsiveness), therefore, may be either allergic or nonallergic in origin. As asthma is largely an atopic, allergen-driven disease, sputum from an asthmatic patient may reveal eosinophils after staining with methylene blue dye, because sputum from atopic individuals typically demonstrates higher levels of eosinophils than in the nonatopic population.

Type 2 Response Rh testing of blood during pregnancy is the initial test to determine prospective Rh incompatibility. With reference to immune-mediated hemolytic anemia, an elevated indirect bilirubin level indicates hemolysis. Red blood cell (RBC) hemolysis is further associated with decreased serum haptoglobin levels. AIHA is also associated with a positive Coombs' test, which detects RBC-specific antibodies in the blood.

Type 3 Response Initial tests are employed to detect complement activation. A complement ELISA will give specific evidence of complement activation and consumption of complement proteins. For example, the ELISA might show lower levels of C_3 and/or C_4, which are two elements of complement that may be diminished if an allergic inflammatory reaction has activated complement. Similarly, the CH50 test, which is a measure of overall complement protein levels, will also be low in this setting. Skin manifestations in type 3 immune responses may be biopsied and stained for immune complex deposition, which is a hallmark of such reactions.

Type 4 Response Skin testing is the initial test of preference for cell-mediated hypersensitivity, e.g., tuberculin skin testing. Allergens are either injected intradermally or applied topically onto patches of skin. Results are then read 48 hours after application. Positive responses consist of induration (for injected allergens) and erythema and papules (for topically applied skin patch testing).

Antigen-specific serum IgE levels may aid in distinguishing allergic from nonallergic immune responses. For example, classic type 1 hypersensitivity reactions are IgE mediated, whereas cell-mediated type 4 responses are not. Although both type 2 and type 3 responses are antibody mediated, the IgE immunoglobulin class is not typically involved. An elevated peripheral eosinophil count may also provide secondary confirmation of recent IgE-mediated atopic disease.

Differential Diagnosis

Clinical history is the mainstay of differentiating allergic disease. Allergies are triggered by exposure to environmental antigens. The history, therefore, must support allergenic exposure proximal to the onset of symptoms and may often reveal partial or temporary relief of symptoms from OTC allergy remedies, as well as possible familial allergic patterns. Additional differentiation of classical allergic disease from other types of immune responses comes from skin test results, antigen-specific IgE levels, and other diagnostic tests aimed at identifying antibody-mediated immune responses.

Alternatively, irritants that enter the body but do not initiate classical immune-mediated hypersensitivity responses include nonallergic sources, such as air pollutants and tobacco smoke. In addition, some research has suggested that susceptible asthmatic patients may experience worsening of symptoms associated with barometric changes in the atmosphere, although it is unclear whether this weather-related phenomenon may actually be due to increases in airborne pollen levels associated with atmospheric pressure changes.

Management

Allergy management requires both symptomatic relief and prevention of exposure to specific allergens. Following the initial diagnosis and treatment of acute symptoms, priority should be given to identifying and avoiding triggering allergens, whether with respect to respiratory symptoms (asthma, allergic rhinitis), cutaneous manifestations (urticaria), ocular allergies, or systemic allergic reactions (anaphylaxis). (Atopic dermatitis, another core atopic disorder, is covered in detail in Chapter 7.) For both allergic rhinitis and asthma patients, long-term immunomodulatory therapy with allergy vaccines (i.e., allergen immunotherapy) offers both effective prophylaxis and attenuation of future atopic symptoms.

Initial Management

The patient must become vigilant in avoiding further allergenic exposure. After clinical history, skin testing, and antigen-specific IgE levels have identified likely triggering allergens, avoidance behaviors should be initiated. For example, individuals diagnosed with hypersensitivity to penicillin must avoid not only penicillin but also cephalosporins, given the likelihood of cross reactivity. However, although penicillin remains one of the most common triggers of antibiotic hypersensitivity, penicillin allergy is typically overdiagnosed on the basis of limited self-reported history. Thus, a detailed patient history should focus on whether an anaphylactic reaction to penicillin truly occurred, as research involving confirmatory skin testing and antibiotic challenge has consistently demonstrated that the majority of patients who report penicillin allergies do not have true penicillin hypersensitivity reactions or contraindicating anaphylaxis. Moreover, when use of a specific antibiotic class is deemed essential in an allergic patient, desensitization to penicillin or other antibiotics can be performed in a controlled clinical environment with the capacity to treatment anaphylaxis and other forms hypersensivity (e.g., intensive care unit).

Along the same lines, bee venom reactions can be avoided in venom-allergic patients by not disturbing beehives or wasp nests. Dust mite–allergic patients may use specially designed mattress and pillow covers that seal in dust mites and their allergenic fecal matter, avoid dust-collecting ceiling fans, remove carpets from bedrooms to limit dust mite exposure during sleeping hours, and regularly wash plush toys and any other potential dust reservoirs in hot water. Patients with pollen allergies should keep windows closed in favor of using air conditioning in both the home and car, as well as bathe soon after outdoor exposure to pollen, which can adhere to clothes and hair. Air conditioning filters should be changed regularly, although high-efficiency particulate air (HEPA) filters and chemical agents purported to reduce the concentration of aeroallergens have not been shown to be consistently effective.

Subsequent Management

Subsequent management consists of ongoing symptom control and immunotherapy. Symptom control can be achieved either through prescribed or OTC agents for common respiratory, ocular, and cutaneous manifestations. There are many classes of drugs that have demonstrated efficacy for symptom management in allergic disease, for example, sympathomimetics (used as decongestants), antihistamines (both oral and topical), corticosteroids (topical, inhaled, or systemic), cromolyn, and theophylline. Newer generation antihistamines have been designed to have less anticholinergic effects and central nervous system penetration and, therefore, cause less tachycardia and sedation than first generation agents.

Of special note, in addition to future allergen avoidance, the most severe form of allergic disease, anaphylaxis, requires emergent treatment (e.g., epinephrine, IV fluids) for immediate life-threatening manifestations caused by preformed inflammatory mediators, as well as prophylactic treatment (e.g., corticosteroids) for delayed, late phase manifestations caused by de novo, newly formed immune mediators, as described in Advanced Practice Nursing Interventions 17.2. Because late phase anaphylactic reactions may occur up to 24 hours following allergen exposure and can prove fatal, prophylactic corticosteroids should be given although they are ineffective in treating acute symptoms, given their slow onset of action.

Symptom Control   Many OTC agents are sympathomimetic (alpha-receptor agonist) in activity. Common examples of oral drugs in this class include pseudoephedrine (Sudafed), chlorpheniramine (Chlor-Trimeton), and oxymetazoline (Afrin). In addition, epinephrine (Primatene Mist) was previously available OTC as an inhalational therapy in the same class of sympathomimetic drugs. However, sale of the chlorofluorocarbon (CFC)–containing formulation of inhaled epinephrine was prohibited by the U.S. Food and Drug Administration (FDA) in 2012.

Sympathomimetic agents may display both alpha-adrenergic and beta-adrenergic properties. They vasoconstrict engorged mucosa (alpha-adrenergic property) and dilate the bronchioles by relaxing smooth muscle (beta-adrenergic property). Therefore, they support antihistamines in drying secretions while opening up the airways of the nasopharynx and bronchial tree. In addition, however, they also typically increase heart rate and may lead to palpitations (beta-adrenergic effect). Because of their low molecular weight and solubility, sympathomimetics may cross the blood–brain barrier, resulting in irritability, anxiety, and addiction potential, particularly when combined with other psychoactive substances such as ethanol. In addition, topical intranasal agents such as oxymetazoline are well known to induce tachyphylaxis (decreased response to the drug following frequent use over a relatively short period of time), resulting in rebound nasal congestion upon withdrawal after chronic use (rhinitis medicamentosum).

The abuse potential of OTC sympathomimetics remains high for many reasons. They are available for purchase and consumption without professional supervision, are relatively inexpensive, provide rapid symptomatic relief, and are heavily marketed. In addition, sympathomimetic formulations may be readily manipulated to form highly addictive illicit drug substances, such as methamphetamine (which in recent years has resulted in increasing restrictions on the OTC availability of some of these drugs, such as pseudoephedrine). In addition, some studies suggest that regular use of short- and long-acting beta-adrenergic inhalants, such as albuterol (Proventil) and salmeterol (Serevent, Advair) may increase disease morbidity in asthmatic patients, including both exacerbations and asthma-related deaths.

Another class of agents widely used for allergic reactions and chronic atopic disease are the antihistamines. With both first and second generation agents now available OTC, antihistamines are widely used in allergic disease for their ability to block H_1-histamine receptors and thereby reduce the effects of histamine released early on in the inflammatory cascade. The blockade of H_1-receptor sites also contributes to the therapeutic effect of drying secretions. Adverse effects include overdryness and sedation. The risk of sedation, particularly in older adults and children, may require dose reduction or a limited drug trial. Newer generation antihistamines such as desloratadine (Clarinex), fexofenadine (Allegra), and cetirizine (Zyrtec) are typically less sedating than first generation agents (diphenhydramine [Benadryl], hydroxyzine [Atarax]). Thus, at prescribed doses, these second generation agents dry secretions without causing excessive drowsiness in most patients and can be dosed once daily. They are also not associated with untoward cardiac events (QTc prolongation, fatal arrhythmias), which had been observed with other long-acting second generation antihistamines now withdrawn from the market (astemizole [Hismanal], terfenadine [Seldane]), particularly when used in combination with macrolide antibiotics or azole antifungals.

Anticholinergic agents such as intranasal ipratropium (Atrovent) are also very effective at drying secretions.

H₂-receptor antagonists such as cimetidine (Tagamet) and Ranitidine (Zantac) may also be useful in managing mild allergic reactions, although they are primarily used to decrease the production of stomach acid for GI symptoms. In some cases when allergy patients have failed to improve after receiving epinephrine and diphenhydramine, they have responded to cimetidine. However, H₂ blockers are known to cross the blood–brain barrier and may have mood-altering effects, particularly in elderly patients.

Corticosteroids form a third group of drugs used in symptom control. Given their long onset of action (several hours), they have little role in the acute treatment of symptoms. However, they may prevent the recurrence of symptoms in patients with mild allergic reactions, such as urticaria, and they also constitute part of the long-term treatment regimen of life-threatening allergic reactions, such as the manifestations of systemic anaphylaxis, including severe laryngeal edema, bronchospasm, or hypotension. For most hypersensitivity reactions, a dosage of 1 to 2 mg/kg per day of prednisone for 4 or 5 days is usually sufficient to prevent recurrent or late-onset symptoms. Short-term pulse dosing such as this does not require tapering. However, the clinician should consider tapering the regimen if the patient has received corticosteroid therapy in the recent past or if there are plans to continue therapy for more than several weeks. When given as short-term therapy, prednisone and other corticosteroids have fairly benign adverse effect profiles. However, prolonged use of systemic corticosteroids has a number of implications, including the development of Cushingoid syndrome, adrenal insufficiency, and hyperglycemia. Inhaled corticosteroids such as fluticasone propionate (Flovent) are used as standard prophylactic controller medications in allergic asthma (see Chapter 9). Intranasal corticosteroids such as mometasone furoate (Nasonex) are extremely effective for long-term control of both nasopharyngeal and ocular allergic rhinitis symptoms (see Chapter 8). Because corticosteroids are immunosuppressive, anti-inflammatory agents, they effectively downregulate the allergic immune responses characteristic of atopic disease.

Immunotherapy Allergen immunotherapy (allergy vaccine) offers the patient long-term control of atopic disease. Given the small, albeit well documented, risk of anaphylaxis or other hypersensitivity reactions associated with allergen immunotherapy, its use is usually limited in scope to patients with intractable allergic rhinitis or asthma whose disease fails to be controlled with symptom management or for whom consistent allergen avoidance is not possible. Immunotherapy regimens should be prescribed and administered by a qualified specialist with expert knowledge in allergic diseases as the first step is the proper identification of key allergens, which serve as the patient's most troublesome environmental triggers.

Depending on the number of allergens identified, these extracts are combined into one or more allergy vaccine mixtures, taking into account both cross-reactivity of individual allergens and the reduced stability of certain allergen extracts (e.g., plant pollens, animal dander) in combination with others, given the presence of proteolytic enzymes in many fungal and insect (e.g., dust mite, wasp or bee venom) extracts.

Injections of commercially prepared extracts of these allergens are given subcutaneously in 0.5 mL allotments of diluent that progress from minimal dilutional strength to higher concentrations. The weekly injections continue, increasing in concentration until symptoms are controlled and/or the maximum concentration of allergen extract is achieved, at which time the frequency of injections may be decreased to a goal of once monthly. Of note, immunotherapy may require more than 12 months of treatments before maximal effects are observed. There are also "rush immunotherapy" protocols that are being evaluated, which are shorter course regimens that escalate a patient to maximal allergen extract concentrations more quickly than traditional regimens. Current guidelines recommend continuing allergen immunotherapy for 3 to 5 years, after which many individuals experience lasting suppression of allergic hypersensitivity, allowing for the tapering and eventual cessation of extract injections. However, many patients experience recurrence of allergic symptoms when they attempt to stop or even taper the frequency of maintenance immunotherapy. Thus, although not generally recommended, some patients may continue immunotherapy for life.

Injection allergen immunotherapy has been used for over a century. However, a newer development is sublingual formulations, in which liquid extract is administered in drops under the tongue. The concept behind these regimens is the same as traditional subcutaneous and intradermal injection immunotherapy although the convenience of this dosing route is self-evident, particularly given the potential for self-administration in nonclinical settings. Although sublingual immunotherapy (SLIT) has gained acceptance in Europe, its use is not widespread in the United States because evaluations of its safety and efficacy are ongoing.

Other forms of biological immunotherapy exist for allergic diseases. For extremely refractory cases of atopy, such as severe allergic asthma with atopic dermatitis, Xolair (omalizumab; anti-IgE–specific monoclonal antibody immunotherapy) may be effective. Xolair is FDA approved for moderate to severe persistent asthma in persons 12 years and older. This therapy acts by binding up circulating IgE and preventing its interaction with cell-surface molecules on blood cells that mediate allergic hypersensitivity responses, including mast cells, basophils, and eosinophils, thereby preventing initiation of the allergic cascade.

One clinical scenario, which offers insight into a patient who might benefit from immunotherapy, would be that of a 55-year-old woman diagnosed with severe and persistent allergic rhinitis refractory to both OTC and prescription controller medications. Her primary triggering allergens are dust mites, ragweed pollen, egg, and *Aspergillus*. Food-based allergen immunotherapy is not considered an acceptable therapeutic strategy, given the relatively higher risk of anaphylaxis to food antigens. Thus, she completely avoids egg in her diet. To avoid dust mite exposure, she has removed all carpeting from her bedroom and replaced her curtains with window blinds. However, she cannot relocate from her home in the midwestern United States, where ragweed pollen levels are elevated between July and October. Her husband cleans the bathroom tiles and kitchen cabinets where *Aspergillus* might grow. For the past 3 months, she has consulted the clinician on six occasions. Her medication regimen includes a prescribed inhaled intranasal corticosteroid and both long- and short-acting antihistamines. Nonetheless, her symptoms keep her awake at night, and recently she has started to wheeze, requiring use of an albuterol metered-dose inhaler. Her primary care clinician referred her to an allergist, who made the specific allergen diagnoses and recommended allergen immunotherapy on the basis of the severity and recurrence of her symptoms, as well as her refractoriness to other medications. Of note, given the risk of anaphylaxis associated with allergen immunotherapy, the risk–benefit ratio of this approach will have to be discussed extensively with the patient before she initiates the allergy vaccine regimen.

Follow-up and Referral

Follow-up consists of both regular visits and increased consultations during seasonal allergy periods, depending on symptoms. Follow-up tests include a CBC to evaluate for leukocytosis and eosinophilia, as well as fasting blood sugar tests to assess for hyperglycemia, should systemic corticosteroids be required.

An allergist should be consulted if the symptoms cannot be controlled. The allergist is responsible for ordering and evaluating skin tests and for prescribing, administering, and evaluating the effectiveness of immunotherapy.

Patient Education

Depending on the patient's clinical manifestations, she or he must know what foods or other environmental allergens to avoid. The patient and clinician should decide together how to identify and control exposure to triggering allergens that may have been unknown by the patient before the diagnosis. For example, few patients know the places that dust mites hide or understand how to kill *Aspergillus* with simple household chemicals.

Patients with significant respiratory symptoms may need to learn how to use nasal inhalants for significant rhinitis symptoms or metered-dose inhalers (MDIs) for bronchial/pulmonary symptoms. Initial use under the

clinician's supervision can provide both the patient and clinician with reassurance that the drug will be delivered correctly. The use of spacers for MDIs should be discussed and encouraged as a means of maximizing medication delivery (see Chapter 9). The patient should learn which drugs may be taken together without significant risk of interaction and which should be administered alone or with food to facilitate absorption. The narrow therapeutic index of some drugs, such as theophylline, will require vigilance on the part of the patient to report the early symptoms of drug toxicity.

Patients with a history of anaphylaxis must have epinephrine available at all times for emergencies should they come in contact with the offending allergen. The immediate use of epinephrine after any exposure to a known anaphylactic triggering agent is crucial.

The clinician should prescribe a self-administered epinephrine kit and have the patient demonstrate understanding of its use before leaving the office. There are several brands of epinephrine available in kit form (Ana-Kit, AnaGuard, EpiPens, TwinJect). The expiration date for most kits is 1 year, and some kits contain more than one dose of epinephrine, which the patient injects IM for rapid delivery in a postexposure setting. The patient should be instructed that whenever a dose is self-administered, emergency department care should be sought in case the reaction worsens or recurs, requiring more advanced therapy such as IV epinephrine or crystalloids. Given the life-threatening nature of anaphylaxis, susceptible individuals with a history of systemic hypersensitivity reactions to environmental triggers must always have access to a readily available source of epinephrine.

Many patients will take OTC agents to help with allergy symptoms and should be taught to read and interpret drug labels correctly to check for ingredients that might cause tachycardia, drowsiness, or other adverse effects. Patients should be cautioned to be alert for any OTC formulations containing ephedrine, phenylephrine, phenylpropanolamine, or pseudoephedrine.

■ RHEUMATOID ARTHRITIS

Rheumatoid arthritis (RA) is a chronic, progressive, systemic inflammatory disease that primarily affects the synovial joints although it may affect many organ systems. Joints are destroyed over a long course of disease remissions and exacerbations. Structural deformities, which create emotional as well as physical trauma for the patient, are common as the disease progresses. *Healthy People 2020* has three objectives related to this chronic debilitating condition: (1) increasing the proportion of adults with chronic joint symptoms who have seen a health-care provider for their symptoms, (2) increasing the proportion of adults with physician-diagnosed arthritis who have had effective evidence-based arthritis education as an integral part of the management of their condition, and (3) reducing the proportion of adults with physician-diagnosed arthritis who find it "very difficult" to perform specific joint-related activities.

Epidemiology and Causes

In the general U.S. population, RA is the second most common connective tissue disease and the most destructive to the joints. Women with the disease outnumber men at a ratio of 2.5 to 3.1:1, with a worldwide incidence of approximately 3 in 10,000 persons. Prevalence increases with age, with a peak of cases occurring between ages 40 and 60 years after an onset of disease between ages 20 and 40 years. RA has been observed across all racial and ethnic groups, but familial patterns have been observed, with first-degree relatives of affected patients having approximately a twofold to threefold higher risk of developing disease. Characterizing the genetic predispositions for disease remains an area of active research, and an association between rheumatoid arthritis and the human leukocyte antigen (HLA) system, a series of linked genes on the sixth chromosome, has been observed. Although genetic risk factors have been identified, the cause of the disease is as yet unknown. In turn, most therapies target the inflammatory pathways that mediate disease manifestations. Other potential etiological factors that have been implicated include infection, autoimmunity, environmental triggers, and hormonal influences.

Pathophysiology

Rheumatoid arthritis causes joint destruction through a number of immunopathogenic mechanisms. Proteolytic enzymes, known as proteases, digest the tissue components of affected joints. This is speculated to occur due to local antigens that evoke the inflammatory cascade in the joint space; however, the source of these antigens is not fully characterized. These antigens may be autoimmune targets (e.g., type II collagen found only in articular cartilage and the vitreous of the eye, glycoprotein-39 found in cartilage, citrulline-containing peptides [CCPs] including citrullinated fibrin, and glucose-6-phosphate isomerase), which activate self-reactive T cells that initiate the inflammatory cascade.

T cells comprise nearly half the immune cells in an inflamed rheumatoid joint and are characterized by an activated T-helper phenotype based on the cell surface expression of HLA-DR (MHC class II) antigens, CD27, CD4, as well as the costimulatory molecules CD28 and CD40. However, it has been difficult to characterize the antigenic specificity of the initial set of T cells that trigger this immune response, because the inflammatory cascade is characterized by widespread recruitment of so-called "bystander T cells" that do not express autoantigen specificity but nonetheless proliferate and contribute to the destruction of the affected joint through cytokine expression. Interestingly, some evidence indicates that it may not be the antigens themselves that trigger self-reactive T cells, but rather genetic mutations that

alter specific amino acids within MHC class II antigen-presenting molecules (such as HLA-DRβ1) found on antigen-presenting cells. Other work has implicated superantigen interactions, in which several different T cell clones are activated independent of their association with MHC class II molecules.

Cells of the synovial (joint) lining including joint endothelium, T cells, and fibroblast-like cells proliferate, producing cytokines (e.g., interleukin-1 [IL-1], IL-6, IL-8, IL-15, IL-18, IFN-γ), neuropeptides such as substance P, and chemotactic factors that induce expression of cell adhesion molecules (e.g., intercellular adhesion molecule [ICAM]–1, vascular cell adhesion molecule [VCAM]–1, P-selectin, E-selectin). This leads to increased recruitment of an array of immune cells into the affected joint, including mast cells that produce histamine, tryptase, leukotrienes, cytokines, and chymase; multinucleated cells and macrophages which are the main source of potentially toxic nitric oxide and destructive matrix metalloproteinases (MMP) (e.g., collagenase [MMP-1], stromelysin [MMP-3], macrophage elastase [MMP-12]); and self-reactive plasma cells capable of producing autoantibodies (e.g., rheumatoid factor). Synovial fibroblasts further produce MMP-13, which has great specificity for type II collagen and is primarily responsible for soft tissue invasion in the affected joint.

Particularly noteworthy in the pathogenesis of RA is the production of rheumatoid factor—polyclonal antibody species typically of the IgM class that have specificity for the constant Fc region of IgG. Rheumatoid factor thus forms large immunocomplexes capable of activating complement proteins that themselves are cytolytic and chemotactic. The production of these antibodies is enhanced by cytokines secreted by regulatory CD4+ T helper cells. The plasma cell genes that encode rheumatoid factor undergo somatic mutations that increase their affinity for IgG, a process known as affinity maturation. Although rheumatoid factor is not pathognomonic of RA (as it may also be present in scleroderma, systemic lupus erythematosus [SLE], and even some viral infections) and may be absent in up to 25% of cases, the presence of these antibodies in the peripheral circulation correlates with invasive disease of greater severity.

Another type of autoantibody found in the blood of RA patients, anti-CCP antibodies (primarily specific for the protein filaggrin), are considered more specific for RA than rheumatoid factor and are now widely used in the diagnosis of early RA. However, they do not appear to play as significant a role in joint destruction and immunopathogenesis of RA as rheumatoid factor, because citrullinated peptides (which are the target of anti-CCP antibodies) are not typically found in the synovium of affected joints.

Tumor necrosis factor–alpha (TNF-α) is one of the main cytokines that trigger the proliferative rheumatoid synovium, which explains the efficacy of anti–TNF-α immunotherapies in treating RA. However, in addition to TNF-α, a wide array of cytokines have been implicated in the pathophysiology of the rheumatoid joint, including granulocyte-macrophage colony-stimulating factor (GM-CSF), IL-2, IL-13, IL-17, and transforming growth factor–beta (TGF-β). Moreover, cells of the synovial lining undergo transformation into a rapidly proliferating state (although incapable of true metastasis) in which several types of transcription factors (NF-κB, Fos, Jun, Raf, Myc) and intracellular kinases (e.g., mitogen-activated protein kinase [MAPK]) are upregulated.

As these various inflammatory pathways elaborate over time, joints are progressively destroyed by an invasive rheumatoid pannus. Similar to a destructive malignancy, the rheumatoid pannus is a creation of the inflamed synovium. It consists of granulated vascular tissue extending from the vascular bed into the joint space and is characterized by increased angiogenesis (new blood vessel formation), which is mediated by the upregulation of several angiogenic cytokines and growth factors, including hypoxia-inducible factor (HIF)–1, vascular endothelial growth factor (VEGF), heparin-binding growth factors, macrophage angiogenic factor (MAF), epithelial neutrophil activating peptide-78 (ENA-78), TNF-α, PGE_1, PGE_2, and IL-8. Nevertheless, this increased vascularity is often inadequate for the exaggerated level of cellular proliferation in the rheumatoid synovium. In addition, the increased intra-articular pressure within the affected joint resulting from this cellular proliferation, fibrin and clotting factor deposition, and fluid accumulation may tamponade articular vessels, resulting in progressive joint ischemia.

Mutations and overexpression of certain cell cycle regulatory proteins such as the *p53* tumor suppressor gene have been identified in cells of the rheumatoid synovium, which may render them less susceptible to apoptosis (programmed cell death). As discussed, cells in the pannus release proteolytic enzymes (e.g., MMP, glycosidases) that destroy the connective tissue matrix, including glycosaminoglycans, fibronectin, proteoglycans such as chondroitin sulfate, collagen, and eventually subchondral bony structures. Moreover, certain components of the rheumatoid pannus, such as regulatory T cells and bone marrow stromal cells, induce differentiation and proliferation of bone osteoclasts, which leads to further joint destruction. Fortunately, however, the pannus remains responsive to antiproliferative immunosuppressant treatments.

Within the synovial fluid, an inflammatory response also ensues but with a notably different distribution of immune cells. Polymorphonuclear neutrophils are the most prominent cellular infiltrate, numbering upwards of one billion in severely inflamed joints. These cells secrete a host of proteolytic enzymes into the joint fluid (e.g., myeloperoxidase, collagenase and other MMPs, elastase, and lysozyme), as well as inflammatory cytokines (e.g., prostaglandins, IL-1β), and chemotactic factors (e.g., leukotriene B4, platelet activating factor). Because

accumulation of joint fluid distends the joint capsule and contributes greatly to articular pains, aspiration of this exudative fluid may provide instant relief.

The immunopathology of RA is widespread and extends well beyond the joint synovium. Constitutional signs and symptoms including fever, anorexia, weight loss, and fatigue may be prominent during acute flares, reflecting the systemic nature of the disease, which may involve layers of the heart muscle, cardiac valves, pulmonary visceral pleura, spleen, larynx, dura mater, and sclera (extra-articular manifestations). In turn, other organ manifestations of RA may include pericardial effusions, cardiac dysfunction (including myocardial infarction), and rarely pericarditis. Lung manifestations may include pleural effusion, pleuritis, interstitial fibrosis, and bronchiolitis obliterans with organizing pneumonia (BOOP). Hematological findings are not uncommon and may include anemia of chronic disease or thrombocytosis, whereas RA associated with both splenomegaly and neutropenia is termed *Felty's syndrome.* Ocular manifestations include keratoconjunctivitis associated with dry eye syndrome (sicca), as well as episcleritis, uveitis, and nodular scleritis, which can be sight-threatening.

Another common extra-articular manifestation of RA is rheumatoid nodules, which typically appear on the elbows but may be found on any extensor surface of the body that is subject to repeated mechanical stress, pressure, or irritation. Found in up to 25% of RA patients, these initially microscopic nodules are subcutaneous and may form into larger granulomas, characterized by a central section of fibrinoid necrosis, which is surrounded by a palisade of radially arranged and elongated connective tissue cells that are enveloped by chronic granulation tissue.

Clinical Presentation
Subjective

In the early stages of the disease, the RA patient may complain of malaise, diffuse arthritis, weight loss, anorexia, and low-grade fever. In addition, the patient may complain of neuropathic pain in the extremities, painful eyes, and chest pain upon deep inspiration.

The patient typically awakens with joint pain and stiffness but reports that it improves as the day progresses. Not only does pain subside, but the swelling associated with joints in the early morning also abates with moderate activity, thereby leading to decreased joint stiffness. If left untreated, however, as the disease progresses over time, recurrent pain and swelling in both small and large peripheral joints form the subjective picture that is ultimately associated with diminished activity and a downward spiral of worsening pain and immobility.

Objective

The key physical findings are peripheral symmetric polyarthritis and morning stiffness, which typically lasts longer than 1 hour. The clinician will note that some joints demonstrate more involvement than others. These include the proximal interphalangeal (PIP) and metacarpophalangeal (MCP) joints in the hands and wrists, as well as the knees. The toes and ankles also tend to be affected. The clinician should expect the affected joints to be tender (painful to pressure), edematous, and partially immobile. Radiographic x-ray changes in early disease may be nondescript or absent even though synovial changes have already begun, although advanced magnetic resonance imaging (MRI) has shown promise as an imaging modality capable of detecting early joint manifestations with increased sensitivity compared with x-ray studies.

As the disease progresses, affected joints will appear more deformed and rigid, with diminished range of motion. Characteristic findings of advanced disease include the boutonnière deformity of affected fingers, in which the PIP joint is in a nonreducible state of flexion, along with hyperextension of the distal interphalangeal (DIP) joint, as well as the complementary swan neck deformity, in which the PIP joint is hyperextended and the DIP joint is in a constant state of flexion. The most severe form of structural joint damage in the hands is known as arthritis mutilans, which is characterized by extensive bone resorption, complete loss of the joint space, shortening and malpositioning of the fingers, and almost complete loss of function. In contrast to small joint involvement, monoarticular arthritis of a large joint is a far less common presentation in RA and is more suspicious for reactive arthritis, which does not typically manifest with morning stiffness.

Physical examination may also reveal additional significant findings associated with extra-articular organ manifestations of the disease. A cardiac rub associated with pericarditis may be detected. A pulmonary friction rub or diminished respiratory excursion may suggest inflammation in the visceral pleura, as well as involvement of the bony structures of the ribs and sternum. Dry crackles may reflect an interstitial pulmonary process in advanced chronic disease. A finding of injected sclera suggests scleritis. Loss of sensation, especially in the lower extremities, indicates peripheral neuropathy, and ecchymotic lesions may appear on the arms and legs. Rheumatoid nodules are commonly observed over the olecranon process or other extensor surfaces of the limbs and may be tender.

Diagnostic Reasoning
Diagnostic Tests

The initial test of preference for diagnosis is peripherally circulating rheumatoid factor (RF), which is an IgM class autoantibody that binds to the FC portion of IgG. The test result provides both qualitative and quantitative information that is useful in correlating with physical markers of RA. For example, a positive titer of greater than 1:150 indicates a poorer prognosis and is often accompanied by findings of severe disease such as rheumatoid nodules. It is necessary to interpret both the presence of RF (qualitative) with the dilutional titer

(quantitative) because rheumatoid factor may be present in other diseases and its incidence increases with age. It is estimated that only 75% of RA patients are positive for RF.

Because RF alone is not diagnostic of RA, a more specific test is for circulating anti-CCP antibodies in the peripheral blood. This autoantibody species is more specific for RA than rheumatoid factor is and may be detected earlier in the disease process. However, anti-CCP titers correlate less well with severity of disease or prognosis, compared with rheumatoid factor.

Initial testing should also include an erythrocyte sedimentation rate (ESR), which will be elevated if the disease is active. C-reactive protein (CRP) is an acute-phase reactant, which, like ESR, is reflective of a heightened inflammatory state. Thus, CRP may be evaluated in addition to or in place of ESR as a nonspecific indicator of inflammation. Other tests include a complete blood count (CBC) to rule out anemia as a potential cause of fatigue and to evaluate for an associated leukocytosis or, alternatively, neutropenia. A platelet count (showing normal or high values) will become more elevated as joints become more inflamed. In addition, joint fluid analysis may aid in distinguishing rheumatoid arthritis from other causes of joint inflammation, such as infection. Aspirates from rheumatoid joints will show between 2,000 and 50,000 WBCs/mcL and a pronounced neutrophil component. Advanced Assessment 17.1 compares the typical results of synovial fluid analysis in RA and other inflammatory and infectious disorders.

Subsequent laboratory tests may be used as markers of disease progression. For example, ESR and CRP act as markers of inflammation, which may be helpful in charting the course of disease and response to therapy. Quantitative antinuclear antibodies (ANAs) may also help in differentiating rheumatoid arthritis from SLE, because lower titers suggest rheumatoid disease. If the diagnosis is in doubt, a comprehensive autoantibody panel may be drawn to help distinguish RA from other autoimmune connective tissue disorders, such as Sjögren's syndrome, although interpretation of such panels typically requires expert rheumatologic knowledge.

Radiographic x-ray changes in the joints may not be evident in the initial phases of the disease. However, after the disease has run its course for 6 months or more, radiographs will reveal bone erosions in the joints of the hands and feet. Plain films may show bony erosions in up to 30% of patients within 1 year of diagnosis and up to 90% of cases after the first 2 years. MRI has gained wider acceptance in recent years as a more sensitive (albeit significantly more expensive) detection method for joint changes in early disease. Research is ongoing into the cost-benefit assessment of early disease detection with MRI as a trigger for earlier medical intervention that could potentially lead to decreased disease progression and subsequent complications over time, thereby off-setting the initial expense.

Advanced Assessment 17.1   Analyzing Synovial Fluid

	Normal	Noninflammatory	Inflammatory	Purulent	Hemorrhagic
Clarity/color	Clear, yellow	Transparent, xanthochromic	Opaque, white or translucent	Opaque, white	Opaque, hemorrhagic
Leukocytes/mL	<200	200–2000	2,000–50,000	50,000–300,000	Variable
Percent of PMN	<25%	<50%	>75%	50%–100%	Variable
RBCs	Low	Low	Low	Low	High
Possible causes	Normal	Osteoarthritis Trauma SLE Polyarteritis nodosa Scleroderma Corticosteroid therapy	Rheumatoid arthritis Rheumatic fever Reactive arthritis Crystal synovitis	Septic arthritis Bacterial infection Fungi Tuberculosis	Trauma Blood dyscrasias Tumor Anticoagulants Sickle cell disease Myeloproliferative diseases

Differential Diagnosis

In general, an array of connective tissue diseases must be considered in the differential diagnosis. These include osteoarthritis, gout, chronic Lyme disease, SLE, infection by human parvovirus B19, polymyalgia rheumatica, Sjögren's syndrome, sarcoidosis, and various neoplasms. Osteoarthritis almost never affects the wrists and the metacarpophalangeal joints. Osteoarthritis is classically known for affecting the DIP joints with Heberden's nodes (hard, bony swellings) in the fingers. In contrast, these distal joints are less commonly affected in RA, and there are typically no Heberden's nodes in the hands. Within the thumb, the carpophalangeal joint is typically affected in osteoarthritis, whereas the interphalangeal joint is more often affected in RA.

Gout is distinguished by its gold standard test, which is a synovial aspirate revealing urate crystals. For crystalline arthritides, gout crystals are negatively birefringent, whereas pseudogout has positively birefringent calcium pyrophosphate crystals. Chronic Lyme disease usually involves only a single joint and is not polyarthralgia. A characteristic expanding bull's-eye rash known as erythema migrans is typical, and positive serological markers against the causative agent *(Borrelia burgdorferi)* distinguish Lyme disease from RA.

In reference to infection by human parvovirus B19, which may also manifest with joint pain, serological evidence of antiparvovirus B19 IgM antibody and a characteristic rash with an erythematous "slapped cheek" appearance distinguish this infection from RA. When considering acute viral polyarthritis, other causative infections include hepatitis C and rubella (rubeola virus), which may be distinguished from RA via specific immunoassays and organism-specific antibody titers.

SLE arthritic changes are almost never deforming, nor would one typically expect erosive changes on radiographs. Patients with polymyalgia rheumatica are usually negative for rheumatoid factor or have low titers. In addition, this disease usually strikes persons older than 50 years. Whereas qualitative RF positivity increases with age and may be nonspecifically present in older adults, patients with polymyalgia rheumatica suffer from myalgias but not distinctive arthralgias or arthritis.

A more challenging disease to distinguish from RA is psoriatic arthritis, because joint manifestations may not occur concurrently with cutaneous psoriatic findings in these patients. However, if psoriatic lesions are not present at the time of evaluation, a family history of psoriasis and joint manifestations in one or more relatives usually supports this diagnosis. Finally, some neoplasms can mimic rheumatoid disease, but again, RF is typically negative or quantitatively low in this setting.

Management

Management of RA progresses from conservative interventions to aggressive symptom management. Although the disease is debilitating over time, clinicians have recognized the potential adverse effects of immunosuppressive and anti-inflammatory therapies, including increased infection risk and hepatotoxicity. Thus, systemic therapy is typically initiated in response to symptom manifestations, thereby sparing the liver and GI tract from early use of potentially toxic agents.

The overall goals of management are to reduce pain and inflammation and to spare joint function. It is possible to achieve these goals in early management without pharmacological agents. This section on management, therefore, includes nonpharmacological interventions as therapy for RA, particularly early in the disease process.

Initial Management

Joint swelling and immobility on rising, which abate or diminish throughout the day, characterize early rheumatoid disease. Early disease symptoms can be managed by one or a combination of the following: physical and occupational therapies, heat and cold applications, exercise, rest, assistive devices, splints, meditation, chiropractic adjustments, and weight loss.

Physical and occupational therapists are educated to identify strategies that promote function and prevent immobility. Their special skills in motivating patients to remain active should not be underestimated in early disease management. Often patients attend therapy sessions and derive accompanying educational and emotional benefits from associating with other patients diagnosed with RA.

Heat and cold applications provide analgesia and relaxation to muscles and connective tissue. It is usually necessary to try both heat and cold therapy with individual patients because some respond better to one than the other. Application in anticipation of exercise may enhance joint mobility during exercise. Particularly helpful to some patients is to remain seated in warm water for 10 to 30 minutes.

Exercise reduces pain and inflammation only if the affected joints are not stressed during an inflammatory period. Outside an inflammatory event, the joints may undergo judicious stress through an increase in resistance exercises to promote strength and endurance. Thus, isometric exercises should be prescribed for inflamed joints, and isotonic exercises should be done at other times. Patients may also benefit from low resistance aerobic exercise at the shallow end of a swimming pool.

Rest reduces pain and inflammation by controlling joint movement. However, one must distinguish between systemic rest and resting the joints. Systemic rest signifies a prescribed period of relaxation that may involve sleep. Patients with mild inflammation may benefit from systemic rest in the prone position for 1 to 2 hours per day; the rest period may extend upwards to 2-hour periods three or four times daily during waking hours, as necessitated by severe inflammation. Like systemic rest, resting the joints should be done in a prone position to avoid hip contractures; however, the duration of rest is much shorter than systemic rest, usually lasting only 20 to 40 minutes. In either case, the patient should prepare a method for awakening to prevent excessive systemic rest, because excessive rest may signal depression or other underlying disease.

Assistive devices include those that the patient requires to complete activities of daily living. Canes or crutches can relieve stress to affected weight-bearing joints during periods of acute inflammation. Once the inflammation subsides, the patient may walk free of the device. When the clinician or physical therapist recommends using a cane or crutches, it is important to the patient's self-esteem and inner hope to explain that these may be required only temporarily. Other assistive devices for the home include bars for gripping the inside of a shower or bathtub or beside the toilet, a raised toilet seat, retrieval–extension devices for picking up items from the floor or at a distance, and an electronic chair lift to help the patient manage stairs.

Splints reduce pain, promote function, and stabilize involved joints. The hands and wrists are the preferred regions for splints, which are usually applied at night. Splints of the hips and knees are usually not preferred over lying prone. The position of optimal function should be considered when applying the splint. Moreover, the material of the splint should be lightweight, unabrasive, and durable enough to withstand frequent applications. Because self-application is preferred, the splint should be structured so that the patient can apply it without assistance.

Meditation relieves depression and anxiety associated with chronic disease and disability. In addition, it promotes self-care practices and self-efficacy. Meditation may follow traditional spiritual paths, whereby patients learn from teachers in traditional religious communities. Alternatively, meditation may involve guiding the attention through the use of restful music, images, spiritual charms, and breath-work. Patients with RA should meditate in a prone position to prevent postmeditation joint stiffness and pain.

The role of chiropractic adjustment remains controversial among traditional Western medicine practitioners; however, its benefits to the patient with RA must be considered. Chiropractors can relieve pressure to unaffected joints that compensate for decreased weight-bearing or activity in the affected joints. Although adjustments may require repeated manipulations and therapeutic benefits may be short lived, other benefits include an increased sense of well-being and improved quality of life.

Weight loss reduces pressure on weight-bearing joints in the lower extremities and enhances activity. Alternatively, overeating may be a sign of depression. Thus, weight gain must be addressed in an overall plan of encouraging weight reduction (if applicable) to achieve ideal body weight.

Subsequent Management

Drug therapies include analgesics, NSAIDs, corticosteroids, nonbiological and biological disease modifying antirheumatic drugs (DMARDs), and older therapies as described in the sections that follow.

Analgesics Analgesics such as acetaminophen (Tylenol) or capsaicin cream, gel, lotion, or roll-on may be effective even though they have no anti-inflammatory effects. Though aspirin has been the mainstay of therapy for RA, acetaminophen as a nonopioid pain reliever may help for mild pain. Of note, opioid analgesics have also been used for more significant pain although these agents are addictive and are not disease modifying in RA. Given the public health risks associated with the overuse of prescription opioids, reliance on narcotic analgesics as primary RA therapy is strongly discouraged and presents a significant danger for the patient.

NSAIDs Subsequent management begins with a consideration of cyclooxygenase inhibitors, which include aspirin and other NSAIDs. Drugs of this class need not be used daily during the early stages of disease. Rather, the patient can employ them only when there is pain that is unrelieved by nonpharmacologic means. Patients may be individually more responsive to one type of NSAID than another, and trial courses are sometimes required to determine the most effective agent although simultaneous use of multiple NSAIDs is discouraged. Different NSAIDs may also differ in their side effect profiles (e.g., sulindac 150 mg PO 2 times daily conferring fewer GI side effects than other NSAIDs). However, the adverse effects of NSAIDs as a class are well documented, including renal toxicity, GI side effects, platelet inhibition, and idiosyncratic hypersensitivity reactions. Thus, they should not be used indiscriminately.

Extra-strength (1,000 mg) aspirin can be used up to three to four times per day if baseline liver function studies, platelet count, renal function studies, and Hct are within normal limits. Caution must be exercised when prescribing 4 g of aspirin per day to persons older than age 65, however, as their liver and renal functions may be impaired by age. Dosage reductions are warranted should adverse effects ensue or laboratory markers dictate.

Aspirin should always be taken with 8 ounces of water or milk to avoid pill erosion or ulceration of the gastric mucosa. Enteric-coated aspirin is preferred to prevent gastric erosion. Concurrent anticoagulant therapy is a relative contraindication to aspirin and other NSAID use, which means that they should either be avoided altogether or prescribed in lower doses, relative to coagulation studies and clinical history.

Other NSAIDs may be substituted for aspirin should adverse effects or diminishing therapeutic efficacy warrant the switch. Notably, over time and with chronic use, individual drugs of the same class of NSAIDs can lose their effectiveness in an individual patient; therefore, NSAIDs provide a wide range of therapeutic options, and clinicians can recommend another drug in the class if treatment effects diminish with a given agent.

The primary adverse effect of the NSAIDs is GI upset. Their inhibition of gastric prostaglandin E (a natural protectant) predisposes the gastric mucosa to erosion. Most of the NSAIDs can be taken with an H_2-blocker such as ranitidine (Zantac) to reduce dyspepsia; however, H_2-blockers do not reduce hemorrhage or mucosal erosion. Proton pump inhibitors such as omeprazole (Prilosec) OTC or esomeprazole magnesium (Nexium) suppress gastric acid secretion and may be preferred to H_2-blockers for GI prophylaxis.

With reference to liver function, minimal elevations in serum transaminases are to be expected at daily doses of 2,400 mg ibuprofen (Motrin, Advil) for adults younger than age 65 years; the maximum dose may go as high as 3,200 mg/day if no adverse effects are apparent, but prolonged use of such doses may confer significant renal, hepatic, or GI toxicity, as well as iatrogenic hypertension. Should transaminase levels exceed two times normal, a dose reduction is indicated along with laboratory evaluation for infectious causes, such as hepatitis B and C.

Toxicity from prolonged NSAID use may result in renal impairment and present with acute renal failure requiring emergent care, as patients are prone to overuse NSAIDs, given their OTC availability and highly marketed nature. Thus renal toxicity is as important a consideration as are gastritis and ulcer formation. A rise in serum creatinine or blood urea nitrogen after starting NSAID therapy is an indication for further testing and a possible dose reduction or cessation. Fortunately, should renal failure develop, it is usually reversible after withdrawing the agent, given the proper supportive care.

Corticosteroids Corticosteroids (up to 7.5 mg of PO prednisone daily or injected intra-articularly, such as triamcinolone) may be helpful. However, side effects of prolonged corticosteroid use include adrenal insufficiency, hyperglycemia, osteoporosis, increased infection risk, and skin discoloration, which explains why maximal daily therapy is not recommended for more than 6 months. In addition, calcium, vitamin D, and bisphosphonates are indicated with prolonged corticosteroid use to mitigate bone demineralization. (The adverse effect profile of corticosteroids is thoroughly covered in the atopic dermatitis section of Chapter 7.)

Disease-Modifying Antirheumatic Drugs Disease-modifying antirheumatic drugs (DMARDs) include immunosuppressants and immunomodulators of various types, many of which have been used for decades. However, the newest class of DMARDs are biological immunotherapeutic agents, including anticytokine immunotherapies (TNF-α inhibitors, IL-1 inhibitors, IL-6 inhibitors) and anti–B-cell and anti–T-cell agents (see Drugs Commonly Prescribed 17.1: Disease-Modifying Anti-Rheumatic Drugs). Active disease should be treated early with DMARDs within 3 months of disease onset and even more aggressively in severe disease. Potential side effects of these therapies include the risk of reactivating latent or dormant TB infection with anti–TNF-α therapy, given the inhibition of cell-mediated immunity; therefore, TB screening should be instituted in all patients before starting biological immunosuppressive agents (Level I; Singh et al, 2012).

Combination therapy with DMARDs is more effective than monotherapy, and several different combinations have been tested. There is strong evidence for the efficacy of the combination of three DMARDs—methotrexate, sulfasalazine, and hydroxychloroquine—versus methotrexate monotherapy or dual therapy with only sulfasalazine and hydroxychloroquine (Level I;

Drugs Commonly Prescribed 17.1   Disease-Modifying Antirheumatic Drugs (DMARDs)

Drug	Adverse Reactions and Prescribing Considerations
Aminoquinoline	
hydroxychloroquine (Plaquenil)	May cause irreversible retinopathy, alopecia, blood dyscrasias.
Immunosuppressant	
cyclosporine (Neoral)	Indicated only in patients who have not responded to methotrexate. Pregnancy Category C. Monitor renal and hepatic function. Reduce dose if hypertension occurs.
Pyrimidine Synthesis Inhibitors	
leflunomide (Arava)	Monitor LFTs. May cause GI upset, leukopenia, thrombocytopenia.
Salicylate Sulfonamides	
sulfasalazine (Azulfidine)	Monitor LFTs. May cause GI upset, leukopenia, thrombocytopenia, urine or skin discoloration.
Folic Acid Antagonist	
methotrexate (Rheumatrex)	Monitor LFTs. May cause blood dyscrasias, GI upset, hepatotoxicity, opportunistic infections, fatal skin reactions.
Tumor Necrosis Factor (TNF)-α Blockers	
	Caution with all TNF-α blockers against reactivation TB and hepatitis B, predisposition to serious infection, development of lupus-like syndrome, development of selective cytopenias and pancytopenias, worsening of demyelinating syndromes, worsening of heart failure, increased malignancy rates, and cautious use in patients at risk for hepatic injury or with elevated liver function tests.
adalimumab (Humira)	May be used with or without methotrexate in moderate to severe RA.
etanercept (Enbrel)	May be used with or without methotrexate in moderate to severe RA.
infliximab (Remicade)	Should be used in combination with methotrexate for moderate to severe RA.
certolizumab (Cimzia)	May be used with or without methotrexate in moderate to severe RA.
golimumab (Simponi)	Should be used in combination with methotrexate for moderate to severe RA.
Interleukin-1 Receptor Antagonists	
anakinra (Kineret)	May cause predisposition to infections, headache, GI upset, neutropenia.
Interleukin-6 Antagonists	
tocilizumab (Actemra)	May be used with or without methotrexate in patients with an inadequate response to one or more DMARDs, including TNF-α blockers. May predispose to infections, hyperlipidemia, GI perforation in at-risk patients.
Anti–B-cell Agents	
rituximab (Rituxan)	Indicated for use with methotrexate in patients who do not respond to TNF-α blockers. Stop hypertension medications during treatment. May cause angioedema, GI upset, blood dyscrasias.
Anti–T-cell Agents	
abatacept (Orencia)	May be used as monotherapy or with other DMARDs, other than TNF-α blockers. May predispose to infections, headache, or respiratory adverse events in COPD patients.
Tyrosine Kinase Inhibitors	
tofacitinib (Xeljanz)	May be used as monotherapy or with other DMARDs, other than TNF-α blockers or potent immunosuppressants such as azathioprine or cyclosporine. May predispose to infections, hepatic enzyme elevations, neutropenia, anemia, GI perforation in at-risk patients.

O'Dell et al, 2002). There is also a high level of evidence for adding a TNF-α blocking agent to methotrexate therapy in patients with moderately or highly active disease after 3 months of methotrexate monotherapy (Level I; Singh et al, 2012; Maini et al, 1999). In turn, although the anti–TNF-α agents are considered first-line biological DMARDs, other biological agents have been approved for use in patients with an inadequate therapeutic response or intolerance to anti–TNF-α agents (e.g., abatacept, rituximab, tocilizumab), as well as the small molecule tyrosine kinase inhibitor tofacitinib. It is not recommended, however, that immunosuppressive biological agents with different mechanisms of action be used in combination, given the heightened risk of serious infection. Thus, therapies should be crafted based on the tolerance of side effects and the presence of comorbid conditions.

Older Therapies Many other DMARDs are possible options in the event of treatment failure with aspirin and other NSAIDs, but these are used less often now, given their low therapeutic index (higher toxicity risk) and the development of the newer agents discussed previously. These include azathioprine (Imuran), gold sodium thiomalate (Myochrysine), antimalarials, penicillamine (Depen), sulfasalazine (Azulfidine), and minocycline hydrochloride (Minocin). Hydroxychloroquine is an antimalarial usually used in milder disease, compared with sulfasalazine, which is used more often in moderate disease. Most of the COX-2 inhibitors, which were a mainstay of therapy in the past, are no longer marketed because of their cardiovascular risks. Celecoxib (Celebrex) is one of the last remaining.

Methotrexate is an older agent that is also used in many common chemotherapeutic regimens for the treatment of cancer. In contrast to many other older DMARDs, methotrexate remains highly effective in RA, including early on in the disease process (Level I; Singh et al, 2012) at low-dose regimens. It may be administered in adults younger than age 65 years at an initial weekly dose of 7.5 mg PO. The dosage may be doubled the second week if tolerance and therapeutic aims necessitate, although its full therapeutic effect may take 4 to 6 weeks to manifest. Maximum dosage is typically 25 mg per week.

Toxic effects of methotrexate include interstitial pneumonitis, hepatic cirrhosis, and teratogenicity. It is therefore not used in women at risk of pregnancy or in patients with chronic liver disease or elevated hepatic function tests. Combined use of methotrexate with NSAIDs, sulfonamides (e.g., sulfamethoxazole/trimethoprim [SMX/TMP]), or sulfonylureas such as glipizide (Glucotrol) increases the chance of hepatotoxicity, so concurrent use of these drugs is discouraged. Increased risk of hepatotoxicity is also seen with diabetes, obesity, and renal disease, in association with methotrexate use. Initiation of therapy, therefore, must be weighed against its potential risks and the availability and appropriateness of alternative therapeutic options.

Follow-up and Referral

Follow-up of patients with RA requires routine clinical laboratory evaluation and episodic adjustments in interventions. Routine clinical laboratory evaluation is performed every 90 days and includes CBC, platelet count, serum liver and renal function studies, and fasting blood sugar. Most of the adverse effects of drugs used in the management of RA can be monitored with this routine panel. If methotrexate is used, a serum albumin level should be added to the routine panel of tests to monitor for hepatic synthetic function.

The CRP blood test is a nonspecific method for evaluating the severity and course of the inflammatory process. CRP is normally less than 0.8 mg/dL and is, therefore, typically elevated in RA before treatment. Failure to decrease the CRP level after initiating treatment may thus indicate a lack of efficacy of the therapeutic agent or the presence of underlying infection or tissue necrosis; therefore, CRP should be monitored to determine the effectiveness of therapy. ESR may follow this same pattern during the course of treatment and may serve as a less technically involved, and therefore more widely available, alternative test compared with CRP.

Following scheduled laboratory evaluations, each visit to the clinician should address the clinical history since the last visit. Attention focuses on the efficacy of relief measures and the onset, duration, and frequency of pain and swelling of the joints. Standardized and validated disease assessment tools may be completed by the clinician at each visit to assess how well treatment interventions have achieved the targeted goals of low disease activity and complete disease remission, commonly known as "treating to target."

The clinician should refer the patient to a rheumatologist if initial management (including aspirin or NSAID therapy) fails. The rheumatologist is responsible for initiating therapies such as methotrexate and other DMARDs, including newer biological agents. Comanagement may mean that the rheumatologist will evaluate the patient twice each year once stable or more frequently, as signs and symptoms necessitate. In particular, specialist input is typically required to effectively "treat to target."

Patient Education

Patient education focuses on the goals of therapy, which are reduction of pain, control of inflammation, and preservation of function. Many of the key patient education topics were covered under Initial Management. In addition, education should address the therapeutic and adverse effects of any drugs employed. Finally, because RA is a chronic disease, education should also envelop the emotional, social, and spiritual sequelae of living with recurrent bouts of pain and disability.

The goals of therapy are best realized by promoting self-care. Education concerning self-care should include caregivers who must share common therapeutic goals for the patient before they can support self-care practices. To help keep the patient from sinking into a cycle of seeking secondary gains from the "sick" role, the caregiver should support normal social role behaviors by encouraging self-care. The caregiver, therefore, becomes integral to achieving the goals of therapy. In turn, these therapeutic goals should be reviewed at each visit. This is an ideal context to employ the *Circle of Caring* model involving all medical modalities, nursing modalities, complementary therapies, and the patient's family.

■ INFECTIOUS MONONUCLEOSIS

Infectious mononucleosis is a viral syndrome characterized by prolonged malaise and fatigue, fever, sore throat, tender cervical lymphadenopathy, and a predominant monocytosis with a reactive lymphocytosis on peripheral blood smear. Also present may be GI manifestations including nausea, vomiting, and anorexia; abdominal organomegaly; headache; and, occasionally, a morbilliform viral exanthem (rash). Infectious mononucleosis results from acute infection with Epstein-Barr virus (EBV) or, less commonly, cytomegalovirus (CMV). Saliva is the most common source of infectious virions, which explains the traditional adage that refers to this condition as the "kissing disease."

Epidemiology and Causes

Infectious mononucleosis occurs predominantly among sexually active individuals aged 10 to 35 years. Sexual activity, in this sense, implies the exchange of bodily fluids between sex partners, particularly the exchange of saliva. Although the disease can occur outside of this age range, case reports are rare. Its distribution is equal among genders, economic classes, and educational levels, although the incidence of clinical infection is up to 30 times higher in whites than blacks.

The cause of the disease is recent infection by EBV (90% of all cases, with an incubation period of 30–50 days) or, to a much lesser extent, CMV, toxoplasmosis, human herpesvirus–6 (HHV-6), or acute HIV infection. Even certain medications such as isoniazid, phenytoin, or carbamazepine may induce a mononucleosis-like illness. However, it is EBV infection that has been best characterized, associated with a prolonged recovery period with persistent symptoms lasting up to a year, and is connected most consistently to the significant sequelae of infectious mononucleosis.

Pathophysiology

Both EBV and CMV are members of the Herpesviridae family of viruses. Infection by these viruses is particularly widespread, with up to 95% of adults being seropositive for EBV-exposure. Humans are the major reservoir for latent EBV infection, which typically spreads through intimate contact with asymptomatic viral shedders. EBV infection may result in a number of conditions, given its tropism for (ability to infect) B and T lymphocytes.

EBV typically enters the body via oropharyngeal epithelial and lymphoid cells, which explains the ability of the virus to be shed in saliva. Migration of B cells throughout the lymphoreticular system allows for widespread dissemination of this virus. Circulating antibodies are soon formed against viral antigens, as well as against unrelated RBC-specific antigens, the latter being termed heterophile antibodies. These IgM antibodies serve as a primary means of early detection of EBV infection, although they are not highly specific, given that they may also be present in HIV infection, lupus, or with underlying lymphoma. In addition, up to 20% of EBV-infected adults and teens may not produce heterophile antibodies.

An atypical peripheral lymphocytosis occurs 1 to 3 weeks after the onset of clinical symptoms, which is characterized largely by an activated set of HLA-DR+, CD8+ T cells, as well as nonspecific CD16+ natural killer (NK) cells. These cells are key to preventing the acute lysis of virally infected cells (lytic phase of infection) and establishing nonlytic, subclinical lifelong infection (latent phase of infection). Acute symptomatic manifestations of EBV infection such as infectious mononucleosis are believed to result from suboptimal lymphocytic immune responses, rather than from ongoing viral replication. In turn, antiviral therapies are ineffective in the treatment of infectious mononucleosis.

Although the majority of EBV infections are subclinical, significant manifestations include not only infectious mononucleosis but also relatively benign cases of upper respiratory infection, otitis media, and even potentially fatal cases of Hodgkin's and non-Hodgkin's lymphoma. Sequelae of EBV infection are largely determined by the age of the infected host, with adolescents and young adults being most susceptible to infectious mononucleosis. The precise reasons for these differential manifestations are not fully understood. However, they are thought to relate to the size of viral inoculum and the extent of the host B cell immunoresponse, both of which vary with age. In turn, patients with infectious mononucleosis due to EBV may develop serious sequelae affecting virtually any organ system. In contrast, infectious mononucleosis caused by CMV is typically a self-limited condition without significant complications, except in significantly immunosuppressed individuals.

Clinical Presentation
Subjective

Patients present with an acute history of fever, neuropathies, headache, photophobia, dysphagia, sore throat, diffuse chest pain, dyspnea, cough, nausea, anorexia, myalgias, and arthralgias. They usually cannot identify a known contact with EBV before the onset of symptoms.

Objective

Patients may report fevers as high as 39°C (greater than 102.5°F) among children and teenagers. Cervical and postauricular lymphadenopathy may be painful on examination. Nuchal stiffness associated with painful lymph nodes may be present although not as rigid as in meningitis. The pharynx is typically injected, and there may be exudate across the tonsils or in the tonsillar crypt. Tachycardia may be accompanied by other arrhythmias, in particular premature atrial contractions. The lungs may reveal fine, scattered inspiratory crackles (rales). Splenomegaly is present in up to 60% of patients. Although splenic rupture is rare (2 in 1,000), it is a potentially fatal sequela. The liver may also be enlarged and tender to deep palpation.

A maculopapular rash may be evident across the trunk and upper extremities although this finding is infrequent. More commonly, antibiotics may be inadvertently started because of a suspicion of bacterial infection. This often results in a characteristic maculopapular or morbilliform rash, seen most commonly with concurrent use of beta-lactam antibiotics such as amoxicillin or ampicillin, or occasionally with antibiotics of other classes, such as azithromycin and fluoroquinolones. Such rashes can be particularly concerning for parents because they may be mistaken for an antibiotic allergy. Although the pathophysiology of these antibiotic-induced rashes is unclear, they are likely related to circulating non-IgE antibodies specific for the antibiotic but are not typically associated with immediate hypersensitivity reactions such as anaphylaxis.

Diagnostic Reasoning

The diagnostic reasoning for infectious mononucleosis should progress in stepwise fashion, according to the complexity of its presentation. The symptoms of mononucleosis mimic those of many diseases; therefore, laboratory findings play an important role in the differential diagnosis.

Diagnostic Tests

The first set of laboratory tests to be ordered includes a complete blood count (CBC), heterophile antibody test (Monospot), rapid plasma reagin (RPR) test (which may be positive in infectious mononucleosis, as well as syphilis infection), throat cultures, serum liver transaminases, and serum bilirubin. The goal of initial testing is to establish a pattern of results that would indicate infectious mononucleosis. Lymphocytosis predominates—atypical lymphocytes account for at least 10% of total lymphocytes. Mild thrombocytopenia and neutropenia are frequent transient findings. Liver enzyme levels, particularly serum transaminase levels, are mild to moderately elevated in about 90% of patients with infectious mononucleosis.

The Monospot test detects heterophile antibodies, and although not highly sensitive, is the most commonly run laboratory test in the work-up of EBV infection. These antibodies are found in 80% to 90% of patients with acute infectious mononucleosis although the test may take up to 3 weeks to become positive. Thus, retesting may be necessary if the first test was done early on in the disease process. Heterophile antibodies usually disappear by 3 months but are sometimes present for up

to a year. The test is less sensitive in younger patients (75% sensitivity in children aged 24–28 months and 25% in children aged 10–24 months). EBV-specific serologies should therefore be checked in children. In fact, further testing of serum IgM antibodies to EBV may prove useful in adult patients as well, if a diagnosis based on initial testing is questionable. Anti-EBNA and anti-VCA are two specific anti-EBV serology tests that are widely available, although they are also less sensitive in younger patients (60% sensitivity in infants, but up to 100% sensitivity in young adults). False-positive results for EBV have been noted in HIV-infected individuals but are considered rare.

During the first 20 to 30 days after EBV infection, the CBC could show a granulocytopenia but no rise in lymphocytes. By the fourth week after infection, however, the CBC could reveal a lymphocytic leukocytosis, with more than 10,000 WBCs/mcL and more than 30% of those being lymphocytes. Under microscopic examination, lymphocytes are larger than normal and typically stain more darkly using standard cell microscopy preparations.

In isolated infectious mononucleosis, throat cultures will be negative for *Streptococcus* and other bacteria. Although RPR will be negative in most cases, a transient false-positive RPR result may occur in up to 10% of cases. Serum levels of liver transaminases and bilirubin will likely be elevated.

Differential Diagnosis

Many diseases present similarly to infectious mononucleosis; however, careful assessment of the patient's signs and symptoms as well as diagnostic tests will assist in making the diagnosis. Table 17.3 presents a comparison of the signs and symptoms of EBV-related syndromes. Glandular variant infectious mononucleosis, in which lymphadenopathy is out of proportion to the pharyngitis, differs from systemic variant mononucleosis, which presents with fever and fatigue and typically has mild or absent lymphadenopathy and pharyngitis.

A positive result on the heterophile antibody (Monospot) test will distinguish infectious mononucleosis from other diseases of similar presentation. In the differential of exudative pharyngitis, streptococcal, adenoviral, diphtherial, gonococcal, and herpes simplex infections should all be considered. HIV-infected or otherwise myelosuppressed teenagers and young adults may present with findings similar to those of EBV mononucleosis if they are infected with CMV or toxoplasmosis, but the heterophile (Monospot) test is more likely to be negative in these cases. In addition, peritonsillar abscess should be ruled out by an adequately collected throat culture.

Management

Symptom control is the mainstay of management for someone with infectious mononucleosis. The overall plan of care, therefore, involves supportive measures, including providing a quiet atmosphere for prolonged rest and recovery.

Table 17.3   Epstein-Barr Virus–Related Syndromes

	Infectious Mononucleosis	Oral Hairy Leukoplakia	Duncan's Disease (X-linked Lymphoproliferative Disorder)
Malaise	+	+/–	+
Lymphadenopathy	+	+	+
Fever	+	+/–	+/–
Splenomegaly	+ (50% of cases)	+/–	+
Pharyngeal exudate	+	–	–

+ present; – absent.

Antivirals are not available for either initial or subsequent therapy as symptom manifestations are largely unrelated to active viral replication. Rather, initial management focuses on symptom relief with rehydration, NSAIDs, gargling with warm salt water for throat pain, and OTC throat lozenges. Acetaminophen may be used for supportive, analgesic, and antipyretic treatment, although it will not confer anti-inflammatory benefits. In cases in which the airway is in danger of obstruction due to significant lymphadenopathy or mucosal swelling, corticosteroid therapy (prednisone) should be introduced over the course of 5 days (40 mg/day PO, potentially followed by a longer tapering period for persistent symptoms). Steroids may reduce viral shedding but do not affect symptom duration or the duration of convalescence.

Complications may arise in some patients over the course of the disease. Although peritonsillar abscess is rare, the soft palate and tonsils may become so edematous that the airway may be threatened. Therefore, the risk of airway obstruction should be assessed. In addition, a mild hepatitis may be seen in 90% of cases and requires cessation of any hepatotoxic medications if possible, and in extreme cases, interferon-alpha injections. Impending splenic rupture due to significant splenomegaly necessitates surgical resection of the spleen, and the wearing of an abdominal guard is often recommended as a presurgical preventive measure.

Acyclovir may reduce the severity of the lytic phase of active viral replication, but it does not affect the latent phase and therefore has no clear therapeutic role in infectious mononucleosis. Results of human vaccine trials against specific viral proteins (gp350/220) that target the B cell surface receptor for the virus (CD21) have been mixed; however, research is ongoing on novel vaccines, including vaccinia-based recombinant vaccine constructs.

Follow-up and Referral

Patients should be followed-up to monitor for the development of serious sequelae. Neurological complications may include Guillain-Barré syndrome, facial nerve palsy, meningoencephalitis, aseptic meningitis, transverse myelitis, or optic neuritis. Hematological complications may include hemolytic/aplastic anemia, thrombocytopenia, thrombotic thrombocytopenic purpura (TTP), hemolytic uremic syndrome, disseminated intravascular coagulation, or potentially fatal splenic rupture (spontaneous or traumatic). Cardiovascular complications may include myocarditis. Renal and genitourinary complications may include glomerulonephritis or genital ulceration, and GI complications may include pancreatitis.

It is important to provide the patient with a full clinical picture of the disease, including its prolonged course of recovery, so that the patient may play an active role in self-assessment during the follow-up period. Referrals are rare unless significant complications ensue. Patients with hemolytic anemia and TTP should be referred to a hematologist. Any patient with encephalitis will require an immediate neurology consultation. Patients with pericarditis must be referred to a cardiologist.

Patient Education

Young, school-age patients must be warned of the dangers of contact sports and rough-housing for at least 4 weeks after the onset of symptoms, because splenic rupture occurs predominantly within 3 weeks of symptom onset and may occur in the absence of frank splenomegaly (50% of splenic rupture cases). In addition, up to half of all splenic rupture cases may occur without any preceding trauma, and rupture does not correlate with symptom severity or abnormal laboratory results. A good rule of thumb is that the patient's energy level must be at baseline before the resumption of strenuous or risky physical activity, and this must not occur before 4 weeks. However, strict bedrest is required during this entire period and will be driven largely by the patient's energy level.

Patients must learn that their recurrent fevers will typically disappear long before they feel recovered; fevers will typically subside after 10 to 14 days although energy level will not rebound to baseline until 1 to 3 months postinfection. Therefore, teenagers and young adults who typically manage busy schedules and active lives will need to accept that they require rest for a prolonged recovery period that will last weeks, rather than days.

Other elements to consider in patient education include giving information about prescribed drugs, including appropriate dosage and adverse effects. The clinician should also caution patients to avoid alcohol and cigarette use because they will aggravate coughing and nausea. Alcohol should be avoided for a minimum of 3 months after liver function tests return to normal. Appropriate follow-up and patient education should also include age-appropriate counseling regarding sexual practices, given that, unlike infectious mononucleosis, some sexually transmitted infections may be fatal or significantly affect future fertility.

CHRONIC FATIGUE SYNDROME AND FIBROMYALGIA SYNDROME

Chronic fatigue syndrome (CFS) remains poorly understood, despite abundant attention in the scientific and lay press. The lack of agreement as to its cause, laboratory markers, and clinical course may explain why the syndrome is not discussed in some medical texts. There appears to be significant overlap between CFS and fibromyalgia syndrome (FMS), another controversial chronic pain syndrome. The majority of patients with CFS meet criteria for FMS, and at least 70% of patients with FMS meet criteria for CFS. Moreover, both these disorders have been widely recognized in persons with comorbid psychiatric illness, because nearly two-thirds of CFS patients and one-third of FMS patients meet criteria for depression, dysthymia, or anxiety disorders. Many authors have criticized the historical and physical diagnostic criteria for both conditions as having a strong potential for overlap with somatization disorders. See the Iceberg figure for additional fibromyalgia syndrome information.

Epidemiology and Causes

Without a generally accepted working definition of CFS, it is difficult to systematically ascertain its epidemiology. Chronic fatigue is a presenting complaint in up to 25% of patients presenting to ambulatory care settings, and it is estimated that approximately 10% of these individuals meet diagnostic criteria for CFS. Numerous books in the popular press have advanced the belief that women are affected two times more often than men. The same references tend to agree that younger women are more often affected. Causes of CFS have been hypothesized to be autoimmune and infectious in etiology; however, the causes for the syndrome have yet to be determined. Importantly, it is a diagnosis of exclusion. The incidence of CFS ranges from 4 to 8.6 cases per 100,000 adults.

More epidemiological data for FMS exist in the medical literature. An estimated 11 million people in the United States have FMS, and 80% to 90% are women. The prevalence of FMS has been estimated at 0.5% for men and 3.4% for women, with some studies claiming an increased prevalence in women compared with men of up to 10:1. Prevalence is higher in older patients, at more than 7% for women aged 60 to 79 years.

These numbers are reflected in the clinical impact of FMS as up to 20% of all patient visits to rheumatology practices are for FMS. It is now considered the most common cause of generalized musculoskeletal pain in women aged 20 to 55 years. FMS may occur with greater frequency in patients with disorders characterized by systemic inflammation, including rheumatoid arthritis (RA), systemic lupus erythematosus, and hepatitis C infection. However, an underlying inflammatory etiology to FMS is unclear, because relatives of patients with fibromyalgia are seven times more likely than relatives of patients with RA to have FMS. In addition, several studies have shown that up to 50% of patients with FMS have a history of sexual and/or physically violent abuse, suggesting the importance of psychological factors in the development of FMS.

Pathophysiology

Despite extensive investigation, the pathophysiology of CFS and FMS are not clear. It has been hypothesized that both syndromes may be disorders of muscle energy metabolism, inflammatory or immunopathological diseases of muscle, generalized disorders of pain perception, neuronally mediated hypotension, neuroendocrine disturbances, dysregulated serotonin secretion, sleep disturbances, or a sequela of sexual abuse or domestic violence. However, it is important to note that none of these etiologies has been consistently confirmed through randomized and controlled prospective studies. Although depression and anxiety disorders demonstrate great overlap with both CFS and FMS, it is controversial as to whether these conditions occur concurrently, whether CFS and FMS lead to psychiatric sequelae, or whether these chronic conditions are somatic manifestations of underlying mood disorders. In turn, patients commonly experience accusations of malingering (intentionally fabricating symptoms for secondary gain), which, by definition, would be unfounded if any of the aforementioned etiologies are confirmed.

Extensive work has explored a potential infectious etiology for CFS, focusing on EBV, retroviruses, and human herpesvirus–6 (HHV-6) as causative agents. However, there has been difficulty in reproducing positive results across different laboratories. Moreover, no consistent serological profile has been identified that distinguishes patients with CFS from control groups across multiple studies.

Several studies, however, have demonstrated qualitative and quantitative differences in immune function between patients with CFS and controls, including reduced numbers of NK cells with depressed function, reduced levels of immunoglobulin and immune complexes, and increased numbers of cell surface adhesion molecules, among others. However, the differences are of questionable clinical significance and have been inconsistent and even conflicting between different studies.

Studies that have examined neuroendocrine differences between affected patients and controls have produced similarly inconclusive results. Although some evidence points to undersecretion of adrenocorticotropic hormone (ACTH) and reduced serum cortisol levels, these findings are not specific for CFS and have also been observed in FMS, as well as in healthy subjects with altered sleep patterns related to overnight work shifts.

Studies attempting to clarify the etiology of FMS have also not been definitive. For many years, FMS was considered a disorder of muscle metabolism, possibly related to chronic hypoxia of muscular tissue. However, studies of lactate levels, muscle force studies, and postexertional pain have demonstrated a marked similarity between patients with FMS and sedentary controls. Thus, the most current theories suggest that patients with FMS suffer from disproportionate perceptions of pain, exacerbated by muscle inactivity and deconditioning. In fact, lower pain perception thresholds have been documented in first-degree relatives of patients with FMS.

Although no studies have been conclusive, altered pain perception is more likely to be a central rather than peripheral nociceptor (pain receptor) phenomenon. This is supported by observations in FMS patients of altered patterns of sleep and mood, decreased blood flow to pain centers in the brain, and alterations in serotonin secretions and the pituitary-hypothalamic-adrenal neuroendocrine axis. In addition, autonomic dysregulation of heart rate and systemic blood pressure has also been implicated on the basis of tilt-table testing for orthostatic hypotension; however, again, these findings have not been consistently reproduced. An anti-inflammatory component to the myalgias of FMS has never been shown, which likely explains the lack of efficacy of NSAID and corticosteroid therapies in this condition.

Clinical Presentation

Subjective

The symptomatic presentation of CFS and FMS may overlap considerably. Patients may report postexercise malaise, fatigue, multiple joint pains, headaches, impaired memory and concentration, depressed mood, cognitive disturbances, sore throat, restless and disordered sleep, and myalgias. Often the patient will also report having consulted one or more specialists concerning these vague symptoms.

Objective

The onset of CFS is sudden and may be preceded by a mononucleosis-like illness or by significant gastrointestinal findings. This same type of preceding event may also herald the onset of FMS.

The patient will appear tired. The skin may be pale. Cervical lymph nodes, if enlarged, will be shotty and nontender. Otherwise, the examination may be unremarkable. Despite complaints of impaired memory and concentration, the results of objective mental status assessments may vary with reference to recent recall and problem-solving abilities.

For a diagnosis of FMS to be made, the patient must have widespread muscular pain that has been present for at least 3 months; the pain should be present in 11 of 18 trigger points (also called tender points) on digital palpation with an applied pressure of 4 kg/cm (enough force to whiten the examiner's nailbed). The 18 trigger points are bilateral sites at nine key locations (see Table 17.4). Pain at these sites should be significantly greater than at

Table 17.4	Diagnostic Criteria for Fibromyalgia*
History Criteria	Pain is considered widespread when ALL of the following are present: Pain in the left side of the body Pain in the right side of the body Pain above the waist Pain below the waist Axial skeletal pain (cervical spine, anterior chest, thoracic spine, or lower back)
Pain Criteria	Pain exists in 11 of 18 tender points (trigger points) on digital palpation (at a force of at least 4 kg): Occiput: Bilateral, at the suboccipital muscle insertions Low cervical: Bilateral, at the anterior aspects of the intertransverse spaces at C5–C7 Trapezius: Bilateral, at the midpoint of the upper border Supraspinatus: Bilateral, at origins above the scapula spine near the medial border Second rib: Bilateral, at the second costochondral junctions, just lateral to the junctions on upper surfaces Lateral epicondyle: Bilateral, 2 cm distal to the epicondyles Gluteal: Bilateral, in upper quadrants of buttocks in anterior fold of muscle Greater trochanter: Bilateral, posterior to the trochanteric prominence Knee: Bilateral, at the medial fat pad proximal to the joint line For a tender point to be "positive," the client must state that the palpation was painful. A statement of "tender" is not considered "painful."

*Client must have a history of widespread pain (present for at least 3 months) in specific anatomic areas and must exhibit this pain during an examination of tender points.

Source: Running, AF, and Berndt, AE: *Management guidelines for nurse practitioners working in family practice.* FA Davis, Philadelphia, 2003, p 586.

The Iceberg of Fibromyalgia

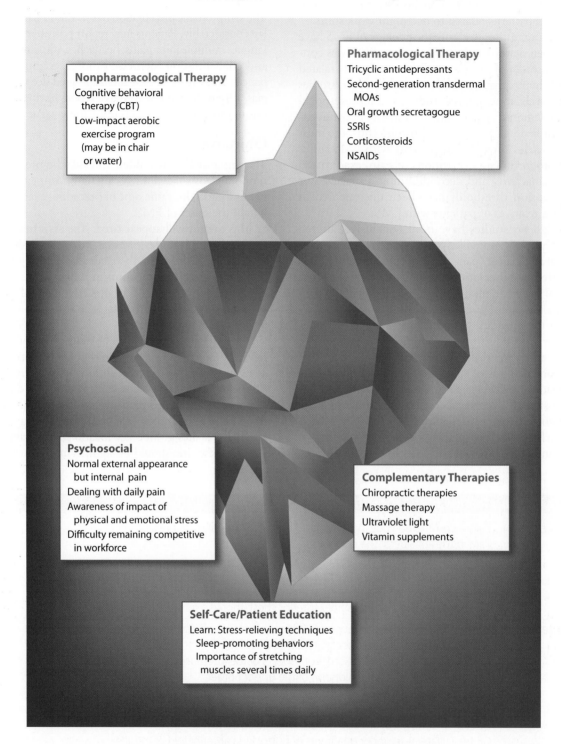

Nonpharmacological Therapy
Cognitive behavioral
  therapy (CBT)
Low-impact aerobic
  exercise program
  (may be in chair
  or water)

Pharmacological Therapy
Tricyclic antidepressants
Second-generation transdermal
  MOAs
Oral growth secretagogue
SSRIs
Corticosteroids
NSAIDs

Psychosocial
Normal external appearance
  but internal pain
Dealing with daily pain
Awareness of impact of
  physical and emotional stress
Difficulty remaining competitive
  in workforce

Complementary Therapies
Chiropractic therapies
Massage therapy
Ultraviolet light
Vitamin supplements

Self-Care/Patient Education
Learn: Stress-relieving techniques
  Sleep-promoting behaviors
  Importance of stretching
    muscles several times daily

control sites, which are not expected to be tender, such as the patient's thumbnail or midforearm.

Diagnostic Reasoning
Diagnostic Tests

Chronic fatigue syndrome tends to strike once active, highly functional adults. The physical exam for CFS is typically normal. Advanced imaging tests such as CT and MRI are not indicated in the absence of significant physical findings. In addition, virus-specific serologies against EBV or Lyme disease are also not recommended without a strong suspicion by history or physical exam findings, because any positive result is likely to be a false positive in the setting of low suspicion.

Laboratory testing for FMS should include the same screening tests as for CFS, as well as muscle enzymes (creatine kinase, aldolase). ANA is often not helpful unless an autoimmune disorder such as systemic lupus erythematosus (SLE) is highly suspected because it may provide a false-positive result that incorrectly labels these patients as having lupus.

Differential Diagnosis

There is a wide differential diagnosis for both CFS and FMS. The majority of alternative diagnoses can be ruled out via the basic laboratory studies mentioned in the preceding text. The differential includes rheumatic disease, such as SLE, rheumatoid arthritis, and polymyalgia rheumatica; endocrinological diseases, such as thyroid disease and parathyroid disease, metabolic myopathies, and neuropathies; infectious diseases, such as Lyme disease; mood disorders and psychiatric diseases, including depression, dysthymia, personality disorders, and psychotic illness; malingering; and other conditions such as irritable bowel syndrome, cancer, and parkinsonism.

Myofascial pain syndrome involves a more limited number of tender muscular trigger points than FMS, as well as involuntary constrictions of muscular fascia (fibrous connective tissue that surrounds muscles), which has been considered as either a separate clinical entity or a regional variant of FMS.

The patient should be classified as having CFS or idiopathic chronic fatigue if severe fatigue persists or relapses for 6 months or longer. It should be classified as CFS if the fatigue criterion is met and four or more of the following symptoms are concurrently present for 6 months: impaired memory or concentration, sore throat, tender cervical or axillary lymph nodes, muscle pain (myalgia), multiple joint pains (arthralgias), new headaches, restless sleep, and postexertion malaise.

The Centers for Disease Control and Prevention (CDC) diagnostic criteria for CFS are based on clinically evaluated persistent or relapsing fatigue without explanation with at least four of the following self-reported symptoms (but no criteria for physical exam findings): impaired concentration/short-term memory, sore throat, tender cervical/axillary nodes, muscle pain, arthralgias without redness or swelling, poor sleep, new-onset headache or headache of a new and worsening pattern, and malaise after activity that lasts at least 24 hours. For patients with chronic fatigue who do not fit these criteria, the term *idiopathic chronic fatigue* is used, but these criteria are still being evaluated for validity. Sjögren's syndrome should also be considered as a differential diagnosis as many CFS patients also present with anhydrosis.

Management

Management of CFS and FMS remains controversial. The goal of therapy is to enable the patient to have the best quality of life possible within the limitations of chronic disability related to pain.

The two therapies that have been shown to be beneficial in terms of symptom relief and increased function (albeit not curative) are cognitive-behavioral therapy (CBT) that changes beliefs and behaviors that are barriers to recovery, and graded exercise. Increased bedrest should not be encouraged. A supportive approach to the patient–clinician relationship is critical. This reinforces that CFS or FMS is a genuine diagnosis and, thus, avoids the debate between psychological and "organic" etiologies.

The following pharmacotherapies have been tried with little consistent success: the Alzheimer's drug galantamine (Reminyl), intravenous immune globulin (IVIG), acyclovir (Zovirax), and selective serotonin reuptake inhibitors (SSRIs) such as citalopram (Celexa), fluoxetine (Prozac), and paroxetine (Paxil). Corticosteroids have shown some benefit in uncontrolled studies but come with the risk of adrenal suppression. Moreover, controlled, blinded studies have not confirmed these benefits.

Positive Lyme titers should not be taken as a definite sign of infection unless IgM is positive with a strong suspicion of this disorder, because false positive rates will be high otherwise. Thus, antibiotics should not be given indiscriminately, based solely on positive Lyme titer results.

The long-term prognosis of CFS is better than the short-term prognosis. However, certain factors have been cited as predicting a poor prognosis: (1) having more than eight medically unexplained physical symptoms other than the ones cited as CFS diagnostic criteria, (2) lifetime history of dysthymia, (3) chronic fatigue lasting more than 1.5 years, (4) less than 16 years of formal education, and (5) age greater than 38 years at the onset of disease.

For FMS, acetaminophen (650 mg 4 times daily) and tramadol (Ultram; 75 mg 4 times daily) as combination therapy may be helpful analgesics, but there is little to no evidence that NSAID or corticosteroid therapy is beneficial. As a narcotic, tramadol carries abuse potential, but this is generally considered less than for higher potency narcotic pain medications, such as oxycodone, hydrocodone, or morphine. Amitriptyline (Elavil), 75 mg daily in divided doses, remains one of the medications most frequently prescribed. Although it helps some patients, research has shown that after 3 months it has no greater effect than placebo. Additionally, this and other tricyclics have anticholinergic side effects. A similar transient therapeutic effect has also been seen with cyclobenzaprine (Flexeril), which appears effective for the first 3 months, initially taken at 5 mg three times daily and then increasing to 10 mg three times daily. The adage of "start low and go slow" applies to this medication as well. Desipramine (Norpramin) is an alternative tricyclic agent with fewer side effects and may work in patients who respond to amitriptyline but cannot tolerate it. Of all the SSRIs, fluoxetine has been most promising when taken in doses from 20 to 80 mg daily. Dual norepinephrine and serotonin reuptake inhibitors such as duloxetine (Cymbalta) (40–60 mg daily) have shown some benefit as well. Although management guidelines are not well established, tramadol should probably be added only after psychotropic medications are tried first. In addition, low-dose clonazepam (Klonopin, 0.5 mg at bedtime) may be helpful, and research is also being done on the usefulness of antiseizure medications. One of the most recently approved agents for FMS is pregabalin (Lyrica), which may be started at 75 mg two times daily and increased to a maintenance dose of 150 to 225 mg 2 times daily. Pregabalin may cause dizziness or somnolence, however, and has the potential to cause severe allergic reactions.

An ongoing low-impact aerobic (cardiovascular) exercise program (walking, swimming, biking, water aerobics) with CBT, hypnotherapy, or electromyogram biofeedback therapy may be a useful adjunct in certain patients, because these therapies have been shown in limited trials to increase quality of life (although not affect symptom severity). Chiropractic and massage therapies are only weakly supported. Trials with ultraviolet light (especially blue light) exposure have shown mixed results. Vitamin supplementation also has received mixed results in small clinical trials.

Follow-up and Referral

Follow-up should occur according to the symptoms reported. Because many of these patients have been treated for affective psychiatric disorders in the past, they may already know what psychological manifestations should trigger professional assistance.

Typically, patients are referred to rheumatologists initially to assist in confirming the diagnosis by ruling out autoimmune syndromes. Referral to regional specialists who study and treat CFS and FMS may be required. Psychiatric referral could be necessary if mood disorders are apparent or mental status test results warrant.

Patient Education

For both CFS and FMS, management relies on helping the patient cope with a chronic condition by learning methods to deal with the chronicity of the symptoms. While validating its impact on the patient's life, clinicians should stress that the patient does not have a fatal disease. Although symptomatic, it may be relatively benign in terms of the risk of complications, and the patient can live a normal and productive life. Living with the uncertainty of the diagnosis and the chronicity of the problem are continuing challenges for both the patient and clinician. This is illustrated in The Patient's Voice 17.1. Patients may be encouraged to use whatever alternative means they believe might assist them with pain relief such as chiropractic, therapeutic touch, guided imagery, hypnosis, and so on. At present, there are no definitive answers or guaranteed treatments for these conditions. Pain is as the patient perceives it, and any treatment may relieve the pain if the patient believes it to be helpful. Patients should understand that physical and emotional stress can worsen their symptoms. Patient education has been shown in unblinded studies to improve FMS symptoms and quality of life and is a critical component of treatment. The *Circle of Caring* model is tested in cases in which a patient is frustrated and experiences daily pain. It is especially trying when a patient outwardly appears to be fine but is mentally suffering on the inside. Conditions such as these may require multiple resources and for all involved with the patient to focus on finding what works best for each individual patient. Nursing Research–Based Practice Box 17.1 describes the responses of parents and families to the presence of CFS as a chronic parental illness and the challenges that exist.

The Patient's Voice 17.1
Chronic Fatigue Syndrome

I have been chronically tired for years. It started out that I would drive the kids to school in my nightgown, then I'd go back to bed. I had given up my job the year before. Thank goodness we could afford it. My husband thought that I was depressed, so I went to doctor after doctor and tried all sorts of antidepressant medications with no relief. One doctor suggested that I needed to see a psychiatrist because the antidepressants were not working and he said I was obviously depressed. I knew "deep down" that I wasn't depressed, but I also knew that something wasn't right. I knew I had to do something when I overheard one of my kids on the phone telling his friend not to come over because his Mom was just "having another lazy day in her PJ's."

That same week, I heard an ad on the radio inviting participants for a study on chronic fatigue syndrome. I had heard about the syndrome vaguely and thought it was just a "catch-all term" for tiredness. I didn't really think it was a medical condition. I called the phone number given for the study and just answering a few questions over the phone, I felt 200% better! There actually is a medical name for the condition that I know I have. Now, I know I'm not crazy or just lazy. I can't wait to participate in the study. Even if it doesn't help me, I'll feel better knowing that what I have is "real."

Nursing Research-Based Practice 17.1

Donalek, JG. When a parent is chronically ill: Chronic fatigue syndrome. *Nurs Res* 58(5):332–339, 2009.

As chronic illness may reshape not only the life of the ill parent but also that of the entire family, this study was undertaken to describe the responses of parents and the ensuing family system responses to the presence of chronic fatigue syndrome as a chronic parental illness. This qualitative study involved eight ill parents and multiple members of their families. After interviews were conducted, thematic analyses at the individual, intrafamily, and across-family levels were used to explore the phenomena. The parents described the onset of illness, an ongoing struggle to receive diagnosis and care, and the significance of the illness in transforming present and future roles of family members. Multiple members of their family together with the ill parent described how they struggled with the reality of the illness, the shifting roles and responsibilities of the parents and their children, the reduced family income, and the frequent social isolation that could be exacerbated by the controversial nature of the illness. Families described and demonstrated their struggles to maintain a normal family life and make plans in the face of continuing uncertainty. Recommendations are made for future directions in family nursing research exploring the responses of families in which a parent is chronically ill.

■ LYME DISEASE

Lyme disease is a multisystem inflammatory disease of infectious etiology that does not take its name from the spirochete that causes it, *Borrelia burgdorferi.* Instead, it is named for a town in Connecticut (Old Lyme) where it was isolated among residents in the 1970s. It is a tick-borne illness that is prevalent among people who live in wooded areas of the eastern United States, with 96% of cases occurring in the following 13 states: Connecticut, Delaware, Maine, Maryland, Massachusetts, Minnesota, New Hampshire, New Jersey, New York, Pennsylvania, Vermont, Virginia, and Wisconsin. In addition, Lyme disease has been isolated in eastern provinces of Canada, some parts of Europe, and Australia.

Epidemiology and Causes

According to Centers for Disease Control and Prevention (CDC) data, the incidence of Lyme disease rose steadily over 10 years to a peak in 2009, but declined in 2010 and 2011. Some estimates suggest a tripling in the number of cases over the last several decades. However, epidemiological data gathering policies at the state level have been criticized as being imprecise and leading to exaggerated case numbers, with both overreporting and overdiagnosis being cited as potential confounders. For example, although incidence should be correlated with isolates of *B burgdorferi,* spirochete isolates have not been consistently identified in a number of states where cases have been reported.

Vector-borne diseases do not distinguish among races, gender, or other demographic traits. Lyme disease in the United States is limited only to individuals with exposure to *B burgdorferi* via tick bites. In Europe and Asia, other species of *Borrelia* such as *B afzelii* and *B garinii* are also causative agents, but these are not typically isolated in the United States. These differences in bacteriology may underlie the differing clinical manifestations of this disease by geography, for example, a higher frequency of arthritis and erythema migrans (bull's-eye) rash seen in the United States.

Pathophysiology

The likelihood of infection relates to the duration of tick exposure. The infected tick must feed for at least 24 to 48 hours before it passes along the spirochete to the host. Up to 90% of cases are transmitted via bites from ticks in the immature nymph stage, rather than due to bites from adults. Because of the small size of the tick (which is smaller in comparison to the typical wood ticks found on dogs), finding the tick before 24 hours have elapsed may prove difficult. However, vigilant inspection of skin and hair after exposure to wooded areas heightens the success of locating and removing the tick and, thereby, preventing spirochete transmission.

Lyme disease is transmitted primarily by the tick *Ixodes scapularis.* Once hatched from summer leaf clutter blanketing the forest floor, tick larvae acquire spirochetes on taking their first blood meal from infected mice, birds, or other small mammals. The larvae eventually detach from their hosts to molt and emerge the following spring as infected nymphs that are prone to spreading disease when feeding in the late spring, summer, and early fall. After this blood meal, these nymphs detach from their hosts and molt into adult forms later in the fall, in turn, seeking blood meals and transmitting the infection most often to white-tailed deer throughout the rest of the season and into the winter and early spring, before laying another egg mass the following summer to begin the cycle again. Thus, the 2-year tick life cycle and the ability to identify and avoid bites from larger adult ticks help to explain the seasonal preference for Lyme disease being spread by nymphs in the summer months, rather than in the winter.

Half of the ticks that occupy the eastern and midwestern United States in localized hotspots of high disease incidence may be infected with the spirochete; therefore, there is a high likelihood of infection by tick exposure in the wooded areas of these regions. Few ticks along the Pacific Coast of the United States are infected (*Ixodes pacificus*), so tick bites in this region are less likely to pass the spirochete to a human host. Although only 30% of affected persons can clearly recall an antecedent tick bite, blood meals by infected ticks remain the only well-documented mechanism of spirochete transmission to human hosts. Some evidence exists for transplacental transmission from infected mothers to developing fetuses, but this generally results in good outcomes, and the clinical significance of intrauterine infection is questionable.

The causative organisms of Lyme disease are capable of producing systemic tissue injury with a relatively low microbial load. This occurs despite the absence of any excreted microbial toxins or widespread host inflammatory responses, such as a lymphocytic infiltrate. At the initiation of infection, spirochetes are believed to bind fibronectin and epithelial cell–derived proteoglycans in the extracellular matrix (e.g., heparin, dermatan sulfate) via glycosaminoglycan receptors. This initiates a mild local inflammatory response that causes cutaneous erythema at sites of spirochetal invasion and centrifugal spread from the original tick bite. Subsequent spirochetemia and tissue-specific binding allows for the development of neurological sequelae (via glycosphingolipid receptors), a vasculopathy similar to endarteritis obliterans seen in syphilis, and cardiac conduction defects in certain individuals. Arthritis is thought to be due to joint inflammation from localized exposure to spirochetal antigens, such as outer surface protein A (OspA) or the heat shock protein groEL.

B burgdorferi has been shown to exert immunomodulatory influences on host cells, including both decreased MHC class II antigen-presenting molecules on Langerhans cells isolated from late-phase cutaneous skin lesions and upregulation of the class II MHC molecules HLA-DRβ1, HLA-DR2, and HLA-DR4 on synovial endothelial cells in arthritic joints. The role of cytokines in this disease has not been fully elucidated, but several studies have demonstrated increased levels of macrophage-derived tumor necrosis factor–alpha, interleukin-1 (IL-1), and IL-6 in the blood, synovial fluid, and cerebrospinal fluid (CSF) of affected persons.

In addition, an autoimmune pathology has also been implicated in late disease manifestations. Most notably, the predominant T-cell receptor found on activated T lymphocytes after infection is specific for an epitope of OspA presented within certain class II MHC molecules that are upregulated in affected patients. Moreover, this OspA epitope has been shown to be cross-reactive with the leukocyte adhesion molecule human lymphocyte function associated antigen–1 (LFA-1), which is highly expressed on T lymphocytes. Studies of transgenic mice tolerant to OspA suggest that this protein does not fully explain these autoimmune phenomena.

Some evidence has suggested the importance of a *Borrelia*-specific superantigen. In addition, IgM antibodies against the spirochete protein flagellin are cross-reactive with human axonal proteins and myelin; these have been suggested to mediate the neurological sequelae of Lyme disease. Several other types of autoantibodies have been identified in the CSF of Lyme disease patients.

However, it is not known whether these antibodies play a role in the actual pathogenesis of the disease or are simply a benign secondary consequence of infection.

Clinical Presentation
Subjective

Early in the course of the disease, the patient typically complains of a flu-like illness, including fever, chills, and myalgia. The patient may report having discovered a rash or red spot that grew in size. The report of a rash may be accompanied by objective findings on examination.

Later in the course of the disease, malaise, fatigue, headache, neck pain and stiffness, and generalized pains may constitute presenting symptoms. Left untreated, the disease will progress so that complaints will include multiple joint arthritis. Late in the disease trajectory, the patient may complain of memory loss, cognitive disturbances, mood changes, and peripheral neuropathy in addition to arthritis.

Objective

In early-localized disease, occurring days to 1 month after exposure, rash is seen in 90% of cases, accompanied by the nonspecific findings of fatigue, malaise, headache, myalgias and arthralgias, cervical stiffness, and lymphadenopathy. The patient may also present with a low-grade fever. The exanthem is called erythema migrans, which is a rash caused by the tick bite that is typically located on parts of the body where the tick selectively feeds, such as the axilla, groin, and waistband. The bull's-eye–appearing rash grows in size as it spreads ("migrates") from the site of the bite. The classic rash of erythema migrans is occasionally pruritic and/or burning, may develop central clearing, and is typically greater than 5 cm in size. The presence of this rash is essentially diagnostic of Lyme disease in the setting of appropriate clinical findings and may obviate the need for serological confirmation.

In early-disseminated disease, which occurs days to 10 months after infection and often in the absence of erythema migrans, the patient presents with systemic manifestations including carditis (less than 10% of cases) and neurological manifestations (10% of cases) such as lymphocytic meningitis, cranial nerve (CN) palsies (especially of CN VII) and radiculoneuritis. This neurological triad is known as Bannwarth's syndrome and is more common in European cases of Lyme disease than in the United States.

In late disease, which may be months to years after exposure, symptoms are characterized by intermittent arthritis (50%, which responds to oral antibiotic therapy) and arthralgias (20%), with 10% having monoarthritis of the knee. In addition, patients may have neurological manifestations known as tertiary neuroborreliosis, including encephalopathy, neurocognitive impairment, and peripheral neuropathy, as well as cutaneous manifestations such as solitary lymphocytoma and acrodermatitis chronica atrophicans. These cutaneous manifestations are typically seen only in European cases due to *B afzelii.*

Objective findings later in the disease include regional or organ-specific physical abnormalities. Cardiac findings include dysrhythmias and a prolonged P-R interval. A rare finding is third-degree heart block. If the neurological system is involved, objective findings may include nuchal rigidity, sensorimotor disturbances, and paresthesias. Mental status examination may be positive for impaired problem resolution. Skin eruptions resembling the erythema migrans of early infection may recur later, as well. Very late in the disease trajectory, musculoskeletal findings predominate. In particular, joints become edematous and are associated with pain to touch. Gait disturbance may occur in association with encephalopathy. In contrast, upper respiratory or GI symptoms are more consistent with viral syndromes than with Lyme disease.

Diagnostic Reasoning
Diagnostic Tests

The term *chronic Lyme disease* is not preferred because it tends to foster fixation on this diagnosis as a cause of chronic, nonspecific complaints. Cultures of the skin lesion or rash can isolate *B burgdorferi* in half of the cases. Because the culture takes a long time to grow, serological studies are preferred. Histological and immunological staining is low yield in diagnostic testing owing to the low frequency of causative organisms. Positive serologies with ELISA tests against *Borrelia* sonicates containing mixtures of bacterial antigens (which often have suboptimal specificity, giving a number of false positives due to cross-reactivity with normal human proteins, other spirochete infections, EBV infection, or autoimmune disorders such as SLE or RA) must be confirmed by Western blot tests in which specific spirochetal proteins (e.g., heat shock proteins, flagellins) are directly detected by antibody staining. Western blot (or immunoblot) tests have lower sensitivity than the ELISA, but have greater specificity, so they are useful to confirm Lyme disease but may not be preferred for general screening. These tests should be measured against CDC testing standards, however, and not just those of an individual laboratory, as there will be a great deal of variation between laboratories. It may be best to send blood samples to a laboratory associated with an established academic medical center doing research on Lyme disease. A hepatic panel may also be helpful when characterizing the disease, because hepatitis may be apparent.

Patients are often seronegative with early localized disease manifesting only with the characteristic rash (erythema migrans); thus, blood testing may be ineffective as an initial diagnostic method. However, patients are usually positive for *Borrelia*-specific IgM and IgG by the early disseminated phase (6–8 weeks after exposure). Early antibiotic therapy may render serological tests

negative for unknown reasons, as spirochetes may still be detected. In contrast, previous vaccination with LYMErix (a Lyme vaccine that is now off the market) can lead to false-positive ELISA tests for several years after vaccination. Also, antibody tests may stay positive even after Lyme disease has been treated and has fully resolved. IgM levels can remain elevated for more than a year, so they cannot be used to make a diagnosis of active disease, but rather only to confirm a diagnostic suspicion, if suspected for other reasons. These tests are nearly always positive in late stage disease, and a negative ELISA in these patients has strong negative predictive value and should not be followed by a Western blot test, because these will have lower sensitivity. *Borrelia*-specific antibody levels should be measured in the synovial fluid and CSF if there is clinical evidence of localized inflammation in the joints or CNS (closed-space inflammation) to determine whether this inflammation is due to *Borrelia* infection or is merely coincidental.

Lyme disease should never be diagnosed based on laboratory tests alone. Laboratory tests are only confirmatory, not diagnostic, and they should never be used as screening tools, because the false-positive rates are too high. A diagnosis of Lyme disease should also be made only with findings that clearly suggest this disease, rather than with only nonspecific chronic complaints. However, research-based diagnostic criteria for Lyme disease may be too narrow to be used for clinical diagnosis, because these will exclude many cases. For a number of reasons, the following tests for Lyme detection are not widely accepted because they may be considered experimental: variable surface antigen (VlsE) ELISA, PCR, urinary antigen testing, T-cell proliferative responses, and immune complex disruption. Thus, these laboratory tests should not be trusted to confirm a diagnosis of Lyme disease.

Differential Diagnosis

Differential diagnoses for Lyme disease include viral syndromes, Rocky Mountain spotted fever, and relapsing fever. It is important not to confuse FMS or CFS, which are not inflammatory disorders and have never been shown to be clearly infectious in etiology. Although FMS may develop after the onset of Lyme disease, it is important not to simply accept a diagnosis of chronic Lyme disease made previously by another clinician, because there is little evidence that this condition actually exists, as opposed to the late manifestations of the disease, which are considered genuine aspects of the disease process. Human granulocytic ehrlichiosis, caused by *Anaplasma phagocytophila,* is an important consideration as an alternate or a comorbid diagnosis, especially in the setting of high fever and severe constitutional complaints, elevated liver enzymes or leukopenia/thrombocytopenia.

Management

The goal of management is not only to stop the manifestations of the disease at the time of diagnosis, but also to prevent progression of the disease. About 90% of early-localized disease responds to antibiotic therapy, although empiric antibiotic therapy after any tick bite is not recommended. However, if a patient presents with a tick still attached to the skin that is positively identified as one of the known *Ixodes* carriers of Lyme disease from a geographical area confirmed to have high rates of *Borrelia* infection, antibiotic therapy may be initiated immediately after initial laboratory testing and later stopped if the diagnosis is not confirmed. The duration of treatment depends on the extent of involvement. Regimens for early-localized disease should last for 10 to 14 days, whereas 30 days of therapy are required for cardiac, neurological, and arthritic manifestations.

Doxycycline (Vibramycin) 100 mg two times daily may be used in the initial management of erythema migrans. Doxycycline, or any tetracycline, is not recommended for children younger than 8 years of age or pregnant women. The dosage is 2 mg/kg for children older than 8 years. Doxycycline is also effective against ehrlichiosis, however, which is an important differential diagnosis and may present as a comorbid infection. Alternative agents include amoxicillin (Amoxil), cefuroxime (Ceftin), and erythromycin (E-mycin). Cefuroxime is typically more expensive than doxycycline or amoxicillin. The amoxicillin dose is 500 mg three times daily (50 mg/kg per day divided every 8 hours, with this same maximum dose in children). The cefuroxime dose is 500 mg two times daily in adults and up to 30 mg/kg per day divided two times daily with this same maximum dose for children. Up to 15% of patients may display worsening of symptoms with rigors, fever, or hypotension in the first 24 hours of antibiotic therapy due to an acute inflammatory cytokine surge involving TNF-α, IL-6, and IL-8. This is referred to as a Jarisch-Herxheimer reaction and is well documented in tick- and louse-borne relapsing fever conditions. Macrolides such as erythromycin are not as effective as doxycycline, amoxicillin, or cefuroxime and should be used only for patients intolerant to these other first-line choices. A first generation cephalosporin such as cephalexin (Keflex) should not be used because these are not active against *Borrelia*.

Early-disseminated disease with mostly musculoskeletal manifestations should be treated with the same oral agents for 2 to 3 weeks total as long as meningitis or third-degree heart block is not noted. If neurological sequelae (other than isolated facial nerve palsy) or third-degree heart block is noted, IV antibiotic therapy should be started with ceftriaxone (2 g daily) or cefotaxime (2 g three times daily) for 2 to 4 weeks. First- and second-degree heart block and isolated facial nerve palsy can be treated with 3 weeks of oral antibiotics. A lumbar puncture should be done to analyze the CSF for anti-*Borrelia* antibodies or inflammatory cells (WBCs), because neurological manifestations may be subclinical. If subclinical meningitis is suspected with elevated WBCs in the CSF, IV antibiotic therapy is required. Third-degree heart block should be treated with IV ceftriaxone

or cefotaxime, and prednisone 40 to 60 mg/day in divided doses may be added if patients do not respond within 4 days, but this approach has not been validated in randomized trials. Late Lyme disease is treated with amoxicillin or doxycycline for at least 4 weeks if arthritis is the primary manifestation. If patients fail one or two courses of oral antibiotic therapy or if late disease presents with neurological sequelae (or if a lumbar puncture shows subclinical meningitis with WBC or autoantibodies), IV antibiotic therapy of ceftriaxone or cefotaxime for 4 weeks should be used.

All IV antibiotic therapy may be completed on an outpatient basis if the patient has reliable IV access (generally, a peripherally inserted central catheter or a central venous catheter, as opposed to a peripheral IV line) and a stable social situation. In addition, at least the first IV dose should be given in a monitored setting to evaluate for drug hypersensitivity. Weekly CBCs should be done to monitor for leukopenia, which may be seen with ceftriaxone and cefotaxime. Ceftriaxone may cause biliary sludging, which can be monitored with weekly hepatic panels to evaluate for hyperbilirubinemia. If this occurs, the patient should be switched to cefotaxime. GI effects, including *Clostridium difficile* colitis, may also occur. Doxycycline causes photosensitivity, and amoxicillin and cefuroxime can cause drug rashes.

Combination antibiotic therapy, an oral course of antibiotics following IV courses, pulse therapy with weekly IV treatments, and extended regimens lasting beyond 2 to 4 weeks have never been validated through randomized trials and should be avoided. These are only likely to increase drug toxicity. There is also no evidence that pharmacological treatment of asymptomatic seropositivity, found on routine "screening" for instance, is of any benefit. These patients should be thoroughly evaluated, however, to determine whether an asymptomatic phase is actually latent infection that will eventually manifest as late disease, because such individuals typically do not progress through early disease manifestations.

Failure of antibiotic therapy may relate to co-infection with other tick-borne diseases, such as ehrlichiosis. Headache, fatigue, and malaise may persist after treatment, but continued infection or the presence of a comorbid condition should probably be suspected only if symptoms worsen after treatment, if new signs of inflammation develop, or if there are documented changes on neuropsychiatric testing.

Follow-up and Referral

Follow-up for symptomatic presentations, before an actual diagnosis is made, may require weekly sessions. Thus, antibiotic therapy may be started after initial laboratory testing, if Lyme disease is highly suspected, and later stopped if the diagnosis is not confirmed on follow-up.

The rash of erythema migrans begins to resolve after the fifth dose of oral antibiotics, whereas fibromyalgic and CFS-like symptoms (e.g., headache, weakness, fatigue, arthralgias) may persist for years after infection. Actual FMS is also recognized as a postinfectious complication of Lyme disease.

Referral to a specialist may not be required if the diagnosis is straightforward. However, if the diagnosis is unclear, rather than overtreating with antibiotic therapy, a referral to an infectious disease specialist is indicated for further evaluation and recommendations. Neurological, cardiac, and other serious manifestations may necessitate appropriate specialist referrals should these manifestations persist, despite primary care management.

Patient Education

People should be encouraged to avoid foliage, especially at the ankle level, along wooded paths and to walk in the center of the path to avoid low-lying brush. Hikers should wear clothing that can prevent ticks from attaching to skin. When planning an activity in the woods, the patient should wear long pants and boots, and pants should be tucked inside the boot lip. Shirt collars should be closed. Tick repellant should be applied to the exposed skin and scalp. After removing clothing, the patient should inspect the axillae, groin, and waistband areas, in particular, for evidence of attached ticks or bites.

If infection has already occurred, the patient needs to learn the course of the disease and that recurrence of symptoms after initial treatment might occur. Seropositivity does not equal immunity against reinfection. Reinfection is possible with *Borrelia* of a different strain if the patient remains exposed to high-risk environments, although symptoms do not tend to be worse than those of the initial infection.

■ SJÖGREN'S SYNDROME

Sjögren's syndrome (SS) is a chronic inflammatory autoimmune disorder caused by exocrine dysfunction. It presents as dryness in all areas of the body where there are exocrine glands associated with mucous membranes, most notably the salivary and lacrimal glands. However, SS has the potential for affecting a wide array of organ systems including the skin, lung, kidney, and heart. In addition, the hematopoietic system may be affected with a propensity for lymphoma.

Epidemiology and Causes

SS has a worldwide distribution with an annual incidence of 4 in 100,000; 70% of these cases may be primary, whereas the others are associated with comorbid conditions and are considered secondary. Accurate estimates of disease prevalence are complicated by a lack of agreement as to the defining diagnostic criteria of the disease. However, it is generally agreed that SS strikes women nine times more often than men. Rheumatic diseases often accompany it. The typical age range for disease onset is 40 to 60 years. The cause of the syndrome has not been fully characterized, although it is generally considered autoimmune in nature. Because SS typically accompanies underlying rheumatic diseases, investigations evaluating the etiological links among these conditions are ongoing.

Pathophysiology

As an autoimmune disorder, lymphocytic infiltration in all affected organs is the pathophysiologic hallmark of SS. Pooling of lymphocytes and plasma cells in the lacrimal glands causes the characteristic dry eye conjunctivitis of the syndrome called keratoconjunctivitis sicca, while parotid enlargement and diminished salivary excretions result from a similar infiltrate within the salivary glands along with hyperplasia of the ductal epithelium, which produces characteristic dry mouth (xerostomia).

At least three-quarters of these infiltrating cells are T lymphocytes, primarily of the CD4+ T helper subset, with classical TCR αβ receptors and expressing a memory cell phenotype including LFA-1 surface adhesion molecules. About 10% of the infiltrating cells are B-lymphocytes and plasma cells that produce significant amounts of oligoclonal immunoglobulin. The adjacent glandular epithelium expresses high levels of class II MHC (HLA-DR) and costimulatory molecules such as B7, suggesting antigenic T-cell stimulation is central to the pathogenesis of SS. It is unclear whether these stimulatory antigens are autoantigens and/or certain viral antigens.

Evidence for a genetic predisposition to SS is supported by studies that recognize a familial propensity for specific HLA-DR3, HLA-DR5, and HLA-DRβ3 alleles in affected patients and their relatives. Primary SS has also been linked to genetic polymorphisms in regulatory DNA sequences of the IL-10 gene, a cytokine that influences cell-mediated immunity. However, IFN-γ and IL-2 appear to be the primary immunomodulatory cytokines in SS. Produced by ductal epithelium, IFN-γ upregulates the expression of HLA-DR molecules on epithelial antigen presenting cells and potentiates T-lymphocyte cellular cytotoxicity. Cytolytic destruction of exocrine gland tissue does not appear to explain the full pathology of SS, however, because decreased saliva and tear production does not correlate well with the degree of histological damage on glandular biopsies.

The importance of autoantibodies in the pathophysiology of SS has long been emphasized. Autoantibodies specific for acetylcholine receptors in salivary glands have been suggested to impair the secretion of saliva in histologically normal glands. Far more common, however, are autoantibodies to specific nucleoproteins associated with RNA, including anti-Ro (SSA) antibodies seen in up to 90% of SS cases and anti-La (SSB) antibodies seen in up to half of cases. Although the pathogenetic role of these antibodies is unclear, the same antibodies can be found in a variety of other autoimmune disorders, including neonatal lupus, in which they may mediate complete heart block after crossing the placenta from mother to child. Anti-α-fodrin antibodies may be even more sensitive and specific for SS than anti-Ro or anti-La, but their pathological significance is not fully established.

Infection by various viruses, including EBV, retroviruses such as human T-cell lymphotropic virus (HTLV-1), hepatitis C virus, and coxsackievirus, has been suggested to underlie primary SS. In vitro studies and preclinical animal models have demonstrated that infection with these viruses is capable of leading to lymphocytic infiltrates of the salivary and lacrimal glands, recreating many of the same symptoms as SS. Although viral particles are typically not present in high numbers, viral infection has been suggested to break tolerance to autoantigens and lead to SS via autoimmune activation. The relationship between SS and viral infection is not entirely clear, however, because much of the etiological evidence is indirect and does not predominate for any single virus.

Disorders of estrogen have also been indirectly implicated because primary SS is seen predominantly in women. Moreover, postmenopausal women taking estrogen-containing hormone replacement therapy (HRT) have a higher incidence of ocular dryness compared with non-HRT controls. This evidence remains circumstantial, however.

Clinical Presentation
Subjective

A patient may complain of dryness of the eyes and the feeling that a particulate is in them. Keratoconjunctivitis sicca is dryness of the cornea caused by a deficiency of tear secretion in which the corneal surface appears dull and rough and the eye feels gritty and irritated. The patient may also complain of dryness of the mouth (xerostomia) caused by cessation of normal salivary secretions. In addition, the patient may complain of loss of taste and smell, recurrent dental caries, dysphagia, vaginismus, and rectal bleeding. Associated complaints may be those of rheumatoid arthritis (RA), including joint swelling, pain, and malaise, as well as low-grade fever.

Objective

The patient may appear chronically ill, particularly if RA precedes SS. The patient's breath may smell fetid because of dental caries and mucosal dryness, and mucosal beds of the nose and throat will be pale and may reveal small fissures. The tongue could be beefy red because of dryness. Similar findings are associated with the vagina and anus.

Many other systemic, albeit rare, manifestations of SS may be present: a macular, papular, vesicular, or purpuric skin rash; arthralgias and myalgias; cardiopulmonary manifestations such as pericarditis or pulmonary hypertension from lymphocytic interstitial pneumonitis; pulmonary emboli due to circulating antiphospholipid/anticardiolipin antibodies; interstitial nephritis leading to renal tubular acidosis or glomerulonephritis (similar to that of systemic lupus erythematosus [SLE]); gastroesophageal reflux disease (GERD); hypothyroidism due to autoimmune thyroiditis; neurological sequelae including peripheral (mononeuritis multiplex or symmetric neuropathies) and autonomic neuropathies, CNS manifestations mimicking multiple sclerosis, transverse myelitis, optic neuritis, or ischemic strokes that may be due to vasculitis, thrombosis, or demyelination. Fatigue is another important aspect of the presentation, due to disrupted sleep patterns from mucosal dryness or accompanying systemic symptoms such as arthralgias and myalgias.

Diagnostic Reasoning
Diagnostic Tests

SS is diagnosed via clinical and laboratory findings, rather than identification of a single causative agent. Clinical diagnosis of SS includes six defining criteria: (1) inadequate tear production (evaluated using the Schirmer test with filter paper to blot tears on the lateral third of the lower eyelid [less than 5 mm of wetting in 5 minutes is abnormal] or using artificial replacement tears more than 3 times daily); (2) signs of corneal epithelial damage from dry eye using Rose-Bengal or fluorescein staining and slit-lamp examination; (3) decreased saliva production; (4) lymphocytic infiltration of labial salivary gland tissue on histopathology following labial gland biopsy—the closest test to a gold standard for diagnosis (greater than 50 immune cells surrounding an intact glandular lobule); (5) impaired salivary gland function by objective testing via radionuclide technetium scanning (quantitative salivary gland scintigraphy demonstrating poor uptake), parotid sialography with parotid gland cannulation and injection of oil-based contrast material, or spontaneous salivary production of less than or equal to 1.5 mL/15 min; and (6) autoantibodies including anti-Ro (SSA) and/or anti-La (SSB).

Initial lab tests include a CBC, rheumatoid factor, ANA, and gamma-globulin. The CBC might reveal an anemia of chronic disease, which is typically mild, leukopenia, and/or eosinophilia. The eosinophilia is caused by autoimmune factors and not by external antigens. Rheumatoid factor (RF) is positive in three-fourths of samples. ANA is typically elevated, as are gamma-globulin levels.

Electrophoresis studies are required to determine whether SS is present alone or in combination with other rheumatoid disease. SS alone typically manifests more specific autoantibodies—anti-Ro/SSA and anti-La/SSB—whereas SS and rheumatoid disease together may reveal antibodies against exocrine ducts and RA-associated nuclear antigens.

Differential Diagnosis

As patients with SS have a higher prevalence of hypothyroidism, this should be screened via a thorough history and TSH/free T_4 level. Further laboratory work-up includes a basic metabolic panel with hepatic function tests (liver transaminases), RF (to assess for RA), and ANA (to assess for SLE). HIV and hepatitis C testing may also be indicated. Sarcoidosis could be evaluated with a chest x-ray exam to evaluate for hilar lymphadenopathy or interstitial lung disease. An MRI or ultrasound and biopsy should be done if there is unilateral salivary gland enlargement to rule out malignancy or specific glandular pathology, such as acute bacterial sialadenitis. Bilateral salivary gland swelling may be due to acute viral infection (e.g., mumps, coxsackievirus, echovirus, or EBV) or chronic infection with HIV or hepatitis C; granulomatous disease such as sarcoidosis, amyloidosis, or TB; malnutrition; alcoholism; and eating disorders such as bulimia or anorexia with purging features.

Further differentials for SS include other autoimmune disorders that may exist concurrently, such as SLE, scleroderma, or RA. In fact, RF may be positive in up to 75% of cases. It is also critical to distinguish SS from patients with FMS or depression who may have significant anticholinergic toxicities from psychiatric medications, which can lead to dry eyes and especially dry mouth. Dry eyes may also result from impaired blinking due to muscular or neurological disorders, vitamin A deficiency leading to mucin deficiency (xerophthalmia), conjunctivitis, infiltration of the lacrimal glands (from sarcoidosis, lymphoma, or amyloidosis), or blepharitis from Meibomian gland dysfunction. Dry mouth can also result from sialadenitis from obstructing salivary gland stones, chronic viral infections (hepatitis C, HIV), and iatrogenic anticholinergic drug effects. In fact, the following conditions are exclusion criteria in terms of meeting the defining criteria of SS: previous head/neck irradiation or preexisting lymphoma, comorbid infection with hepatitis C or HIV with AIDS, sarcoidosis, graft versus host disease, or recent use of anticholinergic medications. Symptoms of mucosal dryness are also common in liver disease and depression, so these must be considered.

Management

The management of this syndrome consists primarily of symptom-directed supportive care, although research into immunomodulatory therapies is ongoing. To address the primary manifestations of dry eyes and dry mouth, normal saline eyedrops can relieve lacrimal dryness, and hard candies and gum may be used to stimulate salivation but should be sugar-free to avoid worsening dental caries. Dried fruits that contain malic acid may also be helpful in stimulating salivation. In extreme cases of salivary dryness, the patient should be encouraged to apply an artificial salivary gel or use a mouth spray. Fluids can also keep the mouth well lubricated as long as they do not contain caffeine (a diuretic) or ethanol (as used in mouthwash), which can be drying. Special toothpastes and toothbrushes designed for a dry mouth are also available. Quarterly dental evaluations, along with vigorous flossing and regular brushing, may prevent dental caries. Dry lips may be

treated with Vaseline and dry skin with moisturizing lotions, and vaginal dryness may be treated with intravaginal lubricant jelly.

Artificial tears and salivary gels often contain hypromellose (0.3%) or methylcellulose (0.3%) and may be used every 2 to 4 hours if needed. Several of these can be irritating to certain individuals. Pilocarpine (Salagen) 5 mg PO three to four times daily and cevimeline (Evoxac) 30 to 60 mg PO three times daily are specific cholinergic (muscarinic) agonists (parasympathomimetics) for stimulating aqueous secretions. These drugs are contraindicated in persons with narrow-angle glaucoma or iritis, owing to their mydriatic effects. Cevimeline should not be used if a patient has asthma, because it can worsen respiratory secretions. Acetylcysteine can be used as a mucolytic if thick mucous fibers coat the eyes, but this smells like rotten eggs because of its sulfur content. Spreading agents such as polyethylene glycol and dextran-70 0.1% drops are also available for dry eyes. Topical cyclosporine 0.05% 1 gtt every 12 hours is FDA approved to increase tear production, presumably by decreasing T-cell infiltration within the conjunctivae. If these treatments prove ineffective, the patient may undergo punctal occlusion, in which collagen plugs are placed by an ophthalmologist in the lacrimal puncta on the inferior eyelid so that tears (artificial or natural) cannot drain away to the nose.

The following are rarer systemic manifestations of SS, along with specific treatments:

- Macular, papular, vesicular, or purpuric skin rashes may require biopsy and treatment as a form of vasculitis.
- Arthralgias and myalgias may respond to NSAIDs or hydroxychloroquine.
- Inflammatory cardiopulmonary manifestations such as pericarditis or pulmonary hypertension from lymphocytic interstitial pneumonitis may require treatment with corticosteroids (prednisone) or other immunosuppressants (azathioprine, chlorambucil, cyclophosphamide).
- Interstitial nephritis leading to renal tubular acidosis or glomerulonephritis (similar to that of SLE) may require corticosteroid or immunosuppressant therapy (cyclophosphamide, mycophenolate).
- Rare neurological sequelae such as peripheral mononeuritis multiplex or symmetrical neuropathies and autonomic dysfunction (confirmed by tilt-table tests) may require mineralocorticoid therapy.
- Neuropathies and CNS manifestations mimicking multiple sclerosis, transverse myelitis, optic neuritis, or ischemic strokes may be due to vasculitis, thrombosis, or demyelination and require treatment with immunosuppressants.

Follow-up and Referral

Follow-up consists of ongoing evaluation to assess the effectiveness of symptom management and the need for alterations in treatment. If SS presents as an isolated condition, follow-up evaluations may occur as infrequently as twice per year. However, more frequent evaluations are necessitated by concurrent disease. Referrals may not be necessary except when this syndrome accompanies other diseases. The clinician may consult with a rheumatologist initially to differentiate the disease from other rheumatic conditions and to confirm the diagnosis.

During follow-up examinations, it is important to monitor for dental caries or oral candidiasis, which can lead to severe mouth pain and requires antifungal therapy. It is also important to screen for infectious conjunctivitis and complications from nasal dryness and laryngotracheal reflux, which can stimulate vagal responses and mimic allergic or recurrent sinusitis symptoms, including repeated throat clearing and postnasal drip–like symptoms. This type of reflux may be treated with proton pump inhibitors (similar to GERD), with referral to an ear, nose, and throat specialist if needed.

Patient Education

The patient should learn that mucosal dryness can be controlled with conservative interventions. Regular application of artificial lubricants locally can prevent the soreness and untoward effects of dry mucosae. The patient should be encouraged to wear sunglasses to protect the eyes from strong light, wind, and dust, as well as to avoid low-humidity environments that exacerbate dryness. If the patient has sore lesions in the mouth, tobacco, alcohol, and both spicy and salty foods should be avoided. OTC medications that decrease pharyngeal secretions, such as antihistamines, antidepressants, anticholinergics, and atropine derivatives, should be avoided. Patients should be warned that they are at greater risk with surgeries requiring general anesthesia and intubation, given their increased risk for thick, inspissated mucus and atelectasis.

■ SYSTEMIC LUPUS ERYTHEMATOSUS

Systemic lupus erythematosus (SLE) is an inflammatory autoimmune disease. It tends to affect many organ systems. Spontaneous remissions and exacerbations characterize the clinical picture. SLE can be mild or aggressive and even life-threatening in presentation.

Epidemiology and Causes

The prevalence of SLE is 40 to 50 cases per 100,000 and is associated with age, gender, race, and genetics. Nearly 85% of patients with SLE are women, most often in their 20s and 30s. However, 15% of cases present after age 55 years. Juvenile cases are not uncommon, though, with 20% of diagnosed patients being younger than 16 years. In children, the female to male ratio is 3:1; in adults, it is 10 to 15:1. Epidemiological studies have identified sex hormones as potential causative factors for SLE, because

onset of the disease in women typically occurs between menses and menopause. Estrogen has been shown to stimulate T cells, B cells, and macrophages, as well as increase expression of cytokines, endothelial cell adhesion molecules, and antigen-presenting major histocompatibility complex (MHC) molecules. SLE flares have also been associated with hyperprolactinemia. In contrast, androgenic hormones such as testosterone tend to be immunosuppressive, which may also contribute to the gender specificity of SLE. Of note, although men typically experience less photosensitivity than women, they are often considered to have more severe disease manifestations, with a greater incidence of serositis and higher 1-year mortality rate, although tending to present at an older age at onset.

Persons of African descent are four times more likely to develop the disease, compared with Caucasians. SLE also disproportionately affects patients of Asian ancestry, with other studies showing higher rates in Hispanic patients. Several lines of evidence have demonstrated a genetic component to SLE, for example, a high concordance rate between monozygotic twins, a propensity for specific HLA-DR class II MHC genes in affected individuals, and positive gene linkage studies in affected siblings. Poor prognostic factors include concurrent hypertension, male gender, having active disease at a young age, low socioeconomic status, and being African American. In particular, trends related to ethnic background (i.e., higher disease rates in people of color) have been observed with many chronic diseases and are multifactorial in nature. They must not be attributed solely to "genetic differences between the races," because worse outcomes are also associated with the presence of prothrombotic antiphospholipid antibodies (e.g., lupus anticoagulant, anticardiolipin) and highly active inflammatory disease, both of which may be addressed through individualized treatment plans to decrease the risk of morbidity.

Although not causative of SLE, several triggering factors for acute exacerbations have been identified. These include exposure to ultraviolet (UVB and UVA) rays, which is believed to cause increased cytokine and cell adhesion molecule expression; microbial infection (e.g., EBV, *Mycobacteria,* trypanosomes) that may stimulate cross-reacting autoantibodies; emotional stress, which, although controversial, has been tied to mild disease flares; pregnancy and postpartum hormonal fluctuations; and surgery, which may increase the formation of autoantibody-containing immune complexes via the release of intracellular antigens into the circulation from tissue trauma. Exposure to cigarette smoke or silica dust also increases the risk of developing SLE, which implicates inflammatory lung pathology.

Pathophysiology

The pathophysiology of SLE is best understood by a review of the diagnostic criteria. The diagnosis of SLE is made after 4 or more of the following 11 criteria are met in the absence of medications or other disorders known to induce these effects, as defined by the American College of Rheumatology (ACR):

- Arthritis—nonerosive and usually involving two or more joints
- Photosensitivity—often triggering skin rashes, exposure to the sun's UVB rays may be a triggering event for SLE exacerbations
- Oral (or nasal) ulcers—typically painless
- Malar rash—bilateral butterfly formation across the cheeks and nasal bridge
- Discoid rash—red raised patches, sometimes with denuded central areas
- Serositis (inflammation) of the pleura or pericardia
- Renal disease (any one of three indicators): more than 0.5 g/day proteinuria, 3+ or more proteinuria (as detected by dipstick), or cellular casts
- Hematological disorders (any one of four indicators): hemolytic anemia, leukopenia (less than 4,000 WBCs/mcL), lymphopenia (less than 1,500 lymphocytes/mcL), thrombocytopenia (less than 100,000 platelets/mcL)
- Neurological disease (e.g., seizures, psychoses) not otherwise explained by iatrogenic or metabolic causes
- Positive ANA
- Immunological abnormalities (any one of four indicators): positive antiphospholipid antibodies such as anticardiolipin or lupus anticoagulant, antibody to double-stranded native DNA (anti-dsDNA), anti-Sm (Smith) antibody, false-positive serological test for syphilis (VDRL, RPR)

SLE is, at its core, a condition of disordered immunity in which mechanisms that normally prevent immune cell activation by autoantigens are eliminated. A number of factors have been identified that contribute to this autoimmune activation, for example, an inhibition of suppressor T cells that normally downregulate immune responses, an increase in CD4+ T helper cells, increased cytokine production (e.g., IFN-α, IL-4, IL-6, IL-10), polyclonal B-cell activation, and dysregulated intracellular signaling (particularly pathways involving cytosolic calcium). These changes contribute to a significant production of autoantibodies that are considered to be a hallmark of the disease. Mouse models of SLE have demonstrated dysregulated apoptosis in which nuclear antigens (e.g., DNA, ribonucleoprotein, histones) are exposed on the cell surface, capable of recognition by autoreactive lymphocytes. In turn, autoantibodies often appear in the serum years before the actual onset of SLE symptoms.

Autoantibodies are also formed against cell surface antigens, including antibodies specific for red and white blood cells, platelets, and neuronal and renal cells. These antibodies mediate cellular destruction via complement activation, antibody-dependent cellular cytotoxicity, and opsonization. Although not seen universally, autoantibody-derived immune complexes are believed to underlie the pathology of a majority of clinical manifestations of SLE. Histochemical staining has identified immune complex deposition along the basement membrane in nephritic kidneys, at the dermal–epidermal junction in skin lesions, within the choroid plexus, as well as the pleural cavity and pericardium—all major sites of SLE pathology. The biochemical nature of both the autoantigen and autoantibody (e.g., size, charge, binding affinity, rate of phagocytic clearance, ability to be neutralized by complement proteins) determines where these complexes form and the extent of tissue damage after their deposition.

One of the organ systems most severely affected by immune complex deposition is the kidneys. In addition to the deposition of circulating immune complexes along the glomerular basement membrane, autoreactive IgG_1 and IgG_3 anti-DNA antibodies also bind directly to autoantigens in the basement membranes, serving as a nidus for complement activation. These chemotactic complement proteins then attract leukocytes and mononuclear cells that phagocytose the immune complexes, releasing cytokines and clotting factors that lead to fibrinoid necrosis, ongoing inflammation, renal scarring, and kidney dysfunction. Diffuse proliferative glomerulonephritis is the most common histological form of lupus nephritis, which results from this inflammation. In contrast, lupus membranous nephropathy is not associated with inflammation. Rather, in this setting, immune complex activation is separated physically from circulating immune cells by the glomerular basement membrane, resulting in epithelial injury and proteinuria without active inflammation.

A subset of individuals with SLE is also prone to developing antiphospholipid antibodies, including antibodies against the β-2-glycoprotein I complex and cardiolipin, as well as the lupus anticoagulant. These individuals have more severe disease, related primarily to an increased thrombogenic state, which predisposes to both venous and arterial thromboembolism, resulting in a greater incidence of deep venous thrombosis, pulmonary embolism, cerebrovascular accidents (strokes and transient ischemic attacks), and recurrent first-trimester miscarriages due to placental infarcts. Normally, β-2-glycoprotein has an anticoagulant effect, which is abrogated by these antiphospholipid antibodies.

One of the most characteristic physical findings of SLE is a bilateral malar rash. This and other SLE skin rashes are exacerbated by sun exposure, largely due to ultraviolet damage to DNA in skin keratinocytes and alterations in membrane phospholipid metabolism. Thus, anti-DNA, anti-RNA, anti-Ro, anti-La, and antiphospholipid autoantibodies form that mediate keratinocyte destruction and local skin inflammation. IL-1 production from cutaneous keratinocytes and antigen-presenting Langerhans cells potentiates this inflammatory response.

Clinical Presentation

Subjective

The patient may complain of malaise, fever, anorexia, and unplanned weight loss. The patient may also complain of blurred vision and conjunctival swelling. Sleeplessness and depression are also common complaints. Joints may be reported to be swollen and painful by history, but this may not be evident on examination. Shortness of breath and painful inspiration may be present if lung pathology exists. Vague abdominal pains and/or abdominal cramping could also enter into the history.

Objective

Integumentary findings may include the following:

- A characteristic "butterfly" rash, as well as other photosensitive rashes.
- Alopecia and scalp exanthema are typical findings.
- Splinter hemorrhages, periungual erythema, and fingertip lesions may be observed on the fingers and toes.
- Lymphadenopathy in several regions of the body indicates systemic disease.
- Discoid lupus presents with scarring and highly inflammatory (even ulcerating) skin lesions but often does not present with the familiar autoantibodies of SLE, including ANA, anti-dsDNA, and anti-Smith antibodies.
- Raynaud's phenomenon, a vascular condition, may be seen in up to 40% of patients as whitish-blue skin color changes in response to cold temperatures, which then change to red upon rewarming, often predating other symptoms.

Musculoskeletal findings may include the following:

- Musculoskeletal joint pains (asymmetrical, nondeforming, migratory arthritis—often in the hands and fingers) occur in 90% of cases and are often the presenting complaint.
- Swollen joints may not follow a particular pattern, as in other rheumatic diseases; joint inflammation is typically nonerosive on radiographs.

Neurological findings may include the following:

- Cognitive thought processes may be impaired. Therefore, the clinician should carefully listen to the patient's explanations in response to questioning, in order to establish lapses in logic; however, these deficits often are not evident in mental functioning assessments commonly used in primary care settings, such as the Folstein Mini-Mental State Exam.
- Evidence of peripheral paresthesias and diminished deep tendon reflexes may be present.

Cardiac findings may include the following:

- A systolic murmur may be present.
- Distended jugular veins suggest right-sided cardiac failure, which may be seen with pulmonary hypertension or interstitial lung disease.

Gastrointestinal findings may include the following:

- Painless oral and nasal ulcers may be seen.
- Right upper abdominal quadrant tenderness may accompany the finding of hepatomegaly; hepatitis is a common finding.
- Right lower quadrant tenderness suggests right colon enlargement, which may be caused by intestinal vasculitis.

Diagnostic Reasoning

Diagnostic Tests

Initial testing should include a CBC with platelet count, basic metabolic panel (serum electrolytes and kidney function tests), serum albumin (which will be reduced in nephropathy), ANA, urinalysis (UA), and antibody screens for anti-dsDNA (highly specific with 75–95% sensitivity), antiphospholipid antibodies, and anti-Sm antibodies (highly specific but with only 25% sensitivity). Other common autoantibodies include those against single-stranded DNA and nucleoprotein, including antiribonucleoprotein as seen in scleroderma and both anti-Ro (SSA) and anti-La (SSB) as seen in SS.

The CBC may show either anemia or leukopenia or both. If the patient is leukopenic, the differential may reveal lymphocytopenia. One-third of patients with SLE will be thrombocytopenic. ANA results are likely to be elevated in more than 90% of samples; however, this is not specific for SLE. Numerous other inflammatory diseases are also associated with an elevated ANA. Changes in serum levels of autoantibodies (rising anti-dsDNA levels) or complement (decreasing CH50, C3, and C4) correlate with active SLE disease. Elevated ESR and CRP levels are nonspecific markers of active inflammation. Proteinuria is a possible finding from the UA in nephrotic or nephritic patients, with hematuria in the latter. All these tests should be used in conjunction with clinical presentation (history and physical examination) to evaluate for worsening of the disease state and should not be overinterpreted or underinterpreted in isolation. These initial laboratory tests, along with characteristic clinical manifestations, should be sufficient to confirm a diagnosis of SLE. Of note, as reflected in the SLE diagnostic criteria, RPR tests for syphilis may be falsely positive (due to anticardiolipin antibodies or other SLE-related phenomena).

Pertinent imaging tests should be guided by clinical presentation, such as a chest radiography for pulmonary symptoms, renal ultrasound in the face of renal failure, and plain films for arthritic joints. If indicated in the setting of pulmonary findings, pulmonary function tests often have a restrictive pattern, given inflammation and scarring in the lungs. More invasive procedures such as renal biopsy are indicated when histology is needed to determine prognosis and guide therapy. Electrocardiography and echocardiography are indicated to evaluate for pericarditis and other cardiac pathology, and specific tests such as ventilation–perfusion (V-Q) scans or high-resolution spiral CT scans of the lungs are used to evaluate for pulmonary emboli in prothrombotic patients. As with other thrombotic phenomena, a negative D-dimer test may effectively rule out thrombosis; however, the nonspecific nature of this test in inflammatory conditions typically decreases its diagnostic utility in SLE.

As with SS, keratoconjunctivitis sicca may result, as can pathognomonic, although rare, cotton wool retinal exudates from retinal vasculitis. Scleritis and anterior uveitis may occur but are both uncommon. Mild to moderate cytopenias may affect all three major cell lines (i.e., leukopenia, anemia, thrombocytopenia), with thrombocytopenia leading to easy bruising and purpura. Rarely, severe autoimmune hemolytic anemia can also result. In contrast, thrombophilia may also occur, increasing the risk of thrombosis, including deep vein thrombosis and arterial blood clots, especially if antiphospholipid antibodies or lupus anticoagulant are present (the latter being paradoxically named, as it increases the risk of thrombosis). This prothrombotic state is the cause of recurrent miscarriages (abortions) early in pregnancy, usually in the first trimester. Thus, such an obstetric history should always make the clinician think of antiphospholipid syndrome and SLE as a potential underlying diagnosis.

Differential Diagnosis

The differential diagnosis for SLE includes vasculitis, rheumatoid arthritis, scleroderma, SS, juvenile idiopathic arthritis (particularly the systemic form), chronic active hepatitis, drug reactions, drug-induced lupus, and polyarteritis. The diagnostic criteria set forth under pathophysiology in this section should aid in distinguishing SLE from these other diseases. Hypothyroidism also needs to be ruled out as a cause of fatigue; the TSH and free T_4 test should provide this information. Drug-induced lupus has a milder presentation and is associated predominantly with procainamide, hydralazine, and minocycline, as well as anti-TNF biological immunodulators.

Management

The principal goal of therapy is symptom control. Many patients require little or no intervention. Mild joint pain may be managed with nonpharmacological interventions, as provided in the section on RA. Emotional support and referral to SLE support groups are both helpful in establishing control over some symptoms. Dietary modifications should consider the specific clinical presentation. For example, active inflammatory states may require higher calorie diets if weight loss is a concern; in contrast, corticosteroid-induced surges in appetite may call for lower calorie diets, whereas corticosteroid- or NSAID-induced hypertension and hyperlipidemia (or that accompanying lupus nephritis) may call for low-salt and low-fat/low-cholesterol diets, respectively. Likewise, a lack of sun exposure because of photosensitivity may require vitamin D and calcium supplements to prevent

bone loss, especially given chronic corticosteroid use. If conservative management fails, however, the patient may require antimalarials, corticosteroids, immunosuppressants, or immunomodulatory biological agents.

Constitutional symptoms are often the most troubling for patients. Fatigue is the most common symptom and tends to be the most debilitating. It can happen even in the absence of signs of active inflammation. Fatigue may be multifactorial, but if due predominantly to SLE, it tends to respond to treatment with hydroxychloroquine, corticosteroids, or even dehydroepiandrosterone (DHEA). In addition to weight loss associated with hyperinflammatory states, weight gain may also occur due to generalized edema resulting from hypoalbuminemia in nephrotic syndrome (anasarca) if there are kidney manifestations or water retention and increased appetite associated with glucocorticoid use. If fever is present, it is important to deduce whether it is due to the SLE itself, infection (more likely if fever occurs while the patient is on active corticosteroids or immunosuppressive therapies and is episodic), or a drug reaction that may also present with a morbilliform rash and be prolonged, without response to NSAIDs or acetaminophen.

NSAIDs are effective for mild musculoskeletal symptoms and mild serositis (inflammation of serosal layers, such as the pleura or pericardia). Cyclooxygenase-1 (COX-1) inhibitors are used most frequently, as several COX-2 inhibitor NSAIDs have been withdrawn from the market due to serious cardiovascular health risks. In turn, the remaining COX-2 inhibitors should be used with caution.

Cutaneous manifestations of lupus, including discoid lupus, respond well to antimalarials such as hydroxychloroquine (Plaquenil), which are also second-line agents for joint pains and myalgias. Antimalarials are also effective in treating serosal inflammation (pleuritis and pericarditis) and constitutional symptoms including fatigue and fever. Given their association with the long-term reduction of multiple SLE-related complications, their use is recommended in nearly all SLE patients. However, these agents are not without side effects and require appropriate monitoring, including for potential ocular toxicity.

When multiple organ systems are involved or manifestations within a given organ system are moderate to severe, glucocorticoids may be given alone or in combination with another immunosuppressant. Prednisone and other glucocorticoids are effective at treating and preventing relapses if started as soon as a marked rise in anti-dsDNA is observed in the setting of clinical disease manifestations. In turn, it is not uncommon for SLE patients to be maintained on low doses of corticosteroids. However, although they are often considered a mainstay of SLE treatment, the clinician must be aware of the important side effects of systemic (both IV and PO) corticosteroids, which include avascular necrosis (i.e., reduction in blood supply to a major joint such as the knee or hip, which results in joint necrosis), osteopenia and osteoporosis with fractures or vertebral collapse, growth inhibition in children, glaucoma and cataracts, hyperglycemia and diabetes, hypertension, weight gain, early atherosclerosis that can lead to long-term coronary artery disease and heart damage, as well as cognitive dysfunction and behavioral changes, which may be associated with both short-term and chronic use. Thus, although corticosteroid therapy is associated with a delayed time to onset of organ damage after diagnosis, the side effects and health risks of corticosteroids are well documented and result in significant morbidity in SLE patients. In turn, many lupus specialists strive to decrease corticosteroid use whenever possible, particularly through the use of steroid-sparing agents.

One of the newest additions to the SLE treatment armamentarium is the FDA-approved biological immunomodulatory agent belimumab (Benlysta), a monoclonal antibody therapy that binds the soluble B-cell growth factor B-lymphocyte stimulator (BLyS), thereby preventing signaling through its cognate B-cell surface receptor. As BLyS is known to support autoreactive B cells in SLE, belimumab effectively inhibits the production of autoantibodies capable of mediating organ damage and inflammation. Although not a curative therapy for SLE and not indicated to treat acute flares, belimumab has been shown to decrease disease activity, reduce disease flare rates, and improve symptoms in autoantibody-positive lupus patients, as well as lead to reductions in controller corticosteroid therapy.

Persistent evidence of SLE-related organ damage or symptomatic flares in the face of NSAID or antimalarial controller therapy may signal the need for more aggressive immunosuppressive therapy, such as higher-dose glucocorticoid pulse therapy or the addition of other immunosuppressants such as mycophenolate mofetil (Cellcept), azathioprine (Imuran), methotrexate, or cyclophosphamide (Cytoxan). For example, pulmonary manifestations related to lung inflammation may include pleuritis with a pleural friction rub, lung effusions, pneumonitis, interstitial lung disease, alveolar hemorrhage, or eventually pulmonary hypertension.

Of note, GI manifestations often relate to SLE treatments, rather than to the disease itself, such as gastritis and peptic ulcers resulting from chronic NSAID and corticosteroid use. However, SLE-related vasculitis can lead to inflammation of the pancreas, large intestine, and serosal layers of the peritoneum, as well as to esophagitis and GERD. Both hepatomegaly and splenomegaly may also be detected, along with lymphadenopathy.

The cardiovascular system may manifest with pericarditis or a verrucous form of nonbacterial endocarditis known as Libman-Sacks endocarditis. This is associated with antiphospholipid antibodies and can produce emboli due to valvular insufficiency and turbulent blood flow. There is also a well-documented phenomenon of transplacentally delivered anti-Ro (SSA) and anti-La (SSB) anti-single-stranded DNA antibodies from a mother with SLE to her developing fetus, which can result in potentially fatal third degree heart block for the baby. This is known as neonatal lupus, which is not a manifestation of primary lupus in the fetus, however, and is not the same as pediatric SLE.

CNS and psychiatric manifestations of SLE are quite varied and may require aggressive immunosuppressive treatment. These may include cognitive defects, delirium, depression, mania, anxiety, psychosis (which may also result iatrogenically from corticosteroid use), headache, aseptic meningitis, and various neuropathies. Ischemic CNS damage from thromboembolic cerebrovascular accident may underlie these symptoms as well.

Kidney involvement may be clinically apparent in up to half of all SLE patients and is the primary reason for lupus-related hospitalization. Renal biopsy may reveal several histological subtypes of lupus nephritis. Type I is normal. Type II is pure mesangial and carries with it a good prognosis. Type III is segmental and focal proliferative lupus nephritis and usually responds to corticosteroids. Type IV is diffuse proliferative lupus nephritis, which is typically considered to carry the worst prognosis, presenting with hypertension and leading to end-stage renal disease (ESRD) or death in up to 50% of cases. Type IV patients typically require an induction of remission and maintenance treatment regimen with high-dose corticosteroids and immunosuppressants such as azathioprine (Imuran), mycophenolate mofetil (Cellcept), or cyclophosphamide (Cytoxan). Type V is membranous nephritis with a variable presentation that worsens as complement levels decrease due to more immune complex formation and organ deposition. One-third of Type V patients need no treatment other than that for other SLE symptoms, one-third require low to moderate dose corticosteroids, and one-third need high-dose corticosteroids. Type VI is advanced sclerosing lupus nephritis, which nearly always leads to ESRD, given the irreversibility of renal fibrosis.

Although SLE-related organ damage often signals the need for aggressive immunosuppressive therapy, the severity of organ damage does not always correlate with the severity of inflammation. For instance, kidney dysfunction may relate to irreversible scarring from past kidney inflammation that has since resolved and, in turn, may not be effectively treated with immunosuppressants. This is an important distinction for the clinician to make because worsening or ongoing inflammation may be treated with corticosteroids or immunosuppressants, whereas treating noninflammatory organ damage with this same regimen just increases the risks of side effects and iatrogenic complications due to immunosuppression, without improving the underlying organ damage.

Disease progression in the face of potent immunosuppressants, such as cyclophosphamide, portends a particularly poor prognosis. Several immunomodulatory treatments are being explored, including immune system ablation with high-dose chemotherapy, with or without stem cell transplantation. In addition, although not

FDA approved to treat lupus, the anti-B cell (anti-CD20) monoclonal antibody immunotherapy rituximab (Rituxan) is often used in refractory SLE patients, given its familiar side effect profile and relatively long record of clinical use in other indications.

Five-year survival in SLE has greatly improved in recent decades, given the therapeutic advances discussed in this section, and is currently greater than 90%. However, the course of SLE tends to be relapsing and remitting, characterized by recurrent flares with intermittent periods of quiescence, sometimes resulting in prolonged periods of remission lasting several years. In turn, CNS and renal involvement, especially diffuse proliferative nephritis or advanced sclerosing nephritis, portend the worst prognosis. Indeed, most SLE inpatients are admitted for renal issues, whereas patients with isolated cutaneous and joint/muscle manifestations have the best prognosis. Short-term death is also often due to infection related to immunosuppression by multiple classes of SLE medications, in addition to organ involvement associated with active inflammation in the heart, kidney, or CNS.

Follow-up and Referral

Follow-up of SLE patients is critical to track the course of the disease, which is highly variable across patients. SLE patients who require only nonpharmacological management should still be seen at least twice per year to assess for disease progression. Patients requiring medication are typically seen at least every 3 months after stabilization on an optimal controller regimen. Before consultation with a rheumatologist, patients should receive laboratory evaluation in the primary care setting including CBC, UA, CRP, and ANA to follow the course of the disease. In addition, SLE patients have a greater risk of lymphoma. A greater risk of breast cancer, abnormal Pap smears, and squamous cell skin cancer has also been suggested. Thus, appropriate cancer screening in the primary care setting is critical.

Referral to a rheumatologist is indicated if antimalarials, corticosteroids, immunosuppressants, or biological immunomodulators are to be prescribed.

Patient Education

Newly diagnosed patients should receive referrals to information hotlines for SLE and an array of patient advocacy groups, given the potential life-changing impact of this disease. Many organizations, which are listed in the Resources section at the end of this chapter, will provide patients with access to materials that support symptom control. In addition, patients should learn their individualized trajectory of disease and prognosis, depending on their particular clinical manifestations.

Patients should learn that rest is essential during disease exacerbations (lupus flares). The need for increased oral fluids and correct dosing of NSAIDs are also essential parts of the educational plan. Patients should understand the need for professional intervention when their temperature escalates beyond 101.5°F (38.5°C), because fevers can signal the onset of an opportunistic infection or a lupus flare, for which the clinician should be consulted immediately.

Immunizations have not been shown to "bring out SLE" and should not be avoided, except for live attenuated vaccines in immunocompromised hosts. If possible, sulfonamide antibiotics (e.g., trimethoprim/sulfamethoxazole [Bactrim]) and tetracyclines should be avoided, because they may lead to adverse effects in SLE patients, including exacerbation of photosensitivity. Women should be encouraged to avoid pregnancy until the disease is in remission for at least 6 months because there are high miscarriage rates due to thromboembolus. In addition, birth control pills may exacerbate disease manifestations, although low-dose estrogen pills appear to be better tolerated. Corticosteroids, NSAIDs, and hydroxychloroquine are usually used to treat pregnant women, whereas other immunosuppressants such as methotrexate and cyclophosphamide are contraindicated in pregnancy due to potential teratogenic effects.

■ HUMAN IMMUNODEFICIENCY VIRUS INFECTION

Infection by HIV results in eventual destruction of the immune system. HIV binds to the CD4+ T-cell receptor in conjunction with the cellular coreceptors chemokine C-C motif receptor 5 (CCR5) or C-X-C chemokine receptor 4 (CXCR4) to enter and infect immune cells in the human body. In early HIV infection, the patient's CD4+ T-cell (T4 cell, T4 lymphocyte) count remains above 500 cells/mcL of peripheral blood. Over time, the immune system weakens as HIV infection leads to significant immune dysregulation, and the patient's CD4+ T-cell count begins to decline. When this occurs, the patient becomes susceptible to opportunistic infections.

Although there is no cure at this time for HIV infection, viral suppression of HIV to undetectable levels in the peripheral blood can be achieved by a combination of potent antiretroviral (ARV) agents. With early detection and initiation of treatment, HIV infection can be managed as a chronic but controllable infectious disease.

Table 17.5 presents the Centers for Disease Control and Prevention (CDC) HIV classification system for adults and adolescents.

Epidemiology and Causes

HIV was originally identified in homosexual men in the 1980s, but the virus affects men and women of all races, ethnicities, and sexual orientations, as well as infants, children, and adolescents. In 2011, an estimated 34 million people were believed to be infected with HIV worldwide. Although new infections have fallen by more than 20% since 2001, there were still 2.5 million new infections in 2011 or close to 7,000 new cases per day. HIV has affected all regions of the world. According to the Joint United Nations Programme on HIV/AIDS (UNAIDS),

Table 17.5 CDC HIV Classification System for Adults and Adolescents

This system emphasizes the importance of CD4+ T-lymphocyte testing in clinical management of HIV-infected persons. The system is based on three ranges of CD4+ T-cell counts and three clinical categories, giving a matrix of nine exclusive categories.

Criteria for HIV Infection

Persons age 13 years or older with repeatedly (two or more) reactive screening tests (ELISA and specific antibodies identified by a supplemental test such as the Western blot). Other specific methods of diagnosis of HIV-1 include virus isolation, antigen detection, and detection of HIV genetic material by PCR or bDNA assay.

AIDS-Defining Condition

The term *AIDS-defining illness* refers to any of a list of infections, diseases, or conditions that, when occurring in an HIV-infected person, leads to a diagnosis of AIDS, the most advanced stage of HIV infection. AIDS is also diagnosed if an HIV-infected person has a CD4+ T-cell count below 200 cells/mcL, regardless of whether that person has an AIDS-defining condition. Twenty-six conditions were identified and classified as AIDS-defining conditions in 1993 by the Centers for Disease Control and Prevention (CDC).

Clinical Category	CD4+ T-cell Count*	Clinical Manifestations
A1	≥500 cells/mcL	Category A consists of one or more of the conditions listed below in a person with documented HIV infection. Conditions listed in Categories B and C must not have occurred. • Asymptomatic HIV infection • Persistent generalized lymphadenopathy (noted in two or more extrainguinal sites, at least 1 cm in diameter for ≥3 months) • Acute (primary) HIV infection with accompanying illness or history of acute HIV infection
A2	200–499 cells/mcL	See A1.
A3	<200 cells/mcL	See A1.
B1	≥500 cells/mcL	Symptomatic HIV infection (but not A or C conditions) Examples include but not limited to: • Bacillary angiomatosis • Candidiasis, vulvovaginal: Persistent >1 month, poorly responsive to treatment • Candidiasis, oropharyngeal • Cervical dysplasia, severe, or carcinoma in situ • Constitutional symptoms such as fever or diarrhea >1 month (The above must be attributed to HIV infection or have a clinical course or management complicated by HIV.)
B2	200–499 cells/mcL	See B1.
B3	<200 cells/mcL	See B1.
C1	≥500 cells/mcL	Category C includes the clinical conditions listed below; for classification purposes, once a Category C condition has occurred, the person will remain classified as category C: • Bacterial pneumonia, recurrent (≥2 episodes in 1 year) • Candidiasis: Esophageal, tracheal, bronchi, lungs • Cervical cancer, invasive • Coccidioidomycosis, disseminated or extrapulmonary • Cryptococcosis, extrapulmonary • Cryptosporidiosis, chronic intestinal (>1 month) • Cytomegalovirus disease in other than liver, spleen, nodes (e.g., CMV retinitis) • Encephalopathy, HIV-related • Herpes simplex with mucocutaneous ulcer >1 month, bronchitis, pneumonia, esophagitis • Histoplasmosis, disseminated or extrapulmonary • Isosporiasis, chronic intestinal >1 month

Table 17.5 CDC HIV Classification System for Adults and Adolescents—cont'd

		• Kaposi's sarcoma • Lymphoma: Burkitt's, immunoblastic, primary central nervous system • *Mycobacterium avium* complex or *M kansasii,* disseminated or extrapulmonary • *M tuberculosis,* pulmonary or extrapulmonary • *Mycobacterium,* other species, disseminated or extrapulmonary • *Pneumocystis jiroveci* pneumonia (PCP) • Progressive multifocal leukoencephalopathy (PML) • *Salmonella* bacteremia, recurrent • *Toxoplasma gondii* (brain) • Wasting syndrome due to HIV (involuntary weight loss >10% of baseline body weight) with either chronic diarrhea (≥2 loose stools per day for ≥1 month) or chronic weakness and fever ≥1 month
C2	200–499 cells/mcL	See C1.
C3	<200 cells/mcL	See C1.

*There is diurnal variation in CD4+ counts, averaging slightly higher in the afternoon, in HIV-positive persons. Blood for sequential CD4+ counts should be drawn at about the same time each day.

Source: Public Health Service Revised Classification System for HIV Infection (Adolescents and Adults) 1993 Revised. In C. Kirton (Ed.), *ANAC's core curriculum for HIV/AIDS nursing,* ed 2. SAGE, Thousand Oaks, CA, pp. 351–353.

two-thirds of all people living with HIV are in sub-Saharan Africa (23 million), with 58% of these cases being women.

Significant epidemiological changes have occurred in the United States with respect to HIV infection. In 1992, the majority of cases in the United States were among white, non-Hispanic individuals. In more recent years, the face of the epidemic has changed, as minorities and women have been disproportionately affected. Reports from the CDC note that African Americans accounted for nearly half of all new HIV infections in the United States in 2010, despite comprising only 12% to 14% of the population. Reflective of this disproportionate impact, the rate of new infections among African American men was seven times as high as in white men, and the rate in African American women was nearly 20 times that of white women. Hispanics/Latinos have also been disproportionately affected, representing 20% of all new HIV infections in 2009, despite comprising only 16% of the population, with an overall infection rate nearly three times as high as whites. Latina women, in particular, are affected at even higher rates, estimated at four times the rate of white women. These trends may reflect differences in socioeconomic factors, such as income, education, and health-care access, rather than only racial or ethnic background.

The largest decline in reported cases has occurred among men who have sex with men (MSM). In contrast, the greatest increase in HIV infection is now seen in individuals with heterosexual contact. Also of concern is the increasing rate of HIV infection in persons older than 50 years. Concerns have similarly been raised about the incidence of HIV infection in adolescents and young

adults. CDC data indicate that in 2009, 39% of all new HIV infections were in young people aged 13 to 29 years, with most having been acquired sexually. In contrast to the larger gay community, infection rates appear to be increasing among MSM in this younger age-group, with disproportionately higher rates among young people of color. In 2010, HIV disease was the sixth leading cause of death among people aged 25 to 34 years in the United States.

HIV-1 is the type of virus found predominantly in the United States. HIV-2 is relatively rare in the United States, except among immigrants from West Africa, where the predominance of cases originate. HIV-2 is biologically similar to HIV-1 but shows reduced virulence, with a slower rate of CD4+ T-cell decline. Blood banks now routinely test for both HIV-1 and HIV-2. Co-infection with both HIV-1 and HIV-2 may occur, and HIV-2 should be considered in patients who were born in Africa, have traveled in Africa, or have had sexual contact or shared needles with someone from Africa.

Transmission

HIV is transmitted through the exchange of blood and body fluids and cannot be transmitted by casual contact (e.g., handshakes, closed or open-mouth kisses, and hugs). HIV is considered a sexually transmitted disease (STD; sexually transmitted infection) because both the human immunodeficiency virus and CD4+ T cells may be present in semen and vaginal secretions. During vaginal or anal sex, friction can cause minute tears to these highly vascular mucous membranes. These minute tears can allow systemic exposure to HIV-infected bodily fluids during penetrative intercourse, particularly on ejaculation. The use of latex condoms can help prevent the exchange of secretions. Anyone who has had unprotected sex (without a condom or other adequate form of barrier protection) is considered potentially at risk for HIV infection. The risk of HIV transmission from a single episode of unprotected receptive vaginal intercourse with a known HIV-positive sexual partner is estimated to be between 0.08% and 0.2%, and the infection risk associated with a similar episode of receptive anal intercourse is 0.1% to 0.3%. The risk of HIV transmission from oral sex (mouth to genital or mouth to anal contact) is difficult to determine, because most people who practice oral sex also practice other forms of sex during the same encounter. Oral to vaginal (cunnilingus), oral to anal (anilingus), and receptive oral to penile (fellatio) sex carry little risk of HIV transmission. However, the highest risk of HIV transmission from oral sex would be to a person performing fellatio on an HIV-infected man who ejaculates. Factors that increase the risk of HIV transmission from oral sex include oral or genital ulcers or cuts, bleeding gums, and concurrent sexually transmitted infections.

HIV can also be transmitted through the sharing of needles with an HIV-infected person; therefore, injection drug users (intravenous [IV] drug abusers) are a high-risk group for HIV infection. Of particular relevance to health-care workers, needle-stick injuries are the most common cause of occupational exposure to HIV. Treatment Standards/Guidelines 17.1 presents the postexposure prophylaxis guidelines for health-care workers, and The Patient's Voice 17.2 presents one health-care worker's perspective when faced with such a situation. The risk of HIV transmission from a single episode of needle-sharing during injection drug use with a known HIV-positive partner has been estimated at 0.67%, and the risk from an occupational needle stick from an HIV-positive patient is estimated at 0.3%.

Before blood banks began universal testing for HIV, people who had blood transfusions were at risk for HIV infection, as were hemophiliacs who might have been given contaminated blood products. Routine testing of all blood products for HIV-1 and HIV-2 has now virtually eliminated this route of transmission in the United States and other developed nations with universal blood testing standards. However, given the potential of an HIV-positive individual to donate blood during the asymptomatic and undetectable window period before HIV-specific seroconversion has occurred, transmission rates as low as 1 in 1,000,000 to 1 in 2,000,000 are typically cited during informed consent procedures for transfused blood products.

HIV can be maternally transmitted from mother to newborn. The AIDS Clinical Trials Group (ACTG) 076 study, which provided oral zidovudine (Retrovir; ZDV;

Treatment Standards/Guidelines 17.1 · Postexposure Prophylaxis for Health-Care Workers

Postexposure Prophylaxis (PEP) Regimens

Three-drug combination regimens lasting 1 month are recommended in all cases of occupational exposure. In contrast to prior guidelines, two-drug regimens are no longer recommended, unless in consultation with an HIV specialist.

Preferred regimen: *Integrase inhibitor PLUS 2-NRTI backbone*

• Raltegravir (Isentress, RAL) 400 mg twice daily PLUS Truvada (tenofovir DF 300 mg + emtricitabine 200 mg) 1 tablet once daily

Alternative regimens: *Integrase inhibitor or NNRTI or PI (ritonavir-boosted) PLUS 2-NRTI backbone*

Alternative Integrase inhibitor
• Elvitegravir (EVG) 150 mg once daily; available as a fixed-dose combination (Stribild/Quad Pill) with cobicistat (cytochrome P450 3A enzyme inhibitor) 150 mg, tenofovir DF (TDF 300 mg), and emtricitabine (FTC) 200 mg taken once daily

Alternative NNRTI
• Etravirine (Intelence, ETR) 200 mg (comes as 100 and 200 mg tablets) twice daily
• Rilpivirine (Edurant, RPV) 25 mg once daily (comes as 25 mg tablet); also available as a fixed-dose combination

(Complera) with tenofovir DF (TDF 300 mg) + emtricitabine (FTC) 200 mg taken once daily

Alternative PI (ritonavir-boosted)
• Darunavir (Prezista, DRV) 800 mg (comes as 400 mg tablets) once daily with ritonavir (Norvir; RTV) 100 mg (comes as 100 mg capsule) once daily
• Darunavir (Prezista, DRV) 600 mg (comes as 75, 150, and 600 mg tablets) once daily with ritonavir (Norvir; RTV) 100 mg (comes as 100 mg capsule) twice daily
• Atazanavir (Reyataz; ATV) with ritonavir (Norvir; RTV): ATV 300 mg (comes as 100, 150, and 300 mg capsules) with ritonavir (Norvir, RTV) 100 mg twice daily; may be taken as ATV 400 mg (comes as 200 mg capsules) without ritonavir once daily, but not if taken with tenofovir DF (TDF)
• Saquinavir (Invirase; SQV) with ritonavir (Norvir; RTV): SQV 1,000 mg (comes as 500 mg tablet) with RTV 100 mg (comes as 100 mg capsule) twice daily

Alternative 2-NRTI Backbone
• Zidovudine (Retrovir; AZT; ZDV) 600 mg daily with food (300 mg twice a day or 200 mg three times a day) PLUS lamivudine (Epivir; 3TC) 300 mg (300 mg once a day or 150 mg twice a day); can be dosed as Combivir (combination drug of Retrovir 300 mg and Epivir 300 mg) taken as one tablet twice a day

Treatment Standards/Guidelines 17.1   Postexposure Prophylaxis for Health-Care Workers—cont'd

Begin PEP:

After occupational exposure:

• Begin PEP promptly, as quickly as possible, preferably within hours, rather than days, after exposure, according to the regimens listed above.

• If possible, determine HIV status of exposure source to assist in guiding HIV PEP, but PEP should not be delayed while awaiting test results. It is also unnecessary to rule out whether an exposure source that tests negative is within a seronegative window period, unless acute antiretroviral syndrome is suspected clinically.

• Consultation with an HIV specialist should not delay initiation of HIV PEP but may be indicated in the following situations: delayed exposure reporting (>72 hours); unknown exposure source (e.g., used needle in sharps container); pregnancy or breastfeeding in exposed health-care provider; suspected HIV drug-resistance in exposure source; concurrent illness in exposure source (e.g., hepatitis B or C co-infection).

• Contraindicated in PEP: nevirapine (hepatotoxicity, rhabdomyolysis, hypersensitivity).

• Generally not recommended in PEP: didanosine (serious and life-threatening adverse events); nelfinavir; tipranavir (serious and life-threatening adverse events); stavudine + didanosine (peripheral neuropathy, pancreatitis, lactic acidosis).

• Recommended only with expert consultation: abacavir (requires negative HLA B57–01 testing before use); efavirenz (teratogenic, neuropsychiatric effects, serious or life-threatening drug interactions); enfuvirtide (subcutaneous dosing, significant side effects, antidrug

antibodies may develop and lead to false positives on HIV testing); fosamprenavir; maraviroc (requires Trofile assay to confirm R5 HIV strain tropism before use); saquinavir; stavudine.

• All health-care workers (HCWs) with occupational exposure to HIV will need follow-up, even if they do not start PEP, including short-term follow-up 72 hours after initial exposure and HIV antibody testing at baseline.

• Perform drug-toxicity monitoring, including a complete blood count and renal and hepatic function tests, at baseline and 2 weeks after starting PEP. If toxicity is noted, dose reduction or drug substitution should be considered with expert consultation, with further diagnostic studies as indicated.

• Provide follow-up counseling and medical evaluation periodically for 6 months postexposure (at 6 weeks, 12 weeks, and 6 months). Follow-up may be shortened to 4 months postexposure (at 6 weeks and 4 months) if a fourth generation combination p24 antigen-HIV antibody detection assay is used. Observe precautions (barrier contraception, avoidance of blood/tissue donation, avoidance of pregnancy and breastfeeding) to prevent secondary transmission of HIV throughout the entire follow-up period.

• Provide appropriate medical care for HCWs who become infected with HIV. An occupational exposure is an emotionally charged event for most HCWs and can have a severe psychological impact. Psychological support is needed to help deal with the stress of awaiting HIV test results and to assist in coping with the side effects of PEP.

The Patient's Voice 17.2

HIV Infection

I am furious! I've been a nurse for 20 years and have always been proud of my skills and techniques. I have been stuck by needles, but only a few times during my career . . . usually when a patient suddenly moved and not through negligence on my part. I thought nothing of it, until last month when I went to my doctor because I was feeling so tired and run down. He asked if I had been tested for HIV, and I said no. Just to appease him, I had the test done, and it was positive.

The only thing I can relate it to is a needle stick that occurred when I was working in home health several years ago. I didn't even think anything of it at the time, and I didn't even fill out an incident report. I don't have any recourse now since I can't prove I was infected "on-the-job." Now, I hear about the needleless syringes and all the safe guards in place. If I had them back then, I probably wouldn't be in the situation I am now! I am angry! What do I do now?

AZT) to HIV-infected women during pregnancy, with IV AZT during labor and liquid AZT to the newborn postnatally, demonstrated a dramatic decrease in HIV maternal transmission from 25% to 30% to as low as 8%. Current guidelines that employ elective cesarean section to avoid birth canal exposure, thorough STD screening and treatment, as well as updated prenatal and perinatal ARV regimens for both mother and child, have decreased this rate even further to less than 1% in some centers. However, HIV is present in the breast milk of infected mothers, so breastfeeding by an HIV-infected woman is still considered a potential route of transmission and is not recommended in the United States and other countries where adequate formula feeding is a readily available alternative.

HIV-infected women have poorer survival rates than men, but no difference has been found in the rate of disease progression. Some studies indicate, however, that survival is not necessarily related to sex or race; rather, it is related to unequal socioeconomic status and thus unequal access to care and appropriate drug therapy, among other factors.

In response to the changing HIV epidemic, in 2003 the CDC proposed new strategies for advancing HIV prevention: (1) Make voluntary HIV testing a routine part of medical care. (2) Implement new models for diagnosing HIV infection outside of medical settings. (3) Prevent new infections by working with persons diagnosed with HIV and their partners to minimize risk of transmission. (4) Further decrease perinatal HIV transmission. As discussed in more detail under Diagnostic Reasoning, opt-out HIV testing has become increasingly common as a strategy to increase overall HIV testing rates.

Pathophysiology

HIV is a member of the Lentivirinae subfamily of "slow" retroviruses, known for their prolonged latent infectious period, persistent viremia, species-specific infectivity, tropism for cells of the immune and nervous systems, and subsequent destruction of host immune defenses including the triggering of autoimmune responses. Evolutionarily conserved members of this family include simian immunodeficiency virus (SIV) and feline immunodeficiency virus (FIV).

HIV was identified as the causative agent of AIDS in 1984. As the predominant strain worldwide, HIV-1 has been genetically divided into groups or subtypes M, N, and O. Accounting for the majority of HIV-1 cases, group M has been further subdivided into subclasses known as clades, designated A through J. In the United States, nearly all HIV infections are due to HIV-1 clade B, with estimates of up to 98%. Clades A, C, D, and E are most common in developing nations, with some studies indicating that clade E has a greater propensity for heterosexual transmission. HIV-2, found predominantly in West African nations, Angola, Mozambique, France, and Portugal, results in slower disease progression and appears less readily transmissible.

Studies utilizing quantitative assays of plasma HIV RNA have provided new insights into the pathogenesis of HIV infection. Molecular genetic studies have resulted in a better understanding of the viral genome and its complex replication process, which has led to multidrug therapy that attempts to suppress viral replication at different stages of the HIV life cycle. The HIV genome consists of several regulatory genes (*nef, rev, tat, vif, vpu,* and *vpr*) and three structural genes called *gag* (encoding several core capsid proteins), *pol* (encoding reverse transcriptase and integrase), and *env* (encoding several outer viral envelope surface proteins involved in binding of the HIV virion to target host cells).

These gene products produce an HIV virion consisting of a nucleoprotein core with two copies of single-stranded genomic RNA and several key proteins, including p6 and p7 (nucleocapsid proteins bound directly to genomic RNA), p24 (a capsid protein forming a shell around the genomic core), and p17 (a matrix protein that lines the inner surface of the virion's outer lipid bilayer, providing structural integrity). Also included in the core are several enzymes involved in viral replication including reverse transcriptase, integrase, and protease. This nucleoprotein core is surrounded by an outer lipid bilayer studded along its surface by two major glycoproteins named for their molecular mass in kilodaltons, gp120 and gp41.

The sequence of events in HIV infection begins with the transfer of the virus from one host to another. Once the virus is transmitted across the mucocutaneous barrier and into the bloodstream, HIV attaches to cells at the CD4+ receptor site via gp120. CD4+ receptors are found on many cells of the body, including cells of the central nervous system, GI tract, and immune system (e.g., CD4+ T cells, monocyte-derived macrophages, and tissue dendritic cells). At the onset of HIV infection, the average number of CD4+ T cells is about 1,000/mcL (normal range: 500–1,500/mcL).

Although CD4+ T cells were first identified as the primary target of HIV infection, it is now known that tissue dendritic cells called Langerhans cells found within the genital mucosal epithelium are believed to be the earliest targets of HIV infection, given their proximity to the initial site of HIV exposure. After infection, dendritic cells bind to CD4+ T cells and subsequently migrate to draining lymph nodes via regional lymphatic channels. Within these lymph nodes, HIV further infects follicular dendritic cells capable of presenting virus to circulating hematopoietic cells. Thus, the lymph nodes are a major site of viral replication and a focus of HIV infectivity.

After attaching to the target host cell, HIV enters the cell by fusion at the plasma membrane. This is a sequential process, which first involves a conformational change in HIV after gp120 binding to CD4 that allows the virion to interact with chemokine receptors on the host cell surface. This initiates another conformational change, which exposes the gp41 viral envelope protein and brings the virion into even closer proximity to the plasma membrane.

Thus, in addition to interactions with gp41, viral adhesion requires the aid of secondary coreceptors, most notably the chemokine receptors CXCR4 (also known as fusin), which binds T-cell–tropic HIV strains called X4 viruses, and CCR5, which binds macrophage-tropic strains or R5 viruses. Tissue dendritic cells express CCR5 and less commonly CXCR4. In turn, R5 viruses are more common early on in HIV infection, whereas X4 viruses predominate in the later stages of symptomatic infection. Studies of people who have had multiple exposures to HIV yet remain uninfected have shown that these people have defects or polymorphisms in these coreceptors, which may explain why they have not become infected. In turn, investigational studies are addressing each step in the viral fusion process as a potential target for pharmacological intervention, for example, the CCR5 antagonist maraviroc (Selzentry) and the gp41 fusion inhibitor T-20 (enfuvirtide [Fuzeon]).

Once HIV enters the healthy CD4+ T cell, the cell becomes infected, and HIV begins its replication activities by converting its own genetic material (RNA) into complementary DNA strands, using the RNA-dependent DNA polymerase enzyme reverse transcriptase (RT)—the hallmark of retroviruses. Viral DNA then becomes double stranded and is incorporated into the host cell genome by viral integrase, and the RNA template is digested by viral RNAse. This new DNA acts as a blueprint for replication, directing the infected host cell to make new viral particles. In recent years, ARV medications have been developed to inhibit the genomic integration step in the viral replication process, for example, the integrase inhibitor raltegravir (Isentress).

Because mammalian cells do not express reverse transcriptase, this enzyme was the first retrovirus-specific therapeutic target for HIV medications in the form of nucleoside (and nucleotide) RT inhibitors (NRTIs), as well as the nonnucleoside RT inhibitors (NNRTIs). These agents either serve as competitive chain terminators of elongating viral DNA strands or interfere with the DNA template-primer activity of RT.

Importantly, RT lacks the histone repair enzymes characteristic of mammalian DNA polymerases. This results in a high rate of uncorrected mutations during each cycle of viral DNA replication. In turn, this leads to the rapid development of resistance by HIV to most ARV agents, particularly if used suboptimally as monotherapy or, alternatively, as combination therapy with a high degree of patient noncompliance.

In addition to genomic replication, a large portion of viral DNA is transcribed and subsequently translated into a large polyprotein, which must then be activated. The HIV protease enzyme, acting like "chemical scissors," catalyzes the cleavage of polyproteins into mature structural proteins and enzymes. This process results in formation of a large number of infectious viral particles, which bud from the host cell and seek out new cells to infect. Given its effect on such a large number of viral proteins, HIV-specific protease serves as a critical target for one of the most potent classes of ARV agents—the protease inhibitors.

Once HIV enters the body, a series of stages occur in the infectious process:

- The acute retroviral stage or syndrome (or primary infection period)
- The asymptomatic stage (including a "window" period before seroconversion)
- The symptomatic stage of HIV infection, which may result in opportunistic infections and acquired immunodeficiency syndrome (AIDS)

The initial period of infection, or acute retroviral syndrome, resembles infectious mononucleosis and is accompanied by high HIV viremia, often in excess of 1 million viral copies/mL. Primary HIV infection refers to the 4- to 7-week period of rapid viral replication immediately following exposure and infection by the virus. About 30% to 60% of individuals with primary infection develop an acute syndrome characterized by fever, malaise, lymphadenopathy, pharyngitis, headache, myalgia, and sometimes rash. Importantly, common cold symptoms including rhinorrhea and congestion are typically absent during acute retroviral syndrome.

There is spontaneous recovery from these flu-like symptoms in 1 to 3 weeks. Within days after the initial infection, however, there is extension of virus to the regional lymph tissue, presumably by dendritic cells. This is followed by massive viremia with extensive involvement of lymphatic tissue. Within a few weeks, there is an immune response resulting from the complex interplay of HIV-specific cytotoxic T-cell responses, plasma and B-cell–mediated humoral antibody formation, and cytokine production. Seroconversion (the development of antibodies to HIV in the blood) usually occurs 1 to 3 months after viral transmission. Once seroconversion has occurred, the ELISA test used to diagnose HIV will be positive in infected individuals. However, from the point of initial infection before detectable seroconversion, there is a variable "window period," which may last anywhere from 2 to 14 weeks. Although the infected person will have a negative antibody blood test during this asymptomatic period, the patient is already infectious to others and may transmit the virus.

HIV infection is a dynamic process characterized by a high rate of viral replication and significant immune dysregulation. Complete viral latency, a "quiet time" for the virus, does not exist. Initially, in individuals with acute HIV infection, the viral load is extremely elevated (10^5–10^7 copies/mL). Once the host immune response begins, plasma HIV RNA levels decline rapidly. Without treatment, this level fluctuates for the initial 6 months of infection until a set point is reached. The "set point" refers to a steady state of the plasma HIV RNA level that persists for years. During this time, the immune system is actually in a hyperactivated state known as immune activation, in which markers of cellular immune activity such as proliferation, changes in cell surface proteins, and cytokine production are all increased, as are overall levels of immunoglobulin. However, these processes are not coordinated or effectively directed toward clearing the virus, and eventually, plasma HIV viral load begins to increase progressively. At that time patients begin to deteriorate clinically as CD4+ T-cell counts decline even further. Studies have demonstrated that the rate of CD4+ T-cell decline is not fully accounted for by the direct viral infection and destruction of these cells. Rather, the dysregulated state of immune activation, which directly correlates to HIV viral load, is a major contributing factor. Thus, it is important to understand that HIV-associated immune activation does not result in an effective immune response against the virus, but actually contributes to progressive immune suppression in the setting of HIV viral replication and a detectable viral load.

In turn, the magnitude of the viral set point predicts the rapidity of disease progression, and chronic therapy is designed to drive this set point down as far as possible.

Through the use of HIV detection assays to determine the level of viral activity in the peripheral blood (called viral load tests), it has been shown that the level of plasma HIV RNA is proportional to the rates of viral replication and CD4+ T cell destruction. Viral load is one of the most useful tests for predicting the risk of progression to AIDS. Because the natural history of HIV infection varies from one patient to another, the plasma HIV viral load can help predict the rapidity with which clinical immunodeficiency will develop. Fortunately, with the initiation of appropriate ARV therapy, the immune system appears to retain the capacity for cellular recovery even at later stages of HIV infection. Thus, therapeutic strategies were developed that avoided the rapid initiation of ARV medications at the time of diagnosis in favor of more conservative treatment approaches based on low CD4+ T-cell count thresholds, which sought to minimize the long-term side effects and genetic resistance that developed as a consequence of ARV medication exposure. However, more recent evidence has indicated that the regeneration of the immune system that results after initiating ARV treatment is more complete if therapies are started earlier in the course of the disease, such as when CD4+ T-cell counts reach 500 cells/ml. Thus, the optimum stage for initiating ARV therapy has yet to be firmly established, because several factors must be weighed simultaneously.

The half-life of a free HIV virion is less than 1 hour, whereas the half-life of an acutely infected T cell is approximately 1 day. In HIV infection, an estimated 1 to 10 billion viral particles are produced and cleared each day. Studies suggest that billions of CD4+ T cells may be destroyed every day, eventually overwhelming the immune system's capacity to regenerate. This rapid turnover of virus and CD4+ T lymphocytes occurs throughout the course of HIV infection. An additional pool of longer-lived macrophages and follicular dendritic cells infected with HIV may persist for up to several weeks. However, it is a smaller, long-lived pool of memory lymphocytes that numbers approximately 1 million, which may persist for several years in a latent infected stage, creating a viral reservoir within the host. These cells may be localized to tissue, rather than present in the peripheral circulation, and may be located in immune privileged sites, protected from both host defense systems and therapeutically effective medication levels. Thus, by avoiding the antiretroviral activity of current pharmacotherapies, these cells may enter into an active lytic stage of viral replication up to several decades later, exposing the immune system to rapid viral proliferation. Research suggests that the inability to clear HIV from the body in full and cure the infection is a function of this pool of long-lived HIV-infected reservoir cells, which current pharmacotherapies are unable to destroy completely.

Over a period of time, the replication activities of the virus eventually supersede the capacity for CD4+ T-cell regeneration. As the CD4+ T-cell count declines, patients become increasingly susceptible to opportunistic infections and malignancies. Falling below a CD4+ T-cell count of 200 cells/mcL due to HIV infection is the laboratory definition of developing AIDS. In some patients, the rate of CD4+ T-cell loss is extreme, with counts dropping below 200 cells/mcL within 2 years, whereas in a small subset of patients—called long-term nonprogressors—CD4+ T-cell counts above 500 cells/mcL may be maintained up to 10 years after infection, in the absence of any ARV medication. In addition, many of these patients are also able to suppress HIV RNA viral load without the use of ARV medications to less than 50 copies/mL of peripheral blood (often called "elite controllers"), which is the current lower limit of detection of most diagnostic HIV viral load tests used clinically in the United States. Extensive research programs are currently focused on this subset of long-term nonprogressors, whose individual immune responses may be critical to developing effective therapies to control viral replication and attenuate immunosuppression.

Clinical Presentation
Subjective

A careful history should be done to determine the patient's risk of HIV infection, because certain behaviors place a patient at higher risk of exposure to HIV than others. Focus on History 17.1 lists questions the clinician should ask to assess these risks. Although this list is not exhaustive, these questions can generate discussion and open the door to a more detailed history or clarify the patient's misconceptions regarding HIV infection.

In acute HIV infection, more than 8% of patients have symptoms such as fever (90%), sore throat (70%), myalgia (60%), headaches (60%), cervical lymphadenopathy (50%), and night sweats (50%). However, the majority of patients with acute HIV infection are asymptomatic.

Across the disease spectrum, the HIV-positive patient may present with symptoms reflecting any of the following clinical presentations: flu-like symptoms (acute retroviral syndrome typically seen in the early stage of HIV infection, anywhere from 6 days to 6 weeks after viral transmission); darkish colored purple spots on the skin (indicative of Kaposi's sarcoma); nonproductive cough, shortness of breath, and fever that has been present for several days or weeks, suggesting *Pneumocystis jiroveci* pneumonia (PCP, a fungal infection formerly known as *Pneumocystis carinii*), *Mycobacterium tuberculosis,* or other bacterial pneumonia, typically seen in patients with CD4+ T-cell counts below 200 cells/mcL; and/or constitutional symptoms such as weight loss, night sweats, chronic fever, and/or chronic diarrhea (usually seen in patients with advanced HIV infection, or AIDS, with CD4+ T-cell counts below 200 cells/mcL).

Focus on History 17.1 Evaluating Risk of HIV Infection

Sexual History and Sexually Transmitted Diseases

- Describe your sexual relationships.
- Describe your sexual orientation.
- Describe your sexual practices. Have you ever had anal sex?
- Have you ever had a sexually transmitted disease (STD)?
- Have you ever had vaginal discharge or problem (for women)? Penile discharge or problem (for men)?
- Have any of your sexual partners been tested for STDs?
- Do you practice safer sex, such as using condoms or other forms of barrier protection?
- What form of birth control do you use, if any?
- Have any of your sexual partners been told that they were HIV positive or had AIDS?
- Would you expect any of your sexual partners to have been exposed to a STD or HIV? Why or why not?

Substance Abuse

- Have you ever injected drugs (legal or illegal [street])?
- Have you ever shared needles, such as for injections, piercings, or tattoos?
- Have you ever used (in any form) illegal or street drugs?
- Do you drink alcohol? If so, how much?

Transfusion History

- Did you receive any blood or blood products between 1977 and 1985?
- Are you or your partner a hemophiliac?
- Have you ever received any donor sperm during artificial insemination?

Infection History

- Have you or a sexual partner ever had any form of hepatitis?
- Have you or anyone close to you been diagnosed with tuberculosis (TB)? If so, what is (or was) the treatment?
- Have you ever had a positive test for TB?
- Have you ever taken medications for TB?

Occupational History

- Do you work in the health-care field? In a long-term residential facility? In a jail or prison?
- Are you exposed to blood or other body fluids while on the job?
- Have you ever had a needle-stick injury?

Objective

The most common clinical signs and physical exam findings of HIV infection include the following:

- Persistent generalized lymphadenopathy: This is a relatively common feature early in HIV infection when the patient is often asymptomatic. During the assessment, the clinician must be alert for enlarged lymph nodes involving two noncontiguous sites, other than inguinal nodes. The clinician should measure and record the size of nodes if palpable, although significant nonpalpable lymphadenopathy may also be evident on imaging exams.

- Pulmonary symptoms: These are seen with community acquired pneumonia, PCP, tuberculosis, and bacterial pneumonia. The clinician should be alert for decreased breath sounds and reports of shortness of breath, nonproductive cough, fever, or night sweats.

- Localized *Candida* infections: Thrush is a common finding in HIV infection. The presence of thrush indicates advanced immunosuppression, with a high probability of a serious or opportunistic infection within 3 years. The clinician should carefully assess the oral cavity, using a high-quality flashlight. Look for the presence of white plaques (thrush), darkish purple lesions (possibly Kaposi's sarcoma), or a whitish, hair-like growth on the tongue (oral hairy leukoplakia caused by Epstein-Barr virus, seen in advanced states of immunosuppression). If white plaque is found, attempt to lightly scrape a portion with a tongue blade. If thrush is present, the plaque will bleed as it is scraped off. *Candida* esophagitis is a late complication of HIV infection; the usual presentation is thrush with odynophagia. *Candida* vaginitis in women with HIV infection is more likely to be recurrent or refractory to therapy.

- Kaposi's sarcoma: These lesions may be flat macules or raised, nodular papules—purple in color in light-skinned patients and dark brown to black in darker-skinned patients. The lesions can be found on any part of the skin or mucous membranes. Thus, the clinician should perform a thorough dermatological examination of the back, buttocks, extremities, hands, and feet. Transmitted by human herpesvirus–8 (HHV-8), Kaposi's sarcoma has become less common in the United States, with the advent of more effective ARV medications and an increased understanding of the fecal-oral route of transmission of HHV-8.

- Sexually transmitted diseases: STDs increase the likelihood of HIV transmission or acquisition. The clinician should do a thorough examination of the rectal and genital area, inspecting for perianal and genital herpes simplex lesions, as well as penile or vaginal discharges reflective of gonorrhea or other sexually transmitted infection.

- Neurological and ophthalmic signs and symptoms: Headache is a common complaint in acute retroviral syndrome, whereas neck stiffness and pain along with malaise and impaired cognition may be signs of smoldering meningitis, such as that caused by *Cryptococcus*, which, in contrast to bacterial meningitis, typically has an insidious onset. The clinician should also conduct a careful funduscopic exam to check the retina for signs of cytomegalovirus (CMV) infection or fungal endophthalmitis in patients with late-stage HIV infection.

- Weight loss: The clinician should document height and weight at the time of the examination and record the patient's description of weight loss (amount lost over what period of time), because this is a common presenting sign in patients with undiagnosed HIV infection and may herald progressive immunosuppression.
- Cytopenias: Anemia, leukopenia, and/or thrombocytopenia often complicate HIV infection. The clinician should check the overall complete blood count (CBC) with leukocyte differential, in addition to specific T-lymphocyte subset (CD4+ and CD8+) counts to assess the level of HIV-associated immunosuppression.

Diagnostic Reasoning

Diagnostic Tests

A diagnosis of HIV infection is based on the presence of antibodies to HIV in the blood. Most commercially available HIV test kits in the United States were developed specifically for HIV-1 detection; HIV-2–specific antibodies may also be detected by these tests but with much less sensitivity. Thus, it is important for the clinician to order diagnostic tests developed specifically for HIV-2 detection, if suspected either alone or as a co-infection with HIV-1.

Historically, for many years HIV testing was performed only after mandatory pretest counseling with informed consent, in which the implications of both positive and negative test results were discussed in detail, as well as privacy restrictions regarding test results. In recent years, however, public health measures have moved toward opt-out HIV testing in the United States as a more effective means of screening larger numbers of people (Level I; Branson et al, 2006). In opt-out strategies, pretest counseling is no longer mandated, although patients are informed that confidential HIV testing may be done in the course of normal health-care delivery (such as at prenatal clinics or during emergency department visits), unless patients specifically refuse (i.e., "opt-out" of) such testing.

Some jurisdictions also require that a patient be informed of his or her right to anonymous versus confidential testing. In anonymous testing, the patient is issued an identification number, and test results are associated with this number only. No names are used, and the results cannot be traced back to any personal identifier, regardless of result. In turn, anonymous test results are not typically reportable to health departments. In confidential testing, the patient's name is used, but the results may not be released without a patient's permission, except under certain circumstances as a matter of law. If the test result is positive, the patient's name and positive HIV status may be reported to the health department, as is done with other sexually transmitted and communicable diseases. Some jurisdictions only mandate reporting of AIDS cases, rather than all HIV infections. In turn, primary care providers should be aware of federal, state, and local HIV reporting requirements

(which often change over time), educate the patient about them, and ensure that the patient is aware of the extent and limits of HIV test result confidentiality.

The preferred method for diagnosis of acute HIV infection is an HIV RNA viral load or cellular DNA assay, because HIV DNA and RNA may be detected before seroconversion. In contrast, the ELISA test cannot detect HIV infection during the window period (the time between transmission and seroconversion), when HIV-specific antibodies have not yet formed. It is important to understand that a cellular HIV DNA assay detects HIV viral DNA that has been integrated into the host cellular genome and is more sensitive than antibody-based tests or plasma HIV RNA viral load assays. Thus, despite their higher cost, cellular HIV DNA assays are the preferred diagnostic test in the immediate postpartum period for children born to HIV-infected women. Plasma viral load is typically suppressed by prenatal or perinatal ARV therapy, which may lead to false-negative results on HIV RNA viral load assays in HIV-infected neonates. HIV-specific antibody tests are also problematic in infants born to HIV-infected women, because maternal antibodies typically cross the placenta, potentially leading to false-positive results.

Some state, federal, and managed care companies do not perform a viral load test until after a serological diagnosis is made, given its greater expense. A viral load test costs approximately 15 to 20 times more than an ELISA test. For this reason, clinicians typically use an ELISA test to screen for HIV-specific antibodies. If the ELISA test is positive, a second, more sophisticated test, the Western blot, is done on the same sample of blood. The Western blot test involves the separation of individual HIV viral proteins into defined bands within a polyacrylamide gel matrix to which a patient's serum is then applied; any HIV-specific antibodies in the serum will then adhere to the HIV viral proteins in the gel matrix. The presence of any two of the following antibody specificities in the patient's serum—p24, gp41, or gp 120/160 bands—constitutes a positive Western blot result and serves as a more specific confirmatory test for diagnosing HIV infection. In many states, positive Western blot test results must be reported to health departments. Studies have shown that the frequency of false-negative test results in a high-prevalence population is about 0.3%. The usual cause of false-negative test results is testing during the window period, although Western blot tests also tend to be more sensitive than ELISA tests.

In recent years, commercial self-testing kits designed to be used at home, as well as rapid testing kits designed to be used in high-throughput clinical settings (such as emergency departments, labor and delivery units, or obstetric/gynecological clinics), have become increasingly common. For example, OraQuick Advance HIV-1/HIV-2 Rapid Antibody Test is a point-of-care diagnostic test designed for use with oral fluids (swabbing between the teeth and gums) or plasma specimens. After 20 minutes, the test device indicates if HIV-specific antibodies are present in the sample by displaying two reddish-purple lines in a small window on the device. Several other rapid HIV tests for use with serum or plasma are also available (e.g., Uni-Gold Recombigen HIV, Reveal G3 Rapid HIV-1 Antibody Test, and MultiSpot HIV-1/HIV-2). A reactive result on a rapid HIV diagnostic test is typically considered a preliminary positive and should be confirmed by a Western blot test. The recently FDA-approved Alere Determine HIV-1/2 Ag/Ab Combo is able to detect simultaneously both HIV-1 p24 antigen and antibodies to HIV-1 and HIV-2 from serum, plasma, or whole blood samples, allowing the clinician to distinguish between acute onset (p24 antigen alone) and established (p24 antigen and HIV-specific antibodies) infection.

At the time of initial diagnosis, a T-cell subset blood test should be done to determine the patient's CD4+ T-cell count. A viral load test, which is a quantitative assay of HIV RNA concentration in the peripheral blood, should also be drawn to determine the patient's viral replication activity. These two tests are evaluated together to determine the stage of illness and as a predictor of disease progression. As mentioned earlier, the viral load test is the preferred method of diagnosing acute HIV infection, given its greater sensitivity at this early stage.

A discussion of these test results may be the beginning of a dialogue between the clinician and the HIV-infected client on the need for HIV prevention behaviors, to decrease the probability of an HIV-infected patient transmitting HIV to other persons, as well as acquiring additional strains of HIV from infected partners. It is unrealistic to assume that all HIV-infected persons will subsequently practice lifelong abstinence. Thus, a discussion of behaviors to minimize viral transmission via sexual activity or otherwise is a critical component to every patient visit.

Although over time with effective treatment, a plasma HIV RNA viral load assay may become undetectable (i.e., below the lower limit of detection, which is typically 50 copies/mL), the clinician and patient should understand that this test only reflects the level of cell-free virus in the peripheral blood. Thus, it is still possible that latently infected cells might transmit infection in the absence of detectable viremia.

Additional baseline laboratory evaluations in a newly diagnosed individual should include a CBC with differential to check for other cytopenias; a complete serum chemistry profile including hepatic transaminases, blood urea nitrogen (BUN), and creatinine levels; and a complete urinalysis. Additional studies for concurrent infections include the Venereal Disease Research Laboratory (VDRL) or rapid plasma reagin (RPR) tests for syphilis; serum anti-toxoplasmosis IgG titer; hepatitis A, B, and C serologies; and a Pap smear for female clients. A tuberculin skin test (TST; purified protein derivative [PPD]; Mantoux test) should be done unless the patient has a documented history of tuberculosis or positive TB skin test in the past. Other tests for sexually transmitted diseases should be done as determined from the clinical presentation and typically include evaluations for gonorrhea and chlamydia.

If a patient presents with pulmonary symptoms, vital signs should be assessed for fever and tachycardia. The clinician should also check the oxygen saturation level and obtain a chest x-ray examination and arterial blood gas analysis. Hypoxemia and bilateral pulmonary infiltrates on an x-ray film indicate a pulmonary process but may not differentiate between PCP and TB in the HIV-infected patient. Differentiating between the two requires additional diagnostic testing, such as pathogen-specific culture or staining assays of respiratory samples, for example, sputa or bronchial alveolar lavage fluid obtained via bronchoscopy. A TST may also assist in the work-up of TB, with or without the placement of one or more anergy controls to commonly encountered antigens, such as *Candida* or tetanus toxoid (in a vaccinated individual). Anergy testing may allow the clinician to disregard a negative TST result as excluding TB infection, because it is common for individuals with advanced immunosuppression to have impaired cell-mediated immunity. However, it is also possible that defects in cell-mediated immune responses may be selective for particular antigens over others. Thus, some clinicians feel that anergy testing is unhelpful in the setting of advanced immunosuppression and discount negative diagnostic test results based on cell-mediated immunity altogether.

Differential Diagnosis

Immunosuppression can be noted in a variety of situations besides HIV infection, such as the patient on chemotherapy, radiation therapy, or long-term corticosteroids. Certain cancers can also cause a decrease in the CD4+ T-cell count. Differential diagnosis for acute retroviral syndrome includes Epstein-Barr virus (EBV) mononucleosis, CMV mononucleosis, toxoplasmosis, rubella, viral hepatitis, syphilis, or drug reactions. Cytopenias including lymphopenia may be due to a primary or infiltrative bone marrow disorder and may require bone marrow biopsy if an HIV test is negative.

Management

Principles of management for early HIV infection include (1) initial disclosure of HIV status, (2) initiation of drug therapy to suppress the virus, and (3) monitoring of viral activity to determine any need to modify or revise drug therapy.

Key components of HIV infection management include prevention of transmission, preserving immune function, prophylaxis against opportunistic infections in the face of low CD4+ T-cell counts, early diagnosis and treatment of opportunistic infections, and optimizing quality of life. Figure 17.1 presents an algorithm for the management of early HIV infection.

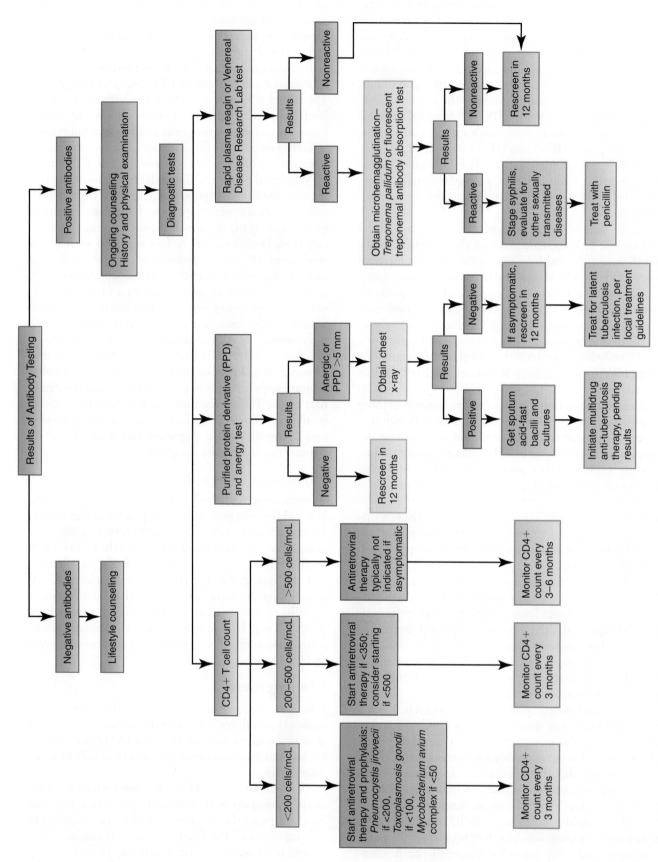

Figure 17.1 Treatment flowchart for management of early HIV infection.

Initial Disclosure

With the advent of rapid HIV testing and the CDC's emphasis on integrating HIV prevention into standard medical care, HIV test results may now be obtained during regular clinic visits. However, the disclosure of HIV test results is a critical event in the clinician–patient relationship. Disclosure counseling sets the tone and foundation for the patient's acceptance, knowledge base, and attitudes about his or her HIV infection. Disclosure of HIV test results is typically a stressful period for the patient, who may experience significant denial toward a positive test result. Even with a confirmatory Western blot test, some agencies offer to repeat the test to ensure that the diagnosis is correct and help the patient accept the reality of the diagnosis in a timely fashion. Some guidelines and concepts for disclosure counseling are summarized here:

- Disclosure counseling should be done face to face. In planning the disclosure of the patient's HIV status, the clinician should assess the degree to which the patient or parent/guardian is prepared to receive the results. The clinician should also assess the patient's social, demographic, cultural, and psychological characteristics, which may relate to coping with a positive HIV test. During the disclosure session, the provider should discuss the natural history of HIV infection, the potential effects of HIV infection on physical and mental health, the role of health maintenance practices, the availability of treatment, and the need to practice HIV prevention behaviors.
- The disclosure counseling process is an opportunity to provide immediate interventions and involve the patient in ongoing medical, mental health, social, and family support networks. Immediate interventions may include the following: assessing the patient for the risk of inflicting violence to themselves or others; ensuring that the patient will receive a thorough medical evaluation for staging and initial care; informing the patient of ongoing availability of services; scheduling the next appointment; addressing prevention of further HIV transmission; assessing the availability of an immediate support person and other care providers; providing available local and national resources of information on HIV infection; and making appropriate referrals for any ongoing services that cannot be provided on site.
- The patient should be informed of the potential for discriminatory practices against persons with HIV. Clinicians should assist patients in understanding the advantages and disadvantages of disclosing their HIV status to others by providing counseling, factual information regarding legal aspects of disclosure, opportunities for patient education and dialogue, and referrals as needed.
- The patient should be strongly advised and encouraged to disclose their HIV status to significant others,

particularly sexual and needle-sharing partners. Some local and state health departments will do partner notification without disclosing the name of the HIV-positive person, providing partners with the knowledge that they have been exposed to a sexually transmitted disease and that HIV testing is advised.

The prevention of HIV transmission must be discussed at the time of the initial diagnosis of HIV infection. The patient's blood and semen become infectious to others shortly after the patient is initially infected, so risky sexual behaviors need to be addressed immediately. The patient should also be advised against donating blood, plasma, tissue, body organs, and sperm.

The patient must also understand that the virus mutates or changes within each person; therefore, the HIV-infected person is at risk of acquiring a slightly different HIV virus from another HIV-infected individual—a phenomenon known as superinfection. The existence in the patient of a second virus can complicate the selection of an appropriate ARV regimen, increase the likelihood of infectious complications, and hasten the progression of disease. Patients from West Africa are also at risk of co-infection with strains of both HIV-1 and HIV-2.

Initiation of Drug Therapy

Although HIV infection in the 1980s was almost universally associated with death within several years, it is crucial to emphasize to the patient that improved and simplified ARV regimens have prolonged survival and improved quality of life for many persons who are infected with the virus. In fact, some recent studies have suggested that with early and attentive medical care, optimized medication adherence, and healthy lifestyle habits, HIV-infected patients may enjoy nearly the same life expectancies as noninfected individuals in the United States. Thus, the importance of beginning appropriate drug therapy and the need for continual follow-up with a health-care provider must be stressed.

Concepts of Medication Therapy Fundamental concepts that underlie the foundation of ARV treatment for HIV infection include the following:

- Eradication of HIV infection cannot be achieved with current HIV drug therapy.
- Complete viral latency does not exist. Some level of viral activity is present throughout the course of the infection.
- The level of plasma HIV RNA is proportional to the rate of viral replication and the rate of CD4+ T-lymphocyte destruction. The plasma HIV RNA level can help predict the rapidity with which clinical immunodeficiency will develop.
- Treatment-induced changes in HIV RNA levels (and, to a lesser extent, changes in CD4+ T-lymphocyte counts) correlate with clinical outcome. Studies have demonstrated that greater reductions in viral load are associated with greater improvements in clinical

outcomes. These two markers have been shown to strongly predict the likelihood of disease progression, including death.

- Viral replication leads to the generation of viral mutants. Some of these mutants will be resistant to one or more ARV drugs. Therefore, the greater the immediate suppression of the virus, the fewer drug-resistant strains will be available to reproduce. Incomplete inhibition of viral replication leads to the emergence of drug-resistant populations and to resumption of disease progression. Therefore, emergence of drug resistance may be delayed by optimized suppression of viral replication.
- Complete immune reconstitution, particularly for those who have advanced HIV disease, may not be possible. Regeneration and increases in CD4+ T-cell counts are typically seen in patients receiving ARV therapy; however, the loss of CD4+ T-lymphocyte clones as the disease progresses may not be entirely reversible. Early intervention with ARV therapy is therefore a strategy to preserve immune function.
- An important sequela of ARV therapy is immune reconstitution inflammatory syndrome (IRIS; immune restoration disease), which is an exuberant immune response in a previously immunosuppressed individual, presumably due to the reduction in immune activation and dysregulated immune responses after the initiation of ARV treatment and HIV viral load suppression. Thus, IRIS may manifest as paradoxical worsening of infectious symptoms, due to a previously treated and clinically improved opportunistic infection. Alternatively, new opportunistic infections may spontaneously arise after starting ARVs in a form known as unmasking IRIS, believed to be due to subclinical opportunistic infection at the time of ARV initiation. Other manifestations of IRIS include autoimmune or malignant phenomena. Although the pathogenesis of this syndrome is not fully understood, IRIS may affect 10% to 40% of patients, ranging from mild to life-threatening presentations. Treatment usually involves anti-inflammatory medications (e.g., NSAIDs, corticosteroids) and supportive care, but in its most severe form, IRIS may require stopping ARV therapy.
- There are both benefits and risks to deferring HIV drug therapy. In the United States, the initiation of ARV therapy is recommended for all HIV-infected persons with CD4+ T-cell counts of 350 cells/mcL or lower (Level I; Emery et al, 2008; HIV Trialists' Collaborative Group, 1999; Zolopa et al, 2009). This treatment threshold is lower in some developing nations where health-care resources are more limited, but treatment delay is inversely correlated with a patient's ability to achieve maximal immune reconstitution after starting treatment. Some research suggests that initiating ARVs at even higher CD4+ T-cell counts (350–500 cells/mcL or greater

than 500 cells/mcL) is more likely to restore the immune system to preinfection status. In turn, the question of when to initiate ARV treatment based on CD4+ T-cell count remains unsettled. However, regardless of CD4+ T-cell count, ARV treatment is recommended for HIV-infected individuals with AIDS-defining illnesses (see following section on AIDS), HIV-associated nephropathy, hepatitis B co-infection in whom antiviral treatment against hepatitis B is also indicated, or who are pregnant.

- Some benefits of deferring therapy include avoiding treatment-related side effects that may have a negative impact on quality of life, avoiding drug-related toxicities, preserving future treatment options, delaying the development of drug resistance related to incomplete viral suppression, and allowing time for the patient to understand the demands of drug treatment.
- Some risks of deferring therapy include potential irreversible damage to the immune system; potential progression to AIDS; and the potential for increased risk of transmission of untreated virus to others.
- Although HIV drug therapy has dramatically improved survival time, the long-term impact of drug therapy has not been established. Patients on drug therapy have experienced a wide variety of side effects, including increased cholesterol levels, hyperglycemia, metabolic acidosis, lipodystrophy, and wasting of the face and extremities (lipoatrophy). Drug-related lipodystrophy and lipoatrophy are also typically not improved by exercise or dietary modification. In turn, close and continual clinical monitoring of patients on HIV drug therapy is essential.

Drug Categories There are currently six FDA-approved drug categories of ARV therapy: nucleoside reverse transcriptase inhibitors (NRTIs), nonnucleoside reverse transcriptase inhibitors (NNRTIs), protease inhibitors (PIs), fusion inhibitors, integrase inhibitors, and chemokine (C-C motif) receptor 5 (CCR5) antagonist. Some clinicians further divide the drugs by using the category of nucleotide reverse transcriptase inhibitors (NtRTIs) to describe the unique characteristics of the NRTI drug tenofovir (Viread, TDF), which chemically is a nucleotide analog, rather than a nucleoside analog. In addition, fusion inhibitors are sometimes considered an overarching category that encompasses drugs with diverse mechanisms of action, including inhibition of gp41 fusion (e.g., enfuvirtide or T-20) and CCR5 antagonism (e.g., maraviroc). Combination drug therapy (also known as an HIV drug cocktail) is termed *highly active antiretroviral therapy* (HAART). These regimens consist of both base and backbone components, which together include at least three active ARV agents from at least two different drug categories, as described at the end of this section (see Treatment Standards/Guidelines 17.2: Antiretroviral Therapy).

Treatment Standards/Guidelines 17.2 Antiretroviral Therapy

Initiation of Therapy

- HIV drug therapy should be immediately started for all patients with a history of an AIDS-defining illness or severe symptoms of HIV infection regardless of CD4+ T-cell count.
- Therapy is now recommended for counts less than 350 cells/mcL; even stronger evidence for starting at T-cell counts <200 cells/mcL.
- The principles for initiation of ARV therapy and the goals of treatment are the same for HIV-infected women as for all adults and adolescents (Level I; Panel on Antiretroviral Guidelines for Adults and Adolescents, 2013). Therapy should be started in pregnant women with the goal of maximal viral suppression to prevent perinatal transmission to the fetus and newborn (Level I; Panel on Antiretroviral Guidelines for Adults and Adolescents, 2013) but may be stopped postpartum if not indicated in the mother herself.
- Therapy should also be started in patients with HIV-associated nephropathy or co-infection with hepatitis B virus (HBV) when anti-HBV treatment is indicated. In the HIV and HBV co-infected patient, the ARV regimen should include agents active against both HIV and HBV, such as emtricitabine, lamivudine, and tenofovir (Level I; Panel on Antiretroviral Guidelines for Adults and Adolescents, 2013). In patients co-infected with HIV and hepatitis C virus (HCV), ARV therapy should be considered regardless of CD4+ T-cell count (taking into account potential drug interactions of anti-HIV and anti-HCV therapy), because this may slow the progression of liver disease.
- Therapy is recommended for patients older than 50 years, regardless of CD4+ T-cell count, given the risk of non-AIDS related complications and the potential for a reduced immunological response in older HIV-infected patients.

Preferred Regimen (Level I; Panel on Antiretroviral Guidelines for Adults and Adolescents, 2013)

NNRTI base: Efavirenz OR PI base: ritonavir-boosted atazanavir, ritonavir-boosted darunavir (once daily),

OR Integrase inhibitor base: raltegravir PLUS 2-NRTI backbone: tenofovir and emtricitabine

Alternative Regimen

- NNRTI base: efavirenz PLUS 2-NRTI backbone: abacavir and lamivudine
- NNRTI base: rilpivirine (only if pretreatment HIV RNA ≤ 100,000 copies/mL) PLUS 2-NRTI backbone: abacavir and lamivudine OR tenofovir and emtricitabine
- PI base: ritonavir-boosted atazanavir, ritonavir-boosted darunavir, ritonavir-boosted fosamprenavir (once or twice daily), ritonavir-boosted lopinavir (once or twice daily) PLUS 2-NRTI backbone: abacavir and lamivudine (OR tenofovir and emtricitabine for boosted-fosamprenavir or boosted-lopinavir)
- Integrase inhibitor base: raltegravir PLUS 2-NRTI backbone: abacavir and lamivudine OR cobicistat-boosted elvitegravir in fixed combination daily dosing with 2-NRTI backbone: tenofovir and emtricitabine

Therapy Not Recommended

- Efavirenz in the first trimester of pregnancy or in women at risk for pregnancy
- Efavirenz in people with unstable psychiatric disease
- Nevirapine in people with hepatic impairment, or women/men with pre-ARV CD4+ T-cell counts >250/400 cells/mcL, respectively
- Atazanavir in patients on proton pump inhibitors equivalent to 20 mg/day of omeprazole
- Once-daily boosted lopinavir in pregnant women
- Nevirapine with tenofovir/emtricitabine or fosamprenavir with delavirdine, given reports of early virological failure with these combinations
- Unboosted atazanavir with tenofovir or didanosine PLUS lamivudine/emtricitabine
- Tenofovir in patients with renal insufficiency
- Abacavir in patients with HIV VL >100,000 copies/mL or at high risk for cardiovascular disease
- Didanosine in patients with pancreatitis or peripheral neuropathy
- Zidovudine in patients with anemia or neutropenia

NRTIs were the first effective class of ARV drugs developed for HIV infection and are active against both HIV-1 and HIV-2. The nucleoside analogs work by incorporating themselves into elongating DNA strands of the virus during its replication cycle. Given their unique chemical structure, they cause a termination of the growing DNA strand immediately after incorporation. Because the resulting DNA is incomplete, it cannot contribute to a new viral particle. Drugs in this category include zidovudine (Retrovir; ZDV; AZT), lamivudine (Epivir; 3TC), didanosine (Videx; ddI), ddI-EC (Videx EC), zalcitabine (Hivid; ddC), stavudine (Zerit; d4T),

Combivir (combination drug containing AZT and 3TC), abacavir (Ziagen; ABC), Epzicom (combination drug containing ABC and 3TC), Trizivir (combination drug containing ABC, 3TC, and AZT), emtricitabine (Emtriva; FTC), tenofovir (Viread; TDF), and Truvada (combination drug containing FTC and TDF).

Abacavir has been associated with a hypersensitivity syndrome characterized by influenza-like symptoms, including fever, malaise, rash, myalgias, headache, nausea, vomiting, and diarrhea. This syndrome is not mediated by drug-specific IgE antibodies and is not considered an immediate hypersensitivity reaction, although it typically manifests within days of starting abacavir and the medication must be stopped immediately. In addition, abacavir hypersensitivity syndrome may manifest with severe and life-threatening symptoms such as hypotension, particularly on drug reexposure. Thus, abacavir should never be restarted in these patients. Genetic testing has revealed that the B*5701 allele of the human leukocyte antigen (HLA) gene complex has a strong association with this syndrome. Testing for this allele is indicated before starting abacavir, and presence of the allele is a contraindication for this drug (Level I; Mallal et al, 2008).

NNRTIs are called nonnucleoside inhibitors because, even though they work at the same stage as nucleoside analogs, they act in a completely different manner. NNRTIs stop HIV-1 production by binding directly to the reverse transcriptase enzyme and preventing the transcription of viral DNA from RNA (i.e., the unique action of the HIV reverse transcriptase enzyme). The NNRTIs are generally effective in crossing the blood–brain barrier and may be useful in managing HIV-associated dementia. The drugs included in this category include nevirapine (Viramune), delavirdine (Rescriptor), and efavirenz (Sustiva; contraindicated in pregnancy, due to teratogenicity). At present, agents in this category are considered specific for the reverse transcriptase enzyme of HIV-1 and are ineffective against HIV-2 infection.

PIs work at the end of the viral replication cycle by restricting the action of the HIV protease enzyme, which processes viral parent proteins into smaller functional component proteins. Thus, PIs prevent the successful assembly and release of new HIV virions from infected CD4+ T cells. The development of this class of drugs gave rise to HAART, as combination regimens containing agents from three distinct ARV classes were shown to be effective in reducing HIV viral load to below the limit of detection of currently available HIV viral load tests. The drugs in this category include saquinavir (Invirase; SQV), indinavir (Crixivan; IDV), ritonavir (Norvir; RTV), nelfinavir (Viracept; NFV), fosamprenavir (Lexiva; LXV; prodrug of amprenavir [Agenerase]), atazanavir (Reyataz; ATV), tipranavir (Aptivus; TPV), and Kaletra (lopinavir/ritonavir; LPV/r). PI drugs are typically given in conjunction with low-dose ritonavir, a practice known as "boosting" the PI. This is because ritonavir is a strong inhibitor of the cytochrome p450 enzymatic degradation pathway, which is the primary means of PI metabolism. In turn, PI drug levels are markedly increased in the presence of ritonavir, and lower doses of the primary (boosted) PI may be administered in order to minimize PI-related toxicities, such as GI upset. Kaletra is a fixed combination formulation of boosted lopinavir developed to minimize pill burden. PIs are active against both HIV-1 and HIV-2.

Fusion inhibitors work by stopping the virus from attaching to target cells. Enfuvirtide (Fuzeon; T-20) was the first FDA-approved drug in this category and, in contrast to other ARVs, is administered in adults via twice daily subcutaneous injection. An additional category of fusion inhibitors is the CCR5 antagonists, which prevent the binding of macrophage-tropic HIV R5 virions to the cellular coreceptor CCR5. Maraviroc (Selzentry) is the first drug to be FDA approved in this category. Clinical trials are ongoing of other CCR5 antagonists, as well as fusion inhibitors that block binding of T-cell–tropic HIV X4 virions to the other major cellular coreceptor, CXCR4. Of note, before initiating CCR5 antagonist therapy, a patient must undergo a test of viral tropism (Level I; Panel on Antiretroviral Guidelines for Adults and Adolescents, 2013) to determine whether M-tropic R5 viruses, T-tropic X4 viruses, or a mixture of the two predominate, known as dual tropism. This assessment is critical, as CCR5 antagonists will be effective only in the former setting and, in fact, may lead to treatment failure and contribute to disease progression in the presence of X4 viral strains. Given the cost of commercial tropism tests such as the Trofile Assay, this therapeutic option may be impractical in resource-limited settings.

One of the newer categories of ARV drugs to be developed is the integrase inhibitors, of which raltegravir (Isentress) is the first agent to be FDA approved. Another member of this class, elvitegravir, was recently approved for use with the cytochrome p450 inhibitor cobicistat (a drug with no anti-HIV activity of its own) in a fixed combination pill with the NRTIs tenofovir and emtricitabine. Integrase inhibitors directly inhibit the DNA strand transfer function of the HIV integrase enzyme, which allows incorporation of newly transcribed HIV DNA into the host cell genome. Inhibition of this critical step in the HIV replication cycle prevents the production of new HIV virions. As with other newly developed ARV drugs, integrase inhibitors were first evaluated for their potential role in multidrug salvage regimens given to patients who experience ARV treatment failure while on HAART, with reemergence of detectable viral loads. However, these drugs are gaining increased acceptance as first-line ARV agents.

HAART regimens have been successful in suppressing HIV viral load to below the limit of detection of commercial viral load tests (less than 50 copies/mL), although these drug cocktails are unable to clear the virus completely. The HAART base typically consists of either one NNRTI (preferably efavirenz) (Level I; Gulick et al, 2006), a PI boosted with low-dose ritonavir to allow for once daily dosing, or an integrase inhibitor (raltegravir); the HAART backbone usually consists of two NRTI agents (preferably tenofovir and emtricitabine) (Level I; Panel on Antiretroviral Guidelines for Adults and Adolescents, 2013). Drugs Commonly Prescribed 17.2: Highly Active Antiretroviral Therapy presents key prescribing information on these drugs.

Clinical Guidelines   Clinical practice guidelines have been developed for the use of ARV therapy for

Drugs Commonly Prescribed 17.2 Highly Active Antiretroviral Therapy (HAART)

Drug	Adverse Reactions and Prescribing Considerations
Nucleoside Reverse Transcriptase Inhibitors (NRTIs)	Lactic acidosis and severe hepatomegaly with steatosis have been reported for individual and combination therapy. Immune reconstitution inflammatory syndrome is a potential sequela of any HAART regimen.
abacavir (Ziagen, ABC)	Take with or without food. Has caused severe allergic reactions resulting in death; occurs in about 8% of all patients, usually during the first 6 weeks of taking abacavir but can occur at any time. Patients should be screened before dosing for the presence of the HLA-B*5701 allele and not receive abacavir, if positive. Hypersensitivity syndrome to abacavir is a multiorgan syndrome usually characterized by at least two of the following manifestations; fever; rash; malaise, fatigue, or achiness; GI symptoms of nausea, vomiting, diarrhea, or abdominal pain; or respiratory symptoms including dyspnea, cough, or pharyngitis. Less common signs and symptoms of hypersensitivity include myolysis, edema, abnormal chest x-ray, and paresthesia. Anaphylaxis, liver failure, renal failure, hypotension, acute respiratory distress syndrome, respiratory failure, and death have occurred in association with hypersensitivity reactions. Inform patients to stop taking the drug and to seek medical care immediately if patients develop a skin rash or any two or more of the following symptoms; sudden fever; severe tiredness or achiness; diarrhea, nausea, vomiting, or stomach pain; sore throat, shortness of breath or cough; or generally ill feeling. These symptoms should be listed on a warning card included with the prescription, which patients should carry with them at all times. If these symptoms are caused by an allergic reaction, the patient should never take abacavir or an abacavir-containing medicine (e.g., Epzicom, Trizivir) again because death may occur within hours. If abacavir treatment is stopped for a period of time, it is important that the clinician be notified before the individual resumes dosing. Use with caution in patients with cardiovascular disease.
didanosine (Videx, ddl) ddl-EC (Videx EC)	May cause pancreatitis (alcohol exacerbates toxicity), peripheral neuropathy, retinal depigmentation, optic neuritis, hyperuricemia. Take on an empty stomach, at least 30 minutes before or 2 hours after eating. Monitor uric acid levels. If using buffered powder for oral solution, do not mix with fruit juice. Drugs such as ketoconazole or dapsone, whose absorption can be affected by the level of acidity in the stomach, should be administered at least 2 hours before didanosine. Use with caution in patients with impaired renal or hepatic function. Do not give with tetracycline.
emtricitabine (Emtriva, FTC)	Most common adverse effects: mild to moderate headache, nausea, diarrhea, and skin rash. Skin discoloration on palms and soles may occur. Rarely (1%), patients may develop elevated triglycerides >750 mg/dL or creatine kinase over five times the upper limit of normal. Take with or without food. In patients co-infected with HIV and hepatitis B virus (HBV), severe acute exacerbations of hepatitis B may occur after stopping drug; hepatic function should be monitored closely for at least several months after discontinuing emtricitabine in such patients.
lamivudine (Epivir, 3TC)	Generally well tolerated, but may cause GI distress or rarely peripheral neuropathy.
stavudine (Zerit, d4T)	May cause neuropathy, pancreatitis, nausea, vomiting, chills, fever, diarrhea. Take with or without food. Adjust dose if renal function is impaired.
tenofovir (Viread, TDF)	Nucleotide reverse transcriptase inhibitor (NtRTI); most common adverse effects: asthenia, diarrhea, nausea, and vomiting. Less common adverse effects: hepatotoxicity, lactic acidosis, abdominal pain, anorexia, flatulence, allergic reaction, dyspnea, Fanconi's syndrome, hypophosphatemia, pancreatitis, proximal tubulopathy, renal failure or insufficiency, and acute tubular necrosis. Follow renal function periodically. Studies have also shown decreases in bone mineral density and increases in serum levels of bone-specific alkaline phosphatase, osteocalcin, C-telopeptide, and urinary N-telopeptide, although it is not clear if long-term administration of tenofovir (greater than 1 year) causes bone abnormalities. Take with or without food. Closely monitor patients taking didanosine and tenofovir; suspend tenofovir if signs or symptoms of pancreatitis, symptomatic hyperlactemia or lactic acidosis develop;

(Continued)

Drugs Commonly Prescribed 17.2   Highly Active Antiretroviral Therapy (HAART)—cont'd

Drug	Adverse Reactions and Prescribing Considerations
	stop didanosine in patients who develop didanosine-associated adverse events. In patients co-infected with HIV and HBV who stop tenofovir, hepatic function should be monitored closely with both clinical and laboratory follow-up for at least several months, given the anti-HBV activity of tenofovir. If appropriate, initiation of anti–hepatitis B therapy may be warranted after stopping tenofovir.
zalcitabine (Hivid, ddC)	May cause peripheral neuropathy, pancreatitis (rare). Advise patient to watch for abdominal pain, nausea and vomiting, ulcers, mouth sores. Do not give with didanosine. Avoid simultaneous use with antacids.
zidovudine (Retrovir, ZDV, AZT)	May cause headache, GI distress, mild macrocytosis with or without anemia or neutropenia (bone marrow suppression). Take with food or antacids. Check CBC on ongoing basis. Hold if WBC falls to below 750 cells/mcL or with evidence of neutropenia. May take acetaminophen for headache, if not contraindicated. Stop if severe anemia develops; persistent anemia may respond to erythropoietin. Long-term use may result in myalgias, muscle wasting and weakness, increased creatine phosphokinase.
Combivir (combination of AZT and 3TC)	See information on zidovudine and lamivudine.
Epzicom (combination of ABC and 3TC)	See information on abacavir and lamivudine. Greater risk of early virological failure compared with Truvada (FTC and TDF) in patients with high HIV viral loads >100,000 copies/mL.
Trizivir (combination of ABC, AZT, and 3TC)	See information on abacavir, zidovudine, and lamivudine.
Truvada (combination of FTC and TDF)	See information on emtricitabine and tenofovir.
Nonnucleoside Reverse Transcriptase Inhibitors (NNRTIs)	Immune reconstitution inflammatory syndrome is a potential sequela of any HAART regimen.
delavirdine (Rescriptor, DLV)	May cause a skin rash on the upper body and arms. Take with water. Advise patient that skin rash usually lasts less than 2 weeks; use diphenhydramine or topical cortisone. Advise the patient with achlorhydria to take with an acidic beverage (orange or cranberry juice). Use with caution in patients with impaired renal function. Do not give at same time as antacids. If patient is also on didanosine, separate administration by 1 hour. Do not give if patient is on phenytoin, phenobarbital, carbamazepine, rifabutin, rifampin, cimetidine, famotidine, nizatidine, or ranitidine. Plasma concentrations of the following drugs are increased: indinavir, saquinavir, clarithromycin, dapsone, rifabutin, ergot derivatives, alprazolam, midazolam, triazolam, dihydropyridines (nifedipine, amlodipine, felodipine), quinidine, and warfarin. Do not use with fosamprenavir, given risk of early virological failure.
efavirenz (Sustiva, EFV)	May cause CNS symptoms (light-headedness, inability to concentrate, anxiety, dysphonia) or rash. Combination therapy may cause nausea, vomiting, diarrhea, headache. Do not give to women at risk of becoming pregnant; contraindicated in pregnancy.
etravirine (Intelence, ETR)	Approved in patients with resistance to other ARVs, including other NNRTIs. Contraindicated in lactose-intolerant patients. Reported cases of Stevens-Johnson syndrome, toxic epidermal necrolysis, erythema multiforme, hypersensitivity reactions, and hepatic failure.
nevirapine (Viramune, NVP)	May cause a rash (may decrease after initiation of therapy). Considered alternative NNRTI therapy compared with efavirenz, given risk of early virological failure in patients with high HIV viral loads. Do not use in men with pre-antiretroviral CD4 T cell counts greater than 400 cells/mcL or women with pre-antiretroviral CD4 T-cell counts greater than 250 cells/mcL, given risk of severe hepatotoxicity (including liver failure) in these individuals. Do not use in patients with moderate to severe hepatic impairment.

Drugs Commonly Prescribed 17.2 Highly Active Antiretroviral Therapy (HAART)—cont'd

Drug	Adverse Reactions and Prescribing Considerations
rilpivirine (Edurant, RPV)	Not recommended in patients with HIV RNA >100,000 copies/mL, given increased risk of virological failure. Not recommended for use with rifampin and its derivatives, proton pump inhibitors, St. John's wort, and antiepileptic drugs, including carbamazepine, phenobarbital, and phenytoin. Adverse events include rash, hepatotoxicity, depression, insomnia, and headache.
Protease Inhibitors (PIs)	May be boosted with low-dose ritonavir to increase drug levels. All PIs inhibit the CYP3A metabolic pathway to various extents. GI distress is significant class effect. May cause hypertension or diabetes mellitus. Not recommended for use with rifampin or its derivatives, given reduced PI levels. Caution against coadministration of PDE_5 inhibitors (sildenafil, tadalafil), because PIs may potentiate adverse effects of PDE_5 inhibitors (hypotension, visual changes, priapism). Caution when coadministering with HMG-CoA reductase inhibitors (statin drugs), because PIs may potentiate adverse effects of these drugs (myalgias, rhabdomyolysis). Immune reconstitution inflammatory syndrome is a potential sequela of any HAART regimen.
atazanavir (Reyataz; ATV)	Convenient once-daily dosing regimen. Do not coadminister boosted atazanavir and nevirapine. Atazanavir may cause headache, nausea, skin rash, allergic reaction, new onset or exacerbation of diabetes mellitus or hyperglycemia, asymptomatic hyperbilirubinemia, lactic acidosis, PR-interval prolongation, abdominal pain, back pain, increased cough, depression, diarrhea, lipodystrophy, nausea, vomiting, or microscopic hematuria. Take with food. Unlike other PIs, has minimal effect on lipid levels. Coadministration is contraindicated with drugs that are highly dependent on CYP3A for clearance, and specifically with rifampin, irinotecan, bepridil, lovastatin, simvastatin, indinavir, proton-pump inhibitors (e.g., pantoprazole, esomeprazole, omeprazole), and St. John's wort. Consider risk–benefit in patients with preexisting AV conduction abnormalities, given potential for PR interval prolongation. Concurrent administration with amiodarone, lidocaine, or quinidine may increase antiarrhythmic drug concentrations, resulting in serious or potentially life-threatening adverse events; caution and concentration monitoring is suggested. Risk–benefit should also be considered in patients with obesity, diabetes mellitus, or hyperglycemia, hepatic function impairment, elevated transaminase levels, hepatitis B or C, or type A or B hemophilia.
darunavir (Prezista, DRV)	Most common adverse effects: diarrhea, nausea, headache, and nasopharyngitis. May also cause abnormal liver and pancreatic function tests, abnormally high lipid levels, or decreases in WBC counts. Primarily metabolized by liver; use with caution in patients with hepatic impairment.
fosamprenavir (Lexiva; LXV)	Common adverse reactions include mild to moderate diarrhea, nausea, vomiting, headache, oral paresthesia, abdominal pain, depressive symptoms or mood disorders, or mild to moderate skin rash. Rarely (less than 1%), patients may develop severe or life-threatening skin reaction, including Stevens-Johnson syndrome; stop in patients with severe or life-threatening rash or with moderate rash accompanied by systemic reactions. Take with or without food. Use with caution in patients with known sulfonamide allergy. Concomitant use with lovastatin or simvastatin is not recommended. Coadministration with dihydroergotamine, ergonovine, ergotamine, methylergonovine, pimozide, rifampin, midazolam, triazolam, or products containing St. John's wort (*Hypericum perforatum*) is contraindicated. Serious or life-threatening drug interactions could occur between fosamprenavir and amiodarone, systemic lidocaine, bepridil, tricyclic antidepressants, or quinidine. Do not give with ritonavir, flecainide, or propafenone. Carbamazepine, phenobarbital, and phenytoin should be used cautiously in combination with fosamprenavir, because they may decrease fosamprenavir effectiveness. Do not use with delavirdine, given risk of early virological failure.

(Continued)

Drugs Commonly Prescribed 17.2   Highly Active Antiretroviral Therapy (HAART)—cont'd

Drug	Adverse Reactions and Prescribing Considerations
indinavir (Crixivan; IDV)	May cause nephrolithiasis, transient increases in bilirubin, abdominal pain, fatigue, weakness, flank pain, feeling unwell, nausea, diarrhea, vomiting, acid regurgitation, loss of appetite, dry mouth, back pain, headache, trouble sleeping, dizziness, taste changes, rash, upper respiratory tract infection, dry skin, or sore throat. Take on empty stomach and with plenty of fluids; do not take with grapefruit juice. Keep dry in container. May cause kidney stones due to crystallization of drug within the kidneys.
lopinavir (LPV)	May be at increased risk for pancreatitis or elevated triglyceride levels. Take with food. Risk–benefit should be considered if patients also have diabetes mellitus, hepatic function impairment, hepatitis B or C, or a history of pancreatitis. Do not use with rifampin, because it may lead to loss of virological response and possible drug resistance, including with other PIs or any other coadministered antiretroviral agent.
nelfinavir (Viracept; NFV)	May cause mild to moderate diarrhea, nausea, or flatulence. Take with meals or light snack. Contraindicated with drugs dependent on CYP3A for clearance, if serious or life-threatening reactions may result from elevated drug levels.
ritonavir (Norvir; RTV)	May cause nausea, vomiting, diarrhea, stomach pain, taste change, fatigue, mild to severe skin sensitivity, or numbness around the mouth. Take with meals (full stomach) to improve absorption of the drug. Keep in refrigerator. May mix oral solution with 8 oz. chocolate milk, Ensure, or Advera (nutritional supplement drink). Patients on birth control pills (ethinyl estradiol) may need to increase dosage. Also may need to increase dosage if on theophylline.
saquinavir (Invirase; SQV)	Take with meals. Do not give with rifampin, rifabutin, phenobarbital, phenytoin, dexamethasone, or carbamazepine.
tipranavir (Aptivus; TPV)	Most common adverse effects: diarrhea, nausea, vomiting, fatigue, and headache. Coadministration with ritonavir has been associated with clinical hepatitis and hepatic decompensation, including death. Vigilance warranted in individuals with advanced HIV disease or those with chronic hepatitis B or C co-infection. Individuals with hemophilia may have increased risk of bleeding. Women using estrogens may have an increased risk of rash. Other side effects include skin reactions, elevated lipid levels, and fat redistribution. Absorption increases when taken with a high-fat meal. Antacids reduce absorption. Contraindicated in individuals with moderate to severe hepatic insufficiency. Like other PIs, net inhibitor of CYP3A and may increase plasma concentration of agents primarily metabolized by this enzyme. Alternate methods of nonhormonal contraception should be used with women on estrogen-based birth control pills.
Kaletra (combination of lopinavir and ritonavir; LPV/r)	See information on lopinavir and ritonavir. Contraindicated in patients with known hypersensitivity to any component, including ritonavir. Contraindicated with drugs that are highly dependent on CYP3A for clearance and for which elevated plasma concentrations are associated with serious and/or life-threatening events, such as cardiac arrhythmias, prolonged or increased sedation, or respiratory depression. These drugs include some antihistamines, ergot derivatives, pimozide, and some sedatives. Do not use with rifampin, because it may lead to loss of virological response and possible drug resistance, including with other PIs or any other coadministered antiretroviral agent.
Fusion Inhibitors	Immune reconstitution inflammatory syndrome is a potential sequela of any HAART regimen.
enfuvirtide (Fuzeon; T-20)	Adverse side effects include local injection site reactions, hypersensitivity reactions, increased rate of bacterial pneumonia, peripheral neuropathy, sinusitis, conjunctivitis, pancreatitis, anxiety, decreased appetite, asthenia, cough, depression, herpes simplex, pruritus, insomnia, myalgias, and weight loss.
maraviroc (Selzentry, MVC)	CCR5 antagonist; before beginning therapy, patient must undergo test of viral tropism to determine if R5 (CCR5-binding M-tropic) viruses predominate, in the absence of X4 (CXCR4-binding T-cell–tropic) viruses.

Drugs Commonly Prescribed 17.2 Highly Active Antiretroviral Therapy (HAART)—cont'd

Drug	Adverse Reactions and Prescribing Considerations
Integrase Inhibitors	Immune reconstitution inflammatory syndrome is a potential sequela of any HAART regimen.
Elvitegravir (EVG)	See information on Stribild/Quad Pill. CYP3A4 inducers or inhibitors may alter blood levels. When combined with cobicistat, may lead to more drug interactions than raltegravir.
raltegravir (Isentress, RAL)	Common adverse reactions include headache, nausea, asthenia, and fatigue. Use with caution in patients at increased risk of myopathy or rhabdomyolysis, e.g., patients receiving concomitant medications known to cause these conditions such as HMG-CoA reductase inhibitors (statins).
Multiclass Combination Therapies	Immune reconstitution inflammatory syndrome is a potential sequela of any HAART regimen. Convenient once-daily HAART dosing regimen: 1 pill per day.
Atripla (combination of EFV, FTC, and TDF)	See information on efavirenz, emtricitabine, and tenofovir.
Complera (combination of RPV, FTC, and TDF)	See information on rilpivirine, emtricitabine, and tenofovir. Not recommended in patients with HIV RNA >100,000 copies/mL, given greater risk of virological failure. Take with meal.
Stribild/Quad Pill (combination of elvitegravir, cobicistat, FTC, and TDF)	See information on elvitegravir, emtricitabine, and tenofovir. Cobicistat has no antiviral activity but is a potent inhibitor of the CYP3A4 degradation pathway and, thus, boosts ARV levels. Not recommended to start in patients with creatinine clearance ≤70 mL/min; may increase risk of proximal renal tubulopathy. Adverse events include diarrhea, nausea, and headache. Not recommended for use with HMG CoA-reductase inhibitors, rifampin and its derivatives, anxiolytics (e.g., midazolam, triazolam), ergot derivatives, St. John's wort, and PDE_5 inhibitors.

HIV-1–infected adults and adolescents. These guidelines are revised on an ongoing basis by the Panel on Clinical Practices for Treatment of HIV Infection, convened by the U.S. Department of Health and Human Services, and are considered "living documents" that may be obtained online at www.AIDSinfo.nih.gov, a public access Web site maintained by the National Institutes of Health. Treatment Standards/Guidelines 17.2 presents the most current version of these HIV treatment guidelines for adults and adolescents. Clinical practice guidelines have also been developed by expert panels on HIV care for pediatric patients and pregnant women and may be accessed at this same website. It is critical for the clinician providing HIV care to be familiar with these guidelines, as specific recommendations exist regarding the timing of HAART initiation in different patient populations.

In contrast to HIV-1, far less is known about effective treatments against HIV-2. Given the slower progression and decreased virulence of HIV-2 compared with HIV-1, treatment guidelines regarding when to initiate therapy for HIV-2 infection are less established, and treatment decisions regarding HIV-2 infection should be referred to an infectious disease specialist.

Designing a Compatible Medication Regimen
The patient's ability to adhere to a potent combination drug cocktail must be discussed in detail before initiating therapy. Once a client is started on drug therapy, there is a risk of developing drug resistance if viral suppression is not maintained. Viral mutations causing drug resistance can rapidly occur within 2 weeks to as little as 2 days of a patient stopping medication or failing to take the full set of prescribed doses. ARV medications all have varying requirements regarding dosing, dietary restrictions, numbers of pills to be taken each day, and drug interactions. The clinician must prescribe a HAART regimen that is compatible with the patient's day-to-day activities, including lifestyle, eating habits, social habits, and work and home environments.

Nursing Research–Based Practice Box 17.2 discusses an alternative methodology for the prediction of adherence to anti-HIV treatment, because effective treatment is fundamental to controlling the progression to AIDS. Helping the patient to live with HIV requires a multidisciplinary approach. See the Iceberg figure for additional suggestions.

Monitoring HIV Viral Load The HIV viral load test directly measures the concentration of viral particles in the patient's plasma. Thus, viral load test results are reported as either copies or units per milliliter of plasma. If the test result is below the detection threshold of the assay, the viral load is considered undetectable. This means that the amount of virus in the blood is so minimal that it cannot be measured by the test being used (i.e., below the level of detection), rather than indicating the virus has

The Iceberg of Living with HIV

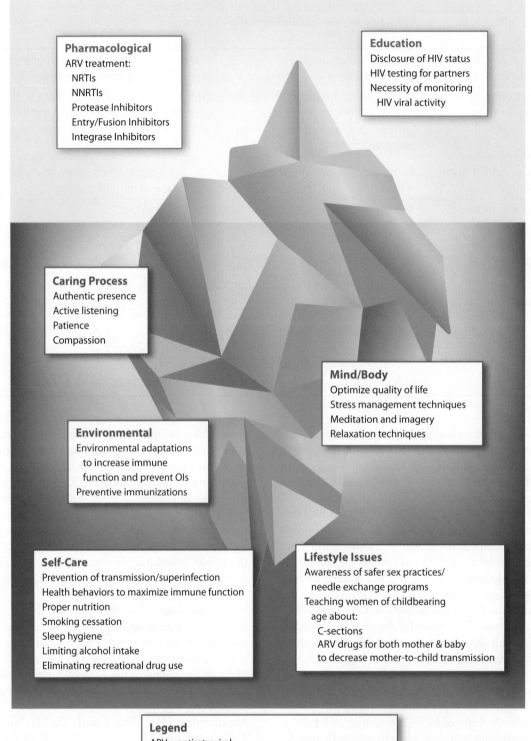

Pharmacological
ARV treatment:
  NRTIs
  NNRTIs
  Protease Inhibitors
  Entry/Fusion Inhibitors
  Integrase Inhibitors

Education
Disclosure of HIV status
HIV testing for partners
Necessity of monitoring
  HIV viral activity

Caring Process
Authentic presence
Active listening
Patience
Compassion

Mind/Body
Optimize quality of life
Stress management techniques
Meditation and imagery
Relaxation techniques

Environmental
Environmental adaptations
  to increase immune
  function and prevent OIs
Preventive immunizations

Self-Care
Prevention of transmission/superinfection
Health behaviors to maximize immune function
Proper nutrition
Smoking cessation
Sleep hygiene
Limiting alcohol intake
Eliminating recreational drug use

Lifestyle Issues
Awareness of safer sex practices/
  needle exchange programs
Teaching women of childbearing
  age about:
    C-sections
    ARV drugs for both mother & baby
    to decrease mother-to-child transmission

Legend
ARV = antiretroviral
NRTIs = nucleoside reverse transcriptase inhibitors
NNRTIs = non-nucleoside reverse transcriptase inhibitors
OIs = opportunistic infections

Nursing Research–Based Practice 17.2

Thompson, IR, and the EuResist Network Study Group et al. An alternative methodology for the prediction of adherence to anti-HIV treatment. *AIDS Res Ther* 6:9, 2009. doi:10.1186/1742-6405-6-9

Successful treatment of HIV-positive patients is fundamental to preventing progression to AIDS. Treatment failure may be related to drug resistance and/or insufficient drug levels in the blood. Severe side effects, coupled with the intense nature of many drug regimens, can lead to treatment fatigue and consequently to periodic or permanent medication nonadherence. Although nonadherence is a recognized problem in HIV treatment, it is poorly detected in both clinical practice and health outcomes research and is often based on unreliable information such as self-reports, or in a research setting, Medication Events Monitoring System pill bottles or prescription refill rates. To meet the need for objective information on adherence, this study proposes a method using viral load and HIV genome sequence data to identify nonadherence among patients.

With nonadherence operationally defined as a sharp increase in viral load in the absence of drug resistance mutations, it was hypothesized that periods of nonadherence can be identified retrospectively based on the observed relationship between changes in viral load and HIV mutations. It was suggested that validation of the hypothesized approach would serve as a first step on the road to clinical practice. The information inferred from clinical data on adherence would be a crucial feature of treatment prediction tools to aid practitioners in daily clinical practice. In addition, distinguishing characteristics of biological markers routinely used to assess the progression of HIV disease may be identified in the adherent and nonadherent groups. This latter approach would directly help clinicians to differentiate between nonresponding (albeit adherent) versus nonadherent patients.

been completely eradicated from the body. Several different commercial assays measure HIV viral load, varying in cost and sensitivity (i.e., with lower detection limits). At present, the standard commonly adopted in the United States is a lower detection limit of 50 copies/mL, although less expensive assays with decreased sensitivity (detection limits of 400–500 copies/mL) are commonly used in developing countries, given resource limitations. Highly sensitive detection assays capable of measuring HIV viral load down to a single copy per milliliter have been developed for research purposes.

A baseline viral load is determined by taking two separate viral load tests, approximately 2 to 3 weeks apart. If the results of the two tests are similar, a stable baseline is established and used to monitor the effects of drug therapy. The viral load should be repeated 4 to 6 weeks after initiation of drug therapy or after any alteration in an ARV regimen is made. The initiation of ARV therapy should correspond with a decrease in viral load, typically by a factor of 10 after 2 to 4 weeks. Effective HAART will often suppress viral load fully after 8 to 12 weeks of therapy. Thus, if viral load is about the same or higher than the baseline level after initiating treatment, changes in the drug regimen are likely needed. It should be noted that reestablishment of complete suppression of the virus to below the detection limit of established viral load assays (e.g., HIV RNA less than 48 copies/mL) should remain the primary goal of ARV therapy (Level I; Panel on Antiretroviral Guidelines for Adults and Adolescents, 2013). Once an effective drug regimen has been established, the viral load should be repeated every 3 to 4 months to confirm chronic viral suppression. Of note, changes in viral load of less than threefold are not considered significant.

Because the tests measure viral activity, anything that affects the production of virus can influence the results. A sudden rise in viral load can occur after an active infection, such as from influenza or a herpes outbreak, as previously inactive HIV-infected CD4+ T cells may become activated by these infections and begin producing HIV. A viral load test can also be affected by the administration of a vaccine, so a test should not be done until 4 to 6 weeks after an acute illness or vaccination.

At present, there are at least three distinct assay methods commercially available to assess viral load: polymerase chain reaction (PCR), branched DNA (bDNA) test, and nucleic acid sequence–based amplification (NASBA). Because the methods of each test are slightly different, results may not be equivalent. Table 17.6 presents key information on several common HIV viral load tests.

CD4+ T-cell count is typically followed with similar frequency to assess for adequate immune reconstitution after initiating HAART, although cellular immune reconstitution typically lags behind decreases in viral load, with an expected increase in CD4+ T cells of 100 to 150 cells/mL annually in adequately treated patients. Immunological nonresponders who fail to undergo adequate cellular immune reconstitution on HAART, despite viral load suppression, remain at increased risk for opportunistic infection and may require alterations in their ARV regimen, as directed by an HIV specialist. Studies are currently underway to evaluate various immunostimulant therapies in this specific patient population.

Follow-up and Referral

Follow-up for a patient infected with HIV will be required for the rest of the patient's life. However, even if the results of an HIV antibody test are negative, the

Table 17.6   Viral Load Tests

- Viral load monitoring can establish the prognosis of a patient with HIV infection. Rising viral load indicates disease progression; falling viral load indicates a favorable prognostic trend.
- Plasma viral load may range from a few hundred virions (also called viral copies or viral equivalents) to more than a million per mL, a 10,000-fold range. Such large ranges are easiest to express in logarithms (logs).
- To express a number in logarithmic form, a base is raised to a power. The latter is the logarithm, or exponent. The base 10 is commonly used in medicine without being explicitly specified; often only the power (the exponent, or log) is shown. A viral load of 10,000 copies/mL, or 10^4 copies/mL, is 4 logs. A viral load 10 times as high, or 100,000 copies/mL, is 10^5 copies/mL, or 5 logs.
- Changes in viral load are commonly expressed in either numerical or logarithmic terms. For example, a twofold change is equal to approximately a 0.3-log change.
- In viral load measurements, the sum of the laboratory and biological variation is generally assumed to be 0.3–0.5 log (twofold to threefold). Therefore, only changes greater than this are considered meaningful. The following table gives further information on several of these exams.

Type	Manufacturer	Name	HIV Range
Polymerase chain reaction (PCR)	Roche Diagnostics	Amplicor HIV-1 Monitor Test 1.5	400–750,000 copies
PCR	Roche Diagnostics	Amplicor HIV-1 Monitor Test 1.5 Ultra Sensitive	50–75,000 copies
Branched DNA PCR	Chiron/Bayer	VERSANT HIV-1 RNA 3.0 Assay (bDNA)	<50–500,000 copies
Nucleic acid sequence–based amplification (NASBA)	Organon Teknika	NucliSens HIV-1 QT	80–10,000 copies

clinician should still discuss risk reduction behaviors with the patient to mitigate the chance of future infection. Moreover, the patient also needs to understand that the test may be negative if the patient is still in the window period before seroconversion. Thus, the HIV antibody test should be repeated in 3 to 6 months, without intervening risky behaviors, in order to confirm initial negative results. If any risky behaviors occur before the test is repeated, the time period for retesting will need to be recalculated, because the window period may last up to 3 months after initial infection.

For the patient who tests positive, the pros and cons of beginning ARV medications should be discussed thoroughly. The patient's present clinical condition, HIV viral load, and CD4+ T-cell count will need to be considered to determine the timing and composition of the most appropriate HAART regimen. Moreover, the patient should be educated regarding the major aspects of HAART so that he or she can actively participate in determining what ARV choices would be most compatible with his or her lifestyle and ability to adhere to different therapeutic regimens. Importantly, the patient may need time to accept the diagnosis in order to make the most informed decisions regarding future medical care. Thus, although these issues should be raised in a timely fashion, it may not be beneficial to the patient to discuss the choice of HAART regimens or other major

medical decisions at the time of diagnosis. A follow-up visit should therefore be scheduled to discuss strategies for coping with the diagnosis, as well as specifics regarding the patient's choice of HAART regimen, if applicable. Follow-up will also be necessary to monitor the effects of drug therapy on HIV viral load and to discuss any factors affecting medication adherence.

In general, a primary care practitioner should refer the patient to an immunology or infectious disease specialist for follow-up HIV care, although in resource-limited settings where specialty physicians may not be available, many primary care practitioners are providing general HIV care as well. This becomes particularly important with regard to the appropriate management of prophylactic medications against common opportunistic diseases, including PCP and mycobacterial infections (see following section on AIDS). In addition, concurrent chronic viral infections, such as hepatitis B or hepatitis C, require specialty referral to an appropriate clinical specialist (such as a hepatologist), because these infections are typically more aggressive with a worse prognosis in the setting of concurrent HIV infection.

If the patient is having severe pulmonary symptoms, he or she may need to be admitted to the hospital to rule out PCP, TB, or community-acquired pneumonia. If Kaposi's sarcoma is suspected, the patient may need to be referred to an oncologist if the condition is severe or affecting any internal organs. If there is a suspicion of

CMV retinitis, the patient should be immediately referred to an ophthalmologist for a thorough eye exam because uncontrolled infection can lead to blindness.

In addition to appropriate therapeutic and prophylactic regimens, modifications in unhealthy lifestyle behaviors can have an enormous impact on the health and well-being of an HIV-infected client. Thus, the clinician should seize this opportunity to counsel the client on smoking cessation, limiting alcohol intake, and eliminating recreational drug use. Health maintenance of the HIV-infected patient also requires close attention to preventive immunizations, including pneumococcal vaccine (23-valent polysaccharide Pneumovax vaccine) that may be readministered after 5 years, annual influenza vaccination (but not the intranasal attenuated live virus vaccine, which is contraindicated in immunocompromised patients), tetanus toxoid boosters every 10 years, quadrivalent HPV vaccine, and vaccination for both hepatitis A (two vaccinations spaced 6 months apart) and hepatitis B (three vaccinations spaced 1 and 6 months apart). Importantly, attenuated live virus vaccines including measles, mumps, rubella (MMR), oral polio virus (OPV), bacillus Calmette-Guérin anti-TB vaccine (BCG), intranasal influenza vaccine, and those for varicella (chickenpox) and yellow fever are contraindicated in HIV-infected patients with advanced disease and significant immunosuppression. However, the MMR and varicella vaccines may be given early in the course of the disease to nonimmunosuppressed HIV-infected individuals.

Patient Education

HIV infection is a lifelong chronic disease. Education may facilitate self-care activities that can decrease the risk of superinfection with other HIV strains, hepatitis viruses, and opportunistic pathogens. The patient requires extensive personalized education for his or her specific medical conditions and therapeutic regimen, including specific drug contraindications and interaction warnings. It is also critical to provide adequate support to facilitate adherence to what may be a demanding HAART regimen. Likewise, the patient will need continual reinforcement and education on the need to attain and maintain effective HIV preventive behaviors, such as safer sex practices to decrease the potential of transmitting HIV to others or acquiring new HIV strains. A wide variety of patient education materials are available from pharmaceutical companies, AIDS support organizations, and government and health-care agencies (see Resources section at the end of this chapter). Educational programs for clinicians are also available through the Association of Nurses in AIDS Care (ANAC) at 1-800-260-6780.

◼ ACQUIRED IMMUNODEFICIENCY SYNDROME

If left untreated, HIV infection will eventually undermine the immune system. Once the CD4+ T-cell count is below 200 cells/mcL, opportunistic infections become more frequent, and these can be life-threatening unless diagnosed and treated in a timely manner. Once the CD4+ T-cell count falls below 200 cells/mcL or the patient develops an opportunistic infection or other AIDS-defining illness, the HIV-positive patient is classified as having progressed from HIV infection to AIDS.

Epidemiology and Causes

AIDS, which is the advanced stage of HIV infection, is a leading cause of death in sub-Saharan Africa. In contrast, early detection of HIV infection and improved HIV drug therapy have dramatically decreased the death rate from AIDS in resource-rich nations.

There is tremendous variation in the natural history of HIV infection from one patient to another. Thus, it is impossible to predict precisely when AIDS will occur in a person infected with HIV, but studies from the 1980s to the mid-1990s indicated the usual survival time after the diagnosis of AIDS was just 3 years. In more recent years, however, the impact of early HIV diagnosis and treatment, including HAART initiation before the development of AIDS and prophylactic medications to prevent opportunistic infections, has increased the survival time and quality of life for many HIV-infected persons, including those with full-blown AIDS.

Unfortunately, some HIV-infected persons do not respond to drug therapy with adequate viral load suppression (referred to as treatment failures or virological failures) or CD4+ T-cell restoration (referred to as immunological nonresponders). These clients require close monitoring for opportunistic infections, malignancies, and other life-threatening conditions as their immune status deteriorates, despite standard treatment. Evidence suggests that these patients still benefit from HAART, although regimen changes should be considered as newer agents become available, particularly those from different categories of ARV agents.

Pathophysiology

HIV is well recognized for its lengthy latency period after acute infection, in which infected persons remain relatively asymptomatic in the absence of HAART, despite persistent low level viremia and progressive CD4+ T-cell destruction (approximately 40–80 CD4+ T cells/L per year in untreated patients). However, among individual patients, there is wide variability in length to progression to clinical AIDS. Although the average latency period in untreated individuals has been estimated at 9 years, a subset of HIV-infected persons known as rapid progressors will clinically deteriorate to AIDS within a period of months to less than 2 years after initial infection. This is in stark contrast to approximately 5% of infected persons known as long-term nonprogressors, who show little to no progression of disease for more than a decade, despite the absence of ARV therapy. A complex interplay of multiple environmental and genetic factors of both the host and the infecting virus underlies this variation.

Anti-HIV immune responses include both humoral and cell-mediated mechanisms. HIV-specific antibodies form in the majority of individuals within several weeks to 3 months of initial infection; however, these antibodies are insufficient to prevent disseminated infection. These neutralizing antibodies appear to play a role in natural killer (NK) cell destruction of HIV-infected cells via antibody-mediated cellular cytotoxicity. In addition, CD8+ cytotoxic T cells also target HIV-infected cells for destruction. However, these mechanisms are unable to fully eradicate HIV infection from long-lived cellular compartments (e.g., follicular dendritic cells, memory T lymphocytes) or cells that are physically sequestered from the lymphatic system (e.g., central nervous system [CNS] cells).

Given HIV's tropism for cells of the hematopoietic and immune systems, CD8+ killer T-cell activity, which is key in clearing the high levels of viremia associated with initial HIV infection, also contributes significantly to CD4+ T-cell destruction and eventual progression to clinical AIDS. This can occur via single cell killing of infected host cells, resulting from an accumulation of unintegrated viral DNA and eventual cell lysis or via disruption of normal host cell protein synthesis. However, in vitro studies have also revealed that HIV-infected cells are capable of fusing with large numbers of uninfected CD4+ T cells to create large, multinucleated syncytia or multicellular aggregates. This process has been theorized to contribute to the rapid depletion of the helper T-cell compartment in advanced stages of HIV infection.

Shared structural homology between the HIV envelope glycoproteins gp120 and gp41 and MHC class II molecules is thought to underlie the cross-reactivity and autoimmune destruction of T lymphocytes and antigen-presenting cells in the HIV-infected individual. However, even before significant CD4+ T-cell depletion occurs, dysregulated B-cell activity and autoantibody production caused by regulatory T-cell dysfunction may lead to autoimmune damage of additional cell lineages and organ-specific tissues, including primary HIV-associated thrombocytopenia, HIV nephropathy, and HIV cardiomyopathy.

In addition to destruction at the cellular level, advanced HIV infection is also characterized by destruction of the gross lymphatic architecture over a period of months to years. This includes disruption of the lymph node follicular network, which is critical for immune cell trafficking and exposure to circulating antigens, both of which are necessary to mount effective immune responses.

Qualitative defects in immune cell function are also important to the pathogenesis of advanced HIV infection. Binding studies with gp120-specific immunoglobulins demonstrated that T-cell anergy (inactivation) could be induced by antibody binding of CD4+ T-cell surface receptors. In addition, increased rates of apoptosis

(nonnecrotic programmed cell death) have been demonstrated in T cells repeatedly stimulated by a specific antigen; this mechanism may be particularly relevant to chronic HIV infection with persistent low level viremia.

Given this progressive immunosuppression, the patient with AIDS is at high risk for developing viral, bacterial, fungal, and/or protozoal opportunistic infections. Common viral infections include CMV, herpes simplex virus, varicella zoster virus, and progressive multifocal leukoencephalopathy (PML, due to the John Cunningham or JC virus). Common bacterial infections include *Mycobacterium avium* complex (MAC; due to *M avium* and *M intracellulare*) and TB. Common fungal infections include candidiasis, PCP, histoplasmosis (*Histoplasma capsulatum),* and cryptococcosis (*Cryptococcus neoformans).* Common protozoal infections include cryptosporidiosis, which causes chronic diarrhea, and cerebral toxoplasmosis (*Toxoplasma gondii* infection of the CNS), which can be life-threatening. Other potential problems include malignancies and AIDS wasting syndrome (involuntary loss of more than 10% of body weight with more than 30 days of either diarrhea or weakness and fever).

Clinical Presentation
Subjective

In assessing the patient with AIDS, it is important to realize that symptomatic manifestations of opportunistic infections are varied and may affect any organ system.

The patient may complain of visual problems, such as a loss of central or peripheral vision, blurring of vision, loss of visual acuity, eye pain, photophobia, or the development of "floaters." Such complaints should raise suspicion for CMV retinitis or fungal endophthalmitis (ocular histoplasmosis).

Neurological symptoms or alterations in mental status, including headaches, confusion, mood swings, personality changes, dizziness, neck stiffness, fever, lethargy, malaise, nausea, vomiting, photophobia (intolerance of light due to resulting eye pain), neurological deficits, hemiparesis, ataxia, cranial nerve palsies, or seizures, may be the result of herpes encephalopathy, PML, cryptococcal meningitis, or cerebral toxoplasmosis.

Gastrointestinal (GI) problems such as diarrhea and abdominal pain may present concurrently with unintentional weight loss, fever, chills, or night sweats, as a result of CMV enterocolitis, viral gastroenteritis, pancreatitis, AIDS wasting syndrome, MAC, *Salmonella* or other enteric bacterial infection, cryptosporidiosis, giardiasis, isosporiasis, or histoplasmosis. The clinician should note whether GI symptoms are of sudden onset or insidious, because chronic diarrhea may result not only from the more rapid onset of opportunistic infections, but also from progressive malabsorption syndromes or as a direct effect of HIV infection in the gut known as AIDS enteropathy.

Dermatological problems may develop, such as stinging or burning papules or bumpy rashes in a linear or clustered pattern, which may be indicative of herpes simplex or HPV infection, particularly if located in the anogenital region. Other painless lesions, such as the purplish plaques of Kaposi's sarcoma, may go unnoticed in areas poorly visible to the patient (e.g., the back).

The patient may also complain of pulmonary symptoms, such as shortness of breath or a persistent cough. These symptoms may be accompanied by fever, chills, night sweats, weight loss, purulent or blood-tinged sputa, or chest pain, which may be indicative of PCP, bacterial pneumonia, or active TB. The clinician should determine the onset of pulmonary symptoms, because PCP and TB are usually insidious in presentation, with worsening of symptoms over days to weeks, whereas pulmonary toxoplasmosis progresses more rapidly.

In addition, nonspecific complaints of fatigue, weakness, and fever with anemia and leukopenia could signify disseminated MAC with bone marrow involvement.

Objective

A complete physical exam is indicated for the patient with AIDS because an array of opportunistic infections and malignancies may affect literally any organ system (Level I; Panel on Opportunistic Infections in HIV-Infected Adults and Adolescents, 2013). Some of the most common physical presentations are presented in this section by organ system.

With CMV retinitis, retinal changes are seen on ophthalmoscopic exam. With toxoplasmosis encephalitis (the most common presentation of *Toxoplasma* infection), the clinician should check for altered level of consciousness, impaired cognition, and any stroke-like symptoms. Of note, the physical examination findings of cryptococcal meningitis are typically not as striking as the fulminant meningitic symptoms of bacterial meningitis.

Oropharyngeal examination may reveal erythematous mucosal ulcers, which should raise suspicion for herpes simplex or CMV, or if patchy white lesions are present, candidiasis or EBV-associated oral hairy leukoplakia, which is typically limited to the tongue, gingivae, and/or buccal mucosa.

A wide variety of skin lesions may present with AIDS. Herpes simplex lesions are initially papulo-vesicular (fluid-filled), painful, and pruritic; these clustered lesions become progressively erythematous and ulcerated, eventually crusting over before healing. The lesions of shingles are exquisitely painful papules and vesicles, which present with a burning sensation and are distributed over a well-demarcated region of the skin known as a dermatome, corresponding to the cutaneous area innervated by a single spinal nerve. Venereal warts associated with HPV infection (condyloma acuminata) appear as raised, flesh-colored papules, with or without stalks, in isolation or in clusters. Cutaneous Kaposi's sarcoma presents with

one or more raised, darkish colored lesions that may occur anywhere on the body, whereas cutaneous cryptococcosis usually presents as a single ulcerated nodule at the site of infection. Papular pruritic eruption of HIV (PPE) is a highly pruritic rash that presents as widespread papular to nodular skin lesions; as a diagnosis of exclusion, the etiology of PPE is unclear but has been suggested to be due to a dysregulated immune response to arthropod bites, because it often improves after initiating HAART. Eosinophilic folliculitis is an overlapping diagnosis with PPE in which biopsy confirms perifollicular eosinophilic infiltration that has been suggested to be of autoimmune etiology.

Findings on pulmonary examination may be nonspecific in the setting of a wide variety of infectious processes, such as PCP, TB, or community-acquired pneumonia. Therefore, physical exam findings should be considered within the context of a careful medical history detailing clinical presentation and timing of symptom onset, along with appropriate diagnostic imaging and laboratory studies. Advanced Assessment 17.2 presents additional history and physical exam information to be gathered from the HIV-positive patient.

Diagnostic Reasoning
Diagnostic Tests

Ideally, the patient with AIDS should have had all initial diagnostic testing done when he or she was first diagnosed with HIV infection. However, a significant number of patients are initially diagnosed only after they progress to AIDS (particularly in resource-limited areas), as extreme physical manifestations typically lead patients to seek medical care. Once the peripheral CD4+ T-cell count falls below 200 cells/mcL, the patient is formally diagnosed with AIDS. Outside of the United States, in resource-limited settings without access to reliable HIV diagnostic testing or T-cell counts, clinical criteria are typically used empirically to determine a diagnosis of AIDS and initiate therapy.

HIV drug resistance testing is typically done for all patients before initiating HAART to help guide the choice of ARV regimen. Resistance testing is also typically repeated for clients who have been on HIV medications but do not respond to drug therapy or experience treatment failure with reemergence of a detectable viral load greater than 1,000 copies/mL (virological failure) (Level I; Panel on Antiretroviral Guidelines for Adults and Adolescents, 2013). The most common form of resistance testing is known as HIV genotyping, in which specific viral mutations are detected via DNA sequence analysis compared with a "wild type" (nonmutated) HIV reference sequence. Based on large epidemiological data sets of viral sequences from HIV-infected patients, mutations are classified as to their potential for leading to ARV drug resistance. Of note, the full array of HIV mutations detected in an individual typically does not represent a

Advanced Assessment 17.2   HIV-Positive Patient

History

Present Illness	When did you take the HIV antibody test?
	Why did you take the HIV antibody test?
	What brought you to the clinic today?
Past Medical History	Have you been to a health-care provider for HIV care?
	Do you know what your viral load is? What your CD4+ count (T-cell count) is? When were these tests last done?
	Have you had any opportunistic infections such as PCP or thrush? Were you ever hospitalized for these infections?
	What is your past medical history? Surgical history?
	Are you using any nontraditional (alternative or complementary) therapies? If so, please explain.
	Have you ever had heart problems or a history of high cholesterol?
Social Support History	What is your living situation (e.g., home life, support system [friends, relatives], financial situation, emotional situation, occupational situation, sexual relationships)?
	What do you know about HIV infection?
	If you are sexually active, do you practice safer sex? If so, please explain.
Medication History	What HIV drugs have you taken in the past? How long were you on them? How long have you been off them?
	Have you been taking any medications for prophylaxis? Do you take them all or just some of the time?
	What other medications are you taking (prescription, over-the-counter, herbal)?
Nutritional History	Tell me about your usual diet.
	Do you eat raw eggs or raw fish?
	How do you cook your meat?
	Do you take any appetite enhancers?
	Do you take any nutritional supplements?
Travel History	Do you travel often? If so, where?
	Have you traveled or lived in other states or out of the country? If so, when, where, and for how long?

Physical Examination

General Overview and Mental Status	Level of consciousness
	Confusion
	Difficulty in remembering
	Change in mental status or mood
	Fatigue
	Change in activities of daily living
Neurological System	Headaches and associated signs and symptoms
	Neurological exam; cranial nerve exam
Respiratory System	Shortness of breath or dyspnea and associated signs and symptoms
	Cough and associated signs and symptoms
	Hiccups
	Lung sounds
	Respiratory rate, rhythm, characteristics; use of accessory muscles
Cardiovascular System	Heart sounds
	Pulse rate, rhythm, characteristics
Hematological and Lymphatic System	Swollen, enlarged, or tender glands
	Night sweats, fever

Advanced Assessment 17.2   HIV-Positive Patient—cont'd

Gastrointestinal System and Nutrition	Sores or white spots in mouth or lips; dental assessment
	Problems eating or swallowing
	Nausea/vomiting
	Change in weight or appetite
	Change in bowel habits (diarrhea, constipation)
	Nutritional intake
	Anorectal symptoms

single HIV viral strain, but rather characterize a population of viral strains present in a given patient. Thus, ARV medications do not actually cause HIV genetic mutations to occur, but rather, these medications exert pressure on the viral population to enrich or select for strains that developed drug resistance mutations due to the background mutational error rate of the viral reverse transcriptase enzyme.

HIV phenotyping assays also exist in which drug resistance is measured by growing viral isolates from a patient in the presence of individual ARV agents and comparing these growth rates to those of a wild type HIV strain. Given the higher cost of HIV phenotyping tests, however, these are done much less frequently than HIV genotyping tests.

Table 17.7 includes additional laboratory tests to perform and how to interpret them, as guided by the patient's presenting signs and symptoms. For clients with suspected TB or PCP, the clinician should order a PPD, arterial blood gas (ABG), chest x-ray, and sputum examination for smear and culture. Tests for acid-fast bacilli (AFB) are done for TB, and a silver stain will detect fungal forms in PCP. In addition to sputa, bronchoalveolar lavage fluid (from bronchoscopy) may be examined, as well as specific blood cultures. For patients with neurological symptoms, a referring physician should order a computed tomography scan or magnetic resonance imaging of the brain to check for the presence of ring-enhancing lesions, which could be associated with *Toxoplasma gondii* or CNS lymphoma, or nonenhancing areas of white matter (demyelination), which could indicate PML.

If diarrhea is present, with or without other GI symptoms, the clinician should send stool cultures for infectious organisms, including examination for protozoal forms, ova, and parasites. Viral infections such as CMV colitis may require colonoscopic biopsy of the GI mucosa for definitive diagnosis.

Differential Diagnosis

The differential diagnoses for AIDS-associated illnesses are quite extensive, particularly with regard to pulmonary, neurological, and GI manifestations. In the pulmonary differential, consider TB, PCP, MAC, histoplasmosis, or other bacterial, viral, fungal, or protozoal infections of the pulmonary system, as well as internal Kaposi's sarcoma affecting the lungs. Regarding the neurological system,

the clinician should consider CNS lymphoma or other malignancy, in addition to the cerebral infections discussed earlier of toxoplasmosis and PML. In the GI system, CMV and disseminated MAC infection must be considered, as well as protozoal infections (cryptosporidiosis, isosporiasis, giardiasis) and malabsorption syndromes. Pan-cytopenias should raise suspicion of disseminated MAC infection in the bone marrow.

Management

In addition to prophylactic treatment and ARV medication, therapy for the person with AIDS is both supportive and educational, geared toward maximizing both the quantity and quality of life. In contrast to the early years of the HIV epidemic, given the effectiveness and availability of current ARV treatments, most HIV-infected patients are now able to live in a state of chronic, relatively stable infection for many years, rather than progressing to full-blown AIDS, provided treatment guidelines are adhered to and healthy lifestyle behaviors are followed. In turn, long-term medical management of HIV-infected patients in the United States and other developed nations is largely focused on the prevention and treatment of many of the same chronic diseases seen in the general population, such as cardiovascular disease (see Chapter 10).

However, opportunistic infections still affect a substantial number of HIV patients, even in resource-abundant settings, given factors such as therapeutic nonadherence, barriers to health-care accessibility, and comorbid medical conditions that interfere with effective HIV treatment. Thus, correctly identifying the causative organism of a presenting opportunistic infection is crucial to initiating appropriate treatment in a timely fashion. Because CD4+ T-cell count serves as the major clinical indicator of immunocompetence in HIV-infected individuals, when CD4+ T-cell count falls below 200 cells/mcL, the HIV-positive client becomes increasingly prone to opportunistic infections. PCP prophylaxis is required for CD4+ T-cell counts less than 200 cells/mcL, *Toxoplasmosis gondii* prophylaxis for counts less than 100 cells/mcL, and MAC prophylaxis for counts less than 50 cells/mcL.

Candidiasis

Oral candidiasis can be treated with fluconazole (Diflucan) 3 to 6 mg/kg (maximum of 100 mg/day) PO daily

Table 17.7   Diagnostic and Screening Tests to Evaluate the HIV-Positive Patient

Test	Interpreting the Results
Complete blood count (CBC)	Anemia is common, may be related to HIV, infection, or medication (particularly AZT). Explore to find cause: Bone marrow biopsy may be done; check for fungi, *M avium* or tuberculosis, CMV, parvovirus, and malignancy. If anemia is related to medication, may need to prescribe erythropoietin (ProCrit).
Platelets	Thrombocytopenia is often seen: In early infection idiopathic thrombocytopenia purpura may be seen; in later infection the thrombocytopenia may be because of marrow suppression. Thrombocytopenia may also be seen with Kaposi's sarcoma.
Differential white blood cell (WBC) count	Leukopenia is common; WBC counts less than 2,000 cells/mcL are common and by themselves are not a cause for alarm. If using medications that cause neutropenia, may need to prescribe colony-stimulating factors such as filgrastim (Neupogen).
Clinical chemistry	Renal function may be impaired because of HIV nephropathy, volume depletion from diarrhea, or wasting. Elevated LDH may be nonspecific or related to PCP, lymphoma, hemolysis, or muscle wasting, or may be caused by HIV or AZT. Elevated triglycerides may be a response to cytokine activation. Low albumin levels may indicate malnutrition. Elevated pancreatic enzymes may indicate pancreatitis due to certain NRTIs (didanosine, stavudine)
Interferon-gamma release assay or purified protein derivative (PPD), tuberculin skin test (TST)	Positive interferon-gamma assay result or PPD induration of 5 mm or more is considered a positive reaction (no reaction may be caused by anergy); evaluate for signs/symptoms of active TB with physical examination and chest x-ray.
CD4+ T-cell count	>500 cells/mcL: at low risk for opportunistic infections. 500–200 cells/mcL: low to moderate risk for opportunistic infections <200 cells/mcL: high risk for opportunistic infections; prophylaxis for PCP, MAC may be needed while awaiting increase in T-cell count in response to effective antiretroviral therapy To calculate absolute CD4+ count: number of WBC × % lymphs × % CD4+ = absolute CD4+ T cell count
HIV viral load	A decrease in the HIV viral load indicates effective response to antiretroviral therapy; an increase in the viral load indicates disease progression.

or itraconazole 200 mg PO daily for 14 days. Antifungal prophylaxis is not typically initiated until after an AIDS patient is treated for his or her first fungal infection and recurrent episodes become apparent.

Chronic Diarrhea

Infectious diarrhea may require specific antibiotic therapy. Often, however, chronic diarrhea will improve after starting suppressive HAART, as CD4+ T-cell count increases. For symptomatic relief of diarrhea, the patient may try loperamide (Imodium) 4 mg PO to start, then 2 mg every 6 hours or after each bowel movement, up to 16 mg/day. Other options are diphenoxylate-atropine (Lomotil) 2.5 to 5 mg three times daily; paregoric 5 to 10 mL four times daily; or tincture of opium 0.3 to 1.0 mL four times daily and as needed, up to 6 mL/day. Alternative/complementary therapies, including acupuncture and moxibustion, have been reported to decrease diarrhea and associated abdominal discomfort.

Cryptococcosis

For acute treatment of *Cryptococcus neoformans* infection, use amphotericin B deoxycholate (Fungizone) 0.7 to 1.0 mg/kg IV daily for 14 days, with or without 5-flucytosine 100 mg/kg PO divided four times daily, then fluconazole (Diflucan) 400 mg daily or itraconazole 200 mg PO two times daily for 8 weeks. In milder cases, fluconazole 400 to 800 mg daily for 8 to 12 weeks may be used, although inadequate treatment may lead to antifungal resistance. CNS infection (cryptococcal meningitis) should be treated with an initial period of IV induction therapy. Serum cryptococcal antigen (CRAG) titers should be followed, as well as cerebrospinal fluid (CSF) titers if applicable, to evaluate response to therapy. Secondary antifungal prophylaxis with fluconazole 200 mg PO daily is typically continued for life or until the CD4+ T-cell count is greater than or equal to 200 cells/mcL for at least 6 months.

Cryptosporidiosis

There is no definitive cure for *Cryptosporidium* infection. Patients typically improve with supportive care (rehydration) and resolve the infection after starting HAART. In severe cases, nitazoxanide 500 to 1,000 mg PO two times daily given with food for 14 days may help to clear the infection.

Cytomegalovirus

Several options are available for the acute treatment of CMV infection, which may affect diverse organ systems, causing enterocolitis, pneumonitis, or sight-threatening retinitis. Ganciclovir (Cytovene) may be given at 5 mg/kg IV every 12 hours for 14 days (discontinue zidovudine during this induction phase) or foscarnet (Foscavir) 90 mg/kg IV every 12 hours for 14 days. The dose of either drug should be reduced in patients with renal failure. In addition, cidofovir (Vistide) 5 mg/kg IV may be given with probenecid (Benemid) for 1 week, then reduced to every 2 weeks. Cidofovir should not be used in patients with renal insufficiency. Also, a combination of foscarnet/ganciclovir, or intravitreal injections or implants of ganciclovir (which treat only the affected area), may be tried. For maintenance, ganciclovir 5 mg/kg IV daily or foscarnet 90 to 120 mg/kg IV daily may be given. Oral ganciclovir 1 g PO three times daily is not as effective but should be considered for systemic CMV coverage for patients with ocular implants.

Herpes Simplex

For treatment of acute herpes simplex virus manifestations, the clinician should prescribe acyclovir 200 to 400 mg PO three times daily for 7 to 10 days, famciclovir 250 mg PO three times daily, or valacyclovir (Valtrex) 1 g PO two times daily for 7 to 10 days. For suppressive treatment, acyclovir 400 mg PO two times daily for 3 to 7 days per week should be given. Foscarnet 40 mg/kg IV every 8 hours for 10 days can be used for acyclovir-resistant herpes.

Herpes Zoster

Herpes zoster (varicella zoster virus, shingles) should be treated with acyclovir (Zovirax) 800 mg PO five times daily for 7 to 10 days or famciclovir (Famvir) 500 mg PO three times daily for 7 days plus topical silver sulfadiazine for skin lesions. In severe cases, the patient may require IV acyclovir (10 mg/kg per dose) every 8 hours. Valacyclovir (Valtrex), a prodrug of acyclovir, may also be used at 1 g PO every 8 hours for 7 days; although more expensive than acyclovir, its simplified dosing regimen may result in greater adherence.

Histoplasmosis

Primary prophylaxis with itraconazole 200 mg PO daily is indicated for patients with CD4+ T-cell counts less than 150 cells/mcL who live in endemic areas. Disseminated *Histoplasma capsulatum* infection is treated with a 2-week induction period of liposomal amphotericin B 3 mg/kg IV daily (5 mg/kg for meningitis), followed by itraconazole 200 mg PO three times daily for 3 days and then two times daily for at least 1 year. Secondary prophylaxis with itraconazole 200 mg PO daily, initiated after resolution of initial histoplasmosis infection, is often continued for life.

Kaposi's Sarcoma (Human Herpesvirus–8)

Although Kaposi's sarcoma has been associated with underlying HHV-8 infection, herpes-specific antiviral therapies are not utilized in current treatment regimens. Rather, cutaneous Kaposi's sarcoma typically improves on HAART, as HIV viral load is suppressed and immune status improves. However, disseminated disease may require more aggressive treatment, particularly if any internal organs are affected. Local treatment consists of cryotherapy, excision, intralesional vinblastine, or radiation. Systemic chemotherapy for more severe disease may include vinblastine, vincristine, doxorubicin, liposomal doxorubicin, liposomal daunorubicin, bleomycin, or paclitaxel. For more severe cases requiring chemotherapy, treatment is typically guided by a qualified oncology specialist.

Mycobacterium avium Complex

At CD4+ T-cell counts less than 50 cells/mcL, three drugs may be used for MAC prophylaxis: azithromycin (Zithromax) two 600-mg tablets together (1,200 mg) once a week; rifabutin (Mycobutin) 300 mg/day; or clarithromycin (Biaxin) 500 mg two times daily. However, prophylactic regimens readily induce multidrug resistance in MAC strains. Thus, MAC prophylaxis should never be initiated until active MAC infection has been thoroughly ruled out in any patient who presents with suggestive constitutional symptoms, such as fever, malaise, fatigue, or chills. MAC prophylaxis may be stopped if CD4+ T-cell counts increase above 100 cells/mcL for more than 3 months.

For acute treatment, use clarithromycin 500 mg PO two times daily or azithromycin 500 to 600 mg PO daily plus ethambutol 15 mg/kg PO per day, with or without rifabutin 300 mg PO daily. If the patient fails to respond, the provider should consider adding amikacin (Amikin) 10 mg/kg per day IV/IM for 1 to 2 months, or try ciprofloxacin or ofloxacin.

Mycobacterium tuberculosis

Several ARV drugs are contraindicated or require dosage adjustments when coadministered with TB medications capable of affecting the cytochrome p450 enzymatic pathway, such as rifampin and rifapentine. Thus, it is critical to review current guidelines for each HIV drug the patient is prescribed using a frequently updated resource such as AIDSinfo (www.aidsinfo.nih.gov), the official Web site sponsored by the National Institutes of Health, which posts national treatment and prevention guidelines for HIV infection. To reduce the risk of secondary reactivation TB, patients with latent TB infection (LTBI) diagnosed as a positive tuberculin skin test (PPD) greater than or equal to 5 mm or a positive interferon-gamma release assay in the absence of active pulmonary disease (i.e., negative radiological imaging, absence of clinical signs and symptoms) should take isonicotinoylhydrazine (INH) (Isoniazid, Laniazid) 300 mg daily with pyridoxine 500 mg PO daily for 9 months. LTBI treatment with rifapentine is contraindicated for patients on PIs and most NNRTIs.

For active TB infection, patients should be started on INH 300 mg daily plus rifampin 600 mg plus pyrazinamide 15 to 30 mg/kg daily plus either ethambutol (Myambutol) 15 mg/kg daily or streptomycin 15 mg/kg IM daily (maximum 1 g), although ARV regimens should be modified to avoid potentially dangerous drug interactions between certain agents, such as rifampin and PIs/NNRTIs. In turn, rifabutin may be used as an alternate to rifampin, given its improved drug interaction profile. Patients on pyrazinamide should undergo regular serum uric acid monitoring, whereas ethambutol use requires periodic visual acuity and red-green color perception testing, given risks of ocular toxicity. Pyrazinamide and ethambutol may be discontinued after 2 months in order to minimize toxicity, depending on TB susceptibility testing. Thus it is critical to send sputum acid-fast bacilli (AFB) cultures as soon as possible. Combination treatment for active TB infection should be continued for at least 6 months after conversion to negative sputum cultures.

Oral Hairy Leukoplakia (Epstein-Barr Virus Infection)

These common oral lesions found mainly on the tongue typically improve after the initiation of effective HAART.

Pneumocystis jiroveci Pneumonia

There are several options for prophylaxis of PCP at CD4+ T-cell counts less than 200 cells/mcL. The first is trimethoprim-sulfamethoxazole (TMP/SMX, Bactrim, Septra) one double-strength (DS) tablet daily or three times per week. Prophylaxis may be better tolerated when begun with small doses leading to incremental increases, such as TMP/SMX suspension 1 mL PO daily for 3 days, then 2 mL PO daily for 3 days, then 5 mL PO daily for 3 days, then 10 mL PO daily for 3 days, then 20 mL PO daily for 3 days, and then 1 DS TMP/SMX tablet daily. Between 10% and 40% of all patients on this oral course will develop an allergic reaction with fever and a pruritic morbilliform rash and will have to stop treatment. However, this reaction is typically not IgE mediated nor is it considered an immediate hypersensitivity reaction. It may be mediated by an allergic reaction to the sulfa moiety, particularly in individuals of the slow acetylation phenotype who metabolize sulfonamides at slower rates. Given the effectiveness of TMP/SMX for PCP prophylaxis, rechallenge with TMP/SMX may be attempted at a later date. Dapsone (Avlosulfont) 100 mg PO daily, inhaled nebulized pentamidine (NebuPent) 300 mg every

month, or atovaquone 1,500 mg PO daily can also be used for prophylaxis, although these regimens are not as effective as TMP/SMX prophylaxis. PCP prophylaxis may be stopped if CD4+ T-cell counts increase above 200 cells/mcL for more than 3 months.

For the treatment of mild to moderate PCP, the clinician may prescribe TMP/SMX 15 mg TMP/kg total daily dose, divided three times daily PO or IV. A typical adult dose is 2 tablets of DS TMP/SMX PO every 8 hours. Other treatments include pentamidine 4 mg/kg daily IV; dapsone 100 mg daily (check G-6-PD level before dosing, given the risk of anemia) plus TMP 15 mg/kg daily divided three times daily; clindamycin 600 mg PO or IV three times daily plus primaquine 30 mg daily; atovaquone (Mepron) 750 mg PO two times daily with meals plus pyrimethamine (Fansidar) 50 to 75 mg PO daily; or trimetrexate (Neutrexin) plus dapsone plus leucovorin (folinic acid; Wellcovorin), with continuation of therapy for 3 weeks before switching to maintenance therapy. Patients with acute PCP who develop respiratory distress will require hospitalization. If patients develop hypoxia as documented on a room air arterial blood gas with a PaO_2 of less than 70 mm Hg or an arterial-alveolar O_2 gradient greater than 35 mm Hg, patients should also be started on corticosteroids (prednisone 40 mg PO 2 times daily for 5 days, then 40 mg PO daily for 5 days, then 20 mg PO daily for 11 days; all doses given 30 minutes before TMP/SMX dosing) to reduce pulmonary inflammation associated with PCP.

Progressive Multifocal Leukoencephalopathy

There is no treatment for this progressively deteriorating disease caused by JC virus infection of the CNS. Some patients improve on ARV therapy for the underlying HIV infection, which adequately suppresses HIV viral load. In advanced or progressively deteriorating cases, however, the clinician and referring physician should consider discussing hospice care with the patient, family, or significant others, because the prognosis is nearly uniformly fatal.

Toxoplasmosis

For prophylaxis against *Toxoplasma gondii* at CD4+ T-cell counts less than 100 cells/mcL, use DS TMP/SMX 1 tablet PO daily or three times per week or dapsone 50 mg PO daily plus pyrimethamine 50 mg PO every week with folinic acid (Wellcovorin) 25 mg PO per week. Prophylaxis may be stopped if CD4+ T-cell counts increase above 200 cells/mcL for more than 3 months.

For acute treatment, use pyrimethamine 75 to 100 mg PO daily plus folinic acid 10 to 20 mg PO daily plus either sulfadiazine 1 to 1.5 g PO four times daily or clindamycin 600 to 900 mg PO four times daily for 6 to 8 weeks. For maintenance suppressive therapy, use pyrimethamine 25 to 50 mg PO daily plus either sulfadiazine 1 g PO two times daily or clindamycin 300 to 450 mg PO four times daily.

Follow-up and Referral

Clinical status, medication adherence, and the availability of social supports all determine how often the patient will need follow-up appointments. Follow-up visits tend to be more frequent on initiation of HAART or any new medications in order to assess for response to therapy, as well as drug tolerance. A CD4+ T-cell count should be obtained every 3 to 6 months. HIV viral load should be determined when initiating or switching ARV regimens, and a follow-up viral load must be done in 2 to 8 weeks to determine effectiveness of the medication regimen; viral load should fall by at least a factor of 10 after 2 weeks of HAART. Resistance testing should be considered if a therapeutic response is not noted with HAART or HIV viral rebound occurs despite adequate medication adherence. In stable patients, HIV viral load may be checked every 3 to 4 months. The goal of HAART should be complete viral suppression to below the limit of detection on standardized commercial HIV viral load assays.

Specialty referrals are unique to each patient and are guided by HIV-related complications, such as opportunistic infections and malignancies, which develop in the immunosuppressed individual. For example, in addition to periodic visits to an infectious disease or HIV specialist, a referral should be made to an ophthalmologist whenever the patient complains of visual problems, whereas unresolved diarrhea or GI problems may require referral to a gastroenterologist. Similarly, an oncology referral may be necessary for patients with Kaposi's sarcoma or if there is a suspicion of malignancy.

Patient Education

Patient education is an ongoing process and does not end with counseling after the initial diagnosis. Patient-centered education should include an ongoing review of health maintenance and HIV prevention behaviors, because sexual abstinence should not be assumed for any patient, regardless of HIV status. Patient education is particularly important regarding the early detection of visual problems. Other healthful behaviors, such as smoking cessation and limiting alcohol intake, should be discussed within the larger context of HIV infection, given the increased morbidity and mortality risk imparted by these behaviors. The clinician should also work with the client to convey the risks of drug interactions, given the complicated nature of HAART metabolism and both prophylactic and treatment regimens for opportunistic infections. Because blood levels of ARV medications may be increased or decreased by several other common medications, the client must understand the need to discuss any other medications being taken simultaneously. In addition, a thorough understanding of self-care practices to avoid opportunistic infections is critical. Table 17.8 presents household infection precaution guidelines.

Because AIDS has taken on a "female face," as an increasing number of women have become affected, the

Table 17.8	Household Infection Precaution Guidelines
Food and Cooking	• Sharing dishes and silverware is fine; wash them with hot soapy water between uses. • Do not eat or drink raw or unpasteurized milk products (because of risk of *Salmonella* infection [food poisoning]). • Do not eat raw or undercooked meat (because of risk of toxoplasmosis or other infections); cook all meat to a temperature of at least 140°F. • Use a separate cutting board for raw meat and fish; all cutting boards should be plastic and have no nicks or scratches. • Cook or peel organic fruits and vegetables; many organic foods are composted with substances such as manure that can contain infectious organisms. Avoid organic lettuce. • When cooking for other people, do not lick your fingers or taste food from the cooking spoon. Use a separate spoon to taste and use it only once.
Kitchen Cleaning	• Common mold and fungi found in the kitchen can be very dangerous to people with an impaired immune system. Use a cleansing agent to clean the kitchen counter; rinse area thoroughly. • Keep separate sponges for kitchen and bathroom. Always use clean sponges for washing counters and dishes; disinfect sponges by soaking them in a bleach solution (9 parts water to 1 part bleach) for 5 minutes. • To prevent mold from growing, frequently clean the inside of your refrigerator; use baking soda and water. • Mop the kitchen floor at least once a week and immediately clean up after spills. Pour mop water down the toilet, not the kitchen sink. • Keep the house well ventilated to prevent the spread of airborne infections. • Keep garbage in covered trash cans lined with plastic bags.

(Continued)

Table 17.8   Household Infection Precaution Guidelines—cont'd

Bathroom Cleaning	• Use a bleach solution (9 parts water to 1 part bleach) to clean the shower, bathtub, and sink; mop the bathroom floor at least once a week and immediately clean up after any spills. • If any body fluids are spilled (blood, urine, feces, vomit, semen) clean them up first; then use a bleach solution (9 parts water to 1 part bleach). Do not use the bleach solution directly on body fluids (it may cause a terrible-smelling gas). • Use full-strength bleach to disinfect the toilet. • Do not share washcloths or towels without washing them in between uses. • Never share toothbrushes, razors, or other personal equipment.
Pets	• If someone who does not have HIV cannot clean up after the pet, then wear gloves and wash hands thoroughly in hot soapy water afterward. • Change a cat's litter box every day. • Avoid handling turtles or cleaning their cages because of the risk of *Salmonella*.
Gardening	• Always wear gloves and wash hands thoroughly afterward.

need for women to use effective contraception and infection prevention methods has taken on a new urgency in recent years. In addition, affected women should be encouraged to get a Pap smear every 6 months because there is a higher prevalence of vaginal and cervical abnormalities among HIV-infected women. If abnormalities are present, they tend to be more severe and progress more rapidly in HIV-infected women.

All patients should be encouraged to complete advance directives early in the course of the HIV infection. If the clinician broaches this topic at a later stage of the disease (i.e., after a patient has developed AIDS), the patient may mistakenly assume that the clinician has additional information regarding his or her prognosis of which the patient is unaware. Thus, lines of communication need to be kept open between the clinician, the patient, significant others, and family members, depending of the extent of diagnosis disclosure by the client.

Complementary Therapies 17.1 lists complementary therapies that may be useful for some conditions discussed in this chapter.

Complementary Therapies 17.1*

Condition	Agent	Adverse Reactions and Considerations
Allergy	Methyl-sulfonyl-methane (MSM)	May cause bloating, diarrhea, difficulty concentrating, fatigue, GI discomfort, insomnia.
	Vitamin E	May cause abdominal pain, diarrhea, blurred vision, fatigue, headache. When given with anticoagulants/antiplatelets, may increase risk of bleeding. May interfere with chemotherapy effectiveness. When given in high doses, monitor coagulation panel.
Anemia	Vitamin A	May cause nausea, vomiting, anorexia, weight loss, weakness, alopecia, amenorrhea, arthralgia, blurred vision, bone pain, epistaxis, headache, rash. May increase risk of bleeding when given in high doses in conjunction with anticoagulants. Monitor vitamin A levels.
	Folic acid	May cause paresthesia, somnolence, diarrhea, polycythemia vera. May mask pernicious anemia. Antagonizes levodopa, phenytoin.
Pernicious anemia, sickle cell disease *Fatigue*	Vitamin B_{12}	Do not give with aminosalicylic acid, chloramphenicol, or colchicine. Monitor vitamin B_{12} levels.
Rheumatoid arthritis	Pantothenic acid	May cause diarrhea, dyspepsia, nausea. May increase risk of bleeding when given with antiplatelet agents/anticoagulants. Additive effect when given with cholinesterase inhibitors.

Complementary Therapies 17.1*—cont'd

Condition	Agent	Adverse Reactions and Considerations
	Selenium	May cause nausea, vomiting, hepatorenal dysfunction, irritability, garlic/metallic odor/taste, tremor, weakness. Prolongs sedation when given with barbiturates. Increases effectiveness of erythropoietin. Decreases efficacy of niacin and HMG-CoA reductase inhibitors.
	Feverfew	May cause nausea, bloating, constipation, diarrhea, dyspepsia, flatulence, headache, arthralgia, insomnia, muscle stiffness, photosensitivity. May increase risk of bleeding when given with antiplatelet agents/anticoagulants. Stop 2 weeks before surgery.
	Vitamin D	May cause nausea, vomiting, anorexia, constipation, dehydration, weakness, headache. Vitamin D may increase calcium levels, use with caution in patients with hypercalcemia, hyperparathyroidism, lymphoma, renal disease, sarcoidosis, or tuberculosis.
Fibromyalgia	Vitamin E	See above.
	Sam-e (*S*-adenosylmethionine)	May cause nausea, vomiting, diarrhea, anxiety, decreased blood glucose, dizziness, flushing, headache, insomnia, palpitations, skin rash. When given with SSRIs, may increase serotonergic effects; may increase risk of hypoglycemia when given with antidiabetic agents. Monitor blood glucose, LFTs.
	Magnesium (Mg)	May cause areflexia, asthenia, cardiac arrhythmias, drowsiness, hypotension, loss of tendon reflexes. Increases absorption of antidiabetic agents; additive effects when given with antihypertensive agents. Monitor blood pressure, blood glucose, LFTs.
Chronic fatigue syndrome	Coenzyme Q_{10}	May cause nausea, vomiting, diarrhea, dizziness, flu-like symptoms, hypotension, irritability, rash, thyroid hormone alterations. Additive effects when given with antihypertensives and antihyperlipidemic agents. Decreases effects of corticosteroids. Monitor LFTs, lipid profile, blood glucose, blood pressure.
HIV/AIDS	Vitamin A	See above.
	Vitamin B_{12}	See above.
	Vitamin C	May cause abdominal cramps, diarrhea, nausea, rash.
	Coenzyme Q_{10}	See above.
	Beta-glucan	May cause nausea, vomiting, flushing, dizziness, headache, keratoderma, urticaria. When given with antidiabetic agents, may increase risk of hypoglycemia. Additive effects when given with antihypertensive agents and antihyperlipidemic agents. Monitor blood glucose, BP, lipid profile, WBC count.
General Immune System Boosters	Vitamin A	See above.
	Vitamin B_6	Prolonged excessive use may cause neuropathy. May decrease levels of phenobarbital and phenytoin.
	Vitamin C	See above.
	Vitamin D	See above.
	Vitamin E	See above.

*Many patients use these agents and are convinced of their effectiveness. However, there is no Level I Evidence (high-quality randomized controlled trials) to support the use of these supplements.

This table may not be all-inclusive.

Source: Ulbricht, C. *Davis's pocket guide to herbs and supplements.* FA Davis, Philadelphia, 2011.

References

Evidence-Based Practice

Branson, BM, et al. Revised recommendations for HIV testing of adults, adolescents, and pregnant women in health-care settings. National Guidelines Clearinghouse. 2006. Retrieved from www.guidelines.go/summary/summary.aspx?doc_id=9799&nbr=005246&string=

Emery, S, et al. Major clinical outcomes in antiretroviral therapy (ART)–naive participants and in those not receiving ART at baseline in the SMART study. *J Infect Dis* 197(8):1133–1144, 2008.

Gulick, RM, et al. Three- vs four-drug antiretroviral regimens for the initial treatment of HIV-1 infection: A randomized controlled trial. *JAMA* 296(7):769–781, 2006.

HIV Trialists' Collaborative Group. Zidovudine, didanosine, and zalcitabine in the treatment of HIV infection: Meta-analyses of the randomised evidence. *Lancet* 353(9169):2014–2025, 1999.

Maini, R, et al. Infliximab (chimeric anti-tumour necrosis factor monoclonal antibody) versus placebo in rheumatoid arthritis patients receiving concomitant methotrexate: A randomised phase III trial. ATTRACT Study Group. *Lancet* 354:1932–1939, 1999.

Mallal, S, et al. HLA-B*5701 screening for hypersensitivity to abacavir. *N Engl J Med* 358(6):568–579, 2008.

O'Dell, JR, et al. Treatment of rheumatoid arthritis with methotrexate and hydroxychloroquine, methotrexate and sulfasalazine, or a combination of the three medications: Results of a two-year, randomized, double-blind, placebo-controlled trial. *Arthritis Rheum* 46:1164–1170, 2002.

Panel on Antiretroviral Guidelines for Adults and Adolescents. Guidelines for the use of antiretroviral agents in HIV-1 infected adults and adolescents. Department of Health and Human Services (DHHS). Last updated and reviewed February 12, 2013. Retrieved from http://aidsinfo.nih.gov/ContentFiles/AdultandAdolescentGL.pdf

Panel on Opportunistic Infections in HIV-Infected Adults and Adolescents. Guidelines for prevention and treatment of opportunistic infections in HIV-infected adults and adolescents; recommendations from the Centers for Disease Control and Prevention, the National Institutes of Health, and the HIV Medicine Association of the Infectious Diseases Society of America. Retrieved from http://aidsinfo.nih.gov/contentfiles/lvguidelines/adult_oi.pdf

Singh, JA, et al. 2012 update of the 2008 American College of Rheumatology recommendations for the use of disease-modifying antirheumatic drugs and biologic agents in the treatment of rheumatoid arthritis. *Arthritis Care Res* 64(5):625–639, 2012.

Zolopa, A, et al. Early antiretroviral therapy reduces AIDS progression/death in individuals with acute opportunistic infections: A multicenter randomized strategy trial. *PLOS One* 4(5):e5575, 2009.

Bibliography

General

Longo, DL, et al. *Harrison's principles of internal medicine*, ed 18. McGraw-Hill, New York, 2012.

Papadakis, MA, et al. *Current consult medicine*. Lange Medical Books/McGraw-Hill, New York, 2007.

Anemias

Flamm, MJ. New strategies for diagnosing iron overload. *Clin Advis* 10(11):59–64, 2007.

Gunder, LM. What you can learn from RBC analysis. *Clin Advis* 11(12):19–23, 2008.

Platt, A, and Eckman, JR. Diagnosing anemia. *Clin Rev* 16(12):43–50, 2006.

Sen, S. Anemia in a patient previously treated for renal insufficiency. *Clin Advis* 11(8):72–74, 2008.

Fibromyalgia/Chronic Fatigue Syndrome

Donalek, JG. When a parent is chronically ill. *Nurs Res* 58(5):332–339, 2009.

Gupta, NE, et al. Respect for chronic fatigue long overdue. *Clin Advis* 11(2):50–58, 2008.

Jain, R, and Jain, S. Fibromyalgia: Management strategies for the primary care practitioner. *Adv Primary Care Med Clin Update* 15–18, 2008.

Marter, A, and Agruss, JC. Solving the riddle of fibromyalgia: An evidence-based practice protocol for the advanced practice nurse. *J Nurse Pract* 4(6):424–437, 2008.

Mease, P, and Seymour, K. Fibromyalgia syndrome: Guidelines for effective care. *Consultant* 48(7):525–532, 2008.

Mease, P, et al. A closer look at diagnosing and treating fibromyalgia. A Pfizer CME/CE monograph sponsored by the North American Center for Continuing Medical Education, November 2008.

HIV/AIDS

Armington, KJ. How to recognize and prevent HIV infections. *Clin Advis* 10(12):36–42, 2007.

Branson, BM, et al. Revised recommendations for HIV testing of adults, adolescents, and pregnant women in health-care settings. *CDC MMWR* 55:RR-14, 2006.

Campbell, W, et al. Complementary therapies for HIV. *Adv Nurse Pract* 16(8):41–43, 2008.

Epstein, R, et al. Four types of Kaposi sarcoma. *Consultant* 48(11):848–850, 2008.

Guberski, TD. Nurse practitioners, HIV/AIDS, and nursing in resource-limited settings. *J Nurse Pract* 3(10):695–702, 2007.

Kalayjian, RC, et al. Suppression of HIV-1 replication by antiretroviral therapy improves renal function in persons with low CD4 cell counts and chronic kidney disease. *AIDS* 22(4):481–487, 2008.

Kuhar, DT, et al. Updated U.S. Public Health Service guidelines for the management of occupational exposures to human immunodeficiency virus and recommendations for postexposure prophylaxis. *Infect Control Hosp Epidemiol* 34(9):875–892, 2013.

Smith, DK, et al. Antiretroviral postexposure prophylaxis after sexual, injection-drug use, or other nonoccupational exposure to HIV in the U.S.: Recommendations from the U.S. Department of Health and Human Services. *MMWR Recomm Rep* 54(RR-2):1–26, 2005.

Swan, AM. Acute HIV infection in primary care. *Adv Nurse Pract* 17(9):49–54, 2009.

Thompson, IR, et al, and the EuResist Network Study Group. An alternative methodology for the prediction of adherence to anti-HIV treatment. *AIDS Res Ther* 6:9, 2009. doi:10.1186/1742-6405-6-9. Retrieved from www.aidsrestherapy.com/content/6/1/9

U.S. Preventive Services Task Force. Behavioral counseling to prevent sexually transmitted infections. U.S. Preventive Services Task Force recommendation statement. *Ann Intern Med* 7(149):491–496, 2008.

Rheumatoid Arthritis

Blumenauer, B, et al. Etanercept for the treatment of rheumatoid arthritis. In *The Cochrane Library*, Issue 2, 2005. John Wiley & Sons, Chichester, UK.

Furfaro, N. Rituximab for rheumatoid arthritis—Practical guidance for optimizing treatment. *Adv Nurse Pract* 16(1):61–64, 2008.

Maini, R, et al. Infliximab (chimeric anti-tumour necrosis factor monoclonal antibody) versus placebo in rheumatoid arthritis patients receiving concomitant methotrexate: A randomised phase III trial. ATTRACT Study Group. *Lancet* 354:1932–1939, 1999.

O'Dell, JR, et al. Treatment of rheumatoid arthritis with methotrexate and hydroxychloroquine, methotrexate and sulfasalazine, or a combination of the three medications: Results of a two-year, randomized, double-blind, placebo-controlled trial. *Arthritis Rheum* 46:1164–1170, 2002.

Osiri, M, et al. Leflunomide for treating rheumatoid arthritis. In *The Cochrane Library*, Issue 2, 2005. Chichester, UK: John Wiley & Sons.

van de Putte, LB, et al. Efficacy and safety of adalimumab as monotherapy in patients with rheumatoid arthritis for whom previous disease modifying antirheumatic drug treatment has failed. *Ann Rheum Dis* 63:508–516, 2004.

Resources

Fibromyalgia/Chronic Fatigue Syndrome
National Fibromyalgia Association
www.fmaware.org
American Fibromyalgia Syndrome Association, Inc.
www.afsafund.org
Chronic Fatigue and Immune Dysfunction Syndrome Association
    of America (CFIDS)
www.cfids.org
National Fibromyalgia Research Association (NFRA)
www.nfra.net
HIV/AIDS
AIDSinfo: US Department of Health and Human Services
www.AIDSinfo.nih.gov
Office of National AIDS Policy: The White House
www.whitehouse.gov/onap/aids.html
Centers for Disease Control and Prevention (CDC)
National Prevention Information Network
www.cdcnpin.org
AIDS Resource List
www.specialweb.com/aids
The Center for AIDS
www.centerforaids.org
HIV Consumer Council
www.hivcouncil.org
The H.O.P.E. Foundation
www.hopedc.org
National Pediatric AIDS Network
www.npan.org

Allergies and Infectious Diseases
National Institute of Allergy and Infectious Diseases, National Institutes
    of Health
www.niaid.nih.gov
Autoimmune Diseases
American Autoimmune Related Disease Association
www.aarda.org
Arthritis Foundation
www.arthritis.org
Lupus Foundation of America
www.lupus.org
S.L.E. Lupus Foundation
www.lupusny.org
Lupus Research Institute
www.lupusresearchinstitute.org
American College of Rheumatology
www.rheumatology.org
Pain
American Pain Society
www.ampainsoc.org
International Association for the Study of Pain
www.iasp-pain.org
Sickle Cell Anemia
Sickle Cell Disease Association of America
www.sicklecelldisease.org

Psychosocial Problems

Chapter 18

Dianne M. Loomis, DNP, FNP-BC •
Kim S. Griswold, MD, MPH, AS, RN •
Patricia A. Pastore, MS, FNP-BC

OVERVIEW OF PSYCHOSOCIAL PROBLEMS

Psychosocial and mental health problems constitute 22% of primary-care visits. In the last decade there has been a substantial increase in the number of people living with serious mental illness and substance abuse disorders who receive care from primary-care providers and emergency department services. This increase is often related to the long wait times for initial evaluation by mental health providers and the nationwide shortage of such providers, particularly in rural communities. The chronic debilitating nature of serious mental health disorders places a heavy emotional and financial burden on the individual, his or her family, and society. A mental health disorder affects the patient's functional capacity, family relationships, and economic stability and can often lead to the development of comorbid chronic diseases and premature mortality.

The lifetime risk for a mental health disorder for individuals living in the United States is 50%. An estimated 26.2% of Americans aged 18 and older—about one in four adults—suffer from a diagnosable mental disorder in a given year. The main burden of illness is concentrated in a much smaller proportion—about 6%, or 1 in 17—who suffer from a serious mental illness. Serious mental illnesses include schizophrenia, bipolar disorder, severe depression, and other psychoses that lead to persistent functional impairment.

The economic impact of treating these disorders has increased over the last decade during which U.S. spending on mental health services has increased from $25 billion to $60 billion. These disorders comprise one of the five most costly medical conditions, extracting a severe cost burden on the nation and on the families and systems that provide support and care for people with a serious mental illness. Moreover, results from the National Comorbidity Survey funded by the National Institute of Mental Health revealed that major mental disorders cost the nation an additional $193 billion annually in lost earnings alone.

Psychological and physical health influence each other greatly and can be approached effectively in an integrated manner. The signs and symptoms of mental disorders exist on a continuum and affect patients, families, and society, each in a unique way. What determines the burden of illness is the severity of symptoms, their duration, and the level of functional impairment they cause. The *Diagnostic and Statistical Manual of Mental Disorders, Fifth Edition* (DSM-5) emphasizes the relevance and significance of cultural factors and their influence on the expression and management of psychosocial illness. The Cultural Formulation Interview in the DSM-5 provides a mechanism for assessing the impact of culture on an individual's clinical presentation and course.

In this chapter, common complaints and the most prevalent mental health diagnoses are presented, with an emphasis on integrated management and collaboration. For individuals and families who do not have English as their first language, it is crucial that a bicultural, appropriately trained interpreter be provided for all interviews. Furthermore, it is optimal if the interpreter has specialized expertise and additional training in interpreting mental health issues. Management of mental health disorders during and after pregnancy is discussed in a separate section, accompanied by evidence-based recommendations for treatment, follow-up, and appropriate consultation during the prenatal and postnatal periods.

All primary-care clinicians should be familiar with the DSM-5. (See Advanced Assessment 18.1 for an overview of the DSM-5 diagnostic classification system.) For purposes of this textbook, the primary behavioral health diagnoses will be discussed; various clinical subtypes can be referenced directly from the DSM-5.

Advanced practice registered nurses (APRNs) are in an ideal situation to diagnose and manage patients whose psychosocial issues cause great suffering, yet are amenable to treatment. Patients may present to primary care with a constellation of signs and symptoms that have medical and psychological underpinnings. It is important both to consider previously identified psychosocial issues and to evaluate for undiagnosed mental health disorders. Patients benefit from continuity of care and from the nursing emphasis on patient-centered care.

Persons with serious mental illness are now dying 25 years earlier than the general population, which may be partially related to their mental illness or to side

Advanced Assessment 18.1 The Diagnostic and Statistical Manual of Mental Disorders, Fifth Edition *(DSM-5)*

The DSM-5 is a descriptive manual of mental disorders authored by the American Psychiatric Association. The DSM-5 was recently released, and it addresses the scientific and practice advances witnessed since it was last published nearly 15 years ago. It provides the diagnostic criteria for each mental disorder. These descriptions enable clinicians to diagnose, communicate about, and treat people with various mental disorders. It has been demonstrated that the use of such criteria enhances agreement among clinicians.

Precise DSM-5 criteria have been defined for each diagnosis with the addition of and reorganization of some previously identified conditions. This manual is divided into three sections: Section I contains user information, Section II contains the diagnostic criteria, and Section III addresses cultural aspects and conditions that need further research, including emerging measurement tools.

Previously, the diagnostic codes provided in the DSM-IV-TR paralleled the official World Health Organization's International Classification of Diseases ICD-9-CM codes. This consistency in coding does not persist with the changes to the DSM-5 and ICD-10-CM but should be incorporated by the 2015 roll-out of the ICD-11-CM. Providers of mental health will need to become knowledgeable of both sets of codes.

Nonaxial System

The five-part clinical axis of the DSM-IV-TR has been changed to include a three-category, nonaxial system. The first category combines the clinical disorder(s) and/or the personality and/or the developmental disorder with the known medical conditions; category two identifies the applicable environmental and psychosocial stressors; and category three provides a global assessment of functioning. In previous editions, a companion resource for primary care was developed. There are no plans to provide such a companion, because one of the goals of the DSM-5 revision was to reorganize the text to incorporate clinical decision making for the disciplines of psychiatry and primary care, where many individuals seek and receive mental health care. Accurate identification and treatment has the potential to improve morbidity and mortality from mental health disorders.

Using DSM-5 Symptom Criteria

Specific symptom criteria are listed and defined for all DSM-5 disorders and problems. In most cases, these criteria include symptom type, number, intensity, and duration. To meet the symptom criteria for a particular disorder, the patient must have experienced the minimal number of specified symptoms for a defined period of time, and the symptoms experienced should be sufficient to cause distress or impair psychosocial functioning. Persons who have fewer symptoms of less duration or less intensity may have an atypical form of the disorder, or their condition may be described as subclinical. The term *subclinical* does *not* imply that treatment is unnecessary. Atypical symptoms and subclinical symptoms can cause significant distress.

Using DSM-5 Distress Criteria

Symptomatic patients typically report subjective distress. However, a patient's distress may also be observed by others or assessed by the practitioner. There are no absolute measures of symptom-induced distress: Symptoms that are highly distressing to one person may be only mildly distressing to another. The experience of distress should not be confused with the manner in which a person expresses his or her distress. It is possible for a highly distressed person who is suffering a great deal to have trouble expressing his or her distress, whereas others may be able to describe their distress in painful detail. Whether or not a distressed person is expressive should not overly influence the assessment. Often, simple verbal statements of symptom-related discomfort and suffering are sufficient.

---

effects of treatment. However, their increased morbidity and mortality is largely due to treatable medical conditions that are caused by modifiable risk factors such as smoking, obesity, substance abuse, and inadequate access to medical care.

Models of integrated and collaborative care are effective and lead to better outcomes for patients with mental health problems. Primary Care Medical Homes have assumed prominence in our health-care delivery system, and the Medical Home lends itself to the precepts of combined care. The collaborative method is based on Wagner's Chronic Care Model and emphasizes behavioral change, use of information systems such as the electronic health record, and a team approach, utilizing high-level expertise for illness management and strong community linkage.

When comparing chronic care collaborative models (CCCM) versus other care conditions, it has been found that in practices using the CCCM, patients scored higher on scales for quality of life and social role function, as well as for management of specific illnesses. The collaborative model is one with which APRNs are familiar and in which they can use to best advantage a combination of their clinical and relationship skills.

■ ANXIETY DISORDERS

Anxiety affects approximately 40 million adults; thus, it is the most common psychiatric disorder in the United States. It most commonly presents in the 20- to 45-year-old age-group and affects women more frequently than it does men. For most people, anxiety is an unpleasant state of physical and psychological arousal that interferes with effective psychosocial functioning. Mild anxiety is a normal fact of life and can be positive; however, severe or chronic anxiety can become debilitating.

Anxiety symptoms are typically manifested in several dimensions: affective, cognitive, behavioral, and somatic. Affectively, anxiety is an experience of dread, foreboding, or panic, often accompanied by autonomic hyperactivity—primarily sympathetic—manifested as bodily symptoms. The affective component is typically countered by cognitions that seek to make sense of or minimize the discomfort. Some other affective symptoms of anxiety are apprehension, fear, irritability, intolerance, frustration, and overreaction or hypersensitivity to personal feelings of shame. Behaviors such as avoidance, distractibility, and restlessness reflect the anxiety

or may evolve in response to it. Behavioral symptoms of anxiety may include apathy, compulsions, rigidity, overreactions, preoccupation, and repetitive actions such as hair pulling or nail biting. Somatic symptoms of anxiety range in intensity from a loss of appetite, dry mouth, and fatigue, to diarrhea, sweating, chest pain, hyperventilation, vomiting, and paresthesias. Highly anxious persons may experience the full range of anxiety symptoms or may have only one or two symptoms. The classification of *anxiety disorders* is largely based on clinical presentation (Table 18.1).

Differential Diagnosis

The primary-care provider must differentiate between patients with a relatively mild and transient anxiety state, often externally situated, and patients with a pervasive and more debilitating anxiety disorder. A variety of psychiatric disorders, such as mood disorders, certain psychoses, dementias, and substance-abuse disorders present with anxiety as a prominent part of their constellation of symptomatology. This can pose considerable diagnostic and treatment challenges for the primary-care clinician. For example, anywhere from 42% to 100% of depressed patients (average 67%) have anxiety symptoms, and 33% of depressed patients have panic attacks. In addition, 17% to 65% (average 40%) of anxious patients and 33% of patients with panic disorder have depressive symptoms.

Table 18.1 Classification of Anxiety Disorders	
Generalized Anxiety Disorder (GAD)	• Occurs more days than not, for at least 6 months. • Excessive anxiety and worry about a number of things. • Inability to control worry. • Associated with three or more symptoms: Easily fatigued, difficulty concentrating, muscle tension, sleep disturbance, feeling "hyper," feelings of restlessness.
Anxiety Disorder due to a general medical problem	• General anxiety, panic, other manifestations as a direct physiological consequence of a general medical problem.
Substance-Induced Anxiety Disorder	• General anxiety, panic, other manifestations directly related to medication usage, intoxication, or withdrawal.
Anxiety Disorder Not Otherwise Specified	• Prominent and persistent anxiety and/or phobic avoidance that does not meet full criteria of any other anxiety disorder.
Post-Traumatic Stress Disorder (PTSD)	• Exposure to traumatic events that involved actual or threat of severe injury to self and/or others. • Response involves terror, helplessness, intense fear. • Event is consistently reexperienced by upsetting dreams, acting/feeling as if event is reoccurring, physiological reactivity, intrusive image re: event, intrusive thoughts re: event, intense distress on exposure to certain triggers. • Numbing. • Increased arousal from sleep, sleep disturbances, angry outbursts/instability, hypervigilance, exaggerated startle response. • Lasts longer than 1 month.

Source: Adapted from American Psychiatric Association. *Diagnostic and statistical manual of mental disorders, fifth edition* (DSM-5). American Psychiatric Association, Arlington, VA, 2013.

Many medical conditions in which there is stimulation of the sympathetic nervous system mimic anxiety, complicating the diagnosis. For example, undiagnosed arrhythmias and metabolic conditions, as well as drug reactions, may all manifest as anxiety (Table 18.2). In all cases, potential physical explanations for anxiety symptoms should be evaluated first. The extreme variability of anxiety presentations in primary care makes it one of the most commonly seen complaints.

Anxiety disorders are the most prevalent psychiatric conditions in the United States. Data from the National Comorbidity Survey indicate a 24.9% lifetime and an 18.2% 1-year prevalence rate for any anxiety disorder. Although anxiety disorders were once thought to be of minor clinical significance, it is now clear that they are serious illnesses, responsible for substantial morbidity and, possibly, mortality.

The anxiety disorders, like the mood disorders, can also be viewed on a continuum. Anxiety disorders encompass diagnoses of Panic Disorder, Panic Attack Specifier, Agoraphobia, Specific Phobia, and Generalized Anxiety Disorder. Several of these more common anxiety disorders are discussed next.

■ GENERALIZED ANXIETY DISORDER

Generalized anxiety disorder (GAD) is characterized by excessive worry (over 6 months) about multiple concerns that are difficult to control. Persons with GAD experience a range of upsetting physical symptoms, along with hyperarousal and insomnia. A diagnosis of GAD requires evidence of disrupted or impaired occupational or social functioning. GAD is more disruptive than normal anxiety, which is characterized by apprehension and mild physical symptoms of upset such as headache. From 50% to 90% of patients with GAD have another comorbid mental disorder, most commonly depression.

Epidemiology and Causes

Epidemiological studies indicate that in general, the yearly prevalence of anxiety disorders in adults is approximately 15%. Women tend to be diagnosed with anxiety disorders more often than men are. Individuals with a history of trauma—recent, childhood, or adolescent—can be more vulnerable to anxiety disorders, including panic disorder and specific phobias, as well as depression. Exposure to childhood trauma and its effects in health and behavioral outcomes have been well documented in the Adverse Childhood Experience (ACE) Study available at www.acestudy.org. Onset of GAD often occurs during childhood or adolescence. Prevalence in the general population is 5% to 6%, but this proportion rises to approximately 25% in primary-care populations.

People suffering from GAD have about a 60% chance of a comorbid psychiatric diagnosis, most often depression; this is associated with a poorer prognosis. A mixed anxiety and depressive disorder has become common enough that a new disorder—mixed anxiety and depression—has been identified. From 30% to 50% of individuals diagnosed with GAD also have a current depressive disorder.

There is solid evidence that at least some genetic component contributes to the development of anxiety disorders. For example, children of parents with an anxiety disorder have higher rates of anxiety disorders themselves. Data from twin registries support the hypothesis

---

Table 18.2 Physiological Causes of Anxiety

- *Cancers:* Carcinoid syndrome, pancreatic cancer, lung cancer, pheochromocytoma
- *Cardiac:* Mitral valve prolapse, arrhythmia, congestive heart failure, ischemic heart disease
- *Pulmonary:* Asthma, chronic obstructive pulmonary disease, sleep apnea, pulmonary embolism, hypercapnia, hypoxia
- *Neurological:* Ménière's disease, cerebrovascular accident (stroke), transient ischemic attack, multiple sclerosis, encephalopathy, subdural hematoma
- *Hematological:* Anemia
- *Metabolic:* Thyroid disease, hyperparathyroidism, Cushing's syndrome, Addison's disease, hypoglycemia, hyperglycemia, hyponatremia, hypokalemia
- *Nutritional:* Folate deficiency, vitamin B_{12} deficiency, iron deficiency

Medications and Medication Side Effects

Significant anxiety can develop as an adverse effect of prescribed or over-the-counter (OTC) medications. Medications commonly associated with drug-induced anxiety include:

- *Prescription drugs:* Aminophylline, digitalis, dopamine, epinephrine, levodopa, lidocaine, neuroleptics, NSAIDs, steroids, SSRIs, theophylline, sympathomimetics, thyroid preparations
- *OTC drugs:* Certain decongestants containing ephedrine and pseudoephedrine, caffeine, certain cough syrups, salicylates (in large doses), nicotine, monosodium glutamate, phenylpropanolamine
- *Herbal preparations:* Ephedrine, ginseng, yohimbine
- *Illicit drugs:* Amphetamines, marijuana, cocaine, ecstasy, methamphetamine, hallucinogenics
- *Others:* Alcohol, caffeine, organic solvents

that anxiety disorders are at least partially genetically determined. No anxiety disorders, however, are likely to result from a simple Mendelian abnormality. Anxiety disorders commonly coexist with depression and substance-abuse disorders.

Pathophysiology and Psychodynamics

It is well established that the autonomic nervous system of some patients with anxiety disorder, especially those with panic disorder, demonstrate increased sympathetic tone, adapt slowly to repeated stimuli, and respond excessively to moderate stimuli. The three major neurotransmitters associated with anxiety are norepinephrine, serotonin, and gamma-aminobutyric acid (GABA).

Functional brain-imaging studies, including positron emission tomography, single-photon emission computed tomography, and electroencephalography, of patients with anxiety disorders have variously reported abnormalities in the frontal cortex, the occipital and temporal areas, and, in one study of panic disorder, the parahippocampal gyrus.

Clinical Presentation

The primary symptoms of GAD are anxiety, motor tension, autonomic hyperactivity, and cognitive vigilance (see Table 18.1). The anxiety is excessive and interferes with other aspects of the patient's life. Shakiness, restlessness, and headaches are common manifestations of motor tension. Autonomic hyperactivity is commonly manifested by excessive sweating, various gastrointestinal symptoms (increased acidity, nausea, and epigastric pain), palpitations, tachycardia, headaches, and shortness of breath. Irritability and a quick-to-startle response are typical of cognitive vigilance. Often these patients seek help for their somatic symptoms.

The distinction between GAD and normal anxiety is emphasized by the specification that the symptoms of GAD must cause significant impairment or distress.

It is important to screen for anxiety, and a variety of questionnaires are available (see Table 18.4 later in the chapter). These include the Beck Anxiety Inventory, the Hamilton Anxiety Rating Scale, the Anxiety Disorder Interview Schedule, and the Primary Care Evaluation of Mental Disorders (PRIME-MD) (see Advanced Assessment 18.2), which asks about somatic symptoms such as stomach, back, and chest pain; dizziness; and sweating; as well as mood-related symptoms such as depressed feelings and loss of interest in activities.

Numerous epidemiological and survey studies have demonstrated high rates of comorbid psychiatric conditions in children and adults with anxiety disorders. Therefore, aggressive measures to diagnose anxiety disorders and comorbid depression or other mental disorders are essential because, left untreated, they can significantly disrupt an individual's life. Moreover, because of familial correlations, consider screening children of parents with anxiety disorder, as well as parents with children who have been diagnosed with panic or other anxiety disorders (Level II; Beidel and Turner, 1997).

Diagnostic Reasoning

The differential diagnosis of GAD includes all medical disorders that may cause anxiety and typically a medical work-up is necessary, including standard blood chemistry, electrocardiogram, and thyroid function tests specifically. Caffeine intoxication, stimulant abuse, and alcohol, sedative, anxiolytic, and hypnotic withdrawal must all be ruled out. A complete list of all medications, both prescribed and over the counter, must be reviewed, including all herbal agents. An environmental/occupational assessment

---

Advanced Assessment 18.2   Screening and Diagnostic Tool

PRIME-MD

The PRIME-MD is a two-stage instrument that assesses common mood, anxiety, eating, alcohol, and somatoform disorders. It has a self-report *screening/case finding* component, the Patient Questionnaire (PQ) to be administered *before* the clinical encounter. It consists of 25 Yes/No questions about signs and symptoms present during the previous month and one question about the patient's overall health. The questions are divided into five groups corresponding to the five categories of mental disorders assessed by the PRIME-MD.

A current version of the PRIME-MD, the Patient Health Questionnaire (PHQ), increases the efficiency of PRIME-MD by making the entire screening and diagnostic process largely self-report and taking only 3 minutes of the clinician's time. The PHQ is four pages long and contains questions similar to those in PRIME-MD-CEG (Clinical Evaluation Guide). However, the PHQ contains questions specific to women, with questions dealing with menstruation, pregnancy, and childbirth. The completed PHQ provides the clinician with most of the symptom-based information required to make the diagnoses at the beginning of the interview. This then allows more time for an assessment of the patient's life-situation and personal history. This tool was designed for a low-health-literacy population, but the tool may still prove difficult for some patients to fill in by themselves. This is especially so for elderly patients, immigrants, refugees, and persons with low educational attainment. These populations are all at risk for mental disorders. Information from the PHQ can provide baseline data for some disorders and may prove useful in tracking the patient's response and progress over time with repeated administrations.

might also be called for as inhalation of volatile gases—such as gasoline, paint, insecticides, carbon monoxide, and carbon dioxide—may all cause symptoms of anxiety.

The history and mental status exam should explore the diagnostic possibility of panic disorder, phobias, and obsessive-compulsive disorder. Distinguishing GAD from major depressive disorder and dysthymic disorder is difficult because of the frequency of co-occurrence. In patients with comorbid depression and anxiety, the symptomatic profile may be balanced or either symptom can predominate. Patients may meet all the criteria for one disorder and only partially those for the other; they may meet the criteria for both disorders; or they may demonstrate symptoms of both disorders but may not meet the full diagnostic criteria for either.

Any patient who has symptoms of anxiety or depression should be evaluated for current symptoms of both disorders. Both GAD and social anxiety disorder are commonly comorbid with major depressive disorder. Identification and treatment of depression in this group of anxious patients can lead to improved outcomes and quicker recovery. The practitioner needs to perform a thorough suicide and/or homicide risk assessment in all patients who present with significant or alarming psychosocial issues.

Management

Education and Self-Care Management

Planning care for the patient with GAD begins with education. All too often, the person with GAD lacks sufficient general information about GAD and has little understanding about his or her personal GAD symptoms. Patient education includes symptom recognition, effective interpretation of physical symptoms, a decrease in the intake of stimulants such as caffeine and nicotine, and relaxation training. Changes in coping should focus on developing more effective self-awareness and relaxation skills. Patients who develop routine methods of preventing acute anxiety and promoting relaxation are more successful than patients who attempt to cope with their GAD on an as-needed basis.

Areas of patient functioning that have been affected by anxiety should be well defined, and clear goals of improvement should be developed for each area. Some areas of functioning may be less affected by anxiety than others; however, improvement in major areas of functioning, such as being able to function at work or to maintain personal relationships, should be included.

Pharmacological Management

Some benzodiazepines (alprazolam and diazepam) can be helpful in the acute management of GAD, but it is important to remember that if the patient has comorbid depression, use of a benzodiazepine may exacerbate depressive symptoms. Dependence may also occur in those patients with predisposing factors and with long-term

use. Nonetheless, unrelieved GAD symptoms can lead to additional new problems, such as substance abuse and severe social withdrawal.

Antidepressants, typically a selective serotonin reuptake inhibitor (SSRI), can be efficacious for the longer-term treatment of GAD and are particularly helpful if the patient has a coexisting depression. Escitalopram (Lexapro), paroxetine (Paxil), sertraline (Zoloft), and the serotonin-norepinephrine reuptake inhibitor (SNRI) venlafaxine (Effexor) are effective in the acute treatment of GAD as is the partial agonist buspirone (Buspar) (Level I; Baldwin et al, 2005). Treatment up to 24 weeks is associated with greater response rates (Level I; Baldwin et al, 2005). When a sedating medication is needed, moderately sedating tricyclic antidepressants (TCAs; [imipramine]) can be considered. One helpful regimen is to start the patient on both a benzodiazepine and an SSRI and then to taper the benzodiazepine as the SSRI reaches full effect. The goal of medication treatment for GAD should be to reduce or relieve symptoms sufficiently to enable effective self-care and to promote satisfactory levels of functioning. (See Drugs Commonly Prescribed 18.1: Antianxiety Agents.) Additional medications that have proven efficacy are the antipsychotic trifluoperazine (Stelazine), the antihistamine hydroxyzine (Vistaril), and the antiseizure medication pregabalin (Lyrica) (Level I; Baldwin et al, 2005).

Nonpharmacological Management

In acute management of GAD, nonpharmacological management has similar efficacy to pharmacological therapy (Level I; Baldwin et al, 2005). Cognitive-behavioral therapy (CBT; Table 18.3) has proven effective in dealing with GAD, as well as other disorders. Cognitive-behavioral treatment has a lower relapse rate in contrast to other forms of psychological modalities (Level I; Baldwin et al, 2005). It is unknown if combining drug and nonpharmacological treatments results in greater long-term improvements (Level I; Baldwin et al, 2005).

Follow-up and Referral

Monthly follow-up appointments may be needed until the patient with GAD has established alternative resources for support and assistance. A clear follow-up plan decreases the problem of excessive or ineffective appointments. Ongoing assessment includes evaluation of the primary symptoms, as well as assessment of the current risk of suicide/homicide. Complete documentation of the evaluation and plan is essential. Practitioners may wish to make themselves available to anxious patients, and referrals to patient education and support groups may be helpful for some patients with GAD. The plan should include strict criteria for seeking emergency services. The goal is to protect the patient from unknowingly becoming overreactive to his or her GAD symptoms. Improvement can become more obtainable when a realistic understanding of the illness is

Drugs Commonly Prescribed 18.1   Antianxiety Agents

Drug	Indication	Adverse Reactions and Prescribing Considerations
Classification Benzodiazepines: Short Half-life (<12 hours)		
alprazolam	Anxiety, GAD, panic disorder	C-IV controlled substance. All benzodiazepines are associated with potential anterograde amnesia, CNS depression, and paradoxical reactions. Sedation, memory deficits, ataxia, narrow-angle glaucoma. Association with falls and injury in the elderly. Caution with depressed patients and substance abuse, impaired hepatic or renal function. Most contraindicated in obstructive sleep apnea (OSA). Many drug–drug interactions (CYP pathways, CYP3A4-mediated). Withdrawal symptoms with abrupt discontinuation. The onset of withdrawal symptoms is usually seen on the first day without drug and lasts 5–7 days—slow taper. Treatment longer than 4 months should be reevaluated to determine the patient's need for the drug. Avoid valerian, St. John's wort, kava kava, gotu kola. Potential severe allergic reactions (anaphylaxis, angioedema) and complex sleep-related behaviors, which may include sleep-driving, cooking and eating food while asleep, and making phone calls while asleep.
oxazepam	Anxiety and ETOH withdrawal	See above.
temazepam	Insomnia, short-term	See above. Administer 30 minutes before bedtime. Lack of active metabolites; excellent option for the elderly.
triazolam	Insomnia, short-term	In elderly, higher incidence of CNS adverse reactions not a drug of first choice.
Classification Benzodiazepines: Intermediate Half-life (12–24 hours)		
alprazolam XR	GAD, panic disorder, anxiety with depression	Extended-release tablet: Should be taken once daily in the morning; do not crush, break, or chew. Onset 1 hour and duration 12 hours
estazolam	Insomnia short-term	No active metabolites
lorazepam	Amnesia induction Anxiety sedation induction Status epilepticus	
Classification Benzodiazepines: Long Elimination Half-life (>24 hours)		
chlordiazepoxide	Anxiety, ETOH withdrawal	The onset of withdrawal symptoms is usually seen after 5 days, with a duration of 10–14 days.
clonazepam	Absence seizures Lennox-Gastaut syndrome Myoclonic seizures Panic disorder	Less sedating than other anxiolytics; onset of full anxiolytic effect can take 3–6 weeks; less dependence. Risk of suicide ideation when used for seizures. Monitor complete blood count (CBC), liver function tests (LFTs).
clorazepate	Anxiety, ETOH withdrawal, partial seizures (adjunctive)	Increased risk of suicidal ideation when used for seizures. Long-acting metabolites; do not use in elderly. Monitor CBC, LFTs.
diazepam	Amnesia induction, anxiety, drug-induced seizures, ETOH withdrawal, muscle spasms, partial seizures, sedation induction Status epilepticus, tetanus, tonic-clonic seizures	Monitor CBC, LFTs.

Drugs Commonly Prescribed 18.1 Antianxiety Agents—cont'd

Drug	Indication	Adverse Reactions and Prescribing Considerations
flurazepam	Insomnia short-term	Avoid in elderly and debilitated. Active metabolites with extended half-lives may lead to delayed accumulation and adverse effects.
quazepam	Hypnotic	Long-acting; daytime sedation and fatigue, but this may prevent withdrawal symptoms when stopped.
Classification Nonbenzodiazepines		
Azapirones buspirone	Anxiety, GAD	Low risk of cognitive or motor impairment, may cause dopamine-related movement disorders (restlessness). Avoid St. John's wort, valerian, gotu kola, kava kava. May take 2–3 weeks to see full effect, little potential for abuse, needs continuous use, does not potentiate the effects of alcohol.
SSRIs escitalopram		See Drugs Commonly Prescribed 18.2.
SNRIs duloxetine venlafaxine		See Drugs Commonly Prescribed 18.2.

Source: Clinical pharmacology [database online]. Gold Standard, Inc., Tampa, FL, 2013. http://cp.gsm.com

Table 18.3 Cognitive-Behavioral Strategies

Assumptions
• Alterations in content of underlying cognitive processes alter affective states and behavioral problems, i.e., thinking alters feeling and doing.
• Correction of these faulty constructs ("stinking thinking") can lead to clinical improvement.
• A person's appraisal/perception of situations is reflected in his or her cognitions (both thoughts and visuals).
• Through therapy, patients become aware of these faulty constructs and learn to alter them.

Processes
• Identify and alter cognitive distortions that maintain symptoms
• Time-limited, usually 15–25 weeks, once weekly
• Collaborative empiricism
• Structured and directive
• Assigned readings
• Homework and behavioral techniques
• Desensitization in some patients
• Identification of irrational beliefs and automatic thoughts
• Identification of attitudes and assumptions underlying negative thoughts

Source: Adapted from Kaplan & Sadock's *Synopsis of psychiatry,* ed 9. Lippincott Williams & Wilkins, Philadelphia, 2009.

maintained. Referral to a specialist is most useful when the patient needs this level of assistance in order to develop effective self-care skills.

Patient Education

Education about antianxiety medications should be reviewed with the patient and family members, including issues of overuse and dependency on medications, as well as potential adverse effects. The need to avoid combining antianxiety medications with alcohol should be addressed. The clinician should provide written instructions if the patient appears to have limited ability to concentrate. The practitioner should also discuss with the patient and family the causes and treatment of anxiety.

The provider may want to suggest to the patient and family complementary methods of anxiety management, such as relaxation techniques (see Complementary Therapies 18.1), guided imagery, music therapy, physical activity, yoga, and acupuncture. If appropriate, nutritional practices may need to be changed to include a healthier diet.

GAD cannot be managed with medication alone. Consistent and active patient self-care is required. At the same time, the highly symptomatic patient, no matter how motivated, is unlikely to be able to engage in self-care when his or her GAD symptoms are poorly controlled. GAD symptoms can increase the difficulty of learning new information, including learning new

Complementary Therapies 18.1 Relaxation Therapy Techniques

This breathing technique will help you relax, as well as provide increased energy, health, and concentration. Try using this technique for at least 15 minutes each day, on an empty stomach. Do not stand up suddenly after performing these exercises, because they can lower blood pressure, making you dizzy.

Step 1: Sit in a comfortable chair and in a quiet location to minimize distractions.

Step 2: Close your eyes.

Step 3: Begin by taking a slow, deep breath in through your nose and breathe out through your mouth slowly and deeply, like blowing out a candle.

Step 4: Breathe in slowly for a count of 4, hold for a count of 7, and breathe out for a count of 8. Repeat this several times.

Step 5: The following techniques may also help you to relax while doing the breathing exercise:

  a. Visualize a favorite, peaceful setting, such as a beach, forest, desert, or meadow.

  b. Play peaceful music in the background.

  c. Begin at your feet and repeat to yourself that your feet are warm and heavy. Once you have achieved that, move up to your legs, your torso, and then your arms and hands. The sensation of heaviness and warmth should spread throughout your entire body.

  d. Repeat a favorite phase, or mantra, with each breath.

  e. Tighten different muscles while inhaling and relax them while exhaling (start with you feet and move systematically up your body.

self-care skills. Many primary-care settings now have access to comprehensive patient education programs in which the nurse practitioner can play a pivotal role. Giving patients enough time to practice newly adopted self-care skills, such as mindfulness-based stress reduction programs and meditation, may assist patients to cope with ongoing symptoms.

■ PANIC DISORDER

Panic disorder, which typically presents in young adulthood, is a disabling condition. It can impair the social, family, and working lives of the patient suffering from it. Panic disorder symptoms are recurrent, intense, short episodes of panic-level psychological and physical symptoms of anxiety. The initial panic episode must be spontaneous and unexpected, and it cannot occur when the person is the focus of others' attention, such as when speaking in front of an audience. A combination of sudden panic-symptom onset and panic-symptom severity

creates secondary symptoms of fear. These secondary fear symptoms essentially define this disorder. Fear compels the patient with panic disorder to seek emergency health-care services repeatedly. To the patient, panic symptoms are life-threatening and signal a serious health problem or an impending nervous breakdown. Patients endure an unshakable sense of doom and danger that they cannot define.

Patients who have lived with panic disorder for a while come to associate the onset of their symptoms with specific circumstances. They may or may not be accurate in their assessment, but they may nevertheless believe that a given situation or set of circumstances triggers their panic symptoms. When this is the case, the patient may develop methods of avoiding the trigger situations and circumstances. Panic symptoms can be triggered by a wide variety of stimuli such as substance use, a change in daily routine, or exposure to feared situations, such as being in crowds or closed-in spaces. Panic triggers may or may not be easy to avoid. An episode of panic typically lasts about 10 minutes or less; however, the secondary distress that follows a panic episode can last for hours.

The frequency and severity of panic episodes and the triggered emotional and behavioral responses to panic symptoms can vary from patient to patient. Individual patterns also may vary. Panic disorder differs from occasional panic attack, now defined in DSM-5 as Panic Attack Specifier. The main distinction is that a diagnosis of panic disorder is based on a pattern of recurrent, unexpected panic attacks. At least one of these attacks must have been followed by 1 month or more of persistent worry and/or maladaptive changes in behavior. Persons with severe panic disorder become highly fearful of future panic episodes and may become preoccupied with searching for the "true meaning" of their panic symptoms. They are likely to make significant changes in their behavior and routines in the hope of avoiding future panic episodes. Without evidence of panic avoidance, it is difficult to confirm a diagnosis of panic disorder. Persons with panic disorder may become vigilant in their efforts to anticipate and thus avoid future panic episodes. Evidence of this anticipatory anxiety clarifies the diagnosis of panic disorder.

Epidemiology and Causes

The prevalence of panic disorder is generally believed to be 1.5% to 3%, although perhaps 10% of the population has had at least one isolated panic attack. Panic disorder is more common also in persons with medical conditions. For example, in pulmonary clinics (where patients with asthma and other conditions that cause shortness of breath seek treatment) 10% to 20% of patients may be affected by panic disorder. Ten percent to 20% of patients who present to the emergency department with chest pain are in actuality suffering from a panic disorder.

Panic disorders typically appear in late adolescence or young adulthood, with a peak at 25 years of age. There is a second peak between 35 and 44 years. Panic disorder affects women approximately twice as often as men. Empiric research indicates that approximately 70% of patients with panic disorder have at least one major depressive episode during their lifetime. These patients also suffer from social anxiety or social phobia; they may also be generally anxious, chronic worriers, with high rates of post-traumatic stress disorder (PTSD) and obsessive-compulsive disorder (OCD).

Panic disorders appear to have a genetic component. Several studies have suggested that patients with panic disorder are at high risk for suicidal ideation and attempts. Comorbidity with major depression can increase the rate of attempted suicides. Further, panic disorder patients have a propensity to self-medicate with alcohol and drugs. These facts should alert the clinician to the serious nature of this disorder.

Pathophysiology and Psychopathology

Structural brain-imaging studies, such as magnetic resonance imaging, have demonstrated pathological involvement in the temporal lobes, particularly the hippocampus, in patients with panic disorder. Some studies use specific panic-inducing substances (such as caffeine, lactate, or yohimbine) to assess effects of panic on cerebral blood flow. Anxiety disorders and panic attacks are specifically associated with cerebral vasoconstriction. This in turn may cause central nervous system symptoms such as dizziness and peripheral nervous system symptoms such as hyperventilation and hypercapnia.

Genetic predisposition to panic disorders, especially in those with agoraphobia, has been established in a number of studies. First-degree relatives of those with panic disorder have a fourfold to eightfold higher risk for the development of the disorder than first-degree relatives of other psychiatric patients. Twin studies have demonstrated a higher concordance for panic disorder in monozygotic twins than in dizygotic twins. No data indicating association between a specific chromosomal location or mode of transmission and panic disorder exist at this time.

Studies have shown that patients with panic disorder typically experience greater distress about life events than control subjects, and that in the months before the onset of panic, they demonstrate a higher incidence of stressful life events. What was primarily a mild feeling of anxiety suddenly becomes an overwhelming feeling of apprehension and dread, replete with somatic symptoms.

The pathogenesis of the panic attacks may be related to neurophysiological factors triggered by psychological reactions that are likely precipitated by the unconscious meaning assigned to stressful events. When assessing a patient with panic disorder, the practitioner should conduct a complete assessment of possible triggers, including inquiry about current or past abuse, loss of significant others, and other stressful life events.

Clinical Presentation

As with anxiety disorders, consider screening certain at-risk patients for panic disorder (Level II; Beidel and Turner, 1997; Biederman et al, 2001). Patients more at risk include those patients with a family history of panic and/or anxiety disorders and patients who have a comorbid psychiatric disorder, such as major depression, bipolar disorder, or substance-use disorders.

Ask the patient to describe the panic/anxiety episodes in detail, noting frequency, duration, and precipitating events. Panic disorder is marked by recurrent and unpredictable panic attacks. The panic attacks come on unexpectedly, developing suddenly within 10 minutes and usually resolving within the hour. These attacks are distinct episodes of intense fear and discomfort associated with four or more specific physical symptoms. Frequency and severity of attacks vary from once a week to clusters of attacks separated by months of well-being. The first attack often occurs outside of the home.

Spontaneous panic attacks have no obvious stimuli, whereas situational panic attacks are in response to a phobic stimulus. Limited symptom attacks are spells manifesting one or two symptoms such as dizziness, tachycardia, or respiratory distress. Often limited symptom attacks occur early in the course of panic disorder or between panic attacks. Although panic disorder may occur without any obvious causative events, it can occur in early adult life after a loss, threat of a loss, physical illness, or an episode of drug abuse.

After having several panic attacks, as many as 80% of patients begin to fear the next attack. They also experience phobic avoidance of circumstances associated with attacks. This is called anticipatory anxiety, which may become more disabling than the panic attacks themselves. Patients may become agoraphobic, culminating in increasingly circumscribed lives; some patients eventually become completely homebound.

The risk factor with the best predictive power for panic disorder is a positive family history. Other types of mood and anxiety disorders often are comorbid in patients who experience panic disorder. It is important to look not only for panic disorders in the family history but also for other mental disorders.

Perform a comprehensive physical examination to rule out organic causes for the patient's symptoms. If the history suggests that significant organic disease is unlikely, the physical examination should be focused primarily on the organ system of most concern (e.g., the heart in a patient with chest pain). Consider laboratory tests to rule out physical causality.

DSM-5 symptom criteria for panic attack include the following: fear of losing control, dying, or going crazy; chills or hot flushes; paresthesias; palpitations; choking sensations; shortness of breath; and gastrointestinal distress.

Diagnostic Reasoning

Diagnosis is generally clinical in nature. Tools that may provide a fairly accurate assessment in a relatively short time include the Mini-International Neuropsychiatric Interview (M.I.N.I.) and the PRIME-MD. Diagnosis will then structure appropriate treatment and follow-up. Consider the array of medical, cultural, or other psychiatric conditions that may mimic symptoms/signs of panic disorder, especially with the onset of any anxiety disorder (Level II; Simon and Fischmann, 2005). Panic symptoms are common, for example, in patients with schizophrenia, bipolar disorder, and depression. Cultural expression of panic may include headache, tinnitus, and sobbing.

Assess for medical conditions that may accompany, contribute to, or cause panic symptomatology; these conditions include pheochromocytoma, hyperthyroidism, seizure disorder, and cardiac arrhythmias that may originate from an acute myocardial infarction. Consider that the use of or withdrawal from therapeutic or recreational drugs may cause panic attacks. Therapeutic drugs include theophylline and steroids. Recreational drugs include cocaine, amphetamines, and caffeine. Drug withdrawal symptoms are typically associated with drugs such as alcohol, barbiturates, and benzodiazepines. As described previously, the differential diagnosis of panic disorder is complicated by a high rate of comorbidity with other psychiatric conditions, especially abuse of alcohol and benzodiazepines, which patients may initially use in an attempt to self-medicate.

Distinguish panic disorder from other anxiety disorders based on the patient's history as well as patient behavior and symptoms and the contexts in which they occur. To be diagnosed with panic disorder, the patient needs to satisfy the following four criteria:

1. A history of recurrent, unexpected panic attacks.
2. At least one of the attacks has been followed by at least 1 month by (a) a persistent concern about having additional attacks, (b) worry about the implications of an attack, or (c) a significant change in behavior related to the attacks.
3. The panic attacks are not due to effects of a substance (e.g., drug abuse, medication) or a general medical condition (e.g., hyperthyroidism).
4. The panic attacks are not better accounted for by another mental disorder, such as social phobia, OCD, PTSD, or separation anxiety disorder.

Management
Pharmacological Management

The pharmacological treatment of panic disorder is relatively straightforward and effective. The major recent advances in the treatment of panic disorder have been the advent of SSRIs and SNRIs and their recognition as powerful antipanic drugs. Generally, they are recommended as first-line pharmacological therapy in panic disorder (Level I; American Psychiatric Association, n.d.). Patients with panic disorder are often very sensitive to the pharmacological effects of various medications. When initiating pharmacological therapy, the practitioner may consider starting the drug at half of the recommended dose and gradually increasing the dose over several days. This strategy assists patients to slowly become acclimated to the effect of the medication. It is important to monitor and increase the dose until full therapeutic dosage is achieved. If the response to the initial SSRI is inadequate, the clinician may consider changing the drug, switching to another antidepressant, or adding a second medication (Level I; American Psychiatric Association, n.d.). Additional medications shown to be effective include the tricyclic antidepressants (TCAs), benzodiazepines, valproic acid (Depakote), or gabapentin (Neurontin). One should avoid extensive use of the benzodiazepines, except in specific circumstances where the patient is unable to tolerate an SSRI/SNRI or TCA, and they should not be utilized in a depressed patient as monotherapy (Level II American Psychiatric Association, n.d.). When they are used, a long-acting preparation is preferred, on an around-the-clock basis. When shorter-acting benzodiazepines are used "as needed," the risk is increased for greater tolerance and possible abuse or addiction. These particular anxiolytics can also exacerbate the depression that may coexist with panic disorder. After panic attacks have ceased, patients are maintained on medication for a minimum of 6 months. Pharmacological blockade of panic generally leads to a decrease in both anticipatory anxiety and phobic avoidance. A common approach is to use benzodiazepines for immediate relief. Other medications may be added, either concurrently or after symptoms are attenuated. Once these medications become effective, the benzodiazepine treatment may be tapered and discontinued.

Nonpharmacological Management

Cognitive-behavioral therapy (Table 18.3) is the first-line treatment for panic disorder, and useful adjuncts are self-help CBT-based books and self-help programs (Level I; American Psychiatric Association, n.d.). Patients who receive CBT have longer periods of remission and longer-term benefits. CBT is also useful to facilitate the gradual withdrawal from benzodiazepines (Level I; American Psychiatric Association, n.d.), which are often used for immediate symptom relief in panic disorder. CBT is aimed at altering the unproductive and dysfunctional thinking that helps to generate and maintain anxiety. Patients with panic disorder learn to face their fear, so that attacks are avoided. CBT is effective in treating maladaptive behaviors associated with anxiety, mainly by gradual exposure to more adaptive situations. CBT encompasses a range of treatments, each consisting of several elements, including breathing techniques (Level I; American Psychiatric Association, n.d.), education, continuous panic monitoring, development of anxiety management skills, cognitive restructuring, and in vivo exposure. Some sources recommend brief, highly focused behavioral and cognitive psychotherapeutic techniques for panic. Hypnosis and alternative therapies (yoga, meditation) are sometimes useful as part of combined therapies but are not as effective as CBT. Some patients find relief in chiropractic treatment and acupuncture.

Follow-up and Referral

Patients with panic disorder can be managed in primary-care settings once a plan of care has been agreed to. Generally, pharmacological follow-up is scheduled every 1 to 2 weeks when initiating therapy, and then every 2 to 4 weeks until therapeutic dosage is achieved. Appointments can be spaced further apart as the dosage is stabilized and the symptoms reduced (Level I; American Psychiatric Association, n.d.). (See Advanced Practice Nursing Interventions 18.1.) As with any serious psychological condition, referral to specialist consultation or to hospital care should be made as appropriate. This includes *mandatory* inquiry about suicidal history, ideation, or intent. Also the practitioner should consider referring the patient to a psychiatrist if he or she fails to respond after 6 to 8 weeks of standard treatment. Similarly, patients should be referred to an appropriate medical specialist if an occult underlying organic disorder is suspected. The practitioner should assess the patient's response to treatment and symptom intensity and reinforce patient education at every visit, as well as review strategies to manage panic attacks. The ongoing therapeutic alliance with the primary-care clinician is crucial for long-term successful treatment.

Patient Education

For treatment to be effective, the patient and family must understand panic disorder and work together aggressively as active participants in the treatment plan. Moreover, the patient and family must be aware of the potential adverse effects of any drugs prescribed and work toward using relaxation techniques, deep breathing, and cognitive-behavioral strategies to control panic.

■ AGORAPHOBIA

A person can be agoraphobic without having a diagnosis of panic disorder. However, 30% to 50% of individuals with agoraphobia report panic attacks or are diagnosed with panic disorder.

The DSM-5 defines *agoraphobia* as marked fear about two or more of the following:

- Using public transportation
- Being in open spaces
- Being in enclosed spaces
- Standing in line or in a crowd
- Being outside of the home alone

Research of treatment options for agoraphobia without panic disorder has not been done. Currently it is recommended to follow the treatment guidelines for panic disorder with agoraphobia.

■ POST-TRAUMATIC STRESS DISORDER

Post-traumatic stress disorder (PTSD) is a syndrome that develops after a person witnesses, participates in, or hears of an extreme traumatic stressor. The reaction to this experience is typically fear and helplessness, reliving the event over and over, and trying to avoid being reminded of it. The symptoms must be severe enough to last for more than a month after the event and must significantly affect critical areas in the person's life such as interpersonal relationships and occupational roles.

PTSD symptoms are responses to experiences that are overwhelming, for example, war, torture, natural disasters, terrorism, assault, rape, serious accidents, fires, and the like. Typically, persons reexperience the trauma in their dreams and daily thoughts, and they try to evade anything that reminds them of the event. Patients can also undergo a "numbing" of responsiveness along with a physiological state of hyperarousal. This is usually accompanied by depression, anxiety, cognitive difficulties, and often substance abuse. Comorbid disorders make persons more vulnerable to developing PTSD (see Case Study 18.1).

Advanced Practice Nursing Interventions 18.1 Panic Disorder

Management

Goal: Full remission, elimination of panic attacks, anxiety, phobias, and disability; restoration of well-being.

Institute treatment with low-dose selective serotonin reuptake inhibitors (SSRIs); increase dose as tolerated to target dose.

Monitor closely for adverse effects.

Continue treatment for 12–24 months; phase out treatment slowly (over 4–6 months).

Refer to an anxiety disorder specialist if response is not satisfactory or if comorbid conditions are present.

Patient and Family Education

Teach the patient and family about panic disorder.

Advise patient not to abruptly stop medication.

Source: American Psychiatric Association. Practice guideline for the treatment of patients with panic disorder. Updated January 2009. Retrieved from www.guideline.gov/summary/summary.aspx?ss=15&doc_id=14230&nbr=007124&string=panic

CASE STUDY 18.1 Post-Traumatic Stress Disorder

Jennifer, a 45-year-old nurse and married woman with two children, presented to the Veteran's Administration Medical Center (VAMC). . . . She lived in a rural community and served a total of 24 years in the military (13 years active duty in the U.S. Army and 11 years in the U.S. Army Reserves). She was deployed for 7 months during the Gulf War and for 19 months to Kuwait and Iraq. The deployment to Kuwait and Iraq was extended several times and her support system was also affected when various individuals of the medical team were reassigned to different locations. Jennifer denied any previous psychiatric history but reported a random sexual assault at age 20 for which she never received treatment.

During her Operation Iraqi Freedom (OIF) deployment, she was at Abu Ghraib prison for 4 months and experienced mortar attacks, multiple casualties, prolonged working hours, and exposure to horrific injuries and death. She became adept at dissociating herself from these conditions until her fourteenth month of deployment. At that time, she lost interest in activities she normally enjoyed and became isolated from colleagues; her communication with family members also decreased. After redeployment, she began to have panic attacks, and she had intrusive symptoms and nightmare. Sensory experiences such as hearing helicopters, seeing blood, or smelling seared meat would provoke intrusive symptoms. She became increasingly isolated and alienated.

Jennifer's recovery encompassed the three stages of PTSD recovery. Providing a safe environment is a prerequisite to begin the process. During empowerment, the survivor can choose to speak about the experience, to remember, and to mourn. Narrative reconstruction and reconnection allows the survivor to reprocess the traumatic events into a tolerable form. And third, reconnection allows the individual to confront the traumatic past, accept the personal changes, and to reengage with the world and actively recreate a future.

Jennifer sought treatment at a VAMC outpatient psychiatric clinic 3 months after redeployment with the initial diagnoses of major depression and panic attacks. Her initial treatment included an SSRI and trazodone for sleep. On her third appointment, after utilizing a validated tool for PTSD, she was diagnosed with mild-moderate PTSD. As her medications began to improve her symptoms, she began to verbalize the traumatic experiences she had witnessed and could then reframe those experiences. Unfortunately, after four sessions her psychiatrist retired, and Jennifer was referred to group therapy, which she was unable to do. She sought care at a community health provider for the next year and continued the medications. Jennifer continued to heal through family support, retiring from the military, and receiving new career training.

Many veterans receive treatment outside of the VA system, and it is important for APRNs to be aware of the evidence-based pharmacological and nonpharmacological treatments for PTSD.

Source: Adapted from Feczer, D, and Bjorklund, P. Forever changed: Posttraumatic stress disorder in female military veterans, a case report. *Perspect Pscyhiatr C* 45(4):278–291, 2009.

Epidemiology and Causes

The lifetime prevalence of PTSD in the general population is approximately 8% to 9%, and it is twice as common in women. Women are most likely to suffer from PTSD as a result of rape or sexual molestation. Men are more commonly affected by military combat or witnessing other forms of extreme violence. The prevalence of the disorder can therefore be higher among specific groups, such as war veterans, victims of terrorist attacks, or survivors of disasters. Thus the development of PTSD varies with the degree of exposure, the type of traumatic event, and the severity of the precipitating cause. For example, most studies of adult survivors of disaster have found a PTSD prevalence of 30% to 60% after a disaster.

Recent immigrants from areas of social and/or political instability can be highly susceptible to PTSD. However,

for many reasons, immigrant patients may choose not to share their traumatic experiences with a practitioner. This reluctance may have to do with significant feelings of vulnerability that a recent immigrant may feel.

Other risk factors include female gender, age (the very young and the very old are especially susceptible), race, education, socioeconomic status, education, family history, reported abuse in childhood, reports of other adverse childhood factors or trauma, poor social and/or family support, and comorbidities. Comorbidities with PTSD include an increased association with anxiety, substance abuse, and mood disorders. There is at least one psychiatric disorder present in more than 70% of men and women diagnosed with PTSD and an increased incidence of depression and mania in patients with PTSD, compared with the general population. (See Risk Factors 18.1.)

- Physical or sexual childhood abuse
- Sexual or other life-threatening assault/accident
- Combat exposure
- Being involved in fire, flood, hurricane, or other natural disaster
- Witnessing someone being badly injured or killed

The prognosis for patients suffering from PTSD is influenced by multiple factors, including whether the disorder is acute, chronic, or delayed; the presence or absence of previous mental disorders; the patient's premorbid personality; available support resources; compliance with treatment; and the patient's ability and desire to learn new coping mechanisms.

The adaptive person who suffers from acute PTSD after exposure to a traumatic event has a better chance for full recovery, especially if his or her family is supportive. Untreated, about 30% of patients recover completely, 40% continue to have mild symptoms, 20% continue to have moderate symptoms, and 10% remain unchanged or become worse.

Pathophysiology and Psychopathology

A number of biological variables have been implicated in PTSD. There is strong evidence, for example, for altered function in the noradrenergic system. Specifically, soldiers with PTSD-like symptoms may experience nervousness, high blood pressure, increased heart rate, palpitations, sweating, flushing, and tremors—all symptoms associated with adrenergic drugs. Veterans with PTSD demonstrate increased epinephrine concentrations in 24-hour urine samples, and increased urine catecholamines have been found in 24-hour urine samples of sexually abused girls. Some studies have revealed cortisol hypersuppression in trauma-exposed patients who develop PTSD, compared with patients exposed to trauma who do not develop PTSD.

A personal predisposition may be necessary for symptoms to develop after a traumatic event, and individuals apt to develop PTSD may have a preexisting mood or anxiety disorder or a family history of anxiety or other psychiatric disorder. Patients with existing serious mental disorders are at risk for victimization and, at times, assault, and they may be more likely to develop PTSD.

Clinical Presentation

The principal clinical features of PTSD are painful reexperiencing of the event, a pattern of avoidance, and emotional numbing. Typically, a combination of a trauma, the personal characteristics of the person experiencing the trauma, and a variety of post-traumatic factors all must coalesce for the person to develop PTSD. A diagnosis of PTSD will rarely be made unless the patient exhibits at least one symptom from each symptom category.

- Intrusive symptoms: The first category includes reexperiencing the traumatic event or having intrusive symptoms. This experience can manifest itself as a nightmare, a flashback, or simply sudden, vivid memories that are accompanied by painful emotions or images related to the trauma.
- Avoidance symptoms: The patient avoids any situation or activity that might revive memories of the trauma. This symptom can severely impair the patient's relationships with others because close emotional ties with family, friends, and colleagues may be included among the situations that the patient intentionally avoids. Patients suffering from PTSD commonly complain that they cannot feel emotions, especially emotions toward those who are closest to them.
- Hyperarousal symptoms: The third category includes hyperarousal symptoms. As a result of being hypersensitive or on edge, patients may experience episodes of unprovoked anger, jumpiness, and seem to be "on guard" most of the time. Patients may behave as though they are facing constant threats of danger or further trauma. They can become hyperreactive to unexpected sounds or encounters. Problems with concentrating or remembering current information are common, and terrifying nightmares can lead to severe insomnia.

In addition to hearing the patient's complaints, the practitioner needs to assess other pertinent factors to help establish goals for the patient as part of the planning process and to determine level of insight and functional status. A short diagnostic tool can help quickly assess if the patient is experiencing PTSD (see Table 18.4).

To meet the official DSM-5 criteria for a diagnosis of PTSD, symptoms must have persisted for more than 1 month and must have caused clinically significant distress in social, occupational, or other areas of functioning. PTSD is considered *acute* if symptoms have been present for less than 3 months; *chronic* if the symptoms have been present for more than 3 months; and *delayed* if symptom onset occurs 6 months or longer after the trauma.

Diagnostic Reasoning
DSM-5 Symptom Criteria

The DSM-5 symptom criteria for PTSD are as follows:

- Exposure to actual or threatened death, serious injury, or sexual violence by direct experience, witnessing an event, or being closely related to a person who has suffered a traumatic event.
- Presence of one or several of the clinical symptoms mentioned previously.

Table 18.4 Screening Tools for Primary Care*

		Comments
Primary Care—Brief Tools	Staab, JP, and Evans, DL. A streamlined method for diagnosing common psychiatric disorders in primary care. *Clin Corn* 3(3):1–7, 2001. doi:10.1016/S1098-3597(01)90057-2	Screening tools for depression, anxiety, PTSD, stress, substance use, and cognitive functioning
Behavioral Screening	Pediatric Symptom Checklist www2.massgeneral.org/allpsych/psc/psc_home.htm	Goal is to identify behavioral and psychosocial problems. Free and available in various languages
ADHD—Pediatric	ADHD Rating Scale-IV Conners' Parent Rating Scales (SNAP-IV) Swanson, Nolan, and Pelham-IV Teacher and Parent Rating Scale www.adhd.net/snap-iv-form.pdf (SWAN) Strengths and Weaknesses of ADHD-Symptoms and Normal-Behavior Rating Scale www.adhd.net/SWAN_SCALE.pdf Parent/Teacher Disruptive Behavior Disorder Rating Scale http://ccf.buffalo.edu/pdf/DBD_rating_scale.pdf Impairment Rating Scale http://ccf.buffalo.edu/pdf/Impairment_scale.pdf	Sensitivity (92%) and specificity (94%)
	Vanderbilt Assessment Scales www.nichq.org/adhd.html	Developed for use in primary care Validated in preschool-age children Reliable clinical and research tool Parent and teacher evaluations
ADHD—Adult	(ASRS-v1.1) Adult ADHD Self-Report Scale Symptoms Checklist www.hcp.med.harvard.edu/ncs/ftpdir/adhd/18%20Question%20ADHD-ASRS-v1–1.pdf (WHO)	Internal consistency and test-retest reliability (one page) 6 questions
	Childhood ADHD Symptoms Scale Self-Report http://healthnet.umassmed.edu/mhealth/ADHDSelfReport.pdf	Retrospective report of childhood symptoms
	(CAARS) Conners' Adult ADHD Scales (CSS) Current Symptoms Scales Wender Rating Scale	Self-report and Observer-report forms Self-report and Observer-report forms 61 questions. Self-retrospective symptom report
Anxiety	GAD-7[1]	Sensitivity 89%; specificity 82% (5 = mild, 10 = mod, 15 = severe)
	Consider just asking, "Are you bothered by nerves or worrying a lot over the last month?" Anxiety Disorder Interview Schedule Primary Care Evaluation of Mental Disorders (PRIME-MD) Beck Anxiety Inventory HADS-Hospital Anxiety and Depression Scale www.nwph.net/lifestylesurvey/userfiles/mental/things/HAD.pdf Hamilton Anxiety Rating Scale	These longer scales are available, but sensitivity and specificity are no better than the brief scales. Some contain evaluation of depression also.

Table 18.4   Screening Tools for Primary Care*—cont'd

		Comments
	(PSWQ) Penn State Worry Questionnaire https://outcometracker.org/library/PSWQ.pdf	Useful to evaluate excessive worry (16 questions)
Alcohol	AUDIT	The Alcohol Use Disorder Identification Test (AUDIT) consists of 10 questions regarding the quantity of alcohol consumed combined with the individual's experience in using alcohol www.who.int/substance_abuse/activities/sbi/en
	AUDIT-C (3 questions) www.thenationalcouncil.org/galleries/business-practice%20files/tool_auditc.pdf	Both AUDIT and AUDIT-C scales perform similarly to detect heavy drinking and/or active drinking or abuse or dependence. The AUDIT-C has been validated for white, African American, and Hispanic populations.
	CAGE Single-Question Alcohol Screening Test[2] www.ncbi.nlm.nih.gov/pubmed/19247718 TWEAK www.projectcork.org/clinical_tools/html/TWEAK.html	Cut down, annoyed, guilty, eye opener "How many times in the last year have you had X (number) or more drinks in a day?"
		TWEAK is excellent for women with heavy drinking or abuse and for dependence in various ethnic groups.
	Multiple tools available www.project-cork.org/clinical_tools/s	
Pregnancy	Pregnancy Validated Screening Tools Alcohol, depression, substance use, IPV	Summary of various screening tools with source citation and available links www.dbhds.virginia.gov/documents/scrn-perinatal-instrumentschart.pdf
SUD	NMASSIST available at: www.drugabuse.gov/nidamed/screening	(NIDA: Modified Alcohol, Smoking, and Substance Involvement Screening Test) Resource guide and online tool available.
	Multiple tools available www.project-cork.org/clinical_tools/s	
Gambling	"Lie/Bet" www.npgaw.org/2005/041.htm South Oaks Gambling Screen (SOGS)	Ever had to lie to significant other about how much you gambled? 100% sensitivity, 85% specificity Most extensively studied (20 questions)
Bipolar	Mood Disorder Questionnaire (MDQ) [2006]	
Depression	PHQ-9[3] http://patienteducation.stanford.edu/research/phq.html	PHQ-9 score ≥10 had a sensitivity of 88% and a specificity of 88% for major depression. PHQ-9 scores of 5 = mild, 10 = moderate, 15 = moderately severe, and 20 severe depression.[3]
	PHQ-2 FEELING DEPRESSED OR LITTLE INTEREST IN THE PAST MONTH	Administration time 5 minutes. Administration time 1 minute.[4]

Continued

Table 18.4   Screening Tools for Primary Care*—cont'd

		Comments
	Beck Depression Inventory (BDI)	21 items. Administration time 5–10 minutes. Can be utilized in geriatric population older than age 65.
	QIDS www.ids-qids.org	Available in self-report and clinician format with the identical 16 questions. Multiple languages available.
	Geriatric Depression Scale (GDS) www.stanford.edu/~yesavage/GDS.html	Available in short and long format; multiple languages. Score greater than 10 most likely depression, greater than 5 warrants further evaluation. 30 questions. Administration time 10–15 minutes. Self-report—20 items
	CES-D Center for Epidemiologic Studies Depression Screen http://dionysus.psych.wisc.edu/Lit/Articles/RadloffL1977a.pdf	Administration time 5–10 minutes. Reliable in geriatric population older than age 65.
	Zung Self Rating Depression Scale http://healthnet.umassmed.edu/mhealth/ZungSelfRatedDepressionScale.pdf	Twenty items. Takes 5–10 minutes to complete.
Eating Disorders	Scoff Questionnaire	5 questions
	Eating Disorder Screen for Primary Care (ESP)	5 questions
	Eating Attitudes Test (EAT-26)	26 item self-report
IPV	One question: Have you ever been threatened, hit, or kicked?	Allows clinician to ask further questions. www.massmed.org/AM/Template.cfm?Section=Home6&CONTENTID=7356&TEMPLATE=/CM/ContentDisplay.cfm
	SAFE[5,6]	S = Stress/Safety: Are you **safe** in your current relationship? A = Afraid/abused: Ever in a relationship where you felt **afraid**, threatened, or abused? F = Do your **family/friends** know what is happening, and could you tell them? E = Do you have an **emergency** plan (place to go and resources)? (Adapted from Massachusetts Medical Society Committee on Violence. *Partner violence: How to recognize and treat victims of abuse. A Guide for Physicians and other Health Professionals,* ed 4. Massachusetts Medical Society, Waltham, MA, 2004.)
Panic	MINI[7]	Sheehan, DV, et al
	Prime MD[8]	Multiple modules for various conditions.
PTSD	(PCL) PTSD checklist www.ptsd.va.gov/professional/pages/assessments/ptsd-checklist.asp and www.mirecc.va.gov/docs/visn6/3_PTSD_CheckList_and_Scoring.pdf	Military and civilian versions (sensitivity 69%–94%; specificity 83%–99%)

Table 18.4	Screening Tools for Primary Care*—cont'd	
		Comments
	SPAN[9] doi:10.1016/S0165–1781(99)00070–0	Startle, physical reaction when event relived, anger, numbness/detachment
	Primary Care PTSD (PC-PTSD)[10]	Four yes-or-no items. Scoring positive if 2 or more yes answers or hyperarousal alone.

*All tools were validated using the DSM-IV criteria.

Sources:

[1]Spitzer, RL, et al. A brief measure for assessing generalized anxiety disorders. GAD 7. *Arch Intern Med* 166:1092–1097, 2006. http://archinte.ama-assn.org/cgi/reprint/166/10/1092

[2]Smith, PC, et al. Primary care validation of a single-item alcohol screening test. *J Gen Intern Med* 24(7):783–788, 2009.

[3]Kroenke, K, et al. The PHQ-9: Validity of a brief depression severity measure. *J Gen Intern Med* 16(6):606–613, 2001.

[4]Whooley, MA, et al. Case-finding instruments for depression. Two questions are as good as many. *J Gen Intern Med* 12:439–445, 1997.

[5]Ashur, ML. Asking about domestic violence: SAFE questions. *JAMA* 269:2367, 1993.

[6]Neufeld, B. SAFE questions: Overcoming barriers to the detection of domestic violence. *Am Fam Physician* 53:2575–2580, 1996.

[7]Sheehan, DV, et al. The MINI-International Neuropsychiatric Interview (M.I.N.I.): The development of a structured psychiatric interview for DSM-IV and ICD-IO. *J Clin Psychiatry* 59(Suppl 20):22–23,1998.

[8]Spitzer, RL, et al. Utility of a new procedure for diagnosing mental disorders in primary care: The PRIME-MD study. *JAMA* 272:1749–1756, 1994.

[9]Meltzer-Brody, S, et al. Derivation of the SPAN: A brief diagnostic screening test for post-traumatic stress disorder. *Psych Res* 88:63–70, 1999.

[10]Prins, A, et al. The primary care PTSD screen (PC-PTSD): Development and operating characteristics. *Prim Care Psych* 9(1):9–14, 2003. www.ptsd.va.gov/professional/articles/article-pdf/id26676.pdf

Management

In general, there is a lack of well-designed, randomized clinical trials to inform the pharmacological or nonpharmacological management of PTSD. There are gaps in the study of PTSD in subgroups, such as those individuals with traumatic brain injury, combat-related symptoms, or comorbid psychiatric disorders. There needs to be more rigorous research undertaken with veterans and an agreed-on "recovery" definition of the disorder.

Nonpharmacological Management

Crisis intervention immediately after the traumatic event may lead to avoidance of this disorder. However, critical incident debriefing, previously thought to be a helpful approach, was found to increase symptomatology when used with survivors of the September 11, 2001, terrorist attacks and is no longer recommended. Cognitive-behavioral therapy (CBT) has proven helpful for symptom relief when used individually and with groups.

Several specific CBTs for PTSD include prolonged exposure (PE), stress inoculation therapy (SIT), and image rehearsal therapy (IRT). PE was developed for women with rape trauma and is an effective first-line treatment with sustained benefit over time. One technique called "imaginal exposure" has the patient imagine and describe trauma and associated emotions and can be effective in reducing PTSD symptom severity. In vivo exposure uses systematic desensitization to triggers of trauma. With desensitization, the patient is exposed to his or her trauma "trigger" in a controlled environment.

Improvement is achieved by gradually increasing the time of exposure to the trigger until the patient no longer reacts with panic.

SIT may be considered a "toolbox" for managing anxiety and focuses on correcting the patient's intrusive symptoms by teaching relaxation techniques, such as breathing exercises, that can be used to help self-manage intrusive symptoms when they occur. IRT is a brief approach—three sessions—that was found to decrease chronic nightmares and improve sleep quality. All of these approaches are specialized forms of care, but practitioners in primary-care settings can refer patients to providers who can offer these services.

Another intervention for PTSD is psychodynamic psychotherapy. This method focuses on helping the patient to examine personal values and how the experience of the traumatic event violated them. The goal is to resolve the conscious and unconscious mental conflicts that were created by the trauma. The patient works on strengthening his or her self-esteem as a way of increasing the ability to cope with the trauma.

Family therapy can be helpful when family relationships have been affected by the patient's symptoms. When family members complain that the patient does not communicate and is difficult or unpredictable, a family therapist can help the family accomplish positive changes in their relationships and functioning and help them learn to cope with their own feelings about the patient's experiences.

Group therapy or peer-counseling groups are also effective interventions for PTSD. Health groups can encourage members to share similar traumas and symptoms safely. Through participation in these groups, individuals with PTSD can learn that they are worthy and that they are not somehow guilty for their trauma. Patients may find it easier to learn new coping techniques from other group members. Relaxation therapy and other forms of complementary therapies are also helpful for persons with PTSD. Massage, positive imagery, meditation, and yoga have all been shown to be beneficial.

Pharmacological Management

Various medications can improve symptoms. The SSRIs paroxetine (Paxil) and sertraline (Zoloft) are approved for use in PTSD, and they are at times effective in its acute treatment (Level II; Stein et al, 2006). They have been shown to improve all core PTSD clusters (numbing, intrusions, hyperarousal), and are effective in both genders, all trauma types, and in patients with comorbid disorders.

A review of pharmacological treatment for PTSD by the Institute of Medicine (IOM) in 2007 found insufficient evidence for the efficacy of most medications, including SSRIs, prazosin (Minipress), anticonvulsants, benzodiazepines, and second generation antipsychotics. Since 2012, an ongoing review process for the treatment of PTSD in war veterans has been undertaken by the IOM. One study demonstrated that prazosin improved global functioning, decreased PTSD symptoms, decreased nightmares, and improved the quality of sleep in in combat-related PTSD. For some patients, TCAs may be effective. Anxiolytic medications can be used for acute or short-term symptom management only. Buspirone (Buspar) may reduce intrusive symptoms for some patients and is a relatively safe anxiolytic.

Follow-up and Referral

If a patient is not fully recovering from a traumatic experience, he or she should be referred to a behavioral health specialist. The symptoms of PTSD can be very disturbing, and most patients will require more time and support than is available in primary-care settings. Pharmacological management may also require specialized management, especially if an SSRI has been tried and the patient proves refractory to treatment. Patients will most likely wish to continue with their primary-care practitioner for some aspects of their care. Recovery from trauma is a slow process; patients may stop and start treatment for years. When this is the case, their relationship with their primary-care practitioner becomes a stabilizing force.

Patient Education

It is important that the patient with PTSD and his or her family have a good understanding of the disorder, the chronic nature of PTSD, and the potential adverse effects of any medications prescribed. For some patients, interventions of a holistic nature may prove beneficial.

Regular physical activity, good nutritional practices, and other self-care interventions can help to control symptomatology. Disease progression could lead to suicidal ideation and/or violence. The patient and family should be counseled regarding danger signs and the need for close follow-up and possible intervention.

■ OBSESSIVE-COMPULSIVE DISORDER

Epidemiology and Causes

Obsessive-compulsive disorder (OCD) is diagnosed when a person has obsessions (recurrent or intrusive thoughts) or compulsions (conscious, standardized, recurrent behaviors) severe enough to cause the person marked distress. OCD is a chronic disorder, with lifetime prevalence estimated at 2% to 3%. The disorder has its onset in childhood, late adolescence, or early adulthood. There is a male preponderance in earlier onset of the disorder, whereas females predominate when diagnosed at a later age. In many cases, there is an acute onset of the disorder, possibly after a significant stressful life event.

In childhood, a unique presentation is the Pediatric Autoimmune Neuropsychiatric Disorders Associated with Group A Beta-hemolytic Streptococcal Infection (PANDAS). Still to be fully explained, this subtype occurs before adolescence and is characterized by the acute onset of at least two episodes of OCD behaviors or tics and a documented group A beta-hemolytic streptococcal infection. OCD is a familiar disorder, and first-degree relatives of persons diagnosed with OCD or with Tourette's syndrome are at increased risk for development of OCD.

Pathophysiology and Psychopathology

There is a commonality between OCD and depressive disorder, evidenced by similarities in sleep electroencephalograph studies and in neuroendocrine dexamethasone testing. Recent studies of adults with OCD have elucidated particular symptom complexes that have some correlations with both genetic and neuroimaging modalities and may have treatment implications. These complexes are contamination/washing, symmetry/ordering, checking, and hoarding.

Behaviorally, obsessions may represent a conditioned response to anxiety, and the compulsions relieve or reduce the anxious symptoms and become an ingrained behavior. Psychiatric comorbidities in patients with OCD include eating, anxiety, and mood disorders. Children may also exhibit tics and attention-deficit disorder. Children presenting with coexisting OCD and bipolar disorder may have a poorer response to treatment.

Clinical Presentation

Patients may present in primary care with either depression or anxiety because of the distress and inability to function caused by their symptom complex. However, it is quite likely that patients can keep their symptoms secret for many years and may not be diagnosed until quite late. Some patients may have already sought psychiatric care. Inquiry can be made about family psychiatric history, as well as the specific symptom complex exhibited by the patient. Common obsessions include concern with bodily wastes or germs, fear of death, a need for symmetry, forbidden or intense sexual thoughts, or intrusive sounds. Reported compulsions include excessive hand washing or bathing, repeated rituals, touching, checking, counting, and hoarding.

Diagnostic Reasoning

For a diagnosis to be made in the adult, the DSM-5 requires that symptoms must caused marked distress and cause interference with social and occupational functioning. The neurological differential includes Tourette's syndrome and temporal lobe epilepsy. Psychiatric considerations are schizophrenia, depression, phobic disorder, GAD, and PTSD. Remember that the patient with OCD has good insight into his or her symptomatology, which is not often the case in the psychotic disorders.

Rating scales for the severity of the disorder include the 10-item Yale-Brown Obsessive-Compulsive Scale (Y-BOCS) and in children the Children's Yale-Brown Obsessive-Compulsive Scale (CY-BOCS). A seven-item self-report OCD screen (SOCS) has a high sensitivity (0.97) and specificity (0.88) for differentiating patients with OCD from healthy controls. This questionnaire is available online (http://ocdyouth.iop.kcl.ac.uk/downloads/socs.pdf).

Children brought to the attention of the family nurse practitioner should be diagnosed and treated in concert with specialized psychiatric care. If PANDAS is suspected, appropriate clinical and laboratory testing should be performed (throat culture, ASO titers, judicious blood work).

(DSM-5 Symptom Criteria for OCD are presented in Table 18.1.)

Management

In general, due to the shame that the obsessions and compulsions can induce in patients, a strong therapeutic alliance and the building of trust are crucial for ongoing care. Families should be involved and given appropriate education and resources, such as information from the OCD Foundation Web site.

Pharmacological Management

SSRIs are recommended as first-line pharmacological management of OCD in children and adults (Level I; Soomro et al, 2008). Generally, higher doses of the SSRIs are required to treat OCD than are needed for depression or anxiety. Although use of SSRIs in children and adolescents carries a warning to be aware of a possible increase in suicidal ideation, studies have shown that in OCD, the benefits of treatment outweigh the risks. Clomipramine (Anafranil), a tricyclic, can be used as a second-line therapy; however, the risks of seizures, weight gain, and cardiovascular events must be carefully considered.

Nonpharmacological Management

CBT is also regarded as first-line management, either alone or in combination with an SSRI. CBT can be delivered individually, in group sessions, or with families. Exposure with response prevention (ERP) is another widely used counseling method, effective in both the adult and pediatric populations. This technique involves exposing patients to their obsessions, triggering their anxiety/discomfort, and working with them to overcome their compulsions.

Follow-up and Referral

The primary-care practitioner should address medical concerns coexisting in the patient with OCD and be mindful of medication side effects or interactions. When a medication is begun, the patient should be seen weekly for the first month, and a response should be seen within the first 6 weeks. Symptom severity can be assessed through the use of the aforementioned rating scales. OCD can be difficult to treat, because patients respond to treatment modalities quite differently with improvement responses of 40% to 60%. It is recommended that care be given in coordination with mental health specialists. Patients should be followed regularly, with attention paid to health maintenance issues. Referrals may be necessary for consequences of compulsive behaviors, such as to a dermatologist for trichotillomania, to a neurologist for coexistent Tourette's syndrome, or for dental care for excessive gum cleaning.

Patient Education

Education of the patient, family, and parents of the child with OCD is extremely important. Web sites provide information and links to support groups (e.g., http://familydoctor.org/online/famdocen/home/common/mentalhealth/anxiety/133.html; www.ocfoundation.org). Being educated and informed about the condition helps treatment compliance as well.

DISORDERS THAT MAY INCLUDE DEPRESSIVE SYMPTOMATOLOGY

■ OVERVIEW

The following sections include major depression, dysthymia, bipolar disorders, and schizophrenia. Major depressive disorder is the hallmark diagnosis in this

The Iceberg of Depression

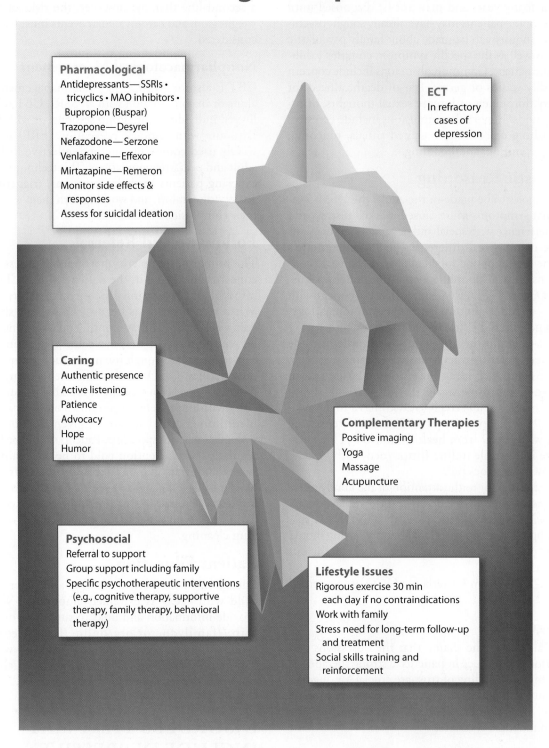

Pharmacological
Antidepressants—SSRIs •
   tricyclics • MAO inhibitors •
   Bupropion (Buspar)
Trazopone—Desyrel
Nefazodone—Serzone
Venlafaxine—Effexor
Mirtazapine—Remeron
Monitor side effects &
   responses
Assess for suicidal ideation

ECT
In refractory
cases of
depression

Caring
Authentic presence
Active listening
Patience
Advocacy
Hope
Humor

Complementary Therapies
Positive imaging
Yoga
Massage
Acupuncture

Psychosocial
Referral to support
Group support including family
Specific psychotherapeutic interventions
   (e.g., cognitive therapy, supportive
   therapy, family therapy, behavioral
   therapy)

Lifestyle Issues
Rigorous exercise 30 min
   each day if no contraindications
Work with family
Stress need for long-term follow-up
   and treatment
Social skills training and
   reinforcement

category, and in DSM-5 a more chronic form, Persistent Depressive Disorder or Dysthymia, is included.

■ MAJOR DEPRESSIVE DISORDER

A common psychosocial symptom seen in primary-care settings is depression. Depression is common for many reasons.

People use the term *depression* to describe a wide variety of negative emotional experiences, ranging from sadness to disinterest in pleasurable activities to self-hate. The hallmarks of major depression are sadness and apathy. In most cases, the sadness and apathy associated with major depression can be distinguished from ordinary changes in mood.

No description of depression, whether as a symptom or disorder, is complete without addressing the psychological pain and suffering of depression. The pain of depression can become so severe that some depressed persons are willing to go to any length to obtain even a moment of relief. Depression-related thoughts of death or suicide are not uncommon. Yet the pain of depression can be difficult to articulate: The depressed person may only be able to make vague references to "hurting" or "feeling bad." (See Nursing Research–Based Practice 18.1.)

Individual variations in the clinical presentation of depression can be great, sometimes making the condition difficult to recognize. The more common patient presentation of depression in primary-care settings is the person who has moderate to severe feelings of sadness or apathy that he or she attributes to depression. Common presentations also include complaints of unexplained fatigue, irritability, anger, anxiety, and hyperactivity. Many deeply depressed persons are unaware of their depression. Slowed thinking and emotional numbness—two severe symptoms of depression—can contribute to minimal self-awareness of depression. Gender can affect presentation, but gender should not influence assessment.

Cultural variations in the presentation of depression are also individualized, based on how traditional or nontraditional the individual's attitudes and behaviors are. Patients may focus less on personal experiences and more on physical aches and pains. Ethnic and cultural norms concerning privacy, embarrassment, and disclosure will have an impact on the patient's presentation.

Major depressive disorder is characterized by severe negative changes in mood, thinking, and behavior. A person who is severely depressed will have intense feelings of sadness, irritability, or apathy. These feelings may persist at all times and are unrelieved by circumstantial changes. At home, at school, at work, or in recreational situations, the mood of the depressed person basically varies little. In some cases, the mood of the depressed person may vary slightly but without improving significantly.

Negative changes in thinking associated with depression are common. Depressed thinking can be described as global, distorted, and circular. Rather than dealing with today, the depressed person may instead focus on distant events or think about the future as if it is a singular, knowable event. With depression, the balance between positive and negative thoughts about self, about life, and about the future becomes distorted. Negative views can seem more valid than positive views. Global negative thinking can take on a ruminative or circular pattern, so that the depressed person's negative thinking seems to always depart from and arrive at the same painful conclusions.

Major depression interferes with decision making and concentration. The smallest decision, such as whether or not to make a phone call, becomes difficult. Depression-related negative changes in thinking can be very upsetting. The depressed person may become alarmed by his or her inability to make choices or to concentrate. Although others may recognize negative changes in the depressed person's thinking, the onset of negative thinking can also develop without warning to the patient. The negative thinking associated with major depression may include thoughts of death and suicide. Some people make a clear distinction between passive thoughts of death and active thoughts of suicide, but both patterns are disturbing.

Changes in behavior associated with major depression may occur. The person's behavior may become uncharacteristic. For this reason, significant others may become aware of the depression before the depressed person does. Depression-related changes in behavior range from changes in grooming and in interpersonal interactions

---

Nursing Research–Based Practice 18.1   Postpartum Depression

Beck, CT. Teetering on the edge: A substantive theory of postpartum depression. *Nurs Res* 42(1):42–48, 1993.

This classic, grounded theory study utilized a qualitative approach to develop theory regarding women's perceptions of postpartum depression. Drawing a sample of 12 from a postpartum support group, the researcher conducted in-depth interviews with the women about their experiences of postpartum depression. What emerged was a rich description of the nature of postpartum depression and how these women managed their depression. "Teetering on the edge" was the hallmark metaphor that the researcher extracted to describe the process that the participants confronted during their depression. They felt "between" sane and insane, and the researcher identified several stages: "Encountering the terror" described the unpredictable nature of feelings that overwhelmed them, anxiety and panic attacks, obsessions, and loss of concentration. In the next stage, called "the dying of self," the women experienced isolation, withdrawal, and feelings of dissociation and depersonalization. Most had suicidal ideation. In the next stage, "struggling to survive," they began to grapple with their feelings. They searched out support groups, used prayer and faith to manage the depression, and began, hesitantly, and with some steps forward and some steps backward, to recover.

Women are at highest risk of developing postpartum depression from a few days to 6 months following childbirth. APRNs need to be aware of this type of depression and be alert to it. They need to educate others about the phenomenon and truly understand the meaning of the experience to these women.

to substance abuse, irritability, aggression, and social withdrawal.

Epidemiology and Causes

It is estimated that between 5% and 20% of the population will experience a significant depression at some time during their lives. The lifetime prevalence of a major depressive disorder (MDD) is 16.5% with a 6.7% 12-month prevalence rate. The prevalence of depression in older adults (over age 65) can be as high as 40% in hospitalized and nursing home patients and as high as 30% in community-dwelling elders or in adults living with chronic medical conditions. Older adults have many risk factors for depression because of the frequent losses experienced within this age-group. There is a higher incidence of depression in women (21%) than in men (13%). Researchers have studied this phenomenon for decades, but there does not appear to be a single, universal explanation for women's greater susceptibility to depression.

Once a person experiences a depressive episode, he or she is at high risk for a recurrence. As many as 50% of these individuals go on to experience a recurrence; after two episodes, there is an 80% chance of another recurrence.

One out of seven patients with recurrent depressive illness commits suicide, and of those who do, 70% have seen their primary-care provider within 6 weeks before committing suicide, often for somatic complaints. In the absence of systematic screening, usual care by primary-care providers fails to detect between 30% and 50% of depressed patients. This makes it imperative that primary-care practitioners learn to inquire sensitively about depression and to utilize evidence-based screening tools appropriately (see Table 18.4). Risk factors for depression are presented in Risk Factors 18.2.

Depression is also an independent risk factor for morbidity and mortality from cardiac disease. In patients with coexisting atrial fibrillation and congestive heart failure who received optimal treatment, a higher rate of depressive symptoms correlated with increased cardiovascular mortality. The World Health Organization (WHO) estimates that by 2020, depression will rank second only to cardiovascular illness in terms of disease burden and as a worldwide cause of disability. Similarly, patients with comorbid diabetes mellitus and depression face increased mortality in comparison to those patients without concomitant disease.

Pathophysiology and Psychopathology

A correlation between the hypersecretion of cortisol and depression is one of the oldest observations in biological psychiatry. Neurovegetative signs and symptoms of depression may correlate with various neuroendocrine abnormalities.

Approximately 5% to 10% of all patients with depression have a coexisting thyroid disorder. Recent research has focused on the theory that a subset of depressed

Risk Factors 18.2	Major Depression
Age	Adolescent or older adult
Gender	Female
Family History	Strong family history of depression, suicide or attempt, alcohol abuse, or other substance abuse
History	History of migraine headaches, back pain, recent myocardial infarction, and/or peptic ulcer disease
Current Medical Condition	Current chronic disease (especially multiple diseases) Insomnia
Lifestyle	Stress Poverty Less than high school education Recent traumatic event Parent or caregiver of a child or children with behavioral disorders, especially hyperactivity Retired

patients may have an unrecognized autoimmune disorder that affects the thyroid gland. Some depressed patients benefit from liothyronine. A thyroid level should be obtained on all depressed patients.

Alterations in sleep, appetite, and sexual behavior, as well as biological changes in endocrine, immunological, and chronobiological measures in depressed patients, all suggest dysregulation of the hypothalamus. The stooped posture of depressed patients, motor slowness, and minor cognitive impairments are similar to the signs of disorder of the basal ganglia, such as Parkinson's disease and other subcortical dementias.

Genetic factors are strongly implicated in the development of depressive disorder, although it is impossible to rule out psychosocial factors, as well as other nongenetic factors. Adoption studies have also provided supporting data to the idea that there is a genetic basis for the inheritance of mood disorder. For major depression, the concordance rate in monozygote twins is about 50%, arguing strongly for a genetic disposition. A recent study indicated that a functional polymorphism in the serotonin transporter gene (5-HTT) may interact with stressful life events to markedly increase the risk for depression and suicide.

Psychosocial factors also contribute to depression. Stressful life events have been demonstrated to precede first episodes of mood disorders. Some speculate that the stress accompanying the first episode results in long-lasting changes in the brain's biology. Thus, the person is at high risk for subsequent episodes of mood disorder, unrelated to an external stressor. The external psychosocial factors most often associated with the onset of a major depressive episode is the loss of a spouse or losing a parent, especially if it occurs before age 11. Another risk factor is unemployment; persons out of work are three times more likely to report symptoms of an episode of major depression than those who are employed. However, what may seem to be a relatively mild stressor from an outside perspective may be devastating to the person because of whatever idiosyncratic meaning that he or she assigns to the event.

Clinical Presentation

Assessment of major depression need not be overly complicated, but the focus of the assessment should include more than the presence or absence of significant sadness or apathy. The sadness and apathy that characterize major depression may be reported by the patient, observed and reported by significant others, or observed by the practitioner. Two quick questions that provide a preliminary screen for depression are recommended by the U.S. Preventive Services Task Force. The patient is first asked if he or she has felt down or hopeless over the past month and then asked if there has been little interest in doing things over the past month. A positive response to one or both questions in this screen indicates possible major depression, but the test has a high false-positive rate. Thus, confirmatory testing should be performed using a validated screening instrument or a clinical interview.

The Patient Health Questionnaire–9 (PHQ-9) consists of a checklist of nine symptoms. The patient is asked to indicate the frequency with which these symptoms have occurred over the preceding 2 weeks. The test is scored based on symptom frequency. This instrument can be filled out quickly either in the waiting room or exam room before a primary-care visit and provides an effective supplementation to the two-question screening. A similar measure of symptom severity, the self-rated Quick Inventory of Depressive Symptomatology (QIDS-SR), can be used for the same purpose and has the additional benefit of including symptom severity and may thus provide a sensitive measure of change with treatment (see Table 18.4).

Programs aimed at enhancing public awareness of depression have been effective, in that more patients are likely to seek professional health care for major depression as a result of having accurately self-assessed their symptoms. Patients may bring in depression self-assessment surveys published in popular magazines or local newspapers. When patients have self-assessed their depression symptoms, practitioners can determine symptom intensity, symptom duration, and symptom impact on functioning. It can also be helpful to ask patients to identify which symptoms they consider treatment priorities.

Some patients with major depression may, as a result of the disorder, find it difficult to list their symptoms. In this case assessment, screening assessment tools such as the Zung Self-Rating Depression Scale (SDS) or Beck Depression Inventory (BDI), checklists, direct observations,

or yes-or-no questions may be substituted. When yes-or-no assessment questions are used, all yes responses should be explored. Extremely depressed patients may not tolerate assessment in any form that requires effort on their part. They can become irritable and impatient with the practitioner for asking questions that, to the patient, seem unnecessary. This situation can sometimes be improved by indicating that the purpose of asking questions is to understand fully the patient's depression and not to qualify or disqualify the patient for treatment.

The Geriatric Depression scale (GDS) is a widely validated screening tool for use in older adults (see Table 18.4). Depression is one of the five major health problems confronted by older adults. Clinicians need to be aware of the common presenting symptoms (see Table 18.5).

Diagnostic Reasoning
DSM-5 Symptom Criteria

The DSM-5 symptom criteria for major depression state that five (or more) of the following symptoms have been present during the same 2-week period and represent a change from previous functioning. At least one of the symptoms is either (1) depressed mood or (2) anhedonia, meaning loss of interest or pleasure:

- Depressed mood expressed as feelings of sadness or hopelessness. Irritability may be the primary symptom in adolescents and children.
- Markedly diminished interest (apathy) in most activities.
- Change in appetite.
- Insomnia or hypersomnia.
- Behavioral agitation or retardation.
- Loss of energy.
- Feelings of worthlessness or guilt.
- Loss of concentration.
- Recurrent thoughts of death or suicide.
- These symptoms cause significant functional impairment and are not related to a medical illness or from the effects of a substance.

Table 18.5 Components of Depression in Elderly Persons
• Vegetative—poor appetite, disrupted sleep, early morning awakening
• Somatic—pain throughout body or out of proportion with underlying pathology
• Psychological—obsessive feelings of guilt and worry, ruminations throughout the night; suicidal ideation; memory problems
• Psychomotor—anxiety; psychomotor agitation
• Diurnal variation in symptoms—cannot "get moving" in morning, or specific time of day when depression is worst

The depressive episode can be further "specified" as follows: with anxious distress, with mixed features, with melancholic features, with atypical features, with psychotic features, with catatonia, with peripartum onset, and with seasonal pattern.

In patients with comorbid anxiety and depression, the symptom profile may be balanced or either symptom can predominate; in addition, some patients with so-called mixed anxiety and depression may demonstrate symptoms of both disorders but may not meet the full diagnostic criteria for either. Any patient who has symptoms of either depression or anxiety should be evaluated for current symptoms of both disorders. Consensus recommendations from a panel of experts who represent psychiatry, primary care, pharmacy, and managed care state that every patient suspected of having unipolar depression be evaluated for bipolar disorder using a quick screening tool before being treated with antidepressants. It is also necessary initially to rule out other medical conditions and substance use. Then, it must be determined if the patient has ever experienced symptoms of mania or hypomania. Then the patient's depressive symptoms must be assessed for severity, duration, recurrence, and the like to differentiate among the depressive disorders. One consideration is persistent depressive disorder or dysthymia, which is distinguished by time course without episodes of mania or hypomania.

Differential Diagnosis

All patients must be carefully evaluated for underlying medical conditions. Many medical and neurological disorders and pharmacological substances can produce symptoms of depression. Careful medical history and physical examination should be done on all patients, including a neurological exam and routine blood work and urinalysis. The history needs to include the patient's personal as well as family history of depression and suicide. Tests for thyroid and adrenal function should be included because disorders of both of these endocrine systems can mimic depression. Cardiac drugs, antihypertensive agents, sedatives, hypnotics, antipsychotics, antiepileptics, antiparkinsonian drugs, analgesics, antibacterials, steroids, and antineoplastics are all commonly associated with depressive symptomatology. A careful medication review, including over-the-counter drugs and herbal agents, as well as evaluation of alcohol and substance use, is imperative. The most common neurological disorders that may manifest depressive symptoms are Parkinson's disease (50%–75% of patients have depressive symptoms that do not correlate with physical disability), dementing illnesses (including Alzheimer type), epilepsy, cerebrovascular disease, and tumors. The interictal changes associated with temporal lobe epilepsy can mimic a depressive disorder, especially if the epileptic focus is on the right side. There is increasing evidence of linkages between depression and cardiovascular disease, not limited to sequelae but actually preceding the event. In brain tumors, depression is more common in cases of anterior lobe tumor as opposed to posterior lobe lesions, and in both cases it responds to antidepressants. The pseudodementia of MDD can be differentiated from true dementia with regard to onset (sudden in the case of pseudodementia), and guilt and self-reproach are common features of MDD, but not of dementias. Patients with depression will sometimes not answer questions, whereas those with dementia may confabulate. Depressed patients may be "coaxed" into remembering during an interview; those with primary dementia cannot.

In terms of mental disorders, depression can be a feature of virtually any disorder listed in the DSM-5. Depression has a high comorbidity with the anxiety disorders, as well as alcohol-use disorders, eating disorders, schizophrenia, schizophreniform disorder, and somatoform disorder, especially somatization disorder. Bereaved patients also need careful assessment.

Management

Remission of symptoms should be the standard for successful treatment of depression. Remission is defined as an absence of depressive symptoms or a PHQ-9 score of less than 5, and this is the goal of therapy. Alternatively, response can be defined as a reduction on the PHQ-9 score of 25% to 50%. In clinical trials, only 25% to 35% of patients experience complete remission of depressive symptoms. Clinical practice guidelines are available at https://www.icsi.org/_asset/fnhdm3/Depr-Interactive0512b.pdf. Achievement of remission is important because incomplete relief of symptoms may increase the risk of relapse and further impairment. The mainstays of treatment are the use of appropriate antidepressants and/or psychotherapy (Level I; Institute for Clinical Systems Improvement, 1996; Michigan Quality Improvement Consortium, 2012). For mild to moderate depression, either medication or psychotherapy is recommended; if the depression is more severe, evidence-based guidelines support the simultaneous use of both (Level I; Institute for Clinical Systems Improvement, 1996; Michigan Quality Improvement Consortium, 2012). When the patient expresses suicidal intent or plan or has a history of suicidal attempt, consultation with a behavioral specialist or psychiatrist is important. In addition, treatment of a mood disorder such as major depression requires a *Circle of Caring* (see Chapter 2). For patients from differing ethnic groups or cultures, discussion of acceptable treatments should form the basis of therapeutic management (Level I; Institute for Clinical Systems Improvement, 1996; Michigan Quality Improvement Consortium, 2012).

Pharmacological Management

With pharmacological therapy, about 7 out of 10 patients with severe major depression will obtain symptom relief. Medications that are effective in the front-line treatment of MDD are the selective serotonin reuptake inhibitors (SSRIs), serotonin-norepinephrine reuptake inhibitors (SNRIs), norepinephrine reuptake inhibitors (NRIs), tricyclic antidepressants (TCAs), and dopamine agonists (DAs) (Level I; Kaiser Permanente Care Management Institute, 2012). Prescribing antidepressant medication begins with patient education. Each patient should be given as much information as is necessary to ensure that he or she understands the potential benefits of taking medication, the specific medication being prescribed, anticipated effects, possible adverse effects and how to handle them, and what to do in an emergency. When possible, this information should be made available in writing. Effective patient education makes it possible for patients to participate in their care and decreases the risks of having a patient agree to take medications without being fully informed of the medication risks and benefits.

The process of prescribing medications begins with building a patient symptom profile. A comprehensive list of current and recent patient symptoms is developed. This symptom list includes the symptoms, their intensity, duration, and effects on day-to-day functioning and role performance. From this list, two to four target symptoms are selected. Target symptoms should be identified and used to determine the most appropriate antidepressant medication.

The side-effect profiles for the newer neurotransmitter receptor–specific antidepressant medications are less severe than those for the TCAs. The receptor-specific antidepressants also have a lower risk of lethal overdose, but significant adverse reactions can occur. The advantages of fewer adverse effects and greater patient safety are significant, but many patients will experience initial adverse effects from the newer antidepressants.

Patients who are sensitive to the powerful serotonin activity produced by the SSRIs may be better able to tolerate antidepressants that have serotonin and norepinephrine (NE) activity, NE activity only, less specific serotonin activity, or an atypical antidepressant. Depressed patients who cannot tolerate SSRIs or the atypical antidepressants may be able to obtain excellent symptom relief from TCAs. TCAs are not less effective than newer antidepressant medications, but they can produce more side effects, take longer to work, and are more lethal in overdose.

Antidepressant medications can be prescribed based on their half-life, neurotransmitter activity, side-effect profile, and clinical efficacy. The half-life for newer antidepressant medications ranges from hours to several days. Neurotransmitter activity accounts for the significant differences in medication effects, including sedation, activation, anxiolytic (antianxiety), and anticompulsive effects. Important common side-effect risks with serotonin-specific antidepressants include decreased sexual desire, decreased sexual response, headache, stomach upset, sedation, fatigue, or nervousness. Absolute medication-dose limitations have been defined for patients with seizure disorders, renal disease, and liver disease. Some newer antidepressants are contraindicated for persons with bulimia, and some drugs have significant liver P450-interaction effects. There appear to be fewer age-related dose limitations; thus, newer antidepressants tend to be well tolerated by depressed older adults and adolescents. Ongoing clinical trials with pregnant women suggest that for some women, antidepressant medication can be a safe option.

Individual reactions to antidepressant medications are unique, but in general, antidepressant medications with significant NE effects (e.g., bupropion) tend to be activating. Antidepressant medications with multiple neurotransmitter effects (e.g., venlafaxine) may be effective when serotonin-specific antidepressants are not. Patients who have difficulty adjusting to the short-term side effects of antidepressants with a short half-life (e.g., sertraline, paroxetine) may experience milder short-term side effects with longer half-life antidepressants (e.g., fluoxetine). For some patients, dramatic decreases in adverse effects can be obtained by adjusting the time of day the medication is taken. Patients who are bothered by adverse effects when they take an antidepressant in the morning may experience only mild side effects if they take the same medication with dinner or at bedtime. Extremely low starting doses may be necessary when it is clear that a patient seems able to benefit from an antidepressant but cannot tolerate medication side effects during the early stages of treatment. According to a meta-analysis by Cipriani et al (2009) comparing efficacy and acceptability of second generation antidepressants, sertraline and escitalopram should be considered for initial therapy for adults with moderate to severe depression. Barriers to adherence to pharmacological guidelines can be intolerable side effects, efficacy, and cost. Switching between classes of antidepressants is common. Maximizing the dosage by a systematic stepwise approach is recommended to achieve a full therapeutic effect. When an agent does not seem to be effective, switching agents or classes is recommended. Switching between SSRIs and SNRIs can be done by prescribing the new drug at equivalent dosage. Switching from SSRI to TCA or SNRI can be accomplished through cross-tapering, where SSRI is gradually reduced over a 1- to 2-week period as the new drug is introduced and gradually increased to therapeutic levels. Cross-tapering is also recommended for mirtazapine. Because paroxetine possesses the most distressing discontinuation symptoms, one approach may be to switch to fluoxetine and then slowly taper. Discontinuation symptoms are generally not a problem for bupropion because it does not possess strong serotonergic properties. It is recommended to taper bupropion over a 1-week period while initiating the new drug at full dosage. Paroxetine, fluvoxamine, and fluoxetine are metabolized by the liver and could potentially increase the blood level of bupropion and increase risk of seizure, especially at high doses of bupropion. Refer to specific prescribing considerations and patient information regarding monoamine oxidase inhibitors. The most important aspect is to warn patients about abrupt cessation and formulate a plan to discontinue by tapering over a 2- to 3-week period.

Providers are advised to identify all supplements or medications the patient is currently taking before starting an antidepressant medication, particularly if the patient has not taken a psychotropic medication before. This list should include all compounds—prescribed and self-administered. Many people now medicate themselves with over-the-counter (OTC) products—vitamins, minerals, herbal remedies—that they may not consider medications. The high number of such products now available makes this information vital. Patient use of megadose vitamin and mineral supplements, weight-loss or weight-gain products, and nutritional supplements should also be noted. At present, the standard of practice regarding the use of prescribed and herbal compounds is that the two treatments should not be used simultaneously. For example, there is no

compelling evidence for the efficacy of St. John's wort in either mild or moderate depression; neither is the herb recommended in cases of more serious major depressive disorder (Level I; Institute for Clinical Systems Improvement, 1996; Michigan Quality Improvement Consortium, 2012). For information on specific drugs for major depression, see Drugs Commonly Prescribed 18.2.

Nonpharmacological Management

Both interpersonal and cognitive-behavioral therapy have been shown to be effective for the treatment of depression, and there is evidence that the combination of psychotherapy and pharmacotherapy may be more effective than either alone. Patients with major depression need hope and reassurance. Both are particularly important with patients who may have lived with untreated depression. Informing a person that his or her disorder is major depression and that the disorder can be treated sets the stage for patients to define goals for improvement and begin to combat the secondary demoralization that can develop after months of untreated depression. False reassurances and unrealistic expectations must be avoided, however. The support needs of patients with

Drugs Commonly Prescribed 18.2	Selective Serotonin Reuptake Inhibitors (SSRIs)	
Drug	**Indication**	**Adverse Reactions and Prescribing Considerations**
All SSRIs		Common to most SSRIs: Response rates—60%–70% Remission rates—20%–35% Lowest risk of overdose Avoid sudden discontinuation Do not prescribe with monoamine oxidase inhibitors (MAOIs) Hepatic excretion: monitor LFTs Agitation, weakness, dizziness, headache, drowsiness (dose in evening), insomnia (dose in morning), nausea/vomiting (self-limiting 1–3 weeks), and xerostomia. SIADH, serotonin syndrome (caution with "triptans") SSRI-induced mania If anxiety/panic disorder develops or history of such, start low and adjust dose slowly. Risk factor for suicide. No to slight weight gain except paroxetine Sexual dysfunction that resolves in 1–3 days after medication discontinued; no MAOIs for 2 weeks after discontinuing SSRIs; wait 2 weeks after discontinuing MAOIs to start (except fluoxetine).
citalopram (Celexa)*	Depression SAD,† panic disorder,† PTSD†/ OCD† hot flashes*†/PMDD†	Higher acceptability. Tolerability similar to sertraline. Monitor weight, TSH
escitalopram (Lexapro)*	Depression, generalized anxiety disorder Depression in children ages 12–17	Higher efficacy and acceptability Shortest onset of action 1–2 weeks Monitor TSH, weight Insomnia that increases 50% with 20 mg dose

Drugs Commonly Prescribed 18.2   Selective Serotonin Reuptake Inhibitors (SSRIs)—cont'd

Drug	Indication	Adverse Reactions and Prescribing Considerations
fluoxetine (Prozac)*	Bulimia Depression OCD Panic disorder PMDD Depression and OCD in children	Less severe discontinuation syndrome due to long half-life. Nausea (20%), headache, GI complaints (10%), anxiety, nervousness, insomnia, drowsiness, fatigue, dizziness, tremor Monitoring parameters: Weight, LFTs, thyroid function tests (TFTs), and growth rate Must wait 5 weeks after discontinuing before initiating MAOI
fluvoxamine (Luvox)*	OCD Social anxiety disorder	More side effects than other SSRIs Monitor growth rate and weight
paroxetine (Paxil)*	Depression Generalized anxiety Hot flashes Menopause OCD Panic PTSD PMDD SAD	Most severe discontinuation syndrome Weight gain variable Nausea/vomiting occur in 25%, xerostomia, sedation, insomnia, tremor Monitor renal function and LFTs and TSH
sertraline (Zoloft)*	Depression OCD Panic PTSD PMDD SAD	High efficacy. Nausea, vomiting, diarrhea, drowsiness, headache Monitor LFTs, TSH, weight
fluoxetine/olanzapine (Symbyax)	Bipolar depression Treatment-resistant depression (failed two separate antidepressants)	Remission rate of 25.5% Same as each individual medications
Serotonin-Norepinephrine Reuptake Inhibitors (SNRIs)		
All SNRIs		Common to most SNRIs: Response rates—60%–70% Remission rates—up to 50% Risk of overdose intermediate between low SSRI to high TCA Avoid sudden discontinuation. Do not prescribe with MAOIs Hepatic excretion: Monitor LFTs. Agitation, weakness, dizziness, headache, drowsiness, insomnia, nausea/vomiting (self-limiting 1–3 weeks), and xerostomia. SIADH, serotonin syndrome (caution with "triptans") SNRI-induced mania If anxiety/panic disorder develops or history of such, start low and adjust dose slowly. Contraindicated in uncontrolled closed-angle glaucoma. Sexual dysfunction that resolves in 1–3 days after medication discontinued. Monitor BP for onset induced hypertension and orthostatic hypotension, no MAOIs for 5 days after discontinuing SNRIs; wait 2 weeks after discontinuing MAOIs to start.

Continued

Drugs Commonly Prescribed 18.2   Selective Serotonin Reuptake Inhibitors (SSRIs)—cont'd

Drug	Indication	Adverse Reactions and Prescribing Considerations
desvenlafaxine (Pristiq)*	Depression	No monitoring required.
duloxetine (Cymbalta)*	Depression Diabetic neuropathy Fibromyalgia GAD Musculoskeletal pain Osteoarthritis	Do not use with hepatic impairment or seizure disorder. May cause hepatic failure. May cause symptomatic orthostatic hypotension. May cause hypertension.
venlafaxine (Effexor)*	Depression GAD Panic disorder Social anxiety disorder	Monitor BP due to potential emergent hypertension. Insomnia, nervousness. Associated with weight loss. Monitor cholesterol.

*Black Box Warning:** Children, suicide ideation.
†Non–FDA approved.
PMDD, premenstrual dysphoric disorder; SAD, social anxiety disorder; SIADH, syndrome of inappropriate antidiuretic hormone secretion.

Tetracyclics

Drug	Indication	Adverse Reactions and Prescribing Considerations
mirtazapine (Remeron)*	Depression	Response and remission rates—53%–63% Somnolence (high incidence) and weight gain. Precautions include dizziness, increased cholesterol levels, elevated liver transaminase, and orthostatic hypotension. Risk of seizures at higher doses. Can cause agranulocytosis. Monitor glucose, liver transaminases, lipids, BUN/creatinine (Cr), and ECG.
maprotiline (Ludiomil)*	Depression	Contraindicated with MAOIs. Seizure precaution; caution with CVD. Monitor liver transaminases, TFTs, and ECG

Serotonin Modulator

Drug	Indication	Adverse Reactions and Prescribing Considerations
nefazodone (Serzone)*	Depression	Risk of hepatic failure. Response rate—35%–67% Remission—35%–52% Modest antidepressant; used mainly for hypnotic and anxiolytic effects. Allow washout period when discontinuing fluoxetine and starting nefazodone (at least 1 week). Monitor liver transaminases
trazodone (Desyrel)*	Depression	Avoid electroconvulsive therapy (ECT); do not give after myocardial infarction; potentiates alcohol, other CNS depressants; sedative effect; avoid use before or after discontinuation of MAOIs without adequate period. Monitor ECG, liver transaminases, BUN/Cr

Miscellaneous: Aminoketone Derivative

Drug	Indication	Adverse Reactions and Prescribing Considerations
bupropion (Wellbutrin)*	Depression Nicotine withdrawal SAD	May decrease weight. Less sexual side effects. Avoid use in known seizure disorders. Avoid use with history of eating disorders. Response rate—52%–70%

Drugs Commonly Prescribed 18.2   Selective Serotonin Reuptake Inhibitors (SSRIs)—cont'd

Drug	Indication	Adverse Reactions and Prescribing Considerations
		Effective in smoking cessation; less sexual dysfunction; safe in overdose Increased risk of seizure

TCAs

Drug	Indication	Adverse Reactions and Prescribing Considerations
All TCAs	In addition to major indications may be used in conjunction with mood stabilizers and antipsychotics to treat concomitant depression	Common to most TCAs: Response rates—43%–70%. Remission rates—25%–60% Narrow therapeutic index; high lethality with overdose Analgesic, anticholinergic, and antimuscarine actions; high side-effect burden Risk of cardiotoxicity Variable depending on specific drug Wait 2 weeks after discontinuation of fluoxetine, MAOIs. Do not use with history of seizures, glaucoma, urinary retention. Monitor for suicidality, drug levels helpful to monitor. Monitor ECG and BP. Treat constipation with fiber and exercise.
amitriptyline (Elavil)*	Depression	Monitor TFTs, liver transaminases, ECG, serum concentrations
amoxapine (Asendin)*	Depression	Moderate sedation. Monitor orthostatic BP, may cause tardive dyskinesia and NMS Monitor TFTs, liver transaminases, ECG, serum concentrations
clomipramine (Anafranil)*	OCD	Strong anticholinergic effect and sedation, hypotension Monitor ECG and liver transaminases
desipramine (Norpramin)*	Depression	Less sedating Monitor ECG and liver transaminases, TFTs
doxepin (Sinequan)*	Anxiety Atopic dermatitis Depression Eczema Insomnia Lichen simplex	Strong sedation and orthostatic hypotension Monitor ECG and liver transaminases, serum concentration
imipramine (Tofranil)*	Depression Enuresis	Moderated effect on sedation and hypotension Monitor ECG and liver transaminases, serum concentrations
nortriptyline (Pamelor)*	Depression	Monitor TFTs, liver transaminases, ECG, serum concentrations
protriptyline (Vivactil)*	Depression	Strong anticholinergic effects, mild sedation ECG, liver transaminases
trimipramine (Surmontil)*	Depression	Strong sedation effect, monitor orthostatic blood pressure ECG, liver transaminases, TFTs

*__Black Box Warning:__ Children, suicide ideation.

Continued

Drugs Commonly Prescribed 18.2   Selective Serotonin Reuptake Inhibitors (SSRIs)—cont'd

MAOI

Drug	Indication	Adverse Reactions and Prescribing Considerations
isocarboxazid (Marplan)*	Depression	60%–70% remission rates; may be better in atypical depression; requires dietary restrictions. Common foods to avoid, cheese, dried fruits, bananas, chocolate, raspberries. Dextromethorphan potential for serious adverse effects and necessity of dietary restrictions, MAOIs (e.g., phenelzine, tranylcypromine) generally are not used as initial therapy for major depressive disorder. Monitor liver transaminases and renal function
tranylcypromine (Parnate)	Depression	Monitor liver transaminases and renal function
phenelzine (Nardil)*	Depression	Monitor liver transaminases and renal function

*Black Box Warning: Children, suicide ideation.
Source: Clinical pharmacology [database online]. Gold Standard, Inc., Tampa, FL, 2013. http://cp.gsm.com.

major depression can be significant. It is unlikely that, in a primary-care setting, practitioners will be able to meet all of a patient's support needs. For this reason, new sources of support should be identified. Friends, relatives, and spouse or partners are important potential sources of information, comfort, and assistance. Professional-led support groups and peer self-help groups are also highly effective.

Support is an important resource for all depressed patients, but patients who are anxious or irritable may require a great deal of practitioner patience. Anxious, irritable patients can be indecisive, critical, and demanding and can appear uncooperative or uninterested. Every effort must be made to avoid getting into a power struggle or challenging upset patients. In the long run, reassuring acceptance is easier and more effective.

Establishing a routine and focusing on activities and behaviors rather than feelings may be a constructive approach. Massage, relaxation therapies, exercise, good nutrition, and a variety of forms of self-care should be initiated and supported.

For some patients, the only important outcome of treatment for major depression is symptom relief. Normalized sleep, appetite, mood, energy, and concentration should, however, be viewed as minimal patient outcomes. Symptom relief and symptom remission are necessary patient outcomes, but if the patient's risk for future episodes of depression is to be significantly lowered, additional outcomes need to be addressed. Improved patient depression awareness is important. Patients treated for major depression should, as a stated outcome of treatment, increase their understanding of major depression and improve their personal methods of coping with depression. The most important outcome is that the patient will immediately seek help

should symptoms of major depression return. Recurrent episodes of major depression or major depression that has continued unrelieved for months or is characterized by extremely high symptom levels requires referral and specialized care, sometimes in an inpatient setting.

Follow-up and Referral

Follow-up during treatment of depression and/or anxiety is absolutely necessary to ensure adherence to therapy. The patient must be monitored to ensure that the prescription was filled and that the medication was taken. Treatment outcome should be assessed regularly using formal diagnostic assessment tools. Target symptoms are used to evaluate the effectiveness of medication during early stages of treatment and until full symptom remission is obtained. In moderate to severe depression, follow-up is determined by the severity of the initial PHQ-9.

A reasonable criterion for extending the initial treatment is to assess whether the patient is experiencing a 25% or greater reduction in baseline symptom severity at 6 weeks of therapeutic dose. If the patient's symptoms are reduced by 25% or more, but the patient is not yet at remission, and if medication has been well tolerated, continue to prescribe. Raising the dose is recommended. In the acute phase of treatment and recovery, the patient should be seen or contacted every 1 to 2 weeks within the first month of therapy and at least once in the succeeding 4 to 8 weeks. For persons who can be treated effectively with antidepressant medication, satisfactory symptom remission often is achieved within 4 to 8 weeks. Many patients begin to feel better in 2 to 3 weeks. When the patient reports target symptom relief or the assessment indicates symptom remission has been achieved, the practitioner and patient develop a treatment and discontinuation plan. The duration of medication treatment for uncomplicated major depression is at a minimum 6 to 12 months at the treatment dose (Level I; Institute for Clinical Systems Improvement, 1996; Michigan Quality Improvement Consortium, 2012; Kaiser Permanente Care Management Institute, 2012). The treatment duration algorithm is available from https://www.icsi.org/_asset/fnhdm3/Depr.pdf. A longer treatment period is recommended for patients with complicated or multiple disorders or patients who have a history of one or more years of untreated depression. In these instances, treatment duration should extend from 15 months to 5 years. Short half-life antidepressants are discontinued gradually over a period of 2 to 3 weeks. Persons who experience significant serotonin withdrawal syndrome may report flu-like symptoms that last a few days. Consultation with a specialist should be considered if withdrawal symptoms appear to be significant or persistent.

Patient Education

It is vital for the provider to teach the patient and significant other(s) to report signs of increased agitation, irritability, and suicidality. Emergency phone numbers (such as crisis services) and tertiary care sites need to be given to the patient and significant others should such symptoms emerge. It has been known for some time that in some cases, starting a severely depressed patient on antidepressants may, after 1 to 2 weeks of treatment, provide the boost in energy needed for the patient to design and carry out a suicide plan. Danger signs and symptoms include the following:

- Hallucinations or delusions
- Severe adverse effects from antidepressant medications (e.g., severe urinary retention, fluctuation in blood pressure, seizures, cardiac complications)
- Suicidal thoughts
- Extreme self-care deficits (e.g., not able to care for basic needs)

The person and his or her family need to understand that depression generates feelings of helplessness, powerlessness, and pessimism; major decisions should be delayed. The practitioner should reassure the patient that current feelings will change. All side effects of drugs should be clearly understood, and the provider should stress the importance of taking medication daily as ordered for maximum effect. The clinician should advise the patient and family that drugs to offset adverse effects are available, or that medication can be changed. Patients should be encouraged to maintain a schedule of activities and to maintain their regularly scheduled visits with their primary-care clinician.

■ BIPOLAR AND RELATED DISORDERS

Bipolar disorder (BD) is commonly seen in the primary-care setting and is frequently mistaken for other conditions, most commonly major depressive disorder (MDD).

The spectrum of bipolar disorder includes bipolar I (BD I), bipolar II (BD II), cyclothymic disorder, substance/medication-induced bipolar, and bipolar and related disorders due to another medical condition. The three major categories—BD I, BD II, and cyclothymic disorder—will be discussed here.

Defining the length of the manic episode helps to differentiate between the various disorders. Patients with BD I have had at least one episode of true mania preceded by or followed by hypomanic or a major depressive episode. BD II is characterized by recurrent depression and hypomania. Cyclomania involves symptoms of hypomania and depression that do not meet the full criteria for any one disorder. Symptom criteria for BD I, BD II, and cyclomania with descriptions of mania and hypomania are presented in Table 18.6.

Clinicians must be able to distinguish between depressive episodes occurring in the context of unipolar depression and bipolar mood disorders because patients suffering from BD require mood-stabilizing pharmacological therapy, and their symptoms may worsen with antidepressant monotherapy. Emerging data from a variety of sources have confirmed a typical delay between symptom onset and diagnosis of 5 to 10 years, with patients seeing an average of four health-care providers before the correct diagnosis is given. MDD is a common misdiagnosis, the treatment for which (e.g., antidepressant monotherapy) may induce mania in BD patients. Over a 5-year period, 85% of patients with BD will have a relapse after one affective episode. During interepisodic periods, half of the patients may experience subsyndromal symptoms, such as cognitive impairment and impulsivity; the length of interepisode intervals progressively diminishes with each recurrence. Inappropriate pharmacological treatment for BD is associated with increases in morbidity and mortality and with suicide. BD is frequently encountered in primary care; therefore, for optimal outcomes, an accurate history, assessment, and diagnosis are required (see Table 18.6).

Epidemiology and Causes

The pathogenesis of bipolar disorder is as yet unknown, but biological, psychological, and social factors are thought to contribute. Depression and BD differ significantly in their genetics, prognosis, and treatment. BD is the sixth leading cause of disability worldwide in patients aged 15 to 55. The financial burden of this disorder eclipses that of diabetes, and the impact on occupational function due to BD is more extensive than in major depressive disorder. Two-thirds of patients with BD are substantially adversely affected by their illness; but the negative impact of BD goes beyond its morbidity rate. Twenty-five percent to 50% of patients with BD have a lifetime risk of suicide attempt; up to 15% of patients will complete the attempt. Suicide attempts can occur in patients in the manic, hypomanic, depressive, and mixed phases of BD but are most likely to occur in patients in a depressive or mixed state.

Table 18.6   Symptom Criteria for BD I, BD II, and Cyclothymic Disorder

BD I: To meet symptom criteria identification of at least one lifetime mania episode must have occurred (see description below). Often mania episodes are preceded by or followed by hypomania or major depressive episodes. A major depressive episode is not required for the diagnosis. Various specifiers can also be included. Refer to the DSM-5 for further information.

BD II: To meet symptom criteria identification of at least one hypomania episode and one major depressive episode must have occurred (see description below). NO history of a mania episode. Various specifiers can also be included. Refer to the DSM-5 for further information.

Cyclothymic Disorder—numerous episodes of depressed mood that do not meet full criteria for major depression, mania, or hypomania that have occurred over a 2-year period for adults or 1 year in children and adolescents. There have been no symptom-free periods for greater than 2 months. Specifier may include anxious distress. These patients have a 15%–50% chance of developing BD I or BD II.

Mania

A distinct period of abnormally elevated or irritable mood lasting at least 7 days and accompanied by either three of the symptoms below with euphoria **or** four of the symptoms below with irritability: grandiosity, psychomotor agitation or an increased involvement in planning or executing multiple activities, high-risk behavior with adverse consequences, a decreased need for sleep, incessant talking or pressured speech, racing thoughts, and distractibility. In addition, the symptoms cause significant functional impairment and are not related to a medical illness, therapeutic drug, or a drug of abuse. May include psychotic features in as many as 50%–80% of patients, but this is not a necessary criterion. Symptoms are marked and often require hospitalization.

Hypomania

A distinct period of persistently elevated, expansive or irritable mood, lasting for at least 4 days, that is clearly different from the usual nondepressed mood. Symptoms can include grandiosity, psychomotor agitation or an increased involvement in planning or executing multiple activities, high-risk behavior with adverse consequences, a decreased need for sleep, incessant talking or pressured speech, racing thoughts, and distractibility. Symptoms are not severe enough to cause marked impairment in occupational or social functioning and do not require hospitalization, but the changes are noticeable by others and clearly differ from the person's baseline functioning. No psychotic features are present, and the symptoms cause significant functional impairment and are not related to a medical illness, therapeutic drug, or a drug of abuse.

Major Depressive Episode

The symptom criteria for major depression state that five (or more) of the following symptoms have been present during the same 2-week period and represent a change from previous functioning. At least one of the symptoms is either (1) depressed mood or (2) loss of interest or pleasure: Depressed mood expressed by the patient as feelings of sadness or hopelessness. Depressed mood may also be reported by significant others and may be reported as tearfulness. These symptoms need to be present nearly every day and for most of each day. Irritability may be the primary symptom in adolescents and children, markedly diminished interest or pleasure (apathy) in most activities, change in appetite nearly every day or a weight loss defined as greater than 5% of body weight loss over a 1-month period, insomnia or hypersomnia, observable behavioral agitation or retardation, loss of energy nearly every day, feelings of worthlessness or guilt, loss of concentration or indecisiveness, recurrent thoughts of death or suicide. The symptoms cause significant functional impairment and are not related to a medical illness, therapeutic drug, or a drug of abuse.

Adapted from American Psychiatric Association. *Diagnostic and statistical manual of mental disorders, fifth edition* (DSM-5). American Psychiatric Association, Arlington, VA, 2013.

BD I has a lifetime prevalence of 1% to 3%; when the entire spectrum of bipolar disorder is included, the prevalence may approach 7% to 10%. Men and women are equally affected, although BD II is more common in women. The mean age of onset of BD I is 18 years of age, and for BD II it is 20 years of age. It can occur in early childhood, adolescence, or as late as the sixth or seventh decade. New onset of mania after age 40 is rare and should prompt consideration of a medical condition, such as frontotemporal neurocognitive disorder, thyroid dysfunction, or substance abuse or withdrawal.

Genetic components appear to play a significant role in transmitting BD II. On average, there is a 10-fold risk

for first-degree relatives with MDD; they are 1.5 to 2.5 times more likely to have BD I than first-degree relatives of control subjects. The fact that about 50% of all BD I patients have at least one parent with a mood disorder (most often MDD) further supports inheritability. If one parent has BD I, the child has a 25% chance of developing a mood disorder. When both parents have BD I, the odds of their child developing a mood disorder range from 50% to 75%. Support of the genetic basis of mood disorder is also found in twin and adoption studies, which show a strong genetic component for the inheritance of BD I. It is unknown how culture affects the expression of bipolar disorder. Transcultural validation of screening tools is unknown and therefore difficult to evaluate.

Pathophysiology and Psychopathology

Depression and mania are affective states on a continuum of mood disorder. As such, many current biological theories of depression also apply to mania. Several genetic variants were associated with bipolar disorder in genome-wide association studies. Clinical consequences of BD have profound effects on the quality of life for patients living with BD. Understanding of the complex gene–environment interactions is likely to emerge in the future and holds great promise for clearer understanding of affective illness.

Clinical Presentation

BD may be viewed as a disorder of "elevated mood" that may manifest itself as euphoria or irritability or dysphoria, characterized by a depressed mood with or without irritability. Approximately 25% of all patients experience episodes of pure mania, 40% demonstrate mixed (dysphoric) mania, and 10% to 25% are called "rapid cyclers," manifesting rapid shifts from mania to depression. Onset of a BD mood episode typically begins with depression. Descriptions of mania, hypomania, and cyclomania are presented in Table 18.6.

Onset of BD occurs in prepubertal years, in adolescence, or in adulthood. An initial manic episode may be related to an adverse life event or stressor; however, subsequent episodes may occur without an identifiable trigger. Seasonal changes may result in fall or winter depression and spring or summer mania. Light exposure may trigger manic episodes. Many women with BD report mood changes related to the menstrual cycle. Manic episodes usually last 3 to 6 months if untreated, and the symptoms typically escalate rapidly during a period of days. Psychotic symptoms may be present in the acute manic phase or in the depressive phase. Psychotic depression should raise an index of suspicion that the patient may have an underlying bipolar disorder. Older adult patients may manifest irritability rather than elated mood. Untreated depressive episodes may last 6 to 12 months, and some treatment-resistant patients suffering from depression may actually have BD. Almost 90% of all persons with BD experience depression, and most BD patients present for treatment during a depressive episode. In *all* patients presenting with depression, clinicians should inquire specifically about symptoms of past manic or hypomanic episodes, past treatment and responses, and family history. Patients may be asymptomatic during interepisode periods.

Over a 5-year period, 85% of patients with BD will have a relapse after one affective episode. Though some patients experience limited functional recovery despite successful syndrome treatment, early intervention is associated with improved outcomes. Most commonly these patients present for treatment for a depressive

episode than for the euphoria associated with a manic or hypomanic episode. Only one lifetime manic or hypomanic episode is required for a patient to be diagnosed with BD. Often patients, for a variety of reasons, may leave out this episode when reviewing their medical history and clinicians may fail to query or recognize previous hypomanic or manic symptoms. Some patients may even identify periods of normal mood as depressed when compared with mania.

Diagnostic Reasoning
DSM-5 Symptom Criteria

The DSM-5 symptom criteria for the spectrum of bipolar disorders are presented in Table 18.6.

The following mnemonic, DIGFAST, is useful for identifying BD:

- Distractibility
- Insomnia (decreased need for sleep)
- Grandiosity (inflated self-esteem)
- Flight of ideas (racing thoughts, negative for rumination)
- Activities (increased, goal directed)
- Speech (pressured, increased talkativeness)
- Thoughtlessness (pleasure-seeking activities that show poor judgment such as spending sprees, sexual indiscretions, reckless driving, arguments if irritable)

Differential Diagnosis
Bipolar I

The differential diagnoses to consider are the following: MDD, other bipolar disorder, anxiety disorders, attention-deficit/hyperactivity disorder (ADHD), personality disorders, and substance use. It is essential to obtain a full psychiatric history and also, if the patient consents, to interview family and friends to corroborate information and establish the diagnosis of BD (Level II; Suppers et al, 2001). Patients with mania often lack insight into their symptoms and often do not report them. They feel euphoric during a manic episode and value their productivity during an episode of hypomania. Family members and friends may be able to report historical clues, personal factors, and suicidal ideation that may be associated with increased suicide risk and may point to a diagnosis of BD that the patient has not revealed to any clinician. As part of the history, ask specifically about the onset, frequency, and duration of symptoms, distractibility, seasonality, and other characteristics of a depressed patient's high and low moods, to help differentiate between bipolar and unipolar depression (see Table 18.7).

Bipolar II

In addition to the differential diagnoses listed for BP I, schizophrenia spectrum disorders need to be considered. It is essential to inquire about suicide, because most suicide attempts are associated with depressive episodes or during depressive features of mixed episodes.

Table 18.7 Distinguishing Between Bipolar and Unipolar Depressive Episodes

- Ask all depressed patients about history of mania and hypomania.
- Ask about family history of bipolar disorder—"loaded" family history is a clue to bipolarity in "unipolar" patients.
- Involve family member and/or significant other in screening process.
- Administer a screening instrument for bipolar disorder, such as the Mood Disorder Questionnaire.
- Early age at onset (<25 years) is another clue for bipolarity.
- Psychotic features are another clinical clue for bipolarity in the seemingly unipolar patient, as is seasonal pattern.
- Adverse and/or inadequate antidepressant response such as treatment-emergent hypomania or agitation, erratic or uneven antidepressant responses, multiple antidepressant failures, or "treatment-resistant depression."

Source: Adapted from Hirschfeld, RM, and Vornik, LA: Recognition and diagnosis of bipolar disorder. *J Clin Psychiatry* 65(Suppl 15):5–9, 2004; and Loganathan, M, et al. When to suspect bipolar disorder. *J Fam Pract* 59(12):682–688, 2010.

Cyclothymic Disorder

Differentiating between the various bipolar disorders can be a major challenge, especially in determining the length of previous episodes. In addition, borderline personality disorders and substance-induced disorders need to be considered.

Overall Considerations for All Bipolar Disorders

The two diagnoses most likely to be confused with bipolar disorders are substance abuse and cluster B personality disorders, and there may be comorbidities with these entities. However, in substance abuse, euphoria/dysphoria is temporally related to drug intoxication and withdrawal state. In cluster B personality disorders, "mood swings" last from minutes to hours to days, not weeks to months, and are typically closely associated to interpersonal disruptions or alliances.

Inquire about chronic or recurrent nonspecific physical symptoms (e.g., fatigue, headache, or gastrointestinal distress) and about depressive or manic feelings and behaviors. Consider medical disorders that may coexist or appear similar to BD. Medical disorders to consider are thyroid dysfunction, vasculitis, chronic infection, malignancies, and metabolic disorders. Clinical and laboratory findings may help to exclude these causes. Review family history, particularly of first-degree relatives. Ask about recent medications, including hormonal contraceptives, and about treatment during prior episodes. Evaluate any suspected temporal association between drugs and symptoms because many drugs can induce or exacerbate manic or depressive symptoms. Levodopa and corticosteroids are the most common causes of

drug-induced mania; these agents can also cause depressive symptoms.

Patients with BD may choose to self-medicate with drugs and alcohol to relieve anxiety, insomnia, agitation, and excessive fatigue. Drugs, alcohol, and some medications may also contribute to these symptoms. Over half of those patients who meet the criteria for bipolar disorder have an alcohol or substance-use disorder or other mental health disorder, increasing the risk for suicide attempt. Assess the severity, frequency, and longitudinal course of depressive and manic episodes and determine whether the symptoms meet the specific diagnostic criteria for bipolar or another psychiatric disorder. Ask about deterioration in the baseline level of functioning at work or school or in personal relationships.

Patients with BD appear especially sensitive to sleep deprivation, which may occur in conjunction with stressors such as bereavement, childbirth, vacation, longer work hours, and shift changes. They may experience periods of decreased need for sleep. Specific details about sleep–wake periods, including daytime naps, meal times, social activities, hobbies and other areas of interest, interpersonal attitudes, and ability to work and perform household tasks are helpful. Inquire about a typical day.

Patients with mania or depression usually do not report characteristic psychological descriptors (e.g., elation, grandiosity, inflated self-esteem, racing thoughts, irritability or agitation), so activities may provide diagnostic clues. For example, grandiose thinking may manifest as reckless gambling, spending sprees, or sexual promiscuity. Conversely, increased productivity, enhanced perceptual ability, altered view on interpersonal relationships, and fluctuating symptoms without substantial negative social or occupational consequences suggest hypomania.

Routine screening for depression is advised in primary-care settings, but little attention has been focused on screening for past episodes of hypomania or mania. The Mood Disorder Questionnaire (MDQ) is a validated screening tool for BD (Fig. 18.1). The likelihood of underdiagnosis or a missed diagnosis is greatly lessened by the routine use of a screening instrument such as the MDQ. Use of the MDQ can identify 70% of persons with BD while eliminating the diagnosis for 90% of persons without the predilection. More recently, there has been some question whether the MDQ may underdiagnose BD II disorder because of the requirement for moderate to severe impairment of functioning as many patients feel that during a hypomanic episode they actually function better. The Bipolar Spectrum Diagnostic Scale is better for ruling out the diagnosis of BD than for giving a positive diagnosis. If a patient scores positive for BD on this scale, further clinical evaluation is necessary to make the diagnosis.

Always assess for suicide risk. It is essential to inquire about suicide ideation and intentions, and about extent of plans or preparations for, prior attempts at, family history of, and recent exposure to suicide. This is essential

1. Has there ever been a period of time when you were not your usual self and...	YES	NO
...you felt so good or so hyper that other people thought you were not your normal self, or you were so hyper that you got into trouble?	❏	❏
...you were so irritable that you shouted at people or started fights or arguments?	❏	❏
...you felt much more self-confident than usual?	❏	❏
...you got much less sleep than usual and found that you didn't really miss it?	❏	❏
...you were much more talkative or spoke faster than usual?	❏	❏
...thoughts raced through your head or you couldn't slow your mind down?	❏	❏
...you were so easily distracted by things around you that you had trouble concentrating or staying on track?	❏	❏
...you had much more energy than usual?	❏	❏
...you were much more active or did many more things than usual?	❏	❏
...you were much more social or outgoing than usual; for example, you telephoned friends in the middle of the night?	❏	❏
...you were much more interested in sex than usual?	❏	❏
...you did things that were unusual for you or that other people might have thought were excessive, foolish, or risky?	❏	❏
...spending money got you or your family into trouble?	❏	❏

2. If you checked YES to more than one of the above, have several of these ever happened during the same period of time? *Please circle one response only.*

YES   NO

3. How much of a problem did any of these cause you — like being unable to work; having family, money, or legal troubles; getting into arguments or fights? *Please circle one response only.*

No problem   Minor problem   Moderate problem   Serious problem

Figure 18.1 The Mood Disorder Questionnaire (MDQ). *(Source: Hirschfeld, RM, et al. Development and validation of a screening instrument for bipolar spectrum disorder: The Mood Disorder Questionnaire. Am J Psychiatry 157:1873–1875, 2000).*

both at presentation and during subsequent mood episodes because the lifetime risk for suicide in patients with BD is up to 15%. Most suicide attempts are associated with depressive episodes or during depressive features of mixed episodes.

Diagnostic Work-up

A complete physical exam is needed, as well as a neurological assessment to exclude other etiologies of mood symptoms or psychosis. The patient's mental status should be assessed, including general appearance, attitude, behaviors, mood, affect, speech, thought processes and content, concentration, and memory. Focus the physical and neurological exam (cranial nerves, reflexes, muscle tone, gait) on identifying or excluding a medical cause of the patient's symptoms, comorbidity, and the possibility of precipitating factors such as thyroid disorder, head injuries, or substance abuse.

Diagnostic testing may include a complete blood count (CBC) with differential, platelet count, comprehensive blood chemistry panel, thyroxine (T_4), thyroid-stimulating hormone (TSH), rapid plasma reagin (RPR), HIV antibody test, urinalysis, urine toxicology screen, and pregnancy test. In the setting of HIV/AIDS, hepatitis C, and other infectious causes, new-onset mood or bipolar-like symptoms require further studies to exclude organic causes of mood changes. Consider conducting a Mini-Mental State Exam to assess cognition. Refer to neurology or infectious disease to assist with diagnosis if indicated. Brain magnetic resonance imaging (MRI) or computed tomography (CT) scans may be helpful if clinical findings suggest an underlying organic central nervous system (CNS) disorder.

Management
Pharmacological Management

The ideal treatment goal for patients with BD is complete remission of current symptoms, prevention of future affective episodes, and return to premorbid function.

Mainstays of therapy are mood-stabilizing medications. Drug therapy is used to achieve symptom remission and return function in patient with BD. Mood stabilizers, second generation antipsychotics, first generation antipsychotics, and adjunctive anxiolytics and antidepressants are used to treat BD. Factors in determining which medication will most likely result in treatment remission depend on the diagnosis—BD I or BD II, manic versus depressed, acute or maintenance, rapid cycling versus nonrapid cycling, and whether psychotic symptoms exist. Attempts should be made to use the lowest possible dose to minimize side effects, particularly with first generation agents.

Considerations before initiating therapy include the patient's age, because the elderly may be more sensitive to side effects of antipsychotic medications. It is essential to prescribe the lowest possible dose and monitor for side effects. Always consider the possibility of pregnancy in women of childbearing age before initiating psychotropic medications. Knowledge of past treatment history, effectiveness, tolerability, failures, and side effect profiles allows the practitioner to provide individualized, patient-centered care. It is likely there will be a need to change treatment modalities over time. Several weeks are required to assess the effects of a new treatment.

Collaboration with a psychiatrist will aid the clinician in selecting appropriate drug therapy to treat acute manic episodes in patients with BD (Levels I, II; Akiskal et al, 2005). The mainstays of BD drug treatment are those with mood-stabilizing properties. Treatment options for patients with BD I and acute hypomania, mania, or mixed episodes should begin with lithium, valproic acid (Depakote), or antipsychotic agents. Carbamazepine (Tegretol) or oxcarbazepine (Trileptal) may also be used. If there is no response or a partial response, combination therapy such as lithium plus valproic acid, lithium plus an atypical antipsychotic, or an atypical antipsychotic plus valproic acid may be considered. If still not effective, clozapine (Clozaril) may be added or electroconvulsive therapy (ECT) may be introduced.

It is important that lithium be prescribed at a therapeutic dose. Valproic acid is now usually preferred, however, for patients with multiple manic episodes, mixed episodes, and rapid cycling. Carbamazepine, another anticonvulsant agent, is a good alternative. Combinations of these agents may be used if patients do not respond to a single agent. If the patient does not respond fully, atypical antipsychotics may be added to one or more mood stabilizers. Lamotrigine (Lamictal) has proved particularly effective for rapid cycling, particularly in patients with severe depression. Lamotrigine should not be initiated in primary care. Long-acting benzodiazepines, such as clonazepam and lorazepam, may be used for rapid treatment of manic symptoms and to calm and sedate patients until acute mania or hypomania has subsided and the mood stabilizer has taken effect. In the case of psychotic symptoms, antipsychotics may be

added. ECT may be used for patients with severe BD with drug treatment–resistant mania or psychotic depression.

Episodes of depression pose particular challenges. There are fewer approved treatments for bipolar depression. Overall, antidepressant medications do not control depression as effectively in bipolar as in unipolar depression and may trigger mania. Mood stabilization is still the primary goal, however, and mood stabilization therapy (lithium, carbamazepine, and valproic acid) should be optimized (in the case of lithium, serum level of 0.8 mEq/L or above) before starting antidepressant therapy. If depression persists 2 to 4 weeks after optimization of the mood stabilizer, it is recommended that either bupropion (antidepressant), lamotrigine (anticonvulsant, mood stabilizer), or an SSRI (antidepressant) should be added. These agents are not mood stabilizers. They are effective against depression but can precipitate mania and should not be given to a bipolar patient without a transitional mood stabilizer. Venlafaxine may also be useful in some cases of severe depression that have not responded to other therapy. Any patient developing symptoms of hypomania while taking an antidepressant should stop taking it; in addition, he or she should be slowly tapered after a period of sustained remission. Severely depressed or delusional patients may benefit from an antipsychotic.

Lithium remains the gold standard for treatment of BD and has been shown to be uniquely effective in decreasing suicidal behavior. Lithium appears to be most effective early in the course of the illness, for classic manic symptoms, in patients in whom depression immediately follows mania, and in patients with a strong family history of BD. However, lithium also has a number of potential adverse effects, including a life-threatening neurotoxicity that can occur at serum levels higher than 2.0 mEq/L. Lithium levels should be obtained twice weekly until the patient's clinical status and levels are stable at which time they may be obtained every 1 to 3 months. Serum trough lithium levels are drawn 8 to 12 hours after the last dose.

Adverse drug interactions can occur with such commonly used drugs as thiazide diuretics, NSAIDs, angiotensin-converting enzyme (ACE) inhibitors, diltiazem (Cardizem), verapamil (Calan, Verelan), and antipsychotics. Additional potential adverse effects include nausea, diarrhea, tremor, polyuria, and polydipsia. Lithium may exacerbate psoriasis and acne, cause hypothyroidism (5% to 35%), and in 20% of patients (usually after 15 or more years of treatment) lead to renal insufficiency. Lithium takes several weeks to become effective and may contribute to weight gain of at least 7% of baseline. Owing to potential adverse effects, lithium therapy should be preceded by an evaluation of renal, cardiac, and thyroid function, as well as a pregnancy test. Most patients demonstrate residual symptoms during maintenance therapy. If depression persists, the patient may need an adjunctive antidepressant. Many patients do not stay on lithium. Some regret the loss of the exhilaration that occurs during a manic episode; some patients are concerned about weight gain or tremor. In one study, 50% of patients acknowledged some degree of medication nonadherence in the previous 2 years, and 32% reported only partial adherence in the preceding month.

Anticonvulsant medications are not mood stabilizers; however, some of these agents have proven effective for the treatment and/or maintenance of mania and/or BD. These agents have become alternative treatments for patients who need a mood-stabilizing agent but who do not fare well with lithium; additionally, these medications also may be used in combination with lithium. Anticonvulsant agents work by enhancing the inhibitory activity of the neurotransmitter gamma-aminobutyric acid (GABA).

Divalproex/valproic acid is considered first-line pharmacological treatment for acute mania or mixed episodes and maintenance. There is some evidence of antidepressant effect as well. Divalproex appears to be most effective for rapid cycling and mixed episodes, in patients who have had more than three manic episodes, and in patients with comorbid alcohol abuse. Valproic acid is comparable to lithium, and generally better tolerated, during the maintenance period. The most frequently observed side effects when valproic acid is used in the treatment of acute mania are nausea, vomiting, weight gain, tremor, dizziness, and sedation. Serious adverse effects include hepatotoxicity, pancreatitis, thrombocytopenia, and teratogenicity. Serum valproate levels, liver function tests, and CBCs should be monitored closely during treatment with valproic acid.

Valproic acid is a cytochrome 450 enzyme inhibitor and may engender metabolic interaction with other drugs. Valproic acid can induce menstrual irregularities and a higher risk for polycystic ovary syndrome (PCOS), which affects 2% to 7% of women in their reproductive years and is characterized by chronic anovulation and hyperandrogenism.

Carbamazepine is approved for the treatment of acute mania and mixed episodes associated with bipolar disorder. Therapeutic serum levels for BD have not been established; usually concentrations used for seizure disorders (4–12 mcg/mL) are applied. Serum levels as well as CBC, platelets, and liver function must all be monitored as potential side effects include agranulocytosis, aplastic anemia, hepatic failure, Stevens-Johnson syndrome, and pancreatitis. Carbamazepine reduces levels of other drugs, however, such as oral contraceptives and dihydropyridine calcium-channel blockers.

Lamotrigine received approval as maintenance therapy for BD in 2003. This agent appears to have antidepressant effects and has been found to be effective in rapid-cycling BD. The most significant adverse effects are Stevens-Johnson syndrome and toxic epidermal necrolysis, both of which can be fatal.

Typical antipsychotic agents such as haloperidol (Haldol) have been frequently used to treat bipolar mania as a class. These agents work well in reducing symptoms such as paranoia, hallucinations, delusions, and thought disturbances. However, they have not been studied for efficacy in treating BD and carry the risk of extrapyramidal symptoms (EPS), such as akathisia, dystonia, torticollis, parkinsonism, and tardive dyskinesia.

Newer second generation, or atypical, antipsychotics have a lower propensity to induce EPS. Both classes of drugs block dopaminergic transmission, but the newer drugs also act through various receptors such as dopamine, histamine, and alpha-adrenergic. These are standard agents for schizophrenia and are approved for use as monotherapy for mania and with mood stabilizers. See the section of this chapter on psychotic disorders for further discussion of typical and atypical antipsychotics.

Maintenance drug therapy should be based on the patient's response to initial treatment and in conjunction with a psychiatrist. Patients at high risk for recurrence should consider lifelong therapy, generally with mood stabilizers. Lithium and valproic acid are first-line agents used in maintenance therapy, alone and in combination. Although there are some differences in side effects, the dropout rates are similar, and both agents demonstrate equal effectiveness. Carbamazepine may be used as an alternative.

Adjunctive drug therapy should be considered for comorbid disorders. For example, if a patient with BD is compliant with medication yet has persistent symptoms, he or she may have a concurrent anxiety or substance use disorder. Antidepressants with mood stabilizers or antipsychotics as adjunctive agents may be used for treatment of depression. If a patient is persistently anxious, most psychiatrists will assess for a mixed state, occult substance abuse, or a medical condition. In summary, management options are based on the patients' primary symptoms of mania, depression, or mixed states (see Table 18.8). In addition, treatment algorithms can be accessed at www.dshs.state.tx.us/mhprograms/pdf/TIMABDman2007.pdf.

Nonpharmacological Management

Patients living with BD may have difficulty discussing unusual events or thoughts and often have poor insight regarding symptoms or the need for treatment. They respond best to proactive, collaborative, and individualized treatment, as exemplified in the *Circle of Caring* model. Developing a therapeutic alliance is imperative, because BD is chronic and needs long-term management. Establishing a trusting relationship with a medical home will provide patients the opportunity to experience continuity of care, to attend to health maintenance and any chronic medical problems, and to maintain a collaborative connection with their behavioral health providers and supports.

Obtain a consultation with a psychiatrist if you suspect BD once you have excluded medical etiologies. Accurate

Table 18.8   Management of Bipolar Disorder

Symptomatology—Manic/Mixed	Management Strategies
First-line	Lithium plus an antipsychotic Valproate plus an antipsychotic (Second generation antipsychotics are preferable) Carbamazepine Electroconvulsive therapy (may be used if preferred by the patient, patients with severe illness, or if patient is pregnant) For less ill patients, monotherapy with lithium, valproate, or an antipsychotic may be preferable
Adjunctive treatments	Benzodiazepine Gabapentin Topiramate
Nonresponse	Optimize the initial medication dose Add or change mood-stabilizing drug Add or change antipsychotic Add lamotrigine

Symptomatology—Depressed	Management Strategies
First-line	Lithium or lamotrigine Electroconvulsive therapy (for patients with life-threatening inanition, suicidality, or psychosis; severe depression/pregnancy)
Nonresponse	Optimize the initial medication dose Add another mood stabilizer Add an antipsychotic Add an antidepressant Electroconvulsive therapy

Source: Adapted from American Psychiatric Association. *Diagnostic and statistical manual of mental disorders, fifth edition* (DSM-5). American Psychiatric Association, Arlington, VA, 2013; and St. John, D. Bipolar affective disorder. *Clin Rev* 15(6):47, 2013.

diagnosis can be complicated because other psychiatric disorders may appear similar. Consultation will provide clinicians with a more accurate diagnosis as well as assistance with managing pharmacological regimens and acute crisis should it be necessary. Consider referral to an integrated treatment provider for dual-diagnosed patients with substance and/or alcohol dependence. Hospitalization is necessary for patients with BD who may be a danger to

themselves or others or who are unable to care for their needs. Patients with mood disorders, particularly mania, are often unwilling to enter a hospital voluntarily and may require involuntary commitment.

A supportive primary-care provider can help in monitoring the patient's overall status, as well as encouraging adherence to the medication regimen. The clinician can also provide referral for specific psychosocial interventions for patients with BD (Levels I, II; Miklowitz et al, 2003; Colom et al, 2003). Along with a psychiatrist, a behavioral health specialist may aid recovery by relieving depression, delaying episodes, and improving function and treatment adherence. Psychoeducation is aimed at providing information about BD and treatment and is an important resource for patients, families, and supports. The goals of psychoeducation are to increase knowledge and acceptance of the disorder and to address denial and nonadherence to the treatment plan. Meta-analysis has shown that patient education combined with drug treatment helps to improve adherence (Level II; Gonzalez-Pinto et al, 2004).

Psychotherapy, although not effective as monotherapy, can significantly enhance treatment response and prevent relapse. Interpersonal, family-focused, cognitive-behavioral, supportive, and psychoeducational approaches increase illness awareness, improve collaboration with health-care professionals and supportive family and friends, and may assist in lifestyle regulation. There is good evidence that cognitive-behavioral therapy (CBT) protects against relapse. CBT has proved efficacious, resulting in greater acute treatment response and supporting greater maintenance of treatment gains.

The onset of manic and depressive episodes is often associated with psychosocial stress. Patients should be encouraged to pace their activities at work and to maintain a regular schedule. A change in sleep patterns often heralds the onset of a manic or depressive episode. Insomnia may be a precipitant or a prodromal warning sign. Maintenance of regular sleep habits helps prevent escalation of mood symptoms into a full-blown episode. Educate BD patients and their families about the risks of stress, substance abuse, and irregular and inconsistent sleep patterns, meals, and other daily habits.

Follow-up and Referral

Education is a key component to effective adherence to therapy and to family support. Open discussion of all treatment options, side effects, and their management is critical and is a hallmark of patient-centered care. Monitoring and managing symptoms over time, including triggers and early warning signs, is essential. Self-monitoring and better symptom recognition are desirable goals. The prevalence of nonadherence with mood stabilizers ranges from 18% to 52%. Reasons include denial of diagnosis, unwillingness to take medication long term, perceived improvement in health, and adverse side effects of medications. Patient adherence to the medication regimen can make a difference in patient outcomes. In one 18-month study, 81% of partially adherent patients required hospitalization versus just 9% of adherent patients. Patients may ask if they will need to continue taking the same medication for life. The specific medications prescribed may change as new agents are introduced and as the individual's treatment needs are reassessed. What will remain constant is the need to monitor the patient with BD over his or her lifetime.

The practitioner can help the patient and family develop realistic treatment goals by actively listening and being responsive to patient needs and by regularly addressing mixed feelings about adherence to treatment. Patients with BD struggle with a variety of interpersonal and/or occupational issues. As stabilization management and supervision are lessened after an acute affective episode, patient attendance at follow-ups may decrease. During this postacute period, intensive collaboration with the patient and family can be invaluable for establishing the framework for long-term interactions that build on the therapeutic *Circle of Caring.*

Involvement of family and friends is critical to successful follow-up because progression of BD may be difficult to validate via self-report. Sensitivity to early warning signs of potential mood destabilization is important. Many patients do not try to achieve treatment goals. Symptoms of illness often preclude sound judgment, and patient unwillingness to tolerate medication side effects are some of the causes of apparent nonadherence.

Regularly reviewing with the patient "quality of life" versus "effects of treatment" and emphasizing the improved prognosis associated with maintenance therapy may improve medication compliance. CBT, family therapy, or interpersonal therapy should all target self-monitoring, treatment adherence, communication skills, and coping strategies to complement pharmacotherapy.

If a patient presents with early manifestations of relapse, promptly assess the clinical scenario and review the drug regimen. It is essential to investigate possible medication nonadherence, drug–drug interaction, and substance use and to obtain a drug level before initiating a change in the current regimen. If the cause of relapse is unclear or the symptoms fail to respond to standard treatment, a psychiatrist should be consulted. Periodically the patient should be reevaluated for known or new medical conditions or medication use that may complicate management; at every encounter, he or she should also be assessed for suicide risk.

Patient and Family Education

Educate the family and patient about the nature of bipolar illness and about the importance of medication compliance, regular visits for clinical and laboratory monitoring, and contacting their health-care provider before stopping or starting any medication (prescribed or over the counter). Patients should avoid complementary therapies such as St. John's wort, because they may interfere with some psychotropics. Educating the patient and family about potential side effects of all medications is important, as is informing them of the many options available to minimize or eliminate side effects. Patients and their families need to understand the importance of maintaining adequate blood levels of medication in prevention of relapse and of contacting the health-care provider in the event of unpleasant side effects rather than stopping the medication.

At follow-up visits, the practitioner can counsel the patient and family about coping with stressors that may precipitate manic or depressive episodes, about maintaining a consistent lifestyle, about signs of relapse, and about medication adherence. Written patient instructions can reinforce the following recommendations:

• Limit "everyday" stimulants such as coffee, alcohol, and over-the-counter medications that contain these substances because they can trigger mood episodes.
• Maintain regular sleep patterns.
• Avoid taking unnecessary or illegal drugs because they can trigger mood episodes; they can also prevent the benefits or increase the adverse side effects of necessary medications.
• Try to maintain a regular work schedule. If necessary, take time off rather than "tough it out" if mood symptoms hinder your ability to work.

As patients learn more about the stress of their illness on family members, it may help them reduce both their own stress and the disruption that it can cause. Patients may develop such insights by learning more about bipolar illness and by joining a bipolar support group or a mental health organization for lay people. Educate patients and families to watch for early signs of relapse, including changes in sleep patterns, grooming habits, energy or sexual interest, concentration problems, mood instability, or changes in self-esteem. Most patients experience a change in sleep patterns early in the development of an episode of mania or depression. Even small amounts of stimulants may interfere with sleep patterns or mood and possibly trigger a relapse. Insomnia may be either a precipitant or a warning sign. Early recognition of these signals, promptly followed by contacting the primary-care provider, can help prevent relapse. Maintenance of regular sleep patterns (including a prescription for benzodiazepine to promote regular sleep patterns) may prevent escalation of early symptoms into full episodes.

BD patients tend to minimize their limitations and vulnerabilities and may decide to discontinue treatment. There should be an individual action plan for coping and seeking assistance whenever the patient or family members suspect the patient is experiencing early manifestations of relapse. Knowing their assigned roles in the patient's action plan may be an important resource when the patient is tempted to stop therapy. They should feel free to contact their psychiatrist, counselor, or primary-care provider for advice whenever necessary, especially in light of self-destructive, aggressive behavior or any changes in daily routine that cause concern.

■ ACUTE SUICIDE RISK

Annually, more than 30,000 Americans complete a suicide. *Completed suicide* refers to self-inflicted death; *attempted suicide* refers to potentially lethal acts that do not result in death and nonlethal, attention-seeking gestures such as superficial cuts on wrists. Each person who attempts suicide is unique, but if there is a shared personal characteristic, it is likely to be a profound sense of hopelessness—hopelessness in the sense that the individual perceives there is no future, or that the future that he or she envisions is somehow unacceptable. Suicidal patients may be angry, sad, or confused. They may be quite honest about their suicidal plans or may refuse to disclose their true thoughts and feelings. Suicidal thoughts and feelings commonly are associated with mood disorders, principally BD, schizophrenia, and alcoholism. Persons who are overwhelmed by severe psychosocial problems and/or medical problems may also experience suicidal thoughts. Suicidal thoughts can have an acute onset, meaning that for a period of time, the person is at risk for acting on thoughts of suicide. Chronic suicidal thoughts are also common. In this case, the person never feels completely free of thoughts of taking his or her life. Impulsive suicidal behavior is the most difficult to assess, in that—by definition—this type of suicidal behavior is likely to occur without warning. Patients who are troubled by thoughts of suicide but are clear about their determination not to act on their suicidal thoughts may be appropriate candidates for primary-care management. For example, a patient who is in a great deal of pain associated with a serious physical illness may develop acute suicidal thoughts when overwhelmed by physical pain. Any suggestion of impulsive or chronic suicidal thoughts or evidence of actual suicidal behavior is an indicator for emergent evaluation by a specialist. (See The Patient's Voice 18.1.)

The Patient's Voice 18.1
The suffering of the suicidal is private and inexpressible, leaving family members, friends, and colleagues to deal with an almost unfathomable kind of loss, as well as guilt. Suicide carries in its aftermath a level of confusion and devastation that is, for the most part, beyond description.
Kay Redfield Jamison

Epidemiology and Causes

Suicide is the eleventh leading cause of death in the United States and the fourth leading cause of death among adolescents and young adults. Every 17 minutes another life is lost to suicide, as every day 86 Americans take their own lives and more than 1,500 attempt

suicide. For every two victims of homicide in the United States, there are three deaths from suicide, and there are now twice as many deaths due to suicide than due to HIV/AIDS. More than half of all suicides occur in adult men aged 25 to 65. In the month before their suicide, 75% of elderly persons had visited a physician. Males are four times more likely to die from suicide than are females, and sadly, many who make suicide attempts never seek professional care immediately after the attempt. About 10% to 20% of all persons who attempt suicide eventually take their own lives.

Older white men who are widowed or unmarried have the highest suicide rate, as they are most likely to commit suicide with a firearm. Usually these men are living alone and lack social support. Unemployment, a fall in economic status, medical illness, family history, previous suicide attempt, and anniversary of a loss are all risk factors for suicide. Males are three times more likely than females to successfully complete a suicide, although elderly women (75 and older) account for 20% of the suicide deaths among those 65 and older; this number is expected to rise as the population of older women increases. Single and widowed persons of both sexes have a higher incidence of suicide. Adolescent (15–24 years) and geriatric (65 years and older) populations are at highest risk, especially Native Americans and Caucasian males. Attempted suicide is 10 times more frequent than completed suicide. One study indicated that 91% of suicide acts involving firearms result in death, whereas drug overdoses—thought the most common method—lead to fatality only 2% of the time. Fatality rates associated with drowning were found to be 84%; hanging, 82%; and poisoning with gases, 64%. The prime suicide site of the world is the Golden Gate Bridge in San Francisco.

Special at-risk occupations include physicians (especially women physicians and/or psychiatrists), musicians, dentists, law enforcement officers, firefighters, lawyers, and insurance agents. Thirty-two percent of persons who commit suicide have sought medical attention within the prior 6 months. A number of CNS diseases increase the risk of suicide, specifically, epilepsy, multiple sclerosis, head injury, cardiovascular disease, Huntington's disease, dementia, and AIDS. All of these diseases are associated with mood disorders. Loss of mobility, disfigurement, and intractable pain are also associated with an increased risk of suicide. Certain drugs such as reserpine (Serpasil), corticosteroids, antihypertensive agents, and some antineoplastic agents can produce depression that may lead to suicide.

Pathophysiology

It is well documented that suicidal behavior, like other psychiatric disorders, tends to run in families. A family history of suicide increases the risk of attempted suicide and of completed suicide in most diagnostic groups. Twin studies suggest a genetic component in suicide. Over several studies, monozygotic twin pairs had a significantly higher concordance for both attempted and completed suicide than dizygotic twins did. Danish American adoption studies also yielded strong evidence that adoptees who had committed suicide had, on further investigations, a strong family history in biological relatives compared with no evidence of suicide in the adopting relatives. A further study of adoptees with mood disorders demonstrated that adoptee suicide completers with a situational crisis or impulsive suicide attempt, or particularly both, had more biological relatives who had committed suicide than controls had. It was suggested that the genetic factors lowering the threshold for suicidal behavior may lead to an inability to control impulsive behavior. Environmental stress, or the presence of a psychiatric disorder, may be a potentiating mechanism that triggers or fosters the impulsive behavior in the direction of suicide. The risk for suicide in patients with mental disorders is highest for those diagnosed with mood disorder.

Clinical Presentation

Clinicians must assess an individual patient's risk for suicide on the basis of clinical examination. Acute risk factors may include severe psychic anxiety, anxious ruminations, global insomnia, depression with delusions, and recent alcohol or other substance use. Suicidal behavior is multidimensional, with complex factors contributing to the overall risk of a future suicide attempt. Suicide screening tools often focus on previous attempts or intent to commit suicide, with various supportive items such as demographic information, level of social support, and coexisting mental health disorders. Because the goal of a suicide scale is to prevent completion, the sensitivity of the scale must be high so as not to miss a potential suicide. The risk of high sensitivity is overidentification of potential attempts. The Modified SAD PERSONAS Scale (see Risk Factors 18.3) has an administration time of 1 to 2 minutes, and the authors recommend this as a rapid screening tool for nonpsychiatrists to obtain the objective information necessary to make an initial assessment of suicidality.

Hopelessness about the future is a "red flag" for possible suicidal intent, as well as suicidal thoughts, especially if accompanied by a plan and intent. Giving away personal possessions, quitting a job, and an appearance of peace may all signal that the person has made the

Risk Factors 18.3   Acute Suicide Risk

The mnemonic "SAD PERSONAS" (Campbell, 2004; Patterson, 1983) may be used to evaluate a person's suicide risk. Consider risk factors within the context of the clinical presentation.

- S = Sex
- A = Age
- D = Depression
- P = Previous attempt
- E = Ethanol abuse
- R = Rational thinking loss
- S = Social support loss
- O = Organized plan
- N = No spouse
- A = Availability of lethal means
- S = Sickness

The following table presents a detailed description of acute suicide risk factors.

Gender	Males complete suicide (about one-half kill themselves using a gun) at a 3:1 ratio compared with females. Females are more likely to attempt suicide (usually by overdose) and act impulsively without warning than males.
Age	The risk of suicide increases with age, with persons aged 65 and older being more likely than younger persons to take their own lives (women peak at age 55; men at age 75). Older adults tend to use more lethal means and are less likely to voice their suicidal intent to others. Bereavement, social isolation, and deteriorating health status are thought to contribute to the high suicide rate in this group. Recent trends indicate that the suicide rate among young persons, aged 25–34, is increasing. Adolescents are a high-risk group, with suicide the second leading cause of death in this group. Gay adolescents who have been the victims of hate crimes or bullying, who fear social rejection, or who are socially isolated can be at increased risk for developing suicidal thoughts.

Continued

Risk Factors 18.3 Acute Suicide Risk—cont'd

Race and Ethnicity	Caucasians are at the greatest risk for suicide; however, suicide is one of the leading causes of premature death in minority groups.
Employment Status	Unemployed persons are at higher risk, although social class has not been shown to correlate strongly with increased risk for suicide.
Marital Status	Single, divorced, and widowed persons are at a significantly higher risk.
Immigration Status	Persons who migrate within the United States are at higher risk for suicide, as are those who immigrate to the United States. Social isolation appears to be a significant risk factor for immigrants.
Substance Abuse Problems	Persons with alcohol and drug problems are at extremely high risk for suicide, particularly when their substance abuse is complicated by other risk factors. More than one-third of persons who take their own lives are intoxicated at the time of their deaths. Alcoholism and substance abuse problems of a chronic nature account for 25% of all completed suicides.
Comorbidities	Major depression and bipolar disorders account for approximately 50% of all suicides. Schizophrenia and other psychotic disorders account for approximately 10% of completed suicides. Seventy percent of patients with borderline personality disorder will have at least one suicide attempt.
Medical Conditions	Chronic, life-threatening, or painful physical illness is associated with increased risk for suicide. Specific high-risk illnesses include AIDS, Huntington's disease, cancer, peptic ulcer, spinal cord injury, head injury, renal disease requiring dialysis, chronic intractable pain, uncontrolled diabetes with amputation, multiple sclerosis, numerous psychosomatic illnesses.
Medications	Certain medications increase suicidal risk: Steroids, antihypertensives (reserpine, methyldopa, clonidine), corticosteroids, opiates, antituberculosis drugs (isoniazid, ethionamide, cycloserine), anabolic steroid withdrawal, barbiturates, benzodiazepines, antidepressants, cocaine and amphetamine withdrawal.
Other	Additional suicide risk factors include recent bereavement, legal and financial problems, recent arrest or impending court dates, and being a victim of abuse or sexual assault.

*Campbell, WH. Pearls: Revised "SAD PERSONS" helps assess suicide risk. *Curr Psychiatry* 13:3, 2004.

decision to commit suicide. Self-mutilation, suicide threats and attempts, hallucinations, and delusions all indicate high risk for suicide.

Patients who are suicidal may state their intentions, but many will find it hard to volunteer this information. The impulsive person will often appear to be so and will give information that shows a great deal of recent poor judgment. The determined person may refuse to answer questions or may give information freely, thinking that his or her plan cannot be interfered with. The confused patient is more likely to seem unable to protect himself or herself from harm. Confused patients include persons suffering from auditory hallucinations instructing them to commit suicide and patients who are under the influence of drugs and alcohol. Suicidal patients may also express extreme anger and rage and may also have thoughts of homicide, as though taking their own life permits them to consider taking someone else's life first.

Management

Suicide prevention is carried out at two levels—interpersonal and community. Interpersonal prevention includes risk assessment, intervention (e.g., medications, counseling, hospitalization), and referral to a specialist. Community prevention is based on the crisis model of 24-hour community hotline services and walk-in crisis counseling services. Crisis counseling services should include a crisis response team that is dispatched immediately to schools or locations where assistance may be needed. These response teams can intervene to reduce the risk of suicide contracts among peers or "copycat" suicides. One systematic review found that physician education and programs to reduce access to lethal means (especially firearms) were effective in reducing the risk of suicide. In 2001, the Surgeon General organized the National Strategy of Suicide Prevention, under the auspices of the National Institutes of Health (NIH). Because suicide is such a serious public health problem, the *National Strategy* proposes public health methods to address it. The public health approach to suicide prevention represents a rational and organized way to marshal prevention efforts and ensure that they are effective. Only within the last few decades has a public health approach to suicide prevention emerged with good understanding of the biological and psychosocial factors that contribute to suicidal behaviors. Its five basic steps are to clearly define the problem; identify risk and protective factors; develop and test interventions; implement interventions; and evaluate effectiveness.

Careful assessment of suicide risk factors, willingness to consult with other practitioners and specialists, and planning are the hallmarks of effective suicide risk management. Most completed suicides are associated with psychiatric disorders, and the combination of depression and use of alcohol or other substance abuse is strongly correlated with suicide attempts. Assess suicidal ideation, intent, and risk to determine the severity of depression (Level II; Institute for Clinical Systems Improvement, 2012).

The assessment should cover the patient's recent personal history and pay special attention to recent stressful life events and changes in mental status. Reports of recent losses, humiliations, demoralizing experiences, substance use and abuse, and relationship problems should be explored. Persons who have been abusing drugs and/or alcohol can suddenly become highly motivated to end their lives when they first realize that they are no longer in control of their substance use. Even a person who is recovering from substance abuse and has stopped using the substance can be at high risk for suicide when faced with the painful consequences of substance abuse, including withdrawal or severe drug cravings.

All suicidal statements should be considered *seriously,* but no one can predict the actual behaviors of a suicidal patient. One of the most valuable assessment tools for practitioners is the willingness to question a patient directly about his or her suicide risk. Two good general questions are "How long can you go on the way you are?" and "Are you feeling so badly that you sometimes wish you could go to bed and not wake up?" Examples of more specific questions are "What is your plan for suicide?" and "Have you assembled what you need?" Suicide plans are assessed on their *specificity, availability,* and *lethality* (SAL): The more specific and detailed the plan and the more available and lethal the method, the higher the risk of suicide.

Once it is determined that the patient is suicidal, the level of risk will determine the direction of the intervention. A major decision to be made is whether the patient needs to be hospitalized. The absence of a strong social support system, history of impulsive behavior, a suicidal plan of action, or the availability of weapons are indications for hospitalization. If hospitalization is deemed necessary but the patient has no way of getting there, or if he or she refuses to go, it will be necessary to call 911 to dispatch someone from the police or sheriff's department to escort the patient to the hospital. The primary goal of the intervention is to maintain the patient's safety. Therefore, the following considerations are important:

- Reduce or eliminate imminent danger.
- Never leave a patient alone who is actively suicidal.
- Involve family members or significant others who care so that they can stay with the patient until the crisis has passed.

The best predictor of suicide risk is a history of previous suicide attempt. All persons with suicide gestures, attempts, and threats should be thoroughly screened for suicide risk factors and referred to a specialist for a full mental status exam, as well as psychiatric consultation. It is important to diagnose and treat any underlying psychiatric and/or substance-abuse disorders. The clinician and the patient's family or significant others should ensure the patient's safety by the least restrictive method, starting with removing potentially lethal objects and providing very close supervision. Some patients at acute high risk will require inpatient hospitalization for constant one-to-one supervision (including use of restraints, if indicated) and ongoing treatment. ECT may provide rapid, safe, and effective treatment for severely depressed, acutely suicidal patients.

Sometimes a no-suicide contract can be initiated. In the case of an angry or manipulative patient, this is usually not advisable. If a patient who is considered seriously suicidal cannot make the commitment to abide by a no-suicide contract, immediate hospitalization is necessary. A no-suicide contract is not a guarantee that a suicide will not happen, nor is it a substitute for clinical judgment. A mental health professional should be the person to implement a no-suicide contract. When it is appropriate to use them, no-suicide written contracts should include the following components:

- An agreement from the patient not to harm himself or herself
- An agreement that the patient will contact a mental health professional if the patient's suicidal impulses become unmanageable
- An agreement from the mental health–care provider to be available to the patient for a specified period of time, usually until the patient returns for a follow-up visit or another part of the intervention has taken place (e.g., when the patient has met with a psychotherapist for evaluation or therapy)
- Contact numbers for the mental health–care provider

Both the patient and mental health–care provider sign the contract. A copy is given to the patient, and the original is kept in the agency records.

After this, it is essential to implement an ongoing program of help. This should involve the following:

- Treatment of the presenting symptoms
- Referral for individual or group therapy
- Referral for support groups
- Referral to a community program

If the patient is not hospitalized and until the treatment program is in effect, the clinician must continue to monitor the patient to ascertain his or her safety.

Appropriate documentation is critical. Follow the agency guidelines for documenting situations involving suicidal risk. Records should include statements made by the patient; the decision-making process followed; potential ramifications of nontreatment; what has been shared with the patient and the family; and the consultation process. To avoid malpractice litigation, practitioners need to perform and document a complete assessment addressing both the risk and the precautions taken and follow evidence-based guidelines. A standard of care exists for assessment of suicide risk but not for the prediction of suicide. Complete and accurate documentation is key (Table 18.9).

Follow-up and Referral

Safety plans for patients who are not acutely suicidal include a follow-up appointment within 24 hours of assessment and a follow-up telephone call for missed appointments. Patients and involved family and friends should be given the local 24-hour crisis telephone number and information regarding access to emergency services. Practitioners must take responsibility to ask patients about weapons and pill stashes, and then take steps to have these items located and removed for safekeeping. If medications are prescribed, the amount should not exceed a 1-week supply, with no refills. Patients who are at risk should be seen at least weekly, and social support systems must be mobilized. Be aware that caring for a patient contemplating suicide can be very difficult (see Table 18.10).

Patient Education

Patient and family education includes providing suicide crisis hotline numbers to the patient and/or family members. Patients should be instructed to avoid alcohol. Encourage the patient to seek out adequate treatment for uncomfortable symptoms of physical illness, possibly including a prescription for analgesics to reduce suffering. Teach the patient that options appear narrowed when a person is feeling depressed and suicidal, and review alternative ways of thinking. Encourage the patient to reach out for support and to reach out immediately when feeling the urge to harm himself or herself. Teach the patient to use specific, more constructive outlets for anger rather than self-destructive ones. Mobilize a social support system for the patient and educate significant others regarding suicidal risk and danger signs. Educate the patient and family that as the patient's mood "lifts" in response to antidepressant treatment, there is an increased risk of suicide related to increased energy. At these times, patients must be monitored closely for increased risk.

In the event that the patient does commit suicide, the clinician should prepare the family for a complex

Table 18.9	Suicide Assessment and Management

Suicide Assessment

1. Psychiatric evaluation that includes the following:
   • Specific psychiatric signs and symptoms
   • Psychiatric history, including current treatment
   • Past suicidal or other self-injurious behaviors (including intent of such acts)
   • Family history of suicide, mental illness, and dysfunction
   • Current psychosocial situation and nature of crisis
2. Inquire about suicidal thoughts, plans, behaviors (elicit presence of suicidal ideation, suicide plan, intent, and lethality of plan including access to weapons, pills)
3. Suicide risk estimation to include demographic factors, major psychiatric syndromes (primary and comorbid conditions), specific psychiatric symptoms, other aspects of psychiatric history and physical illness

Management

1. Attend to patient's safety.
2. Establish and maintain a therapeutic alliance.
3. Determine a treatment setting (e.g., involuntary hospitalization, partial hospitalization, and intensive outpatient programs, ambulatory settings).
4. Develop a plan of care.
5. Coordinate care and collaborate with other providers.
6. Promote adherence to treatment plan.
7. Provide education to the patient and the family.
8. Reassess safety and suicide risk (include suicide crisis and chronic suicidality).
9. Monitor psychiatric status and response to treatment.
10. Obtain consultation if needed.

Documentation and Risk Management

1. Documentation issues specific to suicide
2. Be aware of own emotions and reactions, particularly when responding to those with severe or recurring suicidality or self-injurious behaviors—for difficult-to-treat patients, consultation and supervision from a colleague, as well as documentation of same, is recommended.
3. Suicide prevention contracts: limitations and clinical usefulness—not recommended in patients who are psychotic, agitated, impulsive, or using intoxicating substances.
4. Management of a suicide in one's practice.
5. Mental health intervention for surviving family and friends after suicide.

Source: Abstracted from American Psychiatric Association, 2003. http://psychiatryonline.org/content.aspx?bookid=28&sectionid=1673332

grief reaction that may follow. Suicide is particularly tragic because of the fallout that the death bequeaths to survivors. Edward Shneidman coined the term *postvention*, which refers to an intervention strategy that attempts to minimize the impact of patient suicide and to ensure that survivors of suicide have adequate services and support available to them.

Table 18.10 Support for Health-Care Providers Caring for Patients at Risk for Suicide

- Be aware of your personal and professional limits and honor them.
- Know the legal standards about suicide, duty to report, confidentiality, and liability.
- Consult with others so that you are not the only decision-maker assessing the risk of the suicidal patient.

Postsuicide interventions by the clinician include the following:

- Educating the family members about suicide
- Allowing the family members to share their grief, including any burdens or other factors that the family members may feel (e.g., guilt, shame, anger, inability to do anything, situation out of their control)
- Encouraging family members to attend support groups, such as Survivor of Suicide (SOS) groups, which are available in most communities

The typical SOS group is sponsored by a mental health or social services agency and is facilitated by mental health professionals, survivor peers, or a combination of both. Referrals to such groups following a completed suicide are essential.

SCHIZOPHRENIA SPECTRUM DISORDERS

Psychotic disorders are disturbances of thought and signal a departure from reality with some combination of hallucinations and delusions. Abnormalities may occur in one or more of five domains: delusions, hallucinations, disorganized thinking (speech), grossly disorganized or abnormal motor behavior (including catatonia), and negative symptoms. A person with psychosis may exhibit difficulties with communication, insight, behavior, and relationships. Psychosis may be the direct result of medication effects, such as illicit drugs or prescribed steroids. It may also be confused with delirium, which most often signals overwhelming infection or other medical causes. Psychotic disorders may coexist with other psychiatric disorders. Schizoaffective disorder exhibits symptoms of both schizophrenia and mood disorders and most likely represents a continuum of illness within the psychotic grouping. Psychotic disorders can be classified into several categories as outlined in Table 18.11. Schizophrenia is among the most chronic disabling and economically catastrophic medical disorders of the severe

Table 18.11 Psychotic Disorders

Psychotic Disorder	Description
Schizophrenia with several subtypes	Onset: Acute or insidious. Symptoms present for at least 6 months with at least two or more + or – symptoms present for at least 1 month. Social, employment, or self-care impairment.
Mania with psychosis	Onset: Variable. Signs and symptoms must be present for 1 week or if hospitalization is required. Psychotic signs and symptoms present only during mood disorder. Social and employment impairment during episode.
Mixed episode with psychoses	Onset: Variable. Signs and symptoms must be present for 1 week or if hospitalization is required. Meets criteria for depression and mania. + Signs and symptoms only with mood symptoms. Social and employment impairment during episode.
Major depression with psychotic symptoms	Onset: Variable. Lasts 2+ weeks. + Signs and symptoms occur only during mood episode. Impairment during episode (includes postpartum).
Schizoaffective disorder	Often viewed on a continuum of schizophrenia–mood disorder with psychotic symptoms or psychosis without mood disorder. Impairment similar to schizophrenia.
Brief psychotic disorder	Onset: Acute. Full expression within 2 weeks and complete remission 1–3 months, lasts at least 1 day but less than 1 month. May have an acute stressor.
Schizophreniform	Usually acute onset of symptoms. Criteria of schizophrenia are met, but <6 months symptoms.
Delusional disorder	Criteria for schizophrenia are not met. Onset subtle, nonbizarre delusions, symptoms last >1 month.

Sources: American Psychiatric Association. *Diagnostic and statistical manual of mental disorders, fifth edition* (DSM-5). American Psychiatric Association, Arlington, VA, 2013; and Fochtmann, LJ, et al. Other psychotic disorders. In Sadock, BJ, et al, *Kaplan and Sadock's comprehensive textbook of psychiatry.* Lippincott Williams & Wilkins, Philadelphia, 2009.

mental illnesses. The WHO ranks it as one of the top 10 illnesses contributing to the global burden of disease. People with schizophrenia often suffer terrifying symptoms such as hearing internal voices not heard by others, or believing that other people are reading their minds, controlling their thoughts, or plotting to harm them. These symptoms may leave them fearful and withdrawn. Because of its disconcerting symptoms, a diagnosis of schizophrenia has serious implications for patients and families and can lead to significant medical comorbidities secondary to pharmacological treatments and unhealthy lifestyles.

Epidemiology and Causes

The lifetime risk for schizophrenia is estimated between 0.3% and 0.7%, although there are reported variations related to race and ethnicity, immigration status, and socioeconomic and geographical factors. In the Epidemiologic Catchment Area Study, the lifetime prevalence of schizophrenia among adults aged 30 to 44 years was 2.3%; persons older than age 65 years have a lifetime prevalence of 0.3%. Age at onset occurs earlier in men, commonly in the early twenties; women may present in their late 20s to early 30s. However, in both males and females, subtle symptoms may occur long before a definitive diagnosis is made, and males tend to have a worse prognosis and more difficult course. The prevalence of schizophrenia in adolescents is low, but it can occur in childhood before age 13. Early onset points to a poor prognosis although research is evolving. Developmental pathways are poorly understood. Family history of schizophrenia, obstetric complications and developmental difficulties, abuse, major life events, and parental loss may contribute to the development of the disease.

The disease course is variable, with some patients exhibiting mild symptoms only; but the majority of patients with schizophrenia follow a chronic course with some signs of functional impairment. These characteristics are barriers for employment and financial stability; moreover, they may interfere with stable housing and the patient's ability to navigate and maintain access to quality medical care. Poor engagement in health maintenance initiatives such as cancer screenings, exercise, nutrition, tobacco cessation, and identification of other comorbid chronic medical diseases play a role in poor outcomes.

Pathophysiology and Psychodynamics

A certain cause of schizophrenia is not known. It is most likely a multifactorial disorder consisting of biological, psychological, and social factors. Urban birth and rearing, social adversity and trauma, heavy cannabis use, migration, and stressful life events all suggest increased risk of schizophrenia. Migrant populations experience raised rates of schizophrenia. Increased rates of social adversity and family disruption experienced by some migrant populations may be thought to contribute to increased occurrence.

Clinical Presentation

The onset of schizophrenia may be abrupt or insidious. The majority of individuals have a slow and gradual development of clinical symptoms. Depressive symptoms occur in approximately half of cases. Schizophrenia presents with four symptom clusters that are used to describe the disorder, and each has implications for therapeutic treatment. Positive symptoms, negative symptoms, cognitive impairments, and affective disturbances comprise these clusters.

Positive symptoms refer to the "active" qualities of these symptoms that are abnormal and are synonymous with psychosis. Positive symptoms include delusions, hallucinations, disorganized thinking (speech), and grossly disorganized or abnormal behavior (catatonia). Delusions are the hallmark of positive symptoms, occurring in more than half of patients. Delusions are fixed beliefs not amenable to change despite conflicting evidence. They can include persecutory, referential, somatic, religious, or grandiose themes. Hallucinations are sensory impressions without basis of reality, prompting thought disorganization. They are vivid and clear to the individual experiencing them and may occur in any sensory modality such as auditory, visual, somatic, olfactory, or gustatory. Auditory hallucinations are distinct from the individual's own thoughts and are the most common type of hallucination. They must occur in the context of a clear sensorium. Disorganization is seen in behavior and/or thinking. Disorganized thinking is typically inferred from speech and must substantially impair effective communications. Commonly observed forms of abnormal speech are as follows:

- Tangentiality—getting off topic without answering questions appropriately
- Circumstantiality—will answer question in markedly roundabout manner
- Derailment—switching topics without a logic sequence
- Neologisms—creation of new, idiosyncratic words
- Word salad—words are placed together without any sensible meaning.

Grossly disorganized or abnormal motor behavior (including catatonia) may occur with schizophrenia with problems noted in goal-directed activities and activities of daily living. Positive symptoms can be experienced in combination, and most do respond to pharmacological treatment, although remission may be incomplete.

Negative symptoms represent a diminished or lack of normal characteristics—diminished emotional expression and avolition. *Diminished emotional expression* encompasses reductions in expression of the face, eye contact, intonation of speech, and movements of the hands, head, and face that contribute to emotion of speech. *Avolition* represents decline in motivated self-initiated purposeful activities. This encompasses loss of affective responsiveness, verbal expression, and communication, personal and social motivation, and enjoyment. Primary negative symptoms can be resistant to treatment and closely related to functional outcome. Secondary negative symptoms may be routed in other manifestations of the illness or treatment.

Cognitive impairments in schizophrenia often are seen early in life, with steady decline after the onset of the illness, and correlate with functional impairment. Affective disturbances, which are difficulties with mood and affect, are seen with schizophrenia and affect how society perceives patients. Depression and anxiety can be detected during or after a psychotic episode, and providers must be alert for risk of suicide, particularly at the initiation of treatment, immediately after an acute psychotic crisis, and throughout outpatient encounters (see Table 18.12).

The DSM-5 symptom criteria for schizophrenia are as follows:

- Two or more of the characteristic *positive symptoms* (delusions, hallucinations, disorganized speech, grossly disorganized or catatonic behavior) or *negative symptoms* (diminished emotional expression or avolition). At least one of the *positive symptoms* must be delusions, hallucinations, or disorganized speech. Must be present for the greater part of 1 month or less if treated.
- Difficulties experienced with social skills such as interpersonal relationships, work, or self-care.
- Continuous symptoms for 6 months and at least 1 month of characteristic symptoms.
- Exclusion of other medical or psychiatric disorders.
- Disturbance not attributed to effects of substance abuse or other medication.
- If there is a history of autism spectrum disorder or childhood communication disorder, the diagnosis of schizophrenia is made only if prominent delusions or hallucinations in addition to the other required symptoms for schizophrenia are present for at least 1 month.

Schizoaffective disorder appears to be one-third as common as schizophrenia with an estimated prevalence of 0.3%. The incidence is higher in females than in males. Age of onset is typically early adulthood, although it may occur in adolescence to adulthood. The basis of a diagnosis of schizoaffective disorder entails an uninterrupted period of illness during which the individual continues to display active or residual symptoms of psychotic illness. During this period of psychosis, symptom criteria for schizophrenia have to be met. Social dysfunction and exclusion of autism spectrum disorder or other communication disorders of childhood onset required for schizophrenia do not have to be met. Occupational function and

Table 18.12	Symptom Clusters of Schizophrenia

Positive Symptoms—exaggeration of normal processes
- Hallucinations: Perception of a sensory process in the absence of an external source; can be auditory, visual, somatic, olfactory, or gustatory, alone or in combination.
- Delusions: Fixed false belief despite evidence that it is not true. Classified as bizarre delusion—clearly implausible; or nonbizarre delusions—although not true, is understandable with possibility of being true. Categorized as grandiose, paranoid, nihilistic, and erotomanic.
- Disorganization: Manifested in speech and behavior, loose or illogical thoughts lacking connectivity.
- Movement disorders: Grossly disorganized or abnormal motor behavior including catatonia.

Negative Symptoms—absence or diminution of normal processes
- Flat or blunted affect
- Alogia: Poverty of speech, thought blocking, increased latency of response
- Asociality/anhedonia: Loss of pleasurable feelings, failure to engage with peers socially
- Apathy: Lack of self-motivation, poor grooming and hygiene, anergy

Cognitive Impairments
- Poor executive functioning, concrete thoughts, diminished processing speed
- Difficulty focusing, maintaining attention
- Verbal and visual learning and memory deficits
- Verbal comprehension
- Social cognition

Affective Disturbances
- Blunt, odd expressions or actions that are interpreted as such and affect societal impression of the individual
- Stigmatization, poor self-esteem
- Depression and anxiety
- Increased risk of suicide

Source: American Psychiatric Association. *Diagnostic and statistical manual of mental disorders, fifth edition* (DSM-5). American Psychiatric Association, Arlington, VA, 2013. Adapted from www.surgeongeneral.gov/library/mentalhealth/chapter2/sec2.html#manifest

social functioning is often impaired but need not be a defining criterion for diagnosis. This is in contrast to schizophrenia. There may be restricted social contact, anosognosia (poor insight), and difficulties with self-care; however, *negative symptoms* may be less severe and less persistent. Alcohol and substance abuse can be associated with schizoaffective disorder. Individuals may go on to a diagnosis of schizophrenia, major depressive disorder, or bipolar disorder. As with schizophrenia, schizoaffective disorder carries a 5% lifetime risk of suicide, and assessment regarding suicide lethality must be always addressed.

The DSM-5 symptom criteria for schizoaffective disorder are as follows:

- Uninterrupted period of illness during which there is a major mood episode (depressive or manic).
- Delusions or hallucinations for 2 or more weeks in the absence of a major mood episode (depressive or manic) during the lifetime duration of the illness.
- Symptoms that meet criteria for a major mood episode are present for the majority of the active and residual portions of the illness.
- Disturbance not attributed to effects of substance abuse or medical condition.

Table 18.11 briefly identifies other psychotic disorders for consideration.

Initial presentation may occur in the primary-care setting. The role of the primary-care provider is to identify and refer any suspected or new cases of schizophrenia for urgent psychiatric evaluation. In some settings, especially in rural settings, this may be difficult owing to a paucity of mental health services and psychiatric providers. The primary-care provider is responsible to evaluate the patient's current risk to self and others. Any person presenting with psychosis for the initial or "first break" should be fully evaluated for underlying medical conditions. Consideration of substance abuse should be one of the primary differentials, and toxicology testing should be performed. Alcohol, opioids, cocaine, amphetamines, barbiturates, and hallucinogens are some of the most common offenders. In addition, it is not only consumption of these agents, but also withdrawal from them, that may precipitate symptoms. Commonly prescribed medications such as anticholinergic agents, phenytoin, steroids, H_2 blockers (cimetidine), and anxiolytics may produce similar symptoms. Other differentials to consider include delirium, in which the onset of symptoms occurs more rapidly and in which visual hallucinations are more common, versus schizophrenia, in which symptoms occur over a longer time period and auditory hallucinations occur more frequently. Medical illnesses such as hepatic encephalopathy, hyponatremia, hypoglycemia, hypoxia, intracranial bleed, infection, meningitis/encephalitis, and so forth should also be considered. A complete history and physical exam with attention to neurological and mental status exam are essential. Laboratory evaluation should include CBC with differential, electrolytes, renal function, liver profile, thyroid function, drug and alcohol toxicology, and pregnancy. Attention should be paid to potential infectious diseases processes with screening for syphilis, HIV, and hepatitis C. It may be determined that further testing for heavy metals, EEG, or brain imaging with MRI or CT is warranted.

Management

Schizophrenia is a chronic illness that influences virtually all aspects of life for patients and their families.

Treatment goals should address reducing or eliminating symptoms, maximizing quality of life, improving function, and promoting and maintaining recovery within the context of an early intervention model of care. Treatment involves a multidisciplinary approach: assertive outreach approaches, family involvement and interventions, psychological interventions and psychologically informed care, vocational and educational interventions, and antipsychotic medication and monitoring (Level I; Scottish Intercollegiate Guidelines Network, 2013).

Pharmacological intervention is the mainstay for treatment of schizophrenia (Level I; Scottish Intercollegiate Guidelines Network, 2013; American Psychiatric Association, 2006). Early therapeutic intervention is important. Pharmacological intervention is quite effective in addressing the *positive symptoms* of schizophrenia. The negative symptoms are best addressed in a more multifaceted approach including cognitive-behavioral therapy (CBT) (Level I; Pitschel-Walz et al, 2001). Strategies to prevent relapse and encourage medication adherence are essential. The Expert Consensus Guideline Series determined that adherence problems in patients with serious mental illness primarily stem from poor insight and lack of illness awareness or distress associated with specific side effects or a general fear of potential side effects.

The *Circle of Caring* (see Chapter 2) is essential in helping the patient navigate the complex system of primary care and mental health services, as well as providing education for patients and significant others to access available community resources. Understanding the lived experience of the patient, family, and community of those living with schizophrenia, as well as their definition of wellness and recovery, helps to foster insight and adherence to the treatment plan. Of critical importance is the establishment of the therapeutic alliance, providing a supportive environment, maintaining continuity of provider when possible, and developing a trusting relationship where the patient is the active participant in his or her care. Recovery includes wellness and provision of primary care. Management of comorbid conditions is central to that effort.

Targets of Treatment

The goals of therapy include management of the positive and negative symptoms; evaluation of community issues such as employment, homelessness, justice issues, and victimization; and assessment of co-occurring illnesses such as PTSD, substance abuse, and depression (Level I; Scottish Intercollegiate Guidelines Network, 2013; American Psychiatric Association, 2006). In addition, it is essential to provide education to significant others in an attempt to enhance the therapeutic alliance and compliance with the treatment plan (Level I; Scottish Intercollegiate Guidelines Network, 2013).

Pharmacological Management

Antipsychotic medications are considered primary treatment for psychotic symptoms (Level I; Scottish Intercollegiate Guidelines Network, 2013; American Psychiatric Association, 2006; National Institute for Health and Clinical Excellence, 2009). These medications help to alleviate the positive symptoms and decrease hospital days and relapse rates. In addition, a greater response to medication is often seen when it is started early in the course of the disease (Level I; American Psychiatric Association, 2006; National Institute for Health and Clinical Excellence, 2009). Initiation of early and effective doses of antipsychotic medication is important, because it may influence the effect on the patient and family, as well as the risk of injury to self or others.

Because medication-naive patients are more sensitive to the psychotropic effects of medications (they respond to lower doses), initiation at the lower end of standard dose is recommended. Response rates are variable; slow titration of antipsychotic medication is recommended to help reduce the risk of intolerable side effects that may affect long-term adherence. Patients who experience a first episode are very responsive to treatment; remission is achieved within 3 to 4 months for 70% of patients, and 83% have a stable remission by 1 year. Accessing treatment may be difficult due to the alarming symptoms and the impaired thinking process.

The antipsychotic medications can be divided into two categories: (1) first generation, conventional, or "typical"; and (2) the second generation "atypical" antipsychotic medications. The typical, or conventional, antipsychotics have been used since the 1950s. These medications are very effective; however, the side effects can be troubling, and nonadherence has been attributed to these side effects (see Table 18.13). All antipsychotic medications work to reduce the positive symptoms. The negative symptoms have not diminished with the use of the conventional antipsychotics, but the "atypicals" seem to address some of these issues. The Clinical Antipsychotic Trials of Intervention Effectiveness project (CATIE) sponsored by the National Institute of Mental Health looked at the various drug regimens, comparing the conventional antipsychotic perphenazine and various "atypicals." This study found no difference in discontinuation rates for the conventional versus the atypical antipsychotics. Depot medications are particularly important for patients with compliance issues. Adjunctive medications help with controlling side effects and assisting with comorbid illnesses such as anxiety and depression.

Extrapyramidal symptoms (EPS) are among the most troubling for the conventional agents and can occur in 75% of patients prescribed these agents. It is theorized that these symptoms are related to blockage of the dopamine receptors and thus the decreased availability of dopamine. This reduction can generate alteration in a person's movement and functioning. These symptoms can be categorized as akathisia, dystonia, pseudoparkinsonism, and tardive dyskinesia and are summarized in Table 18.14. Anticholinergic medications are utilized to manage the symptoms experienced by many patients treated with antipsychotic medications. Prophylactic treatment with anticholinergics may be utilized to diminish EPS. Patient education is essential in discussing EPS in order to identify and treat these symptoms and to ensure adherence to the pharmacological regimen. In addition, if anxiety and/or assaultive behaviors are present, treatment with benzodiazepines may be used. Clozapine has been found to be helpful in management of suicidal behaviors and treatment-resistant symptoms (Level I; American Psychiatric Association, 2006; National Institute for Health and Clinical Excellence, 2009). Treatment of coexisting depression with antidepressants may prevent worsening of psychotic symptoms and improve overall functioning.

Individuals with serious mental illness particularly benefit from a consistent source of care, a comprehensive medical record, and continuity of provider. Primary care

Table 18.13 Comparison of the First Generation Antipsychotics and Risk of Side Effects		
High Potency	**Low Potency**	**Shared Side Effects**
High risk of extrapyramidal effects	Lower risk of extrapyramidal effects	Moderate risk of weight gain
Moderate risk of sedation	High risk of sedation	Low risk of metabolic effects
Low risk of orthostatic hypotension and tachycardia	High risk of orthostatic hypotension and tachycardia	High risk of sexual dysfunction
Low risk of anticholinergic and antiadrenergic effects	High risk of anticholinergic and antiadrenergic effects	Seizures
Higher risk of neuroleptic malignant syndrome	Lower risk of neuroleptic malignant syndrome	Allergic and dermatological effects

Sources: American Psychiatric Association. *Practice guideline for the treatment of patients with schizophrenia,* ed 2. Feb 2004. Arlington, VA. Retrieved from www.guideline.gov/summary/summary.aspx?doc_id=5217&nbr=003572&string=schizophrenia; and National Collaborating Centre for Mental Health Schizophrenia. Core interventions in the treatment and management of schizophrenia in primary and secondary care: Complete summary. National Institute for Health and Clinical Excellence (NICE), London, UK, 2002, updated March 2009. Retrieved from www.guideline.gov/content.aspx?id=14313&search=schizophrenia

Table 18.14 Extrapyramidal Symptoms, Description, and Treatment

Movement Disorder/Timing	Description	Treatment
Akathisia Occurs a few days to a few weeks after initiation of medication.	Restlessness Subjective: Impaired concentration, unable to remain calm Objective: Pacing, foot-tapping, shifting weight from foot to foot	Discontinue medication Benzodiazepines: lorazepam, diazepam, alprazolam Beta blockers such as propranolol
Dystonia May occur after a single dose of medication to several days later.	Involuntary muscle contractions affecting the head and neck (hoarseness, laryngeal spasms, oculogyric crisis) May involve the torso and extremities (torticollis, opisthotonos)	Anticholinergics Antiparkinsonian medication
Pseudoparkinsonism May occur after a single dose, but typically usually seen a few weeks later as the dosage is increased.	Slow pill-rolling movement of hands, cogwheel rigidity, shuffling gait, mask-like facies, loss of arm swing, and bradyphrenia After prolonged use "rabbit syndrome": tremor of lips characterized by constant chewing motion	Anticholinergics
Tardive Dyskinesia Late appearing manifestation, months to years.	Involuntary rapid movements of the face (lip smacking, grimacing, facial distortions), torso and extremities 6% irreversible	Prevention and screening tools for movement disorders every 3–6 months Anticholinergic agents Antiparkinsonian agents Removal of agent

Adapted from Courey, TC. Detection, prevention, and management of extrapyramidal symptoms. *J Nurse Pract* 3(7):464–469, 2007; and Schultz, SH, et al. Schizophrenia: A review. *Am Fam Physician* 75:1821–1829, 2007.

plays a fundamental role in promoting healthy behaviors such as physical activity, smoking cessation, and health maintenance screening. The primary-care provider should evaluate cardiac risk factors including hypertension, hyperlipidemia, and QT prolongation, as well as endocrine disorders such as metabolic syndrome, diabetes, and hyperprolactinemia. The weight gain seen with the "atypical" antipsychotics can be modified by lifestyle interventions such as exercise, dietary education, psychoeducation, and the administration of metformin (Glucophage). In a randomized controlled trial, metformin was more effective, but lifestyle intervention also reduced weight gain; the strongest effect was seen in patients who combined lifestyle intervention and metformin (Level I; Scottish Intercollegiate Guidelines Network, 2013). Myocarditis is a potential adverse reaction to clozapine (Clozaril). Patients presenting with fatigue, tachypnea, chest pain, fever, and dyspnea need emergent evaluation with an electrocardiogram, white blood cell count, and serum troponin levels. If myocarditis is diagnosed, clozapine must be stopped.

Currently the manufacturer recommends evaluation of cataracts at baseline and every 6 months for patients taking quetiapine (Seroquel). Ongoing education that builds on previous medical encounters is essential to assist the patient and family with methods to reduce the increased risk of cardiac- and pulmonary-related events. An increased risk of mortality from cancer has been demonstrated in patients with schizophrenia, especially for women with breast cancer and for men with lung cancer.

Monitoring for diabetes and dyslipidemia is especially important in patients with a positive family history of those conditions and in those receiving a second generation antipsychotic (Level II; American Psychiatric Association, 2006; National Institute for Health and Clinical Excellence, 2009). Recommendations include sequential measurement of body mass index, waist circumference, blood pressure, fasting glucose, and fasting lipid profile at baseline, 1 month, 3 months, and annually. Assess individual and family medical history at baseline and annually.

In addition, the clinician can help encourage the patient to remain compliant with the antipsychotic medication regimen, as well as all nonpharmacological therapies, to prevent relapse (Level I; American Psychiatric Association, 2006; National Institute for Health and Clinical Excellence, 2009). Persons experiencing a first episode should remain on the antipsychotic medication for at least 18 months. Olanzapine (Zyprexa) has been shown to be slightly more effective than haloperidol although the difference is only slight statistically. Discontinuation rates for haloperidol are slightly higher due to side effects (Level I; Scottish Intercollegiate Guidelines Network, 2013). Generally the second generation antipsychotics have a lower risk of tardive dyskinesia. It is important to note that each medication carries its own side-effect profile and metabolic risks. Adverse effects of medications should be discussed as choice of medication is agreed on. (See Drugs Commonly Prescribed 18.3 and 18.4.)

Drugs Commonly Prescribed 18.3 Typical Antipsychotics

Drug	Indication	Adverse Reactions and Prescribing Considerations
High Potency		
perphenazine*	Psychosis Severe behavioral disturbances due to cognitive impairment Nausea/vomiting	Highest risk for neuroleptic malignant syndrome Monitor for movement disorder (AIMS), CBC, LFTs, annual eye exam, renal function, serum prolactin, photosensitivity Administration 2–3x/day
fluphenazine (Prolixin)*	Psychosis	Monitor for movement disorder, CBC, LFTs, annual eye exam, serum prolactin, skin exanthems Administration 2–3x/day
trifluoperazine (Stelazine)*	Psychosis Anxiety disorder	Monitor for movement disorder, CBC, LFTs, annual eye exam, serum prolactin Administration 2–3x/day
haloperidol (Haldol)*	Acute psychosis Schizophrenia ADHD Tourette's disorder	Significant EPS, prolactinemia QT prolongation risk: Mild if oral, high if IV administration. Sedation, weight gain, rare photosensitivity. Monitor for movement disorder, CBC, LFTs, annual eye exam, serum prolactin, and urinalysis
thiothixene (Navane)*	Schizophrenia	Monitor for movement disorder, CBC, LFTs, annual eye exam, serum prolactin, TFTs and urinalysis Photosensitivity CBC, ophthalmological exam, TFTs, and urinalysis
Medium Potency		
loxapine (Loxitane)*	Bipolar Schizophrenia	Photosensitivity, seizures CBC, ophthalmological exam, TFTs and urinalysis
molindone (Moban)*	Schizophrenia	AIMS assessment
Low Potency		
chlorpromazine (Thorazine)*	Acute intermittent porphyria Acute psychosis Nausea/vomiting Tetanus Schizophrenia Hiccups	Photosensitivity, sulfite sensitivity AIMS assessment, CBC, ophthalmological exam, and prolactin

*Dementia: Black Box.
AIMS, Abnormal Involuntary Movement Scale; EPS, Extrapyramidal symptoms
Sources: Clinical pharmacology [database online]. Gold Standard, Inc., Tampa, FL, 2013. http://cp.gsm.com.
Courey, TC. Detection, prevention, and management of extrapyramidal symptoms. *J Nurse Pract* 3(7):464–469, 2007.
Jibson, MD. Antipsychotic medications: Classification and pharmacology. Retrieved from www.utdol.com/online/content/topic.do?topicKey=psychiat/13184view=print
Jibson, MD. Antipsychotic medications: Treatment issues. Retrieved from www.utdol.com/online/content/topic.do?topicKey=psychiat/13586&view=print
U.S. National Guideline Clearinghouse. Schizophrenia: Complete summary. 2006. Retrieved from http://web.ebscohost.com/nrc/detail?vid=1&hid=111&sid=523710bf-789a-4f70-af4c-3c6d37d858a5%40sessionmgr113&bdata=JnNpdGU9bnJjLWxpdmU%3d#db=nrc&AN=5000006519

Drugs Commonly Prescribed 18.4   Atypical Antipsychotics

Drug	Indication	Adverse Reactions and Prescribing Considerations
clozapine (Clozaril)*	Schizophrenia Schizoaffective disorder	Agranulocytosis, lowered seizure threshold† Rare myocarditis Anticholinergic effects, no EPS, postural hypotension, prolong QT interval, sedation Metabolic effects: monitor weight gain++, increased lipids++, FPG++ CBC with differential, LFTs and AIMS
olanzapine (Zyprexa)*	Bipolar depression Bipolar disorder Depression Mania Schizophrenia	Anticholinergic effects, dizziness/hypotension Sedation Metabolic effect: weight gain++ Monitor AIMS assessment, glucose, LFTs, neurological function, lipid profile
quetiapine (Seroquel)*	Bipolar depression Bipolar disorder Depression Mania Schizophrenia	Anticholinergic effects, postural hypotension somnolence Metabolic effects: weight gain+, FPG+ Ophthalmological exam Monitor AIMS assessment, glucose, LFTs, neurological function, lipid profile
risperidone (Risperdal)*	Autism Bipolar disorder Mania Schizophrenia	Anxiety, agitation, hypotension, sedation EPS+++ Metabolic effects: Weight gain+, increased lipids +, FPG+, hyperprolactinemia++ Monitor: AIMS assessment, glucose, LFTs, neurological function, lipid profile
aripiprazole (Abilify)*	Autism Bipolar disorder Depression Mania Schizophrenia	Rarely significant side effects of EPS, weight gain, or prolactin elevation Monitor: AIMS assessment, glucose, LFTs, neurological function, lipid profile
ziprasidone (Geodon)*	Bipolar disorder Mania Schizophrenia	May prolong QT interval Rarely significant side effects of EPS, weight gain, or prolactin elevation Monitor: ECG, AIMS assessment, glucose, LFTs, neurological function, lipid profile
paliperidone (Invega)*	Schizoaffective disorder Schizophrenia	May prolong QT interval, EPS, tachycardia Metabolic effects: weight gain+, prolactinemia Monitor AIMS, ECG
iloperidone (Fanapt)*	Schizophrenia	Anticholinergic+, dizziness, tachycardia, orthostatic hypotension+, sedation, EPS+ Prolong QT interval+++ Metabolic effects: Weight gain++, prolactinemia+ Monitor AIMS and ECG

*Dementia: Black Box.
†Doses greater than 600 mg.
EPS, Extrapyramidal symptoms.
+ mild, ++ moderate, +++ high risk.
Adapted from the following sources:
Clinical pharmacology [database online]. Gold Standard, Inc., Tampa, FL, 2013. http://cp.gsm.com.
Courey, TC. Detection, prevention, and management of extrapyramidal symptoms. *J Nurse Pract* 3(7):464–469, 2007.
Jibson, MD. Antipsychotic medications: Classification and pharmacology. Retrieved from www.utdol.com/online/content/topic.do?topicKey=psychiat/13184view=print
Jibson, MD. Antipsychotic medications: Treatment issues. Retrieved from www.utdol.com/online/content/topic.do?topicKey=psychiat/13586&view=print
U.S. National Guideline Clearinghouse. Schizophrenia: Complete summary. 2006. Retrieved from http://web.ebscohost.com/nrc/detail?vid=1&hid=111&sid=523710bf-789a-4f70-af4c-3c6d37d858a5%40sessionmgr113&bdata=JnNpdGU9bnJjLWxpdmU%3d#db= nrc&AN=5000006519

Nonpharmacological Management

Because schizophrenia is characterized by remissions and relapses, looking at a variety of strategies to optimize functional status is important. Stigmatization, which represents a chronic negative interaction with the environment that most persons living with schizophrenia deal with on a regular basis, must be recognized. Stigmatization reduces schizophrenia to a stereotyped set of negative attitudes, fears, and incorrect beliefs that affects how the disease is understood. Harmful effects of stigma may increase the schizophrenia liability and have negative effects on the clinical course of the disease. Labels and social disapproval may result in patient anxiety and contribute to negative discrimination. This negativity can influence health-care access, damage self-esteem and self-efficacy, and increase depressive symptoms. Increased likelihood of the misuse of alcohol and drugs may be related to the prejudice and discrimination related to schizophrenia.

The *Circle of Caring* model, encompassing the concepts of authentic presence, advocacy, knowing, commitment, and patience, is the essence of humanistic, quality, medical care for all populations but is critically important for those living with schizophrenia and other serious mental illnesses. This model must be fostered in staff training and incorporated into the culture of your health-care setting to reduce the negative effects of stigma.

There is some evidence that practicing active coping strategies and sharing stories with peers may reduce stigma and facilitate attendance at primary care. Peers have the unique lived experience of being mental health consumers themselves who are in recovery. With peer support training, they are able to share experiences and coping strategies that support recovery for those living with mental illness. Services run by trained peers also include assistance with housing and benefits advisement, employment and career counseling, justice issues, advocacy, and independent living skills. Peer-delivered services have been shown to diminish feelings of isolation, to improve coping skills, and often to decrease the need for hospitalization.

Social skill training improves social adjustment and coping skills (Level I; American Psychiatric Association, 2006; National Institute for Health and Clinical Excellence, 2009). Supportive individual and group psychotherapy along with medications can reduce relapses and enhance occupational and vocational functioning (Level II; American Psychiatric Association, 2006; National Institute for Health and Clinical Excellence, 2009). Employment may destigmatize a person coping with both psychiatric disability and a criminal record, and paid employment may aid in community integration. Family education helps to improve communication between the patient and mental health services and subsequently helps to reduce relapse rates and improve family functioning (Level I; American Psychiatric Association, 2006; National Institute for Health and

Clinical Excellence, 2009). Social centers aim to address isolation experienced by most patients. Social centers, sometimes called "club houses," provide a voluntary semistructured program wherein patients can meet in a safe environment to share conversation and participate in activities with others having similar concerns. For patients with persistent positive symptoms, CBT has been found to be helpful in the reduction of both symptoms and relapse rates (Level I; American Psychiatric Association, 2006; National Institute for Health and Clinical Excellence, 2009). Patients who have experienced a high incidence of relapse may benefit from an assertive community treatment (ACT) team approach (Level I; Scottish Intercollegiate Guidelines Network, 2013). ACT is an evidence-based program that provides culturally sensitive services for individuals with severe and persistent mental illnesses who have not benefited from traditional outpatient mental health programming and who also have a significant history of hospitalizations for mental health reasons. ACT is a comprehensive, multidisciplinary, team-based approach to treatment, with a strong emphasis on recovery principles individualized to meet the patient's needs. Services include case management, medication management, vocational counseling and placement, family counseling and psychoeducation, mental health and substance abuse counseling, and wellness management education. Services are provided in the community in the consumers' natural settings. Services are provided 24 hours a day, 7 days a week, for as long as needed. ACT participation is either voluntary or court mandated. The team approach includes a psychiatrist, psychiatric nurse, counselors, case manager, and peer support. The original ACT model included a nurse practitioner who provided medical care, but this is no longer an integral part of the ACT model. A hallmark of ACT is to develop a positive, trusting relationship with each client to improve his or her compliance with mental health treatment and focus on mental health and recovery.

■ CARE IN PREGNANCY FOR PATIENTS WITH PSYCHIATRIC DISORDERS

When pregnancy coexists with a psychiatric disorder, women need to be informed of all pharmacological and nonpharmacological treatment options so that they may make informed decisions. The decision to continue or withhold pharmacological treatment can pose a risk to the mother, the developing fetus, and the pregnancy outcome. Shared decision making between the woman, her primary-care provider, her obstetrician or midwife, and her mental health provider should be undertaken to minimize risk to the developing fetus and to enable the mother to have few or no psychiatric symptoms during pregnancy and the postnatal and lactation periods. A key concept is to treat these women as individuals, taking into consideration each woman's particular history, personal situation, and all available resources. All women of childbearing age should be encouraged to take appropriate daily amounts of folic acid; not only is this routinely recommended for prevention of neural tube defects in the fetus, but it may also serve to mitigate the effects of other medications taken during prepregnancy and gestational phases.

Limitations exist in the current evidence-based literature regarding pregnancy outcomes and psychiatric disorders. For example, not all studies on the use of antidepressants have included analysis of the mothers' psychiatric condition; further, confounding variables, such as poor prenatal care and use of tobacco or illicit substances, may alter study findings if not adequately controlled for. It has been documented that use of tobacco and alcohol by pregnant women can result in psychotic symptomatology in their offspring. In general, the mother's history of any psychiatric disorder and severity of symptom expression should be a guiding principle regarding observation and treatment during pregnancy. In addition, the primary-care clinician has in his or her armamentarium not only pharmacological treatment but also person-centered modalities ranging from cognitive-behavioral therapy (CBT) to social supportive care. When the mother's psychiatric condition is intractable to treatment and/or her symptoms place her or the fetus in jeopardy, electroconvulsant therapy (ECT) may be the treatment of choice and is approved for use during pregnancy and postpartum.

Epidemiology

The incidence of depression in pregnancy is estimated between 15% and 25%, but there is insufficient evidence to recommend routine depression screening. A joint report from the American College of Obstetricians and Gynecologists (ACOG) and the American Psychiatric Association advises close monitoring of a woman's emotional health during the prenatal and postnatal periods.

Management

For women who have an existing psychiatric diagnosis, treatment should be guided by the woman's prior pregnancy and medical history, as well as by the safety of pharmacological agents. Studies on the use of pharmacological agents during pregnancy offer the basis for treatment guidelines covering specific pharmacological agents and drug classes. There are pharmacological guidelines for depression in pregnancy endorsed by the American Psychiatric Association and ACOG, as well as available through the governmental National Clearinghouse Guidelines. One set of guidelines can be accessed at www.guideline.gov/content.aspx?id=36811&search=depression+and+pregnancy. Guidelines suggest that providers use a standardized tool for assessment of depression in pregnancy. Tools that have been validated in pregnancy are the PHQ-9 and the Edinburgh Postnatal Depression Scale. Screening should minimally occur at

the initial prenatal visit, at the four to 6-week postpartum visit, and again at three to 4 months after delivery. For women who have an active diagnosis of depression or a previous history of depression, evaluation for depression should occur at each visit. Positive screening requires further evaluation. This evaluation includes the duration and intensity of symptoms, suicide ideation, anxiety, substance use, and psychotic symptoms. Treating depressive disorders in pregnancy can affect the health of the mother and fetus. Untreated depression has been linked to altered fetal growth, interrupted prenatal care, miscarriage, preterm birth, substance use and abuse, infant temperament and behavioral issues, and mother-attachment issues. Women with a history of mania or hypomania are at risk for severe postpartum depression. Treatment of depression in the perinatal period involves a multidisciplinary, stepped-care approach based on the depression severity. For mild depression, CBT or interpersonal psychotherapy is indicated. For moderate depression, CBT (individual, group, or computer-assisted) or interpersonal psychotherapy is recommended. For women with symptoms that persist for greater than 8 weeks, an antidepressant should be considered. Psychiatric referral is indicated for women with severe depression, suicide ideation, psychotic symptoms, bipolar disorder (or a history of mania or hypomania), a current or recent episode of severe depression, no response to pharmacotherapy or psychotherapy, a history of schizophrenia or postpartum psychosis, severe coexisting anxiety, obsessive-compulsive disorder, panic disorder, eating, disorder, or substance abuse. In addition, ECT may be indicated for resistant depression during both the prenatal and postpartum periods.

Several psychiatric/psychotropic medications appear safe in pregnancy. For mood disorders, neither the tricyclic agents (TCAs) nor fluoxetine (an SSRI) has proven teratogenic, based on observational studies. There are limited data on the use of other SSRIs and SNRIs in pregnancy; most have shown no adverse outcomes, except for paroxetine, which has been associated with cardiac malformations. Guidance regarding the safety of medications during lactation is also limited. Generally, it is recommended to use agents that have shorter half-lives and greater protein-binding. Low infant serum levels of paroxetine and sertraline have been reported. Doxepin and clozapine should be avoided in lactating women. Women should be informed of the potential risks of the pharmacological agents, as well as the risks of untreated depression.

If a patient exhibits signs and symptoms of anxiety or panic disorder, the first choice of pharmacological agent during pregnancy should be an SSRI, because benzodiazepines are associated with an increased risk of orofacial clefting and cardiac malformations. In the case of bipolar disorder, a major problem occurs when considering the use of mood-stabilizing drugs. All of these agents are associated with teratogenesis, including valproic acid and carbamazepine (neural tube defects) and lithium (Ebstein's anomaly or hypoplasia of the right ventricle).

In women who suffer from psychotic disorders during pregnancy, a first generation agent with higher potency, such as haloperidol, should be used. Although this may seem paradoxical, use of lower-potency drugs, such as chlorpromazine, has been associated with teratogenicity during the first trimester. Newer "atypical" agents such as risperidone and olanzapine have not yet been adequately studied in pregnancy to offer any recommendations as to their use.

A further consideration is the postpartum period, when rapid transitioning of hormones may influence psychiatric presentations. Women with bipolar disorder are at highest risk postpartum for relapse into depression, mania, or rapid cycling. Other conditions with a higher risk of recurrent symptoms include women newly diagnosed with major depression during pregnancy, with recurrent major depression, or with a history of psychosis. There is limited evidence to guide the recognition and management of postpartum psychosis. A Cochrane review in 2013 concluded that further research is necessary before concrete guidelines can be developed. In these cases, medication should be considered immediately postpartum, whether it be an antidepressant or a mood-stabilizing agent. In addition, all providers should discuss medication effects on lactation and carefully explore with the woman her feelings about and experience with breastfeeding. Here as well, the *Circle of Caring* and nonpharmacological therapies can be offered.

Management of psychiatric disorders during pregnancy can be challenging but can be achieved with person-centered care, attention to available evidence, and well-coordinated, shared care with obstetric and mental health professionals.

■ GRIEF

Grief, mourning, and *bereavement* are terms that define a universal human response to loss.

Pathophysiology and Psychodynamics of Grief

Grieving is both an emotional and a physiological response. In acute grief, as in cases of other stressful events, there may be a disruption of biological rhythms. It is well documented that grief is accompanied by impaired immune function, specifically decreased lymphocyte proliferation and impaired functioning of natural killer cells, although it is not known how clinically significant these changes are. Manifestations of grief reflect cultural context, the individual's personality, previous life experiences, the significance of the loss, past psychological history, the relationship with the deceased, existing family and social networks, other life events, resources, educational level, and general state of health.

The stages of grieving, identified in the classic work of Elisabeth Kübler-Ross, are as follows:

- Denial
- Anger
- Bargaining
- Depression
- Acceptance

Grief is identified when the onset of a patient's symptoms is associated with the death of a loved one, either recent or past. Grief, however, may not be limited to the physical death of a loved one. Grief can also result from the loss of a significant relationship or the loss of an important aspect of one's identity.

Clinical Presentations

Each person grieves in a manner that is, for him or her, meaningful and effective. With normal grief, there is consistent progress toward acceptance.

Grief consists of three distinct phases: avoidance, confrontation, and accommodation.

- Acknowledging the loss
- Reacting to the separation—feeling the pain, expressing reactions
- Recollecting and reexperiencing the deceased and the relationship—realistically reviewing and remembering the deceased
- Relinquishing attachment to the deceased while still acknowledging a loving connection to the deceased
- Readjusting to move adaptively into the new reality without forgetting the old
- Reinvesting; redirecting one's energy to new goals, pursuits, hopes, causes, beliefs, activities

Grief can be understood as a journey along a well-marked psychological path: Each person travels in his or her own way and at his or her own speed. The way a person grieves, and, consequently, the amount of time a person needs to move from agony to acceptance is heavily influenced by personal, social, cultural, religious, and spiritual norms.

Lifestyle is also a factor to be considered. Individuals who live in social isolation may find it more difficult to grieve a loss without close significant others who can offer comfort and assistance. Grieving for a loss alone can drain psychosocial resources that are needed for day-to-day functioning. An equally difficult modern problem is the overvaluation of immediacy. Living with technology has increased our cultural expectations for speed. Human experiences that require time may appear suspect in this context. Busy employers, families, and friends may support grieving, as long as (in their perceptions) it does not take too long—the implication being that personal grief should not take too much time, or demand too many valuable social resources. After a year has passed, family and friends may begin to ask why the grieving person is not "over" his or her loss yet.

Grief can present in a number of different ways. It can range from absent or delayed grief to excessively intense and prolonged emotions, or to complicated grief associated with suicidal ideation or frank psychosis. The risk factors for a more complicated grief reaction include (1) sudden and/or violent death, (2) social isolation, (3) individuals who believe that they are in some way responsible for the death (real or imagined), (4) individuals with a history of traumatic losses, and (5) individuals who had an intensely ambivalent or dependent relationship with the deceased. In some instances, reduced or absent grief may be an appropriate reaction.

Differential Diagnosis

Cultural, ethnic, religious, and social beliefs, community and family traditions, and personal characteristics all determine how and when a person, a couple, or a family will mourn a loss. For some people, grieving is a well-defined, highly satisfying ritual. For others, particularly those who have never suffered a major loss before, grief can be confusing and disturbing. In terms of psychosocial health and well-being, the process of mourning should allow the person to experience pain but achieve acceptance. Grief reactions that are harmful to self or others or that persist without progressing toward acceptance require specialized care. Because of the pain and disturbance associated with extreme grief, some individuals may present their mourning as an illness that requires treatment rather than as a process.

Grief and depression share many of the same characteristics, and it can sometimes be difficult to evaluate exactly when the scope of normal grieving has slipped into a pathological realm. It is important to distinguish the grieving process from a major depressive episode. DSM-5 points out several features that help to define each process.

An individual with a history of depression is at risk for becoming depressed at times of major loss. The mood disturbance in depression is typically pervasive and unrelenting, whereas fluctuations of mood in grief are common. Grief is often described as "coming in waves, washing over" the individual affected; even in intense grief, moments of happy reminiscence can surface. In contrast, people suffering from major depression feel hopeless—they cannot imagine ever feeling better. Nonpathological grief, on the other hand, is a normal, although intensely painful, state that is responsive to support, empathy, and the passage of time. The emergence of a major depressive disorder associated with grief is a medical emergency and should be treated as such.

Management

All too often, treatment for bereavement occurs within the realm of tertiary intervention, when grief has already emerged as complicated. Early detection and preventive interventions could alleviate suffering and lead to earlier and more effective treatment. Primary-care clinicians can assist in the attainment of those goals by doing the following:

• Validating pain and distress related to loss
• Providing appropriate pharmacological therapy
• Making bereaved patients aware of the many supportive therapies available and having ready a list of referrals

In the case of terminal illness, early and ongoing bereavement assessment and a collaborative process are essential components of a preventive approach to bereavement care. Interventions include bereavement education and counseling that assist in facilitating communication with the dying person. There is strong evidence that involvement and caregiving benefits survivors.

Management of grief includes preparing (if possible) the person and family for the normal stages of grieving—normalizing grief. The practitioner should let the person know that feelings of guilt and anger are normal and counsel patience. Encouraging expression of feelings may be helpful. Offering comfort is important, but the practitioner must recognize that he or she cannot "fix" things for the patient—efforts to remove emotional pain can actually hinder the grieving process. Utilizing the *Circle of Caring* model, community services that focus on grief, especially traumatic grief (miscarriage, death of a child at birth, death from violence or war), church resources, family support, and other support services to deal with special issues, for example, single parenting, may all be beneficial. Provide medical therapy as indicated depending on symptomatology and past history. A brief course of a short-acting sedative may be appropriate during acute grief to induce sleep or to get through the funeral and burial, especially when supportive interventions have not succeeded. The use of drugs such as tranquilizers or alcohol, which numb emotions, should be discouraged over time. Narcotizing patients with drugs interferes with the normal process of grieving. Antidepressant therapy may be considered for patients with particularly prolonged or complex grief reactions, even when it may be difficult to differentiate depression from a normal grief response. Clinical data suggest that SSRIs may be beneficial and assist the patient to mobilize the energy necessary to progress through the stages of mourning and grief.

Specific counseling sessions for the bereaved may be extremely valuable and may assist in the prevention of pathological mourning or depressive reactions. These sessions, with trained counselors, can assist the grieving person in recognizing and expressing angry or ambivalent feelings toward a deceased person. Group counseling, as well as self-help groups, can be important adjunctive therapies. More than 30% of widows and widowers reported feeling isolated from friends and withdrawing from social activities; self-help groups offer companionship, social contact, and emotional support.

This is particularly important given the contraction of the family unit in modern times. Have a referral list available to assist the patient in seeking such psychosocial support.

The goals for treating complicated grief reactions include facilitating mourning and helping the patient to find new activities and relationships to substitute for the loss. Studies have found that effective treatment of depressive syndromes, even as early as 6 to 8 weeks after the death of a loved one, reduces suffering and facilitates the work of grief. The outworn notion that medications or psychotherapy impede the process of grief is unsubstantiated and may, at times, serve to prolong suffering and disability. Obviously, elements of psychosis clearly indicate a need for more aggressive treatment: Some patients may even become suicidal and should be monitored closely.

Follow-up

The manifestations of grief usually subside over time. Typically, acute grief reactions gradually lessen and within 1 to 2 months the grieving person is able to eat and sleep normally, beginning to return to normal functioning. Traditionally, grief lasts from 6 months to 1 year as the grieving person experiences the calendar year at least once without the lost person. This varies from person to person and is dependent on circumstances. The normal grieving process can extend up to 2 years.

Patient Education

It is important to prepare the person and family for the emotional "triggers" that will exacerbate the sense of loss—holidays, birthdays, or the anniversary of the death or traumatic event. The clinician should encourage good nutrition and health habits, especially in elderly patients. Grieving persons should be encouraged to maintain self-care and not to neglect any active medical problems of their own. The clinician can encourage physical activity as a positive way of dealing with the stress of grieving.

■ SUBSTANCE-RELATED AND ADDICTIVE DISORDERS

The chapter for substance-related and additive disorders in the *Diagnostic and Statistical Manual of Mental Disorders, Fifth Edition* (DSM-5) has undergone several changes. To eliminate the confusion between the terms *substance abuse* and *dependence,* these terms were removed and replaced with specific symptom criteria for each disorder. One important deletion is the criterion for recurrent legal issues. In addition, several behavioral addictions were added. These additions include gambling and Internet gambling. Evidence for other behavioral addictions such as hypersexuality, shopping, or exercise is less clear and is not included.

The primary-care provider has an obligation to inquire about, provide information about, and make appropriate referrals for substance-related or behavioral addictions. All agents in the substance-use disorder (SUD) category can cause tolerance, habituation, and physical dependence. The legal substances that fall into this category include tobacco and alcohol; illicit substances including cannabis, cocaine, opioids, hallucinogens, inhalants, stimulants, sedatives, hypnotics, and anxiolytics. Caffeine is unique in that it is not classified as an SUD agent, but symptom criteria for intoxication and withdrawal are provided. The science of addictions has grown over the last 20 years, and it appears that a neurophysiological basis is common to all addictive behaviors. These disorders are considered chronic and relapsing because despite significant negative consequences, the behaviors continue. It is now recognized that dopamine is vital in this process, and thus pharmacological agents have been introduced to target certain areas of the brain. Targeted treatments for tobacco, alcohol, and opioids are now available.

Substance-Related Disorders

It is important to note that in the United States, the term *addiction* has been replaced by the term *substance-use disorder.* The core features of SUDs include a triad of behavioral, physiological, and cognitive symptoms. A basic understanding of several terms is essential. Soon after consuming an agent, *intoxication* occurs. This process is considered reversible; as the effect of the substance wears off, a return to baseline generally occurs. Intoxication can occur in individuals without an SUD as well as in individuals with an SUD. Several symptoms of intoxication include impaired judgment, psychomotor and interpersonal behavioral changes, and alertness. Substance *withdrawal* is characterized by functional impairment related to the cessation or reduction of a substance, which is demonstrated in physiological, cognitive, and behavioral symptoms.

Use is defined as sporadic or intermittent utilization of alcohol or drugs with no adverse consequences. *Abuse* is defined as utilization of drugs or alcohol that causes the user some type of adverse consequence. *Dependence* involves physiological and/or psychological components. *Physical dependence* refers to the physiological effects of withdrawal from rapid dose reduction, abrupt cessation of the drug, or administration of an antagonist. *Psychological* or *behavioral dependence* emphasizes pathological use patterns and substance-seeking activities; it is a subjective need for the substance. *SUD* is a chronic illness characterized by impaired control, social impairment, and use despite significant consequences, tolerance, and withdrawal.

The risk of SUD is directly related to the properties of the drug of choice, such as availability, cost, how quickly the brain perceives the substance, and its ability to produce gratification or pleasure, as well as various environmental factors. A person may initially consume a drug for any number of reasons. However, people continue using a drug based on the actual or perceived rewards of substance use. Denial and rationalization of substance use, substance effects, or consequences of substance use make it possible for an individual to continue to use a substance as though he or she is immune to unexpected or dangerous consequences. Substance-related disorders that may be seen in a primary-care setting and that are included in this chapter are nicotine, alcohol, cannabis, hallucinogen, inhalant, opioid, sedative and hypnotic, and stimulant disorders. Caffeine is discussed in the intoxication and withdrawal section.

Epidemiology and Causes

The highest prevalence rates for substance use occur in persons aged 18 to 24 years. The current statistics are derived from the 2012 National Survey on Alcohol and Drug Dependence, which can be accessed from www.samhsa.gov/data/NSDUH/2012SummNatFindDetTables/NationalFindings/NSDUHresults2012.htm. In 2012, 26.7% of adults in the United States reported tobacco use. Use over the last 10 years has declined slightly. Tobacco use is the leading preventable cause of death and disability. The total direct and indirect costs incurred by the United States are nearly $200 billion. Nicotine and tobacco contribute to deaths from cancer, heart and lung disease, and infant mortality attributable to maternal smoking. More than 52% or 135.5 million persons aged 12 and older reported current alcohol use (one or more drink in the last month). Alcohol remains the primary substance of abuse and dependence; 14.9 million persons are dependent on or abuse alcohol alone, and 2.8 million persons are dependent on or abuse alcohol plus illicit drugs. For persons aged 12 years and older, 23.9 million persons had utilized an illicit substance in the previous month. Current illicit drug use among persons aged 12 years and older increased from 8.1% in 2008 to 9.2% in 2012. Substance dependence or abuse is estimated at 8.5% or 22.2 million in persons aged 12 or older. The total annual cost to society of substance use problems is estimated at almost $559 billion (health costs, loss of productivity, and crime-related costs).

Among all classifications—alcohol, alcohol plus illicit drugs, and illicit drugs alone—levels of dependence and abuse have remained stable from 2002 to 2012. The survey further identified that male sex, ethnicity, and education level seem to correlate with current alcohol use. Caucasians (57.4%) followed by individuals belonging to more than two races (51.9%) reported the highest alcohol use. The rates of alcohol use for other groups, in declining order, were as follows: African Americans 43.2%, American Indians or Native Alaskans 41.8%, Hispanics 41.7%, and Asians 36.9%. With increasing levels of education in adults age 18 or older, alcohol use increased; in addition, among adults with less than 12 years of education only 36.6% currently used alcohol versus 68.6% of college graduates. College students were more likely to use alcohol, binge drink, and drink heavily

than their peers who were not full-time students and those not in college; these rates did not change from 2002 to 2012. Binge alcohol use peaks in 21- to 25-year-olds with rates of 45%. More men aged 18 to 25 years (62.9% of males) reported alcohol use than women (57.5%). Increased volume of alcohol consumption correlates with increased use of illicit substances and tobacco use. Drinking and driving has declined over the last 10 years but was essentially unchanged from 2011 to 2012. The number of persons who drove under the influence of alcohol at least once in the past year was estimated to be 11.2%. Underage drinking (aged 12–20) is of particular concern, with current drinking rates estimated to be 9.3 million persons. These values have slowly declined over the past 10 years.

Marijuana was found to be the number one illicit substance used in 2012, followed by psychotherapeutic agents (pain relievers, stimulants, tranquilizers, and sedatives), cocaine, hallucinogens, and inhalants. The least used illicit substance was heroin. Marijuana's current use increased from 5.8% to 7.3% from 2007 to 2012. It is estimated that 4.3 million persons aged 12 years or older were classified as dependent on or an abuser of marijuana; 2.1 million persons aged 12 years and older were classified as dependent on or an abuser of pain relievers; and 1.1 million persons were classified as dependent on or an abuser of cocaine.

Age is a factor. In youths aged 12 to 17 years, concurrent use of illicit substances was greater in those who used tobacco or alcohol. The rate for substance dependence or abuse is highest for adults aged 18 to 25 years at nearly 18.9%, compared with youth aged 12 to 17 years at 6.1% and adults older than age 26 years at 7.0%. In addition, rates of nonmedical use of prescription drugs increased from 4.1% to 4.6% in young adults aged 18 to 25 years. In adults aged 26 to 59 years, there has been a gradual increase in illicit use, with marijuana and nonmedical use of prescription drugs being the most prevalent. This increase is suspected to be related to the aging baby boomers, who are known to have had increased exposure. Male sex, ethnicity, education, employment status, and criminal justice population seem to correlate with illicit substance use. In summary, national statistics indicate that the most commonly used legal substances are caffeine, alcohol, and nicotine; the most commonly used illegal substances are marijuana, prescription pain relievers, and cocaine.

Different population-based causes for substance abuse have been described. As with all psychiatric disorders, the initial causative theories evolved from psychodynamic models; subsequent models include behavioral, genetic, and neurochemical explanations. According to one National Institute on Drug Abuse (NIDA) survey, family transmission is a core risk factor for substance abuse. Both social learning and genetic models have been developed to explain the increased risk and incidence of substance abuse in the children of substance-abusing parents. Compared with earlier generations, however, Americans today are more likely to seek the immediate gratification and immediate solutions offered by drugs.

Comorbidities (also known as "dual diagnosis") are common in persons with substance abuse. The most common comorbidities are substance abuse with more than one substance and mood disorders including bipolar disorder, anxiety disorders, antisocial personality, and schizophrenia. People who abuse substances are about 20 times more likely to die from suicide than are those in the general population. About 15% of people with alcohol abuse or dependency commit suicide. The frequency of suicide among individuals in this group is second only to that among patients with major depression; many individuals with alcohol abuse or dependency may have underlying depression, further increasing their suicide risk.

Neurophysiological Basis of Addiction

Knowledge of the basic neurophysiological concepts of addiction is essential. Deleterious effects are seen in all individuals exposed to substance abuse. In infants exposed in utero, prematurity and developmental issues are seen; adolescents demonstrate poor school performance and high dropout rates, as well as an increased risk of violence and infectious diseases. Further, adults demonstrate poor concentration, coping, and interpersonal skills, which adversely affects employment, family dynamics, and parenting skills. In the past, many clinicians felt that addiction was a moral weakness, and this engendered negative perceptions about the patient; however, current knowledge helps to identify the differences in the brains of those with addiction and those without addiction. This research has helped to provide targeted treatments for specific diseases.

Anatomical pathways, neurotransmitter dysregulation, and imbalance and neuroadaptation are important neurophysiological components of addiction. The dopaminergic pathways located in this area of the brain are believed to be essential for the feelings of pleasure, reward, motivation, and incentive salience (whereby exposure to a stimulus is transformed from a pure sensory experience to one that brings it to the forefront of consciousness and causes it to be sought out). In addition, this area is essential for learning and memory, executive decision making, and behavior control.

Tolerance and dependence are believed to be related to the alteration of the neurochemical pathways, as well as overall cellular changes of the brain. This process of neuroadaptation can be persistent and permanent. These changes affect how the brain functions and have been the focus of research to describe the compulsive and harmful effects of addiction.

Diagnostic Reasoning
DSM-5 Symptom Criteria

The DSM-5 divides the substance-related disorders into two groups: *Substance Use Disorders* (those pathological behaviors associated with substance seeking activities) and *Substance-Induced Disorders* (intoxication, withdrawal, and mental disorders caused by a medication or a substance). The severity of substance-use disorders is identified as mild, moderate, or severe. Mild SUD occurs when there is a presence of two to three symptoms; moderate SUD is when there are four to five symptoms; and severe SUD is identified by six or more symptoms.

Substance-Use Disorders

The substance-use disorders are identified by the major symptom criteria listed below, taking into account the inherent properties of the specific substance. These behaviors need to occur within the previous 12 months with at least two of the following symptoms:

Impaired Control
- Use of a substance in greater amounts than intended or for more prolonged periods of time
- Persistent desire to use a substance or unsuccessful efforts aimed at decreasing or controlling substance use
- Extensive amounts of time spent obtaining, using, or recovering from the substance
- Intense desire or craving for the substance

Social Impairment
- Recurrent substance use results in work, school, or home obligation failures
- Continued substance use despite persistent interpersonal or social problems
- Continued substance use results in social isolation and/or withdrawal from recreational and family activities

Risky Use
- Recurrent substance use in physically hazardous situations
- Continued use despite physical or psychological problems

Tolerance
- Characterized by a marked increase in the amount needed to achieve the desired effect or intoxication, or a marked decrease in the effect achieved with the same amount of substance

Withdrawal
- Symptoms that occur when a substance has not been used; or the substance is used to relieve the symptoms of withdrawal

The existence and prevalence of significant comorbidities may make the "primary" disorder difficult to identify.

However, it is always necessary to concurrently treat the substance-abuse and dependence issues, regardless of the comorbidity. Evidence shows that unless the comorbid condition is also addressed and treated, recurrence of the substance abuse is likely.

Nicotine Disorders

Nicotine is the addictive substance in tobacco and is present in cigarettes, cigars, chewing tobacco, pipes, and snuff. Nicotine is readily absorbed and causes the adrenal glands to produce epinephrine. The epinephrine then stimulates the central nervous system (CNS), producing increases in heart rate, blood pressure, and respiration. At the same time, nicotine suppresses insulin output from the pancreas, leading to chronically high levels of blood glucose. Nicotine increases levels of the neurotransmitter dopamine as well, which accounts for a feeling of pleasure and relaxation. Thus, the immediate effects of nicotine are a brief period of stimulation and mild improvements in alertness, mood, and memory. The immediate brain dopaminergic and acetylcholine effects make the drug highly self-reinforcing. The half-life of nicotine is approximately 2 hours. Two hours after smoking, the chronic smoker experiences irritable nicotine cravings. As a mild stimulant, nicotine causes alterations in metabolism that can suppress appetite. Adolescent girls may intentionally become smokers with the hope that using nicotine will help them to stop the normal weight gain associated with puberty or improve their ability to control their appetite. Fear of weight gain keeps many young female smokers from stopping: A temporary weight gain of about 10 pounds is not uncommon when smokers first quit.

The biochemistry of nicotine withdrawal is complex, and nicotine withdrawal symptoms make quitting difficult. Management of withdrawal symptoms is the first and foremost goal of smoking cessation treatment. Nicotine withdrawal symptoms start within 2 hours of the last dose of nicotine, peak within 48 hours, and can last for weeks. Symptoms include severe cravings, irritability, decreased concentration, drowsiness, insomnia, decreased heart rate, decreased blood pressure, impaired motor skills, muscle tension, and increased appetite.

Treatment for tobacco dependence is effective, so all patients presenting for care should be asked about use of tobacco on a regular basis (Level I; U.S. Department of Health and Human Services, 2008). This should include regular questioning of and discussion with children and adolescents. Advice about smoking cessation increases rates of abstinence when done by primary-care providers (Level II; U.S. Department of Health and Human Services, 2008). Telephone, personal, and group counseling about tobacco cessation are all effective. There is a dose response seen for the clinical interventions and abstinence. Higher abstinence rates are associated with session length (more than 10 minutes), face-to-face treatment sessions (4–8 sessions OR 1.9; more

than 8 sessions OR 2.3), and the total amount of intervention contact time up to 90 minutes (Level I; U.S. Department of Health and Human Services, 2008). It is crucial that clinicians continue to provide guidance and counseling as patients move through their abstinence journey. The reference guide to utilizing the five As (ask, advise, assess, assist, and arrange) for treating tobacco use and dependence is available at www.surgeongeneral.gov/tobacco/tobaqrg.htm. Pharmacotherapy should be encouraged, and first-line effective therapies include nicotine replacement agents (gum, inhaler, nasal spray, and patch), bupropion SR (Wellbutrin SR), and varenicline (Chantix) (Level I; U.S. Department of Health and Human Services, 2008). There is evidence also suggesting that combination nicotine therapy is more effective than a single form of nicotine replacement (Level II; U.S. Department of Health and Human Services, 2008). Second-line therapies for tobacco cessation include clonidine (Catapres) (Level I; U.S. Department of Health and Human Services, 2008) and nortriptyline (Pamelor, Aventyl) (Level II; U.S. Department of Health and Human Services, 2008). At this time, there is not sufficient evidence available to rate the long-term efficacy of varenicline. See Drugs Commonly Prescribed 18.5 for available pharmacological agents.

Alcohol Disorders

According to the National Institute on Alcohol Abuse and Alcoholism (NIAAA), the younger the age at drinking onset, the greater the chance that at some point in life an individual will develop an alcohol disorder. The person who begins drinking before age 15 is four times more likely to develop an alcohol disorder as an adult. Researchers have found that the risk of adult alcohol disorders *decreases* by 14% for each additional year of age drinking onset is delayed. Individuals who start drinking at age 21 to 22 years have significantly lower risks for developing adult alcohol dependence. Alcohol disorders are family disorders. It is estimated that one in five adults in the United States has lived with an alcoholic while growing up. Children who grow up with alcoholism are at risk for being abused and becoming adult problem drinkers. Concurrent depression, anxiety, or personality disorder; evidence of a family history of alcohol disorder; or evidence of early age at drinking onset are critical risk factors for alcohol disorder. Although there is little debate that alcohol is an addictive drug, there is a great deal of debate regarding the nature of alcoholism. The core of the debate has to do with significant evidence of alcoholism as a genetic disorder, a biological disease, and as a maladaptive behavior. Alcoholism cannot be fully explained by any one of these models. What is not clear is how these different factors interact. What is clear, however, is that significant exposure to high blood alcohol levels increases the risk of uncontrolled, compulsive, or problem drinking.

The unique biochemical effects of alcohol are related to the drug's ability to produce both short-term and

Drugs Commonly Prescribed 18.5   Smoking Cessation

Drug	Indication	Adverse Reactions and Prescribing Considerations
Nicotine Replacements	Smoking cessation	Do not use concurrently with other nicotine products. Not indicated immediately after myocardial infarction, significant arrhythmias, or unstable angina. Not recommended for pregnant or nursing mothers; attempt nondrug treatment first. Pregnancy Category D for patch and inhalers and Category C for gum. Common side effects include tachycardia, nausea.
Transdermal patch		Apply topically to trunk or upper outer arm. Firmly press patch for at least 10 seconds (may need to shave area). Apply one patch per day for 16–24 hours, usually in the a.m. Use for 24 hours if symptoms of withdrawal occur in a.m. If vivid dreams occur, remove at bedtime and reapply on awakening. Skin reaction may be reduced by rotating sites.
Gum/lozenges		Gum must be chewed until a "tingling" sensation is felt and then "parked" in the buccal mucosa until the sensation dissipates and then chewed again. Repeat process; usually total of 30 minutes. Lozenge is to be sucked slowly over 30 minutes and not swallowed. For success with either agent: Use at least 9 pieces a day. Do not drink anything other than water for 15 minutes before and during gum chewing. Use in response to nicotine craving and decrease over time.
Nasal spray		Nasal spray: Prime pump, and administer intranasally by tilting head back and spraying into each nostril with meter-dose pump. Do not sniff, inhale, or swallow.
Inhalers		Inhaler method mimics smoking behavior. Must insert cartridge for each use. With the inhaler in place, use rapid shallow sucking method (preferred) or inhale slowly and deeply (requires effort). Cartridge used up in 20 minutes of active puffing.
Bupropion		Prescribe at 150 mg/day for 3 days; then increase to 150 mg twice daily. Do not take second dose sooner than 8 hours, and do not take later than 5:00 p.m. Do not use in patients with seizure disorder or eating disorder. Monitor for hypertension, especially if used with nicotine replacement. **Black Box Warning:** Increased risk of suicidal thinking and behavior. Counsel patients to stop medication if any changes in mood or behavior occur. Pregnancy Category C
Varenicline		If symptoms of depressed mood, agitation, or suicide occur, discontinue. **Black Box Warning: bipolar disorder, depression, schizophrenia, suicidal ideation.** Pregnancy Category C

Source: Clinical pharmacology [database online]. Gold Standard, Inc., Tampa, FL, 2013. http://cp.gsm.com.

long-term changes in neuron membranes and the enhancement and inhibition of critical ion channels. As a CNS depressant, alcohol compares to drugs such as barbiturates and benzodiazepines. Alcohol is readily absorbed from the stomach and small intestine into the bloodstream and is metabolized by the liver.

Alcohol intoxication is greatest when blood alcohol levels are increasing. In other words, alcohol intoxication is a manifestation of the rate at which alcohol is consumed.

- A blood alcohol level of 0.05 causes disruptions in thinking, judgment, and inhibition.
- A blood alcohol level of 0.1 produces obvious intoxication.
- A blood alcohol level of 0.2 results in depression of motor functioning and emotional/behavioral dyscontrol.
- A blood alcohol level of 0.3 produces stupor and confusion. Blood alcohol levels of 0.4 and higher produce coma.

Several terms are utilized in the literature to describe alcohol disorders, and it is important to have an understanding of the various definitions. The NIAAA defines *low-risk drinking* for men as less than 4 drinks per day and no more than 14 drinks per week, and for all women and men aged 65 and older no more than 3 drinks per day and no more than 7 drinks per week. *At-risk drinking* is consuming volumes greater than these guidelines. *Harmful drinking,* on the other hand, occurs when alcohol is causing physical, psychological, or social harm exhibited by zero to two dependence criteria and zero to one abuse criteria. The DSM-5 categorizes disorders as alcohol-use disorder, alcohol intoxication, and alcohol withdrawal (see Diagnostic Reasoning).

Other terms are frequently seen in the literature. The term *problem drinker* refers to persons who do not meet the diagnostic criteria for abuse or dependence but who experience problems related to alcohol, and the World Health Organization (WHO) uses the term *harmful use,* which can be defined as drinking that is causing either physical or psychological harm. In addition, the term *hazardous drinking* is characterized by the risk of harmful consequences (physical, mental, or social) related to alcohol use. Binge drinking (i.e., consuming 5 or more alcoholic beverages within 2 hours for men and more than 4 alcoholic beverages for women) often results in acute impairment and causes a large portion of alcohol-related deaths.

Alcohol affects circulation and cardiac functioning and dilates skin blood vessels, thereby producing flushing and a drop in body temperature. Reduction in risk of coronary artery disease has been proposed as a benefit of light to moderate consumption. The rationale for this proposal is based on the finding that in low doses, alcohol can increase high-density lipoprotein and decrease low-density lipoprotein. This benefit is canceled out, however, by common unhealthy behaviors such as poor diet or smoking or excessive use.

Alcohol-use disorder typically has a slow, progressive course; persons generally present for care after 10 to 20 years of use. At-risk drinking may progress to an alcohol-use disorder with its attendant morbidity and mortality. Components of the history can include driving under the influence (DUI), work issues, and relationship issues. Alcohol disorders have several deleterious health consequences. Manifestations of involvement of the cardiovascular system include hypertension, arrhythmias, dyslipidemia, cardiomyopathy, and stroke; gastrointestinal system involvement can be seen initially with dyspepsia and progress to gastritis, peptic ulcers, abnormalities of the liver enzymes, alcoholic hepatitis, fatty liver, pancreatitis, esophageal varices, and cirrhosis. Neuropsychiatric changes include peripheral neuropathy, memory impairment, suicidality, cortical atrophy, and dementia. Cancer risk is also increased, with oral, pharyngeal, laryngeal, esophageal, and possibly breast and colon cancers being the most prevalent. Safety issues are substantiated by an increased number of motor vehicles accidents, falls, burns, episodes of violence, and risky sexual behaviors.

It is important to understand that gender plays a part in alcohol disorders. Recommendations on daily use of alcohol for women are less than for men because of women's smaller body mass and less efficient ability to metabolize alcohol. Among heavy drinkers (men and women), women develop problems with alcohol at an accelerated rate and are at greater risk for cirrhosis; in addition, increased rates of miscarriage are seen.

Knowledge of alcohol withdrawal symptoms and appropriate therapy is essential. Abrupt cessation of alcohol in dependent persons can range from mild (characterized by symptoms such as irritability, tremulousness, and insomnia) to severe symptoms (characterized by withdrawal seizures, delirium tremens [disorientation, diaphoresis, visual hallucinations, tachycardia, hypertension, and agitation]); if left untreated, death is a potential complication. Treatment may occur in both the outpatient setting and the inpatient setting. Pharmacological therapy of withdrawal includes the intermediate- or long-acting benzodiazepines such as lorazepam, oxazepam, diazepam, or chlordiazepoxide. Carbamazepine has also been shown to be effective in mild to moderate symptoms of withdrawal and has the added advantage to decrease craving. In addition, adjunctive medications include antipsychotic medications such as haloperidol, which is utilized in patients with significant hallucinations and agitation. Cardiovascular stabilization with beta blockers needs to be considered in patients with coronary heart disease. When beta blockers are used with oxazepam, stabilization of vital signs and decreased craving have been demonstrated. In addition, clonidine has been found helpful in controlling hypertension and tachycardia. Phenytoin may be appropriate for patients with an underlying seizure disorder, but it is not effective for withdrawal seizures.

Screening It has been estimated that one in five patients presenting to primary care has a current problem or past problem with alcohol abuse. Primary care provides an excellent opportunity to address alcohol-related issues, provide education and information, and offer therapeutic modalities. Screening and behavioral interventions for alcohol disorders are recommended by the U.S. Preventive Services Task Force (USPSTF) (Level II; USPSTF, 2013) for all adults. NIAAA recommends screening as part of routine evaluations and in response to medical conditions that are affected by alcohol, as well as before prescribing medications that may interact with alcohol.

Several screening tools are available such as CAGE, Audit, and so forth (see Table 18.4). More recently, asking one question, "How often in the past year have you exceeded the maximum daily limit (specific for men and women as previously identified)?" has been found to be comparable in sensitivity and specificity to more involved tools. This question not only provides information to the clinician, but it also informs the patient of safe amounts of alcohol consumption. The clinician may use a more specific tool or refer the patient to a specialist to properly identify the severity of the disorder. Proper identification of at-risk drinking and alcohol abuse is important so that proper treatment can be initiated. Brief counseling is recommended for at-risk drinkers (Level II; USPSTF, 2013). Pharmacological therapy has been found to be helpful for dependent and chronic dependent drinking.

Cannabis Disorders

The psychoactive effects of marijuana are produced by cannabinoids, of which tetrahydrocannabinol (THC) is the active ingredient. Specific receptors for cannabis have been identified in the brain, particularly in the basal ganglia, hippocampus, and cerebellum. Tolerance and psychological dependence on cannabis have been reported, and abrupt discontinuation of high daily doses can produce withdrawal symptoms that include irritability, insomnia, and mild nausea. The euphoric effects of marijuana can last for hours. These effects include distortions of time, sound, color, and taste; changes in the ability to concentrate; and dreamlike states. Studies of the mental status changes produced by smoking marijuana indicate that the drug affects behavior by increasing brain cell–receptor sensitivity to dopamine. THC can create a mellow mood state by increasing gamma-aminobutyric acid (GABA) activity. THC impairs short-term memory by decreasing brain acetylcholine activity. High doses of marijuana are associated with red eye; mild increases in heart rate; orthostatic hypotension; increased appetite; dry mouth; and disruptions in recall, memory storage, and sensory-input coding. Memory impairment appears to be the most significant long-term effect of marijuana use.

Marijuana is most commonly smoked either through cigarettes (joints, nails, and reefer) or pipes (bongs or bowls); a potent marijuana resin (hashish) is also smoked. Ingestion is not as common but may be seen in foods and teas. Because marijuana is commonly smoked, it is very well absorbed from the pulmonary system to the circulatory system to the brain. Behavioral effects tend to develop immediately. Absorbed THC is distributed throughout the body but concentrates in body fat. THC crosses the blood–brain barrier with ease and efficiency. THC also crosses the placenta and affects the fetus. Ingested THC is slowly metabolized and eliminated by the liver over a period of 1 to 4 days. Chronic marijuana smokers can test positive for THC metabolites for weeks, despite brief drug-free periods.

Smoked marijuana has been shown to improve appetite in persons with HIV and AIDS and to reduce nausea and vomiting in chemotherapy patients. In recent years, the potency of THC in marijuana has increased from a low of 0.5% in the 1970s to levels from 6% to 10% in 2000. No longer a "Sixties symbol" of social rebellion, marijuana today may be equated by smokers with tobacco, alcohol, and caffeine. As with long-term users of nicotine, alcohol, and caffeine, long-term marijuana smokers who wish to stop usually find it extremely difficult to do so. Heavy daily users of marijuana experience significant withdrawal symptoms and cravings.

Significant health risks are associated with inhalation of marijuana. Fifty to seventy percent more carcinogens are present in cannabis than in tobacco, and thus patients may present to primary care with common respiratory complaints of cough, asthma, and respiratory infections. In addition, there is an increased incidence of head and neck cancers (twofold to threefold increase), as well as lung cancer. Circulatory changes seen include variability of blood pressure, arrhythmias, and cerebellar infarction. Immune system dysfunction and fertility issues of erratic ovulation and reduced sperm count have also been reported. Overall the most significant changes are in mood and cognition. Exacerbation of panic attacks, anxiety, and depression has also been reported. Other behavior changes may include a lack of desire to participate in activities; persistent cognitive and memory impairment, especially if abuse began in adolescence; and psychotic symptoms. In genetically predisposed adolescents, exposure to cannabis has been associated with onset of psychosis and worsening outcomes of schizophrenia. Medical marijuana use for various conditions such as glaucoma, AIDS wasting, neuropathic pain, spasticity, and nausea from chemotherapy has been proposed, but the Food and Drug Administration (FDA) and Drug Enforcement Administration (DEA) do not support its use at this time, although marijuana use for medical purposes is legal in some states. Limitations currently are related to a lack of valid studies with consistent THC dosage. In addition, the physical risks related to inhalation may further limit its use.

Hallucinogen-Related Disorders

The phencyclidines are synthetic agents that produce a range of feelings from dissociation to stupor and death. The dissociative agents can be smoked, consumed orally, or snorted. These agents include PCP, or angel dust. In addition, several other substances produce similar effects: ketamine (vitamin K, Special K, and Valium K) and *Salvia divinorum*. Persons taking these substances may present with various injuries from falls and accidents. Memory loss and deficits in cognition can last for months with chronic use.

The "other" hallucinogen use disorders involve the following substances: LSD, or lysergic acid diethylamide (acid, blotter, cubes, microdot yellow sunshine, blue heaven); mescaline (buttons, cactus, mesc, peyote); MDMA or ecstasy; and psilocybin (magic mushrooms, purple passion, shrooms, little smoke). These agents can produce hallucinations, nausea, and altered perceptions. These substances are usually taken orally but can be smoked, snorted, or taken by injection. Duration of effect can vary from hours to days depending on the substance. Flashbacks can occur with LSD. Ecstasy possesses stimulant properties and long-term neurotoxic effects in addition to the hallucinogenic properties. Withdrawal symptom criteria have not been established for any of the hallucinogenic agents.

Inhalant-Related Disorders

The exposure to volatile hydrocarbons from solvents (paint thinners, gasoline, glues); gases (butane, propane, aerosol propellants, nitrous oxide); nitrites (isoamyl, isobutyl, cyclohexyl) with street names such as laughing gas, poppers, snappers, and whippets comprise these disorders. These substances can produce neurocognitive problems, as well as pulmonary and cardiac issues. Inhalants have been associated with sudden death related to cardiac arrhythmias but also through respiratory depression and aspiration.

Opioid-Related Disorders

Opioid abuse can include both prescription and/or illicit drugs such as heroin. The most frequent prescription drugs of abuse include hydrocodone, fentanyl, oxycodone, oxymorphone, morphine, and methadone. Opioids can both relieve pain and cause euphoria. The pain relief effect by opioids is achieved by the drug attaching to the opioid receptor and thus blocking the subjective feeling of pain. The statistics of prescription abuse continue to escalate. Particular populations at risk for prescription opioid abuse include women, adolescents and young adults, and older adults. Attention to adequate pain management has become recognized as the standard of care. It is the clinician's responsibility to adequately evaluate, assess, and prescribe appropriate therapy for pain. This can be a daunting task in primary care. Several strategies may be helpful. Current guidelines are available

in dealing with chronic nonmalignant pain (see www. jpain.org/article/S1526-5900%2808%2900831-6/ abstract).

Heroin (also known as smack, H, ska, junk) abuse results in significant costs related to medical care, criminal justice, and lost productivity; it is estimated to cost the United States billions of dollars annually. Heroin can be injected, snorted, or smoked. Medical issues related to heroin use involve HIV/AIDS, hepatitis B and C, and tuberculosis, to name a few; social issues involve justice issues, the interference with education and employment, and significant family distress. More information about heroin abuse and addiction may be obtained at www. drugabuse.gov/publications/research-reports/heroin-abuse-addiction. Neonatal issues such as low birth weight and abstinence (withdrawal) symptoms can be addressed during pregnancy, with the mother receiving prenatal care in addition to comprehensive drug treatment and methadone maintenance.

Overall the number of new nonmedical users of pain relievers has not changed over the last 10 years. In 2012, 2.1 million persons were dependent on or abusers of prescription pain relievers. For the most recent use, over 54% of users obtained pain relievers free from family or friends, followed by 14.9% who bought the substance from a friend or relative.

Sedative-Hypnotic– or Anxiolytic-Related Disorders

The substances used in this disorder include barbiturates, carbamates such as muscle relaxers, and benzodiazepine and benzodiazepine-like agents. These substances are CNS depressants that can be utilized for legitimate medical conditions, but the behaviors of early refills and obtaining prescriptions from multiple providers helps to define this disorder. These agents can cause various neurological deficits in memory, coordination, autonomic depression, and cognition, and they produce many of the same effects as alcohol.

Stimulant-Related Disorders

Cocaine and amphetamine-related substances are included in this disorder. These substances are typically smoked, snorted, or injected. Diversion of stimulant attention-deficit/hyperactivity disorder medications also contributes to this disorder.

Cocaine Disorders

Cocaine acts as a CNS stimulant by blocking the reuptake of dopamine, thereby increasing dopamine activity in several areas of the brain. Cocaine may also have dopamine-agonist effects. The dopamine effects of cocaine account for most of the immediate and long-term effects of the drug. Biochemical studies of cocaine have shown that cocaine has extremely self-reinforcing, self-rewarding properties, and thus is highly addictive. The euphoria of cocaine intoxication, combined with the dysphoria of cocaine crashing and craving, can lead to compulsive consumption.

Cocaine is available in several forms: the hydrochloride salt that is inhaled or injected; the alkaloid solid, rock crystal (crack) made by combining the salt with baking soda or ammonia that is usually smoked; and freebase that is manufactured by heating the salt form and combining it with ether and then inhaling (freebasing). Intravenous administration and smoking have the most rapid pharmacological and euphoric onset of action (within 10–30 minutes), as well as discontinuation effect, whereas the onset for intranasal usage is 30 to 60 minutes. Compulsive and abusive use is associated with IV and smoking routes of administration.

One of the most important studies of cocaine's effects on the brain and emotional states successfully used functional magnetic resonance imaging (fMRI) to study the rush, high, low, and craving experiences of cocaine-dependent adults. Maximum cocaine blood levels were reached in an average of 7 minutes after infusion, dysphoria and paranoia developed about 11 minutes after infusion, and cravings for more cocaine occurred about 12 minutes after infusion. One of the most impressive indicators of the speed and scope of cocaine's effects on the brain was that subjects reported maximal feelings of euphoria as cocaine was being infused, before maximal cocaine blood levels had been reached. Cocaine intoxication is characterized by elation, significant increases in self-esteem, and the perception of improved task performance. Intoxication can also produce agitation, irritability, impaired judgment, impulsive sexual behavior, aggression, hyperactivity, and mania. Chronic cocaine use has been associated with the onset of symptoms of thought, personality, and mood disorders and with paranoid psychosis.

Tolerance to cocaine occurs as users are unable to achieve the euphoric effects of the first episode of use and subsequently escalate the dosage. In addition to its stimulant effect, cocaine also has anesthetic and convulsant effects; and sensitization develops even without a change in dosage. It is believed that this has contributed to deaths by cardiac arrest or seizure followed by respiratory arrest that may occur with the first use episode and precipitately with any use thereafter. Cardiovascular conditions such as hypertension, angina, myocardial infarction, and cerebrovascular accident may also be seen. In addition, pulmonary edema and respiratory depression may occur. Potential complications of pregnancy include abruptio placentae, uterine rupture, and hypertension. Higher rates of sudden infant death syndrome have been reported in infants exposed to cocaine prenatally.

Cocaine withdrawal is typically characterized by irritability, depression, and anxiety and generally decreases after the first few weeks of abstinence. Currently, there are no FDA-approved pharmacological agents to assist withdrawal. In early abstinence, insomnia may be problematic, as evidenced by memory and attention deficits

that may place the individual at higher risk of relapse. Some infants manifest symptoms such as tremulousness and irritability during the neonatal period.

Over the past few decades, smoked cocaine (crack), an extremely rapid-acting form of the drug, became cheap and easy to obtain. Cocaine has consistently been linked with severe social problems and antisocial behavior, such as gang violence and prostitution. Harmful behaviors such as driving while impaired, sexually transmitted disease exposure, and violence are also reported.

Amphetamine-Type Disorders

Substances include amphetamines, dextroamphetamine, methamphetamine, and methylphenidate. After having been a relatively popular and cheap drug of abuse, amphetamines quickly came to be associated with violent, bizarre behavior at a time when mellow "highs" were more socially acceptable. Decades later, amphetamines, particularly methamphetamine ("crank"), have once again become popular among older adolescents and young adults.

Methamphetamine is a synthetic agent also known as speed, meth, chalk, ice, and crystal. Users describe being high as being "amped" (amplified) or "tweaked." Methamphetamine is a potent, easy-to-make, inexpensive stimulant, which can be snorted or injected. "Crystal-meth" is methamphetamine in a free-base form; "ice" is a high-grade form of "crystal-meth" that is sold in rocks, like crack cocaine. Because of its purity and potency, "ice" is expensive; one hit can deliver an extreme amphetamine high that can last for hours. A methamphetamine rush is intense. Intoxication includes elation, increased self-esteem, increased physical endurance, insensitivity to fatigue, and feelings of being invulnerable. Methamphetamine half-life is 11 hours or more, which far exceeds that of cocaine. This long half-life contributes to the longer neurological changes. But like cocaine, amphetamine increases dopamine activity, is self-reinforcing, and is a highly efficient addictive agent. Several side effects of methamphetamine use are hyperthermia, dehydration, a significant anxiety, insomnia, mood disturbances, and violent behavior, as well as psychosis. These symptoms can persist even after the behavior of abuse has stopped. Additional physical signs and symptoms include dermatological changes such as sores and dental issues, including tooth decay and tooth loss.

Chronic users experience acute episodes of euphoria and dysphoria that can mimic bipolar disorder. Other medical issues that can occur with stimulant use include nasal septum perforation, respiratory and cardiovascular issues such as chest pain, myocardial infarction, arrhythmias, and stroke. Stimulant use produces several adverse pregnancy outcomes.

Clinical Presentation

Patients who ask questions about their personal substance use may have used substances for a relatively short period of time; but more often, patient questions are motivated by having recently suffered negative consequences from long-standing substance use. Routine substance use and abuse screening has become a standard of practice in primary care. The most consistent identifier for substance abuse may be the numerous health consequences of abusing drugs and alcohol. Personal characteristics are not reliable indicators. Persons of all ages, races, religions, and every socioeconomic status are susceptible to substance abuse, and substance dependence typically follows substance abuse.

Substance-Induced Disorders

Substance-induced disorders are divided into intoxication, withdrawal, and mental disorders caused by a medication or a substance. The clinical presentation of a person with substance intoxication, abuse, or withdrawal will vary depending on the substance abused. Table 18.15 presents a summary of the clinical presentation of an individual with cannabis, cocaine, amphetamine, nicotine, caffeine, or alcohol intoxication and withdrawal. The DSM-5 symptom criteria are listed below.

Substance Intoxication

- Symptoms are reversible and are directly related to recent ingestion of a substance.
- The substance causes substance-specific induced behavioral or psychological changes. These behaviors can include issues associated with judgment, wakefulness, interpersonal skills, and the like.
- The symptoms cannot be explained by another medical or psychological problem.

Withdrawal

- Substance-specific physiological, psychological, and cognitive changes associated with the absence of or decreased use of the substance usually associated with intense craving to diminish the symptoms.
- The syndrome causes functional impairment.
- The symptoms cannot be explained by another medical or psychological problem.

Caffeine-Related Disorders

Caffeine is present in many products. The average daily U.S. consumption over the last 10 years has remained

---

Table 18.15   Clinical Presentation: Selected Substance Intoxication and Withdrawal

Cannabis-Related Disorders

- *Cannabis-Use Disorder:* Two or more of the symptom criteria should be present within the previous 12 months.
- *Intoxication:* Intoxication typically includes euphoria, grandiosity, impairment of complex mental processes; user perceives self and experiences as occurring in slow motion. Symptoms occur within **2 hours** of cannabis use. Two or more of the following should also be present: conjunctiva injection (red eye), increased appetite, dry mouth, and tachycardia. The above symptoms are not attributable to any other substance or medical condition.
- *Cannabis Withdrawal:* Occurs after stopping cannabis after prolonged use. Within 1 week three or more of the following symptoms are present: anxiety, depression, anorexia, irritability, insomnia or disturbing dreams, agitation, or various physical symptoms such as headache, tremors, fever, or chills. The above symptoms cause significant sociocognitive impairment and are not attributable to any other substance or medical condition.

Stimulant-Related Disorders

- *Stimulant-Use Disorders:* Two or more of the symptom criteria should be present within the previous 12 months.
- *Intoxication:* Intoxication typically includes a sudden change in behavior, which can include hypervigilance, euphoria, etc., accompanied by two or more of the following: pupil dilation, either an increase or decrease in heart rate, blood pressure, or motor activity. Chest pain, nausea and/or vomiting, weight loss, or neurological changes such as seizures, dystonias, or confusion. Symptoms occur either during or shortly after use. The above symptoms are not attributable to any other substance or medical condition.
- *Withdrawal:* Occurs within hours or days of last use. There is intense dysphoria and weariness. Suicidal thoughts and behavior can develop. Characteristic withdrawal includes severe dysphoria and two or more of the following: fatigue, vivid nightmares, insomnia or hypersomnia, increased appetite, and psychomotor retardation or agitation. Some people may have only mild withdrawal symptoms. Experienced heavy users may plan their drug use to include substances that can prevent or minimize withdrawal. The above symptoms cause significant sociocognitive impairment and are not attributable to any other substance or medical condition.

Tobacco-Related Disorders

- *Tobacco-Use Disorder:* Two or more of the symptom criteria should be present within the previous 12 months.
- *Tobacco Intoxication:* No characteristics for intoxication.
- *Tobacco Withdrawal:* Cessation of daily tobacco use will produce symptoms within 24 hours. Four or more of the following symptoms must be present: depressed mood, sleep disturbances, impaired concentration, anxiety, restlessness, appetite increase, and irritability. The above symptoms cause significant sociocognitive impairment and are not attributable to any other substance or medical condition.

Table 18.15   Clinical Presentation: Selected Substance Intoxication and Withdrawal—cont'd

Hallucinogen-Related Disorders

- *Phencyclidine- or Other Hallucinogen-Use Disorder:* Two or more of the symptom criteria should be present within the previous 12 months.
- *Phencyclidine or Other Hallucinogen Intoxication:* Several behavioral symptoms occur shortly after use of phencyclidine. These symptoms can include impulsiveness, aggressiveness, confrontational and psychomotor agitation, etc. Two of the following signs and symptoms will generally occur within 1 or 2 hours following ingestion of the substance: nystagmus, increased heart rate or blood pressure, decreased sensitivity to pain, ataxia, sensitivity to sound, muscle rigidity, and seizures or coma. For other hallucinogens the psychological symptoms that occur shortly after use include significant depression, anxiety or paranoia, "fear of losing one's mind," accompanied by significant perceptual changes. Shortly after use, two or more of the following signs and symptoms will occur: pupil dilation, increased heart rate and blood pressure, tremors, sweating, and incoordination. The above symptoms are not related to any other substance or medical condition.
- *Phencyclidine or Other Hallucinogen Withdrawal:* There are no established withdrawal symptoms.

Inhalant-Related Disorders

- *Inhalant-Use Disorders:* Two or more of the symptom criteria should be present within the previous 12 months.
- *Inhalant Intoxication:* Problematic behaviors occur after exposure to an inhalant. Intoxication typically includes a sudden change in behavior, which can include belligerence and impaired judgment accompanied by two or more of the following: neurological symptoms such as nystagmus, dizziness, slurred speech, incoordination, unsteady gait, tremor, muscle weakness and decreased reflexes, vision changes, lethargy, and euphoria. The above symptoms are not related to any other substance or medical condition.
- *Inhalant Withdrawal:* Generally mild and not recognized as a specific disorder.

Opioid-Related Disorders

- *Opioid-Use Disorder:* Two or more of the symptom criteria should be present within the previous 12 months.
- *Opioid Intoxication:* Intoxication typically includes a sudden change in behavior, which can include euphoria, change in motor activity, indifference, etc., with pupillary constriction and accompanied by either slurred speech, impaired concentration, or altered mental alertness. Symptoms occur either during or shortly after use. If hallucinations are present, a specifier with perceptual disturbances is required. The above symptoms are not related to any other substance or medical condition.
- *Opioid Withdrawal:* Can occur either on interruption in use or with the administration of an opioid antagonist. Characteristic withdrawal begins within minutes to days after last use. At least three of the following symptoms need to be present: severe dysphoria, gastrointestinal symptoms of nausea and/or vomiting or diarrhea, eye tearing or rhinorrhea, diaphoresis or pupillary dilation, fever, yawning, and sleep disturbances. The above symptoms cause significant sociocognitive impairment and are not related to any other substance or medical condition.

Sedative, Hypnotic, or Anxiolytic Disorders

- *Sedative-, Hypnotic-, or Anxiolytic-Use Disorders:* Two or more of the symptom criteria should be present within the previous 12 months.
- *Sedative, Hypnotic, or Anxiolytic Intoxication:* Intoxication typically includes a sudden change in behavior, which can include significant and frequent changes in mood, aggression, or impaired judgment. In addition, one or more of the following symptoms: nystagmus, change in sensorium, change in gait, garbled speech, or coma. Symptoms occur either during or shortly after use. The above symptoms are not related to any other substance or medical condition.
- *Sedative, Hypnotic, or Anxiolytic Withdrawal:* Symptoms can occur within hours to days of last use. Symptoms can include tremor, palpitations, increased blood pressure, nausea and vomiting, motor hyperactivity/restlessness, nervousness, insomnia, hallucinations, and grand mal seizures. At least two of the above symptoms must be present. The above symptoms cause significant sociocognitive impairment and are not related to any other substance or medical condition.

Caffeine-Related Disorders

- *Caffeine Intoxication:* Recent ingestion of a caffeinated product (usually greater than 250 mg). In addition, five of the following symptoms occur shortly after ingestion: agitation, excitability, diuresis, facial flushing, an increase in motor activity, insomnia, tachycardia, etc. The above symptoms cause significant sociocognitive impairment and are not related to any other substance or medical condition.
- *Caffeine Withdrawal:* Sudden cessation or decreased use of daily caffeine generally results in symptoms within 24 hours. Three or more of the following symptoms must be present: headache, fatigue, impaired concentration, mood changes, and various physical symptoms such as muscle aches and nausea and vomiting. The above symptoms cause significant sociocognitive impairment and are not related to any other substance or medical condition.

Source: American Psychiatric Association. *Diagnostic and statistical manual of mental disorders, fifth edition* (DSM-5). American Psychiatric Association, Arlington, VA, 2013.

stable at 300 mg per person per day. At low doses, caffeine causes symptoms such as insomnia and restlessness. At high doses (greater than 1,000 mg/day), caffeine may induce arrhythmias, and psychomotor agitation can occur. Death from caffeine can occur with ingestion of 5 to 10 g. Well-known products that contain caffeine are coffee, tea, soft drinks, over-the-counter medications, energy drinks, some snack foods, some ice creams and yogurts, and chocolate. There is great variability in the amount of caffeine present in products as well as the individual's response to a particular dosage. The primary source of caffeine for adults and youths comes from beverages. The caffeine content of coffee can range from 95 to 330 mg depending on the size of the beverage. Even decaffeinated coffee contains small amounts of caffeine ranging from 3 to 12 mg/serving. The caffeine content of tea ranges from 15 to 74 mg/serving. Caffeinated soft drinks include colas, Mountain Dew, and some root beers. The caffeine content of these beverages can range from 22 to 69 mg per 12 ounce serving. Energy drinks can contain anywhere between 33 and 400 mg of caffeine per serving. Over-the-counter medications that contain caffeine include analgesic and weight loss products, as well as agents used to inhibit sleep; caffeine contained in these products can range from 30 to 130 mg/serving. For further information on various or specific products, see the FDA report at www.fda.gov/downloads/AboutFDA/CentersOffices/OfficeofFoods/CFSAN/CFSANFOIA-ElectronicReadingRoom/UCM333191.pdf. Nowadays, youth are exposed to caffeine products at younger ages. The impact of long-term, higher caffeine exposure at younger ages poses many unanswered questions.

Gambling Disorder

To meet the DSM-5 criteria for a gambling disorder, four of following symptom criteria need to be present for 12 months and the disorder must be causing significant distress:

- The amount of money used to gamble increases to achieve same level of excitement
- Displays symptoms of irritability when attempting to decrease or stop gambling
- Attempts to stop or decrease gambling have failed
- Spends significant amount of time trying to figure out how to get money to gamble or planning next episode
- Gambling often occurs when feeling distressed
- Attempts to break even by returning to gamble after a loss
- Lies to others
- The behavior has harmed relationships with significant others (family, friends, employer, etc.)
- Is unable to manage financial responsibilities independently

Severity of the disorder is rated as mild with 4 to 5 criteria met, moderate with 6 to 7 criteria met, and severe with 8 to 9 criteria met.

Management

The first treatment goal in substance abuse is abstinence. Research for many years has shown that moderation in usage is rarely effective for those with a substance abuse problem. The second goal is restoring the physical, psychological, and social well-being of the person and family. Significant damage has often been done to the patient's support system. The family may have additional codependent and enabling issues to address and also may need treatment. Sometimes relationships that have remained intact during the substance-abuse phase ultimately falter and disintegrate when one partner becomes engaged in treatment.

Although some patients with substance-related problems recover without formal treatment, especially as they age, most require a variety of interventions. Approaches include specific procedures or techniques such as individual therapy, family therapy, group therapy, relapse prevention, pharmacotherapy, and treatment programs. Treatment programs tend to be multidisciplinary and often include a specific set of procedures. However, there is no standardization of terminology for categorizing treatment programs and procedures, and their effects are difficult to measure. Broadly, some programs focus on controlling acute withdrawal (detoxification), and others aim at long-term behavioral change. Some use pharmacological interventions, and others are based on individual psychotherapy, Alcoholics Anonymous (AA) or other 12-step principles, or therapeutic community principles. Publicly funded treatment programs for drug dependence are categorized as methadone maintenance (mostly outpatient), outpatient drug-free programs, therapeutic communities, or short-term inpatient programs. Substantial reduction in illicit drug use, antisocial behaviors, and psychiatric distress among patients dependent on cocaine or heroin are much more likely following treatment lasting at least 3 months. Such a time-in-treatment effect is seen across very different modalities, from residential therapeutic communities to ambulatory methadone maintenance programs.

After an initial period of detoxification, persons in treatment for substance abuse will need a period of sustained rehabilitation that includes education, support, and, in some cases, psychotropic drugs to discourage them from using the substance involved or to treat any underlying psychiatric disorder.

Patients with substance-use disorders may be resistant and fearful or lack the will and motivation to confront their behavior. In addition to primary care, specialized substance treatment services are needed if the patient's disorder is to be addressed adequately and his or her risk for substance-related disability, morbidity, and mortality are to be decreased. Primary-care practitioners are often the first health-care professionals to observe the health and psychosocial impact of substance abuse; sometimes the practitioner is the only health-care professional the patient is willing to talk to. Clinicians can take advantage of this by striving to help patients recognize their substance abuse and take the first steps toward improvement. Several options are available from brief advice, printed information, brief intervention (FRAMES) (see Resources), professional intervention, peer intervention, and referral to treatment and/or self-help groups. Brief intervention has been most helpful for the "at-risk" drinker; for the dependent drinker, its role is less clear.

An *intervention* is a strategy to get a person who has been resistant to treatment to confront the reality of his or her drug and/or alcohol problem. In a private location, close family and friends confront the individual with the facts of his or her substance abuse and the consequences of actions the individual has taken or failed to take. The intervention is an attempt to hold the person accountable for his or her actions, using a "tough love" approach. The end result sought is for the person to willingly choose to seek treatment. Patients with poor physical health or severe legal and interpersonal problems will need improvement in these areas in order to feel able to change their substance-abuse behaviors. Substance-related mental disorders should be treated as well. Patients often already have a great deal of information about their substance abuse and the benefits of stopping. The most useful patient education will address the process of stopping. Some people are able to stop on their first try, but the more typical pattern is repeated efforts to stop until the individual is finally substance free.

Specific management of each case will depend on the substance being abused. General indications for the need for inpatient treatment of substance abuse are presented in Table 18.16. Specific interventions and assessment tools the clinician may use for nicotine or alcohol disorders can be accessed from www.surgeongeneral.gov/tobacco/tobaqrg.htm and www.ahrq.gov/legacy/clinic/tobacco/tobaqrg.htm. Clinical tools can be accessed at www.projectcork.org.

Pharmacological therapies are available for nicotine, alcohol, and opioid disorders. Nicotine agents are listed in Drugs Commonly Prescribed 18.5. Pharmacological options for maintenance of alcohol abstinence in dependent drinkers include disulfiram (Antabuse), oral and extended-release injectable naltrexone (Revia), and acamprosate (Campral) (Level I; Anton et al, 2006). For most, naltrexone is the primary drug choice unless co-occurring opioid use is present (Level II; Rösner et al, 2010).

Treatment options for opioid disorders may include detoxification (managed opiate withdrawal), behavioral strategies, and pharmacological intervention. Long-term maintenance of abstinence can be achieved by methadone maintenance and buprenorphine (Subutex, Buprenex) alone or with naltrexone. It is imperative for all disorders that behavioral therapies are ongoing

---

Table 18.16   Indications for Inpatient Treatment of Substance Abuse

Several factors need to be considered when identifying the best treatment placement for patients with substance-use disorders. Of particular concern is withdrawal from alcohol and from the sedative, hypnotic, and anxiolytic agents. Withdrawal from these agents can cause cardiovascular collapse, delirium, and death. Withdrawal from opiates does not impart the same risk. Cardiac monitoring may be indicated in cocaine intoxication. Assessing medical stability requires evaluation of several factors. These factors include the following:

Current Situation
- Severe illness—unable to tolerate oral medications
- Suicidal and homicidal ideation—either in ideation or intent
- Lengthy and heavy substance abuse
- Prior unsuccessful attempts at ambulatory medically supervised withdrawal
- Social conditions such as homelessness with decreased chance to complete ambulatory medically supervised withdrawal
- Active psychosis or severe cognitive impairment
- Medical conditions—cardiovascular disease, pregnancy, liver disease
- Withdrawal symptoms for the substance OR taking the same (or closely related) substance to relieve symptoms of withdrawal
- Alcohol withdrawal symptoms as defined by DSM-5. Objective measurement of alcohol withdrawal symptoms is recommended. The Clinical Institute Withdrawal Assessment of Alcohol (CIWA-Ar) is commonly utilized. Scores of greater than 20 are considered severe; 10–19 moderate withdrawal; and scores less than 10 are interpreted as mild. Consider inpatient management for scores greater than or equal to 10.
- Severely dependent on sedative, hypnotic, and anxiolytic agents

Past History
- History of withdrawal
- History of withdrawal seizures or delirium tremens

Source: VA document. Assess level of physiological dependence and indications for stabilization including risk of withdrawal. VHA/DoD clinical practice guideline for the management of substance use disorders. 2009. Retrieved from www.guideline.gov/summary/summary.aspx?doc_id=3169&nbr=002395&string=VHA%2fDoD.

(Level II; Lieber et al, 2003; Willenbring et al, 1995; Willenbring & Olson, 1999).

Treatment of the severely mentally ill who are also drug dependent continues to pose problems; specialized addiction agencies have trouble treating such patients. Generally, integrated treatment of both the psychiatric disorder and the addiction is more effective than either parallel or sequential treatment. Integrated models of care are limited but increasingly recognized in local and state mental health agencies. A related issue is the funding of treatment programs for substance-related disorders in general. Managed care organizations tend to assume that the relatively brief course of outpatient counseling will be effective with patients who are dependent on illicit drugs, perhaps suffer from significant comorbidities, and who have minimal social supports. At present, the trend is a short-term view that provides the care that costs the least, ignoring studies that show that more services can produce better long-term outcomes.

Follow-up and Referral

In addition to primary care, patients being treated for substance abuse will need access to several information and support resources, which should include education services, treatment programs, and support groups. It is unlikely that any single program or support group will be sufficient, so patients are encouraged to make repeated contact with several different types of programs and groups (see Case Study 18.2).

Referral to a specialist should be made immediately when the patient's behavior represents a danger to self or others. Substance abuse, particularly alcohol abuse, is a factor in motor vehicle accidents, family violence, and suicide. It can also be very helpful for patients to have at least one appointment with a specialist, in order to develop a comprehensive assessment of the patient's substance use and abuse. For the patient, this assessment is a critical source of information that can reduce his or her ambivalence toward making needed changes in substance-related behaviors. Seeing a specialist can also be motivational, in that one of the most common reasons for failing to try to make required changes in behavior is the patient's unspoken fears of failure.

Patient Education

Individuals who have developed psychological and physical needs for a substance often have also formed strong attachments to their substance-use lifestyle and substance-based relationships. It may be impossible to effectively address a person's substance abuse without taking into account his or her substance-based relationships and attachments. A person can become strongly attached to the people, places, and community that make up his or her substance-abuse lifestyle. From friendships among coworkers that develop at designated smoking areas to football parties and alternative lifestyles, for many people, the thought of giving up their attachments may be more painful than the thought of giving up their actual substances of abuse. The fear of losing these valued attachments is frequently used to rationalize continued substance abuse.

Personal losses may increase or decrease the motivation to significantly change substance-use behaviors. Individuals who have not suffered substance-abuse–related losses may nevertheless have to deal with significant interpersonal conflicts related to their substance-abuse behaviors. Years of substance abuse can result in the loss of all non–substance-based relationships, significant loss of self-esteem, financial losses, and loss of physical and mental health. These personal losses can have a devastating psychological impact on the individual. The patient may feel that he or she is in a no-win situation: Feelings of hopelessness may manifest as ambivalence about making needed changes in substance-use behaviors or bravado about continued substance abuse.

CASE STUDY 18.2 Substance Abuse and the *Circle of Caring*

The following vignette, abstracted from L. Smith-Battle, M.A. Drake, and M. Diekemper, "The Responsive Use of Self in Community Health Nursing Practice," *Advances in Nursing Science* 20(2):85, 1997, addresses a person with substance abuse. It is a story that highlights the skills of involvement, coordination, and advocacy that helped to reintegrate this mother into the community and the child into the family. The mother's eventual reintegration was contingent on the APRN's responsiveness and perseverance in a situation with an uncertain outcome, which demonstrates practice within a *Circle of Caring*.

In this situation, an unreceptive new mother tested positive at the birth of her baby for cocaine abuse. The infant was severely injured at 2 months of age in a car accident when, unrestrained, he hit his head against the dashboard. The infant was removed from the mother's care and placed with an aunt. The following account is from a nurse involved with the family:

> [In the year after the accident], I saw the baby at the aunt's house and we got him involved with developmental programs . . . I hooked them up with all that . . . Meanwhile, I was visiting mom. [Describes how the mother was in and out of treatment programs.]

CASE STUDY 18.2 Substance Abuse and the *Circle of Caring*—cont'd

I got a phone call from her one morning. She told me that a drug dealer had beat her up and put a gun to her head over a 5-dollar debt. "I'm going to die. I'm either going to get killed or I'm going to die of using cocaine." So I worked with the social worker and we got her into a long-term, 3-month treatment [program] away from the entire environment. And when she came back, I will never forget, I cried when I called her. She had make-up on. She had gained weight . . . I didn't even recognize her . . .

A year later, when she came back, she started visiting with her son at the aunt's house, and gradually the whole team, the social worker, myself, the aunt, and all other interventionists, we had huge meetings and we basically started reintegrating the child into the home. And now she has him full-time. And she's been clean . . . She keeps up with all [her son's appointments] and she goes to Narcotics Anonymous three times a week. She wants to become a treatment counselor and . . . she finished her GED. She's just a total success story . . .

. . . She told me once, "Everyone that ever cared about me has left me or treated me like crap." . . . [it] was the first time in her life where [although] she was down-right obnoxious and hateful [to me], I never bit back or quit coming. I mean, I accepted her behavior because I knew it was the drug use and it wasn't her.

The clinician should educate patients regarding the effects of drugs, especially during pregnancy, and provide information on substance abuse and treatment to patients and their families. Practitioners should provide information regarding danger of exposure to HIV, hepatitis, and other infections, and to obtain appropriate testing if there is suspicion of exposure. Care providers should teach family members about the dynamics that may continue to enable substance abuse; often they are unaware of these. The clinician can give family members specific feedback in this area about behaviors that he or she has observed; it is also important to discuss the strategy of using an intervention with the family and how to set up one if indicated.

Codependence is a term that has come to mean the behavioral patterns of family members who have been significantly affected by another family member's substance use or addiction. Related concepts of enabling and denial may characterize family members of patients who abuse substances. Twelve-step programs should be encouraged—for example, Narcotics Anonymous (NA) or Alcoholics Anonymous (AA) for the individual with the substance-abuse problem and Al Anon for family members. As noted earlier, family members and significant others need treatment also. The *Circle of Caring* model may be utilized in caring for those with addictions.

■ SLEEP–WAKE DISORDERS

Description and classification of sleep–wake disorders has been expanded in DSM-5 to reflect the important diagnostic overlay of medical conditions that affect normal sleep patterns. Of particular importance to primary care are Insomnia Disorder, Obstructive Sleep Apnea Hypopnea Syndrome (OSAHS), Substance/Medication Induced Disorder, and Restless Legs Syndrome (RLS). Insomnia disorder will be presented in detail, because insomnia is an underpinning of each of these disorders. The criteria and important contributing factors for OSA, RLS, and substance-induced sleep disorder will be discussed.

Insomnia disorder, or difficulty sleeping, is an extremely common problem, yet it is one that is etiologically complex. It is defined as difficulty in falling asleep or maintaining sleep, early morning wakefulness, or any combination of these. It must cause clinically significant distress or functional impairment, occur at least 3 nights per week, be present for at least 3 months, and not be a consequence of a substance.

Epidemiology and Causes

It is estimated that 10% to 17% of the primary-care population report daytime insomnia symptoms and that 6% to 10% meet criteria for the disorder. Women appear to be slightly more affected than men are, and up to 50% of sufferers have a comorbid mental disorder.

Acute insomnia may be precipitated by physical or emotional discomfort. Examples include pain, acute illness, and environmental disturbances such as noise, light, and temperature. Sleeping at a time that is inconsistent with daily biological (circadian) rhythms because of plane travel across time zones (jet lag) or shift work may also precipitate acute insomnia. Any number of underlying medical conditions may contribute to insomnia. Pain may contribute to wakefulness; indeed, often the question, "Does the pain awaken you at night?" is an important piece of information in determining the severity of pain. Examples of painful conditions that commonly affect sleep are arthritis and muscle cramps. Insomnia is also associated with some types of delirium and dementias (e.g., "sundowning"). Acid reflux and duodenal ulcers may also cause insomnia. Fibromyalgia is closely associated with insomnia and is classified by some as a sleep disorder. Additional risk factors for insomnia include chronic illnesses, thyroid disorders, obesity (also correlated with sleep apnea), and drug usage. Insomnia related to discomfort in certain sleeping positions is common during pregnancy; it may also occur during the postpartum period because of caregiving that interrupts sleep, along with postpartum hormonal shifts.

A variety of psychosocial problems may also contribute to insomnia: Anxiety, mania, and schizophrenia specifically are associated with insomnia. Traumatic events can precipitate an acute, transient insomnia that may become chronic if not properly managed. Chronic stress, hyperarousal of the type associated with PTSD, poor sleep hygiene, and behavioral conditioning may contribute to primary insomnia—insomnia that cannot be related to any specific underlying factors.

Pathophysiology

Normal sleep is a periodic state of rest accompanied by varying degrees of unconsciousness and relative inactivity. It is normally an easily reversible, regular, recurrent state. The functions of sleep are restorative and hemostatic, critical for normal thermoregulation and energy conservation. Sleep disturbance is often an early symptom of impending mental illness.

Two physiological states compose sleep: non–rapid eye movement (NREM) and rapid eye movement (REM) sleep. In NREM sleep most physiological functions are markedly lower than in wakefulness although there may be episodic, involuntary body movements during NREM sleep. In contrast, REM sleep is characterized by physiological activity levels similar to those in wakefulness and a high level of brain activity and is sometimes called *paradoxical sleep*. NREM sleep is composed of stages 1 through 4, with stages 3 and 4 being the deepest portions. Typically, NREM sleep is punctuated with an REM cycle typically every 90 to 100 minutes during the night. The first REM period tends to be the shortest, lasting less than 10 minutes; later REM periods may last 15 to 40 minutes each. Most REM periods occur in the last third of the night; most stage 4 sleep occurs in the first third of the night.

These sleep patterns change over the course of a person's life. In young adulthood, REM comprises about 25% of sleep, and NREM approximately 75%. These figures remain fairly constant in normal sleep, although there is a reduction in both slow-wave sleep and REM sleep in older persons. NREM sleep increases after exercise and starvation and is thus thought to be associated with satisfying metabolic needs.

Daily variations in a variety of physiological functions affecting the endocrine, thermoregulatory, cardiac, pulmonary, renal, gastrointestinal, and neurobehavioral systems, as well as sleep–wake cycles, are governed by the 24-hour rhythm in humans. The timing and internal architecture of sleep are coupled directly to the output of the endogenous circadian pacemaker. Misalignment

of the output of the endogenous circadian pacemaker with the desired sleep–wake cycle can, therefore, induce insomnia, decrease alertness, and impair performance of shift workers, and accounts for the phenomenon of jet lag. Sleep deprivation for prolonged periods can lead also to hallucinations, ego disorganization, and delusions, and REM-deprived patients may exhibit irritability and lethargy.

Clinical Presentation

Insomnia may not be the chief reason for an office visit. It may be detected, however, by incorporating sleep-related questions into the general review of systems. Direct inquiry is important because patients with chronic insomnia often have never discussed their problem or have lived with it for so long that they do not think that anything can be done about it. The primary consequences of acute insomnia are sleepiness, negative mood, and impairment of performance. The severity of the components is related to the amount of sleep lost on one or more nights. Patients with chronic insomnia frequently complain of fatigue, mood changes (e.g., depression, irritability), difficulty concentrating, and impaired daytime functioning.

The assessment should include questions about sleep, as well as questions about daytime functioning, where the full effects of altered sleep are manifested. The actual number of hours of sleep required for each individual to subjectively feel refreshed varies markedly. Although the ability to maintain sleep alters with age, the individual's need for sleep does not change significantly. The patient's medical history and comorbidities are other important parameters that should be documented. Many medical problems, such as gastroesophageal reflux disease (GERD), worsen at night because they may be aggravated by recumbency.

It is necessary to rule out all underlying causes, for example, pain and the disease or condition that is the cause of the pain. A thorough drug history must be taken, including all over-the-counter drugs such as decongestants and cough syrups that contain decongestants, which act as stimulants. In addition, a complete history of all herbal remedies used, especially teas that may contain caffeine or ginseng and a variety of other CNS stimulants, should be obtained. When patients buy products in health food stores, they often do not think of them as "drugs." Screen for any illicit drug and alcohol use. (See Focus on History 18.1).

It may also be helpful for the patient to keep a sleep diary (see www.sleepeducation.com/EvaluateSleep.aspx). A sleep diary is a useful tool to track exactly when and under what conditions the patient sleeps, as well as diet, exercise, and drug habits that may help reveal the underlying problem. In addition, a record of all exercise and physical activity may prove helpful. The sleep diary also helps to further define the nature of the sleep problem. The delayed sleep phase type of circadian

Questions to ask:

- How has the person been sleeping recently?
- How long has the problem existed?
- Does the person have any underlying psychiatric or medical conditions?
- Is the person's sleep environment conducive to sleep? For example, are there any problems that would make sleeping difficult, such as noise, temperature, light, or space?
- Does the person work shift work or odd hours? What time does the person usually go to sleep? Get up? Are these hours the same on the weekday as well as the weekend?
- Does the person travel frequently?
- Does the person use caffeine, alcohol, drugs, or tobacco? If so, how much, and what are the specifics concerning the patient's use?
- Does the person have difficulty staying awake or report dozing off during normal daily activities?
- Does the person report any daytime consequences of not sleeping?
- Does the person (or partner) report:
  - Loud snoring, gasping, or stop breathing at night? (Suggests sleep apnea)
  - Legs or arms jerking during sleep? (Suggests periodic limb movement)
  - Creeping, crawling, or uncomfortable feelings in the legs that are relieved by moving them? (Suggests restless legs syndrome)

rhythm sleep disorder, for example, manifests itself with difficulty falling asleep at the desired time and difficulty waking at the desired time. The advanced sleep phase pattern, in contrast, is characterized by difficulty staying awake in the evening and by early awakening. Some persons awaken during the night and cannot fall back to sleep. Consider screening for insomnia as part of regular patient care (Level II; Schutte-Rodin et al, 2008).

Diagnostic Reasoning
DSM-5 Symptom Criteria

The DSM-5 symptom criteria for insomnia disorder are as follows:

1. Dissatisfaction with sleep quantity or quality associated with
   - Difficulty initiating sleep.
   - Difficulty maintaining sleep
   - Early-morning awakening with inability to return to sleep.
2. The sleep disturbance occurs at least three times per week for at least 3 months and causes clinically

significant distress or impairment in social, occupational, educational, academic, behavioral, or other important areas of functioning.
3. Co-occurring mental disorders and medical conditions do not adequately explain the predominant complaint of insomnia.

There may be objective corroboration by a family member of acute or chronic insomnia, but basically insomnia is a subjective complaint. In cases of suspected sleep apnea, it may be necessary for the patient to undergo polysomnography. Reserve laboratory evaluation for confirmation of medical or other sleep disorders that may underlie insomnia, such as obstructive sleep apnea (Level II; Schutte-Rodin et al, 2008).

Management
Nonpharmacological Management

The first National Institute of Health "state of the science" conference on insomnia since 1983 was held in June 2005. One important finding was recognition of the tendency of insomnia to be a chronic, potentially lifelong illness. Given the chronic nature of this problem, long-term treatment is often advisable. The panel stated that evidence supports the efficacy of cognitive-behavioral therapy (CBT) for the treatment of chronic insomnia (Level I; Schutte-Rodin et al, 2008), but it noted that there is very little evidence to support the efficacy of other treatments (including antidepressants, antipsychotics, and antihistamines), despite their widespread use.

Nonpharmacological treatment is therefore recommended in the initial management of insomnia (Levels I, II; Schutte-Rodin et al, 2008). The clinician should review and explain sleep hygiene "violations" expressed by patients (Level I; Schutte-Rodin et al, 2008). Recommendations include keeping sleeping and waking times regular, spending less than 8 hours in bed, maintaining adequate nutrition and exercise regimens, and avoiding sleep-altering substances such as caffeine and alcohol. All underlying causes of insomnia, such as pain, must be treated. Any drugs and/or herbal supplements that may be contributory should be discontinued. The patient should be encouraged to avoid daytime napping and to develop bedtime rituals that are conducive to sleep. Recommendations for appropriate sleep parameters include associating the bedroom with "sleepiness," not staying in bed for longer than 20 minutes when wakeful, and leaving the bedroom until tired, before returning (Level II; Schutte-Rodin et al, 2008). An exercise schedule may prove beneficial, although evening exercise may be stimulating. Alcohol should be avoided after 5:00 p.m., as should heavy evening meals (a light evening snack may sometimes be conducive to sleep). Reassurance and supportive counseling are essential; insomnia is not a complaint that should be taken lightly. Issues of caregiving for young children or older adults living in the home may be a part of the clinical picture. Again, diversionary lifestyle changes and situational support may be more effective than pharmacological measures for these patients. Sleep parameters can be reviewed and reemphasized several times during return visits before resorting to pharmacological measures. (See Advanced Practice Nursing Interventions 18.2.)

Pharmacological Management

Some evidence suggests that for some patients with persistent insomnia, adding a short course of a medication to CBT produced an additive benefit. Advantages of the sedative-hypnotics are that they hasten sleep onset, decrease the number of nighttime awakenings, increase total amount of sleep time (varies with medication duration of action), and make sleep more refreshing. Some of the disadvantages are that they may alter sleep architecture over time by decreasing slow-wave sleep and REM sleep and that they may cause residual sedation, psychomotor and cognitive impairment, psychological dependence in vulnerable individuals, and rebound insomnia. Medications indicated for insomnia include five older benzodiazepines (estazolam, flurazepam, quazepam, temazepam, and triazolam) and three newer nonbenzodiazepine medications (eszopiclone, zaleplon, and zolpidem).

The elimination half-lives of the sedative-hypnotics (see Drugs Commonly Prescribed 18.6) vary tremendously, and as a result, so does their duration of action. The advantages and disadvantages of a given duration of action must be assessed in light of each patient's individual needs. All agents in this class have some potential for abuse although the newer agents may have less. All are classified as Schedule IV by the DEA. Clinical trials have provided some evidence that sleep can improve to some degree without the use of any medication, because patients receiving placebo often reported as much improvement during the study as those taking medication. In sleep studies, a placebo is not an "inactive" treatment in that all study participants must adhere to nonpharmacological regimens (such as going to bed and getting up at regular hours, not napping, avoiding caffeine and alcohol) that are recognized as effective remedies for insomnia. Depression is the most common comorbid psychiatric diagnosis with chronic insomnia; however, medications such as the SSRIs should be utilized only in the setting of depression and not solely for the treatment of insomnia (Level II; Schutte-Rodin et al, 2008). Concurrent treatment of both insomnia and an underlying psychiatric comorbidity may result in greater improvements for the patient.

Advanced Practice Nursing Interventions 18.2   Insomnia

Behavioral Treatment	Relaxation therapy (progressive muscle relaxation therapy), autogenic training, electromyogram, biofeedback.
Sleep Restriction Therapy	Poor sleepers often increase their time in bed. Sleep restriction therapy curtails this time. For example, if a person reports sleeping only 5 hours per night, he or she should be counseled to stay in bed only 5 hours per night. As sleep improves, increase time in bed in 15- to 30-minute intervals. It works best to alter bedtime and keep rising time constant. Do not reduce sleep to less than 5 hours per night.
Stimulus Control Therapy	Functions on premise that insomnia is a conditioned response to temporal (bedtime) and environmental (bed/bedroom cues). Objective is to reassociate the bed and bedroom with rapid sleep onset. Stimulus control therapy counsels: (1) Go to bed only when sleepy. (2) Use the bed only for sleep. (3) Get out of bed and go into another room when awake; go back into the bedroom only when sleepy. (4) Maintain a regular rise time, regardless of sleep deprivation during the night. (5) Avoid daytime napping.
Cognitive Therapy	Identify dysfunctional ideas about sleep and replace them with more functional approaches, e.g., 8 hours of sleep is not necessary for everyone; insomnia and less sleep does not have to destroy one's life. This approach helps minimize anticipatory anxiety around sleep.
Physical Therapy	Exercise: Regular physical activity will assist with sleep. Advise the patient not to exercise too close to bedtime. Massage: Weekly massage may assist with relaxation.
Pharmacological Therapy	Hypnotics, antidepressants, antihistamines, melatonin.
Reassurance and Support	Active listening and patience; encourage ventilation of feelings, especially if stress is a component of the insomnia.

Drugs Commonly Prescribed 18.6 Sedatives and Hypnotics

Drug	Indication	Adverse Reactions and Prescribing Considerations
Benzodiazepines		C-IV controlled substance. All benzodiazepines are associated with potential anterograde amnesia, CNS depression, and paradoxical reactions. Sedation, memory deficits, ataxia. Caution with narrow-angle glaucoma. Association with falls and injury in the elderly. Caution with depressed patients and substance abuse, impaired hepatic or renal function. Most contraindicated in obstructive sleep apnea (OSA). Many drug–drug interactions (CYP pathways). Withdrawal symptoms with abrupt discontinuation. The onset of withdrawal symptoms is usually seen on the first day without drug and lasts 5–7 days—slow taper. Treatment longer than 4 months should be reevaluated to determine the patient's need for the drug. Avoid valerian, St. John's wort, kava kava, gotu kola. Potential severe allergic reactions (anaphylaxis, angioedema) and complex sleep-related behaviors, which may include sleep-driving, cooking and eating food while asleep, and making phone calls while asleep.
estazolam (ProSom)	Insomnia, short-term	Intermediate acting. No active metabolites
flurazepam (Dalmane)	Insomnia, short-term	Long acting. Avoid in elderly and debilitated. Active metabolites with extended half-lives may lead to delayed accumulation and adverse effects.
temazepam (Restoril)	Insomnia, short-term	Intermediate acting. Administer 30 minutes before bedtime. Lack of active metabolites—excellent option for the elderly.
triazolam (Halcion)	Insomnia, short-term	Short acting. In elderly, higher incidence of CNS adverse reactions; not a drug of first choice.
quazepam (Doral)	Insomnia	Long-acting daytime sedation and fatigue, but may prevent withdrawal symptoms when stopped.
Benzodiazepine Like		CV IV controlled substance. Daytime sedation, anterograde amnesia, rebound insomnia. Less anxiolytic properties than the benzodiazepines. All patients should be advised of residual morning effects and of complex sleep-related behaviors. This may include sleep-driving, cooking and eating food while asleep, and making phone calls while asleep. All patients should be advised to get at least 4 hours of sleep after taking a short-acting agent and at least 7 hours of sleep with a long-acting agent.
eszopiclone (Lunesta)	Insomnia, long-term	Long half-life of 6 hours; good for sleep initiation and maintenance. Advise to get 8 or more hours of sleep. No hangover effect; may have metallic taste. Headache, dizziness, and somnolence. Potentiates CNS depressants.
zaleplon (Sonata)	Insomnia, short-term	Short half-life, about 1 hour. Good for patients that have difficulty falling asleep, not for sleep maintenance. Advise to get at least 4 hours of sleep. Dosage adjustment for hepatic impairment.
zolpidem (Ambien)	Insomnia, short-term	Half-life 1.4–2.4 hours. Good for patients that have difficulty with falling asleep. Headache, dizziness, and somnolence. Take with liquid—food can delay absorption; CNS depression. No known rebound insomnia or hangover effect. Reduced dosage in women and geriatric populations.

Continued

Drugs Commonly Prescribed 18.6 Sedatives and Hypnotics—cont'd

Drug	Indication	Adverse Reactions and Prescribing Considerations
zolpidem CR (Ambien CR [extended release])	Insomnia, long-term	Half-life 1.4–2.4 hours, but released over a longer duration. Headache, dizziness, and somnolence. Sleep may be impaired after discontinuation. Abuse potential low. Reduced dosage in women and geriatric populations. Complex sleep-related behaviors, which may include sleep-driving, cooking and eating food while asleep, and making phone calls while asleep.
Melatonin Receptor Agonist		
Insomnia	Ramelteon (Rozerem)	Indicated to promote sleep onset. Peak concentrations within 1 hour if fasting, avoid high fat meal. No withdrawal or rebound insomnia. Does not affect REM sleep. May affect testosterone and prolactin levels. Somnolence, dizziness, fatigue, nausea, and exacerbated insomnia. Monitor liver transaminases.
OTC		
diphenhydramine (Benadryl)	Insomnia, short-term use less than 2 weeks	May have next day sedation, dry mouth, decreased cognitive function. Potentiates CNS depression; caution with asthma, other respiratory disorders; glaucoma; hyperthyroidism.

Source: Clinical pharmacology [database online]. Gold Standard, Inc., Tampa, FL, 2012. http://cp.gsm.com.

Follow-up and Referral

Transient insomnia may turn into chronic insomnia. For this reason, treatment is essential. Insomnia should resolve with patience, counseling, and treatment, and patients should be followed until the situation is resolved (Level II; Schutte-Rodin et al, 2008). A concern is daytime sleepiness (sleep apnea, for example, is highly correlated with car accidents). The patient may need to be referred for supportive counseling, especially if insomnia is related to a traumatic event. The entire environmental situation of the patient and family should be assessed. Are there caregiver issues involved, and can external and additional support be provided or arranged for? Is there a need for diversionary activities, or a need to increase the individual's physical activity level? If sleep apnea is suspected, a polysomnogram should be ordered.

■ OBSTRUCTIVE SLEEP APNEA/HYPOPNEA

This is the most common sleep-related manifestation of medical illness, defined as repeated episodes of upper pharyngeal obstruction during sleep. *Hypopnea* refers to reduced airflow, and *apnea* to a total restriction of airflow. Symptoms are most prominently daytime sleepiness and nighttime snoring. Associated medical conditions include GERD, hypertension, headache, reduced libido, and erectile dysfunction.

Epidemiology

Obstructive sleep apnea (OSA) is a common disorder, occurring in 1% to 2% of children, 2% to 15% of middle-aged adults, and in over 20% of older adults. The condition is very strongly associated with obesity and with male gender. There is also a genetic basis, with a twofold risk among first-degree relatives of probands.

Diagnosis and Management

The differential diagnosis includes ruling out other sleep-related disorders such as narcolepsy, hypersomnia, and circadian rhythm disorders. Polysomnography (PSG) is the hallmark of diagnosis and treatment of OSA. The test uses respiratory effort and peripheral pulse oximetry to quantify episodes of hypopnea and apnea. This is reported as the apnea-hypopnea index (AHI). PSG records brain electrical activity, eye movements, and muscle potentials, indices that may help to identify and diagnose restless legs syndrome and other disturbances of the sleep–wake cycle.

Continuous positive airway pressure (CPAP) machines tend to mitigate symptoms and enhance patients' quality of life, but no long-term studies have demonstrated a long-term reduction in mortality. Individuals with OSA have an increased risk of occupational accidents and an almost sevenfold increase in motor vehicle accidents. There may be state-by-state restrictions for commercial drivers suffering from OSA. Associated morbidities range from hypertension and heart failure to neurological disease and depression. Lifestyle modifications most important to the long-term control of symptoms secondary to OSA include weight control, tobacco cessation, exercise, and avoidance of sleep-disruptive agents such as sedatives and alcohol.

DSM-5 Symptom Criteria

The DSM-5 symptom criteria for OSA include either of the following:

1. Evidence by PSG of at least five obstructive apneas or hypopneas per hour of sleep and either of the following sleep symptoms:
   - Nocturnal breathing disturbances: snoring, snorting/gasping, or breathing pauses during sleep.
   - Daytime sleepiness, fatigue, or unrefreshing sleep despite sufficient opportunities to sleep that is not better explained by another mental disorder (including a sleep disorder) and is not attributable to another medical condition.
2. Evidence by PSG of 15 or more obstructive apneas and/or hypopneas per hour of sleep regardless of accompanying symptoms.

■ RESTLESS LEGS SYNDROME

RLS is a neurological, sensorimotor condition that is typified by uncomfortable sensations in the lower extremities such as burning, tingling, crawling, or itching and an uncontrollable desire to move the legs. One result is the inability to obtain or maintain an appropriate sleep pattern.

Usually a development in older adults, the syndrome does have a familial component, which manifests at younger ages. Important differential diagnoses are arthritis, peripheral neuropathy, ischemia, and radiculopathy. A complete neurological examination and appropriate laboratory testing will help to focus the diagnosis.

Diagnosis is difficult because it is mainly by self-report of symptomatology. There is an overlay of comorbidities including depression, anxiety, panic, and PTSD.

Patient Education

The patient and family members need to be reassured and counseled regarding the transient nature of RLS, including the lifestyle measures that can be instituted to assist with sleep. The establishment of healthful sleep rituals, increasing physical activity and regular exercise, the need to refrain from alcohol consumption and smoking later in the day, and the need to eat lighter in the evening should be discussed. Care should be used with all pharmacological therapies because of the possible adverse effects and their potential for drug dependency, especially in elderly patients.

■ EATING DISORDERS

Eating disorders, which include both anorexia nervosa and bulimia nervosa, are not routinely assessed in primary care, although they can be a significant health problem. Eating disorders occur on a continuum; the number of individuals with subclinical symptoms exceeds those with full disorder symptomatology. Being female is a risk factor for developing an eating disorder. At present the incidence of eating disorders among males is low, but there is evidence of persistent increases. DSM-5 characterizes feeding and eating disorders as persistent disturbances from altered consumption or restriction of food intake, resulting in significant functional impairment. Included in the DSM-5 classification are Rumination Disorder, Avoidant Food Intake Disorder, Anorexia Nervosa, Bulimia Nervosa, and Binge-Eating Disorder.

Bulimia Nervosa

Recurrent episodes of binge eating, followed by compensatory methods to prevent weight gain, and self-evaluation unduly influenced by body shape are the three essential features of *bulimia nervosa* (BN). Persons with BN undergo feelings of loss of control during bingeing episodes, and their self-esteem is excessively influenced by their body shape and weight.

There are two types of bulimia—purging and nonpurging. A person with BN who purges regularly will engage in self-induced vomiting and/or misuse of diuretics, laxatives, or enemas. With nonpurging BN, persons compensate for their food intake with excessive exercise or fasting. In extreme cases, individuals may abuse thyroid hormone replacement medication or try other types of stimulant medication.

Some individuals with BN alternate between cycles of strict dieting or fasting and cycles of binge eating and purging, whereas others may compensate for binges with excessive (several hours every day) exercise patterns. Persons with BN who cycle between bingeing and fasting or extreme food restricting have a poorer prognosis. The daily number of times the person with BN purges tends to increase over time and can lead to serious medical complications. In the primary-care setting, it is not unusual for persons with BN to refuse to disclose their symptoms.

Individuals with BN experience a sense of lack of control over eating during an episode and tend to misperceive themselves on the basis of their body weight and shape. Comorbidity with other psychological disorders is common, especially depression, anxiety, and substance abuse. Periods of food, calorie, and fat restrictions are often followed by bingeing and purging. The individual may feel an intense sense of shame about this behavior and may go to great lengths to keep it secret from others, including health-care providers.

Anorexia Nervosa

Anorexia nervosa (AN) is characterized by a refusal to maintain a minimally normal body weight and an intense fear of gaining weight. In early adolescence, the patient may also fail to achieve expected weight and height gains. There are two types of AN—restricting and binge-eating/purging AN. With restricting AN, weight loss is usually accomplished by reducing or restricting all food intake or restricting dietary fat. With binge-eating/purging AN, there is binge eating followed by self-induced vomiting and chronic and excessive use of laxatives or diuretics. Providers can expect patients to resist changes in their diet or weight, and patients may put a great deal of effort toward frustrating the practitioner's efforts to help.

Anorexia can be accompanied by serious physiological consequences, including amenorrhea, signs and symptoms of starvation, and electrolyte abnormalities.

One in 10 patients with AN dies suddenly from starvation, cardiac arrest, or suicide. AN is associated with depression in 65% of cases; social phobia in 34%; and obsessive-compulsive disorder in 26% of cases. AN is a serious medical disorder, with estimates of mortality ranging up to 20%. Patients with anorexia nervosa rarely self-identify and often demonstrate poor insight into their condition. Clinicians therefore have a responsibility to help patients recognize their diagnosis and work with them to assess their readiness to change and their integration with additional elements of care.

Epidemiology and Causes

The lifetime prevalence estimate for AN is 0.6% and for BN is 1.0%. For each disorder, the risk is up to three times higher in women than in men, with a median age at onset between 18 and 21 years. An exact cause of eating disorders is not known but is considered to be a possible multifactorial combination of genetic, neurochemical, and sociocultural factors. Recent work indicates that childhood obesity may be a risk factor for bulimia, and there is evidence that familial transmission may occur. The state of starvation itself initiates dramatic physiological changes in a variety of body systems leading to a cascade-like cycle that makes it difficult to discern which biological change may have precipitated the process; nonetheless, it becomes self-perpetuating.

Pathophysiology and Psychopathology

There appears to be a constellation of factors that include biological, social, and cultural forces that contribute to eating disorders. Recent studies point to some genetic differences in the major groups of eating disorders, AN and BN. When families of individuals with a high incidence of bulimia are examined, family members with an increased risk for obesity are found; however, in families of individuals with the restricting subtype of anorexia, there is no increased risk for obesity. So although these are two genetically related disorders, there clearly may be important differences between them. There is an increased frequency of BN in first-degree relatives of patients with this disorder. Some evidence points to higher concordance rates in monozygotic twins than in dizygotic. Sisters of patients with AN are more likely to be affected, but the causality involved may be more social than genetic. Cultural factors may be difficult to ascertain, because few studies have looked at eating disorders and their occurrence in different countries. Certain populations who may not have appropriate access to care may therefore not be accurately diagnosed.

Clinical Presentation

Eating disorders are characterized by intense feelings of shame, guilt, and embarrassment. It is important to know key warning signs of eating disorders to provide care early in the disease process; early intervention has a better prognosis. (See Focus on History 18.2.)

Focus on History 18.2   Anorexia and Bulimia

Anorexia Nervosa

Warning signs	To assess for warning signs of anorexia, it is important to obtain answers to the following questions: • Has the patient had any *substantial weight loss*? • Does the patient have signs or symptoms of *depression or mood swings*? • Does the patient have a *preoccupation with weight, calories, and food*? • Does the patient *wear baggy clothes*? • Does the patient have a history of *excessive exercise*?
Signs	Hypotension, hypothermia, dry skin, bradycardia, edema, lanugo
Symptoms	Amenorrhea, constipation, abdominal pain, hypothermia, lethargy or fatigue, anxious energy, headaches

Bulimia Nervosa

Warning signs	To assess for warning signs of bulimia nervosa, it is important to obtain answers to the following questions: • Has the patient had any significant *weight loss or gain*? • Does the patient have signs or symptoms of *depression*? • Does the patient have a *great concern for weight*? • Does the patient *visit the bathroom after meals*? • Has the patient alluded to *strict dieting/bingeing cycles*? • Does the patient have *marked criticism of his or her body*?
Signs	Tooth enamel erosion, enlarged parotid glands, periodontal disease
Symptoms	Irregular menses, abdominal pain, fatigue or lethargy, peripheral edema, bloating, depression

Individuals with eating disorders typically do not present with that as a key symptom or problem but with other somatic complaints. Therefore, the clinician must be alert to screen for these disorders among adolescents and young adults, particularly those thought to be at high risk. Assessment should be comprehensive and include physical, psychological, and social needs and a comprehensive assessment of risk to self. The primary-care provider should take responsibility for initial assessment and the initial coordination of care. This includes the determination of the need for emergency medical or psychiatric assessment. Where management is shared between primary and secondary care, there should be a clear agreement in writing as to who should be monitoring the patient on a regular basis. It should be shared with patient and family so all lines of responsibility are clear.

Screening for eating disorders may use brief screening methods such as questionnaires and clinical presentation. Available screening instruments include the SCOFF Questionnaire, the Eating Disorder Screen for Primary Care (ESP), Eating Attitudes Test (EAT-26), and Eating Disorders Inventory–Second Edition (EDI-2). The SCOFF consists of five questions designed to assess the core features of anorexia nervosa and bulimia. It is a mnemonic, with each letter based on a keyword in each question of the screening tool: Sick, Control, One, Fat, and Food. It was designed to be brief, to be administered in primary care, and to be answered with yes-and-no responses. The EAT-26 is better validated but takes longer to administer and score. The EDI-2 is a standardized measure of symptoms associated with anorexia, bulimia, and other eating disorders. Although reliable and valid with good psychometrics, it does not yield a specific diagnosis but has utility as a screening instrument. Assessment of body mass index (BMI), height, weight, and centile charts for age should be done on all patients. When AN or BN is suspected, a complete physical examination is needed to rule out other diseases or disorders that could produce severe weight loss.

Other physical assessments such as pulse, blood pressure, core temperature, cardiovascular and peripheral examination, and sit-ups/squat test for muscle power should be done on all patients. Laboratory investigations include complete blood count, endocrine testing, erythrocyte sedimentation rate, blood urea nitrogen (BUN) and electrolytes, creatinine, liver function tests (LFTs), random blood glucose, urinalysis, and electrocardiogram.

Anorexia Nervosa

Assessment for AN should include a weight history, including highest and lowest weight, and the frequency with which the person experiences significant weight fluctuations. Ask about ideal weight goals. Persons with AN tend to have extremely unrealistic goals for a low ideal weight. Excessive weight loss is often the most obvious sign of AN, but individuals with AN rarely complain of weight loss. Persons with AN are likely to deny that a problem exists although as they lose more weight, their fear of becoming fat intensifies. Severe weight loss eventually results in electrolyte imbalance and dehydration, with significant risks of serious medical complications such as cardiac arrhythmias. Individuals with AN who purge may experience electrolyte imbalances, edema, and enlarged parotid glands. Long-standing amenorrhea can leave females at risk for developing osteopenia and osteoporosis.

Individuals with AN may complain of hypothermia, constipation, lethargy, or excess nervous energy. APRNs may find evidence of significant hypotension, dry skin, and dull hair. Hypertrophy of the salivary glands may be present if the person with AN purges. Chronic dehydration can result in impaired renal function, cardiovascular problems, and osteoporosis. Positive laboratory findings in AN include leukopenia, anemia, elevated BUN, elevated LFTs, hypomagnesemia, hypophosphatemia, and elevated thyroid-stimulating hormone. Hypercholesterolemia and sinus bradycardia are also common findings in patients with AN.

Bulimia Nervosa

Persons with BN vary in their weight and appearance, but most have a normal BMI score. Many persons with BN have an extensive history of dieting. Assessment of dieting history, including both weight gain and loss as well as dieting, is important. BN is considered less life-threatening than AN; however, serious health complications can also develop with BN.

Dental erosion (from gastric acid) and periodontal disease are common in patients with BN, as are complaints of swollen salivary glands, especially the parotid glands, GERD, sore throat, and esophageal irritation. Persons who regularly engage in self-induced vomiting can develop scars or calluses on the backs of their hands from repeated trauma from the teeth.

Laboratory findings may indicate many abnormalities, including hypokalemia, hyponatremia, hypochloremia, increased serum bicarbonate, and/or elevated levels of serum amylase. In severe cases of purging, electrolyte imbalance and dehydration may lead to cardiac arrhythmias, which can lead to heart failure and sudden death. Esophageal bleeding, tears, and gastric rupture can also occur.

Diagnostic Reasoning
DSM-5 Symptom Criteria

The DSM-5 symptom criteria for anorexia nervosa are as follows:

- Restriction of energy intake resulting in *significantly low weight*.
- Intense fear of gaining weight or of becoming fat.
- Lack of recognition of the seriousness of the current low body weight.

DSM-5 Symptom Criteria

The DSM-5 symptom criteria for bulimia nervosa are as follows:

- Recurrent episodes of binge eating.
- Recurrent inappropriate compensatory behaviors (self-induced vomiting; misuse of laxatives, diuretics, or other medications; fasting; or excessive exercise).

Management

The therapeutic relationship is central to management of the person with an eating disorder. Using the readiness to change model can help the patient and their family set realistic and safe goals. If the patient's condition does not require hospitalization, outpatient treatment of eating disorders can be effective. A multidisciplinary team, including the primary-care practitioner, nutritionist, and a psychiatric nurse specialist, is needed. Good communication between team members is essential because even motivated patients will have strong urges to resist treatment.

There are certain danger signals that mandate hospitalization. These include the following:

- Weight less than 85% of healthy body weight for that individual
- Signs that the person is suicidal
- Evidence of physiological instability such as hypokalemia or dehydration
- Lack of response to outpatient treatment

Evidence of psychotic thinking, hallucinations, or severe obsessions is also grounds for inpatient treatment, as are signs of other addictive behaviors, such as substance abuse. When there is severe family and/or staff conflict over the proposed treatment plan, hospitalization might also be indicated, preferably at a specialty treatment center.

Inpatient Management

Goals for the patient who is hospitalized are fairly specific and include the following:

- Prescribed bedrest with supervised meals until the person has obtained a weight greater than 80% to 85% of his or her healthy body weight.
- A 300-calorie stepwise gradual increase in calories consumed (as the calories consumed are increased and weight increases, there is a stepwise increase in activity as well).
- Work to establish the target weight.
- Weigh daily at first; as the weight gain progresses, this may be reduced to three times per week.
- Medicate for symptom relief.
- For the patient with AN, the goal is to achieve a weight gain of 1 to 2 pounds (0.45–0.91 kg) per week, with tube feedings used only as a last resort.
- For the patient with BN, meals and bathroom privileges should be supervised, with no access to the bathroom for 2 hours after eating.

The patient's psychological and nutritional status should be continuously assessed. A supportive, structured environment and programs should be provided, preferably in a specialized center, or the patient should be admitted to a specialized eating disorder unit. If purging is involved, the clinician should identify the triggers and precipitants and help the patient work to establish alternative behaviors. Focused individual, group, and family therapies are also indicated.

Outpatient Management

On an outpatient basis, therapy revolves around building trust and a therapeutic alliance. The practitioner should involve the person with AN or BN in setting the target weight. The weight gain can be achieved gradually unless any danger signals surface.

The clinician should weigh the patient weekly at first and later monthly if progress is being made. The focus should be on overall indices of health, not just on weight. The practitioner should prescribe medication if necessary for symptom relief and challenge any fear of uncontrollable weight gain. If purging is involved, precipitants should be identified and alternative behaviors should be established. A cognitive-behavioral approach combined with education is often effective. Interpersonal therapy or CBT should be offered to patients with BN and binge-eating disorder (Level I; William et al, 2008), although self-help programs are helpful for some patients (Level II; William et al, 2008).

Family therapy as well as individual therapy may be necessary; the person should be referred to specialists in these areas. These may be APRNs who specialize in eating disorders and/or family therapy and social workers, psychologists, or psychiatrists who have expertise in those areas. The primary-care provider can, however, continue to play an important role on the interdisciplinary team and should maintain contact with the person being treated for an eating disorder.

Pharmacological therapy has been found to be effective in some cases, slightly more so with patients with BN (Level II; William et al, 2008). Antidepressant medications (especially SSRIs) have become mainstays of treatment of eating disorders. Fluoxetine (Prozac) 10 to 80 mg daily is the only FDA-approved drug for bulimia. It is sometimes necessary to use higher than normal doses for effective treatment of bulimia.

Follow-up and Referral

Treatment of AN and BN requires specialized care. Providers play the key role in helping patients to accept referral to an eating disorders program. Making this decision is extremely difficult; patients may fail to follow through repeatedly before they actually accept treatment. Persons may appear to wish to have this decision made for them, but this is rarely the case. Involuntary treatment for an eating disorder is rarely effective. Persons who are dangerously malnourished and in need of emergency weight regain must be hospitalized.

The course of illness with an eating disorder is long and highly variable. In a recent study of AN patients, about 50% achieved complete recovery, 21% had an intermediate outcome, and 26% had an outcome that was poor, with an overall mortality rate of 9.8%. Half of BN patients were reported to have recovered fully, 30% experienced occasional relapse, and almost 20% maintained the full criteria for BN. Relapse is common, especially during times of stress (e.g., marriage, childbearing). There is significant morbidity from cardiac arrest and eventual suicide. Poor prognosis is indicated by repeated hospitalizations, initial low weight, being married, and poor maturation. Depression is often a sequela of recovery. Both eating disorders are best approached as chronic conditions marked by improvement and relapse. Older women appear to reach a stage of development at which they have the psychological skill to establish control over their food and weight-related behaviors. Recovered persons may continue to have complex feelings about food and their weight, but their self-care behaviors are more effective.

Patient Education

Information must be provided on the long-term effects of anorexia and/or bulimia. This may be especially important for the person with the disorder, because she (or he) may simply be unaware of some of the long-term health consequences. The provider can take the following steps: (1) Provide information on appropriate programs if dealing with addictions is involved in the treatment plan. (2) Review nutritional information and recommended dietary program. (3) Teach stress management and relaxation techniques for persons and families involved, especially at mealtimes, which are always tense. (4) Provide education on health effects of laxatives and diuretics. (5) Reinforce the long-term nature of these disorders and the need for long-term follow-up and treatment. (6) Point out that under stress, regressive behaviors occur. Involve the family in what symptoms to identify and report. For persons who have used self-induced vomiting, encourage better dental care. It is important to teach strategies for dealing with self-destructive behaviors in ways that do not reinforce them.

■ ATTENTION-DEFICIT/ HYPERACTIVITY DISORDER

Attention-deficit/hyperactivity disorder (ADHD) is a persistent pattern of inattention, gross motor hyperactivity, and impulsivity that interferes with social, school, and work functioning. The disorder typically manifests itself in childhood, but symptoms may continue into adolescence and adulthood. Adults must show a childhood onset of symptoms to receive a diagnosis of ADHD.

Inattentiveness in school and work activities is evidenced in difficulty following through on instructions, as well as distractibility, performing work carelessly, and moving from one uncompleted task to another. In social activities, inattentiveness is expressed as frequent shifts in conversation, inability to concentrate, and not following the rules of games or activities.

Hyperactivity is usually expressed through fidgetiness or squirming while seated, not remaining seated when expected to do so, and excessive running or climbing in situations when it is inappropriate. In adolescents and adults, symptoms of hyperactivity take the form of feelings of restlessness and difficulty engaging in quiet sedentary activities. Impulsivity manifests itself as impatience, difficulty in delaying responses, blurting out answers before questions have been completed, difficulty awaiting one's turn, and frequently interrupting or intruding on others to the point of causing difficulties in social, academic, or occupational settings. Impulsivity may lead to accidents and engagement in potentially dangerous activities without consideration of possible consequences.

Symptoms typically worsen in situations that require sustained attention or mental effort or that lack intrinsic appeal or novelty. Signs of the disorder may be minimal or absent when the person is under very strict control or in a one-to-one situation. The behaviors of ADHD are more likely to occur during group situations.

Epidemiology and Causes

The prevalence of ADHD is estimated at 5% in school-age children and 2.5% of adults. The disorder is much more frequent in males than in females. In children the male-to-female ratio is 2:1 and for adults the male-to-female ratio is 1.6:1. Although early onset is common (50% meet diagnostic criteria for ADHD by age 4), some patients have later onset, and it is not uncommon for the disorder to persist into adulthood. There are limited data on prevalence in adolescence and adulthood, but the persistence of symptoms into adulthood has been estimated from 30% to as high as 70% of children who were diagnosed with ADHD.

To date, no single etiology for ADHD has been identified. Data from biological, environmental, and psychosocial research suggest several risk factors or causes for the disorder. Data from various family, twin, and adoption studies suggest a genetic origin for some forms of this disorder. In addition, children with parents or siblings with ADHD are at increased risk.

Recent work suggests that maternal smoking, alcohol abuse, and exposure to toxins during pregnancy are related to hyperkinetic-impulsive behavior in children. Perinatal influences that are thought to contribute to ADHD include prematurity, intrauterine growth retardation, precipitous or prolonged labor, and perinatal asphyxia. In addition, postnatal CNS abnormalities resulting from trauma, infections, cerebral palsy, and lead exposure have been linked to the development of ADHD in childhood. Common comorbidities include Tourette's syndrome, learning disability, genetic disorders, and other psychiatric disorders. There is no strong scientific evidence that food additives, colorings, preservatives, or sugar contributes to ADHD.

Pathophysiology

Currently, there is no known neurophysiological or neurochemical basis for the disorder. Imbalances among the levels of norepinephrine, dopamine, and epinephrine all seem to be involved. Behavior and attention are best controlled when optimal balance is achieved. Computed tomography head scans of children with ADHD showed no consistent pathological findings. Studies using positron emission tomography have found diminished cerebral blood flow and lower metabolic rates in the frontal lobe areas of children with ADHD than in controls. It is theorized that the frontal lobes are not adequately performing their inhibitory function.

Clinical Presentation

Parents may be the first to note excessive motor activity (hyperactivity) during the toddler years. The disorder is not usually diagnosed during this time, however, because that is the normative developmental stage. Toddlers and preschoolers may have difficulty participating in sedentary activities, such as sitting still while listening to a story in preschool. Parents may describe the child as "always on the go," and the child may appear to constantly run, jump, and not sit still. There may also be excessive talking and interrupting of others.

ADHD is most often diagnosed during the childhood years (especially during elementary school) when the child's decreased attention span affects classroom work and academic performance. The school-age child with ADHD will usually have difficulty remaining seated, be unable to complete assignments and turn them in, and talk out of turn. Hyperactive behaviors in these children may include constantly tapping their hands; shaking of their feet or legs; getting up during meals; and talking excessively while watching television, doing homework, or in other quiet activities.

In childhood and adolescence, impulsive symptoms associated with ADHD often lead the individual to break family, interpersonal, and educational rules. Disruptive behaviors and few social skills can make bonding with peers difficult and may lead to association with deviant peer groups and substance and tobacco abuse. In adulthood, restlessness may lead to difficulty in participating in sedentary activities, as well as to avoiding occupations, such as desk jobs, that provide limited opportunity for spontaneous movement. Adults with ADHD often complain of boredom and frustration with job and life routines.

Various medical, psychological, and genetic conditions need to be assessed. Medical disorders such as thyroid disease, lead toxicity, and iron deficiencies (ferritin levels less than 30 ng/mL) have been associated with increased behavioral symptoms. Physical findings of microcephaly, growth retardation, and facial anomalies coupled with the behavioral findings may suggest fetal alcohol syndrome. Although patients and family may report a history of a higher rate of physical injury (because of excessive motor activities and impulsivity), there are no specific physical features associated with ADHD. It is important for the clinician to be able to distinguish symptoms of ADHD from developmentally age-appropriate behaviors in active children. It is also important to differentiate ADHD from symptoms of inattention in children with learning disabilities or those with pervasive developmental disorders. The clinician should be aware that ADHD may not be the sole diagnosis; comorbid problems such as learning disorders, autism, conduct disorders, oppositional defiant disorders, genetic disorders, mood disorders, anxiety, and substance abuse, particularly in adults and adolescents, can coexist. Genetic conditions to consider include neurofibromatosis and fragile X, Turner, Prader-Willi, and Williams syndromes.

During a structured assessment in the practitioner's office, symptoms may not be evident, because they are most often seen in a less structured environment, such as school or work. Children with ADHD may not be able to report their own symptoms accurately because of their age; therefore, information should be gathered from parents or guardians and supplemented by reports from teachers. The DSM-5 provides guidance for diagnosis of ADHD for individuals aged 17 and older. It may be necessary to review early academic records or report cards for the presence of impulsivity, hyperactivity, and inattentive symptoms during the early school years. Additional questions related to family history of ADHD should be conducted. Adult patients may need to question their parents regarding ADHD behaviors that were evident from childhood. Key areas for questioning relate to complaints of boredom, disorganization or frustration in work, and a tendency for impulsive, impatient, and restless behavior.

Generally, diagnostic tests are not indicated, but a serum lead, ferritin, and/or thyroid level may be considered. Electroencephalography (EEG), diagnostic imaging, and genetic testing may be indicated for those patients who present with anomalies or soft neurological signs.

Diagnostic Reasoning/Differential Diagnosis
DSM-5 Symptom Criteria

Some hyperactive and impulsive or inattentive symptoms must have been present before 12 years of age, and some impairment from the symptoms is present in one or more settings (home, work, school, or social interaction). In addition, there must be clear evidence of clinically significant impairment in social, academic, or occupational functioning, as well as evidence that the symptoms are not caused by another disorder.

ADHD is characterized by six or more of the following symptoms of inattention that have persisted for at least 6 months to a degree that is maladaptive and inconsistent with developmental level.

Inattentive
• Pattern of careless mistakes
• Difficulty sustaining attention in tasks or play activities
• Does not listen when spoken to
• Does not follow through on instructions
• Has difficulty organizing tasks and activities
• Loses things necessary to complete tasks
• Avoids, dislikes, or is reluctant to engage in sustained mental activity
• Easily distracted by external stimuli
• Forgetful

Hyperactivity and impulsivity can occur with or without inattentive symptoms. When six or more of the following symptoms are present and have persisted for at least 6 months to a degree that is maladaptive and inconsistent with developmental level, the diagnostic criteria are met for hyperactivity/impulsivity disorder.

Hyperactivity
• Often fidgets with hands and feet, squirms
• Leaves classroom or refuses to remain seated when it is expected
• Runs or climbs excessively
• Difficulty playing or engaging in quiet activities
• Acts as if "driven by a motor"
• Talks excessively
Impulsivity
• Blurts out answers
• Difficulty waiting turn
• Interrupts, intrudes

For individuals aged 17 and older, at least five (not six) of the inattention and/or hyperactivity-impulsivity symptom criteria listed must be present.

Screening

Screening for psychosocial issues has become more common as providers become increasingly aware that 13% of preschoolers and 12% to 25% of school-age children exhibit emotional/behavioral problems. Utilizing a tool at regular well-child visits may help to identify this chronic condition, particularly in children with academic and behavioral issues (Level II; Wolraich et al, 2011). The Pediatric Symptom Checklist is a one-page questionnaire that is completed by the parent. This tool is free and is available in multiple languages and a pictorial format. The tool and scoring instructions are available from www2.massgeneral.org/allpsych/psc/psc_forms.htm. If screening is positive, assessment with an ADHD-specific tool should occur (Level II; Wolraich

et al, 2011). Various tools are available and need to be completed by both the parents or guardians and the teacher (Level I; Wolraich et al, 2011) (see Table 18.4).

Early diagnosis and treatment are associated with improved school performance, behavior, and social interaction (Level I; MTA Cooperative Group, 1999). For adults, assess prior history of ADHD, previous school performance, history of mental health diagnoses, substance abuse, and current or past medication use. Assess current symptoms with inquiry into their effect on current school performance, work, and home. Various adult screening tools are readily available (see Table 18.4). For patients who do not specifically meet the criteria for ADHD or whose history and behavior are not consistent with ADHD, referral to a neurodevelopmental specialist, behavioral health specialist, or neurologist is warranted. (See Nursing Research–Based Practice Box 18.2.)

Management

A comprehensive plan needs to address the chronic nature of the disorder, including developmental challenges throughout the life span, treatment options (pharmacological and nonpharmacological), and community and school resources (Level II; Wolraich et al, 2011). Reappraisal of the plan with medication reassessment needs to be done periodically and appropriate changes made.

Pharmacological Management

Pharmacotherapy is generally not recommended for preschool children unless the symptoms have not responded to behavioral therapy, the symptoms have persisted for more than 9 months, and the symptoms are present in more than one setting. Pharmacotherapy can help improve symptoms in the areas of school, work, social interaction, and family life. If the diagnostic criteria are met, it is recommended to initiate pharmacological treatment with an FDA-approved medication for ADHD for individuals aged 6 to 11 years (Level I; Wolraich et al, 2011). The evidence is strongest for use of dextroamphetamine (DEX), D- and D,L-methylphenidate (MPH), mixed salts amphetamine, and less for atomoxetine (Strattera), extended-release guanfacine (Intuniv), and extended-release clonidine (Kapvay) (Level I; Wolraich et al, 2011). For adolescents aged 12 to 18 years, pharmacological treatment should be offered with the assent of the teen (Level I; Wolraich et al, 2011).

The core symptoms are best managed by stimulant medications, which have shown response rates of 75% to 80%. The stimulant agents (MPH or amphetamine) should be considered first-line therapy (Level I; Wolraich et al, 2011). Both immediate-release and sustained-release formulations are available. The advantages for once-daily dosing include compliance, convenience, and confidentiality (school). Management includes beginning the stimulant at a low dose and titrating upward until symptoms are controlled, generally every 1 to 3 weeks, until optimal treatment outcome is achieved or

Nursing Research–Based Practice 18.2   Attention-Deficit/Hyperactivity Disorder

Lobar, SL, et al. Parents', physicians', and nurse practitioners' perceptions of behaviors associated with attention deficit hyperactivity disorder. *J Am Acad Nurse Pract* 11(6):237–242, 1999.

This exploratory descriptive study conducted a survey to identify parents', nurse practitioners', and physicians' perceptions of behaviors most commonly associated with attention-deficit/hyperactivity disorder (ADHD). A convenience sample of 29 physicians, 23 nurse practitioners, and 41 parents who were members of a parent support group was obtained. The study utilized the ADHD Rating Scale, which highlights symptomatology consistent with hyperactivity, inattention, and impulsivity. In addition, qualitative data were collected from parents regarding their reasons for seeking health care for their children. This study arose in part because of the recurrent changes and revisions in nomenclature and defining criteria and the use of multiple subjective observers in a child's behavioral evaluation that may confound the identification of ADHD. It was important to assess whether there was consistency in perceptions of ADHD in the varied reports.

This study found that there was no significant difference between nurse practitioners, parents, and physicians in their perceptions. All respondents were familiar with ADHD and were aware of the DSM criteria for the disorder. The researchers note that the similarity in responses may have been a function of shared knowledge. The parents in the support group were all well educated as to the definitions of ADHD. The addition of teachers, who are often involved in the observation of children with ADHD, might have been useful. The study supported the fact that collaboration between parents and health-care providers was important in enhancing the accurate formulation of a diagnosis of ADHD, which is based largely on subjective criteria.

the side-effect profile prohibits further titration (Level II; Wolraich et al, 2011). It is not necessary to begin with a short-acting agent before using a sustained-release agent. If the maximum dosage does not control the symptoms, switching to another stimulant is indicated. Stimulants may increase levels of seizure drugs, SSRIs, tricyclics, and warfarin. (See Drugs Commonly Prescribed 18.7.)

Atomoxetine is not a stimulant and may be used if the stimulant drugs are not tolerated or contraindicated. Atomoxetine has an effect both on ADHD and on co-morbid anxiety. Some situations where this may be the drug of choice are active substance abuse, tics, comorbid anxiety, or mood lability. Less appetite (weight loss) and less insomnia are seen with atomoxetine. Full clinical

Drugs Commonly Prescribed 18.7   Attention-Deficit/Hyperactivity Disorder (ADHD) Medications

Drug	Indication	Adverse Reactions and Prescribing Considerations
methylphenidate		
D,L-methylphenidate D-methylphenidate (MPH)	ADHD: Age 6 years and older Narcolepsy	C-II controlled substance. Available in short and extended-release formulations. Age 6 years and older. Caution administration with history of drug or alcohol dependence. Administer short-acting forms every 4 hours during daytime hours only because administration after late afternoon is associated with insomnia. Extended-release typical duration 8–12 hours Monitor growth parameters and weight Laboratory testing: CBC with differential and platelet count. Long-acting formulations available. 2009 FDA notification of potential of sudden death in healthy children treated with stimulants. Do not use in severe cardiac disease. May improve driving performance in adolescents and adults Transdermal preparation and OROS methylphenidate (Concerta) less abuse potential

Drugs Commonly Prescribed 18.7   Attention-Deficit/Hyperactivity Disorder (ADHD)
Medications—cont'd

Drug	Indication	Adverse Reactions and Prescribing Considerations
Amphetamine		
d-amphetamine (DEX) mixed amphetamine salts lisdexamfetamine dimesylate	ADHD Narcolepsy Age 3 years and older (mixed amphetamine salts) Extended-release age 6 years and older *Lisdexamfetamine age 6 years and older	C-II-controlled substance. **Black Box Warning:** High potential for abuse Sudden death and CVD events Available in short-acting and extended-release formulations Insomnia, weight loss, tics, tachycardia, and elevated BP Give on awakening Stop slowly, not suddenly Stimulant medication with less abuse potential May cause anorexia, insomnia, GI upset, emotional lability Avoid in cardiovascular disease Rare cardiomyopathy 2009 FDA notification of potential of sudden death in healthy children treated with stimulants. Monitor height and weight for all agents
SNRI		
Atomoxetine (Strattera)	ADHD: Age 6 years and older *FDA approved indication for adults	Once daily in a.m.; interacts with MAOIs; GI upset; weight loss; mood swings Sedation, GI distress Decreased appetite Potential CYP2D6 interactions Black Box for suicide ideation

The following medications are approved by the U.S. Food and Drug Administration (FDA) for the treatment of ADHD: dextroamphetamine (DEX), D- and DL-methylphenidate (MPH), mixed salts amphetamine, and atomoxetine.

*Stimulants do not have an indication in adults, and dosing guidelines are based on clinical studies rather than FDA-reviewed material. Doses of stimulants should advance slowly every several days until appropriate response is obtained.

Drug	Indication	Adverse Reactions and Prescribing Considerations
Alpha-agonist		
clonidine (Catapres) guanfacine (Tenex, Intuniv)	ADHD ADHD	More effective in treatment of impulsivity/hyperactive symptoms vs. inattention symptoms; must be tapered on discontinuation Beneficial in comorbid Tourette's and tics Sedation, dizziness Monitor BP and heart rate Treatment of stimulant-induced insomnia Treatment of tics and insomnia Advantages of guanfacine over clonidine: less sedation and longer duration of action
TCAs*		
imipramine (Tofranil)* desipramine (Norpramin)*	ADHD ADHD	ECG recommended at baseline and with dose increases Monitoring blood levels is useful in guiding dosing Black Box warning suicide ideation Anticholinergic effect Sudden death; use only if other TCAs not effective
Other		
bupropion (Wellbutrin)*	ADHD	Insomnia, decreased appetite Seizure risk

Source: Clinical pharmacology [database online]. Gold Standard, Inc., Tampa, FL, 2006. http://cp.gsm.com
*Off-label use.

effect may take up to 6 weeks, and thus educating the child, parent, and teachers is essential. Considerable attention has been given to the comorbid occurrence of SUD and ADHD and whether it is related to the use of amphetamines. Meta-analysis has shown that stimulant use in childhood actually reduced the risk of SUD by 50%. Medication diversion among adolescents, especially to improve academic performance, is a consideration when prescribing for patients with ADHD. The alpha-2 agonists, such as clonidine and guanfacine, can be utilized for ADHD treatment, as well as used adjunctive to the other stimulant medications. Clonidine is particularly helpful for insomnia.

Stimulant medications may not be effective in up to 30% of children, or adverse drug reactions prevent compliance. Side effects are common, occurring in about 70% to 90% of patients, but are usually mild and transient. Common side effects include weight loss, appetite suppression, abdominal pain, insomnia, and headache. Irritability and tics may develop. The practitioner needs to be aware of the common side effects and have strategies to offset them, including dose reduction, changing medication, and prescribing adjunctive medications. Insomnia can be managed with clonidine, antihistamines, and trazodone (Desyrel). Other agents that may be helpful for insomnia include melatonin and cyproheptadine (Periactin). Randomized controlled studies regarding tics have shown that patients with comorbid disease (tic plus ADHD), the tic disorder actually decreased with stimulant medications. For patients with medication-induced tics, reduction of dose or alternative medication may be necessary. Consideration of comorbidities is important because it may alter the treatment regimen, especially with cardiac disease. Congenital heart disease including hypertrophic cardiomyopathy or significant cardiac-related symptoms should prompt cardiac evaluation before initiating pharmacological therapy. Stimulants are contraindicated in Tourette's syndrome, monoamine oxidase inhibitor use, hereditary fructose intolerance, and glaucoma.

If all FDA-approved agents have been utilized without response, reevaluation of the diagnosis, as well as consultation, is essential. Non–FDA-approved drugs utilized are bupropion and tricyclic antidepressants.

For adults, three medications are FDA approved for treatment of ADHD. These three medications are extended-release amphetamine (Adderall), extended-release methylphenidate (Focalin XT), and nonstimulant atomoxetine. In adults, multimodal therapy is more effective than pharmacological therapy alone. Considerations in females of childbearing age and pregnancy must be also considered. See Drugs Commonly Prescribed 18.7.

Nonpharmacological Management

Behavioral techniques can include parental training, classroom management techniques, and peer interventions. Evidence-based group parent training programs and early educational programs are recommended as the initial step for children ages 4 to 5 years. In children aged 6 years and older, behavioral therapy may be initiated alone or adjunctively with medications (Level II; Wolraich et al, 2011). Combined therapy seems to be helpful in patients with comorbid anxiety and conduct disorders, as well as those who are economically disadvantaged and members of minority groups (Level I; MTA Cooperative Group, 1999). Patients who receive both medications and behavioral therapy have shown improvement in social interaction and academic achievement, but not in ADHD symptoms. Adolescents without comorbid conditions who respond well to pharmacological therapy (ADHD tool assessment) may not need additional therapy (Level I; Wolraich et al, 2011; MTA Cooperative Group, 1999). In addition, children with other psychosocial issues are more likely to benefit from combined therapy (Level I; MTA Cooperative Group, 1999). Information on parental education about ADHD, behavioral management, public behavior management, school reports, and dealing with persistent behavioral issues can be accessed at www.aacap.org/galleries/PracticeParameters/JAACAP_ADHD_2007.pdf.

There is no evidence to support the use of CBT, play therapy, dietary modifications, or EEG feedback in the treatment of ADHD in children (Level II; Wolraich et al, 2011). Involvement of the educational system is imperative. Teachers need to implement classroom behavior management strategies to help children with ADHD improve their focus and find modalities that enhance self-control (Levels I, II; Daly et al, 2007). Another strategy to improve academic performance is peer tutoring. Peer tutoring allows immediate feedback, one-to-one as well as continuous interface, and shows improved test scores and engagement in learning. Many other resources are available (see Resources).

ADHD may persist into adolescence and adulthood. Reevaluation and continued support educationally and occupationally may be needed. Adults can benefit from CBT in addition to drug therapy (Level I; Safren et al, 2005). Organizational skills training including time management, study strategies, and empowerment to minimize distractions may increase function.

Follow-up and Referral

Follow-up for patients diagnosed with ADHD includes performing a validated ADHD rating and monitoring scale for core symptoms (see Table 18.4) and a behavioral report or teacher narrative report for target symptoms. A 40% to 50% reduction in core symptoms or achieving targeted goals is considered an adequate response. Titration of medications can occur every 1 to 3 weeks. Medications used for ADHD may cause headaches, abdominal pain (which can be avoided by taking medication with meals), and growth delay. Office visits should be scheduled initially at 2 to 4 weeks, followed by every month for 6 months and then every 3 to

6 months thereafter. The focus of these visits includes physical parameters (height, weight, cardiac evaluation including blood pressure and pulse), assessment on behavioral progress (utilizing an ADHD scale helps to objectively identify behavioral changes from the parent and teacher), monitoring of medication compliance and side effects, and continued education and referral to support services if indicated. A reduction in growth of 2% as seen on the growth chart signifies a potential problem, and adjustment of the treatment plan can include a drug holiday or changing the medication. Specific laboratory tests are not generally indicated. Targeted endpoints include improved grades and ADHD rating scales, acceptable family interactions, and improved peer interactions.

Children with ADHD are at increased risk for abuse, depression, and social isolation and should be monitored for these. Parents will need regular support and advice and may need referral for family therapy to cope with the added demands. The provider should establish contact with the child's teacher every school year. Parents, teachers, and advisors should encourage career choices that allow autonomy and mobility. There is no increased frequency of delinquency unless other comorbid features (such as oppositional defiant disorder or conduct disorder) exist.

Adolescence offers new challenges, and the practitioner needs to address these issues both with the adolescent and the family. Increased independence, decision-making, and risk-taking behaviors need to be addressed. In addition, discussion about the continued need for and benefit of medication may ensue. In general, if the patient has been symptom free for longer than 1 year with no adjustment in medication dosage despite increases in weight and height, consideration about remission should occur. Summer vacation or prolonged vacation may be a good time to trial a drug holiday. Several concerns arise during adolescence. Driving needs to be discussed, stressing the importance of symptom control. Monitoring for diversion of controlled substances is essential. If there are concerns regarding this, use of atomoxetine, extended-release guanfacine, or extended-release clonidine should be considered. In some situations, treatment with a stimulant agent that possesses a smaller risk for abuse could be utilized.

Patient Education

Adherence to the treatment plan is improved when the patient and family understand the chronic nature of ADHD and its potential impact on school, social life, and occupational functioning. Continued education about medications and management of side effects may improve adherence. Utilization of various community support groups may also assist families and adults to deal with developmental challenges. There are a number of interventions that parents, family members, and teachers can do in addition to administering medication (Table 18.17). They must be educated to be aware of all potential adverse effects of medications but also should be counseled

Table 18.17	Patient Education: Attention-Deficit/Hyperactivity Disorder (ADHD)

Teach parents to do the following:
• Have the child do one task at a time.
• Use "time-out" periods for bad behavior.
• Make eye contact each time they are making a request.
• Reinforce good behavior or tasks the child does well with rewards and attention.
• Use behavior therapy such as token systems.
• Stop unacceptable behavior before it escalates.
• Make use of parent support and advocacy groups.
• Deal with negative feelings and unrealistic expectations.
• Incorporate family therapy, anger-management training, and social training.
• Coordinate homework with teachers.
• Work closely with teachers for consistent behavioral plan.

Teach teachers to do the following:
• Make sure the child has a second set of books at home.
• Make work sessions short.
• Help the child deal constructively with negative feelings.
• Provide immediate consequences for bad behavior.
• Reinforce good behavior.
• Coordinate homework with parents.
• Work closely with parents for a consistent behavioral plan.

extensively in behavioral techniques. Parents should be educated regarding realistic expectations and should be made aware of support groups for themselves as well as child advocate groups. They must be helped to deal with whatever negative feelings may emerge as a result of the diagnosis of ADHD.

■ INTIMATE PARTNER VIOLENCE

Intimate partner violence (IPV) is defined as a pattern of assaultive and coercive behaviors that may include inflicted physical injury, psychological abuse, sexual assault, progressive social isolation, stalking, deprivation, intimidation, and threats perpetrated by someone who is, was, or wishes to be involved in an intimate relationship with an adult or adolescent, and aimed at establishing control by one partner over the other. IPV is not associated with any ethnic group, religion, income level, level of education, employment, or sexual orientation. However, typically the victim is a child, a woman, or an elderly person, and the typical perpetrator is a man (in the case of partner abuse), a parent or other trusted adult (in the case of child abuse), or an adult child or other caregiver (in the case of elder abuse). More than one type of violence may occur in any given family; for example, in one study, 45% to 70% of battered women reported that their batterer also abused their children. In 2013, the World Health Organization (WHO), the U.S. Preventive Services Task Force (USPSTF), and Cochrane Reviews released identification and treatment recommendations for IPV. All guidelines encourage clinicians to be alert to physical and behavioral signs of abuse such as trauma or somatic symptoms.

Epidemiology and Causes

Estimates of the prevalence of IPV in the United States are that 1 to 4 million women per year are physically, sexually, or emotionally abused by their partners. Thirty-one percent of women report IPV at some point in their life. Violence by women against men also occurs although women are 7 to 14 times more likely to be battered. More than 1 million children are abused each year, and approximately 550,000 elderly individuals suffer abuse and/or neglect. Thousands of women and children die as a result of IPV each year. Annual health-care costs are estimated to be $44 million annually, not including money lost from work absenteeism, turnover, and decreased productivity.

Examples of IPV include punching, slapping, kicking, burning, pushing, dragging, choking, restraining, and sexual assault. In one study, 68% of domestic assault incidents involved weapons; in 15% of these cases the assault resulted in serious injury. Recent research indicates that 82% of women killed in their homes are killed by someone they knew, 55% in the context of a quarrel, physical domestic fight, or assault by a spouse, lover, or close relative. Statistics on violent crime indicate that three out of every four American women murdered die at the hands of their male partners. Recurrent violence is common; in one study, 89% of victims reported previous episodes of injury; 34% of these victims were battered on a daily basis.

Additional risk factors that increase the potential for violence include financial instability, pregnancy (15%–25% of pregnant women are abused physically while pregnant, with the abuse often leading to birth defects), the birth of a child, and job loss by either partner. Women are at great risk when they leave an abusive relationship. They have a 75% greater chance of being killed by their batterers than women who stay.

Numerous studies have documented that women with a history of IPV have greater rates of physical symptoms, a higher prevalence of unexplained physical symptoms, a greater number of symptoms, and poorer overall health status than nonabused controls. Similarly, IPV survivors have higher rates of mental health problems, including major depressive disorders, depressive symptoms, dysthymia, generalized anxiety disorder, phobias, PTSD, suicidality, and substance abuse. IPV survivors have been found to have higher health-care costs and increased utilization.

Psychodynamics and Pathophysiology

Intimate partner violence occurs in families of every racial and religious background and in every socioeconomic stratum. Although alcohol/substance abuse and a history of childhood abuse are important correlates of IPV, they do not cause or explain IPV.

Violent individuals use fear, pain, injury, humiliation, and suffering to establish power and control over their victims. The pattern for IPV is often unpredictable. In some cases, the only predictable element of the violence may be the offender's use of violence to establish power and control over the person he or she wants to dominate. This includes stalking behaviors that are intended to display the violent person's skill, strength, and determination. In other cases, with no warning at all, or after repeated threats, a violent individual can become intent on killing his or her victim. The abused individual often is forced into isolation, which prevents anyone from observing the violence or assisting the victim. The psychologically isolated victim typically is convinced that he or she is alone and that no one cares or is willing to help. A common pattern, known as the *cycle of violence,* starts with an episode of violence, followed by reconciliation, increasing tension, and the next episode of violence. Typically, the periods of tension and episodes of violence increase in duration while the reconciliation periods become shorter.

Victims of IPV often develop strong dependency needs and may deny the violence. About 50% of battered wives grew up in violent homes, and their most common trait is dependency. Victims may rationalize the violence by thinking that they can change the violent individual's behavior by making changes in their own behavior. For example, women with small children and women who are unemployed may deny the violence exists because they feel escape is impossible. Victims of domestic violence, particularly adolescents who feel they cannot escape, may first try to escape psychologically by abusing alcohol or drugs. However, all too often the violence is then blamed on the victim's substance abuse.

Clinical Presentation

Routine screening for IPV is recommended by the USPSTF for all women of childbearing age at initial visits and periodically (Level II; Moyer, 2013); this is in contrast to the WHO and Cochrane recommendations in which universal screening is not recommended. The USPSTF found insufficient evidence to routinely screen the elderly or other vulnerable populations. The WHO's premise for not recommending universal screening is based on studies that demonstrate that although an increased number of women experiencing IPV were identified, the outcomes were unchanged. Of utmost importance is that safety and confidentiality are established before asking questions about abuse (Level II; Moyer, 2013). Always preface IPV questioning with an appropriate and nonthreatening explanation such as, "I ask all of my patients these questions because these problems affect many people's health." Avoid using stigmatizing words such as *domestic violence* or *abuse.* In some instances, a patient may disclose a past experience with violence that may provide useful information in providing appropriate care.

Women who end an abusive relationship are usually at greater risk for serious injury—and therefore in greater need of intervention—than women who are still involved in an abusive relationship, but these individuals are less likely to seek help. Men should also be screened if signs of abuse are evident (Level II; Moyer, 2013). Men who have sex with men and men who are disabled may be at a higher risk and should be screened as part of the social and sexual history.

It is difficult to know when to include violence in the differential diagnosis. Recognition of IPV continues to be difficult because the victim and the abuser often conspire to conceal it. The partner, if present, may be suspicious. Look for symptoms or behaviors that may signal abuse such as exacerbation or poor control of chronic illness, sleep disturbances, chronic pain, or frequent unexplained appointment changes. Behavioral red flags are (1) a patient who is reluctant to speak in front of her partner or gives evasive answers and (2) an overly protective or controlling partner. Any patient presenting with multiple complaints or whose symptoms are not consistent with her history should be assessed for violence at least once and reassessed if she fails to respond to therapy appropriately. Exposure to IPV is frequently linked with mental health issues such as depression, anxiety, suicide attempts, and/or substance abuse. Problems or injuries during pregnancy should raise the level of suspicion, as should delays in seeking medical care. The first goal of assessment is to determine whether or not an individual is a target of violence. The second goal is to evaluate the level of danger. The patient must be seen alone.

Ask the partner, children, and family members to leave the room. If an interpreter is needed, use a gender concordant professional interpreter rather than a family member. If the partner refuses to leave, do not confront him or her; instead, strategize a way to get the patient alone later. Requesting a urinalysis or chest x-ray exam is often an effective approach.

The clinician must communicate concern and caring and tell each woman that all women are assessed for abuse. The seriousness of the issue cannot be underscored enough. Although it may be necessary to obtain specific information, the clinician should try to limit data-gathering to essentials. Some sources suggest "funneling," beginning with innocuous questions and progressing to more directed approach. Consider the utilization of a validated instrument. (See Focus on History 18.3.) Many patients will disclose emotional abuse long before they are comfortable disclosing physical abuse, even if both are occurring. A key component of the abuse experience is intrusion; many patients who are in an abusive relationship may perceive questioning as intrusive. Again, sensitivity is crucial.

Do not jump to conclusions too quickly. One sign or symptom alone is not sufficient to make a "diagnosis" of abuse. The clinician should be aware that a traumatic experience such as abuse, especially over an extended period of time, will have an impact on the victim's thought processes and belief systems. This must be taken into consideration during the assessment. It is imperative for clinicians to remain objective and nonjudgmental. Maintaining contact with a patient in the primary-care

---

Focus on History 18.3   Intimate Partner Violence (IPV): Three Questions to Ask

By asking the following three questions, the APRN may be able to identify approximately 75% of women at risk for IPV. A positive response to any of the three questions represents a positive screen.

• Have you been hit, kicked, punched, forced to have sex, or otherwise hurt by someone within the past year? If so, by whom?
• Do you feel safe in your current relationship?
• Do you feel threatened or controlled by a partner or ex-partner or anyone else in your life?

(Source: Reprinted with permission from Feldman, K, et al. Accuracy of three brief screening questions for detecting partner violence in the emergency department. *JAMA* 277:1357–1361, 1997.)

At this point, ask the patient what change, if any, he or she wants to make. Do *not* expect or even try to "fix" the situation. An abusive relationship is most often a chronic condition. As with any condition that threatens a patient's health, an important step is to determine the urgency of the situation. If there is any recent violence or threat, it is essential to assess the level of danger. Listen first to the women's own assessment; if she feels she is in danger, she most likely is. But her assessment that she is not in danger may be a misperception. There are a variety of Danger Assessment tools such as the Danger Assessment–2 (DA-2), which is a 20-question instrument; another validated tool is the Spouse Abuse: Assessing Level of Violence in the Home, which includes a revised form of that instrument and its use. Ask if the patient feels safe in the primary-care office; if the abuser is in the waiting room or likely to return, ask the patient what she would like you to do. Inquiring whether the abuser has access to weapons is critical. The clinician should aid patients in assessing the risk of future harm (Level II; Moyer, 2013).

If the patient responds with a "no" to all questions but there is still a suspicion of abuse, avoid confrontation. Make a note of the concerns on the chart, offer resources, and leave the issue open for future discussion. Ask again on future visits. Note that this is a "concern for possible abuse," not the leading diagnosis if unconfirmed.

environment and working within a *Circle of Caring* may help the clinician make this difficult assessment, as well as a viable plan for dealing with the difficult situation.

Management

The overarching goals of therapy include safety, empowerment, perpetrator accountability, and social policy change. Careful documentation of assessment findings is critical to effective management of the health-care needs of victims of domestic violence. The clinician should record the history using specific, plain language, in the patient's own words when possible. Record all physical findings, use a body map, and take photographs only if the patient consents. The clinician should preserve physical evidence, if appropriate. Thorough, well-documented medical records may prove to be crucial in a legal case. Psychiatric hospitalization may be indicated if the patient is actively suicidal, acutely psychotic, unable to care for herself, and does not have any safe alternatives for care.

Treatment for a victim of abuse involves more than treating the injuries and providing telephone numbers and referrals. Developing a caring relationship with the patient is essential. It is important to validate the lived experiences of IPV, offer support, and assist in safety planning. This is truly a patient who needs a *Circle of Caring.* Advanced Practice Nursing Interventions 18.3 lists some general interventions clinicians can make, including a danger assessment and counseling concerning the individual danger assessed. For some patients, even accepting printed material about domestic violence or abuse can be a dangerous act. False reassurance is to be avoided. Victims of IPV typically look for professionals they feel they can trust, and individuals who are planning their escape may require a great deal of time and support before they act.

Refer to appropriate law enforcement or social services agencies and develop a patient "safety plan," although there is no guarantee that the patient will comply with the plan or be willing to contact law enforcement or social services. In some practice settings, the health-care provider may need to take these actions unilaterally; in others, a team approach is more facilitative.

Follow-up and Referral

Any evidence of IPV requires full compliance with local reporting and referral laws. Local and state agencies for victims have established protocols and systems for providing services that include emergency housing, health care, foster care, and displacement counseling. Despite the significant incidence of IPV, there is still a shortage of referral services for violent offenders. Violent individuals who are motivated to stop their violence may benefit from community support groups. Local crisis services and police hotlines should be contacted to protect victims of domestic violence. Victims of IPV should have the phone number and address for local emergency services, legal

Advanced Practice Nursing Interventions 18.3
Intimate Partner Violence

Prevention:
- Teach conflict resolution skills.
- Create a safety plan to remove the individual(s) from the violent situation.
- Inquire about the abuse. Questions to ask include the following:
  1. Has the physical violence increased in frequency/severity over the past year?
  2. Have you ever been choked?
  3. Has a weapon or threat with a weapon been used?
  4. Have you been threatened with death, or do you believe the individual could kill you?
  5. Is there a gun in the house?
  6. Have you ever been forced to have sex when you did not wish to?
  7. For women, have you ever been abused while you were pregnant?
  8. Is alcohol or substance abuse a factor? How often is the alcohol or substance used?
  9. Have your daily activities been controlled?
  10. Is the individual violent and constantly jealous of you?
- Provide community resources.
- Provide counseling and other therapy as indicated (for example, crisis intervention, post-traumatic stress disorder therapy, physical rehabilitation).
- Document findings and interventions.

Source: Adapted from Jezierski, M. Abuse of women by male partners: Basic knowledge for emergency nurses. *J Emerg Nurs* 20(5):361–368, 1994.

advocacy programs, and support groups, or at least be informed regarding how to obtain this information.

Consider referral for mental health evaluation for associated psychiatric problems. Those living with abuse may have associated major depression, panic disorder, PTSD, suicidal thoughts, and co-occurring substance abuse. A patient who may refuse referrals for domestic violence services may accept a referral to obtain help with abuse-related depression and anxiety.

Participate in prevention by working with local and state coalitions against domestic violence, child abuse, and elder abuse. In addition, the work environment should have clear policies and procedures defining abuse-reporting procedures. This is important in every office, because primary-care clinicians are often the "first stop" for victims of abuse.

Patient Education

Education regarding who is at risk and information about the cycle of violence is a crucial step. One way to initiate dialog is to display information about IPV in your practice site, including waiting areas, exam rooms, and restrooms. Local, state, and national agencies have available patient education materials that are also available in many languages. Professional development on domestic violence in many states is mandated on an annual basis. It is important to remember that much knowledge in this area is new. The concept of battering as a social problem did not become widely accepted until the 1960s.

Overcome clinician barriers to addressing IPV. Professional development should include the provision of knowledge and skills to address IPV (Level I; Moyer, 2013). Establish a referral base with local providers with expertise in IPV. Include training for support staff about IPV. Incorporate screening for IPV into primary care by creating a safe environment and integrating routine inquiry.

Education about the fact that a woman may be *more* at risk *after* she leaves an abusive relationship is also very important (Level II; Moyer, 2013). Options for help need to be made available and accessible to the individual at risk. Instrumental support for new mothers, for example, may be important in limiting child abuse or other forms of domestic violence. Careful attention to the risk factors for violence in a relationship is necessary, and most important, the practitioner should provide information on where and how to get help.

■ SEXUAL ASSAULT

Sexual assault (SA) is defined by the National Crime Victimization Survey (NCVS) (www.nida.nih.gov/DirReports/DirRep906/DirectorReport11a.html) as forced sexual intercourse involving physical force or psychological coercion, with vaginal, anal, or oral penetration by the offender(s), including the use of foreign objects. The three key components of sexual assault are these:

- Lack of consent
- Threat or use of force
- Vaginal, anal, or oral penetration by body part or object

Sexual assault is a violent act, one of conquest and control. The offender's intent is to dominate, humiliate, and degrade the victim. For the victim, sexual assault is a highly traumatic event that can have long-term effects on the physiological and psychological well-being of the survivor. It is important to note that victims of sexual assault can be female or male.

Rape can be a life-threatening situation. The victim experiences shock and panic. Rapists may urinate or defecate on their victims, ejaculate into their faces and hair, force anal intercourse, insert foreign objects into the vagina and/or rectum, and cause other physical injury, including death. After the rape, the victim experiences shame, confusion, humiliation, fear, and rage. Many become phobic about sex. Few emerge from the assault completely unscathed. The degree of damage usually depends on the violence of the attack, the vulnerability of the victim, and the support system available to him or her immediately after the attack. Many victims

go on to develop post-traumatic stress disorder (PTSD), depression, or alcohol and/or drug abuse and are more likely to contemplate suicide.

Date rape, or acquaintance rape, is far more common than rape by strangers and may lead to serious health and adjustment problems for girls and women. Research has suggested that more than 50% of the women who have vaginal, oral, or anal intercourse against their will do not label these experiences as sexual assault or rape. Other forms of sexual assault and rape include child sexual abuse, sexual hate crimes, incest, male sexual assault, sexual harassment, stalking, partner rape, and sexual exploitation by trusted professionals including health-care clinicians, therapists, teachers, priests, and police officers.

Epidemiology and Causes

It has been estimated that every minute in the United States, an adult woman is sexually assaulted. According to the Federal Bureau of Investigation, over the last decade there has been a 15% decrease in the number of forcible rapes reported to local police departments. In 2010, there were 84,767 forcible sexual assaults reported to local police departments. The U.S. study of sexual assault titled "Rape in America" estimated that only one in six sexual assaults is actually reported to law enforcement. Prevalence of sexual assault has been reported at 255,630 incidents in the 2006 NCVS by the U.S. Department of Justice (www.nida.nih.gov/DirReports/DirRep906/DirectorReport11a.html). Of those incidents, 39.1% were committed by strangers, whereas 60.9% were committed by perpetrators known to the survivors. One out of 6 women and 1 out of 33 men will experience an attempted or completed sexually assault or rape at some point in their lifetimes. The vast majority of sexual assaults occur before age 18. In 2008, according to the U.S. Department of Justice, the number of forcible rapes was 89,000, which represented a 1.6% decline from 2007 estimates. This is an estimated 57.7 offenses per 100,000 females (www.ovw.usdoj.gov/sasp.htm).

According to the NCVS, women who are young, unmarried, and in a low-income group are the most frequent victims of sexual assault. The highest victimization rate for women is in the 16- to 19-year-old age-group, with the second highest rate occurring in the 20- to 24-year-old age-group. Divorced and single women experience higher rates of sexual assault than married or widowed women, and women in low-income groups experience higher rates of assault than women in moderate or high-income groups. In addition, women of color report sexual assault twice as frequently as do white American women, with African American, American Indian/Alaskan women, and women of mixed race reporting the highest lifetime rates of rape or attempted rape. Sexual assault is more likely to occur in the survivor's home (43%) or in the home of a friend (15%). Most sexual assaults (65%) occur in the evening and during the summer months. Finally, most sexual assault survivors

(78%) know their rapists. When the sexual assault is committed by a stranger, 31% of the time the sexual assault takes place in the home of the survivor or a friend's home. In some cases, sexual assault is part of the larger picture of intimate partner violence.

Men who commit rape, according to crime statistics, are typically between 25 and 44 years of age; 51% are white and tend to rape white victims; 47% are black and tend to rape black victims; the remainder are mixed. Thirty-four percent of all forcible rapes involve alcohol. The Violence Against Women Act of 2005 created the Sexual Assault Services Program (SASP; www.ovw. usdoj.gov/sexassault.htm), which is federally funded and dedicated to direct intervention and related assistance for survivors of sexual assault. State and local communities have responded as well to combat sexual assault.

Pathophysiology and Psychopathology

Sexual assault, typically a rape, is an act of violence and humiliation that happens to be expressed through sexual means. Power and anger are expressed through rape and are often part of another crime. Rapists typically threaten their victims with fists, a knife, a gun, and frequently harm them in other ways. Victims may experience beatings, sustain injuries emotionally and physically, and may be killed.

Clinical Presentation

Through their work with sexual assault survivors, experts have identified a set of immediate and long-term effects of sexual assault called the *rape trauma syndrome.* Rape trauma syndrome is considered a normal response to sexual assault. There are two identified phases of survivor responses—the *initial* or *acute phase,* characterized by a period of disorganization, and the *long-term phase,* characterized by a period of reorganization.

Initial or Acute Phase

During the initial or acute phase, many sexual assault survivors experience both physical symptoms and emotions such as fear, shock, and disbelief. Four major categories of physical symptoms have been identified:

- Physical trauma: Symptoms include soreness and bruising from the physical attack on the hands, throat, neck, breasts, thighs, legs, arms, back, buttocks, head, and face.
- Skeletal muscle tension: Symptoms include tension headaches, fatigue, and sleep disturbances.
- Gastrointestinal irritability: Symptoms include stomach pains, nausea, and a decreased appetite.
- Genitourinary disturbance: Symptoms include vaginal and/or anal bleeding and bladder and vaginal infections.

In the first few hours after the assault, survivors of a sexual assault often experience shock or disbelief. Several researchers have observed in their study of sexual assault survivors that survivors tended to have one of two emotional response patterns—expressed or controlled. The expressed style is the expression of fear, anger, and anxiety through behaviors such as crying, sobbing, paradoxical smiling, restlessness, and tenseness. The controlled style masks the psychological distress with a calm, composed, subdued affect. There were equal numbers of both expressed and controlled response styles among sexual assault survivors.

Long-Term Phase

In the long-term phase, psychological symptoms such as depression, anxiety, and fear are prominent. This phase has three components:

- Motor activity: Sexual assault survivors often exhibit an increase in motor activity with a range of activities, such as changing their residence and telephone number and adopting a variety of personal safety and security measures. They may turn to family and friends for assistance with these activities. Survivors may make special trips home or to some location that symbolizes safety and social acceptance.
- Nightmares: Nightmares after sexual assault are often upsetting, and violent dreams can occur for months after the sexual assault. The nightmares may contain images that are clearly connected to the sexual assault, but nightmare content may also fail to be obviously related to the sexual assault.
- Trauma-phobia: As the term implies, *trauma-phobia* is a phobic reaction to trauma in which the phobia develops as a psychological defense against the sexual assault experience. The more common phobias are fear of being indoors, fear of being outdoors, fear of being alone, fear of being in crowds, fear of having people behind the individual, and sexual fears. Fear of sexually transmitted disease (STD), including HIV, is also a powerful source of psychological trauma. It has been estimated that 4% to 30% of sexual assault survivors are diagnosed with an STD as a result of the sexual assault.

Some victims of sexual assault have what has been called a "silent rape reaction"; these survivors have not reported the assault to anyone. They experience psychological burdening and are not able to resolve their thoughts and feelings about the sexual assault. Consider unreported sexual assault as a basis for atypical psychological symptoms such as atypical anxiety; abdominal pain not otherwise specified; sexual relationship problems; significant changes in sexual behavior patterns; unexplained, sudden onset of phobias; and chronic low self-esteem.

Diagnostic Reasoning

The diagnosis of sexual assault is made by patient complaint and confirmed by forensic evidence.

Management

During the initial or acute phase, sexual assault survivors may be seen in emergency departments, rape crisis centers, primary-care offices, or police stations. If the sexual assault has occurred within the last 72 hours, forensic physical evidence should be collected. If the survivor chooses to remain anonymous, a "Jane Doe Rape Kit" enables forensic evidence to be collected without revealing identifying information. Survivors are given a code number that can be used to identify themselves if they choose to report later. The Violence Against Women and Department of Justice Reauthorization Act of 2005 (and reauthorized in 2013) provides that states may not require those who have experienced sexual assault to participate in the criminal justice system or cooperate with law enforcement in order to be provided with a forensic medical exam. Under this provision, a state must ensure access to an exam free of charge even if the survivor chooses not to report to the police or otherwise cooperate with the criminal justice system.

The use of a Sexual Assault Nurse Examiner (SANE), if one is available, is highly recommended. These nurses receive special training in collecting forensic evidence and providing crisis intervention and offer a number of advantages over emergency department practitioners. For example, the survivor is seen by one specialist rather than by several practitioners, which decreases the time a sexual assault survivor spends in the emergency department and ensures that she (or he) receives sensitive, nonjudgmental care by a practitioner who is an SA specialist. Equally important, the nurse is skilled in the collection of forensic evidence, resulting in higher conviction rates of sexual assault.

Care for survivors is not always consistent when they present to emergency departments. A retrospective study of care received in the emergency department from the 2003 National Hospital Medical Care Survey showed that the majority of sexual assault patients did not receive sufficient care in accordance with national treatment guidelines. Consider consultation with an expert in forensic examination (Level II; Sievers et al, 2003). Law enforcement should be involved; however, patients may decline to discuss the assault with police. Conversely, in some cases, patients may choose to cooperate so that testing costs will be paid by law enforcement. Initial treatment for sexual assault survivors includes the sexual assault interview, physical exam for physical assessment and forensic evidence collection, and crisis intervention.

The Sexual Assault Interview

Ascertain the capacity of the patient to consent to a forensic examination. Evaluate understanding and appropriate responses when obtaining the diagnostic history. Drugs, alcohol, developmental disability, or young age may cause a delay in obtaining the patient's consent. In the case of severe head or critical injury, law enforcement may provide a court order to proceed with forensic evidence collection. Before doing a diagnostic physical exam, it is imperative to address psychological issues related to the examination itself (Level II; Campbell & Raja, 1999). Patients presenting after sexual assault have undergone an experience that denied them the right to consent. There are important psychological and legal implications with obtaining forensic evidence, and the patient's consent and opportunity for a family member, friend, or patient advocate to be present should not be undervalued.

The sexual assault interview is performed in a room away from the waiting areas and exam rooms, while the survivor is still fully clothed, often with a police officer present. It should be done unrushed and with sensitivity. The sexual assault interview begins with general health information, including drug allergies, current medications including birth control, surgical history, tetanus and hepatitis B immunization if relevant, major health problems, pregnancy status if known, first day of last menstrual period, gravidity, parity, history of STDs, and most recent consensual sexual contact.

Questions about the sexual assault follow the general health information questions. Although this history is difficult for the patient to report, it is important to obtain an accurate history for collection of forensic evidence in order for the examiner to locate all points of physical contact and penetration, as well as documenting the survivor's activity immediately following the sexual assault.

The sexual assault survivor is asked the date, time, and place of the sexual assault and all events surrounding the sexual assault. Inquire about the use of force or threats of force, including threats of future harm to the patient or acquaintance, presence of a weapon, or threats to expose a personal secret. Notation of the type of force; use of restraints; number of assailants; and type of assault such as fondling, kissing, licking, penetration or attempted penetration of the mouth, vagina, or anus by finger, object, or penis need to be documented. "Drug-facilitated sexual abuse" associated with gamma-hydroxybutyrate (GHB) or alcohol may be suspected when the patient also reports lapses in consciousness, and GHB may be detected in urine up to 96 hours after consumption. Ask whether a condom was used. Ask about activities since the assault such as bathing, urinating, defecating, douching, gargling, eating, brushing teeth, and washing or wiping self.

A complete physical exam should be performed, assessing for injury and potential evidence. All physical exam and forensic evidence collection procedures should be fully explained with ample opportunities for clarification if needed. The physical examination can be traumatic for survivors; thus, survivors should be allowed to control the exam as much as possible. This can be accomplished by letting the survivors know they can refuse any part of the exam or stop the procedure at any time.

Sexual assault survivors should also be encouraged to have a support person such as a friend, spouse, or family member with them during the exam. In addition, a counselor or patient advocate from the local rape crisis center may also be available to support the sexual assault survivor during the exam. Although sexual assault survivors may decline such support, they should be offered and encouraged to accept it.

Physical Examination and Forensic Evidence Collection

The practitioner needs to be aware of state guidelines for evidence collection. The physical exam begins with the removal of all items of clothing. Each item of clothing worn at the time of the sexual assault is placed in a separate bag and then signed over to a law enforcement officer as forensic evidence. Physical forensic evidence that can be found on clothing includes hair, blood, semen, and saliva. Gloves should be worn throughout the physical exam to preserve evidence.

The sexual assault kit, available in most states, should contain all materials needed. Become familiar with the forms before doing the sexual assault exam. Document the general appearance of the patient and complete a head-to-toe assessment for signs of trauma, including an oral exam, skin exam for lacerations, swelling, broken fingernails, and foreign material such as leaves, grass, fibers, dried blood, and dried secretions anywhere on the body. Forensic evidence includes samples of the individual's hair (head and pubic) and saliva; oral, vaginal, and rectal swabs; and fingernail scrapings. It is important to label specimens accurately, noting the collection time and date and the signature of each person who provided and received them.

A detailed anogenital exam is performed to assess for injury (Level II; Sugar et al, 2004; Read et al, 2005). Pelvic, vaginal, and rectal exams are completed at the end of the exam. Colposcope and/or toluidine blue dye can be used to assess genital injury and provides permanent documentation of injuries that may heal very quickly and avoids having the patient subjected to reexamination or potential loss of evidence. Toluidine blue dye is a nuclear stain that adheres to the areas of injury on subepithelial nucleated cells but not to intact epithelial cells; therefore, it is not useful for mucosal surfaces such as the vagina or anus. Almost half of genital exams done with a colposcope of women who have been raped will have a normal exam. Anoscopy is utilized to view extent of rectal injuries. Genital injuries can also be detected when women participate in consensual intercourse. Although forensic evidence should be collected as soon as possible, exams performed several days after the sexual assault can still produce findings.

Laboratory testing for STDs is recommended only if treatment is deferred. STD testing at this time would detect only preassault infection. Consider testing in minors, because they are unable to give consent to engage in intercourse. However, serological testing for HIV, hepatitis B, and syphilis is recommended, because the efficacy of prophylactic treatment is not complete. Seroconversion that is attributed to the assault may be covered by the Victims of Violent Crimes Fund. Further collection of blood, buccal, and urine specimens is recommended for crime lab testing for DNA, pregnancy testing for all women of childbearing age, and toxicology analysis if indicated (Level II; Nelson et al, 1996). A 6-year, retrospective study of 1,421 sexual assault patients who presented to the emergency department found that 12% reported drug-facilitated sexual assault. This group had a longer delay in presentation to the emergency department, less often had police involvement, and had a decreased occurrence of genital and other injury. Hospitalization may be necessary to treat unstable medical conditions or to provide surgical intervention or psychiatric stabilization.

Nonpharmacological Treatment

Crisis intervention with sexual assault survivors includes encouraging them to talk about their feelings, validating these feelings, educating survivors about rape trauma syndrome, and identifying concerns related to the sexual assault. Psychological support is necessary to address the patient's needs and should be done before the sexual assault interview. These concerns include prevention of pregnancy and/or STDs, physical safety, and the need for specialized sexual assault psychotherapy and community support groups. Physical safety becomes a focus of concern for anyone who has just been assaulted. Sexual assault survivors can become preoccupied with the fear that their attacker will try to hurt them again. This is especially true when the survivor knows the identity of the attacker or the assault occurred in the survivor's home. Clinicians can help survivors start to problem-solve safety concerns and help to meet the survivor's immediate needs for safety. Some individuals may elect to live with friends or family until they begin to feel safe again.

A supportive approach and focusing on restoring the victim's sense of adequacy and control over his or her life are the best means for supporting the survivor provided there is no severe underlying pathology that might warrant a different treatment plan. Group therapy with homogeneous groups has been found to be effective for many. A rape victim fares best when he or she receives immediate support and can ventilate her feelings of rage and fear to loving family members and to supportive clinicians and law enforcement officials. A longitudinal study of sexual assault survivors showed that negative social reactions and blame of the victim were associated with worsened PTSD symptoms. Socially acceptable means of recourse, such as the arrest and conviction of the rapist, can help the victim. (See Advanced Practice Nursing Interventions 18.4.)

Advanced Practice Nursing Interventions 18.4 Crisis Intervention

Persons Amenable to Crisis Intervention	• History of recent, specific crisis situation (may be an event, e.g., sexual assault, natural disaster; or developmental, e.g., death, divorce, job loss). • Clear-cut evidence of psychological incapacitation, specifically, severe anxiety related to the event. • High motivation to overcome the crisis. • Previously demonstrated ability to cope.
Processes	• Practitioner must rapidly establish psychological rapport with the person and develop psychological insight on part of the person; speed is essential. • Person must actively participate. • Person and practitioner must work together to overcome the crisis.
Methods	• Main task is to decrease anxiety through reassurance, suggestion, environmental manipulation, psychotropics. • Review steps that have led to crisis and promote understanding of the maladaptive response to the crisis. • Focus on developing more adaptive ways of coping with the crisis situation. • Length of intervention may vary from 1–2 sessions to 1–2 months. • Brief hospitalization may be part of the plan.
Outcomes	• Patient better equipped to deal with future stressors. • Intervention ended as soon as possible, hopefully at a higher developmental level than before crisis. • Intervention may be viewed as both therapeutic and preventive.

Source: Adapted from Kaplan, H, and Sadock, BJ. *Synopsis of psychiatry*, ed 8. Williams & Wilkins, Baltimore, MD, 2002.

Pharmacological Therapy

Medications to treat STDs and pregnancy should be offered. A tetanus booster is necessary if patients who experienced lacerations or abrasions have not been adequately immunized. HIV counseling, as well as testing and prophylaxis, should be offered to all survivors. Provider encouragement was shown to have an association with the patient's decision to start HIV prophylaxis treatment. Consider referral to an infectious disease specialist to guide antiretroviral therapy. Offer hepatitis surface antibody testing with vaccination. Administer HBIG if there is a high risk of exposure by a known hepatitis B–positive assailant. Emergency contraception should be offered to female patients after penile-vaginal assault, especially to those patients who have not had a tubal ligation or do not have an intrauterine device (Levels I, II; von Hertzen et al, 2002). Referral to an obstetrician/gynecologist and a urology specialist may be needed for treatment for specific traumatic injuries that require further care.

Follow-up and Referral

Sexual assault survivors should be encouraged to use the support services available from community rape counseling centers, such as individual therapy, group therapy, and self-defense training, as well as legal follow-up. The majority of rape counseling centers offer 24-hour crisis hotlines. Many individuals may not feel they need this support or that their family and friends are there for

them. Survivors continue to be at risk for long-term problems, however, and to have grief and mourning needs long after the immediate crisis has passed and significant others have come to believe that the crisis is over. Rape counseling center personnel understand the long-term course of events of sexual assault. Some rape counseling centers are also able to provide advocates to support survivors as they deal with the legal and judicial systems. These services are often offered free of charge or at greatly reduced rates.

Medical follow-up after the initial visit is important to reassess any traumatic injuries, review laboratories, advise post-HIV test counseling, and reassess psychological status and recovery. Consider retesting for pregnancy if the patient has not had the expected menstrual cycle. Repeat HIV, hepatitis B, and STD testing as indicated.

Patient Education

Education begins with the first patient encounter, allowing the survivor to regain control and become an active participant in her recovery, incorporating patient-centered care. Include education about the diagnostic work-up, management, psychological and medical recovery, and advice about community support services, as well as discussion of the long-term effects of sexual assault. Impress on the patient the need to engage with psychological evaluation early on. The most common long-term effect of sexual assault is the development of PTSD. Recent research has indicated that sexual assault survivors may be the largest single group of PTSD sufferers. PTSD was originally defined to explain the set of symptoms observed in survivors of natural disasters and military combat and includes symptoms such as anxiety, depression, nightmares, flashbacks, and sleep disturbances. Researchers have found that 94% of the women who had been sexually assaulted met the criteria for PTSD 12 days after the sexual assault and that 46% of these women still met the criteria 3 months later.

In addition to having higher rates of PTSD, sexual assault survivors reported higher rates of drug and alcohol problems, depression, attempted suicide, anxiety, obsessive-compulsive disorder, and medical care use. Sexual assault survivors were 13.4 times more likely to have had alcohol-related problems and 26 times more likely to have had problems with drug abuse, compared with women who were not sexually assaulted. Survivors were three times more likely to have had a major episode of depression, four times more likely to have had thoughts about suicide, and 13 times more likely to have attempted suicide compared with other women. Finally, survivors of sexual assault report more symptoms of illness across all body systems and perceive their health less favorably than do other women. Symptoms that are diagnosed at a much higher rate in sexual assault survivors include chronic pelvic pain, gastrointestinal disorders, headaches, general pain, and premenstrual symptoms. Every effort should be made to encourage the patient to initiate long-term support for dealing with the trauma of sexual assault. The health-care provider, practicing within a *Circle of Caring*, may be in the best position to maintain contact with the patient and facilitate growth and healing.

Davis*Plus* | For additional resources please visit
http://davisplus.fadavis.com

References

Evidence-Based Practice

Akiskal, HS, et al. Reassessing carbamazepine in the treatment of bipolar disorder: Clinical implications of new data. *CNS Spectr* 10(Suppl): 1–11, 2005.

American Psychiatric Association. Practice guideline for the treatment of patients with panic disorder. Retrieved from http://psychiatryonline.org/content.aspx?bookid=28&sectionid=1680635

American Psychiatric Association. *Practice guideline for the treatment of patients with schizophrenia,* ed 2. Complete summary. 2006. Retrieved from http://psychiatryonline.org/content.aspx?bookID=28&sectionID=1665359

Anton, RF, et al. Combined pharmacotherapies and behavioral interventions for alcohol dependence: The COMBINE study: A randomized controlled trial. *JAMA* 295(17):2003–2017, 2006.

Baldwin, DS, et al. Evidence-based guidelines for the pharmacological treatment of anxiety disorders: Recommendations from the British Association for Psychopharmacology. *J Psychopharmacol* 19: 567–596, 2005.

Beidel, DC, and Turner, SM. At risk for anxiety: I. Psychopathology in the offspring of anxious parents. *J Am Acad Child Adolesc Psychiatry* 36:918–924, 1997.

Biederman, J, et al. Further evidence of association between behavioral inhibition and social anxiety in children. *Am J Psychiatry* 158: 1673–1679, 2001.

Campbell, R, and Raja, S. Secondary victimization of rape victims: Insights from mental health professionals who treat survivors of violence. *Violence Vict* 14:261–275, 1999.

Cipriani, A, et al. Comparative efficacy and acceptability of 12 new-generation antidepressants: A multiple-treatments meta-analysis. *Lancet* 373(9665):746–758, 2009.

Colom, F, et al. A randomized trial on the efficacy of group psychoeducation in the prophylaxis of recurrences in bipolar patients whose disease is in remission. *Arch Gen Psychiatry* 60: 402–407, 2003.

Daly, BP, et al. Psychosocial treatments for children with attention deficit/hyperactivity disorder. *Neuropsychol Rev* 17(1):73–89, 2007.

Gonzalez-Pinto, A, et al. Psychoeducation and cognitive-behavioral therapy in bipolar disorder: An update. *Acta Psychiatr Scand* 109: 83–89, 2004.

Institute for Clinical Systems Improvement. Major depression in adults in primary care. January 1996 (revised May 2013). Retrieved from https://www.icsi.org/_asset/fnhdm3/Depr.pdf

Institute for Clinical Systems Improvement. Major depression in adults in primary care. January 1996 (revised May 2012).

Retrieved from www.guideline.gov/content.aspx?id=37277&search=depression

Kaiser Permanente Care Management Institute. Adult depression: Clinical practice guidelines. Kaiser Permanente Care Management Institute, Oakland, CA, 2012. Retrieved from www.providers.kaiserpermanente.org/info_assets/cpp_cod/cod_depression_guideline_0712.pdf

Lieber, CS, et al. Veterans Affairs Cooperative Study of polyenylphosphatidylcholine in alcoholic liver disease: Effects on drinking behavior by nurse/physician teams. *Alcohol Clin Exp Res* 295(17): 1757–1764, 2003.

Michigan Quality Improvement Consortium. Primary care diagnosis and management of adults with depression. Updated January 2012. Retrieved from www.guideline.gov/content.aspx?id=36621&search=depression

Miklowitz, DJ, et al. A randomized study of family-focused psychoeducation and pharmacotherapy in the outpatient management of bipolar disorder. *Arch Gen Psychiatry* 60:904–912, 2003.

Moyer, VA; U.S. Preventive Services Task Force. Screening for intimate partner violence and abuse of elderly and vulnerable adults: U.S. Preventive Services Task Force recommendation statement. *Ann Intern Med* 158(6):478–486, 2013.

MTA Cooperative Group. A 14-month randomized clinical trial of treatment strategies for attention-deficit/hyperactivity disorder. The MTA Cooperative Group. Multimodal treatment study of children with ADHD. *Arch Gen Psychiatry* 56:1073–1086, 1999.

National Institute for Health and Clinical Excellence. Schizophrenia: Core interventions in the treatment and management of schizophrenia in adults in primary and secondary care. March 2009. Retrieved from www.nice.org.uk/nicemedia/pdf/CG82NICEGuideline.pdf

Nelson, MS, et al. Validation of probe EFD52 (D17S26) for forensic DNA analysis. *J Forensic Sci* 41:557–568, 1996.

Patterson, WM; Dohn, HH; Patterson, J; Patterson, GA (April 1983). "Evaluation of suicidal patients: the SAD PERSONS scale." *Psychosomatics* 24 (4): 343–5, 348–9. doi:10.1016/S0033-3182(83)73213-5. PMID 6867245.

Pitschel-Walz, G, et al. The effect of family interventions on relapse and rehospitalization in schizophrenia—a meta-analysis. *Schizophr Bull* 27:73–92, 2001. Retrieved from www.ncbi.nlm.nih.gov/pubmed/11215551?dopt=Abstract

Read, KM, et al. Population-based study of police-reported sexual assault in Baltimore, Maryland. *Am J Emerg Med* 23:273–278, 2005.

Rösner, S, et al. Opioid antagonists for alcohol dependence. *Cochrane Database Syst Rev* 8(12):CD001867, 2010. doi:10.1002/14651858.CD001867.pub2

Safren, SA, et al. Cognitive-behavioral therapy for ADHD in medication-treated adults with continued symptoms. *Behav Res Ther* 43(7):831–842, 2005.

Schutte-Rodin, S, et al. Clinical guideline for the evaluation and management of chronic insomnia in adults. *J Clin Sleep Med* 4(5): 487–504, 2008.

Scottish Intercollegiate Guidelines Network (SIGN). Management of schizophrenia: A national clinical guideline. Management of schizophrenia. (SIGN publication no. 131.) Edinburgh, Scotland, SIGN, March 2013. Retrieved from www.sign.ac.uk

Sievers, V, et al. Sexual assault evidence collection more accurate when completed by sexual assault nurse examiners: Colorado's experience. *J Emerg Nurs* 29:511–514, 2003.

Simon, NM, and Fischmann, D. The implications of medical and psychiatric comorbidity with panic disorder. *J Clin Psychiatry* 66(Suppl 4):8–15, 2005.

Soomro, GM, et al. Selective serotonin re-uptake inhibitors (SSRIs) versus placebo for obsessive compulsive disorder (OCD). *Cochrane Database Syst Rev* 23(1):CD001765, 2008. doi:10.1002/14651858.CD001765.pub3

Stein, DJ, et al. Pharmacotherapy for post traumatic stress disorder (PTSD). *Cochrane Database Syst Rev* 1, 2006. Doi:10.1002/14651858.CD002795.pub2

Sugar, NF, et al. Physical injury after sexual assault: Findings of a large case series. *Am J Obstet Gynecol* 190:71–76, 2004.

Suppes, T, et al. The Stanley Foundation Bipolar Treatment Outcome Network. II. Demographics and illness characteristics of the first 261 patients. *J Affect Disord* 67:45–59, 2001.

U.S. Department of Health and Human Services. Treating tobacco use and dependence: 2008 update. Rockville, MD. Retrieved from www.guideline.gov/summary/summary.aspx?ss=15&doc_id=12520&nbr=6444&string=

U.S. Preventive Services Task Force. Screening and behavioral counseling interventions in primary care to reduce alcohol misuse. May 2013. Retrieved from www.uspreventiveservicestaskforce.org/uspstf/uspsdrin.htm

von Hertzen, H, et al. Low dose mifepristone and two regimens of levonorgestrel for emergency contraception: A WHO multicentre randomised trial. *Lancet* 360:1803–1810, 2002.

Willenbring, ML, et al. Integrated outpatient treatment for medically ill alcoholic men: Results from a quasi-experimental study. *J Stud Alcohol* 56(3):337–343, 1995.

Willenbring, ML, and Olson, DH. A randomized trial of integrated outpatient treatment for medically ill alcoholic men. *Arch Intern Med* 159(16):1946–1952, 1999.

William, PM, et al. Treating eating disorders in primary care. *Am Fam Physician* 77(2):187–195, 196–197, 2008.

Wolraich, M, et al; Subcommittee on Attention-Deficit/Hyperactivity Disorder, Steering Committee on Quality Improvement and Management. ADHD: Clinical practice guideline for the diagnosis, evaluation, and treatment of attention-deficit/hyperactivity disorder in children and adolescents. *Pediatrics* 128(5):1007–1022, 2011.

Bibliography

General

American Psychiatric Association. *Diagnostic and statistical manual of mental disorders, fifth edition.* American Psychiatric Association, Arlington, VA, 2013.

Carlat, DJ. The psychiatric review of symptoms: A screening tool for family physicians. *Am Fam Physician* 58:1617–1624, 1998. Retrieved from www.aafp.org/afp/981101ap/carlat.html

Kaplan, HI, et al. *Kaplan and Sadock's synopsis of psychiatry*, ed 9. Lippincott Williams & Wilkins, Philadelphia, 2009.

Kern, DE, et al. Teaching the psychosocial aspects of care in the clinical setting: Practical recommendations. *Acad Med* 80(1): 8–20, 2005.

Kessler, RC, and Merikangas, KR. The National Comorbidity Survey Replication (NCS-R): Background and aims. *Int J Methods Psychiatr Res* 13:60–68, 2004.

Kübler-Ross, E. *On death and dying.* Basic Books, New York, 1965.

Loretz, L. *Primary care: Tools for clinicians.* Mosby, St. Louis, 2005.

Maier, W, et al. The Hamilton Anxiety Scale: Reliability, validity, and sensitivity to change in anxiety and depressive disorders. *J Affect Disord* 14:61–68, 1988.

Russell, L. *Mental health care services in primary care: Tackling the issues in the context of health care reform.* Center for American Progress, Washington, DC, October 2010. Retrieved from www.americanprogress.org/issues/2010/10/pdf/mentalhealth.pdf

Soni, A. Top 10 most costly conditions among men and women, 2008: Estimates for the U.S. civilian noninstitutionalized adult population, age 18 and older. Statistical Brief #331. July 2011. Agency for Healthcare Research and Quality, Rockville, MD. Retrieved from www.meps.ahrq.gov/mepsweb/data_files/publications/st331/stat331.pdf

Spitzer, RL, et al. Health-related quality of life in primary care patients with mental disorders. Results from the PRIME-MD 1000 study. *JAMA* 274:1511, 1995.

Spitzer, RL, et al. Validation and utility of a self-report version of PRIME-MD: The PHQ primary care study. *JAMA* 282:1737, 1999.

U.S. Department of Health and Human Services. Mental health: A report of the Surgeon General—Executive summary. U.S. Department of Health and Human Services, Substance Abuse and Mental Health Services Administration, Center for Mental Health Services, National Institutes of Health, National Institute of Mental Health, Rockville, MD, 1999. Retrieved from www.surgeongeneral.gov/library/mentalhealth/summary.html

Wagner, EH, et al: Organizing care for patients with chronic illness. *Milbank Q* 74:511–544, 1996.

Woltmann, E, et al. Comparative effectiveness of collaborative chronic care models for mental health conditions across primary, specialty, and behavioral health care settings: Systematic review and meta-Analysis. *Am J Psychiatry* 169:790–804, 2013.

Zimmerman, GL, et al. A "Stages of Change" approach to helping patients change behavior. *Am Fam Physician* 61:1409–1416, 2000.

Anorexia Nervosa and Bulimia Nervosa

American Psychiatric Association. *Treatment of patients with eating disorders*, ed 3. May 2006. Retrieved from www.psychiatryonline.com/pracGuide/pracGuideTopic_12.aspx

Cotton, M, et al. Four simple questions can help screen for eating disorders. *J Gen Intern Med.* 18:53, 2003.

Crowther, JH, and Sherwood, NE. Assessment. In Garner, DM, and Garfinkel, PE (Eds.), *Handbook of treatment for eating disorders,* ed 2. Guilford Press, New York, 1997, p 34.

Davison, GC, and Neale, JM. *Abnormal psychology*, ed 6. John Wiley & Sons, New York, 1994.

Jacobi, C, et al. Coming to terms with risk factors for eating disorders: Application of risk terminology and suggestions for a general taxonomy. *Psychol Bull* 130(1):19–65, 2004.

Morgan, JF, et al. The SCOFF questionnaire: Assessment of a new screening tool for eating disorders. *BMJ* 319:1467–1468, 1999.

National Collaborating Centre for Mental Health. Eating disorders. Core interventions in the treatment and management of anorexia nervosa, bulimia nervosa and related eating disorders. British Psychological Society, Leicester, UK, 2004. Retrieved from www.nice.org.uk/nicemedia/pdf/cg9fullguideline.pdf

Striegel-Moore, RH, and Bulik, CM. Risk factors for eating disorders. *Am Psychol* 62(3):181–198, 2007.

Vitousek, KB, and Orimoto, L. Cognitive-behavioral models of anorexia nervosa, bulimia nervosa, and obesity. In Kendall, P, and Dobson, KS (Eds.), *Psychopathology and cognition*. Academic Press, San Diego, CA, 1993, p 191.

Walsh, T, and Garner, DM. Diagnostic issues. In Garner, DM, and Garfinkel, PE (Eds.), *Handbook of treatment for eating disorders,* ed 2. Guilford Press, New York, 1997, p 27.

Williams, PM, et al. Treating eating disorders in primary care. *Am Fam Physician* 77(2):187–195, 2008.

Anxiety

American Psychiatric Association. *Practice guideline for the treatment of patients with panic disorder,* ed 2. American Psychiatric Association, Washington, DC, 2009.

Anda, RF, et al. The enduring effects of abuse and related adverse experiences in childhood: A convergence of evidence from neurobiology and epidemiology. *Eur Arch Psychiatry Clin Neurosci* 256:174, 2006.

Baker, SL, et al. The Liebowitz Social Anxiety Scale as a self-report instrument: A preliminary psychometric analysis. *Behav Res Ther* 40:701–715, 2002.

Baldwin, DS, et al. Evidence-based guidelines for the pharmacological treatment of anxiety disorders: Recommendations from the British Association for Psychopharmacology. *J Psychopharmacol* 19(6): 57–59, 2005.

Bonadonna, R. Meditation's impact on chronic illness. *Holist Nurs Pract* 17(6):309–319, 2003.

Fava, M, et al. Zolpidem extended-release improves sleep and next-day symptoms in comorbid insomnia and generalized anxiety disorder. *J Clin Psychopharmacol* 29(3):222–230, 2009.

Kim, SW, et al. The Yale-Brown Obsessive-Compulsive Scale: A reliability and validity study. *Psychiatry Res* 34:99–106, 1990.

Kim, SW, et al. The Symptom Checklist–90: Obsessive-compulsive subscale: A reliability and validity study. *Psychiatry Res* 41:37–44, 1992.

Mishel, MH, and Braden CJ. Finding meaning: Antecedents of uncertainty in illness. *Nurs Res* 37(2):98–103, 1998.

Pollack, M, et al. Eszopiclone coadministered with escitalopram in patients with insomnia and comorbid generalized anxiety disorder. *Arch Gen Psychiatry* 65(5):551–562, 2008.

Rivas-Vazquez, RA, et al. Current issues in anxiety and depression: Comorbid, mixed, and subthreshold. *Prof Psychol Res Pr* 35(1): 74–83, 2004.

Susman, JL. Differentiating between depression and anxiety in family practice: The challenges in managing depression and anxiety. Retrieved from www.medscape.org/viewarticle/498450

Zung,WW. Prevalence of clinically significant anxiety in a practice family setting. *Am J Psychiatry* 143:1471–1472, 1986.

Zung, WWK. A rating instrument for anxiety disorders. *Psychosomatics* 12:371–379, 1971.

Attention-Deficit/Hyperactivity Disorder

American Academy of Pediatrics. Steering Committee on Quality Improvement and Management, Subcommittee on Attention-Deficit/Hyperactivity Disorder. Appendix to ADHD Clinical Practice Guideline: Implementing the key action statements—An algorithm and explanation for process of care for the evaluation, diagnosis, treatment, and monitoring of ADHD in children and adolescents. *Pediatrics* SI1–21, 2011. Retrieved from http://pediatrics.aappublications.org/content/suppl/2011/10/11/peds.2011-2654.DC1/zpe611117822p.pdf

American Academy of Pediatrics. Subcommittee on Attention-Deficit/Hyperactivity Disorder, Steering Committee on Quality Improvement and Management, Wolraich, M, et al. ADHD: Clinical practice guideline for the diagnosis, evaluation, and treatment of attention-deficit/hyperactivity disorder in children and adolescents. *Pediatrics* 128(5):1007–1022, 2011.

Biederman, J, et al. Impact of psychometrically defined deficits of executive functioning in adults with attention deficit hyperactivity disorder. *Am J Psychiatry* 163(10):1730–1738, 2006.

Burgess-Champoux, T, et al. Perceptions of children, parents, and teachers regarding whole-grain foods, and implications for a school-based intervention. *J Nutr Educ Behav* 38(4):230–237, 2006.

Daly, BP, et al. Psychosocial treatments for children with attention deficit/hyperactivity disorder. *Neuropsychol Rev* 17(1):73–89, 2007.

Dobie, C, et al. Institute for Clinical Systems Improvement (ICSI). Diagnosis and management of attention deficit hyperactivity disorder in primary care for school age children and adolescents. Retrieved from https://www.icsi.org/guidelines_more/catalog_guidelines_and_more/catalog_guidelines/catalog_behavioral_health_guidelines/adhd/March 2012

McCabe, SE, et al. Medical use, illicit use and diversion of prescription stimulant medication. *J Psychoactive Drugs* 38(1):43–56, 2006.

McDonnell, MA, and Dougherty, M. Righting a troubled course: Diagnosing and treating ADHD in adults. *Adv Nurse Pract* 8:53–56, 2005.

Monastra, VJ. Overcoming the barriers to effective treatment for attention-deficit/hyperactivity disorder: A neuro-educational approach. *Int J Psychophysiol* 58(1):71–80, 2005.

MTA Cooperative Group. Moderators and mediators of treatment response for children with attention-deficit/hyperactivity disorder: The Multimodal Treatment Study of children with attention-deficit/hyperactivity disorder. *Arch Gen Psychiatry* 56(12):1088–1096, 1999.

Pelham, WE, Jr, and Fabiano, GA. Evidence-based psychosocial treatments for attention-deficit/hyperactivity disorder. *J Clin Child Adolesc Psychol* 37(1):184–214, 2008.

Pliszka, S. Practice parameter for the assessment and treatment of children and adolescents with attention-deficit/hyperactivity disorder. *J Am Acad Child Adolesc Psychiatry* 46(7):894–921, 2007.

Rabiner, DL, et al. The misuse and diversion of prescribed ADHD medications by college students. *J Atten Disord* 13(2):144–153, 2009.

Safren, SA, et al. Cognitive-behavioral therapy for ADHD in medication-treated adults with continued symptoms. *Behav Res Ther* 43(7): 831–842, 2005.

Salmeron, PA. Childhood and adolescent attention-deficit hyperactivity disorder: Diagnosis, clinical practice guidelines, and social implications. *J Am Acad Nurse Pract* 21:488–497, 2009.

Waite, R. Women and attention deficit disorders: A great burden overlooked. *J Am Acad Nurse Pract* 19:116–125, 2007.

Bipolar Disorder

Akiskal, HS, et al. Reassessing carbamazepine in the treatment of bipolar disorder: clinical implications of new data. *CNS Spectr* 10(6):Suppl 1–11, 2005.

American Psychiatric Association. *Practice guidelines for the treatment of patients with bipolar disorder,* ed 2. 2002. Retrieved from http://psychiatryonline.org/content.aspx?bookID=28&sectionID=1669577

Bowden, CL, et al. Bipolar disorder: Keys to diagnosis—strategies for effective management. *Consultant* 45:S2–S33, 2005.

Craddock, N, and Sklar, P. Genetics of bipolar disorder. *Lancet* 381: 1654–1662, 2013.

Crismon, ML, et al. Texas medication algorithm procedural manual: Bipolar disorder algorithms. 2007. Retrieved from www.pbhcare.org/pubdocs/upload/documents/TIMABDman2007.pdf

Das, AK, et al. Screening for bipolar disorder in a primary care practice. *JAMA* 293(5):956–963, 2005.

Gonzalez-Pinto, A, et al. Psychoeducation and cognitive-behavioral therapy in bipolar disorder: An update. *Acta Psychiatr Scand* 109:83–90, 2004.

Griswold, KS, and Pessar, LF. Management of bipolar disorder. *Am Fam Physician* 62(6):1343–1353, 1357–1358, 2000.

Hirschfeld, RM. Development and validation of a screening instrument for bipolar spectrum disorder: The Mood Disorder Questionnaire. *Am J Psychiatry* 157:1873, 2000.

Hirschfeld, RM, et al. Screening for bipolar disorder in the community. *J Clin Psychiatry* 64:53–59, 2003.

Hirschfeld, RM, et al. Screening for bipolar disorder in patients treated for depression in a family medicine clinic. *J Am Board Fam Pract* 18(4):233–239, 2005.

Jamison, KR. *An unquiet mind.* Vintage Books, New York, 1995.

Kahn, D, et al. Treatment of bipolar disorders: A guide for patients and families. *Postgrad Med Rep* 209–116, 2004.

Kaye, NS. Is your depressed patient bipolar? *J Am Board Fam Pract* 18(4):271–281, 2005.

Kessler, RC, et al. Prevalence and effects of mood disorders on work performance in a nationally representative sample of U.S. workers. *Am J Psychiatry* 163(9):1561–1568, 2006.

Management of Bipolar Disorder Working Group. VA/DoD clinical practice guideline for management of bipolar disorder in adults. Department of Veterans Affairs, Department of Defense, Washington, DC, 2010. Retrieved from www.guideline.gov/content.aspx?id=16314&search=bipolar

Miklowitz, DJ, et al. A randomized study of family-focused psychoeducation and pharmacotherapy in the outpatient management of bipolar disorder. *Arch Gen Psychiatry* 60:904–912, 2003.

Reiger, DA, et al. Comorbidity of mental disorders with alcohol and other drug abuse. Results from the Epidemiologic Catchment Area (ECA) Study. *JAMA* 264:2511–2518, 1990.

Depression

Beck, AT, et al. *Cognitive therapy of depression.* Guilford Press, New York, 1979.

Cipriani, A, et al. Comparative efficacy and acceptability of 12 new-generation antidepressants: A multiple-treatments meta-analysis. *Lancet* 373(9665):746–758, 2009.

Daniel, EF. Optimizing outcomes for patients with depression and chronic medical illnesses. *Am J Med* 121(11):S38–S44, 2008.

Frasure-Smith, N, et al. Elevated depression symptoms predict long-term cardiovascular mortality in patients with atrial fibrillation and heart failure. *Circulation* 120(2):134–140, 2009.

Hazell, P, et al. Tricyclic drugs for depression in children and adolescents. *Cochrane Database Syst Rev* 6, 2013. Art. No.: CD002317. doi:10.1002/14651858.CD002317.pub2

Kessler, RC, et al. The epidemiology of major depressive disorder: Results from the National Comorbidity Survey Replication (NCS-R). *JAMA* 289:3095–3105, 2003.

Kroenke, K, et al. The PHQ-9: Validity of a brief depression severity measure. *J Gen Intern Med* 16:606–613, 2001.

Mitchell, J, et al. Institute for Clinical Systems Improvement. Adult depression in primary care. National Guideline Clearinghouse, updated September 2013. Retrieved from https://www.icsi.org/_asset/fnhdm3/Depr-Interactive0512b.pdf

Lin, EH, et al. Depression and increased mortality in diabetes: Unexpected causes of death. *Ann Fam Med* 7(5):414–421, 2009.

Major depressive disorder among adults. National Institute of Mental Health Web site. Retrieved from www.nimh.nih.gov/statistics/1mdd_adult.shtml

Richard, LK, and Daniel, EF. Introduction: Chronic medical conditions and depression. The view from primary care. *Am J Med* 121(11):S1–S7, 2008.

Robert, MC, and Kenneth, EF. Depression in patients with coronary heart disease. *Am J Med* 121(11):S20–S27, 2008.

Sobczak, JA. Managing high-acuity-depressed adults in primary care. *J Am Acad Nurse Pract* 21(7):362–370, 2009.

Wayne, JK. The comorbidity of diabetes mellitus and depression. *Am J Med* 21(11):S8–S15, 2008.

Intimate Partner Violence

Brown, KB, et al. Effectively detect and manage elder abuse. *Nurse Pract* 29(8):22–27, 2004.

Feldhaus, K, et al. Accuracy of three brief screening questions for detecting partner violence in the emergency department. *JAMA* 277:1357–1361, 1997.

Moyer, VA; U.S. Preventive Services Task Force. Screening for intimate partner violence and abuse of elderly and vulnerable adults: U.S. Preventive Services Task Force recommendation statement. *Ann Intern Med* 158(6):478–486, 2013.

National consensus guidelines on identifying and responding to domestic violence victimization in health care settings, 2004. Retrieved from www.futureswithoutviolence.org/section/our_work/health/_health_material/_consensus_guidelines

Taft, A, et al. Screening women for intimate partner violence in healthcare settings. *Cochrane Database Syst Rev* 4(4):CD007007, 2013. doi:10.1002/14651858.CD007007.pub2

World Health Organization. Responding to intimate partner violence and sexual violence against women: WHO clinical and policy guidelines. Retrieved from http://apps.who.int/iris/bitstream/10665/85240/1/9789241548595_eng.pdf

Grief

Kübler-Ross, E. *On death and dying*. Basic Books, New York, 1965.

Obsessive-Compulsive and Related Disorders

American Psychiatric Association. Practice guideline for obsessive compulsive disorder. November 2007 (reaffirmed 2012). Retrieved from www.guideline.gov/search/search.aspx?term=obsessive+compulsive

Gilbert, AR, and Malouf, FT. Pediatric obsessive-compulsive disorder: Management in primary care. *Curr Opin Pediatr* 20:544–550, 2008.

Raskind, MA, et al. A trial of prazosin for combat trauma PTSD with nightmares in active-duty soldiers returned from Iraq and Afghanistan. *Am J Psychiatry* 170(9):1003–1010, 2013.

Soomro, GM, et al. Selective serotonin re-uptake inhibitors (SSRIs) versus placebo for obsessive compulsive disorder (OCD). *Cochrane Database Syst Rev* CD001765, 2008. doi:10.1002/14651858.CD001765.pub3

Panic Disorder

American Psychiatric Association. *Practice guideline for the treatment of patients with panic disorder,* ed 2. American Psychiatric Association, Washington, DC, 2009.

Post-Traumatic Stress Disorder

American Psychiatric Association. *Practice guidelines for the treatment of patients with acute stress disorder and posttraumatic stress disorder.* American Psychiatric Association, Arlington, VA, 2004 (reviewed 2008). Retrieved from www.guideline.gov/content.aspx?id=5954&search=posttraumatic+stress

Feczer, D, and Bjorklund, P. Forever changed: Posttraumatic stress disorder in female military veterans, a case report. *Perspect Psychiatr C* 45(4):278–291, 2009.

Galea, S, et al. The epidemiology of post-traumatic stress disorder after disasters. *Epidemiol Rev* 27(1):78–91, 2005.

Institute of Medicine. *Treatment of PTSD: An assessment of the evidence report brief.* October 2007. Retrieved from www.iom.edu/Reports/2007/Treatment-of-PTSD-An-Assessment-of-The-Evidence.aspx

Kaiman, C. PTSD in the World War II combat veteran. *Am J Nurs* 103(11):32–41, 2003.

Pregnancy

Austin, M-P, and Highet N; *Guidelines Expert Advisory Committee. Australian clinical practice guidelines for depression and related disorders—anxiety, bipolar disorder and puerperal psychosis—in the perinatal period. A guideline for primary health care professionals.* Melbourne, Australia, Beyondblue: The National Depression Initiative, February 2011.

Van Mullem, C, and Tillett, J. Psychiatric disorders in pregnancy. *J Perinat Neonatal Nurs* 23(2):124–130, 2009.

Vesga-Lopez, O, et al. Psychiatric disorders in pregnant and postpartum women in the United States. *Arch Gen Psych* 65(7):805–815, 2008.

Ward, RK, and Zamorski, MA. Benefits and risks of psychiatric medications during pregnancy. *Am Fam Physician* 66:629–636, 2002.

Yonkers, KA, et al. The management of depression during pregnancy: Report from the American Psychiatric Association and the American College of Obstetricians and Gynecologists. *Gen Hosp Psychiatry* 31(5):403–413, 2009.

Schizophrenia Spectrum Disorders

Arango, C, et al. A comparison of schizophrenia outpatients treated with antipsychotics with and without metabolic syndrome: Findings from the CLAMORS study. *Schizophr Res* 104(1-3):1–12, 2008.

Arseneault, L, et al. Causal association between cannabis and psychosis: Examination of the evidence. *Br J Psychiatry* 184:110–117, 2004.

Bartels, SJ, and Pratt, SI. Psychosocial rehabilitation and quality of life for older adults with serious mental illness: Recent findings and future research directions. *Curr Opin Psychiatry* 22(4):381–385, 2009.

Bebbington, PE, et al. Psychosis, victimisation and childhood disadvantage: Evidence from the second British National Survey of Psychiatric Morbidity. *Br J Psychiatry* 185:220–226, 2004.

Cantor-Graae, E, and Selten, JP. Schizophrenia and migration: A meta-analysis and review. *Am J Psychiatry* 162:12–24, 2005.

Clemmensen, L, et al. A systematic review of the long-term effects of early onset schizophrenia. *BMC Psychiatry* 12:150, 2012. doi:10.1186/1471-244X-12-150

Courey, TC. Detection, prevention, and management of extrapyramidal symptoms. *J Nurse Pract* 3(7):464–469, 2007.

Davidson, L, et al. Peer support among adults with serious mental illness: A report from the field. *Schizophr Bull* 32(3):443–450, 2006.

Eric, TR, et al. Cancer mortality in patients with schizophrenia. *Cancer* 115(15):3555–3562, 2009.

Fearon, P, et al. Incidence of schizophrenia and other psychoses in ethnic minority groups: Results from the MRC AESOP Study. *Psychol Med* 36:1–10, 2006.

Gough, SA, and Robert, P. Diabetes and its prevention: Pragmatic solutions for people with schizophrenia. *Br J Psychiatry Suppl* 47:S106–S111, 2004.

Griswold, KS, et al. Primary care after psychiatric crisis: A qualitative analysis. *Ann Fam Med* 6(1):38–43, 2008.

Hunter, RE, et al. Risperidone versus typical antipsychotic medication for schizophrenia. *Cochrane Database Syst Rev* 2:CD000440, 2003. doi:10.1002/14651858.CD000440

Kamble, P, et al. Use of antipsychotics among elderly nursing home residents with dementia in the US: An analysis of National Survey Data. *Drugs Aging* 26(6):483–492, 2009.

Kendler, KS, et al. Lifetime prevalence, demographic risk factors, and diagnostic validity of nonaffective psychosis as assessed in a US community sample. The National Comorbidity Survey. *Arch Gen Psychiatry* 53:1022–1031, 1996.

Kessler, RC, et al. Prevalence and treatment of mental disorders, 1990 to 2003. *N Engl J Med* 352(24):2515–2523, 2005.

Kessler, RC, et al. The individual-level and societal-level effects of mental disorders on earnings in the United States: Results from the National Comorbidity Survey Replication. *Am J Psychiatry* 165:703–711, 2008.

Kirkbride, JB, et al. Heterogeneity in incidence rates of schizophrenia and other psychotic syndromes: Findings from the 3-center AeSOP study. *Arch Gen Psychiatry* 63:250–258, 2006.

Lieberman, JA, et al. Effectiveness of antipsychotic drugs in patients with chronic schizophrenia. *N Engl J Med* 353(12):1209–223, 2005.

Lumby, B. Guide schizophrenia patients to better physical health. *Nurs Pract* 32(7):30–37, 2007.

McIntyre, RS. Understanding needs, interactions, treatment, and expectations among individuals affected by bipolar disorder or schizophrenia: The UNITE global survey. *J Clin Psychiatry* 70(Suppl 3):5–11, 2009.

Morden, NE, et al. Health care for patients with serious mental illness: Family medicine's role. *J Am Board Fam Med* 22(2):187–195, 2009.

Moore, THM, et al. Cannabis use and risk of psychotic or affective mental health outcomes: A systematic review. *Lancet* 370:319–328, 2007.

Murray, CJL, and Lopez, AD. *The global burden of disease.* Harvard University Press, Cambridge, MA, 1996.

National Association of State Mental Health Program Directors (NASMHPD) Medical Directors Council. *Morbidity and mortality in people with serious mental illness.* NASMHPD, Alexandria, VA, 2006. Retrieved from www.nasmhpd.org/docs/publications/MDCdocs/Mortality%20and%20Morbidity%20Final%20Report%208.18.08.pdf

National Collaborating Centre for Mental Health Schizophrenia. Core interventions in the treatment and management of schizophrenia in primary and secondary care: Complete summary. National Institute for Health and Clinical Excellence (NICE), London, UK, 2002, updated March 2009. Retrieved from www.guideline.gov/content.aspx?id=14313&search=schizophrenia

Newcomer, JW. Comparing the safety and efficacy of atypical antipsychotics in psychiatric patients with comorbid medical illnesses. *J Clin Psychiatry* 70(Suppl 3):30–36, 2009.

Perkins, DV, et al. Gainful employment reduces stigma toward people recovering from schizophrenia. *Community Ment Health J* 45(3):158–162, 2009.

Read, J, et al. Childhood trauma, psychosis and schizophrenia: A literature review with theoretical and clinical implications. *Acta Psychiatr Scand* 112:330–350, 2005.

Sadock, BJ, et al. *Kaplan and Sadock's comprehensive textbook of psychiatry.* Lippincott Williams & Wilkins, Philadelphia, 2009.

Sartorius, N. Lessons from a 10-year global programme against stigma and discrimination because of illness. *Psychol Health Med* 11:383–388, 2006.

Schooler, N, et al. Risperidone and haloperidol in first-episode psychosis: A long-term randomized trial. *Am J Psychiatry* 162(5):947–953, 2005.

Schultz, SH, et al. Schizophrenia: A review. *Am Fam Physician* 75:1821–1830, 2007.

Selten, JP, and Cantor-Graae, E. Social defeat: Risk factor for schizophrenia? *Br J Psychiatry* 187:101–102, 2005.

Tran, EF, et al. Cancer mortality in patients with schizophrenia: An 11-year prospective cohort study. *Cancer* 115(15):3555–3562, 2009.

Tungpunkom, P, and Nicol, M. Life skills programmes for chronic mental illnesses. *Cochrane Database Syst Rev* (2):CD000381, 2008. Retrieved from http://onlinelibrary.wiley.com/doi/10.1002/14651858.CD000381.pub3/abstract;jsessionid=D60C655F00DC99A768737C86CD920D13.f03t01

Van Os, J, et al. The schizophrenia enviroment. *Curr Opin Psychiatry* 58:141–145, 2005.

Velligan, DI, et al. The expert consensus guideline series: Adherence problems in patients with serious and persistent mental illness. *J Clin Psychiatry* 70(Suppl 4):1–46, 2009.

Warner, R. Recovery from schizophrenia and the recovery model. *Curr Opin Psychiatry* 22(4):374–380, 2009.

Willhite, RK, et al. Gender differences in symptoms, functioning and social support in patients at ultra-high risk for developing a psychotic disorder. *Schizophr Res* 104(1-3):237–245, 2008.

Wu RR, et al. Lifestyle intervention and metformin for treatment of antipsychotic-induced weight gain: A randomized controlled trial. *JAMA* 299(2):185–193, 2008.

Sexual Assault

Campbell, R, et al. Responding to sexual assault victims' medical and emotional needs: A national study of the services provided by SANE programs. *Res Nurs Health* 29:384–398, 2006.

Du Mont, J, et al. HIV postexposure prophylaxis use among Ontario female adolescent sexual assault victims: A prospective analysis. *Sex Trans Dis* 35:973–978, 2008.

Kahn, AS, et al. Calling it rape: Differences in experiences of women who do or do not label their sexual assault as rape. *Psychol Women Q* 27:233–242, 2004.

Sievers V, et al. Sexual assault evidence collection more accurate when completed by sexual assault nurse examiners: Colorado's experience. *J Emerg Nurs* 29:511–514, 2003.

Straight, JD, and Heaton, P. Emergency department care for victims of sexual offense. *Am J Health Syst Pharm* 64(17):1845–1850, 2007.

Sugar, NF, et al. Physical injury after sexual assault: Findings of a large case series. *Am J Obstet Gynecol* 190:71–76, 2004.

Ullman, SE, et al. The role of victim-offender relationship in women's sexual assault experience. *J Interpers Violence* 21:798–819, 2006.

U.S. Department of Justice. Frequently asked questions: Anonymous reporting and forensic examinations. Updated September 2013. Office on Violence Against Women. Retrieved from www.ovw.usdoj.gov/faq-forensic-examinations.html

von Hertzen, H, et al. Low dose mifepristone and two regimens of levonorgestrel for emergency contraception: A WHO multicentre randomised trial. *Lancet* 360:1803–1810, 2002.

Workowski, K, and Berman, S. Department of Health and Human Services: Centers for Disease Control and Prevention. Sexually transmitted diseases treatment guidelines, 2010. *MMWR* .59(RR 12):1–116, 2010. Retrieved from www.cdc.gov/std/treatment/2010/STD-Treatment-2010-RR5912.pdf

Sleep–Wake Disorders

Benca, RM. Diagnosis and treatment of chronic insomnia: A review. *Psychiatr Serv* 56:332–343, 2005.

Buscemi, N, et al. Manifestations and management of chronic insomnia in adults. June 2005. Agency for Healthcare Research and Quality, Rockville, MD. Retrieved from www.ahrq.gov/clinic/tp/insomntp.htm

Gutierrez, C, and Brady, P. Obstructive sleep apnea: A diagnostic and treatment guide. *J Fam Pract* 62(10):565–572, 2013.

NIH State-of-the-Science Conference statement on manifestations and management of chronic insomnia in adults. Retrieved from http://consensus.nih.gov/2005/2005InsomniaSOS026html.htm

Palmer, LJ, and Redline, S: Genomic approaches to understanding obstructive sleep apnea. *Respir Physiol Neurobiol* 135(2-3):187–205, 2003.

Roth, T. Comorbid insomnia: Current directions and future challenges. *Am J Managed Care* 15:S6–S13, 2009.

Schutte-Rodin, S, et al. Clinical guideline for the evaluation and management of chronic insomnia in adults. *J Clin Sleep Med* 4(5):487–504, 2008.

Substance-Related and Addictive Disorders

Addiction science: From molecules to managed care. National Institutes of Health, National Institute on Drug Abuse Web site. 2008. Retrieved from www.drugabuse.gov/publications/addiction-science-molecules-to-managed-care/introduction/drug-abuse-costs-united-states-economy-hundreds-billions-dollars-in-increased-health

Allen, JP, et al. A review of research on the Alcohol Use Disorders Identification Test (AUDIT). Alcoholism. *Clin Exp Res* 21:613, 1997.

American Academy of Family Practice. Tobacco-use prevention and cessation (position paper). March 2009. Retrieved from www.aafp.org/about/policies/all/tobacco-prevention.html

Anton, RF, et al. Combined pharmacotherapies and behavioral interventions for alcohol dependence: The COMBINE study: A randomized controlled trial. *JAMA* 295(17):2003–2017, 2006.

Babor, TF, and Higgins-Biddle, JC. Brief intervention: For hazardous and harmful drinking: A manual for use in primary care. 2001. Retrieved from http://whqlibdoc.who.int/hq/2001/who_msd_msb_01.6b.pdf

Bayard, M, et al. Alcohol withdrawal syndrome. *Am Fam Physician* 69(6):1443–1450, 2004.

Beckham, N. Motivational interviewing with hazardous drinkers. *J Am Acad Nurse Pract* 19(2):103–110, 2006.

Blow, FC, et al. Brief screening for alcohol problems in elderly populations using the Short Michigan Alcoholism Screening Test–Geriatric Version (SMAST-G). *Alcoholism Clin Exp Res* 22(Suppl):131A, 1998.

Bradford, T, et al. Methamphetamine abuse. *Am Fam Physician* 76:1169–1176, 2007.

Bradley, KA, et al. Screening for problem drinking: Comparison of CAGE and AUDIT. Ambulatory Care Quality Improvement Project (ACQUIP). Alcohol Use Disorders Identification Test. *J Gen Intern Med* 13:379–388, 1998.

Caulker-Burnett, I. Primary care screening for substance abuse. *Nurse Pract* 19(6):42–48, 1994.

Centers for Disease Control and Prevention. Current cigarette smoking among adults—United States, 2011. *Morb Mortal Wkly Rep* 61(44): 889–894, 2012. Retrieved from www.cdc.gov/mmwr/preview/ mmwrhtml/mm6144a2.htm?s_cid=%20mm6144a2.htm_w

Clemens, SL, et al. A review of the impacts of health and health behaviors on women's alcohol use. *Am J Health Behav* 33(4):400–415, 2009.

Dasgupta, A. False-positive DOA testing results due to prescription medications. *MLO* 24–26, 2009.

Ewing, JA. Detecting alcoholism. The CAGE questionnaire. *JAMA* 252:1905–1907, 1984.

Fiellin, DA, et al. Screening for alcohol problems in primary care: A systemic review. *Arch Gen Psychiatry* 160:1977–1989, 2000.

Food and Drug Administration. Caffeine intake by the US population. 2010. Retrieved from www.fda.gov/downloads/ AboutFDA/CentersOffices/OfficeofFoods/CFSAN/ CFSANFOIAElectronicReadingRoom/UCM333191.pdf

Gassman, RA. Practitioner-level predictors of alcohol problems detection and management activities. *J Subst Use* 12(3):191–202, 2007.

Gawin, FH. Cocaine addiction: Psychology and neurophysiology. *Science* 251:1580–1586, 1991.

Griswold, KS, et al. Adolescent substance use and abuse: Recognition and management. *Am Fam Physician* 77(3):331–336, 2008.

Harwood, GA. Alcohol abuse screening in primary care. *Nurse Pract* 30(2):56–61, 2005.

Hedlund, JL, and Vieweg, BW. The Michigan Alcoholism Screening Test (MAST): A comprehensive review. *J Operat Psychiatry* 15:55, 1964.

Johnson, BA, et al. Topiramate for treating alcohol dependence: A randomized controlled trial. *JAMA* 298(14):1641–1651, 2007.

Knight, JR, et al. Validity of brief alcohol screening test among adolescents: A comparison of the AUDIT, POSIT, CAGE, and CRAFFT. *Alcohol Clin Exp Res* 27:67–73, 2003.

Mann, K, et al. The efficacy of acamprosate in the maintenance of abstinence in alcohol-dependent individuals: Results of a meta-analysis. *Alcohol Clin Exp Res* 28(1):51–63, 2004.

McGuinness, P. Update on marijuana. *J Psychosoc Nurs Ment Health Serv* 47(10):19–22, 2009.

McCusker, RR, et al. Caffeine content of energy drinks, carbonated sodas, and other beverages. *J Anal Toxicol* 30:112–114, 2006.

Reinert, DF, and Allen, JP. The Alcohol Use Disorders Identification Test (AUDIT): A review of recent research. *Alcohol Clin Exp Res* 26:272–279, 2002.

Rösner, S, et al. Opioid antagonists for alcohol dependence. *Cochrane Database Syst Rev* 12:CD001867, 2010. doi:10.1002/14651858. CD001867.pub2

Smith, P, et al. Primary care validation of a single-question alcohol screening test. *J Gen Intern Med* 24(7):783–788, 2009.

Srisurapanont, M, and Jarusuraisin, N. Naltrexone for the treatment of alcoholism: A meta-analysis of randomized controlled trials. *Int J Neuropsychopharmacol* 8(2):267–280, 2005.

Manubay, J. Essentials 387: Addiction medicine. AAFP Web site. 2009. Retrieved from www.aafp.org/fpe/2011/0800/387.html#KeyPractice

U.S. Department of Health and Human Services. Results from the 2007 National Survey on Drug Use and Health: National findings, 2007. Retrieved from www.drugabusestatistics.samhsa.gov/nsduh/ 2k7nsduh/2k7results.cfm#Ch7

U.S. Department of Health and Human Services. Treating tobacco use and dependence: 2008 update. U.S. Department of Health and

Human Services, Public Health Service. Retrieved from www. surgeongeneral.gov/tobacco/treating_tobacco_use08.pdf

U.S. Department of Health and Human Services, National Institutes of Health, NIDA. Addiction science: From molecules to managed care. 2008. Retrieved from www.drugabuse.gov/publications/ addiction-science-molecules-to-managed-care/introduction/ drug-abuse-costs-united-states-economy-hundreds-billions-dollars-in-increased-health

U.S. Department of Health and Human Services, National Institutes of Health, NIDA. Commonly abused drugs chart. March 2011. Retrieved from www.drugabuse.gov/drugs-abuse/commonly-abused-drugs/commonly-abused-drugs-chart

U.S. Department of Health and Human Services, National Institutes of Health, NIDA. Epidemiologic trends in drug abuse, National Institute on Drug Abuse. 2011. Retrieved from www.drugabuse. gov/sites/default/files/cewgjune2011_vol_ii_508.pdf

U.S. Department of Health and Human Services, National Institutes of Health, NIDA. Prescription drugs: Abuse and addiction. July 2001 (revised 2011). Retrieved from www.nida.nih.gov/ ResearchReports/Prescription/prescription7.html

U.S. Preventive Services Task Force. *Guide to clinical preventive services*, ed 2. International Medical Publishing, Alexandria, VA, 1996.

VHA/DoD clinical practice guideline for the management of substance use disorders. 2009. Retrieved from www.guideline.gov/ summary/summary.aspx?doc_id=3169&nbr=002395&string= VHA%2fDoD

Willenbring, ML, et al. Helping patients who drink too much: An evidence-based guide for primary care clinicians. *Am Fam Physician* 80(1):44–50, 2009.

Zammit, S, et al. Maternal tobacco, cannabis and alcohol use during pregnancy and risk of adolescent psychotic symptoms in offspring. *Br J Psychiatry* 195(4):294–300, 2009.

Suicide Risk

Beck, AT, et al. Hopelessness, depression, suicidal ideation and clinical diagnosis of depression. *Suicide Life Threat Behav* 23:139, 1993.

Blumenthal, S, and Kupfer, D (Eds.). *Suicide over the life cycle: Risk factors, assessment, and treatment of suicidal patients.* American Psychiatric Press, Washington, DC, 1990, p 177.

Campbell, WH. Pearls: Revised "SAD PERSONS" helps assess suicide risk. *Curr Psychiatry* 13:3, 2004.

Eaton, DK, et al. Youth risk behavior surveillance—United States, 2007. *Morb Mortal Weekly Rep* 57:SS-4, 2008.

Gaynes, BN, et al. Screening for suicide risk. Systemic evidence review no. 32. Rockville, MD, 2004. Retrieved from www.ahrq.gov/ downloads/pub/prevent/pdfser/suicidser.pdf

Holkup, P. Evidence-based protocol. Elderly suicide: Secondary prevention. University of Iowa Gerontological Nursing Interventions Research Center, 2002. Retrieved from www.guideline.gov/ summary/summary.aspx?ss=15&doc_id=3308&nbr=2534& string= suicide

Mackenzie, T, and Popkin, M. Medical illness and suicide. In Blumenthal, S, and Kupfer, D (Eds.), *Suicide over the life cycle: Risk factors, assessment, and treatment of suicidal patients.* American Psychiatric Press, Washington, DC, 1990, p 205.

U.S. Department Health and Human Services. Summary of national strategy for suicide prevention: Goals and objectives for action. SMA01–3518. Retrieved from http://mentalhealth.samhsa. gov/publications/allpubs/SMA01–3518/default.asp#summary

U.S. Preventive Services Task Force. Screening for suicide risk: Recommendation and rationale. *Am J Nurse Pract* 9(3):46, 2005.

Resources

Academy of Child and Adolescence Psychiatry
www.aacap.org
Academy of Experts in Traumatic Stress
http://aaets.org
Brief Interventions
www.addictionadvisor.co.uk/THLmedicalguidelines/A3.pdf
How Do I Deliver a Brief Intervention?
www.dryoutnow.com/alcohol-treatment/pdf_a007.shtml
Alcohol Use Disorders Identification Test: Guidelines for Use in Primary Care
www.who.int/substance_abuse/publication/alcohol/en
American Psychological Association
www.apa.org

Association for Marriage and Family
www.aamft.org
Children and Adults with Attention-Deficit/Hyperactivity Disorder
www.chadd.org
Measuring Violence-Related Attitudes, Beliefs, and Behaviors Among Youths: A Compendium of Assessment Tools
www.cdc.gov/ncicp/pub-res/measure.htm
National Center on Elder Abuse
www.elderabusecenter.org/default.cfm
National Clearinghouse for Drug and Alcohol Information
www.health.org
National Institute on Alcohol Abuse and Alcoholism
www.niaaa.nih.gov

National Institute of Mental Health suicide facts
www.nimh.nih.gov/research/suifact.cmf
National Institute on Drug Abuse
www.nida.nih.gov
National Hospice and Palliative Care Organization
www.nho.org
Nursing Network on Violence Against Women
www.nnvawi.org/assessment.htm
Partnerships Against Violence Network
www.pavnet.org
Peace at Home
www.peaceathome.org
Project Cork information on substance abuse
www.projectcork.org
Sexual Assault Resource Service
www.sanesart.com/Default.asp

SleepNet
www.sleepnet.com
Treatment Improvement Exchange—Treatment Improvement
   Protocols (TIPs)
www.treatment.org/Externals/tips.html
U.S. Department of Justice Office on Violence Against Women
www.usdoj.gov/ovw
World Health Organization
www.who.int/health_topics/en
National Institute of Mental Health
www.nimh.nih.gov/health/trials/schizophrenia.shtml
National Alliance of Mental Health
www.nami.org

Emergency Problems

Jill E. Winland-Brown, EdD, APRN, FNP-BC •
Brian Oscar Porter, MD, PhD, MPH

Chapter 19

In the United States in a typical year, there are approximately 130 million emergency department (ED) visits. Thirty-eight million of those are injury-related visits. Falls are the most common reason for an injury-related visit. Almost 43% of all Americans will visit an ED this year; 35% of ED visits will involve a patient being x-rayed, and 17% will involve computed tomography or magnetic resonance imaging scans.

COMMON PROBLEMS

■ PNEUMOTHORAX AND HEMOTHORAX

Pneumothorax refers to the abnormal presence of air in the potential space between the parietal and visceral pleura in the thorax. *Hemothorax* refers to the abnormal presence of blood in the same region. For this potential space to become occupied by air or blood, there must be an injury to one of the pleurae. A pneumothorax is described as *closed* if the chest wall is intact or *open* if the chest is violated and communicates with the atmosphere.

Epidemiology and Causes

Pneumothorax and hemothorax are usually the result of a trauma that penetrates the chest wall and violates the parietal pleura or of a blunt force trauma that fractures ribs, which violate the parietal or visceral pleura. Pneumothorax may be procedurally related; for example, during placement, a central line or arterial catheter may accidentally puncture the lung. Most patients (60%) who have suffered a penetrating or high-energy blunt trauma to the chest will have a hemothorax and/or pneumothorax. A pneumothorax (in 25% of patients) or other extrathoracic injuries (in 13%) will usually accompany a hemothorax. The etiology of pneumothorax can be traumatic (ribs piercing the pleura as a result of a motor vehicle accident, for instance), iatrogenic (as a complication of a central-line insertion), idiopathic (spontaneous), or related to an underlying disease process (such as a ruptured emphysematous bleb in the lung apices in a patient with chronic obstructive pulmonary disease [COPD]). With the increased incidence

of COPD, pneumothorax is becoming more common in the primary-care setting.

A spontaneous pneumothorax, which accounts for two-thirds of all pneumothoraces, occurs most commonly, and this type is more prevalent in tall, slender young men. It is usually the result of a rupture of a superficial bleb. A *bleb* is a defect on the lung surface that appears as an outpouching. Such defects may be inherited or related to forces placed on the lung during growth, development, and remodeling of inflammatory lung tissue. Cigarette smoking clearly predisposes an individual to bleb formation and spontaneous pneumothorax with a clear dose–response relationship, likely due to repeated inflammatory insults to the lung parenchyma. Patients with connective tissue disorders, such as Marfan syndrome or homocystinuria, are also susceptible to spontaneous pneumothoraces. In addition, women with thoracic endometriosis may suffer from recurrent catamenial pneumothoraces or hemothoraces, which are related to their menstrual cycles and bleeding from extrauterine endometrial implants. Catamenial pneumothorax occurs within 72 hours before or after the menstrual cycle. Surgical exploration of the diaphragm should be done in females with repeated pneumothorax. Rare, heritable genetic conditions also exist that predispose individuals to primary pneumothorax, such as the familial cancer condition characterized by renal cancer and benign skin tumors known as Birt-Hogg-Dube syndrome. However, such conditions are typically not suspected without a strong family history. Thirty percent to 50% of patients with a history of spontaneous pneumothorax will have a recurrence of this condition.

Secondary pneumothoraces are most often due to underlying emphysematous COPD or HIV-associated *Pneumocystis jiroveci* (formerly known as *Pneumocystis carinii*) pneumonia. Other etiologies for the clinician to consider include asthma, neoplasms, as well as pulmonary infarction.

Other common predisposing conditions include cystic fibrosis and other conditions that cause significant bronchiectasis, as well as any cavitary lung infection, such as tuberculosis, in which cavities may rupture through the parietal pleura, leading to gas escape into the pleural space. Hemothoraces may similarly result when cavitary lung lesions invade both blood vessels and the parietal pleura; however, penetrating chest trauma remains the primary cause of hemothorax.

Pathophysiology

Although the underlying etiology of pneumothorax and hemothorax varies widely as described in the preceding text, the collection of either gas or blood within the pleural space ultimately results from a similar pathophysiological mechanism. The thorax contains the lungs, heart, and major blood vessels. A visceral pleural layer surrounds the outer surface of the lungs, and the chest wall is lined with a parietal pleural layer. The pleural space is a potential space resulting from the apposition of the two pleural membranes. The pleural cells that line the lungs and chest wall continually absorb any gas or fluid that collects in the pleural space, which maintains a negative pressure of −10 to −12 mm Hg. This thoracic pressure differential allows the lungs to expand during inspiration. Any trauma or membrane rupture that results in violation of either pleura can eliminate this negative pressure and allow fluid or air to collect in this space. In turn, this will have a negative impact on the ability of the lungs to expand effectively.

Clinical Presentation

Subjective

The most frequent presenting symptoms of patients with pneumothorax and hemothorax are dyspnea and chest pain. The severity of the symptoms depends on the size of the pneumothorax or hemothorax. Typically, these conditions are associated with other injuries, which may mask the dyspnea or chest pain. For example, a patient who has a head injury or is unconscious may have altered breathing patterns related to a cerebral event. If the clinician is not alert to the possibility of chest pathology, a pneumothorax or hemothorax may be missed. Fractured ribs may mimic the type of pain encountered with a pneumothorax or hemothorax. If rib x-ray studies are the only type (view) ordered, the technique used to perform this type of x-ray exam correctly will obscure the subtle radiographic findings of a pneumothorax. A chest x-ray film with both posterior-anterior and lateral views should be ordered for any patient who may have suffered chest trauma. A high index of suspicion is needed when considering a pneumothorax or hemothorax.

Objective

Because of decreased lung volume, patients with pneumothorax or hemothorax will usually have a lower than normal oxygen saturation and may present with cyanosis and varying levels of tachypnea and tachycardia. Lung sounds can be used to help determine the presence of a pneumothorax or hemothorax: Auscultation of absent breath sounds on the affected side has a high-positive predictive value for these conditions, but a normal auscultation does not rule out the presence of pneumothorax or

hemothorax. A patient with a large hemothorax can present with frank hypovolemic shock.

Diagnostic Reasoning

Diagnostic Tests

Any patient who has sustained blunt chest trauma and/or penetrating chest trauma must have an upright chest x-ray film to rule out pneumothorax or hemothorax. A supine chest x-ray film can miss many significant thoracic injuries and should not be relied on to rule out these conditions. The clinician should review the x-ray film, comparing the lung fields bilaterally and looking for any differences in lung markings on one side. When a pneumothorax is present, a subtle light line will be noted—this is the edge of the lung tissue. Beyond that point, the pleural cavity will have absent lung marking. Depending on the technique used, the amount of fat, clothing, or other objects visible on the film, the difference in the pathological and normal pleural cavity can be very difficult to visualize. It is helpful to use a bright viewing box, position the x-ray film horizontally, and focus on the lateral and lateral-superior aspects of the pleural cavity, where most pathology is found.

If a pneumothorax is suspected but not found on an inspiratory chest x-ray study, the clinician should request an expiratory chest x-ray exam. During the expiratory phase, the thoracic volume is decreased; the relative size of the pneumothorax is increased and thus may be more easily detected.

If a hemothorax is suspected, the clinician should order a lateral decubitus view, which will reveal the shifting of blood to the lowest part of the pleural cavity. If doubt still exists or a more accurate determination of size of the defect is required, a computed tomography (CT) scan is the definitive test.

Differential Diagnosis

Differential diagnoses for pneumothorax and/or hemothorax include pneumonia, pulmonary embolism, myocardial infarction, angina, and intercostal muscle strain.

Management

Emergency Management

The patient with a pneumothorax or hemothorax is usually cared for and managed in the ED; therefore, if the clinician suspects that a patient presenting to a primary-care setting has a pneumothorax and/or hemothorax, emergency medical services (EMS) should be called, the patient's respiratory and cardiovascular status should be evaluated and supported as indicated, and then the patient should be transported to the ED immediately.

General Management

A pneumothorax is measured as a percentage of thoracic volume. A mild pneumothorax is less than 15%, a moderate one is 15% to 60%, and a severe one is more than

60%. Most mild and some small to moderate pneumothoraces (fewer than 20%–30%) can be treated conservatively with observation if the patient is not experiencing any untoward effects. The patient should be admitted for continuous observation and serial chest x-ray films. Patients should be placed on supplemental oxygen (up to 100% for a significant pneumothorax), even if the O_2 saturation is normal on room air, as this helps resorption of the pneumothorax. If the size of the pneumothorax remains unchanged over 8 hours, it is usually safe to allow the body to absorb the air. Any patient with a moderate or severe pneumothorax will require a tube thoracostomy (chest tube).

A hemothorax of even mild to moderate size requires insertion of a chest tube. Any patient who presents with significant dyspnea or who is too unstable for ancillary studies and has a high risk of having a pneumothorax or hemothorax should receive a chest tube immediately. The tube should be inserted in the fourth to fifth intercostal space, at the anterior or midaxillary line. Directing the tube posteriorly and toward the apex can effectively remove both air and fluid. Because 2% to 20% of patients with chest tubes usually have infectious complications, antibiotic prophylaxis may be warranted in some patients.

Most pneumothoraces can be treated in a nonurgent manner. Patients with significant respiratory distress will respond quickly to insertion of a chest tube. Patients with a tension pneumothorax, however, require immediate stabilizing treatment (Box 19.1).

Follow-up and Referral

After a period of observation, patients with a mild pneumothorax who do not require a chest tube can be discharged with continued follow-up in 1 to 2 days. Patients with a large pneumothorax, a tension pneumothorax, or a hemothorax requiring a chest tube should not be discharged until the pleura has been drained of blood, and the lung has been reexpanded for at least 24 hours. Strenuous exercise should be limited until the patient has fully recovered; it is possible to reopen and aggravate the pleural defect until it has fully healed. The patient should be advised to follow up with a primary-care provider in 1 week for repeat chest radiograph to evaluate for percent of reexpansion. If the pneumothorax is not fully expanded at this time, the clinician should consult a cardiothoracic surgeon.

Patient Education

Patients who have been diagnosed with a spontaneous pneumothorax should be counseled that up to 23% to 30% will have a recurrence at some point. An explanation of the signs and symptoms to watch for—dyspnea, persistent cough, and chest pain—should be given to all patients, regardless of the type of pneumothorax. The clinician should consider consulting respiratory therapy before discharge for incentive spirometry teaching, as an aid in recurrence prevention.

■ POISONING

Because most adult poisonings are intentional and self-inflicted (the second highest cause of suicide at 24%), the goal is to treat the immediate event and get the patient into counseling as soon as possible to determine precipitating factors and prevent recurrence. During childhood, poisonings are most often due to accidental ingestions.

Epidemiology and Causes

It has been estimated that more than 2 million poisoning accidents occur each year. The majority of these involve children. More than 90% of all poisonings occur in the home. Children younger than age 6 years account for approximately 60% of all poisonings reported. Adult poisonings account for 80% to 90% of all hospital admissions from poisoning. Most adult poisonings involve intentional ingestions, such as recreational drug exposures or suicidal gestures or attempts by overdose. Table 19.1 presents common poisonings. The American Association of Poison Control Centers

---

Box 19.1   Tension Pneumothorax

Patients with a tension pneumothorax usually have some type of penetrating trauma such as a gunshot or knife wound. A *tension pneumothorax* develops when air in the potential space between the parietal and visceral pleura is under pressure. The defect in the pleura allows air to enter the potential space during inspiration, but because of a flap mechanism (which functions like a one-way valve), air does not escape. This mechanism increases the pressure on the affected lung and, if not corrected, will lead to a complete collapse of that lung. If the defect is left untreated, the pressure will continue to increase and force the mediastinum to the unaffected side. This will cause the major blood vessels to kink and restrict normal blood flow to and from the heart, which can cause death within minutes.

A tension pneumothorax is a true medical emergency and must be treated immediately. There is no time for x-ray exams to diagnose this condition. The emergent stabilizing treatment involves performing a needle thoracostomy. This is accomplished by inserting a large-bore (18-gauge or larger) needle into the chest. The needle should be inserted between the second and third rib intracostal space at the midclavicular line. The needle should be inserted just over the third rib to avoid penetrating the neurovascular bundle that runs parallel to the rib on the inferior border.

Table 19.1	Common Poisonings		
Name/Type	**Signs and Symptoms**	**Diagnosis**	**Management**
Drugs acetaminophen (Tylenol)	Nausea, vomiting After 24–48 hours postingestion—hepatic necrosis with jaundice, hepatic encephalopathy, renal failure, possible death	Acetaminophen level	Activated charcoal acetylcysteine (Acetadote) for 36 hours after ingestion
Barbiturates: phenobarbital (Phenobarb) pentobarbital sodium (Nembutal)	Decreased level of consciousness Drowsiness Confusion Ataxia Vertigo Slurred speech Shallow respirations Bradycardia Headache Cyanosis Hypothermia Cardiovascular collapse	Toxicology screen	Gastric lavage with activated charcoal and cathartic Airway maintenance Ventilatory assistance
Benzodiazepines: clorazepate potassium (Tranxene) diazepam (Valium) alprazolam (Xanax)	CNS depression Drowsiness Dizziness Headache Ataxia Hypotension Memory impairment Salivation changes	Toxicology screen	Gastric lavage Symptomatic treatment Airway maintenance Ventilatory assistance
CNS stimulants: methylphenidate (Ritalin, Concerta), amphetamine mixture (Adderall)	Vomiting, emotional lability, nervousness, fever, dizziness, hypertension, tachycardia, psychosis, dyskinesias, Tourette's syndrome, seizures	Toxicology screen	
Cocaine	Nervous system stimulation Restlessness Hallucinations Tachycardia Dilated pupils Chills Fever Abdominal pain Vomiting Muscle spasms Irregular respirations, progressing to death	History of cocaine use Toxicology screen	diazepam (Valium) IV Emetic Gastric lavage Oxygen Symptomatic treatment
Heroin	Euphoria Flushing Pruritus Miosis	History of heroin use Toxicology screen	Maintain patent airway Oxygen Symptomatic treatment naloxone (Narcan) 2 mg IV

Table 19.1	Common Poisonings—cont'd		
Name/Type	Signs and Symptoms	Diagnosis	Management
	Decreased level of consciousness Bradycardia Shallow, slow respirations Hypotension Hypothermia		nalorphine HCl IV Respiratory stimulant: 3–5 mL doxapram hydrochloride
lithium (Lithobid, Lithotabs, Duralith)	Vomiting, diarrhea, slurred speech, decreased coordination, drowsiness, muscle weakness or twitching	CSF lithium level Toxicology screen	Induced emesis Gastric lavage Osmotic and saline diuresis (if renal function is normal) Urine alkalization Hemodialysis
Salicylates (aspirin, methylsalicylate)	Nausea, vomiting, gastritis, hypercapnia, tachycardia, tinnitus, agitation, confusion, coma, seizures, cardiovascular collapse, pulmonary edema, hyperthermia, possible death	Elevated prothrombin time Toxicology screen with a level >100 mg/dL Arterial blood gases reveal respiratory alkalosis with an underlying metabolic acidosis	Activated charcoal Gastric lavage IV NaBicarb Possible hemodialysis
Tricyclic antidepressants (SSRIs are relatively safe, even in overdose): amitriptyline (Elavil) imipramine (Tofranil) nortriptyline (Pamelor)	Confusion Dizziness Decreased level of consciousness Hypotension Tachycardia Hyperthermia Mydriasis Dry mucous membranes Cardiac dysrhythmias Seizures	Toxicology screen	Gastric decontamination with activated charcoal and cathartic Symptomatic treatment
Foods General food poisoning: Foods consumed with toxins present	Vomiting, afebrile, abdominal cramping	Toxins: *Staphylococcus aureus, Bacillus cereus, Clostridium perfringens, Shigella, Salmonella.* Toxin can be detected in food or stool specimens.	Fluids and electrolyte replacement Ciprofloxacin (use with caution) Disease usually self-limiting Antimotility drugs
Poisonous fish	Abdominal cramps Nausea Vomiting Diarrhea Paresthesia Hypotension Respiratory paralysis	History of ingesting fish	Supportive treatment for symptoms

Continued

Table 19.1   Common Poisonings—cont'd

Name/Type	Signs and Symptoms	Diagnosis	Management
Scombroid fish poisoning (bacteria producing scombrotoxin)	30 minutes to 2 hours after ingestion: Peppery sensation on tongue Urticarial pruritic rash Headache Dizziness Periorbital edema Nausea Vomiting	History of ingesting fish	Gastric lavage Antihistamines Symptomatic treatment
Other Substances			
Arsenic	Metallic taste Garlic odor to breath Burning pain throughout GI tract Vomiting Dehydration Shock Seizures	Order toxicology screen and/or attempt to discover type of material ingested by investigating all suspect containers	Gastric lavage Fluid and electrolyte management Treat shock and pulmonary edema Possible blood transfusions
Carbon monoxide	Deep respirations Pink (cherry red) tissues and skin (with COHb ↑ 30%) Initial bradycardia, progressing to tachycardia Pounding pulse Dizziness Paresis Tinnitus Headache Faintness Nausea Dilated pupils	Carboxyhemoglobin (COHb) ↑	100% oxygen, under hyperbaric pressure Symptomatic treatment
Corrosive materials: Lysol, tincture of iodine, carbolic acid (phenol)	Burned tissues along GI tract Brownish stains on lips and tongue Stridor from laryngeal swelling Nausea Vomiting Abdominal cramps Hematemesis Watery, mucoid, or bloody stools Violet or black mucous membranes Carbolic acid—white or gray mucous membranes Hydrochloric acid—grayish mucous membranes Nitric acid—yellowish mucous membranes Sulfuric acid—tan or dark-stained mucous membranes	As above	Opiates for pain Possible tracheostomy Aggressive fluid and electrolyte resuscitation Antibiotics and corticosteroids

Table 19.1	Common Poisonings—cont'd		
Name/Type	Signs and Symptoms	Diagnosis	Management
Iodine	Brown stains on lips and mouth Burning pain in mouth and throat Yellow emesis (blue if starch is present)	Diagnosis based on symptoms and open or empty container found at scene	Cornstarch or flour solution: 15 g in 2 cups of water given orally if patient is conscious, or gastric lavage if patient is comatose Morphine sulfate for pain
Lead: lead-based paints, lead-contaminated dust, hobbies (e.g., stained-glass windows)	Colicky abdominal pain, constipation, headache, irritability, coma, convulsions Chronic poisoning—learning disorders in children, motor neuropathy (wrist drop)	Blood levels: 10–50 mcg/dL—mild toxicity 50–70 mcg/dL—moderate toxicity 70–100 mcg/dL—severe toxicity Microcytic anemia	*Up to moderate toxicity:* Edetate calcium disodium (EDTA) Oral chelator—succimer (dimercaptosuccinic acid, DMSA) *Severe toxicity:* Edetate calcium disodium continuous IV, dimercaprol (BAL) IM
Strychnine	Sense of suffocation Cyanosis Dyspnea Tachycardia Muscle rigidity Contractions Seizures	As above	Gastric lavage Oxygen Sedatives

has a Toxic Exposure Surveillance System (TESS), which is a database of detailed toxicological information on more than 24 million poison exposures reported to U.S. poison control centers. The Web address where annual reports are published is listed at the end of the chapter.

Pathophysiology

The pathophysiology of poisonings varies widely, depending on the substance inhaled or ingested. Most poisonings are dose related, and the diagnosis is usually clinically based. However, the clinician should consider the toxicity of the poison and utilize blood and urine toxicity screens when indicated. Discussion of a representative sample of potential toxins emphasizes this point. For example, with the inhalation of motor vehicle exhaust, the chemical binding of carbon monoxide (CO) to the hemoglobin component in blood results in the formation of carboxyhemoglobin (COHb), which prevents the binding of oxygen to hemoglobin with subsequent transport to bodily tissues. In contrast, with a tricyclic antidepressant overdose (e.g., amitriptyline, nortriptyline, imipramine), the toxic cardiovascular and central nervous system (CNS) effects are secondary to the anticholinergic effects of the medication and the alteration in cardiac cells, which results in conduction disturbances such as QTc prolongation.

With a barbiturate overdose (e.g., phenobarbital), there is decreased neuronal activity, depressed central sympathetic tone, and inhibition of cardiac contractility. These medications act directly on inhibitory gamma-aminobutyric acid (GABA) receptors by increasing the affinity of the GABA ligand to its cognate receptor and increasing the average opening time of chloride ion channels. Benzodiazepines such as lorazepam (Ativan), alprazolam (Xanax), and diazepam (Valium) are also CNS depressants that enhance GABA receptor activity but at a molecularly distinct portion of the receptor. Benzodiazepines increase ligand affinity and the frequency of ion channel opening, but not the duration of open channel time. Thus, given this difference in mechanism, benzodiazepines have less potential for toxicity than barbiturates because their effects are saturable.

Clinical Presentation

Signs and symptoms of various types of poisoning are listed in Table 19.1.

Subjective

The history is an essential component of the diagnosis and treatment plan when a patient is being evaluated for a possible ingestion of a poisonous substance. Interviewing the patient, family, and significant others will give the practitioner valuable information regarding what may have been ingested, as well as the amount ingested and time since the exposure. A lack of symptoms does not preclude the possibility that ingestion has occurred. The history may be very unreliable because poison ingestion is usually associated with the pediatric population and suicidal gestures.

Objective

The physical exam should include an assessment for evidence of trauma and neurological symptoms. The clinician should also assess for odors that may give a clue as to what was ingested. The neurological exam should include a mental status exam; an assessment for seizure activity; and assessments of pupils, the gag reflex, and any focal signs. Additional cardiac, respiratory, gastrointestinal (GI), and renal assessments may be required, depending on the type of poison ingested.

Diagnostic Reasoning

Diagnostic Tests

The diagnostic tests ordered will vary depending on the poisoning situation. Laboratory testing should include toxicology screening. If the specific drug ingested is known, quantitative levels of that agent should be obtained (mg/kg of body weight), along with routine chemistry testing, which includes electrolyte levels. COHb levels should be monitored to detect evidence of carbon monoxide poisoning.

Differential Diagnosis

Differentials for poisoning may range from a bipolar disorder to a transient ischemic attack. Because many substances produce GI symptoms, GI tract disorders should also be ruled out. In addition, overdose of many substances produce CNS symptoms, so vascular and cerebral pathology must also be ruled out. The clinician should always consider head injury in any patient arriving in the ED with altered mental status.

Management

Emergency Management

Poisonings are usually managed in the ED; therefore, if the patient presenting to a primary-care setting has a complaint of poisoning, emergency medical services should be called, the patient's respiratory and cardiovascular status should be evaluated and supported as indicated, and then the patient should be transported to the ED immediately. Emergency management in this scenario includes the A, B, C, Ds, for airway control, breathing, circulation, and drugs.

Because aspirin and acetaminophen are commonly overdosed substances, many clinicians check acetylsalicylic acid and acetaminophen levels with any overdose or potentially intentional toxin ingestion so as not to miss this diagnosis.

General Management

For management of common poisonings, refer to Table 19.1. If there is any question about treatment, the local poison control center should be consulted. The Poison

Help Line (1-800-222-1222) of the American Association of Poison Control Centers can direct individuals to local control centers.

Management may also include gastric lavage and the administration of activated charcoal. A protected airway is essential before initiating lavage and is contraindicated in the presence of caustic ingestions. Gastric lavage may be performed to prevent the poison from reaching the stomach or intestinal tract, where many chemicals are commonly absorbed. Gastric lavage is accomplished by the insertion of a large-bore orogastric tube and lavaging the stomach with normal saline solution. Gastric lavage should be performed only in a conscious patient in order to avoid aspiration of stomach contents. Activated charcoal is often given after gastric lavage, especially after acute ingestions, to absorb the toxins. However, it does not absorb heavy metals, alcohol, caustics, or cyanide. The dose of activated charcoal for children is 1 to 2 g/kg; for adults, the dose is 50 to 100 g/kg. The activated charcoal may be given with or without sorbitol. Sorbitol is a cathartic and may produce dehydration and electrolyte imbalance in young children; therefore, it should be used with caution.

Aside from gastric lavage and GI decontamination, another method of eliminating toxins from the body is whole bowel irrigation by administering cathartic solutions such as Go-Lytely. Forced diuresis and alteration of urine pH can be used to remove certain toxins. Acidic toxins can be trapped in alkaline urine, and alkaline toxins trapped in acidic urine. Sodium bicarbonate administration can be used to alkalinize urine to a pH greater than 7.0.

Extracorporeal removal—for example, through dialysis, plasmapheresis, and exchange transfusion—is capable of removing almost any toxin from the bloodstream. Chelation is used to remove heavy metals such as lead, and hyperbaric oxygen is used for carbon monoxide poisoning.

Adults who are comatose should be given dextrose, thiamine, and naloxone. If hypoglycemia can be diagnosed, 50 to 100 mL of 50% dextrose should be given by IV bolus, as hypoglycemia can cause irreversible brain damage. In malnourished patients or patients with suspected alcohol abuse, 100 mg of thiamine should be given. Naloxone, 0.4 to 2 mg given intravenously may reverse opioid-induced respiratory depression and coma. Additional doses of up to 5 to 10 mg may be required.

Follow-up and Referral

Follow-up and referral will depend on the nature of the poisoning or overdose and the patient's response. If the poisoning or overdose was a suicide attempt or a call for attention, a psychiatric referral is indicated. The patient with suicidal ideation or attempts should never be discharged home without having a psychiatric evaluation clearly documented.

Patient Education

When teaching the patient's family about poisonings, the clinician should advise parents to call the Poison Help Line (1-800-222-1222) of the American Association of Poison Control Centers if a poisoning occurs. Historically, syrup of ipecac was used by parents to induce vomiting, but it is no longer recommended by the American Academy of Pediatricians owing to its potential for misuse and the regurgitation of corrosive ingested substances, which may cause more damage.

General teaching points for preventing poisonings include the following:

- Keep all medications and hazardous products locked up and out of the reach of children.
- Keep all medications in child-resistant containers.
- Never call medication "candy."
- Dispose carefully of all unused or old medications.
- Do not leave medications on countertops or tables, especially if children are present.
- Never transfer a hazardous material into another container.
- Do not mix chemicals unless you know what the reaction will be.

■ HEAT-RELATED ILLNESSES

Heat-related illnesses include heat cramps, heat syncope, heat exhaustion, and heat stroke. It is important to understand that heat-related illnesses are actually a continuum of conditions that range from mild to severe. Heat-related deaths are preventable. Heat response plans should be established before they are needed.

Heat cramps occur in hot weather when a person performs strenuous tasks and drinks large volumes of water, causing an electrolyte imbalance. Sodium chloride is lost from excessive perspiration.

Heat syncope is a heat-related fainting episode. This may occur because of vasodilation and peripheral pooling of blood, volume deficit, and sluggish vasomotor tone. Venous return does not support the required cardiac output, and syncope occurs. Heat syncope can result from inadequate cardiac output and postural hypotension. Recovery is immediate once the patient faints and lies flat.

Heat exhaustion occurs when there is a prolonged period of fluid loss (e.g., perspiration, diarrhea, or use of diuretics) and exposure to warm ambient temperatures without adequate fluid and electrolyte replacement. It is more common in younger persons and older adults.

A core body temperature of at least 104.9°F (40.5°C) characterizes *heat stroke*. Heat stroke occurs when heat production is greater than heat loss. There may be damage to multiple organ systems, and mortality may be as high as 10%. Heat stroke may be classic or exertional and is a true medical emergency. It must be rapidly assessed and treated.

Epidemiology and Causes

On average, 650 persons die each year of heat-related illnesses in the United States. Heat stroke is ranked third—behind head and neck trauma and cardiac disorders—as a cause of death among high school athletes in the United States. Factors associated with an increased risk of heat-related illnesses include age (both very young children and older adults are at higher risk); a history of a chronic illness, such as a cardiovascular, endocrine, nervous system, or psychiatric disease; use of certain medications, such as antihistamines, beta blockers, and diuretics, to name a few; fever or dehydration; a previous history of heat stroke; and heavy clothing. Many drugs possess anticholinergic side effects that may result in the inability to perspire. Individuals on beta blockers may have a diminished ability to cope with heat, thus resulting in a heat-related illness. Monoamine oxidase inhibitors and sympathomimetics can cause core temperature disturbance, leading to rapidly occurring muscle rigidity, extensive rhabdomyolysis, and electrolyte disorders that can prove fatal. Autonomic neuropathy of diabetes cause heat-related illnesses. Because diabetes is prevalent within the population, this is an important cause of faulty heat dissipation. The conditions of autonomic neuropathy of diabetes and beta-adrenergic and cholinergic blockade are often unrecognized contributors to heat-related illness that clinicians need to be alert to. Certain living conditions, such as living in an urban setting, living alone, and not using air conditioning during hot weather, are other risk factors. Exertion-related heat stroke may be a complication of unconditioned amateurs involved in strenuous athletic competitions.

Pathophysiology

Human beings are homeothermic, with a core temperature ranging from 97.0°F (36.1°C) to 99.5°F (37.5°C). When the body temperature reaches 107.6°F (42°C), oxidative phosphorylation occurs, and multiple key enzymes cease to function. Thermal regulation is controlled in the anterior hypothalamus, which receives information from the temperature of the circulating blood and from skin sensors. When the hypothalamus is stimulated, the respiratory rate increases to enhance heat loss via expired air; cardiac output is increased to facilitate cutaneous and muscular blood flow, which helps dissipate heat; and sweat glands become active in their role of sustaining evaporative heat loss.

Heat loss is dependent on radiation, convection, conduction, and evaporation. Radiation and conduction result in direct transfer of heat to the environment. When environmental temperatures reach 95°F (35°C), these mechanisms for heat transfer are no longer effective.

Convection is heat loss related to air circulation. This process relies on wind velocity. Evaporation of sweat is the only physiological mechanism for eliminating heat in an environment hotter than 95°F. The body's ability to sweat is affected by skin conditions (such as sunburn), systemic diseases that affect sweating (such as cystic fibrosis), and drugs that inhibit sweating (such as phenothiazines). Increased core temperatures stimulate peripheral vasodilation and sweating. Venous return to the heart increases, resulting in increased cardiac output and heart rate. A concurrent sympathetic response is decreased blood flow to the kidneys. The kidneys are damaged if this process continues; myoglobin is produced as a by-product. If this condition is not aggressively treated, it will lead to rhabdomyolysis. Respiratory function may be compromised by pulmonary edema. Hepatic function is often decreased because of the general decrease in perfusion. Clotting abnormalities can range from thrombocytopenia to disseminated intravascular coagulation. Such abnormalities usually occur in severe heat illness. The metabolic rate increases and sweat production can increase to 1.5 L/hr, which may result in dehydration.

Acclimatization is a term that refers to the body's ability to adapt to heat stress. This adaptation primarily involves the sweating mechanism. In the unacclimatized person, each liter of sweat contains 30 to 50 mEq of sodium. This sodium level decreases to as little as 5 mEq/L in the fully acclimatized person, and the rate of sweating can be increased to 1.5 to 3 L/hr. This means that the acclimatized person doubles sweat production, losing one-third to one-fifth the total amount of sodium. Potassium wasting compensates for sodium loss. Therefore, a fluid and electrolyte imbalance can develop quickly in an unacclimatized person. Cardiac output increases with acclimatization, as does muscle aerobic metabolism, which is more efficient. As the heart muscle responds, cutaneous circulation improves, and heat dissipation is augmented. The body develops a new, lower point at which sweating begins. Finally, increased secretion of aldosterone aids in sodium conservation by the kidneys and sweat glands. The additional sodium enhances extracellular fluid volume, which plays a part in the accelerated cutaneous blood flow and heat dissipation.

Clinical Presentation
Subjective

For any heat-related illness, a complete history of the circumstances preceding the incident should be obtained. Any past history that may assist with the differential diagnosis is crucial. Medications that the patient is currently taking should be reviewed.

Objective

A complete physical examination, including monitoring the patient's cardiac status, vital signs, and core temperature, should be performed.

The clinical presentation may include hot dry skin, decreased level of consciousness, tachycardia, tachypnea, decreased urinary output, hyperpyrexia of greater than 104.9°F (40.5°C), hypotension, seizures, nausea and vomiting, decerebrate posturing, diarrhea, and dilated, nonresponsive pupils.

Table 19.2 describes the signs and symptoms and recommended management of the various types of heat-related illnesses.

Diagnostic Reasoning
Diagnostic Tests

There are no specific diagnostic tests performed. Management follows good assessment techniques (see Table 19.2).

Differential Diagnosis

The differential diagnosis of heat stroke should include CNS infections, cerebrovascular accident, and diabetic ketoacidosis. If the patient has recently traveled outside the country, the clinician should consider malaria or typhoid fever. In addition, the clinician should consider thyroid storm, meningitis, encephalitis, or brain abscess. Some toxicological issues to consider include salicylate, anticholinergic, phencyclidine (PCP), cocaine, or amphetamine toxicity.

Management
Emergency Management

Heat stroke is a medical emergency, with core body temperature reaching greater than 105°F (40.5°C). If the patient presenting to a primary-care setting has heat stroke, emergency medical services should be called, the patient's respiratory and cardiovascular status should be evaluated and supported as indicated, and then the patient must be transported to the ED immediately.

General Management

Specific management of heat-related illnesses is presented in Table 19.2. General management includes cooling the patient. The safest and most practical method is to remove all clothing and spray warm water over the body surface. Evaporation can be increased with fans, which should circulate air over as much body surface as possible. If ice packs are used, they should be placed in the axilla and groin, with the skin protected from local injury by a wrapping over the pack. Extremities should not be packed in ice, especially in older patients, because this treatment is poorly tolerated in older adults. Cooling of the internal core temperature can also be achieved by gastric or peritoneal lavage with cold saline. In extreme cases, hemodialysis can be used to cool blood. The goal is to reduce the temperature to 102°F (38.8°C) within the first hour. To avoid hypothermia, further active cooling should cease when a

Table 19.2   Types of Heat-Related Illnesses

Type of Illness	Signs and Symptoms	Management
Heat Cramps Heat cramps occur in hot weather when a person performs strenuous tasks and drinks large volumes of water, causing an electrolyte imbalance. Sodium chloride is lost from excessive perspiration.	Cramps, especially in the large muscle groups, such as shoulders, thighs, and abdominal wall muscles; weakness; nausea; tachycardia; pallor; profuse diaphoresis; cool, moist skin; and/or a history of ingestion of large amounts of hypotonic solution	Sodium chloride PO or IV (depending on the degree of discomfort and the clinical status of the patient). An oral saline solution of 4 tsp of salt per gallon of water may be used. Salt tablets are absorbed very slowly and should not be given. If IV therapy is indicated, 1,000 mL 0.9% NaCl infused over 1–3 hours is preferred. Cool environment Rest
Heat Syncope Heat syncope is a heat-related fainting episode. This may occur because of vasodilation and peripheral pooling of blood, volume deficit, and sluggish vasomotor tone. Venous return does not support the required cardiac output, and syncope occurs. Heat syncope can result from inadequate cardiac output and postural hypotension. Recovery is immediate once the patient faints and lies flat.	Orthostatic syncopal episode, dizziness	Place the patient in a supine position. Oral fluid replacement Cool environment Rest
Heat Exhaustion Heat exhaustion occurs when there is a prolonged period of fluid loss (e.g., from perspiration, diarrhea, or use of diuretics) and exposure to warm ambient temperatures without adequate fluid and electrolyte replacement. Heat exhaustion is more common in young patients and older adults.	Thirst, anxiety, anorexia, cramps in muscles, malaise, syncope, headache, dehydration, tachycardia, muscle weakness, orthostatic hypotension, nausea and vomiting, cutaneous flushing and/or possible elevated temperature above 37.8°C	Remove the patient from the hot environment into an air-conditioned room or a shady or cool place. Treat symptomatically; for example, elevate legs for postural hypotension Oral fluid replacement if no GI symptoms are present and if patient is alert and oriented; replace fluids and electrolytes at about 1 L/hr for several hours. Recovery should be rapid, within 2–3 hours. If not, patient may need additional interventions.
Heat Stroke Heat stroke occurs when heat production is greater than heat loss. Mortality rates from heat stroke may be as high as 10%. There may be damage to multiple organ systems. Heat stroke may be divided into classic and exertional. Heat stroke is a true medical emergency—it must be rapidly assessed and treated.	Core body temperature of at least 104.9°F (40.5°C), acute mental status changes, absent sweat, tachypnea, decreased urinary output, hypotension, seizures, nausea and vomiting, diarrhea, dilated nonresponsive pupils, decerebrate posturing	Rapid cooling; if ice packs are used, place them in groin and axillary region. Monitor rectal temperature. Supplemental oxygen, including possible intubation, may be necessary. IV fluids (usually 0.9% normal saline).

core temperature of 101°F (38.3°C) is achieved. Antipyretics are ineffective in lowering the temperature in heat-related illnesses. IV fluids, such as normal saline or dextrose and half normal saline are usually given. Chlorpromazine (Thorazine) 25 to 50 mg IV or diazepam (Valium) 5 to 10 mg IV may be given initially to control shivering and then every 4 hours. In addition, the patient's urinary output, rectal temperature, and cardiac status should be monitored. Supplemental oxygen is also often administered.

Follow-up and Referral

A patient is discharged after a complete recovery. Other than teaching to prevent further episodes (see next section), no special follow-up or referral is necessary.

Patient Education

Heat-related illnesses, with their devastating effects, can be avoided or at least reduced in severity through simple preventive measures. These include the following:

- Becoming acclimatized
- Avoiding alcohol consumption during exposure in hot, humid areas
- Wearing protective, light-colored clothes and a hat when outdoors in hot weather
- Ingesting adequate amounts of balanced liquids (e.g., Gatorade) to maintain fluids, electrolytes, and homeostasis
- Pacing personal activities

If a patient has suffered from a heat-related illness in the past, he or she will be more prone to heat-related illnesses in the future.

Patients should be taught to gradually build up time spent in hotter conditions (acclimatization). It should be stressed that the higher the temperature and greater the humidity, the greater the risk for heat injury. Fluids must be consumed before there is an urge to drink. If exercising, prehydration is important. The best fluids are simply water or a low-sugar electrolyte drink.

Education about heat-related illnesses should be a part of health maintenance. The clinician should remind parents not to leave children in cars unattended. Older adults should be cautioned about the increased risk of heat-related illnesses, especially if they have medical conditions or are taking medications that increase the risk of heat-related illnesses. Athletes should drink more fluids and exercise during the coolest part of the day.

COLD-RELATED ILLNESSES

■ FROSTBITE

Because of the growing number of homeless persons and the increasing numbers of individuals participating in outdoor activities during cold weather, frostbite is becoming a growing concern.

Frostbite is freezing of an exposed area, usually the ears, cheeks, nose, fingers, and toes. If a previously frostbitten area becomes frostbitten again after it has healed, permanent tissue damage can occur, resulting in necrosis to that body part.

Epidemiology and Causes

The individuals at greatest risk for frostbite are adults aged 30 to 49. The anatomical regions at greatest risk for injury are the hands and feet, which account for 90% of frostbite injuries. The ears, nose, cheeks, and penis are also prone to frostbite.

There are many predisposing factors that can contribute to frostbite. Cold is the most prevalent factor, but it is not the only factor. In addition, the duration of contact, humidity, wind, clothing, and preexisting medical conditions also contribute to the incidence of frostbite. Although both the actual temperature and duration of exposure affect frostbite severity and resultant tissue injury, it is the duration of exposure that has the greater impact.

Although prolonged contact with a cold object can produce frostbite, it is the cold humidity that contributes to evaporative heat loss. Wet skin is more conducive to ice crystal formation. Wind contributes to an increasing loss of heat (exposure in relation to the wind-chill factor). Inadequate clothing or overly constrictive clothing can contribute to an increased incidence of frostbite. Constrictive clothing can reduce circulation to extremities. Diseases such as atherosclerosis, diabetes, and previous cold-related injuries predispose individuals to frostbite. In addition, individual behaviors such as alcohol consumption and smoking, poor self-care, immobility, drug abuse, and altered mental status increase the risk of frostbite.

Pathophysiology

The pathophysiology of frostbite occurs in several stages: tissue freezing, hypoxia, and release of inflammatory mediators. As tissues cool, the circulation slows, allowing ice crystals to form, first extracellularly and then intracellularly, which damages the cell membrane. Crystals that form extracellularly exert osmotic force and pull fluid from the intracellular space, resulting in cellular dehydration. As this process continues, the cell membrane is damaged. Intracellular crystals cause more damage to the cell as they expand within it.

Hypoxia results from cold-induced local vasoconstriction. This vasoconstriction leads to acidosis and increased local blood viscosity as well as hypoxia. Although the body has a natural defensive mechanism against the cold (called *cold-induced vasodilation*—the "hunting response," which prevents rapid freezing of the skin), prolonged exposure to cold eventually causes this response to fail, and freezing takes place. As capillary blood flow ceases, arterioles and venules thrombose, leading to the release of inflammatory mediators. The release of prostaglandins and thromboxane promotes vasoconstriction, platelet aggregation, and blood vessel thrombosis, which worsen endothelial damage. If left unchecked, this process will lead to cell death and widespread tissue necrosis.

Clinical Presentation

Subjective

Initially, the patient complains of a tingling sensation of the body part, followed by pain and eventual numbness.

Objective

Classically, the clinical presentation of frostbite has been categorized according to four degrees of injury. The classification should be applied after some rewarming has been done because all victims of frostbite present similarly at first, with tingling and redness followed by pallor and numbness.

- **First-degree frostbite (partial skin freezing):** Erythema, edema, hyperemia, no blisters or necrosis, occasional skin desquamation (5–10 days later), transient stinging and burning, and possible throbbing and aching; the patient may also have hyperhidrosis (excessive sweating).
- **Second-degree frostbite (full-thickness injury):** Erythema, substantial edema, vesicles with clear fluid, blisters that desquamate and form blackened eschar, numbness, and vasomotor disturbances (in severe cases).
- **Third-degree frostbite (full-thickness injury and subcutaneous freezing):** Violaceous/hemorrhagic blisters; skin necrosis and blue-gray discoloration; initially, no sensation (tissue feels like a block of wood) but shooting pains, burning, throbbing, and aching develop later.
- **Fourth-degree frostbite (full-thickness injury and subcutaneous tissue, muscle, tendon, and bone freezing):** Little edema is present. Initially, skin is mottled, deep red, or cyanotic; later, skin becomes dry, black, and mummified; possible joint discomfort.

Diagnostic Reasoning

Diagnostic Tests

There are no definitive diagnostic studies for frostbite, especially within the first week of injury. Doppler studies may be helpful to assess blood flow.

Differential Diagnosis

Differential diagnoses for frostbite may include the following:

- Frostnip—a mild form of cold injury.
- Chilblain (erythema pernio)—tender red to red-blue itchy nodules on extremities triggered by cold weather

and thought to result from chronic vasospasm. There is no actual freezing of the tissue.
- Immersion foot—hyperhidrosis (excessive perspiration) of the feet causing thickening, maceration, and tenderness of the skin due to prolonged submersion in water or cold (also called trench foot, because it affected soldiers camped for days in trenches during times of war).
- Hypothermia.

Management

Emergency Management

Frostbite is a medical emergency because of the potential for extensive tissue necrosis and loss of limb. If the patient presenting to a primary-care setting has frostbite, the area should be rewarmed as stated below. Hot liquids such as coffee, tea, or broth should be administered.

General Management

The basis of treatment for frostbite is reversing the pathological effects of the ice-crystal formation, vasoconstriction, and the release of inflammatory mediators. Treatment should not be started if there is a possibility of refreezing. If it is suspected that the patient has second- to fourth-degree frostbite, hospitalization should be considered.

The first measure is to rewarm the affected area. Rewarming is accomplished by using warm water (104°F [40°C] to 108°F [42.2°C]). Care must be taken not to rub the affected area. The affected part should be placed in water for 10 to 30 minutes until the tissue is pliable and red. This process can be very painful; therefore, narcotics should be administered and titrated for comfort.

Blister management in patients with frostbite is somewhat controversial. Blisters containing clear or milky fluid should be debrided and covered with aloe vera every 6 hours. Aloe vera is a potent antiprostaglandin agent. Hemorrhagic blisters should be left intact and covered with aloe vera. The affected area should be wrapped with a sterile dressing, splinted, and elevated. Silvadene and Bacitracin have proved to be effective as antibacterials; however, use of these topical ointments may interfere with the aloe vera.

It is unclear whether prophylactic antibiotic use is warranted for frostbite. The use of penicillin G 500,000 units IV every 6 hours for the first 72 hours has proven effective. Ibuprofen 400 mg PO every 4 to 6 hours should be administered for its antiprostaglandin activity. Ibuprofen is a potential inhibitor of thromboxane— more potent than other anti-inflammatory drugs. The patient's tetanus status should also be assessed. Patients who are being treated for frostbite should not be allowed to smoke.

Patients may need daily hydrotherapy to debride devitalized tissue. In some instances, referral to a surgeon for a fasciotomy or escharotomy may be needed if there is limited range of motion in an extremity or if the possibility of "compartment syndrome" develops. Compartment syndrome occurs when any structure such as a nerve or tendon is being constricted in a space. The sheath or tendon is enlarged because of the inflammation and no longer able to move freely in the compartment. This results in a cut-off of the circulation, a critical condition, and may result in loss of a limb. It may take up to 3 to 4 weeks for full demarcation of the tissue damage to occur; therefore, amputation should not be considered before this time.

Follow-up and Referral

The majority of patients with frostbite injuries should be admitted to the hospital for 2 to 4 days. If dressings are in place, the patient should be monitored every 2 to 3 days to assess the healing potential. If debridement or grafting is necessary, the patient should be referred to a dermatologist or a vascular surgeon.

Patient Education

Patients should be taught to watch for signs of infection, to take medication as prescribed, and to use extreme care regarding further exposure to cold. The following preventive measures should also be recommended:

- Do not go outdoors for prolonged periods of time.
- Wear a hat or earmuffs, mittens, and dress in layers.
- Keep dry and change out of wet clothing.
- Dress in natural materials such as cotton or wool.
- Avoid caffeine, tobacco, and alcohol when going out in the cold, because these substances leave the skin more prone to thermal injury.
- Check the skin every 12 to 20 minutes for signs of frostbite.

■ HYPOTHERMIA

Accidental hypothermia is a medical emergency that can threaten life and limb and is defined by a core temperature of less than 95°F (35°C). If not treated promptly and accurately, the diagnosis carries a high mortality rate. In the United States alone, hypothermia is responsible for hundreds of deaths each year. The outcome depends on the underlying medical conditions and length of exposure to the elements.

Epidemiology and Causes

The incidence and prevalence of hypothermia are difficult to quantify, because not all cases are reported. The hypothermic patient is more likely to be older (with a mean age of 45 years), to be uninsured, and to consume more critical care than most other ED diagnoses. Approximately 700 people die in the United States from accidental primary hypothermia each year (Level I; Li et al, 2013). The condition of hypothermia tends to

affect disadvantaged patients and is preventable with community involvement. Problems with alcoholism, homelessness, and mental illness are common to patients in this category. The other category of affected individuals includes adventure-seekers, including hunters, skiers, climbers, boaters, and swimmers. Despite treatment in a hospital, 40% of patients with moderate to severe hypothermia die.

Pathophysiology

The reduction in body core temperature starts with a cascade of events. First, there is a loss of heat from the body. This can involve evaporation, convection, conduction, respiration, and, most importantly, radiation through which 50% of the body heat is lost rapidly. Common causes of hypothermia are prolonged exposure to lower extremes of outdoor temperature without protective clothing. Alcohol, drug abuse, homeless status, and being elderly are all potential contributing factors. The prognosis is highly dependent on the length of exposure, as well as the provider's recognition of and rapid intervention for the condition. For example, progressive organ failure increases as the core body temperature decreases; however, this situation is potentially reversible with adequate rewarming. The clinician should be aware of the pathophysiological changes in acid–base balance; during rewarming, the pH remains constant until the core body temperature reaches 89.6°F (32°C). At this temperature, there is a decline in calcium (Ca^{2+}) and magnesium (Mg^{2+}), accompanied by an increase in the pH. Observation of arterial blood gases (ABGs) and electrolytes is essential to monitor acid–base balance.

Clinical Presentation
Subjective

The hypothermic patient may arrive with a core body temperature ranging from less than 82.4 to 95°F (28–35°C). Depending on the core temperature, the patient may or may not be conscious enough to give a subjective history. If conscious, the primary complaint is coldness accompanied with a feeling of exhaustion.

Objective

Typically, the initial presentation consists of evolving signs and symptoms of hypothermia. Moreover, it is usually categorized by the level of the core body temperature.

1. *Mild hypothermia* is defined as a core temperature of 89.6 to 95°F (32–35°C).
   - The cardiopulmonary response is by vasoconstriction, hypertension, tachycardia, and tachypnea.
   - The renal response is cold diuresis and defective distal tubular absorption of water and sodium.
   - The neurological response involves shivering, ataxia, slowed mental processes, and an apathetic affect.

2. *Moderate hypothermia* is defined as a core temperature of 82.4 to 89.6°F (28–32°C).
   - The cardiopulmonary response is evidenced by hypotension, bradycardia, respiratory depression, and a J-wave on the electrocardiogram (ECG). Atrial fibrillation and junctional bradycardia are both associated with a high mortality rate, as noted in a prospective multicenter study by researchers.
   - The renal system clamps down, and urine output decreases.
   - The neurological responses are now diminished level of consciousness, dilated pupils, decreased reflexes (including gag reflex), and an inability to mount a shivering reflex.
3. *Severe hypothermia* is defined as a core temperature of less than 82.4°F (28°C).
   - The cardiopulmonary response may now reveal profound bradycardia with ventricular dysrhythmias or asystole, accompanied by pulmonary edema and/or apnea.
   - Renal blood flow is greatly diminished, leading to oliguria.
   - Neurologically, the patient loses consciousness, and coma rapidly ensues; pupils are nonreactive.

Diagnostic Reasoning

Diagnostic Tests

Initial laboratory tests consist of ABGs, complete blood count (CBC), basic metabolic panel with blood urea nitrogen (BUN) and creatinine, alcohol and drug levels along with coagulation studies, prothrombin time (PT), partial thromboplastin time (PTT) and international normalized ratio (INR), chest x-ray, and ECG. The advanced practice registered nurse (APRN) should also consider that all tests might need to be repeated frequently during rewarming because the pathophysiology may change.

Differential Diagnosis

The clinician should consider head injury, stroke, myocardial infarction, diabetic hypoglycemia or hyperglycemia, drug or alcohol involvement, sepsis, and hypothyroidism.

Management

Emergency Management

The initial management consists of assessing airway, affirming breathing, and monitoring circulation. The clinician should intubate and ventilate if needed. In addition, warmed IV fluids of normal saline and rewarming the body at 1° to 2°C (1.8°–3.6°F) an hour should be initiated. Caution should be taken to prevent shivering because this action depletes glycogen stores. Further treatment should consist of gradually rewarming the internal and external temperatures, supportive treatment with warm fluids and oxygen, and monitoring acid–base balance with treatment accordingly.

General Management

General management should include gradually rewarming the body, supportive care with warm IV fluids, cardiac monitoring, frequent vital signs, and repeating electrolytes, ABGs, and ECG as needed.

Follow-up and Referral

The clinician will need to consider the patient's age, psychological and medical status, and his or her living situation to plan appropriate follow-up care. If the patient is homeless, a wide social network must be cast to prevent recurrence of hypothermia, and a case manager should be consulted. The clinician may have to discern if the patient has a home or a shelter during the winter and whether he or she has a coat to wear and food to eat.

Patient Education

Each patient will have different needs for education from the clinician, who must consider the audience or receiver of the educational information. Basic education is best and includes advice on dressing appropriately for winter weather, keeping the body dry and well covered when outdoors. The clinician should warn the patient to avoid alcohol and overexertion during extremely cold temperatures.

COMMON INJURIES

■ WOUNDS AND LACERATIONS

Wounds and lacerations result in a disruption of the continuity of the skin commonly related to trauma. The mechanism and energy of the force causing the defect determines the type and severity of the wound. Wounds can range from trivial lacerations or abrasions, which occur daily in children on playgrounds, to more severe injuries such as stabbings or shootings that may require immediate surgical care. All wounds have the potential of becoming infected and should be evaluated for occult injury and retained foreign bodies. Proper evaluation and care will reduce the morbidity associated with wounds.

Epidemiology and Causes

In a recent year, 12% of all visits to the emergency department (ED)—that is, 11.5 million visits—were related to wounds. The average laceration seen in the ED is 1 to 3 cm in length; 13% of the wounds seen are considered "dirty." In one study, scalp and face lacerations accounted for 51% of wounds seen in the ED, upper extremity lacerations accounted for 34%, and lower extremity lacerations accounted for 13%. Adult wounds become infected about 5% of the time, whereas wounds in children become infected 1.2% of the time. Almost 75% of the patients with wounds were men with an average age in the early 20s.

Wound care is a highly litigious area of health care. Missed fractures, missed foreign bodies, and wound infections are common reasons for medical practitioners to be named in a lawsuit. Although wound-care litigation is not associated with the highest payouts, it is prudent in any case for the clinician to perform a thorough assessment and maintain complete documentation of wound care. Wound management accounts for 5% to 20% of ED malpractice claims. Although culturing the wound can subsequently guide the treatment and identify infectious complications, it is essential that the clinician visually appraise the wound for signs of infection before more invasive action and stronger antibiotics are required.

Pathophysiology

The skin is made up of several layers, which are divided into the epidermis and dermis. The skin acts as a barrier, regulates body temperature, aids in elimination of waste, and helps prevent dehydration. It also contains the cutaneous nerves, is a reservoir for nutritional stores and water, and is a source of vitamin D when exposed to sunlight. The ability of bacteria and other substances to penetrate the skin is related to the depth of the wound. Wounds that do not penetrate the stratum germinativum—the basement layer of the skin—do not leave scars.

The healing process is a complicated one and involves many processes that occur simultaneously:

- *Injury phase.* This phase involves coagulation and platelet release. This process enhances the inflammatory response in the wound.
- *Inflammatory phase.* This phase is characterized by increased capillary permeability, which allows white blood cells (WBCs) to migrate into the wound. Neutrophils and monocytes act as scavengers and rid the wound of debris and bacteria. In addition to providing wound defenses, inflammation stimulates other monocytes to promote fibroblast replication and neovascularization.
- *Epithelialization phase.* This phase involves migration of fibrils across the wound. These fibrils are a result of collagen synthesis. This process requires tissue lactate and ascorbic acid and is directly related to local arterial PO_2. Of note, lacerations may heal by primary intention when the edges of the wound are approximated with sutures and allowed to heal together. Suturing techniques that allow for maximal eversion of the wound edges once approximated facilitate healing by primary intention. Alternatively, open wounds may heal by secondary intention, as granulation tissue fills in open lacerations whose edges are not approximated. Collagen synthesis in the healing wound peaks at day 7 post-trauma, and the tensile strength (which determines the ability of the wound to remain intact) increases rapidly at this stage. Typically, the wound will have only 15% to

20% of its normal tensile strength at 3 weeks and 60% by 4 months.
- *Remodeling phase.* In this final phase, the process involves wound contraction and tissue formation. This process begins on the third day after the injury and continues for up to 6 months. The appearance of the wound can change during this period; for this reason, plastic surgeons will usually wait 6 months before considering revising a scar.

Clinical Presentation

Subjective

A thorough history of the injury must be obtained and documented. Information regarding how the wound occurred is important. The mechanism of wounding is useful in determining the likelihood of deep structure injury, infection risk, extent of tissue damage, and likelihood of associated injuries. For example, a laceration that occurred when a glass shattered in the hand has a high likelihood of having a retained foreign body. A wound that occurred when a hand became caught in a machine has a high likelihood of having an associated fracture. Questions regarding medical history should also be included. For example, a patient with diabetes or a history of vascular problems has a higher possibility of infection (see Focus on History 19.1).

Focus on History 19.1 Wounds and Lacerations

History

- Mechanism of injury
- Potential for foreign body
- Potential for underlying injury
- Potential for infection
- Type of injury
- Age of wound
- Delayed or immediate presentation
- Tetanus immunization status
- Allergies
- Comorbidities (especially vascular problems)

Physical Examination

- Vital signs
- General examination
- Vascular injury
- Nerve involvement
- Located over joint
- Tendon damage
- Associated with fracture (open or closed)
- Range of motion
- Wound contamination
- Foreign body
- Avulsion injury
- Puncture

Objective

A description of any wound should include the length and depth (in centimeters) and the type of defect found. The depth of the wound is described as *partial thickness* if all layers of the skin have not been violated. If any subdermal tissue can be seen in the wound, it is considered a *full-thickness* defect. Wounds this deep may involve injuries to deeper structures; further evaluation is necessary.

Different types of wounds are associated with specific types of associated injuries and special considerations. Refer to Advanced Assessment 19.1 for various types of wounds and special considerations associated with their assessment and treatment.

Any wound to an extremity should be evaluated for distal circulation and sensation. Circulation should be assessed by determining if the distal extremity has a strong pulse. For fingers or toes, the clinician should

Advanced Assessment 19.1 Wounds and Lacerations

Type	Special Considerations
Abrasion	
A partial-thickness defect to the skin, usually associated with an abrasive force being applied to the skin.	• Ensure that the wound is thoroughly cleansed (this may require anesthesia). For cleansing larger areas of abrasion, consider using topical viscous lidocaine. Use caution with children because the amount of medication applied to large wounds may cause lidocaine toxicity. Allow about 10–15 minutes after administration of lidocaine for sufficient absorption. • Remove all embedded dirt because it can lead to "tattooing" of the skin. Tattooing can occur when the skin has healed and the epidermis has grown over the embedded dirt—the dirt is visible through the thin epidermis layer of skin. • Examine the entire area of the wound. Look for any deep lacerations, which may be hard to find because of the size of the wound. Any deep lacerations within an abrasion must be closed with sutures after thorough exploration, debridement, and irrigation. The goal of closure is to loosely approximate the edges. If the wound is deep, use a subcutaneous suture to allow the wound to heal without having to disturb the granulation tissue to remove the stitches later.
Stellate or Flap Laceration	
When the defect in the skin involves a flap or stellate defect; this usually occurs with a ripping mechanism or blunt trauma to a bony structure such as the skull.	• During exploration, fully retract the flap to allow for visualization to the base of the defect. Typically, this is the deepest part of the laceration. It is important to examine the area under the flap carefully for possible injuries to deeper structures. • Scalp lacerations should be explored for galeal injury. The galea is a fibrous fascia that covers the skull. If the galea has a large defect (more than 3 cm), it should be closed with deep sutures. • If a flap laceration has a nonviable portion, it should be excised. When closing these types of defects, the first suture should bring all the sections of the flap or star together. Following the initial stitch, closure of the remaining defect can be accomplished using normal interrupted sutures.
Linear Laceration	
Single linear or near-linear defect in the skin; usually caused by a sharp instrument.	• Thorough wound exploration is required to ascertain deep structure involvement. If tendons are involved, orthopedic consultation is recommended. • If muscular fascia are violated, these defects must be closed with deep sutures. If these wounds are not repaired, the possibility of muscular herniation is increased.

Continued

Advanced Assessment 19.1   Wounds and Lacerations—cont'd

Type	Special Considerations
	• If a joint is violated, an orthopedic consultation is highly recommended. Depending on the mechanism of injury and how dirty the wound is, surgical exploration and irrigation may be necessary. • Wounds in regions with low cosmetic significance, such as the scalp, can be closed using staples, which are faster and easier to place and remove than conventional sutures. Staples have a lower tissue inflammatory response and are well tolerated. Staples must be removed with special instruments, however, so follow-up must be considered when the decision regarding type of wound closure is made. If the patient's primary-care provider is not familiar with staple removal or does not have the correct instrument, placement of stitches is recommended. • Wounds with low tension that do not cross a joint can be closed using tissue adhesive. This eliminates the need for suture removal and has been found to have similar or better cosmetic results than stitches. Using tissue adhesive to close wounds is much faster and decreases the amount of pain associated with wound closure. Before closing the wound, it is important to make sure that the wound has been thoroughly explored and cleaned. This may require infiltration with local anesthesia. Tissue adhesive can be used over wounds that have had subcutaneous sutures placed. Tissue adhesive can also be used to hold fingernails and toenails in place after nailbed repair. • Wounds under high tension must be closed with subcutaneous stitches or mattress sutures to reduce the tension on the skin edge. High-tension wounds will produce a larger scar and have a higher risk of dehiscence. To avoid this, sutures should remain in place longer in these types of wounds.
Crush Injury	
A defect caused by a high-pressure force, such as a dog bite.	• These wounds have diminished vascularization related to the tissue disruption and swelling. Debriding devitalized tissue is necessary to decrease the bacterial load and eliminate that potential nidus of infection. • The practitioner should consider whether delayed primary closure or allowing the wound to heal by secondary intention is appropriate. Consultation with the referring primary-care provider is recommended.
Tendon Injury	
A force applied that is great enough to cause a disruption to a tendon; this could be a penetrating or blunt force.	• All wounds near tendons must be explored for possible tendon injuries. If tendon damage is found, consultation with an orthopedist is recommended. • Extensor tendon injuries may be closed by the primary-care practitioner, providing he or she has been properly trained in the technique. Early antibiotic prophylaxis is indicated. • Flexor tendon injuries usually require primary wound closure by an orthopedic specialist. There is a high morbidity associated with flexor tendon injuries. Early antibiotic prophylaxis is indicated.

Advanced Assessment 19.1   Wounds and Lacerations—cont'd

Type	Special Considerations
Joint Violation	
A force, usually applied by a sharp, penetrating injury, that disrupts the joint capsule.	• All wounds near joints must be explored for potential violations of the joint capsule. If any such injury is found, consultation with an orthopedist is recommended. • If the wound is near a joint and a violation of the joint capsule cannot be ruled out, the saline-load test can be used to assess whether penetration of the capsule has occurred. • If the metacarpophalangeal (MCP) joint is injured and any possibility of an injury from a bite (open mouth) exists, immediate follow-up by an orthopedist is needed. The area should be surgically irrigated to avoid joint morbidity.
Cellulitis	
An infection of deeper tissue, usually caused by a defect to the integrity of the skin that was inoculated by bacteria. The infection usually involves *Staphylococcus aureus* and/or *Streptococcus* bacteria.	• Placing patients with simple, noncomplex wounds on antibiotic prophylaxis does not affect the incidence of infection. Typically, 2%–10% of wounds in adults will be infected. • Mild cellulitis should be treated with an oral course of a first or second generation cephalosporin. Although the infection can be treated on an outpatient basis, it is important to have the patient return for wound check within 24–48 hours, depending on the extent of cellulitis, to determine if the antibiotic therapy is effective. The region of erythema should be outlined with a tissue marker on initial examination; this demarcation can be used to assess treatment effectiveness or failure if the erythema continues to increase. Wounds that exhibit fluctuance (palpable fluid under the skin) should be incised and drained to reduce the tension on the wound and decrease the bacterial load. • Patients with diabetes or other conditions that may involve vascular compromise need to be treated more aggressively. Treat the initial findings of cellulitis or wounds that appear dirty with parenteral antibiotics and place the patient on oral antibiotics. Close follow-up is required. These patients may need to be seen daily in the office, depending on the extent of cellulitis. • Patients who present with cellulitis should receive a thorough history and physical to determine the possible mechanism of injury. All hand and foot wounds that become infected should be x-rayed to rule out foreign bodies. Any wound that, based on the history and/or physical exam, has a high potential of having a foreign body should be x-rayed. • If fluctuance is felt, the wound should be incised and drained. The placement of a drain or packing is dictated by the size of the site and clinical judgment. • Patients with wound infections involving angioedema or accompanied by fever or chills should receive parenteral antibiotics. Inpatient treatment should be considered for these patients.

assess blanching. A normal blanch response (capillary refill time) is considered to be less than 2 seconds. Distal sensation should be checked to rule out nerve injury. A gross neurological screening exam should be done on all patients who present with wounds to the extremities: This involves lightly touching the extremity or digit distal to the injury and comparing the response with sensation in uninjured extremities or digits. If the patient states that the sensation is similar, the clinician should document it. If the sensation is decreased, different, or if the patient complains of paresthesias, a two-point discrimination test should be performed to rule out nerve injury.

All wounds must be explored to identify any deep structure injuries or foreign bodies and to help determine the type of closure required. After the wound is anesthetized, a bright light should be used to illuminate the wound. Wound edges should be retracted, but it is important not to cause trauma to the tissue that may impede normal healing. Blindly probing a wound can cause additional tissue destruction or nerve or vascular injury. Using an Adson forceps with teeth or tissue retractors, the clinician should hook the wound edge and retract it to expose deep structures. The clinician should probe the wound with gloved fingers only.

For large wounds, it is important to examine the full length of the wound because only a small section of the wound may be deep enough to cause deep structure injury. The defect should be examined for any tendon injury. Exposed tendon will appear as a shiny white structure in the wound. Any wound that involves the extremities must be assessed for tendon and nerve injuries. The range of motion of the affected extremity or digit should be tested carefully against resistance in all planes in which the extremity can be moved. During the movement, the clinician should ask the patient if the resistance causes a pain in the wound. If a partial tendon laceration is present, movement against resistance will cause pain at the site. The wound needs to be explored, and deep structures should be examined during the full range of motion to the involved extremity. A tendon injury may be hidden because the defect may not be visible in the wound at the position in which it is being examined. The injury may have occurred at a different degree of flexion.

Examination for injuries to underlying muscular fascia is required. If a large defect is found, the fascia must be closed to prevent herniation of the muscle in the future.

If the wound is near a joint, violation of the joint capsule must be ruled out. The joint capsule is lined with a synovial membrane and contains synovial fluid, which lubricates the joint and also provides cushioning for the joint. If the synovial capsule is violated, the joint is seeded (contaminated) with bacteria, and the possibility of developing a septic joint is likely. The joint capsule is a shiny white structure; if it has been penetrated, bone ends are palpable and can be visualized. Again, the joint must be examined through the full range of motion to look for a defect. If a joint violation is suspected but cannot be confirmed by visualization, the clinician should order an x-ray film, which may show air in the affected joint. This is a rare finding, however, and should not be relied on to rule out the presence of joint violation.

A *saline-load test* can be performed to accurately determine if a joint violation has occurred. The practitioner should (using sterile technique) inject sterile saline in the joint, in a place away from the defect, and assess whether any saline escapes through the wound. The amount of saline to be injected is dictated by the size of the joint. Findings are considered negative when the saline injection causes distention of the joint without evidence of leakage or, in a conscious patient, distends the joint capsule to the point of discomfort.

Diagnostic Reasoning
Diagnostic Tests

X-ray films should be taken of wounds that may be associated with a bony abnormality or that raise suspicion of a retained foreign body. Wounds that may have a retained foreign body should be assessed before anesthesia by palpating over the defect and margin of the wound to determine whether the patient can feel a foreign body in the wound. This sensation should be documented. X-ray studies can help to rule out foreign bodies, even fragments of glass of 1 mm in size. Foreign bodies will appear either radiopaque (white) or radiolucent (black), depending on the substance. Some materials, specifically plant-type material (including wood and thorns), will not be visible on x-ray film. As an alternative imaging modality, the clinician may consider ultrasound to rule out radiopaque or radiolucent foreign bodies. Most x-ray exams are now digital, just as mist cameras are being replaced with digital technology. With digital cameras, there is no film to process, which involves noxious chemicals and requires vast amounts of expensive storage areas. The benefit of this technology is that the images can be examined within seconds of completion of the radiograph and the view can be greatly enlarged for better viewing. The images are in a computer database and can be instantly viewed by the clinician or a radiologist on the other side of the world. The clinician can consult with an orthopedist regarding the treatment of a complicated fracture while both providers view the x-ray from their different locations.

The presence of a fracture near the wound defect must be treated as an open fracture. Treatment requires consultation with an orthopedic surgeon and close follow-up. Depending on the type of wound and its size and location, surgical irrigation and closure may be necessary. Prompt antibiotic prophylaxis is indicated—within 2 to 3 hours of injury, if possible. All open fractures require prophylactic antibiotics to prevent infection and osteomyelitis, and antibiotics should be utilized in all closed long bone fractures as well. There is no indication for laboratory studies in the initial treatment of wounds and lacerations. One caveat is that if the patient is taking anticoagulants and the wound is bleeding profusely, the clinician should consider PT and INR, as the bleeding may be related to hypocoagulopathy. Moreover, a CBC would be indicated if the clinician suspects excessive blood loss. If the patient presents with cellulitis or if an abscess develops, a wound culture is indicated.

Differential Diagnosis

A differential diagnosis for wounds is usually not indicated because the diagnosis is usually obvious. Associated injuries include fractures, foreign bodies, sprains, and strains.

Management

Emergency Management

If the primary-care setting has suturing capabilities, a simple wound or laceration may be treated in the office. A patient with a large wound, however, especially one that needs major debridement or appears to be infected, should be referred to the ED. All patients with wounds should be asked about prior tetanus immunization. If more than 5 years have elapsed, a tetanus booster should be administered.

General Management

Wound Cleansing After a thorough history and physical examination, all wounds must be cleansed. The most effective way to lower the bacterial count in a wound is through irrigation with a high-pressure stream of solution aimed directly into the wound. Irrigation with a syringe and needle/catheter is more effective than bulb syringe irrigation for laceration cleansing and irrigation. (Level I; ENA Emergency Nursing Resources Development Committee, 2011). Although traditionally, most providers use normal saline, potable tap water is equivalent and may be superior to normal saline for laceration cleansing and irrigation. (Level I; ENA Emergency Nursing Resources Development Committee, 2011). The amount of solution needed is dictated by the size and level of contamination of the wound. A good rule of thumb is to infuse 50 to 100 mL of solution per centimeter of wound length.

The clinician may want to consider the use of a splash shield. The device has a luer-lock for any size syringe and allows for a high-pressure stream of fluids to irrigate the wound effectively, while protecting the clinician.

Saline irrigation or even soapy water is preferred to a dilute povidone-iodine (Betadine) solution, because Betadine can be irritating and cytotoxic to lacerated tissue. The clinician should avoid hydrogen peroxide (H_2O_2), because it can be very irritating to the wound.

Scrubbing, if employed, needs to be done gently to ensure that the mechanical force applied does not cause damage to the tissue. Scrubbing with an ionic polymer solution such as Shur Cleanse may also be done because it has been shown to loosen up debris and remove superficial foreign bodies.

Wound Debridement The wound needs to be debrided of devitalized tissue. Devitalized tissue is any tissue that is devascularized or extremely macerated. This type of tissue is a nidus for bacterial growth and disrupts tissue defenses. Debridement should be done using a sharp scalpel or scissors so that the debrided edge will be clean and sharp. Using a sharp instrument will cause less tissue trauma and vascular damage at the wound margin. It is important to remove only devitalized tissue. A wound with jagged edges should not be debrided unless the edges are devitalized tissue. Jagged wound margins give the clinician landmarks to use when closing the defect. The jagged edges also increase the surface area of the wound edge and decrease the amount of tension on the wound margin, which can decrease the size of the scar.

Wound Closure Wound closure is done to reduce the size of scarring and decrease the risk of infection or other morbidity. The closure technique used is dictated by the type of wound. Depending on the size and location of the wound, the clinician should consider using sutures, staples, Steri-strips, or 2-octylcyanoacrylate tissue adhesives, such as Dermabond.

2-Octylcyanoacrylate tissue adhesives can be utilized for superficial lacerations less than 6 cm long and in low tension areas. It should not be used over a joint or on any grossly contaminated wounds. Caution should be exercised when repairing wounds near the eye because the adhesive is very fluid and can run into the eye, essentially gluing it shut. If this happens, the clinician must apply an antibiotic eye ointment to aid in slowly dissolving the adhesive. If it cannot be removed for an eye examination, the patient should see an ophthalmologist immediately.

For 2-octylcyanoacrylate tissue adhesive application, the skin must be clean and dry. The wound is approximated with sterile fingers or tissue forceps, taking care not to injure the tissue with the forceps. Once the wound is well approximated, and the fingers are at least 1 cm away, apply the adhesive in concentric circles, allowing 15 seconds in between applications. Advise the patient not to scrub the adhesive and not to apply any antibiotic ointment, because this can dissolve the adhesive. Adhesive tape should not be placed directly over the site.

Another application for the cyanoacrylate tissue adhesive is in the repair of skin tears. Once the skin tear has been cleansed, the torn skin should be unfurled, which is teasing the curled up pieces of skin back to their previous locations. Under no circumstances should the clinician cut the torn skin off because it actually can be used as an allograft. Then the cyanoacrylate adhesive can be applied with excellent results. This tissue adhesive can also be a barrier against common bacterial microbes, including certain staphylococci, pseudomonads, and *Escherichia coli* (Level I; Gaffey et al, 2012).

To decrease tension in high-tension areas, subcutaneous stitches or a mattress technique will be helpful. To close a flap or stellate laceration, the half-buried horizontal mattress technique should be used. To avoid obvious scars and poor cosmetic results, landmarks must be meticulously aligned and skin layers placed in good alignment, with the first suture being placed in the center of the wound. Suturing techniques are illustrated in Therapeutic Procedure 19.1. Remember to "approximate, not strangulate."

Wound Dressings The wound should be kept clean, dry, and covered. For sites that are difficult to keep bandaged, a thin layer of antibiotic ointment should be applied to provide protection to the wound. The bandage should be changed daily or if it becomes wet or dirty. It is helpful to apply antibiotic ointment to the wound when the dressing is changed.

Antibiotic Therapy Antibiotic prophylaxis for most wounds is not indicated. A clean, recently injured wound in a well-vascularized area has a very low chance (only 3%–5%) of becoming infected. Antibiotic prophylaxis does not affect the infection rate. Dog, cat, or human bite wounds, however, have been shown to respond to antibiotic prophylaxis. Early antibiotic therapy, especially if initiated within 2 hours of wounding, has been shown to decrease the chance of infection from bite wounds. Typically, animal bites have a high rate of infection and are not closed with sutures unless they are

Therapeutic Procedure 19.1 Suturing Techniques

Technique	Advantages	Disadvantages
Buried suture	Allows good approximation of wound edges.	Minimal eversion occurs.
Buried vertical mattress suture	Has prolonged eversion; allows early removal of top layers of sutures.	If too superficial, more likely to split.

Therapeutic Procedure 19.1 Suturing Techniques—cont'd

Technique	Advantages	Disadvantages
Running continuous suture	Quick, good for children; even tension.	Entire suture must be removed.
Interrupted suture	Permits precise adjustments between sutures; allows selection of sutures.	Increased risk of uneven tension over the suture line; higher incidence of "railroad track" scarring.
Vertical mattress suture	Good dead-space wound closure; increased wound eversions; increases wound strength.	Time consuming; increased risk of suture marking; difficult to approximate wound edges.
Corner (half-buried) suture	Used in skin-flap suturing; decreases risk of obstruction of blood supply to sutured skin flap.	Edge approximation more difficult; risk of trauma to skin flap; increased risk of dead space.

Continued

Therapeutic Procedure 19.1   Suturing Techniques—cont'd

Technique	Advantages	Disadvantages
Subcuticular suture	Lower incidence of scarring; best for edge approximation.	Poor tensile strength; time consuming; poor wound eversion.
Horizontal mattress suture	Good for dead-space closure; good wound eversion; some hemostasis occurs.	Increased risk of scarring; increased risk of epidermal necrosis.
Wound-closure strips 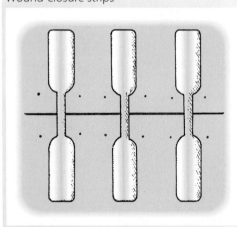	Minimal wound trauma; more resistant to wound infections.	Poor wound eversion; more difficult wound-edge approximation.

Source: Colyar, MR, and Ehrhardt, CR. *Ambulatory care procedures for the nurse practitioner.* FA Davis, Philadelphia, 2004, with permission.

Suture Materials

Nonabsorbable

Silk	Not recommended due to frequent tissue reaction
Nylon	Most common
Polypropylene	Best for subcuticular and continuous type suturing
	Easiest to pull out

Therapeutic Procedure 19.1   Suturing Techniques—cont'd

Suture Materials

Absorbable (metabolized after about 3 weeks—used in inner tissues)

Synthetic polymers	Synthetic for deep layers
	Absorbed by hydrolysis (not for skin)
Surgical catgut	Dissolves in an unpredictable time frame
	Excites tissue reaction during its destruction

Tissue Adhesives

A "glue"-type adhesive of *n*-butyl 2-cyanoacrylate monomers is used in combination with, or as an alternative to, sutures in wound closure.

Suture Size

Smallest size   Largest size

10/0—9/0—8/0—7/0—6/0—5/0—4/0—3/0—2/0—0—1—2—3—4—5—6—7—8—9—10

6/0 is thinner than a human hair; use, for example, in eye surgery.

Family practice clinicians use primarily 3/0 and 4/0.

Suture Choices

Fine sizes	Plastic surgery
	Ophthalmic surgery
	Pediatric surgery
	Vascular surgery
Medium sizes	All other kinds of surgery
Heavy sizes	Retention
	Anchoring bone

disfiguring. If sutures are placed, they should be loose to allow for drainage. Grossly contaminated wounds or wounds that involve areas of diminished vascular supply, such as fingers, toes, and ears, may also benefit from prophylactic antibiotics. Wounds that have an increased risk of infection include the following:

- Crushing injuries
- Dirty wounds
- Jagged wounds
- Wounds with devitalized tissue
- Wounds that are more than 12 to 19 hours old
- Bite wounds, especially from humans (if they are meat eaters), cats, and dogs
- Wounds with retained foreign bodies
- Wounds closed with subcutaneous stitches

Patients with diabetes or a history of vascular compromise should be started on antibiotics prophylactically. Parenteral administration of ampicillin/sulbactam, cephalexin, or ceftriaxone is the initial treatment of choice. This should be followed by oral therapy with amoxicillin/clavulanate, cephalexin, or cefadroxil. If the patient has allergies to penicillin or cephalosporins, the practitioner should consider prescribing doxycycline, with or without clindamycin, or ciprofloxacin.

When treating cellulitis or established infections, the clinician should consider initial parenteral therapy with

ampicillin/sulbactam, cefoxitin, cephalexin, or ceftriaxone. The clinician should consider wound cultures before starting antibiotics on grossly infected wounds. If the bacterial cultures prove to be resistant to the prescribed antibiotic, it should be changed to one to which the bacterium is sensitive. If the patient has allergies to penicillin and cephalosporins, the clinician should consider using doxycycline, clindamycin, or ciprofloxacin. All parenteral therapy should be followed with oral antibiotic therapy for 7 to 10 days. Appropriate choices for oral therapy include cephalexin or cefadroxil for most infections. Wounds that have a high chance of being infected with anaerobic bacteria (i.e., wounds involving contamination with mucus or feces) need to have additional antibiotic coverage with clindamycin or amoxicillin-clavulanate. Close follow-up is important for the first 8 to 24 hours after therapy has been started. If the infection appears to be responding to the therapy, the clinician should continue oral therapy, with additional follow-up as indicated by the extent of the injury and infection. Severe infections require inpatient IV therapy. Outlining the area of erythema with a tissue marker during the initial visit will allow subsequent practitioners to assess treatment response more easily. Any extremity or digit that is infected should be immobilized to reduce the inflammatory response related to mechanical movement of the cellulitic region.

Follow-up and Referral

Patients should be followed up in the office every few days to check the status of wound healing. Home health-care nursing is an effective mode of wound care follow-up in the outpatient setting. Many hospitals also have wound management clinics that have board-certified wound specialist RNs, clinicians, and physicians who are well equipped to care for difficult wounds or patients with many comorbidities, such as insulin-dependent diabetes mellitus and peripheral vascular disease.

Suture or Staple Removal Sutures must remain in place long enough to allow adequate tensile strength to develop during the healing process. The amount of time before suture removal varies with the location of the wound and the cosmetic importance of the wound site. Sutures that are left in too long can cause scarring, and the healing tissue can cover the sutures if left in too long; however, sutures over joints or areas of high skin tension must remain in longer. If staples are used, follow-up will need to be with a clinician who has a staple remover.

The following are the recommended times for suture removal:

- Face: 4 to 6 days; after suture removal, reinforce wound closure with Steri-strips
- Scalp: 6 to 10 days
- Trunk: 7 to 10 days
- Arms and legs: 10 to 14 days
- Joints: 14 days

Patient Education

The patient may take a shower 12 to 24 hours after the initial wound repair. Studies have shown that wound healing has formed a protective barrier that will prevent bacterial invasion after as little as 8 hours. The wound should not be submersed in water, however, until after suture removal or scar formation.

The clinician should explain to the patient that up to 6% of wounds do become infected. Patients should watch for signs of infection, including redness surrounding the area (cellulitis), red streaks coming from the wound (angioedema), and any purulent discharge from the wound (wound infection). Other secondary signs of infection include increasing pain, fever, and chills. Patients with high-risk wounds should be instructed to follow up with the clinician who treated the wound or another provider in 1 to 2 days so that the wound can be evaluated for healing and signs of infection. As of September 2014, 15% of Americans still lack health insurance. These individuals will not be able to afford to go anywhere but back to the ED for follow-up and suture removal.

Patients may ask whether placing vitamin E ointment on the wound will promote healing. Topical vitamin E should be avoided because it is a weak steroid that can delay healing and cause dehiscence in high-tension wounds. Oral intake of vitamin E during the healing process is beneficial; a good diet will provide the needed amounts.

Aloe vera is a weak salicylate-containing gel. Patients may ask if applying this compound is useful to wound healing. Aloe vera may provide mild pain relief, but it does not improve wound healing or help reduce wound infections. Patients should be advised that taking ibuprofen (Motrin) or another NSAID will serve the same function.

Box 19.2 presents discharge instructions for patients with wounds and lacerations.

■ BURNS

Approximately 450,000 patients with burn injuries receive medical treatment each year in EDs. According to the 2012 Fact Sheet of the American Burn Association, there was an average per year of 40,000 hospitalizations related to burn injury, with 30,000 of those occurring at specialized burn centers. In that same year, there were 3,400 fire and burn deaths. This included 2,550 deaths from house fires, 300 from vehicle crash fires, and 550 from other sources including electrical fires and hot liquids or objects. The survival rate for a burn injury is 96%. Because the majority of patients with burn injuries are treated as outpatients, it is important for clinicians to possess the knowledge and skills to treat burns. If a patient with a major burn is brought to an outpatient setting, it may be necessary to assess and stabilize the patient so that he or she can be safely transported by EMS to a hospital ED or burn center. Therefore, all practitioners should know how to perform a primary and secondary survey in the initial treatment of a burn victim.

Although thermal injury is the most common etiology of burn wounds, several other etiologies of burns exist. Various agents that can cause burn injuries are listed in Table 19.3.

Box 19.2   Discharge Instructions: Wounds and Lacerations

- Keep the injured extremity elevated above the level of the heart if possible.
- Cleanse the wound daily with warm, soapy water. Gently remove debris and any scab that is present.
- Lacerations over joints should be immobilized until the sutures are removed to prevent further injury from mechanical irritation.
- For lower extremities, the patient should be advised to do isometric exercises to prevent a deep vein thrombosis while wearing a splint.
- Watch for signs of infection: redness, increased pain, swelling, fever, red streaks progressing up the extremity, any purulent discharge (pus) from the wound.
- Check wound as needed for any signs of infection. For high-risk wounds, routine checks every 24 hours are recommended.

Table 19.3	Burn Injuries
Type of Injuries	**Characteristics**
Chemical	• *Damage:* Destruction of tissues from coagulation or desiccation of tissue protein; action continues until agent is removed; skin penetration by many chemicals leads to systemic toxicity • *Effects:* Injury is generally deeper than it appears; small percentage of admissions to burn units
Cold Liquids/Gases	• *Damage:* Frostbite (freezing of tissues) results in ice crystal formation, which draws water out of the cells into the extracellular space; crystals expand, causing mechanical destruction of cell membranes and organelles • *Effects:* Cell destruction, electrolyte imbalances
Electrical	• *Damage:* Destruction of tissues from heat generated by electric current passing through tissues; arc burn or thermal injury • *Effects:* Injury is usually more extensive than it appears; cardiac conduction system may be affected, leading to sudden death or arrhythmias; severe muscle contraction can produce long-bone or vertebral fractures; severe muscle destruction leads to release of myoglobin, which can affect kidney function
Radiation	• *Damage:* Occurs primarily by gamma/x-ray particles; affects the reproductive mechanisms of tissue cells, leading to cellular death • *Effects:* Proportional to extent of injury and depth
Thermal	• *Damage:* Destruction of tissues from flames, scalding liquids, or steam • *Effects:* Proportional to extent of injury and depth. Thermal burns account for highest percentage of admissions to burn units.

Chemical burns occur in industrial, military, home, agricultural, school, and research laboratory settings. For clinicians working in these settings, especially in a student health-care setting where there is a chemistry laboratory, it is important to have knowledge of the initial care of chemical burn injuries.

People living in the United States spend increasing amounts of time outdoors, working, playing, and exercising, often in clothing that exposes a large area of skin to the sun. Few people know the degree of risk posed by overexposure to the sun and that the risks go beyond skin cancer. Overexposure to ultraviolet (UV) radiation not only results in painful sunburn but also causes malignant melanoma, basal cell carcinomas, squamous cell carcinomas, actinic keratoses, premature aging of the skin, cataracts, immune-system suppression, sun poisoning (phototoxicity), and contact photodermatitis. *Sun poisoning (phototoxicity)*, also called *sun sensitivity,* is considered a systemic or allergic reaction to overexposure to the sun, usually in conjunction with sunburn. *Contact photodermatitis* is an acute or chronic inflammatory skin reaction resulting from the combined effects of a photosensitizing substance (drugs or another chemical) plus UV light (immunological/delayed hypersensitivity).

Epidemiology and Causes

The risk of all types of burns is highest in people 18 to 35 years of age. The male-to-female ratio is 2:1 for both injury and death. Burns are the second most common cause of accidental death in the United States. The death rate in patients older than age 65 is three times greater than that of the overall burn population. According to the 2012 Fact Sheet of the American Burn Association, the ethnicity of burn victims on average for a year was as follows: 59% Caucasian, 19% African American, 15% Hispanic, and 7% other. For burn patients admitted to hospitals, 44% received burns from fire/flame, 33% from scalding (hot liquids), 9% from contact with hot items, 4% from electrical sources, 3% from chemical sources, and 7% from other sources. Mortality rates from burns have significantly decreased over the last four decades. In the 1950s, a 50% total body surface area (TBSA) burn was associated with a 50% mortality rate. Now, a young, previously healthy person can survive almost any size burn. This improvement in mortality rates is the result of a better understanding of early resuscitation, metabolic support after the injury, early wound excision and closure, and control of infection.

More than 25,000 products are capable of producing chemical burns. About 40% of all reported occupationally related injuries concern the skin, and about 25% of these are caused by chemical burns. Common household chemical burns are caused by lye (drain cleaners, paint removers), sodium hypochlorite (disinfectants, bleaches), sulfuric acid (toilet-bowl cleaners), and phenols (deodorizers, sanitizers). The body sites most often burned by chemicals are the face, eyes, and extremities.

Health problems resulting from overexposure to sunlight are caused by UV radiation, which is commonly split into three bands: UVA, UVB, and UVC. UVA radiation is not absorbed by the Earth's ozone layer, which is in the atmosphere. The ozone layer protects the Earth by absorbing most UVB rays coming from the sun. UVB is particularly effective at damaging DNA. This damage is a cause of melanoma and other types of skin cancer. UVC radiation is extremely dangerous but is completely absorbed by ozone and normal oxygen. Researchers have estimated that individuals get 80% of their lifetime sun exposure by age 18. Malignant melanoma is one of the fastest-growing forms of cancer in the United States. New cases of melanoma have more than doubled over the past two decades. There may be a link between childhood sunburns and malignant melanoma later in life.

Sunburn can alter the distribution and function of WBCs up to 24 hours after exposure to the sun. Repeated exposure to UV radiation may cause more long-lasting damage to the body's immune system. No matter what a person's skin type or susceptibility to burns may be, sun exposure makes the body more vulnerable to infections and cancers. This is why diseases such as chickenpox, systemic lupus erythematosus, and herpes simplex become worse with sun exposure. Ultraviolet light therapy is used to treat psoriasis, however, because UV radiation decreases epidermal proliferation.

Overexposure to the sun can also change the texture of skin, giving it a tough, leathery appearance. The sun also causes discoloration in skin tone, including brown, red, yellow, or gray spots. Excess exposure to UV radiation can cause a painful burn of the cornea. Chronic eye exposure to UV radiation may increase the incidence of cataracts, pterygium (in which a fleshy membrane covers the eye), and possibly macular degeneration.

Risk for sun poisoning is increased in persons who take medications that cause photosensitivity, such as oral contraceptives, tetracycline antibiotics, amoxicillin, sulfa drugs, and thiazide diuretics. Risk of sun poisoning also increases with metabolic disorders such as diabetes mellitus or thyroid disease and underlying infection. Patients who have had previous episodes of sun poisoning or who use immunosuppressive drugs are also at increased risk. Other contributing factors include medical disorders such as discoid lupus erythematosus, systemic lupus erythematosus, or porphyria. Exposure to industrial light sources, such as welding arcs, places people at greater risk for phototoxicity.

Agents that may photosensitize the skin include oral antidiabetic agents, NSAIDs, antibiotics, phenothiazines, sulfones/sulfonamides, chlorothiazides, and griseofulvin. The PABA (*p*-aminobenzoic acid) in sunscreen lotion may also cause photosensitivity dermatitis.

Pathophysiology

Local Response

Cellular injury by heat results in the release of cellular enzymes and vasoactive substances, such as histamine, kinins, serotonin, prostaglandins, leukotrienes, and interleukin-1. The activation of complement also occurs. As a result, vascular permeability is altered; and significant hemodynamic, metabolic, and immunological effects occur locally and systemically. The magnitude of the response is proportionate to the extent of injury. At the capillary level, there is a significant shift of protein molecules, fluid, and electrolytes from the intravascular space to the extravascular space. Lymph flow increases initially but subsequently decreases or ceases because the lymphatic vessels become blocked by the serum proteins leaking through the walls of the damaged capillaries. In extensive burn injury (involving more than 25% TBSA), edema forms in both burned and unburned areas because of a generalized increase in capillary permeability and hypoproteinemia. The edema may also be caused by the volume and oncotic pressure effects of the large fluid resuscitation volumes. Maximum edema is seen 18 to 24 hours after burn injury. A decrease in cell transmembrane potential also occurs in extensive burns, causing a shift of extracellular sodium and water into the cell, which results in cellular swelling. With adequate resuscitation, the membrane potential is restored within 24 to 36 hours.

Systemic Response

The response of all organ systems to burn injury occurs in a biphasic pattern of hypofunction followed by hyperfunction. The degree of physiological change is proportionate to the extent of burn; it appears to reach a maximum response in the patient with burns over 50% of the TBSA. As the burn wound heals or is closed, organ function returns to normal.

The metabolic response is one of the most significant alterations after burn injury. Hypermetabolism begins as resuscitation is completed and is probably mediated by the secretion of catecholamines. The extensive healing process requires a rapid metabolic rate to support tissue anabolism and reaches its peak between the sixth and tenth days after burn injury. When the wound is closed, oxygen consumption slowly returns to normal. Protein wasting and weight loss are other elements of the metabolic response to a severe burn.

Wound Healing

When a burn injury disrupts the integumentary system, the body automatically responds with a series of overlapping physiological changes to repair and restore epithelial continuity. The *inflammatory response* begins at the moment of injury and lasts from 3 to 4 days after injury. Localized edema, erythema, heat, and tenderness are characteristic signs of the inflammatory response. During the *fibroblastic phase,* which occurs approximately 4 to 20 days after the injury, cells needed for tissue repair and reconstruction proliferate. Fibroblasts at the wound site migrate over the new capillary network, laying down a bed of granulation tissue (collagen) to fill the wound space. During *wound contraction,* which occurs as granulation tissue forms, myofibroblasts cause the wound edges to pull toward the center. Epithelial cells from the burn margins then migrate across the wound and eventually reproduce to form a protective barrier. This process is called *epithelialization.* Epithelial cells also migrate from the hair follicles and sweat glands, forming small islands of cells known as *epithelial buds.* Newly forming epithelial cells are easily damaged by mechanical trauma and desiccation. If allowed to dry, the wound will form *neo-eschar,* retarding the healing process. The epithelial cells must secrete enzymes to dissolve the eschar in their path. The *maturation phase* occurs when immature granulation tissue is highly organized and serves to restore tissue strength. This phase begins approximately 20 days after burn injury and continues beyond 1 year. Contractures can occur if a burn wound heals with extensive scar tissue formation over a joint. A *contracture* is the fixation of a joint or area of skin into a flexed or fixed position. This is caused by atrophy and shortening of muscle fibers or by scar formation and the loss of the normal skin elasticity.

Under optimum conditions, a partial-thickness burn heals in 2 to 6 weeks. The persistence of eschar on a full-thickness burn may delay healing; if the area involved is large, this will cause the patient to remain hypermetabolic. As bacteria proliferate beneath the eschar, there is a possibility of infection. Approximately 2 weeks after burn injury, the eschar begins to separate from underlying tissue as a result of microbial and leukocytic action on subeschar collagen fibers. Separation generally occurs from the wound margins inward but may occur in patches. Eschar may also be removed earlier by surgical excision.

Clinical Presentation

Sun poisoning may present with urticaria, a red rash accompanied by edema, fever, fatigue, dizziness, gastrointestinal symptoms, or malaise. Hematuria, casts, and proteinuria may occur. Contact photodermatitis results in pruritic papules with erythema and occasionally vesicles 24 hours or more after sun exposure. The skin rash will occur in the area where the chemical was applied and sun exposure occurred.

Burn injuries have been classified traditionally from first through third degree. Currently second- and third-degree burns are classified as either partial-thickness or full-thickness. Partial-thickness injuries can be further categorized as superficial or deep. The signs and symptoms of the various depths of burn are as follows:

- *Superficial (first-degree) burns.* These burns involve the epidermal layer only. The patient presents with pain, hyperemia, and erythema. The surface is dry, with no vesicles or blisters, and blanches with pressure. The wound heals in approximately 5 days, without scarring. The prototype of a first-degree burn is a mild sunburn. If it occurs over a large surface area, it can result in fever, weakness, chills, and vomiting.
- *Superficial partial-thickness (second-degree) burns.* These burns involve the epidermis along with the upper layer of dermis. Signs and symptoms include erythema, hyperemia, pain, moist skin, and hypersensitivity to touch. Vesicles and blisters appear several hours after injury. The healing time is within 21 days, with minimal scarring.
- *Deep partial-thickness (second-degree) burns.* These burns produce destruction of epidermis with most of the dermis. Epidermal cells lining hair follicles and sweat glands remain intact. This level of burn may convert to full-thickness injury. The burn wound may be pale, mottled, pearly white, mostly dry, often insensate, and difficult to differentiate from a full-thickness burn. The burn will heal by wound contraction and reepithelialization within 3 to 6 weeks. Often excision and grafting are done to provide a better functional cosmetic result and to decrease length of healing time.
- *Full-thickness (third-degree) burns.* These burns result in destruction of all layers of skin down to or past the subcutaneous fat, sometimes involving fascia, muscle, and bone. The nerves are also destroyed. Hair pulls easily out of the follicles, and the patient does not feel pain when this is done. The clinical picture is of thick, dry, leathery eschar; white, cherry red or brown/black in color; the tissue is insensate, with blood vessels thrombosed. The wound will require skin grafting.

Diagnostic Reasoning
Diagnostic Tests

Initial laboratory studies for a patient with a major burn should include a CBC, electrolytes, BUN, creatinine, and glucose. Pulse oximetry and arterial blood gas determinations should be done, including a COHb level to determine the percentage of hemoglobin bound to carbon monoxide.

The COHb levels listed below correlate with the following clinical symptoms:

- Less than 10% COHb: No symptoms
- 20% COHb: Headache, nausea, vomiting, loss of dexterity
- 30% COHb: Confusion, lethargy, ST-segment depression on ECG
- 40% to 60% COHb: Coma
- More than 60% COHb: Death

If the COHb level is less than 40%, treatment should consist of 100% oxygen administered by high-humidity flow mask. A patient who has a COHb level of 40% or higher should be considered for transfer to a hyperbaric chamber.

Differential Diagnosis

Photodermatitis must be differentiated from contact dermatitis that may develop from one of the many substances in suntan lotions and oils. Sensitivity to the sun's rays may also be part of a more serious condition such as erythropoietic protoporphyria, systemic lupus erythematosus, pellagra, or porphyria cutanea tarda.

Management

Emergency Management: Major Burns

A patient with a major burn should be taken immediately to a burn center. A *major burn* is defined as follows:

- Partial-thickness burn greater than 25% TBSA in a person 10 to 50 years of age, or greater than 20% TBSA in a child younger than 10 years of age or in an adult older than age 50
- Full-thickness burn greater than 10% TBSA in any individual
- Serious burn involving the hand, face, foot, or perineum
- A burn complicated by inhalation injury
- An electrical burn
- A burn in an infant, an immunocompromised patient, or an elderly patient

Primary Survey   Initial management of the patient with a major burn injury should include maintaining the patient's airway, breathing, and circulation. For airway management, the clinician should assess the patency of the patient's airway while maintaining the head and neck in a neutral position. If a spinal cord injury is probable, the APRN should apply a cervical collar, sandbags, and backboard as appropriate.

For breathing management, while the clinician is maintaining the patient's breathing, the clinician should simultaneously observe the patient's skin color, monitor the oxygen saturation via pulse oximetry (SpO_2), and auscultate the lungs to ensure bilateral effective ventilation. The clinician should be alert for signs of smoke inhalation and thermal airway injury if the patient has a history of being in a fire in an enclosed space. Signs and symptoms include facial burns; presence of soot around mouth and nose and in sputum; singed nasal hairs; coughing of carbonaceous black sputum; difficulty swallowing; signs of hypoxemia, such as tachycardia, dysrhythmias, anxiety, or lethargy; increased or decreased respiratory rate; increased use of accessory muscles for breathing; intercostal or sternal retractions; inspiratory stridor; hoarseness; and expiratory stridor. Once an airway injury has occurred, no measures can be taken to limit its progress, and complete airway obstruction can occur. If signs of airway injury are present, the patient will need to be intubated. After extensive swelling has occurred, intubation will be very difficult. Humidified oxygen at 5 to 10 L/min should be administered by face

mask along with a bronchodilator (albuterol 5 mg unit dose nebulized or 50 mcg/puff, four to eight puffs by metered-dose inhaler with a spacer, every 15–20 minutes as needed). If the patient has signs of carbon monoxide poisoning (headache, nausea, vomiting, dizziness, loss of manual dexterity, confusion, lethargy, unconsciousness, and cherry-red skin color), 100% oxygen should be administered via a nonrebreathing mask.

For circulation management, if the patient presents in the outpatient setting with thermal injuries that involve more than 20% TBSA, the patient will need to be transported to a hospital emergency department or burn center. If there is evidence of burn shock, the clinician should provide for oral rehydration using balanced salt solutions. The patient should be encouraged to drink enough fluid to keep the urine clear and copious. If this is not possible, a large-bore (16- or 18-gauge) IV catheter should be inserted in an upper extremity vein, preferably through unburned skin. The clinician should infuse lactated Ringer's solution at an initial rate of 500 mL/hr. The specific hourly rate can be calculated later during the secondary assessment. Because the cell membranes leak even large molecules for the first 24 hours after a burn, the initial fluid of choice remains Ringer's lactate rather than protein solutions. If an indwelling urinary catheter is available, the clinician should insert a 16-French indwelling urethral catheter and measure the patient's urinary output. A urine output of 1 mL/kg per hour or 30 to 50 mL/hr should be maintained. A patient with an extensive burn injury can be expected to develop an ileus, so, if an 18-French nasogastric tube is available, it should be inserted and connected to low, continuous suction to prevent aspiration.

Secondary Survey   The clinician should obtain a complete set of vital signs, including a rectal temperature. The airway and breathing should be continually reassessed, and the oxygen administration adjusted as indicated. Signs of pulmonary injury can be delayed for 12 to 24 hours after the initial exposure to noxious gases. After the patient's airway, breathing, and circulation are under control, management should include a secondary survey. If there is time for a secondary survey before transportation to the hospital or burn center, the patient's clothing should be removed. Jewelry should also be removed and secured in a safe place. The patient should be placed on and covered with a clean, warm sheet and clean blankets with overhead warmers if available. No other wound care is required until the patient reaches the hospital or burn center.

At this point a head-to-toe systematic survey can be performed, checking for neurological injuries and any fractures that need to be stabilized. The depth and extent of burn can now be estimated, using the "rule of nines," as shown in Figure 19.1. When the burns are scattered, a rule of thumb is that the size of the patient's palm is equal to approximately 1% TBSA.

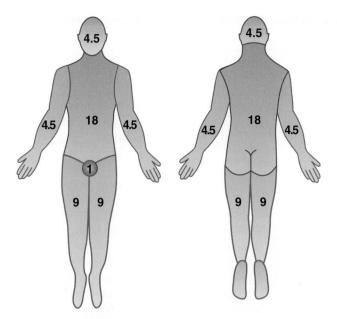

Figure 19.1 The rule of nines. *(Source: Richard, RL, and Staley, MJ. Burn care and rehabilitation: Principles and practice. FA Davis, Philadelphia, 1994, p 109.)*

The weight of the patient should be obtained, either from a scale or from the patient or family, and recorded in kilograms. At this point, the volume of fluids required for resuscitation can be calculated. The clinician should administer 4 mL/kg of body weight per percent TBSA over a 24-hour period. One-half of the calculated amount should be administered during the first 8 hours after the burn injury occurred—not after the time the IV line was first established. The remaining half of the fluid should be administered over the next 16 hours. Patients transferred to burn centers from outpatient settings often arrive overloaded with fluids. Pulmonary edema and hypoxia are exacerbated by overly vigorous fluid administration. Care must be taken to calculate the appropriate volume of fluids correctly and to monitor the patient's response to fluid resuscitation carefully.

During the secondary survey, the peripheral pulses should be evaluated every 15 minutes whenever patients have a burn injury over a large percentage TBSA. The clinician should observe the patient for edema formation as fluids are administered. There is the potential for the pressure of the edema fluid to obliterate arterial blood flow. This is especially true in extremities with circumferential full-thickness burns. The patient may need surgical removal or debridement of eschar to relieve the pressure. Blood pressure measurements should be taken every 15 minutes although they are often somewhat misleading in this phase.

Pain medication should be administered. Prostaglandin inhibitors, such as ibuprofen, can be used to suppress or reduce the systemic inflammatory response that occurs with burns of all severity. A short-acting narcotic, such

as IV morphine or dilaudid, can also be administered if not contraindicated. The patient will need a tetanus immunization during the secondary survey, but administration of this medication and laboratory evaluations can be done once the patient reaches the hospital or burn center.

General Management: Minor Burns

A patient with minor burn injuries can usually be treated in an outpatient setting. Minor burn injuries include a burn of less than 15% TBSA in patients 10 to 50 years of age, or less than 10% in a child younger than age 10 years or an adult older than age 50 years.

Superficial (First-Degree) Burns These burns should be cooled with wet compresses. Ice should not be placed directly on the skin. Aloe vera gel can be applied topically to the burn. Remedies (anesthetic sprays) with benzocaine or lidocaine may provide relief from pain, but these medications produce sensitivity reactions in some people. The patient can be given ibuprofen (Motrin), 800 mg every 8 hours or aspirin or another NSAID. NSAIDs work by blocking the production of prostaglandins, which are thought to be important mediators of pain in sunburned skin. If sunburn is severe, the clinician should administer oral prednisone in a rapid taper: day 1, 80 mg; day 2, 60 mg; day 3, 40 mg; day 4, 20 mg; day 5, 10 mg. There are no benefits to prescribing topical corticosteroid ointments or creams.

Superficial Partial-Thickness and Deep Partial-Thickness (Second-Degree) Burns These burns should be irrigated gently with cool water or saline solution to remove all loose dirt and skin. If the burn is chemical, the caustic agent should be washed off with large amounts of water. Any necrotic skin should be peeled off or trimmed. Small, thick blisters should be left intact. Thin, fluid-filled blisters, greater than 1 inch in diameter, should be drained and the dead skin trimmed off using aseptic technique.

There are at least three different methods for the outpatient management of superficial partial-thickness burns. The first method is to apply a topical antimicrobial to the wound. Agents commonly used are presented in Drugs Commonly Prescribed 19.1. Silver sulfadiazine (Silvadene) is the most frequently used topical agent although it cannot be used in patients with sulfa allergies or on the face because of silver staining. Alternative topical agents for burns on the face are ophthalmic gentamicin ointment, neosporin, or bacitracin. When these ointments are applied to the face, no overlying dressing should be used. If antibiotic creams are unavailable, such as in an outdoor setting or in the home, aloe vera gel can be applied to the burn.

Burn wounds on areas other than the face should be covered with a dressing, which should be removed twice a day at home. The burn should be washed with mild antiseptic soap and water, then more antibiotic ointment and a clean dressing should be applied. This regimen

Drugs Commonly Prescribed 19.1   Burns

Topical	Indications	Dosage and Comments
Antimicrobial Agents		
Bacitracin ointment	Antimicrobial, especially for sensitive areas (e.g., lips, eyelids)	Apply to cleansed area 2–3 times daily. Does not penetrate eschar.
clotrimazole cream (Lotrimin)	Fungal infections of burn wounds	Apply thin coat to wound; wait 20 minutes before applying dressing. Not for ophthalmic use. May cause skin irritation and blistering.
mafenide acetate (Sulfamylon)	Active against most gram-positive and gram-negative organisms Drug of choice for electrical and ear burns	Apply 1–2 times daily using sterile gloves; do not use dressings (may reduce effectiveness and cause maceration). Monitor for signs of acidosis; intake and output; and for signs of allergic skin reaction. Penetrates eschar better than other agents. Pain occurs on application to partial-thickness burns and for 30 minutes thereafter. Allergic maculopapular skin rash may occur. Use with caution in patients with impaired renal or pulmonary function. Hyperchloremic metabolic acidosis may occur. Superinfection with fungi possible.
silver nitrate	Active against wide spectrum of bacterial pathogens and fungal infections Used for patients with sulfa allergy or diseases such as toxic epidermal necrolysis syndrome	Apply 0.5% solution wet dressings 2–3 times a day; ensure dressings stay moist. Preserve solution in a light-resistant container. Protect area with plastic to prevent staining from solution spills and splashes; stains everything black (including unburned skin). Poor penetration of eschar. Electrolyte imbalances may occur; methemoglobinemia may occur.
silver sulfadiazine (Silvadene)	Active against wide spectrum of microbial pathogens Most frequently used agent for partial- and full-thickness thermal injuries	Apply once or twice a day using sterile gloves; leave wounds exposed or apply gauze dressing over wound. Do not use if cream is dark in color. Transient neutropenia may occur after 2–3 days. Only moderate penetration of eschar. Bone marrow depression may occur. Use with caution in patients with impaired hepatic or renal function.

should continue for 7 to 10 days until the burn is healed. This particular method of therapy has some disadvantages in the outpatient setting. Some antimicrobial agents (such as Sulfamylon) encourage wound maceration and therefore cannot be used under a dressing. Also, most topical agents lose their potency in 6 to 24 hours after application, making frequent dressing changes necessary.

An alternative dressing for the superficial partial-thickness burn is to cover the burn with a fine-mesh gauze, such as Xeroform gauze, without a topical antibiotic. This gauze is covered with gauze pads, then a bulky absorbent dressing such as Kerlix is wrapped around the wound to provide some protective bulk. The clinician should inspect the wounds and change the dressings the following day because the maximum amount of wound seepage occurs within the first 24 hours; the burn wound should also be assessed for infection, which should be aggressively treated. The same type of dressing is reapplied. The burn is reevaluated after 4 days, and the bulky dressing removed. If a fluid collection has occurred beneath the Xeroform gauze, the dressing will need to be removed, the wound cleansed, and a new Xeroform gauze applied. If the Xeroform gauze is still in place without any fluid collection, it should be left in place, and the burn rewrapped. Another follow-up visit should be scheduled for a reexamination in 5 days. At that time, the Xeroform gauze, impregnated with the crust from the burn, should separate from the epithelium, revealing healed epithelium. Once the wound is left open, it must be kept clean and protected from extremes of temperature. The wound should epithelialize in approximately 3 weeks. Epithelialization, however, may not occur for 2 to 3 months if the wound is a deep partial-thickness burn in which the only skin remnants are the hair follicles or sweat glands.

A third method for outpatient burn-wound management is to place a semisynthetic occlusive dressing such as Biobrane, xenografts, Op-site, or DuoDerm over the wound. These dressings are less readily available and are expensive. They are most useful for the immunocompromised patient because they minimize the risk of infection. They can be used on flat-surface superficial partial-thickness burns of the extremities and trunk. The goal is for the dressing to adhere to the wound surface and for there to be no exudate or fluid between the dressing and the burn. The dressing is usually removed after 7 to 10 days because the wound is typically healed by then. If there is leaking or nonadherence at any time, the dressing must be changed. Superficial partial-thickness burn wounds heal faster using this method, and patients find this method easier and more comfortable.

Hydrocolloid dressings have been found to significantly decrease the number of required dressing changes compared with chlorhexidine paraffin gauze dressing (Level I; Wasiak & Cleland, 2009).

The clinician should administer oral antibiotics only if the burn becomes infected. The current evidence does not support prophylactic antibiotic therapy in acute burns (Level I; Lee et al, 2009). Any partial-thickness burn will convert to a full-thickness burn if it becomes infected, especially with *Streptococcus* organisms; if infection occurs, the patient may have to be admitted for IV antibiotics. Signs of infection include pus, foul odor, cloudy blisters, increased swelling and redness in the normal skin around the burn, and fever greater than 101°F (38.3°C). Antibiotics prescribed for infections include oxacillin, mezlocillin, and gentamicin. All patients with infected burns should receive tetanus prophylaxis.

Chemical Burns

Consultation from physicians at a burn center should be obtained for treatment of chemical injuries. When a patient with a chemical burn is assessed, the clinician should don protective clothing and gloves. The first priority is to stop the burning process. Any of the patient's garments that have become saturated with the chemical should be rapidly removed, and the patient should be transported rapidly to a shower irrigation area. All other garments should be removed from the patient before the irrigation is complete. If the agent is a powder-like material, such as lime, the clinician should brush off as much as possible before irrigating the burned area. The hair and the areas under the nails and between the toes should be checked for collections of the chemical. The patient may be more comfortable on a chair in a running shower, but any patient who is unstable should be kept horizontal during the irrigation. A chemical burn should be irrigated with water for no less than 30 minutes and preferably for 60 minutes. Irrigation may need to be continued for hours in the case of alkali burns. Irrigation decreases the concentration of the chemical agent and physically removes it from the wound; the rate and amount of reaction between the chemical and the tissue will thus be decreased. Following irrigation in the outpatient setting, the clinician should place wet towels over the patient and arrange for transportation to the hospital. Although wet towels help to relieve pain and continue to dilute the chemical, caution is needed to prevent hypothermia if the burn (TBSA) is extensive. If possible, the clinician should take samples of the chemical agent with a product label to the ED. Use of pH litmus paper may help determine continued presence of alkali or acid in burn wounds. After irrigation and debridement of remaining particles and devitalized tissue, antimicrobial agents should be used and tetanus immunization updated as needed.

For moderate to large burns caused by hot tar or asphalt, the wound should be rapidly cooled with large volumes of water. The tar can then be removed using a petrolatum-based product such as Neosporin ointment. When a large body surface area is involved, an unopened jar of mayonnaise will suffice. The wound can be dressed with a petrolatum-based dressing such as Xeroform gauze. The dressings can be changed, and the wound should be washed with water every 6 to 8 hours until the tar dissolves. Tar can be removed from the cornea or conjunctiva with polysorbate-containing neomycin sulfate; consultation with an ophthalmologist is recommended.

If a patient presents with fingers that are adhered together with a fast-setting epoxy glue, the glue can be removed with acetone. If the glue is on the mucous membranes, the area can be swabbed with vegetable oil until the glue is removed. For glue in the eyes, the clinician should use an ophthalmic antibiotic ointment. Care must be taken or else the drying glue can cause corneal abrasion. Once the glue is removed, the eye should be examined with fluorescein and a Woods lamp with a black light to discern corneal abrasion.

If exposure to hydrofluoric acid (used in glass etching) or oxalic acid has caused a chemical burn, the affected area should be irrigated with water and then neutralized with subcutaneous injections of 10% calcium gluconate. This should be done only after consultation with physicians at a burn center.

If phenol (an acidic alcohol used in sanitizers and disinfectants) is the causative agent, the area should be irrigated with water only if a high-density shower is available. Phenol is more soluble in polyethylene glycol; therefore, a 50% solution of this agent should be used to irrigate the skin as soon as possible.

Follow-up and Referral

Although dressing changes may not have been recommended until 5 to 7 days after injury, all patients with a burn injury must still be reassessed in 24 hours to reevaluate the depth and extent of the burn.

Patient Education

Patients should be advised to elevate the burned area, especially if it is an extremity, and to return to the clinician's office or the ED if signs of an infection appear. Patients should also be given a prescription for analgesic medication.

Patients with sunburns should be informed that sunscreens with PABA may cause photosensitivity dermatitis. Photoplex broad-spectrum sunscreen lotion not only provides protection from UVB radiation but also offers absorbent protection from UVA rays and may be beneficial for patients who experience photosensitivity activated by UVA. Other useful substitutes are sunshades that contain titanium dioxide, zinc oxide, or talc. The patient should notify the health-care provider if pain and fever persist for more than 48 hours. Patients should be informed about the sunscreen protective factor index (SPF), a system of evaluating the effectiveness of various formulations for protecting the skin from the sun. Protective agents are rated 1 to 50 by the Food and Drug Administration (FDA). A sun-protective factor (SPF) of 15 means that the sunscreen provides 15 times the protection of unprotected skin.

The patient should also be informed about the Ultraviolet (UV) Index, which was developed by the National Weather Service and the Environmental Protection Agency. The UV Index provides a forecast of the expected risk of overexposure to the sun and indicates the degree of caution individuals should take when playing, working, or exercising outdoors. The UV Index predicts exposure levels on a 0 to 10+ scale, where 0 indicates a low risk of overexposure and 10+ means a very high risk of overexposure. A patient information sheet on sun safety tips should be given to patients, especially those who have sustained a sunburn severe enough to require treatment. See Table 19.4 for patient information for patients with sunburns.

Table 19.4   Patient Information: Sunburn

- Always wear sunscreen when outside on a sunny day. A sunscreen with a sun-protection factor (SPF) of at least 15 will block most harmful UV radiation. For the average adult, the recommended dose is 1 ounce, or one-quarter of a 4-ounce bottle, per application. Reapply every 2 hours, after being in the water, or after exercising and sweating.
- Use broad-spectrum sunscreens—those that contain active ingredients that absorb at least 85% of the UVA and UVB rays of the sun.
- Protect sensitive areas such as the nose and rims of the ears. Use a lip balm containing a sunscreen. This can help keep some people from getting cold sores.
- Minimize exposure to the sun during the hours when the sun is directly overhead, when exposure is most damaging, from 8 a.m. to 4 p.m. Sun (UV) exposure before 8 a.m. or after 4 p.m., when the sun is lower on the horizon, is typically only one-third that at midday. If your shadow is shorter than you are (around midday), you are being exposed to high levels of UV radiation.
- Wear sunglasses that block 99%–100% of UV radiation. Babies and children should also be protected with sunglasses in order to prevent cataracts that may develop later in life.
- Wear a hat with a wide brim to provide protection to your eyes, ears, face, and the back of your neck.
- Wear tightly woven, loose-fitting clothes during prolonged periods in the sun.
- Avoid sunlamps and tanning parlors.
- Watch for the UV Index:
  - UV Index 0–2 (minimal): Precautions include wearing a hat.
  - UV Index 3–4 (low): Precautions include wearing a hat and using a sunscreen with an SPF of at least 15.
  - UV Index 5–6 (moderate): Precautions include wearing a hat, using a sunscreen with an SPF of at least 15, and staying in shady areas when outside.
  - UV Index 7–9 (high): Precautions include wearing a hat, using a sunscreen with an SPF of at least 15, staying in shady areas when outside, and staying indoors between the hours of 10 a.m. and 4 p.m.
  - UV Index 10+ (very high): Precautions include staying indoors as much as possible and taking other precautions when outdoors.
- Be aware that UV radiation increases 5% for every 1,000 feet of altitude. In North America, the sun is closest to the Earth on June 21, so spring skiing in the Rocky Mountains without protection is very dangerous. Snow and water can also reflect the sun's rays, making sun exposure more intense.

■ ANIMAL AND HUMAN BITES

An animal bite is a bite wound to humans from dogs, cats, or other animals, including other humans. In most cases, bites result in puncture wounds, possible lacerations, and, in some cases, crush injuries. All bites, regardless of the source, are considered to be contaminated wounds and have a substantial risk for infection.

Dogs inflict 60% to 90% of mammalian bites, with an overall infection rate of 15% to 20%. Risks of infection from dog bites are greatest for puncture wounds, crush injuries, and bites to the hand. Dog bites in general have a 5% infection rate, but a dog bite to the hand has a 40% infection rate. The most common infectious agents isolated from dog bites are *Staphylococcus aureus, Pasteurella multocida, Corynebacterium* species, and alpha-hemolytic streptococci.

Cats inflict 5% to 20% of mammalian bites. The needle-like teeth of the cat result in puncture wounds with a high incidence of infection—around 50%. In more than 50% of these wounds, *Pasteurella multocida* is isolated; this bacterium causes wound infections that develop within 24 hours of the bite, resulting in an intense inflammatory response. Serious bone and joint infections may be caused by *P multocida*.

The third most common cause of mammalian bites is from human beings: These bites account for 2% to 3% of bites reported. Common infectious agents isolated from human bite wounds include *S aureus,* streptococci, *Corynebacterium* species, *Bacteroides* species, and *Eikenella corrodens.* Two percent of reported bites are from rodents.

Epidemiology and Causes

Two to five million animal bites occur annually in the United States. Of these bites, 80% result in only minor injury. Researchers have reported that 1% of all patient visits to the ED are the result of bite wounds, and 1% to 2% of these wounds result in hospitalization. About 900 victims of dog bite injuries are treated in the ED every day. Bite wounds occur in all age-groups but are most common in children. Half of dog-bite victims are children younger than age 15. The majority of bite wounds are from a domestic pet known to the victim, with large dogs being the most common source of injury. Cat bites are more common in women, although, in general, men receive more bite injuries than women do. Human-bite injuries from fistfights are common in teenagers and in alcohol-intoxicated men aged 30 to 35 years. Accidental human bites occur most commonly in children, usually as a result of poorly supervised interactions. Approximately 10% of bite wounds in the ED require suturing and follow-up care. Animal bites cause 10 to 20 deaths annually in the United States and involve mostly infants and small children.

Some of the causes of animal bites include separating fighting animals; chasing wild animals; fist-fighting; disturbing a sleeping, feeding, unfamiliar, or injured animal; and kissing, teasing, or playing recklessly with an animal. Individuals who are more likely to be bitten by animals include those who work in animal control, mail delivery, farming, hunting, police work, and veterinary medicine. Some sick or injured wild animals—such as squirrels, skunks, or bats—will attack humans without provocation and may carry rabies. The clinician should be familiar with state laws and regulations regarding bite wounds from mammals and rabies prophylaxis, especially in areas where rabies is endemic. If the animal can be captured, it should be observed for 10 days for signs of rabies. Unfortunately, if the animal is killed and not reported or if it escapes, the incidence of potential rabies goes undocumented and may continue to pose a threat to the community.

Pathophysiology

The risk of bite-wound infection depends on the wound location, tissue damage, patient characteristics, time elapsed before treatment, and the type of animal that inflicted the bite. Wounds should be classified as low risk or high risk to facilitate decision making regarding antibiotic therapy and wound suturing. *Low-risk wounds* include lacerations involving the extremities, face, and body. Wounds at low risk for infection include bites on the face, ears, scalp, and mouth. Large, clean lacerations and bites by rodents are at low risk for infection. *High-risk wounds* include those in the distal extremities (hand, wrist, or foot), the scalp of an infant, a wound over a joint, or a penetrating wound of the cheek. Puncture wounds and nondebridable crush injuries are of high risk. Patients at high risk for infection are those older than age 50 years and individuals with prosthetic joints or valves, asplenia, chronic alcoholism, diabetes mellitus, altered immune status, or peripheral vascular disease, or patients who are on chronic corticosteroid therapy. Bites from domestic cats, large cats, primates, pigs, or humans (especially hand wounds) present the highest risk of infection.

Human bites in locations other than the hand, if treated promptly, have no greater risk of infection than a dog bite. Most human bites are sustained in fights, but 15% to 20% of bites reported in one study were secondary to "love nips" (related to sexual activity). A closed-fist injury ("fight bite") occurs from a laceration over the metacarpophalangeal (MCP) joint caused by striking an opponent's tooth. When this occurs, infectious organisms from the mouth are inoculated directly into the bone or joint, which can lead to septic arthritis or osteomyelitis. Also, when the fingers of the closed fist are extended, the injured extensor tendons retract proximally, sealing off the tissues. This sets the stage for a rapidly progressive infection of the tendon and adjacent tissue layers.

Clinical Presentation
Subjective

The circumstances of the bite injury should be determined. These include the area(s) of the body injured, time elapsed since the injury, type of animal (including breed), current location of the animal, relationship of the animal to the victim, vaccination and health status of the animal, and whether the attack was provoked or unprovoked. The patient should be asked about his or her occupation, medication allergies, tetanus immunization status, any history of immunological compromise, and any specific musculoskeletal, neurological, or vascular complaints resulting from the bite. If the bite is on the patient's hand, the clinician should ask the patient which hand is the patient's dominant hand. Any comorbid conditions should also be determined.

Objective

Seventy-five percent of the bite wounds seen in the ED or practitioner's office will be located on the extremities where the victim handled or attempted to avoid the animal or another person. Injuries to the head and neck are the next most common bite wounds. The clinician should inspect the skin and soft tissues, noting the presence or absence of lacerations, punctures, scratches, abrasions, swelling, crush injuries, and/or devitalized tissue. All puncture wounds should be examined carefully, and the likelihood of injury to structures beneath the skin must be considered. A vascular examination should be performed, noting skin temperature, capillary refill time, and relevant pulses.

The range of motion of all affected areas should be assessed, evaluating the functional status of potentially involved tendons. Motor and sensory nerve function should also be evaluated. To assess sensory function of the hand, the clinician must note sensation to light touch and two-point discrimination on the volar pads of the fingertips. The patient should be able to detect stimuli less than 5 mm apart in the axis of the digit; the response should be compared with the uninjured side. The patient should be evaluated for a skeletal injury and carefully assessed for neurovascular, joint, tendon, and osseous injury.

If the patient does not present with the bite wound until several hours to several days following the injury, the clinician should perform a careful search for evidence of local or systemic infection and regional adenopathy. Infection will be evidenced by increased pain, swelling, erythema, warmth, decreased range of motion at joints, or drainage from a puncture-wound site. A high index of suspicion should always be maintained for the possibility of a retained foreign body in the wound, especially when an infection develops at a puncture-wound site.

Diagnostic Reasoning

Diagnostic Tests

A radiograph of the affected area should be obtained if a fracture is suspected; if a foreign body is present (e.g., tooth fragment, with a higher risk of tooth fragments in bites from older animals); if a bone, joint, or tendon has

been penetrated; or if a puncture wound has become infected. In general, two-view x-ray films should be taken. A culture and Gram stain are not useful before the onset of clinically apparent infection. The examination of purulent material may show a predominant organism in an established infection, but culture is not warranted unless the results will change the treatment. If the patient presents with a localized wound infection several hours or days after the bite, the clinician should obtain a site Gram stain and both aerobic and anaerobic cultures after superficial decontamination of the wound but before debridement of devitalized tissues. Cultures of wounds are also indicated in cases in which an immunocompromised patient is infected, where there is sepsis, or when antibiotic therapy has failed. To obtain optimal cultures, the clinician should perform percutaneous or deep wound aspiration. If significant blood loss has occurred, it is important to obtain a CBC.

If the patient is seriously ill with a bite-wound infection, diagnostic tests should include a thorough laboratory evaluation (including CBC with platelets, electrolyte panel, glucose level, BUN and creatinine levels, and PT/PTT), at least two blood cultures, wound-site Gram stain and cultures, and appropriate x-ray studies.

Differential Diagnosis

The diagnosis is typically straightforward by history; no differential diagnoses are indicated. However, to properly direct management, it is critical that the type (source) and extent of the bite wound be characterized as much as possible.

Management

Emergency Management

The clinician may treat bite wounds in the office using the following protocol.

General Management

Analgesia   Pain management is commonly provided with analgesic agents such as NSAIDs and acetaminophen (Tylenol). If nonnarcotic oral agents are not effective and the patient is in severe pain, ketorolac (Toradol) 30 to 60 mg IM or meperidine (Demerol) 1 mg/kg IM with hydroxyzine (Atarax) 25 to 50 mg IM may be tried. **Wound Cleansing**   Bites and scratches should be cleansed with mild soap and water or 1% povidone-iodine (Betadine) solution, removing the animal's saliva from the wound. Rid the wound of any particulate matter. If the bite was caused by a potentially rabid wild or domestic animal (e.g., skunk, raccoon), the clinician, wearing protective gloves, should thoroughly irrigate the wound with 1% benzalkonium chloride, which has been demonstrated to be capable of inactivating the rabies virus. **Local Anesthesia**   Using a 25-gauge or smaller needle, the clinician should infiltrate the wound edges with 1% lidocaine (without epinephrine). The maximum dose of lidocaine for local infiltration is 4 mg/kg (0.4 mL/kg of a 1% solution).

Wound Irrigation The wound should be irrigated with 500 to 2,000 mL of normal saline. For wounds considered to be at high risk for infection, the clinician can use a 1% povidone-iodine (Betadine) solution. For irrigation, a 30-mL syringe with an 18- to 20-gauge plastic catheter should be used to achieve an irrigation pressure of 5 to 8 psi. This method of irrigation has been shown to reduce wound infection.

Wound Debridement The clinician should remove foreign material, devitalized tissue, and eschar. Margins of puncture wounds should be debrided to an approximately 1- to 2-mm rim to allow for better drainage and improved cleansing.

Wound Closure Fresh facial bites without signs of inflammation should be closed with sutures after thorough wound cleansing and preparation. Bite wounds of the hand should not be sutured. For bites to other areas in need of closure or bites greater than 24 hours old, one may consider using delayed primary closure. A layer of fine-mesh gauze can be applied to the wound, which should be packed open, dressed, and followed closely. If there is no purulence or wound-margin erythema at 3- to 5-day follow-up, wound closure may be performed.

Tetanus Immunization Bite wounds are tetanus-prone injuries. If the patient has received a primary immunization series but not a booster within the past 5 years, a tetanus booster should be administered. For patients with absent or incomplete primary immunization, 250 units of tetanus immune globulin should be given in addition.

Antimicrobial Therapy Patients should receive antibiotic prophylaxis for 3 to 5 days if the wound is a fresh bite wound; if they were bitten by a cat; have a hand bite; have moderate to severe tissue damage; have a wound that may involve a tendon, bone, or joint; have one or more puncture wounds; or have a suppressed immune system. Patients with infected wounds should be given antibiotic therapy based on the results of aerobic and anaerobic culture. The most common causative organisms isolated in wound infections after animal attacks are *Staphylococcus* and *Streptococcus*. Antibiotics prescribed should also cover the less common pathogens such as *Pasteurella* and *Eikenella*. Antimicrobial prophylaxis for cat bites, high-risk dog bites (to the hand, or bites with considerable tissue damage), and human bites can be provided with amoxicillin and clavulanate for 3 to 5 days. An alternative that has fewer GI side effects is cefuroxime, also for 3 to 5 days. Hospital admission and parenteral antibiotic therapy will be necessary for all significant human bites to the hand, especially closed-fist injuries and bites involving penetration of the bone or joint. Cefuroxime IV or ampicillin-sulbactam IV, or ticarcillin-clavulanate IV, should be used for these high-risk bites.

Positioning The injured area should be elevated for several days after injury. For bites located over joints, the joint should be immobilized for 3 to 5 days in proper position depending on the bite location: 20 degrees wrist extension, 70 to 90 degrees flexion for metacarpophalangeal joints, and 10 degrees flexion for proximal interphalangeal and distal interphalangeal joints.

Rabies Prophylaxis Rabies is caused by a rhabdovirus that can be found in the saliva of many mammals. The rabies virus is highly neurotoxic and can be fatal. The clinician should refer questions about postexposure prophylaxis to the local health department or an infectious disease specialist. If a dog or cat is healthy and available for 10 days of observation, showing no development of rabies, no treatment of the exposed person is necessary. At the first sign of rabies in the dog or cat that inflicted the bite, begin treatment. About 85% of all cases of animal rabies in the United States now occur in wildlife. Skunks, foxes, bats, raccoons, coyotes, bobcats, and other carnivores should be considered rabid unless proven negative by laboratory test. The risk of rabies in lagomorphs (rabbits) and rodents (e.g., mice, rats, chipmunks, and squirrels) is minute.

If postexposure rabies is indicated, both rabies immune globulin (RIG) and human diploid-cell rabies vaccine (HDCV) or rabies vaccine, adsorbed (RVA) should be given as soon as possible. The clinician should discontinue the vaccine if fluorescent-antibody tests for rabies of the sacrificed animal's neural tissue are negative. Dosing is as follows:

- RIG: 20 IU/kg. If anatomically possible, one-half the dose should be infiltrated around the wound and the other half given IM (in the gluteal muscle).
- HDCV: 1 mL IM in deltoid region on days 0, 3, 7, 14, and 28 if the patient has not been previously vaccinated.
- RVA: 1 mL IM in deltoid region on days 0, 3, 7, 14, and 28 if the patient has not been previously vaccinated.

Individuals who have been previously vaccinated with either HDCV or RA should not receive RIG; they should, however, receive 1-mL "booster" doses IM of either HDCV or RVA on days 0 and 3.

The clinician should also evaluate the potential for transmission of hepatitis B or C virus (HBV or HCV) in human bites. If HBV or HCV prophylaxis is indicated, hepatitis B immune globulin (HBIG), 0.06 mL/kg IM, should be administered immediately and repeated in 30 days. Also, the practitioner must consider whether the human bite was by a known HIV carrier.

Postexposure HIV Prophylaxis Health-care workers working with combative HIV-positive patients may be victims of human bite wounds; these workers may also be exposed to a needle stick or mucous membrane exposure involving an HIV-positive patient and should refer to the section on this topic in Chapter 17 that covers postexposure HIV prophylaxis, which is an emergency problem.

Follow-up and Referral

The patient should be discharged to home after thorough and meticulous wound management, with follow-up within 48 hours. Infection, cellulitis, abscess, osteomyelitis, septicemia, tenosynovitis, septic joint (suppurative arthritis), rabies, and the loss of an injured body part are all potential complications of bites. Other systemic diseases that can occur as complications are bubonic plague, cat-scratch disease, rat-bite fever, leptospirosis, tularemia, tetanus, and sporotrichosis.

Patients with severe cellulitis, systemic manifestations of infection, failure to respond to appropriate outpatient treatment within 48 hours, or bite-wound infections that involve a bone, joint, tendon, or nerve should be admitted to the hospital. The practitioner should obtain early consultation with an infectious disease specialist if needed. Septic arthritis, osteomyelitis, and closed-fist injuries ("fight bites") will require orthopedic consultation.

Patient Education

If the bite was inflicted by a wild animal or in an unprovoked attack by a domestic animal, the practitioner should ask the patient to have the animal that inflicted the bite checked for rabies. The patient or his or her family should contact the local health department and consult with the animal control officer about the patterns of rabies among the animals in the local area. Individuals should be taught the importance of not petting or feeding strange or wild animals.

Patients will need to be reminded to elevate injured extremities to prevent swelling and to return for follow-up if signs of fever, redness, or swelling occur. The clinician should instruct patients to watch for red streaks, increased warmth at the wound site, increasing pain, foul odor, or increased drainage.

■ ARTHROPOD BITES AND STINGS

Arthropods are members of Arthropoda, a large phylum of animal life characterized by an external body support structure known as an exoskeleton, which includes lobsters and crabs, as well as mites, ticks, spiders, and insects. Arthropod bites and stings involve penetration of the skin by some part of the animal accompanied by release of venoms that can cause local or systemic symptoms. Some arthropods, such as ticks, also transmit disease. The majority of disorders caused by bites and stings of arthropods are from spider bites; bee, wasp, and ant stings; caterpillar spine irritation; interactions with sucking bugs, beetles, flies, and other winged insects; bites from lice, fleas, mites, and ticks; and stings from scorpions.

The venoms produced by venomous insects and other arthropods can be classified according to their effects:

- Vesicating toxins (e.g., from blister beetles, certain stinging caterpillars, and millipedes) produce blisters.
- Neurotoxins (e.g., from black widow spiders, bark scorpions, certain ticks, wheel bugs, and Hymenoptera [honey bees, bumblebees, wasps, hornets, yellow jackets, and fire ants]) attack the CNS.
- Cytotoxic and hemolytic toxins (e.g., from Hymenoptera, ground scorpions, mites, chiggers, wheel bugs, and the brown recluse spider) destroy tissue.
- Hemorrhagic toxins (e.g., from lice, fleas, ticks, mites, true bugs, and biting flies) prevent blood from clotting.

Of the Hymenoptera, the yellow jacket is the major cause of insect-sting reactions. The yellow jacket, hornet, and other wasps feed on sugary sources and are attracted to foods commonly found in garbage cans and at picnics. Yellow jackets, wasps, and hornets nest under logs, in the ground, or in walls; care should be taken to avoid disturbing them during gardening and lawn mowing. When a wasp stings, it injects a venomous fluid under the skin.

The imported fire ant is a small, light reddish brown to dark brown, nonwinged stinging insect that is responsible for increasing numbers of acute allergic reactions. This insect attaches itself to its victim by biting with its jaws; then it pivots around its head, stinging in multiple sites in a circular pattern with its stinger, which is located on its abdomen. The two species of imported fire ants (originally from Brazil) are found predominantly in nine southern states, particularly along the Gulf Coast, and are gradually spreading westward and northward. Fire ants inhabit loose dirt and make nests that produce up to 200,000 ants during a 3-year period. Fire ants swarm if provoked and may attack in great numbers. The fire ant's venom causes hemolysis, the depolarization of cellular membranes, activation of the alternate complement pathway, and general tissue destruction.

The brown recluse spider's (*Loxosceles reclusa*) natural habitat is along the Mississippi River Valley, especially in northwestern Arkansas and southern Missouri. Because this spider can live in old boxes and furniture, it is easily transported to other states. The brown recluse spider prefers warm, dry locations such as woodpiles, cellars, and abandoned buildings; it is generally nocturnal in activity. The "fiddleback" spider has a characteristic violin-shaped marking on the dorsum of its cephalothorax (head and body section). The spider's venom contains sphingomyelinase D; it is chiefly cytotoxic, causing local tissue destruction. The necrosis is caused by an aggregation of leukocytes and platelets that forms a hemostatic plug in venules and arterioles.

Black widow spiders *(Lactrodectus mactans)* are relatively aggressive. They are found throughout the United States, predominantly in the South. Around houses, the black widow spider is found in protected places such as garages, storage sheds, crawl spaces under buildings, and rainspouts. Female spiders of the genus *Lactrodectus* carry the characteristic orange-red hourglass-shaped marking on the ventral abdomen. Black widow spiders are the most feared of all spiders because they injure their victims by injecting one of the most potent venoms secreted by any animal. The *Lactrodectus* venom is a neurotoxin that acts on the myoneural junction and exerts its damage by releasing acetylcholine and norepinephrine.

Scorpions are found throughout the world. They are nocturnal and spend the day under rocks, logs, and floors. The only species that is particularly dangerous, *Centruroides exilicauda* (the bark scorpion), is found mostly in the southwestern United States. This small Mexican scorpion is usually less than 2 inches long, yellow to brown, and possibly striped. The last segment of the scorpion's tail-like structure contains the venom glands and stingers. Most scorpions are relatively harmless, producing only local reactions, but the venom of *Centruroides exilicauda* has effects similar to those of black widow spider venom, producing severe systemic toxicity. The venom is predominantly a neurotoxin that causes repetitive firing of axons by activation of sodium channels.

Some of the more common ticks in the United States are the brown dog tick and the American dog tick. Ticks are frequently encountered by hikers and people who work outdoors. When feeding, ticks make a small hole in the skin, attach themselves with a modification of one of the mouthparts (which has teeth that curve backward), and insert barbed, piercing mouthparts to remove blood. The American dog tick *(Dermacentor variabilis)* may transmit Rocky Mountain spotted fever (caused by the intracellular bacteria *Rickettsia rickettsii*), tularemia (caused by the coccobacillus *Francisella tularensis*), and other diseases from animals to people. This tick has also been reported to cause paralysis if it attaches at the base of the skull or along the spinal column. Paralysis is caused by a toxic secretion produced by the feeding tick. Lyme disease (caused by the spirochete bacterium *Borrelia burgdorferi*) is also transmitted by ticks. Most disease transmission occurs in the New England states, where the primary vector is the deer tick/black-legged tick *(Ixodes scapularis)*. Species that are close relatives to the deer tick, such as the western black-legged tick *(Ixodes pacificus)*, are also capable of transmitting the disease.

Fleas are wingless, blood-sucking insects, some species of which transmit arboviruses to humans by acting as host or vector for the organism. Certain species of fleas transmit plague, murine typhus, and tularemia. If a house has been previously occupied by pets that were infested with fleas, the abandoned hungry fleas may form a welcoming party for the newly arrived "human guests."

Chiggers, or "red bugs," are the larvae of harvest mites. Infestations due to chiggers are caused by mite larvae that feed on the host skin cells. In other parts of the world such as India, Central and Southeast Asia, and Australia, chiggers may transmit scrub typhus (caused by the rickettsial bacteria *Orientia tsutsugamushi*). Chiggers become active in the spring, although in southern states, such as Florida, they may be active all year. Chiggers attach themselves to the skin of humans or frequently to hair follicles or pores by inserting their piecing mouthparts. They prefer to attach themselves to parts of the host's body where clothing fits tightly or where the flesh is thin, tender, or wrinkled. During feeding chiggers inject digestive enzymes into the skin, which dissolves tissue. Chiggers feed by sucking up the liquefied tissues; they do not burrow in the skin. After 3 days, when the larva is engorged, it drops off. Chiggers are most often found in low, damp areas where vegetation is heavy, although some species prefer dry areas. They are most abundant in areas covered with shrubs and small trees, where rodents are numerous.

Mosquitoes are blood-sucking arthropods attracted to hosts by moisture, carbon dioxide, estrogens, sweat, or warmth. They are vectors of many infectious diseases.

The species of blood-sucking flies that can produce allergic reactions are deerflies, blackflies, horseflies, and sandflies. Fly bites can also result in cutaneous myiasis in which parasitism by fly larvae occurs. When a fly, such as the human botfly, deposits an egg on human skin, the egg hatches immediately, and the larva enters the skin through the bite or through another small break in the skin. The larvae grow to 15 to 20 mm under the skin, as a growing red, pruritic papule develops into a tender furuncle, with eventual emergence of the fly larvae.

Some of the stinging caterpillars are the puss caterpillar, saddleback caterpillar, and the hag moth caterpillar. These caterpillars are found primarily in the southeastern states, especially in Texas and Florida. These caterpillars have spines that are hollow hairs containing poison sacs. When the spines break off, a toxin flows from the spines onto the victim's skin, causing a burning sensation.

Epidemiology and Causes

Millions of people in the United States are injured by venoms produced by insects and other arthropods each year, with a notable number of deaths. In one 10-year period, 65 deaths were reported to be caused by spiders in the United States. Of these, 63 deaths were from black widow spider bites. Bee and wasp stings cause more deaths than any other venomous animal. There are 40 to 50 fatalities each year from Hymenoptera stings. These insect stings result in a rapid progression of toxic effects: 80% of the deaths result from anaphylactic shock less than 1 hour after the sting. Spider bites, however, have a longer time interval between bites and time of death, with 89% of victims dying more than 12 hours after being bitten. Ninety-five percent of all venomous animal fatalities occur from April to October, when animals and potential victims are most active. The risk of insect bites increases with lack of protective measures and in areas with heavy insect infestations. Previous exposure to venom can predispose the victim to anaphylaxis.

Pathophysiology

The normal or usual reaction following an insect sting is local erythema, pain, pruritus, and swelling. Insect stings always cause pain. This normal reaction should subside in 1 to 2 hours. The more significant reactions to insect bites can be categorized as large local reactions, toxic reactions, systemic or anaphylactic reactions, delayed reactions, and unusual reactions.

A *large local reaction* could spread more than 6 inches beyond the sting, consisting of prolonged and marked edema at the site of the sting injury, peaking at 48 hours and lasting as long as 1 week. This reaction may be accompanied by nausea, vomiting, and fatigue. A large local reaction can involve one or more neighboring joints and may even produce airway obstruction if the sting was in the mouth or throat. The history of a large local reaction is typically not associated with the risk of anaphylaxis upon future stings.

A *toxic reaction* occurs when there is a history of multiple stings, often more than 10. Toxic reactions are caused by nonantigenic properties of Hymenoptera venom. They resemble systemic reactions but have a greater frequency of gastrointestinal disturbances. Diarrhea, nausea, vomiting, light-headedness, and syncope are common signs. The patient may also have headache, drowsiness, fever, involuntary muscle spasms, edema without urticaria, and occasionally seizures. Urticaria and bronchospasm are not present, and the symptoms usually subside within 48 hours.

Systemic or anaphylactic reactions may range from mild to fatal. The majority of such reactions occur within the first 15 minutes, and nearly all will occur within 6 hours after the insect sting, but some may not occur until 24 to 36 hours later. The shorter the interval between the sting and the onset of symptoms, the more severe the reaction. Fatalities that occur usually result from either hypotension or airway obstruction. The patient will present initially with generalized urticaria, itching eyes, dry cough, and facial flushing. These symptoms may progress rapidly to chest or throat constriction, dyspnea, wheezing, laryngeal stridor, frothy sputum, cyanosis, diarrhea, abdominal cramps, nausea, vomiting, chills and fever, vertigo, shock, loss of consciousness (LOC), and involuntary loss of bowel and bladder function.

When an individual predisposed to Hymenoptera allergy is initially stung, there is an increase in the production of antigen-specific IgE antibodies. The antibodies become attached to mast cells and basophils, and the individual becomes sensitized to undergo an anaphylactic reaction after a subsequent sting. Anaphylaxis is a type I immediate hypersensitivity immune response to a triggering antigen/allergen found in insect venom. In this type of reaction, once introduced into the body, the circulating venom antigen binds to antigen-specific IgE molecules that are bound to mast cells and basophils. Binding of two or more cell membrane–bound IgE molecules to the same antigen (a process known as antibody cross-linking) leads to the degranulation of mast cell and basophil cytoplasmic contents and the release of preformed vasoactive mediators including histamine and tryptase. These substances are potent systemic vasodilators, accounting for the immediate flushing and life-threatening symptoms of hypotension, angioedema, and mucosal swelling with potential airway compromise.

Infusion of histamine into normal subjects causes the following effects and can be diminished by antagonists of specific histamine receptors: flushing (H_1 plus H_2), hypotension (H_1 plus H_2), tachycardia (H_1), headache (H_1 plus H_2), pruritus (H_1), rhinorrhea (H_1), and bronchospasm (H_1). Honeybee venom contains histamine. Wasp venom contains histamine and serotonin. Hornet venom contains histamine, serotonin, and acetylcholine. The fact that histamine acts through both H_1 and H_2 receptors emphasizes the importance of administering both H_1 and H_2 antihistamines during allergic reactions. However, the only reliable method of countering the life-threatening hypotension and mucosal edema associated with anaphylactic histamine release is with immediate administration of epinephrine, a potent vasoconstrictor.

Following this immediate response, through complex lymphocyte (e.g., T cell) and granulocyte interactions, other inflammatory vasoactive cytokines, including prostaglandins, leukotrienes, and bradykinin, begin to form several hours after exposure. These substances contribute to a second, later phase of anaphylaxis that typically occurs 6 to 12 hours after acute exposure to the triggering antigen. Leukotrienes and prostaglandins are responsible in part for vascular permeability, vasodilation, smooth-muscle contraction, and mucus secretion. Downregulation of the inflammatory response by these de novo–formed mediators is the goal of steroid treatment in anaphylaxis because steroids such as hydrocortisone and methylprednisolone exert their peak effects 4 to 8 hours after administration and are ineffective against the immediate life-threatening anaphylactic response. In turn, steroids are more helpful for severe, prolonged allergic reactions and to manage delayed, late-phase responses. Of note, late-phase anaphylactic reactions may be as severe as early-phase reactions. Thus, corticosteroids are a cornerstone of extended management for 24 to 48 hours after the onset of the initial acute reaction.

Another type of *delayed reaction* to insect venom can appear 10 to 14 days after an insect bite or sting; this reaction is also antibody mediated, but by IgG or IgM, rather than by IgE. This type of reaction presents as a serum sickness–like illness, which is a type III antigen–antibody response in which immune complexes are deposited in the various tissues of the body. The patient's signs and symptoms include malaise, headache, fever, urticaria, lymphadenopathy, and polyarthritis. Additional unusual reactions may be neurological or vascular in nature. They include nephrosis, vasculitis, serum sickness, encephalitis, and neuritis. Their etiology varies but may be due to an immunological pathogenesis.

Clinical Presentation
Subjective
The clinician should determine the history of the sting or bite, including the exact time of injury, and an exact description of the arthropod or species of insect, if possible. As the skin is inspected for signs of the insect or spider bite, the patient should first be evaluated for any anaphylactic symptoms or signs of a systemic reaction. The clinician should also determine if the patient has had previous allergies to insect bites, a history of allergies or asthma, or any known allergies to horses or horse serum. A family history of anaphylaxis to bites or stings should also be elicited.

With stinging insects, the patient will usually remember the insult because the sting induces immediate pain. For biting insects, there may be some delay between the actual bite and the itching that follows. The patient's history should be carefully pursued to identify the probable source of exposure. For indoor exposure, fleas are common offenders although spider bites are also responsible for indoor bites. The clinician should inquire about whether pets have recently occupied the dwelling or if the patient has been to a home with pets.

Objective
Hymenoptera (bee and wasp) stings produce immediate pain and a red papule surrounded by a pale zone of edema, with varying amounts of local swelling. Large local reactions are common, spreading more than 6 inches (15.2 cm) beyond the sting, peaking at 48 hours, and lasting as long as 1 week. A mildly sensitive person will experience hives, malaise, wheezing, conjunctivitis, rhinitis, fever, and nausea. A severely sensitive person will suffer diffuse urticaria, facial swelling, laryngeal edema, bronchospasm, vomiting, cyanosis, abdominal pain, arrhythmias, and hypotension. Most fatalities occur within 1 hour of the sting.

Fire ant stings produce vesicles that become sterile pustules; these pustules subsequently become necrotic within several hours and may take up to 10 days to heal.

If broken, the pustules may become infected. Systemic symptoms include nausea, vomiting, faintness, headache, fever, numbness, and muscle spasms.

Brown recluse spider bites are unusual in that persons bitten usually do not feel pain for 2 to 3 hours. A single necrotic lesion occurs, usually measuring 0.5 to 2 cm in size, self-limited in spread, and lacking adenopathy or sustained general toxicity. The typical bull's-eye lesion is created when the red blister is encircled by a pale, irregularly shaped and ischemic halo, which in turn is surrounded by extravasated blood. The pustule may gradually grow to form a crater-like lesion over 3 to 4 days, with associated lymphadenopathy and low-grade fever. Rarely, there is a generalized systemic reaction 24 to 48 hours after the bite, with fever, malaise, arthralgias, rash, and hemolysis.

Black widow spider bites create an initial puncture wound that disappears rapidly, leaving a local swelling where tiny red spots appear. Symptoms of envenomation occur within 10 to 60 minutes, including severe pain in the bitten extremity and muscle spasms of the abdomen and trunk. Diffuse paresthesias, ptosis, and hyperactive deep tendon reflexes may be noted. Victims are in agonizing pain and may develop hypertension, headache, muscular rigidity and spasm, hyperreflexia, vomiting, abdominal pain, agitation, or psychosis. Symptoms peak at 2 to 3 hours after the bite and may last up to 24 hours.

Scorpion stings are immediately intensely painful, with little or no erythema or swelling. Generalized reactions may occur within 1 hour and progress to maximum severity in 5 hours. The reactions can be graded as follows:

- Grade I: Local pain and paresthesias at the site of envenomation
- Grade II: Pain and paresthesias remote from the sting bite, along with local findings
- Grade III: Either somatic skeletal or cranial nerve neuromuscular dysfunction, including blurred vision, wandering eye movements, hypersalivation, difficulty swallowing, upper airway obstruction, slurred speech, jerking of the upper extremities, restlessness, arching of the back, severe involuntary shaking and jerking
- Grade IV: Both cranial nerve and somatic skeletal neuromuscular dysfunction

Hypertension, nausea, vomiting, hyperthermia, tachycardia, and respiratory distress may also occur. Children younger than 10 years of age are more likely to have severe or prolonged reactions to scorpion stings. Older children and adults usually recover within 10 to 12 hours.

Tick bites can produce lesions that vary from small pruritic nodules to extensive ulceration, induration, and erythema. The lesions may be accompanied by malaise, fever, and chills. Tick-induced paralysis occurs more frequently during the spring and summer, when ticks are feeding. Symptoms occur 5 to 6 days after the adult female tick attaches and include irritability, restlessness, and paresthesias in the hands and feet. Over the next 24 to 48 hours, ascending, symmetric, and flaccid paralysis, with loss of deep tendon reflexes, occurs. Within 1 to 2 days, severe generalized weakness is possible, accompanied by respiratory paralysis.

Flea bites produce lesions that are so similar to those of lice and scabies that diagnosis is often difficult. Flea bites produce itching papules, found in zigzag lines, especially on the legs and in the waist area. The lesions present as central hemorrhagic puncta surrounded by erythematous and urticarial patches. Pruritus is intense. Once the lesions clear, dull red spots may persist. Impetigo may develop as a complication. If the fleas remain in the environment, new lesions continue to appear.

Itching from *chigger bites* is usually noticed 4 to 8 hours after chiggers have attached or have been accidentally removed. Initially, a papule develops and ultimately enlarges over 24 to 48 hours to form a nodule. Pruritus peaks on the second day. The fluid injection causes nodules to appear, which may last for 2 weeks. Patients who exhibit an allergic reaction to the fluid injected (saliva) will develop severe soft tissue edema, itching, and fever. Chigger bites usually occur around the ankles, waistline, knees, or in the armpits. Mite infestations may be associated with an erythema multiforme–like rash and fever.

An immediate skin reaction to *mosquito bites* includes erythema, wheal, and itching. A delayed reaction 12 to 24 hours later consists of redness, edema, and a burning pruritus. Blistering and necrosis can also occur. The immediate reaction is of short duration, whereas a delayed reaction may persist for hours, days, and even weeks. Some individuals have a history of allergy to mosquito saliva, consistent with an increasing reaction to seasonal exposures accompanied by progressively more pronounced edema and pruritus. The allergic response can be accompanied by fever, generalized malaise, nausea, vomiting, and necrosis, with resulting scarring.

Blood-sucking flies can cause pain and subsequent pruritus when they pierce the skin. Allergic reactions can occur; if flies inject their eggs under the skin, the patient can also develop myiasis. As the fly larvae hatch and grow under the skin, the initial pruritic papule becomes a furuncle with a central opening that exudes serosanguineous fluid. The tip of the fly larva may even protrude from the central opening, or bubbles produced by its respiration may be seen.

The *puss caterpillar's sting* causes intense, immediate pain, often in spasms. This is followed by local edema, pruritus, and a rash of red blotches and ridges. The lesions consist of red or white papules and vesicles, often forming a perfect grid like mark where the caterpillar made contact. Ordinarily no systemic manifestations occur; the localized symptoms typically subside within 24 hours. In some patients, however, the intense pain may cause nausea and vomiting, as well as headache, fever, and lymphadenopathy. The papular or urticarial rash usually subsides within a few hours to 1 to 2 days after contact, but it may persist for up to 1 week.

Diagnostic Reasoning
Diagnostic Tests

In an arthropod bite or sting that results in systemic involvement, the APRN should order blood type and crossmatch, coagulation studies, CBC, electrolytes, BUN, creatinine, and urinalysis. ABGs and pulse oximetry may also be necessary. For suspected tick-borne diseases such as Rocky Mountain spotted fever and Lyme disease, further laboratory studies are in order. For example, spirochetes can be seen in the blood smear in 70% of cases of tick-borne relapsing fever. Lyme disease, Rocky Mountain spotted fever, and tularemia, which also occur from tick bites, are diagnosed by antibody titer. However, results from these antibody titer assays are often not available for days to weeks, with empiric treatment often initiated before this. Thus, these tests are usually sent for confirmation only when a strong suspicion already exists and should not be sent indiscriminately.

Differential Diagnosis

Consultation with a regional poison control center may be indicated to correctly identify, diagnose, and/or treat arthropod bites and stings. It is very helpful to know which arthropods are indigenous to the local area, especially which ones have been causing recent infestations and injuries.

Bites of fleas, lice, and scabies mites produce lesions that are so similar that diagnosis is often difficult. Cercaria or nonhuman schistosomes cause similar lesions, which appear after the patient has been in infected water. Scabies has a more gradual onset but should also be considered in the differential diagnosis. The diagnosis of chigger infestation can usually be made on the basis of probable outdoor exposure and typical skin lesions. Patients who present with a "bull's-eye" rash following a suspected deer tick bite should be tested for Lyme disease.

When examining an urticarial reaction to an insect bite, other causes of urticaria should be considered; but if the hive (wheal) has a central punctum, its cause is likely an insect bite. Other foreign bodies can produce pruritic papules in the skin. Dermatitis herpetiformis should be included in the differential diagnosis, particularly when only excoriations are found. Eruptions associated with other viruses or with atopic dermatitis, allergic or irritant contact dermatitis, and drug sensitivity must also be considered. An uncommon idiopathic disorder, Mucha-Habermann disease, also presents with scattered necrotic papules and vesicles, but this type of rash is usually more generalized and symmetric. Some of the other skin conditions that may be confused with local or systemic reactions to arthropod stings and bites include streptococcal necrotizing fasciitis, focal cutaneous necrosis, various infections, local thromboses, punctures, trauma, drug reactions, vasculitis, purpura, Arthus (type III, serum sickness) reactions, emboli to the skin, other bites that leave small puncture wounds, and artifacts.

Anaphylaxis from an insect sting may be confused with a vasovagal reaction, which is a disorder of central vasoregulation caused by increased parasympathetic tone mediated by the vagus nerve (cranial nerve X). A vasovagal reaction typically produces pallor, nausea, bradycardia, extreme diaphoresis, and hypotension that may result in syncope, whereas flushing, hypotension, tachycardia, and mucosal edema with severe bronchoconstriction are seen in anaphylaxis. Severe reactions to scorpion stings may present with symptoms similar to those of insecticide poisoning, with direct CNS effects.

Confirmation of stinging insect allergy is made by the detection of venom-specific IgE. This can be performed through an immediate reaction skin prick test, which measures the cutaneous histaminic response to dilute doses of allergen after scratching the skin surface with an antigen-coated needle tip, allowing for binding to IgE on skin mast cells with subsequent degranulation. Yellow jacket, honeybee, yellow hornet, bald-faced hornet, and wasp extracts are available for diagnosis and treatment of stinging insect allergies. A patient is considered sensitive if a skin reaction of 1+ or greater occurs at a venom concentration of 1 mg/mL or less, provided that the 1+ reaction is greater than that of the diluent control. This is the most sensitive test for picking up allergic states and is commonly used as an allergy screening tool. However, it lacks specificity and may thus overestimate allergic states.

IgE antibodies reacting with venom also may be measured by serum assay known as the radioallergosorbent test (RAST). In this test, a patient's serum is applied to a culture plate surface coated with the specific allergen of interest, allowing for specific antibody-binding to the plate. After excess serum is rinsed away, a second fluorescent-labeled antibody specific for the constant region of IgE is applied to the plate to reveal any of the patient's antigen-specific IgE that bound to the plate during the first step of the assay. Thus, the greater the amount of fluorescence, the higher the concentration of antigen-specific IgE in the patient's serum. The RAST is not as sensitive as the skin test although it is more specific and is thus more effective in ruling out, rather than ruling in an allergic state.

Management
Emergency Management
Anaphylactic shock and respiratory distress are true emergencies; the clinician should focus on stabilizing

the patient while arranging for immediate transport to the ED.

Systemic or Anaphylactic Reactions It should be stressed that anaphylaxis may be triggered by etiologies other than bites and stings. Anaphylactic reactions are extreme emergencies and may be a reaction iatrogenically caused by medications, environmental exposures, and especially food allergies, which are quite common. The treatment for anaphylaxis is standard and is included here.

The clinician should place a conscious patient in a comfortable position, ensuring unimpeded ventilation. Hypotensive patients should be placed supine or in a modified Trendelenburg position if respiratory status allows.

The clinician must maintain an adequate upper airway and give supplemental oxygen by mask or nebulizer with inhaled racemic epinephrine (0.5 mL of 2.25% epinephrine in 2 mL of normal saline), not to exceed three treatments in 60 minutes. However, racemic epinephrine should not be considered an adequate substitute for systemic epinephrine in the case of a life-threatening attack. Thus, in the case of impending upper airway compromise, inadequate oxygenation, or profound shock, the clinician must prepare for immediate administration of systemic epinephrine (as described below) and endotracheal intubation if necessary to maintain an open airway. Cricothyrotomy is to be performed if severe angioedema precludes intubation via the oral route.

In the case of airway edema, bronchospasm, and/or cardiovascular instability (with or without cutaneous manifestations of urticaria or angioedema), the clinician should immediately administer aqueous epinephrine 1:1,000 IM into the upper outer thigh region, which provides the most rapid entry into the systemic circulation. The dose is 0.3 to 0.5 mg every 10 to 20 minutes as indicated. One can inject 0.1 to 0.2 mg of the epinephrine dose directly into the sting bite, causing vasoconstriction and reduction of swelling. If the reaction is limited to urticaria and pruritus, there is no wheezing or facial swelling, and the victim is more than 45 years old, one should reserve epinephrine for a worsened condition. Epinephrine maintains the blood pressure, causes bronchial dilation, and antagonizes adverse actions of the mediators of anaphylaxis. It also reduces the subsequent release of mediators through its action on mast cells and basophils.

In the setting of vasodilatory anaphylactic responses with hypotension, laryngeal edema, or severe bronchospasm, when there is no response to IM epinephrine, IV administration is a more appropriate route. Epinephrine is the single most life-saving treatment in the reversal of hypotension, airway edema, and bronchoconstriction associated with anaphylaxis. The clinician should place 0.1 mg (1 mL of 1:10,000 solution epinephrine) in 10 mL of normal saline (NS) and administer as a slow IV push over 10 minutes. This dose is to be repeated once or twice every 10 minutes as required. Alternatively, a continuous infusion of IV epinephrine at 1 to 5 mg/min can be started. This is constituted by adding 1 mg of 1:1,000 aqueous epinephrine (1 mL) to 250 mL NS, creating a concentration of 4 mg/mL.

Excessive infusion rates may be associated with cardiac ischemia and arrhythmias. One-half of the above recommended doses should be used initially in elderly patients or those with cardiovascular disease, diabetes mellitus, thyroid disease, cerebral arteriosclerosis, or Parkinson's disease. Patients who are taking beta-adrenergic blocking agents may be refractory to treatment with epinephrine. Glucagon (5–15 mg/min IV) may be a useful agent in the treatment of anaphylaxis in the presence of beta blockade.

Antihistamines are included in the treatment regimen. With H_1-blocking antihistamines, the clinician may administer diphenhydramine IV or PO as needed (in severe anaphylaxis, administer 100 mg IV initially); or hydroxyzine IM as needed. The newer generation H_1 blockers such as cetirizine, fexofenadine, and desloratadine are less sedating and may be just as effective if the patient may be treated with oral medications. For H_2-blocking antihistamines, the clinician may administer cimetidine IV or ranitidine IV. If available, cimetidine is the preferred H_2 blocker because it has greater peripheral effects than does ranitidine, which is more specific for the gastrointestinal tract.

In addition to immediate epinephrine as described previously, albuterol may be used to treat bronchospasm, administered via nebulizer every 20 minutes as necessary. A loading dose of aminophylline 6 mg/kg IV (if the patient is not currently taking aminophylline or theophylline) may be administered over 20 to 30 minutes, followed by a continuous IV infusion (0.7 mg/kg per hour) in otherwise healthy nonsmoking adults.

Circulatory support should be provided as necessary. The clinician may infuse 0.5 to 1 L of either NS or lactated Ringer's solution every 20 to 30 minutes as needed to support the blood pressure at a level above 90 mm Hg systolic. The need for further fluid resuscitation should be determined by monitoring blood pressure, cardiac rhythm, and urine output. Usually, a total of 3 L can be given rapidly to an adult without ill effect. The clinician should be cautious with patients with congestive heart failure or the elderly, given the risk of pulmonary edema. Hypotension that is refractory to epinephrine and IV fluids may be treated with norepinephrine (Levophed) via IV infusion. Phenylephrine (Neo-Synephrine) as an IV bolus every 10 to 15 minutes as necessary or as a continuous IV infusion may also be used. The infusion should be decreased once blood pressure has stabilized. Glucagon is also useful in patients on beta-adrenergic blocking agents because it stimulates cardiac inotropic and chronotropic function independent of beta blockade. Patients taking beta blockers may also benefit from terbutaline SC.

If the allergic reaction is prolonged or severe or if the patient is regularly medicated with corticosteroids, the clinician should administer hydrocortisone, methylprednisolone, or dexamethasone IV, with a 10-day oral taper to follow. If the therapy is initiated orally, the clinician should administer prednisone 60 to 100 mg daily. Even in the case of reactions that do not appear to be prolonged, systemic corticosteroid therapy should be administered for 24 to 48 hours after the onset of the initial reaction to minimize the chance of late-phase anaphylactic reactions, which may manifest up to 24 hours after the initial reaction and may be as severe as early-phase reactions.

General Management

Normal Reactions Normal reactions to arthropod bites and stings do not require treatment other than local applications of cold compresses (ice) and analgesics. NSAIDs such as ibuprofen PO are effective if given immediately because they block prostaglandins. Secondary infections are common; therefore, a topical antimicrobial ointment such as mupirocin 2% (Bactroban) ointment should be applied to the area.

Large Local Reactions Large local reactions to arthropod bites or stings are treated with antihistamines, such as diphenhydramine IV or PO and cimetidine IV or PO. Intramuscular administration of diphenhydramine is not usually done because of the pain involved and the fact that the drug is absorbed very rapidly PO. A corticosteroid such as methylprednisolone PO the first day, then tapered over 5 days, will hasten resolution of a large local reaction to a bee or wasp sting. Tapering slowly prevents a rebound flare-up of symptoms. Some clinicians also administer IV calcium gluconate. Importantly, large local reactions are not associated with the risk of anaphylaxis on future stings by the same type of insect.

Delayed Serum Sickness-Type Reactions Delayed serum sickness-type reactions in response to multiple bee, wasp, or fire ant stings can be managed with a corticosteroid such as prednisone (Deltasone) 60 to 100 mg, tapered over 2 weeks. The pruritus caused by insect bites can be controlled by a variety of oral antihistamines. Hydroxyzine is commonly prescribed because its dosage is very flexible, and it produces few anticholinergic adverse effects. If patients are driving and working during the day, they should reserve the hydroxyzine for nighttime use to help with sleep. Treatment of urticaria may also require an antihistamine that is an H_2 blocker, such as cimetidine.

For arthropod bites, when topical steroids are needed, class I (e.g., betamethasone dipropionate) or class II (e.g., fluocinonide) topical steroids may be administered 2 times daily. Lesions may take weeks to resolve. Topical antipruritics include lotions with 0.25% menthol, 1% phenol, or both (Sarna lotion) and topical anesthetics such as pramoxine (Pramosone).

Topical antihistamines and benzocaine are not recommended because of their potential for allergic sensitization. Topical doxepin (Zonalon) is now available and is effective. Infected insect bites can be treated with topical 2% mupirocin or neomycin. Extensive impetigo will need treatment with oral antibiotics, dicloxacillin, or erythromycin.

Hymenoptera Stings   When a patient is stung by a honey bee, the stinger should be removed by scraping it with a dull object. The stinger should not be grasped and pulled because this contracts the venom sac, thus releasing more toxins. Wasps and other bees do not leave a stinger and are capable of stinging many times. One should cleanse the site and apply antiseptic. Blisters from fire ant stings should not be broken. Ice should be applied with a pack, with or without a paste of papain (unseasoned meat tenderizer), and the body part should be elevated.

There is no specific antivenin for Hymenoptera stings. If the reaction is extensive or if there is envenomation from multiple stings, more aggressive therapy may be indicated. This includes administering IV calcium gluconate with an antihistamine such as diphenhydramine, IV or orally. Oral prednisone, 40 mg daily for 2 to 3 days, can be very helpful in reducing the local swelling. Appropriate tetanus prophylaxis should be completed. In severe envenomations, an IV corticosteroid such as hydrocortisone, 2 mg/kg should be administered at the earliest opportunity (see also the section on systemic or anaphylactic reactions).

Brown Recluse Spider Bite   The patient should apply cold compresses intermittently for the first 4 days after the bite, over a sterile dressing. Administer an oral antibiotic, such as dicloxacillin, cephalexin, or erythromycin for 10 days. Elevation of the affected part may be beneficial. Drug treatment is controversial; many brown recluse spider bites are minor and heal without specific treatment other than tetanus prophylaxis. One current treatment for a severe wound is to obtain a glucose-6-phosphate dehydrogenase (G6PD) screen and if negative, immediately give dapsone (Avlosulfon) 50 mg (adult dose) orally 2 times daily for 10 days. If G6PD enzyme deficiency is documented, the patient should discontinue dapsone to avoid hemolysis.

Black Widow Spider Bite   The natural course of the envenomation is to resolve completely after a few days, with pain persisting for a week or more. Ice should be applied judiciously to the bite wound. The clinician should administer a narcotic analgesic, such as morphine. All opioids may have a histaminic agonist effect, so these medications should be avoided in cases with significant histaminic responses. Muscle relaxants such as diazepam (Valium) may also be given. The patient should be monitored for hypertension and administered a centrally acting or vasodilating antihypertensive if necessary. An alternative, more controversial treatment for black widow spider bites would be to add calcium

gluconate 0.1 to 0.2 mL/kg IV given slowly to alleviate muscle spasm. Reserve antivenin for seriously ill infants and older patients and proceed with horse serum sensitivity testing. One vial of antivenin is sufficient for most patients.

Scorpion (Centroides exilicauda) Bite   The patient should apply ice for 30 minutes each hour to relieve local pain. Intense cooling should be avoided, and the affected part should be immobilized. Do not apply a tourniquet. Opiate analgesics should be avoided because they potentiate the toxicity of the venom and may lead to apnea. The clinician should administer diazepam or phenobarbital to control seizures, along with sympathetic antihypertensive agents to control hypertension. Hyperthermia from uncontrolled muscular activity can be managed with cooling. The administration of antivenom (antivenin) is controversial because it is derived from horse serum and thus carries a risk of anaphylaxis. Horse serum sensitivity testing is done to screen against anaphylaxis, which is a risk with many of the antivenin medications. Antivenin should be administered only in a hospital critical care setting.

Tick Bite   The clinician should always remove ticks. The tick can be covered with alcohol, machine oil, mineral oil, salad oil, or gasoline on a tissue or gauze pad. This blocks the tick's breathing pores and causes it to withdraw from the skin. It may take 30 minutes for the tick to disengage its mouthparts. Ticks should not be removed manually because squeezing the tick's body may inject more viral or bacterial pathogens into the victim. The clinician should observe for a local reaction or infection at the site. Most victims of tick paralysis will show improvement within hours of tick removal and return to normal in several days. Patients with Rocky Mountain spotted fever or Lyme disease will require further treatment, including antibiotics and follow-up monitoring for chronic health problems.

Flea Bites   The patient should clean the lesions well with soap and water and apply a topical antiseptic ointment. To relieve pruritus and discomfort, calamine lotion with phenol can be applied. A systemic antihistamine, such as hydroxyzine (Atarax), can be administered to control itching.

Chigger Bites   Chiggers are easily removed from the skin by taking a hot bath or shower and lathering with soap several times. The bath will kill attached chiggers. For moderate to severe cases, topical steroid creams and oral antihistamines may provide some relief. Systemic steroids will also provide relief for severe pruritus. Topical antibiotic therapy is indicated for secondary infection.

Mosquito Bites   Immediately after the person is bitten, he or she should apply a cold (ice) pack. A topical steroid ointment can be applied to the site. Oral steroids such as prednisone should be used only when the reaction is prolonged and severe, given their potential adverse effects.

Fly Bites Fly bites are treated the same as mosquito bites. In addition, if the patient presents with cutaneous myiasis, the clinician should exert pressure to extrude the organism (fly larva). The larva may emerge if its breathing hole in the skin is occluded with heavy oil, nail polish, or bacon fat. Alternatively, the clinician can inject 2 mL of local anesthetic into the base of the lesion, thus extruding the larva by fluid pressure. Take care not to rupture the larva because an inflammatory reaction may result.

Caterpillar Spine Irritation Broken-off spines can be removed by applying adhesive tape, a commercial facial peel, or a thin layer of rubber cement. Then an oral antihistamine and/or NSAID can be administered. If the dermatitis is persistent and severe, the clinician should prescribe oral prednisone 60 to 100 mg for adults, to be tapered over 10 days.

Follow-up and Referral

After a severe allergic reaction, further delayed reactions and recurrence of symptoms are possible, particularly as the effects of the medication decrease. Patients may benefit from repeated doses of antihistamines and glucocorticoids over the next several days. All patients with severe allergic reactions who are discharged home should have follow-up in 24 to 48 hours. All such patients should be referred to an allergy specialist.

Individuals who have experienced a serious anaphylactic reaction should be prescribed three kits for the self-administration of epinephrine by injection or nebulization (EpiPen or Ana-Kit) and instructed on its use. These patients should also keep in each kit oral diphenhydramine and cimetidine. One kit should be kept in a bag or purse that is carried with the individual at all times, a second in the school or work setting, and a third kit should be kept in the home. Many individuals also keep a kit in the glove compartment of a personal vehicle. However, it is important to explain to the patient that extremes of heat and cold can affect the stability of many medicines, including life-saving epinephrine. Thus, storing a kit in the glove compartment is not recommended.

Individuals with a history of an acute allergic reaction (including systemic cutaneous reactions) with positive venom skin tests or a serum sickness-type reaction after an insect sting are considered at risk for subsequent sting reactions. Venom immunotherapy to prevent IgE-mediated allergic reactions may be recommended, and referral to an allergist is required for specialized assessment, including allergy testing (venom skin testing and venom-specific serum IgE–RAST testing). Of note, venom immunotherapy will not prevent future type III immune complex-mediated serum sickness reactions, which do not involve the IgE allergic antibody. In addition, patients with large local reactions are not considered candidates for venom immunotherapy and do not require venom skin tests, because these reactions are not associated with the risk of anaphylaxis on future stings. Patients who have been treated for anaphylaxis and who use beta-adrenergic blocking agents should be switched to alternative medications.

Patient Education

Patient education information regarding arthropod bites and stings is provided in Table 19.5.

■ HEAD TRAUMA

Head traumas that may be encountered by the clinician in a primary-care setting include cerebral contusions, concussions, skull fracture, and epidural or subdural hematomas. In contrast, subarachnoid hemorrhage typically results from the spontaneous rupture of intracranial aneurysms (greater than 80% of cases), rather than a traumatic etiology.

Epidemiology and Causes

Head trauma is a leading cause of morbidity and mortality in the United States. It affects approximately 2 million persons per year, with about one head injury occurring every 15 seconds. About 30% of all visits to the ED are for treatment of head-related injuries. The vast majority of head traumas result from motor vehicle crashes in young adults aged 15 to 24 years. The next most common causes are football and wrestling in men and soccer and basketball in women. Although it is estimated that approximately 3.8 million concussions occur in the United States annually during competitive sports and recreational activities, half of those go unreported. In people older than age 65 years, falls account for the majority of head injury deaths. Falls are the most common reason for an injury-related visit to an emergency department. Traumatic brain injury (TBI) may also be the result of drugs and alcohol, violence, and sports-related injuries.

Pathophysiology

Mild head trauma is usually the result of a sudden deceleration injury or rotation force that causes shearing forces within the brain. These forces cause axonal and blood vessel disruptions. Injury to small blood vessels can manifest themselves as petechial hemorrhages; or, if the bridging veins connecting the cortex to the venous sinuses are involved, acute subdural hematomas may occur, which are potentially fatal. In contrast, subarachnoid hemorrhages, with their resultant meningeal findings including extreme headache and neck stiffness, result far more commonly from ruptured intracranial saccular aneurysms, also called berry aneurysms (greater than 80% of cases), rather than from trauma.

The area of cerebral injury becomes ischemic and edematous. As edema increases, the autoregulatory control of intracranial vessels is lost. The blood–brain barrier breaks down, resulting in increased loss of fluid into the brain parenchyma, which in turn results in increased

Table 19.5	Patient Education: Arthropod Bites and Stings

- Avoid mowing lawns or working with flowering ornamentals when bees and wasps are collecting nectar.
- Stand still if a stinging insect is near you. If it attacks, brush it off (do not slap at it) to prevent a sting.
- Do not walk in the yard in bare feet.
- Wear gloves when gardening.
- Keep garbage cans covered outdoors. Sweet items like soft drinks, ripened fruits, and watermelons attract bees and wasps.
- Avoid perfumes, hair sprays, and colognes.
- Pick fruit as it ripens and dispose of rotten fruits.
- If you are attacked by a swarm of bees, wasps, yellow jackets, or hornets, leave the area immediately, using your arms to protect your face.
- Control wasps by applying insecticides to the nest.
- Avoid areas where insect exposure is likely to occur and always wear shoes when outdoors.
- Avoid wearing perfumes, after-shave lotions, and brightly colored clothing outdoors because these attract insects.
- If you are severely allergic to bee or wasp stings or to any medication, wear medical identification jewelry indicating the anaphylaxis-causing substance or event.
- Check bathrobes and bed sheets for spiders if you are about to use them after a long absence.
- When you enter an attic or storeroom to open cardboard boxes, give the brown recluse spiders a chance to vacate, because they will avoid you if they can.
- Have someone try to capture the spider for identification. Immediately seek health care, and contact the local poison control center.
- Treat pets for ticks by using dusts, dips, or sprays.
- When you enter tick-infested areas, keep clothing buttoned, shirts tucked inside trousers, and trousers inside boots.
- Wear light-colored clothing because this makes it easier to spot ticks; lighter clothing is also less attractive to biting flies.
- Do not sit on the ground or on logs in brushy areas.
- Keep brush cleared or pruned along frequently traveled areas. Use repellents to protect exposed skin; however, ticks will crawl over treated skin to untreated parts of the body.
- For treatment of flea infestations, treat not only the pet, but also professionally fumigate the house.
- If you are going into areas suspected of being infested with chiggers, wear protective clothing and use repellents.
- Apply a repellent containing *N,N*-diethyl-3-methylbenzamide (commonly known as DEET) and wear permethrin-impregnated fabric.
- Apply repellents to legs, ankles, cuffs, waist, and sleeves, either to clothing or directly to the body as directed by the repellant's label.
- Avoid unnecessary use of lights at campsites, and camp in a site that is high, dry, open, and uncluttered.

intracranial pressure (ICP). As ICP increases, cerebral blood flow decreases, leading to tissue hypoxia, a decrease in the serum pH level, and an increase in the carbon dioxide level. This process leads to cerebral vasodilation and edema, which further increases the ICP (a vicious cycle). The increased ICP causes compromise in cerebral perfusion that, if not treated and reversed, leads to increasing hypoxia and secondary brain injury. If the condition remains untreated, the brain herniates downward toward the brainstem, causing irreversible brain damage. A summary of the clinical features of ICP and management guidelines is provided in Table 19.6.

Cerebral Contusion

A *cerebral contusion* is a focal brain injury involving cortical bruising, and, at times, vessel lacerations. This is one of the most common cerebral injuries; it is associated with hemorrhage, edema, and brain swelling. Contusions are classified as *coup* (injury directly beneath the

point of impact) or *contrecoup* (injury directly opposite the point of impact). Temporal and frontal lobes are the most common sites affected. Contusions are graded as mild or severe and superficial or deep. Superficial contusions usually involve the cortical and subcortical tissue, whereas deep contusions penetrate the white matter.

Concussion

A *concussion* involves diffuse brain injury. It is associated with a transient loss of consciousness that occurs immediately following nonpenetrating blunt head trauma. Most patients with only a brief loss of consciousness (less than 5 minutes) are not admitted to the hospital if their subsequent neurological exam remains within normal limits. However, close observation by a responsible adult educated in the warning signs of neurological deterioration is critical for at least the next 24 hours.

A mild concussion is associated with a slightly longer loss of consciousness. It classically presents with confusion,

Table 19.6   Clinical Features and Management of Increased Intracranial Pressure (ICP)

0–15 mm Hg: normal
>15 mm Hg: increased

Clinical Features	Management to Reduce ICP
Decrease in level of consciousness	Elevation of head
Headache	Restriction of fluids
Nausea	Acetazolamide (Diamox) 250 mg 4 times daily
Vomiting	Induced hyperventilation
Amnesia	IV mannitol (Osmitrol) infusion
Agitation, restlessness	IV furosemide (Lasix)
Increased BP with a widening pulse pressure	Possible surgical evacuation of hematoma
Decreased pulse rate	
Changes in respiratory rate and pattern	
Papilledema, one or both eyes	

Pupil Assessment

PERL—pupils equal and react to light
PERRL—pupils equal, round, and react to light
PERRLA—pupils equal, round, react to light and accommodation

disorientation, and, at times, retrograde amnesia (inability to recall events surrounding the injury) or post-traumatic amnesia. The confusion and disorientation usually last only minutes, but recurrent dizziness, headache, and difficulty concentrating may last for months.

A classic concussion, resulting from a loss of consciousness of less than 6 minutes, typically produces retrograde and post-traumatic amnesia and mild neurological impairment. The duration of amnesia can be a predictor of severity: The longer the amnesia, the more severe the concussion. Severe concussions usually have a normal head computed tomography (CT) scan and neurological exam; however, these patients are typically admitted to the hospital for close observation.

Postconcussion syndrome is usually associated with mild head trauma. The syndrome consists of the following signs and symptoms, which can start as early as 1 day post-trauma and persist up to 6 months after injury: headaches, dizziness, fatigue, irritability, insomnia, anxiety, impaired concentration, and loss of memory. Loss of consciousness does not have to occur for postconcussion syndrome to develop, and it is estimated that up to 50% of patients who suffer mild head trauma will develop this syndrome.

Skull Fracture

Skull fracture may occur with a severe blow to the head. Skull fracture increases the risk of underlying epidural or subdural hematoma. Basilar skull fractures (fracture of the base of the skull) can occur as an extension of fracture in another area of the skull. Basilar skull fractures can cause leakage of cerebrospinal fluid (CSF), an entry point for bacteria leading to meningitis, or pneumocephalus (air entry into the CSF-filled spaces within the head). Key

clinical manifestations associated with basilar skull fracture are hemotympanum (blood behind the tympanic membrane), ecchymosis over the mastoid process ("Battle's sign"), or periorbital ecchymosis ("raccoon sign"). Routine x-ray films may not reveal skull fracture; therefore, radiographs are usually nondiagnostic and can cost precious minutes of critical-care time. The clinician should be aware that basilar skull fracture is a clinical diagnosis and proceed immediately with a head CT. CSF may leak through the cribriform plate region of the skull causing nasal CSF rhinorrhea. Patients with suspected skull fracture require careful examination of the cranial nerves. Cranial nerves (CNs) that are likely to be injured include the olfactory nerve (CN I), optic nerve (CN II), oculomotor nerve (CN III), trochlear nerve (CN IV), trigeminal nerve (CN V), abducens nerve (CN VI), facial nerve (CN VII), and acoustic nerve (CN VIII).

Epidural Hematoma

Severe head trauma can cause intracranial bleeding that can put pressure on the brain tissue. The brain is surrounded by the *meninges,* three layers of protective membranes. The layers from the cranial bone going interiorly consist of the dura mater, arachnoid membrane, and pia mater (see Fig. 19.2). Between each membrane is a compartment or space where blood from ruptured vessels can collect. Between the cranial bone and dura mater is the epidural space. The middle meningeal artery courses through this space and can rupture when the cranium (skull) is fractured. The middle meningeal artery runs tightly along the wall of the cranial bone, forming grooves in the bone. With a skull fracture, this artery is easily ruptured and bleeds rapidly within the epidural space, resulting in an *epidural hematoma.* The volume of

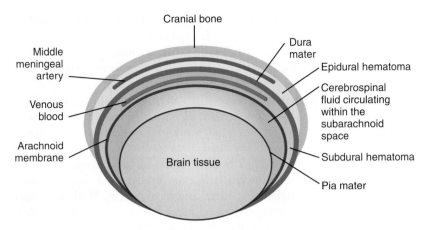

Figure 19.2 The layers of the meninges, cranial circulation, and location of hematomas. *(Courtesy of Teri Capriotti, DO, MSN, CRNP.)*

blood may be large enough to displace the brain, causing neurological deficits and coma within hours after skull injury. Skull x-ray films reveal a fracture line that passes through a groove on the cranium. A head CT scan can visualize the region of the bleed, and brain dysfunction is due primarily to parenchymal compression, which can be relieved with evacuation of blood from the epidural space. A head CT should be considered by the clinician in any head injured patient who meets any of the following criteria:

• Is on anticoagulants, or those with a history of bleeding dyscrasias
• Has sustained loss of consciousness
• Has an altered mental status
• Is suspected of alcohol or drug ingestion
• Has vomited repeatedly
• Has a Glasgow coma scale below 15
• Is older than age 60
• Has a Battle's or raccoon sign
• Is an infant with suspected shaken baby syndrome

Subdural Hematoma

Head trauma can also cause a *subdural hematoma,* which is a venous bleed. Venous bleeding occurs within the subdural space—the compartment between the dura mater and arachnoid membrane (see Fig. 19.2). A venous bleed is slow and will clot off in a short amount of time. Thus, a subdural hematoma may develop slowly over days to weeks and can be due to relatively mild head trauma. Thus, subdural hematomas may be acute (less than 72 hours old), subacute (between 3 and 20 days old), or chronic (greater than 20 days old). Acute subdural hematomas most commonly result from traumatic rupture of the bridging veins, which span the cortex and the dural venous sinuses. If such acute bleeds require surgical intervention and are not rapidly treated within several hours after injury, mortality rates are strikingly high (up to 90%).

In contrast, chronic subdural hematomas pose less of a mortality threat. The majority originate from subdural hygromas, which are potential spaces formed between the dura mater and the brain surface following separation of the dura–arachnoid interface due to ischemic or traumatic brain injury or atrophy resulting in a loss of brain parenchyma. These spaces become filled with CSF. A neomembrane eventually forms that lines the space, becoming a site of neovascularization by fragile intracranial vessels prone to rupture and formation of the chronic subdural hematoma.

Neurological deficits may not be noted until a large volume of blood is present. Brain dysfunction is due primarily to parenchymal compression, which can be relieved with evacuation of blood from the subdural space. CT scans and x-ray studies may not clearly reveal a subdural hematoma, making it difficult to diagnose. Magnetic resonance imaging (MRI) can show displaced brain tissue away from the skull, which is a key finding of subdural hematoma. Patients on anticoagulants, with coagulation deficiencies, or with liver impairment are particularly susceptible to subdural hematomas. Alcohol abusers are also susceptible to subdural hematomas, which may be a subacute as well as an acute condition. It can be a slowly evolving source of increased intracranial pressure.

Clinical Presentation
Subjective

A full history of the event causing the head injury is needed. This should include the mechanism of injury, an approximation of the amount of force involved with the trauma (if the event was witnessed), and whether the patient experienced loss of consciousness (LOC). Epidural hematomas are especially characterized by the patient losing consciousness briefly, then a brief "lucid" moment when the patient may be awake and talking, followed by a momentary unconsciousness occurring minutes after the injury, then becoming increasingly symptomatic, possibly progressing to coma. If a family member or friend is with the patient, the clinician should ask that person if the patient appears normal; a person close to the patient can identify subtle changes that the clinician may not recognize. Patients may complain of headaches and confusion. When a patient complains of "the worst headache of my life," the clinician should suspect a subarachnoid bleed or subarachnoid hemorrhage.

Clinical presentation depends on the structures involved. General symptoms include behavior, motor, and speech deficits. Intoxicated patients present clinical challenges. Signs and symptoms of cerebral injury can be masked by alcohol intoxication. These patients require a head CT scan, close monitoring, and serial neurological exams until they are sober because their history and initial physical exam will be unreliable.

Objective

A patient presenting with a head injury should receive a rapid neurological exam to rule out significant cerebral injury. This exam should include checking mental status, cranial nerves, extremity strength, deep tendon reflexes, and cerebellar function. Hypoactive reflexes may result from damage to the spinal cord.

The Glasgow Coma Scale (GCS) may also be used to rapidly evaluate the level of consciousness (see Advanced Assessment 19.2). The GCS establishes baseline data in each of three areas; eye opening, motor response, and verbal response. A numerical score is assigned according to the chart. A score of 15 represents normal neurological function; a score of 7 usually indicates an unconscious patient, and a score of 3 represents a deep coma state. With any head trauma, the GCS should be done at least every 2 hours to assess for any changes.

The clinician may note bradycardia, hypotension, somnolence, seizures, and focal deficits. With a cerebral hemorrhage, these clinical features generally develop immediately after the trauma. These symptoms develop several hours after the injury with an acute epidural hemorrhage. An acute subdural hemorrhage may occur in a day or months after the head trauma.

All patients should be monitored for signs of increased ICP (see Table 19.6). The early signs of increased ICP are headache, nausea and vomiting, amnesia, altered

---

Advanced Assessment 19.2   Rapid Neurological Exam

Level of Consciousness

Glasgow Coma Scale

Motor response	6	Follows commands
	5	Localizes pain on stimulus
	4	Withdraws from painful stimulus
	3	Shows abnormal flexion in response to pain
	2	Shows abnormal extension in response to pain
	1	No response
Verbal response	5	Oriented
	4	Confused
	3	Inappropriate words
	2	Unintelligible sounds
	1	No responses
Eye-opening	4	Spontaneous
	3	Opens eyes on verbal command
	2	Opens eyes on painful stimulus
	1	No response

Score: 15 = normal; <7 = coma.

Mental Status

FOGS

Family story
Orientation
General information
Spelling

Calculations

Count backward from 100 by 7s or repeat a three-digit number.

Recall

Recall two objects.

Advanced Assessment 19.2   Rapid Neurological Exam—cont'd

Cranial Nerves

CN I	Olfactory	Smell (not usually assessed during acute exam)
CN II	Optic	Visual acuity, gross visual fields, funduscopic exam
CN III	Oculomotor	Pupillary response, eye movement (upward and medial gaze)
CN IV	Trochlear	Eye movement (downward and medial gaze)
CN V	Trigeminal	Teeth clenching, corneal reflex
CN VI	Abducens	Eye movement (lateral)
CN VII	Facial	Frown, smile, and puff cheeks; assess symmetry
CN VIII	Acoustic	Hearing
CN IX	Glossopharyngeal	Gag reflex
CN X	Vagus	Swallowing, gag reflex
CN XI	Spinal accessory	Shrug shoulders and turn head; assess strength and symmetry
CN XII	Hypoglossal	Articulation and tongue movement

Gross Motor Strength and Symmetry

Upper and lower extremities	Look for symmetry and strength.

Cerebellar Function

Romberg's test	Look for stability and pronator drift.
Coordination	Finger to nose and heel to shin
Reflexes	Biceps, triceps, patellar, Achilles, Babinski

level of consciousness, changes in speech, drowsiness, agitation, restlessness, and/or loss of judgment. Any of these signs should prompt the caretaker to take the patient to the ED immediately.

Late signs of increased ICP are dilated, nonreactive pupils (from pressure on the oculomotor nerve), unresponsiveness to verbal or painful stimuli, abnormal posturing patterns (e.g., flexion, extension, or flaccidity), increased systolic blood pressure resulting in a widening pulse pressure, decreased pulse rate, and changes in respiratory rate and pattern. The last three are known as the *Cushing response or reflex.* The late signs are usually observed in patients who are hospitalized and currently being monitored.

In addition, a patient with a basilar skull fracture should be assessed for the following:

Hemotympanum—blood behind the tympanic membrane
Battle's sign—ecchymosis over the mastoid process
Raccoon sign—periorbital ecchymosis
Rhinorrhea with CSF, or ear drainage with CSF
Alterations with cranial nerve function:
- CN I, olfactory nerve—anosmia, may experience loss of smell, or hyposmia
- CN II, optic nerve blindness, field cuts

- CN III, oculomotor nerve—assess for PERL problems indicative of increased ICP, loss of eye movements, diplopia, ptosis, dilated or unreactive pupil
- CN IV, trochlear nerve—impaired downward gaze, diplopia
- CN V, facial nerve—loss of sensation, absent blink/corneal reflex, muscle atrophy
- CN VI, abducens nerve—eye fails to abduct, diplopia
- CN VII, facial nerve—if lower motor neuron affected—ipsilateral (same side) weakness of entire side of face, loss of corneal reflex. If upper motor neuron affected—contralateral (opposite side)
- Weakness of lower half of face
- Lost, delayed, or metallic taste
- CN VIII, acoustic nerve—dizziness, hearing loss

Diagnostic Reasoning
Diagnostic Tests

For mild head injuries, if the patient did not have a loss of consciousness and did not exhibit focal neurological signs or have a history of significant mechanism of injury, close monitoring by a responsible adult is appropriate.

Patients with a history of LOC, significant mechanism of injury (which includes a fall that is equal to their height), a GCS score of 14 or less, impaired alertness or memory, a palpable depressed fracture, signs of increased ICP, positive findings on a rapid neurological exam, or a documented skull fracture should have a head CT scan. A plain CT scan is indicated; CT with contrast is not indicated for minor head trauma. If a cerebral hemorrhage is found, emergent surgery is indicated.

Electroencephalography (EEG) may be helpful when a post-traumatic seizure disorder is suspected. A lumbar puncture may be done for support in diagnosing subarachnoid hemorrhage as indicated by the presence of red blood cells, elevated proteins, and a moderate reduction in glucose. A lumbar puncture is contraindicated in an intracerebral hemorrhage because it may precipitate a herniation syndrome in patients with a large hematoma. MRI can show displaced brain tissue away from the skull, a key finding with a subdural hematoma.

Differential Diagnosis

Typically, a patient with a head trauma will present following an injury, making the diagnosis obvious. However, if a closed head injury occurred and the patient is comatose, other conditions that can result in coma must be ruled out, such as drug overdose, cerebrovascular accident, diabetic ketoacidosis, neuromuscular disorders, and so on.

Management

Emergency Management

A thorough history and physical exam are necessary for any patient who presents with a head injury. Immobilization should be maintained until the patient is fully awake and CT findings are negative. It cannot be stressed enough that a head CT needs to be ordered on any head-injured patient who is on anticoagulant medication such as warfarin or clopidigrel. (See Nursing Research–Based Practice 19.1 for a study related to CT orders.)

General Management

A patient with a minor head injury may be sent home with a competent caregiver who is able to follow the instructions listed under Patient Education. Management of patients with traumatic brain injuries is presented in Table 19.7.

Patients with temporal cerebral injury can be problematic because these structures are close to the tentorium and midbrain. Progressive edema can lead to elevated ICP and herniation. It is important that the clinician repeat neurological assessments often to look for subtle changes that represent early signs of increased ICP. The earlier these signs are identified and treatment is begun, the better the prognosis for the patient.

An abstract of an article on using healing touch as a complementary therapy for traumatic injuries in general is provided in Nursing Research–Based Practice 19.2.

Follow-up and Referral

A patient with a mild head injury who is sent home with a competent caregiver may not need any follow-up unless problems develop. The patient and caregiver must be alert to signs and symptoms of increased ICP. Very small bleeds may not be revealed on the initial head CT and can bleed insidiously. Patients and family members should verbalize understanding of discharge instructions and return accordingly. (See Patient Education.)

The patient with a severe head injury will be followed by a neurosurgeon. The patient may be discharged from the hospital directly to a rehabilitation facility and will be followed by their staff.

Research has shown that the prevalence of any psychiatric illness in the first year after moderate to severe TBI approached 49%, and it approached 34% after mild TBI. Persons with a mild TBI with prior psychiatric illness had evidence of persisting psychiatric illness. Patients with any TBI should be followed closely and monitored for any affective disorders to determine the need for early postinjury psychiatric intervention.

Patient Education

The patient with a mild head injury should be with a responsible adult for the first 24 hours after injury. Decreased activity and light diet are recommended for the first 24 hours. The patient should be awakened every 2 to 4 hours during the first 24 hours. The patient should report back if he or she develops vomiting, an inability

---

Nursing Research–Based Practice 19.1

Brown, R, and Furyk, J. Racial disparities in health care—emergency department management of minor head injury. *Int J Emerg Med* 2(3):161–166, 2009.

International research has demonstrated disparities in the emergency department (ED) care of patients of certain racial or ethnic backgrounds. The management of minor head injuries requires a careful clinical assessment to determine the requirement of a CT scan of the head. This study used a retrospective, structured, medical record review of 270 patients presenting to an ED with minor head injury. The findings showed no statistically significant disparity based on race in the management of minor head injuries with regard to decision to perform a CT head scan. There is some evidence that indigenous patients waited longer to be seen.

Table 19.7	Traumatic Brain Injuries (TBIs)		
Injury	Clinical Features	Diagnosis	Management
Concussion	Brief loss of consciousness (<5 minutes) Mild concussion—slightly longer loss of consciousness, confusion, disorientation, retrograde amnesia, recurrent dizziness, headache, dizziness, vertigo, difficulty concentrating, bradycardia, hypotension, transient neurological deficits, visual disturbances	History MRI Positron emission tomography	Close observation for 24 hours Nonnarcotic pain medications
Cerebral Contusion	Longer loss of consciousness Changes in personality, behavior, and speech deficits Intracranial pressure (ICP) elevation	History	Monitor Glasgow Coma Scale (GCS) Neurological consultant
Basilar Skull Fracture	Hemotympanism—blood behind tympanic membrane Battle's sign—ecchymosis over mastoid process Raccoon sign—periorbital ecchymosis CSF rhinorrhea Alterations in cranial nerve functioning CSF otorrhea	Cranial nerve examination Skull x-ray films CT	Monitor GCS Neurological consultant Antibiotics if infection present Rare—intracranial surgical repair Monitor intracranial pressure
Epidural Hematoma	Brief loss of consciousness → lucid moment → longer period of loss of consciousness Headache, confusion, somnolence, seizures, focal deficits, pupil abnormalities (unilateral and eventual bilateral pupil dilation and decreased reactivity to light) Hemiparesis or hemiplegia, flexion or extension posturing	CT scan	Monitor GCS Neurological consultant With a significant mass effect—immediate surgical evacuation and ligation of bleeding vessels; if not possible, burr holes to evacuate hematoma
Subdural Hematoma (SDH)	Extreme headache, neck stiffness Progressive decrease in level of consciousness, ataxia, seizures, incontinence, and eventual pupil and motor function alterations With severe SDH, GCS usually <8	MRI	Neurological consultant Monitor ICP Monitor GCS Surgical intervention

---

Nursing Research–Based Practice 19.2

Burr, JP. Jayne's story: Healing touch as a complementary treatment for trauma recovery. *Holistic Nurs Pract* 19(2): 211–216, 2005.

 Trauma recovery is a complex process. Present research acknowledges the difficulties of trauma recovery and limited conventional treatment options. Human biofield therapies are used successfully in a variety of settings for various patient complaints. The practices of human biofield manipulation; healing touch; and its predecessor, therapeutic touch, are effective holistic therapies that treat body, mind, and spirit to improve physiological and psychological complaints, health perception, and well-being. Jayne's story illustrates the beneficial integration of healing touch as a complementary therapeutic option in recovery from motor vehicle collision trauma. Support for incorporating healing touch therapy in the recovery regimen of individuals recuperating from trauma is suggested.

to move his or her arms or legs equally well, a temperature of 100°F (37.7°C), a stiff neck, pupils of unequal size or shape, convulsions, severe headache that does not go away with acetaminophen or ibuprofen, confusion, disorientation, or a change in personality or behavior. These signs and symptoms are indicative of increased ICP and demand immediate attention in the ED.

■ MUSCULOSKELETAL TRAUMA

Musculoskeletal trauma refers to injuries involving the musculoskeletal system. These injuries may present as minor innocuous wounds or with obvious deformities. The clinician needs to resist the urge to treat the obvious deformity or fracture and neglect looking for the occult injury. Musculoskeletal sequelae can be associated with or caused by problems in other systems—neurological, endocrine, nutritional, or psychological. A thorough history and physical examination are required to rule out other bodily system involvement. This section discusses the musculoskeletal trauma of sprains, strains, and fractures.

Epidemiology and Causes

Musculoskeletal injuries are one of the most common injuries seen in the office and emergency/urgent care setting. Patients of all ages are susceptible to injury. The annual cost of caring for people with musculoskeletal system injuries is in the billions of dollars. The loss of productivity to industry is staggering. Musculoskeletal disorders as a frequent cause of work disability account for productivity losses equivalent to 1.3% of the gross national product. There is an increase in the incidence of injuries among the younger population that can be attributed to a higher participation in sports and riskier recreational activities such as in-line skating (rollerblading) and skiing.

Fitness classes and field sports are the most common culprits associated with musculoskeletal injuries in the younger population. Racket sports, walking, and low-intensity sports are associated with injuries in older adults. Usually the lower extremities are involved, especially the knees and ankles. Older patients tend to have more overuse injuries, such as metatarsalgia, plantar fasciitis, and meniscal knee injuries. Younger patients tend to have more patellofemoral syndromes and stress fractures.

Knees and ankles are the most common sites injured in high school athletes. Sprains and strains are by far the most common type of injuries.

Occupational strains occur more often in the morning hours and in the first 4 hours of the work shift. Days earlier in the week, especially Monday, have a higher incidence of injury. Married workers aged 30 to 50 years are injured more frequently than other individuals. The occupations associated with a higher than average risk include nurses and truck drivers.

Americans have a fracture rate of approximately 21.1/1,000 per year (23.5 per year per 1,000 males and 18.8 per year per 1,000 females), which is very similar to the rate in other industrialized countries. Males aged 15 to 49 years are almost three times more likely to sustain a fracture than females of the same age. There are three main peaks of fractures distribution—first among young adult males, second among older adults (affecting elderly men and women equally), and last, an increase in fractures, especially of the wrist, in women older than age 40 years.

Pathophysiology
Sprains and Strains

A *strain* involves microscopic and macroscopic tears or stretching of muscle fibers. These injuries require more than just muscle contraction to occur; excessive stretching or stretching while the muscle is being activated is required. The injury usually occurs within the muscle's normal range of motion. The portion of the muscle that is typically injured is at the muscle–tendon junction. Research has shown that muscles that cross multiple joints or have a complex architecture are more susceptible to strains. Muscles most frequently injured include the hamstring, rectus femoris, gastrocnemius, and adductor longus muscles. A severe strain to the rectus femoris, hamstring, or abdominal wall muscles has been shown to have a poor prognosis for rehabilitation and may benefit from surgical repair.

A *sprain* is caused by stretching or twisting beyond the normal range of motion of a joint or musculo–ligamentous unit. A sprain can be impossible to differentiate from a strain during the physical exam. Injuries involving joints are usually sprains because ligaments are more prominent around joint capsules. A history of overuse and/or excessive force, as opposed to a fall, hyperextension, or twisting of a joint, is more likely related to a strain. If bony tenderness at the injury site is found during the physical exam, x-ray films are required to rule out fractures. A high suspicion of fracture is required, especially in the young and in older adults. The young are not able to provide an accurate history and full cooperation during the physical exam. Many minor fractures (such as a torus fracture) are missed because the child does not complain and the parents or guardians are not aware of an injury. Older adults can have blunted pain sensation, especially to the extremities, related to neuropathies. The clinician should be aware of this and should be very astute when considering x-ray studies on these populations.

Fractures

A *fracture* is a break in the continuity of a bone; a fracture is usually associated with a blunt force. Fractures are classified as *open* or *closed,* depending on whether they communicate with the atmosphere. Open fractures have an increased incidence of infection and must be aggressively treated. Many need to be surgically irrigated.

Fractures can also be partial or complete. A *partial fracture* involves disruption of only a portion of the cortex, whereas a *complete fracture* involves circumferential disruption in the cortex. Complete fractures are unstable; inappropriate initial stabilization can lead to additional injuries to the muscles or neurovascular structures.

When assessing the patient, the clinician should ask about the mechanism of injury. Fractures can occur at locations other than the obvious site of injury. The force can be transmitted to other areas of the body, causing fractures. A person who fell off a roof and landed on his or her feet may have an obvious calcaneus (heel bone) fracture, but fractures of the hips, pelvis, and back must also be ruled out.

The goal of fracture management is to align the bones in a near-normal plane in order to allow the fragmented ends to heal together and return to normal function. The initial phase of healing starts with hematoma formation. This bridges the fractured fragments. The inflammatory phase follows, and granulation tissue is formed on the fracture surfaces. During this process, the hematoma is reabsorbed, which provides the first continuity between the fragments. This takes place approximately 10 to 14 days after injury. During this time, the bone surrounding the fracture line becomes less dense. This makes the fracture line easier to identify. Callus is then formed on both the periosteal and endosteal surfaces of the bone; the callus acts as a biological splint. The calcification of the bone then begins: First, calcium phosphate is deposited, and then the bone undergoes osseous metaplasia. It takes approximately 2 to 3 weeks for the callus to be visible on x-ray film. The callus is then slowly reabsorbed, and the fracture surfaces develop a firm bony union. During this phase, the calcified region undergoes organization, and the peripheral margins begin to smoothen. The process ends with remodeling, then consolidation.

In a healthy adult, the whole process takes approximately 2 months for smaller long bones (such as the humerus) and up to 4 months for large bones (such as the femur). Oblique fractures typically heal more quickly than transverse ones. Children tend to heal more quickly, and older patients more slowly.

Radiologic (x-ray) evidence of abundant callus formation at the fracture site that is organized, and bone ends that have remained stable on serial films, means the fracture should be stable enough to remove the cast. Limited activity is recommended until full strength is returned.

Clinical Presentation
Subjective

The signs of any musculoskeletal injury involve one or more of the following: pain, swelling, deformity, disability, abnormal motion, and tenderness. The history and mechanism of injury will help guide the physical exam. It will help to focus on obvious and occult areas of injury.

Documentation of the mechanism in the history is important. It is imperative that occult injuries are identified.

Objective

The importance of performing a thorough and complete physical exam cannot be emphasized enough. Life-threatening injuries must be identified quickly. This is facilitated by completing a quick primary survey, which can be accomplished in 90 seconds by an experienced practitioner. Following the primary survey, the more complete and thorough secondary survey can be performed. This is when fractures should be identified.

Diagnostic Reasoning
Diagnostic Tests

It is imperative that suspected sites of musculoskeletal trauma be radiographed to rule out fractures. Radiographic (x-ray) studies are the mainstay of orthopedic care. It is important that the clinician order the correct x-ray exam for the injury suspected. There are evidence-based guidelines to help clinicians choose the most appropriate imaging exam for patients' clinical conditions. The latest version of the American College of Radiology (ACR) Appropriateness Criteria is located at www.acr.org/Quality-Safety/Appropriateness-Criteria. Many x-ray studies will include views of several joints and bones. The clinician must resist ruling out fractures in regions other than the area the specific x-ray exam ordered is intended to reveal. Each x-ray study has a specific technique that ensures that the correct angles, bony structures, and other information are included to allow the practitioner to rule out pathology to that specific region. If a patient has pain in the foot and the ankle, an ankle x-ray film will miss foot pathology, and a foot x-ray film will miss ankle pathology. Advanced Assessment 19.3 presents tips on reading an extremity x-ray film.

Many providers will order routine comparison views of the uninjured extremity, especially in children with open growth plates. This may be helpful on rare occasions. Unfortunately, many x-ray technicians have this as "standing orders" from their facility. This practice should not be condoned, because it exposes a growing child to unnecessary radiation when a thorough exam usually pinpoints the location of the injury. When examining an infant or a child who will not move or bear weight on an extremity, the clinician should palpate the entire extremity while observing the patient's facial expressions. Once the injury is palpated, the patient's face will reveal discomfort, which will assist the clinician in localizing the injured site.

Differential Diagnosis

The goal of differential diagnosis in musculoskeletal trauma is to distinguish more serious bony fractures from strains and sprains, because these injuries are

Advanced Assessment 19.3   Reading an Extremity X-Ray Film

- Conduct a thorough history and determine the mechanism of injury. This will help to determine the location and type of injury to expect. The area of injury should be examined. These procedures will focus your attention to the area of suspicion on the film. Always review the x-ray film after the exam, even if you viewed it before examining the patient.
- Using a well-lighted viewing box, follow the cortex of the injured area, looking for any defects. The cortex should be smooth and crisp; any area of haziness or any defect needs to be scrutinized using a bright (hot) light.
- Look at the soft tissue surrounding the area of concern. Injuries will cause soft tissue swelling. This may help focus your attention on the injured area. Scrutinize this region with a bright (hot) light.
- Several regions of the body, especially joints, have certain signs to look for that may reflect an occult injury. Confer with the collaborating physician or refer the patient to an orthopedic physician.

treated differently. As joint swelling and tenderness is a common presentation of such injuries, it is also critical to consider a variety of rheumatological and infectious disorders, such as a septic joint, rheumatoid arthritis, or osteoarthritis. An appropriate history that seeks to characterize any preceding musculoskeletal trauma typically readily differentiates these conditions. However, if suspected, basic laboratory tests such as a CBC may also be helpful.

The differential diagnosis for fractures also includes *reflex sympathetic dystrophy.* Also known as Sudeck atrophy and causalgia, this is a post-traumatic syndrome with three clinical stages—*early, dystrophic,* and *atrophic.* Early in the condition, a constant aching or burning occurs in the affected limb. Motion or external stimulation increases the symptoms, usually out of proportion to the original injury. The dystrophic stage follows in which the skin of the affected extremity becomes glossy and cold and range of motion is limited. Finally, the atrophic stage is marked by skin atrophy and contracture. No correlation exists between incidence or symptom severity and the extent or type of the original musculoskeletal injury. Thus, early diagnosis of this syndrome is difficult, especially after an apparently trivial injury. Early diagnosis is extremely important, however, because the earlier treatment is initiated, the better the response. Treatment is aimed toward restoration of function through physical therapy. Antidepressant therapy may be beneficial, as may prednisone.

Management

Emergency Management

Emergency management of the patient with musculoskeletal trauma initially consists of RICE therapy discussed below. If the patient can be seen immediately in the primary-care office with radiographic capabilities, the patient may choose to see the clinician. If not, the patient should go directly to the ED.

General Management: Sprains and Strains

After appropriate stabilization and 2 to 3 days of rest and elevation, the injury site can be examined more easily.

The pain and swelling typically will be reduced, which will facilitate a better physical exam. Injuries that had negative x-ray studies initially but were extremely painful or were suspicious for fracture can be reradiographed in 10 to 12 days. Because of the healing process, the fracture line can be more easily visualized at that time.

RICE Therapy   Rest, ice, compression, and elevation (RICE) are the mainstay of all musculoskeletal injury treatment. The amount of rest needed depends on the severity of the injury.

Rest means no use of the affected limb or joint, for minor injuries or sprains for 1 to 2 days, then slow progression as tolerated by the patient. If the activity being performed causes pain to the injury site, the level of activity needs to be reduced to levels that do not cause pain. Mild discomfort after activity is considered normal during the rehabilitation phase.

Ice, a potent anti-inflammatory, should be applied 30 minutes on and 30 minutes off, three to five times per day, to the injury site. Ice is also recommended during the rehabilitation phase if mild pain after activity is experienced. Ice therapy for 24 to 48 hours after the injury is recommended. After that period, warm, moist heat to the region is advocated to increase the circulation to the area, which promotes reabsorption of blood and edema that has collected at the injury site.

Compression by elastic wrap or other splinting material is used to provide counterpressure at the site of injury to help tamponade bleeding to the region. This will help decrease the amount of swelling and blood at the injury site. The influx of blood causes localized inflammation, which leads to leaking of plasma and other substances into the area. Instruct the person applying the compression wrap to always include the distal extremity—the foot or hand—to prevent a tourniquet effect.

Elevating the affected limb above the level of the heart will decrease bleeding into the tissue surrounding the injury and help to reduce the pain. After the first 48 hours, when bleeding into the area has stopped, elevation will facilitate reabsorption of blood and fluids at the injury site.

Pain Management   The use of an NSAID for pain management is also recommended in conjunction with RICE therapy. Muscle relaxants such as cyclobenzaprine

(Flexeril) may be indicated for the management of acute painful musculoskeletal conditions associated with muscle spasm. They reduce tonic somatic muscle activity at the level of the brainstem.

General Management: Fractures

Initial fracture care involves stabilization of the bone ends to avoid further injury or damage to neurovascular structures. During the secondary survey, when possible fractures are identified, immediate temporary splinting should be instituted. Severely angulated long bone fractures should be straightened before they are splinted. Splints should be applied in such a way as to immobilize the joints above and below the fracture site to avoid motion of the bone ends involved. Commercially available metal and plastic splints are used for this purpose.

After the radiograph and confirmation of a fracture, a more permanent splint should be applied. During immobilization, the clinician must consider the fact that fracture sites will continue to swell in the first 24 to 48 hours. Placing a rigid circumferential cast on the patient in the first 24 to 48 hours can lead to vascular compromise and compartment syndrome. To avoid this, the patient should be placed in a plaster splint. A plaster splint is placed on only half of the splinted limb and can be adjusted or molded to allow optimal stabilization of certain fractures. The skin should be padded to avoid local necrosis, and the splint should be secured by an elastic bandage. This type of splint allows the extremity to swell without affecting distal circulation.

Even with good technique, some fractures are not visible initially and will not appear until 7 to 10 days after the injury. At that time, the margins of the fracture absorb and will widen the radiolucent line at the fracture site. New bone will also be produced beneath the periosteum at the margins of the fracture, which will accentuate the fracture line. This will allow fractures that were not identified initially to be visualized. If a fracture is suspected but not visible at the initial visit, the injury should be treated as a fracture and reexamined clinically and radiographically in 7 to 10 days. The patient should be informed of the rationale for this treatment. Always add this to the discharge instructions in writing and have the patient sign his or her understanding.

Follow-up and Referral

The patient should be reexamined by an orthopedic surgeon in 3 to 4 days after application of a cast or splint to evaluate his or her neuromuscular status. In addition, the patient should be instructed to report any of the following signs and symptoms, which may reflect compartment syndrome—intense pain, hypoesthesia (a dulled sensitivity to touch), paresthesia (numbness, prickling, or tickling), muscular weakness, or paralysis. The patient with these signs should be referred to an orthopedic surgeon immediately. In 6 weeks to 2 months, a follow-up

with the orthopedic surgeon and an x-ray film will determine whether bone consolidation has occurred and if the cast can be removed.

Patient Education

Any site of a previous bony fracture will be weakened no matter how long after healing, and this site will always be more prone to a second fracture. Patients should always take this into account when deciding on what type of exercise or musculoskeletal activity to engage in.

In the future, it may be possible to predict which patients are at higher risk for fractures. Single bone mineral density measurement may be able to predict the risk of fragility fractures (distal radius, proximal humerus, hip, and vertebra) in women. This would help identify populations who would benefit from teaching and prevention strategies.

To avoid musculoskeletal injury, good physical conditioning is important. Consistent activity and exercise will strengthen muscles and reduce the chance of injury. See Chapter 15 for patient education about ways to prevent musculoskeletal injuries.

■ LOWER BACK PAIN

Up to 80% of the population experiences lower back pain at some time in their lives. A common problem in the workplace due to muscular or ligamentous strain, lower back pain accounts for one of the most frequent causes of days lost from work. Only about 15% of patients have a specific injury.

Pathophysiology

Lumbar spinal nerve impingement is a common cause of lower back pain. Disk herniation produces the deficits predictable for the site involved as listed in Table 19.8.

Clinical Presentation

Subjective

If no accident or trauma is involved, the patient will usually complain of a time-sequence history of symptoms which may be gradual or sudden and may be localized in the lumbosacral area or radiating. If a disc syndrome is present, the patient may complain of radiation into the leg, sensory changes, motor weakness, or difficulties with bowel or bladder function.

Objective

The clinician should perform a neurological examination of the lower extremities that will detect the small deficits produced by disc disease and the large deficits produced by such problems as cauda equina tumors. Performing a straight-leg-raising test may indicate nerve root irritation if radicular pain is produced when the leg is raised 60 degrees or less.

The disc herniation and radiculopathy of lumbar spinal nerves L4 to L5 and L5 to S1 are particularly

Table 19.8	Lumbar Spinal Nerve Impingement/Herniated Disc Signs		
Spinal Nerve Affected	Dermatome; Sensory Deficit	Myotome; Weakness Shown	Reflex Affected
L4	Anterior thigh, medial shin	Quadriceps; knee extension weak	Patellar
L5	Great toe, dorsum of foot	Anterior tibial and extensor hallucis; dorsiflexion of great toe (walking on heels)	
S1	Lateral border of foot, small toe	Gastrocnemius; plantar flexion of foot (walking on toes)	Achilles

Any L4–S1 root irritation can cause "sciatica": pain from buttock down lateral leg; + straight leg raising sign; if patient develops acute bladder, bowel problems, bilateral leg involvement = medical emergency.

Source: Teri Capriotti, DO, MSN, CRNP.

common sources of acute back pain often due to trauma. L4 to L5 and L5 to S1 radiculopathy ("sciatica") may be objectively assessed in terms of dermatome sensory deficit, myotome muscle weakness, and deep tendon reflex deficits as depicted in Table 19.8. The clinician should assess for the inability to walk on toes, inability to walk on heels, and the inability to dorsiflex the great toe, which may relate to specific lumbar spinal nerve involvement.

Classic lower back pain that is less serious involves pain in the lower back with or without pain radiating down one leg.

Diagnostic Reasoning

Diagnostic Tests

In the majority of cases, a precise diagnosis cannot be made. Usually the initial history and physical examination will lead to the diagnosis. The challenge is to identify patients who require more extensive or urgent evaluation. Diagnosis is usually not confirmed by palpation of the spine. Lumbar x-ray films are usually not indicated for patients with acute low back pain unless there is evidence of a possible fracture or a possible tumor or infection. Magnetic resonance imaging (MRI) is reserved for patients who are surgical candidates or who have evidence of systemic disease.

Differential Diagnosis

The differential diagnoses for lower back pain include muscular strain; primary spine disease such as disc herniation or degenerative arthritis; systemic disease, such as metastatic cancer; and regional diseases, such as aortic aneurysm. Patients with systemic disease such as vertebral osteomyelitis typically have a history of smoking, weight loss, age older than 50 years, diabetes mellitus, a history of recurrent urinary tract infections, and cancer. The clinician should be aware of a potential spinal abscess, which is very rare; however, any patient presenting with low back pain, radiculopathy, and fever should have an MRI immediately, because pressure on the

spinal cord may be causing irreversible damage. Low back pain at night, unrelieved by rest of lying supine, may suggest a malignancy, either vertebral body metastasis, multiple myeloma, or a cauda equina syndrome, which is a serious complication of herniated disk and needs emergency medical treatment. Cauda equina syndrome, multiple lumbar nerve root compressions, is a medical emergency; the patient would present with leg weakness or saddle area anesthesia, bowel or bladder incontinence, or impotence.

Low back pain that worsens with rest and seems to improve with activity is usually caused by ankylosing spondylitis or other seronegative spondyloarthropathies, especially with an insidious onset after age 40.

Patients with penetrating peptic ulcer disease may present with back pain, and this should be ruled out as a diagnosis. Patients with endocarditis may present with a cardiac murmur in addition to back pain, and this should be further evaluated. In addition, referred back pain may be a result of renal stones.

Management

The majority of patients with lower back pain will improve in 1 to 4 weeks. Conservative therapy is indicated if all the differential diagnoses are ruled out. Treatment consists of NSAIDs, unless severe pain requires opioids or muscle relaxants, for 1 to 2 weeks. NSAIDs have proven to be as effective as opioids and muscle relaxants, and the latter should be avoided if at all possible. The adage of "let pain be your guide" refers to keeping the patient mobile and ideally staying at work. Patients should not stay in bed for longer than 2 days, unless the pain is due to sciatica, which may require a week in bed. A program of exercise should be developed that allows the patient to return to a normal regimen as soon as possible.

Some patients benefit from heat therapy and some from ice therapy. It is individualistic. When heat is preferred, moist heat for 20 to 30 minutes at least four times per day may be effective. When cold therapy is preferred, ice over the affected area for 10 to 15 minutes every 1 to

2 hours may be effective. Some patients prefer heat alternated with ice.

Intensive rehabilitation for chronic back pain is more cost-effective and results in a reduction of disability and fewer complications than surgery, although research shows that it is slightly less effective than spinal fusion surgery.

Follow-up and Referral

If patients cannot be managed by a general clinician, a specialist may be needed depending on the radiographic or MRI results. Physical therapy may be ordered by the general clinician or by a specialist. Patients should be followed up in 1 week to verify that the injury was in fact lower back pain and not more serious.

Patient Education

All patients should be taught good body mechanics. These include the following:

- Ask for help if the weight is too great to lift by oneself.
- Keep the back straight; lift with the legs.
- Push rather than pull objects.
- Do not twist sideways; face the object to be lifted.
- Use a footstool to lessen back strain.
- Do not sit or stand for prolonged periods of time; move or stretch at least every 30 minutes.
- Sleep on a firm mattress, and sit in a supportive chair.
- Maintain good posture.
- Wear flat, supportive shoes.

An exercise program should be developed to strengthen the back, relieve pressure on compressed nerves, and help protect the patient's back from reinjury. Although most exercises should not be attempted until the episode of acute back pain is resolved, therapeutic exercises may relieve pain.

■ FOREIGN BODY OBSTRUCTIONS

This section discusses ear, nose, throat, vaginal, and rectal foreign body obstructions. Common foreign body obstructions and their treatment are discussed in Table 19.9.

Epidemiology and Causes

Foreign body obstructions are common problems seen in the primary-care setting. Most of these problems involve children. Foreign body obstructions most commonly result from the patient inserting a foreign body into a body orifice.

Pathophysiology

The pathophysiology of a foreign body obstruction depends on which orifice is obstructed. Otic (ear canal) occlusion may contribute to otitis externa or otitis media, especially if the tympanic membrane is ruptured. Nasal occlusion may predispose to rhinitis, sinusitis, or epistaxis (nosebleed). Moreover, nasal, pharyngeal, tracheal, or even esophageal occlusion may all result in varying degrees of respiratory compromise if the respiratory tract is at all obstructed either internally or via external compression on the airway.

Table 19.9   Common Foreign Body Obstructions

Ears

Foreign bodies in the auditory canal are common problems, especially in children. Foreign bodies can be vegetative, inanimate, or animate objects. Foreign bodies in the ear are usually asymptomatic unless they are left in the ear for a prolonged period of time and an infection develops. The clinician should obtain a complete history to elicit whether there is a possibility of multiple foreign bodies. The practitioner should assess both ears to obtain a comparison view. It is important to try to ensure that there is no perforation of the tympanic membrane before trying to remove the foreign body.

Children can have a foreign body in the ear for such a long period that cerumen will eventually mask the foreign body. The clinician will need to have clear views of the tympanic membrane in any child with repeat otitis media symptoms to rule out foreign body.

A live insect trapped in the ear canal usually causes great distress. The patient will present with agitation, nausea, and tearing. The initial therapy is to immobilize the insect. This can be done by placing 2% lidocaine in the external ear canal, which will terminate the movement of the insect. The insect can then be removed.

Removal of inanimate objects is not always straightforward. If the patient is uncooperative or the foreign body is difficult to grasp, ear, nose, and throat (ENT) consultation is suggested. If the object becomes lodged too deeply, it will be difficult to remove, and the patient may need general anesthesia for successful removal. If the object is small, irrigation is an option.

If the object is appropriately shaped and accessible, alligator or bayonet forceps may be used to grasp and remove it. Suctioning may also assist in the removal of an object. A Yankauer suction catheter has a small orifice and a firm catheter tip that may facilitate foreign body removal.

After successful removal of the object, the ear canal needs to be checked for infections, superficial scratches, and tympanic-membrane perforation. If there is no evidence of infection, the patient may be discharged home. If an infection is present, it should be treated as an otitis.

Continued

Table 19.9	Common Foreign Body Obstructions—cont'd

Nose

Nasal foreign bodies are most commonly seen in children. They are usually discovered after purulent discharge is noticed. The history is important, but children are usually reluctant to admit to what or how much they have placed in their nose.

The diagnosis is made by direct visualization. If the patient or child is uncooperative, a restraining device or sedation may be needed. If the patient is cooperative, the following steps may be used to remove the foreign body:
• Help the patient to blow his or her nose to see if the foreign object will come out.
• If the mucosa appear swollen, soak a pledget in Neo-Synephrine and insert it into the nare; care should be taken not to push the foreign body further into the nose.
• Using a nasal speculum and alligator or bayonet forceps, visualize the foreign body and gently remove it. Other methods include using an ear curette, single skin hook, or right-angle ear hook. Another method that has been used is to pass a small urinary catheter superior to (beyond) the object, inflate the balloon, and pull the object out.

All of these methods can be successful if the patient is cooperative. Care must be taken not to push the foreign body down the back of the patient's throat, where it may be aspirated into the trachea.

After successfully removing the object, the clinician should inspect the nares for other foreign bodies. No further treatment is necessary.

If removal is unsuccessful, referral to an ENT specialist may be necessary.

Throat

Swallowed objects are commonly seen by the primary-care provider. Usually, they are not life-threatening, but any object that becomes lodged in a position where it can obstruct the airway is a true emergency. Although most swallowed objects will pass spontaneously, up to 10%–20% require some type of intervention. There are several physiological narrow spaces in the esophageal-gastrointestinal tract that may restrict movement of objects. In the pediatric population, the cricopharyngeal area is the most common site for obstruction, followed by (in order of frequency) the thoracic inlet, aortic arch, tracheal bifurcation, and hiatal narrowing. The majority of obstructions in adults occur at the distal end of the esophagus. Usually once the object has passed through the pylorus, it will pass through the rest of the GI tract without problems. If the object has sharp edges, however, it can injure the intestines and/or become lodged anywhere in the GI tract. Ingested foreign bodies can also cause airway obstruction or perforation.

If the object becomes lodged in the esophagus, the adult patient may present with the feeling of something in the throat, pain, and the inability to swallow secretions. Pediatric patients may present with vomiting, gagging, choking, stridor, inability to swallow, increased salivation, and a sensation of a foreign body in the chest.

If there is a possible foreign body ingestion, a chest x-ray study should be ordered to see if the object is lodged in the esophagus. Foreign bodies will show up only if they are radiopaque. If the object is in the stomach, the patient should be monitored for passage of the object through the GI tract. The stool will need to be examined. If the object is not found, an abdominal flat-plate x-ray film can be used to determine the location of the object. Objects that fail to be expelled may have to be removed by invasive procedures such as colonoscopy or surgery.

A food bolus is usually the cause of ingested foreign bodies in the adult population. Typically, inadequately chewed meat is the main culprit. If the patient is unable to swallow saliva secretions, a chest x-ray film should be obtained. Glucagon, a smooth-muscle relaxant, may be administered intravenously to relax the esophagus. A 1-mg dose is given IV; the dose may be repeated after 20 minutes if the object has not passed. The patient will usually vomit, which causes the foreign body to be expelled; it is important to ensure that the patient does not aspirate the vomitus. If glucagon has not produced a successful effect, a GI consultation should be obtained. Some references recommend a barium swallow to visualize where the obstruction is located; however, most GI specialists prefer that no barium be given because it can obstruct their view of the bolus during endoscopy.

If a coin becomes lodged in the esophagus, it should be removed by endoscopy. Two other methods that may be tried include passing an indwelling urinary catheter behind the object, inflating it, and pulling the object out. Objects that become lodged in the esophagus can be safely pushed into the stomach by a small urinary catheter.

Ingestion of button batteries is a true emergency situation. The batteries can cause burns to the GI mucosa and must be removed quickly.

The treatment for ingestion of a sharp object is controversial. Most practitioners recommend that sharp objects be removed so that they do not cause a perforation before they pass into the intestine.

Vagina

Vaginal foreign bodies can be the result of children exploring their sexuality or an incident of child abuse; in adults, the foreign body may be a forgotten tampon or diaphragm. The only treatment necessary is removal of the foreign body. Most of the discharge and odor will disappear after the foreign body is removed. If the foreign body is lodged in the side

Table 19.9	Common Foreign Body Obstructions—cont'd

wall of the vagina, the clinician should irrigate the area with normal saline to gently remove the object from the wall. If a foreign body is suspected in a small child, general anesthesia for exploration should be considered if the object is not visible and cannot be removed by gently pulling on the labia. Emotional support and reassurance is important to patients. Privacy must be maintained to avoid undue embarrassment.

Rectum
A variety of objects have been inserted into the rectum. They are usually found in the rectal ampulla and are usually palpable with digital examination. All patients presenting with the chief complaint of foreign body in the rectum need x-ray exams of the abdomen to show the position, shape, and number of foreign bodies in the rectum. The x-ray film will also show if free air is present in the abdomen. This is indicative of a perforation of the bowel, which is the most serious potential complication.

Removal of the foreign body from the rectum requires that the rectal sphincter be relaxed. If a brief attempt at removing the foreign body is unsuccessful, the practitioner should consider conscious sedation to relax the sphincter muscle. Conscious sedation requires close monitoring and is best carried out in an inpatient or emergency setting. If there is any possibility of perforation, an emergency GI consultation is needed.

A vaginal occlusion, if unattended, can lead to toxic shock syndrome (mediated by infection with *Staphylococcus aureus* or *Streptococcus pyogenes*) or pelvic inflammatory disease. A bowel obstruction may result from a foreign body occluding the rectum if the object inserted is high enough. Obviously, early diagnosis and intervention will best protect against adverse effects from prolonged obstruction.

Clinical Presentation

Subjective

The patient will present with a complaint of a foreign body, with signs and symptoms specific to the bodily orifice involved. However, if the individual is unaware of the presence of a foreign body, such as in the case of a forgotten tampon left in place, the patient may complain of a foul-smelling vaginal discharge. Alternatively, a nasal or otic occlusion may lead to a feeling of head fullness or headache. Of note, many of these affected patients are children who may or may not be able to fully express their discomfort or pain verbally.

Objective

Based on the patient's complaint and the orifice involved, the signs will vary. A rectal occlusion may cause abdominal cramping, an increase in bowel sounds, and abdominal distention. A vaginal occlusion may result in a foul-smelling vaginal discharge. An insect or piece of cotton caught in the ear may cause equilibrium problems, dizziness, tinnitus, and diminished hearing on the affected side. A foreign body in the nose of an adult is rare.

Diagnostic Reasoning

Diagnostic Tests

Diagnostic tests are usually not indicated, but radiological studies may be appropriate if physical examination is insufficient to fully characterize the obstructing organism. However, because the majority of foreign bodies are not radiopaque, x-ray findings may be quite subtle, requiring formal interpretation by a radiologist. In some cases, direct endoscopy of the nasopharyngeal, respiratory, or gastrointestinal tracts may be required to identify the obstructing object.

Differential Diagnosis

The diagnosis is usually obvious because of the patient's complaint.

Management

Emergency Management

The clinician may attempt to remove the foreign body in the office. If the attempt is unsuccessful, the patient should be sent to the ED.

General Management

See Table 19.9 for general management of ear, nose, throat, vaginal, and rectal foreign body obstructions.

Follow-up and Referral

Follow-up is usually not indicated once the foreign body is removed. The patient should be alerted to signs and symptoms of an infection should one occur after discharge. If a rectal perforation has occurred as a result of a foreign body, an emergency gastroenterology referral is indicated.

Patient Education

Because children are usually involved in foreign body incidents, prevention is essential. Parents should be encouraged to buy age-appropriate toys and to keep small objects out of the reach of children. Also, children should be taught not to put objects in the various orifices of their bodies.

DISASTER PLANNING AND THE JOINT COMMISSION'S STANDARDS

Disaster preparedness has always been a foremost concern for the medical community; however, recent events including natural disasters and acts of terrorism have triggered increased concern. Whether in cities or rural settings, communities rely on the local hospital to be organized and equipped to meet their needs. Unfortunately, some community hospitals are insufficiently staffed in times of need (Level I; The Joint Commission, 2006).

Communications between the ED and other agencies, for example, can be a formidable challenge to effective disaster management. Coordination between departments, agencies, and organizations should focus on exchanging current information, working together for a common cause, and maintaining a clear flow of information. In addition, relief assistance may not arrive for several days, employees may not be willing or able to get to the hospital, and communication disruptions with outside agencies are possible. Recent catastrophes have put hospitals on notice to develop standards; disaster research must be retrospective and applied to reduce future disaster-related morbidity and mortality.

The Joint Commission has required disaster planning for more than 30 years. According to The Joint Commission, disaster planning for hospitals must include critical standards for effectiveness, standards based on lessons learned, and realistic strategies. Each hospital should have these guidelines in the ED, as well as a current reference text on disaster preparedness and management. An emergency planning guide is available online from The Joint Commission (2006), and the World Health Organization also has a Hospital Emergency Response checklist.

 DavisPlus | For additional resources please visit http://davisplus.fadavis.com

References

Evidence-Based Practice

ENA Emergency Nursing Resources Development Committee. Emergency nursing resource: Wound preparation. Emergency Nurses Association, Des Plaines, IL, 2011. Retrieved from www.guideline. gov/content.aspx?id=36844&search=emergency+department

Gaffey, MM, et al. 2-Octyl cyanoacrylate (Dermabond) wound adhesives. Updated April 19, 2012. Retrieved from http:// emedicine.medscape.com/article/874047-overview

Lee, F, et al. Evidence behind the WHO guidelines: Hospital care for children: What is the role of prophylactic antibiotics in the management of burns? *J Trop Pediatr* 55:73–77, 2009.

Li, J, et al. Hypothermia. Updated April 9, 2013. Retrieved from http://emedicine.medscape.com/article/770542-overview

The Joint Commission. Standing together: An emergency planning guide for America's Communities. May 17, 2006. Retrieved from www.jointcommission.org/Standing_Together__An_Emergency_ Planning_Guide_for_Americas_Communities

Wasiak, J, and Cleland, H. Burns: Hydrocolloid dressing. *BMJ Clin Evidence* (10), 2009. Retrieved from www.clinicalevidence.bmj. com/ceweb/conditions/wnd/1903/1903_13.jsp

Bibliography

General

American College of Radiology. American College of Radiology appropriateness criteria for ordering DX tests. Retrieved from www.acr.org/Quality-Safety/Appropriateness-Criteria

Colyar, MR, and Ehrhardt, CR. *Ambulatory care procedures for the nurse practitioner*, ed 2. FA Davis, Philadelphia, 2004.

Kristof, K. Many Americans still lack health insurance. *Moneywatch*. Sept. 24, 2014. http://www.cbsnews.com/news/many-americans- still-lack-health-insurance/ Accessed October 19, 2014.

Spettel, CA. Anaphylaxis alert. *Adv Nurse Pract* 17(1):45–52, 2009.

U.S. Department of Health and Human Services, Centers for Disease Control and Prevention. National Center for Health Statistics. 2012. Retrieved from www.cdc.gov/nchs/fastats/ervisits.htm

Animal and Human Bites

Endom, EE. Initial management of animal and human bites. Updated October 25, 2012. Retrieved from www.uptodate.com/contents/ initial-management-of-animal-and-human-bites

Hahlbohm, D. Stinging insect allergy. *Adv NPs PAs* 4(4):20–22, 2013.

Burns

America Burn Association resources page. Retrieved from www. ameriburn.org/resources_factsheet.php

Lee, F, et al. Evidence behind the WHO guidelines: Hospital care for children: What is the role of prophylactic antibiotics in the management of burns? *J Trop Pediatr* 55:73–77, 2009.

Wasiak, J, and Cleland, H. Burns: Hydrocolloid dressing. *BMJ* (10), 2009. Retrieved from www.clinicalevidence.bmj.com/ceweb/ conditions/wnd/1903/1903_13.jsp

Disaster Preparedness

Beach, M. *Disaster preparedness and management*. FA Davis, Philadelphia, 2010.

Spain, KM, et al. When disaster happens: Emergency preparedness for nurse practitioners. *J Nurse Pract* 8(1):38–44, 2012.

The Joint Commission. Standing together: An emergency planning guide for America's Communities. May 17, 2006. Retrieved from www.jointcommission.org/Standing_Together__An_ Emergency_Planning_Guide_for_Americas_Communities

Head Trauma

Harmon, KG, et al. American Medical Society for Sports Medicine position statement: Concussion in sport. *Clin J Sport Med* 23(1): 1–18, 2013.

Temperature-Related Illnesses

Fowler, DR, et al. Heat-related deaths after an extreme heat event. *Morb Mortal Wkly Rep* 62(22):433–436, 2013. Retrieved from www.medscape.com/viewarticle/806946

James, L, et al. Hypothermia. 2013. Retrieved from http://emedicine. medscape.com/article/770542

Pneumothorax

Gillespie, PT, and Cassivi, SD. Catamenial pneumothorax [Abstract]. US Natl LibMed NIH. *Mayo Clin Proc* 80(5):677–680, 2008.

Sange, M, and Langrish, CJ. *Respiratory disease and its management: Pneumothorax in the critically ill.* Springer, London, 2009.

Sprains and Strains

DuBois, J. Evaluating and treating sprains and strains. *Clin Rev/Conven Care* 2(2):4–7, 2009.

Wounds and Lacerations

Anonymous. Wound infection: Primary considerations. *Consultant* 53(4):268–270, 2013.

Blankenship, RB, and Baker, T. Imaging modalities in wounds and superficial skin infections. *Emerg Med Clin North Am* 1:223–234, 2007.

ENA Emergency Nursing Resources Development Committee. Emergency nursing resource: Wound preparation. Emergency Nurses Association, Des Plaines, IL, 2011. Retrieved from www.guideline.gov/content.aspx?id=36844&search=emergency+department

Moore, GP, and Pfaff, JA. Malpractice cases in wound care and a legal concept: Special defense. *West J Emerg Med* 9:238–239, 2008.

Slobogean, GP, et al. Single-versus multiple dose antibiotic prophylaxis in the surgical treatment of closed fractures: A meta-analysis. *J Orthop Trauma* 22:264–269, 2008.

Strauss, EJ, et al. A prospective, randomised, controlled trial of 2-octylcyanoacrylate versus suture repair for nail bed injuries. *J Hand Surg Am* 33:250–253, 2008.

Resources

Poisonings

National Center for Injury Prevention and Control
www.cdc.gov/ncipc.org (through this site access TESS—Toxic Exposure Surveillance System)
American Association of Poison Control Centers
www.aapcc.org

Heat- and Cold-Related Injuries

MEDDAC Preventive Medicine Climatic Injury Awareness and Prevention Site
http://iach.amedd.army.mil/departments/prevmed.asp

Burns

The Burn Resource Center
www.burnsurvivor.com

Insect Bites

West Nile Virus
www.emedicine.com/westnile.htm
Internet Sources on Insect Bites
www.lib.uiowa.edu/hardin/md/insectbites.html

Head Trauma

American Association of Neurological Surgeons/Congress of Neurological Surgeons (AANS)
www.aans.org
MedlinePlus: Traumatic Brain Injuries
http://nlm.nih.gov/medlineplus/headandbraininjuries.html

Caring-Based Nursing: The Practice

All segments of our profession need to work together toward a common goal, a future in which legal and professional regulation and education of nurses at the graduate level are aligned so that one educational product, the advanced practice nurse, is prepared to fill a variety of roles in the health care system. —Linda R. Cronenwett: Molding the future of advanced practice nursing. Nursing Outlook 43:112–118, 1995.

Palliative Care

Susan Derby, RN, MA, GNP-BC, ACHPN •
Mary Layman Goldstein, RN, MS, ANP-BC, ACHPN

Chapter 20

■ DEATH AND DYING IN AMERICA

At present, in the United States, the total number of deaths from all causes is more than 2.5 million per year. The leading causes of death in the United States continue to be heart disease and cancer, accounting for nearly 50% of overall deaths, followed by stroke and respiratory disease (Centers for Disease Control and Prevention, 2010).

In 1900, the average life expectancy in the United States was about 50 years; by 2011, this had increased to approximately 78.7 years according to the Organization for Economic Cooperation and Development (OECD), slightly lower than the OECD worldwide average of 80.1. Use of antimicrobials, improved sanitation, and technological advances have all significantly increased life expectancy for the average American. Cancer has long been known to be a disease of aging. Changes in demographics occurring in the United States will increase the number of cancer cases and cancer deaths for the population aged 65 and older. Currently, 60% of all cancers and 70% of deaths from malignant tumors occur in this age-group. Thus, there will be a substantial increase in the numbers and proportions of Americans in this age-group, who are at highest risk and most vulnerable to cancer.

Significantly, however, although cancer accounted for the largest number of hospice admissions when hospice care in the United States was first established in the 1970s, today, cancer diagnoses account for less than half of all hospice admissions (36.9%). Along with an increased lifespan has come oftentimes many years of slow death from chronic, progressive diseases. According to the National Hospice and Palliative Care Organization (NHPCO, 2013), the top four noncancer primary diagnoses for patients admitted to hospice in 2012 were debility unspecified (14.2%), dementia (12.8%), heart disease (11.2%), and lung disease (8.2%).

Where Death and Dying Occur

Discussions of where people die shed little light on how they die, how physical symptoms are managed, how psychological and spiritual issues are addressed, the level of training and education the staff has in end-of-life care management, and how suffering is relieved. The site where death occurs is influenced by many factors including age, marital status, family support, finances, reimbursement issues, cultural beliefs, and cause of death.

Until the 20th century, most people died at home, cared for by family and close friends. Over the past century, death has become institutionalized, with a shift from the home to the hospital or health-care institution. Statistics for 2011 regarding deaths in the United States reveal that about 25% of deaths occurred at home, about 25% in a nursing facility, and about 50% in a hospital—15% in the emergency department and 35% in acute care. The National Hospice and Palliative Care Organization (NHPCO, 2013) estimated that more than 44.6% of all deaths in the United States involved patients who are receiving hospice care, a distinct increase. However, often these patients are receiving hospice care for just a few days before they die. Additionally, people continue to be hospitalized more frequently in the last 3 months of life and often spend time in an intensive care unit, subject to technological and life-saving measures, and spend a disproportionate amount of healthcare dollars (Institute of Medicine [IOM], 2014).

Hospice Care

Barriers to utilization of hospice care include the following:

- Difficulties in estimating prognosis
- Criterion that the patient have a life expectancy of 6 months or less
- Primary management at home with intermittent respite of care available for symptom control
- Need for a caregiver in the home
- Patient and family fear
- Communication problems
- Lack of knowledge and access to services
- Problems with funding mechanisms of insurers

Prognosticating a life expectancy of 6 months or less in non–cancer-related diseases has been especially difficult.

Medicare hospice eligibility criteria are that (1) the patient be eligible for Medicare Part A (Hospital Insurance); (2) the patient's doctor and the hospice medical director certify that the patient is terminally ill and has 6 months or less to live if the illness runs its normal course, (3) the patient must give informed consent to the hospice care; and (4) the patient receive care from a

Medicare-approved hospice program (U.S. Department of Health and Human Services, 2008).

A new program from the Centers for Medicare and Medicaid Services may change this. Until now, to receive hospice care, patients had to agree to forego any further attempts at curative treatment. The new Medicare Choices Model will soon offer an option for Medicare beneficiaries to receive hospice care services while still receiving treatment for curative care.

A PARADIGM SHIFT TO PALLIATIVE CARE

Hospice and *palliative care* are terms that are often used interchangeably. Both provide supportive medical, social, emotional, and spiritual services to patients and their caregivers. Both services rely on the combined knowledge and skill of interdisciplinary teams of professionals. Hospice care provides care to patients at the end of life. Palliative care provides comfort care and a support system to both the family and patient, integrating the psychological and spiritual aspects of patient care, throughout the trajectory of illness, from the time of diagnosis until death, and encompasses end-of-life care. This includes offering help to bereaved family members after the death of a loved one. The hospice movement in the United States has been greatly influenced by the work of Dr. Elisabeth Kübler-Ross, who researched the dying process and advocated changes in the way society views death. In the United States, the first hospice opened in 1974 in New Haven, Connecticut. It was based on St. Christopher's Hospice, founded in Great Britain in 1967. Since that time, hospital-based hospice programs have been primarily replaced by home-based and nursing home–based hospice programs.

Primary practitioners who provide care to chronically ill patients with terminal conditions are expected to incorporate the basic elements of palliative care into their practice, regardless of setting. These elements are defined by the eight domains of palliative care as outlined in the *Clinical Practice Guidelines for Quality Palliative Care, Second Edition* (2009) (National Consensus Project for Quality Palliative Care [NCP], 2009) (Table 20.1).

Five national palliative care organizations formed a consortium to oversee the National Consensus Project for Quality Palliative Care (NCP). These include the American Academy of Hospice and Palliative Medicine, Center to Advance Palliative Care, Hospice and Palliative Care Nurses Association, Last Acts Partnership, and National Hospice and Palliative Care Organization. Together, these five organizations, came to consensus, issuing the following statement: "The goal of palliative care is to prevent and relieve suffering and to support the best possible quality of life for patients and their families, regardless of the stage of the disease or the need for other therapies. It can be delivered concurrently with life-prolonging therapies

Table 20.1	Domains of Palliative Care: The National Consensus Project for Quality Palliative Care

1. Structure and Processes of Care
2. Physical Aspects of Care
3. Psychological and Psychiatric Aspects of Care
4. Social Aspects of Care
5. Spiritual, Religious, and Existential Aspects of Care
6. Cultural Aspects of Care
7. Care of the Imminently Dying Patient
8. Ethical and Legal Aspects of Care

Source: *Clinical practice guidelines for quality palliative care,* ed 2. National Consensus Project for Quality Palliative Care, Pittsburgh, PA, 2009

or as the main focus of care. Leadership, collaboration, coordination, and communication are key elements for effective integration of these disciplines and services" (NCP, 2009). Other definitions include patient- and family-centered care that optimizes quality of life by anticipating, preventing, and treating suffering. Palliative care throughout the trajectory of illness involves addressing physical, emotional, psychosocial, religious, and spiritual needs of patients and their families.

Suffering and Spirituality

Receiving a diagnosis of an incurable disease can be one of the most frightening experiences for any human being. Fear of potential suffering and pain as well as fear of loss of control, of relationships, and of existence itself are some of the issues that confront the patient. Psychosocial distress may significantly influence treatment decisions, quality of life, and disease progression. All care providers and clinicians on the front lines of cancer care can improve the recognition and management of cancer-related distress. Up to 43% of patients with cancer report measurable levels of psychosocial distress, and this is most likely a gross underrepresentation.

The diagnosis of suffering is often missed by healthcare providers, perhaps because suffering is an experience of the whole person and is highly personal and subjective. Cassell (1999) suggests that suffering is the state of distress caused by the threat of the loss of intactness or the disintegration of a person from whatever the cause. In serious illness, all aspects of the individual are affected: physical, mental, spiritual, emotional, and social. Suffering involves an eroding of the normal defenses that help us to keep intact, to relate to others, and to have purpose in life. Human suffering is a complex, multidimensional experience that often goes beyond physical pain. To this point, the National Comprehensive Cancer Network (NCCN) 2014 guidelines include 72 pages of clinical guidelines on "Distress Management" (NCCN, 2014).

When a life-threatening disease is first diagnosed, the individual may be terrified but must often quickly make decisions regarding his or her treatment. During this phase, the patient often seeks counsel, support, and advice from others including friends, relatives, and health-care professionals. Characteristic of this phase is an information-gathering period, in which the patient becomes knowledgeable about the disease, treatment, and adverse effects. The patient's exploration may extend to religious and/or spiritual aspects of being. After treatment, the patient may experience ongoing anxiety and depression related to fear of disease relapse. With disease relapse and progressive illness and disability, the patient may become more depressed and verbalize feelings of hopelessness. In one study (Flaming, 1995) that evaluated nurses' perspectives of patient suffering, four domains of suffering were identified: to bear it, to stay in control, to protect themselves, and to strengthen.

Ferrell and Coyle (2008) describe nurse suffering that occurs when nurses witness the suffering of their patients. The relationship among the nurse, the patient, and the patient's family can be close and intense; and each party is vulnerable to each other. Nurses who care for cancer patients and palliative care staff who deal with cancer patients are at great risk for suffering given the percentage of patients who die or who are close to death.

Spirituality is concerned with the transcendental, the inspirational, and existential way we live our lives. From his experience in Auschwitz, Victor Frankl (1959) came to believe that suffering can be helpful if a meaning to suffering is identified. He used the terms *existential frustration* to define the confusion felt from a lack of meaning in one's situation and *existential vacuum* as the absence of meaning in one's life. When one is faced with unavoidable suffering, according to Frankl, the individual is free to choose how to respond and may either be master or victim. Finding meaning in suffering, says Frankl, comes from transcendence, or rising above the self, and finding meaning. Meaning encompasses three domains: creativity, experience, and attitude. Meaning can be found in creating something or accomplishing a task; experiential meaning involves finding pleasure or nourishment of the soul in ordinary things; and attitudinal meaning involves finding courage or experiencing joy despite a terrible, unalterable situation.

Providing care to people who are suffering is an awesome task that often challenges religious or spiritual beliefs. It calls for the highest level of knowledge, sensitivity, and empathy. Patients who are ill or dying report that they want nurses and doctors who are caring. We often hear stories from patients about "uncaring" health professionals who seem cold and indifferent to the suffering of their patients, and we all too frequently see some of these individuals in our daily practice. Palliative care encompasses the basic tenets of caring, including respect for the individual, empathy, and compassion. It calls for a *Circle of Caring* (see Chapter 1).

Medical and Nursing Education in Palliative Care: A Recent History

Education of health-care professionals in palliative and end-of-life care was not routinely a part of medical and nursing curriculums. In many clinical settings, including both inpatient and ambulatory care, there were no established guidelines for pain and symptom management for patients with cancer, including terminal or end-of-life care. Even in settings in which guidelines existed, there was variable support for or assurance that these guidelines were adhered to in practice.

A growing recognition of the need to provide better care for dying patients, many of whom were in pain and suffering, led the Robert Woods Johnson Foundation to fund a landmark study. Funded with $28 million dollars, the study was conducted over a 4-year period and included 9,000 participants suffering from life-threatening illnesses in five U.S. teaching hospitals across the country. In 1995, the reports of this study were published in the *Journal of the American Medical Association.* Named the Study to Understand Prognoses and Preferences for Outcomes and Risks of Treatment, it became known by the acronym SUPPORT.

Some disturbing findings in the study were as follows:

- Forty-six percent of patients with do-not-resuscitate (DNR) orders had the order written 2 days before death.
- Fewer than 50% of physicians understood their patients' preferences.
- Fifty percent of patients who could communicate had moderate to severe pain during the last 3 days of life.

A 1997 study by an Institute of Medicine (IOM) panel concluded that physicians and other caregivers in the United States fail to provide competent palliative and supportive care to dying patients. It also concluded that a significant number of terminally ill patients experience serious pain and other discomforting symptoms such as dyspnea. These findings were dismally reconfirmed in a recently published IOM report (September 2014) on care of the dying. This report, prepared by an appointed committee of 21 experts and released on September 17, 2014, concluded that the United States needs to overhaul its "broken" end-of-life care system to improve patient's quality of life in their final days and to cut rising health care costs. The 507-page report, titled *Dying in America,* was funded by a $1.5 million anonymous donation (Belluck, 2014). The conclusions of this study were that physicians and other caregivers in the United States *still* fail to provide competent palliative and supportive care to dying patients.

Multiple studies document deficiencies in knowledge about pain and palliation of symptoms associated with progressive disease. In a 1997 survey of medical residents in a university-based surgical program, a significant number of deficits existed in the knowledge of how to provide care for common symptoms of advanced cancer, including management of opioid-related nausea, vomiting, and terminal dyspnea (Oneschuk et al, 1997). Other surveys have documented deficiencies in physicians during their residencies in the areas of opioid selection, conversion, and management of opioid toxicities and addiction. In a 2003 survey of approaches of medical oncologists toward palliative care for patients with advanced cancer, only a minority of physicians collaborated with a palliative care specialist, a palliative home service, an inpatient hospice, or a psychologist. Overall, 88.4% of respondents supported the belief that medical oncologists should coordinate the end-of-life care, but a substantial minority, 42%, felt that they were inadequately trained for this task (Cherny & Catane, 2003).

Nurses' knowledge of and attitude toward pain and symptom management strongly parallel those of physicians, although there is some evidence that educational efforts have been beneficial. McCaffery and Ferrell (1997) compared the results from surveys in 1995 and 1998 of nurses' knowledge of pain assessment, opioid dosing, and likelihood of addiction. They found improvements in the nurses' assessment and titration upward of opioid dose as well as a decrease in concerns about addiction, although a clear association still existed between time on opioids and concerns about addiction. In another study of nurses' knowledge and attitudes of cancer-related pain, O'Brien et al (1996) found that experienced nurses who have cared for cancer patients are more knowledgeable and have more liberal attitudes toward pain management than nurses who have not cared for cancer patients.

Professional Educational Efforts to Improve the Practice of Pain Management and Palliative Care

Major educational efforts have been made by health-care professionals to improve professional knowledge deficits. A variety of approaches and specific programs have been identified to address these knowledge deficits. The Joint Commission standards on pain management have been helpful in making institutions accountable for assessment and management of pain across practice settings (Berry & Dahl, 2000). Efforts at the academic and clinical level provide a framework for care of patients with advanced disease and for patients who are dying. Curriculum changes for both nurses and physicians in many schools now include comprehensive palliative care. In many hospitals, services of palliative care experts or pain and symptom management specialists are being incorporated into the routine care of patients, and the number of training centers nationally is increasing. Many hospitals now provide programs for nurses offering education or clinical mentors. Quality assurance and improvement programs examining pain and symptom management now exist in many institutional settings.

Directives now exist from major professional organizations advocating pain and symptom management. These organizations include the American Nurses Association, American Pain Society, American Board of Internal Medicine, Oncology Nursing Society, American Geriatric Association, American Society of Pain Management Nurses, International Society of Nurses in Cancer Care, International Association for the Study of Pain, European Oncology Nursing Society, and the American Society of Clinical Oncologists. These clinical practice guidelines and directives, as well as major national professional educational efforts on end-of-life-care (End of Life Nursing Education Consortium [ELNEC] and Education for Physicians on End of Life Care [EPEC]), are addressing the problem of inadequate control of pain and knowledge deficits.

In addition, clinical practice guidelines have recently been established by the National Comprehensive Cancer Network (NCCN), which recommends (among other things) routine screening for cancer-related *distress* on diagnosis and admission and at pivotal times in the disease process. These guidelines (NCCN, 2014) also promulgate the use of approved distress assessment tools for screening and the use of clinical pathways based on assessment results. And the ELNEC core curriculum for undergraduate, graduate, and specialty tracks now includes adult, pediatric, geriatric, critical care, veteran, and public hospital foci.

The 2014 IOM report reiterated yet again that medical schools and groups that accredit and regulate health-care providers still need to *greatly* increase training in palliative care and set standards so the clinicians know how to compassionately and effectively treat patients who want to be comfortable but avoid extensive medical procedures.

■ PALLIATIVE CARE

Palliative care focuses on the management of disease in patients with active, progressive disease. The focus of care is on the quality of life. Palliative care furthers the World Health Organization's (WHO's) definition of health, affirming dying as a normal life process. Palliative care as defined by the WHO (2010) is an approach that improves the quality of life of patients and their families facing the problems associated with life-threatening illness through the prevention and relief of suffering by means of early identification and impeccable assessment and treatment of pain and other problems—physical, psychosocial, and spiritual. The goals of care are to alleviate symptoms in a compassionate way, to neither hasten nor postpone death, and to provide a support system to both the family and patient, integrating the psychological and spiritual aspects of patient care throughout the trajectory of illness.

Specifically, according to the WHO (2010), palliative care does all of the following:

• Provides relief from pain and other distressing symptoms

- Affirms life and regards dying as a normal process
- Intends to neither hasten nor postpone death
- Integrates the psychological and spiritual aspects of care
- Offers a support system to help patients live as actively as possible until death
- Offers a support system to help the family cope during the patient's illness and in their own bereavement
- Uses a team approach to address the needs of patients and their families, including bereavement counseling, if indicated
- Will enhance the quality of life and may also positively influence the course of illness
- Is applicable early in the course of illness, in conjunction with other therapies that are intended to prolong life, such as chemotherapy or radiation therapy, and include those investigations needed to better understand and manage distressing clinical complications

If we examine the characteristics of the most prevalent chronic illnesses, including coronary artery disease, chronic lung disease, cancer, cerebrovascular disease, and diabetes mellitus, similarities are apparent. For all chronic illnesses, there is the initial diagnostic period when symptoms become present. This may be over a period of days, weeks, or months and is generally a highly stressful period, with disruption in function and routine. Once a treatment plan is initiated, symptoms may resolve, and the patient may enter a period of remission or stability lasting months or years. What follows are periods of exacerbation, often with hospitalizations, and periods of remission. During this time the patient usually experiences signs and symptoms of disease; alterations in lifestyle, role, family, and job relationships; and often psychological and spiritual distress. As time progresses, if the patient is not cured of the disease or stability is not long lasting, there comes a time of downward progression of disease with a decline in function and worsening symptoms. It is during this time most patients are referred for palliative care. Americans struggling with chronic illnesses and their associated disabilities are often in greatest need of assistance during the last months to year of life. About 30% of Medicare expenditures arise in the patient's last year of life.

The goals of treatment for all chronically ill patients need to be clearly defined by the health-care provider, communicated to the patient and family at the time of diagnosis, and reinforced throughout the trajectory of illness. Broadly, these goals, which parallel the trajectory of disease, can be classified as curative, slowing progression of disease, and palliative control of symptoms or comfort care only. The terminal phase includes the management of symptoms at the end of life. Throughout all phases of illness, emphasis should be placed on palliative control of symptoms either from disease or treatment and maintaining optimum quality of life for the patient.

Expert opinion and qualitative research have characterized priority concerns for patients in late life. Important topics including pain management, family support,

ensuring continuity, making informed decisions, providing for emotional and spiritual support, sustaining function, and increasing survival (Hanson et al, 1997; Singer et al, 1999; Steinhauser et al, 2008; Weinrich et al, 2003).

The Palliative Care Plan

The WHO (2010) has indicated the need for integration of palliative care services throughout the trajectory of illness and stages of cancer from diagnosis to death, and providing support and bereavement counseling for the family after the death of the patient. Devising a palliative plan of care should be part of the ongoing plan of care for the chronically ill patient. Appropriate care depends on several factors, including ongoing communication with the patient and family; assessment of the patient's and family's understanding of goals of care; religious, cultural, and spiritual beliefs; access to community agencies; psychological assessment and coping strategies; and preferences regarding advance directives. Dimensions of a palliative care plan for the health-care provider are outlined in Advanced Practice Nursing Interventions 20.1.

Palliative Cancer Care

In 2014, the American Cancer Society estimated that about 1,665,540 new cases of invasive cancer will be diagnosed in the United States in the next year (American Cancer Society, 2014). This does not include carcinoma in situ (noninvasive cancer) or certain types of skin cancers. Among women, the most commonly diagnosed cancers are those of the breast, lung and bronchus, and colon and rectum. Among men, the most common cancers are cancers of the prostate, lung and bronchus, and colon and rectum. Preliminary data suggest that overall cancer mortality has begun to decline; however, the number of deaths has continued to increase because of the aging population. Cancer is a disease of aging and a prominent cause of overall morbidity and death. From 2002 to 2006, the median age at diagnosis for cancer of all sites was 66 years of age (Horner et al, 2009); 585,720 people are expected to die of cancer this year (2014), which equates to almost 1,600 per day. Relative survival rates have increased for a variety of reasons. Between 2003 and 2008 the relative survival rate was 68%, as contrasted with a 49% relative survival rate from 1975 to 1977 (American Cancer Society, 2014).

The Role of the Primary-Care Provider in Palliative Cancer Care

The health-care provider, as the primary-care provider of record, is critically important. There are a number of important points in the continuum of care for the patient with a chronic, irreversible disease process, most commonly a diagnosis of cancer, which call for a careful, comprehensive response. Often the primary-care provider is the first clinician to see the patient and because of this plays a crucial role. Although many patients are referred to specialists, the primary-care provider commonly provides a

Advanced Practice Nursing Interventions 20.1   Dimensions of a Palliative Care Plan

1. Assess the extent of disease documented by imaging studies, laboratory data.
2. Assess and provide interventions for physical signs and symptoms including pain, dyspnea, delirium.
3. Assess coping strategies and psychological symptoms including presence and absence of depression, suicidal ideology.
4. Determine level and quality of support provided by family and friends. Is additional assistance needed in the home and can it be put into place? Determine community resources and identify what kind of assistance is available.
5. Identify coping strategies and psychological symptoms in family members or caregivers.
6. Perform a religious and spiritual assessment including degree of comfort from beliefs.
7. Evaluate the impact of disease on functional status. What can the patient do, and what assistance is needed with bathing, dressing, ambulation, meal preparation?
8. Evaluate what advance care planning has been done. Have the patient's wishes and preferences for resuscitation, artificial feeding, and hydration been discussed? Has the patient identified a surrogate decision-maker who knows the patient's wishes? Is there documentation on advance directives in the medical record?
9. Evaluate overall quality of life and well-being. Does the patient feel secure that all that can be done is being done? Does the patient feel that physical and psychological symptoms are being satisfactorily addressed? Does the patient feel there is meaning to his or her life?
10. Identify the family burden of caring for the patient. Is attention being paid to support the caregiver so that burnout does not occur? What is the financial burden to the caregiver, and can he or she manage bill paying and reimbursement issues?
11. Determine the level of care needed in the home and provision for that care. What reimbursement issues affect obtaining the level of home care needed?
12. Is there a system in place for ongoing support and assistance to family members and caregivers after the death of the patient?
13. Has the patient identified his or her desire for their place of death? Has he or she communicated these wishes to the family, partner, caregiver?
14. Provide for bereavement counseling and support for the family beyond the life of the patient.

number of essential functions over many years of care, such as teaching about risk factors for many diseases (e.g., avoiding ultraviolet light exposure to prevent skin cancer), detecting occult disease in asymptomatic patients, or diagnosing disease in those with suspicious symptoms. In patients who have a strong family history of some malignancies, the primary-care provider has a responsibility to educate and make appropriate referrals to specialists for genetic testing and/or counseling. NCCN (2014) also provides comprehensive cancer guidelines on screening and prevention of disease. The Patient-Centered Medical Home as identified in the Affordable Care Act should increase the primacy of the role of primary-care provider. This should be a person that knows the patients *the best*.

Discussing the diagnosis and its associated options, as well as arranging for specialty care, is critical. This may be especially difficult in the diagnosis of cancer, which most patients and families still perceive as a death sentence. It may be helpful to set a special appointment time for this discussion and encourage the patient to bring along a family member or advocate. A good understanding of the diagnosis and the potential prognosis is essential to the discussion, as well as awareness of the potential treatment options. There is a whole body of literature on the art of sharing difficult news with patients and families. Again, this often falls to the primary-care provider,

who may not be as used to these types of conversations. Nonetheless, they are important aspects of the primary-care provider's role. The 2014 IOM report, drafted by an interdisciplinary panel that included doctors, nurses, insurers, religious leaders, lawyers, and experts on aging, again emphasizes the need for insurers to create financial incentives for primary-care providers to support ongoing conversations with patients and families on advanced care planning. These, they say, should start as early as major teenage milestones, such as getting a driver's license and deciding if one wants to be an organ donor.

Because the therapeutic window for treatment of certain cancers is small, advice given during this first discussion may be crucial in determining the patient's and family's course of action. Utilizing caring processes and active listening skills during this time is important. It is essential to the subsequent care of the patient that as much information about the patient—biological, emotional, and spiritual—be provided to the specialty care provider.

The patient should be referred for ongoing emotional and/or spiritual support at the time of diagnosis. As a trusted care provider, the primary care provider is the ideal member of the team to recommend and implement this and provide for ongoing follow-up care. This involves being knowledgeable of the appropriate time intervals for certain follow-up tests and knowing what to look for and when. The American Cancer Society is an excellent source for all health-care providers for state-of-the art information on cancer treatment.

The recognition and management of complications, either during or after treatment, is another responsibility of the primary-care provider. Some of these complications may represent metastatic spread of the original cancer, and a high index of suspicion must be vigilantly maintained. In some cases, complications may be life-threatening. Advanced Practice Nursing Interventions 20.2 summarizes the role of the APRN in palliative cancer care.

■ PRINCIPLES OF PALLIATIVE CARE

The health-care provider who delivers primary care is often the one who provides care at the end of life; therefore, having a baseline knowledge of symptom management is crucial. Seriously ill patients with chronic disease and multiple comorbid medical conditions often cross practice settings from emergency department to home and from home to hospital. Because the Medicare hospice benefit is limited to patients with a 6-month prognosis, many patients with long-standing chronic illnesses, including cancer, are ineligible for hospice care, which for many patients has led to unrelieved suffering.

Principles of palliative care useful for the primary-care provider include the following:

1. Careful evaluation of the patient's symptoms
2. A clear understanding of the pathophysiological mechanisms involved in each symptom
3. A judicious approach to diagnostic testing (with an aim of avoiding "overtesting" and testing that does not affect management). Diagnostic testing should always be consistent with a clear understanding of the goals of care for each patient.

4. Establishment of a treatment plan that is simple and subject to continual reevaluation
5. Determining what the patient's and caregiver's expectations are regarding the patient's care at this stage of illness
6. Determining if the patient has special wishes regarding end-of-life care, including place of death and if advance directives have been discussed and documented
7. Referral to a pain and palliative care specialist for aggressive management of these symptoms if routine interventions are inadequate

Pain control is paramount. Pain is the symptom most feared by dying patients. Although usually the manifestation of physical distress, pain may be exacerbated by anxiety, fear, loneliness, and depression. Patients differ vastly in the extent of clinical disease that yields pain, as well as in their ability to tolerate, accept, or cope with pain. Pain expected to be transient may be treated on an as-needed (prn) basis, but chronic pain needs to be treated via a scheduled regimen. The section of this chapter on pain discusses this in greater detail.

Clinical problems frequently seen in terminally ill patients include pain, dyspnea, fatigue, depression, anorexia, weight loss, constipation, and anxiety. Initial evaluation of symptoms must begin with determining the etiology of the symptom evaluated. This is usually done as part of the initial work-up. If the etiology of pain is secondary to the treatment, one should ask whether the treatment can be adjusted or whether it should be discontinued. Goals of care should be reviewed on a routine basis, especially at intervals when treatment decisions need to be made. Other challenges are the ethical dilemmas that may be faced by the health-care provider whose own beliefs may conflict with or be different from the patient's and the family members' or caregiver's. It

---

Advanced Practice Nursing Interventions 20.2   The Role of the Advanced Practice Nurse in Palliative Cancer Care

1. Teaching about risk factors for cancer and lifestyle change to decrease risk
2. Coordination of screening tests in asymptomatic patients (mammogram, colonoscopy)
3. Detecting cancer in asymptomatic patients or those with specific symptoms
4. Informing patient and family of diagnosis and prognosis; it is helpful if this is done in collaboration with the physician involved in the care of the patient
5. Arranging for follow-up care, including psychosocial and spiritual support
6. Being an active participant of the interdisciplinary team
7. Providing follow-up care for ongoing symptom detection and management
8. Identifying and managing complications of care
9. Providing follow-up care and early detection of possible recurrences
10. Providing palliative care
11. Providing referral to a palliative care specialist as indicated
12. Providing for assistance with advance care planning
13. Providing for bereavement counseling and support

is important for health-care providers to recognize that their beliefs are just that, and may frequently differ from those of the patient. For example, one of the most common and controversial clinical issues at the end of life is the need for hydration. Differences of opinion may exist not only between health-care providers and the patient or caregiver, but between family members. When there are concerns about nutrition and hydration at the end of life, the amount of food or fluid given to a dying person should be guided by the patient's desires and his or her ability to tolerate nourishment orally, rather than by calculated nutritional or fluid requirements. It is also important to understand that cultural differences often play a role and should be respected. At the end of life, small amounts of fluids, ice chips, or mouth swabs— classic nursing interventions—are often beneficial.

Another frequent challenge is determining the best way to deliver medication, especially in the home or hospice setting, when the patient is unable to swallow. Routes of administration to consider for the dying patient who cannot swallow include sublingual, intravenous, transcutaneous, subcutaneous, and spinal (e.g., intrathecal, epidural). Creativity is frequently called for, as well as the ability to work in concert with a team of providers, such as pharmacists, clergy, and home-care nurses.

■ PALLIATIVE CARE OF SYMPTOMS IN DYING PATIENTS

Numerous studies have evaluated symptoms during the last weeks of life and indicate that patients experience a high degree of symptom distress and suffering. Ingham and Portenoy (1996) suggested that symptom assessment should be multidimensional, involving determination of the incidence, duration, severity, amount of distress, and impact on function and quality of life. A variety of symptoms in the last year and weeks of life have been identified in the literature including pain, distress, weakness, fatigue, cognitive impairment, and dyspnea.

The Patient's Voice 20.1

Palliative Care

The Patient

"The pain was intolerable, every time I moved my back hurt. The morphine tablets made me sleepy and constipated. The pain of trying to have a bowel movement was almost as severe as the back pain. My doctor basically told me to bear it as these side effects were common."

The Son

My father was clearly dying and was confused at times. The nursing staff gave him injections for pain, but they did not seem to help. When I questioned the nurses, they told me they could not give him more because they did not want to slow his breathing. I thought, "He's dying. Make him comfortable."

Several studies have demonstrated that the most difficult end-of-life symptoms to manage are pain, respiratory distress, and confusional states. In a retrospective review of 100 patients in an inpatient palliative care unit, Fainsinger et al (1991) identified 16% of the patients required sedation to control pain and delirium. In another evaluation of patients during the last week of life, Conill and colleagues (1997) assessed patients at two intervals—their initial consultation and then during the last 7 days of life. Asthenia, anorexia, and dry mouth were the three most common symptoms in both periods, but the incidence of confusional states doubled during the last week of life (30.1% and 68.2%, respectively). Potter et al (2003) assessed 400 patients referred to palliative care services and found the most prevalent symptoms in the cancer population were pain (64%), anorexia (34%), constipation (32%), weakness (32%), and dyspnea (31%).

Needs of nursing home patients at the end of life have also been identified. In one study during the last month of life of nursing home and residential care/assisted living residents, the most common symptoms include pain, dyspnea, fatigue, problems with cleanliness, and symptoms affecting intake. Seventy-seven percent of those studied were cognitively impaired (Hanson et al, 2008). Identification and management of pain and distress in these patients can be especially difficult.

The suffering that patients experience at the end of life is not necessarily related to the severity of the symptom(s). Mild symptoms may cause severe distress, especially if the meaning of that symptom is frightening—if it signifies that death is near. Unrelieved symptoms at the end of life are extremely devastating; they can rob patients and their loved ones of valuable time and meaningful interaction. During this time nurses have a responsibility as patient and family advocates to ensure that symptoms are addressed and treated appropriately.

Palliative management of three of the most difficult symptoms—pain, dyspnea, and delirium—are discussed in the sections that follow. Accurate assessment and diagnosis of these symptoms is assumed. The reader is referred to appropriate sections of this textbook for more information on assessment and diagnosis of these problems.

■ PALLIATIVE MANAGEMENT OF PAIN

According to the International Association for the Study of Pain (1979), pain is identified as a subjective experience and is described as "an unpleasant sensory or emotional experience related to actual or potential tissue damage." Pain is a subjective symptom; there is no test to measure pain. The patient should be actively involved in establishing the goals of pain management, and family members should be involved, when possible. Table 20.2 presents a review of the various types of pain.

The American Society for Pain Management Nursing (2013) issued a position paper on pain management in palliative care. They noted that pain at the end of life *continues to be a substantial concern* and has been estimated

Table 20.2 Types of Pain

Pain may be described as an unpleasant sensory and/or emotional experience related to actual or potential tissue damage. The perception of pain is the result of tissue injury leading to the origination and conduction of pain signals by the central nervous system. Peripheral stimulation occurs when free nerve endings, or nociceptors, found in various parts of the body (e.g., skin, blood vessels, viscera, muscles) are stimulated, which in turn stimulates action potentials to be transmitted along afferent nerve fibers to the spinal cord.

When thinking of a person with pain, it is useful to think about whether the pain is acute or chronic. Sometimes the person may have chronic pain with a new acute pain added.

Acute Pain
- Well-defined temporal pattern of onset.
- Transient, may be associated with hyperactivity of the autonomic nervous system.
- Increased blood pressure, pulse rate, respiratory rate, and perspiration.
- Patients may look like they are in pain and may cry or moan.

Chronic Pain
- Syndrome that is defined by a pattern of pain that persists beyond healing of the acute lesion or recurs over periods of months, or is associated with a lesion not expected to improve.
- Patients experience a decrease in observable signs of pain.
- Blood pressure and pulse rate are normal.
- Sleep disturbance, decreased appetite, depression, and lassitude may be present.

Because of therapeutic implications, it can be helpful to clinicians to determine whether an individual's pain is classified as nociceptive, neuropathic, or both.

Nociceptive Pain
Nociceptive (organic) pain results from activation and sensitization of nociceptors, or pain receptors, located throughout the body. Nociceptive pain may be further subdivided into somatic and visceral pain
1. Somatic pain
   - May be constant, aching, throbbing.
   - Examples include bone metastases, postsurgical incisional pain, musculoskeletal inflammation, or spasm.
2. Visceral pain
   - Results from inflammation, compression, distention, or stretching of thoracic or abdominal viscera (e.g., intra-abdominal metastases, liver metastases).
   - May be diffuse, gnawing, or cramping.

Neuropathic Pain
Neuropathic pain refers to syndromes that may be related to damaged peripheral or central neural structures as a result of tumor progression or infiltration or from chemical injury to the peripheral nerve or spinal cord from surgery, irradiation, or chemotherapy.
- May be continuous or lancinating.
- May be burning, shooting, electric shock–like, squeezing, vise-like.

to still occur in 46% of patients in the last month of life. Concerns about shortening life continue to worry clinicians who use the double-effect argument, although studies demonstrate that adequate pain control may actually extend and prolong life in some cases. To address this concern, they make the following recommendations:

- Enhance evidence-based education for providers in this area.
- Promote accountability for all health professionals to support patient preferences.
- Foster the concept that pain management is a core health care right.
- Recognize that all pain should be treated.
- Improve public understanding of barriers, harmful effects of pain, and need for appropriate treatment.

- Improve accessibility to effective pharmacological, nonpharmacological, and advanced technological treatment modalities.
- Decrease legal, regulatory, and reimbursement obstacles (American Society for Pain Management Nursing, 2013).

The findings of the IOM's report, *Dying in America* (2014), confirms that there is a long way to go to begin to implement and meet these recommendations.

Assessment

Pain management begins with accurate assessment of the patient's pain. This assessment should be incorporated across practice settings into all routine bedside and ambulatory visits, as well as when there is a report of worsening pain or new pain. Inadequate pain assessment was identified as one of the most frequently mentioned barriers hindering adequate cancer pain management (Oldenmenger et al, 2009). Adequate assessment should enable the healthcare provider to determine the cause of the pain, assist in determining treatment, and evaluate the effectiveness of therapeutic interventions and their impact on the quality of life. Assessment of pain is subjective and relies heavily on the patient's report. The use of a multidimensional assessment tool can facilitate understanding and assist in determining treatment efficacy. Validated assessment tools include the Brief Pain Inventory (Daut et al, 1983) and the McGill Pain Questionnaire (Graham et al, 1980). However, it is sometimes difficult to utilize these tools when evaluating a fragile, medically ill person at the end of his or her life. A 10-point (0–10) scale is commonly used to measure pain intensity. If the patient cannot use a numerical scale, a categorical scale of none, mild, moderate, and severe is recommended. Pain assessment should include a detailed history of the pain (including intensity, quality, temporal factors, aggravating and relieving factors, and its effect on activity, mood, and ability to eat) and characteristics, a comprehensive physical examination, a psychosocial evaluation, and a thorough diagnostic work-up to determine the underlying cause of the pain. Table 20.3 outlines the basic principles of pain assessment.

Table 20.3   Basic Principles of Pain Assessment

- Believe the patient's complaint of pain. The patient is the expert in determining the level of pain he or she is experiencing.
- Take a careful history of the pain complaint and incorporate into the overall plan and goals of care.
- If the patient has difficulty communicating because of cognitive or physical impairments, obtain a history from the family or caregiver.
- Observe for nonverbal cues (e.g., crying, grimacing).
- Assess for other symptoms (e.g., agitation, delirium, dyspnea) that may cloud the pain assessment.
- Assess for onset, timing, temporal characteristics, pattern of referral, and aggravating and relieving factors.
- Assess for breakthrough or incident-related pain.
- Examine the site of pain on every patient encounter.
- Facilitate work-up that clarifies the etiology of the pain and extent of disease.
- Evaluate the psychological state of the patient and assess for depression, anxiety, delirium, or suicidal ideation.
- Determine appropriate opioid and route of administration. Consider the cost of medications and economic burden on the patient and family. Consider use of adjuvant analgesics, especially for neuropathic pain.
- Assess and reassess response to treatment and monitor for presence of side effects.
- Treat side effects aggressively.

Management

Palliative management of the patient in pain includes pharmacotherapy, interventional techniques, and non-pharmacological pain management interventions.

Pharmacotherapy

In 2005, the American Pain Society (APS) published guidelines for the management of cancer pain in adults and children; these guidelines promote a systematic and comprehensive approach to cancer pain management. The recommendations are based on a review of the literature rating each one on the strength and consistency of evidence. In its approach to pharmacotherapy, APS recommends that the initial treatment of cancer pain be based on the severity of the pain reported by the individual patient and follows the WHO Three-Step Analgesic Ladder (WHO, 2009). (See Fig. 20.1.) Despite the fact that the WHO treatment principles are widely accepted as the main prescribing guide in cancer pain management, there is insufficient information regarding their level of implementation (Hakonsen et al, 2008). Since 1990, the WHO Three-Step Analgesic Ladder advocates use of analgesics corresponding to three levels of pain intensity and utilizing nonopioid analgesics (NSAIDs and acetaminophen), opioids, and adjuvant analgesics as follows. These recommendations have remained relatively consistent in principle.

Step 1. Pain Persisting or Increasing Patients with mild to moderate pain should be treated with a nonopioid analgesic and, if indicated, an adjuvant drug. Examples of nonopioid analgesics are acetaminophen and the NSAIDs such as aspirin, ibuprofen, indomethacin, and naproxen. Examples of adjuvant drugs include tricyclic antidepressants (TCAs) such as amitriptyline or imipramine and anticonvulsants such as gabapentin, pregabalin, and lamotrigine.

Step 2. Pain Persisting or Increasing Patients who are opioid naive and present with mild to moderate pain or who fail to have adequate analgesia from a nonopioid should be treated with a mild opioid (previously called "weak opioids") and a nonopioid, as well as an adjuvant drug as appropriate. Examples of opioids that can be utilized at this level are codeine, hydrocodone, and oxycodone, with or without acetaminophen. Additionally, adjuvant therapy may be added for fear and anxiety.

Step 3. Freedom From Cancer Pain Patients who present with moderate to severe pain or who fail to have adequate analgesia from the second level of intervention should receive an opioid (previously called "strong opioids") and a nonopioid and/or an adjuvant medication as appropriate. As with mild pain, adjuvant medications are selected on the basis of the underlying pain etiology of an individual patient. Examples of opioids appropriate for moderate to severe pain include morphine, hydromorphone, fentanyl, oxymorphone, levorphanol, and methadone. Opioids are frequently used in combination with a nonopioid if not contraindicated by an

Figure 20.1 Three-step analgesic ladder.

individual's clinical situation. Additionally, adjuvant therapy may need to be added for fear and anxiety.

Health-care providers are advised to place patients receiving opioid therapy on bowel regimens to prevent opioid-induced constipation (Dy et al, 2008). Important considerations when providing pharmacotherapy for an individual's pain management include previous opioid experiences, determining the appropriate opioid (including the route of administration and dosage schedule), and calculating an equianalgesic dose if switching to another opioid (American Pain Society, 2005). Of practical concern is whether a particular medication is covered by an individual's drug plan. Documentation of dose-limiting side effects or treatment failures can help when advocating for prior authorizations for formulary exceptions.

Selecting the Appropriate Opioid When given properly, opioids are among the safest medications available, because adverse effects are predictable and generally controllable. The potency of opioids varies, but they are generally interchangeable with appropriate dose and dosing interval adjustments (Knotkova et al, 2009).

Numerous factors, both patient and drug related, must be considered in the selection of an appropriate opioid. The opioid should be compatible with the patient's age, pain severity, dosing needs, and route of administration requirements. Often financial considerations need to be taken into account, especially when the patient is receiving multiple drugs and the cost of medications needs to be limited. This is another example of the skills and knowledge that advanced practice nurses bring to this endeavor. They are skilled at seeing the *whole* of the iceberg—the concrete manifestations "above the waterline," so to speak, but also informed and sensitive awareness to things unsaid, concerns "below the surface," including psychosocial, economic, spiritual, and concrete issues. At the end of life, certain routes of administration may be preferable owing to patient comfort, ease of administration, ability to swallow, pain severity, and need to titrate rapidly (American Pain Society, 2005). The *Circle of Caring* approach to care supports the multifaceted responses to the patient and family.

When evaluating an opioid for chronic use, renal and liver function should be assessed before initiation of the

opioid. Opioids with long half-lives may not be tolerated in many elderly patients because of clearance or metabolism issues. Renal function declines in older adults. It is also helpful to remember that in elderly patients, normal serum creatinine concentrations do not exclude renal impairment. If patients have underlying renal or liver insufficiency, they should be monitored for signs of toxicity.

For patients with moderate to severe pain who have limited prior treatment with opioids, begin with a short half-life agonist (such as morphine, hydromorphone, or oxycodone). Morphine is the preferred drug because it is widely available, is relatively low in cost, can be administered via a variety of routes, and comes in a variety of formulations including controlled- or sustained-release products that allow for tablets at 8- to 12-hour dosing intervals. Morphine should be used judiciously in patients with renal impairment because of the accumulation of morphine-3-glucuronide and morphine-6-glucuronide. It is easier for clinicians to initiate and titrate an opioid with a shorter half-life than one with a longer half-life (such as levorphanol or methadone). Meperidine is not recommended for the management of chronic cancer pain because of its potential for central nervous system excitability, with possible tremors, myoclonus, and seizures due to the accumulation of the metabolite normeperidine from repeated administration. This effect is pronounced when administered orally (Andersen et al, 2003).

Selecting an Appropriate Route of Administration Both the National Comprehensive Cancer Network (NCCN) cancer pain guidelines for adults (2014) and pediatric patients (2013) and the Clinical Practice Guidelines for the Management of Cancer Pain Panel (Jacox et al, 1994) advocate that the clinician begin with the most available, least invasive route. The oral route is generally preferred. In general, when drugs are administered orally, they have a slower onset of action, a delayed peak time, and a longer duration of effect than drugs administered parenterally. Drugs administered parenterally have a rapid onset of action but a shorter duration of action. This route can be an advantage when dealing with severe incidental pain or rapidly escalating pain.

If the oral route is unavailable, the rectal, sublingual, transdermal, or parenteral route may be used. Rectal suppositories containing morphine, hydromorphone, and oxymorphone are available, and controlled-release morphine sulfate may be administered rectally.

The transdermal fentanyl patch is useful for patients who cannot tolerate oral drugs or for patients for whom compliance with an around-the-clock schedule is difficult to maintain. The fentanyl patch is contraindicated in the management of acute pain. Because analgesic effects are often not appreciated by a patient until 12 to 24 hours after initiation of therapy, an initial titration should not occur before 3 days of fentanyl patch initiation. It is difficult to rapidly titrate using this delivery system. A hospitalized patient may be more safely and efficiently titrated using a fentanyl patient-controlled analgesia (PCA) pump to determine fentanyl requirements. When the fentanyl patch is removed, serum concentrations fall slowly. The fentanyl patch is not recommended for use in patients who have varying levels of pain or who have severe effects such as sedation or confusion from opioids, because these effects may persist for long periods after the patch is removed. A short-acting opioid for breakthrough pain should be prescribed for patients using the fentanyl patch.

Parenteral routes of administration should be considered for patients who require rapid onset of analgesia or high doses of opioids that cannot be administered orally. Parenteral routes include intermittent IV, intramuscular (IM), or subcutaneous (SC) injections and continuous SC or IV infusions. Intermittent SC injections may be administered with the placement of an indwelling 27-gauge butterfly needle, which will eliminate the need for painful intermittent injections. Studies suggest that SC administration is equipotent to the IV dose. Continuous SC or IV infusion devices may also provide patient-controlled rescue doses as an adjunct to the continuous, or basal, rate.

As its name implies, in patient-controlled analgesia, the patient is the only one who should push the prn dose button. This helps to ensure patient safety and prevent overdose situations. However, for patients at the end of life, it may not be possible because of debilitated state, cognitive ability, or neuromuscular impairment for the patient to activate the rescue dose feature (Anghelescu et al, 2005). In this situation, the American Society for Pain Management Nursing (ASPMN, 2006) advocates for the use of authorized agent–controlled analgesia (AACA). AACA is defined as "a method of pain control in which a consistently available and competent individual is authorized by a prescriber and properly educated to activate the dosing button of an analgesic infusion pump when the patient is unable, in response to that patient's pain" (Wuhrman et al, 2007). The authorized agent may be the nurse who is responsible for that particular patient. In that case, AACA could be nurse-controlled analgesia (NCA). Or, in another situation, the authorized agent could be a nonprofessional person such as a parent or significant other, and the method could be referred to as caregiver-controlled analgesia (CCA). The proper use of CCA by a designated proxy can allow for patients to die comfortably at home, without the need to transfer to another setting. The expression "PCA by proxy" is not encouraged because it implies that a potentially unsafe, uneducated, unauthorized individual is activating an individual's PCA pump. The population suitable for AACA (either NCA or CCA) is usually opioid tolerant. Both the ASPMN and the literature propose AACA as a means of safe, effective pain control when a designated proxy is carefully chosen and educated about appropriate use of a PCA for an individual patient (Anghelescu et al, 2005; Czarnecki et al, 2008; Kenagy & Turner, 2007; Wuhrman et al, 2007). It is important to establish policies and procedures for organizations utilizing AACA in their populations to determine criteria for proxy selection, patient monitoring, and education of proxy and health-care team members. Any organization or institution setting up AACA is referred to the recommendations of the ASPMN along with Kenagy and Turner (2007).

Selecting a Dosing Schedule Patients with continuous or frequent pain generally benefit from around-the-clock dosing, which prevents the pain from recurring. Indeed, in order to achieve freedom from pain, WHO advocates giving drugs around the clock at regular intervals and maintains that this stepped therapy is 80% to 90% effective. Continuous-release formulations of opioids utilize either tablets or transdermal delivery systems such as fentanyl, which may improve patient adherence to opioid regimens. A "rescue" or prn dose provides a means to treat pain that breaks through the fixed analgesic schedule or pain that occurs with specific activities such as changing position or ambulating. The drug used for breakthrough pain is usually the same drug in a shorter-acting, immediate-release formulation than the continuous- or sustained-release opioid that is administered on a regular schedule (American Pain Society, 2005). When using transdermal fentanyl, a short half-life opioid is recommended for breakthrough pain (Hanks et al, 2004). Continuous- or sustained-release formulations should not be used as rescue doses or to rapidly titrate the opioid for patients with severe pain (see Table 20.4). In these settings, short-acting opioids should be used. Often a parenteral formulation allows for rapid onset of analgesic action for patients in pain crisis. After analgesia is obtained and a stable dose has been determined, conversion to a continuous-release formulation can be made.

Switching to Another Opioid Patients with suboptimally controlled pain who develop unmanageable side effects that limit upward dose titration on one opioid can benefit from a switch or rotation to another opioid (de Stoutz et al, 1995; Knotkova et al, 2009). If a switch to another opioid is required, the equianalgesic dose table should be used as a guide to determine a reasonably effective and safe starting dose. Because of the existence of incomplete cross-tolerance between drugs, it is necessary to reduce the equianalgesic dose of the new, alternative

Table 20.4 Rescue Dose and Dose Titration

Rescue Dose

The rescue dose is an additional dose of the opioid that is administered on an as-needed basis to treat break-through pain; a short-acting, immediate-release opioid should be used. Oral rescue doses are usually administered on an every-1-to-2-hour schedule as needed. The dose of the oral rescue should be equivalent to approximately 10%–20% of the total 24-hour dose. The dose of the parenteral rescue opioid should be 50% of the hourly infusion rate for patients receiving continuous infusion, administered on a 15- to 30-minute as-needed schedule. It is generally recommended that patients who require four to six rescue doses in a 24-hour period should have an escalation of the baseline dose.

Dose Titration

All patients with chronic cancer pain should be assessed regularly for pain intensity and relief and for the presence of adverse effects. A stepwise escalation of the opioid dose should be done until adequate analgesia or intolerable adverse effects develop. Generally, it is safe to titrate opioids 25%–50% every 24–48 hours. The severity of the pain should determine the rate of dose titration. Doses can become extremely large as a result of titration. It is important to remember that there is no ceiling to opioid doses and titration needs to be based on pain intensity and relief. Caution should be employed when titrating opioids with long half-lives, such as levorphanol or methadone, because accumulation of drug can occur with subsequent toxicity.

dose table, Table 20.6 gives an example of switching routes using the same opioid, and Table 20.7 shows an example of switching from one opioid to another.) Clinicians need to be aware that the science underlying

Table 20.6 Example of Switching From One Route of Administration to Another (Same Drug)

The following example illustrates how to switch from one route of administration to another using the same drug. A 42-year-old woman with metastatic ovarian cancer is receiving morphine sulfate 15 mg/hr IV. She is going to be discharged in 2 days and would prefer to go home with an oral medication. Her parenteral morphine dosage needs to be converted to an oral morphine dosage, e.g., morphine sulfate 15 mg/hr IV to MS Contin PO.

1. Calculate the 24-hour dose of the opioid (including around-the-clock [ATC] and prn rescue doses).
   - Morphine sulfate 15 mg/hr IV = 15 mg × 24 hr = 360 mg IV/24 hr
2. Convert the 24-hour dose of the drug (at prior route of administration) to 24-hour dose of drug (at new route of administration) using the equianalgesic table.
   - Morphine sulfate 10 mg IV = 30 mg PO or 1:3
   - 360 mg IV × 3 = 1,080 mg PO
3. Determine the dosing interval of the new drug. Using sustained-release morphine given q8–12hr, the patient needs 1080 mg PO over 24 hours; therefore, 500 mg every 12 hours.
4. Calculate the prn rescue dose as 5%–15% of the total 24-hour mg dose of the drug. (It may be necessary to adjust the dose because it is commercially available.)
   - 5% of 1,080 mg = 54 mg
   - Therefore, the decision was made to give 60 mg PO q2hr prn as a rescue dose.

opioid by one-half to two-thirds for patients on higher doses of the initial opioid. If switching to an opioid with a long half-life, such as methadone, accumulation of the drug can occur, and the methadone dose should be decreased by 90%. (Table 20.5 presents an equianalgesic

Table 20.5 Equianalgesics

Drug	IV/IM/SC	PO	IV:PO	Half-life	Duration
Morphine sulfate	10 mg	30 mg	1:3	2–3 hours	2–4 hours
Codeine	130 mg	200 mg	—	2–3 hours	2–4 hours
Hydromorphone	1.5 mg	7.5 mg	1:5	2–3 hours	2–4 hours
Levorphanol	2 mg	4 mg	1:2	12–15 hours	4–6 hours
Meperidine	75 mg	300 mg	1:4	3–4 hours	2–4 hours
Methadone	10 mg	20 mg	1:2	12–15 hours	4–8 hours
Oxycodone	—	20 mg	—	2–3 hours	2–4 hours
Oxymorphone	1-mg or 5-mg suppository	—	—	2–3 hours	2–4 hours
Fentanyl	100-mcg patch/IV	4-mg morphine sulfate IV/hr			

Adapted from American Pain Society. *Principles of analgesic use in the treatment of acute pain and cancer pain,* ed 6. American Pain Society, Glenview, IL, 2008.

Table 20.7   Example of Switching From One Oral Opioid to Another

A 65-year-old man with metastatic prostate cancer to bone is receiving sustained-release oral morphine 60 mg PO q12hr and is experiencing severe uncontrollable nausea and vomiting. The decision is made to switch him to oral hydromorphone.
  Calculate the 24-hour dose of the prior opioid (including ATC and prn rescue doses).
• Sustained-release morphine 60 mg PO q12hr = 120 mg PO/24 hr
1. Convert the 24-hour dose of the prior drug to the 24-hour dose of the new drug using the equianalgesic table.
  • Hydromorphone 7.5 mg PO = Morphine sulfate 30 mg PO
  • Hydromorphone 7.5 mg/X = Morphine sulfate 30 mg/120 mg
  • Cross multiply to get 30X = 900 mg
  • Divide both sides by 30 to get X = 30 mg hydromorphone PO/24 hr
2. Calculate the adjusted total 24-hour dose of the new drug.
  • Adjust the dose of new drug as follows:
  a. Reduce the total 24-hour dose of new drug by 25%–50% to account for incomplete cross tolerance. 50% of hydromorphone 30 mg PO q24hr = 15 mg hydromorphone PO q24hr.
  b. If the patient has inadequate analgesia and no side effects from the prior drug, it may not be necessary to reduce the dose of the new drug.
  c. Reduce the drug more if the patient had significant side effects from the prior drug.
  d. If the patient is frail, reduce the dose of the new drug more (75%).
  e. Reduce the dose of the new drug more if the dose of the prior drug was high (>75 mg IM morphine equivalent/day).
  f. If the new drug is methadone, reduce the total 24-hour dose by 90%.
  • Determine the dosing interval of the new drug.
  • Hydromorphone 15 mg PO/24 hr = 2.5 mg PO q4hr. (It may be necessary to adjust the dose because it is commercially available. Hydromorphone 2 mg PO q4hr.)
3. Calculate the prn rescue dose as 5%–15% of the total 24-hour mg dose of the drug being switched. 15% of hydromorphone 15 mg PO q24hr = 2.25 mg hydromorphone PO q24hr. (It may be necessary to adjust the dose because it is commercially available. Rescue dose = hydromorphone 2 mg PO q2h prn.)

relative potency continues to evolve (Knotkova et al, 2009).

Table 20.8 outlines common adjuvants for specific types of pain (e.g., neuropathic and bone pain). A 2009 study that reviewed the prospective database of 1,038 patients with bone metastasis who were referred to a rapid response radiotherapy program found that a significant proportion of patients were undermedicated for pain each year from 1999 to 2006 (Kirou-Mauro et al, 2009). Individuals with an anticipated life expectancy of more than 4 months; a Karnofsky Performance Status of greater than 60; an adequate bone marrow reserve; and no pending or actual pathological fracture, hypercalcemia, or spinal cord compression were identified as suitable candidates for radiopharmaceuticals. Individuals with more limited bone involvement could be referred for possible focal or wide-field (hemibody) external beam radiation. Dy et al (2008), in their evidenced-based standards for cancer pain management, proposed that individuals with metastatic bone pain be offered single-fraction radiotherapy as a treatment option.

The recommendations for the treatment of neuropathic pain are evolving. In 2007, the Fourth International Conference on the Mechanisms and Treatment of Neuropathic Pain (an independent expert panel) and the International Association for the Study of Pain (a multidisciplinary medical specialty society) developed comprehensive evidence-based guidelines for the pharmacological management of neuropathic pain (Dworkin et al, 2007). After a diagnosis of neuropathic pain is established, it is recommended to initiate therapy of the disease that may be causing the neuropathic pain (if possible) and to start first-line symptom treatment with either a secondary amine TCA (e.g., nortriptyline or desipramine) or a selective serotonin and norepinephrine reuptake inhibitor (SSNRI; e.g., venlafaxine or duloxetine). Another option would be to initiate either gabapentin or pregabalin (calcium channel alpha-2-sigma ligand). In addition, patients with a localized peripheral neuropathic pain could use a topical lidocaine alone on the painful area or use it in combination with a TCA, SSNRI, or calcium channel alpha-2-sigma ligand agent. Opioid analgesics and tramadol have been shown to have analgesic efficacy in multiple randomized controlled trials (RCTs) in patients with neuropathic pain and can be utilized for those with severe pain or to assist with pain relief during titration of the first-line medications. Opioid analgesics and tramadol should also be considered for first-line treatment when there is acute neuropathic pain or for treatment of neuropathic cancer pain. If a patient experiences only partial pain relief on one agent and does not experience intolerable side effects, another first-line agent can be added to the original agent. If, however, the pain relief on the original first-line agent is inadequate after an adequate titration trial, the patient should be switched to an alternative first-line agent. Patients with neuropathic pain need

Table 20.8 Adjuvant Drugs for Specific Types of Pain

Neuropathic Pain

Tricyclic antidepressants
- amitriptyline
- desipramine
- imipramine
- nortriptyline

Antiepileptics
- gabapentin (Neurontin)
- carbamazepine (Tegretol)
- oxcarbazepine (Trileptal)
- topiramate (Topamax)
- levetiracetam (Keppra)
- sodium valproate (Depacon)
- tiagabine (Gabitril)
- lamotrigine (Lamictal)
- zonisamide (Zonegran)

Local anesthetics
- EMLA (topical eutectic mixture of local anesthetics lidocaine and prilocaine)
- Epidural and IV lidocaine
- Oral local anesthetics: mexiletine (Mexitil), tocainide (Tonocard)
- Topical lidocaine 5% patches (Lidoderm)

Glucocorticoids

Alpha-2-adrenergic agonists
- tizanidine (Zanaflex)
- clonidine

NMDA receptor antagonists
- ketamine
- dextromethorphan
- amantadine

GABA agonists
- baclofen

Bone Pain

Glucocorticoids

Bisphosphonates
- pamidronate disodium (Aredia)
- zoledronate (Zometa)

Other osteoclast inhibitor
- calcitonin

Radiopharmaceuticals
- Strontium-89
- Strontium-153

Other

Skeletal muscle relaxants
- tizanidine (Zanaflex)
- Benzodiazepines: diazepam benzodiazepines: diazepam (Valium), clonazepam (Klonopin), lorazepam (Ativan)
- Antihistamines
- Antispasmodics: baclofen

Topical agents
- Capsaicin cream
- Lidocaine 5% patch (Lidoderm)
- EMLA cream

to be continually reassessed for pain relief and quality-of-life issues. Those who fail the first-line agents or who did not meet criteria initially can try opioid analgesics or tramadol as a second-line agent. Third-line agents to be considered include certain antiseizure medications (such as carbamazepine, lamotrigine, oxcarbazepine, topiramate, and valproic acid); antidepressants (such as bupropion, citalopram, paroxetine); mexiletine; N-methyl-D-aspartate (NMDA) receptor antagonist; or topical capsaicin. These medications have shown inconsistent results. A referral to a multidisciplinary pain center or a pain specialist is recommended if an individual does not obtain relief from second- or third-line medications (Dworkin et al, 2007). In general, clinicians need to be aware that long-term studies comparing one medication to another, head to head, and those comparing combination regimens still need to be done and must be a priority for research in the treatment of chronic neuropathic pain (O'Connor and Dworkin, 2009). As noted in the 2014 IOM report, pain control continues to be an ongoing area of challenge.

Guidelines that evaluate the clinical practice of using gabapentin and TCAs in the treatment of neuropathic pain in cancer patients found that there is little evidence to demonstrate the superiority of either TCAs or gabapentin over one another in the treatment of neuropathic pain. Both can be effective and are recommended for use in this population. Within the class of TCAs, amitriptyline may have some beneficial effectiveness but may not be as well tolerated in some individuals (Librach et al, 2006).

The Quality Standards Subcommittee of the American Academy of Neurology in 2004 reviewed the literature and made recommendations for another specific neuropathic pain population—those with pain from postherpetic neuralgia. They found TCAs, gabapentin, pregabalin, topical lidocaine patches, and opioids to be effective in the treatment of postherpetic neuralgia pain. They also found epidural morphine, epidural methylprednisolone, acupuncture, benzydamine cream, lorazepam, vitamin E, dextromethorphan, iontophoresis of vincristine, lorazepam, or indomethacin to be of benefit. They noted that at present there is insufficient evidence to make recommendations regarding the long-term effects of the treatments evaluated (Dubinsky et al, 2004). Two updates were added to these guidelines from the National Guideline Clearing House. First, as of December 16, 2008, the U.S. Food and Drug Administration (FDA) is requiring that all manufacturers of antiepileptic drugs include a warning in the labeling of these drugs advising patients prescribed these drugs that there is an increased risk of suicidality. Second, on January 16, 2009, the FDA issued a public health advisory reminding both health-care professionals and patients and their families about the potentially serious hazards of using topical anesthetics. Their concern is that when applied to large areas of skin, or when the area of application is covered, there is a potential for these products to produce an irregular heartbeat, breathing difficulties, seizure, coma, or even death. Their advisory group made recommendations for the safe use of these products (Dubinsky et al, 2004).

Invasive Interventional Pain Management Techniques

There is a small subgroup of patients with pain who may benefit from invasive pain management techniques. Specifically, this group includes individuals who have pain that is localized to one or two areas that is expected to persist. These anesthetic and neurosurgical approaches are indicated when conservative measures utilizing opioids and adjuvant analgesics have failed to provide adequate analgesia or when the patient is experiencing intolerable, unmanageable side effects. These procedures include regional analgesia (spinal, intraventricular, and intrapleural opioids), sympathetic blockade and neurolytic procedures (celiac plexus block, lumbar sympathetic block, cervicothoracic [stellate ganglion] block), or pathway ablation procedure (chemical or surgical rhizotomy or cordotomy). In evaluating patients for these invasive approaches, it is important to ascertain that all other conservative measures have been adequately tried and have failed. Other factors to consider include presence of infection, coagulopathy or use of anticoagulant drugs, functional state, prognosis, coexisting medical conditions, spinal cord disease, and the possibility of rapid progression of disease outside of site that is going to be blocked or ablated (Cherny et al, 1996). Availability of experienced, local health-care providers who can monitor and manage the intervention is essential. A procedure performed by an inexperienced surgeon or anesthesiologist on a medically ill patient may have a suboptimal or an unpredictable outcome (Hassenbach & Cherny, 2004). Readers are directed to other references for a more detailed discussion of interventional pain management techniques (Layman-Goldstein & Coyle, 2010).

To summarize, the APRN should treat according to evidence-based guidelines, which includes keeping abreast of the latest literature in these areas, as well as the limitations of that literature. A good beginning is to treat according to the NCCN guidelines for adult cancer pain (2014). If the patient is thought to be weeks or days from expected death, do not reduce opioid dosage related to a falling blood pressure, respirations, or level of consciousness, and titrate for optimal comfort. This is the goal in palliative care. The clinician should be able to recognize and treat opioid-induced neurotoxicity such as myoclonus and hyperalgesia. If the opioid must be reduced, it should be reduced gradually by 50% within a 24-hour period to prevent acute withdrawal or pain crisis. Patient preference regarding analgesia versus decreased level of consciousness must be a priority. Routes of administration should be modified as needed, applying equianalgesic dose conversions. Specialist consultation may be necessary for management of refractory pain.

Nonpharmacological Pain Management Techniques

Nondrug or nonpharmacological pain management interventions are used to address aspects of an individual's pain that have not responded to other pain management techniques. Selection of a particular nondrug intervention is based on the underlying etiology of the pain and can complement the pharmacological interventions. Nondrug techniques are not to be used as a substitute for pharmacological interventions. Although nondrug interventions cover a broad spectrum of approaches, the three main approaches to nondrug pain management are (1) psychological interventions, (2) physiatric and neurostimulatory interventions, and (3) complementary/integrative interventions. Some interventions may fall into more than one approach. At present, the evidence for the use of nondrug pain management techniques is limited by the lack of large, well-designed, rigorous studies. It is encouraging to see that the evidence-based literature supporting use of these techniques continues to grow (Deng et al, 2004, 2007; Lorenz et al, 2008; Wiffen & Eccleston, 2009).

Psychological interventions for pain management can include patient and family education, distraction, self-statements, relaxation techniques, guided imagery and hypnosis, patient pain diaries, and cognitive-behavioral therapy. Cognitive and behavioral interventions are helpful in reducing emotional distress, improving coping, and offering the patient and family a sense of control. A meta-analysis by Devine (2003) reviewing the effects on pain of nonpharmacological interventions (such as educational, psychosocial, and cognitive-behavioral interventions) in adults with cancer supported the use of these interventions as an adjuvant to analgesic therapy. The Clinical Practice Guidelines for the Management of Cancer Pain Panel (Jacox et al, 1994) and the National Comprehensive Cancer Network (NCCN) cancer pain guidelines for both adults (2014) and pediatric patients (2013) encourage the use of psychosocial interventions for pain management early in the course of disease, as part of a multimodal approach. Clinicians may find that an individual with a life-threatening illness is well versed in using specific psychological approaches and is open to using these techniques to aid in coping with pain and other symptoms. On the other hand, the person may be too weak, debilitated, and cognitively impaired to be taught or even to use a simple, previously utilized, relaxation technique. Assessment is key to developing a realistic plan. The intervention must match the specific problem with an appreciation for the patient's and caregiver's abilities and motivations. Also, nurse practitioners need to be aware of which experts are available in their practice community to facilitate referrals.

Education about pain and its management is an important component of any pain management plan. Oldenmenger et al (2009) found that in 5 out of 11 RCTs patient education decreased pain intensity in a statistically significant way. However, pain control may not be enhanced by additional education without a systematic approach that addresses other barriers, such as inadequate analgesic titration or untreated side effects. The PRO-SELF pain control program "uses education along with repeated reinforcement, skill building, and ongoing nursing support to improve self-care pain management in patients with cancer and their family caregivers" (West et al, 2003). It has been successful in improving the management of cancer pain (American Pain Society, 2005).

In 1996, the National Institutes of Health (NIH) Technology Panel evaluated the effects of relaxation on pain and sleep. This review provided strong evidence for the use of relaxation techniques to reduce pain. The panel divided relaxation techniques into brief and deep methods. In general, the brief methods take less time to acquire or practice. Very often brief methods are abbreviated forms of a corresponding deep method. The brief methods include deep breathing, focused breathing, paced respiration, and self-control. Deep methods include such techniques as progressive muscle relaxation (PMR), autogenic training, and meditation. To use autogenic training, the patient is taught to imagine a peaceful environment and to focus on a "heaviness in the limbs, warmth in the limbs, cardiac regulation, centering on breathing, warmth in the upper abdomen, and coolness in the forehead" (NIH Technology Assessment Panel, 1996, p. 314). The use of PMR involves the tensing and then relaxing in sequence of each of the 15 major muscle groups.

In 2003, Devine performed a meta-analysis on the effect of nondrug interventions such as educational, psychosocial, and cognitive-behavioral interventions on adults with cancer-related pain by reviewing 25 interventional studies published from 1978 through 2001. Six of these studies tested the effect of education. A homogeneous small-to-moderate statistically significant beneficial effect on pain was found. In her discussion Devine pointed out that with the widely accepted strong mandate to educate patients about their pain and its management, there may not be much of a difference between experimental and control content (Devine, 2003).

Physiatric and neurostimulatory modalities include cutaneous stimulation, exercise, immobilization, acupuncture, and transcutaneous electrical nerve stimulation. Referral to a professional who specializes in these modalities may be indicated as appropriate.

Some of the nondrug approaches to pain management that have been discussed are considered mainstream, traditional Western medicine. Other nonconventional therapies fall under the heading of complementary or alternative. Although complementary and alternative therapies are often grouped together under the heading of complementary and alternative medicine (CAM), they are very different. Complementary therapies are used *in addition to* conventional therapies and in some settings are labeled "integrative." Alternative therapies are used *in place of* traditional, mainstream treatment and are not encouraged in the setting of utilizing evidence-based interventions (Berenson, 2005; Cassileth & Gubili, 2009). *Integrative interventions* is becoming the preferred term for these approaches that complement or augment traditional approaches. The National Center for Complementary and Alternative Medicine (NCCAM) groups the CAM modalities into five main areas:

- Alternative medical systems
- Mind–body interventions
- Biologically based therapies
- Manipulative and body-based therapies
- Energy-based therapies

The nondrug interventions that are discussed in this chapter, either traditional or complementary/integrative, are considered a part of the overall pain management plan. Acupuncture, mind-body therapy, and massage therapy are shown in studies to have the strongest evidence for their clinical use in pain control (Deng et al, 2004).

In Traditional Chinese Medicine (TCM), it is thought that good health depends on the balance of energy in the body. Energy—called *chi* or *qi*—is thought to be constantly circulating in the body. Acupuncture attempts to promote circulation of this vital energy. *Acupuncture,* a holistic, energy-based treatment from TCM, has been shown to effectively treat health problems including pain, depression, and nausea (Deng et al, 2004, 2007; NIH Consensus Conference, 1998). Despite building evidence in the literature supporting the use of acupuncture, it still is underutilized in end-of-life palliative care (Standish et al, 2008). In this approach, thin, disposable needles, usually stainless steel, are placed in precise anatomical points (365 specific locations) to balance energy movement along the body's 12 meridians (Berenson, 2005; Decker, 2000). *Acupressure* is the application of finger pressure to the acupuncture points. *Moxibustion* is the stimulation of an acupuncture point by heat. This is done by burning a special compressed combustible substance near the acupuncture point. Other variations in acupuncture stimulation of sites include the use of electrical stimulators or lasers. The NIH Consensus Conference (1998) found that the data in support of acupuncture are as strong as those for many accepted Western medicine–based therapies, and the incidence of adverse effects from acupuncture is substantially lower than for many standard medical procedures or medications used for the same conditions. Adverse effects from acupuncture can include an occasional drop of blood or bruise at the needle insertion site, mild discomfort at site, infection, or, depending on insertion site, pneumothorax. The latter two effects are rare and depend on the experience and training of the acupuncturist (Berenson, 2005).

Based on high-quality evidence, the Integrative Oncology Practice Guidelines recommend acupuncture as "a complementary therapy when pain is poorly controlled" (Deng et al, 2007). Some studies indicate that it may be helpful as an adjunct treatment in painful situations such as headache, menstrual cramps, fibromyalgia, myofascial pain, osteoarthritis, and low back pain. Its effectiveness in relieving musculoskeletal pain remains controversial (Deng et al, 2004). Controlled studies using acupuncture in palliative care patients are in the process of development. Ideally, as more research is done and acupuncture is further incorporated into the mainstream health-care system, more informed decisions regarding the appropriateness of acupuncture for patients in varying situations will be made (NIH Consensus Conference, 1998). As health-care professionals, it is important to guide patients from a perspective of evidence, not marketing. A more detailed discussion of acupressure and acupuncture is beyond the scope of this text. At this time, most insurance policies do not cover acupuncture or other integrative approaches, and most patients and families have to pay out of pocket for these interventions.

Music, a mind–body technique, has been shown to be an effective intervention for pain control through a variety of physiological and psychological effects. Affective, cognitive, and sensory processes can be engaged, activated, and altered by music. In palliative care, music therapy "strives to promote well-being and quality of life for patients and caregivers" (Magill, 2009). This is done by processes such as use of prior skills, alteration of mood, distraction, relaxation, and improved sense of control. Physical effects include increasing or decreasing pulse and blood pressure (Magill-Levreault, 1993; Tuls Hallstead & Tuls Roscoe, 2002). Music therapy, as defined by Spross and Wolff Burk (1995), is "the scientific and systematic use of music to effect beneficial changes in physiological and psychological processes that influence experiences of pain and illness" (p. 175). The use of music therapy in the medically ill can reduce mood disturbance (Cassileth et al, 2003) and affect the suffering and total pain that a sick individual experiences. Tuls Halstead and Tuls Roscoe (2002) offer many concrete examples of how to use music to assist patients as listeners and performers.

Music should not be considered the first-line treatment for pain relief. Fifty-one RCTs of adults or children met criteria to look at the effect of music on acute, chronic, or cancer pain. There was a small but positive finding that music reduced pain and reduced requirements for morphine-like analgesics. The types of pain included in the studies (acute postoperative, chronic, labor, procedural, or experimental pain with the majority involving procedural or postoperative pain) may not readily generalize to pain in individuals at the end of life. More rigorous, well-designed studies looking at the use of music as part of a pain management plan for individuals at the end of life are needed.

Cognitive interventions such as relaxation, guided imagery, and hypnosis discussed earlier fall under the NCCAM category of mind–body methods that may also be helpful in the management of chronic pain.

Reiki, a form of energy therapy, is a Japanese term for universal life energy. Current studies are underway to evaluate its role in symptom management, including that of pain. *Reiki* is defined as a vibrational or subtle energy most commonly facilitated by light touch, the

use of which is thought to balance the biofield and strengthen the body's ability to heal itself. Reiki practitioners gently place their hands on a fully clothed individual's head, back, front, and the site of discomfort (if the person desires) to promote relaxation and decrease pain (Berenson, 2005; Vitale, 2007). A phase 2 study of Reiki in the management of pain in individuals with advanced cancer showed improved pain control and improved quality of life using this noninvasive intervention but no overall reduction in opioid use (Olson et al, 2003).

A Cochrane Database review of touch therapies for pain relief in adults looked at the effectiveness of Reiki, Therapeutic Touch, and Healing Touch (So et al, 2008). Of the studies evaluated for this review, only three studies met criteria for inclusion for Reiki, five for Healing Touch, and seventeen for Therapeutic Touch. The review found that these touch therapies may have a modest effect on pain relief. Of interest, it found that studies that utilized more experienced practitioners had greater reduction of pain. It concluded that more studies, especially those looking at the effect of touch therapies in children, are needed to provide sufficient evidence to promote the use of these interventions for pain relief.

Patients often initiate nondrug interventions, such as application of heat or use of vibration, and frequently choose a technique based on previous use of a particular intervention or on their personal knowledge of home remedies. The technique chosen may or may not be an optimal method to relieve a particular type of pain. In 2002, the National Center for Complementary and Alternative Medicine (NCCAM) released a study that showed that six of the top nine reasons that people use complementary medicine are pain related (Gray et al, 2002). Although pharmacological interventions are usually a well-thought-out part of a pain-management plan, the use of nondrug interventions often is not. There may be little input from an individual's doctor or nurse in initiating an intervention (Rhiner et al, 1993). Many insurance plans do not currently cover nondrug methods, even when prescribed by a licensed provider as part of a well-thought-out pain management plan. The literature continues to evolve as to which specific nondrug interventions will be most effective in helping to control pain at end of life.

Evidence-based standards promoting high-quality management of cancer pain call for screening for the presence of pain and subsequent assessment if pain is identified (Dy et al, 2008). Successful pain management is based on ongoing assessment and reassessment of the patient. It is important to evaluate the individual carefully and apply what is appropriate for that individual in a particular situation, bearing in mind the individual's goals of care. After the initiation of systemic analgesic therapy (based on the WHO analgesic ladder approach) and treatment of underlying disease (if appropriate), the next step would be to consider the addition of psychological, physiatric and neurostimulatory, or integrative techniques to improve pain control and possibly improve the balance between analgesia and side effects (American Pain Society, 2005; Cherny & Portenoy, 1994; Dy et al, 2008; Rhiner et al, 1993). If these measures are ineffective, the consideration of the use of invasive techniques is appropriate (Hassenbach & Cherny, 2004; Miguel, 2000). Finally, if it is impossible to balance pain relief and side effects, sedation at the end of life must be considered.

■ PALLIATIVE MANAGEMENT OF DYSPNEA

Dyspnea may be one of the most frightening and difficult symptoms a patient can experience and can be more difficult to treat than pain. Dyspnea is a subjective feeling of breathlessness, the sensation of labored or difficult breathing, which contributes to severe disability and impaired quality of life. It occurs before death in an estimated 20% to 70% of patients with advanced cancer (Bruera et al, 2000; Ripamonti, 1999; Solano et al, 2006). Patients often describe feelings of suffocation, tightness, congestion, air hunger, choking, or heavy breathing. A review of the literature on management of dyspnea at the end of life reinforces the growing recognition that dyspnea and fear of dyspnea produce profound suffering for patients who are dying and their families. The causes of dyspnea are numerous and related to pulmonary disease, cardiac disease, cancer, metabolic abnormalities, radiation therapy, and surgery. Anxiety is always a component. Higginson and McCarthy (1989) reported that dyspnea prevalence increases in terminally ill patients and is the major uncontrollable symptom. The American Thoracic Society strongly endorses the concept that palliative care for dyspnea be available to patients in all stages of illness and should be individualized based on the needs and preferences of the patient and his or her family (Lanken et al, 2008). It further supports the use of invasive or noninvasive home ventilators and other equipment; the use of oxygen, when appropriate; noninvasive positive pressure ventilation for hypercapnic adults; use of a fan; and opioids and anxiolytics in the management of dyspnea at the end of life.

The 2013 NCCN Guidelines Version 2 includes two new algorithms for palliative management of dyspnea. They stress the importance of prioritizing patient preferences and educating and supporting the family and friends who may be in attendance. These guidelines note that ongoing emotional and spiritual support may be needed for both patient and family to manage this most distressing symptom.

Assessment

Dyspnea is a multidimensional symptom, having both physical and psychological components. For most patients with organic disease, the respiratory distress gets worse with progression of disease. It is highly distressing for families and caregivers, who often feel helpless.

Various tools to measure dyspnea have been documented in the literature and include use of a visual analog scale, structured interviews, self-report questionnaires, and numerical rating scales. Clinical assessment of dyspnea should include a complete history of the symptom, its onset and duration, and precipitating and relieving factors; associated symptoms; and response to medications, oxygen, and behavioral interventions. In cancer patients, data suggest that the frequency and severity of dyspnea increase with progression of disease and, when death is approaching, may be seen as a poor prognostic sign (Booth, 2006). In patients with COPD, intractable breathlessness develops late in the course of the disease, gradually progressing over years.

Etiology and Management of Dyspnea in the Patient With Advanced Cancer

The possible causes of dyspnea in the patient with advanced cancer are multiple and detailed in Table 20.9. Often the etiology is multifactorial, and more than one etiology may be present, especially at the end of life. Relief of dyspnea is aimed at treatment of the underlying disease process, whether malignant or nonmalignant in origin. Symptomatic interventions are used when the process is not reversible.

A variety of sources advocate the use of morphine to manage intractable dyspnea. Jennings et al (2002) completed a systematic review of the use of opioids in breathlessness. They reviewed 18 studies, and the meta-analysis showed a statistically significant positive effect of opioids on the sensation of breathlessness. In another systematic

Table 20.9	Common Causes of Dyspnea in the Advanced Cancer Patient

- Anemia
- Infection
- Pneumonia
- Congestive heart disease
- COPD
- Obstruction of airway by tumor
- Lymphangitic tumor spread in lung
- Pleural effusion
- Asthma
- Pulmonary emboli
- Superior vena cava syndrome
- Fluid overload
- Chronic debility and deconditioning
- Cachexia
- Chemotherapy toxicity (Adriamycin, Bleomycin)
- Radiation fibrosis
- Rib, bone fractures
- Anxiety
- Hepatomegaly
- Ascites
- Excess secretions

review of randomized controlled trials assessing all pharmacological and nonpharmacological interventions for dyspnea in cancer patients, Ben-Aharon et al (2008) analyzed the results of 18 trials. Fourteen evaluated pharmacological interventions included opioids, oxygen, helium-enriched air, and furosemide. Four trials evaluated nonpharmacological interventions. The administration of subcutaneous morphine resulted in a significant reduction of dyspnea using a Visual Analog Scale compared with placebo. No difference was observed in dyspnea when nebulized morphine was compared with subcutaneous morphine. The addition of benzodiazepines to morphine was significantly more effective

than when morphine was administered alone, without additional adverse effects. Table 20.10 outlines the opioid trials and describes the effect of interventions.

The use of oxygen to relieve dyspnea has been examined. Oxygen was not superior to room air for alleviating dyspnea except for patients with hypoxemia. Oxygen has shown no benefit in alleviating dyspnea in patients without hypoxemia (Ahmedzai et al, 2004; Bruera et al, 2003; Bruera, de Stoutz, et al, 1993; Philip et al, 2006). Hypoxemic patients may not be dyspneic, and if they are, reversing the hypoxemia does not always lessen dyspnea. Patients who are dyspneic should be taught how to use a fan before using inhaled oxygen or air (Booth

Table 20.10	Interventions for Dyspnea
Interventions	**Comments**
Oxygen	3–5 L/min via nasal cannula In addition to supplemental oxygen, temporary supplemental support such as CPAP or BiPAP may be considered for severe, acute dyspneic episode that is considered reversible
Pharmacotherapy Morphine sulfate	SC: 50% higher than regularly scheduled dose SC: 5 mg bolus or 2.5 times regular dose every 4 hours SC: 10 mg every 4 hours IV: 1–5 mg/hr
Bronchodilators	Nebulized: Adrenergic and anticholinergic agents 4 times/day (ipratropium bromide [Atrovent], albuterol [Proventil], isoproterenol HCl [Isuprel], or metaproterenol sulfate [Alupent]) PO or IV: aminophylline PO: theophylline (Theo-Dur) 400 mg daily
Corticosteroids	Inhaler: beclomethasone (Vanceril) 1–2 inhalations 3–4 times/day PO or IV: dexamethasone (Decadron) 8–12 mg daily, then taper PO: prednisone 10–30 mg daily
Anxiolytics	PO: lorazepam (Ativan) 0.5–2 mg every 4–6 hours PO: diazepam (Valium) 2–10 mg 2–4 times daily PO: chlorpromazine (Thorazine) 25–50 mg 3–4 times daily PO: haloperidol (Haldol) 0.5–2 mg 2–4 times daily
Diuretics	PO: furosemide (Lasix) 20–40 mg daily
Anticholinergics to reduce secretions	Scopolamine, atropine, hyoscyamine, and glycopyrrolate (does not cross blood–brain barrier; less likely to cause delirium); scopolamine—transdermal and/or SC
Nonpharmacological Therapies Cognitive-behavioral	Relaxation therapy Guided imagery Music Distraction Stress management
Physical measures	Cooler room Fans Physical comfort measures
Support	Ongoing emotional and spiritual support for both patient and family is needed to manage this most distressing symptom

et al, 2008). Helium-enriched air resulted in dyspnea improvement compared with room air or oxygen-enriched air, but this has been evaluated in only one trial (Ahmedzai et al, 2004).

The Oncology Nursing Society, in its Evidence-Based Interventions for Cancer-Related Dyspnea, recommends the use of oral immediate-release and parenteral morphine in treating dyspnea (DiSalvo et al, 2008). It also supports the use of supplemental oxygen in patients with proven hypoxemia.

Nonpharmacological Interventions

Acupuncture, psychological support, breathing control, and coping strategies for dyspnea have been evaluated. In one study of acupuncture followed by acupressure versus placebo acupuncture followed by placebo acupressure, acupuncture was not beneficial for dyspnea relief in cancer patients (Vickers et al, 2005). Nursing intervention studies showed that support, breathing control, and coping strategies have significantly improved breathlessness (Bredin et al, 1999; Corner et al, 1996; Moore et al, 2002). The Cochrane Database review by Bausewein et al (2008) assessed randomized controlled and controlled clinical trials assessing the effects of nonpharmacological and noninvasive interventions to relieve breathlessness due to advanced stages of cancer, COPD, interstitial lung disease, chronic heart failure, or motor neuron disease. They reviewed 47 studies that were categorized to include single interventions such as walking aids, music, chest wall vibration, acupuncture/acupressure, relaxation, neuroelectrical muscle stimulation, and fan. Cooler temperatures, electric fans, stress management techniques, and a variety of physical comfort measures individualized to that patient may help. Multicomponent interventions included counseling and support, breathing training, counseling and support with relaxation, case management, and psychotherapy. They concluded that breathing training, walking aids, neuroelectrical muscle stimulation, and chest wall vibrations appear to be effective in relieving breathlessness in advanced stages of disease. Additionally, there is emerging evidence that in addition to supplemental O_2, temporary ventilator support such as continuous positive airway pressure (CPAP) or bilevel positive airway pressure (BiPAP) may be helpful for a severe dyspneic episode that is deemed to be reversible. Management of dyspnea is based on the cause and includes pharmacotherapy (e.g., bronchodilators, steroids, diuretics, vasodilators, antibiotics, opioids, and sedatives), oxygen, nonpharmacological therapies (e.g., relaxation and breathing exercises), and other appropriate therapies (e.g., transfusion, thoracentesis, and radiation therapy). For most dying patients, the pharmacological use of benzodiazepines, opioids, and corticosteroids remains the primary treatment (Dudgeon, Kristjanson, et al, 2001; Dudgeon, Lertzman, et al, 2001). There may be much resistance among primary-care providers to the use of opioids and sedatives because of unfamiliarity with these drugs, lack

of experience in treating dyspnea in dying patients, low priority given to this symptom, and fear that these drugs may hasten death. If symptoms are difficult to manage, a consultation with a palliative care expert is recommended, and sedation may be appropriate at the end of life.

Table 20.10 presents interventions commonly used for the management of dyspnea. All interventions should be based on the goals of care, with patient and family included in all decision making.

Based on clinical practice, the use of the mnemonic BREATHES (adapted from Kuebler, 1996) may assist the health-care provider in the symptomatic management of dyspnea:

B: Bronchospasm/persistent cough. Consider nebulized albuterol and/or steroids.

R: Rales/crackles, excess secretions. If present, consider reducing fluid intake. If the patient is receiving IV hydration, reduce the fluid rate or discontinue. Consider gentle diuresis with furosemide 20 to 40 mg PO and spironolactone 100 mg PO daily. If secretions are copious, consider scopolamine patch every 72 hours, atropine 0.3 to 0.5 mg subcutaneous or sublingual every 4 hours prn, or glycopyrrolate (Robinul) 0.1 to 0.4 mg IV/IM/SC every 4 to 12 hours prn.

E: Effusion. Consider thoracentesis or a chest tube, if appropriate and depending on the goals of care. Consider intermittent pleural drainage with an indwelling thoracentesis tube.

A: Anxiety. Manage anxiety with low-dose benzodiazepine such as lorazepam (Ativan) 0.5 to 2 mg every 4 hours prn.

T: Tachypnea and breathlessness. Opioids reduce respiratory rate and feelings of breathlessness and anxiety. If patient is opioid naive, begin with morphine sulfate 10 to 15 mg PO every 4 hours and titrate 25% to 50% daily/every other day as needed. Administer nasal oxygen and/or use of a fan. Coadministration of a benzodiazepine such as lorazepam is useful.

H: Hemoglobin low/anemia. Consider a blood transfusion if anemia is contributing to dyspnea and fatigue. If no improvement, do not continue to transfuse.

E: Educate and empathize. Provide teaching and support to the patient and family during this highly stressful period.

S: Sedate. If dyspnea is intractable despite routine, standard efforts, and the patient is actively dying, consider palliative sedation at the end of life.

In the cancer population, two of the more common causes of dyspnea are airway obstruction from extrinsic compression or endobronchial tumor and malignant pleural effusion. Other options include therapeutic bronchoscopy with stent placement and the use of indwelling catheters for intermittent drainage of pleural effusions.

Case Study 20.1 presents an example of the palliative management of a patient with dyspnea.

CASE STUDY 20.1   Dyspnea

Mr. Rather, a 70-year-old man with lung cancer that has metastasized to bone, has persistent dyspnea. He has received radiation therapy to the mediastinum and completed his last course of chemotherapy 4 months ago. He is still at home receiving morphine sulfate 30 mg PO every 4 hours around the clock for bone pain, which has been very effective. He is also receiving prednisone 30 mg PO two times daily for bronchospasm and has an albuterol inhaler, which he rarely uses. He complains of feeling breathless and anxious. He is also very fatigued and cannot sleep at night. He refuses to go to the hospital and says he wants to die in his own bed. He refuses further aggressive intervention and has signed a home do-not-resuscitate (DNR) order. On physical exam, his breath sounds are decreased bilaterally, with occasional rhonchi and no crackles. He has no distended neck veins, gallop, or peripheral edema. His respiratory rate is 24 per minute at rest.

ASSESSMENT AND INTERVENTION

1. Determine the etiology of dyspnea. In the terminally ill patient, dyspnea often has multiple causes. A thorough history and physical examination should be performed and will assist in determining specific interventions. If excessive fatigue is present, consider obtaining a complete blood count to determine if anemia is contributing to dyspnea. Rule out infection and congestive heart failure as contributing causes. Excessive secretions may be treated with agents such as scopolamine, atropine, hyoscyamine, and glycopyrrolate. If appropriate, use pulse oximetry to determine benefits of oxygen therapy, or try O_2 via nasal cannula at 3 L/min prn.

   Mr. Rather is presently receiving morphine sulfate for pain. Increasing the opioids by 50% to a dose of 45 mg PO every 4 hours should assist with tachypnea and anxiety. He will require assessments daily, and the opioids should be titrated daily or every other day by 25% to 50%. Consider increasing his prednisone dose to treat the bronchospasm and adding a trial of nebulized morphine 2.5 to 5.0 mg every 4 hours prn. Encourage use of an albuterol inhaler three or four times daily for bronchospasm.

2. Consider the benefit versus burden of additional interventions that are employed. Mr. Rather has stated that no further aggressive interventions are to be used. As the goals of care have been identified by the patient, it is important that his family members understand them as well.

3. Assess functional status and reduce the need for physical exertion. Provide for assistance with daily activities, positioning techniques, and frequent rest periods. Use of a fan may reduce feelings of breathlessness.

4. Address anxiety and provide support and reassurance. Determine level of support from family and significant others and from spiritual and religious beliefs. Reassure Mr. Rather that symptoms can be controlled. Provide an anxiolytic.

5. Provide for nonpharmacological interventions (e.g., progressive relaxation, guided imagery) if appropriate to reduce anxiety, handheld fans, and a cool room.

■ PALLIATIVE MANAGEMENT OF DELIRIUM

Delirium is one of the most common neurological complications at the end of life. The probability of developing delirium is determined by factors that both predispose patients to developing delirium and increase their vulnerability. Delirium, according to the *Diagnostic and Statistical Manual of Mental Disorders, Fifth Edition* (DSM-V) (American Psychiatric Association, 2013), is characterized as follows:

- Disturbances in attention (reduced ability to direct, focus, sustain, and shift attention and awareness)
- Changes in cognition (e.g., memory deficit, disorientation, language disturbance, perceptual disturbance) that is not better accounted for by a preexisting, established, or evolving dementia

- The disturbance develops over a short period (usually hours to days) and tends to fluctuate during the course of the day
- There is evidence from the history, physical exam, or lab findings that the disturbance is caused by a direct physiological consequence of a general medical condition, an intoxicating substance, medication use, or more than one cause

Table 20.11 outlines DSM-V criteria for the diagnosis of delirium.

Estimates of the prevalence of delirium range from 25% to 40% for patients with cancer at some point during their disease; in the terminal phases of disease, the incidence increases to 90% (Breitbart et al, 2002). The cause of delirium in the medically compromised and dying patient is often multifactorial and often nonspecific.

Table 20.11   DSM-5 Criteria for Diagnosing Delirium

A. A disturbance in attention (i.e., reduced ability to direct, focus, sustain, and shift attention) and awareness (reduced orientation to the environment).

B. The disturbance develops over a short period of time (usually hours to a few days), represents a change from baseline attention and awareness, and tends to fluctuate in severity during the course of the day.

C. An additional disturbance in cognition (e.g., memory deficit, disorientation, language, visuospatial ability, or perception).

D. The disturbances in Criteria A and C are not better explained by another preexisting, established, or evolving neurocognitive disorder and do not occur in the context of a severely reduced level of arousal, such as coma.

E. There is evidence from the history, physical examination, or laboratory findings that the disturbance is a direct physiological consequence of another medical condition, substance intoxication or withdrawal (i.e., due to a drug of abuse or to a medication), or exposure to a toxin, or is due to multiple etiologies.

Reprinted with permission from the Diagnostic and Statistical Manual of Mental Disorders, Fifth Edition, (Copyright 2013). American Psychiatric Association.

Assessment

Because of the complexity of delirium in palliative care settings, it is often underrecognized and undertreated. Behavioral manifestations of delirium include a variety of symptoms that may be interpreted as depression, psychosis, or dementia and may include physiological manifestations such as dysphagia, dysarthria, tremor, or asterixis in patients with comorbid hepatic encephalopathy or uremia. Multiple factors that need to be assessed in the patient include fluid status, electrolyte balance, infection, and polypharmacy. Symptoms include disordered cognition and alteration in arousal (attention), disturbance in consciousness and impaired attention, cognitive changes (memory deficit, disorientation, language disturbance, perceptual disturbance), nightmares, anxiety, restlessness and agitation, irritability, insomnia and daytime somnolence, hallucinations, delusions, and difficulty concentrating. Other symptoms that are often associated with impairment of consciousness, cognitive failure, and psychotic symptoms include disorders of the sleep–wake cycle, vivid dreams, abnormal thoughts, motor abnormalities, and mood changes (Caraceni & Simonetti, 2009). From a behavioral perspective, delirium can be further categorized as hypoactive or hyperactive, depending on level of motor activity and agitation. Patients with hypoactivity are often not diagnosed or receive late diagnosis, owing to the belief that hyperactivity alone is the hallmark of delirium. In reality, hypoactive delirium is the most common type found in the palliative care setting (Breitbart & Alici, 2008) and is often confused with depression. It is characterized by lethargy, sedation, and decreased level of awareness and is associated with a higher rate of mortality. Other assessment

measures include the Delirium Symptom Interview (DSI) and the Intensive Care Delirium Screening Checklist (IDS). (Table 20.12 outlines the symptoms and signs of delirium.)

Delirium is often undertreated for several reasons, including lack of assessment tools, inadequate knowledge of early signs of confusion, and inadequate time spent with the patient to determine cognitive function. Mental status questionnaires, such as the Mini–Mental State Exam (Folstein et al, 1983), the Confusion Assessment Method (CAM) (Inouye et al, 1990), and the Memorial Delirium Assessment Scale (MDAS) (Breitbart et al, 1997), are tools that are relatively easy to administer. A review by Hjermstad et al (2004) concluded that the Structured Clinical Interview for DSM-III-R (Spitzer et al, 1990), the Delirium Symptom Interview (Albert et al, 1992), and the CAM are most relevant to palliative care. The CAM is used as a screening tool but has not been validated for use in palliative care. Diagnostic tests that may uncover physiological changes in the patient that correlate with decreased cognitive function include electroencephalography and brain imaging studies such as computed tomography and magnetic resonance imaging.

Management

Treatment of delirium usually includes identification of the underlying cause, correction of the precipitating factors, and symptom management. Multiple underlying causes may include infection, organ failure, medication adverse effects, dehydration, and metabolic abnormalities (Breitbart & Alici, 2008). Medications commonly associated with delirium are opioids, corticosteroids, benzodiazepines, and anticholinergics. In the very ill or dying patient, however, there may be multiple, often irreversible, causes. The goal of palliative care of delirium

Table 20.12   Common Signs and Symptoms of Delirium

1. Level of alertness/wakefulness/arousal:
   - Hypoalert (hypovigilant)—*most common type found in the palliative care setting; often confused with depression*—characterized by lethargy, sedation, decreased level of awareness and is associated with a higher mortality rate
   - Hyperalert (hypervigilant)
   - Mixed—features of both hypovigilant and hypervigilant with fluctuations during the course of the day
2. Impaired attention
3. Altered sleep–wake cycle
4. Motor changes—hypoactive or hyperactive
5. Affective changes
6. Hallucinations (auditory, visual, or mixed)
7. Delusions
8. Cognitive deficits on mental status testing
9. Dysphagia, dysarthria, tremor, or asterixis in patient with comorbid condition such as hepatic encephalopathy or uremia

is the promotion of comfort and relief of suffering. Whenever possible, cognitive function should be maintained. In one study of hospitalized cancer patients, the presence of delusions was the most significant predictor of patient distress (Breitbart et al, 2002); distress occurred for patients with either hyperactive or hypoactive delirium.

Interventions that may be helpful include restoration of fluid and electrolyte balance, environmental changes, and supportive techniques such as elimination of unnecessary stimuli, provision of a safe environment, and measures that reduce anxiety. Reorientation to the environment by staff and family members by placing familiar objects such as pictures and a large clock and calendar may be helpful. Careful nutrition and bowel and bladder monitoring may avoid dehydration and agitation caused by discomfort. Pain should be assessed for regularly and treated appropriately. Maintaining good sleep hygiene measures by a quiet area with minimal interventions may prevent alteration in the sleep–wake cycle. Relaxation techniques such as massage, soothing music, and warm drinks are also indicated. If the cause of delirium is pharmacological, nonessential and central nervous system depressant drugs should be discontinued. Pharmacotherapy, using sedatives and neuroleptics, however, may be used to manage delirium.

Breitbart et al (1996) conducted a double-blind three-drug analysis of the effectiveness of chlorpromazine, haloperidol, and lorazepam in 30 hospitalized AIDS patients. The analysis indicated that both chlorpromazine and haloperidol were effective; the lorazepam arm of the study was stopped because of early adverse effects, namely cognitive impairment.

The American College of Critical Care Medicine has stated that haloperidol should be considered the preferred drug for treatment of delirium in critically ill adults (Shapiro et al, 1995). Haloperidol is considered the drug of choice in the treatment of delirium at the end of life by a number of reviews and case reports (Breitbart et al, 1996; Caraceni & Simonetti, 2009; de Stoutz et al, 1995; Fainsinger et al, 1993; Massie & Holland, 1992; Mazzocato et al, 2000; Roth & Breitbart, 1996).

An intervention review by Lonergan et al (2009) compared the efficacy and incidence of adverse effects of haloperidol with risperidone, olanzapine, and quetiapine in the treatment of delirium. A decrease in delirium scores was not significantly different comparing the effect of low-dose haloperidol (less than 3.0 mg per day) with that of the atypical antipsychotics olanzapine and risperidone (Han & Kim, 2004;). Low-dose haloperidol did not have a higher incidence of adverse effects than the atypical antipsychotics. High-dose haloperidol (greater than 4.5 mg per day) in one study was associated with an increased incidence of extrapyramidal effects (Hu et al, 2004).

One study compared haloperidol and placebo in the prevention of postoperative delirium (Kalisvaart et al, 2005). The study showed no difference between haloperidol and placebo in the incidence of postoperative delirium, but the severity of delirium was significantly higher in placebo patients than in haloperidol patients; the duration of delirium was significantly less for haloperidol patients than for placebo patients. These results show a clear benefit for surgical patients who are at risk for delirium who are treated preventively with haloperidol.

Table 20.13 lists drugs commonly used to manage delirium. Table 20.14 gives an overview of the key points in the assessment and management of the patient with delirium.

Table 20.13   Drugs Used to Manage Delirium

Drug	Dosage	Route
haloperidol (Haldol)	0.5–2 mg every 2–12 hours For mild delirium, begin with 0.5 mg 2 times daily; for more severe symptoms begin with 1 mg 2–3 times daily	PO, IV, SC, IM
thioridazine (Mellaril)	10–75 mg every 4–8 hours	PO
chlorpromazine (Thorazine)	12.5–50 mg every 4–12 hours	PO, IV, IM
lorazepam (Ativan)	0.5–2 mg every 1–4 hours	PO, IV May worsen delirium and should not be used as monotherapy, always in addition to a neuroleptic when sedation is required
midazolam (Versed)	30–100 mg/24 hr	IV, SC
risperidone	0.5–2 mg every 2–12 hours	PO
olanzapine (Zyprexa)	2.5–5 mg every 12–24 hours	PO Use if sedation is needed to manage an agitated delirium

Table 20.14	At a Glance: Assessment and Management of Delirium

1. Determine the etiology of delirium including common predisposing factors (fever, infection, tumor, altered metabolism of drugs, alcohol, comorbid conditions, urinary/bowel retention). Cause is most often multifactorial in dying patients.
2. Medications commonly associated with delirium are opioids, corticosteroids, benzodiazepines, and anticholinergics.
3. Obtain a careful history of onset and duration of symptoms. Severity of symptoms should be determined. A Mini–Mental State Exam should be performed at intervals during hospitalization. Other assessment measures include the Delirium Symptom Inventory (DSI) and the Intensive Care Delirium Screening Checklist (ICDSC).
4. Treat the underlying cause if possible.
5. Review the goals of care with the patient and family and document in the medical record.
6. Identify advance directives with the patient and family and document in the medical record.
7. Pharmacological management should always include administration of a neuroleptic as a first-line treatment. Add a benzodiazepine if sedation is needed, but benzodiazepines should not be used as first-line therapy.
8. Incorporate nonpharmacological interventions when appropriate such as maintaining good sleep hygiene by maintenance of a quiet environment with minimal interventions.
9. Relaxation techniques such as massage, soothing music, warm drinks.

The European Association for Palliative Care and other palliative care experts advocate for the use of sedation to manage intractable symptoms at the end of life, including agitated delirium, that are refractory to aggressive measures. Symptoms that are refractory cannot be adequately controlled despite aggressive efforts to identify an acceptable therapy that does not compromise consciousness. When determining that a symptom is refractory, considerations include whether further interventions are incapable of providing adequate relief, are associated with excessive or intolerable morbidity, or are unlikely to provide relief in a timely manner. Inherent in this decision-making process is the informed consent of the patient, if possible, and the health-care proxy. Because loss of interactional function will most likely occur, it is important that the patient and family understand the outcomes of this decision. A pain and palliative care expert clinician should be involved in this process (Cherny et al, 2009).

 DavisPlus | For additional resources please visit http://davisplus.fadavis.com

References

Ahmedzai, SH, et al. A double blind, randomized controlled phase II trial of Heliox28 gas mixture in lung cancer patients with dyspnoea on exertion. *Br J Cancer* 90(2):366–371, 2004.

Albert, MS, et al. The Delirium Symptom Interview: An interview for the detection of delirium symptoms in hospitalized patients. *J Geriatr Psychiatry Neurol* 5:14–21, 1992.

American Cancer Society. *Cancer Prevention & Early Detection Facts and Figures 2014.* American Cancer Society, Atlanta, 2014.

American Pain Society. *Principles of Analgesic Use in the Treatment of Acute Pain and Cancer Pain,* ed. 5. American Pain Society, Glenview, IL, 2005.

American Psychiatric Association. *Diagnostic and statistical manual of mental disorders, fifth edition.* American Psychiatric Association, Washington, DC, 2013.

American Society for Pain Management Nursing. Patient controlled analgesia (PCA). *Pain Manage Nurs* 7(4):134–147, 2006.

American Society for Pain Management Nursing position statement: Pain management at the end of life. 2013. Retrieved from www.aspmn.org/Documents/PainManagementattheEndofLife_August2013.pdf

Andersen, G, et al. Relationships among morphine metabolism, pain and side effects during long-term treatment: An update. *J Pain Sympt Manage* 25(1):74–91, 2003.

Anghelescu, D, et al. The safety of patient-controlled analgesia by proxy in pediatric oncology patients. *Anesth Analg* 101:1623–1627, 2005.

Bausewein, C, et al. Non-pharmacological interventions for breathlessness in advanced stages of malignant and non-malignant diseases. *Cochrane Database Syst Rev* 2:CD005623, 2008. doi:10.1002/14651858.CD005623.pub2

Belluck, P. Panel urges overhauling health care at End of Life. *New York Times,* September 17, 2014 – http://nyti.ms/1u1h21u

Ben-Aharon, I, et al. Interventions for alleviating cancer-related dyspnea: A systematic review. *J Clin Oncol* 26(14):2396–2404, 2008.

Berenson, S. Complementary and alternative therapies in palliative care. In Ferrell, BR, and Coyle, N (Eds.), *Textbook of palliative care nursing.* CV Mosby, St. Louis, MO, 2005, pp 491–509.

Berry, PE, and Dahl, JL. The new JCAHO pain standards: Implications for pain management nurses. *Pain Manage Nurses* 1:3–12, 2000.

Booth, S. Improving research methodology in breathlessness—a meeting convened by the MRC Clinical Trials and Cicely Saunders Foundation. *Palliat Med* 20:219–220, 2006.

Booth, S, et al. The etiology of intractable breathlessness in patients with advanced cancer: A systematic review of pharmacological therapy. *Nat Clin Practice Oncol* 5(2):90–100, 2008.

Bredin, M, et al. Multicentre randomized controlled trial of nursing intervention for breathlessness in patients with lung cancer. *BMJ* 318(7188):901–904, 1999.

Breitbart, W, et al. A double-blind trial of haloperidol, chlorpromazine, and lorazepam in the treatment of delirium in hospitalized AIDS patients. *Am J Psychiatry* 153(2):231–237, 1996.

Breitbart, WS, et al. The Memorial delirium assessment scale. *J Pain Sympt Manage* 13(3):128–137, 1997.

Breitbart, W, et al. The delirium experience: Delirium recall and delirium-related distress in hospitalized patients with cancer, their spouses/caregivers, and their nurses. *Psychosomatics* 43:183–194, 2002.

Breitbart, W, and Alici, Y. Agitation and delirium at the end of life: "We couldn't manage him." *JAMA* 300(24):2898–2910, 2008.

Bruera, E, de Stoutz, N, et al. Effects of oxygen on dyspnoea in hypoxaemic terminal-cancer patients. *Lancet* 342(8862):13–14, 1993.

Bruera, E, et al. The frequency and correlates of dyspnea in patients with advanced cancer. *J Pain Sympt Manage* 19(5):357–362, 2000.

Bruera, E, et al. A randomized controlled trial of supplemental oxygen versus air in cancer patients with dyspnea. *Palliat Med* 17(8):659–663, 2003.

Caraceni, A, and Simonetti, F. Palliating delirium in patients with cancer. *Lancet Oncol* 10:164–172, 2009.

Cassell, EJ. Diagnosis suffering: A perspective. *Ann Intern Med* 131(7): 531–534, 1999.

Cassileth, BR, and Gubili, J. Integrative medicine: Complementary therapies. In Walsh, D, Caraceni, AT, Fainsinger, R, et al (Eds.), *Palliative medicine*. Saunders Elsevier, Philadelphia, 2009, pp 1001–1006.

Cassileth, BR, et al. Music therapy for mood disturbance during hospitalization for autologous stem cell transplantation: A randomized controlled trial. *Cancer* 98(12):2723–2729, 2003.

Centers for Disease Control and Prevention. *National Vital Statistic System – Mortality Tables*. Division of Vital Statistics, National center for Health Statistics. Hyattsville, MD, 2010. www.cdc.gov/nchs/nvss/mortality_tables.htm

Cherny, NI, et al. Invasive techniques in the management of cancer pain. *Hematol Oncol Clin North Am* 10(1):121–137, 1996.

Cherny, NI, and Catane, R. Attitudes of medical oncologists toward palliative care for patients with advanced and incurable cancer. Report on a survey by the European Society of Medical Oncology taskforce on palliative and supportive care. *Cancer* 98(11): 2502–2510, 2003.

Cherny, NI, and Portenoy, RK. The management of cancer pain. *Ca: Cancer J Clin* 44:262–303, 1994.

Cherny, NI, Radbruch, L, and Board of the European Association for Palliative Care. European Association for Palliative Care (EAPC) recommended framework for the use of sedation in palliative care. *Palliat Med* 23(7):581–593, 2009.

Conill, C, et al. Symptom prevalence in the last week of life. *J Pain Sympt Manage* 14(6):328–331, 1997.

Corner, J, et al. Non-pharmacological intervention for breathlessness in lung cancer. *Palliat Med* 10(4):299–305, 1996.

Czarnecki, M, et al. Parent/nurse-controlled analgesia for children with developmental delay. *Clin J Pain* 24(9):817–824, 2008.

Daut, RI, et al. The development of the Wisconsin brief pain questionnaire to assess pain in cancer and other diseases. *Pain* 17(2):197–210, 1983.

Decker, GM. An overview of complementary and alternative therapies. *Clin J Oncol Nurs* 4(1):49–52, 2000.

Deng, G, et al. Complementary therapies for cancer-related symptoms. *J Support Oncol* 2(5):419–429, 2004.

Deng, GE, et al. Society for Integrative Oncology Executive Committee, Abrams, D, et al. Integrative oncology practice guidelines. *J Soc Integr Oncol* 5(2):65–84, 2007.

de Stoutz, ND, et al. Opioid rotation for toxicity reduction in terminal cancer patient. *J Pain Sympt Manage* 10(5):378–384, 1995.

de Stoutz, ND, et al. Reversible delirium in terminally ill patients. *J Pain Sympt Manage* 10(3):249–253, 1995.

Devine, EC. Meta-analysis of the effect of psychoeducational interventions on pain in adults with cancer. *Oncol Nurs Forum* 30(1):75–89, 2003.

DiSalvo, WM, et al. Putting evidence into practice: Evidence-based interventions for cancer-related dyspnea. *Clin J Oncol Nurs* 12(2): 341–352, 2008.

Dubinsky, RM, et al. Practice parameter: Treatment of postherpetic neuralgia and evidence-based report of the Quality Standards Subcommittee of the American Academy of Neurology. *Neurology* 63(6):959–965, 2004. Retrieved from www.guideline.bov/summary

Dudgeon, DJ, Kristjanson, L, et al. Dyspnea in cancer patients: Prevalence and associated factors. *J Pain Sympt Manage* 21(2): 95–102, 2001.

Dudgeon, DJ, Lertzman, M, et al. Physiological changes and clinical correlations of dyspnea in cancer outpatients. *J Pain Sympt Manage* 21(5):373–379, 2001.

Dworkin, RH, et al. Pharmacologic management of neuropathic pain: Evidence-based recommendations. *Pain* 132(3):237–251, 2007.

Dy, SM, et al. Evidence-based standards for cancer pain management. *J Clin Oncol* 26(23):3855–3879, 2008.

Fainsinger, R, et al. Symptom control during the last week of life on a palliative care unit. *J Palliat Care* 7(1):5–11, 1991.

Fainsinger, RL, et al. A perspective on the management of delirium in terminally ill patients on a palliative care unit. *J Palliat Care* 9(3): 4–8, 1993.

Ferrell, BR, and Coyle, N. *The nature of suffering and the goals of nursing*. Oxford University Press, New York, 2008.

Flaming, D. Patient suffering: A taxonomy from the nurse's perspective. *J Adv Nurs* 22(6):1120–1127, 1995.

Folstein, MF, et al. The mini–mental state exam. *Arch Gen Psychiatry* 40(7):812, 1983.

Frankl, VE. *Man's search for meaning. An introduction to logotherapy*. Beacon Press, New York, 1959.

Graham, C, et al. Use of the McGill Pain Questionnaire in the assessment of cancer pain: Replicability and consistency. *Pain* 8(3): 377–387, 1980.

Gray, CM, et al. Complementary and alternative medicine use among health plan members. A cross-sectional survey. *Eff Clin Pract* 5(1): 17–22, 2002.

Hakonsen, GD, et al. Adherence to medication guideline criteria in cancer pain management. *J Pain Sympt Manage* 37(6):1006–1018, 2008.

Han, CS, and Kim, YK. A double-blind trial of risperidone and haloperidol for the treatment of delirium. *Psychosomatics* 45:297–301, 2004.

Hanks, GW, et al. Opioid analgesic therapy. In Doyle, D, et al (Eds.), *Oxford textbook of palliative medicine*, ed 3. Oxford University Press, Oxford, 2004, pp 316–341.

Hanson, LC, et al. What is wrong with end-of-life care? Opinions of bereaved family members. *J Am Geriatr Soc* 45:1339–1344, 1997.

Hanson, LC, et al. Symptom experience of dying long-term care residents. *J Am Geriatr Soc* 56(1):91–98, 2008.

Hassenbach, SJ, and Cherny, NI. Neurosurgical approaches in palliative medicine. In Doyle, D, et al (Eds.), *Oxford textbook of palliative medicine*, ed 36. Oxford University Press, New York, 2004, pp 396–405.

Higginson, I, and McCarthy, M. Measuring symptoms in terminal cancer: Are pain and dyspnoea controlled? *J R Soc Med* 82(5): 264–267, 1989.

Hjermstad, MJ, et al. Methods for assessment of cognitive failure and delirium in palliative care patients: Implications for practice and research. *Palliat Med* 18:494–506, 2004.

Horner, MJ, et al (Eds.). SEER cancer statistics review, 1975–2006, National Cancer Institute. Bethesda, MD, http://seer.cancer.gov/csr/1975_2006, based on November 2008 SEER data submission, posted to the SEER Web site, 2009.

Hu, H, et al. A prospective random control study comparison of olanzapine and haloperidol in senile delirium. *Chongging Med J* 8:1234–1237, 2004.

Ingham, JM, and Portenoy, RK. Symptom assessment. In Cherny, NI, and Foley, KM (Eds.): *Hematology clinics of North America: Pain and palliative care*. WB Saunders, Philadelphia, 1996, pp 21–40.

Inouye, SK, et al. Clarifying confusion: The Confusion Assessment Method. A new method for detection of delirium. *Ann Intern Med* 113:941–948, 1990.

Institute of Medicine. *Dying in America*. National Academies Press, Washington, DC, 2014.

International Association for the Study of Pain, Subcommittee on Taxonomy. Pain terms: A list with definitions and notes on usage. *Pain* 6(3):249, 1979.

Jacox, A, et al. *Management of cancer pain. Clinical practice guideline no. 9*. (AHCPR Publication No. 94–0592). Rockville, MD: Agency for Health Care Policy and Research, U.S. Department of Health and Human Services, Public Health Services, 1994.

Jennings, AL, et al. A systematic review of the use of opioids in the management of dyspnea. *Thorax* 57:939–944, 2002.

Kalisvaart, KJ, et al. Haloperidol prophylaxis for elderly hip-surgery patients at risk for delirium: A randomized placebo-controlled study. *J Am Geriatr Soc* 53:1658–1666, 2005.

Kenagy, A, and Turner, H. Pediatric patient-controlled analgesia by proxy. *AACN Adv Crit Care* 18(4):361–365, 2007.

Kirou-Mauro, AM, et al. Has pain management in cancer patients with bone metastases improved? A seven-year review at an outpatient palliative radiotherapy clinic. *J Pain Sympt Manage* 27(1): 77–84, 2009.

Knotkova, H, et al. Opioid rotation: The science and the limitations of the equianalgesic dose table. *J Pain Sympt Manage* 38(3):426–439, 2009.

Kuebler, KK. *Hospice and palliative care clinical practice protocol: Dyspnea*. Hospice Nurses Association, Pittsburgh, 1996.

Lanken, PN, et al. An official American Thoracic Society clinical policy statement: Palliative care for patients with respiratory diseases and critical illnesses. *Am J Respir Crit Care Med* 177:912–927, 2008.

Layman-Goldstein, M, and Coyle, N. Non-drug pain interventions. In LaPorte Matzo, M, and Witt Sherman, D (Eds.), *Palliative care nursing: Quality care to the end of life*, ed 3. New York, Springer, 2010.

Librach, L, et al, and Supportive Guidelines Group. The use of gabapentin and tricyclic antidepressants in the treatment of neuropathic pain in cancer patients: A clinical practice guideline. Cancer Care Ontario (CCO); October 11, 2006. (Evidence-based series; no. 13–8.) National Guideline Clearinghouse. Retrieved from www.guideline.gov/summary

Lo, Bernard. Improving care at end of life: Why is it so hard? *Journal of American Medical Association, 274* (20): 1634-36 – November 22, 1995 – jama.1995.035302999970042

Lonergan, E, et al. Antipsychotics for delirium. *Cochrane Database Syst Rev* 2:CD005594, 2009. doi:10.1002/14651858.CD005594.pub2

Lorenz, KA, et al. Evidence for improving palliative care at the end of life: A systematic review. *Ann Intern Med* 148(2):147–159, 2008.

Magill, L. The meaning of the music in palliative care music therapy as perceived by bereaved caregivers of advanced cancer patients. *Am J Hosp Palliat Care* 26(1):33–39, 2009.

Magill-Levreault, L. Music therapy in pain and symptom management. *J Palliat Care* 9(4):42–48, 1993.

Massie, MJ, and Holland, JC. The cancer patient with pain: Psychiatric complications and their management. *J Pain Sympt Manage* (2): 99–109, 1992.

Mazzocato, C, et al. Psychopharmacology in supportive care of cancer: A review for the clinician: II. Neuroleptics. *Support Care Cancer* 8(2):89–97, 2000.

McCaffery, M, and Ferrell, B. Nurses' knowledge of pain assessment and management: How much progress have we made? *J Pain Sympt Manage* 14(3):175–188, 1997.

Miguel, R. Interventional treatment of cancer pain: The fourth step in the World Health Organization analgesic ladder? *Cancer Control* 7:149–156, 2000.

Moore, S, et al. (Abstract). Nurse led follow up and conventional medical follow up in management of patients with cancer: Randomised trial. *BMJ* 325(7373):1145, 2002.

National Comprehensive Cancer Network. NCCN clinical practice guidelines in oncology: Pediatric cancer pain. Version 2. 2013. Retrieved from www.nccn.org

National Comprehensive Cancer Network. NCCN clinical practice guidelines in oncology: Adult cancer pain. Version 2. 2014. Retrieved from www.nccn.org

National Comprehensive Cancer Network. NCCN clinical practice guidelines in oncology: Distress management. Version 2. 2014. Clinical Practice Guidelines in Oncology, 2014. Retrieved from www.nccn.org

National Consensus Project for Quality Palliative Care (NCP). *Clinical practice guidelines for quality palliative care*, ed 2. National Guideline Clearinghouse. Retrieved from www.guideline.gov

National Hospice and Palliative Care Organization. Hospice statistics and research. 2013. Retrieved from http://www.nhpco.org/sites/default/files/public/Statistics_Research/2013_Facts_Figures.pdf

National Institutes of Health (NIH) Technology Assessment Panel on Integration of Behavioral and Relaxation Approaches into the Treatment of Chronic Pain and Insomnia. Integration of behavioral and relaxation approaches into the treatment of chronic pain and insomnia. *JAMA* 276:313–318, 1996.

National Institutes of Health (NIH) Consensus Conference. Acupuncture. *JAMA* 280:1518–1524, 1998.

O'Brien, S, et al. The knowledge and attitudes of experienced oncology nurses regarding the management of cancer-related pain. *Oncol Nurs Forum* 23(3):515–521, 1996.

O'Connor, AB, and Dworkin, RH. Treatment of neuropathic pain: An overview of recent guidelines. *Am J Med* 122:S22–S32, 2009.

Oldenmenger, WH, et al. A systematic review on barriers hindering adequate cancer pain management and interventions to reduce them: A critical appraisal. *Eur J Cancer* 45:1370–1380, 2009.

Olson, K, et al. A phase II trial of Reiki for the management of pain in advanced cancer patients. *J Pain Sympt Manage* 26:990–997, 2003.

Oneschuk, D, et al. Assessment and knowledge in palliative care in second year family medicine residents. *J Pain Sympt Manage* 14(5): 265–273, 1997.

Philip, J, et al. A randomized, double blind crossover trial of the effect of oxygen on dyspnea in patients with advanced cancer. *J Pain Sympt Manage* 32:541–549, 2006.

Potter, J, et al. Symptoms in 400 patients referred to palliative care services: Prevalence and patterns. *Palliat Med* 17(4):310–314, 2003.

Rhiner, M, et al. A structured non-drug intervention program for cancer pain. *Cancer Pract* 1:137–143, 1993.

Ripamonti, C. Management of dyspnea in advanced cancer patients. *Support Care Cancer* 7(4):233–243, 1999.

Roth, AJ, and Breitbart, W. Psychiatric emergencies in terminally ill cancer patients. *Hematol Oncol Clin North Am* 10(1):235–259, 1996.

Shapiro, BA, et al. Practice parameters for intravenous analgesia and sedation for adult patients in the intensive care unit: An executive summary. *Soc Crit Care Med Crit Care Med* 23(9):1596–1600, 1995.

Singer, PA, et al. Quality end-of-life care: Patients' perspectives. *JAMA* 281:163–168, 1999.

So, PS, et al. Touch therapies for pain relief in adults. *Cochrane Database Syst Rev* (4):CD006535, 2008.

Solano, JP, et al. A comparison of symptom prevalence in far advanced cancer, AIDS, heart disease, chronic obstructive pulmonary disease and renal disease. *J Pain Sympt Manage* 31:58–69, 2006.

Spitzer, RL, et al. *Structured clinical interview for DSM-III-R.* American Psychiatric Press, Washington, DC, 1990.

Spross, JA, and Wolff Burke, M. Nonpharmacological management of cancer pain. In McGuire, DB, et al (Eds.), *Cancer pain management*, ed 2. Jones & Bartlett, Boston, 1995, pp 159–205.

Standish, LJ, et al. Acupuncture is underutilized in hospice and palliative medicine. *Am J Hospice Palliat Med* 25(4):298–308, 2008.

Steinhauser, KE, et al. Factors considered important at the end of life by patients, family, physicians, and other care providers. *JAMA* 284:2476–2482, 2008.

SUPPORT: A controlled trial to improve care for seriously ill hospitalized patients. The study to understand prognoses and preferences for outcomes and risks of treatments (SUPPORT). The Support Principle Investigators (no authors listed). *Journal of the American Medical Association, 274* (20), 1591-8 – Nov. 22-29.

Tuls Halstead, M, and Tuls Roscoe, S. Restoring the spirit at the end of life: Music as an intervention for oncology nurses. *Clin J Oncol Nurs* 6(6):332–336, 2002.

U.S. Department of Health and Human Services, Center for Medicare and Medicaid Services. CMS Publication No. 02154. September 2008.

Vickers, JA, et al. Acupuncture for dyspnea in advanced cancer: A randomized, placebo-controlled pilot trial. *BMC Palliat Care* 4:5, 2005.

Vitale, A. An integrative review of Reiki touch therapy research. *Holist Nurs Pract* 21(4):167–179, 2007.

Weinrich, MD, et al. Dying patients' need for emotional support and personalized care from physicians: Perspectives of patients with terminal illness, families, and health care providers. *J Pain Sympt Manage* 25:236–246, 2003.

West, CM, et al. The PRO-SELF©: pain control program—An effective approach for cancer pain management. *Oncol Nurs Forum* 30(1):65–73, 2003.

Wiffen, PJ, and Eccleston, C. The Cochrane pain, palliative and supportive care group: An update. *Palliat Med* 23(2):179–180, 2009.

World Health Organization. Cancer pain relief and palliative care. Report of a WHO Expert Committee (World Health Organization Technical Report Series, 804). WHO, Geneva, 2010.

World Health Organization. WHO's pain relief ladder. 2009. Retrieved from www.who.int/cancer/palliative/painladder/en

Wuhrman, E, et al. Authorized and unauthorized ("PCA by proxy") dosing of analgesic infusion pumps: Position statement with clinical practice recommendations. *Pain Manage Nurs* 8(1):4–11, 2007.

Bibliography

Alexander, HR, Jr, and Fraker, DK. Shunting procedures for malignant ascites and pleural effusions. In Lotze, MT, and Rubin, JT (Eds.), *Regional therapy of advanced cancer.* Lippincott-Raven, Philadelphia, 1997, pp 271–280.

Allard, P, et al. How effective are supplementary doses of opioids for dyspnea in terminally ill cancer patients? A randomized continuous sequential clinical trial. *J Pain Sympt Manage* 17: 256–265, 1999.

American Cancer Society. *Cancer prevention and early detection facts and figures 2013.* American Cancer Society, Atlanta, 2013.

American Cancer Society. Surveillance research, 2013.

American Pain Society. *Principles of analgesic use in the treatment of acute pain and cancer pain*, ed. 8. American Pain Society, Glenview, IL, 2010.

Belman, MJ, et al. (Borg Rating of Dyspnea) Variability of breathlessness measurements in patients with chronic obstructive pulmonary disease. *Chest* 99:566–571, 1991.

Booth, S, et al, and Expert Working Group of the Scientific Committee of the Association of Palliative Medicine. The use of oxygen in the palliation of breathlessness. A report of the expert working group of the Scientific Committee of the Association of Palliative Medicine. *Respir Med* 98(1):66–77, 2004.

Breitbart, WS, and Jacobsen, PB. Psychiatric symptom management in terminal care. *Clin Geriatr Med* 12(2):329–347, 1996.

Bruera, E, MacEachern, T, et al. Subcutaneous morphine for dyspnea in cancer patients. *Ann Intern Med* 119:906–907, 1993.

Bruera, E, et al. Nebulized versus subcutaneous morphine for patients with cancer dyspnea: A preliminary study. *J Pain Symptom Manage* 29:613–618, 2005.

Cassileth, BR, and Vickers, AJ. Massage therapy for symptom control: Outcome study at a major cancer center. *J Pain Sympt Manage* 28(12):244–249, 2004.

Cepeda, MS, et al. Music for pain relief. *Cochrane Database Syst Rev* (2): CD004843, 2006.

Chater, S, et al. Sedation for intractable distress in the dying—a survey of experts. *Palliat Med* 12:255–269, 1998.

Cherny, NI, and Portenoy, RK. Sedation in the management of refractory symptoms: Guidelines for evaluation and treatment. *J Palliat Care* 10(2):31–38, 1994.

Cohen, MZ, et al. JCAHO: Cancer pain management and the JCAHO's pain standards: An institutional challenge. *J Pain Sympt Manage* 25(6):519–527, 2003.

Cowan, JD, and Walsh, D. Terminal sedation in palliative medicine—definition and review of the literature. *Support Care Cancer* 9:403–407, 2001.

Davis, C, et al. Single dose randomized controlled trial of nebulized morphine in patients with cancer related breathlessness. *Palliat Med* 10:64–65, 1996.

Dubinsky, RM, et al. Practice parameter: Treatment of postherpetic neuralgia and evidence-based report of the Quality Standards Subcommittee of the American Academy of Neurology. *Neurology* 63(6):959–965, 2004. National Guideline Clearinghouse, www.guideline.bov/summary

Field, MJ, and Cassel, CK (Eds.). *Approaching death: Improving care at the end of life.* National Academies of Practice, Washington, DC, 1997.

Grimbert, D, et al. Dyspnea and morphine aerosol in the palliative care of lung cancer [French]. *Rev Mal Respir* 21(6 Pt 1):1091–1097, 2004.

Hogan, C, et al. Medicare beneficiaries' costs of care in the last year of life. *Health Aff* (Millwood) 20:188–195, 2001.

Jackson, KC, and Lipman, AG. Drug therapy for delirium in terminally ill adult patients. *Cochrane Database Syst Rev* 2:CD004700, 2004. doi:10.1002/14651858.CD004770

Levy, MH, and Cohen, SD. Sedation for the relief of refractory symptoms in the imminently dying: A fine intentional line. *Semin Oncol* 32:237–246, 2005.

Magill, L. The use of music to address the suffering in advanced cancer pain. *J Palliat Care* 17(3):167–172, 2001.

Mazzocato, C, et al. The effects of morphine on dyspnea and ventilatory function in elderly patients with advanced cancer: A randomized double-blind controlled trial. *Ann Oncol* 10:1511–1514, 1999.

Mercadante, S, and Arcuri, E. Opioids and renal function. *J Pain* 5(1):2–19, 2004.

National Comprehensive Cancer Network. NCCN Clinical Practice Guidelines in Oncology: Palliative care. Version 1, 2014. Retrieved from www.nccn.org

National Comprehensive Cancer Network. NCCN Clinical Practice Guidelines in Oncology: Dyspnea. Version 2. 2014. Retrieved from www.nccn.org

Navigante, AH, et al. Midazolam as adjunct therapy to morphine in the alleviation of severe dyspnea perception in patients with advanced cancer. *J Pain Sympt Manage* 31:38–47, 2006.

Rousseau, P. Palliative sedation in the management of refractory symptoms. *J Support Oncol* 2:181–186, 2004.

Seale, C, and Cartwright, A. *The year before death.* Ashgate Publishing, Brookfield, VT, 1994.

Therapeutic Radiopharmaceutical Guidelines Group. Radiopharmaceuticals for the palliation of painful bone metastasis. Cancer Care Ontario (CCO), June 15, 2004. (Practice guideline report, no. 14-1.) Retrieved from www.guideline.gov

Thomas, K. *Caring for the dying at home: Companions on the journey.* Radcliff Medical PR, Abington, UK, 2004.

Veterans Health Administration National Ethics Committee. The ethics of palliative sedation as a therapy of last resort. *Am J Hosp Palliat Care* 23:483–491, 2006.

Wein, S. Sedation in the imminently dying patient. *Oncology* 14: 585–592, 2000.

World Health Organization. *Looking forward to cancer pain relief for all: International consensus on the management of cancer pain.* WHO Collaborating Centre for Palliative Cancer Care, Oxford, 2009.

Resources

Academy of Pain Management
www.aapainmanage.com
Academy of Pain Medicine
www.painmed.org
American Botanical Council
www.herbalgram.org
American Cancer Society
www.cancer.org
American Holistic Nurses Association
www.ahna.org
American Pain Society
www.ampainsoc.org
Cancer Care
www.cancercare.org
Choices in Dying
www.choices.org
Food and Drug Administration
www.fda.gov

Hospice Foundation
www.hospicefoundation.org
Memorial Sloan-Kettering Cancer Center
www.mskcc.org/mskcc/html/11570.cfm
National Cancer Institute
www.nci.nih.gov
National Hospice Organization
www.nho.org
National Institutes of Health
www.nih.gov
Oncology Nurses Society
www.ons.org
Physicians' Desk Reference
www.pdr.net
U.S. Pharmacopeial Convention (USP)
www.usp.org

Ethical and Legal Issues of a Caring-Based Practice

Jill E. Winland-Brown, EdD, APRN, FNP-BC •
Bette K. Idemoto, PhD, RN, ACNS-BC, CCRN

Chapter **21**

■ ETHICAL ISSUES

The American Nurses Association (ANA) has designated 2015 as the Year of Ethics in conjunction with the 2014 Gallup Poll, once again citing nursing as being #1 on the list of professions with the highest ethical standards in their annual survey on honesty and ethics.

With economic, social, and legal constraints present in our everyday practice, it is no wonder that health-care providers face ethical dilemmas daily. This section begins with an overview of what ethics is, what constitutes an ethical dilemma, different theoretical approaches to analyzing dilemmas, and a description of ethical principles. Each of us lives by a moral code, whether or not we have taken the time to reflect on what this means. Some people live by the simple code of "an eye for an eye"; others use the "Golden Rule" that forms the core of major religions (see Table 21.1).

Table 21.1	Golden Rules
Whatsoever ye would that men should do to you, do ye even so to them.	*Christianity (Jesus)*
What is hateful to yourself, don't do to your fellow man.	*Judaism (Rabbi Hillel)*
What you don't want done to yourself; don't do to others.	*Confucius*
Hurt not other with that which pains thyself.	*Buddhism*
May I do to others as I would that they should do unto me.	*Plato*
Do naught to others which if done to thee would cause thee pain.	*Hinduism (Mahabharata)*
Hurt no one so that no one may hurt you.	*Islam (Muhammad)*

It is more and more difficult to practice ethically in health care today for many reasons, including dehumanizing procedures, technological advances that affect the quality of life, and the potential for unauthorized sharing of confidential information and violations of privacy because of easy access to data banks. Patients and providers must contend with these and many other problems. Historically, the "virtuous" man or woman who faithfully followed rules that were largely etiquette could be termed *ethical.* Even the early Code for Nurses of the American Nurses Association (ANA) in 1950 dealt with issues of etiquette as being synonymous with ethics. Today, in view of the questions posed by modern health-care practices, those rules seem simplistic.

Ethics

Ethics is a branch of philosophy that considers what is right and what one ought to do when confronted with moral choices. It is termed *bioethics* when those moral choices involve health care. Personal and professional values influence our daily professional lives. Many of these values are known and explicit; others are hidden and unknown. When involved in a professional practice, providers cannot escape the need to clarify their own values. Many excellent books on values clarification (see Resources) are available that can assist health-care providers in exploring their own values and in deciding what is meaningful or valued to them to facilitate self-understanding.

Ethics is integrally related to nursing because nursing is a practice with an inherent moral sense. Nursing ethics attempts to articulate that moral sense, to assess its fulfillment, to explore new possibilities for its fulfillment, and to appraise its adequacy. A classic saying is, "A patient doesn't care what a nurse knows until he knows a nurse cares." This could not be truer than in any situation with a health-care provider and a patient involving life and death choices. The patient wants to know that the provider is an advocate, a friend, and a trusted expert, not someone who is consumed with billing practices or always watching the clock. In addition, professional nursing is both "valued within U.S.

society and is uniquely accountable to that society" (ANA, 2010).

The Skill of Ethical Action

Ethics is the standards or principles governing one's actions in professional practice. It is what the professional "ought" to do. Ethical behavior serves to protect the rights of human beings; a code of ethics is characteristic of all professions. To apply ethics, there are three basic philosophical skills that clinicians need to foster or acquire. First, the clinician must develop an ability for in-depth questioning, not just taking information at face value. Next, the clinician must develop the ability to understand different points of view and make a reasonable, empathetic effort to understand another person's opposing viewpoint. Finally, the clinician must not be afraid to argue a point logically. A dialectic exchange occurs when both parties learn something; it is a win–win situation. It is similar to a formal debate in that those who do not know their opponents' arguments do not completely understand their own.

Professional Codes

The ANA has a Code of Ethics for Nurses; the American Medical Association (AMA) has a code of ethics titled the Principles of Medical Ethics; and the American Hospital Association has a Patient's Bill of Rights, which delineates the hospital's code of conduct owed to patients. There is also a Code of the International Council of Nurses (ICN). The ANA's Code of Ethics for Nurses (the Code) was first adopted in 1950. It helped to legitimize nursing as a profession because one of the components of a profession is having a code of conduct that governs its actions. The Code was formulated by nurses, for nurses, and was voted on at a national ANA convention that had delegates representing all ANA members. The Code serves as a contract between society and the nursing profession: It explicitly sets forth the values and ethical principles that guide the clinical decisions of all practicing nurses. The Code provides a framework within which nurses and advanced practice registered nurses (APRNs) can make ethical decisions and be held accountable to the public for those decisions. It also provides guidance for carrying out the professional role and aids in justifying differences between personal and professional values.

The primary purpose of the Code of Ethics is promotion of high-quality nursing care and protection of the public from incompetent or unethical nursing practice. The Code, revised in 2014, continues to indicate that the recipient of care is the primary consideration in any conflict of interest. The Code sets the ethical standards for nursing, whereas the Nursing Practice Act of each state establishes the legal standards. The requirements of the Code may often exceed, but are never less than, those of the law. To read about the Code of Ethics and the Interpretive Statements, go to www.nursingworld.org.

One of the provisions of the Code states that part of being a professional, and one who is ethical, is to advance the profession by being a member of the association that represents the professionals. For nurses, this is the ANA. Although there are many specialty nursing organizations, the ANA is the umbrella organization that speaks for all nurses. Yet only about 10% of nurses belong to the organization. Increasing membership, particularly among APRNs, is one of the challenges facing nurses who need to become active to effect legislative change. Involvement in the ANA is essential to assist nurses in participating in setting and monitoring national health objectives as in *Healthy People 2020,* including Health Literacy (see Table 21.2).

Ethical Dilemmas

Ethical dilemmas may stem from conflicts regarding what is "right" and other duties and obligations. These conflicts may be between two ethical principles one holds, between two possible actions that both seem right in some way, between the demand for action and the need for reflection, and between two unsatisfactory alternatives. Socrates said that we "must let reason determine our ethical decisions rather than emotion." This is why nursing students are taught to use ethical dilemma resolution guidelines to assist them in the process. Before we can resolve a dilemma, however, we must explore different theoretical approaches and discuss ethical principles.

Table 21.2 *Healthy People 2020*
Since 1979, *Healthy People* has set and monitored national health objectives that meet a broad range of health needs, encourage collaboration across geographical locations, guide individuals toward choosing informed healthy decisions, and measure the impact of preventive actions. *Healthy People 2010* led the way to achieve increased quality and years of healthy life and the elimination of health disparities.
Every 10 years, the U.S. Department of Health and Human Services uses scientific insights and lessons learned from the past decade, along with new knowledge of current data, trends, and innovations, to develop new guidelines. *Healthy People 2020* reflects assessments of major risks to health and wellness, changing public health priorities, and emerging issues related to the nation's health preparedness and prevention.
Regional public comment meetings across the nation were held to draft objectives and develop the framework for selecting the vision, mission, goals, focus areas, and criteria for prioritizing the objectives for the guidelines.
To keep abreast of the process and to see the guidelines, go to http://healthypeople.gov/HP2020.

Ethical Issues for Health-Care Providers

Although there are endless ethical issues for providers in the health-care arena, the most common ones facing practitioners today include the following:

- End-of-life issues: Do-not-resuscitate (DNR) orders, Allow Natural Death (AND) orders, advance directives, artificial nutrition and hydration
- Health-care reform issues
- Cost-containment issues
- Breaches of patient confidentiality
- Incompetent and/or unethical conduct of other health-care professionals
- Pain management and palliative care
- Informed consent
- Access to care
- Health literacy
- HIV and AIDS issues
- Issues surrounding genetics/genomics

Theoretical Approaches

There are many different ethical theories, from developmentalists such as Kohlberg with an ethic of justice, to a feminist perspective of Gilligan with her ethic of caring. Many studies have been done to examine the ethical reasoning of males and females. At least one study comparing the decision making regarding dilemmas between medical students (mostly male) and nursing students (mostly female) found no difference in reasoning abilities. We all face dilemmas with different value systems. Because each individual may use different ethical theories as a basis for his or her decision making, it is necessary to understand where someone else is coming from. These ethical theories suggest how to think and what to think about in dealing with conflicts that require choices. They do not solve dilemmas but rather suggest ways of structuring and clarifying the process.

Two of the most common approaches to analyzing ethical dilemmas are *deontology* and *teleology*.

Deontology

The term *deontology* literally means "from being." The concept involves the notion that there are specific duties we have as rational beings that cannot be broached without incurring moral evil. Immanuel Kant championed this moral perspective in his work.

- Principle of universalizability: Act the same in similar situations.
- Consider the nature of the act itself and the principles or rules involved.
- "Duties" are based on "rights."
- The means justify the ends.
- "Do unto others as you would have others do unto you."

Teleology

The term *teleology* literally means "the study of goals or ends." The concept here is that there are specific goals or ends that human life is intended to achieve, and the role of living well is to enable a person to achieve those goals or ends. Typically, a teleological approach will claim that a human being ought to achieve happiness. Happiness is defined in different ways. Then the ethicist will provide principles or rules of attaining that end. There are many different forms of teleological ethical positions. The most well known are Virtue ethics (Aristotle), Divine Command theory (Aquinas), and Utilitarianism (John Stuart Mill).

- Utilitarianism: The greatest amount of happiness or the least amount of harm for the greatest number
- Considers consequences; calculates benefits
- Theories that focus on goals or ends
- Ends justify the means
- Community-oriented theory; also thinks of future generations

The two approaches to analyzing dilemmas may be further explained by comparing the ways both could be applied in several situations. In the first situation, the same outcome may occur even though two different approaches are taken. Consider the patient who has just found out he is HIV-positive and does not want his partner to be told. A clinician using the deontological approach would act the same in any similar situation and would never tell a lie: The clinician would tell the partner that the patient was HIV-positive. A clinician using the teleological approach would focus on the ends justifying the means: The clinician would feel that the partner has a right to know because he could become infected. The clinician also would calculate the consequences of telling or not telling and would feel that it is best for everyone involved in this situation to know the truth about the patient's condition. In this situation, both the deontologist and the teleologist came to the same decision.

Another example of a situation in which these two different approaches are used, but with different outcomes, is a situation involving a terminally ill patient who is on life support. The deontologist would consider the nature of the act itself (the sanctity of life), the uniqueness of each individual, and the high sense of duty, and would keep the patient on the ventilator. The teleologist, on the other hand, would consider the consequences of maintaining the dying patient on life support, would recognize and consider the suffering of the patient and family, both now and after long-term ventilator treatment, and would support the family in withdrawing the life support. It is imperative that health-care providers look at both sides of ethical dilemmas and at both approaches to analyzing dilemmas so that they may effectively communicate with someone who is approaching the situation from a different viewpoint. If the clinician is unable to "speak the language" of others involved in the dilemma, there is no communicating, and the dilemma may remain unsolved. Communication among all parties is essential.

Ethical Principles

Just as we use principles of physics, biochemistry, psychology, and body mechanics in our everyday functioning as clinicians, we must incorporate principles of ethics in our everyday reasoning (Table 21.3). In recognizing the relationship between principles in physics and those principles in ethics, one should keep in mind that the nature of the principles of physics govern the motion or properties of physical reality in such a way that explain why some object acts as it does. The principles in ethics usually contain the moral "ought." This is important, because unlike the principles of physics, the principles in ethics can be broken. We cannot violate the principle of gravity, but we can violate the principle of autonomy. In other words, when one thinks about the principles of ethics, these principles not only set a standard of behavior but also identify and explain why some actions fail to uphold the principle. These bioethical principles (relating to health care) help us respond to specific dilemmas despite the diversity of the moral traditions from which they are derived. Each ethical conflict that a clinician faces may call for the application of different principles. A dilemma may occur that requires one principle to be sacrificed in favor of another, depending on the situation. Just because the clinician may be clinically competent does not necessarily mean that he or she has expertise in dealing with ethical dilemmas. Reasoning at a principled level is a skill that each individual must practice in order to become morally competent.

Autonomy

The first ethical principle is *autonomy,* which deals with personal liberty of action and self-determination, along with respect for all persons as individuals. It is one of the most frequently mentioned moral principles in contemporary biomedical ethics. Autonomy, sometimes defined as "free will," is a principle deeply rooted in the liberal Western tradition emphasizing the importance of individual freedom and choice. *Autonomy*

means "the ability to act or choose without outside interference." For example, if someone were persuaded to invest his or her life savings in a shady business venture, there is some real sense that that person acted freely. However, if you were asked to hold your hand over some button that, if pushed, would launch some terrible weapon, then your hand was forced down, it would not be reasonable to say that you acted freely. The main difference here is that someone interfered with your ability to choose and act by forcing your hand. Mayeroff (1971) suggested that autonomy is living the meaning of one's life. A truly autonomous person freely chooses actions that are authentic and in concert with basic values. Clinicians, as well as patients, are autonomous. Professional autonomy includes control over the terms of practice, content of the discipline, and the regulation of standards.

This principle of autonomy in bioethical contexts is the basis for medical decisions and informed consent, along with access to health care. The principle of autonomy involves giving patients options and allowing them to choose their own course of action, thereby nurturing the wholeness of the person. Informed consent addresses the strong advocacy component of the health-care provider role and is a large component of autonomy (see Table 21.4). Lack of informed consent accounts for about 10% of all lawsuits against providers.

Situations requiring informed consent include invasive procedures; treatment with significant risks, such as chemotherapy; clinical trials; and research. Situations that do not require informed consent include those involving therapeutic privilege, in which the provider anticipates harm from the knowledge that would be shared during the consent process, in an emergency situation, or with the therapeutic use of

Table 21.3   Ethical Principles
• Autonomy
• Beneficence
• Nonmaleficence
• Veracity
• Confidentiality
• Fidelity
• Justice

Table 21.4   Elements of Informed Consent
Informed consent has two elements:
1. Informed: Information given to the patient about procedure or treatment
2. Consent: The patient's autonomous agreement
To be informed, the patient must receive, *in terms that he or she can understand,* all the information that would affect a reasonable person's decision to consent to or to refuse the procedure or treatment. The information should include all of the following:
1. Description of proposed procedure or treatment
2. Name and qualifications of person performing the procedure
3. Explanation of the potential for death or serious harm or for the discomforting side effects during or after the treatment
4. Alternative treatments available
5. The effects of not having treatment

placebos. Informed consent at its best helps to ensure that the patient takes an active role in dealing with the medical uncertainties and potential problems associated with any procedure to be performed.

A potential ethical behavior that restricts autonomy is paternalism. Health-care providers may assume that they know what's best for the patient and order what they deem to be appropriate, thus acting in a paternalistic manner toward patients, restricting their autonomy. The overall term is *parentalism,* that is, acting as a parent would toward a child and assuming that one knows what is best. An example of parentalism is the clinician who orders a medication for a patient without obtaining his or her consent and says, "Take this; it's essential." Although the treatment may be the correct one, to respect the patient as a person, we should involve him or her in the care and get the patient's approval for treatment. By giving the patient a vested interest in the outcome of care, he or she may be more likely to adhere to the prescribed regimen.

Parentalism involves both paternalism and maternalism. *Paternalism* is the way a father would act toward a child, a more stern approach. A clinician who says, "Cigarettes will kill you. If you're not going to stop smoking, I can't care for you anymore," is using a paternalistic approach. *Maternalism* is the way a mother would react to a child. The end result is the same as paternalism, but it usually involves gentle coercion. A clinician addressing the same patient in a maternalistic manner might say, in effect, "Please don't smoke; it hurts my feelings when you don't follow my recommendations. I don't want to go to your funeral." The best way a clinician can respect a patient's autonomy is to give him or her all the facts, and let the patient choose.

Parentalistic behavior, regardless of benevolent motives or the magnitude of the benefit to be secured or the harm to be avoided, overrides the right of each adult to be treated as a person. To respect another as a person and to maintain his or her autonomy is to take full account of the patient's values. To disregard these values and act paternalistic toward a patient shows contempt for the individual as a person. It regards the person as a mere object rather than one's equal as a person, even if the provider is trying to do something to benefit the patient or protect the patient from harm.

It is within this principle of autonomy that the patient's competence and capacity are considered when dealing with patients who exhibit mental status changes. *Competence* is a legal status; all adults older than age 18 years are assumed to be competent unless a judge specifically declares otherwise. *Capacity* is judged clinically and has to do with whether or not the patient is capable of understanding the options presented. *Substituted judgment* is a different approach to maintaining someone's autonomy because the patient's own value system is used in making a decision: One

seeks to decide what the patient would have decided if the patient had been able to do so.

There are some instances in which the principle of autonomy may be overridden by the state. These situations include an emergency procedure that is necessary to protect a life, such as a blood transfusion for a child of a Jehovah's Witness or an intervention when the potential for suicide exists. A provider can legally treat a patient without getting his or her consent if the patient needs immediate treatment to save his or her life; to prevent loss of an organ, limb, or function; if the patient is unconscious; or, in the case of a minor, if the family cannot be reached. In such situations, the law assumes that if a patient could decide, he or she would choose to receive treatment. This exception is limited. It does not apply if the provider knows the patient had previously said he or she would refuse such treatment if and when offered, or if the provider can wait for consent to be obtained. In only two instances is it legal to have a consent form signed by someone other than the patient: (1) in the instance of a minor and (2) when the patient has been declared legally incompetent.

Another exception to the need for informed consent is when a patient waives the requirement to be informed. A patient may not want to know the details. Nonetheless, the provider still has two responsibilities. The provider must make sure the patient understands that risks and alternatives do exist, and then the provider must clearly document the patient's waiver of his or her right to receive information. Some facilities assume no responsibility for obtaining informed consent and supply no forms for doing so. Their premise is that even with detailed consent forms, it is impossible to provide all the relevant information and that completing the forms actually lessens the communication between the provider and the patient. The actual process of informed consent is what should be aimed for, rather than the completion of forms.

Beneficence

The second ethical principle is *beneficence,* which is mentioned in the Nightingale pledge. It is the provision of benefits and a balancing of harms and benefits and requires positive action. One must purposefully choose the right action, not merely by omission, and do what is in the best interest of the patient. Positive beneficence requires personal risk-taking. For example, clinicians who care for persons with AIDS are acting beneficently toward those patients by caring for them. Beneficence encompasses the principle of utility or proportionality when one weighs the probability of benefits and harms in order to produce the maximal net benefit (utility).

Nonmaleficence

The third ethical principle is *nonmaleficence,* the idea that a health-care provider should, above all, "do no harm," which is mentioned in the Hippocratic Oath. This principle, the foundation on which health care rests, forms the basis for most medical and nursing codes of ethics. It usually involves omissions and does not require taking positive action; the emphasis is on not taking the wrong action and doing something to harm the patient. Several moral rules, such as the prohibition of killing, are derived from nonmaleficence. It must be stressed, however, that it is almost always impossible to ensure someone's benefit without risking some harm. Consider the patient with cancer who is receiving chemotherapy. Chemotherapy may be considered a positive benefit, but the side effects are definitely deleterious. Paternalism is also deeply imbedded within this principle because it is extremely difficult to respect a patient's autonomy while wanting to resolve the conflicts between beneficence and nonmaleficence. Most clinicians want the patient to choose the "right" decision. Consider the situation in which we know a patient would benefit from chemotherapy, yet the patient refuses because of a bad experience that a relative had with similar therapy. The patient's autonomy overrides our beneficent wish in this situation.

Veracity

The fourth principle is *veracity,* or truth telling. Health-care providers may tell half-truths or may omit information because they feel that the patient cannot "handle" the news. Using the principle of autonomy, it is the right of the patient to know and to decide if he or she wants any further information or not. As practitioners, we cannot make that decision for our patients. Veracity is important for obtaining informed consent. The critical issue here is that the patient understands or comprehends what the procedure will do or will cost. One must not only tell the truth, but also tell it in a manner that is understandable by the listener.

Confidentiality

The fifth principle is *confidentiality,* which involves respecting privileged information. This is becoming more and more of a problem because computers can provide access to all kinds of personal information. Consider the situation of the patient who requests a breast cancer gene test to see if she is a candidate for prophylactic care, and the insurance company cancels her policy because she might develop breast cancer in the future. Confidentiality, as well as veracity, are extremely important components of the provider-patient relationship.

Health-care providers need to be aware of the Health Insurance Portability and Accountability Act (HIPAA), which has been fully implemented since 2003. All health-care providers are responsible for maintaining secure electronic files and for ensuring confidentiality when sharing information between health-care providers and third-party organizations. Mandated development of electronic health records (EHR) or electronic medical records (EMR) increase both the potential ethical dilemmas and the positive aspects of efficiency/communication issues.

Fidelity

The sixth ethical principle is *fidelity,* or keeping promises. How many times have we heard providers say that if treatment A does not work, they will try another drug, or treatment B? When the time comes, however, they change their minds because the referral is not indicated, or it would make a negative impact on the audit that the insurance company will do shortly, or the insurance company will not pay for it. We promise that we are going to do all we can to help a patient, and then, when care is futile, the type of care is changed to custodial caring rather than curative caring. Fidelity is critical also because it avoids setting up false expectations. If a health-care provider claims that he or she will do something but fails to follow through, the patient may later not request needed assistance because the patient is expecting the promise maker to once again fail to follow through. The result may be someone not receiving a needed treatment, not believing what others inform them, and so forth.

Justice

The principle of justice or fairness involves weighing individual rights. Justice is the most complex and difficult principle to apply to health care. We frequently must use this principle to allocate scarce resources. The concept of justice in play here is what philosophers call *distributive justice.* The notion involves the idea of how to be fair to everyone involved while recognizing that some resource is scarce. For example, consider the following ways in which a tax refund could be distributed. If the government receives more revenue than needed, there are several ways to distribute the excess: (1) Anyone who filed a tax form and overpaid could receive the same refund; (2) everyone who submitted a tax form and overpaid would receive back what that person overpaid; or (3) everyone who submitted a tax form and was born on a Sunday would receive the same share, but no one else would receive a share. All three of these possible distribution patterns of tax refunds are possible, but no one would think (unless that person was born on Sunday) that the third pattern was fair. The real debate is between the first and the second pattern of distribution. Typically, distribution patterns that are considered fair are ones in which proportionality of the scarce resource is balanced by the need or the immediacy of receiving the resource. There may be only four hearts available for transplant. Eight patients need these, but one patient may die within a few days without the transplant. The immediacy of the need would weigh into how these resources were distributed if the distribution were just. The decision must be based on principles rather than emotion; to be fair to patients, like cases should be treated alike. For example, if there are only so many patient-controlled analgesia pumps available and several candidates need one, who will get the last one? Who should get the liver transplant, and how many times should it be done before it is considered futile? One of the goals of *Healthy People 2010* was to eliminate health disparities. In *Healthy People 2020,* one of the goals is to identify nationwide health improvement priorities. The principle of justice employed in all situations will help achieve this goal.

If these ethical principles are applied deliberately and consistently in practice, fewer mistakes will be made, less harm will be done to patients, autonomy will be respected, and decisions will be based on ethics. Changes in the health-care system are a challenge to health-care providers. Do these changes present ethical dilemmas? Definitely so! An *ethical dilemma* is a situation in which there is no satisfactory answer, and, although many options are available, one seems to conflict with another. Nursing Situation 21.1 presents an ethical dilemma.

Resolution Guidelines

Although there is no blueprint for analyzing dilemmas, the mnemonic ETHICAL is a framework that can be used to provide a systematic method for acting consistently in ethical dilemmas, thus allowing reason rather than emotion to guide one's actions.

E Examine the data.
T Think about which person(s) should be making the decision.
H Humanize the options by constructing a decision tree.
I Incorporate the ethical principles, legal statutes, standards of care, and so on.
C Choose an option.
A Act.
L Look back and evaluate.

Consider the following situation and use **ETHICAL** as a framework to guide your actions:

Sylvia is an 86-year-old woman who presents with a massive suspicious breast lump and a new cough. She has not had a well-woman exam in years, nor has she done a monthly breast self-exam. The clinician explains that she wants Sylvia to get a mammogram. Sylvia refuses, stating that she does not want to know the results. What if the test is positive? Sylvia does not want surgery at her age. After a lengthy discussion, the clinician broaches the subject of advance directives. Sylvia states that, as a widow, she has nothing to live for, but she does not want to sign "a death sentence." She states, "When God wants me, he'll take me." This implies that she does not want extraordinary measures taken to keep her alive.

When applying the resolution guidelines in this situation, the first aspect to consider is **E**, examine the

---

Nursing Situation 21.1   Ethical Dilemmas

Situation 1

Shelly has been an APRN for a number of years and has been frustrated with the change in the health-care system and the resultant care that patients receive. When Joseph Harms, one of her patients, was cut back to part-time hours at work, he and his wife lost their health insurance. Mrs. Harms has been treated by Shelly for several years now for type 2 diabetes mellitus and has been very erratic in glycemic control. The Harmses cannot afford to come in as frequently as they did in the past and now must pay the office and pharmacy bills out of their own pockets. Shelly gives them free samples whenever possible and feels like she is not giving the best quality care when they insist they cannot afford any blood work—only the Accu-Chek in the office. Each office visit costs $60. Shelly has no control over billing.

1. What may happen if a fasting blood sugar, glycohemoglobin (Hb A1C), and urinalysis are not routinely ordered?
2. What may happen if Mrs. Harms cannot afford to see the ophthalmologist and podiatrist this year?

Situation 2

Jessica is 16 years old and is on birth control pills. Her relationship with her mother is precarious. Jessica's mom accompanies her to the NP's office because of symptoms of bronchitis. Samantha, the NP, wants to order an antibiotic; but Jessica's birth control pills will not be effective during the course of antibiotics. Samantha is not sure if Jessica's mom knows her daughter is taking birth control pills. Jessica's mom won't leave the room.

1. Jessica's mom already stated she would not leave Jessica alone in the room. Should Samantha insist?
2. Even though Jessica's mother is present, should Samantha go ahead and tell Jessica about the interactions between antibiotics and birth control pills and the need to use another form of birth control when/if engaging in intercourse?
3. How far does the principle of confidentiality extend? Does the fact that Jessica is a minor play any part?

---

data. The clinician has detected a breast mass and recommended a mammogram as the next step in the diagnostic process. Sylvia has refused. In this step, all the information should be collected and the key participants identified. When interpreting the data, the conflicts presented in the situation should be identified. Are there conflicting rights and obligations? Is there a conflict between two unsatisfactory choices of action? The clinician should enter the world of the person involved and look at the situation from that perspective. The *Circle of Caring* model is definitely utilized in ethical dilemmas. The clinician should delineate the scope of responsibility and authority of each person. Factors should be identified that could limit each person's ability to participate in the decision making, such as fear, coercion, and pain.

The second step, **T**, refers to thinking about and identifying the person(s) who should be making the decision. We do not know if other family members are involved in Sylvia's care, but because she is coming to the office by herself, the clinician assumes that she is independent, competent, and certainly capable of making her own decisions. Even if there were a daughter nearby, the decision would still be Sylvia's to make, although the clinician might ask Sylvia if he or she could discuss the situation with her daughter and share his or her perspective. In most instances, there are other persons or ethical agents involved in the decision making, such as the patient's family, physician, institution, clergy, social worker, and various therapists and consultants. The rights, duties, and responsibilities of each participant must be clarified and analyzed. In addition, because health-care ethics is a complex subject, there will always be difficult cases that will require consultation with people who have special training in relevant fields.

The third step, **H**, is to humanize the options by constructing a decision tree as shown in Table 21.5. This allows all the options to be considered along with all the consequences of those options. Visualizing the results in this fashion can help narrow down acceptable options.

The fourth step, **I**, stands for incorporating all the extraneous data that must be considered when making ethical and/or legal choices. Certainly the clinician is reflecting on his or her ethical principles. By allowing Sylvia the right to make her own choice, even though it is in disagreement with her own recommendation, the clinician is maintaining Sylvia's autonomy. If the clinician were to be beneficent in his or her actions, he or she might strongly urge (coerce) Sylvia to have the mammogram. But then what? Why pursue the mammogram if Sylvia has already stated that if it shows a problem, she will not consider any further action, for example, a biopsy, or more invasive surgery? Does Sylvia have the right to choose an option that might essentially be signing a "death warrant"? Yes, she does, as long as she is competent and has all the information presented to her. The decision tree allows Sylvia to see all the options and the resulting consequences. Although we cannot predict which branch of the tree this particular scenario will take, Sylvia has the right to consider all branches. In this step in the ethical inquiry, all the basic principles should be considered. How does each ethical principle relate to the decision? The Code of Ethics for Nurses should help guide the action. Although codes by definition are brief and general, when used in combination with exploring the relationship of all the ethical principles to the proposed decision, the outcome will be ethical. This step usually points to the most ethical course of action. The ultimate goal of laws is to protect individual rights without

Table 21.5 Resolution Guidelines: Constructing a Decision Tree

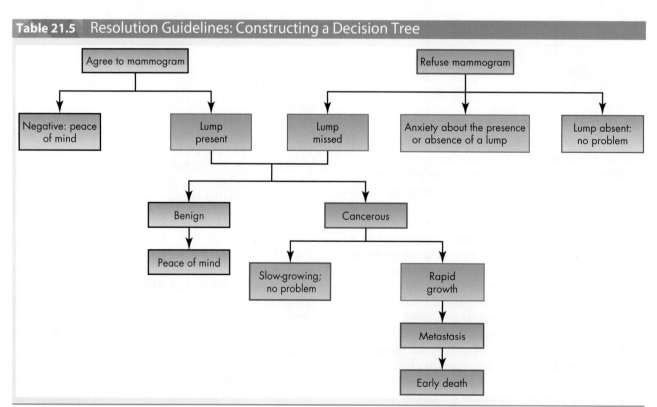

Each state defines the scope of practice within the state Nurse Practice Act. Every state has a Nurse Practice Act.

jeopardizing the welfare of the general population. Laws must be considered in directing action, seeking consultation, and requesting necessary assistance in selected patient-care situations.

The next step, **C**, involves choosing an action, and the following step **A** refers to actually acting on the decision. Sylvia has known all along what her choice would be—taking no action, which is actually choosing an action. The final step, **L**, stands for looking back or evaluating the situation, so that if the clinician were faced with a similar situation in the future, he or she might consider more choices and thus have more "branches" in the decision tree for consideration, or be aware of more legal precedence, and so forth. Especially when we are acting in the role of the primary moral agent, we need to keep abreast of the consequences of our own actions as well as those of others who are acting on behalf of the patient. Previous experience in similar situations can provide a frame of reference for comparisons and assist the clinician in making quality decisions. Although a decision tree is not meant to "lead" the patient to action, it does allow the patient and provider to consider more choices than may have been thought available. Brainstorming should be used; all choices proposed should be taken under consideration, even if they seem unrealistic at the time. Sometimes the first "irrational" choice ends up being the best choice for the patient and his or her family.

Institutional Ethics Committees

When health-care providers have difficult and unclear choices to make, the best course of action is to consult the local Institutional Ethics Committee (IEC). The Standards of The Joint Commission (TJC) state that "the organization has in place a mechanism for the consideration of ethical issues arising in the care of patients and to provide education to caregivers and patients on ethical issues in health care." Although this mandate may be applied loosely and does not mean that the organization will have an ethics committee in place, there is always some help available. A parish nurse may be available for consultation, a bioethicist may be available, or there may be an IEC in place. Some of the larger health-care institutions have ethics consultation services for ethical support to both patients/families and professional staff; the staff for these services may include ethicists who informally address nursing questions and concerns. The purposes of IECs are to serve as a forum for health-care professionals' ethical concerns, as well as for conflict resolution between any of the parties involved. IECs provide advice, education, and consultation to the staff and patients and possibly to the community on actual and potential questions of ethics. They also provide recommendations for and help in developing institutional policies, procedures, and guidelines in areas of bioethical concern; assist in developing formal policies and procedures for identifying, reporting,

and resolving ethical questions and in conducting retrospective reviews of decisions on ethical questions; and offer recommendations for improving policies and procedures used to resolve ethical issues.

IECs are usually multidisciplinary in nature because of the varied amount and types of health-care workers involved in any patient situation. They are composed of physicians, nurses, social workers, clergy, administrative personnel, legal counsel, a patient representative, and someone from the community. The patient representative must actively advocate for the patient, and in doing so, subordinate his or her own needs, opinions, and moral positions to those of the patient or family member. The patient representative works to focus and refocus the committee on the welfare and rights of patients. The ANA and the AMA have developed many position statements (see the ANA Web site for position statements available), such as those on referrals to the most appropriate provider, sexual harassment, and so forth, to assist practitioners in drafting policies. Health-care providers should not hesitate to use their professional organizations as resources.

It is interesting to note that physicians and nurses reason very similarly when faced with ethical dilemmas. (See Nursing Research–Based Practice 21.1.)

Relationship Between Ethics and Law

Although clinicians strive to be ethical in all their actions, they must also think of legalities. Actions that are ethical are not always legal, whereas actions that are illegal are sometimes ethical (Table 21.6). APRNs should

Nursing Research–Based Practice 21.1

Winland-Brown, JE, and Dobrin, AL. A comparison of physicians' and nurses' responses to selected ethical dilemmas. *Forum on Public Policy Online.* Retrieved from http://forumonpublicpolicy.com/spring09papers/papers09spring.html

The purpose of this study was to explore the similarities and differences between physicians' and nurses' responses to four different ethical dilemmas. The dilemmas included surgical error, end-of-life care, possible physician or nurse drug use, and the medical repatriation of an illegal immigrant. Sixty-seven nurses and 26 physicians participated. This study found that physicians and nurses reason more alike than differently on ethical dilemmas. There was only one response to one dilemma where physicians and nurses reasoned significantly differently. Similarly, an equal number of physicians and nurses had experienced moral distress in the past. The variables of religion, gender, education, and ethnicity were significant for some of the responses to the dilemmas. Strategies were suggested to enhance moral reasoning and possibly lessen some moral distress.

Table 21.6	Relationship Between Ethical and Legal Issues*	
	Legal	Illegal
Ethical	Assisting an older patient to complete an advance directive	Assisting in the death of a 99-year-old terminally ill patient
Unethical	Ordering emergency contraception in a Catholic Church–affiliated clinic	Billing for a treatment that was not done

*Although one may not agree with the choices of situations explaining ethical and legal issues, they are presented here for demonstration purposes—to explicate the intricacies of the ethical and legal relationship. Laws represent the minimum ethic governing behavior; compliance with them is mandated. Ethics operate at a higher level; they offer guidelines for resolving ethical dilemmas.

always strive to practice within the ANA Scope of Practice, their State Practice Act, and the Code of Ethics for Nurses, in addition to being cognizant of individual state laws on prescribing authority, signing death certificates, authorizing disabled parking permits, and so on. The circumscribed actions and duties that are allowable in the profession are termed the *scope of nursing practice,* which are defined and guided by each state in the Nurse Practice Act and by common law. Common-law principles govern many interactions affecting nursing and are based on a traditional justice perspective. The state Nurse Practice Act, however, is the single most important piece of legislation for nursing because it is the Practice Act that affects all facets of nursing practice. The Nurse Practice Act cannot grant exceptions, waive the Act's provisions, or expand practice outside the Act's specific provisions.

■ LEGAL ISSUES
Scope of Practice

The scope of practice defines the duties and responsibilities of the APRN and delineates the permissible boundaries of the professional practice. It is defined by statute, rule, or a combination of the two. A major legislative task for the future is for APRNs to define a separate scope of practice within each Practice Act that enables them to act autonomously without barriers to practice, such as limitations on prescriptive authority. Seventeen states allow independent practice as recommended by the Institute of Medicine (IOM) and national consensus statement. Twenty-one states require collaborative agreements with physicians, and 12 require physician supervision, delegation, or team management. Florida is the only state that does not authorize prescriptive authority for nurse practitioners (NPs) for schedule II drugs. With each legislative session, there is hope that all states

will allow APRNs to practice to their fullest scope to benefit the American public.

A model for future APRNs was developed with the collaborative work of the APRN Consensus Work Group and the National Council of State Boards of Nursing APRN Committee. They established clear expectations for licensure, accreditation, certification, and education (known as LACE) for all APRNs, and ultimately these expectations will continue to shape future APRN practice. To download a copy of this report, go to www.aacn.nche.edu/Education/pdf/APRNReport.pdf.

Overview of Nurse Practitioners

There are over 171,000 NPs practicing in the United States today. Approximately 14,000 NPs completed their graduate programs in 2012. With increased demand, the number is estimated to be 244,000 by 2025. According to a 2012 survey from the American Association of Nurse Practitioners, the typical NP has the following characteristics:

- Is female (92%)
- Is white (90.3%)
- Is 48 years old
- Practices as a family NP (48.3%)
- Is actively practicing (89%)
- Has been in practice for 11 years as an NP
- Practices in a primary-care ambulatory setting
- Has an average full-time NP annual income of $98,760
- Sees three or four patients per hour (60%)
- Prescribes medications (97.2%) and writes 19 prescriptions/day
- Is satisfied with his or her practice

Licensure and Certification

Many nonnursing individuals assume that licensing and credentialing are synonymous. It is the responsibility of the clinician to educate other providers and consumers regarding what he or she can and cannot do. Legal authority for all nursing practice, including advanced practice nursing, rests with the individual Board that administers the legal statutes that define nursing practice in each state. Currently for APRNs, this oversight varies. In some states, the Board of Nursing administers and defines advanced nursing practice; in others, it is the Board of Medicine; and in a few states, it is the Board of Pharmacy. The American Association of Nurse Practitioners recommends that state boards of nursing regulate NP practice and prescriptive authority. Legal authority for professional practice was delegated to the states and territories by the U.S. Constitution and is not regulated by federal statutes.

An individual is permitted to practice basic or advanced practice nursing by licensure. *Licensure* protects the public from unsafe practitioners by ensuring a minimal standard for competency. Basic licensure as a registered nurse (RN) is a legal status granted by each state's Board of Nursing. The National Council Licensure Exam that licenses RNs (NCLEX-RN) does not ensure high nursing standards. The NCLEX is designed to assess minimum competency to practice safely. The curriculum of a nursing program, although providing a foundation of nursing knowledge that will graduate a safe and competent practitioner, is not specifically geared to the NCLEX exam. Nursing programs retain autonomy over their own curricula.

Similarly, the NP curriculum is under the control of the graduate faculty and is geared to advancing nursing-based knowledge. On graduation, each prospective APRN applies to the appropriate state board for an advanced nursing license. In some states, the graduate must pass a national certification exam to be eligible for this license. Although the licensing statutes may spell out prescriptive privileges for APRNs, they do not necessarily do that, nor is that the primary purpose of professional licensure. Prescriptive authority for NPs varies from state to state. Some states mandate the filing of a protocol that documents physician oversight, but other states do not. (Table 21.7 shows a sample protocol.) Laws in most states do not mandate physician supervision of NPs. Protocols are similar to standing orders; they can be used as evidence to establish breach of the standard of care if they are not adhered to. The ability to prescribe controlled substances varies from state to state. Restrictions on prescriptive authority limit the ability of NPs to provide comprehensive health-care services.

Credentialing means that the practitioner has met certain criteria through licensure, education, and certification. Criteria for credentialing vary, depending on the credentialing body. A hospital, for example, may use credentialing to grant hospital privileges. Currently 43% of NPs hold hospital privileges, and 15% have long-term care privileges. This number is increasing daily. The

Table 21.7 Sample Advanced Practice Nursing Protocol

I. Requiring authority: Nurse Practice Act, Specific State—list Statutes, Chapters, Administrative Code. Administrative policies pertaining to certification of Advanced Practice Registered Nurses (APRN).

II. Advanced Practice Registered Nurse Certification: _____(name, home address, phone number) is certified as an APRN #_____ by the (list State) Board of Nursing.
  Supervising Professional: Name, address, license number, and DEA number of physician.

III. General Area of Practice: _____ may manage the health care for those patients for which he or she has been educated. His or her master's degree is in _____.
  List practice address, including primary and satellite sites.

IV. Specific Management Areas:
  A. The following measures may be initiated by the APRN:
    1. Conduct a history and physical on patients.
    2. Take medication history, review medication profiles, and suggest necessary revisions.
    3. Order and interpret diagnostic tests necessary to treat, including, but not limited to, lab work, x-ray exams, pulmonary function tests, electrocardiograms.
    4. Diagnose and treat conditions within the scope of practice of a family nurse practitioner.
    5. Instruct patient and families in treatment and medications.
    6. Refer to other providers as appropriate.
  B. The following medications may be prescribed, initiated, monitored, altered, or ordered by the nurse practitioner in accordance with education: antibiotics, antihistamines, antihypertensives, anti-inflammatory agents, antigout agents, anticonvulsants, antimicrobial agents, antifungals, antiarrhythmics, antiparasitic agents, antianginals, antidepressants, antianxiety agents, antipsychotics, beta blockers, calcium-channel blockers, cathartics, laxatives, contraceptives, diuretics, expectorants, muscle relaxants, NSAIDs, optical agents, otic agents, over-the-counter agents, steroids, stimulants, vasodilators, vaccines.
    Controlled substances may be initiated by the APRN only within the facility in which he or she practices, after appropriate federal and state guidelines have been followed by the supervising physician. (Will vary according to state.)
  C. Admit, initiate visits, and discharge patients in hospitals that have granted visiting privileges. Conduct histories and physicals, order diagnostic tests, treatments, and prescribe medications.
  D. Any other measures within the scope of preparation and experience of the APRN.
V. All of the above functions may be performed under the general supervision of the physician.
Signed: _____APRN_____
Date: _____
Signed: _____MD_____
Date: _____

granting of clinical privileges to practice in an institution is influenced by many factors. The primary factors governing the ability of an NP to obtain clinical privileges are the institutional policy, medical staff by-laws, state law, and TJC accreditation standards. Other factors include the desire of the collaborating physician and the NP's education, certification, and continuing education credits, along with his or her eligibility for third-party reimbursement and prescriptive privileges.

Certification is a voluntary process with no legal authority. The primary purpose of certification is to document excellence and specialization. Certification by a nongovernmental agency or association certifies that an individual has met certain predetermined standards for competency and specialization in a particular area. Although some states mandate that an NP pass a national certification exam before granting licensure to practice at an advanced level, not all states do. Currently 97% of all NPs hold national certification. National certification may be necessary to obtain third-party reimbursement; however, that is not the primary purpose of certification. Providing the public with information about the skills of the practitioners is not the primary purpose of certification, either. Other than the specialty organizations, there are two groups that certify APRNs in adult or family practice: the ANA through the American Nurses Credentialing Center (ANCC) and the American Association of Nurse Practitioners (AANP). Both organizations advocate that NPs be nationally certified and obtain annual continuing educational credits in pharmacology.

Prescriptive Authority

Since the mid-1970s, APRNs have had some type of prescriptive authority. Prescriptive authority is an integral component of advanced nursing practice and is regulated from state to state. It is important for APRNs to know the extent of the prescriptive authority they have in the state in which they are practicing and what restrictions, if any, there may be. Restrictions may range from collaborative or supervisory requirements to a need for countersignatures, formulary restrictions, specific protocols, and/or site restrictions. All states grant statutory independent prescribing authority to APRNs; however, three states exclude the authority to prescribe controlled substances. Some states require that APRNs have additional training to gain prescriptive privileges. State-specific regulations affecting prescribing authority severely limit the mobility of nurses who anticipate moving to another state. Both prescriptive authority and the mobility of the APRN's state license are legislative challenges facing APRNs today.

Unfortunately, medication errors accompany prescriptive privileges. At least 44,000 up to as many as 98,000 American deaths annually are due to preventable adverse events as a result of medication errors. Because most patients are taking three or more medications in a 24-hour period, drug–drug interactions are common. APRNs and anyone prescribing medications must ask each patient what medications he or she is taking before ordering a new one and must always consider the potential interactions. It is the clinician's responsibility to empower the patient with knowledge regarding any adverse effects of the medications. The clinician must educate the patient about signs and symptoms to watch for and should provide guidelines regarding when to notify the clinician if a problem arises. Of medical malpractice payments against NPs, 16.5% are a result of medication-related problems. Malpractice rates for NPs remain low, however, with only 2% of NPs named as primary defendants. One policy approach to the problem of medication errors is to implement mandatory reporting of all medical errors.

Reimbursement

Payment standards in the United States are driven by Medicare and Medicaid. APRNs have made great strides in this area and now receive third-party reimbursement in most settings. Payment by private insurance companies is contract specific and varies with each state's insurance commission. Reimbursement has long been a controversial issue. Should APRNs receive equal pay for the same work as physicians? In some areas, these practitioners are reimbursed at 80% of the physician rate. Does this mean they only did 80% of the work or did it only 80% as well as a physician would have? If one asks the recipient of care, the patient will most likely state that the APRN gave the same level of care provided by or expected from the physician. Reimbursement is a moot point, however, in managed care contracts, in which a fixed, predetermined rate is given to all providers, whether APRN or physician. Reimbursement issues are another legislative challenge facing these nurses. When reimbursement issues and practices are addressed, APRNs will be able to practice independently and truly autonomously.

Malpractice

Three components must all be present to establish malpractice: (1) The provider must have a duty to the patient, (2) the standard of care must be deviated from or breached, and (3) harm or damages must occur as a result of the duty and a breach of the standards of care. A plaintiff must prove duty, breach of the duty, damages or injuries, and causation. *Duty* means that a relationship has been established between the defendant and the plaintiff. *Breach of the duty* is the failure to do what the reasonable and prudent person would have done in the same or similar circumstances. *Damages or injuries* include medical expenses; pain and suffering, both physical and mental; lost wages and lost earning capacity; loss of companionship, society, affection, and sexual relations; hedonic damages; and punitive or exemplary damages. *Causation* means that the plaintiff must prove a direct causal connection between the act of negligence and the alleged injuries.

Take the situation of Sally, a clinician caring for Mr. B., who is suffering from congestive heart failure. Sally increases his diuretic but makes no note of his potassium level and orders no replacement potassium. When Mr. B. returns a week later for routine lab testing, his potassium level is found to be low. Sally orders a potassium supplement to begin immediately and a follow-up potassium-level measurement. Is Sally guilty of malpractice? No. Although Sally did have a duty to Mr. B. and she did deviate from the standard of care (which would have been to order a potassium supplement at the beginning), no harm came to Mr. B. Because all the components were not met, malpractice was not established. If patients were aware of this, many false claims would not be filed. If Mr. B. had died from a fatal arrhythmia due to his low potassium level, however, then Sally could be held liable.

In the outpatient office setting, the most common reason for a malpractice suit for both physicians and APRNs is the failure to diagnose correctly. Approximately one-third of the malpractice cases brought against general practitioners involve cases of failure to diagnose in a timely manner. These cases usually involve cancer, particularly cancer of the breast. Failure to diagnose promptly accounts for the highest number of liability cases. Regarding NPs in particular, the most common reason for malpractice suits is related to failure to diagnose or delay in diagnosis. Diagnosing infections that lead to sepsis and diagnosing cancer were top liability issues. APRNs must carry liability insurance to protect themselves and their assets. Each APRN should have a lawyer who will represent him or her rather than the institution the APRN works for. However, nurses are often told that they should not carry their own insurance, and there are typically two reasons for this. The first is that a policy will encourage a lawsuit. There is no evidence to support this, and lack of coverage does not discourage a lawsuit, should there be a legitimate claim. The other reason is that nurses are told that their employer carries liability insurance that will also protect them. Although it is true that employers may provide insurance coverage for their employees, that coverage is subject to the provisions of the insurance agreement, and the employer is the client, not the nurse. Many physicians are "going bare," which means not carrying malpractice insurance. They must post a sign in their office to that effect. Some NPs are considering this as well. One must consider that a malpractice suit can destroy a life, both professionally and financially. As NPs would not consider being without health insurance, so they should not be without liability insurance.

Several different types of policies are available. One type, called the claims-made policy, covers only situations in which the incident occurred and the claim was made while the policy was in effect. Clinicians must review the policy to see if they are to be protected for past incidents, or they should purchase a tail policy that covers future claims. The best type of policy to get is an occurrence policy, which covers liability arising from all acts or omissions during the period the policy was in effect, no matter when the claim is brought. This is the ideal policy, because a claim can be made several years after an incident occurs.

Professional liability policies may be expensive, so the clinician may want to negotiate payment of the policy as part of the employment contract, if he or she is working in a group practice. Malpractice claims against NPs are on the rise, however slowly. The reasons can be attributed to three factors: changes in insurance markets due to fewer carriers, poor litigation laws that have arisen from current tort law practices, and the fact that the scope of practice for NPs has made them more autonomous. Excellent communication skills remain the number one reason why providers avoid a costly judgment or settlement. One study examined whether NPs used a patient-centered communication style or a provider-centered communication style in their patient encounters. Surprisingly, only a minority of NPs used patient-centered communication styles. As the rise in malpractice claims seems to be based on poor communication, NPs must be cognizant of this and consider the positive effects of patient-centered communication styles. (See Nursing Research–Based Practice 21.2.)

Collaboration

Collaboration is a form of interaction among and between providers during their delivery of care. The term implies that there are shared values and that the goal must be directed to what is in the patient's best interest. There is a constructive commitment to work toward that end. There is also mutual trust and understanding and respect of what each participant has to offer in this interdependent relationship. Both the nurse and physician must respect the boundaries of their disciplines and value what the other has to offer and bring to the relationship.

Nursing Research–Based Practice 21.2

Berry, JA. Nurse practitioner/patient communication styles in clinical practice. *J Nurse Pract* 5(7):508–514, 2009.

Nurse practitioners (NPs) spend more than two-thirds of patient-encounter clinical time in intrapersonal communication. The NP literature has little on NP/patient communication styles. The purpose of this study was to examine and document the most common verbal communication style used by NPs in patient interactions. Content analysis was used to analyze 53 NP/patient transcripts for communication style. Based on the transcript analysis, only a minority of NPs used a patient-centered communication style.

The IOM report *The Future of Nursing: Leading Change, Advancing Health* (2010) advocated for nurses to practice to the fullest extent of their education. The IOM emphasizes the importance of collaboration in the relationship of high-quality and safe patient care and suggests that five core competencies be incorporated in all health professionals' education:

- Provide patient-centered care.
- Work in interdisciplinary teams.
- Use evidence-based practice.
- Apply quality improvement.
- Use informatics.

The curricula of APRN programs have included these competencies; in addition, the *Circle of Caring* model emphasizes the essential nature of collaboration between APRNs and all physicians and health-care professionals with whom they work.

Additionally, APRNs must collaborate with physicians because there are many situations APRNs will encounter that are outside their scope of practice. The problem arises when the NP–physician relationship is one of supervision rather than collaboration. Different state boards of nursing delineate the NP's role in different ways. Some states require that physicians supervise or sponsor APRNs, which limits the nurse's scope of practice. Other states require that there be a collaborative relationship. A major challenge for the APRN is to assert his or her autonomy and maintain a professional, collegial, and collaborative relationship with physicians.

The IOM stresses the need for interprofessional education, and many universities and communities are creating opportunities for this to happen among nurses, physicians, social workers, and others. Nursing Research–Based Practice 21.3 illustrates the importance of learning interprofessional skills as a student.

In 1997, when the Oxford Health Plan allowed members to choose NPs as their primary-care providers and paid them the same rate as physicians for the same care, APRNs were finally recognized as independent practitioners who could provide quality care. In a situation such as this, collaboration is key because APRNs are the first to recognize that they are not expert in all areas.

Before being hired, it may be difficult to foresee whether a practice will be truly collaborative or not. There are tools available to assist a new NP in learning the skills of contract negotiation. One such comprehensive tool used to evaluate one's needs and desires in an employment or contractual arrangement is published by the American Academy of Nurse Practitioners, titled "Contract Negotiation for Nurse Practitioners."

Health-Care Reform

The United States is the only industrialized nation in the world without a national health insurance plan in place. The debate over health care reform has centered on the following questions:

- Is there a fundamental right to health care?
- Who should have access to health care and under what circumstances?

Nursing Research–Based Practice 21.3

Machin, AI, and Jones, D. Interprofessional service improvement learning and patient safety: A content analysis of preregistration students' assessments. *Nurse Educ Today* S0260–S0269, 2013.

A culture of continuous service improvement underpins safe, efficient, and cost-effective health and social care. This paper reports a qualitative research study of assessment material from one cohort of final year preregistration health and social care students' interprofessional service improvement learning experience. Initially introduced to the theory of service improvement, students were linked with an interprofessional buddy group and subsequently planned and implemented, if possible, a small-scale service improvement project within a practice placement setting. Assessment was by oral project presentation and written reflection on learning. Summative assessment materials from 150 students were subjected to content analysis to identify the following: service user triggers for service improvement, ideas to address the identified area for improvement, and perceptions of service improvement learning. Triggers for service improvements included service user disempowerment, poor communication, gaps in service provision, poor transitions, lack of information, lack of role clarity and role duplication, and differed between professions. Ideas for improvement included both the implementation of evidence-based best practice protocols in a local context and also innovative approaches to problem solving. Students described both intrapersonal and interprofessional learning as a result of engaging with service improvement theory and practice. Service improvement learning in an interprofessional context has positive learning outcomes for health- and social-care students. Students can identify improvement opportunities that may otherwise go undetected. Engaging positively in interprofessional service improvement learning as a student is an important rehearsal for life as a qualified practitioner. It can help students to develop an ability to challenge unsafe practice elegantly, thereby acting as advocates for the people in their care. Universities can play a key support role by working collaboratively with service organizations; role modeling effective interprofessional working; and supporting research to measure the impact of education on practice.

• What quality is achieved for the high prices currently being spent?

The Patient Protection and Affordable Care Act of 2010

The Affordable Care Act (ACA) was signed into law on March 23, 2010, to reform health care in America. The new health-care law includes reforms to health insurance and the way the health-care industry is run in the United States. The ACA aims to greatly increase the number of Americans who have access to affordable health insurance. This is done by expanding Medicaid to America's poorest, providing tax credits to employers who cover their employees, providing tax credits to individuals who need help paying for insurance, reforming the health-care industry to rein in excess spending, taxing higher earners and the health-care industry, and opening up state-based, competitive, regulated, online health insurance exchanges (Marketplace) where individuals can buy insurance and receive cost assistance. The ACA makes health insurance coverage more secure and reliable for Americans who have it, makes coverage more affordable for families and small business owners, and brings down skyrocketing health-care costs that have put a strain on individuals, families, employers, and the federal budget. The ACA requires that all Americans have access to affordable health care (or pay a tax if they choose to opt out). *Affordable health care* is defined as costing 8% or less of annual income. The ACA also reforms Medicare and Medicaid, as well as the other aspects of the health-care system, including the rates that insurance companies and private health-care facilities receive and patients' rights to health care. (You can read the Affordable Care Act at www.CMS.gov.)

The Congressional Budget Office has determined that the ACA is fully paid for and will provide coverage to more than 94% of Americans while staying under the $900 billion limit that President Obama established. This will bend the health-care cost curve and reduce the health-care deficit over the next 10 years

and beyond. The ACA contains nine titles, each addressing an essential component of reform (www. dpc.senate.gov/healthreformbill/healthbill04.pdf):

1. Quality, affordable health care for all Americans
2. The role of public programs
3. Improving the quality and efficiency of health care
4. Prevention of chronic disease and improving public health
5. Health care workforce
6. Transparency and program integrity
7. Improving access to innovative medical therapies
8. Community living assistance services and supports
9. Revenue provisions

The leading cause of personal bankruptcy in the United States has been medical debt. The ACA will provide health insurance coverage to the almost 46 million people, or the 15% of the U.S. population, without coverage. Many organizations, including the ANA, have examined the potential outcomes of the ACA. Oregon, as an example, is one state with a successful unified health-care program. They accomplished this by rank ordering the community values of persons in the state. Their number-one value is prevention, followed by quality of life. Because nurses are the advocates for patients and persons, our role is to continue to be involved in the development of public policy that will effect change in all aspects of health care. A study of a case involving medical repatriation addressed the issue of an undocumented worker who was not eligible for insurance and the outcome that ensued. This scenario illustrates the need for advocacy and changes in public policy to ensure quality of life for all residents. (See Nursing Research–Based Practice 21.4.)

As the ACA is implemented and APRNs adapt to the public's needs, attention will focus on the concepts of the Medical Home and expansion in both the number and practice of APRNs. See the ANA Web site at www.nursingworld.org.

All health-care providers have an ethical duty to actively engage in legislative efforts that will ensure the best

---

Nursing Research–Based Practice 21.4

Winland-Brown, JE, and Dobrin, AL. Medical repatriation: Physicians' and nurses' responses to a dilemma. *Southern Online Journal of Nursing Research* (SOJNR) 9(4), 2009.

Medical repatriation is an institutional dilemma that affects physicians and nurses. This study analyzed the responses of physicians and nurses to a hypothetical case study involving a young illegal immigrant involved in a truck accident who was deported back to Honduras for lack of medical resources. The only variable that was significant when considering deportation was ethnicity. There was no significant difference between the responses of either physicians or nurses whether the patient should be medically repatriated. When asked about solutions, respondents suggested involving the Hospital Ethics Committee, searching for additional resources to allow this patient to remain in the United States to receive rehabilitation services, and providing ethics training for physicians and nurses to enable them to resolve ethical dilemmas using principled thinking and to (it was hoped) decrease moral distress.

possible condition to optimize the health of the nation. As advocates, providers need to know their state legislators and governors. Information on how to contact each governor is located at the American Academy of Nurse Practitioner's Web site at www.aanp.org, which also includes links to Congressional Legislative Committees.

The ANA strongly believes that APRNs are one of the keys to solving America's health-care crisis. Their current efforts address the important role that APRNs must play in a reformed health-care system. See the ANA Web site for current information on health-care reform (www.nursingworld.org).

 For additional resources please visit
http://davisplus.fadavis.com

References

American Nursing Association. *The essential guide to nursing practicing.* 2010. Retrieved from http://essentialguidetonursingpractice. wordpress.com

Mayeroff, M. *On Caring.* Harper & Row Publishers, New York, 1971

Institute of Medicine. *The future of nursing: Leading change, advancing health.* October 5, 2010. Retrieved from www.iom.edu/Reports/ 2010/The-Future-of-Nursing-Leading-Change-Advancing-Health.aspx

Bibliography

Affordable Care Act. Retrieved from www.hhs.gov/healthcare/ rights/law

Berry, JA. Nurse practitioner/patient communication styles in clinical practice. *J Nurse Pract* 5(7):508–514, 2009.

Buck, JA. The looming expansion and transformation of public substance abuse treatment under the Affordable Care Act. *Health Aff* 30(8):1402–1410, 2011.

CMS.gov. Affordable Care Act in action at CMS. Retrieved from www. cms.gov/about-cms/aca/affordable-care-act-in-action-at-cms.html

Davis, K, et al. How the Affordable Care Act will strengthen the nation's primary care foundation. *J Gen Intern Med* 26(10):1201–1203.

Fairman, JA, et al. Broadening the scope of nursing practice. *N Engl J Med* 364:193–196, 2011.

Green, LV, and Savin, S. Primary care physician shortages could be eliminated through use of teams, nonphysicians, and electronic communication. *Health Aff* 32(1):11–19, 2013.

Hahn, JA, et al. Demystifying state health insurance marketplaces. *Nurs Econ* 31(3):119–143, 2013.

Healthy People 2020. The road ahead. Retrieved from http://healthy-people.gov/HP2020

Inglehart, JK. Despite tight budgets, boosting U.S. health workforce may be policy that is "just right." *Health Aff* 30(2):191–192, 2011. doi:10.1377/hlthaff.2011.0142

Johnson, SR. Controlling costs. *Modern Healthc* 43 7, 12, 2013.

Kocher, KP, and Adashi, EY. Hospital readmissions and the Affordable Care Act: Paying for coordinated quality care. *JAMA* 306(16):1794–1795, 2011.

Kocher, R, et al. The Affordable Care Act and the future of clinical medicine: The opportunities and challenges. *Ann Intern Med* 153:536–539, 2010.

Kohlberg, L. *Philosophy of moral development.* Harper & Row, San Francisco, 1981.

Machin, AI, and Jones, D. Interprofessional service improvement learning and patient safety: A content analysis of pre-registration students' assessments. *Nurse Educ Today* S0260–S0269, 2013.

Mayeroff, M. *On Caring.* Harper & Row Publishers, New York, 1971.

McClellan, M, et al. A national strategy to put accountable care into practice. *Health Aff* 29(5):982–990, 2010.

Medical errors in the USA: Human or systemic? *Lancet* 377(9774):1289, 2011.

Naylor, MD, et al. The importance of transitional care in achieving health reform. *Health Aff* 30(4):746–754, 2011.

O'Connor, JC, et al. Paying for prevention: A critical opportunity for public health. *J Law Med Ethics* 41(Suppl 1):69–72, 2013. doi:10.1111/jlme.12043

Orszag, PR, and Emanuel, EJ. Health care reform and cost control. *N Engl J Med* 363:601–603, 2010. doi:10.1056/NEJMp1006571

Poghosyan, L, et al. Nurse practitioner workforce: A substantial supply of primary care providers. *Nurs Econ* 30(5):268–274, 294, 2012.

Pollack, CE, and Armstrong, K. Accountable care organizations and health care disparities. *JAMA* 305(16):1706–1707, 2011.

Responsible reform for the middle class: ACA. Retrieved from www.dpc.senate.gov/healthreformbill/healthbill04.pdf

Rowe, JW. Why nurses need more authority. *The Atlantic.* May 7, 2012. Retrieved from www.theatlantic.com/health/archive/ 2012/05/why-nurses-need-more-authority/256798

Thorpe, DM. The Affordable Care Act lays the groundwork for a national diabetes prevention and treatment strategy. *Health Aff* 31(1):61–66, 2012.

Van Den Bos, J, et al. The $17.1 billion problem: The annual cost of measurable medical errors. *Health Aff* (Millwood) 30(4):596–603, 2011.

Winland-Brown, JE, and Dobrin, AL. Medical repatriation: Physicians' and nurses' responses to a dilemma. *Southern Online Journal of Nursing Research* (SOJNR) 9(4), 2009.

Winland-Brown, JE, and Dobrin, AL. A comparison of physicians' and nurses' responses to selected ethical dilemmas. *Forum on Public Policy Online.* Retrieved from http://forumonpublicpolicy.com/ spring09papers/papers09spring.html

Zamosky, L. Obamacare's most vexing questions. *Medical Economics.* Retrieved from http://medicaleconomics.modernmedicine.com/ medical-economics/news/obamacares-most-vexing-questions-physicians

Resources

American Academy of Nurse Practitioners
www.aanp.org
National Alliance of NPs
325 Pennsylvania Ave. SE
Washington, DC 20003
(202) 675-6350
American College of Nurse Practitioners
www.acnpweb.org
American Nurses Association
www.nursingworld.org
Healthy People 2020
www.healthypeople.gov/hp2020/objectives/topicareas.aspx

National Organization of Nurse Practitioner Faculties
www.nonpf.com
Web site for NPs
www.webnp.net
National League for Nursing
www.nln.org
NP Central
www.npcentral.net
End of Life Nursing Education Consortium Project (ELNEC)
www.aacn.nche.edu/elnec

The Business of Advanced Practice

Marcella M. Rutherford, PhD, MBA, RN | Chapter **22**

■ INTRODUCTION

Although there is a great deal of dialogue related to the state of the U.S. health-care system, the one thing that everyone agrees on is the need for reform. Too many people are not getting the health care they need—both in quantity and quality. The cost of health care for identical health services varies greatly from state to state. At this time, the path to reform is found in the Patient Protection and Affordable Care Act (PPACA), commonly referred to as the Affordable Care Act (ACA) or "Obamacare," signed into law by President Obama on March 23, 2010. This legislation is focused on expanding coverage, controlling health-care spending, and improving health-care delivery. As health care is being reformed, advanced practice registered nurses (APRNs) have a unique opportunity to be part of the restructuring of the U.S. health-care system. In a system that is looking at cost and quality, APRNs are well positioned to be integral in lowering costs and improving the quality of care. APRNs' costs of care are approximately half of those of the internist and a quarter of costs related to a specialty physician (Porter & Lee, 2013).

To be effective leaders in health care, APRNs need to be knowledgeable about all aspects of the business of health care. APRNs will need the ability to communicate their unique value to the community, to other members of the health-care team, and to the payers. Health care is moving from fee-for-service and toward a performance-based/value-based reimbursement model. In this change-driven environment, providers will need a value agenda that focuses on maximizing the health of their patients.

APRNs have a unique opportunity in this evolving health-care environment. APRNs work in both rural and urban areas and are trained to provide care in various settings, including community health-care centers, public health departments, hospitals and hospital clinics, school/college student health clinics, employee health settings, physician offices, independent medical offices, insurance organizations, rehabilitation and skilled nursing facilities, hospices, home health agencies, the armed forces, Veterans Administration facilities, and schools of nursing. Health-care change has shifted health-care services to the outpatient setting when possible and is moving the primary focus from sick care to wellness care.

This shift fits well with the holistic, social justice focus that is at the heart of all four APRN roles—nurse anesthetist, clinical nurse specialist, nurse midwife, and nurse practitioner. This chapter will focus primarily on the business factors in health-care delivery that affect the role of the nurse practitioner (NP). The PPACA will increase the role NPs play in Accountable Care Organizations and in the medical home. With the growing shortage of primary-care physicians and the rising number of previously uninsured people gaining coverage (15 million through 2014 and increasing to 35 million by 2016), the United States will need more practitioners (Iglehart, 2013).

To be effective advocates for health-care reform and to be successful as industry decision-makers, NPs need business skills. This chapter offers an overview of the current U.S. health-care environment, a review of third-party payers, the basics of PPACA, essentials of business practices, current reimbursement rules, tips for measuring and communicating value, and information for managing a health-care practice. In addition, NP business skills, NP professional choices, and the need for strategic planning are covered. Each section will provide key elements that affect the ability of a practitioner to thrive and achieve professional goals.

■ OVERVIEW OF TODAY'S U.S. HEALTH-CARE ENVIRONMENT

Today's health-care practitioner faces a health-care system in flux. The only sure thing in health-care reform is that it will be reformed. The cost of health care continued to increase despite several decades of aggressive incremental reimbursement policy change initiatives. Both political parties agreed that a new strategy was needed. According to the Kaiser Family Foundation (2012), the health-care portion of the U.S. economy increased from 7.2% in 1970 to 17.9% in 2010. Policy experts attribute a significant portion of the spending to medical technology. In the fall of 2013, there was good news from the government's actuaries, finding total national health spending was growing at the lowest rate ever seen. In August 2013, employer insurance premium increases were averaging just 4% for family policies, whereas in previous years costs commonly increased by 10% to 15% (Altman, 2013). Some of this slowdown in health-care costs can be attributed to the

2008 recession (patients not seeking health services as readily), but some of the slowdown is arguably attributable to the PPACA. In 2010, this bill was signed into law and included "new limits on how much insurance companies can charge for administration and profits (with rebates to consumers if they charge too much), and state review of rates proposed by insurance companies" (Altman, 2013, paragraph 3).

Whether the PPACA is harming or helping the U.S. health-care system is being debated. It is important, however, for all providers to know the main features of the bill that include the following:

- New federal insurance market rules that establish essential standard benefit packages included in all plans
- New health insurance exchanges that will lower administrative costs, pool risk, and offer individuals and small businesses a choice of affordable plans
- A shared responsibility for health care by preserving employer-sponsored insurance and offering tax credits to small businesses
- Improvement of Medicare prescription drug benefits by slowly eliminating the "donut-hole" gap by 2020
- A long-term financing program to support the disabled
- Investment in a stronger primary care foundation by increasing Centers for Medicare and Medicaid Services (CMS) payment for primary care, encouraging patient-centered medical homes, investing in primary-care training, and expanding community health centers
- An innovation center within CMS using payment methods to reward for quality versus volume of services; this innovation also encourages payment based on patient outcomes and provides incentives for productivity
- The creation of an Independent Payment Advisory Board that will make recommendations to reduce cost growth and improve quality
- Investment in the infrastructure that will offer publicly reported information on the quality, costs, and performance of providers; use of information technology in medical care and health insurance carriers; and policies on disease prevention, public health, quality, safety, and the health-care workforce (Goldsteen & Goldsteen, 2013, p. 260)

NPs are poised to gain a prominent role in the implementation of PPACA. Practitioners will be needed in primary care, pediatrics, and obstetrics to offer services to the large numbers of individuals who will gain coverage for health-care services.

■ THIRD-PARTY PAYER RULES

Whether NPs are employed by a hospital or a medical practice or are self-employed, the reimbursement policies that pay their wages will be determined by a third-party payer. Third-party payers fall into seven general categories:

- Medicare
- Medicaid
- Indemnity insurance companies
- Managed care organizations (MCOs)
- Workers' compensation (WC)
- Veterans Administration (VA)
- Auto liability

In addition to these third-party payers, those patients without health insurance are considered private pay.

Each payer has its own policies and fee schedules. All utilize Medicare guidelines as their foundation and make adjustments based on their plan goals. The Centers for Medicare and Medicaid Services (CMS) is the federal agency that administers and provides oversight of both agencies. In 1977, CMS policy gave billing approval for nonphysician practitioners, including NPs. Some payers credential NPs and reimburse them similar to physician billing. Other carriers may either pay NPs based on unique billing rules or may have no specialty for NP billing, instructing NPs to bill under the physician's provider number.

Medicare

Health-care providers wishing to bill the Medicare program can join the program by filling out an application on the Internet-based Provider Enrollment Chain and Ownership System (PECOS) or a using the traditional paper form (CMS-855). Each Medicare provider is assigned a provider number and a unique physician identifying number (UPIN) for billing. As a Medicare provider, the NP agrees to perform services for payment according to the current Medicare physician fee and guidelines. The NP's scope of practice, prescriptive authority, and requirement of physician collaboration are designated by the state legislation. The state gives authority for the nurse licensing board to regulate APRNs.

CMS policy payment is based on yearly published physician and nonphysician provider fee schedules (Medicare Physician Fee Schedule [MPFS]) (CMS, 2013g). For physicians, CMS identifies what services will cost (100% of the physician MPFS) and then stipulates that 80% of the allowed rate will be paid by CMS and 20% is the responsibility of the patient. NPs are reimbursed by CMS at 85% of the physician's fee, with the patient still paying a 20% share. Most patients on the traditional Medicare plan also acquire a secondary insurance plan to cover the 20% patient out-of-pocket expense. In addition to the 20% patient responsibility, Medicare has a yearly deductible. In 2014, the Medicare Part A (hospital services) deductible is $1,216 for each benefit period and the Medicare B (physician/provider, outpatient service) deductible is $147 per year. Information on Medicare beneficiary out-of-pocket expenses can be found at www.medicare.gov/your-medicare-costs/costs-at-a-glance/costs-at-glance.html (CMS, 2013d).

Patient responsibility payment (co-pay and deductible) should be collected in the beginning of the calendar year. These fees, if not precollected, will remain the patient's payment responsibility. Patient billing increases the expense to the practice because of the cost and time involved in collecting funds at a later date. Patients with a Medicare health maintenance organization (Medicare Advantage) plan follow the rules of the commercial carrier. Providers are required by Medicare to make an effort to collect the patient responsibility for services.

Medicare Advantage Plans

Medicare Advantage plans (an umbrella plan under an MCO) must be approved by CMS to become an alternative carrier for Medicare beneficiaries. These plans offer all of the benefits of Medicare and usually offer additional benefits and lower co-payments. Medicare Advantage carriers are paid subsidies by CMS for services rendered by the plan per member. These carriers market their ability to offer traditional CMS service in addition to added health services at a lower cost due to business strategies and economic efficiencies based on their volume of commercial business relationships. Problems have been noted when these plans have not been able to deliver services with greater efficiency than Medicare. Because of the high medical utilization and costs associated in the care of these patients, it became less financially desirable for commercial carriers to offer Medicare Advantage plans. If the plan's payout exceeds the fixed CMS payment, the Medicare Advantage plan incurs a loss.

"Opting Out" Providers

All providers have the option to elect to be a "nonparticipating" provider or to "opt out" of the Medicare program. As a nonparticipating physician, the practitioner can set his or her charge rate at 115% of the Medicare rate but can collect only 95% of the Medicare fee (CMS, 2013f). The Medicare program will pay 75% of the MPFS and the patient must pay the remaining 20% of the allowed (fee) amount, resulting in a 95% payment of the standard CMS fee to the opting-out provider. These physicians, however, are not subject to all of the billing restrictions set by CMS. The physician can elect to be in the Medicare program only one time per year and must provide notice to patients and referring physicians if he or she elects to become nonparticipating.

Patients also must be informed of the physician's status before services are rendered. "Opting out" of the Medicare program limits the ability of participating physicians to utilize referral services. No participating Medicare physicians can refer to physicians who have opted out of the Medicare program. The "opting-out" physician must keep a minimum of $250,000 available at all times to cover any malpractice claims that may arise from health services. An NP working for an "opting-out" physician will not be able to bill for Medicare services. NPs that are employed by or leased by an "opting-out"

physician are at a higher risk for being named in a malpractice case.

Medicaid

Medicaid offers medical assistance for individuals and families with low incomes and resources. Unlike Medicare, it was designed to be jointly funded by both federal and state governments. The federal government assists states in providing medical care to people who meet the program's financial eligibility criteria. Medicaid payments are made directly to the participating providers, who in turn must accept the Medicaid (lower) payment as payment-in-full. Two exceptions are (1) disproportionate share hospital payments (hospitals taking care of a high, disproportionate share of Medicaid-eligible patients) and (2) hospice care.

Under Medicaid, states may impose nominal coinsurance and deductible rates. Emergency and family planning services must be exempt from the co-payment responsibility. The federal contribution matches the individual states' contribution as mandated by law. Reimbursement rates must remain sufficient to enlist enough providers willing to perform services and ensure that medical care is available to the general population in the region.

Guidelines for the Medicaid plan are available at the Medicaid Web site (http://medicaid.gov). Benefits for Medicaid were expanded and enhanced by PPACA and are outlined at http://medicaid.gov/AffordableCareAct/affordable-Care-Act.html (CMS, 2013). There are limitations and criteria for APRN reimbursable services outlined in each state's guidelines that can be located by selecting each state on the Web site.

Other Insurance Plans

Auto liability, workers' compensation, and CHAMPVA (see www.va.gov/hac/forbeneficiaries/champva/champva.asp) are additional health plans. It is important that these plan responsibilities are identified at the time of service (e.g., auto accident injury, injury sustained while on the job, services provided to a veteran, etc.). All of these plans have provisions, billing criteria, and reporting criteria. For auto liability, it is important to identify whether the auto insurance or medical insurance should be billed. When a Medicare patient, for example, receives care that should be paid by his or her auto liability plan, payment will be denied for medical services billed to Medicare. Workers' compensation (WC) claims require notification to the person's employer, use of WC-contracted providers for care, and specific documentation for coverage that must be submitted to the plan. Traditionally these plans limit use of NPs for care delivery, but this should not deter a practitioner from seeking provider status.

Cash/Private Pay

Even with PPACA, there will still remain approximately 20 million people in America who are without health insurance, and many of these individuals will not be

U.S. citizens. Patients who delay seeking health care often enter the health-care system in acute need of care and require higher cost treatment. Despite the fact that the United States invests more than twice the resources in health care as other industrialized nations, it ranks 37th based on health-care outcomes (infant mortality, life expectancy, etc.) compared with the other nations (Roehr, 2008). The nation's return on investment for health care would cause any banker to look for alternative projects!

PPACA

At the core of PPACA are provisions to enhance the outcomes and value of the U.S. health-care system. PPACA legislation is changing the way clinicians are organized and how health care is delivered; it is also focused on reducing cost while improving the quality of services. Because of this law, approximately 60% of the uninsured will gain access to health care. Through PPACA, health-care delivery teams, comprised of both clinicians and nonclinicians, communicate and work together toward the goal of returning the patient to optimum health.

PPACA provisions are detailed at www.HealthCare.gov, a federal Web site managed by the U.S. Department of Health and Human Services. Highlights of the consumer benefits in the bill include the following:

- Consumer assistance programs
- Preventive care
- Children's preexisting conditions coverage
- Preexisting condition cannot affect coverage
- Young adult coverage (under age 26 years can get coverage on parent's plan)
- Affordable insurance exchange plan options
- Small business employees able to purchase insurance from consumer operated and oriented plans (CO-OP).
- Lifetime limits on health plans banned
- Insurance rate increases limited to 10% per year, unless justified
- Provisions for adults aged 65 years or older—preventable care offered with no cost sharing
- Medicare drug discounts—eliminating the "donut hole" by 2020 and offering cost relief starting in 2010

Physician and public support for this legislation remains mixed, with about 50% of the public questioning the benefits of the system. In the autumn of 2013, citizens who had high co-pay and high-deductible plans began getting notices that either their plan premium cost would increase dramatically (plan benefits did not meet the essential standard benefits) or that their plan was being eliminated. These events caused a nationwide negative reaction. In addition, the Web site designed to assist community members to shop for plans on the exchange functioned poorly throughout the month of November 2013. By December, however, the Web site was functioning adequately, and the sign-up period was extended to March 31, 2014.

In addition to the initial problems with enrolling, there are concerns that younger individuals will opt out of health plan coverage. Should this healthy low-risk group decide not to enroll through the exchange or not to sign up for an employer's plan, the financial foundation of this legislation may not be sustainable. For PPACA to work, the younger insured must financially support the older members of society.

PPACA is anticipated to create a surge in patient demand for access to health care. Finding a practitioner will become challenging. The limited number of primary care providers is causing many states to reexamine the scope of practice laws for NPs. NPs are educated to provide primary-care services, but the American Medical Association (AMA) has supported laws that limit NP scope-of-practice, citing concerns for patient safety (Iglehart, 2013). Currently, NPs provide essential primary care; offer disease management; and enhance coordination of care, increase patient care access, and offer high-quality oversight of health care at lower costs. Not only is the MPFS payment for NPs 15% lower than the medical physician's payment, but (as of 2011) the family practitioner's yearly income was approximately $100,000 higher than the average family NP's annual salary (Medical Group Management Association, 2012).

NPs are the largest group of APRNs and function under various degrees of physician supervision depending on the licensing state. Research demonstrates that NPs' primary-care outcomes are equal to or better than physicians' and that NPs gain equal or higher patient satisfaction ratings (National Governors Association, 2012; Newhouse, et al., 2012). The various House and Senate committees involved in implementing PPACA have included NPs as primary providers and acknowledge the shortage of primary-care physicians. In many rural communities and for hospice patients, NPs offer the only access to health care and are critical for reducing health-care costs and meeting the needs of the current underserved citizens. In addition, the Institute of Medicine (IOM) has recommended that nurses be allowed to function to the full scope of their practice. Congress is set to address this issue, but patient demand and need are causing each state to look at this issue as well. Only a few states have fully adopted the APRN Consensus Model, a uniform model supported by the American Nurses Credentialing Center to align licensure, accreditation, and certification in practice. This model must be adopted by all state boards of nursing for implementation planned in 2015. So far, fewer than 20 states allow NPs to practice independently of a physician, based on their training (National Governors Association, 2012).

The PPACA was designed to allow the greatest number of U.S. citizens under age 65 years with employer insurance plans to continue to get insurance coverage as a benefit in their employer benefit package. Employers of more than 50 full-time (working 30 hours or more per week) employees are required to offer the standard

MCO plans. For small businesses (fewer than 50 employees), for employees who work less than 30 hours weekly, and for those not on employer plans, individual plans are available for purchase through state exchanges. The exchange allows citizens to select a plan that meets their financial and health needs. Tax incentives and penalties will be utilized to encourage enrollment. Medicaid eligibility has also been expanded through the Medicaid plan.

The PPACA's goal is to eventually enroll approximately 35 million of the over 50 million U.S. citizens currently without health-care coverage. PPACA legislation eliminates the high deductible, low co-insurance, limited hospital coverage plans of the past. Pharmaceutical costs will be reduced to more affordable rates on PPACA payment formularies. This legislation has changed the health-care game, requiring all MCOs to offer preventive services with no additional cost to beneficiaries. All health plans must now offer the designated minimal benefits, and the beneficiaries can select from a variety of approved plans. Information on the quality of and costs related to the various plans is being disseminated on the Internet. Competition for lower-cost and higher-quality providers and plans will shape health-care reform.

Future reforms for PPACA include the use of telemedicine and other strategies that will offer a competitive advantage for providers. Hospitals and providers are joining Accountable Care Organizations (ACOs) and developing communication networks that will expand their abilities to create efficient teams to treat the full range of patients' health needs. These efficient and effective ACOs will gain higher reimbursements and stimulate carrier and patient demand. Providers who are early adopters will seek out the most talented colleagues to join their ACOs. As a team, this group will focus on offering high-quality, low-cost health care, and the group will financially benefit from this effort. Data reporting and transparency of outcomes will drive health service choices, and those providers who consistently produce desired outcomes at competitive costs will be rewarded.

The use of technology will also offer providers a competitive advantage. Electronic medical records (EMRs) are required and will enhance business practices. EMR utilization will allow improved care communication and care coordination between providers, aligning care offered to patients across the inpatient and outpatient spectrum. NPs' strengths include their holistic approach to patient care, and this technology will enhance their effectiveness in overseeing care delivery.

■ BUSINESS ESSENTIALS

Without adequate funding, providers will be limited in the services and resources they can utilize to support their practice. NPs should understand the importance of maintaining adequate cash flow, obtaining payment for services, overseeing outstanding accounts receivables, implementing a collection policy, controlling overhead costs, utilizing the financial statements, and planning for success by creating and using a realistic operating budget.

Maintaining Cash Flow

Maintaining optimum cash flow is a fundamental goal in all businesses. Without adequate liquid capital, a business will not grow or survive. Today, most health-related services are on a fee schedule determined by a carrier contract. Providers are required to follow the carrier's billing guidelines. A continuous flow of funds is needed to pay for expenses generated in each business cycle.

In today's health-care industry, providers are challenged by payment disbursement interruptions; carrier and patient payments are not guaranteed solely because the service was delivered. Services can be medically indicated and result in healthy outcomes, but if documentation and medical coding do not match approved services' billing guidelines, payment may be initially denied. The number of claims that result in slow payment (greater than 30–45 days) can range between 30% and 50%, and this delay negatively affects provider cash flow.

The profit margin in health care today is very slim. Medicare payment is designed to cover provider costs, and Medicaid payment ranges 15% to 20% lower than Medicare. Net profits for most providers are achieved from the MCOs.

As with any major change in business, PPACA has created a feeling of concern in many providers. Physicians struggle to understand how health-care reform's bundled payment (payment to all providers involved in the complete episode of care) will affect provider cash flow. Bundled payment is designed to cover the services of independent provider units, covering "the full care cycle for acute medical conditions, the overall care for chronic conditions for a defined period of time (usually a year), or primary and preventative care for a defined patient population (healthy children for instance)" (Porter & Lee, 2013, p. 60). Unlike fee-for-service or global capitation, this method aligns payment to care delivery and outcomes under the control of the provider team.

Health-care reform is aimed at bending the cost curve downward; therefore, further cost cutting is predicted and causes concern. Efficiency and quality outcomes will be rewarded in higher reimbursements. Payment models need to include severity adjustments, regional demographic differences, and unavoidable patient complications based on frailty, as well as provisions for unforeseeable high-cost medical events.

Obtaining Payment for Services

All third-party payments are based on the MPFS, referred to as the carriers' "allowed amount" or plan fee schedule. As health-care costs continued to rise, all health-care plans looked for ways to keep insurance payment fees from increasing. Insurance plans implemented higher patient out-of-pocket responsibilities by increasing the deductible and co-payment amounts. In addition, benefits became more limited. Patient out-of-pocket expenses became a larger portion, reducing or not increasing the percent of the medical bill paid by insurance. PPACA has changed this process by eliminating the high deductible, high co-payment plans and stipulating a ceiling of profit that MCOs can realize from unspent premiums. Starting in 2013, overpayments are being refunded annually back to their beneficiaries.

The patient's out-of-pocket responsibility is deducted from the insurance plan's contracted service rate and is reflected on both the insurance plan's statement and the provider's billing; both are provided to the patient beneficiary. For the provider, collecting the patient responsibility for services is a significant portion of accounts receivable. Provider profit margins have also been reducing over the last 10 years. A provider's billing process starts when the patient's demographics are first collected (preadmission or at the time of admission) and continues until the bill is collected. Patients' benefit packages change yearly, and the change in the level of patient responsibility needs to be adjusted by the provider. Because employers change carriers frequently, it is essential that the provider require proof of insurance eligibility at each patient visit. Obtaining patient financial responsibilities creates a collection burden for the provider. Expenses of the practice/organization (accounts payable) are incurred before billing, so if payments are not collected in a timely manner, cash resources to cover payables will become a problem. Slow collection of cash/payment also results in less money to support practice enhancements/resources needed for services. Issues in claims processing that affect cash flow include the following:

- "Unclean" claims—Claims with missing patient demographics, medical coding, and required data elements
- Slow processing of billing records or posting of carrier payment
- Delay or failure to address bill denials and carriers' requests for additional documentation
- Failure to identify underpayments from plan carrier—lower than contract rate
- Changes in software data fields and software interfaces implemented by providers and/or carriers
- Failure to collect patients' responsibility before services

Electronic billing and EMR use reduce labor hours needed for the billing process at both the provider practice and the payer. Reporting tools in the current office software can make billing follow-up more efficient. Providers who ensure that claims are complete, are accurate, and comply with the carrier's guidelines will benefit by timely payment (within 30 days) for the services they provided.

Overseeing Outstanding Accounts Receivables

Accounts receivable (AR) represent the money billed for services rendered to patients that remains unpaid. It is critical that accounts receivable are monitored by financial managers, ensuring that outstanding bills are collected or that changes in payment resulting from new billing requirements and regulations are identified in a timely manner. **The longer money goes uncollected, the less likely it will be collected.** When money goes uncollected beyond 120 days, it is very difficult to obtain payment. Uncollected expected payments (with good practices this remains around 10% of the expected amount) should be kept at the lowest percentage possible.

Accounts more than 30 days old should be reviewed, identifying why the payment has not been received. Hiring knowledgeable coders and offering continuous education to medical billers will be supported by a lower AR. Current and compatible claims software for claim tracking is required, but it is important to select software that enhances provider processes.

Loss of experienced billing employees is a common reason for unanticipated cash-flow delays. Providers need to have a basic understanding of claims-management processes to be able to assist and troubleshoot cash-flow issues and to oversee the training of new billing managers.

Collection Policy

All patients require education as to their payment responsibilities when accessing health-care services. Many patients do not understand their insurance policy benefits and payment responsibility. Patients often feel that they already pay a substantial sum of money in their monthly health premiums and that this should entitle them coverage for needed health services. Co-payments and deductibles are seen as excessive. Explanations of benefits that come after rendered service can cause the patient to become distrustful. In addition, many patients in today's economy are unable to pay the co-payment or deductible portion. Many patients did not pay close attention to the plan benefits when they signed up for the plan. Dedicating employee time to verify and explain eligibility and carrier benefits before treatment is worth the expense. Ensuring patient understanding of payment before services protects the patient–provider relationship.

Controlling Overhead Costs

Increasing practice efficiencies and controlling day-to-day costs enhance a practice's profitability. Implementing cost reduction measures, however, requires careful economic analysis of the impact on the quality of care and on the medical outcomes to patients. If the outcome choices are considered equal, the least costly service should be chosen. Health-care outcomes, however, are often difficult to measure; and, until recently, little emphasis was placed on measuring the cost-effectiveness of care outcomes. Economic analysis should evaluate both the cost benefits and cost-effectiveness of services.

Cost analysis involves understanding the resources/costs needed to provide a service. Direct cost—labor time, supplies, and minor equipment—are easy to identify and should always be evaluated before adding a new service. Indirect costs—administrative, cleaning, electricity, human resources costs, and the like—may be harder to allocate to each service but should be included in the analysis for a valid assessment. In addition, some costs are fixed whereas others are variable—fluctuating with the volume of activity. The office rent or mortgage payment, for example, is a fixed cost; supply expenses (printer paper, record documents, etc.) are variable. To make a profit, payment dollars must cover both direct and indirect expenses related to the services—covering associated variable costs and contributing to fixed expenses.

To maximize financial gain, practitioners and office managers tend to feel that cost shortfalls can be made up with increasing the volume of patients treated. The normal established-patient visit is commonly scheduled as a 15-minute block of time. New patients, however, require more time to gather the patient's history. Established-patient visits are more predictable. Managing scheduling offers some efficiencies to the office; strategies that intermingle established-patient visits between new-patient visits could prevent patient bottlenecks. An appropriate mix of new and established patients is important to ensure a profitable office day.

A nurse practitioner's fee, according to Medicare, is set at 85% of the MPFS. Physician overhead costs commonly hover around 50% of net revenue (CMS, 2013f). An NP's *value* can be linked to the resulting revenue (billed charges) and net revenue (collected payment less expenses associated with the services) generated by the NP. Tables 22.1 and 22.2 provide an example of how to calculate the break-even analysis to demonstrate an NP's impact on practice revenue. Hospital visits, procedures, and other services would need to be added to an estimate. Factors such as the number of new patients, the number of MCO patients (contracted fee rate ranges from 70%–120% of Medicare fees), the length of the visit, the number of private-pay patients, and so forth can affect the profitability of a provider's services. NPs should evaluate their individual patient care practice habits and the impact of these on the overall financial health of the practice.

Utilizing Financial Statements

Financial statements offer a business the ability to monitor the impact of monthly transactions taking place in the practice. The performance of a business can be reviewed using the following accounting reports:

- *Balance Sheet*—Quantify the net worth of the business at a set time (monthly, quarterly, or yearly).
- *Operating or Income Statement*—Compares revenue to expenses in a period of time.
- *Cash-Flow Statement*—Details the movement of cash in and out of the business.
- *Net Income Statement*—Demonstrates whether assets grew as a result of the year's business activities.

An NP should review these documents in order to monitor the health of the company. For example, if the

Table 22.1	Profit/Loss Estimation						
CPT	Vol	% vs	Fee	85%	Overhead	Acct. Receiv.	Collections
99201	69	5%	$43.89	$37.31	$21.95	$1,514.21	$1,362.78
99202	345	25%	$74.51	$63.33	$37.26	$12,852.98	$11,567.68
99203	703.8	51%	$108.91	$92.57	$54.46	$38,325.43	$34,492.89
99204	220.8	16%	$164.67	$139.97	$82.34	$18,179.57	$16,361.61
99205	41.4	3%	$203.80	$173.23	$101.90	$4,218.66	$3,796.79
Total	1380					$75,090.84	**$67,581.75**
99211	0	0%	$20.41	$17.35	$10.21	$—	$—
99212	745.2	18%	$43.89	$37.31	$21.95	$16,353.41	$14,718.07
99213	2484	60%	$72.81	$61.89	$36.41	$90,430.02	$81,387.02
99214	828	20%	$106.83	$90.81	$53.42	$44,227.62	$39,804.86
99215	82.8	2%	$142.90	$121.47	$71.45	$5,916.06	$5,324.45
Total	4140					$156,927.11	$141,234.40
Net Revenue/Yr							$208,816.16

Table 22.2	NP Valuation in the Practice Setting	
NP Cost		
Salary	$95,000	
Benefits	0.27	
Incidental	$1,5000.00	
Total	122,150.00	$(122,150.00)
Practice value		$86,666.16
Assumptions		
Patient visits/day	30	
Productive hours	1,950	
Productive wk/yr	46	
Overhead estimate	50%	
Days/wk	4	
Collection %	90%	

revenue of the company increases dramatically but the costs also increase significantly, the company may not realize additional net profit. These financial statements provide an overview of the company assets, as well as the corresponding liability or debt.

Planning for Success: Using the Operating Budget

Success in business does not just happen; it is a result of research, planning, financial knowledge, and hard work. The rate of rise in health-care costs can be controlled by "developing cost-effective technologies, delivering care in the most cost-effective settings, and using the most cost-effective practice available" (Emanuel, 2008). The APRN role fits well into this prescription for tomorrow's health-care system.

All businesses need direction and boundaries within which sound financial decisions can be made. Budgeting has several very important purposes for those managing a business. Budgets help planning, improve communication, facilitate coordination, improve motivation, help control expenses, and contribute to assessing performance. Budget preparation should involve all members of the business. Gathering all of the anticipated practice needs (expenses) for an upcoming year from all stakeholders will minimize variances to the budget. A successful practitioner sets goals and plans resource needs. The budget projects an estimate of the upcoming year's anticipated revenue and expenses based on obtaining the best information available from all care providers.

■ REIMBURSEMENT RULES

The provider plays an important role in ensuring the success of the business by clearly identifying the diagnosis and service codes that are appropriate for each patient's visit. As a strong business partner, each practitioner who possesses reimbursement knowledge can optimize the billing payment. Specific documentation of key components of care can make a significant difference in the allowed reimbursement.

CPT® Coding (Unlisted Procedures)

Current procedural terminology (CPT®) offers the official procedural coding rules and guidelines required when reporting medical services and procedures performed by physicians and nonphysician practitioners (AMA, 2013). This reference text should be purchased yearly and should be readily available to each practicing provider. Two vendors that publish CPT manuals and other coding references are found on the following Web sites: www.ama-assn.org/ama/pub/category/3113.html and www.ingenix.com. CPT® coding lists and guides are available electronically and can assist in the coding process with algorithms that assist those coding.

In 1977, the Health Care Financing Administration (HCFA) was developed within the Department of Health and Human Services (HHS) to rein in the spiraling costs of health care related to the Medicare program. Originally in 1965, Medicare was the responsibility of the Social Security Administration (SSA). Federal assistance to the Medicaid program was administered by the Social and Rehabilitation Service (SRS). The Department of Health, Education, and Welfare (HEW) oversaw the SSA and SRS. HCFA was created to coordinate Medicare and Medicaid. HCFA was challenged with controlling costs, monitoring services, and updating code references used to uniformly document current care. These codes facilitated assigning descriptors to service delivery as well as assigning reimbursement rates for each service code. HCFA (later to be overseen by CMS) selected CPT® codes developed by the Editorial Board of the American Medical Association. Medicare utilized these codes at an increasing rate in the 1980s. By the early 1990s, commercial insurance carriers (MCOs) were using these codes in their contracts and billing records as well. The Resource-Based Relative-Value Scale (RBRVS) was authorized by Congress to be used to set reimbursement rates (Hsiao, 1987). Today the federal agency is referred to as CMS. This RBRVS scale is discussed later in the chapter.

CPT® Coding Rules

Beginning in the 1990s, physicians were paid for office or surgical procedures based on calculated resource costs, which are designed to reflect the costs needed to provide services. These costs were calculated based on three components:

- The physician's work or medical expertise—makes up approximately 54% of relative value unit (RVU).
- The practice overhead expenses—making up approximately 41% of the RVU.
- Professional liability and malpractice expenses—derived from a formula.

This RVU is multiplied by a conversion factor, which is a monetary value determined yearly by HCFA/CMS and is adjusted for the cost of living/market-basket rates in the geographical region. RVUs are assigned by CMS based on recommendations from the Relative-Value Update Committee of the AMA. Each specialty society in AMA presents detail work and practice expenses to CMS when new CPT® codes or fee rates are requested to be changed. These details are published in the Federal Register before finalization, allowing provider and user comments.

According to the AMA, the purpose of CPT® is to provide a uniform language that describes medical, surgical, and diagnostic services, providing an effective means for reliable nationwide data collection and communications among all stakeholders. In 2000, the CPT® Code Set was designated by the HHS as the national coding standard for physician and other health-care professional services and procedures under the Health Insurance Portability and Accountability Act (HIPAA). Having a common nomenclature allows uniformity in management reporting, medical review, education, outcome measurement, and medical research. CPT® is the accepted nomenclature utilized by all health-care facilities, providers, and vendors. Each service or procedure is represented by a five-digit code. CPT® code inclusion or exclusion does not indicate an endorsement by AMA of the procedure, nor does it indicate that payment will be made.

As of 2005, all CMS billing was required to be sent electronically, unless certain exceptions were granted. The CPT® code set was mandated for all billing records. To improve cash flow and minimize claim denials based on untimely submission, most providers benefit from electronic billing to insurance carriers.

The CPT® manual and Medicare Physician Fee Schedule (MPFS) are published once a year. There are three levels of CPT® codes:

1. Category I—Codes used in contemporary medical practice
2. Category II—Tracking codes used for new or performance measurement
3. Category III—Temporary coding used for new procedures, technology, and services

Yearly code updates are made available in October and implemented in January. Codes without an associated payment fee are commonly related to patient education and nursing services. Transition periods are often extended with reimbursement change.

The CPT® manual Category I codes are presented in six sections:

1. Evaluation and Management
2. Anesthesiology
3. Surgery
4. Radiology
5. Pathology
6. Medicine

CPT® Unlisted Codes

Practitioners should select the code that provides the most specific and accurate match to the services performed. If no code exists that accurately identifies the provided services, an "unlisted" service code is provided in each of the six sections of CPT®. Unlisted codes are discussed later in this chapter.

CPT® Modifiers and Add-on Codes

Specific guidelines for CPT coding are presented at the beginning of each section in the text and should be reviewed before selecting a code. "*Add-on codes*" are at times indicated and should accompany a primary procedure code. Examples of add-on codes for CPTs include "prolonged service" codes that indicate additional time spent with the patient. These codes should never be used alone and must be used with the appropriate primary or level of evaluation and management (E&M) code. A *modifier* provides a means to report that a service or procedure has been altered by the circumstances of its use. It is important that modifiers be used appropriately because proper use may be associated with additional reimbursement. Modifiers are the only means for the practitioner to adjust standard payment rules. Box 22.1 provides an example of the use of modifiers to document services in order to receive the full payment of the proper use of modifiers.

The CPT® and payment fee values are applicable only to CMS services and are regulated and paid by the regional CMS carriers. MCOs can independently determine whether to utilize certain CPT® code rules and/or the reimbursement values for the payment year.

New CPT® Requests

It is important that practitioners participate in and provide CPT® information directly or submit feedback through professional organizations. The CPT® manual

Box 22.1   Modifier Use for Payment

Separately Identifiable Service on the Same Day as an E&M: Modifier 25

A previously treated patient is referred to a gynecological specialist's office following abnormal Pap test results. The patient's pathology is reviewed, and a vaginal exam is performed. From the examination, it is determined that a colposcopy procedure is warranted. The colposcopy procedure is performed on the same day as the evaluation and management (E&M) examination by the same physician. The practitioner will bill a 99213 for an established-patient visit of expanded focused complexity and add a -25 modifier to the CPT code in the bill record. The colposcopy is also billed on the same day of service and was ordered as a result of the E&M findings. Without the -25 modifier on the CPT code, the E&M visit would not be paid.

provides instructions on requesting updates to the CPT® nomenclature. The effectiveness and accuracy of CPT® relies on its ability to reflect actual practice; therefore, practitioners should communicate changes in practice and request coding changes that match provided services. As profit margins shrink, accurate coding becomes essential to maximizing the viability of the business. When requesting a new code, the practitioner should provide supportive information from research articles and medical journals, specific cost information related to the uniqueness of the code, and a specific recommendation concerning the new or existing codes. Suggestions should be submitted to the CPT® Editorial Research and Development of the American Medical Association. Code changes can also be submitted online at the AMA/CPT Web site: www.ama-assn .org/ama/pub/physician-resources/solutions-managing-your-practice/coding-billing-insurance/cpt.page under the area "Applying for CPT® codes."

"Incident To"

"Incident to a physician's professional service" is a billing phrase related to services furnished under the direct supervision of a physician. This does not mean that the physician needs to be in the room, but he or she must be in the same suite or office. The services are related to the course of treatment resulting from an initial visit with the physician and administered by a nonphysician. The nonphysician (often a registered nurses or NP) must be an employee of, or leased by, or performing as an independent contractor of the physician. In this situation, services may be billed under the physician's provider number, obtaining 100% of the physician fee (CMS, 2013f). RNs can provide service "incident to" a physician, but this service is billed under the physician's provider number and is paid at 100% of the contract rate.

NPs may also deliver services "incident to" and generate billing and payment at 100% of the contract rate using the physician's UPIN provider number. CMS provider rules offer guidance under "incident to" billing for services provided under the following circumstances:

- Considered physicians' services when furnished by an allopathic or osteopathic physician
- Performed by a person who meets the definition of an NP
- Not otherwise excluded from coverage by law
- Performed in collaboration with a physician
- State law allows NPs to perform the services

NPs may bill and be reimbursed using their own UPIN when a physician is not on site or in the office. These services, in comparison, are reimbursed at 85% of the MPFS.

Collaboration

Federal law defines the term *collaboration* to mean the following:

A process in which a nurse practitioner works with a physician to deliver health-care services within the scope of the practitioner's professional expertise, with medical direction and appropriate supervision as provided for in jointly developed guidelines or other mechanisms as defined by the law of the State in which the services are performed. 42 U.S.C.S. § 1395x(aa)(6) (Buppert, 2012, p. 154).

The Balanced Budget Act of 1997 approved reimbursement to APRNs for Medicare patients, but it did not alter the language in the law. Some states do not require collaboration whereas others do, and when the term *collaboration* is used, the definition above applies. Regulations vary by state, and collaboration requirements (no collaboration, collaborative relationship, or collaboration with a submitted written protocol) should be verified annually. With PPACA and the IOM report, states are being pressured to allow nurses to practice at their full scope of knowledge.

CPT® Level II Codes

Each year, CMS releases its Healthcare Common Procedure Coding System (HCPCS) code set in the HCPCS Annual Update. The 2014 code set is available on the following Web site: www.cms.gov/Medicare/Coding/HCPCSReleaseCodeSets/Alpha-Numeric-HCPCS.html. HCPCS codes are established by CMS's Alpha-Numeric Editorial Panel and represent primarily items and supplies and nonphysician services not covered by CPT® Level I coding. Drug administration, pharmaceuticals, and durable medical equipment supplies are located in this file. As stated in the previous section, new CPT® codes are often assigned an HCPCS II code and are tracked for a year before a permanent CPT® level code is identified. Demonstration codes used for data collection are also assigned an alphanumeric code. Payment may or may not be associated with these codes, but they are important for data tracking.

ICD-9-CM Codes

CMS and the National Center for Health Statistics (NCHS), two departments within the federal government, provide guidelines for coding and reporting using the International Classification of Diseases, 9th Revision, Clinical Modification (ICD-9-CM), which can be located at www.cdc.gov/nchs/icd/icd9cm.htm or through the vendor Ingenix (Ingenix, 2013). These guidelines have been approved by the AHA, the American Health Information Management Association (AHIMA), CMS, and NCHS. These guidelines are required under HIPAA for all health-care settings. Volumes 1 and 2 are used by all providers, and Volume 3 codes are used exclusively by hospitals for procedural reporting. These codes communicate the diagnosis of the patient's visit or care episode. These codes ensure that consistent and required documentation related to the reasons for care is noted in the medical record. ICD-9-CM coding is used by all insurance carriers to support the services provided in the encounter.

The health-care practitioner is legally accountable for indicating the patient's diagnosis. CMS and many commercial carriers have implemented medical policies that allow computer editing that verifies that the CPT and ICD-9-CM code match. For example, a chest x-ray exam will not be paid as a preoperative screening test unless the patient has a diagnosis indicating respiratory symptoms.

ICD-10-CM

The federal agency NCHS is responsible for and has been challenged with the implementation of a revised ICD-10-CM that will replace ICD-9-CM Volumes 1 and 2. This version was originally presented for a comment period in December 1997. After 60 days, this version of the ICD-10-CM was removed from the NCHS homepage. A new draft version has been available for public viewing since 2003, and the AHA and the AHIMA are conducting joint testing. After this extended testing period, ICD-10-CM has a planned implementation date of October 2014. Many countries have already been using these code sets for several years. This new coding set will extend the number of available codes from 13,600 to over 69,000, adding detail and specificity to current billing and data coding. This change in diagnosis code options will make a significant practice and documentation change for all practitioners. A free Web reference available to providers on this coding can be found at www.icd10data.com. Educational tools and manuals can also be accessed at the CMS Web site: www.cms.gov/Medicare/coding/ICD10/downloads/pcs_refman.pdf.

Providers need to prepare their billing, practice management, and electronic health record vendor for this change and must be sure to verify when all contracted payers are prepared to accept these new codes. In addition, providers and staff will need to be trained on this new coding. Practices should anticipate additional costs associated with the transition to this new data documentation, as well as an initial reduction in productivity.

Medicare Physician and Nonphysician Practitioner Fee Schedule

Each year CMS publishes the *Physician and Non-Physician Practitioner Fee Schedule,* and more information can be accessed at www.cms.gov/apps/physician-fee-schedule/overview.aspx (CMS, 2013b). An MPFS search tool is available at this site.

Electronic billing and automated electronic filing sets have made the implementation of timely transitions to the new MPFS rate possible. This schedule provides a payment rate based on a state local base rate multiplied by the RBRVS, explained earlier in this chapter. The MPFS is the payment rate for all Medicare services provided for that year. When procedures occur that have no CPT, the new code will be paid as a percentage of charge (managed care plans) or at a rate similar to the most

similar CPT code. Unlisted codes are provided in every CPT section; but payment for these nonspecific codes may be delayed, requiring the provider to send medical documentation to detail the services provided. Manual billing, with the supporting documentation to substantiate services, delays payment beyond 45 to 60 days.

MCO plans negotiate contracts with providers based on payment at a percentage of charge or at a percentage of the Medicare fee. Carriers may pay some specialists higher than Medicare does but also can offer fees lower than Medicare rates. In many states, primary-care physicians and internists are paid at a percentage lower than Medicare. General practitioners' and internists' practice volume, or payer mix, is composed of a high percentage of MCO-insured patients. To maintain their patient volume, internists are often financially pressured to sign contracts at rates lower than the MPFS or risk losing a large number of clients. This atmosphere has created an environment where providers are competing for well clients covered by better-paying carriers.

Accountable Care Organizations

Collusion—secretly and collectively sharing rates for the purpose of monopolizing or maintaining a higher payment rate—is prohibited by physician specialties. In addition, MCOs market their plans to employers and clients by demonstrating the large network availability. Periodic trends have surfaced with providers joining various ownership arrangements in order to facilitate fee negotiations, offering MCOs a large number of providers that have a substantial patient base. These large practice groups are often successful in negotiating higher commercial fee schedules. After PPACA became law, this large provider group business model has been rejuvenated in the form of Accountable Care Organizations (ACOs).

ACOs are groups of providers—providers, hospitals, outpatient-care facilities—that come together to coordinate the care of patients. The concept was developed by CMS, and additional information can be found at www.cms.gov/Medicare/Medicare-Fee-for-Service-Payment/ACO/index.html (CMS, 2013e). ACOs are an important part of PPACA success and support the CMS focus of providing care to patients based at both the lowest cost and the highest quality. ACO members work together as a team, and all benefit from the efficiencies and quality of care they can collectively achieve. These low-cost, high-quality provider groups will receiver higher bundled reimbursement shared by the ACO. ACO participation is optional for any provider.

In a geographical area where provider networks are not robust, the MCO provider fee schedule may be higher than the MPFS in an effort to attract specialists in the geographical area. MCOs often bundle CPT® services (e.g., multiple CPT® codes billed on the same day may result in only one CPT® fee paid), so contract rates can be misleading and should be analyzed closely. MCO denials and contract language such as "claims will be paid according to the company's claim processing guidelines" forewarn the provider and allow the carrier to adjust its payment fee. MCO fee schedules should be reviewed yearly to evaluate if the payment fees are updated to the current MPFS (the basis for the MCO's fee rate).

Evaluation and Management Documentation

The encounter form or record is the tool that prompts the clinician to provide proper documentation needed to support billing. Coding not only supports billing but also provides invaluable data, identifies patient trends, and offers data that can help a provider plan for future community needs. These CPT® evaluation and management (E&M) codes require providers to document the extent and complexity of the patient's history, physical exam, and medical decision making. E&M codes relate to the recorded facts, findings, and provider observations and offer a consistent data record for each patient by the carrier.

The level of E&M coding (99201–99205 for new patients and 99211–99215 for established patients) is based on the documentation in the medical record. This documentation provides the following data:

- Reason for consultation
- History of the present illness
- Review of body systems (number of systems involved)
- Physical examination
- Recommendation(s) for testing and treatment

E&M codes differ based on the care setting: hospital inpatient, hospital observation day, hospital outpatient, physician office, and so on. The intensity of care needed in these various settings is provided in the documentation for these E&M codes. The practitioner may also bill using consultation codes. When performing a consultation, the provider is required to document and communicate findings to the referring physician. A consulting provider offers a medical opinion based on the patient findings. Documentation is often requested by the carrier to justify the level of care provided and billed. All practitioners should develop documentation forms/software records that contain the key elements of information for medical record documentation. Table 22.3 offers a chart audit tool that can be used to review the correct assignment of the level codes.

Electronic Medical Record

Electronic medical records (EMRs) are required by all providers in 2014, and penalties will be assessed in 2015 to late adopters. The American Recovery and Reinvestment Act legislation was designed to create a means to store patient medical records and make "meaningful use" of these data. Funding and incentives were made available for providers for several years before the 2014 deadline. In 2015, penalties ranging from 1% to 5% will be levied (Athenahealth, 2012). The importance of all

providers using EMRs is based on the principles of securing patient information and reducing administrative health-care costs. Standardizing EMRs and billing data will also improve provider cash flow, allowing carriers to process claims more efficiently and reduce health-care costs.

EMRs offer the following benefits:

1. Providing a record that can be networked across secure provider systems, providing a longitudinal account of patient care.
2. Developing an information system that allows tracking of care from the acute-care setting to nursing home, retirement home, or clients' private residences.
3. Moving away from an emphasis on episodes of care and toward measurement of care across all settings.
4. Facilitating patient identification that allows providers to track the patient throughout the care delivery system, offering information in a need-to-know environment.

The EMR can offer a system that would store complete documentation across the continuum of providers, collect accurate health data, provide practitioner alerts and reminders, communicate up-to-date resources, link evidence-based bodies of knowledge used for clinical decision support, present real-time cost-effective options, enhance timely reimbursement through interconnectivity to payers offering patient eligibility and authorization requirements, provide accurate identification of patient-to-medication match, present a clean and accurate electronic bill, and electronically transmit payment to providers.

■ VALUE MEASUREMENT

Practitioners should review common policies implemented to control and support practice decision making that falls under fraud and abuse/compliance plans, HIPAA, risk management, and performance improvement. In addition, all providers will benefit from data collection that allows them to demonstrate the value and quality of their performance. A plethora of data and quality indicators are now being generated from health-care delivery practices. To be useful, these data require careful review and analysis. Strategies related to information management, in which nurses are crucial participants, include integration of the electronic health record into all care settings; developing rapid online access to patient records, including information from other clinicians in alternate settings; participating in the creation of a repository of health information and nurse quality indicators; interacting and utilizing online information services, including telemedicine; and use of various technology for health planning and scheduling. In addition, being good stewards of health-care technology should stimulate providers to use the least costly, less invasive technology, if it produces comparable diagnosis and treatment.

Table 22.3	E&M Chart Audit Tool			
CPT	Focus	Elements		
New	*Visits*	*History*	*Exam*	*Medical Decision*
99201	New Patient, Level 1	HPI 1—3 Elements ROS: N/A PFSH: N/A	Single-system: 1–5 Multisystem: 1–5	Straightforward
99202	New Patient, Level 2	HPI: 1–3 Elements ROS: 1 PFSH: N/A	Single-system: 6+ Multisystem: 6+	Straightforward
99203	New Patient, Level 3	HPI: 4+ Elements ROS: 2–9 PFSH: 1	Single-system: 12 Multisystem: 12/2+ organ or 2 from 6 systems	Low complexity
99204	New Patient, Level 4	HPI: 4+ Elements ROS: 10 PFSH: – 3	Single-system: all +1 from each system Multisystem: 2+ organs from 9 systems	Moderate complexity
99205	New Patient, Level 5	HPI: 4+ Elements ROS: 10 PFSH: – 3	Single-system: all +1 from each system Multisystem: 2 from 9 systems	High complexity
Established Visits				
99211	Established Patient, Level 1	Minimal/RN visit	Minimal exam	None
99212	Established Patient, Level 2	HPI: 1–3 Elements ROS: N/A PFSH: N/A	Single system: 1–5 Multisystem: 1–5	Straightforward
99213	Established Patient, Level 3	HPI: 1–3 Elements ROS: 1 PFSH: N/A	Single system: 6+ Multisystem: 6+	Low complexity
99214	Established Patient, Level 4	HPI: 4+ Elements ROS: 2–9 PFSH: 1	Single system: 12	Moderate complexity
99215	Established Patient, Level 5	HPI: 4+ Elements ROS: 10 PFSH: 3	Multisystem: 12/2+ organ or 2 from 9 systems Single system: all +1 from each system Multisystem: 2 elements from 9 systems	High complexity

Note: NEW PATIENTS need all 3 criteria: History, Exam, and Medical Decision, whereas ESTABLISHED PATIENTS require 2 out of 3 criteria (History, Exam, and Medical Decision).

Abbreviations: HPI, history of present illness; ROS, review of systems; PFSH, past, family, and social history.

Fraud and Abuse/Compliance Plans

As health care has evolved and become more sophisticated, the area of health-care ethics has grown. Ethical conflicts arise when providers balance competing pressures affected by professional values, changes in delivery systems, and financial regulations. An example of this is the investigations that the U.S. Department of Justice has pursued when dealing with Medicare fraud allegations. U.S. health-care fraud is estimated to cost $80 billion annually and has caused the federal government to levy high fines and determine the need for whistleblower protection.

The health-care industry has not always been honest about its billing practices, and in response Medicare requires audits of a certain percentage of charts or medical records to prove that the charges are accurate and the proper diagnosis and procedure codes were used. Examples of health-care fraud include up-coding reimbursement claims, billing for medically unnecessary therapy, and billing Medicare and insurance carriers for physician services provided by the nurse practitioner. As of 1996, to willfully and knowingly utilize deceptive billing is a legal violation. The False Claims Act was updated in 2006. Reckless disregard for the rules is auditable and subject to corrective audits and fines. Fines and damages can be levied up to three times the claim amount, with mandatory penalties of $5,000 to $10,000 per claim (CMS, 2009). Tables 22.1 and 22.2 show typical audit forms.

Compliance Plan

All health-care businesses should develop a compliance plan. A compliance officer should be identified and can assist in developing and maintaining an established plan that includes practice safeguards, preventing episodes of fraud and abuse. Antikickback efforts, conflict of interest disclosure, and identification of questionable business practices should be fostered. Adhering to a compliance plan is the responsibility of all employees to ensure that business practices discourage fraud and abuse. One area that needs oversight is the correct assignment of E&M level codes based on history taking, examination, and medical decision making.

HIPAA

HIPAA can mean different policy concerns to different people. The act was separated into two parts, Title I and Title II:

- Title I of the Health Insurance Portability and Accountability Act of 1996 (HIPAA) protects health insurance coverage for workers and their families when they change or lose their jobs.
- Title II addresses administrative simplification and requires the U.S. Department of Health and Human Services to establish national standards for electronic health-care transactions and national identifiers for providers, health plans, and employers. It also addresses the security and privacy of health data. These standards were implemented to improve the efficiency and effectiveness of the nation's health-care system by encouraging the widespread use of electronic data interchange in health care (CMS, 2005).

HIPAA legislation is important to the daily management of the practitioner practice setting. This legislation focuses on password management, workstation security, e-mail and Internet use, and facility/physical security. Password protection is emphasized to ensure the privacy of patients' health-care information. With increased mandatory submission of electronic billing files and EMRs, a provider must take added precautions to protect the patient's electronic personal information.

Risk Management

Risk management is an extension of performance improvement. This program should be organization-wide, with a focus on identifying risks, controlling occurrences,

preventing damage, and controlling legal liability. The goal of risk management is to prevent any undesirable event from happening and to minimize the impact of financial loss due to a malpractice claim. There are eight areas of responsibility for risk management programs:

1. Risk identification
2. Loss prevention and reduction, including incident reports and investigations
3. Insurance claims management
4. Administration of workers' compensation and handling of medical/legal issues
5. Liability assessment of contracts
6. Risk management education
7. Handling product recall and Safe Medical Device Act issues
8. Ensuring compliance with accreditation standards and state and federal laws

Practitioners can be involved with any of the aforementioned areas of risk management. With the rising number and cost of malpractice claims, risk management becomes a powerful tool to demonstrate that prudent care is monitored to ensure appropriate health-care practices.

HEDIS Reporting

Providers should be aware of performance reporting that is required by CMS. The Health-Plan Employer Data and Information Set (HEDIS) is a set of standardized performance measures identified as indicators for consumers so that they can evaluate the quality and cost aspects of the care delivery. Indicators are selected based on current health issues such as cancer, diabetes, asthma, heart disease, and so on, monitoring such indicators as immunization age, mammography frequency, urinary tract infection occurrence, cervical cancer screening, and the like. HEDIS is supported and overseen by the National Committee of Quality Assurance.

Safety and Performance Improvement

Performance improvement initiatives should be part of the day-to-day routine of the medical practice. In some medical offices, the NP is the only professional nursing caregiver. The practitioner should take the lead to encourage office personnel to undertake processes that focus on ongoing improvement. Data analysis of quality monitoring requires the ability to derive trends from statistical data. Once a negative trend is identified, a corrective action plan to address the trend is imperative, demonstrating and monitoring a successful turnaround and improvement.

Both medical and financial errors are not rare, occurring at a rate greater than acceptable to the public and medical community. According to the IOM (2000) study, *To Err Is Human,* a high number of medical errors were identified in the U.S. medical environment, but it took almost 7 years for comprehensive safety and quality outcome changes to be noted throughout the health-care system. Today's health-care leaders are being challenged to decrease errors. The task of reviewing existing medical practices using a systems approach is daunting; however, the benefits are worthwhile.

Other issues that affect the quality of a health-care practice involve actions where the patient feels deperson-alized, perceptions of shorter care delivery time, unwar-ranted denial of coverage, health-care choice restrictions, and overprescribing of unwarranted testing. Many health plans' policy regulations and benefit restrictions have been linked to an increase in malpractice liability claims. Maintaining and fostering a trusted relationship between the provider and the patient has a significant impact on patient participation in care, satisfaction with outcome, timely payment of bill responsibility, and limiting expo-sure to litigation.

APRNs play a valuable role in diligently overseeing health-care outcome improvement efforts, demonstrat-ing accountability in practice. Clinicians are highly val-ued for their ability to recognize familiar patterns and to use their gut instincts in times of complexity, identifying options for interventions (Kerfoot, 2004). A practitioner must not only think through a diagnostic clinical prob-lem, but also provide input on the economic impact of the care delivered in this clinical episode, offering valu-able analysis of the outcome data that are collected from the patients.

Pay for Performance

Stimulated by quality initiatives and the desire to ensure public accountability and public disclosure, the Bush ad-ministration through the Deficit Reduction Act of 2005 required a quality adjustment in the Medicare diagnosis-related group payment for certain hospital-acquired con-ditions. In 2006, CMS identified 19 quality indicators that providers were financially incentivized to track and document. These conditions were identified as resulting in high-volume, high-cost areas of medical care. In 2007, CMS announced a new program called "Hospital-Acquired Conditions (Present on Admission Indicators Reporting) (HACs not POA)" (CMS, 2013b). This new CMS policy was a dramatic payment rule change for Medicare. In 2013, 11 HACs not POA were identified as high-volume preventable patient occurrences and were tracked in all hospitals. The 11 conditions are available at www.cms.gov/Medicare/Medicare-Fee-for-Service-Payment/HospitalAcqCond/Hospital-Acquired_Conditions.html (CMS, 2013b). These HACs not POA result in a decrease in reimbursement from CMS; payment does not cover the costs related to the HAC. Hospitals across the nation have implemented care criteria—often called bundles—aimed at ensuring that these HACs would not occur. CMS undertook this effort because its responsibility required it to safeguard the Medicare Trust Fund by not paying federal monies for preventable medical errors.

Section 3025 of the Affordable Care Act added Section 1886(q) to the Social Security Act establishing the Hos-pital Readmissions Reduction Program, which requires CMS to reduce payments to Inpatient Prospective Pay-ment System (IPPS) hospitals with excess readmissions, effective for discharges beginning on October 1, 2012 (CMS, 2013e). Currently, the policy does the following:

1. Defines *readmissions* as admissions within 30 days to the same or other hospital
2. Includes readmission diagnoses of acute myocardial infarction, heart failure, and pneumonia
3. Establishes a method to calculate the excessive read-mission ratio for each condition and compares it to the ratio of the national hospital data set; uses this to determine the adjustment to the reimbursement rate
4. Establishes a risk adjustment methodology for each diagnosis using National Quality Forum (NQF) data, comparing each facility's readmission ratio to other similar facilities in the United States and adjusting the ratio for clinically relevant factors (demographics, patient frailty, etc.)

Provider Comparison Web Sites

Many states have created Web sites for citizens to query data regarding these identified health outcomes, allowing citizens to compare individual providers and hospitals using common quality indicators. Transparency is being fostered, and providers and payers are being evaluated based on malpractice claims and health outcomes. Finan-cial reward, therefore, is granted to medical providers with quality results. PPACA's legislation includes initiatives to educate the public on both the costs and the quality of their health-care needs and choices. These comparison re-porting sources are designed to create competition, but they also offer providers an opportunity to recapture the trust of the community.

Value-Based Purchasing

The term *value-based purchasing* (VBP) was emphasized as an important initiative of CMS (2013c). This initiative has grown with PPACA. Data collection efforts are pervasive in both the medical and nursing professions. Over 1,000 nursing quality measures are used in hospitals, and many of the quality indicators are directly related to nursing care. Provider quality measures are also focused on indicating value outcomes related to a health-care experience. On August 1, 2013, CMS announced the display of the fiscal year (FY) 2014 IPPS Final Rule, which included a number of policies related to the Hospital VBP Program. In FY 2014, the second year for VBP provider incentives, CMS finalized payment and operational details. CMS also final-ized new policies for FY 2016 that included (1) new VBP measures, (2) performance periods, (3) performance stan-dards, and (4) domain weighting.

The final rule also included policies related to certain measures for FY 2017 through FY 2019, including performance periods and performance standards for those program years, as well as a new domain structure for FY 2017 based on the National Quality Strategy and its priorities of better patient outcomes, quality, safety, and lower cost for Medicare payments (CMS, 2013d).

National Committee for Quality Assurance

The National Committee for Quality Assurance (NCQA) is a nonprofit organization focused on improving the quality of health care by working with providers to foster identifying, measuring, analyzing, and promoting health-care quality. The NCQA seal displayed by a health care facility is a well-known symbol, displayed proudly by a facility and identifying it as well managed and delivering quality health services. NCQA providers must undergo a rigorous review process and submit data annually to maintain the NCQA status (NCQA, 2013). NCQA has developed over 60 standards and requires practices to measure and report annually on over 40 of them.

Medicare's Physician Quality Reporting System

Medicare's Physician Quality Reporting System (PQRS) is a CMS payment incentive program based on reporting provider performance data. Eligible Medicare providers (EP) are identified from their claims and the data provided on quality measures. Beginning in 2015, data will be extracted from EP claims.

■ MANAGING A HEALTH-CARE BUSINESS

The information highway is changing practitioner–client relationships (Bowman-Hayes, 2009). NPs' strengths have always resided primarily in their clinical expertise and their holistic approach to patient care; as a patient advocate, an NP encourages patient independence and offers needed health-care diagnostic and treatment services and self-care teaching. Today's practitioner is also challenged to assist patients as they navigate the Web, coordinate care between networks of providers, and explain information retrieved from a variety of sources. More and more patients are using Internet resources for guidance once medical symptoms arise. NPs need to support patients who do not have access to a computer. Soon those patients will be experiencing knowledge deficits, as well as health-care access deficits.

NP Business Choices

Selecting a business arrangement that offers a practice environment beneficial for NP goals has the greatest prospect for professional success. Business arrangements and clinical expectations should be clearly communicated by all partners and the team of practitioners. Negotiations should include a frank discussion of salary, benefits, hospital privileges, and on-call expectations. In addition, the NP should understand the inherent malpractice risks with the selected specialty and what arrangements are in place to mitigate these risks.

Negotiating Salaries and Benefits

Before signing an agreement with a practice site, the NP should draft a practice agreement as required by the state in which he or she wishes to practice. Each state has detailed criteria defining the level of collaboration that is required between the NP and an oversight physician, if required. Prescriptive authority, still an issue between the AMA and nursing, may require process changes that should be discussed.

The practice specialty, colleague(s) personality, practice environment, patient population, and the current style in the practice setting should be reviewed. Dialogue should be initiated on the degree of autonomy and role of the NP and the other practitioners. Topics to cover during a formal interview with the practitioner include the following:

- Are there any current or pending malpractice claims against the business?
- What is the practice's Medicare and Medicaid status?
- Will I have hospital privileges?
- What number and type of managed care contracts does the practice have? How do these carriers contract and reimburse NP services?
- What is the number of nurses (registered nurses [RNs] and licensed practical nurses [LPNs]/licensed vocational nurses [LVNs]) and support staff available to assist the NP?
- What expectations are there for my net revenue generation?
- What is the expected number of patient visits per day?
- How will I be compensated for services?

There are four base methods by which an NP can negotiate payment:

1. Straight salary
2. Salary based on percentage of payments
3. Salary plus a percentage (bonus) based on payments
4. Hourly rate

There are positives and negatives to each method.
Straight salary is the easiest method of payment. The practitioner is paid a set amount weekly, biweekly, or monthly; the income stream is easily calculated. If the hours or work increase dramatically, however—that is, on-call time, rounds, discharge summaries, dictation, and so forth—there is no additional compensation.

Salary based on a *percentage of payments* is based on an inconsistent dollar amount used to predict and calculate income. A practitioner's salary is calculated on the percentage of payments collected the prior month. Many factors can affect net payment, and the payments collected are often not within the practitioner's control. For example, the type of computer system, number of billing staff, content of managed care contracts, changes in referral sources, and so forth can all create dramatic changes in the cash flow. This payment method has the largest possibility for error and fluctuation.

The *salary plus percentage (bonus)* based on payments allows the practitioner to profit from a higher volume of patients encountered and longer work hours needed to provide service for patients seeking care. This method, however, must be set at a predetermined rate that is achievable. In this method, the practitioner would be paid a set amount weekly, biweekly, or monthly; and, when the payments generated by the practitioner reach a predetermined milestone, additional bonus payments would be provided. In this payment method, the NP should make sure the base salary is adequate to meet the NP's financial commitments.

The last method of payment—*hourly payment*—is a well-understood payment method, and it is similar to how hospital employees and nurses have historically been paid. In this method the practitioner provides time records with the hours worked for payroll payment. This method allows for fluctuations in patient flow and changes in job responsibilities. It also requires the nurse to essentially punch a time card or report hours worked, reducing the level of autonomy the practitioner has in the business.

Employment Benefits

When interviewing for a position, the practitioner should make a list of benefits that are necessary and those that are desired. The benefits that fall into the must-have category usually include health, dental, short-term disability, malpractice, and life insurance; paid vacation time; a retirement plan or 401K; and paid sick time. On-call pay may be seen as a benefit if this allows NPs to enhance their salary based on their availability. Desirable benefits include long-term disability insurance, education allowance, car/parking allowance, investment options, professional meetings reimbursement, and so forth. Each practitioner should survey other NPs to verify the standard benefits packages noted in the area. The NP should fully research all aspects of the practice and communicate needs and wants in writing. Negotiating requested salary and benefits can be supported by the revenue an NP can estimate generating for the practice.

Obtaining Hospital Privileges

All hospitals have credentialing approval processes that require the practitioner to submit and validate his or her educational preparation, licensing, certifications, and clinical competencies. Credentialing usually falls under the allied health validation process established by The Joint Commission and the medical staff hospital bylaws. Practitioners can obtain a copy of the hospital's rules and regulations and familiarize themselves with these regulations, ensuring all guidelines of the facility are achievable.

Practice Insurance

Insurance policies are critical for every business, allowing each business to meet the state's requirements for incorporation. The practitioner should be aware of the insurances needed for all businesses. Some insurance plans are required to obtain the tax identification number (TIN or EIN), and these must be obtained in order to apply for a city, state, and county business license. Table 22.4 provides an overview of optional and mandatory insurance plans selected to protect businesses.

Practice liability insurance provides risk protection for an employer and practitioner against unforeseen events. As an owner, practitioner, or administrative employee of the business, liability value of the practice (capital equipment and resources in the business) should be reviewed annually. As the practice grows and changes, these policies must remain current and reflect the worth of the current equipment and property owned by the practice. For example, significant growth in computers and software in the practice should be added to the practice liability policy, because these resources significantly increase the value of the practice.

A business expense that requires additional consideration includes workers' compensation (WC) insurance. WC insurance coverage has become very expensive over the last decade. With one or two employee claims in the fiscal year, WC coverage and available premiums may become limited and very costly. High-risk businesses may be forced to seek plans through the Joint Underwriting Association, often described as the state's providers of last resort. WC premiums may be high enough to affect the financial health of a business. All practitioners should be aware of the practice policies and make sure employee

Table 22.4	Corporation Insurance Plans
Type of Plan	**Coverage**
Workers' compensation	Medical expenses resulting from on-the-job injury, illness, and death
Unemployment insurance	State and federal coverage; provides payment for loss of employment
Liability insurance insurance	Covers structure, furniture, equipment in the event of a disaster
Business interruption	Covers loss of payments/income in the event of a disaster
Employee fidelity bonds	Verifies employee honesty and deters theft
Life insurance	Many types and should be investigated; covers practitioners
Disability insurance	Risk of disability greater than death and creates financial hardship
Malpractice insurance	Protects practitioner in the event of lawsuit

screenings (protective measures against practice risk) are included in policy, such as drug screening, background verification, and employment screening. Yearly employee education is essential and should include workplace safety processes. Employee actions that deviate from these processes or safety directions should receive documented counseling to protect the practice from avoidable claims.

Malpractice insurance has become a concern and a hotly discussed medical practice expense. Malpractice premiums have doubled and tripled for physicians and NPs over the last few years. The numbers of frivolous lawsuits are increasing, and practitioners are at risk, working in an environment that appears to encourage patients to seek litigation when care outcomes are not as expected or to their liking. Certain physician specialties are more highly litigated, and these specialties have the alternative to "go bare." This option requires the practitioners to declare they will meet the minimum patient compensation payment requirements of the state and to demonstrate an ability to meet liability claims up to a payment limit. Practitioners without malpractice coverage create a concern that the risk will be borne by all those providers required to maintain malpractice insurance—that is, hospitals, hospital-based practitioners, and practitioners who have not opted to "go bare." NPs need to be aware of this business practice, ensuring that they do not end up as the sole insured provider of the business.

If the provider desires to carry insurance protection, he or she should purchase the highest amount of coverage affordable. The ideal coverage is an occurrence policy for $1 million per claim and $3 million in aggregate coverage. Because failure to have proper coverage can be catastrophic, or at least very expensive, it makes good sense to understand the product being purchased and the exposures that are not covered. Several states require that practitioners carry malpractice insurance or post a bond. When investigating choices in malpractice insurance plans, the practitioner should review and compare several different carriers for limits of coverage, whether the policy covers the business and employees, extent of coverage for legal costs, how long the insurance company has been in existence, and the differences between claims-made policies and occurrence policies. The rates can vary greatly, and the stability of each carrier should be examined. It is important to calculate the price of tail coverage when shopping policies and understand the definition of disability for automatic tail provisions. *Tail coverage* is an insurance policy that insures the healthcare providers for malpractice claims reported after a claims-made policy lapses. The status of the malpractice crisis for practitioners will affect how practitioners practice in the future.

Business Planning and Strategies

To compete in the business of health care, practitioners must plan and develop business strategies. Creating a business plan that fits the practice will guide, maintain,

develop, and manage the company. This information should be used to market the efforts of the company to future patients.

A business strategic plan helps the business get organized and provides a roadmap for measureable success. This plan should be developed to guide current and future growth of the business. The business plan will support the needs for funding and will allow lenders to assess the risk involved in investing. It is important that the practitioner review the practice's financial statements. Strategies for business success should be identified, and data sources that will allow the plan to measure success at meeting these goals should be identified. Table 22.5 provides items to include in the business plan.

Table 22.5	Business Plan
Inclusions	Description
Company objectives	Summary of company key ideas
Executive summary	Company leadership and objectives
History of the company	Idea that started the company
Company goals	Short- and long-term goals, as well as identifying the customer • Strengths • Opportunities for growth
Management team	Background and responsibilities of the managers
Vision/mission statement	Unique aspects of your service
Capital and operating expenses	Costs of doing business
Value indicators	Quality measures
Marketing strategy	Convincing lenders and contributors of potential for the business • Analysis of competitors • Demand • Access • Advertisement and promotion
Research and practice evidence	Processes for submission, collection, and reporting
Financial projections	Balance sheet, income statements, cash flow, and units of service
Business risk	Risk management initiatives and monitoring
Change strategy	Benchmarks used to indicate success and failure

Marketing Plan

PPACA will affect the demand for NPs. NPs, however, are traditionally poor at marketing their services to the public and media. Nurse practitioners tend to share their successes and inroads with those within the profession using nursing journals, conferences, and word of mouth communication between colleagues. Consumers, the media, and the general public have been largely overlooked as targets of the NP marketing message.

NPs should identify marketing strategies and then measure the impact of these efforts. First, practitioners can explore opportunities that will inform patients and the public on the role and value of the NP. Print material distributed to patients can offer clarification and differences in roles, as well as highlight educational and practice experiences. Second, practitioners may reach out to the media. Practitioners can seek out local news and broadcasting media that specialize in health. Third, practitioners should share the news regarding faculty, new offices, public health issues, and so forth. This important health outcome data regarding their practice outcomes should be shared with local media via press releases. Fourth, practitioners can make themselves available to news media for commentary and interviews. Fifth, all practitioners should be able to articulate the cost savings they bring to health care. With the health-care industry's increasing need to reduce the costs of health delivery, NPs have an opportunity to establish their role as a leader in the health-care team. Table 22.6 provides a listing of common policies and procedures that guide business managers and employees.

■ CONCLUSION

With the 2014 expansion of health coverage through PPACA legislation, one question looms on the minds of all stakeholders: How will the nation cope with the surge of new patients and their demand for health services? There is already a shortage of primary-care physicians, creating a workforce issue. In addition, the population is growing, as is the percentage of individuals over 65 years of age. Health-care reform will be implemented over the next decade across the United States and will face many challenges. NPs have an opportunity to move past historical limitations and to restructure the delivery system, innovating and taking on tasks that allow them to practice according to their training and to lead this period of change.

NPs who develop a professional vision, articulate their value to the community, demonstrate flexibility, and provide innovative means to create a successful business are needed in today's and tomorrow's health-care system. Knowledge of the financial aspects of health care will be required for NPs to participate in health-care policy

Table 22.6	Common Policies and Procedures
• Hours of practice
• Utilization of space and resources
• Forms and collection of patient information
• Collect co-payments and deductibles at the time of the visit
• Verify eligibility and patient coverage before treatment, on carrier Web site
• Implement frequent billing cycle (e.g., every 15 days)
• Accept credit cards for co-payments and deductible
• Establish payment plans for patients not able to pay in full
• Collecting money, posting money, and depositing money should be handled by different employees
• Verify that billers make daily bank deposits and that receipts are matched daily to the posted payments of that day
• Protect the confidentiality and storage of patient records
• Hazardous waste
• Credentialing of all providers
• Hiring and firing of employees is in accordance with state laws
• Risk management education
• Occupational Safety and Health Administration (OSHA) compliance and HIPAA documentation
• External regulator reporting requirements
• Pharmaceuticals and resources needed for practice
• Quality assurance and effectiveness monitoring
• Compliance forms and yearly verification
• Emergency plans
• Employee education plan
• Equipment monitoring
• Provide general liability for the practice
• Develop a plan for malpractice coverage for all providers
• Business and facility security
• Volunteer policy
• Advertisement and marketing

decisions. Today's practitioners will need knowledge that enhances their ability to analyze and report data that show the quality of their services, that highlight efficiencies related to costs, and that demonstrate their role in increasing access to care for all patients. Clinical and economic expertise will enhance the value-drivers for the profession. Basic business skills will support planning, innovation, and implementation of process changes. NPs are ideally trained to deliver low-cost health care while ensuring that the highest quality is not sacrificed for efficiency. As stakeholders, NPs should play an essential role in overseeing health-care change and ensuring the viability of the health-care system.

References

Altman, D. Obamacare may be holding down costs. September 27, 2013. Retrieved from http://kff.org/health-reform perspective/how-obamacare-may-be-holding-down-costs

American Medical Association. *Current procedural terminology, CPT® 2013.* Standard Edition. American Medical Association, Chicago, 2013.

Athenahealth. Whitepaper: Making a smooth transition: Avoiding the top 5 risks of the ICD 10 conversion. May 2012. Retrieved from www.athenahealth.com/_doc/pdf/whitepapers/ICD-10_Preparing_Your_Practice.pdf

Bowman-Hayes, J. The role of the informatics nurse specialist. *Association of Perioperative Nurses Journal (AORN)* 90(6):922-924, 2009.

Buppert, C. *Nurse practitioner's business practice and legal guide,* ed 4. Jones & Bartlett Learning, Sudbury, MA, 2012.

Centers for Medicare and Medicaid Services. Health Insurance Portability and Accountability Act (HIPAA). 2005. Retrieved from www.cms.hhs.gov/hipaa

Centers for Medicare and Medicaid Services. False Claims Act. 2009. Retrieved from www.coms.hhs.gov/smdl/downloads/SMDO32207Att2.pdf

Centers for Medicare and Medicaid Services. Affordable Care Act. 2013a. Retrieved from http://medicaid.gov/AffordableCareAct/Affordable-Care-Act.html

Centers for Medicare and Medicaid Services. Hospital-acquired conditions. 2013b. Retrieved from www.cms.gov/Medicare/Medicare-Fee-for-Service-Payment/HospitalAcqCond/Hospital-Acquired_Conditions.html

Centers for Medicare and Medicaid Services. Hospital value-based purchasing. 2013c. Retrieved from www.cms.gov/Medicare/Quality-Initiatives-Patient-Assessment-Instruments/hospital-value-based-purchasing/index.html

Centers for Medicare and Medicaid Services. Medicare costs at a glance. 2013d. Retrieved from www.medicare.gov/your-medicare-costs/costs-at-a-glance/costs-at-glance.html

Centers for Medicare and Medicaid Services. Readmission reduction program. 2013e. Retrieved from www.cms.gov/Medicare/Medicare-Fee-for-Service-Payment/AcuteInpatientPPS/Readmissions-Reduction-Program.htm

Centers for Medicare and Medicaid Services. Medicare benefit policy manual. 2013f. Retrieved from https://www.cms.gov/Regulations-and-Guidance/Guidance/Manuals/downloads/bp102c15.pdf

Centers for Medicare and Medicaid Services. Year 2013 Medicare Part B physician and non-physician practitioner fee schedule. 2013g. Retrieved from www.cms.gov/Medicare/Medicare-Fee-for-Service-Payment/PhysicianFeeSched/index.html

Emanuel, E. *Healthcare guaranteed: A simple, secure solution for America.* Perseus Books, Philadelphia, 2008.

Goldsteen, RL, and Goldsteen, KR. *Jonas' introduction to the U.S. healthcare system,* ed 7. Springer, New York, 2013.

Hsiao, WC. The Resource-Based Relative Value Scale: An option for physician payment. *Inquiry* 24(4):360–361, 1987.

Iglehart, JK. Expanding the role of advanced nurse practitioners—Risks and rewards. *N Engl J Med* 368(20):1935–1941, 2013.

Ingenix. *International Classification of Diseases ICD-9-CM standard for hospitals, Volumes 1, 2 & 3.* Ingenix, Chicago, 2013.

Institute of Medicine. *To err is human: Building a safer health system.* 2000. Retrieved from www.iom.edu/iom/iomhome.nsf

Kaiser Family Foundation. Health care costs: A primer. May 1, 2012. Retrieved from http://kff.org/health-costs/report/health-care-costs-a-primer

Kerfoot, K. On leadership: Learning or intuition?—Less college and more kindergarten: The leader's challenge. *Nurs Econ* 21(5):253–255, 2004.

Medical Group Management Association. *Physician compensation and production survey: 2012 report based on 2011 data.* Englewood, CO, 2012.

National Committee for Quality Assurance. About NCQA. 2013. Retrieved from www.ncqa.org/tabid/675/Default.aspx

National Governors Association. The role of nurse practitioners in meeting increasing demand for primary care. 2012. Retrieved from www.na.org/center

Newhouse, RP, et al. Policy implications for optimizing advanced practice registered nurse use nationally. *Policy, Politics, & Nursing Practice, 13,* 2: 81–89, 2012.

Porter, ME, and Lee, TH. Providers must lead the way in making value the overarching goal. *Harvard Business Review,* October 2013. Retrieved from www.acmha.org/content/summit/2014/Strategy_Fix_Healthcare.pdf

Roehr, B. Healthcare in U.S. ranks lowest among developed countries. *BMJ* 337(1):a889, 2008.

Bibliography

American Medical Association. *Healthcare common procedural coding.* HCPC 2014. Level II. Saunders Elsevier, Philadelphia, 2010. Retrieved from www.cms.gov/Medicare/Coding/HCPCSReleaseCodeSets/Alpha-Numeric-HCPCS.html

Buppert, C. Capturing reimbursement for advanced practice nurse services in acute and critical care: Legal and business considerations. *AACN Clin Issues Adv Pract Acute Crit Care* 16(1):23–35, 2005.

Centers for Medicare and Medicaid Services. *ARNP/PA/CNS guidelines.* (First Coast Service Options, Inc.) Medicare Education and Training, Jacksonville, FL, 2005.

Centers for Medicare and Medicaid Services. *Year 2005 Medicare Part B physician and non-physician practitioner fee schedule.* First Coast Service Options, Inc., Jacksonville, FL, 2005.

Centers for Medicare and Medicaid Services. A brief summary. Retrieved from www.cms.hhs.gov/publication/overview-medicare-medicaid

Centers for Medicare and Medicaid Services. The official U.S. government site of Medicare. 2013. Retrieved from www.medicare.gov/forms-help-and-resources/report-fraud-and-abuse/fraud-and-abuse.html

Centers for Medicare and Medicaid Services. ICD-10-PCS reference manual. Retrieved from www.cms.gov/Medicare/coding/ICD10/downloads/pcs_refman.pdf

ICD10Data.com. The Web's free 2014 ICD-10-CM and ICD-10-PCS medical coding reference. Retrieved from www.icd10data.com

The 15-Minute Hour: Practical Psychotherapy for Primary Care

Brandi Parker Cotton, PMHNP-BC, MSN •
Eliezer Schnall, PhD • Marian Stuart, PhD

Chapter **23**

Contemporary advanced nursing practice presents many challenges, not the least of which is being on the frontlines of health management. Patients present for short office visits with complicated chief complaints, often seeking immediate relief from both physical and mental discomfort. In real-world clinical practice, the distinction between psychiatric and medical illness is often blurry, because mental and physical health interconnect. Specifically, psychological problems are often expressed as physical symptoms, and medical problems frequently precipitate psychological distress. Just as medical illness is usually best treated when detected in an early stage, early intervention is critical for psychological problems. Additionally, the emphasis on behavioral health, self-care, and prevention calls for the inclusion of a behavioral health specialist on primary-care teams.

The majority of psychiatric symptomatology will be managed within the primary-care setting. For example, a study by the World Health Organization sampled 1,500 patients around the world, in cities such as Ankara, Athens, Rio de Janeiro, Shanghai, Bangalore, Seattle, Berlin, and Manchester (Üstün & Sartorius, 1995), and found that 25% of patients met criteria for a psychiatric disorder. A more recent study by Smith et al (2014) indicates the need to modify educational curricula for medical students and residents with increased attention to psychiatric diagnoses and treatment. Noting that 25% of patients in outpatient clinics meet criteria for a *Diagnostic and Statistical Manual of Mental Disorders, Fifth Edition* (DSM-5) diagnosis (more common than hypertension and diabetes combined), the authors argue for improved diagnostics and management of psychiatric symptomatology (Smith et al, 2014).

Considering these statistics, it is unsurprising that patients present for primary-care visits reporting psychological concerns. Besieged by psychosocial stressors, patients seek relief for troubled relationships, stressful life events, recent losses, and economic strain. Although most providers agree that a thorough assessment of these contextual influences is important, the pressures of time-sensitive patient encounters create barriers to comprehensive and person-centered care. Given the significant impact of psychosocial factors on the prognosis of disease, building psychotherapeutic skills is critical for primary-care providers. Techniques such as reflective listening, validating emotions, and encouraging patient empowerment are easily utilizable within short office visits. This chapter highlights the various modalities by which providers can assess and address acute stress and maladaptive responses that predict poorer prognosis of disease states; several therapeutic techniques are suggested for routine implementation during brief patient encounters.

■ STRESS

Stress is the physical and mental response that results from having to adapt to demands from the external and internal environments. When under stress, people generally cope less effectively than when they feel comfortable or pleasantly challenged. Distress is experienced when people's resources are overwhelmed by the constant challenges of life, leading to feelings of loss of control. Our understanding of the relationships among stress, coping, and health has been enhanced by the classic, long-term prospective studies of Vaillant (1979), whose findings suggest the following:

- Overwhelmed people regress functionally.
- Poor adaptation is associated with ill health, because risk of disease increases in those with anxiety, depression, and inadequate stress management.
- Offering support to those under stress may facilitate their return to adaptive function and health.

Given this understanding, health promotion and disease prevention require teaching constructive ways of coping with stress. When people become overwhelmed by the circumstances of their lives, whether due to a cataclysmic event, daily hassles, or even personality characteristics, they often become sick and may visit their primary-care provider. It is thus important to screen effectively for stressors and adopt techniques for providing support.

SOCIAL SUPPORT

Social support is a key element in stress management. When one's perception of control over life circumstances decreases, subjective feelings of stress increase dramatically. However, as social support increases, the stress level decreases. Not surprisingly, it has been shown that poor social support is deleterious to health. Health-care providers are in a position to convey essential social support, by providing positive feedback to the patient or by suggesting strategies for handling a particular problem. When people are psychologically stressed or medically ill, they may be particularly vulnerable to negative feelings, namely inadequacy and isolation. A key benefit of social support is that it augments a person's sense of competence and of connection. By reminding patients about their basic strengths, clinicians enhance patients' abilities to function in a healthy way.

COMMONALITIES AMONG PSYCHOTHERAPEUTIC TECHNIQUES

Practitioners by virtue of professional training and commitment to wellness are uniquely positioned to assist their patients in coping, regardless of the specific nature of the problem. Skillfully employed, this professional therapeutic persona alone can decrease stress and enable patients to cope more effectively. After discussions with a health-care provider about their concerns, patients often feel better and may even be able to solve formerly intractable problems. Many providers feel more comfortable calling this "counseling," but such interactions are essentially psychotherapy. Among the elements common to all major schools of psychotherapy noted by Goldfried and Padawer (1982) are (1) patient expectation of receiving help, (2) participation in a therapeutic relationship, (3) obtaining an external perspective, (4) encouraging corrective experience, and (5) repeated reality testing.

TECHNIQUE: "BATHEING" THE PATIENT

Incorporating appropriate questions and responses regarding a patient's psychosocial situation is an acquired skill. The BATHE technique was developed by Stuart, a psychologist, and Lieberman, a medical doctor, in their work with medical students. The technique has been a staple in Rakel's *Textbook of Family Medicine* since the 1990s and published in book form as *The Fifteen Minute Hour* (Stuart & Leiberman, 2008). It is both a quick screening test and an intervention for psychiatric problems, especially appropriate for new patients and those presenting with acute problems and mental distress. It has become an established method of identifying and addressing psychosocial aspects of patients' problems during a brief office visit. It should be utilized early in the interview, usually after elicitation of the chief complaint and the history of the present illness. BATHE has become a standard of primary care. The acronym, intended to complement the "SOAP" method of medical documentation (see Chapter 4 of this volume, pp. 58–59), stands for Background, Affect, Trouble, Handling, and Empathy. Focus on History 23.1 presents the BATHE technique. Although BATHE is not the only technique a clinician can employ, it brings order and efficiency to what may otherwise become a muddled and time-consuming attempt at psychosocial assessment. In the process, it helps tie the biomedical model to the psychosocial in a way that is meaningful for both practitioner and patient. By asking pointed, focused questions that lend themselves to brief but comprehensive answers, the clinician is able to incorporate this very necessary form of assessment into a format that enhances rapport and also helps the patient express feelings, gain insight into the meaning of the situation, and become empowered. Most significantly, it satisfies all the aforementioned elements of psychotherapy: BATHE provides the expectation of help, a therapeutic relationship, an external perspective, the encouragement of new behavior, and the ongoing opportunity to test reality. The clinician must exercise discipline, however, and refrain from a lengthy exploration of the patient's life. BATHE's therapeutic effect derives simply from its focus on the patient's feelings, the subjective meaning of the situation, assessment of how things are being handled, and empathic demonstration of support.

Focus on History 23.1   The BATHE Technique

- **B**ackground The simple question "What is going on in your life?" determines the context of the patient's visit.
- **A**ffect Questions such as "How does that make you feel?" encourage patients to identify and report their emotional reactions to the circumstances described.
- **T**rouble The question "What troubles you most about this?" helps both practitioner and patient focus on the situation's subjective meaning. Even when the patient's affect is positive, a modified version of this question should be asked: "Is there anything about it that troubles you?"
- **H**andling The answer to "How are you handling that?" helps the practitioner assess the patient's level of functioning, helps the patient connect mind and behavior, and communicates the thought that the patient has indeed taken steps toward handling the situation.
- **E**mpathy The statement "That must be very difficult" legitimizes the patient's reaction. Even when the patient is functioning suboptimally, it is important to reflect back the content of the circumstances and support the patient's attempts at resolution.

The BATHE technique has empirical evidence to support its use in increasing patient satisfaction. In 2008, Leiblum published a study exploring the use of the BATHE technique within the primary-care setting. Four experienced family medicine physicians working in a large urban outpatient office, who were trained in the BATHE technique, took part in a study that explored outcomes relating to patient satisfaction with this brief therapeutic intervention. BATHEd patients were more likely satisfied with the information the physician provided and their perception of physician concern for them and were more likely to recommend their physician to others. More recently in 2011, a study explored the use of the BATHE technique within the perioperative setting at Mount Sinai Medical Center in New York. One hundred surgical patients were randomly enrolled in the BATHE group or the control group. The use of the BATHE technique within this setting suggests that it is both clinically effective and practical: Findings suggest that use of the BATHE method increased patient satisfaction but did not increase the length of the physician evaluation (DeMaria et al, 2011).

Ownership

The BATHE technique helps the provider more fully assess the patient's situation and make therapeutic suggestions so the patient can deal with his or her problem more effectively. This is true whether the problem seems predominantly biomedical or psychosocial, because elements of each are invariably involved in the patient's overall situation. Nonetheless, it is crucial that the provider not assume responsibility for resolution of the patient's situation. The patient continues to "own" his or her problem; however, a more comprehensive understanding of the situation and its effect on the patient allows the provider to assist more effectively. Further, as the patient gains confidence that the provider is supportive and able to help, the element of trust in the therapeutic relationship is enhanced.

Applying the BATHE Technique

Practitioners may worry that application of the BATHE technique may uncover unanticipated issues that cannot be adequately addressed within the allotted time. However, BATHE's evaluative component is a *screening tool,* and the clinician must use judgment as to when and how extensively to explore what has surfaced. Sometimes it is important to say, "I am glad you brought this up. Let me examine you to see if there is some physical problem that we need to be concerned about, and afterward we can talk some more." In most cases, BATHEing the patient will take less than a minute and can help prevent the unexpected and time-consuming patient revelations sometimes held until the end of the visit. The essence of psychotherapy consists of making the patient feel competent and connected, and there are numerous additional and complementary techniques that can help

accomplish this. Many such strategies and examples can be found in Stuart and Lieberman's *The Fifteen Minute Hour* (2008). In most cases, however, just "BATHEing" the patient helps to clarify the situation. Once this is complete, patients should have their feelings validated and be supported in expressing those feelings. They should be provided brief information about the effects of stress along with specific suggestions for stress management and relevant problem-solving. If necessary, the patient should be invited to return and explore the situation further. As always, serious problems necessitate referral to a mental health professional, but the practitioner's role in uncovering important issues is invaluable.

■ THE POSITIVE BATHE

The last decade has seen the emergence of a new mental health subfield called positive psychology. Researchers such as Martin Seligman, Edward Diener, and Christopher Peterson are encouraging psychologists to focus on human virtues, character strengths, and the benefits of happiness and personal growth, rather than the traditional exclusive concentration on the study and treatment of mental illness and disturbance. This is very consistent with nursing's emphasis on health promotion and supporting patients' strengths. An impressive and growing literature links positive affect with health and longevity. Positive thought and emotion is believed to bolster the immune system and has even been associated with better health behaviors. One specific area that has garnered attention is gratitude, a trait associated with a sense of well-being and positive feeling. In fact, investigators have shown empirically that related interventions, such as asking subjects to write gratitude letters or keep gratitude journals, lead to decreased physical and mental health symptoms (Peterson, 2006; Stuart & Lieberman, 2008). In keeping with these themes, a new "Positive BATHE" intervention has been developed to help patients focus on autonomy and personal accomplishment, thankfulness, and general positive affect. Practically, learning this additional BATHE repertoire also allows the provider a second form of intervention, especially useful when interacting with the chronically ill or others who may return frequently for follow-up appointments. In this new version, BATHE is an acronym for **B**est, **A**ccount, **T**hankfulness, **H**appen, and **E**mpowerment. Focus on History 23.2 presents the "Positive BATHE" technique.

■ MOTIVATIONAL INTERVIEWING

Motivational Interviewing (MI) is a therapeutic technique supported by a large volume of research. Employed within a wide array of clinical settings, MI is an empirically validated strategy for assisting patients with behavioral change. Developed by Robert Miller, PhD, as a target therapy for substance abuse, the tenets of MI extend to a wide range of clinical audiences. MI asserts that ambivalence is a normal, nonpathological

Focus on History 23.2   The Positive BATHE Technique

- **B**est Asking patients "What's the best thing that has happened to you lately?" encourages recall of positive events, which likely leads to positive affect.
- **A**ccount When patients reflect on the causes of positive events, they discover what they should do to promote recurrence of these events. Questions such as "How do you account for that?" advance this form of contemplation.
- **T**hankfulness The question "What are you most thankful for?" is aimed at triggering gratitude related to the events mentioned and thereby positive feelings and good health.
- **H**appen Asking "How can you make things like that happen again?" suggests that the patient be proactive in attaining positive experiences. It also challenges patients to put character strengths and adaptive traits to use in their day-to-day interactions.
- **E**mpowerment Enthusiastic and empathic practitioner responses, such as "It sounds like you have a fantastic idea!" and "I am sure you can do it!" empower the patient to take the steps necessary for further success and achievement.

component of the change process. Clinicians assist patients in addressing ambivalence by exploring intrinsic motivation, values, and goals. The basic principles of MI promote respect for individual autonomy and belief that the patient is an expert on his or her own behavior. This is a consistent way of supporting the patient's self-care behaviors and taking responsibility for the patient's own health. MI involves empathetic listening and establishing a nonjudgmental, nonconfrontational patient approach. Collaboration and joint decision making encourage "change talk." Techniques of MI include asking open-ended questions, offering affirmative and supportive statements, reflectively listening, and summarizing the patient's situation. MI also encourages clinicians to request permission before offering advice or interventions. Unsolicited advice is likely to promote resistance. If a patient is not yet ready to change a behavior (e.g., beginning a diet, monitoring glucose, adopting an exercise routine, decreasing substance use), it is unlikely that clinicians' advice will be well received (Miller & Rollnick, 2012, pp. 62–72).

The Four Principles of Motivational Interviewing use the acronym RULE (Rollnick et al, 2007, pp. 7–10):

Resist the righting reflex.
Understand your patient's motivation.
Listen to your patient.
Empower your patient.

An important tenet of MI is the use of reflective listening, a key component in helping patients explore ambivalence and resistance to change. Reflective listening ranges from simple to complex: repeating, rephrasing, paraphrasing, and reflecting feeling. Dialogue is strategic; clinicians guide the conversation with reflective statements, not questions, accepting the patient regardless of her or his readiness for change (Rollnick et al, 2007, pp. 7–10).

Consider the following clinical scenarios.

CASE STUDY 23.1

Martin is a 33-year-old man with a history of heavy alcohol use. He presents to his provider and reports a recent job loss due to excessive tardiness. He reports concern that his family faces eviction for failure to pay rent. Martin then discloses that much of his tardiness was a result of hangovers from heavy drinking. He has voiced concerns in the past, specifically reporting: "My wife nags me about spending too much time with my drinking buddies." He expresses concern that an intensive substance abuse program will be too time-consuming but reports several unsuccessful efforts to remain sober when using the 12-step program Alcoholics Anonymous (AA).

Patient: "I know I can really drink a lot after work. It relaxes me, you know. The job thing is tough—my wife has been pressuring me to get treatment or something. I tried AA but it didn't work. A friend of mine did some intensive thing, but I don't have time for that. How am I supposed to spend eight hours at some treatment facility when I need to be out looking for a job?"

The acronym OARS highlights four important components of MI (Miller & Rollnick, 2012):

Open-ended response:
- "What's this been like for you?"
- "What's most important to you at this point?"

Affirming patient:
- "It can be incredibly difficult to acknowledge these things. The fact that you are here today and talking with me about it shows a commitment to making things better."

Reflecting listening:
- "So the drinking is causing strain. It's also a way for you to relax."
- "You want to find a program that is right for you."

Summarizing for patient:
- "From our last few visits, I know you've been thinking about cutting back on the drinking. It seems like today, after the job loss, you are more concerned than you were at our previous visits. You are thinking about treatment options, but it's really important to you to find a program that is going to fit your lifestyle."

Last, providers should **ASK** permission:
- "Do you want any information about alternative treatments in the area?"

CASE STUDY 23.2

Anna is a 43-year-old woman with a body mass index of 35. She is the mother of two and works as a secretary. Anna is diagnosed with hypercholesterolemia and type 2 diabetes. She consumes a high-calorie diet and maintains a sedentary lifestyle.

Patient: "I know I need to lose weight. I keep planning on walking, but it's so cold now."

Open-ended response:
- "Tell me a little more about your goals in this area."

Affirming patient:
- "Implementing an exercise routine can be really difficult. The fact that you are considering how to make it work for you and your lifestyle is an important step."

Reflecting listening:
- "Sounds like you want to exercise, but outdoor exercise isn't realistic in this weather."

Summarizing for patient:
- "You've been monitoring your weight over the past several months, and it seems like you're feeling discouraged with the results. Winter weather makes it even more challenging for you to meet your goals. You want a plan that's going to work for you."

ASK permission:
- "Several of my patients have had a lot of success with a new program—would you like to hear about it?"

The previous clinical examples illustrate how techniques of MI differ from the traditional approach of encouraging behavioral change. MI is rooted in empathic listening and collaborative decision making. Empiric data support these techniques as an effective strategy for increasing adherence to antivirals in HIV-positive patients, decreasing high-risk behaviors, promoting weight loss, treating eating disorders, increasing physical activity, and addressing domestic violence. The diverse application of MI principles suggests its promising role in promoting positive behavioral changes within a broad range of clinical settings (Miller & Rollnick, 2012).

 DavisPlus | For additional resources please visit
http://davisplus.fadavis.com

SUMMARY

Patients' beliefs, values, perspectives, and health behaviors are situated within a broad social and environmental context. Understanding this context is essential to building and establishing rapport between patient and provider and providing holistic, person-centered care. In spite of considerable time constraints, practitioners adopt therapeutic tools to assist patients in changing maladaptive responses and unhealthful behaviors. Utilizing brief psychotherapeutic modalities, such as BATHE, Positive BATHE, and Motivational Interviewing, can improve both patient satisfaction and health outcomes. The 15-Minute Hour indeed lends itself to positive and meaningful interactions.

References

DeMaria, S, et al. Use of the BATHE method in the preanesthetic clinic visit. *Anesth Analg* 113(5):1020–1026, 2011. doi:10.1213/ANE.0b013e318229497b; 10.1213/ANE.0b013e318229497b

Goldfried, MR, and Padawer, W. Current status and future directions in psychotherapy. In Goldfried, MR (Ed.), *Converging themes in psychotherapy: Trends in psychodynamic, humanistic, and behavioral practice.* Springer, New York, 1982, pp 3–49.

Leiblum, SR, et al. To BATHE or not to BATHE: Patient satisfaction with visits to their family physician. *Fam Med* 40:407–411, 2008.

Miller, WR, and Rollnick, S. *Motivational interviewing: Helping people change,* ed 3. Guilford Press, New York, 2012.

Peterson, C. *A primer in positive psychology.* Oxford University Press, New York, 2006.

Rollnick, S, et al. *Motivational interviewing in health care: Helping patients change behavior (applications of motivational interviewing).* Guilford Press, New York, 2007.

Smith, RC, et al. Addressing mental health issues in primary care: An initial curriculum for medical residents. *Patient Educ Counsel* 94(1):33–42, 2014. doi:http://dx.doi.org/10.1016/j.pec.2013.09.010

Stuart, MR, and Lieberman, JA III. *The fifteen minute hour: Therapeutic talk in primary care.* Radcliffe, Oxford, 2008.

Üstün, TB, and Sartorius, N. *Mental illness in general health care: An international study.* Wiley, New York, 1995.

Vaillant, GE. Natural history of male psychologic health: Effects of mental health on physical health. *N Engl J Med* 301:1249–1254, 1979.

Bibliography

Barnett, E, et al. Motivational interviewing for adolescent substance use: A review of the literature. *Addict Behav* 37(12):1325–1334, 2012.

Bartrop, RW, et al. Depressed lymphocyte function after bereavement. *Lancet* 309:834–836, 1977.

Cobb, S. Social support as a moderator of life stress. *Psychosom Med* 38:300–314, 1976.

Cohen, S, et al. Psychological stress and susceptibility to the common cold. *N Engl J Med* 325:606–612, 1991.

Coyne, JC, et al. Nondetection of depression by primary care physicians reconsidered. *Gen Hosp Psychiatry* 17:3–12, 1995.

House, JS, et al. Social relationships and health. *Science* 241:540–545, 1988.

Leiberman, JA, and Stuart, MA. Practicing biopsychosocial medicine. In Rakel, RE (Ed.), *Textbook of family practice,* ed 6. Saunders, Philadelphia, 2002, pp 65–70.

McCulloch, J, et al. Psychotherapy in primary care: The BATHE technique. *Am Fam Physician* 57:2131–2134, 1998.

Miller, WR, and Rose, GS. Toward a theory of motivational interviewing. *Am Psychol* 64(6):527–537, 2009. doi:10.1037/a0016830; 10.1037/a0016830

Rozanski, A, et al. Impact of psychological factors on the pathogenesis of cardiovascular disease and implications for therapy. *Circulation* 99:2192–2217, 1999.

Spiegel, D, et al. Effect of psychosocial treatment on survival of patients with metastatic breast cancer. *Lancet* 334:888–891, 1989.

Putting Caring into Practice: Caring for Self

Mary Lavin, DNP, FNP-BC • Rebecca Carley, DNP, ANP-BC

The importance of self-care for the clinician cannot be overstated. As advanced practice registered nurse (APRN) students confront the demands of graduate school and, later, beginning practice, they realize the necessity of maintaining balance; work and professional responsibilities, family and home life, coursework and clinical practicums—all demand attention. Self-care and health promotion are major components of caring for patients; it is imperative that nurse practitioners care for themselves as well.

A review of the processes introduced in the *Circle of Caring* model provides a valuable starting point for the discussion of self-care of the APRN and indeed any health-care provider. Caring for others makes it incumbent on us all to care for "self." The goal is to actualize the model by directing health-supporting activities toward oneself first, enabling the practitioner to experience and integrate the value gained from self-care, and to use this strength as a source of replenishment in helping others. This chapter provides an introduction to self-care definitions, enumerates some of the challenges to self-care, and makes suggestions for self-assessment and for practical application of healing strategies in advanced practice nursing and primary-care practice in general.

■ BACKGROUND: CARING AND SELF-CARE

Caring has long been considered the domain of nursing, although many other health-care providers care in their own ways. The *Circle of Caring* model presented in Chapter 1 and developed throughout this textbook helps us to deepen our conceptualization of the ways nursing contributes to the process of healing. This model provides for conceptualization instead of simply skills and techniques, and it expands the traditional medical model. The caring processes include patience, courage, advocacy, authentic presence, commitment, and knowing. Caring is central to the profession of nursing and is at the core of many, if not all, nursing theories.

Caring for others has been the usual focus of nursing, but the need to retain nurses within the profession has fostered a new emphasis on self-care of the nurse. Defining *self-care* is a difficult endeavor because there is no single definition that is broadly accepted in the literature. Godfrey et al (2011) conducted an extensive evaluation

of the concept of self-care by examining in detail the definition of self-care through content analysis of 139 definitions that spanned a time period from 1970 through 2009. Seven components of the definition of self-care were identified. These components were stated as aspects related to the following: health, illness and disability, general outcomes, performer of the self-care, action of the self-care, health-care professionals, and the health-care system. Self-care historically has been represented as a low-quality and ineffectual behavior, but the 2000s brought about a broadening of the term and a new appreciation of the importance of self-care.

Some commonly used definitions illuminate these components.

- The World Health Organization defines self-care as "a deliberate action that individuals, family members, and the community should engage in to maintain good health … Self-care includes all health decisions people make for themselves and their family to become and remain physically and mentally fit such as eating healthy foods, exercising regularly, practicing good hygiene, and avoiding health hazards. People in good health, those who are ill or with disability can engage in self-care … Self-care is the ability of individuals, families, and communities to promote health, prevent disease, and maintain health and to cope with illness and disability with or without the support of a health-care provider" (cited in Godfrey et al, 2011, p. 16).

- Wilkinson and Whitehead defined *self-care* as "not involving a health professional … and the individual independently attains and preserves [his or her] desired level of health. Self-care could be understood as people being responsible for their own health and well-being through staying fit and healthy: physically, mentally, and where desired, spiritually" (2009, p. 1,145).

- The American Holistic Nurses Association (AHNA) Standards of Holistic Practice requires the integration of self-care and personal development activities into one's life. Holistic nurses engage in self-assessment, self-care, and personal development and are aware of being instruments of healing. Holistic nurses value themselves and mobilize the necessary resources to care for themselves. They strive to achieve harmony and balance in their own lives and to assist others to do the same. The AHNA describes self-care practices as self-assessment, meditation, yoga, good nutrition, energy therapies, movement or dance, journaling, and creative expression (art, music).

- Orem defines self-care as comprising those activities performed independently by an individual to promote and maintain well-being throughout life (AHNA, 2014).

Regardless of the definition, many helping disciplines are beginning to focus on the issue of self-care for their members. A keyword search will provide an overabundance of literature around this topic across disciplines such as the following: psychology, social work, medicine, education, and emergency medical services. The impact of stress and trauma on optimal functioning and retention of providers is of growing concern amid the changing health-care environment. Many professional associations have developed and incorporated self-care resources that are available on each association's Web site. For example, the American Nurses Association has recently implemented the Healthy Nurse initiative to address self-care issues among nursing professionals (www.ana.org).

Nurse practitioners care for patients with a wide variety of lifestyles, health-care choices, acute-care illnesses, and chronic health-care conditions. To help their patients maintain optimal health, nurse practitioners frequently discuss and advocate for self-care programs with individuals and families. Modeling healthy lifestyle behaviors is an important aspect of patient support and teaching. By caring for himself or herself effectively, the nurse practitioner will promote self-care in patients.

■ CHALLENGES TO SELF-CARE INHERENT IN ADVANCED PRACTICE NURSING

Self-care is an important strategy for nurse practitioners (NPs) for many reasons. There is a great deal of stress inherent in the NP role in primary care. Recent changes in health care in the United States will also greatly affect the role and increase the consequent stress of the nurse practitioner. *The Future of Nursing* (Institute of Medicine [IOM], 2010) suggests that the future of health care will be greatly influenced by nursing and that nurses and nurse practitioners should be allowed to work to the full extent of their education. The Affordable Care Act of 2010 will increase patient access to care and, therefore, increase demand for primary-care practitioners. The Quality and Safety Education for Nurses competencies also demand that nurse practitioners maintain patient safety standards, utilize evidence-based practice strategies, and implement continuous quality improvement. These are all excellent standards of care and will help to provide and maintain comprehensive care for all individuals. However, the demands of new roles combined with the increasing patient population in primary-care practices will continue to stress primary-care providers.

Additional challenges to nurse practitioners include compliance with insurance regulations and maintenance of certifications, the technology explosion, and societal changes. Insurance regulators have a major impact on the time management of, the reimbursement of, and, consequently, the demand for nurse practitioners, as well as other health-care professionals. Reimbursement rates for nurse practitioners' services are often less than the rates for physician providers who are providing the same care. Primary-care practices provide many services that are not covered by insurance carriers such as the completion of prior authorizations for medications and diagnostic tests, as well as forms required for schools and camps.

The introduction and integration of the electronic health record (EHR) during the past decade has created a challenge for all health-care providers to maintain effective communication with patients during office visits. Although the EHR has major benefits for documentation and continuity of care, there is also an increased time demand for documentation during patient visits. Increased time demands are also generated through the adoption of other technology, such as automated appointment scheduling, Web portals for accessing lab results, and texting patient reminders or encouragement for self-care. Although many of these technologies can enhance patient care, new systems must be implemented for the adoption of these practices. In addition, patients frequently search the Internet for answers to health-care questions. Sometimes this patient-conducted research allows for more informed questions for health-care providers, but it often also contributes to patients' anxiety regarding their symptoms.

Social issues such as joblessness, poverty, immigration of undocumented persons, high costs for medications and other treatments, and the aging population all can adversely affect the health care and self-care of patients. Nurse practitioners in primary care are involved in the management of acutely ill and chronically ill patients whose care needs may be challenging and difficult to deal with emotionally. To further complicate matters, APRNs must also deal with confusion about professional boundaries, particularly in light of the emerging doctorate of nursing practice (DNP) and changes in legislation and reimbursement.

There has also been an increasing demand by the IOM and other organizations for the development of interdisciplinary education and health-care teams. This is an overall positive initiative, but it does bring its own stressors. Other health-care professionals are responding to many of these demands, and there is blurring of some roles as different professionals attempt to remain viable and to expand their roles in health care. The roles and responsibilities of the APRN are also changing to reflect these demands. Some of these transitions in scope of care will need legislative action or changes in rules and regulations within licensing/credentialing bodies.

The changing face of health care dictates the need for flexibility as we approach a new era in health care. APRNs have more opportunity to work independently, yet they experience increased risk of legal action. In addition, APRNs may feel squeezed between the conflicting values and roles of being both nurse and primary-care provider, constantly having to negotiate unique interprofessional relationships with other health-care providers. Nurses want to advocate for their patients in a system that does not always appreciate or, at times, even allow them to do their job appropriately and effectively.

Providing excellent care day in and day out can lead to compassion fatigue and/or burnout for individual nurse practitioners. Several authors describe compassion fatigue and burnout as related but separate concepts (Valent, 2002; Lombardo & Eyre, 2011). *Compassion fatigue* occurs when one cannot rescue or save an individual from harm, and this leads to feelings of guilt and distress. Compassion fatigue appears suddenly and resolves quickly. *Burnout* occurs when one cannot achieve his or her goals and results in "frustration, a sense of loss of control, increased willful efforts, and diminishing morale" (Valent, 2002, p. 27). Burnout arises and declines more slowly, but both burnout and compassion fatigue can have negative consequences for both the provider and the client (Sabo, 2006).

■ THE REASON FOR SELF-CARE MANAGEMENT

All nurses experience varying degrees of stress, compassion fatigue, or burnout at some point in their career. Nurse practitioners are easily able to identify problems within others, but frequently avoid dealing with issues that might affect their own well-being. The most important strategy for nurse practitioners is to identify their stressors before they can affect their well-being and that of their clients. Very often nurse practitioners know that something is wrong but avoid taking the time needed to address the concerns in the middle of a highly packed day.

Focusing on personal and professional shortcomings does not lead to optimal health. Nurse practitioners are often able to understand and accept the deficiencies of others, yet they hold themselves to unattainable standards. Self-compassion is the ability to be compassionate to oneself. Emotional intelligence is the ability of the person to recognize emotions, understand the meaning of the emotions, and realize how the emotions affect other people. Characteristics of emotional intelligence include self-awareness, self-regulation, motivation, empathy, and social skills. You can assess your current level of emotional intelligence at www.mindtools.com. Heffernan et al (2010) found a positive correlation between self-compassion and emotional intelligence among nurses. Two overarching principles of a self-care management plan are resilience and positive intentionality. These concepts are interrelated and can enhance the success of self-care practices.

Resilience has been defined by many authors as the ability to keep functioning in the face of continued stress, difficult work conditions, or trauma. Resilience can be seen as a strategy for responding to difficult or adverse situations by positively adjusting to stressors. Resilience can be associated with hope, positivity, and self-efficacy (Sullivan et al, 2012). Some research studies suggest that resilience can actually be strengthened in nurses through the use of different strategies. A review of the literature regarding resilience in health professionals by McCann et al (2013) suggests that laughter/humor, self-reflection, beliefs/spirituality, and professional identity are all related to the characteristic of resilience. Developing positive relationships and encouraging positive attitudes and emotional insight will reinforce resilience.

Positive intentionality is a form of focused consciousness and energy according to Jean Watson. Holding thoughts of caring, loving, kindness, and open receptivity rather than having manipulative intent or seeking power over others leads to healing (Watson, 2002). Focusing on positive intentionality in thoughts and actions enhances caring energy, which leads to healing and improved health.

■ THE PROCESS OF SELF-CARE MANAGEMENT
Self-Assessment

Practicing nurses and experienced nurse practitioners are skilled at assessing a patient's readiness for change and developing plans to improve self-care, but these professionals may not take time to apply a similar process to themselves. The principles discussed in Chapter 3 and the alternative therapies discussed throughout this text can be applied to self-care of the nursing professional. Self-assessment of the provider's current status includes reflection on strengths and identification of areas that need support. This might include time for reflection and appropriate self-evaluation of performance. It might also include identification of strategies that are suggested and validated for stress management. A variety of self-assessment tools are available to assist in the identification of concerns with links to or suggestions for appropriate strategies to make changes. Many organizations have identified professional quality-of-life assessment tools, such as ProQol (http://www.proqol.org).

This self-care assessment can be used to examine the type of self-care strategies that the nurse practitioner is using and identify other areas that might be important for self-care management. Some nurse practitioners will be able to identify stressors and concerns independently. Any method is acceptable as long as it leads to engagement in self-care behaviors.

Goal Setting

Each nurse practitioner can identify individual areas to work on, setting goals depending on his or her perception of balance in life. Specific strategies such as increased exercise and adequate sleep may be important for one person, whereas another may need to focus on prayer or meditation. It is important for the nurse practitioner to evaluate all aspects of the person—physical, psychological, spiritual, and professional and work domains—so that appropriate interventions are utilized to optimize well-being. The APRN engages in self-evaluation concerning clinical practice to monitor and ensure the quality of health-care practice. This is consistent with the National Organization of Nurse Practitioner Faculties (NONPF) core competency for nurse practitioner practice.

Strategies

Strategies for self-care can be divided into categories for all components of well-being of the individual. These include physical aspects, as well as psychosocial and spiritual components. It is important that each professional examine his or her practice to determine whether there are realistic expectations for performance in the clinical area. In addition, other life stressors such as family needs, chronic illnesses, holidays, vacations, and relationships can compound professional stressors.

Physical signs and symptoms of increased stressors such as insomnia, loss of appetite, overeating, and weight gain or loss can require interventions to ensure optimal well-being for the provider. Interventions suggested by personal health-care providers should be followed for optimal physical care. This might include weight loss programs, exercise programs, and strategies for sleep. Occasionally, a practitioner may benefit from some extra personal time for reflection and meditation. Access to and self-referral to treatment programs can be helpful in sustaining interventions.

Professionally, it seems important for nurse practitioners to develop their own "inner circle," a trusted peer group composed of people with similar beliefs, who can mentor them in individual needs. In the literature, the role is referred to as a "coaching" function for professionals (Marshall & Zolnierek, 2012). Discussion of stressors, alternative choices for managing stressors, and debriefing after difficult situations can help to promote self-confidence and self-efficacy. Peers can also be helpful during transition times. Positive, nurturing relationships are imperative for the development of resilience. The focus on positivity is an important strategy because positive feelings increase energy and help one feel more

optimistic about challenging situations. Developing emotional insight and balance in life can also augment a person's resilience. The characteristic of resilience is associated with confidence and self-efficacy. These self-care strategies will help to prevent adverse effects of stress.

Many professionals are involved in various other self-care strategies. Because so many lay publications are devoted to self-care and self-help, there is a plethora of strategies that can be utilized for self-care. Many of these strategies are well researched and validated for effectiveness. But perhaps the most important consideration is that each professional must identify the most appropriate strategies for his or her own self-care. Many professionals participate in exercise programs, yoga, walking and running programs, or weight management programs; many use music, massage, and/or meditation to reduce stress.

Some newer modalities and older Eastern medicine modalities for self-care have also been researched and validated. The Centers for Disease Control and Prevention (CDC) provides ongoing research findings on alternative therapies and serves as an excellent resource of information. Two interesting modalities that are well researched are mindfulness-based stress reduction and energy field strategies.

- **Mindfulness-based stress reduction** is one strategy that has been shown to reduce stress, anxiety, and chronic depression and is recently being utilized for management of other lifestyle problems (see www.umassmed.edu.cfm/index.aspx).
- **Energy field therapies.** *Therapeutic Touch* (TT) is a nursing strategy developed by Dora Kunz and Dolores Krieger. Krieger was a former student of Martha Rogers at New York University, who applied the principles of energy-field interactions, creating a sequential process whereby nurses and caregivers direct their intentionality toward the patient's well-being. Research studies have shown that TT is useful in reducing pain, improving wound healing, aiding relaxation, and easing the dying process (see www.therapeutictouch.org).

Reiki is a form of complementary energy therapy that helps to rebalance the energy field around the person to help restore him or her to a balanced, positive state of energy flow. This therapy helps the individual to feel relaxed and peaceful and has been utilized in a variety of settings to manage stress (Cuneo et al., 2010; Natale, 2010).

CASE STUDY 24.1

Jane R. has been a nurse practitioner for 10 years working in family primary care. Her current salaried position is in an urban community health center that provides care to a multicultural population. During an 8-hour workday, Jane will see 24 to 26 patients. She is the newest provider in the practice and is still building up her case load, so during most days she will see 4 to 6 new patients. Jane admits that most days she completes her EHR documentation at home, spending 2 to 3 hours most workdays and occasionally 1 day on the weekend reviewing and following up on labs and responding to patient e-mails or

CASE STUDY 24.1—cont'd

telephone calls. Jane is constantly worrying about what she is behind on or what she may have missed. Her children are grown and out of the house, but she finds little time to socialize or engage in activities she used to enjoy. She feels guilty that she is not spending more time with her husband. Her husband is concerned about her workload and the constraints work has put on her life.

Jane decided to discuss this issue with the NP who oriented her to this job. She was comforted to find out that her mentor was working as much as she was, but they both wondered if the other providers were having similar experiences. At the next monthly staff meeting, they raised the issue, and Jane was surprised to find that most of the providers were taking work home at night. The group decided to bring this issue to administration as an unacceptable situation. The issue is now being discussed and strategies for improving the situation are being considered. As a result of Jane's contemplation about work stressors, she realized that over time she has stopped exercising, eating well, or having restorative sleep. A colleague suggested that she make an appointment with a nurse who practices Therapeutic Touch. After undergoing several treatments, Jane notes that she is sleeping better, has energy to exercise, and feels less anxious.

CASE DISCUSSION

Jane R. experienced many of the work stressors discussed in this chapter. These stressors compromised her quality of life and her ability to participate in self-care. Reaching out to a colleague and eventually the other providers at her workplace helped Jane to realize that she was not alone. The cooperation and collaboration of her work group provided strength in approaching the administration of the health center. Through this process she realized that she has not been participating in self-care. She was able to seek support from colleagues and to improve her ability to function and participate in self-care.

 For additional resources please visit
http://davisplus.fadavis.com

SUMMARY

In the role of health-care providers in primary care, nurse practitioners are exposed to many stressors and challenges that can lead to frustration and self-criticism, as well as compassion fatigue and burnout. Nurse practitioners are well aware of the importance of self-care strategies and health promotion when caring for patients. It is imperative that nurse practitioner students and APRNs internalize these same concepts of self-care, resilience, and positivity, as well as maintain their sense of intentionality, in order to attain and preserve well-being and professional excellence.

The nurse practitioner must remain open to new strategies and modalities for self-care in the quest to balance personal and professional life. Many professional and other groups advertise conferences, lectures, and webinars on self-care strategies. These strategies, when first utilized by nurse practitioners, can also be taught as self-care strategies for patients.

Nursing is the art and science of human caring. Self-care for practitioners and patients requires continual efforts and openness to new strategies and modalities for health promotion, health education, and patient advocacy. The resilience and positivity developed through self-care strategies will allow APRNs to direct their skill and intentionality toward creating a peaceful, harmonious environment and to share and model excellent care for patients.

References

American Holistic Nurses Association. What is self-care? 2014. Retrieved from www.ahna.org

Cuneo, CL, et al. The effect of Reiki on work-related stress of the registered nurse. *J Holist Nurs* 29:33–41, 2010. Retrieved from http://dx.doi.org/10.1177/089801010377294

Godfrey, CM, et al. Care of self—care by other—care of other: The meaning of self-care from research, practice, policy and industry perspectives. *Int J Evidence-Based Healthc* 9:3–24, 2011. Retrieved from http://dx.doi.org/10.1111/j.1744-1609.2010.00196.x

Heffernan, M, et al. Self-compassion and emotional intelligence in nurses. *Int J Nurs Pract* 16:366–373, 2010. Retrieved from http://dx.doi.org/10.1111/j.1440-172X.2010.01853.x

Institute of Medicine. *The future of nursing: Leading change, advancing health.* 2010. Retrieved from http://iom.edu/Reports/2010/The-Future-of-Nursing-Leading-Change-Advancing-Health.aspx

Lombardo, B, and Eyre, C. Compassion fatigue: A nurse's primer. *Online Journal of Issues in Nursing* 16(1), 2011. Retrieved from http://dx.doi.org/10.3912/OJIN.Vol16No01Man03

Marshall, J, and Zolnierek, C. Supporting nurses through critical practice incidents: The nurse advocate role. *Nurse Leader* 10(2): 34–44, 2012. Retrieved from http://dx.doi.org/10.1016/j.mnl/2011.12.009

McCann, CM, et al. Resilience in the health professions: A review of recent literature. *Int J Wellbeing* 3:60–81, 2013. Retrieved from http://dx.doi.org/10.5502/ijw.v3.i1.4

Natale, G. Reconnecting to nursing through Reiki. *Creative Nursing* 16:171–176, 2010. Retrieved from http://dx.doi.org/10.1891/1078-4535.16.4.171

Sabo, BM. Compassion fatigue and nursing work: Can we accurately capture the consequences of caring work? *Int J Nurs Pract* 12: 136–142, 2006. Retrieved from http://dx.doi.org/10.1111/j.1440-172x.200600562.x

Stamm, BH. Professional Quality of Life: Compassion Satisfaction & Fatigue Scales, RevIV (ProQOL), 1997-2008. http://www.proqol.org.

Sullivan, P, et al. Grace under fire: Surviving and thriving in nursing by cultivating resilience. *Am Nurse Today* 7(12), 2012. Retrieved from www.americannursetoday.com/article.aspx?id=9770#

Wilkinson, A, and Whitehead, L. Evolution of the concept of self-care and implications for nurses: Literature review. *Int J Nurs Stud* 46:1143–1148, 2009.

Valent, P. Diagnosis and treatment of helper stresses, traumas and illness. In Figley, CR (Ed.), *Treating compassion fatigue.* Brunner-Routledge, Hove, UK, 2002, pp 17–37.

Watson, J. Intentionality and caring-healing consciousness: A practice of transpersonal nursing. *Holist Nurs Pract* 16(4):12–19, 2002. Retrieved from http://dx.doi.org/10.1097/00004650-200207000-00005

Bibliography

Henry, J, and Henry, L. *The soul of the caring nurse: Stories and strategies for revitalizing professional passion.* American Nurses Association, Silver Spring, MD, 2004.

Kravits, K, et al. Self-care strategies for nurses: A psycho-educational intervention for stress reduction and the prevention of burnout. *Appl Nurs Res* 23:130–138, 2010.

Lorenz, JM. Making a self-care plan. 2012. Retrieved from www.nursing.advanceweb.com/Continuing-Education/CE-Articles/Making-a-Self-Care-Plan.aspx

Moeini, B, et al. The impact of cognitive-behavioral stress management training program on job stress in hospital nurses: Applying PRE-CEDE model. *J Res Health Sci* 11(2):114–120, 2011.

Thrasher, C. The primary care nurse practitioner: Advocate for self-care. *J Am Acad Nurse Pract* 14(3):113–117, 2002.

Yoder, EA. Compassion fatigue in nurses. *Appl Nurs Res* 23:191–197, 2010.

Resources

American Nurses Association Healthy Nurse Initiative
www.ana.org
Centers for Disease Control and Prevention
www.cdc.gov/feature/handlingstress
www.cdc.gov/features/healthyliving.html
MindTools
www.mindtools.com
Myers-Briggs Type Indicator—transferable skills and personal strengths assessments
www.humannetrics.com
Pumpkin Hollow Retreat Center—Therapeutic Touch
www.pumpkinhollow.org
www.therapuetictouch.org
Robert Wood Johnson Foundation
www.rwjf.org/en/topics/search-topics/S/self-care-management.html

TED Ideas Worth Spreading
www.ted.com/talks
The American Holistic Nurses Association
www.ahna.org/Default.aspx?Tabname=Self-care
The Happiness Project
www.gretchenrubin.com
The Mayo Clinic—Health and Productivity Done Well: Lessons from the Mayo Clinic
www.benefitfocus.com/static/media.HPM_Done_well_final.pdf
University of Buffalo School of Social Work—Community Resources (Self-care Assessment and Resources)
www.socialwork.buffalo.edu/students/self-care/exercises.asp

Physiological Influences of the Aging Process

Age-Related Change	Appearance or Functional Change	Implication
Integumentary System		
Loss of dermal and epidermal thickness	Paper-thin skin	Prone to skin breakdown and injury
Flattening of papillae	Shearing and friction force more readily peels off the epidermis Diminished cell-mediated immunity in the skin	
Atrophy of the sweat glands	Decreased sweating	Frequent pruritus
Decreased vascularity	Slower recruitment of sweat glands by thermal stimulation Decreased body odor Decreased heat loss Dryness	Alteration in thermoregularity response Fluid requirements may change seasonally Loss of skin water Increased risk of heat stroke
Collagen cross-linking	Increased wrinkling	Potential effect on one's morale and feeling of self-worth
Elastin regression	Laxity of skin	
Loss of subcutaneous fat Decreased elasticity	Intraosseous atrophy, especially to back of hands and face	Loss of fat tissue on soles of feet—trauma of walking increases foot problems
Loss of subcutaneous tissue	Purpuric patches after minor surgery	Reduced insulation against cold temperatures; *prone to hypothermia* Check why injury is occurring; be alert—potential abuse or falls
Decreased number of melanocytes	Loss of pigment Pigment plaque appears	Teach importance of using sun block creams; refer to dermatologist as needed
Decline in fibroblast proliferation	Decreased epidermal growth rate Slower re-epithelialization Decreased vitamin D production and synthesis	Decreased tissue repair response
Decreased hair follicle density	Loss of body hair	
Decreased growth phase of individual fibers	Thin, short villus hairs predominate Slower hair growth	
Loss of melanocytes from the hair bulb	Graying of the hair	Potential effect on self-esteem

Continued

Age-Related Change	Appearance or Functional Change	Implication
Alternating hyperplasia and hypoplasia of nail matrix	Longitudinal ridges	Nails prone to splitting
	Thinner nails of the fingers	Advise patient to wear gloves, keep nails short, avoid nail polish remover (cause dryness); refer to podiatrist
	Thickened, curled toenails	May cause discomfort
Respiratory System		
Decreased lung tissue elasticity	Decreased vital capacity	Reduced overall efficiency of ventilatory exchange
	Increased residual volume	
	Decreased maximum breath capacity	
Thoracic wall calcification	Increased anteroposterior diameter of chest	Obscuration of heart and lung sounds
	Displacement of apical impulse	
Cilia atrophy	Change in mucociliary transport	Increased susceptibility to infection
Decreased respiratory muscle strength	Reduced ability to handle secretions and reduced effectiveness against noxious foreign particles	Prone to atelectasis
	Partial inflation of lungs at rest	
Cardiovascular System		
Heart valves fibrose and thicken	Reduced stroke volume, cardiac output; may be altered	Decreased responsiveness to stress
	Slight left ventricular hypertrophy	Increased incidence of murmurs, *particularly aortic stenosis and mitral regurgitation*
Mucoid degeneration of mitral valve	S_4 commonly heard	
	Valve less dense; mitral leaflet stretches with intrathoracic pressure	
Fibroelastic thickening of the sinoatrial node; decreased number of pacemaker cells	Slower heart rate	Increased prevalence of arrhythmias
	Irregular heart rate	
Increased subpericardial fat Collagen accumulation around heart muscle		
Elongation of tortuosity and calcification of arteries	Increased rigidity of arterial wall	Aneurysms may form
Elastin and collagen cause progressive thickening and loss of arterial wall resiliency	Increased peripheral vascular resistance	Decreased blood flow to body organs
		Altered distribution of blood flow
Loss of elasticity of the aorta dilation		Increased systolic blood pressure, contributing to coronary artery disease
Increased lipid content in artery wall	Lipid deposits form	Increased incidence of atherosclerotic events, such as *angina pectoris*, stroke, gangrene
Decreased baroreceptor sensitivity (stretch receptors)	Decreased sensitivity to change in blood pressure	Prone to loss of balance—potential for falls
	Decreased baroreceptor mediation to straining	Valsalva maneuver may cause sudden drop in blood pressure

Age-Related Change	Appearance or Functional Change	Implication
Gastrointestinal System		
Liver becomes smaller	Decreased storage capacity	
Less efficient cholesterol stabilization absorption	Increased evidence of gallstones	
Dental enamel thins	Staining of tooth surface occurs	Tooth and gum decay; tooth loss
Gums recede	Teeth deprived of nutrients	
Fibrosis and atrophy of salivary glands	Prone to dry mucous membranes	Shift to mouth breathing is common
	Decreased salivary ptyalin	Membrane more susceptible to injury and infection May interfere with breakdown of starches
Atrophy and decrease in number of taste buds	Decreased taste sensation	Altered ability to taste sweet, sour, and bitter Change in nutritional intake Excessive seasoning of foods
Delay in esophageal emptying	Decline in esophageal peristalsis Esophagus slightly dilated	Occasional discomfort as food stays in esophagus longer
Decreased hydrochloric acid secretion	Reduction in amount of iron and vitamin B_{12} that can be absorbed	Possible delay in vitamin and drug absorption, *especially calcium* and *iron*
Decrease in gastric acid secretion		Altered drug effect Fewer cases of gastric ulcers
Decreased muscle tone	Altered motility Decreased colonic peristalsis	Prone to constipation, functional bowel syndrome, esophageal spasm, diverticular disease
Atrophy of mucosal lining	Decreased hunger sensations and emptying time	
Decreased proportion of dietary calcium absorbed	Altered bone formation, muscle contractility, hormone activity, enzyme activation, clotting time, immune response	Symptoms more marked in women than in men
Decreased basal metabolic rate (rate at which fuel is converted into energy)		May need fewer calories Possible effect on life span
Genitourinary and Reproductive Systems		
Reduced renal mass	Decreased sodium-conserving ability	Administration and dosage of drugs may need to be modified
Loss of glomeruli	Decreased glomerular filtration rate Decreased creatinine clearance Increased blood urea nitrogen concentration	

Continued

Age-Related Change	Appearance or Functional Change	Implication
Histological changes in small vessel walls	Decreased renal blood flow	
Sclerosis of supportive circulatory system		
Decline in number of functioning nephrons	Decreased ability to dilute urine concentrate	Altered response to reduced fluid load or increased fluid volume
Reduced bladder muscular tone	Decreased bladder capacity or increased residual urine	Sensation of urge to urinate may not occur until bladder is full
Atrophy and fibrosis of cervical and uterine walls	Menopause; decline in fertility	Urination at night may increase
Reduced number and viability of oocytes in the aging ovary	Narrowing of cervical canal	
Decreased vaginal wall elasticity	Vaginal lining thin, pale, friable Narrowing of vaginal canal	Potential for discomfort in sexual intercourse
Decreased levels of circulating hormones	Reduced lubrication during arousal state	Increased frequency of sexual dysfunction
Degeneration of seminiferous tubules	Decreased seminal fluid volume Decreased force of ejaculation Reduced elevation of testes	
Proliferation of stromal and glandular tissue	Prostatic hypertrophy	Potentially compromised genitourinary function; *urinary frequency; increased risk of malignancy*
Involution of mammary gland tissue	Connective tissue replaced by adipose tissue	Easier to assess breast lesions
Neuromuscular System Decreased muscle mass	Decreased muscle strength Tendons shrink and sclerose	Decreased tendon jerks Increased muscle cramping
Decreased myosin adenosine triphosphatase activity	Prolonged contraction time, latency period, relaxation period	Decreased motor function and overall strength
Deterioration of joint cartilage	Bone makes contact with bone	Potential for pain, crepitation, and limitation of movement
Loss of water from the cartilage	Narrowing of joint spaces	Loss of height
Decreased bone mass	Decreased bone formation and increased bone resorption, leading to osteoporosis	More rapid and earlier changes in women
Decreased osteoblastic activity		Greater risk of fractures
Osteoclasts resorb bone	Hormonal changes	Gait and posture accommodate to changes
Increased proportion of body fat	Centripetal distribution of fat and invasion of fat in large muscle groups	Anthropometric measurements required
Regional changes in fat distribution		Increased relative adiposity

Age-Related Change	Appearance or Functional Change	Implication
Thickened leptomeninges in spinal cord	Loss of anterior horn cells in the lumbosacral area	Leg weakness may be correlated
Accumulation of lipofuscin	Altered RNA function and resultant cell death	
Loss of neurons and nerve fibers	Decreased processing speed and vibration sense Altered pain response Decreased deep tendon, Achilles tendon	Increased time to perform and learn Possible postural hypotension Safety hazard
Decreased conduction of nerve fibers	Decreased psychomotor performance	Alteration in pain response
Few neuritic plaques		Possible cognitive and memory changes
Neurofibrillary tangles in hippocampal neurons		Heavy tangle formation and neuritic plaques in cortex of patients with Alzheimer's disease
Neuromuscular System Changes in sleep–wake cycle	Decreased stage 4, stage 3, and rapid eye movement phases Deterioration of circadian organization	Increased or decreased time spent sleeping Increased nighttime awakenings Changed hormonal activity
Slower stimulus identification and registration	Delayed reaction time	Prone to falls
Decreased brain weight and volume		May be present in absence of mental impairments
Sensory System Morphological changes in choroid, epithelium, retina	Decreased visual acuity Visual field narrows	Corrective lenses required Increased possibility of disorientation and social isolation
Decreased rod and cone function		Slower light and dark adaptation
Pigment accumulation		
Decreased speed of eye movements	Difficulty in gazing upward and maintaining convergence	
Sclerosis of pupil sphincter	Difficulty in adapting to lighting changes Increased threshold for light perception	Glare may pose an environmental hazard Dark rooms may be hazardous
Increased intraocular pressure	Increased incidence of glaucoma	
Distorted depth perception		Incorrect assessment of height of curbs and steps; potential for falls
Ciliary muscle atrophy	Altered refractive powers	Corrective lenses often required
Nuclear sclerosis *(lens)*	Presbyopia	Near work and reading may become difficult
Reduced accommodation	Hyperopia	
Increased lens size	Myopia	
Accumulation of lens fibers		

Continued

Age-Related Change	Appearance or Functional Change	Implication
Lens yellows	Color vision may be impaired	Less able to differentiate lower color tones: blues, greens, violets
Diminished tear secretion	Dullness and dryness of the eyes	Irritation and discomfort may result Intactness of corneal surface jeopardized
Loss of auditory neurons	Decreased tone discrimination and voice localization High-frequency sounds lost first	Suspiciousness may be increased because of paranoid dimensions secondary to hearing loss Social isolation
Angiosclerosis calcification of inner ear membrane	Progressive hearing loss, especially at high frequency Presbycusis	Difficulty hearing, particularly under certain conditions such as *background noise, rapid speech, poor acoustics*
Decreased number of olfactory nerve fibers	Decreased sensitivity to odors	May not detect harmful odors Potential safety hazard
Alteration in taste sensation		Possible changes in food preferences and eating patterns
Reduced tactile sensation	Decreased ability to sense pressure, pain, temperature	Misperceptions of environment and safety risk
Endocrine System Decline in secretion of testosterone, growth hormone, insulin, adrenal androgens, aldosterone, thyroid hormone	Decreased hormone clearance rates	Increased mortality associated with certain stresses (burns, surgery)
Defects in thermoregulation	Shivering less intense	Susceptibility to temperature extremes *(hypothermia/hyperthermia)*
Reduction of febrile responses	Poor perceptions of changes in ambient temperature Reduced sweating; increased threshold for the onset of sweating Fever not always present with infectious process	Unrecognized infectious process operative
Alteration in tissue sensitivity to hormones	Decreased insulin response, glucose tolerance, and sensitivity of renal tubules to antidiuretic hormone	
Enhanced sympathetic responsivity		
Increased nodularity and fibrosis of thyroid		Increased frequency of thyroid disease
Decreased basal metabolic rate	Alteration in carbohydrate tolerance	Increased incidence of obesity
Hematological System Decreased percentage of marrow space occupied by hematopoietic tissue	Ineffective erythropoiesis	Risky for patient who loses blood

Age-Related Change	Appearance or Functional Change	Implication
Immune System Thymic involution and decreased serum thymic hormone activity	Decreased number of T cells	Less vigorous and/or delayed hypersensitivity reactions
	Production of anti-self reactive T cells	
Decreased T-cell function	Impairment in cell-mediated immune responses	Increased risk of mortality
Appearance of autoantibodies	Decreased cyclic adenosine monophosphate and glucose monophosphate	Increased incidence of infection
		Reactivation of latent infectious diseases
	Decreased ability to reject foreign tissue	
		Increased prevalence of autoimmune disorders
	Increased laboratory autoimmune parameters	
Redistribution of lymphocytes	Impaired immune reactivity	
Changes in serum immunoglobulin	Increased immunoglobulin A levels Decreased immunoglobulin G levels	Increased prevalence of infection

Source: Kennedy-Malone, L, et al. *Advanced practice nursing in the care of older adults.* FA Davis, Philadelphia, 2014, pp 643–650.

Laboratory Values in the Older Adult

Laboratory Test	Normal Values	Changes With Age	Comments
Urinalysis			
Protein	0–5 mg/100 mL	Rises slightly	May be due to kidney changes with age, urinary tract infection, renal pathology
Glucose	0–15 mg/100 mL	Declines slightly	Glycosuria appears after high plasma level; unreliable
Specific gravity	1.005–1.020	Lower maximum in elderly 1.016–1.022	Decline in nephrons impairs ability to concentrate urine
Hematology			
Erythrocyte sedimentation rate	Men: 0–20 Women: 0–30	Significant increase	Neither sensitive nor specific in aged
Iron Iron binding	50–160 mcg/dL 230–410 mcg/dL	Slight decrease Decrease	
Hemoglobin	Men: 13–18 g/100 mL Women: 12–16 g/100 mL	Men: 10–17 g/mL Women: none noted	Anemia common in the elderly
Hematocrit	Men: 45%–52% Women: 37%–48%	Slight decrease speculated	Decline in hematopoiesis
Leukocytes	4,300–10,800/mm^3	Drop to 3,100–9,000/mm^3	Decrease may be due to drugs or sepsis and should not be attributed immediately to age
Lymphocytes	500–2,400 T cells/mm^3 50–200 B cells/mm^3	T-cell and B-cell levels fall	Infection risk higher; immunization encouraged
Platelets	150,000–350,000/mm^3	No change in number	
Blood Chemistry			
Albumin	3.5–5.0/100 mL	Decline	Related to decrease in liver size and enzymes; protein-energy malnutrition common
Globulin	2.3–3.5 g/100 mL	Slight increase	
Total serum protein	6.0–8.4 g/100 mL	No change	Decreases may indicate malnutrition, infection, liver disease
Blood urea nitrogen	Men: 10–25 mg/100 mL Women: 8–20 mg/100 mL	Increases significantly up to 69 mg/100 mL	Decline in glomerular filtration rate; decreased cardiac output
Creatinine	0.6–1.5 mg/100 mL	Increases to 1.9 mg/100 mL seen	Related to lean body mass decrease
Creatinine clearance	104–124 mL/min	Decreases 10%/decade after age 40 years	Used for prescribing medications for drugs excreted by kidney
Glucose tolerance	62–110 mg/dL after fasting; <120 mg/dL after 2 hours postprandial	Slight increase of 10 mg/dL/decade after 30 years of age	Diabetes increasingly prevalent; drugs may cause glucose intolerance

Laboratory Test	Normal Values	Changes With Age	Comments
Triglycerides	40–150 mg/100 mL	20–200 mg/100 mL	
Cholesterol	120–220 mg/100 mL	Men: increase to 50 mg/ 100 mL, then decrease Women: increase postmenopausally	Risk of cardiovascular disease
Thyroxine	4.5–13.5 mcg/100 mL	No change	Changes suggest thyroid disease; may be seen in euthyroid patients with acute or chronic illness or caloric deficiencies
Triiodothyronine	90–220 ng/100 mL	Decrease 25%	
Thyroid-stimulating hormone	0.5–5.0 mcg/mL	Slight increase	Sensitive indicator for diagnosing thyroid disease
Alkaline phosphatase	13–39 IU/L	Increase by 8–10 IU/L	Elevations >20% usually due to disease; elevations may be found with bone abnormalities, drugs (e.g., narcotics), and eating a fatty meal

Source: Kennedy-Malone, L, et al. *Advanced practice nursing in the care of older adults.* FA Davis, Philadelphia, 2014, pp 651–652.

Common Tests and Their Associations With Diseases and Conditions

Laboratory Test	Increase	Decrease
Acid phosphatase, prostatic	Prostate cancer, prostatic massage, benign prostatic hypertrophy, prostatitis, metastatic bone disease, liver disease, lysosomal storage diseases, sickle cell crisis, thrombocytosis	—
Alanine aminotransferase	Hepatitis, cirrhosis, fatty liver, liver metastases, biliary tract obstruction, infectious mononucleosis, hepatic congestion, pancreatitis, muscular dystrophy, myocardial infarction, renal disease, chronic alcohol abuse	Pyridoxine (vitamin B$_6$) deficiency
Albumin	Dehydration, diabetes insipidus	Overhydration, malnutrition, malabsorption, nephrosis, hepatic failure, burns, multiple myeloma, metastatic carcinomas, acute illness, rheumatic diseases, thyroid disease
Alkaline phosphatase	Bone growth, bone metastases, Paget's disease, osteomalacia, osteoporosis, hyperparathyroidism, hepatic disease, biliary obstruction; cancer of the liver, breast, colon, gallbladder, lung, or pancreas; pulmonary infarction, myocardial infarction, heart failure	Anemia, pernicious anemia, hypothyroidism, hypophosphatasia, hypervitaminosis D, zinc deficiency, magnesium deficiency
Alpha-fetoprotein (in nonpregnant women and men)	Cirrhosis, liver cancer, hepatitis	—
Amylase	Pancreatitis, gastrointestinal obstruction, mesenteric thrombosis and infarction, biliary obstruction, macroamylasemia, parotitis, renal disease, lung carcinoma, acute alcohol ingestion, after abdominal surgery	Severe liver disease, pancreatectomy, pancreatic insufficiency
Aspartate aminotransferase	Myocardial infarction, heart failure, myocarditis, pericarditis, myositis, trauma, hepatic disease, biliary tract obstruction, pancreatitis, infectious mononucleosis, renal infarction, neoplasia, cerebral damage, seizures, hemolysis, alcohol abuse, post–cardiac catheterization, angioplasty or surgery	Pyridoxine (vitamin B$_6$) deficiency, advanced stages of liver disease, uremia, hemodialysis

Laboratory Test	Increase	Decrease
Bilirubin	Hepatic disease, biliary obstruction, hemolytic anemia, pulmonary infarction, Gilbert's syndrome, Dubin-Johnson syndrome, hypothyroidism	—
Calcium	Hyperparathyroidism, acidosis, dehydration, bone cancer, lymphoma, myeloma, sarcoidosis, hyperthyroidism, hypervitaminosis D, milk-alkali syndrome, thyrotoxicosis	Hypoparathyroidism, renal failure, malabsorption, alkalosis, pancreatitis, cirrhosis, hypoalbuminemia, hyperphosphatemia, vitamin D deficiency, overhydration
Cholesterol	High-fat diet, alcoholism, hyperlipoproteinemia, hypothyroidism, biliary obstruction, nephrosis, poorly controlled diabetes mellitus, pancreatitis	Hyperthyroidism, infection, malnutrition, heart failure, malignancies, severe liver disease, chronic obstructive pulmonary disease
High-density lipoprotein cholesterol	Exercise, familial hyperlipoproteinemia, increased clearance of triglyceride, alcohol ingestion, exogenous intake of insulin or estrogens	Malnutrition, obesity, cigarette smoking, diabetes mellitus, hypothyroidism, hypertriglyceridemia, liver disease, renal failure, nephrosis, uremia
Creatine kinase	Myocardial infarction, muscle disease or injury, collagen-vascular disease, meningitis, brain infarction, hyperthermia, after surgery	Sedentary lifestyle
Creatinine	Renal disease, renal calculi, dehydration, muscle disease	Decreased muscle mass, hyperthyroidism, hypopituitarism, liver disease
Glucose	Diabetes mellitus, pheochromocytoma, hyperthyroidism, Cushing's syndrome, acromegaly, brain damage, hepatic disease, renal disease, hemochromatosis, stress (e.g., from emotion, burns, shock, anesthesia), acute or chronic pancreatitis, Wernicke's encephalopathy (vitamin B_1 deficiency), chronic hypervitaminosis A	Excess exogenous insulin, insulinoma, Addison's disease, myxedema, hepatic failure, malabsorption, pancreatitis, glucagon deficiency, extrapancreatic tumors, early diabetes mellitus, postgastrectomy, autonomic nervous system disorders, malnutrition, acute alcohol ingestion
Lactate dehydrogenase	Myocardial infarction, pulmonary infarction, hemolytic anemia, pernicious anemia, megaloblastic anemia, leukemia, lymphoma, hepatic and biliary disease, renal disease, musculoskeletal disease, pancreatitis	—
Lipase	Pancreatic and biliary disease	—
Magnesium	Addison's disease, adrenocortical insufficiency, massive hemolysis, antacid overuse, renal insufficiency	Severe loss of body fluids, malabsorption, renal disease, hyperaldosteronism, hyperparathyroidism, hypercalcemia, uncontrolled diabetes, dietary deficit, hemodialysis, inappropriate secretion of antidiuretic hormone
Phosphorus	Renal failure, hypoparathyroidism, diabetic ketoacidosis, lactic acidosis, respiratory acidosis, acromegaly, hypocalcemia, high phosphate intake (intravenous or oral), vitamin D intoxication, leukemia	Hyperparathyroidism, hypercalcemia, osteomalacia, hypokalemia, disorders that increase renal excretion or decrease renal absorption, vitamin D deficiency, salicylate poisoning, alkalosis, dietary deficit, ingestion of P-binding antacid, alcohol withdrawal, acute gout, hemodialysis

Continued

Laboratory Test	Increase	Decrease
Potassium	Acidosis, hypoadrenalism, hereditary hyperkalemia, hemolysis, acute renal failure, hemodialysis, hypoaldosteronism, thrombocytosis, dehydration, burns, intake of potassium-retaining diuretic, angiotensin-converting enzyme inhibitors, or excessive use of salt substitutes	Malnutrition, vomiting, metabolic alkalosis, diarrhea, nephrosis, hyperaldosteronism, hypomagnesemia, ectopic adrenocorticotropic hormone excess, beta-hydroxylase deficiency, thyrotoxicosis, administration of diuretics, excessive intake of licorice, laxative abuse, excessive sweating
Prostate-specific antigen	Prostate cancer, benign prostatic hyperplasia, prostatic massage, prostatic abscess, prostatitis, cystoscopy	Administration of finasteride
Sodium	Dehydration, vomiting, diabetes insipidus, excessive salt ingestion, diabetes mellitus with diuresis, diuretic phase of acute tubular necrosis, hypercalcemic nephropathy with diuresis, essential hypernatremia due to hypothalamic lesions, hyperaldosteronism, lactic acidosis	Excess exogenous antidiuretic hormone, nephrosis, hypoadrenalism, myxedema, heart failure, diarrhea, vomiting, diabetic acidosis, adrenocortical insufficiency, hyperlipidemia, hyperglycemia, hyperproteinemia
Total protein	Multiple myeloma, myxedema, lupus, sarcoidosis, diabetes insipidus, dehydration, collagen-vascular disease	Burns, cirrhosis, malnutrition, nephrosis, malabsorption, overhydration, gastrointestinal protein loss
Triglyceride	Nephrosis, cholestasis, pancreatitis, cirrhosis, diabetes mellitus, hepatitis, familial hyperlipoproteinemia, alcoholism, glycogen storage diseases, hypothyroidism, metabolic syndrome, nephrotic syndrome, pancreatitis	Malnutrition, hyperthyroidism, hypolipoproteinemia, a-beta lipoproteinemia
Troponin	Myocardial damage	
Urea nitrogen	Renal disease, dehydration, gastrointestinal bleeding, leukemia, heart failure, shock, postrenal azotemia, obstruction of urinary tract, acute myocardial infarction, muscle wasting	Hepatic failure, overhydration, acromegaly, dietary protein insufficiency, prolonged intravenous feedings
Uric acid	Gout, renal failure, diuretic therapy, leukemia, lymphoma, polycythemia, acidosis, psoriasis, hypothyroidism, multiple myeloma, pernicious anemia, tissue necrosis, inflammation, cancer chemotherapy, hemolytic anemia, high-protein weight-reduction diet, lead poisoning, polycystic kidneys, parathyroid hormone imbalance, sarcoidosis, type III hyperlipidemia	Administration of uricosuric drugs, allopurinol, or large doses of vitamin C; Wilson's disease, severe hepatic disease, low-purine diet

Note: Page numbers followed by f refer to figures; page numbers followed by t refer to tables.